American Medical Association

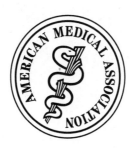

Complete Medical Encyclopedia

American Medical Association

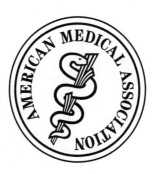

Complete Medical Encyclopedia

Medical Editors

Jerrold B. Leikin, MD

Martin S. Lipsky, MD

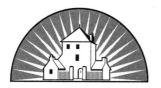

Random House Reference
New York

Published by Random House Reference, New York, New York.
Member of the Random House Information Group,
a division of Random House, Inc.

The recommendations and information in this book are appropriate in
most cases and current as of the date of publication; however, they are
not a substitute for medical diagnosis. For specific information concerning your or your family member's medical condition, the AMA
suggests that you consult a physician. The names of organizations,
products, and alternative therapies appearing in the book are given for
informational purposes only. Their inclusion does not imply AMA
endorsement, nor does the omission of any organization, product, or
alternative therapy indicate AMA disapproval.

Library of Congress Cataloging-in-Publication Data

American Medical Association complete medical
encyclopedia/the American Medical Association.
        1408p. ; cm.
    Includes index.
    ISBN 0-8129-9100-1 (bc)
        1. Medicine, Popular–Encyclopedias. I. Title: Complete medical
encyclopedia. II. American Medical Association.
    [DNLM: 1. Medicine–Encyclopedias—English. W 13 A5118 2003]
RC81.A2 A497 2003
610'.3-dc21

                                                                    2002067340

This book is available for special purchases in bulk by organizations
and institutions, not for resale, at special discounts. Please direct
your sales inquiries to specialmarkets@randomhouse.com or fax
212-572-4961.

Please address inquiries about electronic licensing of reference products, for use on a network or in software or on CD-ROM, to the
Subsidiary Rights Department, Random House Information Group,
fax 212-940-7352.

Random House Reference Web site address:
www.randomwords.com

Printed in the United States of America
987654321
First Edition

New York   Toronto   London   Sydney   Auckland

American Medical Association

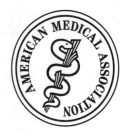

Foreword

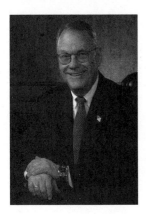

Information about health and medicine is one of the keys to maintaining good health. The patient-physician relationship is strengthened when you, the consumer, take an active role in finding out about health, disease, and medical treatments.

The American Medical Association Complete Medical Encyclopedia contains a wealth of information on diseases and conditions, treatments for diseases (including surgery and medications), medical testing, anatomy, body systems such as the respiratory system, preventive medicine, and food and nutrition. Health concerns of all age groups are included, from infants and children to adults to older people.

An up-to-date home reference book such as this one is essential to today's family. Advances in surgery such as remote surgery, sophisticated new forms of imaging, and new medications are being developed through research, offering new treatment options.

Surveys show that people view the American Medical Association as a trusted source of health information. As part of its mission statement, the AMA provides accurate health information to the public, and this book was prepared to help meet that goal.

We at the American Medical Association hope this book will help you manage your own health and that of family members, within the context of a good patient-physician relationship. In addition, the *American Medical Association Complete Medical Encyclopedia* is intended as a basic home reference on a variety of health and medical topics.

Michael D. Maves, MD
Executive Vice President
American Medical Association

American Medical Association

	Michael D. Maves, MD	*Executive Vice President, Chief Executive Officer*
	Robert A. Musacchio, PhD	*Senior Vice President, Publishing and Business Services*
	Anthony J. Frankos	*Vice President, Business Products*
	Mary Lou White	*Executive Director, Editorial, AMA Press*

Editorial Staff	Jerrold B. Leikin, MD	*Medical Editor*
	Martin S. Lipsky, MD	*Medical Editor*
	Patricia Dragisic	*Senior Managing Editor*
	Eileen Norris	*Senior Editor*
	Dorothea Guthrie Graham	*Contributing Editor*
	Robin Fitzpatrick Husayko	*Contributing Editor*
	Kathryn Nolan	*Contributing Editor*
	Claudia Appeldorn	*Editor*
	Patricia A. Lee	*Editor*
	Susan Duff	*Writer*
	Zoe R. Graves	*Writer*
	Robert McNally	*Writer*
	Shelagh Ryan Masline	*Writer*
	Claudia A. Bauer	*Researcher*
	Bernadette Sukley	*Researcher*
	Phyllis Manner	*Indexer*
	Coralee Montes	*Editorial Assistant*

Illustrations	Mary Ann Albanese	*Art Editor*
	Jayne Azzarello	*Researcher*
	Rolin Graphics, Inc	*General Illustration*

Acknowledgments	Bruce Blehart, JD	
	Claire Callan, MD	*American Medical Association*
	Karen Geraghty	*American Medical Association*
	Thomas Houston, MD	*American Medical Association*
	Audiey Kao, MD	*American Medical Association*
	Rosary Payne, JD	*American Medical Association*
	Joanne Schwartzberg, MD	*American Medical Association*
	Michael J Scotti, Jr, MD	*American Medical Association*

Book Development and Design	Alison Brown Cerier	*Alison Brown Cerier Book Development*
	Irene Carpelis, Sylvain Michaelis, Marianne Palladino	*Michaelis/Carpelis Design Associates*

Medical consultants

Robert Barkin, MD	*Anesthesiology*
Steven N. Blair, PED	*Exercise*
Thomas E. Bournias, MD	*Ophthalmology*
Barbara Burton, MD	*Genetics*
Diane Chen, MD	*Dermatology*
Chris Coogan, MD	*Urology*
Robert M. Craig, MD	*Gastroenterology*
Arthur W. Curtis, MD	*Otolaryngology*
Mike Easton, MD	*Addiction*
Elaine Farrell, MD	*Neonatology*
John Flaherty, MD	*Infectious Disease*
Jeffrey A. Goldman, DDS	*Dentistry*
James Gordon, MD	*Alternative Medicine*
Richard M. Gore, MD	*Radiology*
Stephen Haggerty, MD	*Surgery*
Kathleen A. Havlin, MD	*Hematology*
Tammy Ho, MD	*Nephrology*
Linda Holt, MD	*Gynecology*
Rodney J. Hoxsey, MD	*Reproductive Endocrinology*
Michelle Kambich, MS, CGC	*Genetics*
Karen Koffler, MD	*Alternative Medicine*
Stephen Kozlowski, MD	*Rheumatology*
Jane E. Kramer, MD	*Emergency*
William Leslie, MD	*Oncology*
Arline McDonald, PhD	*Nutrition*
Deeba Masood, MD	*Allergy; Immunology*
Marc S. Micozzi, MD	*Alternative Medicine*
Victor Maris Nora, MD	*Pharmacology*
Peter Orris, MD	*Epidemiology*
Jay Pensler, MD	*Cosmetic Surgery*
Arthur V. Prancan, MD	*Pharmacology*
Joel Press, MD	*Sports Medicine; Physical Therapy*
Daniel Ray, MD	*Pulmonary*
Domeena C. Renshaw, MD	*Psychiatry; Human Sexuality*
Michael Rezak, MD	*Neurology*
Susan Rubin, MD	*Neurology*
Eric Ruderman, MD	*Rheumatology*
Michael Schrift, MD	*Psychology*
Joanne Schwartzberg, MD	*Geriatrics*
Irwin Siegel, MD	*Orthopedics*
Richard Silver, MD	*Obstetrics*
Matthew Sorrentino, MD	*Cardiology*
Mark Stolar, MD	*Endocrinology*
Edward Traisman, MD	*Pediatrics–Neonatalogy*
Punam Verma, PhD	*Microbiology*
Dorothy Wawrose, MD	*Infectious Disease*
Peter Wong, MD	*Surgery*
Vahid Yaghmai, MD	*Biomedical Engineering*

Contents

How to use this book   10

Symptom charts   12

Atlas of the body   65

Twenty-first century medicine   73

Alphabetical encyclopedia
of medicine   97

*Entries on diseases, disorders, conditions,
symptoms, injuries, tests, procedures
including surgery, medications, alternative
therapies, parts of the body, and other
terms*

First aid   1312

Sample legal form   1334

Self-help organizations   1344

HIPAA and confidentiality
of patients' health information   1347

Index   1351

How to use this book

The all-new *American Medical Association Complete Medical Encyclopedia* has been planned to provide the reliable, objective health care information that American consumers have come to expect from the American Medical Association. Featuring more than 5,000 entries and 1,700 illustrations, it is intended to be a comprehensive, concise, and up-to-date source of consumer medical information. This authoritative, single-volume resource will not only help you safeguard and improve your heath, but it will also empower you to communicate more effectively with your doctor. The all-new *American Medical Association Complete Medical Encyclopedia* is positioned as the one book to turn to for definitive information about all of your health-related questions and concerns.

For quick and easy access, the entries in the **Alphabetical encyclopedia of medicine** are arranged alphabetically; many are supplemented with fact-filled charts, medical alerts, and instructive, detailed illustrations. Longer entries are logically divided into subsections. With ease of reading in mind, thumbnail definitions of complex medical terms are provided parenthetically as you encounter them. Terms in SMALL CAPITAL LETTERS are cross-references; these point you to other entries for additional information. If you do not find the main entry topic or term you are looking for, consult the comprehensive **Index** at the back of the book. Many topics are discussed in-depth within medically related entries.

Atlas of the body, featuring full-color illustrations and photographs, is a quick-reference guide to locating the major systems of the human body.

Take charge of your health with the popular AMA **Symptom charts**. These innovative charts outline many possible causes of common ailments, such as diarrhea and sleep problems. As you answer a series of questions with "yes" or "no," arrows in the chart will clearly direct you to further information, a course of action, or recommended medical intervention.

Twenty-first century medicine explores many of the cutting-edge developments in medicine today. From the promise of genetics to new surgical techniques to insights into how the brain works, this lavishly illustrated color section provides vital information about the future of medicine.

First aid is a book within a book, outlining easy-to-follow steps for life's most common emergencies.

Finally, a list of **Self-help organizations** that includes medical societies, voluntary health agencies, government agencies, and other health care groups is included. World Wide Web addresses are featured for those that post reliable Web sites.

The *American Medical Association Complete Medical Encyclopedia* is the ultimate medical reference book for consumers, one you will return to again and again for comprehensive, clear, and authoritative health information.

Symptom charts

Symptom charts help identify the possible causes of many common symptoms, for example, chest pain or diarrhea. After answering "yes" or "no" to the questions on the chart, follow the directional arrows, which lead you to a likely diagnosis. The terms in the boxes that appear in small capital letters (for example, HEADACHE) are cross-references. These cross-references direct you to main entries in the alphabetical encyclopedia of medicine with more information.

WARNING: These symptom charts are designed to help diagnose the most common causes of some common disorders. They are not intended to be exhaustive or to replace medical care by a physician. If any uncertainty remains regarding a diagnosis after consulting a particular chart, be sure to contact your doctor.

To help you determine what to do about various symptoms and whether medical help is needed urgently, the charts use the following language:

■ **EMERGENCY! GET MEDICAL HELP NOW!**
A diagnosis that appears in this box may be life-threatening if prompt medical attention is not obtained. Calling 911 or your local emergency number is usually the best way to secure prompt medical attention.

■ **CONTACT YOUR DOCTOR IMMEDIATELY.**
A diagnosis that appears in this box may be quite serious and require urgent medical attention. Medical advice should be sought immediately. Call your doctor or triage nurse and ask for help in determining the best possible course of action.

■ *Contact your doctor.*
A diagnosis that appears in this box is not usually life-threatening. Nevertheless, medical advice is recommended. Make an appointment to see your doctor for a consultation.

Symptom chart topics

ABDOMINAL PAIN	**14**
ANAL PAIN OR ITCHING	**17**
ANKLE OR FOOT PROBLEMS	**18**
BACKACHE	**20**
BREAST PAIN OR LUMPS	**22**
CHEST PAIN	**24**
CONSTIPATION	**26**
COUGHING	**28**
DEPRESSION	**32**
DIARRHEA	**34**
DIZZINESS	**36**
HEADACHE	**38**
HIP PAIN	**42**
HOARSENESS OR VOICE LOSS	**31**
KNEE PAIN	**44**
MENSTRUAL CRAMPS OR PAIN	**16**
NAUSEA OR VOMITING	**46**
NUMBNESS OR TINGLING	**48**
PENIS, PROBLEMS OF THE	**49**
RASHES IN INFANTS AND CHILDREN	**50**
RASHES IN ADULTS	**52**
SLEEP PROBLEMS	**54**
SWALLOWING DIFFICULTY	**64**
URINATION IN MEN, PAINFUL OR FREQUENT	**56**
URINATION IN WOMEN, PAINFUL OR FREQUENT	**57**
URINE DISCOLORATION	**58**
VISION LOSS OR IMPAIRMENT	**41**
WEIGHT GAIN	**60**
WEIGHT LOSS	**62**

Abdominal pain

Pain experienced in the area of the trunk below the lower edge of the rib cage and above the groin.

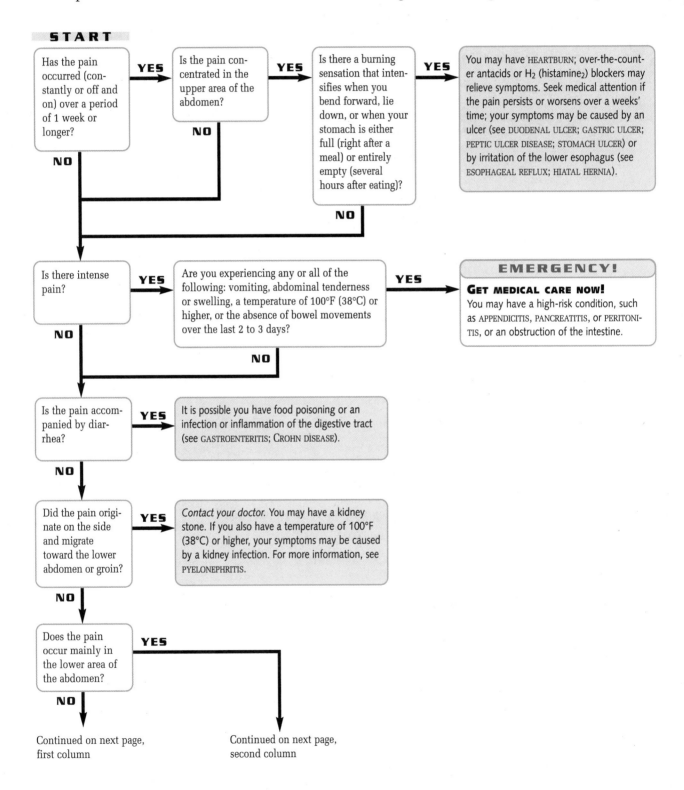

START

Has the pain occurred (constantly or off and on) over a period of 1 week or longer?

YES → Is the pain concentrated in the upper area of the abdomen?

YES → Is there a burning sensation that intensifies when you bend forward, lie down, or when your stomach is either full (right after a meal) or entirely empty (several hours after eating)?

YES → You may have HEARTBURN; over-the-counter antacids or H₂ (histamine₂) blockers may relieve symptoms. Seek medical attention if the pain persists or worsens over a weeks' time; your symptoms may be caused by an ulcer (see DUODENAL ULCER; GASTRIC ULCER; PEPTIC ULCER DISEASE; STOMACH ULCER) or by irritation of the lower esophagus (see ESOPHAGEAL REFLUX; HIATAL HERNIA).

NO (from second box)

NO (from third box)

NO (from first box) ↓

Is there intense pain?

YES → Are you experiencing any or all of the following: vomiting, abdominal tenderness or swelling, a temperature of 100°F (38°C) or higher, or the absence of bowel movements over the last 2 to 3 days?

YES → **EMERGENCY!**
GET MEDICAL CARE NOW! You may have a high-risk condition, such as APPENDICITIS, PANCREATITIS, or PERITONITIS, or an obstruction of the intestine.

NO

NO ↓

Is the pain accompanied by diarrhea?

YES → It is possible you have food poisoning or an infection or inflammation of the digestive tract (see GASTROENTERITIS; CROHN DISEASE).

NO ↓

Did the pain originate on the side and migrate toward the lower abdomen or groin?

YES → *Contact your doctor.* You may have a kidney stone. If you also have a temperature of 100°F (38°C) or higher, your symptoms may be caused by a kidney infection. For more information, see PYELONEPHRITIS.

NO ↓

Does the pain occur mainly in the lower area of the abdomen?

YES →

NO ↓

Continued on next page, first column

Continued on next page, second column

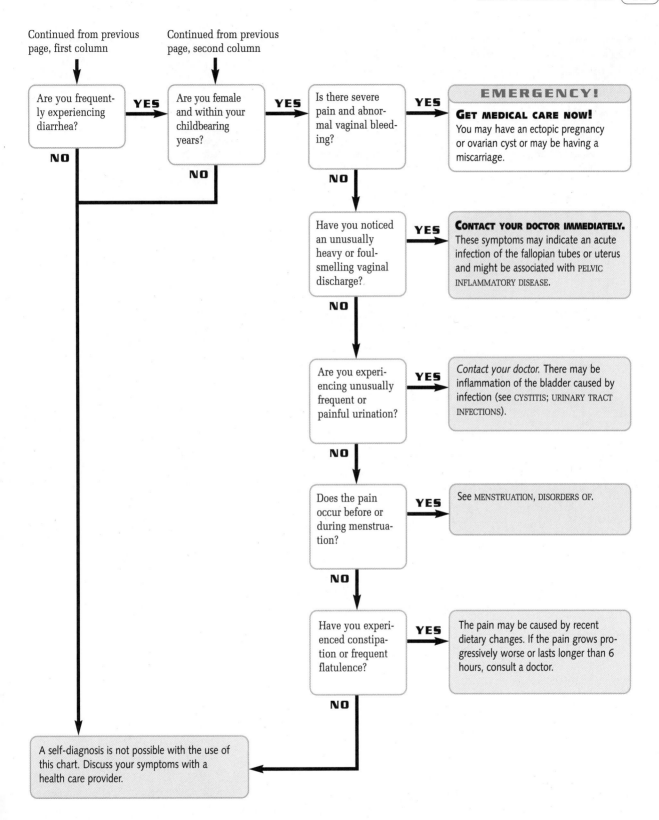

Continued from previous page, first column

Continued from previous page, second column

Are you frequent-ly experiencing diarrhea?

YES → Are you female and within your childbearing years?

NO

YES → Is there severe pain and abnor-mal vaginal bleed-ing?

NO

YES →

EMERGENCY!

GET MEDICAL CARE NOW! You may have an ectopic pregnancy or ovarian cyst or may be having a miscarriage.

Have you noticed an unusually heavy or foul-smelling vaginal discharge?

YES → **CONTACT YOUR DOCTOR IMMEDIATELY.** These symptoms may indicate an acute infection of the fallopian tubes or uterus and might be associated with PELVIC INFLAMMATORY DISEASE.

NO

Are you experi-encing unusually frequent or painful urination?

YES → *Contact your doctor.* There may be inflammation of the bladder caused by infection (see CYSTITIS; URINARY TRACT INFECTIONS).

NO

Does the pain occur before or during menstrua-tion?

YES → See MENSTRUATION, DISORDERS OF.

NO

Have you experi-enced constipa-tion or frequent flatulence?

YES → The pain may be caused by recent dietary changes. If the pain grows pro-gressively worse or lasts longer than 6 hours, consult a doctor.

NO

A self-diagnosis is not possible with the use of this chart. Discuss your symptoms with a health care provider.

Menstrual cramps or pain

Painful muscular contractions associated with menstruation.

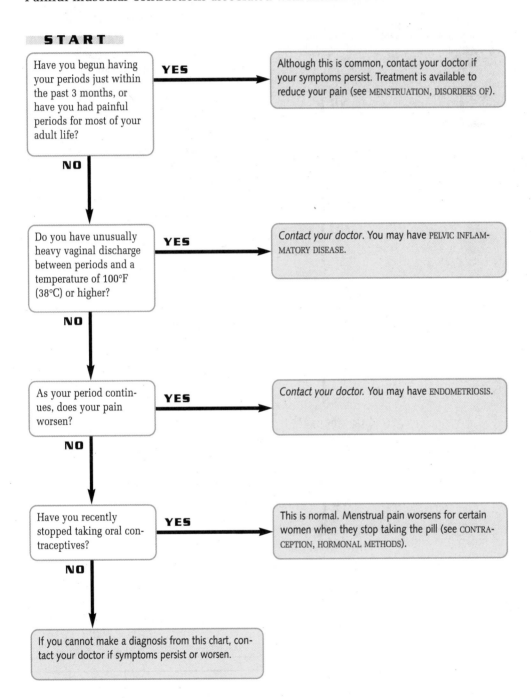

START

Have you begun having your periods just within the past 3 months, or have you had painful periods for most of your adult life?

YES → Although this is common, contact your doctor if your symptoms persist. Treatment is available to reduce your pain (see MENSTRUATION, DISORDERS OF).

NO ↓

Do you have unusually heavy vaginal discharge between periods and a temperature of 100°F (38°C) or higher?

YES → *Contact your doctor.* You may have PELVIC INFLAMMATORY DISEASE.

NO ↓

As your period continues, does your pain worsen?

YES → *Contact your doctor.* You may have ENDOMETRIOSIS.

NO ↓

Have you recently stopped taking oral contraceptives?

YES → This is normal. Menstrual pain worsens for certain women when they stop taking the pill (see CONTRACEPTION, HORMONAL METHODS).

NO ↓

If you cannot make a diagnosis from this chart, contact your doctor if symptoms persist or worsen.

Anal pain or itching

Irritation or discomfort in and around the anus. Itching is usually not serious, but in some cases it can be a sign of an underlying disease.

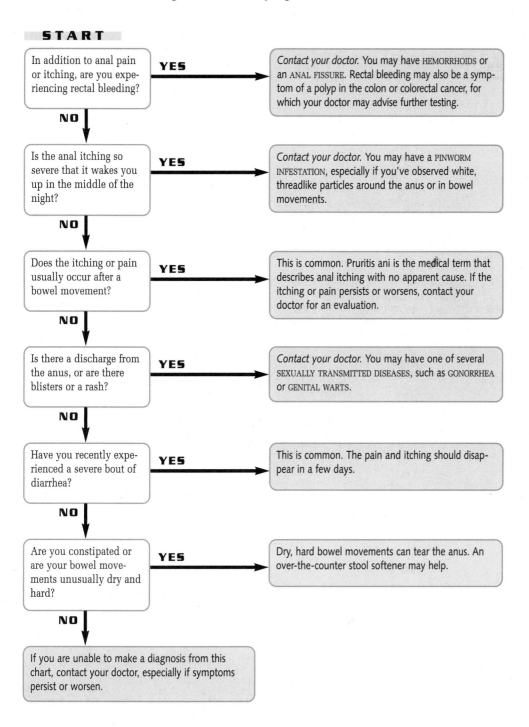

START

In addition to anal pain or itching, are you experiencing rectal bleeding?

YES → *Contact your doctor.* You may have HEMORRHOIDS or an ANAL FISSURE. Rectal bleeding may also be a symptom of a polyp in the colon or colorectal cancer, for which your doctor may advise further testing.

NO ↓

Is the anal itching so severe that it wakes you up in the middle of the night?

YES → *Contact your doctor.* You may have a PINWORM INFESTATION, especially if you've observed white, threadlike particles around the anus or in bowel movements.

NO ↓

Does the itching or pain usually occur after a bowel movement?

YES → This is common. Pruritis ani is the medical term that describes anal itching with no apparent cause. If the itching or pain persists or worsens, contact your doctor for an evaluation.

NO ↓

Is there a discharge from the anus, or are there blisters or a rash?

YES → *Contact your doctor.* You may have one of several SEXUALLY TRANSMITTED DISEASES, such as GONORRHEA or GENITAL WARTS.

NO ↓

Have you recently experienced a severe bout of diarrhea?

YES → This is common. The pain and itching should disappear in a few days.

NO ↓

Are you constipated or are your bowel movements unusually dry and hard?

YES → Dry, hard bowel movements can tear the anus. An over-the-counter stool softener may help.

NO ↓

If you are unable to make a diagnosis from this chart, contact your doctor, especially if symptoms persist or worsen.

Ankle or foot problems

Pain, swelling, tenderness, or bruising of one or both ankles or feet, usually associated with an injury to bones, tendons, or ligaments.

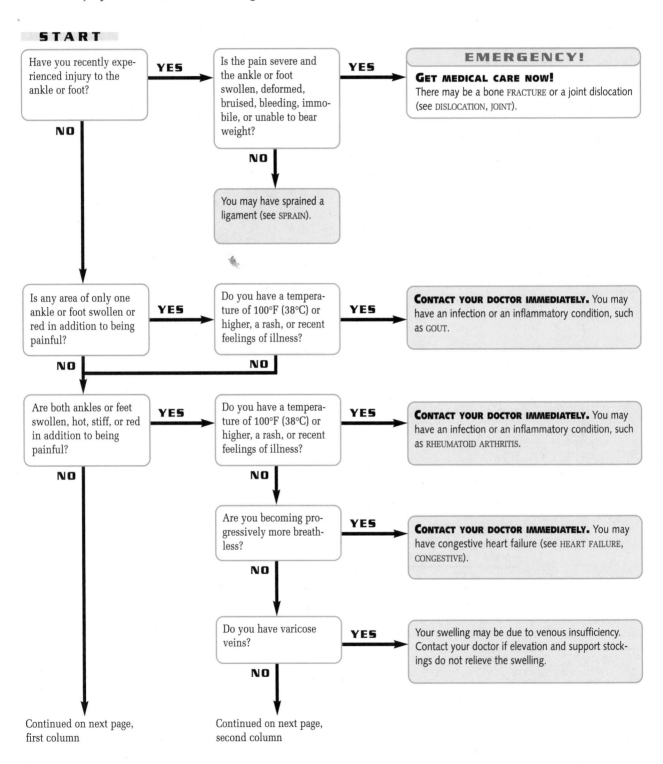

START

Have you recently experienced injury to the ankle or foot?

— **YES** → Is the pain severe and the ankle or foot swollen, deformed, bruised, bleeding, immobile, or unable to bear weight?

— **YES** →

EMERGENCY!

GET MEDICAL CARE NOW! There may be a bone FRACTURE or a joint dislocation (see DISLOCATION, JOINT).

NO ↓ (from pain severe question)

You may have sprained a ligament (see SPRAIN).

NO ↓ (from recent injury question)

Is any area of only one ankle or foot swollen or red in addition to being painful?

— **YES** → Do you have a temperature of 100°F (38°C) or higher, a rash, or recent feelings of illness?

— **YES** → **CONTACT YOUR DOCTOR IMMEDIATELY.** You may have an infection or an inflammatory condition, such as GOUT.

NO / **NO** ↓

Are both ankles or feet swollen, hot, stiff, or red in addition to being painful?

— **YES** → Do you have a temperature of 100°F (38°C) or higher, a rash, or recent feelings of illness?

— **YES** → **CONTACT YOUR DOCTOR IMMEDIATELY.** You may have an infection or an inflammatory condition, such as RHEUMATOID ARTHRITIS.

NO ↓

Are you becoming progressively more breathless?

— **YES** → **CONTACT YOUR DOCTOR IMMEDIATELY.** You may have congestive heart failure (see HEART FAILURE, CONGESTIVE).

NO ↓

Do you have varicose veins?

— **YES** → Your swelling may be due to venous insufficiency. Contact your doctor if elevation and support stockings do not relieve the swelling.

NO ↓

Continued on next page, first column

Continued on next page, second column

Continued from previous page, first column

Continued from previous page, second column

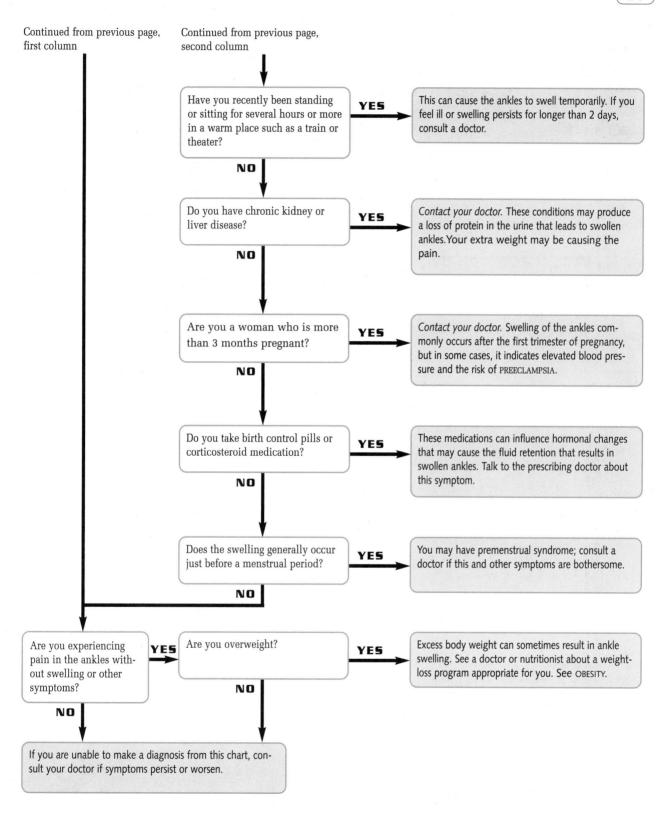

Have you recently been standing or sitting for several hours or more in a warm place such as a train or theater?

YES → This can cause the ankles to swell temporarily. If you feel ill or swelling persists for longer than 2 days, consult a doctor.

NO ↓

Do you have chronic kidney or liver disease?

YES → *Contact your doctor.* These conditions may produce a loss of protein in the urine that leads to swollen ankles. Your extra weight may be causing the pain.

NO ↓

Are you a woman who is more than 3 months pregnant?

YES → *Contact your doctor.* Swelling of the ankles commonly occurs after the first trimester of pregnancy, but in some cases, it indicates elevated blood pressure and the risk of PREECLAMPSIA.

NO ↓

Do you take birth control pills or corticosteroid medication?

YES → These medications can influence hormonal changes that may cause the fluid retention that results in swollen ankles. Talk to the prescribing doctor about this symptom.

NO ↓

Does the swelling generally occur just before a menstrual period?

YES → You may have premenstrual syndrome; consult a doctor if this and other symptoms are bothersome.

NO ↓

Are you experiencing pain in the ankles without swelling or other symptoms?

YES → Are you overweight?

YES → Excess body weight can sometimes result in ankle swelling. See a doctor or nutritionist about a weight-loss program appropriate for you. See OBESITY.

NO ↓

NO ↓

If you are unable to make a diagnosis from this chart, consult your doctor if symptoms persist or worsen.

Backache

Pain or stiffness that may include tenderness and may be experienced continuously or intermittently.

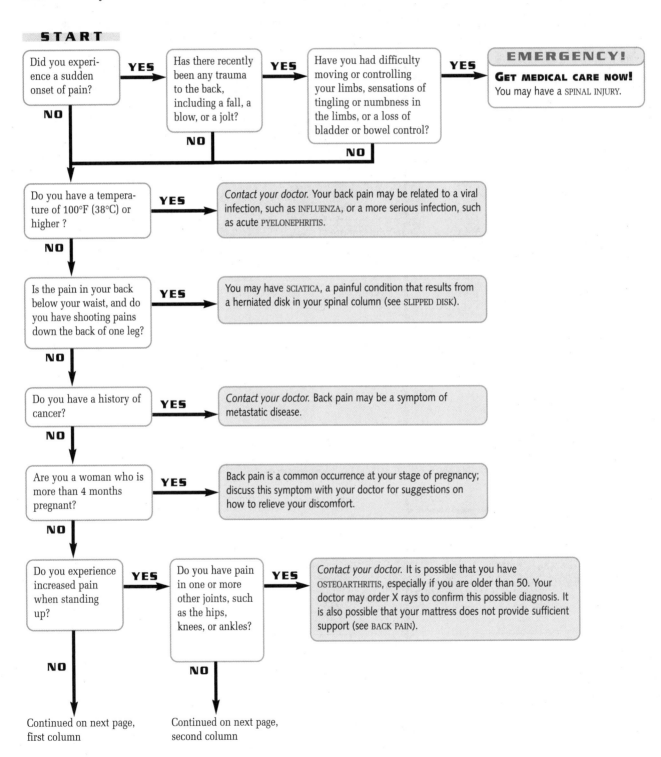

START

Did you experience a sudden onset of pain? — **YES** → Has there recently been any trauma to the back, including a fall, a blow, or a jolt? — **YES** → Have you had difficulty moving or controlling your limbs, sensations of tingling or numbness in the limbs, or a loss of bladder or bowel control? — **YES** →

EMERGENCY!
GET MEDICAL CARE NOW! You may have a SPINAL INJURY.

NO ↓ **NO** ↓ **NO** ↓

Do you have a temperature of 100°F (38°C) or higher? — **YES** → *Contact your doctor.* Your back pain may be related to a viral infection, such as INFLUENZA, or a more serious infection, such as acute PYELONEPHRITIS.

NO ↓

Is the pain in your back below your waist, and do you have shooting pains down the back of one leg? — **YES** → You may have SCIATICA, a painful condition that results from a herniated disk in your spinal column (see SLIPPED DISK).

NO ↓

Do you have a history of cancer? — **YES** → *Contact your doctor.* Back pain may be a symptom of metastatic disease.

NO ↓

Are you a woman who is more than 4 months pregnant? — **YES** → Back pain is a common occurrence at your stage of pregnancy; discuss this symptom with your doctor for suggestions on how to relieve your discomfort.

NO ↓

Do you experience increased pain when standing up? — **YES** → Do you have pain in one or more other joints, such as the hips, knees, or ankles? — **YES** → *Contact your doctor.* It is possible that you have OSTEOARTHRITIS, especially if you are older than 50. Your doctor may order X rays to confirm this possible diagnosis. It is also possible that your mattress does not provide sufficient support (see BACK PAIN).

NO ↓ **NO** ↓

Continued on next page, first column

Continued on next page, second column

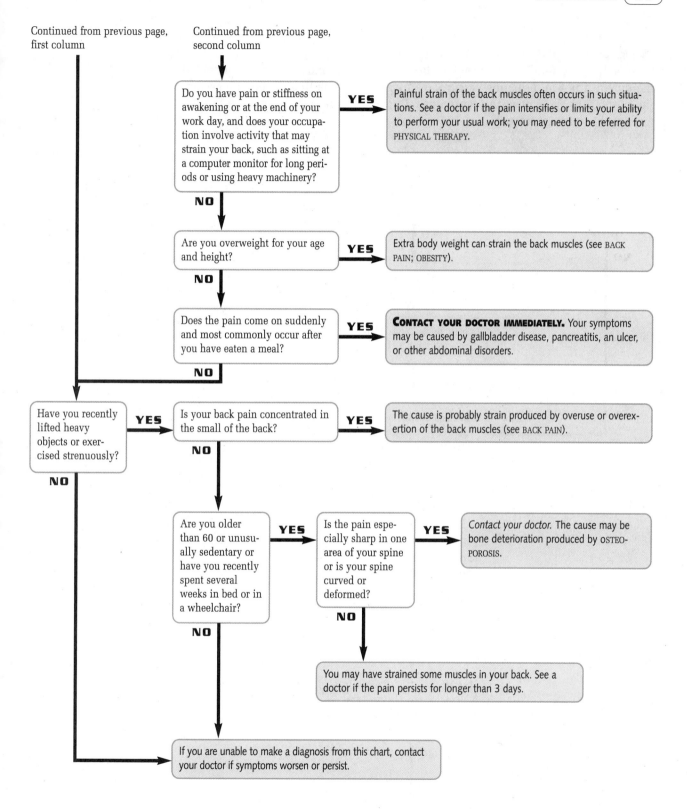

Continued from previous page, first column

Continued from previous page, second column

Do you have pain or stiffness on awakening or at the end of your work day, and does your occupation involve activity that may strain your back, such as sitting at a computer monitor for long periods or using heavy machinery?

YES → Painful strain of the back muscles often occurs in such situations. See a doctor if the pain intensifies or limits your ability to perform your usual work; you may need to be referred for PHYSICAL THERAPY.

NO

Are you overweight for your age and height?

YES → Extra body weight can strain the back muscles (see BACK PAIN; OBESITY).

NO

Does the pain come on suddenly and most commonly occur after you have eaten a meal?

YES → **CONTACT YOUR DOCTOR IMMEDIATELY.** Your symptoms may be caused by gallbladder disease, pancreatitis, an ulcer, or other abdominal disorders.

NO

Have you recently lifted heavy objects or exercised strenuously?

YES → Is your back pain concentrated in the small of the back?

YES → The cause is probably strain produced by overuse or overexertion of the back muscles (see BACK PAIN).

NO (Have you recently lifted...)

NO (Is your back pain...)

Are you older than 60 or unusually sedentary or have you recently spent several weeks in bed or in a wheelchair?

YES → Is the pain especially sharp in one area of your spine or is your spine curved or deformed?

YES → *Contact your doctor.* The cause may be bone deterioration produced by OSTEOPOROSIS.

NO (Is the pain especially sharp...)

You may have strained some muscles in your back. See a doctor if the pain persists for longer than 3 days.

NO (Are you older than 60...)

If you are unable to make a diagnosis from this chart, contact your doctor if symptoms worsen or persist.

Breast pain or lumps

Pain, aching, or tenderness in one or both breasts that may commonly occur during pregnancy, within 4 months postpartum, or during breastfeeding or may be associated with the menstrual cycle or with menopause. Lumps are masses that can be felt during examination of the breast tissues.

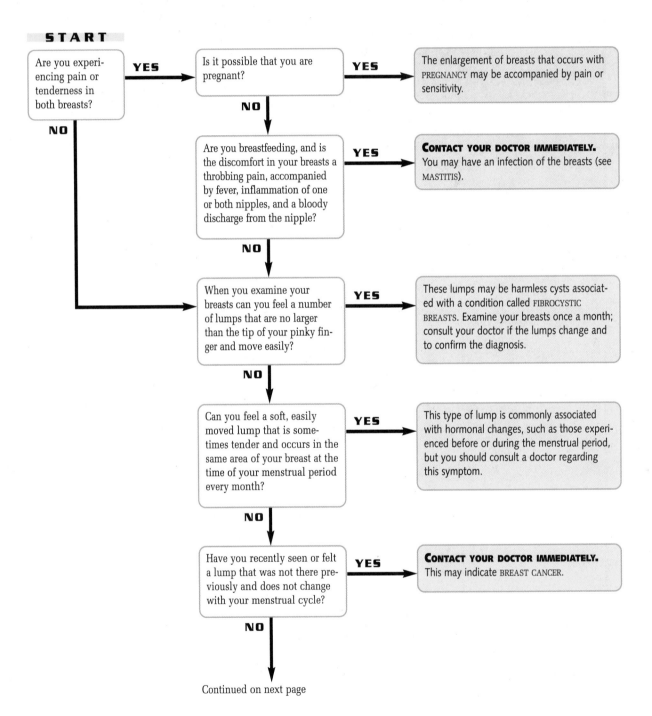

START

Are you experiencing pain or tenderness in both breasts?

YES → Is it possible that you are pregnant?

YES → The enlargement of breasts that occurs with PREGNANCY may be accompanied by pain or sensitivity.

NO ↓

Are you breastfeeding, and is the discomfort in your breasts a throbbing pain, accompanied by fever, inflammation of one or both nipples, and a bloody discharge from the nipple?

YES → **CONTACT YOUR DOCTOR IMMEDIATELY.** You may have an infection of the breasts (see MASTITIS).

NO ↓

When you examine your breasts can you feel a number of lumps that are no larger than the tip of your pinky finger and move easily?

YES → These lumps may be harmless cysts associated with a condition called FIBROCYSTIC BREASTS. Examine your breasts once a month; consult your doctor if the lumps change and to confirm the diagnosis.

NO ↓

Can you feel a soft, easily moved lump that is sometimes tender and occurs in the same area of your breast at the time of your menstrual period every month?

YES → This type of lump is commonly associated with hormonal changes, such as those experienced before or during the menstrual period, but you should consult a doctor regarding this symptom.

NO ↓

Have you recently seen or felt a lump that was not there previously and does not change with your menstrual cycle?

YES → **CONTACT YOUR DOCTOR IMMEDIATELY.** This may indicate BREAST CANCER.

NO ↓

Continued on next page

Continued from previous page

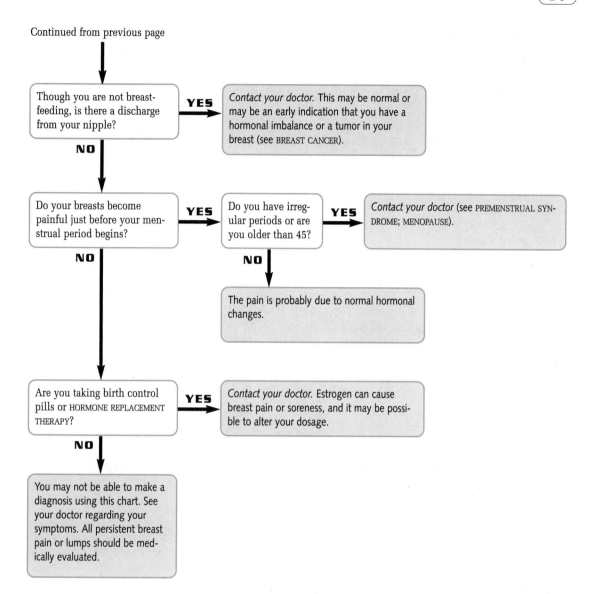

Though you are not breast-feeding, is there a discharge from your nipple?

YES → *Contact your doctor.* This may be normal or may be an early indication that you have a hormonal imbalance or a tumor in your breast (SEE BREAST CANCER).

NO

Do your breasts become painful just before your menstrual period begins?

YES → Do you have irregular periods or are you older than 45?

YES → *Contact your doctor* (SEE PREMENSTRUAL SYNDROME; MENOPAUSE).

NO

The pain is probably due to normal hormonal changes.

Are you taking birth control pills or HORMONE REPLACEMENT THERAPY?

YES → *Contact your doctor.* Estrogen can cause breast pain or soreness, and it may be possible to alter your dosage.

NO

You may not be able to make a diagnosis using this chart. See your doctor regarding your symptoms. All persistent breast pain or lumps should be medically evaluated.

Chest pain

Pain that occurs in the area between the neck and the bottom of the rib cage and may be experienced as mild, aching, dull, and pressing or as severe, stabbing, burning, or crushing.

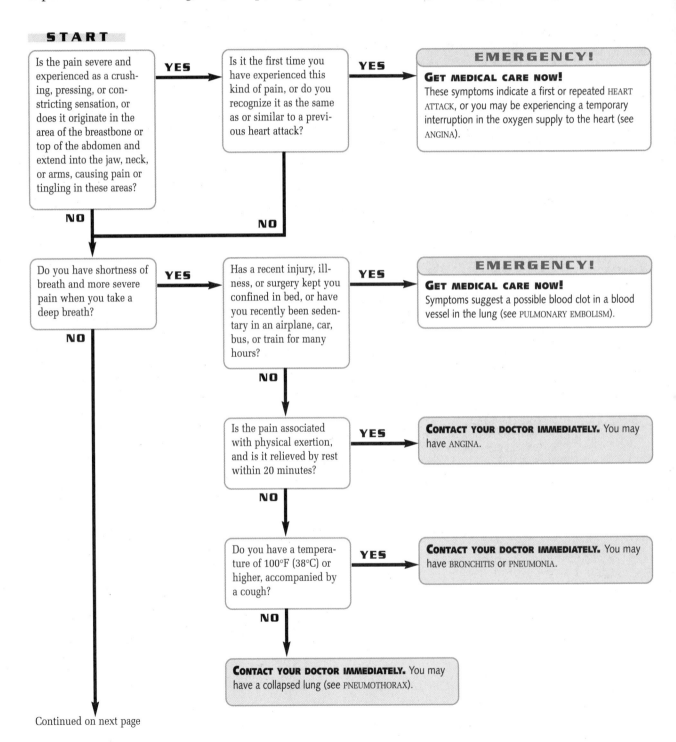

START

Is the pain severe and experienced as a crushing, pressing, or constricting sensation, or does it originate in the area of the breastbone or top of the abdomen and extend into the jaw, neck, or arms, causing pain or tingling in these areas?

YES →

Is it the first time you have experienced this kind of pain, or do you recognize it as the same as or similar to a previous heart attack?

YES →

EMERGENCY!

GET MEDICAL CARE NOW! These symptoms indicate a first or repeated HEART ATTACK, or you may be experiencing a temporary interruption in the oxygen supply to the heart (see ANGINA).

NO ↓ / **NO** ↓

Do you have shortness of breath and more severe pain when you take a deep breath?

YES →

Has a recent injury, illness, or surgery kept you confined in bed, or have you recently been sedentary in an airplane, car, bus, or train for many hours?

YES →

EMERGENCY!

GET MEDICAL CARE NOW! Symptoms suggest a possible blood clot in a blood vessel in the lung (see PULMONARY EMBOLISM).

NO ↓ / **NO** ↓

Is the pain associated with physical exertion, and is it relieved by rest within 20 minutes?

YES →

CONTACT YOUR DOCTOR IMMEDIATELY. You may have ANGINA.

NO ↓

Do you have a temperature of 100°F (38°C) or higher, accompanied by a cough?

YES →

CONTACT YOUR DOCTOR IMMEDIATELY. You may have BRONCHITIS or PNEUMONIA.

NO ↓

CONTACT YOUR DOCTOR IMMEDIATELY. You may have a collapsed lung (see PNEUMOTHORAX).

Continued on next page

Continued from previous page

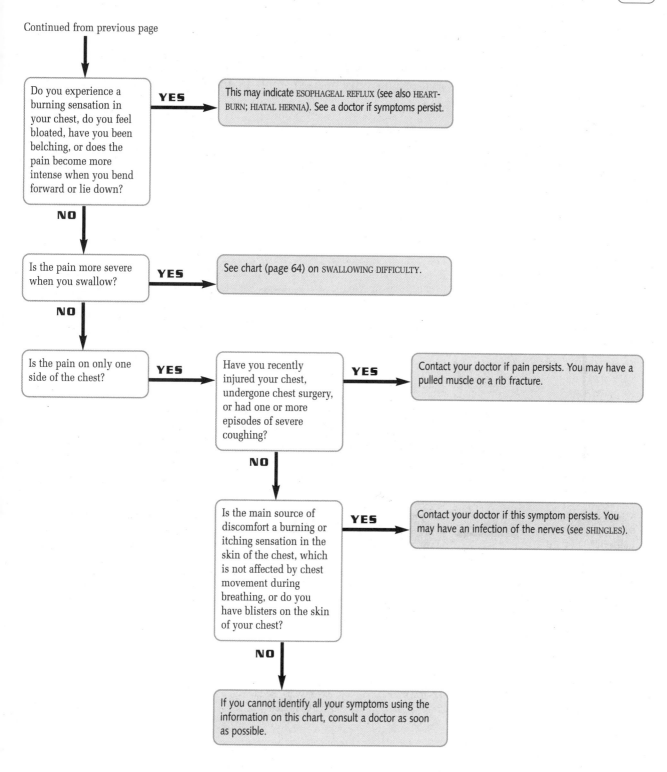

Do you experience a burning sensation in your chest, do you feel bloated, have you been belching, or does the pain become more intense when you bend forward or lie down? — **YES** → This may indicate ESOPHAGEAL REFLUX (see also HEARTBURN; HIATAL HERNIA). See a doctor if symptoms persist.

NO ↓

Is the pain more severe when you swallow? — **YES** → See chart (page 64) on SWALLOWING DIFFICULTY.

NO ↓

Is the pain on only one side of the chest? — **YES** → Have you recently injured your chest, undergone chest surgery, or had one or more episodes of severe coughing? — **YES** → Contact your doctor if pain persists. You may have a pulled muscle or a rib fracture.

NO ↓

Is the main source of discomfort a burning or itching sensation in the skin of the chest, which is not affected by chest movement during breathing, or do you have blisters on the skin of your chest? — **YES** → Contact your doctor if this symptom persists. You may have an infection of the nerves (see SHINGLES).

NO ↓

If you cannot identify all your symptoms using the information on this chart, consult a doctor as soon as possible.

Constipation

Infrequent bowel movements (fewer than 3 per week), painful bowel movements, or uncomfortable bowel movements that produce dry or hard stools in adults.

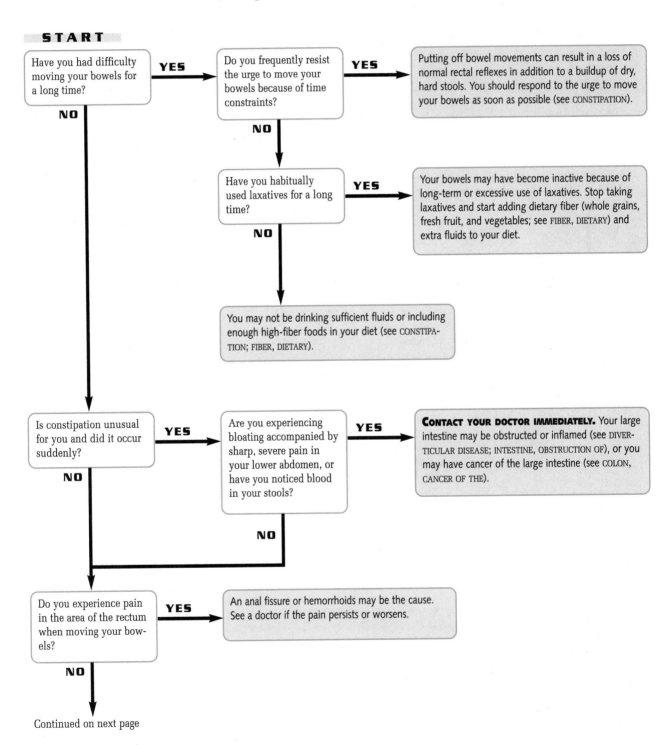

START

Have you had difficulty moving your bowels for a long time? — **YES** →

Do you frequently resist the urge to move your bowels because of time constraints? — **YES** →

Putting off bowel movements can result in a loss of normal rectal reflexes in addition to a buildup of dry, hard stools. You should respond to the urge to move your bowels as soon as possible (see CONSTIPATION).

NO ↓

Have you habitually used laxatives for a long time? — **YES** →

Your bowels may have become inactive because of long-term or excessive use of laxatives. Stop taking laxatives and start adding dietary fiber (whole grains, fresh fruit, and vegetables; see FIBER, DIETARY) and extra fluids to your diet.

NO ↓

You may not be drinking sufficient fluids or including enough high-fiber foods in your diet (see CONSTIPA-TION; FIBER, DIETARY).

NO ↓ (from first question)

Is constipation unusual for you and did it occur suddenly? — **YES** →

Are you experiencing bloating accompanied by sharp, severe pain in your lower abdomen, or have you noticed blood in your stools? — **YES** →

CONTACT YOUR DOCTOR IMMEDIATELY. Your large intestine may be obstructed or inflamed (see DIVER-TICULAR DISEASE; INTESTINE, OBSTRUCTION OF), or you may have cancer of the large intestine (see COLON, CANCER OF THE).

NO ↓

NO ↓

Do you experience pain in the area of the rectum when moving your bowels? — **YES** →

An anal fissure or hemorrhoids may be the cause. See a doctor if the pain persists or worsens.

NO ↓

Continued on next page

Continued from previous page

Are you currently taking any over-the-counter or prescription medications?

YES → *Contact your doctor.* Constipation may be a side effect of a medication you are taking.

NO ↓

Are you pregnant?

YES → Constipation commonly occurs during pregnancy. Discuss possible remedies with your doctor.

NO ↓

Are you experiencing two or more of the following: unexplained weight gain, unexplained fatigue, dry skin or hair, or increased intolerance to cold?

YES → Your thyroid gland may be underactive (see HYPOTHYROIDISM).

NO ↓

Do you have cramping pain in the lower abdomen, usually on the left side?

YES → Have you had constipation accompanied by cramping pain for many years?

YES → Your symptoms may indicate IRRITABLE BOWEL SYNDROME.

NO ↓

Have you had bouts of diarrhea in addition to constipation, and do you sometimes have painful abdominal cramping?

YES → Call a doctor if these symptoms continue or worsen. You may have IRRITABLE BOWEL SYNDROME.

NO ↓

Try taking over-the-counter psyllium fiber or methyl-cellulose to relieve constipation. Consult a doctor if symptoms persist.

NO ↓

If you are unable to make a diagnosis from this chart, contact your doctor if symptoms worsen or persist.

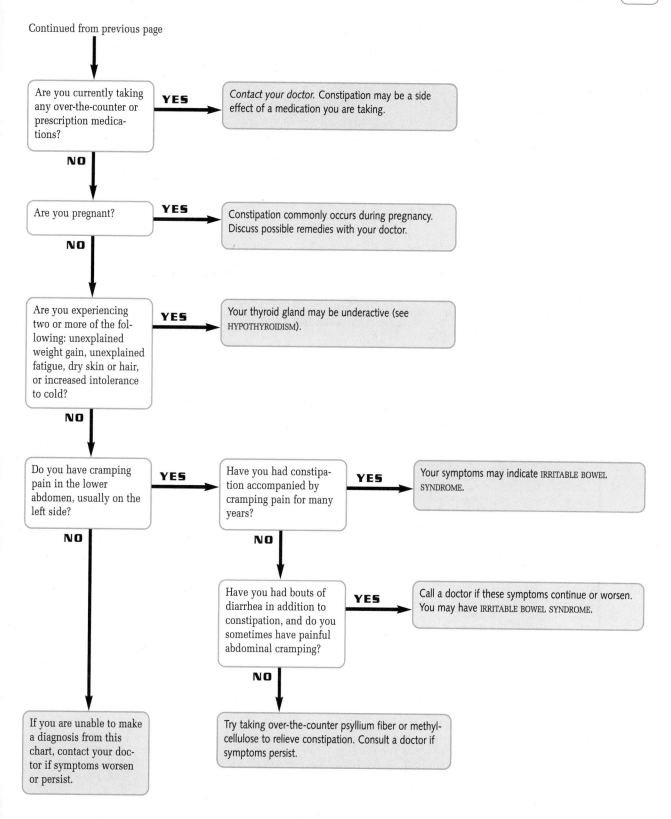

Coughing

A noisy expulsion of air from the lungs.

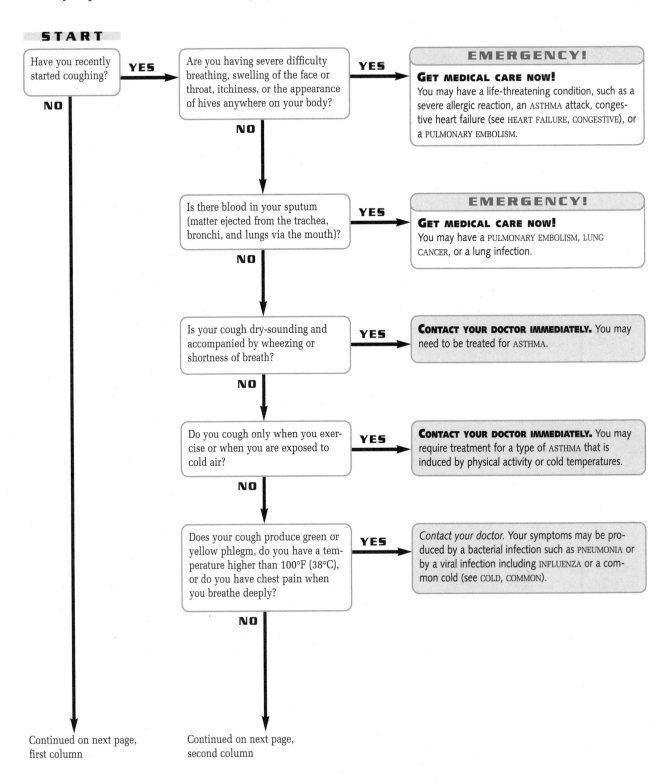

START

Have you recently started coughing? — **YES** → Are you having severe difficulty breathing, swelling of the face or throat, itchiness, or the appearance of hives anywhere on your body? — **YES** →

EMERGENCY!

GET MEDICAL CARE NOW! You may have a life-threatening condition, such as a severe allergic reaction, an ASTHMA attack, congestive heart failure (see HEART FAILURE, CONGESTIVE), or a PULMONARY EMBOLISM.

NO ↓

Is there blood in your sputum (matter ejected from the trachea, bronchi, and lungs via the mouth)? — **YES** →

EMERGENCY!

GET MEDICAL CARE NOW! You may have a PULMONARY EMBOLISM, LUNG CANCER, or a lung infection.

NO ↓

Is your cough dry-sounding and accompanied by wheezing or shortness of breath? — **YES** →

CONTACT YOUR DOCTOR IMMEDIATELY. You may need to be treated for ASTHMA.

NO ↓

Do you cough only when you exercise or when you are exposed to cold air? — **YES** →

CONTACT YOUR DOCTOR IMMEDIATELY. You may require treatment for a type of ASTHMA that is induced by physical activity or cold temperatures.

NO ↓

Does your cough produce green or yellow phlegm, do you have a temperature higher than 100°F (38°C), or do you have chest pain when you breathe deeply? — **YES** →

Contact your doctor. Your symptoms may be produced by a bacterial infection such as PNEUMONIA or by a viral infection including INFLUENZA or a common cold (see COLD, COMMON).

NO ↓

Continued on next page, first column

Continued on next page, second column

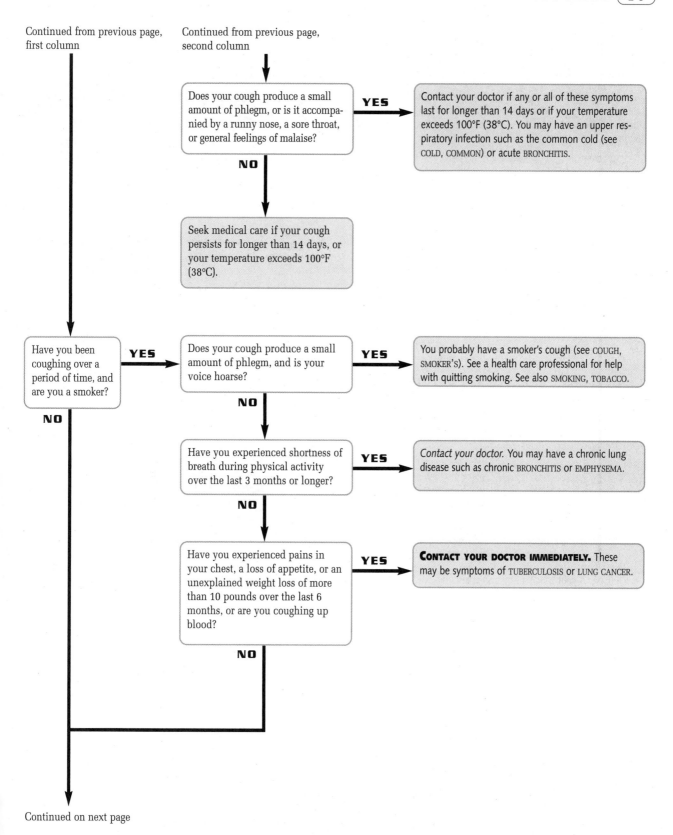

Continued from previous page, first column

Continued from previous page, second column

Does your cough produce a small amount of phlegm, or is it accompanied by a runny nose, a sore throat, or general feelings of malaise?

YES → Contact your doctor if any or all of these symptoms last for longer than 14 days or if your temperature exceeds 100°F (38°C). You may have an upper respiratory infection such as the common cold (see COLD, COMMON) or acute BRONCHITIS.

NO ↓

Seek medical care if your cough persists for longer than 14 days, or your temperature exceeds 100°F (38°C).

Have you been coughing over a period of time, and are you a smoker?

YES → Does your cough produce a small amount of phlegm, and is your voice hoarse?

YES → You probably have a smoker's cough (see COUGH, SMOKER'S). See a health care professional for help with quitting smoking. See also SMOKING, TOBACCO.

NO ↓

Have you experienced shortness of breath during physical activity over the last 3 months or longer?

YES → *Contact your doctor.* You may have a chronic lung disease such as chronic BRONCHITIS or EMPHYSEMA.

NO ↓

Have you experienced pains in your chest, a loss of appetite, or an unexplained weight loss of more than 10 pounds over the last 6 months, or are you coughing up blood?

YES → **CONTACT YOUR DOCTOR IMMEDIATELY.** These may be symptoms of TUBERCULOSIS or LUNG CANCER.

NO ↓

Continued on next page

Continued from previous page

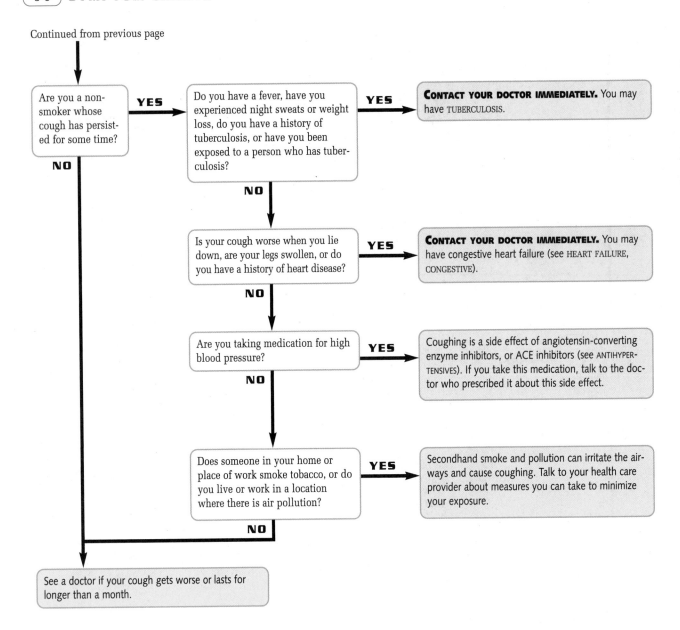

Are you a non-smoker whose cough has persisted for some time?

YES → Do you have a fever, have you experienced night sweats or weight loss, do you have a history of tuberculosis, or have you been exposed to a person who has tuberculosis?

YES → **CONTACT YOUR DOCTOR IMMEDIATELY.** You may have TUBERCULOSIS.

NO ↓

Is your cough worse when you lie down, are your legs swollen, or do you have a history of heart disease?

YES → **CONTACT YOUR DOCTOR IMMEDIATELY.** You may have congestive heart failure (see HEART FAILURE, CONGESTIVE).

NO ↓

Are you taking medication for high blood pressure?

YES → Coughing is a side effect of angiotensin-converting enzyme inhibitors, or ACE inhibitors (see ANTIHYPERTENSIVES). If you take this medication, talk to the doctor who prescribed it about this side effect.

NO ↓

Does someone in your home or place of work smoke tobacco, or do you live or work in a location where there is air pollution?

YES → Secondhand smoke and pollution can irritate the airways and cause coughing. Talk to your health care provider about measures you can take to minimize your exposure.

NO ↓

See a doctor if your cough gets worse or lasts for longer than a month.

Hoarseness or voice loss

Abnormal huskiness in the voice that may range from a slight deepening of the speaking voice to an inability to make the normal sounds of speech.

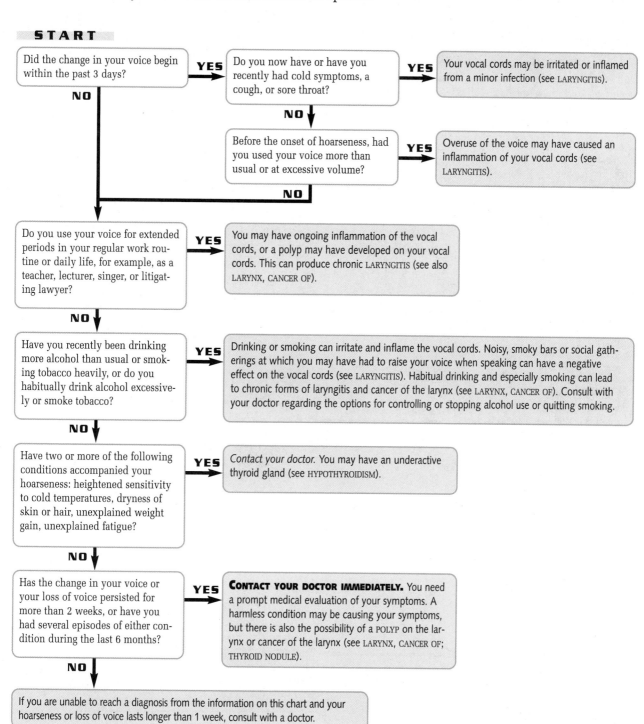

START

Did the change in your voice begin within the past 3 days?

YES → Do you now have or have you recently had cold symptoms, a cough, or sore throat?

YES → Your vocal cords may be irritated or inflamed from a minor infection (see LARYNGITIS).

NO (from cold symptoms) → Before the onset of hoarseness, had you used your voice more than usual or at excessive volume?

YES → Overuse of the voice may have caused an inflammation of your vocal cords (see LARYNGITIS).

NO (from first question and from voice overuse) →

Do you use your voice for extended periods in your regular work routine or daily life, for example, as a teacher, lecturer, singer, or litigating lawyer?

YES → You may have ongoing inflammation of the vocal cords, or a polyp may have developed on your vocal cords. This can produce chronic LARYNGITIS (see also LARYNX, CANCER OF).

NO →

Have you recently been drinking more alcohol than usual or smoking tobacco heavily, or do you habitually drink alcohol excessively or smoke tobacco?

YES → Drinking or smoking can irritate and inflame the vocal cords. Noisy, smoky bars or social gatherings at which you may have had to raise your voice when speaking can have a negative effect on the vocal cords (see LARYNGITIS). Habitual drinking and especially smoking can lead to chronic forms of laryngitis and cancer of the larynx (see LARYNX, CANCER OF). Consult with your doctor regarding the options for controlling or stopping alcohol use or quitting smoking.

NO →

Have two or more of the following conditions accompanied your hoarseness: heightened sensitivity to cold temperatures, dryness of skin or hair, unexplained weight gain, unexplained fatigue?

YES → *Contact your doctor.* You may have an underactive thyroid gland (see HYPOTHYROIDISM).

NO →

Has the change in your voice or your loss of voice persisted for more than 2 weeks, or have you had several episodes of either condition during the last 6 months?

YES → **CONTACT YOUR DOCTOR IMMEDIATELY.** You need a prompt medical evaluation of your symptoms. A harmless condition may be causing your symptoms, but there is also the possibility of a POLYP on the larynx or cancer of the larynx (see LARYNX, CANCER OF; THYROID NODULE).

NO →

If you are unable to reach a diagnosis from the information on this chart and your hoarseness or loss of voice lasts longer than 1 week, consult with a doctor.

Depression

Feelings of sadness, hopelessness, unworthiness, despair, or guilt that may define a passing mood or may be so debilitating that a person becomes unable to cope with everyday life.

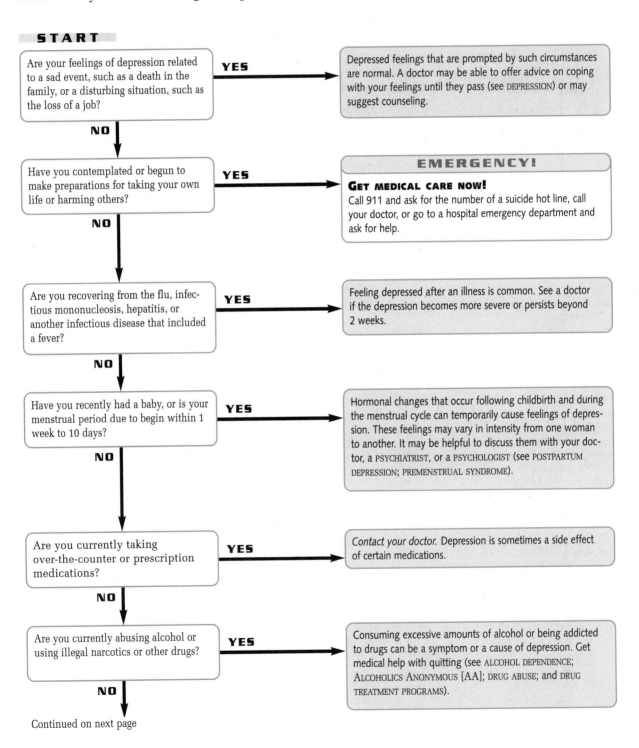

START

Are your feelings of depression related to a sad event, such as a death in the family, or a disturbing situation, such as the loss of a job?

YES → Depressed feelings that are prompted by such circumstances are normal. A doctor may be able to offer advice on coping with your feelings until they pass (see DEPRESSION) or may suggest counseling.

NO ↓

Have you contemplated or begun to make preparations for taking your own life or harming others?

YES → **EMERGENCY!**

GET MEDICAL CARE NOW!
Call 911 and ask for the number of a suicide hot line, call your doctor, or go to a hospital emergency department and ask for help.

NO ↓

Are you recovering from the flu, infectious mononucleosis, hepatitis, or another infectious disease that included a fever?

YES → Feeling depressed after an illness is common. See a doctor if the depression becomes more severe or persists beyond 2 weeks.

NO ↓

Have you recently had a baby, or is your menstrual period due to begin within 1 week to 10 days?

YES → Hormonal changes that occur following childbirth and during the menstrual cycle can temporarily cause feelings of depression. These feelings may vary in intensity from one woman to another. It may be helpful to discuss them with your doctor, a PSYCHIATRIST, or a PSYCHOLOGIST (see POSTPARTUM DEPRESSION; PREMENSTRUAL SYNDROME).

NO ↓

Are you currently taking over-the-counter or prescription medications?

YES → *Contact your doctor.* Depression is sometimes a side effect of certain medications.

NO ↓

Are you currently abusing alcohol or using illegal narcotics or other drugs?

YES → Consuming excessive amounts of alcohol or being addicted to drugs can be a symptom or a cause of depression. Get medical help with quitting (see ALCOHOL DEPENDENCE; ALCOHOLICS ANONYMOUS [AA]; DRUG ABUSE; and DRUG TREATMENT PROGRAMS).

NO ↓

Continued on next page

Continued from previous page

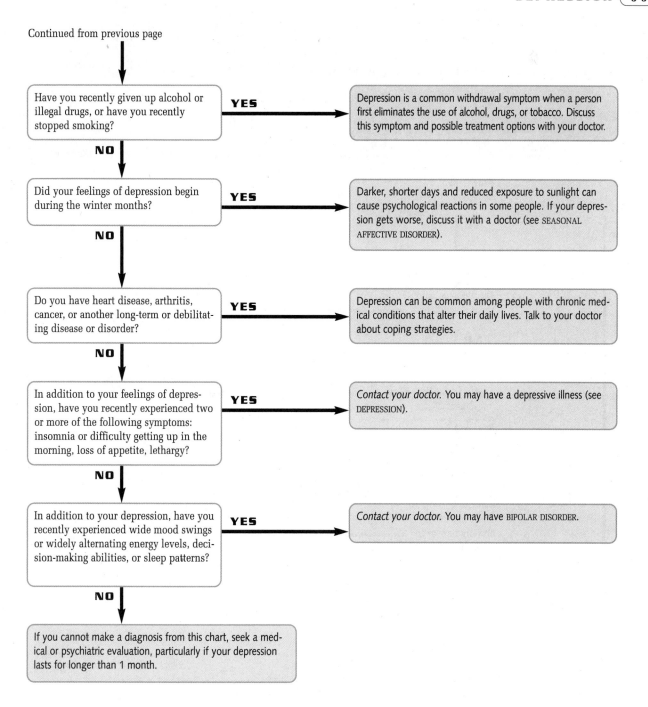

Have you recently given up alcohol or illegal drugs, or have you recently stopped smoking?

YES → Depression is a common withdrawal symptom when a person first eliminates the use of alcohol, drugs, or tobacco. Discuss this symptom and possible treatment options with your doctor.

NO ↓

Did your feelings of depression begin during the winter months?

YES → Darker, shorter days and reduced exposure to sunlight can cause psychological reactions in some people. If your depression gets worse, discuss it with a doctor (see SEASONAL AFFECTIVE DISORDER).

NO ↓

Do you have heart disease, arthritis, cancer, or another long-term or debilitating disease or disorder?

YES → Depression can be common among people with chronic medical conditions that alter their daily lives. Talk to your doctor about coping strategies.

NO ↓

In addition to your feelings of depression, have you recently experienced two or more of the following symptoms: insomnia or difficulty getting up in the morning, loss of appetite, lethargy?

YES → *Contact your doctor.* You may have a depressive illness (see DEPRESSION).

NO ↓

In addition to your depression, have you recently experienced wide mood swings or widely alternating energy levels, decision-making abilities, or sleep patterns?

YES → *Contact your doctor.* You may have BIPOLAR DISORDER.

NO ↓

If you cannot make a diagnosis from this chart, seek a medical or psychiatric evaluation, particularly if your depression lasts for longer than 1 month.

Diarrhea

Frequent passing of loose or watery bowel movements.

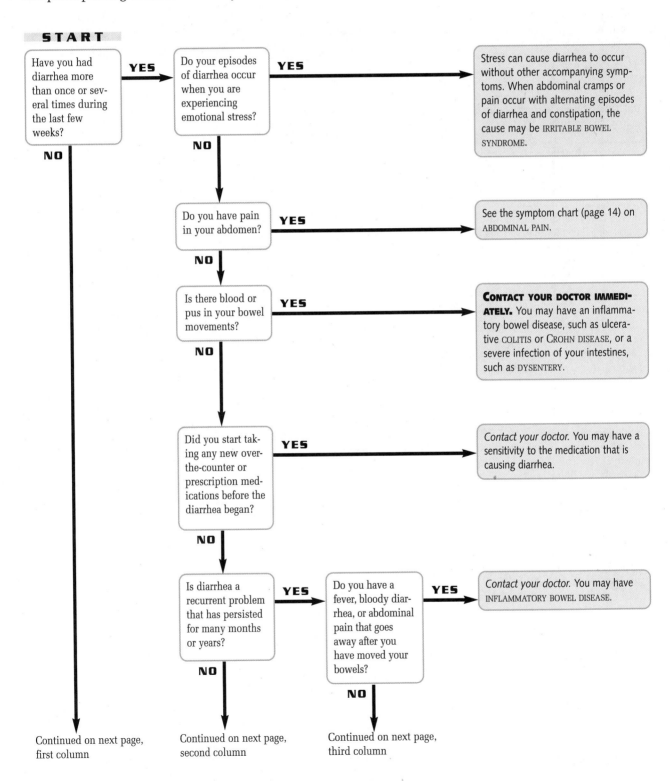

START

Have you had diarrhea more than once or several times during the last few weeks?

YES →

Do your episodes of diarrhea occur when you are experiencing emotional stress?

YES →

Stress can cause diarrhea to occur without other accompanying symptoms. When abdominal cramps or pain occur with alternating episodes of diarrhea and constipation, the cause may be IRRITABLE BOWEL SYNDROME.

NO ↓

Do you have pain in your abdomen?

YES →

See the symptom chart (page 14) on ABDOMINAL PAIN.

NO ↓

Is there blood or pus in your bowel movements?

YES →

CONTACT YOUR DOCTOR IMMEDIATELY. You may have an inflammatory bowel disease, such as ulcerative COLITIS or CROHN DISEASE, or a severe infection of your intestines, such as DYSENTERY.

NO ↓

Did you start taking any new over-the-counter or prescription medications before the diarrhea began?

YES →

Contact your doctor. You may have a sensitivity to the medication that is causing diarrhea.

NO ↓

Is diarrhea a recurrent problem that has persisted for many months or years?

YES →

Do you have a fever, bloody diarrhea, or abdominal pain that goes away after you have moved your bowels?

YES →

Contact your doctor. You may have INFLAMMATORY BOWEL DISEASE.

NO ↓ (from abdomen pain bottom box)

Continued on next page, first column

Continued on next page, second column

Continued on next page, third column

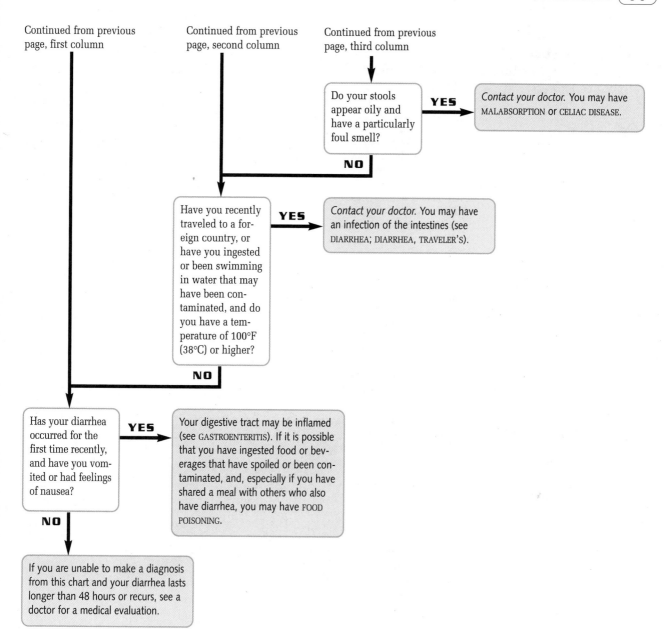

Continued from previous page, first column

Continued from previous page, second column

Continued from previous page, third column

Do your stools appear oily and have a particularly foul smell?

YES → *Contact your doctor.* You may have MALABSORPTION or CELIAC DISEASE.

NO

Have you recently traveled to a foreign country, or have you ingested or been swimming in water that may have been contaminated, and do you have a temperature of 100°F (38°C) or higher?

YES → *Contact your doctor.* You may have an infection of the intestines (see DIARRHEA; DIARRHEA, TRAVELER'S).

NO

Has your diarrhea occurred for the first time recently, and have you vomited or had feelings of nausea?

YES → Your digestive tract may be inflamed (see GASTROENTERITIS). If it is possible that you have ingested food or beverages that have spoiled or been contaminated, and, especially if you have shared a meal with others who also have diarrhea, you may have FOOD POISONING.

NO

If you are unable to make a diagnosis from this chart and your diarrhea lasts longer than 48 hours or recurs, see a doctor for a medical evaluation.

Dizziness

A spinning sensation that may be accompanied by a dazed, unsteady feeling or a sense of light-headedness.

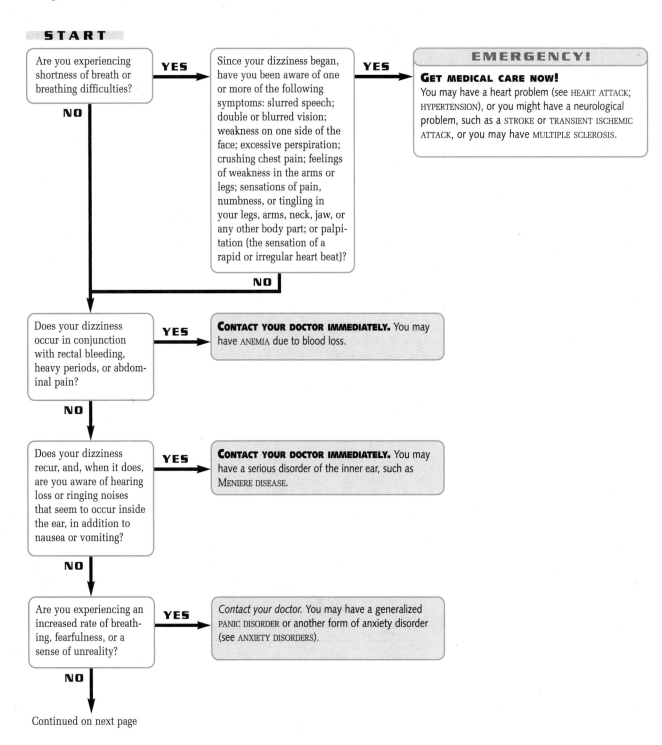

START

Are you experiencing shortness of breath or breathing difficulties?

YES →

Since your dizziness began, have you been aware of one or more of the following symptoms: slurred speech; double or blurred vision; weakness on one side of the face; excessive perspiration; crushing chest pain; feelings of weakness in the arms or legs; sensations of pain, numbness, or tingling in your legs, arms, neck, jaw, or any other body part; or palpitation (the sensation of a rapid or irregular heart beat)?

YES →

EMERGENCY!

GET MEDICAL CARE NOW!
You may have a heart problem (see HEART ATTACK; HYPERTENSION), or you might have a neurological problem, such as a STROKE or TRANSIENT ISCHEMIC ATTACK, or you may have MULTIPLE SCLEROSIS.

NO

NO

Does your dizziness occur in conjunction with rectal bleeding, heavy periods, or abdominal pain?

YES →

CONTACT YOUR DOCTOR IMMEDIATELY. You may have ANEMIA due to blood loss.

NO

Does your dizziness recur, and, when it does, are you aware of hearing loss or ringing noises that seem to occur inside the ear, in addition to nausea or vomiting?

YES →

CONTACT YOUR DOCTOR IMMEDIATELY. You may have a serious disorder of the inner ear, such as MENIERE DISEASE.

NO

Are you experiencing an increased rate of breathing, fearfulness, or a sense of unreality?

YES →

Contact your doctor. You may have a generalized PANIC DISORDER or another form of anxiety disorder (see ANXIETY DISORDERS).

NO

Continued on next page

Continued from previous page

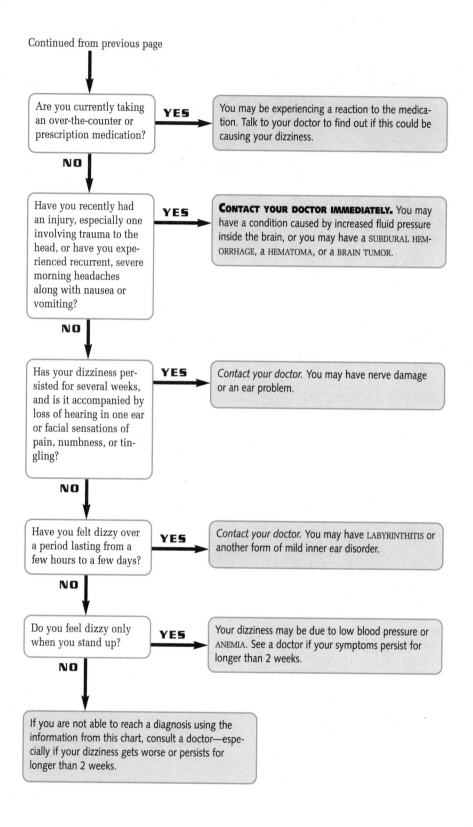

Are you currently taking an over-the-counter or prescription medication?

YES → You may be experiencing a reaction to the medication. Talk to your doctor to find out if this could be causing your dizziness.

NO ↓

Have you recently had an injury, especially one involving trauma to the head, or have you experienced recurrent, severe morning headaches along with nausea or vomiting?

YES → **CONTACT YOUR DOCTOR IMMEDIATELY.** You may have a condition caused by increased fluid pressure inside the brain, or you may have a SUBDURAL HEMORRHAGE, a HEMATOMA, or a BRAIN TUMOR.

NO ↓

Has your dizziness persisted for several weeks, and is it accompanied by loss of hearing in one ear or facial sensations of pain, numbness, or tingling?

YES → *Contact your doctor.* You may have nerve damage or an ear problem.

NO ↓

Have you felt dizzy over a period lasting from a few hours to a few days?

YES → *Contact your doctor.* You may have LABYRINTHITIS or another form of mild inner ear disorder.

NO ↓

Do you feel dizzy only when you stand up?

YES → Your dizziness may be due to low blood pressure or ANEMIA. See a doctor if your symptoms persist for longer than 2 weeks.

NO ↓

If you are not able to reach a diagnosis using the information from this chart, consult a doctor—especially if your dizziness gets worse or persists for longer than 2 weeks.

Headache

Any pain in the head that may range in severity from mild to incapacitating.

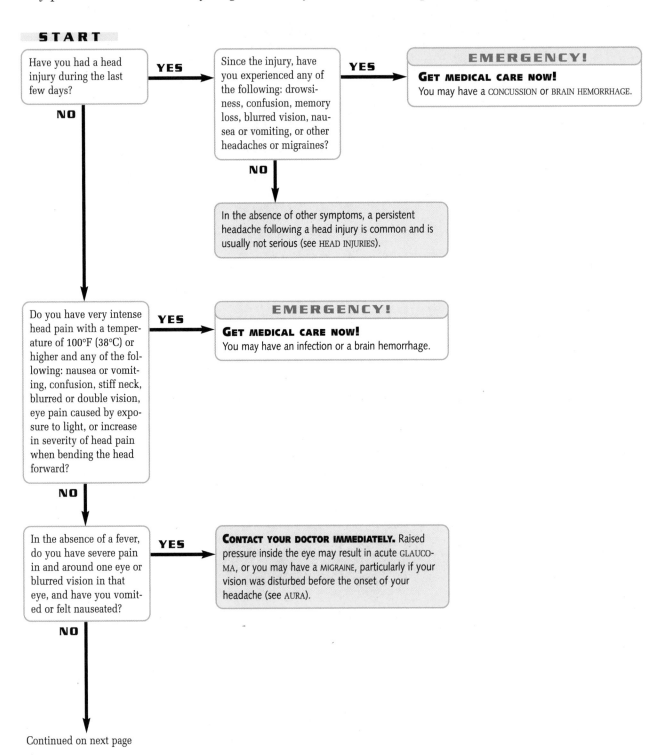

START

Have you had a head injury during the last few days?

YES →

Since the injury, have you experienced any of the following: drowsiness, confusion, memory loss, blurred vision, nausea or vomiting, or other headaches or migraines?

YES →

EMERGENCY!

GET MEDICAL CARE NOW!
You may have a CONCUSSION or BRAIN HEMORRHAGE.

NO ↓

In the absence of other symptoms, a persistent headache following a head injury is common and is usually not serious (see HEAD INJURIES).

NO ↓

Do you have very intense head pain with a temperature of 100°F (38°C) or higher and any of the following: nausea or vomiting, confusion, stiff neck, blurred or double vision, eye pain caused by exposure to light, or increase in severity of head pain when bending the head forward?

YES →

EMERGENCY!

GET MEDICAL CARE NOW!
You may have an infection or a brain hemorrhage.

NO ↓

In the absence of a fever, do you have severe pain in and around one eye or blurred vision in that eye, and have you vomited or felt nauseated?

YES →

CONTACT YOUR DOCTOR IMMEDIATELY. Raised pressure inside the eye may result in acute GLAUCOMA, or you may have a MIGRAINE, particularly if your vision was disturbed before the onset of your headache (see AURA).

NO ↓

Continued on next page

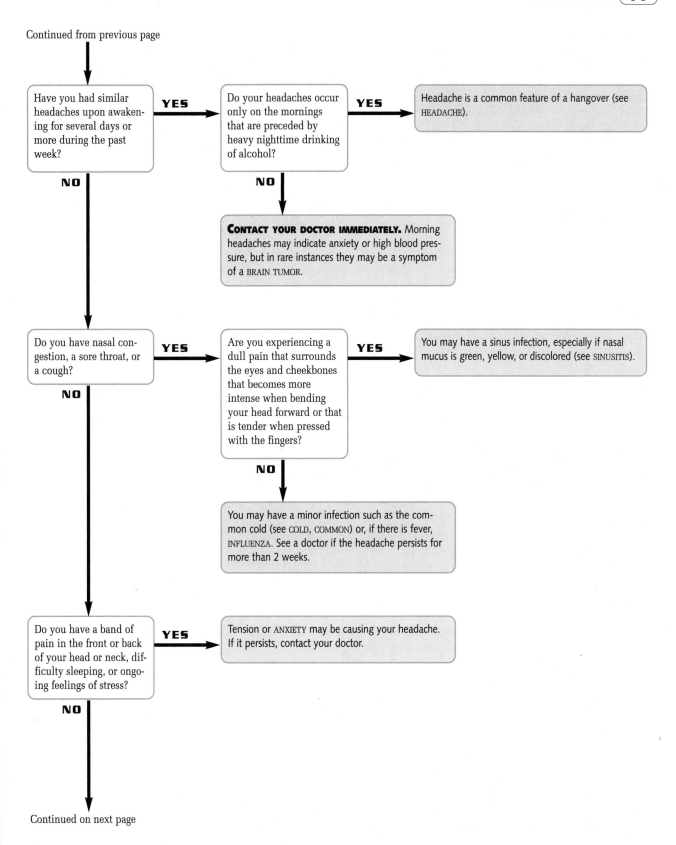

Continued from previous page

Have you had similar headaches upon awakening for several days or more during the past week?

YES →

Do your headaches occur only on the mornings that are preceded by heavy nighttime drinking of alcohol?

YES →

Headache is a common feature of a hangover (see HEADACHE).

NO ↓

NO ↓

CONTACT YOUR DOCTOR IMMEDIATELY. Morning headaches may indicate anxiety or high blood pressure, but in rare instances they may be a symptom of a BRAIN TUMOR.

Do you have nasal congestion, a sore throat, or a cough?

YES →

Are you experiencing a dull pain that surrounds the eyes and cheekbones that becomes more intense when bending your head forward or that is tender when pressed with the fingers?

YES →

You may have a sinus infection, especially if nasal mucus is green, yellow, or discolored (see SINUSITIS).

NO ↓

NO ↓

You may have a minor infection such as the common cold (see COLD, COMMON) or, if there is fever, INFLUENZA. See a doctor if the headache persists for more than 2 weeks.

Do you have a band of pain in the front or back of your head or neck, difficulty sleeping, or ongoing feelings of stress?

YES →

Tension or ANXIETY may be causing your headache. If it persists, contact your doctor.

NO ↓

Continued on next page

Continued from previous page

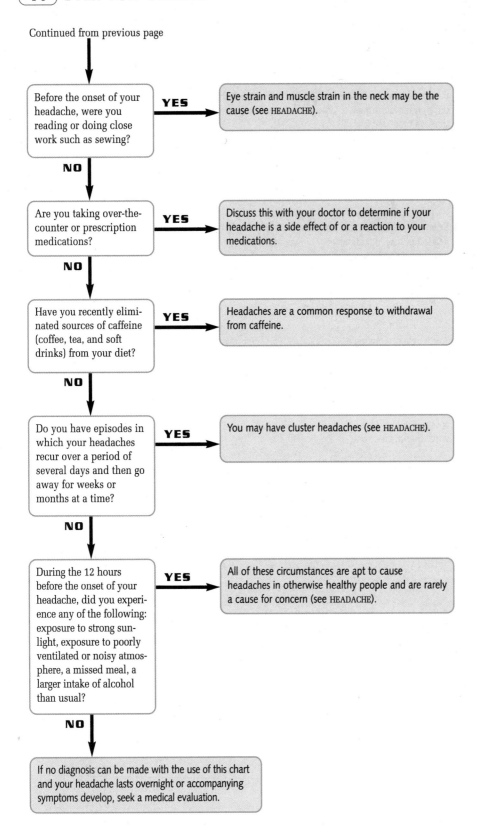

Before the onset of your headache, were you reading or doing close work such as sewing?

YES → Eye strain and muscle strain in the neck may be the cause (see HEADACHE).

NO

Are you taking over-the-counter or prescription medications?

YES → Discuss this with your doctor to determine if your headache is a side effect of or a reaction to your medications.

NO

Have you recently eliminated sources of caffeine (coffee, tea, and soft drinks) from your diet?

YES → Headaches are a common response to withdrawal from caffeine.

NO

Do you have episodes in which your headaches recur over a period of several days and then go away for weeks or months at a time?

YES → You may have cluster headaches (see HEADACHE).

NO

During the 12 hours before the onset of your headache, did you experience any of the following: exposure to strong sunlight, exposure to poorly ventilated or noisy atmosphere, a missed meal, a larger intake of alcohol than usual?

YES → All of these circumstances are apt to cause headaches in otherwise healthy people and are rarely a cause for concern (see HEADACHE).

NO

If no diagnosis can be made with the use of this chart and your headache lasts overnight or accompanying symptoms develop, seek a medical evaluation.

Vision loss or impairment
Problems with one or both of the eyes.

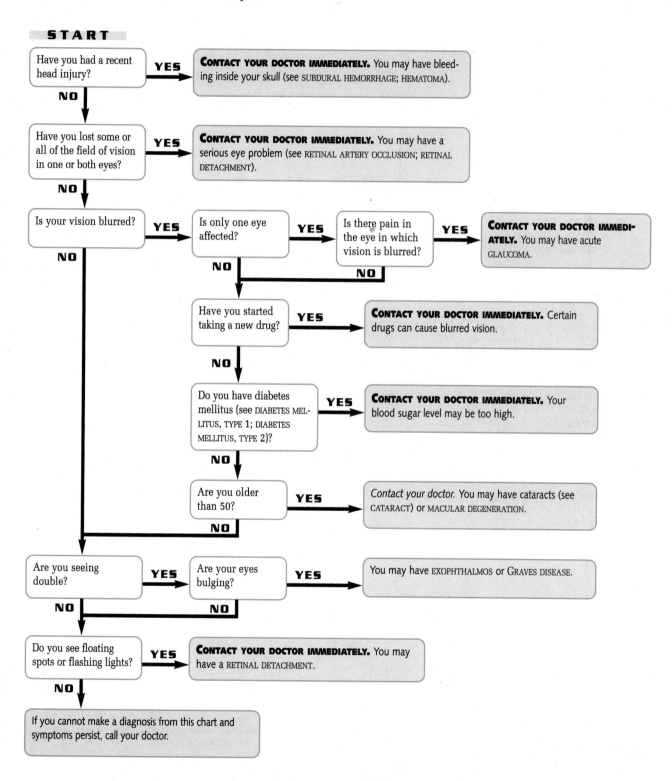

START

Have you had a recent head injury? — **YES** → **CONTACT YOUR DOCTOR IMMEDIATELY.** You may have bleeding inside your skull (see SUBDURAL HEMORRHAGE; HEMATOMA).

NO ↓

Have you lost some or all of the field of vision in one or both eyes? — **YES** → **CONTACT YOUR DOCTOR IMMEDIATELY.** You may have a serious eye problem (see RETINAL ARTERY OCCLUSION; RETINAL DETACHMENT).

NO ↓

Is your vision blurred? — **YES** → Is only one eye affected? — **YES** → Is there pain in the eye in which vision is blurred? — **YES** → **CONTACT YOUR DOCTOR IMMEDIATELY.** You may have acute GLAUCOMA.

NO

NO ↓

Have you started taking a new drug? — **YES** → **CONTACT YOUR DOCTOR IMMEDIATELY.** Certain drugs can cause blurred vision.

NO ↓

Do you have diabetes mellitus (see DIABETES MELLITUS, TYPE 1; DIABETES MELLITUS, TYPE 2)? — **YES** → **CONTACT YOUR DOCTOR IMMEDIATELY.** Your blood sugar level may be too high.

NO ↓

Are you older than 50? — **YES** → *Contact your doctor.* You may have cataracts (see CATARACT) or MACULAR DEGENERATION.

NO

Are you seeing double? — **YES** → Are your eyes bulging? — **YES** → You may have EXOPHTHALMOS or GRAVES DISEASE.

NO

NO ↓

Do you see floating spots or flashing lights? — **YES** → **CONTACT YOUR DOCTOR IMMEDIATELY.** You may have a RETINAL DETACHMENT.

NO ↓

If you cannot make a diagnosis from this chart and symptoms persist, call your doctor.

Hip pain

Pain that may range from mild aching or tenderness to intense, stabbing pains in the area of the hip joint, toward the side of the lower trunk.

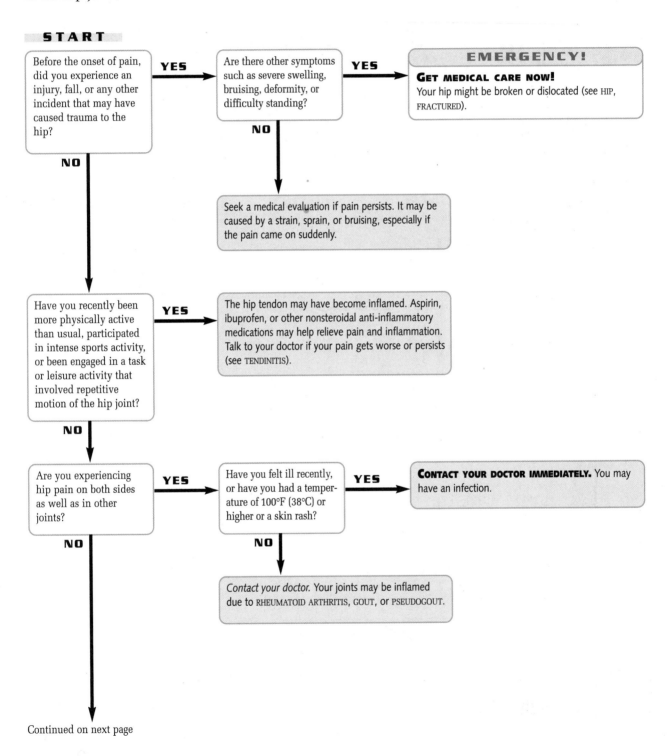

START

Before the onset of pain, did you experience an injury, fall, or any other incident that may have caused trauma to the hip?

YES →

Are there other symptoms such as severe swelling, bruising, deformity, or difficulty standing?

YES →

EMERGENCY!

GET MEDICAL CARE NOW!
Your hip might be broken or dislocated (see HIP, FRACTURED).

NO ↓

Seek a medical evaluation if pain persists. It may be caused by a strain, sprain, or bruising, especially if the pain came on suddenly.

NO ↓

Have you recently been more physically active than usual, participated in intense sports activity, or been engaged in a task or leisure activity that involved repetitive motion of the hip joint?

YES →

The hip tendon may have become inflamed. Aspirin, ibuprofen, or other nonsteroidal anti-inflammatory medications may help relieve pain and inflammation. Talk to your doctor if your pain gets worse or persists (see TENDINITIS).

NO ↓

Are you experiencing hip pain on both sides as well as in other joints?

YES →

Have you felt ill recently, or have you had a temperature of 100°F (38°C) or higher or a skin rash?

YES →

CONTACT YOUR DOCTOR IMMEDIATELY. You may have an infection.

NO ↓

NO ↓

Contact your doctor. Your joints may be inflamed due to RHEUMATOID ARTHRITIS, GOUT, or PSEUDOGOUT.

Continued on next page

Continued from previous page

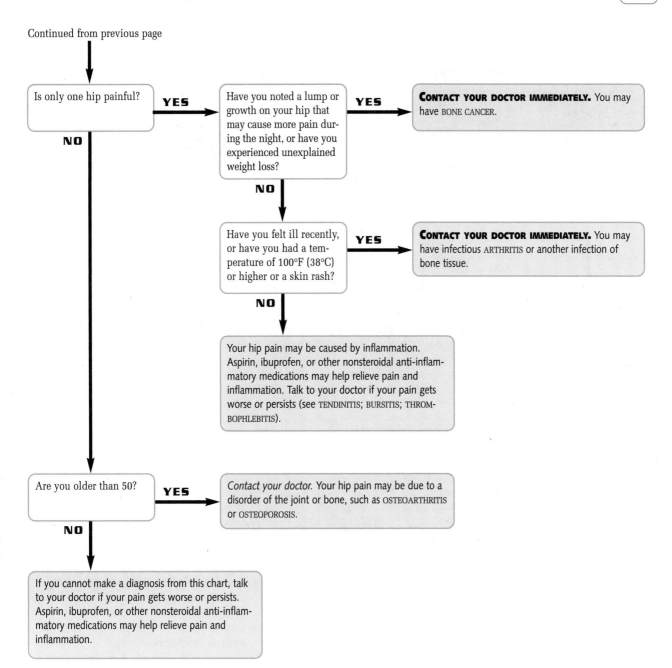

Is only one hip painful?

YES →

Have you noted a lump or growth on your hip that may cause more pain during the night, or have you experienced unexplained weight loss?

YES →

CONTACT YOUR DOCTOR IMMEDIATELY. You may have BONE CANCER.

NO ↓

Have you felt ill recently, or have you had a temperature of 100°F (38°C) or higher or a skin rash?

YES →

CONTACT YOUR DOCTOR IMMEDIATELY. You may have infectious ARTHRITIS or another infection of bone tissue.

NO ↓

Your hip pain may be caused by inflammation. Aspirin, ibuprofen, or other nonsteroidal anti-inflammatory medications may help relieve pain and inflammation. Talk to your doctor if your pain gets worse or persists (see TENDINITIS; BURSITIS; THROMBOPHLEBITIS).

NO ↓

Are you older than 50?

YES →

Contact your doctor. Your hip pain may be due to a disorder of the joint or bone, such as OSTEOARTHRITIS or OSTEOPOROSIS.

NO ↓

If you cannot make a diagnosis from this chart, talk to your doctor if your pain gets worse or persists. Aspirin, ibuprofen, or other nonsteroidal anti-inflammatory medications may help relieve pain and inflammation.

Knee pain

Pain in or around the knee with possible swelling.

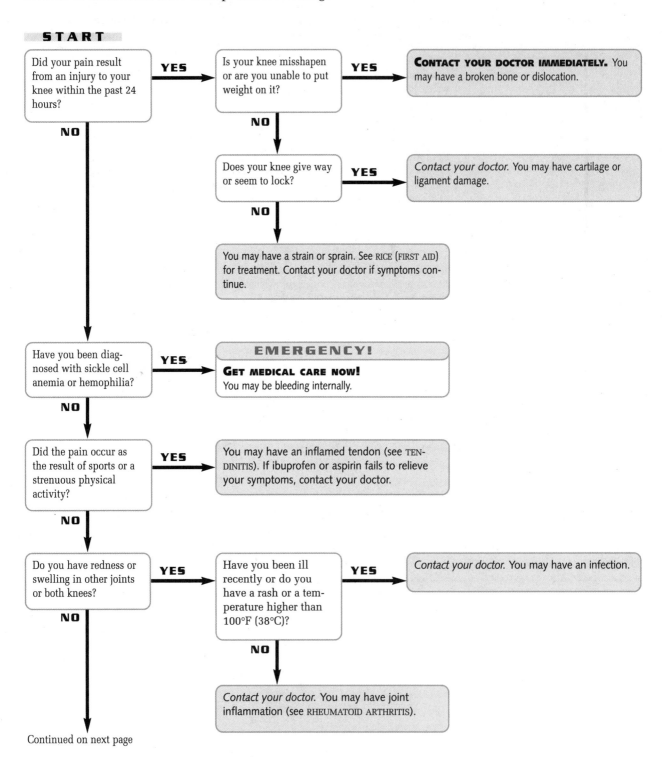

START

Did your pain result from an injury to your knee within the past 24 hours?

YES → Is your knee misshapen or are you unable to put weight on it?

YES → **CONTACT YOUR DOCTOR IMMEDIATELY.** You may have a broken bone or dislocation.

NO ↓

Does your knee give way or seem to lock?

YES → *Contact your doctor.* You may have cartilage or ligament damage.

NO ↓

You may have a strain or sprain. See RICE (FIRST AID) for treatment. Contact your doctor if symptoms continue.

NO ↓ (from first question)

Have you been diagnosed with sickle cell anemia or hemophilia?

YES → **EMERGENCY!**
GET MEDICAL CARE NOW!
You may be bleeding internally.

NO ↓

Did the pain occur as the result of sports or a strenuous physical activity?

YES → You may have an inflamed tendon (see TENDINITIS). If ibuprofen or aspirin fails to relieve your symptoms, contact your doctor.

NO ↓

Do you have redness or swelling in other joints or both knees?

YES → Have you been ill recently or do you have a rash or a temperature higher than 100°F (38°C)?

YES → *Contact your doctor.* You may have an infection.

NO ↓

Contact your doctor. You may have joint inflammation (see RHEUMATOID ARTHRITIS).

NO ↓

Continued on next page

Continued from previous page

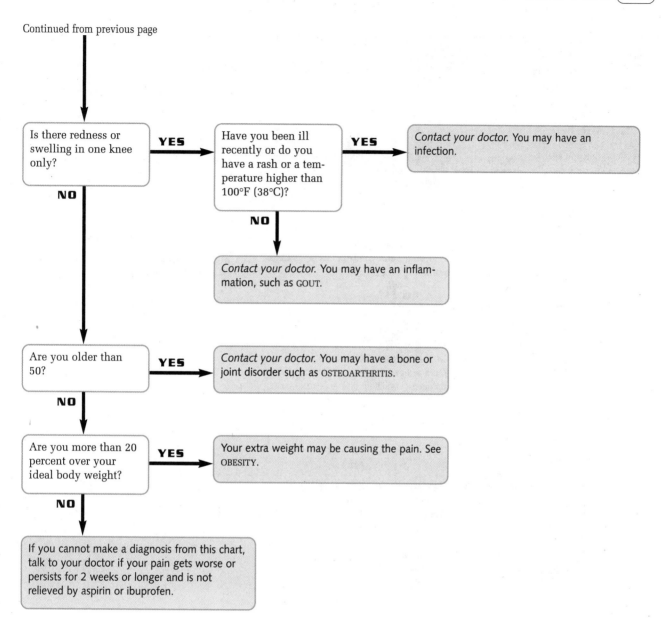

Is there redness or swelling in one knee only?

YES → Have you been ill recently or do you have a rash or a temperature higher than 100°F (38°C)?

YES → *Contact your doctor.* You may have an infection.

NO ↓

Contact your doctor. You may have an inflammation, such as GOUT.

NO ↓

Are you older than 50?

YES → *Contact your doctor.* You may have a bone or joint disorder such as OSTEOARTHRITIS.

NO ↓

Are you more than 20 percent over your ideal body weight?

YES → Your extra weight may be causing the pain. See OBESITY.

NO ↓

If you cannot make a diagnosis from this chart, talk to your doctor if your pain gets worse or persists for 2 weeks or longer and is not relieved by aspirin or ibuprofen.

Nausea or vomiting

Throwing up of the contents of the stomach (vomiting), often preceded by an unpleasant sensation (nausea).

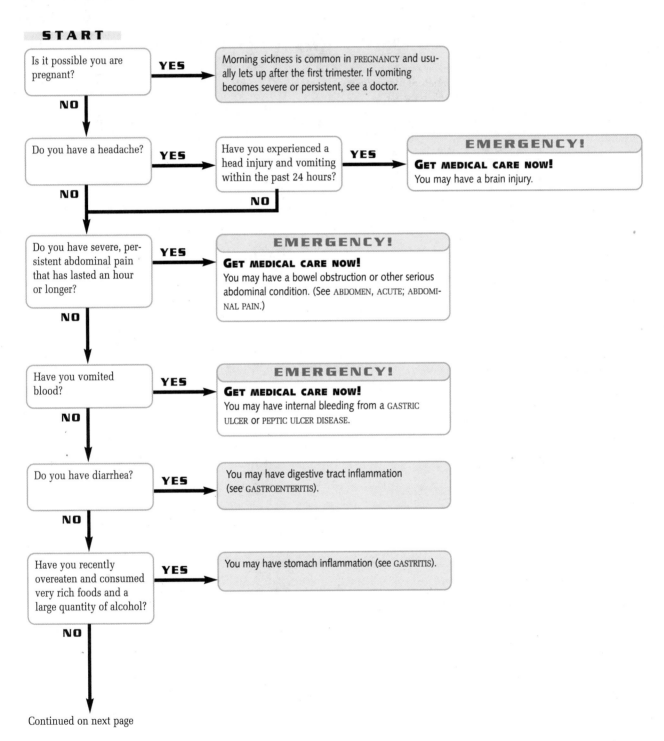

START

Is it possible you are pregnant? — **YES** → Morning sickness is common in PREGNANCY and usually lets up after the first trimester. If vomiting becomes severe or persistent, see a doctor.

NO ↓

Do you have a headache? — **YES** → Have you experienced a head injury and vomiting within the past 24 hours? — **YES** → **EMERGENCY!** GET MEDICAL CARE NOW! You may have a brain injury.

NO ↓ (headache) / **NO** (head injury)

Do you have severe, persistent abdominal pain that has lasted an hour or longer? — **YES** → **EMERGENCY!** GET MEDICAL CARE NOW! You may have a bowel obstruction or other serious abdominal condition. (See ABDOMEN, ACUTE; ABDOMINAL PAIN.)

NO ↓

Have you vomited blood? — **YES** → **EMERGENCY!** GET MEDICAL CARE NOW! You may have internal bleeding from a GASTRIC ULCER or PEPTIC ULCER DISEASE.

NO ↓

Do you have diarrhea? — **YES** → You may have digestive tract inflammation (see GASTROENTERITIS).

NO ↓

Have you recently overeaten and consumed very rich foods and a large quantity of alcohol? — **YES** → You may have stomach inflammation (see GASTRITIS).

NO ↓

Continued on next page

Continued from previous page

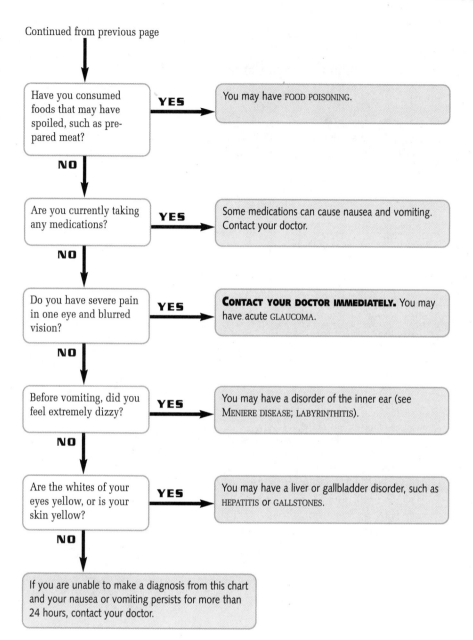

Have you consumed foods that may have spoiled, such as pre-pared meat?

YES → You may have FOOD POISONING.

NO ↓

Are you currently taking any medications?

YES → Some medications can cause nausea and vomiting. Contact your doctor.

NO ↓

Do you have severe pain in one eye and blurred vision?

YES → **CONTACT YOUR DOCTOR IMMEDIATELY.** You may have acute GLAUCOMA.

NO ↓

Before vomiting, did you feel extremely dizzy?

YES → You may have a disorder of the inner ear (see MENIERE DISEASE; LABYRINTHITIS).

NO ↓

Are the whites of your eyes yellow, or is your skin yellow?

YES → You may have a liver or gallbladder disorder, such as HEPATITIS or GALLSTONES.

NO ↓

If you are unable to make a diagnosis from this chart and your nausea or vomiting persists for more than 24 hours, contact your doctor.

Numbness or tingling

Absence of feeling or a "pins and needles" sensation in any part of the body.

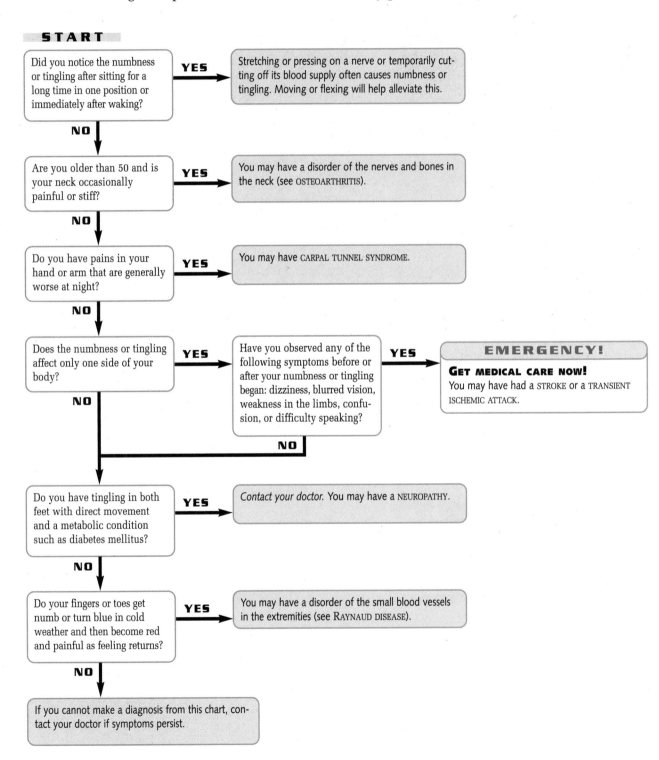

START

Did you notice the numbness or tingling after sitting for a long time in one position or immediately after waking? **YES** → Stretching or pressing on a nerve or temporarily cutting off its blood supply often causes numbness or tingling. Moving or flexing will help alleviate this.

NO ↓

Are you older than 50 and is your neck occasionally painful or stiff? **YES** → You may have a disorder of the nerves and bones in the neck (see OSTEOARTHRITIS).

NO ↓

Do you have pains in your hand or arm that are generally worse at night? **YES** → You may have CARPAL TUNNEL SYNDROME.

NO ↓

Does the numbness or tingling affect only one side of your body? **YES** → Have you observed any of the following symptoms before or after your numbness or tingling began: dizziness, blurred vision, weakness in the limbs, confusion, or difficulty speaking? **YES** → **EMERGENCY!** **GET MEDICAL CARE NOW!** You may have had a STROKE or a TRANSIENT ISCHEMIC ATTACK.

NO (from symptoms box)

NO ↓

Do you have tingling in both feet with direct movement and a metabolic condition such as diabetes mellitus? **YES** → *Contact your doctor.* You may have a NEUROPATHY.

NO ↓

Do your fingers or toes get numb or turn blue in cold weather and then become red and painful as feeling returns? **YES** → You may have a disorder of the small blood vessels in the extremities (see RAYNAUD DISEASE).

NO ↓

If you cannot make a diagnosis from this chart, contact your doctor if symptoms persist.

Penis, problems of the

Pain or discomfort in the penis or testicles.

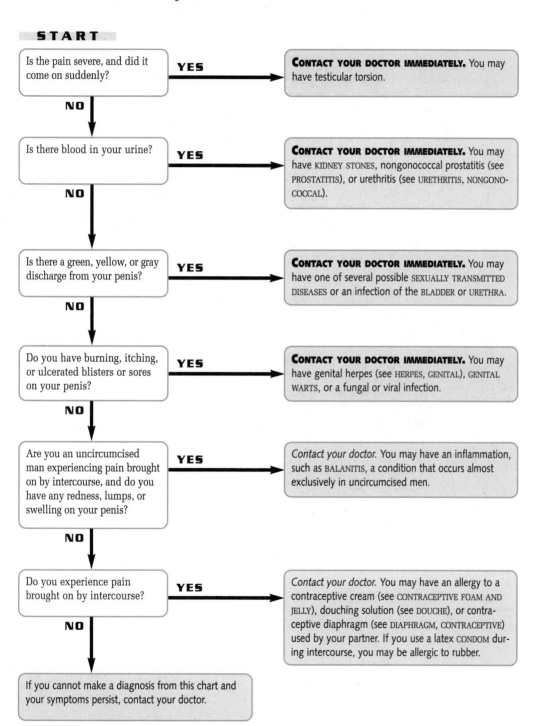

START

Is the pain severe, and did it come on suddenly?

YES → **CONTACT YOUR DOCTOR IMMEDIATELY.** You may have testicular torsion.

NO ↓

Is there blood in your urine?

YES → **CONTACT YOUR DOCTOR IMMEDIATELY.** You may have KIDNEY STONES, nongonococcal prostatitis (see PROSTATITIS), or urethritis (see URETHRITIS, NONGONO-COCCAL).

NO ↓

Is there a green, yellow, or gray discharge from your penis?

YES → **CONTACT YOUR DOCTOR IMMEDIATELY.** You may have one of several possible SEXUALLY TRANSMITTED DISEASES or an infection of the BLADDER or URETHRA.

NO ↓

Do you have burning, itching, or ulcerated blisters or sores on your penis?

YES → **CONTACT YOUR DOCTOR IMMEDIATELY.** You may have genital herpes (see HERPES, GENITAL), GENITAL WARTS, or a fungal or viral infection.

NO ↓

Are you an uncircumcised man experiencing pain brought on by intercourse, and do you have any redness, lumps, or swelling on your penis?

YES → *Contact your doctor.* You may have an inflammation, such as BALANITIS, a condition that occurs almost exclusively in uncircumcised men.

NO ↓

Do you experience pain brought on by intercourse?

YES → *Contact your doctor.* You may have an allergy to a contraceptive cream (see CONTRACEPTIVE FOAM AND JELLY), douching solution (see DOUCHE), or contraceptive diaphragm (see DIAPHRAGM, CONTRACEPTIVE) used by your partner. If you use a latex CONDOM during intercourse, you may be allergic to rubber.

NO ↓

If you cannot make a diagnosis from this chart and your symptoms persist, contact your doctor.

Rashes in infants and children

Childhood rashes may be caused by inflammation of the skin as a result of infection or may occur in conjunction with a childhood illness.

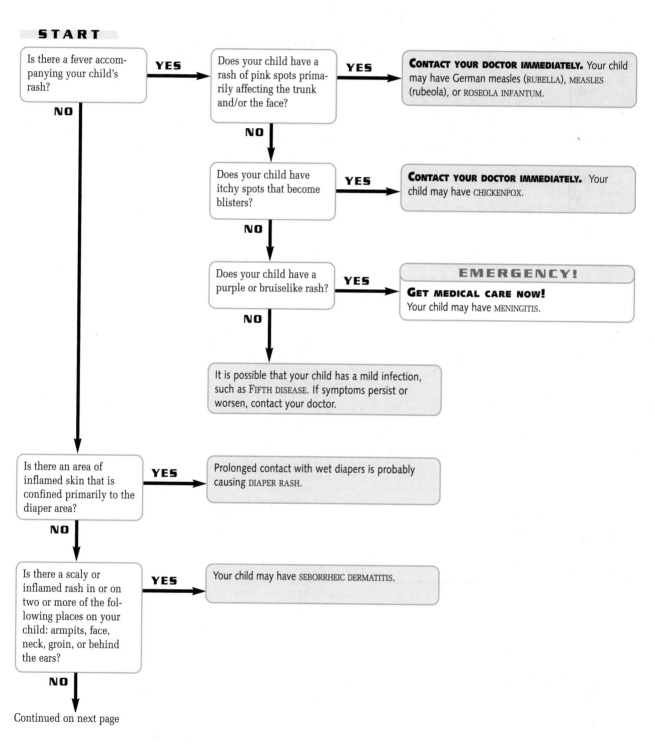

START

Is there a fever accompanying your child's rash?

YES → Does your child have a rash of pink spots primarily affecting the trunk and/or the face?

YES → **CONTACT YOUR DOCTOR IMMEDIATELY.** Your child may have German measles (RUBELLA), MEASLES (rubeola), or ROSEOLA INFANTUM.

NO ↓

Does your child have itchy spots that become blisters?

YES → **CONTACT YOUR DOCTOR IMMEDIATELY.** Your child may have CHICKENPOX.

NO ↓

Does your child have a purple or bruiselike rash?

YES → **EMERGENCY!**
GET MEDICAL CARE NOW!
Your child may have MENINGITIS.

NO ↓

It is possible that your child has a mild infection, such as FIFTH DISEASE. If symptoms persist or worsen, contact your doctor.

NO ↓ (from first question)

Is there an area of inflamed skin that is confined primarily to the diaper area?

YES → Prolonged contact with wet diapers is probably causing DIAPER RASH.

NO ↓

Is there a scaly or inflamed rash in or on two or more of the following places on your child: armpits, face, neck, groin, or behind the ears?

YES → Your child may have SEBORRHEIC DERMATITIS.

NO ↓

Continued on next page

Continued from previous page

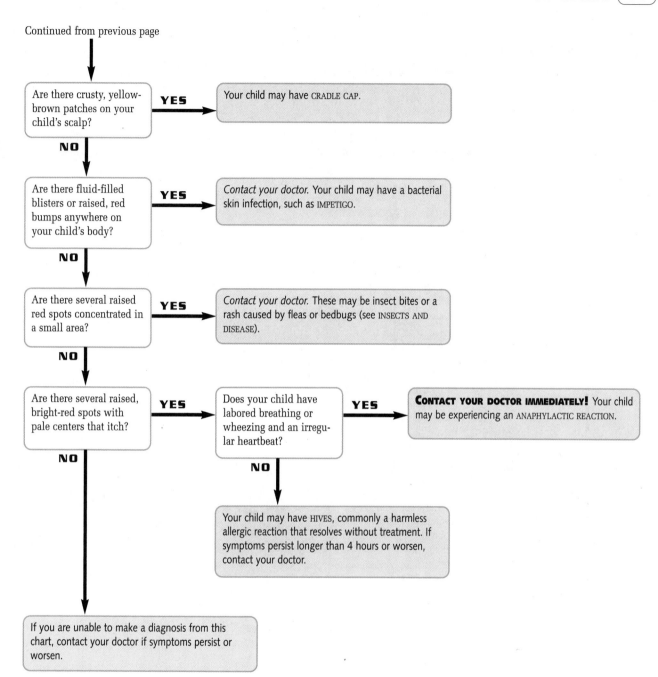

Are there crusty, yellow-brown patches on your child's scalp?

YES → Your child may have CRADLE CAP.

NO ↓

Are there fluid-filled blisters or raised, red bumps anywhere on your child's body?

YES → *Contact your doctor.* Your child may have a bacterial skin infection, such as IMPETIGO.

NO ↓

Are there several raised red spots concentrated in a small area?

YES → *Contact your doctor.* These may be insect bites or a rash caused by fleas or bedbugs (see INSECTS AND DISEASE).

NO ↓

Are there several raised, bright-red spots with pale centers that itch?

YES → Does your child have labored breathing or wheezing and an irregular heartbeat?

YES → **CONTACT YOUR DOCTOR IMMEDIATELY!** Your child may be experiencing an ANAPHYLACTIC REACTION.

NO ↓

Your child may have HIVES, commonly a harmless allergic reaction that resolves without treatment. If symptoms persist longer than 4 hours or worsen, contact your doctor.

NO ↓

If you are unable to make a diagnosis from this chart, contact your doctor if symptoms persist or worsen.

Rashes in adults

Raised, reddened, or discolored areas of skin.

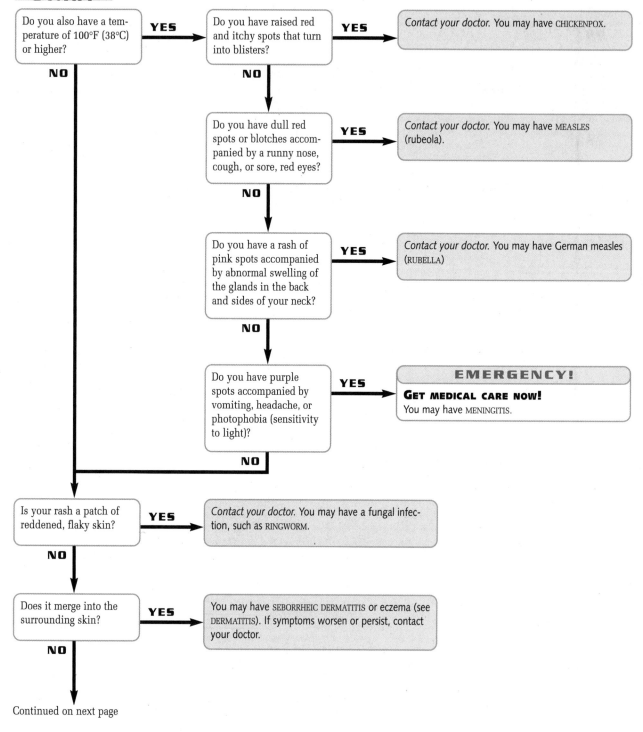

START

Do you also have a temperature of 100°F (38°C) or higher? → **YES** → Do you have raised red and itchy spots that turn into blisters? → **YES** → *Contact your doctor.* You may have CHICKENPOX.

NO / **NO**

Do you have dull red spots or blotches accompanied by a runny nose, cough, or sore, red eyes? → **YES** → *Contact your doctor.* You may have MEASLES (rubeola).

NO

Do you have a rash of pink spots accompanied by abnormal swelling of the glands in the back and sides of your neck? → **YES** → *Contact your doctor.* You may have German measles (RUBELLA)

NO

Do you have purple spots accompanied by vomiting, headache, or photophobia (sensitivity to light)? → **YES** → **EMERGENCY!** **GET MEDICAL CARE NOW!** You may have MENINGITIS.

NO

Is your rash a patch of reddened, flaky skin? → **YES** → *Contact your doctor.* You may have a fungal infection, such as RINGWORM.

NO

Does it merge into the surrounding skin? → **YES** → You may have SEBORRHEIC DERMATITIS or eczema (see DERMATITIS). If symptoms worsen or persist, contact your doctor.

NO

Continued on next page

Continued from previous page

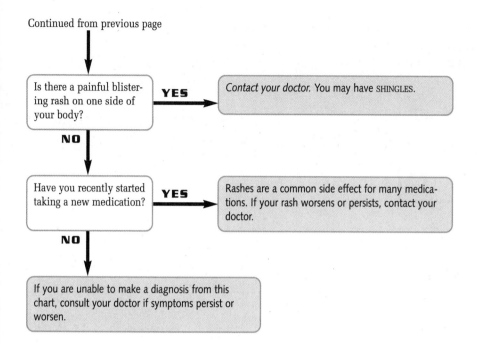

Is there a painful blistering rash on one side of
your body?

YES → *Contact your doctor.* You may have SHINGLES.

NO

Have you recently started
taking a new medication?

YES → Rashes are a common side effect for many medications. If your rash worsens or persists, contact your
doctor.

NO

If you are unable to make a diagnosis from this
chart, consult your doctor if symptoms persist or
worsen.

Sleep problems

Difficulty falling asleep or staying asleep.

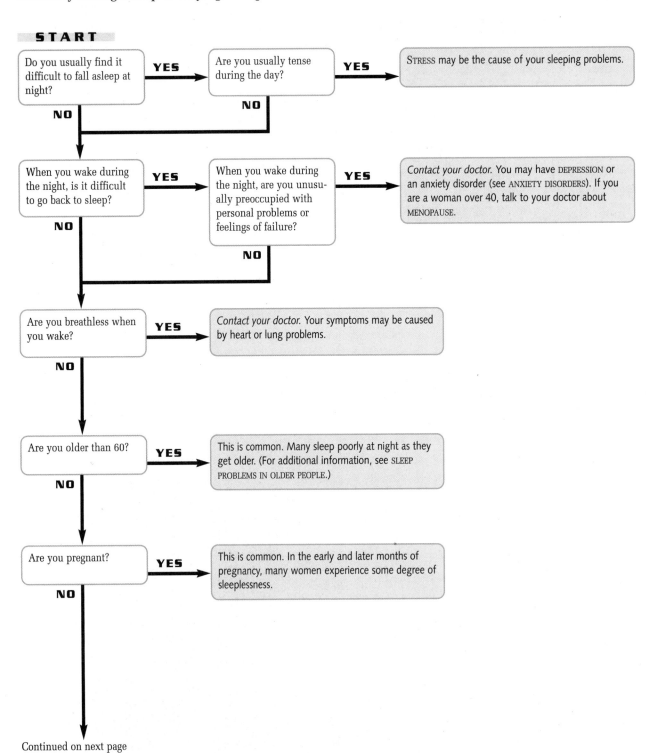

START

Do you usually find it difficult to fall asleep at night? — **YES** → Are you usually tense during the day? — **YES** → STRESS may be the cause of your sleeping problems.

NO ↓ ... **NO** ↓

When you wake during the night, is it difficult to go back to sleep? — **YES** → When you wake during the night, are you unusually preoccupied with personal problems or feelings of failure? — **YES** → *Contact your doctor.* You may have DEPRESSION or an anxiety disorder (see ANXIETY DISORDERS). If you are a woman over 40, talk to your doctor about MENOPAUSE.

NO ↓ ... **NO** ↓

Are you breathless when you wake? — **YES** → *Contact your doctor.* Your symptoms may be caused by heart or lung problems.

NO ↓

Are you older than 60? — **YES** → This is common. Many sleep poorly at night as they get older. (For additional information, see SLEEP PROBLEMS IN OLDER PEOPLE.)

NO ↓

Are you pregnant? — **YES** → This is common. In the early and later months of pregnancy, many women experience some degree of sleeplessness.

NO ↓

Continued on next page

Continued from previous page

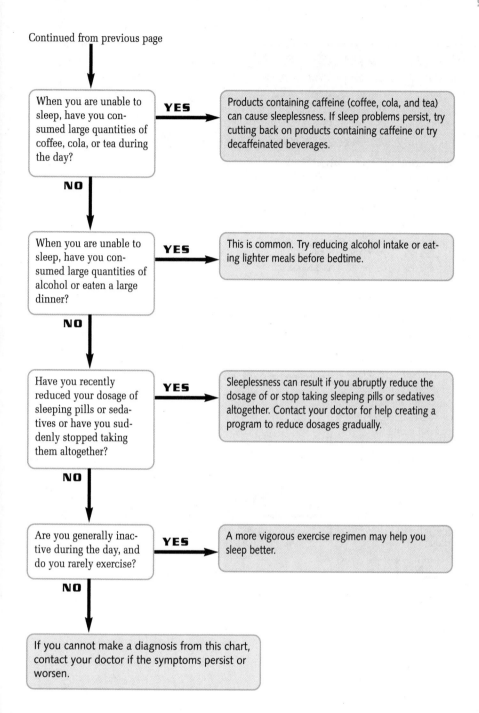

When you are unable to sleep, have you consumed large quantities of coffee, cola, or tea during the day?

YES → Products containing caffeine (coffee, cola, and tea) can cause sleeplessness. If sleep problems persist, try cutting back on products containing caffeine or try decaffeinated beverages.

NO ↓

When you are unable to sleep, have you consumed large quantities of alcohol or eaten a large dinner?

YES → This is common. Try reducing alcohol intake or eating lighter meals before bedtime.

NO ↓

Have you recently reduced your dosage of sleeping pills or sedatives or have you suddenly stopped taking them altogether?

YES → Sleeplessness can result if you abruptly reduce the dosage of or stop taking sleeping pills or sedatives altogether. Contact your doctor for help creating a program to reduce dosages gradually.

NO ↓

Are you generally inactive during the day, and do you rarely exercise?

YES → A more vigorous exercise regimen may help you sleep better.

NO ↓

If you cannot make a diagnosis from this chart, contact your doctor if the symptoms persist or worsen.

Urination in men, painful or frequent

Discomfort when passing urine or excessive urine production.

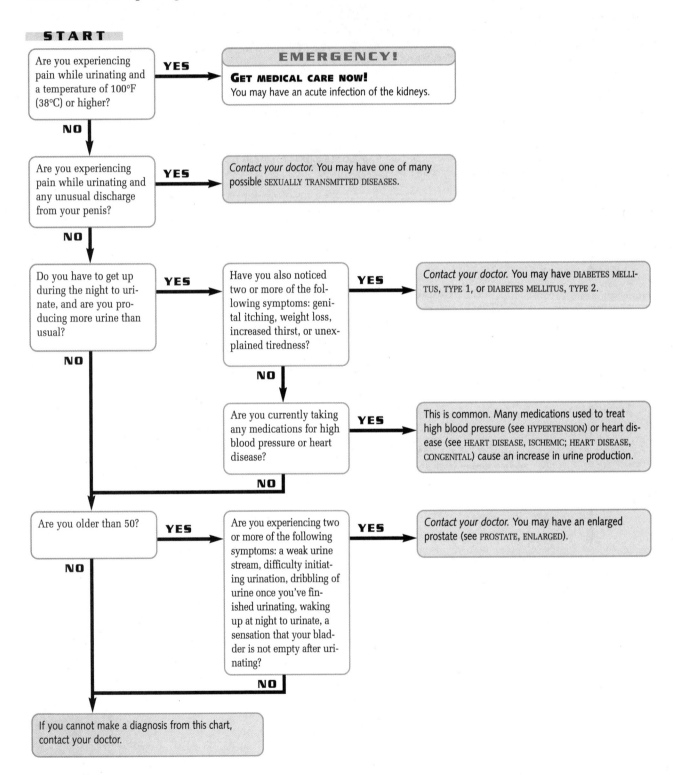

START

Are you experiencing pain while urinating and a temperature of 100°F (38°C) or higher? — **YES** →

EMERGENCY!
GET MEDICAL CARE NOW!
You may have an acute infection of the kidneys.

NO ↓

Are you experiencing pain while urinating and any unusual discharge from your penis? — **YES** →

Contact your doctor. You may have one of many possible SEXUALLY TRANSMITTED DISEASES.

NO ↓

Do you have to get up during the night to urinate, and are you producing more urine than usual? — **YES** →

Have you also noticed two or more of the following symptoms: genital itching, weight loss, increased thirst, or unexplained tiredness? — **YES** →

Contact your doctor. You may have DIABETES MELLITUS, TYPE 1, or DIABETES MELLITUS, TYPE 2.

NO ↓

Are you currently taking any medications for high blood pressure or heart disease? — **YES** →

This is common. Many medications used to treat high blood pressure (see HYPERTENSION) or heart disease (see HEART DISEASE, ISCHEMIC; HEART DISEASE, CONGENITAL) cause an increase in urine production.

NO ↓

NO ↓

Are you older than 50? — **YES** →

Are you experiencing two or more of the following symptoms: a weak urine stream, difficulty initiating urination, dribbling of urine once you've finished urinating, waking up at night to urinate, a sensation that your bladder is not empty after urinating? — **YES** →

Contact your doctor. You may have an enlarged prostate (see PROSTATE, ENLARGED).

NO ↓

NO ↓

If you cannot make a diagnosis from this chart, contact your doctor.

Urination in women, painful or frequent

Discomfort when passing urine or excessive urine production.

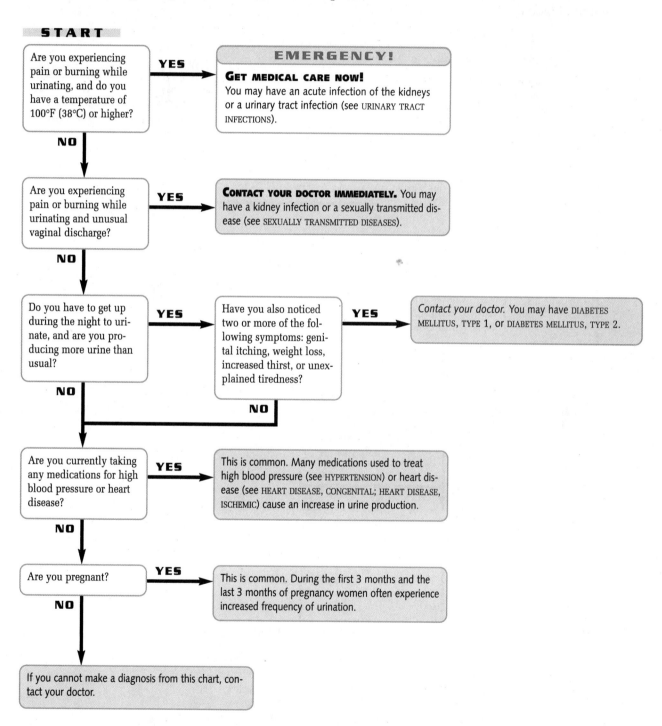

START

Are you experiencing pain or burning while urinating, and do you have a temperature of 100°F (38°C) or higher?

YES →

EMERGENCY!

GET MEDICAL CARE NOW! You may have an acute infection of the kidneys or a urinary tract infection (see URINARY TRACT INFECTIONS).

NO ↓

Are you experiencing pain or burning while urinating and unusual vaginal discharge?

YES →

CONTACT YOUR DOCTOR IMMEDIATELY. You may have a kidney infection or a sexually transmitted disease (see SEXUALLY TRANSMITTED DISEASES).

NO ↓

Do you have to get up during the night to urinate, and are you producing more urine than usual?

YES →

Have you also noticed two or more of the following symptoms: genital itching, weight loss, increased thirst, or unexplained tiredness?

YES →

Contact your doctor. You may have DIABETES MELLITUS, TYPE 1, or DIABETES MELLITUS, TYPE 2.

NO ↓ (returns to main flow)

NO ↓

Are you currently taking any medications for high blood pressure or heart disease?

YES →

This is common. Many medications used to treat high blood pressure (see HYPERTENSION) or heart disease (see HEART DISEASE, CONGENITAL; HEART DISEASE, ISCHEMIC) cause an increase in urine production.

NO ↓

Are you pregnant?

YES →

This is common. During the first 3 months and the last 3 months of pregnancy women often experience increased frequency of urination.

NO ↓

If you cannot make a diagnosis from this chart, contact your doctor.

Urine discoloration

Urine that differs in coloration from the normal pale yellow, appears unclear, or contains any amount of blood.

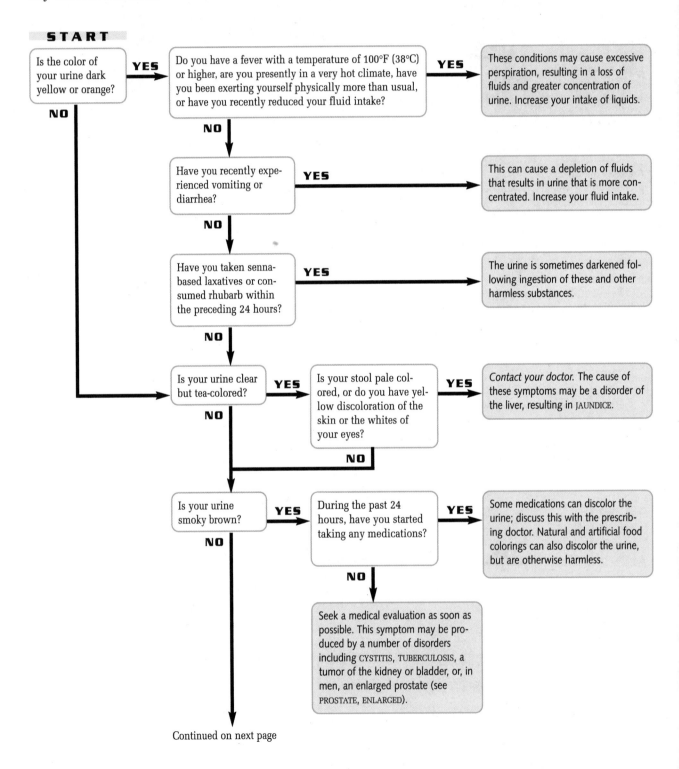

START

Is the color of your urine dark yellow or orange? — **YES** →

Do you have a fever with a temperature of 100°F (38°C) or higher, are you presently in a very hot climate, have you been exerting yourself physically more than usual, or have you recently reduced your fluid intake? — **YES** →

These conditions may cause excessive perspiration, resulting in a loss of fluids and greater concentration of urine. Increase your intake of liquids.

NO ↓

Have you recently experienced vomiting or diarrhea? — **YES** →

This can cause a depletion of fluids that results in urine that is more concentrated. Increase your fluid intake.

NO ↓

Have you taken senna-based laxatives or consumed rhubarb within the preceding 24 hours? — **YES** →

The urine is sometimes darkened following ingestion of these and other harmless substances.

NO ↓

Is your urine clear but tea-colored? — **YES** →

Is your stool pale colored, or do you have yellow discoloration of the skin or the whites of your eyes? — **YES** →

Contact your doctor. The cause of these symptoms may be a disorder of the liver, resulting in JAUNDICE.

NO ↓

Is your urine smoky brown? — **YES** →

During the past 24 hours, have you started taking any medications? — **YES** →

Some medications can discolor the urine; discuss this with the prescribing doctor. Natural and artificial food colorings can also discolor the urine, but are otherwise harmless.

NO ↓

Seek a medical evaluation as soon as possible. This symptom may be produced by a number of disorders including CYSTITIS, TUBERCULOSIS, a tumor of the kidney or bladder, or, in men, an enlarged prostate (see PROSTATE, ENLARGED).

Continued on next page

Continued from previous page

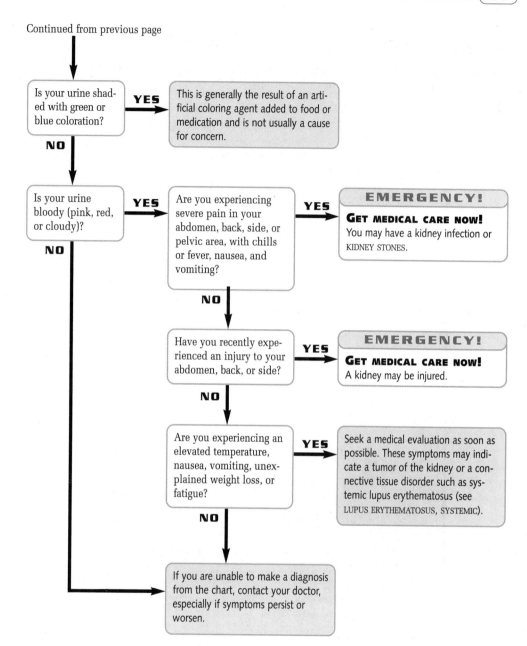

Is your urine shaded with green or blue coloration?

YES → This is generally the result of an artificial coloring agent added to food or medication and is not usually a cause for concern.

NO ↓

Is your urine bloody (pink, red, or cloudy)?

YES → Are you experiencing severe pain in your abdomen, back, side, or pelvic area, with chills or fever, nausea, and vomiting?

YES → **EMERGENCY!**
GET MEDICAL CARE NOW! You may have a kidney infection or KIDNEY STONES.

NO ↓

Have you recently experienced an injury to your abdomen, back, or side?

YES → **EMERGENCY!**
GET MEDICAL CARE NOW! A kidney may be injured.

NO ↓

Are you experiencing an elevated temperature, nausea, vomiting, unexplained weight loss, or fatigue?

YES → Seek a medical evaluation as soon as possible. These symptoms may indicate a tumor of the kidney or a connective tissue disorder such as systemic lupus erythematosus (see LUPUS ERYTHEMATOSUS, SYSTEMIC).

NO ↓

If you are unable to make a diagnosis from the chart, contact your doctor, especially if symptoms persist or worsen.

Weight gain

If your weight exceeds your optimum weight by more than 20 percent, you are overweight and may be endangering your health.

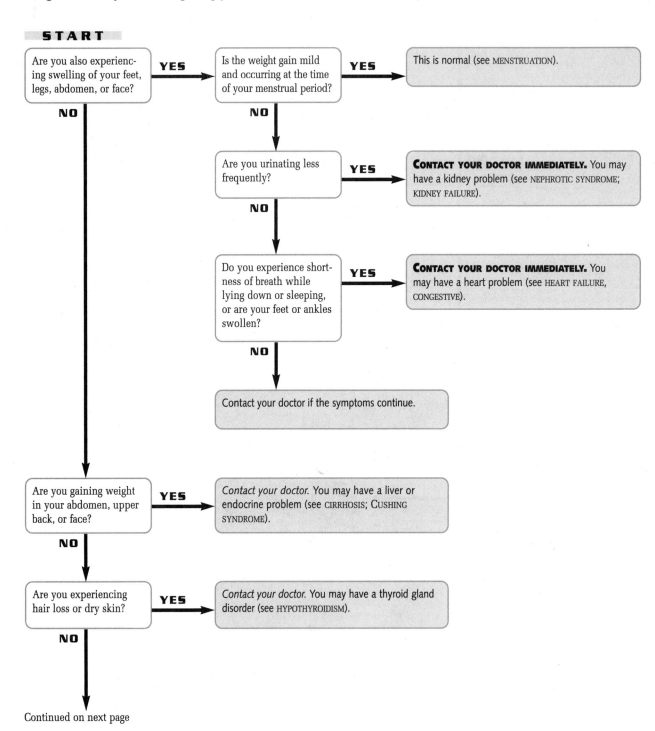

START

Are you also experiencing swelling of your feet, legs, abdomen, or face? — **YES** → Is the weight gain mild and occurring at the time of your menstrual period? — **YES** → This is normal (see MENSTRUATION).

NO (from menstrual question) ↓

Are you urinating less frequently? — **YES** → **CONTACT YOUR DOCTOR IMMEDIATELY.** You may have a kidney problem (see NEPHROTIC SYNDROME; KIDNEY FAILURE).

NO ↓

Do you experience shortness of breath while lying down or sleeping, or are your feet or ankles swollen? — **YES** → **CONTACT YOUR DOCTOR IMMEDIATELY.** You may have a heart problem (see HEART FAILURE, CONGESTIVE).

NO ↓

Contact your doctor if the symptoms continue.

Are you gaining weight in your abdomen, upper back, or face? — **YES** → *Contact your doctor.* You may have a liver or endocrine problem (see CIRRHOSIS; CUSHING SYNDROME).

NO ↓

Are you experiencing hair loss or dry skin? — **YES** → *Contact your doctor.* You may have a thyroid gland disorder (see HYPOTHYROIDISM).

NO ↓

Continued on next page

Continued from previous page

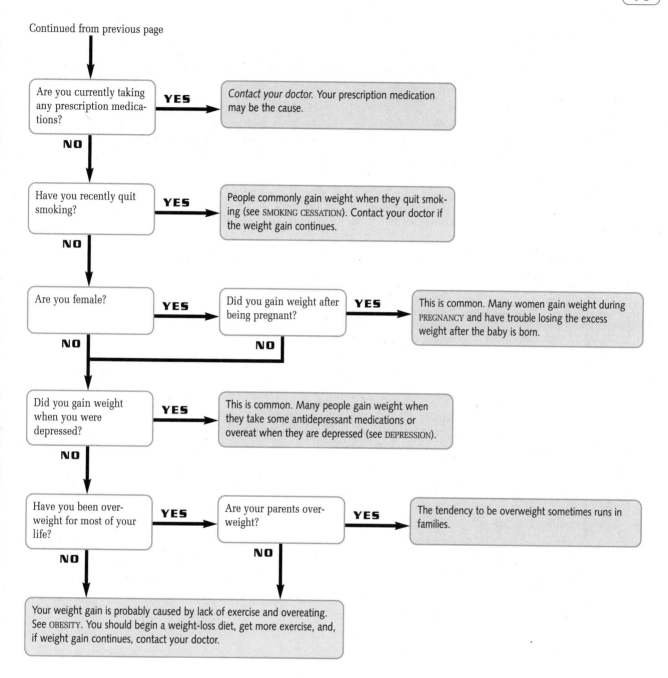

Are you currently taking any prescription medications? — **YES** → *Contact your doctor.* Your prescription medication may be the cause.

NO ↓

Have you recently quit smoking? — **YES** → People commonly gain weight when they quit smoking (see SMOKING CESSATION). Contact your doctor if the weight gain continues.

NO ↓

Are you female? — **YES** → Did you gain weight after being pregnant? — **YES** → This is common. Many women gain weight during PREGNANCY and have trouble losing the excess weight after the baby is born.

NO ↓ / **NO** ↓

Did you gain weight when you were depressed? — **YES** → This is common. Many people gain weight when they take some antidepressant medications or overeat when they are depressed (see DEPRESSION).

NO ↓

Have you been overweight for most of your life? — **YES** → Are your parents overweight? — **YES** → The tendency to be overweight sometimes runs in families.

NO ↓ / **NO** ↓

Your weight gain is probably caused by lack of exercise and overeating. See OBESITY. You should begin a weight-loss diet, get more exercise, and, if weight gain continues, contact your doctor.

Weight loss

Sudden or unexplained loss of weight may be a symptom of a serious underlying condition.

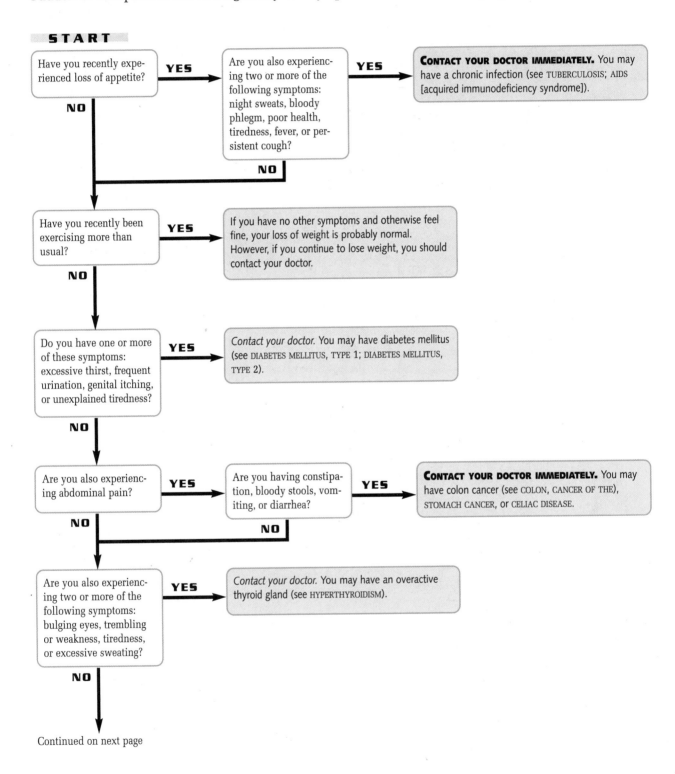

START

Have you recently experienced loss of appetite? **YES** → Are you also experiencing two or more of the following symptoms: night sweats, bloody phlegm, poor health, tiredness, fever, or persistent cough? **YES** → **CONTACT YOUR DOCTOR IMMEDIATELY.** You may have a chronic infection (see TUBERCULOSIS; AIDS [acquired immunodeficiency syndrome]).

NO ↓   **NO** ↓

Have you recently been exercising more than usual? **YES** → If you have no other symptoms and otherwise feel fine, your loss of weight is probably normal. However, if you continue to lose weight, you should contact your doctor.

NO ↓

Do you have one or more of these symptoms: excessive thirst, frequent urination, genital itching, or unexplained tiredness? **YES** → *Contact your doctor.* You may have diabetes mellitus (see DIABETES MELLITUS, TYPE 1; DIABETES MELLITUS, TYPE 2).

NO ↓

Are you also experiencing abdominal pain? **YES** → Are you having constipation, bloody stools, vomiting, or diarrhea? **YES** → **CONTACT YOUR DOCTOR IMMEDIATELY.** You may have colon cancer (see COLON, CANCER OF THE), STOMACH CANCER, or CELIAC DISEASE.

NO ↓   **NO** ↓

Are you also experiencing two or more of the following symptoms: bulging eyes, trembling or weakness, tiredness, or excessive sweating? **YES** → *Contact your doctor.* You may have an overactive thyroid gland (see HYPERTHYROIDISM).

NO ↓

Continued on next page

Continued from previous page

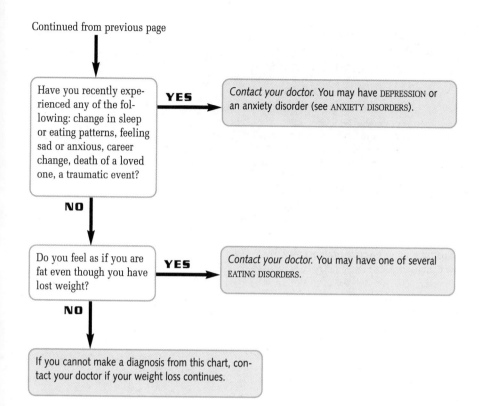

Have you recently experienced any of the following: change in sleep or eating patterns, feeling sad or anxious, career change, death of a loved one, a traumatic event?

YES → *Contact your doctor.* You may have DEPRESSION or an anxiety disorder (see ANXIETY DISORDERS).

NO

Do you feel as if you are fat even though you have lost weight?

YES → *Contact your doctor.* You may have one of several EATING DISORDERS.

NO

If you cannot make a diagnosis from this chart, contact your doctor if your weight loss continues.

Swallowing difficulty

Discomfort when solid food or liquid passes through the esophagus.

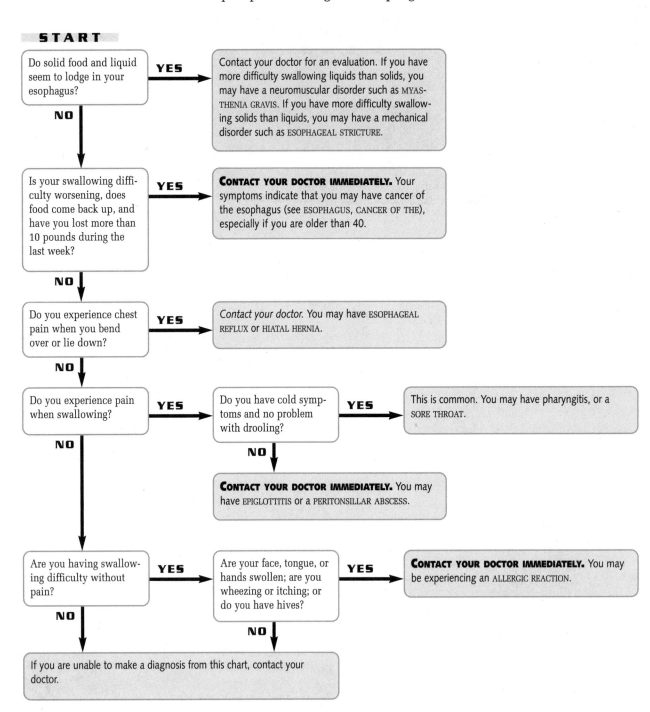

START

Do solid food and liquid seem to lodge in your esophagus?

YES → Contact your doctor for an evaluation. If you have more difficulty swallowing liquids than solids, you may have a neuromuscular disorder such as MYASTHENIA GRAVIS. If you have more difficulty swallowing solids than liquids, you may have a mechanical disorder such as ESOPHAGEAL STRICTURE.

NO ↓

Is your swallowing difficulty worsening, does food come back up, and have you lost more than 10 pounds during the last week?

YES → **CONTACT YOUR DOCTOR IMMEDIATELY.** Your symptoms indicate that you may have cancer of the esophagus (see ESOPHAGUS, CANCER OF THE), especially if you are older than 40.

NO ↓

Do you experience chest pain when you bend over or lie down?

YES → *Contact your doctor.* You may have ESOPHAGEAL REFLUX or HIATAL HERNIA.

NO ↓

Do you experience pain when swallowing?

YES → Do you have cold symptoms and no problem with drooling?

YES → This is common. You may have pharyngitis, or a SORE THROAT.

NO ↓

CONTACT YOUR DOCTOR IMMEDIATELY. You may have EPIGLOTTITIS or a PERITONSILLAR ABSCESS.

NO ↓

Are you having swallowing difficulty without pain?

YES → Are your face, tongue, or hands swollen; are you wheezing or itching; or do you have hives?

YES → **CONTACT YOUR DOCTOR IMMEDIATELY.** You may be experiencing an ALLERGIC REACTION.

NO ↓

If you are unable to make a diagnosis from this chart, contact your doctor.

NO ↓

Atlas of the body

SKELETAL SYSTEM

In addition to providing structural support and protecting the internal body organs, the skeleton is a series of independent levers, which the muscles pull to move different body parts. More than a simple movable frame, however, the skeleton is an artfully designed system that generates bacteria-destroying white blood cells from the marrow of some bones and generates new red blood cells from the marrow of other bones. The bones themselves are self-renewing. In fact, the human skeleton entirely replaces itself about every 7 years.

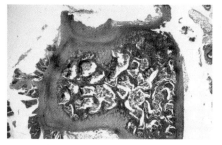

Spongy bone
Although bones appear smooth and hard on the outside, portions of some bones have a spongy interior. The cells of spongy (cancellous) bone have a honeycomblike architecture that is lighter and, when examined microscopically, appears less dense than compact bone.

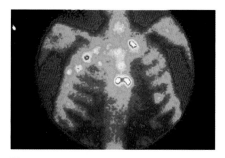

Bone scan
By using a radioactive element, such as technetium, a bone scan is performed to detect bone problems, including infections, tumors, and fractures.

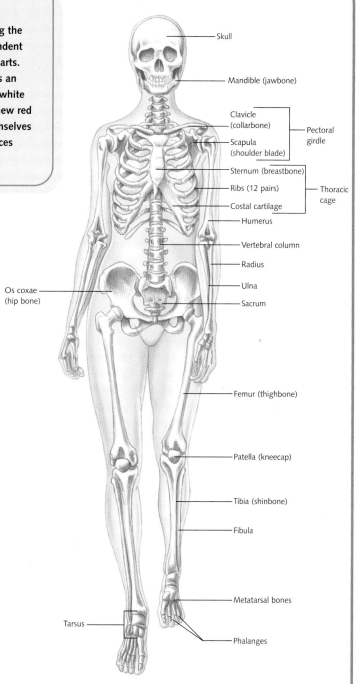

Skull

Mandible (jawbone)

Clavicle (collarbone)

Scapula (shoulder blade)

Pectoral girdle

Sternum (breastbone)

Ribs (12 pairs)

Costal cartilage

Thoracic cage

Humerus

Vertebral column

Radius

Ulna

Os coxae (hip bone)

Sacrum

Femur (thighbone)

Patella (kneecap)

Tibia (shinbone)

Fibula

Metatarsal bones

Tarsus

Phalanges

Bones of the skeletal system

MUSCULAR SYSTEM

The human body has three different types of muscles, each of which is designed to accomplish different tasks. The first type is skeletal muscle, the body's most abundant tissue. Skeletal muscles perform all voluntary movements and make up approximately 40 percent of a man's and 25 percent of a woman's total body weight. The second type is cardiac muscle, which is located in the heart and supplies the force that pumps blood throughout the body. The third type is smooth muscle. Smooth muscle is part of all internal organs.

Striated muscle tissue
Muscles are composed of thousands of long tube-like muscle cells called muscle fibers. The tubelike structure of muscle cells is apparent when viewed microscopically.

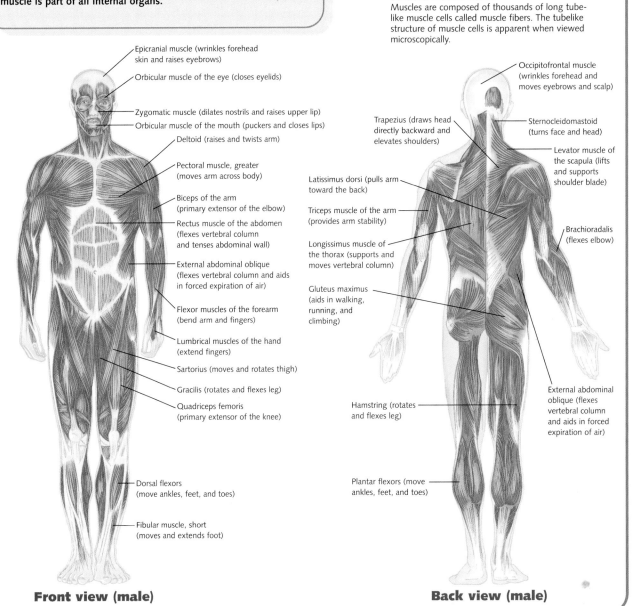

Epicranial muscle (wrinkles forehead skin and raises eyebrows)

Orbicular muscle of the eye (closes eyelids)

Zygomatic muscle (dilates nostrils and raises upper lip)

Orbicular muscle of the mouth (puckers and closes lips)

Deltoid (raises and twists arm)

Pectoral muscle, greater (moves arm across body)

Biceps of the arm (primary extensor of the elbow)

Rectus muscle of the abdomen (flexes vertebral column and tenses abdominal wall)

External abdominal oblique (flexes vertebral column and aids in forced expiration of air)

Flexor muscles of the forearm (bend arm and fingers)

Lumbrical muscles of the hand (extend fingers)

Sartorius (moves and rotates thigh)

Gracilis (rotates and flexes leg)

Quadriceps femoris (primary extensor of the knee)

Dorsal flexors (move ankles, feet, and toes)

Fibular muscle, short (moves and extends foot)

Front view (male)

Occipitofrontal muscle (wrinkles forehead and moves eyebrows and scalp)

Trapezius (draws head directly backward and elevates shoulders)

Sternocleidomastoid (turns face and head)

Levator muscle of the scapula (lifts and supports shoulder blade)

Latissimus dorsi (pulls arm toward the back)

Triceps muscle of the arm (provides arm stability)

Brachioradalis (flexes elbow)

Longissimus muscle of the thorax (supports and moves vertebral column)

Gluteus maximus (aids in walking, running, and climbing)

External abdominal oblique (flexes vertebral column and aids in forced expiration of air)

Hamstring (rotates and flexes leg)

Plantar flexors (move ankles, feet, and toes)

Back view (male)

NERVOUS SYSTEM

The central and peripheral nervous systems are actually systems of systems, which are collectively responsible for gathering information about what is happening to the body, interpreting the information, and triggering appropriate responses to satisfy certain bodily needs. The central nervous system, made up of the brain and spinal cord, regulates functions of the body that are not controlled consciously. The peripheral nervous system is made up of the somatic nervous system and the autonomic nervous system.

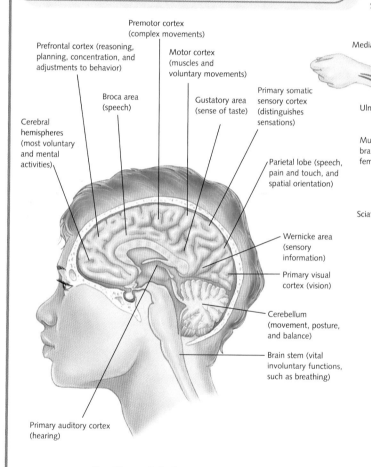

Premotor cortex (complex movements)

Prefrontal cortex (reasoning, planning, concentration, and adjustments to behavior)

Motor cortex (muscles and voluntary movements)

Broca area (speech)

Gustatory area (sense of taste)

Primary somatic sensory cortex (distinguishes sensations)

Cerebral hemispheres (most voluntary and mental activities)

Parietal lobe (speech, pain and touch, and spatial orientation)

Wernicke area (sensory information)

Primary visual cortex (vision)

Cerebellum (movement, posture, and balance)

Brain stem (vital involuntary functions, such as breathing)

Primary auditory cortex (hearing)

Functions of the brain
Since neurons are clustered according to function, it is possible to identify areas of the brain as having specific functions. The brain, however, functions as a whole by the interrelation of its component parts.

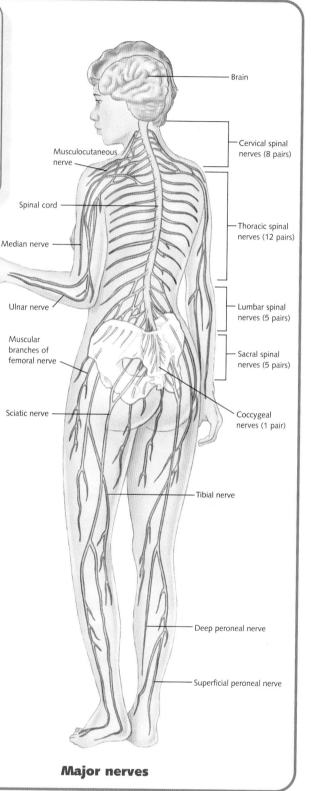

Brain

Cervical spinal nerves (8 pairs)

Musculocutaneous nerve

Spinal cord

Thoracic spinal nerves (12 pairs)

Median nerve

Ulnar nerve

Lumbar spinal nerves (5 pairs)

Muscular branches of femoral nerve

Sacral spinal nerves (5 pairs)

Sciatic nerve

Coccygeal nerves (1 pair)

Tibial nerve

Deep peroneal nerve

Superficial peroneal nerve

Major nerves

HEART AND CIRCULATORY SYSTEM

The heart and blood vessels form the body's circulatory system. Together, they supply a continuous flow of blood to the body. Arteries carry oxygenated blood away from the heart through the main artery, the aorta. Arteries branching from the aorta into arterioles (small arteries) and then into capillaries (tiny vessels between arteries and veins) carry blood throughout the body, where they provide oxygen and nutrients to organs and tissue. Deoxygenated blood is returned to the heart through the veins.

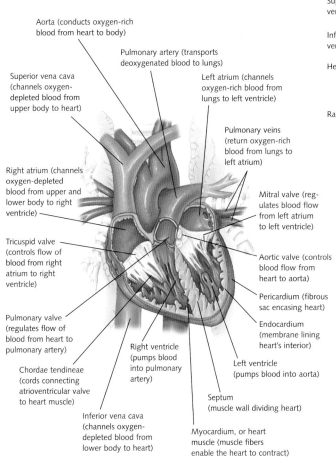

Aorta (conducts oxygen-rich blood from heart to body)

Pulmonary artery (transports deoxygenated blood to lungs)

Superior vena cava (channels oxygen-depleted blood from upper body to heart)

Left atrium (channels oxygen-rich blood from lungs to left ventricle)

Right atrium (channels oxygen-depleted blood from upper and lower body to right ventricle)

Pulmonary veins (return oxygen-rich blood from lungs to left atrium)

Tricuspid valve (controls flow of blood from right atrium to right ventricle)

Mitral valve (regulates blood flow from left atrium to left ventricle)

Aortic valve (controls blood flow from heart to aorta)

Pericardium (fibrous sac encasing heart)

Pulmonary valve (regulates flow of blood from heart to pulmonary artery)

Endocardium (membrane lining heart's interior)

Chordae tendineae (cords connecting atrioventricular valve to heart muscle)

Right ventricle (pumps blood into pulmonary artery)

Left ventricle (pumps blood into aorta)

Inferior vena cava (channels oxygen-depleted blood from lower body to heart)

Septum (muscle wall dividing heart)

Myocardium, or heart muscle (muscle fibers enable the heart to contract)

Structure of the heart
The average adult heart is slightly larger than a clenched fist and weighs about 1 pound.

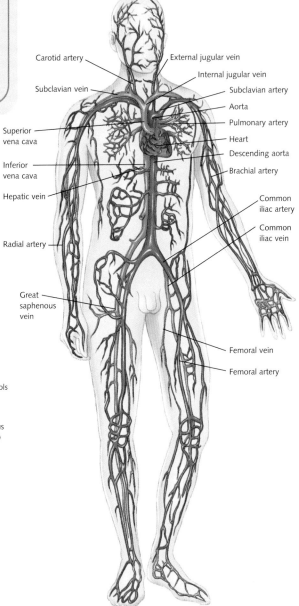

Carotid artery

External jugular vein

Internal jugular vein

Subclavian vein

Subclavian artery

Aorta

Pulmonary artery

Superior vena cava

Heart

Descending aorta

Inferior vena cava

Brachial artery

Hepatic vein

Common iliac artery

Radial artery

Common iliac vein

Great saphenous vein

Femoral vein

Femoral artery

Circulatory system

DIGESTIVE SYSTEM

Overall, four digestive system functions take place to pass food through the digestive tract: ingestion (consumption of food nutrients), digestion (breakdown of food molecules), absorption (absorption of nutrient molecules), and defecation (elimination of undigested residue). These digestive system functions are accomplished by three bodily processes: motility (contractions of the muscles to break down food), secretion (regulation of digestion by producing hormones and digestive enzymes), and membrane transport (method of transporting nutrients to blood and lymph).

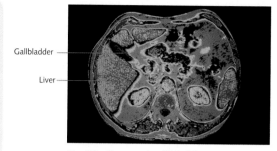

Gallbladder

Liver

Healthy liver and gallbladder
CT scanning (computed tomography scanning) permits doctors to visually examine the organs of the body for signs of disease.

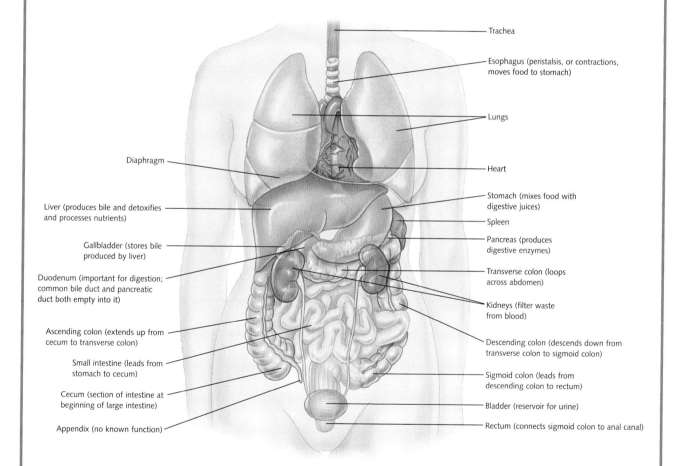

Trachea

Esophagus (peristalsis, or contractions, moves food to stomach)

Lungs

Diaphragm

Heart

Stomach (mixes food with digestive juices)

Liver (produces bile and detoxifies and processes nutrients)

Spleen

Pancreas (produces digestive enzymes)

Gallbladder (stores bile produced by liver)

Transverse colon (loops across abdomen)

Duodenum (important for digestion; common bile duct and pancreatic duct both empty into it)

Kidneys (filter waste from blood)

Ascending colon (extends up from cecum to transverse colon)

Descending colon (descends down from transverse colon to sigmoid colon)

Small intestine (leads from stomach to cecum)

Sigmoid colon (leads from descending colon to rectum)

Cecum (section of intestine at beginning of large intestine)

Bladder (reservoir for urine)

Appendix (no known function)

Rectum (connects sigmoid colon to anal canal)

Digestive organs

FEMALE AND MALE REPRODUCTIVE SYSTEMS

Gonads are the sex glands in which reproductive cells are produced. The female gonads are the ovaries, which produce ova, or eggs. The accessory organs of the female reproductive system include the uterus, two uterine (fallopian) tubes, the vagina, the vulva (genitalia), and the breasts (mammary glands). The male gonads are the testicles, which produce sex cells, or sperm. Additional organs of the male reproductive system include the genital ducts (urethra, ejaculatory ducts, epididymis, and vas deferens), prostate, and the seminal vesicles. The scrotum, penis, and spermatic cord are supportive structures.

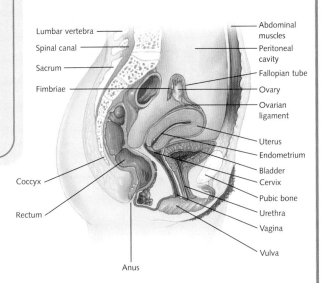

Labels: Lumbar vertebra, Spinal canal, Sacrum, Fimbriae, Coccyx, Rectum, Anus, Abdominal muscles, Peritoneal cavity, Fallopian tube, Ovary, Ovarian ligament, Uterus, Endometrium, Bladder, Cervix, Pubic bone, Urethra, Vagina, Vulva

Female reproductive system

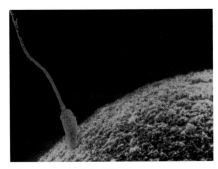

The moment of fertilization
Using its tail to swim to the ovum, or human egg, the sperm penetrates the outer surface of the ovum and the process of cell division begins.

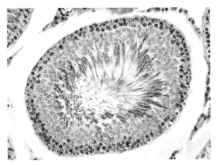

Creation of sperm
With magnification to 80 times, spermatogenesis, the process in which sperm are created in the testis, is visible in a micrograph.

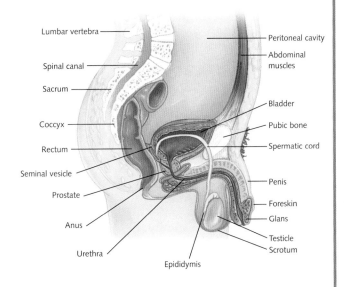

Labels: Lumbar vertebra, Spinal canal, Sacrum, Coccyx, Rectum, Seminal vesicle, Prostate, Anus, Urethra, Peritoneal cavity, Abdominal muscles, Bladder, Pubic bone, Spermatic cord, Penis, Foreskin, Glans, Testicle, Scrotum, Epididymis

Male reproductive system

FEMALE AND MALE URINARY SYSTEMS

The urinary system is made up of six organs: two kidneys, two ureters, the urinary bladder, and the urethra. Because a woman's bladder is located lower in the pelvic area than a man's bladder, the urethra is significantly shorter, which results in urinary tract infections occurring more commonly in women than in men. A man's urethra is the passageway through which both semen and urine pass from the body. The prostate, a gland that produces seminal fluid, is located at the base of the bladder and surrounds the urethra.

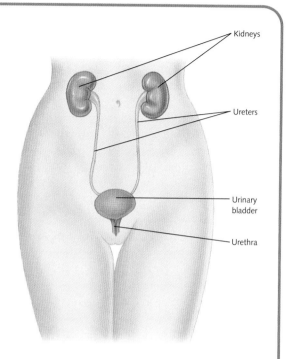

Kidneys

Ureters

Urinary bladder

Urethra

Female urinary system

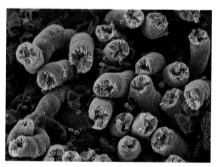

Glomerulus
The glomerulus is the principal filtering device of the nephron. It is here that filtration and purification of the blood takes place.

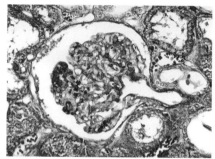

Nephron
The nephron, or uriniferous filtration tubule, is the functional unit of the kidney. There are approximately 1 million nephrons in each kidney.

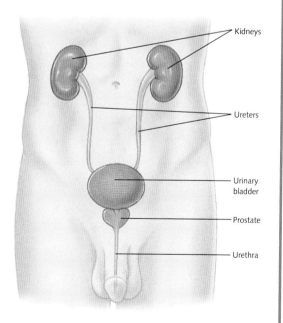

Kidneys

Ureters

Urinary bladder

Prostate

Urethra

Male urinary system

ENDOCRINE AND LYMPHATIC SYSTEMS

Just as the nervous system helps the various components of the body communicate via electrical impulses and neurotransmitters, the endocrine system provides an additional mechanism of internal communication via the movement of hormones through the blood. Even though hormones are carried throughout the body by the blood, they affect only target cells, or cells that have specific receptors to bind particular hormones. In addition to being the body's main defense against infection, the lymphatic system maintains internal fluid balance. The lymphatic vessels act as "drains" that collect excess fluid and return it to the blood before it reaches the heart.

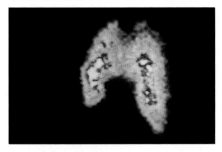

Normal thyroid scan
Thyroid nuclear scans illustrate thyroid function as well as thyroid structure (ultrasound tests show thyroid structure only).

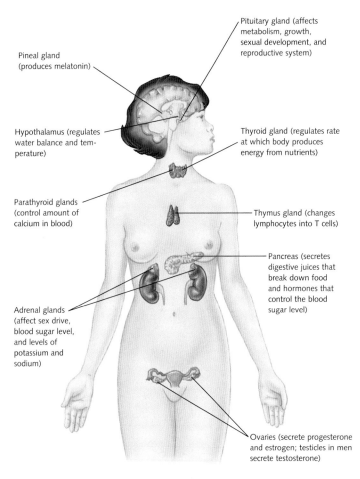

Pineal gland (produces melatonin)

Pituitary gland (affects metabolism, growth, sexual development, and reproductive system)

Hypothalamus (regulates water balance and temperature)

Thyroid gland (regulates rate at which body produces energy from nutrients)

Parathyroid glands (control amount of calcium in blood)

Thymus gland (changes lymphocytes into T cells)

Pancreas (secretes digestive juices that break down food and hormones that control the blood sugar level)

Adrenal glands (affect sex drive, blood sugar level, and levels of potassium and sodium)

Ovaries (secrete progesterone and estrogen; testicles in men secrete testosterone)

Endocrine system

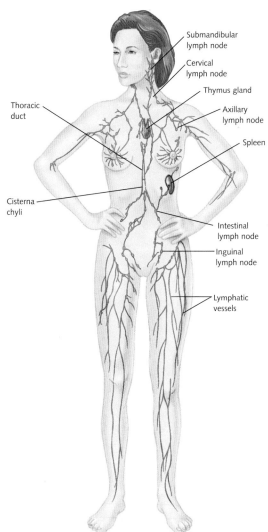

Submandibular lymph node

Cervical lymph node

Thymus gland

Thoracic duct

Axillary lymph node

Spleen

Cisterna chyli

Intestinal lymph node

Inguinal lymph node

Lymphatic vessels

Lymphatic system

Twenty-first century medicine

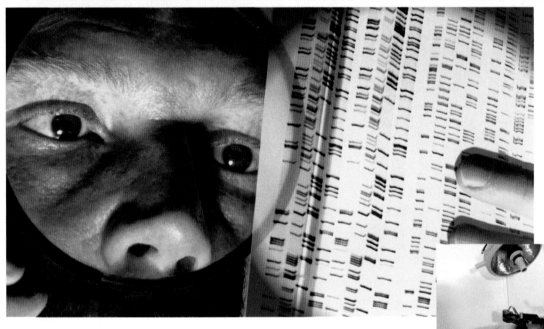

Gene mapping
A scientist studies a person's DNA or "genetic fingerprints" through a magnifying glass.

S till in its infancy, the 21st century has seen medical advancements come along at a staggering pace.

Genetics researchers are beginning to understand how they can cure very serious illnesses by replacing damaged cells with implanted stem cells. In clinical trials, adult stem cell therapy has repaired organs damaged by systemic lupus erythematosus, an autoimmune disease commonly known as lupus. Scientists are studying how they can develop vaccines into plants that can be ingested to prevent viral illnesses.

New digital scanners permit doctors to visualize three-dimensional (3-D) cross sections of interior body areas to help them better diagnose and treat brain tumors, breast cancer, and numerous other disorders. New imaging techniques also enable doctors to observe changes in brain activity that may provide ways to begin treating Alzheimer's disease before it causes severe disability.

Dramatic developments in bionic medicine make possible prosthetic heart valves for people with heart disease. Joint replacements and prosthetic limbs are designed on a computer system to simulate real-life movements. Artificial hands fitted with sensors detect changes in something being held—prompting the "hand" to make an adjustment in the grip. New, implantable nerve stimulators help people who are paralyzed move their hands, stand up, and walk short distances with assistance.

Robotic surgery, in which the surgeon operates controls in front of a computer console to manipulate the surgical instruments in the robot's hands, is making headlines. A camera greatly magnifies the surgeon's vision and provides a 3-D image from inside the area being operated on. The robot's computer program guides surgical knives and at the same time filters out the natural hand tremors that occur occasionally in any surgeon. Patients benefit from smaller incisions, less trauma to the body, and a speedier recovery.

Image-guided surgery permits neurosurgeons to plan brain tumor operations and simulate the procedure on a 3-D grid to avoid damaging delicate healthy brain tissue as cancerous tissue is removed. Virtual surgery simulators being developed include a touch component that permits medical students to "feel" the limbs, organs, and tissues of a virtual patient. They can even practice suturing on virtual skin that is programmed to react in real time as the student stitches the skin closed. Virtual surgery is no substitute for surgery but a valuable method of learning.

Magnified image
A video monitor shows a close-up of what the surgeon sees while maneuvering the surgical controls of the robotic system set up just steps away on the operating table.

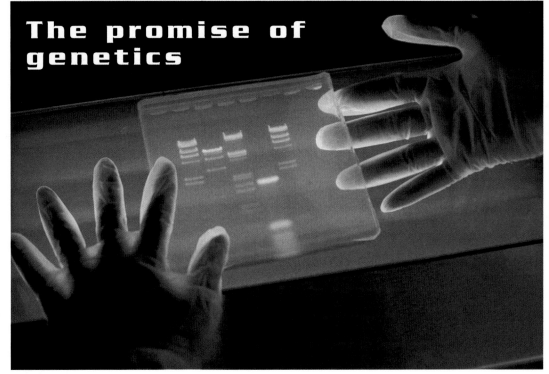

The promise of genetics

Searching for DNA
A scientist with gloved hands works with DNA fragments stained with a fluorescent chemical so that the fragments can be seen as bright bands under an ultraviolet light. Fragments of DNA are separated by size and used during DNA fingerprint analysis or to isolate particular genes.

Perhaps nowhere is the potential for change as exciting as the field of genetics. In the early 1990s, scientists from 18 nations agreed to tackle the gigantic task of itemizing and detailing the complete set of genetic instructions for human beings. In the process of mapping each gene in the human body and learning about all its functions, researchers with the Human Genome Project are now finding exciting new approaches to preventing, diagnosing, and treating disease.

By cracking the code to a person's inherited genetic makeup, researchers and scientists believe clinical research and the practice of medicine in the 21st century will forever be changed as medicine becomes more predictive and prevention-based. Treatment will become more specific and safer, permitting doctors to diagnose disease at earlier, more treatable stages. Genomics-based drug development should lead to new medications for disorders not now treatable and, in some cases, to more effective and safer replacements for current drugs.

This exciting explosion of genetic information revolves around genetic mapping, the technique for locating the site of specific genes on chromosomes. The process of genetic sequencing involves identifying the code of a defective gene in order to compare it with the code of a normal gene so that a particular defect can be identified.

"Genome" refers to the master plan or central set of instructions for the growth, development, and functioning of an organism. It is the body's complete owner's manual or instruction booklet, which is why it has been called the "human blueprint."

Remarkably, people share 99.9 percent of the same coding, which means that the enormous diversity of human beings is encoded at the genetic level by less than a 0.1 percent variation in DNA.

The great accomplishment of the Human Genome Project has been to complete a rough draft of all the approximately 3 billion chemical letters in the human body's DNA, the physical material of inheritance that holds information for all aspects of bodily growth and development. The Human Genome Project is made up of teams of biologists, geneticists, chemists, molecular biologists, physicists, computer scientists, engineers, and mathematicians who are involved in developing computerized data storage and analysis techniques for mapping and sequencing the genome. And, because it is of utmost importance to use new technologies safely and responsibly, specialists involved in the project are also continually evaluating the ethical, legal, and social implications that may arise during human genetics research.

How is this specialized research useful in the ongoing effort to improve human health? Within its first decade of existence, the Human Genome Project identified and sequenced about 7,000 disease genes in humans, a first step in understanding the origin of diseases including cystic fibrosis, some forms of diabetes mellitus and mental retardation, certain metabolic disorders, and severe combined immunodeficiency. Ongoing studies are underway into how these genes function and how changes in the genes, called mutations, cause disease.

Because the genome is the template governing all the body's cellular processes, understanding how genes work has potential applications in several areas. Controlling the formation of blood vessels, for example, may be instrumental in controlling the inflammatory process, which could have direct applications for treating allergies, arthritis, and diseases of the eyes and brain. Promoting blood vessel formation could offer benefits in the treatment of heart attack and stroke.

Abnormalities in genetic sequencing are the cause of all forms of cancer, making cancer the most common genetic disease. A number of dominant and recessive genes involved in the formation and suppression of tumors have been identified. The challenge is to arrive at an understanding of the nature of the abnormality in the cancer cell genes. Gene mapping can provide more precise diagnoses of the many variations in tumor formation.

Variations in the genome sequence also determine differences in a person's level of susceptibility to certain diseases or disorders, as well as the age when a person is afflicted with a particular disease or condition, its severity, and the body's response to medical treatment for the disorder. It is known, for example, that certain variations in what is called the APOE gene are associated with Alzheimer's disease and that a part of the CCR5 gene provides resistance to HIV (human immunodeficiency virus) and AIDS (acquired immunodeficiency syndrome). The mapping of genes known as single nucleotide polymorphisms, or SNPs, can help researchers identify the SNPs that are associated with specific diseases. This approach to medicine is steadily advancing toward an understanding of each individual's genetic uniqueness as a basis for establishing a complete medical blueprint of vulnerabilities and toward the potential for successful prevention and treatment of disease.

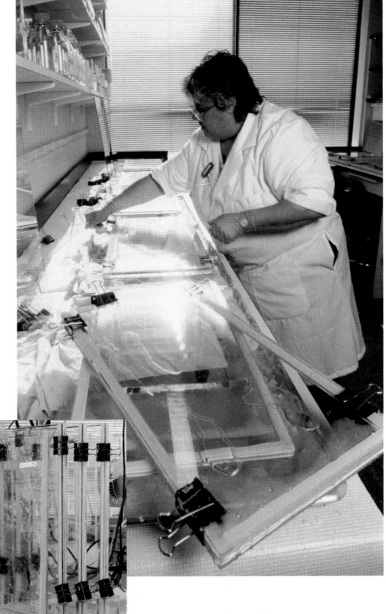

Preparing genetic sequencing plates
A researcher readies glass plates for genome mapping. The plates are coated with a gel that stores genetic sequences that are read with lasers.

Human genome mapping project
A scientist holds a sequencing gel plate used to catalog the genes of mice. Genetic mapping involves determining the sequence of specific genes on chromosomes.

Genetic engineering

Although environmental factors are involved in acquiring illness, human genes determine the basis for the body's defense mechanisms. Genetic engineering is the process of manipulating genes to create medications and vaccines. Because many diseases and disorders are influenced by the functions of genes, genetic engineering offers promise for producing new medications that may be able to treat and cure hundreds of major health problems. One of the primary goals of research is to discover and isolate the genes involved in disease processes and analyze the function of those genes. Insulin that is used to treat diabetes and certain vaccinations against specific viruses, including hepatitis B, can be made in this way. Technical obstacles, as well as responsible resolutions to social and ethical concerns, are being studied so that genetic engineering can continue to advance.

Gene therapy offers disease treatment and prevention methods that use genes to provide the body's cells with the necessary genetic information so they can produce the specific therapeutic proteins needed to treat disease. This therapy may involve correcting genetic disorders and curing life-threatening diseases. Ex vivo gene therapy involves certain blood or bone marrow cells being removed and cultured in a laboratory. The treated genes can be delivered

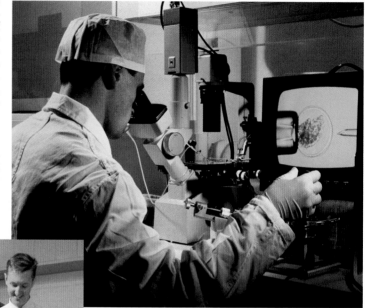

Bovine embryo transfer
A genetics researcher prepares to genetically manipulate the embryo of a dairy cow through a microscope.

into human cells only by means of a carrier, called a vector. The most common vectors are viruses that are unable to reproduce themselves. While these viruses have a unique ability to gain entrance to a cell's DNA, they are also capable of infecting or damaging surrounding tissue when the virus returns to the body.

Disorders such as adenosine deaminase deficiency, a rare genetic disease, have been successfully treated by use of techniques that reengineer cells via gene therapy. Systemic lupus erythematosus (known as lupus) and other autoimmune diseases, in which the body's immune system attacks the body's cells and produces a disease state, cause the body to make antibodies against the cells' DNA. In research settings, scientists have developed the capacity to extract this DNA and attach a toxin to it. When the DNA is reintroduced into the body and antibody-producing cells attack it, the toxin in the engineered DNA destroys the antibody cells that are attacking the body, leaving other cells intact.

The primary challenge of genetic research is to

Genetic cloning
A cow, a goat, and a piglet become the first three species cloned at a veterinary school in Texas.

better understand serious disorders such as heart disease, diabetes, hypertension, psychiatric disorders, and cancer. Some of these are caused in part by many defective genes, all of which must be identified and understood in terms of their function in creating the disease.

In cancer treatment, gene therapy is being studied as a means to enhance the body's natural ability to fight the disease and to make existing cancer cells more responsive to treatments, such as chemotherapy. For example, researchers believe that stem cells, the cells in bone marrow that produce blood cells, can be made more resistant to the side effects of high-dose anticancer treatments and medications.

To treat diseases such as cancer and AIDS effectively, scientists are working on the development of carriers with the ability to target the disease cells throughout the body and integrate the desired gene into the DNA of these cells. The potential of genetic engineering is exciting because it offers the possibility of curing a serious illness by altering a very small number of cells.

Gene splicing

Gene splicing involves taking a gene from one organism and inserting it into the DNA of another. A common gene-splicing technique involves inserting a new fragment of DNA with codes for a specific human protein, like insulin, into a bacterium such as *Escherichia coli (E. coli).* In this process, the gene is initially inserted into a ring of DNA that replicates itself and is involved in the transfer of genes among bacteria. The bacterial cells divide and pass on the new information to the next generation of cells. These bacterial clones can produce large quantities of the new protein, in this case, human insulin.

Gene splicing is a method that has been used to produce adequate supplies of a hormonelike protein, called interferon-alpha, for ongoing research and therapy. (In clinical tests, direct injections of interferon-alpha have been shown to eliminate or significantly reduce genital warts.) In this case, gene splicing is accomplished by introducing a gene that contains the code for interferon-alpha into harmless bacteria, which reproduce to produce large amounts of interferon. This advance in biotechnology has created a process by which enough interferon-alpha can be produced to make it a practical treatment option for medical use. Interferon-alpha is used to treat certain types of leukemia, hepatitis, and genital warts.

Therapeutic proteins

Diseases such as diabetes, hemophilia, and some cancers have traditionally been treated with recombinant proteins. These proteins are produced by genetically modified microorganisms, such as bacteria, that carry the corresponding gene and may be able to stimulate an immune response against tumors or viruses.

Gene therapy, on the other hand, has the potential to use genes as therapeutic agents to enable the body's cells to produce the needed protein, or ther-

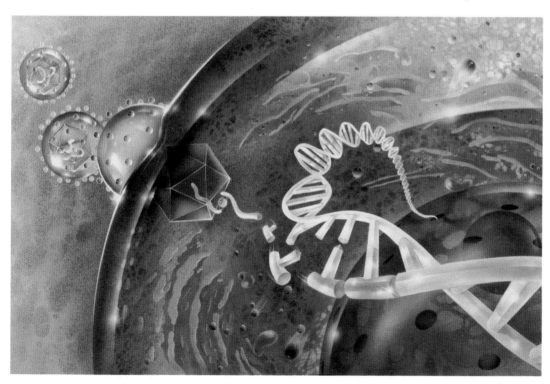

Gene therapy
An artist's rendition shows how gene therapy is accomplished. The virus's genetic material can be altered by scientists so that healthy genes can correct inherited genetic disorders.

apeutic protein, which can provide therapeutic levels of the protein in the blood. When therapeutic proteins are produced at the site of the disease in this way, they may be more effective than recombinant proteins. The therapeutic proteins may provide beneficial effects over a longer period and be less toxic or dangerous to the person being treated.

One aspect of the ongoing research with genetic engineering and therapeutic proteins involves introducing the proteins into plant tissues, from which they can be extracted and administered as medications. There are tests to determine whether these proteins might be expressed in plant tissues that, when eaten, would provide vaccination against disease. There is fascinating potential for deriving vaccines by introducing a virus protein into edible plants so that eating these plants would prevent the viral illness. Human vaccines have already been introduced into, proved to be present in, and extracted from bananas and tomatoes.

Monoclonal antibodies

Monoclonal antibodies are components of the immune system that are exceptionally pure and highly capable of recognizing and binding to a specific disease-causing agent, or antigen. They can be mass-produced in laboratories, which to date have used antibodies from mice for the purpose of targeting specific disease-causing agents. These specialized, manufactured antibodies can be used to diagnose and treat certain malignant tumors, including skin cancer.

The general diagnostic uses of monoclonal antibodies include the ability to measure protein and medication levels in the blood, to type tissue and blood, to identify infectious agents and specific cells within the immune system, and to iden-

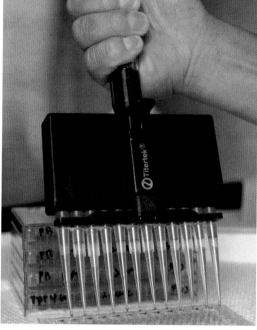

Monoclonal antibodies
A researcher prepares monoclonal antibodies for reproduction. The antibodies can be mass-produced to diagnose and treat certain malignant tumors.

tify human hormones. The monoclonal antibodies also show impressive potential for treating human diseases and disorders, such as for follow-up therapy for leukemia and lymphoma.

Among the goals of research is the attempt to create an antibody that binds exclusively to cancer cells in the body. A powerful radioactive isotope could then be introduced into that antibody and given to a person with cancer to destroy cancer cells without affecting normal cells. Clinical studies have been started with people who have melanoma. Results have shown that monoclonal antibodies can be used safely to reduce the growth of tumors, and generally without toxic effects to the person being treated.

Human therapies have been slow to use monoclonal antibodies because the only ones available have been derived from research with mice, and these "mouse antibodies" are interpreted as "foreign" by the human immune system. The human response against these antibodies is caused by the body's production of antibodies known as HAMAs, or human antimouse antibodies. HAMAs cause the therapeutic antibodies to be rejected by the host and produce immune reactions that can damage the kidneys.

Genetic engineering technology is seeking to discover methods for producing new "designer" monoclonal antibodies that can possibly increase the potency of the antibodies.

Lab mouse and DNA profile
Mice are used frequently for genetic experiments because they produce a large litter of young several times a year, and their size and genetic similarity to humans are ideal for safety tests on chemicals and drugs and to study infectious organisms.

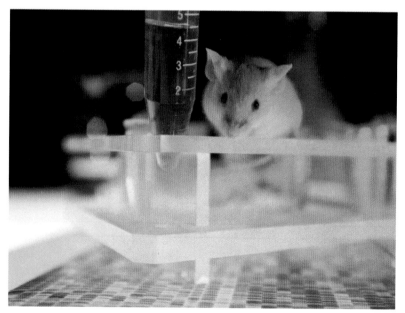

Stem cell research

Stem cells are responsible for creating all the different kinds of blood cells in the body and are usually found in bone marrow but can also circulate in the blood. These cells, which are the subject of much scientific and medical research, have the capacity to renew themselves and form other specialized cells. There is particular interest in the potential of stem cell research to create therapies for treating nerve-related disorders and disabilities such as Parkinson disease.

A severe limitation on stem cell research is the controversy around procuring stem cells from the most useful and abundant source, human embryos. Self-renewing and unspecialized, embryonic stem cells can be multiplied and manipulated by scientists to be transformed into many other types of cells, including brain, heart, and pancreas cells. These cells could be used in the treatment of a wide range of disabling and life-threatening health problems. As of 2002, federal funding of this research has been restricted to the use of a designated 60 existing stem cell lines already obtained from human embryos.

Seeking to find alternative sources, researchers have investigated the possibilities for adult stem cells. These cells, like all stem cells, can make identical copies of themselves over long periods in a process called long-term self-renewal, and they can give rise to mature cell types that have characteristic shapes and specialized functions. For current therapeutic uses, adult stem cells may be obtained from umbilical cord blood, bone marrow, the blood of the person being treated, or a healthy donor. They may also be obtained from animal tissue.

Adult neural stem cells have also been isolated from the brains of mice. These cells could offer potential for treating Alzheimer's and other dis-

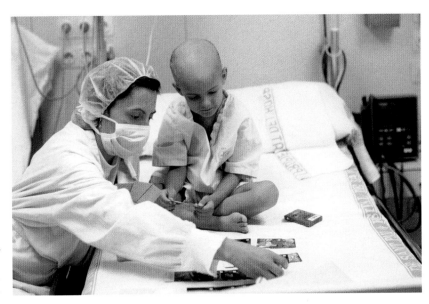

Treating cancer
A child with leukemia is treated with chemotherapy. The anticancer drug stops white bloods cells from multiplying, but the drug acts on all dividing cells, affecting the bone marrow, immune system, the intestinal lining, and even the hair follicles, which is why people undergoing chemotherapy often lose their hair.

eases involving the degeneration of nerve tissues. Encouraging results have been noted when stem cells were extracted from the blood of people who had one of several conditions, including the potentially disabling inflammatory bowel disease known as Crohn disease, multiple sclerosis, and systemic lupus erythematosus. In cases of lupus, adult stem cell therapy was effective at repairing organs that had been damaged by the condition.

Experiments with mice have shown that stimulating the production of stem cells in bone marrow can repair heart damage. Immune system chemicals were injected into the mice to stimulate production of stem cells in their bone marrow. Results indicated improved survival following heart attacks, including repair to heart tissue and recovery of the heart's pumping capacity. Embryonic stem cells from mice have been used to create insulin-secreting cells, an advance that has potential for curing juvenile diabetes. Adult pancreatic stem cells from mice have been harvested and grown in laboratory culture, then injected under the skin of diabetic mice. Within a short time, the injected mice began secreting insulin and the diabetes was reversed. Neural stem cells have been shown to replace and repair damaged brain tissue, indicating potential for treating Parkinson and other central nervous system diseases.

Other advances in stem cell research have included the ability to boost the immune systems in infants with severe combined immunodeficiency by using stem cells removed from the infants' bone marrow. Research is also underway to study the clinical use of stem cells from bone marrow to treat children with a disabling cartilage defect called osteogenesis imperfecta. Adult corneal stem cells have been transplanted into adults for whom traditional cornea implants were not possible, and the transplanted cells restored or improved vision.

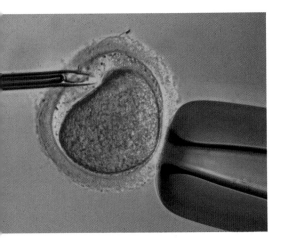

Manipulation of human embryo
A researcher prepares to harvest stem cells from a human embryo for genetic research.

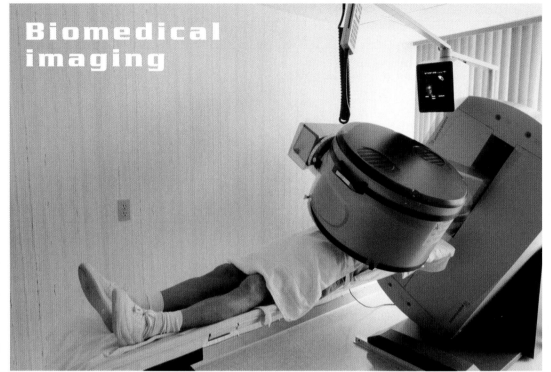

Biomedical imaging

3-D image of the heart
A special technique called SPECT (single photon emission computed tomography) gives a 3-D image of a person's heart after he or she is injected with thallium and then exercises on a treadmill. The dye tracer concentrates only in areas with good blood flow, which helps give an accurate picture of the health of the heart.

In the biomedical engineering field, which seeks to solve medical and surgical problems by applying the principles of engineering, research has led to important new treatment devices in addition to diagnostic tools. Cochlear implants have restored hearing ability to many hearing-impaired people. Implantable defibrillators have been a lifesaving addition for people with certain forms of cardiovascular disease. Kidney dialysis is possible as a result of biomedical engineering research and development. The diagnostic use of noninvasive imaging techniques has resulted in vastly improved treatments for a wide range of health problems.

The scope of biomedical engineering is being expanded by ongoing research into cell and tissue engineering. Technologies are being developed that will permit surgeons to replace or repair the human tissues that make up cartilage, bone, liver, kidney, skeletal muscle, and blood vessels. Tissue-engineering therapies hold great promise and could eventually be applied to diseases such as osteoarthritis, osteoporosis, and atherosclerosis.

New variations to existing biomedical imaging technologies have already made important contributions to diagnostics. Magnetic resonance spectroscopy, for example, is a new variant of MRI (magnetic resonance imaging) that can monitor cell metabolism and detect the changes in metabolism that are caused by degenerative diseases.

A nuclear medicine test called SPECT (single-photon emission computed tomography) uses a radioactive tracer that emits high-energy photons, proven to be an excellent diagnostic tool for coronary artery disease. Sophisticated images can now be used to plan complex surgical procedures in detail. And medical researchers can use images seen through lenses, or on film and computer screens, to aid ongoing research into major health concerns such as heart disease and cancer.

Doctors can now instantly transmit intricate medical images from small, rural hospitals to major medical centers where experts can offer diagnostic collaboration and consultation. Advances in computer technology and data processing are being explored to find ways to manipulate data in order to enhance image quality and transmit the information that creates images to other locations via telephone lines. Comparing and fusing various images into three-dimensional composites is yet another direction explored by researchers developing complex computer software.

More precise mathematical calculations that would sharpen the images produced by PET (positron emission tomography, a scan that permits doctors to look at the chemical and metabolic activity of body tissues) and SPECT have to date been deemed excessively time-consuming. But researchers are now working on algorithms that can offer more detailed and accurate images from PET and SPECT scans in less time.

The ways data are collected by biomedical imaging tools is an important area of research. Many of the contrast media used in CT (computed tomography) scanning and MRI to enhance the blood vessels are rapidly cleared out of the body by the kidneys. The creation of contrast substances that will target a tissue, such as a tumor, just long enough for the imaging procedure and then be immediately eliminated constitutes a current research challenge.

Biomedical engineering researchers are working on developing smaller and less costly imaging machines, such as MRI scanners. The next generation of MRI scanners is expected to be much more compact and effective at monitoring body activities, including blood flow and brain activity. Neuroscientists have already discovered that MRI and PET scanning can be used to observe certain functions of the brain, as well as its structure, and this offers new insights into how memory works.

Modulations in the sound frequency used in ultrasonography (ultrasound) are being studied by scientists with the goal of improving ultrasound images. This research could sharpen the images produced and increase their depth without elevating the ultrasound intensity to higher levels, which carries the risk of overheating body tissues.

Combining imaging techniques is another exciting area of ongoing biomedical research. Measuring heart function and the flow of blood through the heart by coupling MRI and SPECT imaging tools is under study. A combination of CT and PET images is being explored to provide surgeons with more precise images of the body that can be used to guide surgical incisions.

Scientists are also investigating new ways to use their existing imaging tools. They have found that MRI scanners, for example, can report on the presence of sodium, which is information that can help assess a person's kidney function. Data on phosphorus provided by MRI can be an aid to evaluations of muscle function and tumor activity. PET scanning may eventually be capable of distinguishing malignant tumors from benign cysts in the breasts, growths that can be impossible to differentiate with current imaging techniques. There are also studies using ultrasound to measure the strength and flexibility of bones.

Progress in developing bioMEMS (tiny biomicroelectromechanical systems that integrate electrical, mechanical, and optical systems) is likely to set the stage for a new era of what is being called "lab on a chip" diagnostics. This technology has the potential to provide a sensitive analysis of thousands of molecules from a single blood sample and could be performed as routinely as yearly tests for cholesterol. New imaging tools may ultimately offer the ability to understand the molecular mechanisms of disease and their responses to treatments.

Nuclear medicine

Nuclear medicine involves the administration of small amounts of radioactive materials, called radionuclides or radiopharmaceuticals, which are

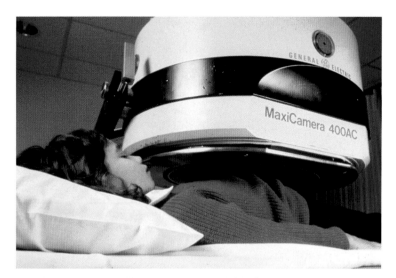

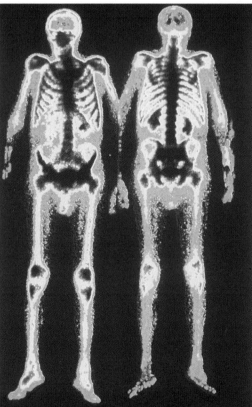

Nuclear medicine scanner
A nuclear medicine gamma scanner takes 3-D images of a girl's lungs.

Full body MRI
The front and back are shown of a person having a full body scan using magnetic resonance imaging, or MRI.

given orally or by injection or inhalation. Each of these materials has a special affinity for a specific type of body tissue or organ so that it can target the designated organ, bone, or other tissue in the body. Once a site in the body has been targeted by a radionuclide, the material emits gamma rays that are picked up by PET cameras to produce an image.

Every major organ and structural system can be imaged by one of the close to 100 different nuclear medicine imaging procedures now available. The procedures can document organ function and provide physicians access to highly sophisticated medical information at a low cost. In many cases, doctors would not be able to acquire this diagnostic information by other means, or they would be able to learn what they needed to know only by performing surgery.

The use of nuclear medicine tools in bone scanning can reveal cancer that has spread and produced secondary tumors on bones. And in addition to structural changes in bone tissue, nuclear scans offer visualization of metabolic changes that occur as a result of very tiny fractures, small tumors, or degenerative bone diseases, such as arthritis.

PET scanning

PET scanning permits a doctor to see cross-sectional images of body functions that can be used to detect subtle changes in the body's metabolism and chemical activities. PET is generally considered a more specific diagnostic technique for certain cancers, brain diseases, and cardiac illnesses and disorders than other techniques such as CT scanning, MRI, or X ray.

Within the last decade, PET has become more routine, especially in diagnosing, evaluating, and treating lung cancer. PET scans are more reliable than traditional imaging techniques for helping a physician detect, identify, and locate lung cancer that has spread.

New uses for PET scanning are being discovered on an ongoing basis as medical specialists find an increasing number of applications for evaluating illnesses. For example, it has the potential for identifying certain brain functions that can be a key aspect in the development of new ways to diagnose and treat brain tumors and mental disorders.

Stereotactic imaging

Stereotactic imaging provides doctors with clear, exacting landmarks that enable them to locate, evaluate, and treat specific but hard to reach sites. The technology is based on three-dimensional (3-D) visualizations of planes or "slices" of interior body areas.

Stereotactic radiosurgery has been used to treat many kinds of malignant tumors that would otherwise be difficult to reach and treat without damaging adjoining or nearby tissues. In addition to brain and spinal cord tumors, the technique is used to treat tumors of the abdomen, prostate, lungs, breasts, and soft-tissue areas surrounding the spine.

Stereotactic technology has been helpful to doctors for evaluating and diagnosing breast abnormalities. The imaging tool can pinpoint the location of growths in the breast that have been discovered on a mammogram but cannot be felt by the doctor during a physical examination. The technique is also used to guide the radiologist in the biopsy procedure. A newer technique using stereotactic imaging involves computer calculations that direct the radiologist in terms of the cor-

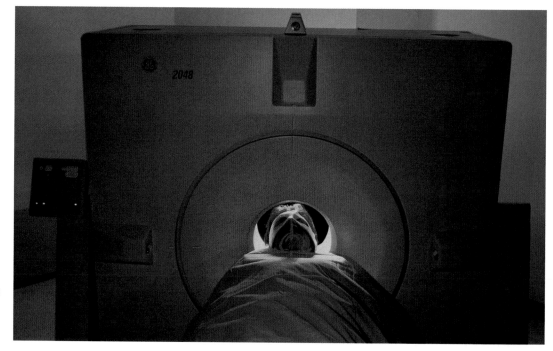

PET brain scanner
Positron emission tomography (PET) scanning permits a doctor to visualize distinct areas of the human brain while the person is comfortable, conscious, and alert.

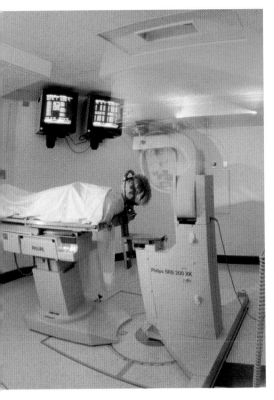

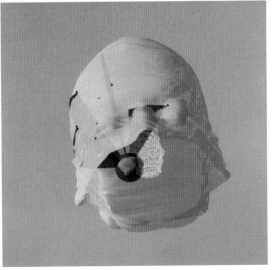

Stereotactic linear accelerator
Stereotactic imaging (far left) provides surgeons a way to pinpoint hard-to-reach spots, such as a brain tumor, as computer-guided beams of radiation are focused directly into the brain tumor.

Computer image of brain tumor
A 3-D computer image of a brain tumor (left) helps doctors precisely pinpoint radiation therapy for inoperable brain tumors.

Optical coherence tomography
OCT uses infrared light waves to reflect the internal microstructure within body tissues, in the case of the scan on the left checking how well a stent angioplasty is working to keep the artery open. The scan of the heart on the right shows that the stent put in after an angioplasty to open up the artery is not working properly, and, thus, blood flow is impeded.

rect angle and depth for the insertion of a core biopsy needle, in which tissue is drawn out of the breast for laboratory analysis. Another procedure, called stereotactic wire placement, involves imaging the abnormality within the breast so that the surgeon can insert a thin wire through a fine needle and identify the location of the growth and obtain a tissue biopsy.

Functional MRI is an exciting new application of magnetic resonance imaging that has great potential for medical research and education. It permits scientists and physicians to observe brain function during specific activities when a person is recovering from a stroke, a head injury, or surgery. The advantages of functional MRI over PET scanning are the speed and resolution of the image and the lack of radiation exposure for the person being tested.

Optical coherence tomography

A method of optical imaging, optical coherence tomography involves the use of near-infrared light pulsed through a device called an interferometer, which aims an "arm" into the tissue to be evaluated. This technique produces shallow, cross-sectional, high-resolution visualizations of the targeted tissue in real time by gathering information that is produced by the interaction of the light collected from the tissue and the light from the interferometer's reference arm.

The resolution of images produced by optical

coherence tomography enables a physician to differentiate microstructures within tissue. This can be very useful in pathology tests in which such tiny distinctions in tissue may indicate disease. Also, because optical coherence imaging has the ability to provide images of living tissue in the body, it can be used to examine tissue that could not be safely removed for traditional surgical biopsy studies. Biomedical scientists are currently striving to use this form of imaging to create "optical biopsies" for a number of diagnostic purposes. In addition to evaluation of tissue that cannot be safely removed surgically, these biopsies could be used to evaluate tissue that may be missed in the usual biopsy procedures. Diseased tissue in the intestines could be evaluated by optical coherence tomography biopsies, for example.

This new technology, which is just in its infancy, offers particularly favorable prospects as a tool for diagnosing and monitoring diseases of the eyes, including glaucoma and certain complications of diabetes, such as macular edema. The images produced can show very early stages of eye disease before they cause loss of vision or other symptoms.

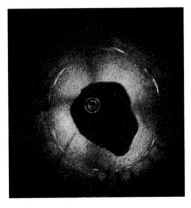

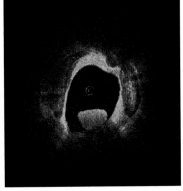

Prenatal scanning and in utero surgery

Prenatal diagnosis for certain serious health problems has generally relied on obtaining and isolating fetal cells for laboratory study. Recently, it has been shown that, in some cases, noninvasive screening techniques may provide equally reliable diagnostic data with less potential risk to the fetus. MRI, for example, can be used to evaluate the brain of a fetus at risk for certain inherited metabolic disorders and can offer important information for a prenatal diagnosis.

Prenatal ultrasound scanning is often performed routinely to visualize the fetus and obtain other related medical information. Ultrasound scans are also commonly used to evaluate the status of a high-risk pregnancy and guide the physician in the performance of amniocentesis, a procedure in which amniotic fluid is drawn out of the woman's uterus to test for fetal birth abnormalities.

Certain serious health risks to the fetus can be

Ultrasound of a fetus
An ultrasound scan shows early movement of a fetus. The colored patches represent the flow of amniotic fluid out of the fetus's mouth so that doctors can observe breathing movements.

detected and surgically treated via prenatal scanning with ultrasound. Hydrocephalus, which is an abnormal accumulation of fluid in the fetus's head, and urinary obstruction and hernias, are conditions that have been successfully treated while the fetus remained in the mother's uterus. For example, surgeons successfully operated on a fetus during a woman's 23rd week of pregnancy to repair a heart defect that most likely would have caused the baby to die soon after birth. The surgery was performed through a needle inserted in the mother's abdomen. Guided by ultrasound images on a monitor, the surgeons were able to widen and repair the narrowed

valve in the baby's heart, which was about the size of a grape.

Virtual colonoscopy

A new procedure is on the brink of replacing the two standard diagnostic tools to help physicians detect polyps, malignant tumors, and other abnormalities in the colon. The recently developed diagnostic tool, called virtual colonoscopy, may eventually be able to serve the same purpose as more invasive procedures such as a sigmoidoscopy and conventional colonoscopy, in which a flexible narrow scope equipped with a tiny camera is inserted through the anus to diagnose cancer or inflammatory bowel disease or to take a biopsy.

Virtual colonoscopy combines CT scanning of the large bowel with virtual reality computer software to provide 3-D images. This advanced visualization technique produces virtual imaging and exploration of the entire colon. In this procedure, after cleansing the colon, the colon is inflated with air to permit examination, and the visualization is produced using an ultrafast CT scanner and a computer.

Some research has demonstrated that this emerging technology has an improved sensitivity over barium enema for detecting polyps and almost matches traditional colonoscopy for sensitivity and diagnostic accuracy. Virtual colonoscopy will offer important advantages over conventional colonoscopy, such as lower cost and reduced physical and emotional discomfort for the person being tested. Further refinements of virtual colonoscopy are being researched, however, because the imaging technique is not yet capable of identifying some of the smaller abnormal growths in the colon.

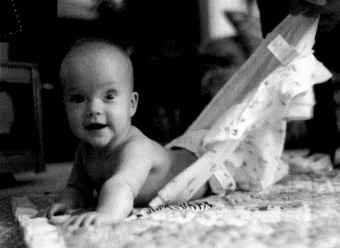

Healthy baby
This baby was diagnosed with spina bifida, a congenital defect in which one or more vertebrae fail to develop completely, and treated while in the uterus. Surgeons were able to perform corrective surgery even before the child was born.

The human brain at work

New technology in brain scanning has enabled scientists to observe and measure the activity of the human brain, an advance that has made possible many new discoveries about how the brain functions. One of the most fascinating applications of PET (positron emission tomography) scanning and functional MRI (magnetic resonance imaging) has been their use to permit observation of the healthy human brain at work. As researchers study increasingly clear electronic images of brain activity taken from a wide range of structural perspectives, their findings have given rise to valuable new insights and a deeper understanding of how human beings learn. Studies have already shown, for example, the changes in brain function that occur as a result of *seeing* words on a video screen as opposed to *hearing* the same words spoken through ear phones.

Neuroscientists' research using functional MRI has demonstrated that the brain becomes more efficient in the ongoing process of learning to do a specific task, using less energy to achieve the same result. It has also been demonstrated via functional MRI studies that the same parts of the brain are activated when a person imagines an object as when the person sees the object.

Brain scans have also been used to investigate the process of remembering. In one study, researchers noted that both halves of the brain are involved in remembering *events*, whereas only one half of the brain is activated in remembering *facts*. This study showed that the activity of remembering an event involves the corpus callosum, which is the brain area that passes information between the two halves. The corpus callosum is not fully developed until a child reaches the age of about 4 years, and this may offer at least a partial explanation for why adults often cannot remember events that occurred before that age.

An interesting aspect of brain activity that has been studied via images produced by the new brain scanning techniques reveals how and where the creation of a memory occurs in the brain. One study demonstrated that specific levels of activity in certain areas of the brain were linked to the formation of a simple verbal memory. The levels of brain activity that were observed in this study offered the scientists clues as to whether a given experience would become part of long-term memory or be forgotten.

Brain activity was recorded by brain scans as people participating in the study read single words. The people were told to analyze the words' meanings and were not told to memorize the words, nor were they aware that their memory was being observed and tested. After an interval of 20 minutes, the same people were shown groups of words and asked which ones they had seen previously (during the brain scanning). The research team then compared the images produced by the brain scans. These images revealed levels of activity in certain parts of the brain when the people remembered the words and activity levels in other areas when they forgot them.

What the researchers discovered was that most of the activity took place in the left frontal lobe and in the left temporal lobe. They were able to identify the location of most of this activity even more precisely to the inner wall of the left temporal lobe, a structure that is positioned on the pathway to the brain's hippocampus. The hippocampus is essential for memory storage and retrieval.

A similar study used brain scans to observe brain function during the activity of forming a visual memory. It was observed that the brain activity that took place in the right frontal lobe and both the left and right temporal lobes predicted which visual images would be recalled.

One medical application for these discoveries is predicting the onset of Alzheimer's disease. An area in the middle of the temporal lobes is one of the first to be affected, resulting in the memory loss typical of Alzheimer's. The ability to observe

Positron emission tomography (PET)
This type of scan permits doctors to look at the chemical and metabolic activity of body tissues, such as this scan (left) of the brain as it processes words. The scan on the right shows the areas of the brain that work to imagine words that are spoken.

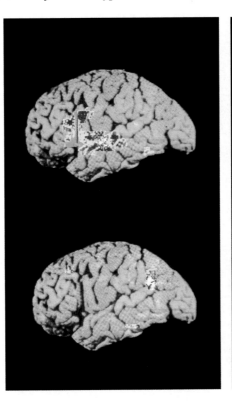
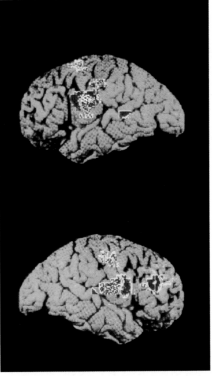

Changes in brain activity
The nuclear medicine scan on top depicts the workings of the normal brain. The scan at the bottom shows the signs of a brain with dementia, a decline in mental ability.

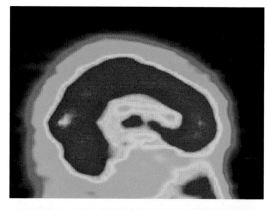

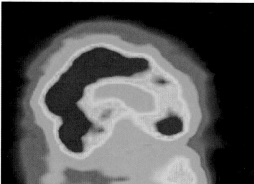

changes in activity in that area of the brain could provide opportunities to begin treating the disease before it causes severe disability. Previously autopsy has been the only way to confirm a diagnosis of Alzheimer's. The ability to study natural repair processes in a brain damaged by stroke is another possible use of this research. Scans of the brain's frontal region taken immediately after a stroke and at progressive intervals from then on could enable physicians to observe functional reorganization activities that contribute to the restoration of speech, for example.

Research related to observing the brain's activity as it relates to memory has dramatic implications for understanding how humans learn, and the memory researchers have expanded their research to an investigation of brain function during learning. One element of learning they have demonstrated is that paying attention to meaning rather than appearance enhances a person's memory of things. Scanning the brains of people assigned to determine either the letter size of written words or the meaning of the words showed that a focus on meaning produced more brain activity and resulted in a better ability to remember the words. Other research using brain scans has shown that repeated practice of a new skill is made more effective when frequent breaks are taken. Further investigations are exploring how to structure learning sessions to optimize the human capacity to learn.

Alzheimer's disease study
A 106-year-old nun, followed up as part of an Alzheimer's disease study that began in 1986, attends ceramics class and exercises daily on a stationary bicycle. Reading and other activities such as crafts may help prevent memory loss.

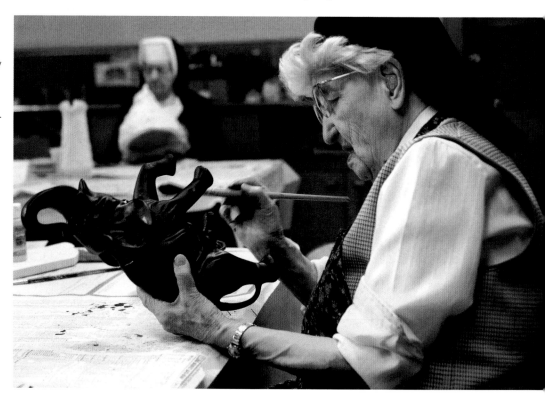

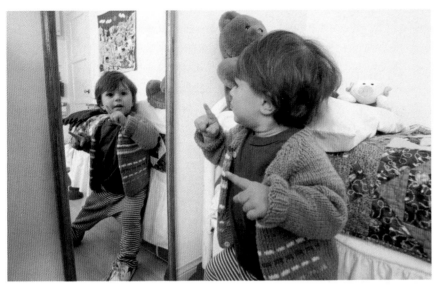

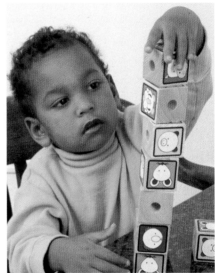

New technologies, and particularly the increased power of brain scanning devices that offer scientists clearer images of the brain's activities, have brought to light new insights about early brain development and its relationship to learning. Brain development establishes the foundation that enables all future learning. Some of this development begins before birth and accelerates immediately after birth. The part of the brain called the cerebral cortex, which controls voluntary actions, thinking, remembering, and feeling, achieves maturation just before a baby's birth.

It is now known that a baby is born with 100 billion brain cells. These cells have not yet created network connections, but will become connected in direct response to the world the baby experiences as the brain matures. For example, since the prenatal brain is programmed to recognize human speech, all babies have the potential to learn language. Yet, a baby who is frequently spoken to can learn approximately 300 more words by the age of 2 years than one who is not often spoken to. The baby's life experiences— what is seen, heard, touched, felt, and understood by the baby—shape the maturation of his or her brain and the baby's ongoing ability to learn.

The networks that are eventually formed by brain cells are essential to thinking and learning. By the age of 3 years, a child's brain has formed about 1,000 trillion connections. This is twice as many connections as adult brains have. It has been discovered that learning ability peaks between the ages of 3 and 10 years. Language, music, and other lifelong skills are most easily learned during this 7-year period. Sometime after the age of 11 years, a child's brain begins to eliminate the unused and unnecessary connections to create a system of networks that is more efficient and more powerful.

The brain's network connections that go

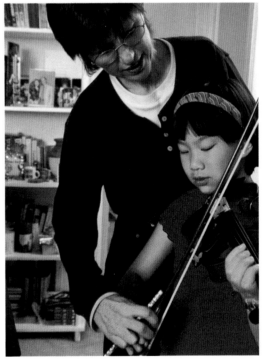

A toddler reflects
By the age of 3 years, children's brains have formed about 1,000 trillion connections, including the ability for toddlers to understand their own reflection in a mirror. A 2-year-old boy begins to learn the motor skills needed to stack and balance blocks. A young girl learns to play the violin. Languages, music, and other lifelong skills are most easily learned between the ages of 3 and 10.

unused do not survive the eventual elimination process, while those that have been used repeatedly during a child's early life are retained. For example, a child who is spoken and read to often during the early years will use the related network connections to quickly master language skills later on. It has been discovered that listening to classical music often during early life stimulates the same neurons in the brain that are used for mathematics and spatial reasoning at a later age.

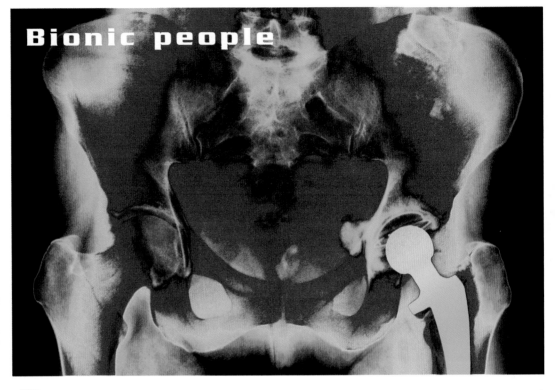

Bionic people

Artificial hip joint
The artificial hip joint can be clearly seen in this X ray of a person with a hip replacement. A prosthetic hip joint is used to replace a diseased hip joint, usually caused by arthritis or by a fracture.

dvances in electronics, DNA discovery, and the newly acquired ability to interpret human genetics have set the stage for amazing advances to be made during the 21st century. A key area is the field of bionics, the meshing of biological science with microelectronic engineering principles, to replace human body parts with what are called cybernetic devices.

Biologists and engineers are combining their knowledge to meld what each specialty group knows about the human gene and the electron. The results could eventually affect almost every aspect of human life. Among the current possibilities are the cloning of human beings, which awaits difficult decisions regarding ethical implications, and the creation of an artificial uterus for women who are unable to achieve pregnancy or do not wish to be pregnant. Other possibilities include the creation of vital organs using a person's own stem cells to replace organs that are diseased or irreparably damaged, including the heart and liver, and bioengineered foods that could resist or counteract serious human health problems, including type 2 diabetes mellitus, cholera, hepatitis B, and high cholesterol levels. There is even a genetic vaccine that could create "buff" body tone in the muscles of a person who does not exercise. These innovations and many more are thought to be inevitable progressions from developments already achieved in research laboratories.

Some engineers believe we are poised to create human machines or robots that will be capable of

human thought, emotion, and consciousness and that the capacity of these machines to instantaneously share knowledge will make them far more advanced intellectually and otherwise than human beings.

While the contemplation of bioengineered robots that are superior in every way to living people is repugnant to some, this technology offers promising implications for creating sophisticated approaches to the treatment of life-threatening genetic diseases and the disabilities of advanced age.

Bionic medicine has already been involved with dramatic improvements in cardiology care. The design of sophisticated prosthetic heart valves has made valve replacement surgery a generally effective treatment with low mortality rates. However, a rare but severe adverse effect caused by infection of the prosthetic material continues to present a challenge to advances in this treatment technique.

Interesting possibilities have been presented by the recent creation of a "cyborg," a mechanical body controlled by the brain of a sea lamprey (a fish that looks like an eel). Light sensors have been positioned in the mechanical robot to feed sensory information to the lamprey's brain. The robot's movements are thus generated in response to the information, or stimuli, received by the lamprey's brain. These stimuli are processed by the lamprey's brain tissue to generate command signals that prompt the robot's motors to move. Although the robot contains only a few of the lamprey's nerve cells, it is able to display complex behaviors in response to simple light stimuli.

This kind of research can help scientists explore the ways brain cells adapt to changing stimuli. The potential for a better understanding of how the brain learns and how memory works could be enhanced by this type of study. It can also offer more information about the possibility of communication between living nerve cells and artificial machines, which could provide a foundation for developing prosthetic limbs and other devices that people who are disabled can control via their own central nervous systems.

Some "cyberneticists" have even predicted that it may eventually be possible to map the entire human brain to a robot, which could involve transplanting the brain of a dying person into a mechanical cyborg. More promising for the immediate future is the possibility of connecting an electronic device, such as a cell phone, directly into the brain.

Joint replacements

Until recently, artificial joints have typically lasted no longer than 15 years. But, the development of prosthetic joints that will last longer and provide the same functions as natural body joints is certain to occur during the 21st century. This is a great boon to people with joint disorders whose limited mobility confines them to wheelchairs and to those who face pain and restricted activity when their joint replacements cease to function. Knee, hip, elbow, shoulder, finger, or any other joint that is damaged by arthritis or other causes can eventually be replaced with a new generation

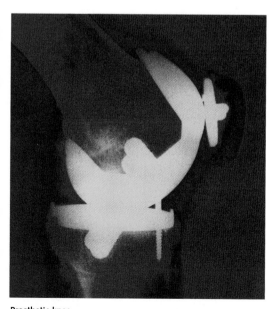

Prosthetic knee
This colored X ray shows an artificial knee joint most likely used for a person whose knee was severely damaged by osteoarthritis or rheumatoid arthritis.

of prosthetics that will last 30 years or more. One area of research is centered on tissue genetics, which is opening up the possibility of improving joint replacement technology by introducing techniques for transplanting the bone and cartilage tissue that make up the joints.

Advances in joint replacement research may also aid those who have chronic back pain. An "intervertebral prosthesis" that replaces disks with metal disk plates combined with a plastic sliding core to cushion spine movement is undergoing clinical trials. One artificial disk device has been under trial at several medical centers throughout the United States and, pending Food and Drug Administration (FDA) approval, could be commercially available by 2004.

Research into possible improvements in joint replacements is aided by the use of digitized, three-dimensional, computerized models that can illustrate the large number and variety of joint movements. Biomechanics and biomaterials laboratories can apply motional axes and loading profiles controlled by specialized software to simulate many different joint movements required by typical human activity. This kind of simulation permits medical researchers to observe and measure, within a mere 7 days, a prosthetic joint's ability to function over a year's time.

Prosthetic limbs

Artificial limbs became more comfortable, stronger, and more mobile during the final decade of the 20th century. Physicians are now able to customize a prosthetic limb to the individual requirements of the person who will be using it. Digitized measurement specifications or an actual cast for an individual prosthetic limb can now be sent to a fabrication center that uses a computer-assisted manufacturing (CAM) system to create a prosthetic model to precise measurements. Computer-assisted design (CAD) systems permit modifications in the dimensions of a device and other manipulations of data on computer screens and provide information that is consistent and storable. Recent advances in the CAD system include the development of handheld tracing pens and scanning digitizers that produce "plaster-free" casts from which prosthetic limbs can be made. Also new are imaging devices that use laser technology and others that are capable of scanning CT (computed tomography) and MRI (magnetic resonance imaging) images and X-ray films directly into a CAD system that can produce exact specifications for a prosthetic limb. The use of digital photo imaging in the design and manufacture of artificial limbs is being developed.

A recent advance in the development of prosthetic feet incorporates a device that uses stored energy. The device functions as a springlike mechanism to propel the user forward. An improved shock-absorption component and ultralightweight materials have enhanced comfort and extended wearability.

Aiming high
A teen with an artificial leg dunks the basketball as he leaps high into the air. A physical therapist teaches a boy with an artificial arm how to master his grip on a trapeze.

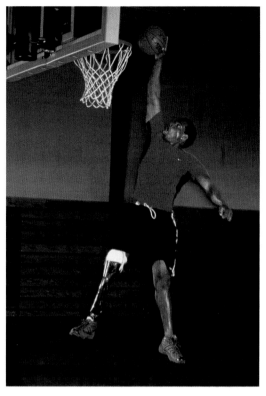

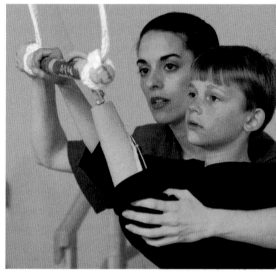

Newly emerging technology in the production of artificial knees has made dramatic improvements in these prosthetics. One advance in this area has resulted in lighter weight prosthetics that provide a shock-absorbing movement to improve the person's comfort and promote a more natural gait. And, a revolutionary upgrade has produced a knee device that is controlled by a microprocessor preprogrammed to precisely match an individual user's natural gait speed in order to adjust the swing speed of the leg. These microprocessors can be driven by pneumatic or hydraulic cylinders. The hydraulic cylinder–driven microprocessor's sensors can interpret changes in movements and weight transfer at the rate of about 50 times per second and then adjust the user's gait speed and improve leg position control so that inclines, steps, and rough terrain may no longer impede walking. Development of a hybrid device that will combine hydraulic stance control with a pneumatic drive for the user's gait is also underway.

While research into microprocessor technology that could be applied to upper limb prostheses is still underway, advances in this area involve the use of myoelectric power, which uses electromagnetic signals from the muscles in the persons' limbs to generate mobility and force in the artificial hand, wrist, or elbow. This technology is based on a phenomenon known as "phantom touch," the perception of sensations and the experience of a sense of control over an absent limb.

Scientists have fashioned prosthetic hands that respond to controls given by the user by developing a silicone sleeve equipped with pressure sensors that fits over the person's forearm. A hard plastic socket on top of the sleeve anchors a mechanical prosthetic hand, which is fitted with electromagnets. Movement in a tendon causes the sensors in the sleeve to transmit a puff of air to a transducer that senses the pressure and transmits an electric signal to the magnets in the artificial hand, triggering movement of the fingers.

This technology has led to such advances as the placement of a sensor in the thumb of a prosthetic hand, which has permitted the person to detect changes in the weight of an object being held, such as a glass being filled with liquid, and can prompt an adjustment in the artificial hand's grip. A new system that combines myoelectric power in the hand with a battery source in the elbow is being developed to permit the elbow and hand to move simultaneously.

The more natural movement provided by these innovations has been enhanced by advancements in a more lifelike appearance of cosmetic coverings for these limbs. Silicone materials can be used to create extremely natural-looking prosthetic "skins," which can be precisely matched to the person's skin color and texture. Because these materials are costly, heavy, and need replacement within a few years, alternatives that are lighter weight and offer more flexibility and longer wear are being sought.

Other relevant emerging research includes the possible use of dental implant technology for the attachment of prosthetic limbs to existing skeletal structures. Just as artificial teeth can be implanted in the jawbone, it is hoped that upper and lower limb prostheses made of titanium could be attached to bone tissue. Clinical trials with the technique have demonstrated superior control over the limb and enhanced sensation perception.

Implantable nerve stimulators

Implantable peripheral nerve stimulators that improve life for people paralyzed by stroke or spinal cord injuries have undergone dramatic improvements in recent years because of new computer chip technology. One version of these devices has helped relieve the severe pain caused by an injured nerve by replacing it with a tingling sensation. People with the device can activate the electrodes required for pain relief and adjust levels to suit their needs.

Nerve stimulators have also been implanted in people who have epilepsy to help them control seizures with little or no need for medication and a reduction in hospitalizations.

FDA-approved versions of implantable nerve stimulators have helped people who are paralyzed by enabling them to move their hands, stand up, and walk short distances with assistance. The devices have also helped restore bowel and bladder control for paraplegics and quadriplegics who have "excitable" muscles available. For people who have been paralyzed by stroke or spinal cord injury, getting back once commonplace abilities is often experienced as nothing short of miraculous.

The device that permits control of the bowel and bladder uses sacral root nerve stimulation to deliver a small current via electrodes, which can be placed around the spinal cord nerve roots in a specialized surgical procedure that permits people to control their functions with a flick of a switch.

An implantable nerve stimulator for the hand stimulates nerve groups so that eight different muscles can be controlled, permitting a person to close the hand and grasp objects. The hand movements are controlled by an external switch worn on the chest that is manipulated by movements of the shoulders.

Still in clinical trials are implantable nerve stimulators that can permit people whose spinal cords have been injured to get up from their wheelchairs and stand. Also being tested are neuroprostheses, which are implanted temporarily under the skin in the forearms of a person who has had a stroke, to retrain the nerves and strengthen muscles. Results offer improved benefits over lengthier sessions of physical therapy. Similar devices may lead to the development of devices that can help improve the gait of people disabled by stroke.

Implanting electrodes in the limbs of people who have had cervical spine injuries (involving the neck vertebrae) has indicated that it may be possible to restore some functional movement to the limbs. In these devices, electricity is used to stimulate the peripheral nerves that are intact in order to transmit signals to the healthy muscles that remain. Development of eight-channel stimulators for the muscles of the lower extremities is in progress with the goal of enabling people with mid-back spinal injuries to stand and take a few steps. Called a mobility system, it has helped a few people stand from their wheelchairs and walk as far as 100 feet.

Researchers believe that nerve regeneration and stem cell studies can produce results that will lead to the re-establishment of neural connections. Combining what is being learned about neural regeneration with the ongoing advances in implantable nerve stimulators offers real hope for people who are paralyzed to regain some functional movement.

Cataract surgery

With advances in equipment, techniques, and anesthesia, the new types of cataract surgery have a near-perfect success rate and are performed as outpatient procedures using eye drops to deliver an anesthetic and surgery that takes 20 minutes and requires no stitches.

The purpose of the surgery is to remove the cloudy cataract that is distorting vision and replace it with a plastic lens implant, called an intraocular lens, or IOL. To do this, the eye surgeon makes a tiny, self-sealing corneal incision using a small diamond blade. Because the incision is so small, the eye heals quickly and eyesight improves.

A new type of implantable lens, called a multifocal lens, can actually correct vision problems including nearsightedness, farsightedness, and astigmatism in people who have had cataract surgery. Most routine activities can be resumed within hours of the surgery.

Ultrasound technology called phacoemulsification, or "phaco" for short, involves the insertion of a probe through the ⅛-inch-long incision made immediately next to the white part of the eye in the clear area covering the iris. An ultrasonic instrument emits sound waves to break up the cataract into minute pieces, which can then be suctioned out through the tip of the probe. The intact portion of the thin membrane that makes up the posterior lens capsule is left in place to support the new implant, and a soft, folded lens is

Seeing clearly after cataract surgery
An ophthalmologist performs cataract microsurgery on a person's eye. The monitor to the left shows the cloudy lens the surgeon is replacing.

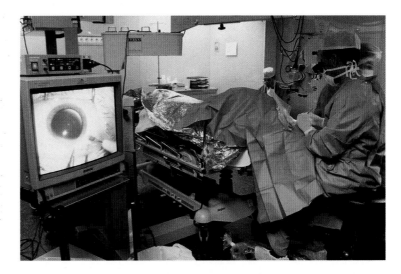

then inserted through the tiny incision. The use of this lens, which provides vision correction, has resulted in many people no longer requiring glasses after cataract surgery.

Stem cell replacement therapy

There is a dazzling array of potential medical applications involving the stem cells that are the source of all the different kinds of cells and tissues that make up the human body. Replacing damaged cells with implanted stem cells holds promise for treating many serious diseases. There is hope that research can lead to using stem cells to generate cells and tissues that could correct damage caused by spinal cord injuries, stroke, Parkinson disease, diabetes mellitus, Alzheimer's disease, arthritis, and various cancers. Stem cell research could lead to using these cells to create new cells that could replace damaged tissues in many of the body's organs, including the brain.

Stem cells have shown remarkable characteristics. They divide into specialized cells to perform specific functions in the body, such as those performed by the heart or the brain. And, at the same time, they replicate themselves, producing exact copies of the original, so that they can remain available to produce the necessary cells when repairs are required throughout the body.

The most common medical use for stem cells is in bone marrow transplants to treat people with certain kinds of cancer, anemia, and some inherited immune disorders. After it was found that certain stem cells, called peripheral blood stem cells, circulate in the blood in addition to being present in the bone marrow, the cells have been collected more routinely from the blood supply rather than from the marrow. Stem cell transplants are considered safer, with decreased possibility of rejection, when a person's own peripheral blood stem cells are used.

Medical uses for stem cells that have already shown promise include the transplantation of corneal stem cells to treat chemical burns to the eye and the transplantation of stem cells to promote cartilage regeneration in certain kinds of damage to the knee. There is the possibility that this technology might be used to replace tissues in the knee that have degenerated because of arthritis.

Bioengineering researchers are investigating the possibility of prompting stem cells to develop into entire organs. One study has discovered how to maintain human embryonic stem cells at their maximum potential to differentiate into any kind of cell in the body. The next step is to understand how to direct the stem cells to form a new kidney or heart that might one day replace a damaged organ.

Laboratory research has shown that certain adult stem cells can differentiate into any one of several different tissues. This sets a new goal of discovering how to direct adult stem cell development so that it favors one type of cell over another. This could lead to the ability to repair damaged tissue in one organ or structure, such as the kidney, with adult stem cells from another site, such as the brain.

If stem cells could be directed in the laboratory to develop into dopamine-producing nerve cells and these cells could be used to replace the neurons that have died in the brains of people who have Parkinson disease, that illness would be

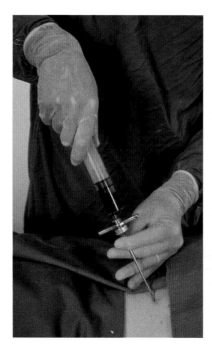
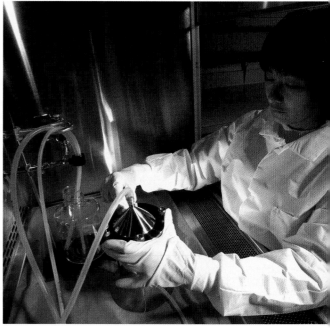

Transplanting cells
A doctor prepares to harvest bone marrow from a healthy person to transplant into a person who has leukemia or aplastic anemia (left). A medical technician isolates insulin cells from a person's pancreas in preparation for transplantation (right).

curable. The challenge has been to find out what is required to transform stem cells into the highly specialized cells, such as neurons in the brain, that need to be replaced. As ongoing research proceeds, stem cells continue to fascinate and confound medical science.

Organ transplants

Medical technology has brought improved success rates to the field of organ transplantation, with heart, liver, kidney, pancreas, lung, and bone marrow transplants becoming much more common surgical procedures. But there is a problem inherent in human-to-human transplants that remains difficult to solve. There are increasing shortages in the supply of donated human organs, and Americans in need of organ transplants continue to die because of the shortage.

But many advancements continue to amaze. An artificial heart has been created out of titanium and a plastic material and developed for use in people whose hearts have irreparably damaged left and right ventricles. This bionic heart is the size of a grapefruit and designed to fully sustain the body's circulatory system so that the person's life can be extended. It is equipped with an internal motor that simulates a natural heartbeat and hydraulically pumps blood through the lungs and throughout the body in response to the physiological needs of the user. The 2-pound device is surgically implanted in the chest and powered by an internal miniaturized electronics package and an external and internal rechargeable lithium battery pack.

Technological innovations in cloning animals have presented scientists with the possibility of finding ways to make organs from animals appropriate for transplantation into humans. The transplantation of animal organs to human beings is referred to as xenotransplantation. Experiments have involved attempts to implant animal hearts, livers, and kidneys into humans. Baboons have often been the animal of choice because of their genetic similarity to humans. However, they also harbor many slow-reproducing viruses that could eventually be lethal to humans.

Pigs have been the most common subjects in cloning experiments because they are easily bred and have humanlike anatomical features. But, pigs have a genetic incompatibility with humans.

Rejection by the human immune system has been an insurmountable barrier to past experiments in xenotransplantation. Nevertheless, pig kidneys have been transplanted into humans on two occasions with some success: in one case, the person survived long enough to receive a human kidney.

The major challenge for biotechnology companies that clone pigs for the express purpose of harvesting organs for human transplants has been to create animals that are missing both copies of the specific gene that prompts organ rejection by the human recipient. Miniature pigs, which are a better size match with humans than full-size pigs,

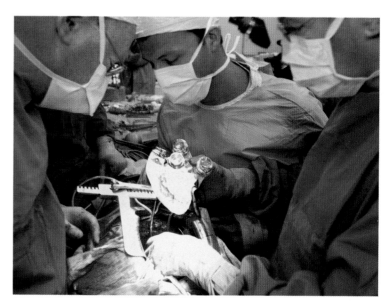

Artificial heart transplant
Surgeons performed the world's first transplant of a battery-powered artificial heart in July 2001.

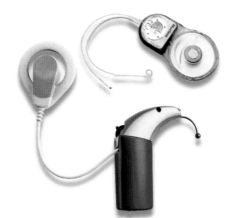

Wonders of hearing
Cochlear implants, shown here with the implant device and the speech processor that is worn outside the ear, are becoming more common as a way to help a person hear.

have been bioengineered to eliminate one copy of the significant gene and have been successfully cloned. This advance set the stage for eliminating the other copy of the gene, but problems remain. One approach under investigation involves genetically altering an animal organ with the human DNA of the recipient to trick the recipient's immune system into recognizing the organ as "human." Animal organs that contain three human genes that will produce human proteins to counter immune rejection have been produced.

Serious concerns persist that organs from pigs could transmit bacteria, viruses, and fungi to humans. These infections may be without symptoms and may be harmless to animals but lethal to people. Many researchers believe, for example, that HIV (human immunodeficiency virus) was introduced into the human population by monkeys. However, this technique can serve as an unlimited supply of transplantable organs.

New surgical techniques

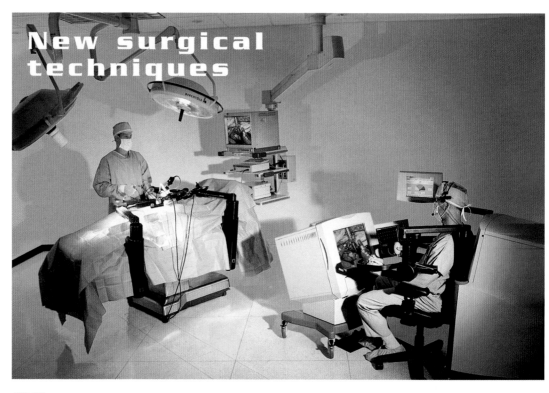

The pluses of robotic surgery
Robotic surgery requires smaller and fewer incisions, often giving the person a faster recuperation rate.

Not the stuff of science fiction anymore, robotic surgery has made its way to the operating room. The Food and Drug Administration (FDA) has to date approved two robotic systems (a form of minimally invasive surgery) to assist surgeons in performing very delicate and complex surgeries to remove gallbladders, prostates, and lung tumors. The robotics systems across the country are part of clinical trials involving cardiac bypass surgery and mitral valve repairs, areas of surgery expected to most benefit from robotic-assisted machines. Some believe FDA approval for robotic brain and spinal cord surgery may not be too far away.

Minimally invasive surgery is not new. For years, doctors have operated with the aid of laparoscopy through tiny holes, for example, in the abdomen to do gallbladder surgery or in the knee to repair torn ligaments. Commonly the surgeon makes several small incisions or ports to manually insert and operate the slim tools, while benefiting from a camera that magnifies the operation on a large video screen.

Many researchers believe robotic surgery will revolutionize traditional heart surgery, in which a long incision is required to enter a patient's chest and a cut in the breastbone is needed to get at the heart. During a coronary bypass, a heart-lung machine takes over the circulation and oxygenation of the blood after surgeons stop the person's heart to perform the procedure. In a minimally invasive procedure, a heart-lung machine is not always used, which leads to far better outcomes. The minimally invasive robotic surgery being tested now requires an incision less than 2 inches long and leaves the breastbone intact, which speeds recovery and lessens postoperative pain. It has long been held that pain, discomfort, and disability following surgery are more frequently due to the trauma involved in gaining access to the body area rather than to the operation itself. Robotic surgery is precise and almost bloodless and inflicts much less trauma to the body, which promotes less risk of infection and shorter hospital stays.

During robotic surgery, the surgeon sits at a console several feet from the patient. One or several small incisions are made, and a tiny camera is inserted into the area to be operated on. The camera uses multiple lenses to provide a three-dimensional (3-D) image from inside the person's body. That image, which magnifies the surgeon's field of vision by 10, making tiny veins and arteries much clearer to see, is displayed in front of the surgeon and on overhead monitors. Surgeons report that the robot helps sharpen their focus to the exact area being operated on and is easier than performing in an operating field cluttered with clamps and other people's hands. The robotic arms hold specially designed surgical instruments that closely mimic the movement of the surgeon's hands as the surgeon operates the robot via a control panel from a computer next to the operating table. The advantage is that a computer program filters out any natural hand tremors that occur occasionally in even the best surgeons. The operation is still totally controlled by the surgeon, who "tells" the robot what to do. The cost of a robotic system is steep, about $1 million, and doctors must be specially trained by the robot's manufacturers, according to FDA rules.

Many believe that in the not too distant future, robotic surgery will involve a surgeon operating on a person remotely, possibly in another hospital, state, or even country. Long-distance robotic surgery may be a way to treat people in remote locations, such as Antarctica, or in states where specialty surgeons are scarce.

Still, there are numerous hurdles to remote surgery, including the lag time that typical long-distance lines hold, which could compromise the patient's outcome when milliseconds count. There are also ethical and legal issues if something goes wrong during the operation and the doctor is not in the room to spring to action. Unexpected complications are not uncommon during surgical procedures because of problems not visible on scans done before surgery or sometimes because of a person's pre-existing condition. Another major drawback to remote surgery is that there has to be a surgical team at the patient's side ready to take over in case of mechanical failure, cardiac arrest, or a severe reaction to the anesthetic.

Image-guided surgery

Computer-based imaging technologies such as CT (computed tomography) and MRI (magnetic resonance imaging) have permitted many diagnostic and therapeutic procedures to be performed in a minimally invasive manner. One of the most fascinating applications of image-guided surgery

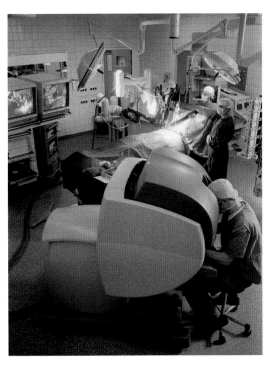

Monitoring the robots
A surgeon peers into a magnified console and manipulates the robotic surgical instruments from a computer console, while the surgical team stands by to monitor the procedure several feet away.

involves the way neurosurgeons approach brain tumors. New digital scanners are able to reconstruct computer-generated images to project the exact location of a tumor that is identified and plotted on a 3-D grid. The computer then can direct the tip of a sensitive instrument, such as a needle or an electrode, to a specific site in the brain. Called stereotactic localization, this innovation has permitted neurosurgeons to precisely biopsy brain tissue or remove tumors through a small opening in the skull instead of through a large incision.

One of the major challenges neurosurgeons faced in the past was how to reach a solid brain mass without cutting through healthy brain tissue. With the stereotactic technique, the surgeon can identify beforehand the least invasive and safest pathway to a deep-seated or centrally located brain tumor. The resulting images can then be used during the procedure to direct the position of the instruments and permit removal of only the abnormal tissue while reducing the risk to healthy surrounding brain tissue. This results in less disability for the person after the operation, less time spent in the intensive care unit, faster overall recovery, shorter hospital stay, and less need for rehabilitative care.

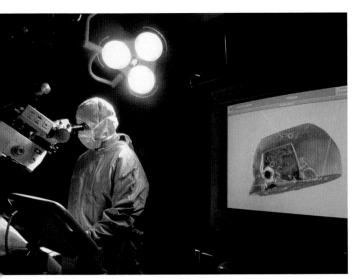

Robotic brain surgery
The image of a brain tumor is magnified on a screen as robotic arms hold surgical instruments that mimic the movement of the neurosurgeon's hands. The surgeon operates the robot from a computer console.

Virtual surgery

Advances in virtual-reality research have spawned a revolutionary new medical tool that has exciting educational and practical applications. Virtual surgery systems that provide highly realistic simulations of surgical procedures have great potential for improving traditional surgical training.

Virtual reality surgical simulators now being developed include a touch component that enables the user to *feel* the limbs, organs, and tissues of a virtual patient in addition to seeing and hearing what is going on during a given procedure. This is possible as a result of new innovations that include force-feedback devices and specialized, real-time computers, which are based on the sense of touch and are equipped with touch-sensitive software.

Virtual surgery can be performed using detachable surgical tools mounted to feedback devices that act as a two-way connection to simulated reality. This system measures the position of the tool being used and applies the corresponding interaction to the user's hand. Real-time three-dimensional images of the surgical tools and the body parts involved are visualized via computer-generated graphic images. A surgery resident can learn standard procedures or new techniques via hands-on experience with a virtual patient. The user can actually use his or her hands to touch, grasp, and manipulate simulated organs.

For the first time, surgical techniques can be practiced without fear of the drastic consequences of error. In fact, surgeons in training can learn from mistakes, and they can repeat procedures until they have mastered the necessary skills. The varying levels of complexity can be adjusted to the doctor's present stage of competence, and the system also offers them objective measures of their ongoing progress as they become more competent.

An application that enables surgeons and medical students to practice suturing with the use of real-time visual and touch-based interaction with

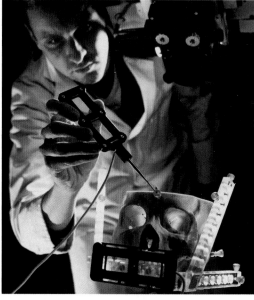

Virtual reality brain surgery
A surgeon uses a handheld pointer to align a virtual reality microscope on a phantom skull. Before the actual surgery, the doctor can see a superimposed image of surrounding brain tissue, find the tumor, and avoid disturbing healthy tissue during surgery.

a photorealistic model is also in development. Models of patient anatomy with a photograph of an actual wound make up the virtual environment for this system. Physical suturing tools attached to a touch-sensitive device can be manipulated as the user looks at virtual counterparts of the same tools on the computer screen.

The software application developed to create these sensations of touching and feeling uses a basic mass-spring model; the skin is approximated to a surface consisting of a network of masses and springs that contours in response to the pressure of the suturing tools on the springs. The degree of contact resistance on the soft tissue surrounding the wound is calculated by the software, which applies commensurate pressure that is experienced by the student via a touch-sensitive device. This resistance pressure is continually adjusted, changing when the suturing needle is inserted into the virtual skin, for example. The software's graphics visualize in real time the changes in the virtual skin's appearance as it is affected by the suturing, providing a highly realistic experience for the trainee.

The challenges in developing these invaluable virtual surgery tools reside principally in fine-tuning the touch-sensation component of the system. Computer graphics are continually improving to create realistic visuals, but the creation of a more realistic tactile experience has lagged behind the advances in imagery. Experienced surgeons report that they rely highly on the sense of touch to identify disease states.

Robotic tools
This close-up of virtual skin shows how a doctor in training can learn to stitch or suture skin by practicing on virtual skin using robotic tools.

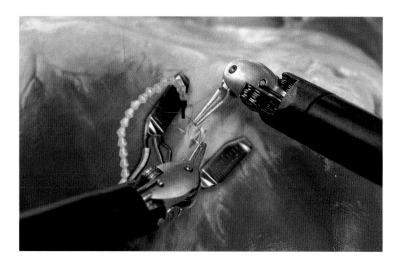

Alphabetical encyclopedia of medicine

Abacavir

An antiviral drug. Abacavir (Ziagen) is used to treat HIV (human immunodeficiency virus) infection, always in combination with another anti-HIV drug. Abacavir works by inhibiting the reproduction of the virus.

Abdomen

The region of the body that lies between the chest (thorax) and the pelvis. The abdomen encloses a cavity that houses organs of the digestive system and urinary tract, and within the bony structure of the pelvis are the organs of the reproductive system (see REPRODUCTIVE SYSTEM, FEMALE; REPRODUCTIVE SYSTEM, MALE). The diaphragm, a sheet of muscle under the ribs, forms the upper boundary of the abdominal cavity. Beneath the diaphragm and to the right lies the liver. To the left lie the stomach, pancreas, and spleen. The small intestine and large intestine are located below the stomach. To the back, behind the digestive organs, are the kidneys, with the bladder and other organs of the urinary tract extending downward. The lining of the abdominal wall is a two-layered membrane, the peritoneum, which encloses, lubricates, and supports the organs within.

Layers of muscle and fat surround the abdomen. In the back and on the sides, the lower ribs and the bones of the spine and hips protect the abdomen; the pelvic bones support and enclose the reproductive organs. In a pregnant woman, the uterus enlarges and extends up into the abdominal cavity.

Abdomen, acute

The medical term for sudden, persistent, and severe ABDOMINAL PAIN. A person with symptoms resembling an

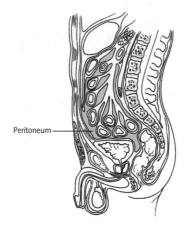

Peritoneum

INFLAMED PERITONEAL MEMBRANE
The most common cause of acute abdomen is inflammation of the peritoneum, the membrane that lines the abdominal cavity. It usually occurs as the result of perforation of the stomach or intestine, which allows bacteria and digestive juices to leak from the digestive tract into the abdominal cavity.

acute abdomen should get an immediate medical evaluation. In addition to conducting a thorough physical examination, the doctor will ask about other general symptoms such as nausea, vomiting, changes in stool, fever, fatigue, and malaise (a general feeling of illness). If the person has a stiff, rigid abdomen, the pain may be caused by PERITONITIS (inflammation of the membrane that lines the abdominal and pelvic walls), which usually requires prompt surgery. Other possible causes of acute abdomen include APPENDICITIS, DIVERTICULAR DISEASE, TUBERCULOSIS, GALLSTONES, and colon cancer (see COLON, CANCER OF THE). Treatment depends on the underlying disorder.

Abdominal pain

FOR SYMPTOM CHART
see Abdominal pain, page 14

Discomfort in the abdominal area or stomach region. Symptoms vary but may include nausea, vomiting, changes in the stool, fever, fatigue, and malaise (a general feeling of illness). Abdominal pain is a symptom that may have a number of different causes. In some cases, it is the result of overeating, eating spicy foods, or alcohol abuse. Abdominal pain may also occur with DIARRHEA or CONSTIPATION. Other times it is due to a more serious underlying problem with a woman's reproductive organs, such as ENDOMETRIOSIS or an ECTOPIC PREGNANCY. Pain from the top center area of a person's abdomen could indicate an ulcer. (See STOMACH ULCER; DUODENAL ULCER; and PEPTIC ULCER DISEASE.) Abdominal pain may indicate a surgical emergency, such as APPENDICITIS. Rarely, pain may have a psychological basis.

Persistent or severe abdominal pain requires prompt medical evaluation. In addition to conducting a thorough physical examination, the doctor will ask questions about other general symptoms. Treatment depends on the diagnosis of the underlying disorder. Immediate treatment must be sought if the abdomen is tender to the touch or rigid and boardlike or if there is vomiting of blood or bloody stools. Abdominal pain that may be a medical emergency and require prompt surgical intervention includes pain accompanied by a stiff, rigid abdomen, which can be a sign of PERI-

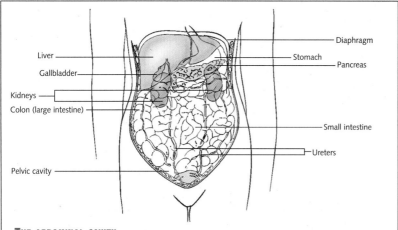

Liver

Gallbladder

Kidneys

Colon (large intestine)

Pelvic cavity

Diaphragm

Stomach

Pancreas

Small intestine

Ureters

THE ABDOMINAL CAVITY
The organs of the digestive, urinary, and reproductive systems are contained in the abdomen. These essential organs are cushioned by layers of muscle and fat and further protected by the bony framework of the ribs, spine, and pelvis.

TONITIS (inflammation of the membrane that lines the abdominal and pelvic walls) or gastrointestinal bleeding of any cause. In addition, pain with nausea and fever may indicate appendicitis or complications of DIVERTICULAR DISEASE, and pain that is accompanied by nausea, fever, and bloating or constipation may indicate a bowel obstruction.

Abdominoplasty

See TUMMY TUCK.

Abduction

Movement of a limb away from the middle of the body. Also, the illegal carrying away of a person by force; a form of kidnapping. Abduction usually involves interfering with a relationship, as in enticing or taking a child away from his or her parent or caregiver.

Ablation

The removal of a growth or harmful tissue. Ablation may refer to the surgical removal of tissue from any part of the body. There are many different ways to ablate tissue including EXCISION (cutting), CURETTAGE (scraping), electrodesiccation (burning with an electric current delivered through a probe), MOHS SURGERY (microscopically controlled surgery removing one layer of skin at a time), CRYOSURGERY (freezing with liquid nitrogen), and LASER SURGERY.

Ablation therapy

A procedure in which a catheter (thin tube) is used to control certain types of abnormally fast, uncoordinated heartbeats, or arrhythmias, by destroying the small areas of tissue causing the abnormality. Destruction of the tissue causing the heart to beat quickly and uncontrollably can prevent arrhythmias from developing and allows the heart to return to a slower, more normal rhythm.

Before the ablation is performed, the area of abnormality is identified by a test known as an electrophysiology study. A catheter is placed in a blood vessel and threaded through the circulatory system to the heart. The electrical activity of the heart is then recorded to identify the precise area of abnormality.

Most ablations are now performed using a catheter in a technique known as radiofrequency ablation. In this procedure, the catheter is inserted through a blood vessel, usually in the groin or thigh but at times in the wrist or mid arm, after the insertion site is numbed with local anesthetic and the person is lightly sedated. The catheter is then threaded through the blood vessels into the heart until it reaches the area of abnormality. Radiofrequency energy emitted from the tip of the catheter heats and destroys the focus of tissue that is causing the fast heartbeat. The catheter is subsequently withdrawn and the insertion site closed. In most cases, the person undergoing the ablation can go home within 24 hours. Complications from radiofrequency ablation are rare, and the success rate in restoring a normal heartbeat is high.

Ablation is occasionally performed surgically. Working through an incision in the chest, the surgeon makes small cuts in the heart to channel its electrical activity, destroys the abnormal tissue by applying cold, or removes a portion of one layer of the heart. Surgical ablation is performed under general anesthesia and requires a longer recovery period than radiofrequency ablation. It may occasionally be performed as a part of another heart surgery, such as valve replacement. See HEART VALVE SURGERY.

Abortion, elective

The voluntary termination of a pregnancy. The 1973 Roe versus Wade decision by the US Supreme Court ruled that American women have a constitutional right to have abortions, legalizing abortion in all 50 states. States may regulate abortions performed after 12 weeks of pregnancy. Some states have passed laws requiring a 24-hour waiting period before an abortion can be performed. Minors must obtain parental consent or approval by a court before an abortion can be performed in some states.

The earlier in pregnancy an abortion is performed, the safer the procedure is for a woman, and the less likely that complications will occur. Most abortions are performed during the first 12 weeks of pregnancy. Sometimes, an abortion is done after 12 weeks because of a maternal illness, or if the fetus dies or has a serious abnormality.

Before an abortion, a doctor will confirm the pregnancy and estimate the gestational age. This is important in determining the appropriate abortion procedure. A pelvic examination is performed to detect possible infection or structural abnormalities. In some situations, an ultrasound examination may be done to pinpoint the age of the fetus (see ULTRASOUND, OBSTETRICAL). The woman is tested to find out her blood type; women with Rh-negative blood are given Rh immunoglobulin as a safeguard to keep them from reacting against possible Rh-positive fetal blood in future pregnancies. Tests for SEXUALLY TRANSMITTED DISEASES may also be done prior to an abortion to facilitate treatment and avoid infectious complications.

ABORTION METHODS

The choice of procedure is usually determined by the stage of the pregnancy. The most common methods of abortion are medical abortion, suction CURETTAGE, D AND E (dilation and evacuation), and labor-induced abortion. Medical abortions utilize drugs to induce the abortion and require a visit to a doctor. Suction curettage and dilation and evacuation procedures can be safely performed in a doctor's office or clinic. Labor-induced abortions are usually performed in hospitals or specialty clinics.

■ *Medical abortion* Two different combinations of drugs can be used to end a pregnancy within the first 6 to 8 weeks of pregnancy. After the medications are given, the embryo dies and is shed later through the vagina. In the methotrexate-misoprostol method, which is available at clinics and doctors' offices, a doctor injects the woman with methotrexate. Several days later, the woman inserts tablets of misoprostol into her vagina. The pregnancy ends within about 2 days, although it can take 3 or more weeks. In the mifepristone-misoprostol method, which is not available everywhere, a doctor gives a woman an oral dose of mifepristone (also known as RU 486). In a few days, she inserts misoprostol tablets into her vagina. The pregnancy ends at home within 4 hours. From 1 to 12 percent of medical abortions fail and require a surgical procedure to end the pregnancy.

■ *Suction curettage* Also called vacuum curettage or vacuum aspiration, it is the most common abortion procedure during the first 12 weeks of pregnancy. For a suction curettage, a doctor performs a pelvic examination to determine the size and position of the patient's uterus and opens the vagina with the use of a speculum. A local anesthetic may be injected into the cervix to numb it. The doctor then dilates (opens) the cervix, by inserting progressively larger wedge-shaped devices called dilators. A woman may feel some slight pressure or cramping as her cervix is dilated. Then, a suction tube is inserted into the uterus. The tube, which is connected to a vacuum pump, is moved around inside the uterus to loosen and empty its contents. A curet, a spoon-shaped instrument, scoops out any remaining tissue. This procedure usually takes 10 to 15 minutes. Afterward, some cramping, nausea, and vaginal bleeding may occur.

■ *Dilation and evacuation* This method most often is performed between weeks 13 and 16 of a pregnancy. The doctor may dilate the cervix with dilators at the start of the procedure or insert thin rods called laminaria into the cervix to dilate it. Laminaria, made from a type of seaweed, absorb moisture and swell over a period of hours, causing the cervix to widen. A woman may be given intravenous fluids, pain medication, or a sedative. A vacuum pump is inserted into the uterus to remove the contents. The walls of the uterus are then scraped to ensure that no tissue remains inside the uterus. A woman may be given a drug called OXYTOCIN to stimulate the uterus to contract. After the procedure, some cramping and vaginal bleeding may occur.

■ *Labor-induced abortion* When a pregnancy has progressed beyond week 16, a doctor can induce contractions to abort the fetus. To initiate LABOR, a woman is given a drug or combination of drugs that will cause her uterus to contract as needed. PROSTAGLANDINS are the most widely used drugs for this procedure; less often, the hormone oxytocin, saline, or UREA may be used. Delivery usually occurs within 24 hours after receiving labor-inducing drugs, which can produce such side effects as fever, nausea, vomiting, and diarrhea.

RECOVERY

Immediately after an abortion, a woman's blood pressure and pulse are monitored, and she is examined for signs of excessive bleeding. The recovery period usually lasts a few hours for an early-term abortion and may extend to an overnight stay in a hospital for a late-term abortion. After any abortion procedure, patients typically experience mild cramping and bleeding that will resemble a normal period. A mild painkiller, such as ibuprofen or acetaminophen, can be taken to relieve any discomfort. Severe complications are rare.

After an abortion, symptoms of pregnancy, such as morning sickness and enlargement of the breasts, should end within a few days. Normal menstruation resumes within 4 to 6 weeks. A follow-up appointment with a doctor is important to ensure that a woman is healing properly and to make certain that no infection is present. A woman should refrain from sexual intercourse for 2 to 3 weeks because pregnancy is possible immediately following an abortion. Before resuming intercourse, a woman should choose a reliable form of birth control to prevent future unplanned pregnancies. Generally, short-term complications from abortion are rare but may include perforations or infection. Long-term concerns include psychological effects and possible uterine scarring, which can lead to infertility. Most abortion centers offer postabortion counseling.

Abortion, missed

Retention of a fetus that has died in the uterus. A missed abortion may have no signs or may be characterized by the absence of a fetal heartbeat, or a uterus that is hard, not growing, or decreasing in size. If a fetal heartbeat is not detected, a fetal electrocardiogram (ECG) and ultrasound are performed to confirm whether the fetus has died. Once a diagnosis is made, the woman and her physician will decide whether to wait and see if a spontaneous abortion (see ABORTION, SPONTANEOUS) will occur or whether to induce labor (see INDUCTION OF LABOR) or perform a dilation and evacuation (D AND E) procedure.

Causes of fetal death can include chromosome abnormalities, inade-

quate oxygen supply to the fetus, RH INCOMPATIBILITY (a reaction of the mother's blood to the fetus' blood), severe infections, and uncontrolled diabetes or high blood pressure in the woman. Sometimes, the cause of death of the fetus is unknown, and maternal blood tests or pathological or genetic studies may be performed to help identify the cause of death.

Abortion, spontaneous

The expulsion of a fetus by the mother's body after the fetus has died in the uterus. Also called a MISCARRIAGE.

Abortion, threatened

Any bleeding during the first half of a pregnancy, before the cervix is dilated (open). Because one in four women may have some spotting or slight bleeding, a threatened abortion is a common diagnosis. With rest, symptoms usually subside, and the pregnancy progresses normally. However, a threatened abortion may proceed to an actual MISCARRIAGE. If vaginal bleeding is accompanied by lower back pain or cramping abdominal pain, a miscarriage is more likely. Even without pain, bleeding can be a sign of a miscarriage or serious complication. A woman who is pregnant should immediately notify her doctor if she has vaginal bleeding or light spotting. A doctor may recommend a fetal ultrasound (see ULTRASOUND, OBSTETRICAL), alone or in conjunction with a hormone level test, to rule out complications and assess the viability of the fetus. When a threatened abortion is diagnosed, a woman may be asked to decrease her level of activity or rest in bed until the bleeding stops.

The symptoms and the stage of the pregnancy offer clues as to the cause of the bleeding. Early in pregnancy, bleeding or light spotting may occur when a fertilized egg implants in the uterus or at the time a woman's period would have been due. However, bleeding in early pregnancy can also be due to an ECTOPIC PREGNANCY, a serious condition in which a pregnancy has developed outside the uterus. Bleeding can also result from an abnormality of the cervix or an inflammation of the vagina. Bleeding late in pregnancy can be a sign of a serious complication, such as a disorder of the placenta, or it may simply signal the beginning of labor.

Abrasion

The scraping or rubbing away of a surface. Abrasions may occur to the skin, teeth, or cornea of the eye. They are often the result of superficial trauma or injury, as in skinned knees or elbows. A surgical form of abrasion is DERMABRASION (removal of the surface layer of skin by high-speed sanding), which results in oozing and crusting of the skin, followed by growth of new skin cells. Over time, most abrasions heal on their own without treatment.

Abreaction

A term describing a controversial process by which repressed emotions, particularly a painful experience or conflict, are brought back to the person's consciousness or awareness. In the process, the person not only recalls, but also relives the material, which is accompanied by the appropriate emotional response. Abreaction may be incorporated into psychotherapy to release blocked feelings surrounding a painful event, such as an instance of sexual abuse. Concerns have been raised about whether the memories are factual or the person was highly suggestible.

Abscess

A collection of pus that accumulates in a body part, usually due to a bacterial infection; the abscess is often accompanied by pain, swelling, and redness. Pus forms from the accumulation of dead tissue, bacteria, and white blood cells, which enter the infected tissue through the walls of the blood vessels to attack the infection. Superficial abscesses (boils) form under the skin, often around a hair follicle in a moist part of the body, such as the groin or armpit. Abscesses can also occur in deeper tissues, such as around a tooth, tonsil, near the vagina or rectum, and in the appendix, breast, kidney, liver, lungs, brain, and bones. Internal abscesses are often accompanied by fever and fatigue. Abscesses are more common in people with diabetes or in people with weakened immune systems. Abscesses are usually caused by bacteria or intestinal parasites.

Superficial abscesses are treated by applying warm, moist compresses, which encourage the infection to break through the skin, relieving the pressure. After the abscess breaks, a dry bandage should be applied. Antibiotics may also be prescribed. If fever develops or the abscess worsens, a doctor may need to drain it. The doctor will open the abscess with a small surgical knife (scalpel), removing as much pus as possible, packing the space left by the abscess with gauze, and covering the site with a dry bandage. The gauze packing is removed after 48 hours, and the skin incision is left open to heal. Superficial abscesses can usually be drained with the use of a local anesthetic in the office of a physician, but deeper abscesses may require surgery and a hospital stay of 1 or 2 days.

Abscess, spinal

Also known as a spinal cord abscess or epidural abscess, a rare but potentially life-threatening disorder characterized by inflammation and an accumulation of infected pus adjacent to the spinal cord. Spinal abscesses are most often caused by a bacterial infection within the spine. They can also occur as a complication of a spinal tap, back surgery, or skin infections that travel into the spine. In developing countries, abscesses are sometimes caused by tuberculosis.

The symptoms of a spinal abscess include backache, fever, chills, loss of movement or sensation, weakness, numbness, and loss of bladder or bowel control. The backache progressively worsens, with pain radiating to other parts of the body. The extent of symptoms corresponds to the location and size of the abscess on the spine. Sometimes only the lower body is involved (as in paraplegia). In other cases, the trunk, arms, and legs are all affected (quadriplegia).

A spinal abscess is diagnosed through physical examination, blood tests, and CT (computed tomography) scanning or MRI (magnetic resonance imaging). The goals of treatment are to relieve the pressure on the spine and cure the infection. An immediate laminectomy (surgical removal of part of a vertebra) is required to relieve compression. Once a laboratory culture identifies the specific

organism responsible for the infection, appropriate antibiotics are prescribed. Prompt diagnosis and treatment are essential. Left untreated, a spinal abscess progresses to spinal cord compression, which can result in permanent paralysis or death.

Absence seizure

Also known as petit mal, a type of seizure characterized by brief episodes of loss of awareness. (See SEIZURE.) Persons having an absence seizure are described as staring or daydreaming. These seizures commonly occur during childhood and often diminish and disappear during adolescence. However, people with absence seizures often develop major motor or grand mal seizures during adolescence or young adulthood. Absence seizures are diagnosed by a characteristic electroencephalogram (EEG) pattern. Some children experience frequent brief seizures throughout the day that impair the ability to concentrate and learn. These seizures respond well to treatment with medications, allowing a return to full participation in school and social activities.

Absorption

The passage of substances across tissues. In intestinal absorption, digested food molecules pass into intestinal cells. In digestion, nutrients are broken down in preparation for absorption. As a series of muscle contractions (peristalsis) moves food through the digestive tract, enzymes and acids secreted by digestive organs break it down into molecules small enough for the body to absorb and use. Absorbed nutrients are subsequently distributed to the organs and cells of the body.

Few nutrients are absorbed directly from the stomach into the bloodstream. Alcohol is one of the few substances that pass from the stomach into the blood. Absorption of most nutrients takes place in the jejunum (the second part of the small intestine) through tiny fingerlike projections called villi.

Fat, carbohydrate, and protein absorption mainly occurs there. Fat globules pass through the villi and into large lymphatic channels, which empty into the bloodstream. Intestinal enzymes break down carbo-

A

hydrates and complex sugars into simple sugars that are absorbed through the wall of the jejunum directly into the bloodstream. Not all carbohydrates can be digested, and some individuals lack the enzymes needed to digest a common sugar such as lactose. Proteins are broken down into amino acids that are absorbed in the jejunum and pass directly into the bloodstream. Fat-soluble vitamins A, D, E, and K and water-soluble vitamins B and C are also absorbed in the jejunum, while the absorption of vitamin B12 takes place in the ileum (the third part of the small intestine). Minerals, especially calcium and iron, are largely absorbed in the duodenum, the site closest to the stomach where the contents are most acidic. Sodium is absorbed throughout the length of the small intestine. Sodium and calcium, with large volumes of fluid, are also absorbed in the large intestine (colon).

Abstinence

The act of refraining from something. Abstinence is a form of deliberate self-denial, such as the avoidance of pleasure obtained from consuming favorite foods or alcoholic beverages or engaging in sexual relations.

Abuse, child

The physical, emotional, or sexual mistreatment or neglect of a child. National studies show that one in 20 American children are physically abused each year. The physical and psychological effects of abuse can be extensive and severe. Abuse can impair brain development and intellect, delay development of skills such as walking and speaking, and cause physical disabilities and other long-term health problems. The psychological damages of abuse outlast the actual episodes of mistreatment. Some abused children develop post-traumatic stress disorder, leading to symptoms such as nightmares and irritability. Low self-esteem and unstable emotions can be the lifelong legacy of abuse. Adults who were abused as children are more likely to need help for depression, anxiety, substance abuse, and eating disorders. They are also more apt to exhibit aggressive behavior and to become abusers themselves.

TYPES OF CHILD ABUSE

As dependent members of society, children are especially vulnerable. Any action taken by an adult that impedes a child's normal healthful development constitutes abuse. Injury to the child can result from physical assault, mental cruelty, and deprivation.

■ *Physical abuse* This type of abuse concerns committing violence against a child. Burns, bruises, broken bones, and other physical injuries are included. Abuse is a leading cause of serious head injury in babies. (See also SHAKEN BABY SYNDROME.) Among the most frequent types of child abuse injuries are burns. Cigarette burns and scalding, in which part of a child's body has been immersed in overly hot water, are common types of burns. Immersion burns leave a characteristic water level mark. Often physical abuse by a caregiver follows his or her unsuccessful attempts to calm a colicky baby or discipline an unruly child. In frustration, the caretaker mistakenly uses inappropriate and unnecessary force. Teaching caretakers how to prevent their anger from turning into physical violence may decrease the frequency of child abuse.

■ *Emotional abuse* Constant bombardment of a child with negative words or behavior can leave deep emotional scars. Criticizing, blaming, isolating, rejecting, and terrorizing a child all are examples of emotional abuse. Withdrawing affection or exposing a child to a violent or sexually inappropriate environment also constitutes emotional abuse. Low self-esteem and feelings of worthlessness that often last well into adulthood typify the outcomes of such abuse. Although emotional abuse can be as harmful as physical abuse, it is much harder to detect. Emotionally deprived or abused children are often withdrawn and listless, and developmentally they may lag behind other children the same age.

■ *Sexual abuse* The involvement of children and adolescents in sexual activities that they do not fully comprehend or for which they are unable to give informed consent is abuse. Activities that violate the social taboos of proper family roles are included. The least reported and most underdiagnosed type of abuse, sexual abuse, may include vaginal,

oral, or anal intercourse; inappropriate touching of a child's breasts or genitalia; an adult exposing his or her genitalia to a child; and involving a child in any activity that gives the abuser sexual gratification. Most sexual abusers are male. Commonly, a family member or close family friend is the sexual abuser.

■ *Neglect* Negligence in caring for a child can take several forms. Physical neglect means depriving a child of basic needs such as food, shelter, and clothing. Emotional neglect includes failing to provide love, support, supervision, and approval necessary for healthy development. Medical neglect consists of withholding necessary medical care. Educational neglect means causing the child to be chronically absent from school. For example, a child may be forced to stay home from school to baby-sit smaller children. Neglected children are often physically smaller than their peers and may lack the nurturing necessary to develop normally.

WARNING SIGNS

Physical symptoms of abuse may include unexplained burns, bruises, or broken bones. In infants and children, abuse or neglect is often shown by a FAILURE TO THRIVE, a condition in which the child does not grow at the expected rate for his or her age and sex. Emotionally abused children can appear unhappy and withdrawn. A child who has been sexually abused may have recurrent infections and be overly explicit in play or conversation. There is reason to suspect abuse if the explanation a parent or caregiver gives for an injury seems inconsistent with the injury or if different caregivers' accounts contradict each other. An inappropriate parental reaction to an injury—either overly concerned or not concerned enough—may be a sign that a child has been abused. Sometimes the child and abuser alike try to hide the abuse. Especially in sexual abuse, children are often confused and ashamed. They may blame themselves, rather than the abuser, and try to conceal the fact that they have been mistreated. Sometimes, children are threatened, intimidated, or bribed into silence by their abusers. They may fear that no one will believe them or not want to get a close family member into trouble. Parents, too, can be in denial or not aware of the symptoms of abuse.

To intervene in child abuse it is important to know how to recognize its less obvious signs. Certain physical and emotional factors may indicate an abusive situation. Unexplained injuries are physical signs of abuse. Puzzling injuries include those on parts of the body that usually do not get injured (the stomach, buttocks, back, face, or backs of hands) and those that were made with an object (cigarette, belt, electric cord, iron, or hand) that leaves a recognizable mark. Sexual abuse may cause physical discharges, sores, injuries in the genital area, and recurrent urinary tract infections.

Psychosocial problems can be emotional indicators of abuse. A child who fears parents or other adults or one who is reluctant to talk about home life or to invite friends over may have been abused. Also a child who shows regressive behavior, such as bed-wetting and soiling, clinging, or thumb-sucking, or one who exhibits inappropriate sexual explicitness may have been abused. Abuse may trigger extreme passivity or aggressiveness or sudden, unexplained changes in behavior. Self-destructive behavior, such as substance abuse, multiple sexual encounters, suicide attempts, crime, running away from home, or poor academic performance, can indicate a problem. Depression, chronic sadness, frequent crying, low self-esteem, feelings of worthlessness, recurrent nightmares, and neglected appearance are also possible signs.

DIAGNOSIS AND TREATMENT

A child who has been abused needs treatment and protection as soon as possible. Early detection and treatment increase the likelihood of a full recovery. Whenever a child may be at risk, it is important to inform a doctor, social services agency, or police department. Parents who suspect their children have been abused should seek help immediately. Seeing the pediatrician or family physician is the first step. Treatment will depend on the type of abuse. The doctor can evaluate the child's condition and treat any physical problems. He or she may also refer the child to a child psychiatrist, child psychologist, clinical social worker, or rape victim advocate. Most abused children benefit from psychological counseling, especially those who have been abused by a parent or other close relative.

Doctors are required by law to report every suspected case of abuse to legal authorities, such as the state child protection agency. Once a case is reported, the agency must investigate it. For his or her own safety, a child is sometimes removed from the home while an investigation takes place. Hospital admission may be required to allow the opportunity for an in-depth medical and social evaluation. Troubled families are then given professional support and guidance. When possible, families are kept together.

RISK FACTORS AND PREVENTION

Abuse can occur in a family of any socioeconomic background, race, ethnicity, or religion. At the greatest risk are children under age 5 and those who require special care and attention. These include premature infants (see PREMATURE BIRTH); babies who cry and fuss a lot (see COLIC); and children who have chronic diseases or disorders, physical or mental disabilities, or behavior problems.

Abusers usually are the child's caregivers: parents and close relatives, stepparents or foster parents, parents' friends, or baby-sitters. Many adults who are abusers were abused when they were children. A violent environment increases the risk of abuse. Abuse occurs in families of all backgrounds but is more common in families that live in poverty. Other risk factors include substance abuse, marital problems, the lack of a strong home support system, limited education, caregiver's youth, unplanned parenthood (singles or couples), and physical or mental illness in the family. Anything that undermines a caregiver's self-control—such as ALCOHOL DEPENDENCE or DRUG ADDICTION—increases the risk of abuse. Parents or other caregivers who are under stress are more apt to engage in impulsive or aggressive behavior. Caregivers who practice techniques to prevent their anger from turning into violence when under stress may be less likely to abuse.

Parents who fear harming their own child should seek help immediately from a doctor, therapist, friend, or member of the clergy. Adults who were abused themselves as children may benefit from counseling. To prevent abuse outside the home, parents should thoroughly investigate the references of childcare facilities. Conversations with other parents are helpful in this regard, as are unannounced visits. When they are old enough to understand (about age 3), children should be taught that it is unacceptable for anyone other than a physician to touch private parts of their bodies.

Abuse, emotional

The intentional use of psychological force to hurt or destroy another person. Emotional abuse can occur between spouses and other sexual partners, between adult children and older parents, or, most commonly, between parents and children. Emotional abuse takes a number of forms, including withholding affection; using threats or terror to control the other; coercive or erratic discipline; scapegoating and rejection; failure to meet such basic physical needs as food, water, and sleep; and failure to provide love, affection, warmth, and security. Emotional abuse can occur alone or along with physical or sexual abuse (see ABUSE, SEXUAL).

Emotional abuse can have severe psychological consequences, particularly for children. Abused children may harbor an unwarranted deep inner feeling that they themselves are to blame for the abusive situation, which continues even though the child consistently attempts to behave well enough to stop the abuse. Eating and digestive disorders, sleep disturbances, compulsive attention seeking, feelings of anxiety and despair, self-mutilation, and suicide attempts are overrepresented in abuse victims, although whether a cause-and-effect relationship exists is controversial. These effects may last into adulthood. It is widely thought that abuse in childhood is one of the main factors leading adults to seek psychiatric help.

Unrealistic expectations of the child are one factor in the cause of emotional abuse by parents, with the venting of frustrations about outside events on the child and ignorance about other ways of parenting. Most abusive parents were abused themselves as children, but there may also be genetic factors, such as temperament traits.

Emotional abuse of children is treated by counseling that helps parents understand their behavior and teaches them alternative ways of dealing with their children. Counseling that addresses the psychological effects of abuse is also needed for children in abusive family settings.

Abuse, of older people

Neglect or physical, psychological, or financial mistreatment of an older person. An estimated one in four older people in the United States is subjected to some form of abuse or neglect. All 50 states have passed legislation to protect older people against abuse. Abuse can occur in the home, a caregiver's home, or a long-term care facility such as a nursing home. A nearly equal number of males and females are abusers. Two-thirds are family members, most often an adult child of the abused person. Close to 70 percent of abused elders are women. The older or more disabled a person is, the more likely a caretaker will abuse her or him. The demands of caring for an infirm person, especially a person with severe mental or physical impairment, can produce stress; stress and frustration sometimes get expressed as violence. For example, incontinence in an older person is a common trigger for abuse. Inadequately trained caretakers and a lack of economic resources are also known contributing factors. In some families, a cycle of violence leads to abuse. People raised in a violent atmosphere may resort to violence in response to stress or conflict (see CAREGIVING FOR OLDER PEOPLE; STRESS).

TYPES OF ABUSE

Physical abuse is the use of physical force that inflicts pain or injury. It can involve slapping, bruising, beating, pushing, shoving, shaking, kicking, pinching, and burning. Intimidation and threatening to inflict physical pain or injury also constitute physi-

cal abuse. Less obvious forms of physical abuse are the inappropriate use of drugs or restraints, force-feeding, physical punishment of any kind, and sexual molestation, which includes all forms of unwanted touching. Sexual contact with a person incapable of giving consent is abuse. Unexplained bruises or fractures, broken eyeglasses, and sudden changes in behavior can be signs of physical abuse.

Psychological abuse is the infliction of anguish, pain, and distress. Also called emotional abuse, it consists of both verbal and nonverbal acts. Verbal abuse may include humiliation, intimidation, threats, and insults. Isolating an older person from family, friends, and normal activities or treating an older person as though he or she were an infant are also abuses.

Financial abuse, while not strictly health-related, refers to preying upon and taking advantage of an older person's vulnerable mental or physical state for financial gain. Financial abuse consists of the illegal or improper use of an older person's assets or property. Examples include forging older people's signatures or cashing their checks without their consent. Deceiving an older person into signing a document, such as a will, is abuse, as is the improper use of a power of attorney or guardianship. Sudden changes in bank accounts and wills may be a sign of financial abuse.

Neglect consists of a caregiver's failure to provide an older person with necessities such as food, shelter, medicine, personal hygiene, and comfort. Weight loss, unkempt appearance, malnutrition, dehydration, untreated health problems, and poor living conditions can be signs of neglect. Abandonment, the most extreme form of neglect, is the desertion of an older person by the person responsible for his or her care. Temporarily leaving a person alone who is unable to care for himself or herself is also neglect. Self-neglect refers to the inability of people living on their own to provide themselves with essential needs, such as food, water, or shelter.

IDENTIFICATION AND INTERVENTION

The appearance of physical injuries,

such as bruises, welts, lacerations, unhealed open wounds, broken bones, or burns, must be investigated. A caretaker's refusal to let visitors see an older person alone may signal an abusive situation. Psychological abuse and neglect are the most difficult to detect because they do not leave obvious signs, and abused older people can be fearful and reluctant to speak up for themselves. Symptoms of psychological abuse may include agitation, withdrawal, and lack of responsiveness. Unusual behavior, such as rocking or biting, or the older person's own reports of mistreatment, are strong indicators of abuse. Dehydration, malnutrition, and lack of personal hygiene are common symptoms of neglect.

Treatment depends on the type of abuse. A doctor will evaluate an older person's condition, treat any physical problems, and report suspected abuse to a local agency. Depending on the nature of the abuse and individual state laws, elder abuse may or may not be considered a crime. In most states, instances of elder abuse should be reported to the adult protective services agency. Every state's attorney general's office is mandated by federal law to establish a Medicare fraud control unit to investigate fraud and patient abuse or neglect in health care programs that participate in Medicare.

RISK FACTORS AND PREVENTION

At greatest risk are older people who are vulnerable because of poor health. Family members or caregivers who have personal problems, such as ALCOHOL DEPENDENCE, DRUG ADDICTION, mental disorders, or financial difficulties, are most likely to become abusers. As an older person's physical or mental status deteriorates, the stress level of caregivers rises and increases the risk of abuse. Training and counseling of caregivers can help prepare them for dealing with incontinence and other stressful aspects of care. This type of help has been shown to reduce the stress that contributes to abuse. Community services and support groups offer help for caregivers dealing with stress. RESPITE CARE is another tension-reliever. A type of substitute care, it provides a break for caregivers. Respite care can last from a few hours up to a few weeks. Day care centers (see DAY CARE, ADULT) and some nursing homes provide this type of temporary care. Also, older persons can spend part of each day in adult day care centers on a regular basis. To prevent abuse outside the home, older people and their families should thoroughly investigate the references and licenses of all care facilities. Research shows that an effective way to prevent or stop abuse is to arrange for services to be provided in the home by outsiders. Home health agencies can arrange for care in the home. For example, hot, nourishing meals can be delivered at low cost by organizations such as Meals-on-Wheels.

Abuse, partner

Physical, sexual, or psychological abuse of one person in a relationship by another. Partner abuse is the most common pattern of domestic or family violence, in which one partner establishes power and control over the other through fear, domination, and intimidation. Although women are most often the victims of domestic violence, women also abuse their male partners. Partner abuse also occurs within same-sex relationships. Partner abuse generally begins with threats, name-calling, and physically destructive acts to objects or pets, escalating to violent behavior such as pushing, slapping, punching, kicking, and breaking of bones.

Partner abuse can take many forms. Physical battering of a partner can range from pushing or bruising to the final violent act of murder. Battering usually starts with relatively small acts of violence that are excused as trivial but that may escalate over time into more frequent and serious attacks. Sexual abuse is a form of physical attack in which one partner is forced to have unwanted sexual intercourse with the other. Psychological battering, which can be just as harmful as physical abuse, can include constant verbal abuse, threats, excessive possessiveness, isolation from friends and family, and destruction of personal items.

In the United States, partner abuse is considered a crime, but laws vary by state.

Abuse, sexual

FOR FIRST AID
see Rape, page 1327

Coercing another person by means of physical force, tricks, bribes, or threats into a sexual activity that gratifies the abuser. Sexual abuse can occur between adults and children or adolescents; between adolescents or older children and young children; and between adults, both heterosexual and homosexual. Sexual abuse between adults or between children or adolescents of different ages is commonly referred to as rape or sexual assault, which includes forced or coerced vaginal, oral, or anal intercourse or penetration with an object. Under the laws of some states, it may also include fondling or erotic touching without the consent of the person being touched. Sexual abuse of children includes not only intercourse or penetration, but also fondling, looking at, or photographing a child's nude body; display of the adult's genitals to the child; and sexual activity in front of a child, including self-stimulation by an adult or intercourse between two individuals. Children are most often sexually abused by members of their own family, which constitutes INCEST. Sexual abuse may cause physical injuries, but most of the damage is psychological and can last long after the abusive incidents. Sexual abuse of all varieties is illegal under state law.

CHILD SEXUAL ABUSE

Abused children, particularly those who have been the victims of family members, typically develop low self-esteem, a feeling of worthlessness, and an abnormal or distorted view of sex. Such children may withdraw and distrust adults and can become severely depressed, anxious, and suicidal. As they mature, victim children may have difficulty relating to others sexually. In many cases, children who have been abused do not understand what has happened to them and do not tell a responsible adult about the experience. If they do tell, they may not be believed. This is most likely when a child is abused by the husband or boyfriend of the mother who cannot believe that her partner would commit such an act. Disbelief adds to the child's emotional distress.

Sexual abuse of a child or adolescent can be difficult to recognize apart from physical symptoms, such as bleeding from the genitals or anus or a sexually transmitted disease. Psychological signs can include unusual hostility or aggression, provocative sexual behavior or extensive sexual knowledge, promiscuity in an adolescent, withdrawal from family and school activities, recurrent nightmares, sleep disturbances, pronounced fear of particular individuals or places, fear or concern about abnormalities in the genitals, and a return to childish behaviors

---

GETTING HELP AFTER SEXUAL ASSAULT

A person who has been sexually assaulted should get help right away. If the doctor's office is nearby, the person should go there. If a hospital is closer, he or she should go to the emergency department.

- Even though the person may feel soiled and dirty, it is vital not to change clothes, shower, wash hands, or brush the teeth. There is a risk of washing away physical evidence of the attack.
- During the examination, the person may be asked to undress on a white sheet or piece of paper to collect hair, dirt, leaves, or other debris that can serve as evidence. Underwear and any torn or stained clothing will be kept as evidence.
- The physician will scrape under the fingernails for samples of the attacker's skin, comb the pubic hair for evidence, and collect visible samples of the attacker's semen, hair, or skin.
- The physician will examine a woman's pelvis and genitals and take samples of fluid from the vagina, anus, and mouth. These samples can help identify the rapist and may also reveal any sexually transmitted diseases to which the person may have been exposed.
- If a woman is at risk of becoming pregnant, the physician may prescribe medication (morning-after pill) that may prevent pregnancy.

such as clinging, bed-wetting, or loss of bowel control.

If a child reports or even hints at abuse, the child should be encouraged to talk freely, be treated with understanding and consideration, and be assured that he or she has done the right thing. Children who perceive that they are listened to may possibly recover better from the experience than those who experience rejection and disbelief.

Abuse within a family should be reported to the local child protective agency. In most states, there is a statutory requirement that health care workers report abuse. Abuse outside the family is a matter for the police or the district attorney. Parents should consult with the child's physician, who may refer them to a doctor who specializes in sexual abuse. The specialist will examine the child and treat any physical problems, gather evidence, and reassure the child. A psychiatric evaluation is usually advised to see how the abuse has affected the child psychologically and to determine whether ongoing counseling is needed.

ADULT SEXUAL ABUSE

Most victims beyond adolescence are women who are sexually assaulted, typically by an acquaintance (so-called date rape), a lover, or a spouse. Rape by a person unknown to the victim is less common but does occur. Sexual abuse is often accompanied or preceded by threats to harm or kill, physical violence, and attempts to control the victim's life.

Sexual abuse can have powerful psychological effects. If the victim does not have the opportunity to heal after the abuse, he or she may develop anxiety, nightmares, feelings of alienation and vulnerability, distrust of others, sexual difficulties, and self-blame. In some cases, victims can develop a severe psychological reaction known as acute stress disorder. If it becomes chronic, it is known as POSTTRAUMATIC STRESS DISORDER.

Victims who do heal from sexual abuse often go through a three-step process. The first emotional reaction to the assault is shock, anger, fear, numbness, and denial that the abuse even occurred. In the second stage, the victim adjusts and resumes normal daily activities, usually by pushing memories of the abuse aside. In the third stage, the victim resolves feelings about the incident and may be able to discuss it without becoming upset. Counseling throughout this process can help the victim to discover and express the emotions connected to the abuse.

CAUSES

Since there are different types of sexual abuse, different causes underlie the actions of abusers. Many causes are highly complex and poorly understood. Recent research shows that almost all adults who abuse children were abused themselves; however, only a minority of abused children grow up to be abusers. Some adults, mostly men, have difficulty connecting intimately with people of their own age and exhibit a strong sexual attraction to children (see PEDOPHILIA). Sexual abuse of women by men can spring from the man's desire to control and dominate the woman and subject her to his will, often seen in people with antisocial personality disorder (SEE PERSONALITY DISORDERS).

Acanthosis nigricans

A dark, velvety thickening of body folds, including the armpits, inner elbows, neck, and groin area.

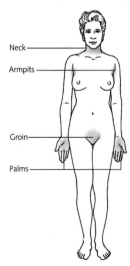

SITES OF ACANTHOSIS NIGRICANS
The darkening and thickening of the skin that characterizes acanthosis nigricans usually occurs where joints flex and the overlying skin folds within the joint. The person may also notice skin tags (small, soft growths), more prominent skin-fold marks, and papillomas (wartlike growths) in these areas.

Hyperpigmentation, or a darkening in the natural color of the skin, may give the appearance that the skin is dirty.

There are benign (not cancerous) and malignant (cancerous) forms of acanthosis nigricans. The benign form may be related to heredity, endocrine disorders, obesity, and use of some medications. Acanthosis nigricans is associated with insulin resistance and has been identified as a risk factor for type 2 diabetes (see DIABETES MELLITUS, TYPE 2). The malignant form is usually associated with cancers of the gastrointestinal tract.

Acarbose

An antidiabetic drug. Acarbose (Precose) is used to treat type 2 diabetes mellitus, also known as adult onset or non–insulin-dependent diabetes mellitus. Acarbose is unlike other antidiabetic drugs because it works in the gastrointestinal tract by slowing the process of carbohydrate digestion. The drug helps to maintain the existing blood sugar level by delaying the absorption of glucose into the blood after meals. It is used as an aid to proper diet and exercise and may be prescribed with other antidiabetic drugs.

Accident prevention

Activities designed to minimize or eliminate hazardous conditions that can cause physical injury; also known as safety awareness. Accident prevention has been considered important only since the 19th century when factory accidents caused so many deaths that public concern in favor of prevention could not be ignored. Today, accident prevention includes occupational safety and public safety, and several international organizations have formed for the development and exchange of information.

Occupational safety addresses the risks encountered in places where people work—offices, factories, farms, construction sites, and commercial and retail facilities. Industrial accidents can occur because of contact with machinery, the lifting of bulk materials, or electrical, chemical, or radiation hazards. The highest rates of severe accidents are reported by the mining, lumbering, agriculture, and fishing industries, while technology industries, such as elec-

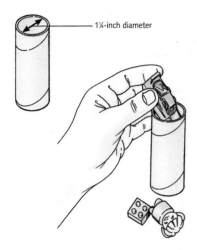

1¼-inch diameter

TOYS WITH SMALL PARTS
To help prevent choking, parents can use a toilet paper tube as a handy indicator of the safe size for toys or toy parts for toddlers. If a toy or toy part fits in the tube, it should be kept out of reach of a child younger than 3 years. Round items (balls, marbles) are particularly hazardous because they can completely block a child's airway.

tronics, have relatively low accident rates.

Public safety addresses the hazards people encounter in the home, during travel or recreation, or in any other situation not covered by occupational safety. Accidents in the home and those involving public or private transportation are the predominant cause of death in people younger than 35 years. Throughout the world, motor vehicle collisions tend to be the primary cause of accidental deaths. In the United States, six times as many people experience nonfatal injuries in accidents at home as in motor vehicle collisions, and twice as many injuries occur at home as occur at industrial sites.

Most accident prevention focuses on education and helping people and industries to identify risks and develop ways to minimize or eliminate them. Examples of such preventive programs include those designed to increase public awareness of the need to wear motor vehicle safety belts and to install smoke detectors.

Accommodation

The eye's shift in focus from far to near. The key process in accommodation is a change in the shape of the lens, the crystalline structure through which light passes into the interior of the eye. When an object is out of focus because it is too close, a nerve signal from the brain causes contraction of the muscles of the ciliary body, a structure that surrounds the lens and is attached to it by small filaments. The contraction of the ciliary body relaxes the filaments and permits the lens to thicken, allowing it to focus on objects closer to the eye. If an object is too far away, the ciliary body muscles relax, and the filaments tighten. As a result, the lens thins and can focus at a greater distance.

If the ciliary muscle is impaired, or if the eye ages and the lens hardens, it loses its flexibility. As a result, accommodation becomes less effective (see PRESBYOPIA). Many people find that they need to start wearing glasses for reading and other close work at about age 40 to 45 years because of this change in accommodation.

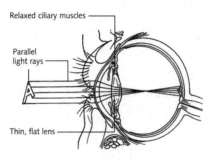

Relaxed ciliary muscles

Parallel light rays

Thin, flat lens

Focus on distant object

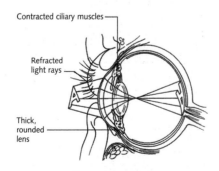

Contracted ciliary muscles

Refracted light rays

Thick, rounded lens

Focus on close object

FOCUSING ON CLOSE OBJECTS
When the eye is focused on a distant object, the ciliary muscles that control the lens relax and the lens thins out and flattens. Light rays are only slightly refracted (bent). To focus on a closer object, the muscles contract and the lens thickens and curves so that it can bend the light rays more—a function called accommodation.

Accreditation

The process by which a professional association grants recognition to a health care organization for its demonstrated ability to meet predetermined standards of medical care. Accreditation may be awarded to teaching institutions, hospitals, health care networks, long-term care facilities, ambulatory care facilities, home care organizations, clinical laboratories, and behavioral health care facilities. Associations that grant accreditation include the Joint Commission on Accreditation of Healthcare Organizations and the Commission on Office and Laboratory Accreditation.

ACE inhibitors

See ANTIHYPERTENSIVES.

Acetaminophen

A pain-reliever (analgesic) and fever-reducer (antipyretic). Acetaminophen (Tylenol is most common, but many drugs contain acetaminophen) is available without prescription to relieve pain and fever associated with a variety of common complaints, including colds, menstrual cramps, flu, headache, toothache, and minor muscular aches. It is associated with less stomach irritation than aspirin, but a person who takes acetaminophen regularly should not drink alcohol, as it can damage the liver. An overdose of acetaminophen can cause liver failure.

Acetylcholine

A NEUROTRANSMITTER, or chemical messenger, that mediates synaptic activity of the nervous system and muscles. Acetylcholine is released from the nerve terminal and travels across the nerve pathways to bind with receptors on the muscle, resulting in muscle activity. After conveying a nerve impulse, acetylcholine is rapidly broken down. MYASTHENIA GRAVIS (an autoimmune disease in which muscles become weak and tire easily) occurs when antibodies block the acetylcholine receptors on the muscles. Acetylcholine is then unable to bind to the muscles and stimulate them. A blood test known as an acetylcholine receptor antibody test is used to diagnose myasthenia gravis.

A

Acetylsalicylic acid
See ASPIRIN.

Achalasia

A rare disorder in which the sphincter muscle at the lower end of the esophagus, a tube that connects the throat and stomach, fails to contract and relax properly. Achalasia causes difficulty in swallowing solids and liquids. Symptoms of achalasia include regurgitation of food eaten in the preceding day or two, chest pain, an unpleasant taste in the mouth, and bad breath.

Diagnosis of achalasia begins with a visual examination of the esophagus, stomach, and duodenum (esophagogastroscopy), using a lighted tube called a gastroscope. An upper GASTROINTESTINAL (GI) SERIES (an X-ray procedure also known as a barium swallow) and esophageal manometry may also be conducted. Manometry, a procedure that measures pressure within the esophagus, is the most sensitive method for diagnosing achalasia. It detects the absence of normal contractions in the body of the esophagus and an increase in pressure at the lower part of the esophagus where it enters the stomach. In some cases, the symptoms of achalasia can be relieved for 6 months to several years by dilating the esophagus in a special procedure that can be repeated as necessary. In resistant cases, surgery may be required. Recently, some relief has been obtained by injection of botulinum toxin into the lower esophageal sphincter.

Achilles tendinitis

A painful inflammation of the tendon that connects the heel bone to the calf muscles of the legs. The Achilles tendon raises the heel and flexes the foot and ankle downward during walking and running. Achilles tendinitis can cause severe pain that inhibits or prevents movement and weight-bearing function in the back of the lower legs. It is usually caused by injury or overuse. The most common contributing factor to this condition is strenuous athletic training, especially jogging and running. Sudden increases in the duration, speed, or level of training may also cause Achilles tendinitis. Lack of flexibility or tightness in the calf muscles and hamstrings may

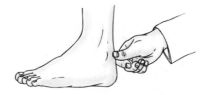

TENDER ACHILLES TENDON
In a person with Achilles tendinitis, the Achilles tendon is inflamed and painful when touched. The painful area can extend along the tendon, but is usually most pronounced just above the heel.

make the problem worse, especially in combination with overtraining. Certain types of athletic shoes can aggravate the condition, specifically when shoes have rigid soles or when there is excessive cushioning in the heel of the shoe.

The most important treatment for this condition is a reduction in the physical training that brought on the symptoms. Gentle stretching of the calf muscles before and after an athletic activity or a workout may be helpful. Applying ice to the painful area after training may also help. The use of orthotics (special shoe inserts) in combination with a heel lift inserted in the shoes may minimize pain by reducing stress on the inflamed tendon. Physical therapy includes the use of whirlpool, electrical stimulation, and ultrasound treatment. If the foot is turned inward, taping the foot may be an element of rehabilitation. Elastic support below the knee, and in severe cases a splint or cast, may be recommended. An anti-inflammatory medication may be prescribed.

Achlorhydria

The absence of HYDROCHLORIC ACID (HCL) in gastric juice, which is formed in the stomach. Hydrochloric acid is a strong acid that helps the body digest proteins and fight infection by killing bacteria that have been ingested. Despite the lack of acid, most digestive processes proceed normally. Achlorhydria is caused by atrophy (shrinking or wasting) of the stomach lining and is frequently associated with pernicious anemia in which there is no absorption of vitamin B12. Less commonly, it is associated with severe iron-deficiency anemia (see ANEMIA, IRON-DEFICIENCY). When achlorhydria occurs in combi-

nation with a GASTRIC ULCER, a malignancy is usually suspected.

Achondroplasia

A common genetic disorder of bone growth that is usually evident at birth. Children with achondroplasia have short arms and legs, particularly upper arms and thighs; large heads with prominent foreheads and noses that are flat at the bridge between the eyes; curved lower spines; bowed lower legs; short stubby fingers; short, flat feet; and poor muscle tone. Other problems include frequent ear infections that can cause hearing loss and back and leg pain and paralysis due to pressure on the spinal nerves from spinal deformities. Achondroplasia affects one in every 10,000 births and equally affects both sexes and all races.

Babies with achondroplasia are delayed in sitting, standing, and walking because of their poor muscle tone, large heads, and short limbs; they eventually catch up with their peers. The disorder generally does not include mental retardation, and the life span is usually normal. Occasionally, infants and small children with achondroplasia die suddenly, usually during sleep. The deaths are thought to result from breathing problems caused by compression of the spinal cord at the base of the skull and in the vertebrae of the neck. Breathing problems can also stem from a small chest, large tonsils, and small facial bone structure.

GENETIC CAUSES

Achondroplasia, a dominant genetic disorder, is caused by an abnormal gene on chromosome 4. Affected individuals have a 50 percent chance of passing it on to their children. However, in 80 to 90 percent of cases, neither of the parents is affected, and the achondroplasia is caused by a mutation in the gene of the affected individual. Paternal age seems to be a factor in these sporadic mutations; men who become fathers when they are 40 years old or older are more likely to have children with achondroplasia than men who are younger. Maternal age is not a factor.

When one or both expectant parents have achondroplasia, prenatal tests can diagnose or rule out the disorder in the fetus. If both parents have achondroplasia, the fetus has a one in four chance of having a much more severe, often fatal, disorder resulting from two copies of the achondroplasia gene. There is no way to predict most cases of achondroplasia. Parents who have the disorder can benefit from genetic counseling.

TREATMENT

There is no current treatment to normalize skeletal development of children with achondroplasia. Infants and children with the disorder should be evaluated by a doctor experienced with the disorder, such as a geneticist or an orthopedist. Detection of spinal abnormalities likely to cause spinal cord compression is particularly important, since breathing difficulties and leg paralysis can result from such compression. Surgery may be necessary to prevent bowed legs or to relieve nerve or spinal cord pressure from surrounding bones. Humps may develop in the middle back that usually go away when the child begins to walk. When the humps fail to go away, surgery may be required. A controversial surgery known as limb-lengthening may increase the ultimate height of a person with the disorder. Treatment may be needed for ear infections to prevent hearing loss, and braces may be used to correct overcrowded teeth.

Acid

A chemical compound capable of neutralizing alkalis and releasing hydrogen ions when in solution. Acids are corrosive and usually have a sour taste. An acid reacts with a base to form a salt, has a pH (a measure of the acidity of a solution) less than 7, and will turn blue litmus red.

Acid reflux

See ESOPHAGEAL REFLUX.

Acid-base balance

A state of equilibrium between acidity and alkalinity of body fluids. The acid-base balance keeps body fluids at or near a neutral pH (neither acidic nor basic) for normal body function. Such a balance is necessary because most of the body's metabolic processes produce acids, while vital cellular activities require a somewhat alkaline, or basic, body fluid. Acid-base balance requires a body fluid pH of between 7.35 and 7.45 if enzyme systems and other metabolic activities are to function normally. If the body fluid pH falls below 7.30, ACIDOSIS is said to exist; if it rises above 7.50, a state of alkalosis exists. Both acidosis and alkalosis are considered serious.

The acid-base balance is achieved through chemical exchanges of hydrogen ions. An acid is a substance capable of giving up a hydrogen ion during a chemical exchange, while a base is a substance that can accept it. The body depends on several mechanisms to maintain body fluid pH at desirable levels, compensating for upward or downward changes in pH. The three major regulatory systems are chemical (buffer systems involving chemicals that either combine with or release hydrogen ions); biological (blood and cellular activity shifts excess acid or base into and out of the cells); and physiological (the lungs compensate for imbalance by regulating the amount of carbon dioxide in the blood, while the kidneys control acidity by reabsorbing or excreting bicarbonate as needed).

Acidosis

A serious metabolic disorder that results from the accumulation of acid or a depletion of the alkaline content of the blood and tissues. The pH of the blood becomes abnormally low, indicating that the blood is excessively acidic. Acidosis occurs in cases of uncontrolled type 1 diabetes (see DIABETES MELLITUS, TYPE 1), severe kidney disorders, and some lung diseases. Respiratory acidosis can result from conditions that prevent the lungs from ventilating properly, causing carbon dioxide to accumulate. Treatment for acidosis depends on the underlying cause. For example, KETOACIDOSIS from uncontrolled diabetes requires administration of intravenous fluids and insulin. In severe cases, sodium bicarbonate to neutralize the acid may be given, or a mechanical ventilator may be used to improve respiration.

Acne

An inflammatory condition characterized by whiteheads, blackheads, and pimples. Acne lesions are seen most frequently on the face but may also develop on the back, chest, shoulders, and neck. Whiteheads—small, hard, painless, white blemishes—commonly occur in clusters on the cheeks, nose, and chin. Blackheads are composed primarily of dried body oils and shed skin cells, while pimples contain pus. In some cases, deeper, boil-like lesions such as nodules (solid masses of tissue) or cysts are present.

CAUSES

Many people mistakenly believe that acne is a result of poor hygiene and eating rich food. However, it is now known that acne is most closely linked with hormonal influences. While acne can occur at any age, it is most common during adolescence. At the onset of sexual maturity, both males and females secrete increased amounts of hormones called androgen hormones, which overstimulate

---

SELF-CARE FOR ACNE

While advanced or chronic acne requires a doctor's care, individuals can take steps to prevent the condition or reduce inflammation:

- Wash face gently twice a day using a mild soap or cleanser.
- Do not excessively scrub the skin.
- Avoid drying astringents and facial scrubs.
- Shampoo hair regularly.
- Do not squeeze or pick at pimples, which can cause scarring.
- Avoid nicking blemishes while shaving.
- Choose skin care products that are labeled noncomedogenic, which means they are less likely to clog pores and lead to blackheads or whiteheads.
- Avoid oil-based skin care products; use makeup that is water-based and oil-free.
- Use flesh-tinted antiblemish lotions or noncomedogenic cosmetics to cover acne.
- Use over-the-counter acne care products that include active ingredients such as benzoyl peroxide, resorcinol, salicylic acid, or sulfur.
- Do not get a suntan in an attempt to conceal acne. Too much sun could cause premature aging of the skin and skin cancer.
- If acne does not respond to self-care, consult a doctor.

A

STAGES OF ACNE

Acne is a disorder of the hair follicles in which blackheads, whiteheads, and other forms of blemishes mar the skin. Hormonal changes cause acne to be most common among adolescents, but acne may occur for the first time in adults as old as 30. Stress and hormonal changes have been proven to cause acne.

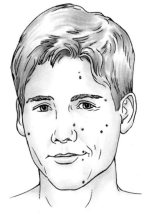

A TEENAGER WITH MILD ACNE
Mild acne takes the form of a few scattered blemishes on the face, neck, and shoulders.

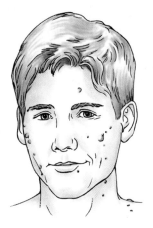

A TEENAGER WITH MODERATE STAGE OF ACNE
Acne is termed moderate when there is an increase in the number of blemishes, as well as the appearance of acne nodules (collections of inflamed cells).

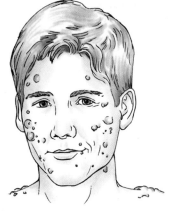

A TEENAGER WITH SEVERE ACNE
Severe acne results when the bacteria population on the skin has gone out of control. Inflamed cysts heal and become reinfected. The face may become pockmarked and permanently scarred. Early treatment may prevent acne from reaching this stage.

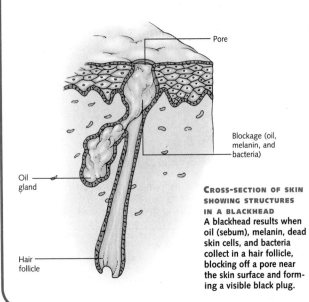

Pore

Blockage (oil, melanin, and bacteria)

Oil gland

Hair follicle

CROSS-SECTION OF SKIN SHOWING STRUCTURES IN A BLACKHEAD
A blackhead results when oil (sebum), melanin, dead skin cells, and bacteria collect in a hair follicle, blocking off a pore near the skin surface and forming a visible black plug.

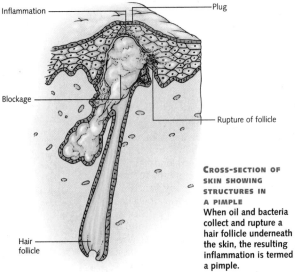

Inflammation

Plug

Blockage

Rupture of follicle

Hair follicle

CROSS-SECTION OF SKIN SHOWING STRUCTURES IN A PIMPLE
When oil and bacteria collect and rupture a hair follicle underneath the skin, the resulting inflammation is termed a pimple.

and enlarge the sebaceous glands (oil glands). Severe acne is much more common in teenage boys than girls, probably because boys secrete more androgens. An oily substance called sebum is produced by the sebaceous glands and is secreted to the surface of the skin through small openings or pores in the skin. When too much sebum is present, the pores can become clogged, and bacteria multiply in tiny blocked channels. These channels become inflamed and swollen and fill with pus.

Acne outbreaks that persist into adulthood are often aggravated by factors such as stress, menstrual periods, or use of corticosteroids. Acne at any age can affect self-image and cause reduced self-esteem, embarrassment, and depression.

TREATMENT

As people age, acne usually disappears on its own. However, if left untreated, it can lead to permanent scarring. Fortunately, there are many antiacne treatments. Topical medications are available both over-the-counter and by prescription. In moderate to severe cases of acne, doctors prescribe oral medications such as antibiotics and isotretinoin. Scars resulting from acne may be improved by procedures including CHEMICAL PEEL, DERMABRASION (removal of the surface layer of skin by high-speed sanding), and LASER RESURFACING.

■ *Topical medications* Lotions and creams are good for treating acne accompanied by dry skin, while alcohol-based gels and solutions are best for treating acne-prone oily skin. These medications are designed to decrease inflammation and limit the formation of new pimples.

Over-the-counter topical medications include benzoyl peroxide, resorcinol, salicylic acid, and sulfur. Benzoyl peroxide has keratolytic (peeling) and antimicrobial (germ-killing) qualities. Resorcinol, salicylic acid, and sulfur help break down whiteheads and blackheads. Side effects of these medications include dry skin, irritation, redness, and burning.

Prescription topical drugs include benzoyl peroxide (in a more powerful concentration than the over-the-counter brands), tretinoin, and antibiotics. Tretinoin, a type of drug called a retinoid, is a derivative of vitamin

A. One of the most effective topical antiacne medications, tretinoin helps penetrate and loosen clogged pores. Tretinoin may enhance the effectiveness of other topical agents, but even low concentrations of tretinoin can leave skin dry, scaly, and red. It is important to use sunscreen during treatment, since using tretinoin heightens skin sensitivity to the sun. Topical antibiotics reduce inflammation and bacteria. Commonly prescribed topical antibiotics include clindamycin and erythromycin, which are used to treat less severe cases of acne.

■ *Oral medications* Antibiotics (such as erythromycin, tetracycline, minocycline, and doxycycline), isotretinoin, and birth control pills are among the oral medications prescribed when topical products fail to control acne. These drugs are effective but can cause side effects. Oral antibiotics may cause increased skin sensitivity to the sun, upset stomach, dizziness, light-headedness, or discoloration of the skin or teeth. Isotretinoin is highly effective for treating acne that results in nodules or cysts or severe acne that has not responded to other methods of treatment. However, it is teratogenic (increases the risk of birth defects), so it must never be used by women who are or may soon be pregnant. Women of childbearing age should stop taking isotretinoin at least 1 month before getting pregnant. In addition, isotretinoin can cause dry mouth, chapped lips, decreased night vision, increased triglyceride levels, and abnormal liver enzyme levels. Periodic blood tests are required to monitor side effects. The risks versus benefits of oral medications must be carefully weighed.

■ *Surgical procedures* Scars resulting from acne may be improved by chemical peels, dermabrasion, or laser resurfacing. In a chemical peel, a mild acid is used to burn off the surface layer of skin, eliminating superficial acne scars and evening out overall skin tone. In dermabrasion, a rapidly swirling wire brush is used to remove damaged skin; dermabrasion is generally a more effective treatment than a chemical peel for deeper scars. In laser skin resurfacing, pulses of laser light vaporize the skin. It is necessary to reduce sun exposure

after undergoing any of these procedures.

Acoustic neuroma

A benign tumor of the eighth cranial nerve (also known as the acoustic nerve, the auditory nerve, and the vestibulocochlear nerve; it is located in the head). The cause of acoustic neuromas is believed to be a defect in a tumor suppressor gene, and bilateral acoustic tumors are associated with a genetic disorder known as NEUROFIBROMATOSIS type 2 (NF2). Acoustic neuromas are almost always noncancerous and do not spread or metastasize to other parts of the body. However, they can grow quite large, causing damage to surrounding structures.

SYMPTOMS

Acoustic neuromas are rarely seen in people younger than 30 years. Acoustic neuromas can press against the hearing and balance nerves, leading to hearing loss, ringing in the ears (tinnitus), and dizziness. Other symptoms include headache, trouble understanding speech, vertigo, loss of balance, and facial numbness or pain. Larger tumors can affect the facial nerve, leading to facial paralysis. Ultimately, if untreated, a large tumor can cause increased pressure on the brain, which may result in lethargy, nausea and vomiting, and a dilated pupil in one eye. In these cases, acoustic neuromas become life-threatening.

DIAGNOSIS AND TREATMENT

MRI (magnetic resonance imaging) of the head is the most effective means of diagnosing an acoustic neuroma. Other helpful tests include CT (computed tomography) scans, hearing tests, caloric stimulation (a test for dizziness or vertigo), electronystagmography (a test of equilibrium and balance), and brain stem auditory evoked response (a test of hearing and brain stem function). The doctor will also take a careful history and perform a neurological examination.

Surgical removal of the tumor is the usual treatment of choice. The goal of surgery, which takes place under general anesthesia, is to remove the acoustic neuroma while preserving as many vital structures as possible. In general, the smaller the tumor, the less the chance of complications. A

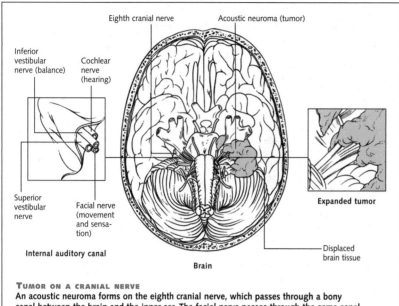

Eighth cranial nerve

Acoustic neuroma (tumor)

Inferior vestibular nerve (balance)

Cochlear nerve (hearing)

Superior vestibular nerve

Facial nerve (movement and sensation)

Internal auditory canal

Brain

Expanded tumor

Displaced brain tissue

TUMOR ON A CRANIAL NERVE
An acoustic neuroma forms on the eighth cranial nerve, which passes through a bony canal between the brain and the inner ear. The facial nerve passes through the same canal. A tumor can exert pressure on these delicate structures and cause problems with hearing, balance, and facial movement and sensation.

Acoustic trauma

A severe injury to the ear caused by a short-duration sound of extremely high intensity such as an explosion or gunfire. One-time exposure to a sufficiently loud noise, sometimes called impulse noise, can cause damage to all the structures of the ear, including the delicate structure of the hearing part of the inner ear, the COCHLEA. The cochlea is the part of the inner ear that is involved with hearing. The resulting hearing loss in one or both ears may be immediate and permanent. Loss of hearing caused by impulse noise is sometimes accompanied by TINNITUS (constant or intermittent ringing, buzzing, or roaring in one or both ears). Loss of hearing and tinnitus due to acoustic trauma are not presently treatable by any medical or surgical procedure, but there can be spontaneous improvement and healing for up to 1 year.

CAUSES

The human ear can perceive sound comfortably up to 100 decibels (dB), the measurement used to measure sound. Human speech averages about 60 dB; a dog's bark or a telephone ring can range from 80 to 100 dB. Impulse noise levels above 140 dB, such as those that may be produced by an airplane engine, firecrackers, explosions, or small firearms, may cause hearing loss from which the ear cannot recover. Individuals differ widely in the amount of hearing loss experienced as a result of identical exposures. Impulse noise is more likely to affect higher frequency (higher

small acoustic tumor is one that is confined within the bony canal between the inner ear and the brain; most small tumors can be completely removed. However, in about half the cases, total loss of hearing results in the affected ear. A medium-sized acoustic tumor is one that extends from the bony canal into the brain cavity, but is not yet putting pressure on the brain itself; sometimes these tumors can be only partially removed. Following surgery, hearing loss is permanent in the affected ear.

Large acoustic neuromas are the most serious. A large acoustic tumor is one that has invaded the brain cavity, producing pressure on the brain and disturbing vital structures. Surgery to remove it is extensive, and the procedure must be terminated before the tumor is completely removed if there are threatening changes in blood pressure, pulse rate, or respiration rate. If this happens, a second operation is usually necessary. Complications from surgery to remove an acoustic neuroma are most common following the removal of large tumors. Often there is permanent hearing loss in the affected ear, and in two of three cases there is also permanent facial weakness or paralysis. Dizziness and balance disturbances are other common compli-

cations, although these problems usually decrease or disappear over time.

Another treatment option is radiation therapy, which slows the growth of the tumor rather than removing it. Radiation may be recommended for older or sick people who cannot tolerate brain surgery or following a procedure in which it was not possible to remove the entire tumor. As with surgery, possible complications of radiation include hearing loss and facial paralysis.

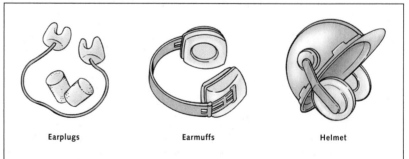

Earplugs

Earmuffs

Helmet

PREVENTING HEARING LOSS
A variety of devices are available to protect hearing in individuals who spend time in situations with strong potential for acoustic trauma—for example, working in an airport. Ear plugs, whether disposable or permanent, reduce sound pressure levels by 10 to 45 decibels. Properly fitted acoustic earmuffs fit over the entire outer ear and form an air seal to block out sound. Simultaneous use of earplugs and earmuffs is recommended when noise levels exceed 105 decibels. A helmet with built-in earmuffs provides hearing protection and also helps prevent head trauma.

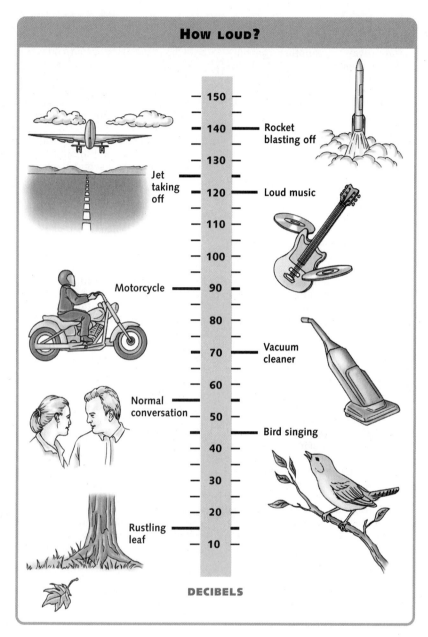

How Loud?

- 150
- 140 — Rocket blasting off
- 130
- Jet taking off
- 120 — Loud music
- 110
- 100
- Motorcycle — 90
- 80
- 70 — Vacuum cleaner
- 60
- Normal conversation — 50
- Bird singing
- 40
- 30
- 20
- Rustling leaf — 10

DECIBELS

pituitary gland. In most cases, the excess production of growth hormone is caused by an ADENOMA, a benign (not cancerous) tumor, which in acromegaly affects the pituitary gland. Middle-aged adults are most commonly affected by acromegaly, which can produce serious illness and premature death. When an adenoma occurs in childhood, the result may be unusually TALL STATURE. If the disorder is properly diagnosed, most people can benefit from treatment, but acromegaly may be difficult to recognize.

One of the most common early symptoms is soft-tissue swelling in the hands and feet, followed by excessive growth in these extremities. Over time, changes in facial bone tissue can produce a protruding brow and lower jaw, an enlarged nose bone, and wide spaces between the teeth. Acromegaly may produce accelerated growth in an adult's height and a thickening of the soft tissues of the hands, feet, heart, liver, spleen, and kidneys. Associated risks include arthritis, carpal tunnel syndrome, diabetes mellitus, sleep apnea, high blood pressure, increased risk of cardiovascular disease, and colon polyps, which could become malignant (cancerous).

Acromegaly is diagnosed by specialized blood tests that measure growth hormone or insulinlike growth factor 1 levels in the blood

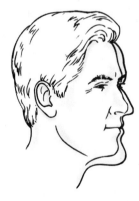

CHARACTERISTIC FEATURES
Some of the most obvious signs of acromegaly occur in a person's facial structure. The bones and soft tissues of the nose and cheeks enlarge and the jaw widens, causing dental problems. The features become more prominent and rounded, a characteristic known as bossing.

pitched) hearing than lower frequency hearing. Pain associated with loud noise (HYPERACUSIS) may also occur.

The use of hearing protectors, such as ear plugs or ear muffs, may prevent damage to hearing when there is potential for exposure to sudden, very loud sounds—for example, at a firing range. Personal hearing protection is also recommended in work situations when possibly hazardous exposure is unavoidable.

Acquired immunodeficiency syndrome

A life-threatening disorder caused by infection with HIV (human immunodeficiency virus) and characterized by a breakdown of the body's immune defenses. See AIDS.

Acromegaly

A rare, slowly progressive, chronic hormonal disorder caused by an overproduction of growth hormone by the and by CT SCANNING (computed tomography scanning) or MRI (magnetic resonance imaging) of the pituitary gland to locate the tumor. Treatment options include surgery to remove the adenoma, medication, and radiation of the pituitary gland.

Acroparesthesia

A sensation of numbness, tingling, or pins and needles at the tips of the extremities (for example, the fingers, hands, and forearms) that most commonly occurs at night. The symptoms of acroparesthesia often awaken the person from sleep and resolve within minutes after vigorously rubbing and shaking the affected extremities. Acroparesthesias are influenced by factors such as activity, rest, posture, congestion, and swelling and are usually associated with carpal tunnel syndrome.

Acrophobia

An abnormal fear of heights. As with other phobias, the fear is excessive and unrealistic. If acrophobia is a symptom of DEPRESSION or if it interferes with the everyday tasks of living, psychological treatment is recommended.

ACTH

Adrenocorticotropic hormone; also known as corticotropin or adrenocorticotropin. ACTH is a hormone that controls the production and secretion of certain other hormones from the ADRENAL GLANDS. The hypothalamus, a regulating region at the base of the brain, is prompted by a number of stimuli and hormones to produce a substance that controls the secretion of ACTH by the pituitary gland, which stimulates the adrenal glands to produce hormones, such as cortisol.

Acting out

A mechanism for dealing with unconscious emotional conflict or stress through behavior rather than in thoughts or feelings. A person who is acting out behaves in a current situation as if it were the setting that originally gave rise to the conflict or stress. For example, a person who experienced a particular kind of conflict with a parent might act out the unconscious feelings aroused by that conflict in a later relationship with another authority figure, such as a

boss or a psychotherapist. Sometimes the term is incorrectly used to show disapproval of another person's impulsive behavior. In psychotherapy, acting out can be valuable as a way of understanding feelings, particularly fear that cannot yet be expressed in words.

Actinic keratosis

A red, scaly, precancerous skin lesion that is the result of years of sun exposure. Actinic keratoses usually occur on parts of the body that experience the most exposure to ultraviolet light, such as the face, ears, and backs of the hands. Most lesions develop in middle age or later; appear as small (less than ¾ inch), dry, scaly bumps on the skin surface; and may be tan, pink, or red. Actinic keratoses are precancerous, meaning that, if left untreated, a lesion may develop into SQUAMOUS CELL CARCINOMA, a serious type of SKIN CANCER. Squamous cell carcinoma is usually not life-threatening if detected and treated early but, if left untreated, it can spread into lymph nodes or internal organs and become incurable.

Early diagnosis and treatment of actinic keratoses are critical. It is important to have a doctor examine any new skin lesions that grow or bleed. Actinic keratoses can be removed by CRYOSURGERY (freezing with liquid nitrogen), topical chemotherapy, CURETTAGE (scraping), electrodesiccation (burning with an electric current delivered through a probe), or CHEMICAL PEEL (use of a chemical agent to remove damaged skin).

Actinomycosis

A rare, chronic infection caused by actinomycetes bacteria and resulting in diseases of the chest, mouth and jaw, and pelvis. Symptoms may include chest pain, lethargy, weight loss, fever, draining sinuses, coughing up sputum, night sweats, and shortness of breath.

CAUSES, DIAGNOSIS, AND TREATMENT

The bacteria that cause actinomycosis are normally found in the mouth and gastrointestinal tract. Poor dental hygiene and dental abscesses may produce the infection in the mouth and jaw and cause facial lesions. When the infection occurs in the

chest, it produces lesions and fluid in the lungs.

The infection is diagnosed by chest X rays, tissue cultures, and bronchoscopy. Actinomycosis is treated by prolonged therapy with penicillin or another antibiotic. The infection is usually cured with antibiotics and occasionally surgery to remove lesions and drain fluid from the lungs. Prompt and thorough treatment is essential: complications from actinomycosis include brain abscess and MENINGITIS.

Acupressure

A noninvasive method to relieve pain and manage stress using the fingertips or hands to stimulate the body's self-curative abilities. Acupressure is an ancient form of Chinese medicine similar to ACUPUNCTURE, but it uses pressure exerted by the hands rather than needles to aid healing. When selected points on the skin are pressed for 3 to 10 seconds, muscular tension is released, blood circulation is stimulated, and the body's natural abilities to heal itself are triggered. The effects of acupressure are seldom long-lasting. Acupressure is intended for short-term symptom relief and self-treatment of tension-related ailments.

Acupressure is used to relieve and prevent sports injuries by improving muscle tone and circulation. As an adjunct to traditional medicine, acupressure is used to speed healing of broken bones after they have been set and to relieve pain associated with cancer. As an adjunct to chiropractic treatment, acupressure is used to relax and tone the muscles of the back to make spinal adjustments easier and more effective. A common application is the acupressure point that is used to relieve nausea. Acupressure is widely practiced in China, but in the United States it is thought to be less effective than acupuncture.

Acupuncture

A technique in which extremely thin needles are inserted into specific points on the body to treat or prevent illness. Acupuncture is an ancient form of traditional CHINESE MEDICINE that has been practiced for 3,000 years. Acupuncture has been known and used in parts of Europe since the

MAPPING OUT ACUPUNCTURE

According to the principles of acupuncture, energy or "qi" flows through the body via 12 main meridians or channels. To strengthen the flow of qi or to remove blockages in the meridians, an acupuncturist inserts a number of tiny, sterile, flexible needles just under the skin at acupoints along the channels.

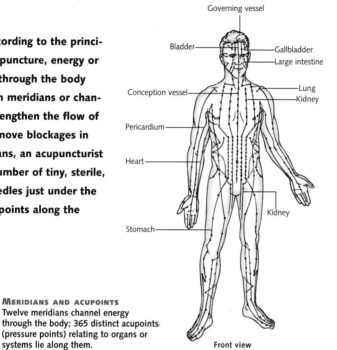

Governing vessel
Bladder
Gallbladder
Large intestine
Conception vessel
Lung
Kidney
Pericardium
Heart
Kidney
Stomach

Front view

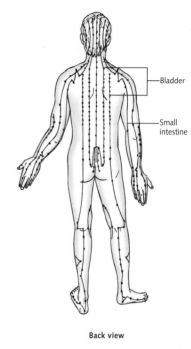

Bladder
Small intestine

Back view

MERIDIANS AND ACUPOINTS
Twelve meridians channel energy through the body; 365 distinct acupoints (pressure points) relating to organs or systems lie along them.

17th century and has been particularly popular in the United States since 1972, when former President Nixon visited China.

PHILOSOPHY OF ACUPUNCTURE

Acupuncture is based on the idea that health is a constantly changing flow of energy, or qi (pronounced "chee"). According to traditional Chinese medicine, imbalances in qi result in disease. Acupuncture is used to restore health by modulating the flow of qi.

Qi is thought to flow through the body by way of channels, called meridians. To strengthen the flow of qi, or to remove blockages in the meridians, the acupuncturist inserts a number of tiny, flexible, sterile needles just under the skin at specific points called acupoints located throughout the body. There are 365 acupoints located along the meridians, each one associated with specific internal organs or organ systems.

ACUPUNCTURE TREATMENT

A visit to an acupuncturist involves

the taking of a complete medical history as well as a physical examination of the body, with particular attention paid to three pulses on the wrist, examination of the tongue, and the smell of the breath and the body. In many cases, the first acupuncture treatment will be given at the first visit, with follow-up visits once or twice a week thereafter.

Acupuncture needles may feel uncomfortable but they rarely hurt. Most needles are extremely thin—about three times the thickness of a human hair—and they enter the skin at the acupoints with little resistance. Anywhere from 1 to 15 needles may be used at a time, and to increase the flow of qi, the acupuncturist may twist the needles or send a weak electrical current through them. The needles are generally left in for 15 to 40 minutes, depending on what is being treated. Some acupuncturists also burn herbs to stimulate acupoints, a process called MOXIBUSTION.

Most people find acupuncture

relaxing; many people fall asleep during the treatment. Some people report feeling a tingling sensation ("pins and needles"), while others feel nothing at all. Many people notice rapid improvement following acupuncture, although long-standing ailments may take many sessions to improve.

USES OF ACUPUNCTURE

In the United States, acupuncture has most often been used to relieve chronic pain caused by arthritis, migraine headache, premenstrual syndrome (PMS), or back pain. Another common use of acupuncture is to assist people in withdrawal from drug and alcohol dependency. Some acupuncturists use it to reduce pain during surgery.

In 1997, the National Institutes of Health (NIH) decided that acupuncture had been demonstrated to be an effective tool for the treatment of various health problems, including the relief of postoperative pain after dental surgery and the treatment of nausea caused by chemotherapy, anesthesia,

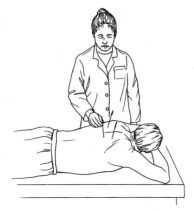

FINE, FLAT NEEDLES
Compared with hypodermic needles, acupuncture needles have flatter points. That is why acupuncture needles usually do not cause bruising when they penetrate the skin.

and pregnancy ("morning sickness"). The NIH also noted that acupuncture had been shown to be a useful adjunctive treatment for headache, CARPAL TUNNEL SYNDROME (a painful condition caused by a compressed nerve in the wrist), and FIBROMYALGIA (pain and tenderness of muscles and associated connective tissue). Acupuncture is also used in the rehabilitation of people who have had strokes.

Acupuncture, ear
A form of acupuncture; auricular therapy. Ear acupuncture is used as an anesthetic for simple operations and has been shown to speed postoperative recovery. The external ear is regarded by acupuncturists as a particularly important indicator of health, because the 12 major meridians, or channels of energy, are thought to cross it. Acupuncturists have identified more than 200 acupoints on each ear, each of which is allied with a body part. Auricular therapy involves the stimulation of acupoints on the ear to treat various conditions. Ear acupuncture is usually practiced alone, although it may be used in conjunction with body acupuncture.

Acute
A term that describes symptoms or disease that begins abruptly and subsides within a relatively short period. In contrast to CHRONIC health problems, the onset of abrupt or acute symptoms is characterized by sharpness, severity, or intensity.

Acyclovir
An antiviral drug. Acyclovir (Zovirax) is used to treat herpesvirus infections, including genital herpes, herpes zoster (shingles), and varicella (chickenpox), as well as other infections. Acyclovir works by interfering with viral DNA, slowing the growth of existing viruses.

ADA
See AMERICANS WITH DISABILITIES ACT (ADA).

Adapalene
An antiacne ointment. Adapalene (Differin) is applied to skin affected by acne once a day (usually 1 hour before bedtime) to reduce inflammation and reddening and to slow the formation of the material that fills acne lesions, or pimples. Using adapalene can make the skin feel itchy, but it is less irritating than other acne medications.

ADD
The acronym for attention deficit disorder. See ATTENTION DEFICIT/HYPERACTIVITY DISORDER.

Addiction
A behavior pursued not for the pleasure or gain it provides but as a way of satisfying a physical or deep-seated psychological compulsion. Characteristically, an addiction dominates the person's life and becomes his or her principal activity or pursuit, often at a high personal cost in terms of family, work, school, financial success, and career. The individual loses

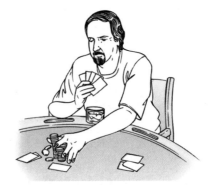

ADDICTIVE BEHAVIOR
As with other addictions, addictive gamblers are unaware of the extent of their loss of control over their behavior. They deny that they cannot quit and go to great lengths to conceal their gambling habit and its financial consequences.

control in regard to the addiction and is incapable of quitting by a simple act of will. He or she may try repeatedly to end the addiction, only to fail and return to the addictive behavior. Addiction often refers to the use of chemicals, such as alcohol (see ALCOHOL DEPENDENCE), tobacco (see SMOKING, TOBACCO), and illegal drugs such as cocaine, crack cocaine, heroin, amphetamines, and marijuana (see DRUG ADDICTION). Addiction can also arise with gambling (see GAMBLING, ADDICTIVE) and sexual activity (see SEXUAL ADDICTION). A person may have more than one addiction and be genetically predisposed to abusing drugs and alcohol.

Addison disease
A rare hormonal disorder that is caused by an inadequate production of cortisol, a hormone produced by the adrenal glands; also known as chronic adrenal insufficiency, hypoadrenocorticism, and hypocorticalism. Addison disease is usually the result of autoimmune disorders. The immune system causes a gradual destruction of the outer layer of the adrenal glands. Less frequently, tuberculosis can cause the adrenal insufficiency leading to Addison disease. Less common causes are fungal infections, the spread of cancer cells to the adrenal glands, AMYLOIDOSIS, surgical removal of the adrenal glands, and failure of the pituitary gland to produce enough ACTH (adrenocorticotropic hormone), the substance that stimulates the adrenal glands to make cortisol. Addison disease affects all age groups and both sexes equally. Symptoms tend to begin gradually and include chronic fatigue, muscle weakness, loss of appetite, weight loss, nausea, vomiting, diarrhea, low blood pressure, a low blood sugar level, and hyperpigmentation. Untreated, this illness can lead to shock and death.

DIAGNOSIS AND TREATMENT
The most specific test for diagnosing Addison disease is the ACTH stimulation test, in which levels of cortisol in the blood or urine are measured before and after a synthetic form of ACTH is injected. The insulininduced hypoglycemia (low blood sugar) test is another diagnostic tool for Addison disease. This test evaluates several specific responses to stress by the hypothalamus, the pitu-

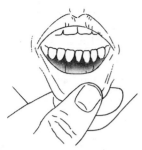

VISIBLE SYMPTOM OF ADDISON DISEASE
Among many general symptoms, Addison disease causes the more specific symptom of darkening of the skin, particularly in the mouth. This so-called hyperpigmentation is caused by excessive secretion by the pituitary gland of the hormone that stimulates the production of melanin (a skin pigment).

itary gland, and the adrenal glands. Checking the ACTH level also helps define the cause of the disorder.

Treatment is aimed at replacing the missing hormones with synthetic forms, such as the oral medication hydrocortisone. Fludrocortisone acetate is a medication taken when ALDOSTERONE, a hormone also made by the adrenal glands, is deficient.

Adduction

Movement of a limb sideways toward the body. Adduction involves the movement of a leg or arm toward the center of the body or the movement of a toe or finger in line with the arm or leg.

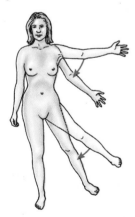

SIDEWAYS MOTION
Adduction of a limb brings the limb back toward the median plane of the body, which bisects the depth of the body; abduction is the opposite motion that brings the limb out from the median plane. These terms can similarly describe sideways motion of other body parts, such as fingers.

Adenitis

An inflammatory condition of a LYMPH NODE; also known as lymphadenitis. Lymph nodes in the neck are commonly affected; the inflammation is usually caused by an infection of the mouth, throat, or ear. Scalp infections, insect bites, and head lice can cause adenitis that affects the lymph nodes at the back of the neck. Swelling and pain occur in the sites where the affected lymph nodes are located.

Respiratory infections sometimes precede mesenteric adenitis or inflammation that affects the lymph nodes located in the mesentery, the membrane that attaches organs to the abdominal wall. Mesenteric adenitis can cause severe abdominal pain and may mimic the symptoms of appendicitis, especially in children. Generalized adenitis, involving all the lymph nodes, may be from a viral infection such as mononucleosis or can be a secondary symptom of syphilis.

Treatment of localized adenitis requires the use of antimicrobial agents to treat the primary infection causing the condition. The application of warm compresses to the affected sites may help relieve discomfort. In severe forms, adenitis is treated surgically to drain the nodes.

Adenocarcinoma

A cancer derived from glandular tissue. Adenocarcinomas develop on the linings or inner surfaces of organs, such as the lung, pancreas, breast, prostate, esophagus, stomach, vagina, urethra, or small intestine. Nearly all colon cancers and about 40 percent of lung cancers are adenocarcinomas.

Adenoidectomy

The surgical removal of enlarged ADENOIDS (clusters of tissue at the back of the nose and throat), usually of a child. Tonsillectomy and adenoidectomy, often done together and called T and A, were routinely performed until the 1960s. Today, it is recognized that the tonsils and adenoids help the body fight infection. Surgery is done only if swollen adenoids or tonsils significantly interfere with a child's ability to breathe, swallow, or speak. An adenoidectomy or tonsillectomy may also be performed to treat a recurring severe sore throat caused by a "strep" infection; an abscess involving the tonsils; a suspected cancerous enlargement of the tonsil; or a middle ear infection that does not respond to other treatments, such as antibiotics or the placement of drainage tubes in the ears (see OTITIS MEDIA). An adenoidectomy is commonly performed when a child is 6 or 7 years of age. Surgery can take place on an outpatient basis, with most children able to go home after 8 to 10 hours of observation. The most frequent complication is bleeding. Children who experience this problem are usually placed on their sides to avoid choking on blood. Acetaminophen or ibuprofen (not

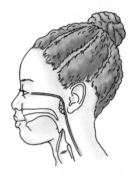

NORMAL ADENOIDS
The adenoids are a pair of glands located at the back of the nasal cavity, above the tonsils. The adenoids begin to grow at about age 3 when a child is most susceptible to infection, start to shrink at about age 5, and disappear at puberty.

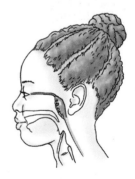

ENLARGED ADENOIDS
In some children, the adenoids keep growing, blocking the airway between the nose and throat and/or between the middle ear and the nose. The child may breathe through his or her mouth, have a runny nose during the day and a cough at night, and have a stuffy-sounding voice. A doctor can see the enlarged adenoids with a mirror and light held at the back of the throat.

aspirin), adequate liquids, and soft food can help relieve the sore throat pain that may persist for 2 weeks following the surgery.

Adenoids

One of two small masses of tissue at the back of the nose above the tonsils. Also known as pharyngeal tonsils, the adenoids are part of the LYMPHATIC SYSTEM, and their function is to stop disease-causing microorganisms from entering the body through the nose or mouth. Adenoids tend to enlarge during childhood and are a frequent site of infections. But adenoids shrink in most children after age 5 and disappear by puberty. Some children are plagued with chronically enlarged adenoids, which may cause snoring, breathing through the mouth, and a nasal-sounding voice. Inflamed adenoids can also cause inflammation in the middle ear (OTITIS MEDIA) and the sinuses behind the nose (SINUSITIS). The doctor can tell whether ear, nose, and throat infections are caused by enlarged adenoids by looking at the back of a person's throat with a light and dental mirror. If the adenoids are infected, the doctor will prescribe antibiotics. When infections reoccur, surgical removal of the adenoids (ADE-NOIDECTOMY) may be recommended.

Adenoma

A benign (not cancerous) tumor of a glandular structure. Adenomas affect many organs such as the pituitary gland, the adrenal glands, and the thyroid glands (see THYROID NODULE).

PITUITARY ADENOMAS

A pituitary adenoma occurs in the pituitary gland, which is located at the base of the brain and produces many hormones that are involved in governing the activity of other glands. Deficiencies of the hormones involved with the thyroid glands and adrenal glands, as well as those involved with growth, balance of water in the body, and sexual function, may result. Small pituitary adenomas are common and, if nonsecreting, rarely produce symptoms. Secreting adenomas give off active hormones and can lead to diseases such as ACROMEGALY and CUSHING SYNDROME.

The rate of growth for a pituitary adenoma varies. It is a benign tumor that may grow gradually, causing few

if any symptoms, or it may show aggressive growth and compress surrounding brain tissues as it expands. The optic nerves or the sinuses may be affected by this compression. Symptoms could include headache and vision disturbances such as loss of peripheral vision, double vision, and drooping of the eyelids. Excessive thirst and urination, fatigue, light-headedness, and intolerance to cold are other symptoms of the presence of a pituitary adenoma. Younger people are affected more often by a fast-growing pituitary adenoma than are older people.

About half of all pituitary adenomas secrete excessive amounts of the hormone prolactin. The abnormally high amount of prolactin may not produce symptoms, or it may result in erectile dysfunction in men and absent menstrual periods in women. Excess prolactin may also cause galactorrhea, the abnormal production of breast milk in women. Pituitary adenomas that secrete excess ACTH (adrenocorticotropic hormone) produce Cushing syndrome.

ADRENAL ADENOMAS

Adrenal cortical adenomas are located on the adrenal cortex (the outer layer of the adrenal glands). These tumors are usually benign, tend to affect women more than men, and are more common in people older than 40 years. If the adenoma secretes cortisol (a hormone produced by the adrenal glands), Cushing syndrome can result. If it produces aldosterone, high blood pressure and low potassium levels can occur. Most adrenal adenomas are nonsecreting and are of concern only if they enlarge.

TREATMENT

Treatment of adenomas usually requires their surgical removal in combination with hormonal therapy to reestablish the proper balance of hormones in the body.

Adenomatosis

An abnormal increase in the number of cells of two or more glands, usually the thyroid gland, adrenal glands, or the pituitary gland, which increases the size of the glands. Adenomatosis is a form of HYPERPLASIA or tumor development affecting these glands and may cause overproduction of various hormones.

Adenomyosis

A condition characterized by abnormal menstrual pain, typically affecting women in their 40s. As a woman ages, endometrial tissue can become embedded in the muscular wall of the uterus. As a result, a woman may experience bleeding and painful menstruation. A doctor may prescribe hormonal medication to control pain and bleeding. If hormonal medications do not alleviate the woman's symptoms, a hysterectomy may be recommended. Menopause usually brings relief.

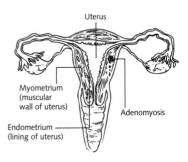

Uterus

Myometrium (muscular wall of uterus)

Adenomyosis

Endometrium (lining of uterus)

FORMATION OF ADENOMYOSIS
Adenomyosis is a condition in which cells of the endometrium (the lining of the uterus) penetrate the muscular wall of the uterus, causing the organ to enlarge and become hard. Although the symptoms may be difficult to tolerate, the condition is benign and does not lead to cancer.

Adenosine diphosphate

See ADP.

Adenosine triphosphate

See ATP.

Adenovirus

A type of virus most commonly associated with respiratory illness. Adenoviruses can also cause gastroenteritis (particularly watery diarrhea), conjunctivitis, cystitis, and rash. When this virus causes respiratory illness, the infection may range from the level of the common cold to more serious illness including pneumonia, croup, and bronchitis. Acute respiratory illness may be caused by infections that occur during conditions of overcrowding and stress.

Adenoviruses are unusually stable and can survive for prolonged periods outside the body. Infections caused by this virus are usually mild, and generally only the symptoms are treated. When serious illness results, it is managed by treating symptoms and complications since no virus-specific therapy is available.

ADH

Antidiuretic hormone; also known as vasopressin. A naturally occurring hormone that regulates fluid balance and blood pressure. ADH is produced by the hypothalamus and has the principal physiological activity of controlling urine volume. It prevents excessive urine production by signaling the kidneys to concentrate the urine, extract water from the urine as it forms, and return the extracted water to the circulation.

ADH is secreted in accordance with the needs of the body. The hypothalamus has receptors that can detect the water concentration in the blood and release ADH accordingly. Conditions such as dehydration or hemorrhaging (in which circulating volume drops below normal) stimulate the hypothalamus to release ADH into the bloodstream. The ADH then stimulates the kidneys to concentrate the urine and conserve the balance of water in the body. ADH also limits the production of perspiration when the body is dehydrated. When the body contains an excessive amount of water, the hypothalamus detects this condition and stops secreting ADH, allowing the kidneys to release a higher volume of urine and normalize body fluids. Certain psychological conditions and substances influence the secretion of ADH. Pain and stress stimulate ADH secretion, as does nicotine, causing less urine to be produced and released. Alcohol inhibits ADH, increasing urine production and possibly contributing to the excessive thirst associated with a hangover.

Vasopressin medication may be administered by injection to control frequent urination and increased thirst in addition to similar symptoms of other disorders, including DIABETES INSIPIDUS. Diabetes insipidus is caused by a lack of ADH in the blood or by the inability of the kidneys to respond normally to this hormone.

ADHD

The acronym for ATTENTION DEFICIT/ HYPERACTIVITY DISORDER.

Adhesions

Bands of scar tissue that form between the loops of the intestines or between the intestines and the abdominal wall. Adhesions develop as tissues heal after abdominal surgery or when there is inflammation of the membrane lining the abdominal wall. Adhesions may cause pain in the abdomen when they are pulled or stretched because scar tissue is not elastic.

Abdominal adhesions rarely cause serious problems. However, at times, a loop of intestine slips under an adhesion and becomes trapped. This can lead to an obstruction of the intestine (see INTESTINE, OBSTRUCTION OF). Gangrene, the death of tissue, can develop if the blood supply to part of the intestine is interrupted. If the trapped intestine is not freed spontaneously or by using techniques such as decompressing the intestine with suction, surgery may be necessary. In this procedure, the abdomen is opened and the adhesions are cut away, releasing the trapped intestine. If part of the intestine has become gangrenous, it is removed and the healthy remaining parts of the intestine are rejoined. Although more adhesions may develop later, most do not cause problems.

Adhesive otitis media, chronic

The end stage of middle ear effusion (accumulation of fluid) that leads to EUSTACHIAN TUBE dysfunction. The eardrum becomes thinner and retracts toward the inner wall of the middle ear. In time, the drum may contact the incus and stapes (small middle ear bones) and even drape over them or touch the inner wall of the middle ear. Early on, this process can be reversed by placement of a drainage tube. In time, the drum may become scarred at the areas of contact, and tubes will become less helpful. The volume of air or fluid in the middle ear will shrink—sometimes down to nothing. The middle ear bones may erode, and sometimes tissue with a grainy texture (granulation tissue) grows from poorly covered bone. The ear may drain, and the tissue growth may resemble a tumor.

Careful examination and cleaning under a microscope, treatment of the inflammation, and CT (computed tomography) scanning will help make the proper diagnosis. Fortunately, hearing loss is usually mild with this condition and usually does not progress. In cases of more severe hearing loss, a hearing aid or surgery is an option, but surgery is difficult and requires a lifetime of tubes to maintain any gain. The condition can progress to a tumor, especially in children and young adults. Examination once or twice a year for a few years by a doctor is needed once this diagnosis is made. See also OTITIS MEDIA.

Adipose tissue

Animal tissue containing fat. Adipose means "fat," and adipose tissue refers specifically to tissue found under the skin or around internal organs that is chiefly made up of fat cells.

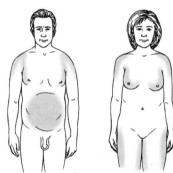

ACCUMULATION OF BODY FAT
Both distribution and proportion of body fat differ between men and women. A man tends to accumulate fat at the shoulders, waist, and abdomen, while a woman has a greater proportion of body fat overall, deposited around the breasts, hips, and thighs. Diet and exercise can substantially alter accumulation of fat.

Adjustment disorder

A mental illness characterized by a disturbing emotional or behavioral reaction to stress that affects the individual's ability to function in work and social life or that greatly exceeds the normal reaction to that type of stress. If adjustment disorder begins in response to a single event, it arises within 3 months of the event and usually improves within 6 months. If the source of stress is ongoing, the disorder may persist for longer than 6 months. A person with adjustment disorder may not be aware of the severity of the stress that underlies the disorder. Adjustment disorder is not usually the diagnosis when an individual is reacting to the death of a loved one (see GRIEVING) or if the person has a history of pre-existing disorders, such as mood or anxiety disorders.

CAUSES AND SYMPTOMS

Adjustment disorder is common; it affects people of all ages. In adults, probable stressors include marital or romantic discord, divorce and separation, financial trouble, loss of a job, work conflicts, life changes such as retirement or menopause, unexpected catastrophes and accidents, a chronic and disabling medical condition, and problems in school. Among adolescents the disorder is likely to be precipitated by parental rejection, family breakup because of divorce, domestic conflict or violence, sexual problems, and trouble with school. The circumstances of an individual's life, such as economic conditions, social and family support, and employment and recreational opportunities, also have a role in the development of the disorder.

Adjustment disorder is often characterized by difficulty meeting the demands of work or school, usually accompanied by a depressed mood. Other symptoms can include hopelessness, frequent crying, agitation, trembling or twitching, heart palpitations, disruptive behavior, vague physical complaints such as headache or stomach pain, anxiety, and sensations of stress or tension.

TREATMENT AND OUTCOME

Adjustment disorder is considered less serious than other psychiatric disorders, but it does increase the risk of suicide and can result in severe depression if left untreated. The goal of treatment is to relieve symptoms and help the individual resolve the emotional conflict so that he or she can return to normal functioning. In most cases, some form of therapy, such as individual psychotherapy, family therapy, behavior therapy, or a self-help group, is recommended.

> Terms in small capital letters—for example, PHYSICAL THERAPY or PAGET DISEASE—indicate a cross-reference to another entry with more information.

Medication may be used, but usually in conjunction with therapy.

Adjuvants

In immunology, substances that are given with antigens to boost a person's immune response. Adjuvants may be classified in two ways: according to their origin (for example, those produced organically or synthetically) or according to their mechanism of action (for example, adjuvants may enhance delivery of the antigen to the immune system or have a direct effect on infection-fighting cells). Some examples of adjuvants include aluminum derivatives, bacterial products, and synthetic polymers.

Adolescence

A period of rapid physical, emotional, social, and intellectual growth from ages 10 through 21. Adolescence begins at PUBERTY with the onset of physical and sexual developments that enable reproduction and ends with the transition into adulthood. Developmentally, adolescence is viewed as beginning at age 10 and proceeding in three stages: early (ages 10 to 13); middle (ages 14 to 17); and late (ages 18 to 21).

The early stage is characterized by the start of puberty (sexual maturation) and a major growth spurt. Girls usually experience puberty a year or two before boys. With the middle stage come intensified sexual desires, increased sociability, and experiments with risky behavior such as smoking, trying alcohol and drugs, and having unprotected sex. Peer pressure becomes a strong influence. In the late stage, the adolescent begins to settle down and focus energies on plans for the future. The psychosocial development of adolescence involves several tasks concerned with transforming the child into an adult. They include establishing independence, achieving a realistic and satisfying self-image, exploring sexuality, and choosing life roles, for example, a career. As the child tries to accomplish these tasks, conflicts often arise.

PHYSICAL HEALTH

As adolescents learn to live independently, they often set their health habits for a lifetime. Establishing healthful behavior such as exercising, eating

right, and not smoking in adolescence can influence lifelong health.

Because of the tremendous growth spurt that takes place during puberty, teenagers require extra calories and good nutrition. Calcium is essential, because half the body's total bone mass is formed during these years. Consuming adequate calcium in adolescence can help protect an individual from the bone-thinning disease osteoporosis in later years. The daily calcium requirement for children over age 10 is 1,300 milligrams a day. The need for iron increases, too. In girls, iron becomes depleted by blood loss during menstruation. Boys need more because of increased muscle growth. Adolescents require at least 15 milligrams of iron per day.

Eating disorders are a serious problem among adolescents, especially girls. ANOREXIA NERVOSA (an intense fear of gaining weight that leads to self-starvation) and BULIMIA (binge eating followed by self-induced vomiting) often become established during the teen years. Both can result in serious chemical imbalances, malnutrition, and many other significant medical problems. An adolescent suspected of having an eating disorder should see a doctor.

Exercise is especially beneficial in the teen years to maintain muscle strength and ensure proper skeletal development. Lack of exercise can lead to weight problems and has been associated with a higher risk of engaging in potentially dangerous behavior. Participating in sports and other physical activities and limiting time spent using the TV or telephone or in other stationary activities can increase overall fitness and maintain proper weight. Adolescents require 9 hours of sleep a night, but often get 6 or fewer. A lack of sleep can contribute to moodiness and depression in teens. Physical changes also heighten the need for attention to personal hygiene. Elevated hormone production causes sweat glands to produce perspiration and body odor and also increases the risk of acne. Daily bathing or showering is suggested for all teens.

BEHAVIOR

Adolescents strive for independence, but at the same time require the love, support, and approval of their parents. Striking the perfect balance is both difficult and rare. It is normal for conflicts to develop about how much independence is appropriate. It is normal for teens to react emotionally when they feel they are not getting their needs met.

In the late stage, adolescents run an increased risk of depression; girls are at twice the risk as boys. Frequency of suicide and attempted suicide is also high among adolescents. Difficulty making the transition from childhood to adulthood, family conflicts, and pressures from school and jobs all can contribute to depression. Symptoms of depression in adolescents include talk of feeling sad, bored, or empty; changes in sleep or eating habits; extreme mood swings; and risky behavior. A child with any of these symptoms needs to see a mental health professional. Treatment of adolescent depression is usually successful, especially when initiated in the early stages of depression.

Hormonal changes in adolescence trigger powerful sexual urges, and most teenagers act on them. However, many teens do not yet possess the maturity to understand the physical and emotional risks of sexual activity. Therefore, adolescent sexual relationships often have negative consequences, including high incidences of emotional stress, unwanted pregnancy, and sexually transmitted diseases. SEX EDUCATION programs have been shown to reduce incidence of pregnancy in teenagers.

HIGH-RISK BEHAVIOR

Adolescents frequently feel invulnerable and do not recognize the consequences of dangerous activities, such as driving too fast, having sex without a condom, or ingesting dangerous chemicals. Motor vehicle collisions are the leading cause of death among 15- to 20-year-olds. Safe driving is an often overlooked and important key to maintaining adolescent health. Because they are learning to be independent, adolescents often try new things, despite inherent dangers. Young people are being exposed to drugs at increasingly younger ages, and it is becoming easier for underage children to obtain alcohol, tobacco, and illegal drugs. Many adolescents experiment with alcohol and drugs. (See also ALCOHOL DEPENDENCE and DRUG ADDICTION.) Adolescent participation in high-risk behavior such as

smoking or drinking is lower for teens whose parents set clear limits and enforce them. Teens whose parents smoke or drink are more likely to do so. Signs of teen substance abuse include drastic mood swings, falling grades, poor hygiene, isolation, and lack of interest in recreational activities. When an adolescent has a substance abuse problem, early intervention has been shown to be effective.

During adolescence, teens begin to seek approval from their classmates and friends rather than their parents. Peers pressure them to participate in behavior that they might ordinarily avoid. There may be pressure to rebel against parental or school authority or to use alcohol or other drugs. Teens may find it difficult to resist a boyfriend's or girlfriend's demands to engage in sexual activity. Teens who participate in clubs, teams, and other extracurricular activities are more likely to resist peer pressure. Such outside interests are believed to help teens resist peer pressure by helping to release stress and build self-esteem.

ADP

Adenosine diphosphate. An organic compound that consists of adenine, ribose, and two phosphate units. ADP is formed when adenosine triphosphate (ATP) is broken down by its reaction with water so that one phosphate unit and one hydrogen ion are removed from the ATP molecule. Most of the reactions that consume energy in the cells are driven by the conversion of ATP to ADP. These reactions include transmitting nerve signals, moving muscles, synthesizing protein, and dividing cells.

Adrenal failure

A sudden, potentially fatal condition that occurs when the adrenal glands do not produce and release a sufficient amount of cortisol; also known as adrenal crisis, addisonian crisis, or acute adrenal insufficiency. Cortisol is a hormone that enables the body to use nutrients, cope with stress, and regulate the immune system. Adrenal failure can also be caused by a sudden withdrawal of corticosteroid medications (see CORTICOSTEROIDS), failure of the pituitary gland, or removal of or injury to the adrenal glands through surgery or infection.

Symptoms include headache, profound weakness, fatigue, lethargic movement, nausea, decreased blood pressure, dehydration, and high fever. Adrenal failure can be diagnosed by the ACTH (adrenocorticotropic hormone) stimulation test, other blood tests, and urine analysis.

Adrenal failure is a medical emergency that requires immediate treatment to avoid shock or even death. Emergency treatment for adrenal failure is an injection of the corticosteroid hydrocortisone. The person must be hospitalized for general observation and for treatment of low blood pressure with intravenous fluids. Antibiotics may be given if infection is involved.

Adrenal glands

The two vital organs that produce and secrete hormones into the bloodstream via veins that drain them; also known as suprarenal glands. Each triangular-shaped adrenal gland is located on top of one of the two kidneys on the right and left sides of the body. The adrenal glands are covered by a thick layer of fatty connective tissue and an outer, thin, fibrous capsule. The adrenal glands have two parts composed of different kinds of cellular tissue and function as separate organs.

The inner portion of an adrenal gland is the smaller portion of the gland. It is called the adrenal medulla and secretes the hormone EPINEPHRINE, which is also called adrenaline. Epinephrine is produced by the sympathetic nervous system at times of stress, and it helps regulate blood pressure and increase heart rate as well as raise the blood sugar level. The adrenal medulla also secretes NOREPINEPHRINE, a hormone that helps maintain normal blood pressure.

The outer layer of the adrenal glands, called the adrenal cortex, makes up the bulk of the gland. The cortex can secrete as many as 30 different steroid hormones in varying amounts. Among the hormones that are secreted in significant amounts, ALDOSTERONE is important for regulating salt and water in the body, and CORTISOL is essential for regulating the response to stress, as well as for regulating the metabolism of fat, carbohydrate, and protein. Adrenal sex steroids are usually the major source of testosterone in women. They are of little importance in men because the testicles make larger amounts of testosterone.

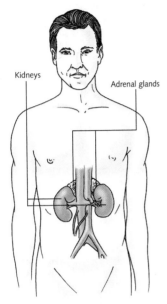

Kidneys

Adrenal glands

LOCATION OF THE ADRENAL GLANDS
The two adrenal glands rest on top of each kidney and receive their blood supply though the renal (kidney) arteries. They release vital hormones directly into the bloodstream, in amounts governed by hormones produced in the pituitary gland and the hypothalamus.

Adrenal hyperplasia, congenital

A group of disorders caused by a deficiency of the enzyme that is essential to the production, by the adrenal cortex (the outer layer of the adrenal glands), of steroid hormones called corticosteroids. The enzyme deficiency in a fetus is the result of inheriting two defective genes, one from the father and one from the mother. Two groups of corticosteroid hormones that are active in the body (glucocorticoids and mineralocorticoids) are affected in the most common form of congenital adrenal hyperplasia. The enzyme deficiency creates a block in the pathway to synthesize the complete hormone. Low levels of the glucocorticoid hormone called CORTISOL can result in an impaired response to stress and other metabolic problems. When there is insufficient circulating cortisol, the pituitary gland secretes an abnormally high amount of ACTH (adrenocorticotropic hormone) to

send a signal to the adrenal glands to produce more cortisol. When congenital adrenal hyperplasia causes a deficiency in the hormone ALDOSTERONE, a potentially life-threatening imbalance between the water and salt in the body results.

Even though the adrenal glands enlarge and work overtime in response to the hormone deficiency, the enzyme deficiency blocks the synthesis of cortisol or aldosterone, resulting in deficient levels of these hormones. Hormone production then shifts toward the sex steroids, especially ANDROGEN HORMONES, which are male hormones. These hormones can produce enlarged external genitalia in male and female infants.

When severe, congenital adrenal hyperplasia produces an inability to respond to stress and properly maintain the balance of salt and water in the body. An affected fetus may become extremely dehydrated, and ADRENAL FAILURE may occur. In milder cases, congenital adrenal hyperplasia may not be diagnosed until after infancy or even until adulthood. Less

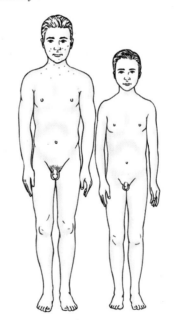

OVERPRODUCTION OF ANDROGEN HORMONES
Of these fraternal twins, age 6, the boy on the left has congenital adrenal hyperplasia. The overproduction of androgen hormones has caused an early growth spurt and prematurely advanced secondary sex characteristics—facial and body hair and a deep voice.

severe forms may result in early sexual development and rapid growth in childhood. Adolescent girls may experience growth of unwanted facial and body hair and irregular menstrual periods. Male and female adolescents may have severe acne. Women who have difficulty getting pregnant because of congenital adrenal hyperplasia may undergo treatment with hormone replacement therapy.

Congenital adrenal hyperplasia is diagnosed by analysis of blood and urine. The condition is generally treated in children by administering hydrocortisone medication, orally or by injection. In adolescents and adults, a more potent, longer-acting corticosteroid, such as prednisone or dexamethasone, may be given. There is also medication to correct salt imbalance. Genital surgery may be necessary for affected females. Psychological counseling is often recommended before puberty, especially for girls.

Adrenal tumors

Abnormal masses of tissue formed by increased cell growth in the adrenal glands; also known as nonfunctioning adrenal adenomas. Adrenal tumors may cause a number of effects or may not produce any symptoms or disorders. Often they are discovered incidentally when the abdomen is scanned for another purpose. Tests can verify that the tumor is producing an excess amount of hormones.

Most adrenal tumors are benign (not cancerous). Malignant (cancerous) adrenal tumors are rare, but cancer may be suspected when the tumor is solid and large or growing. In these cases, surgery may be recommended.

When an adrenal tumor on the adrenal cortex (the outer layer of the adrenal glands) produces excess cortisol, it may cause CUSHING SYNDROME. Tumors of the adrenal cortex may also produce excess sex hormones, causing ADRENOGENITAL SYNDROME. These excess sex hormones are usually the male sex hormones, ANDROGEN HORMONES. In women, androgens may result in menstrual irregularities, deepening of the voice, and hirsutism (excess facial and body hair). In rare instances, female sex hormones may produce erectile dysfunction or enlarged breasts in men. A tumor growing from the adrenal cortex can also produce excess ALDOSTERONE, resulting in high blood pressure.

Tumors of the adrenal medulla (the inner layer of the adrenal glands) cause excessive secretion of the medullary hormones such as EPINEPH-RINE. This can produce high blood pressure, an abnormal blood sugar level, an increased metabolic rate, nervousness, and excessive perspiration. Complications include stroke and cardiovascular disease, such as heart arrhythmias, if the hormone imbalance is not treated.

Adrenaline
See EPINEPHRINE.

Adrenocorticotropic hormone
See ACTH.

Adrenogenital syndrome
A condition, affecting both men and women, caused by the secretion of excess adrenal SEX HORMONES, typically male sex hormones. Adrenogenital syndrome is generally caused by a tumor (see ADRENAL TUMORS) on the adrenal cortex (the outer layer of the adrenal glands). An affected woman will have masculine hair growth patterns (including excess facial hair and sometimes male-pattern hair loss), deepening of the voice, an enlarged clitoris, and a masculine appearance of the skin and muscles. When adrenogenital syndrome occurs in boys before puberty, rapid sexual development may occur at an abnormally young age. In adult males, testosterone may obscure the signs. In rare cases, the adrenal tumor may secrete female hormones, producing enlarged breasts in men.

Advance directives
Legal documents that state how a person's health care should proceed if he or she becomes physically or mentally unable to communicate his or her wishes. Advance directives specify the type of care and who makes the care decisions and may provide instructions on other matters such as ORGAN DONATION. Their primary function is to give a person the option of avoiding aggressive treatments that may cause pain or incur great expense but offer little benefit.

Commonly prepared for older people, advance directives are also used by people with terminal illnesses, those with a condition that has a poor outlook, those who have a strong point of view concerning their care, and parents who do not want to spend their resources on their own terminal care.

TYPES OF DIRECTIVES
An individual usually creates advance directives for future use. Sometimes, as in a do not resuscitate order, a physician can make the order based on medical judgment or previous conversations with the patient or in consultation with a family member or close friend.

■ *Living will* A document made by a mentally competent adult that specifies which medical treatments he or she wants or does not want, in the event that he or she becomes unable to make decisions or communicate them. To be valid, the living will must be witnessed and signed, much like a last will and testament. The will becomes effective when a person loses the ability to express his or her preferences and has become mentally incapacitated or irreversibly unconscious or is in a persistent vegetative state. The living will can specify the nature of life-sustaining treatments to be withheld or withdrawn and the circumstances under which to enact these directives. The treatments specified may include basic measures, such as giving nutrition and fluids (hydration), that may prolong life but provide no comfort.

Almost all states recognize living will statutes. Many states have developed their own living will forms, and sometimes it is possible to sign a preprinted form. However, individuals can create their own personal statements naming the types of life-sustaining surgery or treatments they do or do not want and under what circumstances. Some individuals create living wills to avoid debate within their families over what they would have wanted had they been conscious and also to clarify their beliefs concerning controversial areas such as withholding food and fluids.

■ *Durable power of attorney for health care* A signed, dated, and witnessed document that designates a surrogate decision maker. With a power of attorney for health care, an individual authorizes another person,

or surrogate, such as a family member, close friend, lawyer, or member of the clergy, as an agent to make critical health care decisions when he or she no longer can. The document is designated as durable when it specifies that the agent is empowered to make decisions for the person after he or she becomes incapacitated. An ordinary, or nondurable, power of attorney becomes invalid when the person becomes incapacitated. The agent may be authorized to make decisions about all aspects of health care or only certain ones. Specific instructions about which surgery or medical treatments a person does or does not want can be included, or all decisions can be deferred to the agent. The agent acts as an advocate when a person is incapable of expressing his or her wishes and must try to make decisions the way that the individual would make them if he or she were able. The document can go into effect upon signing or when the person becomes incapacitated. Until the latter, it is possible to revoke the durable power of attorney at any time. Because there are so many options and decisions involved, an attorney usually prepares this type of directive. Another type of durable power of attorney concerns assigning responsibility for business and financial matters to an agent when an individual can no longer manage his or her financial affairs. The agent must follow the wishes of the individual and follow standards mandated by law.

■ *Do not resuscitate order (DNR order)* A directive designating that cardiopulmonary resuscitation (CPR) will not be administered if an individual's heart stops. Usually it is an entry made on a patient's medical record by a physician, based on an evaluation of the patient and the medical judgment that CPR would be futile or that administering CPR is against the patient's wishes. A person can request a DNR order in a living will or durable power of attorney for health care or when entering hospice care. A person may choose to have a DNR order take effect when he or she is irreversibly unconscious or in a persistent vegetative state. Some people may want to forego some types of life support, such as use of a mechanical VENTILATOR, but still may want some type of limited intervention, such as chest compressions. Those instructions can be given in a DNR order.

LEGAL ASPECTS
Federal and state laws regulate advance directives. The federal Patient Self-determination Act compels all hospitals, nursing facilities, hospices, home health agencies, and health maintenance organizations that participate in Medicare or Medicaid to educate their staff and community about health directives. They also must give their patients information about advance directives and about an individual's rights under state law to accept or refuse surgery or medical treatment, regardless of anticipated outcome. Laws concerning advance directives differ from state to state. Most states recognize the validity of advance directives written in another state. Individuals who spend long periods in more than one state are advised to be sure that their advance directives conform to the laws of both states. Persons who have an advance directive should carry a card stating that they have one and where it is. To ensure that advance directives are followed, one copy is usually given to the doctor and another to a family member, friend, or lawyer. No one can be denied admission to a hospital or nursing facility because he or she lacks an advance directive. Any existing health directive must be included in one's medical records. All advance directives can be changed or cancelled at any time.

Adverse drug reaction
An unexpected and potentially harmful response to a drug that is unrelated to its intended effect. Adverse drug reactions can occur because of the nature of the drug taken or because the person taking it is allergic to the drug. In most cases, these responses can occur suddenly or take days, weeks, or even months to appear. The cause of an adverse drug reaction is usually unknown and extremely difficult to predict. Adverse drug reactions are very common; about 10 percent of hospital admissions in the United States are estimated to be related to adverse drug reactions.

RISK FACTORS FOR DRUG REACTIONS

Taking several prescription and over-the-counter drugs contributes to the risk of having an adverse drug reaction. Some people are more at risk for having a drug reaction than others. They include:

- Older people
- Women who are pregnant or breast-feeding
- Babies and children
- People with liver disease or kidney disease
- People with cardiovascular disease
- People taking many medications

Adverse drug reactions can be divided into reactions that represent an excess of the intended effects, reactions that represent an unintended effect and are not understood, and allergic reactions to the drug. An example of an adverse reaction would be when a person with high blood pressure feels dizzy or lightheaded after taking medication; in such a case, the drug has reduced the blood pressure too much. Very small numbers of people develop unpredictable allergic reactions to a drug because of genetic differences in the way their bodies respond to that drug. Such allergic reactions may appear as skin rashes, liver or kidney damage, anemia, reduced white blood cell count, or nerve injury that leads to impaired vision or hearing.

Adverse drug reactions can be mild, moderate, or severe and life-threatening. Because most drugs are taken orally, either as pills or capsules, and are digested in the gastrointestinal tract, the most common reactions are nausea, loss of appetite, and diarrhea. Rashes are also a common adverse drug reaction.

Aerobic
Requiring oxygen. Aerobic is an adjective used to describe activities, life forms, or events that depend on the presence of oxygen.

Aerobic exercise includes brisk physical activities that require the heart and lungs to work harder than they usually do to meet the body's increased demands for oxygen.

Aerobic exercise promotes the circulation of oxygen in the blood. Typical examples of aerobic exercise include running, walking, swimming, dancing, and cycling. Exercise is considered aerobic if the person who is doing the exercise raises his or her heart rate for at least 20 minutes.

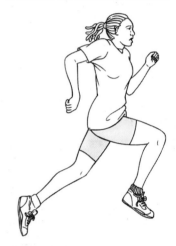

ENERGY WITH OXYGEN
An aerobic workout requires continuous activity that brings the heart rate up to within 70 to 80 percent of its maximum and maintains it at that level for at least 20 minutes. The increased heart rate supplies oxygen to provide energy for the muscles.

Aerodontalgia
Sudden tooth pain caused by changes in the atmospheric pressure; also known as barodontalgia or "flyer's toothache." The pain is usually caused by the change in surrounding air pressure inside an airplane during ascent. Changes in atmospheric pressure can cause a pocket of air within the dental pulp chamber to expand and irritate the nerve in the root. Aerodontalgia is sometimes caused by SINUSITIS, by incomplete dental or root canal treatments, or by dental cysts or abscesses. The condition can usually be avoided by using good oral hygiene practices.

Aerophagia
See AIR SWALLOWING.

Aerospace medicine
The branch of medicine concerned with the physiological and psychological problems of flight, especially those that occur beyond the earth's atmospheric and gravitational forces.

Affect

Refers to the emotion expressed by a person in speech, facial expressions, and behavior. Also refers to the regulation and expression of emotion.

Affective disorders

Another term for mood disorders, which are characterized by a disturbance in emotions and feelings. The disturbance may be expressed as either elation or unhappiness. There are various types of mood disorders, including DYSTHYMIA (a low-grade depression), major DEPRESSION, and BIPOLAR DISORDER.

AFP test

Alpha-fetoprotein test. A measurement of the level of alpha-fetoprotein (AFP) in a pregnant woman's blood; it reflects the amount of AFP produced by a developing fetus. The test is generally offered to women between weeks 15 and 21 of pregnancy and is used to detect birth defects. A high level of AFP in a woman's blood sometimes indicates that the fetus has a neural tube defect, a birth defect in which the skull, brain, or spinal cord does not develop properly. When the test indicates a high level of AFP, an ultrasound may be done to assess the health of the fetus (see ULTRASOUND, OBSTETRICAL). Subsequently, an AMNIOCENTESIS (a test that analyzes the liquid surrounding the fetus) may be done. An amniocentesis can provide a more direct measurement of an AFP level than a blood test and can confirm the presence of neural tube defects that may be missed by an ultrasound or other diagnostic tests. AFP testing combined with other biochemical and hormonal measurements can also screen for other fetal abnormalities, including Down syndrome.

If testing indicates that a fetus may have a genetic disorder, chromosomal abnormality, or serious birth defect, a woman may want to consider whether or not to terminate the pregnancy. In this situation, a woman's doctor may recommend GENETIC COUNSELING to help her make an informed decision.

Afterbirth

The PLACENTA and membranes that are expelled from the mother's body shortly after the birth of the baby. Delivery of the afterbirth commonly occurs within 30 minutes after delivery of the baby and is the final stage of LABOR. After childbirth, a woman's uterus continues to contract, as the placenta separates from the wall of the uterus. The contractions that deliver the afterbirth are not as painful as those that deliver the baby. Once the placenta has moved into the lower uterus or the vagina, a woman can help expel the afterbirth by pushing. The doctor may assist by placing one hand on the woman's abdomen and gently pulling on the umbilical cord with the other hand while the woman pushes.

When contractions of the uterus are not strong enough to deliver the afterbirth, the hormone OXYTOCIN may be given to augment contractions. When a placenta does not separate from the wall of her uterus, it can be removed manually. After the woman receives a mild painkiller, the doctor reaches into the uterus, manually separates the placenta from the uterine wall, and removes it. The afterbirth is carefully examined to verify that the entire placenta and all of the membranes have passed from the woman's body.

Afterpains

Crampy abdominal pains a woman feels after childbirth. After delivery, hormones stimulate contractions that help shrink the uterus to its prepregnancy size. Contractions may last for several days after the birth. When they are painful, the doctor may recommend a pain-relieving medication. Afterbirth pain may increase during breast-feeding because the baby's sucking increases the release of hormones that cause the uterus to contract. Because some medications can pass into breast milk, mothers who are breast-feeding should ask their doctors to recommend a safe pain medication.

Agar

A gelatinlike substance made from red seaweed. Agar is best known as a solidifying component used to culture bacteria for laboratory analysis. Agar is also used as a thickening agent in ice cream and salad dressing and as a substitute for gelatin.

Age spots

Flat gray or brown spots that appear on sun-exposed areas of aging skin (see SUN EXPOSURE, ADVERSE EFFECTS OF); also known as liver spots or solar lentigines. Age spots range from freckle-size to half an inch across. They are caused by cumulative exposure to the sun over the course of a lifetime. Age spots most commonly appear on the face, backs of the hands, chest, and upper back. True age spots are harmless. However, if a person finds them cosmetically disturbing, spots can be lightened with skin-bleaching products. Unlike age spots, large, flat, irregular dark areas can be a form of malignant melanoma (see MELANOMA, MALIGNANT) and require evaluation by a dermatologist.

Agenesis

Absence or lack of development of an organ in an embryo. Examples of agenesis include the absence of ovaries (ovarian agenesis), a defective development of part of the brain (callosal agenesis), or absence of kidneys (renal agenesis).

Agent

Any physical substance capable of producing an effect. An agent can produce a chemical or a biological effect. A pharmacological agent, for example, is one capable of causing a biological response, while a pathological agent is one capable of causing disease.

Agent Orange

An herbicide and a defoliant used by the United States military during the Vietnam War to kill vegetation in forested areas so that enemy guerrilla soldiers would be visible. Agent Orange was a mix of two weed killers developed in the 1940s containing dioxin, a contaminant that is suspected of causing certain cancers in those exposed to it. The name refers to the fact that orange labels were used on the 55-gallon drums in which the product was shipped.

Exposure to Agent Orange has been linked to certain chemical acne, non-Hodgkin lymphoma, HODGKIN DISEASE, and soft-tissue SARCOMA. In 1979, veterans of the Vietnam War filed a class action suit against the manufacturers of Agent Orange that resulted in no admission of liability but ended with a 1987 financial settlement of $180 million, intended to compensate veterans afflicted with disability or disease as a result of exposure to the herbicide.

Ageusia

A loss or impairment of the sense of taste. This can be caused by multiple conditions, including normal aging, smoking, xerostomia (dryness of the mouth), oropharyngeal tumors, malnutrition, and medication reactions. Individuals often assume they have lost their sense of taste when they lose their sense of smell (anosmia).

Aggregation

The ability of the cells known as platelets to clump together to form a clot and stop bleeding. In people who have bleeding problems, aggregation can be measured by taking a sample of blood, mixing it with a substance that causes it to clot, and determining how fast the platelets aggregate.

Aggression

Any form of behavior that entails self-assertion through a domineering, forceful, or assaultive verbal or physical action. Aggression may arise from inborn drives and needs, or it may be a response to frustration. Aggression can be expressed in a variety of ways: a destructive attack, a hostile attitude, or a healthy desire toward mastery.

It also can be directed inward or at inanimate objects or can be triggered by a trivial event, or it may be unprovoked. See EXPLOSIVE DISORDER.

Aging

The decline, over time, of the body's organ systems. Genetics, lifestyle, and disease all influence the rate of aging. Far-ranging physiological changes are a part of aging. Homeostasis, the process through which the body adjusts to external change, becomes impaired. The reserve, or capacity, of many body functions is decreased. For example, growing older diminishes lung capacity, impairing the body's ability to deal with polluted air and making the older individual more sensitive to "smog alert" days. Decreased lung capacity also brings vulnerability to respiratory infections such as PNEUMONIA, which are likely to

cause serious illness or even death. However, chronic disease and disability were once thought to be an inevitable part of aging, and that is no longer the case. Life expectancy in the United States nearly doubled in the 20th century. Today Americans who reach age 60 can expect to live beyond 80. Significant progress has been made in the prevention and treatment of disease. Many serious illnesses that not long ago were life-threatening are now preventable or controllable.

CAUSES OF AGING

The reasons people change as they grow older are not completely understood. In gerontology, the scientific study of the aging process, theories of aging fall into two major overlapping groups. Programmed theories of aging emphasize the notion of internal biological clocks. Meanwhile, damage—or error—theories stress the environmental factors that damage cells and gradually impair organ function.

The programmed theories of aging include programmed senescence, endocrine theory, and immunological theory. Programmed senescence suggests that aging is the result of genetic mechanisms that turn genes on and off, with senescence defined as the period in which genetically programmed changes take place. Endocrine theory holds that, through the actions of hormones, biological clocks control the process of aging. In immunological theory, the programmed decline of the immune system is thought to lead to increasing susceptibility to infectious disease and tumors and, therefore, aging and death.

Damage and error theories of aging suggest that an accumulation of damage from the environment ages the organism. Cells and tissues simply wear out over the years. Some experts believe that the greater the rate of basal metabolism (the rate the body consumes oxygen in the metabolic process), the shorter the life span. Others believe that the accumulation of cross-linked proteins damages cells and tissues. One known example of cross-linked proteins occurs in collagen, a fibrous protein that gives elasticity to the tendons and skin. With age, collagen molecules link, reducing elasticity in those tissues. The theory suggests that similar

cross-linking occurs in other body tissues and affects their functions. Some gerontologists speculate that free radicals, biochemical units that damage DNA, may eventually cause organs to stop working properly.

MANAGING THE AGING PROCESS

People age at different rates. While innate genetic makeup cannot change, lifestyle choices, such as diet, exercise, smoking, and drinking, can modify the aging process. For example, smoking may hasten the aging-related decline in pulmonary function. Recent increases in Americans' calcium intake and the popularity of activities related to weight-bearing exercise may, in the future, result in fewer cases of the aging-related bone disease OSTEOPOROSIS and its consequent bone fractures. Exercise has been shown to preserve balance and increase cardiovascular fitness and muscle strength. Weight-bearing exercise increases bone strength. Hence, a 75-year-old marathoner may be more cardiovascularly fit than a sedentary 20-year-old.

Agitation

Feelings of extreme anxiety accompanied by restlessness of the muscles. Agitation is often shown by repeated twitching or hyperactivity of the face, arms, or legs. Other symptoms of agitation include pacing, hand wringing, head rubbing, fidgeting, or playing with one's fingers. Agitation may be a symptom of a serious underlying psychiatric disorder.

Agnosia

A brain disorder characterized by an inability to interpret sensations correctly. Agnosia can attack any of the five senses. For example, visual agnosia is the inability to identify familiar objects, people, or written words, even though vision is intact. In auditory agnosia, a person can hear but not interpret sounds (such as speech). Olfactory agnosia affects smell, gustatory agnosia affects taste, and ASTEREOGNOSIS is an inability to identify objects by the sense of touch. Time agnosia is a disorder of time awareness, while visual-spatial agnosia reflects an inability to perform simple tasks under visual control or to analyze spatial relationships. A disconnection between the primary sensory auditory or visual input cortex and the related areas in the brain is believed to cause agnosia. Treatment depends on the underlying cause.

Agonal

Involving intense pain; death throes. Agonal is derived from the word "agony." It is used to describe intense pain, particularly that associated with dying.

Agonist

A substance responsible for triggering a response in a cell. Agonist drugs are sometimes called "mimics" because they mimic part of the normal activity within a cell. Agonist drugs work by enhancing or restoring a cell's normal activity.

Agoraphobia

An intense, debilitating fear of open public spaces, such as churches, stores, shopping malls, sports stadiums, and freeways, where escape is difficult or help may not be available if the individual experiences severe anxiety or panic. The word comes from Greek roots that mean "fear of the marketplace." People with agoraphobia often avoid public settings and crowds and may refuse to venture outside the home. The disease impairs the ability of the person to work and have a social life.

Agoraphobia usually begins in a person's 20s, and it affects more women than men. Symptoms include fear of being alone, remaining intentionally housebound for long periods, fear of losing control in public places, feelings of helplessness and dependence, fear of being crazy or dying, feelings that the body or the environment is unreal, and unusual outbursts of anger with twitching. The extreme anxiety or panic is experienced as light-headedness, excessive sweating, heart palpitations, chest pain, difficulty breathing, nausea and vomiting, numbness and tingling, stomach pain or distress, chills or hot flashes, and choking. Agoraphobia may occur alone or with PANIC DISORDER. Untreated, the disease can lead to major depression.

Agoraphobia may be biologically based, but the exact cause remains unknown. Treatment works best when begun early. It consists of medication to alleviate the anxiety along with psychotherapy to teach the person techniques for reducing anxiety. People with agoraphobia should avoid caffeine and other stimulants.

Agraphia

A loss of the ability to write as a result of brain damage. (See DYSLEXIA.) Damage is commonly localized to the posterior part of the brain, although lesions elsewhere have also been associated with difficulty writing. Writing problems most often occur with expressive language problems but can occur in isolation. Agraphia can be divided into the following categories: aphasic agraphia (inability to spell or use correct grammar), constructional agraphia (difficulty spacing or organizing letters correctly), and apraxic agraphia (difficulty coordinating hand movements to write).

AIDS

Acquired immunodeficiency syndrome caused by the human immunodeficiency virus, or HIV. AIDS results when a person's immune system is damaged by HIV infection; this allows other organisms to infect the body, which has become ill equipped to resist them.

A person is diagnosed as having AIDS after developing one of the opportunistic infections that are defined as AIDS-related illnesses. A person who is HIV-positive but has not had an AIDS-related illness such as recurring pneumonia or Kaposi sarcoma, for example, may also be diagnosed with AIDS based on certain blood tests that indicate a severely damaged immune system.

HIV infection usually results in AIDS after a long incubation period during which there are no symptoms. Before it is detected, HIV can weaken the immune system to the extent that the body cannot defend itself against the germs and diseases that become opportunistic infections.

Infections that are generally warded off by a healthy immune system cause serious problems and are often life-threatening for people who have AIDS. Medical intervention may be required to prevent or treat these infections, but AIDS may still result in death due to diseases the body's immune system would normally resist.

SYMPTOMS

The symptoms of AIDS are similar to those of many different illnesses and infections, and each AIDS symptom could also be related to another condition. These symptoms include rapid weight loss; dry cough; recurring fever; profuse night sweats; severe fatigue; swollen lymph glands (located in the armpits, groin, or neck); persistent diarrhea; and memory loss, depression, dementia, and other psychological problems. Certain types of pneumonia or tuberculosis may indicate AIDS. White spots or other lesions in the mouth or on the tongue and in the throat may be symptomatic of AIDS, as are red, brown, pink, or purplish patches under the skin or inside the mouth, nose, or eyelids.

CAUSES

AIDS is caused by HIV, which is passed from one person to another via blood contact or sexual contact. Infection occurs when blood, semen, vaginal fluid, or breast milk from an infected person enters the body of another person. HIV enters the body via the anus or rectum, the vagina, the penis, the mouth, mucous membranes such as those in the eyes or inside the nose, or surface cuts and sores on the skin. The virus may also enter the body through a vein during intravenous injections. Infection occurs most commonly during unprotected vaginal, anal, or oral sex and via needles shared for the injection of illicit drugs. A woman who is infected with HIV and pregnant can pass the virus to her infant during pregnancy, childbirth, or breast-feeding.

Transfusions of infected blood can infect a person with HIV. Since 1985, however, donated blood in the United States is screened for HIV, which makes the risk of infection extremely low. Rarely, health care workers are infected when stuck with needles contaminated with HIV-infected blood or after exposure to infected blood that infects an open cut.

HIV is not transmitted casually and cannot be spread through the air, through water, by insects, or during ordinary social contact such as shaking hands or kissing.

TESTING OPTIONS AND RESULTS

It should not be assumed that symptoms alone indicate a diagnosis of

A

TIMELINE OF THE AIDS EPIDEMIC

Here are some highlights of public health developments regarding AIDS:

June 5, 1981: The *Morbidity and Mortality Weekly Report* publishes a report of five gay men, all previously healthy, with pneumocystis pneumonia.

1982: Centers for Disease Control and Prevention (CDC) officially coins the term acquired immunodeficiency syndrome, or AIDS.

1984: The cause of AIDS is identified as a retrovirus: human immunodeficiency virus.

1985: Food and Drug Administration (FDA) approves first blood test to screen for HIV. Blood banks begin screening the blood supply. Actor Rock Hudson dies of AIDS-related complications.

March 19, 1987: FDA approves zidovudine, or AZT, the first antiretroviral drug for treatment of the disease.

1988: National Institutes of Health (NIH) establishes Office of AIDS Research.

1990: Ryan White, a teen with hemophilia, dies at the age of 18; he had become well-known in the effort to raise awareness after being diagnosed with AIDS contracted from blood products. He successfully sued his school district for the right to attend classes and was the namesake for landmark federal legislation.

1991: Professional basketball player Magic Johnson announces that he is HIV-positive and retires from basketball.

1992: AIDS becomes the number one cause of death for men aged 25 to 44.

1993: CDC expands the case definition of AIDS to include conditions specific to women and those more common among injection drug users.

1994: NIH issues guidelines requiring applicants for grants to address inclusion of women and minorities in clinical research.

December 6, 1995: FDA approves first protease inhibitor, saquinavir. Highly active anti-retroviral therapy (HAART) is born.

1997: AIDS-related deaths in the United States decline by more than 40 percent.

1998: First large-scale human trials for an HIV vaccine begin. First reports of treatment failure and side effects from HAART.

1999: There are 33.6 million people throughout the world living with HIV or AIDS, with two thirds of them residing in Africa.

2000: United Nations Program on HIV and AIDS, World Health Organization, and other groups announce a global initiative to negotiate reduced prices for AIDS drugs in developing countries. The initiative was started because more than 95 percent of those with HIV or AIDS live in developing countries with very limited access to antiretroviral therapy. In Africa, for example, 25 million are infected with HIV or have AIDS, but fewer than 25,000 were able to afford life-sustaining medication before this initiative began.

2001: More than 400,000 Americans have died of AIDS-related complications since 1981. Estimates indicate that between 800,000 and 900,000 people are currently living with AIDS in the United States.

2002: The UN estimates that life expectancy will drop to 45 by 2010 in Africa, due to AIDS.

Adapted by permission of *American Medical News*, Kaiser Foundation, Centers for Disease Control and Prevention, UNAIDS.

AIDS. The medical diagnosis must be made by a doctor based on specific criteria, including a positive result for HIV infection, which is detected by tests for antibodies that combat HIV. These antibodies generally develop within 25 days to 3 months following infection, but may not be detectable for up to 6 months.

Testing for AIDS may be available at a local health department, doctor's office, hospitals, and HIV testing clinics. Many testing sites also provide counseling services to help people understand the test results, their treatment options, and resources available to them in the area.

The enzyme-linked immunosorbent assay, or ELISA blood test, is a complex and highly sensitive test that measures antibodies produced in response to the presence of a viral or other infection. This test is considered especially useful in diagnosing HIV. The enzyme immunoassay, or EIA, is another standard screening test used to determine the presence of antibodies to HIV. This test may be performed as a blood test or an oral swab. A positive ELISA or EIA test result is confirmed by another blood test called a Western blot test. Blood test results are typically available within 1 to 2 weeks. Another test called the polymerase chain reaction, or PCR, is a specialized blood test that offers the advantage of detecting the virus soon after infection, although this test is expensive.

People being tested for AIDS may choose between confidential and anonymous testing options. Confidential testing offers the person tested an official copy of test results with his or her name on it. These confidential results become part of a person's medical records and may be released only with the person's written permission. Anonymous testing provides test results that are identified only by a number, and the person tested is the only one to know the results.

Positive test results indicate an infection with HIV, but may or may not indicate that a person will develop AIDS or HIV-related symptoms and illness. Further evaluation may be necessary to discover damage to the immune system or conditions indicating AIDS. A person with a positive test result is infectious and capable of spreading the HIV virus to others.

Negative test results are not always conclusive; they may indicate that the person is not infected with HIV or that the infection has not yet produced enough antibodies to be detected; this only occurs very early in the course of infection with HIV. Almost everyone with HIV infection

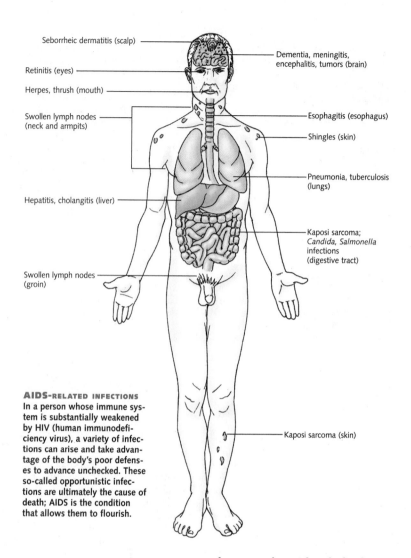

Seborrheic dermatitis (scalp)

Retinitis (eyes)

Herpes, thrush (mouth)

Swollen lymph nodes (neck and armpits)

Hepatitis, cholangitis (liver)

Swollen lymph nodes (groin)

Dementia, meningitis, encephalitis, tumors (brain)

Esophagitis (esophagus)

Shingles (skin)

Pneumonia, tuberculosis (lungs)

Kaposi sarcoma; *Candida, Salmonella* infections (digestive tract)

Kaposi sarcoma (skin)

AIDS-RELATED INFECTIONS
In a person whose immune system is substantially weakened by HIV (human immunodeficiency virus), a variety of infections can arise and take advantage of the body's poor defenses to advance unchecked. These so-called opportunistic infections are ultimately the cause of death; AIDS is the condition that allows them to flourish.

AIDS-related cancers

Cancers associated with AIDS (acquired immunodeficiency syndrome). In AIDS, the destruction of T-helper cells, a type of white blood cell, can severely weaken the immune system. People with AIDS are therefore especially susceptible to infections in which T cells are an important defense. Although AIDS itself is not a cancer, it has been associated with several different cancers, some of which were uncommon or even rare before people with AIDS began to develop them.

Among the cancers associated with AIDS is KAPOSI SARCOMA, a form of skin cancer. Kaposi sarcoma is most common among people with AIDS, although it is seen in people who do not have AIDS, such as kidney transplant recipients. Kaposi sarcoma is triggered by a virus called Kaposi sarcoma–associated herpesvirus (KSHV), also known as human herpesvirus 8 (HHV-8). Other AIDS-related cancers include cancer of the cervix and various lymphomas (cancers of the lymphatic system), such as BURKITT LYMPHOMA and non-Hodgkin lymphoma (see LYMPHOMA, NON-HODGKIN).

Air ambulance

Aircraft used to transport critically ill people to medical facilities from usually remote areas. Air ambulance services operate throughout the United States, and they can provide medical escorts for international flights. Air ambulances are staffed with medical personnel and outfitted

will test positive within 6 months of infection.

TREATMENT
While there is no medically recognized cure for AIDS at this time, early detection offers the best prospects for treatment and preventive care. Treatments are now available to help strengthen the immune system and decrease the usual speed at which HIV weakens it. Antiretroviral therapy (especially combination therapy) is able to slow the progression of the virus, and there are several treatments to prevent or cure some of the opportunistic infections associated with AIDS. Fifteen different antiviral medications are available, which when used in combination, successfully slow the progression of disease,

decrease the risk of death, and improve the quality of life for people with AIDS.

RISKS AND PREVENTION
Avoiding the known circumstances that result in HIV infection is the best approach to avoiding AIDS. Unprotected sexual contact or sharing needles with an HIV-infected person or with a person whose health status is uncertain or unknown carries a strong risk of contracting AIDS via infection with HIV.

AIDS drugs

See ALITRETINOIN; NONNUCLEOSIDE REVERSE TRANSCRIPTASE INHIBITORS (NNRTIS); PROTEASE INHIBITORS; ZALCITABINE (DDC); ZIDOVUDINE.

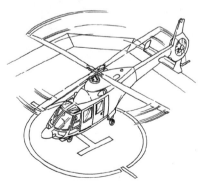

RAPID AEROMEDICAL TRANSPORT
All air ambulances have advanced life support equipment, specially designed to fit the interior of the plane or helicopter. The aircraft also has air-to-ground communication systems so that a doctor can direct and coordinate the medical care the person receives.

as flying intensive care units, carrying cardiac, blood pressure, and oxygen saturation monitors; oxygen; emergency drugs; defibrillators; and other life support systems. Besides the flight crew, the critical care team on board usually consists of a critical care nurse and paramedic, although doctors and respiratory therapists are sometimes included.

Air bags

Inflatable plastic bags mounted under the dashboard of a car that cushion the driver and passengers by inflating automatically in a collision. Some cars are also equipped with side air bags. Air bags are safety restraint systems originally developed to protect drivers and passengers who did not use their seat belts. On impact, air bags are designed to emerge from under the dashboard at up to 200 miles per hour to cushion normal-sized adult males in the event of a collision. Air bags are considered a major auto safety breakthrough and are credited with having saved thousands of lives.

In recent years, air bags have inflated during collisions with sufficient force to injure people and even kill small women and children. The National Highway Traffic Safety Administration has developed rules designed to reduce the risk that air bags will injure or kill, including the development of lower power air bags. Car owners are urged to use seat belts at all times and to have children sit in the back seat, where they are much less likely to be injured. Infant carriers should never be placed in the front seat. See CAR RESTRAINTS.

Air pollution

See POLLUTION, AIR.

Air swallowing

A common cause of gas in the stomach, resulting from excess air taken in, usually when eating or drinking rapidly, chewing gum, smoking, or wearing loose dentures. Air swallowing also commonly occurs when infants cry for a prolonged period. The medical term is aerophagia. Small amounts of air, containing nitrogen, oxygen, and carbon dioxide, are routinely swallowed during eating and drinking. Belching is the way most excess swallowed air leaves the stomach. The remaining gas is partially absorbed in the small intestine. A small amount of air moves into the large intestine where it is released through the rectum.

Airway

The tubular structure in the respiratory system that carries inhaled air through the nose and mouth to the lungs. In the lungs, oxygen is taken up by the blood, while carbon dioxide is eliminated from the tissues and exhaled from the lungs through the airways. The largest airway is the windpipe, or trachea. This structure branches into two smaller airways called the bronchi, which are connected to and supply the lungs. The bronchi repeatedly divide into tiny airways called bronchioles. This system of airways is often referred to as the bronchial tree.

Akathisia

A high state of restlessness characterized by an inability to sit still without fidgeting, an urge to pace about constantly, constant rocking from foot to foot, or muscular quivering, particularly in the legs. Akathisia is often accompanied by feelings of irritability and aggression and can lead to suicide attempts. The condition may be caused by certain medications (strong tranquilizers) prescribed for mental illness, and it can also be a symptom of Parkinson disease, iron-deficiency anemia, and psychiatric disorders, such as manic-depressive illness. Treatment depends on the underlying cause and may include lowering the dose of antipsychotic drugs.

Akinesia

An abnormal slowness and lack of movement. Akinesia may be expressed in different ways, such as a loss of facial expression or a decrease in arm swing. It is a symptom of PARKINSON DISEASE (a progressive, degenerative disease of the nervous system characterized by muscle rigidity, weakness, and tremor). Akinesia associated with Parkinson disease is often treated with levodopa, a chemical precursor of the neurotransmitter dopamine. However, levodopa has many side effects, and over time its use can result in DYSKINESIA (abnormally increased, uncontrollable muscle movement).

Al-Anon

A self-help support group that serves the needs of the families, friends, and partners of people addicted to alcohol. Al-Anon is associated with ALCOHOLICS ANONYMOUS (AA), a self-help group for people recovering from alcoholism who are committed to living sober lives. Al-Anon, like Alcoholics Anonymous, follows the Twelve Steps (see TWELVE-STEP PROGRAM), a series of guidelines for living with alcoholism that emphasize the person's powerlessness over his or her addiction and the need for honesty about the past and the present. Al-Anon stresses the importance of forgiveness and detachment for people whose lives have been affected by

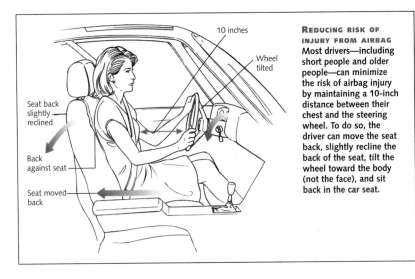

10 inches

Wheel tilted

Seat back slightly reclined

Back against seat

Seat moved back

REDUCING RISK OF INJURY FROM AIRBAG Most drivers—including short people and older people—can minimize the risk of airbag injury by maintaining a 10-inch distance between their chest and the steering wheel. To do so, the driver can move the seat back, slightly recline the back of the seat, tilt the wheel toward the body (not the face), and sit back in the car seat.

alcoholism in family or friends. The support group's main focus is for members to help each other cope with the consequences of a person's addiction and the effects it has on them and the people around them. A similar group called Alateen serves adolescent children of people addicted to alcohol.

Albinism

A group of inherited conditions in which no or little pigment is present in eyes, skin, and hair. Albinism is an inherited metabolic disorder that reduces the usual amounts of a pigment, or coloring agent, called melanin. There are about ten different types of albinism, based on the amount of pigment, that can vary considerably from person to person. Most people with albinism have very light eyes, skin, and hair. All types of albinism lead to problems with vision, usually decreased visual acuity, involuntary eye movements (nystagmus), and increased sensitivity to light. Some people are legally blind, while others have "crossed eyes" or "lazy eye" (STRABISMUS). Some types of albinism involve reduced pigment only in the eyes (ocular albinism). About one person in 17,000 in the United States has some type of albinism, and albinism affects all races. People with albinism live normal life spans.

People with the most severe form of albinism have a total absence of pigment and have white hair, colorless skin, and red irises. They experience photophobia, in which sunlight is painful to their eyes, and they are extremely susceptible to sunburns. Partial albinism (piebaldism) involves patches of unpigmented skin, usually on the forehead, elbows, knees, or other areas. Piebaldism can also occur as a white forelock of hair.

The diagnosis of albinism is usually made through observation of the skin, hair, and eyes. Definitive diagnosis is based on an eye examination, because it is the presence of eye problems that defines the condition. Treatment is intended to reduce symptoms and depends on the extent of the disorder. Skin and eyes must be protected from the sun: sunglasses with UV (ultraviolet) protection should be worn; and skin must always be shielded from the sun by sunscreens with a high

SPF (sun protection factor) and by complete coverage with clothing. Vision problems can be improved with glasses or surgery to correct nystagmus, involuntary movements of the eyeballs. Genetic counseling can help affected individuals or their parents understand the chances of having affected children.

Albumin

A simple protein found in plant and animal tissues. Albumins are water soluble and can be coagulated or made semisolid with the application of heat. Albumins are found in egg white, blood serum, milk, peas, and wheat. In the blood, albumins have an important role in regulating the distribution of water throughout the body and may bind to certain drugs, making them less active. Albumin infusions are often used therapeutically to treat shock, burns, liver failure, and kidney disease.

Albuminuria

Abnormally high amounts of the protein albumin in the urine. Excessive levels of protein in the urine usually result from damage to the glomeruli (the filtering units of the kidneys). Albuminuria may have a number of different causes but is a common problem in people with kidney disease that stems from having diabetes mellitus for an extended period of time. See also MICROALBUMINURIA.

Albuterol sulfate

A bronchodilator drug. Albuterol sulfate (Proventil, Ventolin, Volmax) is used to treat asthma, exercise-induced asthma, emphysema, and bronchospasm by relaxing smooth muscles in the lungs and widening the airways (bronchioles), allowing air to move more freely. Albuterol sulfate can be taken orally, but is most often prescribed as an aerosol inhalant. Although it can cause a mild elevation in heart rate, albuterol sulfate is safer than other bronchodilators for people with heart conditions.

Alcohol and older people

Older people appear to be more vulnerable to the effects of alcohol since changes in their metabolism cause

higher concentrations of alcohol to stay in the bloodstream longer than for younger people. Because alcohol slows down brain activity and affects judgment, alertness, coordination, and reaction time, older people who drink alcohol are at an increased risk for falls and other accidents. Confusion and a slow reaction time due to alcohol use can make it seem as though an older person has ALZHEIMER'S DISEASE. Over time, alcohol abuse damages the central nervous system, liver, heart, kidneys, and stomach.

Many older people regularly take a number of prescription and over-the-counter medications. Mixing alcohol with them can increase the risk of drug side effects. For example, combining aspirin and alcohol increases the risk of stomach bleeding. Taking alcohol with tranquilizers, sleeping pills, or pain medications can intensify their action and can even prove fatal. As people grow older, their ability to metabolize alcohol and other drugs declines. To avoid dangerous interactions, older people should inform their doctors if they drink.

If an older person has a drinking problem, it is especially important to consult a physician. Symptoms of geriatric alcohol abuse are similar to those of other forms of ALCOHOL DEPENDENCE. Drinking to change one's mood, frequent inebriation, and letting drinking take precedence over important needs such as eating are all signs of an alcohol problem. Older adults most vulnerable to developing a problem are men and those who have recently become widowed or have experienced other difficult losses.

Alcohol dependence

A disorder involving addiction to alcohol and characterized by tolerance (the need to consume increasingly larger amounts of alcohol to feel its effects), physical symptoms if alcohol is withdrawn, or both. Alcohol dependence is also known as alcoholism, and alcohol-dependent people are known as alcoholics. Untreated, the disease has severe physical, social, and personal consequences; it is the third leading killer in the United States, following heart disease and cancer.

Alcohol dependence usually develops over a period of 5 to 25 years, although the dependence may take only a few months in adolescents. The disorder may worsen over the course of a person's lifetime (see ALCOHOL AND OLDER PEOPLE). Alcohol dependence affects both men and women of all ages and every ethnic and racial group. The disease cannot be cured, but it can be successfully treated, allowing a person who is alcohol-dependent to live a normal and productive life.

SYMPTOMS AND SIGNS

Alcohol dependence is characterized by constant or periodic preoccupa-tion with alcohol, distorted thinking (particularly denial that alcohol poses a problem), lack of control regarding alcohol use, and continued drinking despite obvious adverse results, such as legal problems, family breakup, health problems, or job loss. Denial is one of the key signs of alcohol dependence. The individual maintains that even when the consequences of drinking are obvious, some factor besides alcohol is at fault. Signs of denial include blaming others, violence directed against family members, arguments over drinking, expressing anger, and continuing to drink while refusing to seek help. Increased tolerance to alcohol is another symptom. Alcohol-dependent people often have to drink larger than normal amounts to feel alcohol's effects, and they may appear sober even after drinking much more than would intoxicate a drinker who is not dependent. They drink excessively and often, gulping drinks or ordering two at a time, and are commonly unable to control drinking, continuing to consume alcohol even after intoxication begins. Alcohol-dependent people typically use alcohol to relieve symptoms such as pain or anxiety, and they commonly forget what happened while they were drinking, a pattern referred to as blacking out. They often feel guilty about what they did or said while drinking.

The majority of alcohol-dependent people who stop drinking experience some anxiety, insomnia, and tremors for a few days; some have few or no symptoms; and a minority have more severe symptoms requiring medical detoxification. Sometimes, withdrawal symptoms appear and last for 3 to 7 days, including hand tremors; increased blood pressure, pulse, and body temperature; nausea or vomiting; and an inability to sleep (insomnia). In some cases, withdrawal causes delirium tremens (DTs), which can involve confusion and altered mental state (delirium), agitation, hallucination, feelings of persecution, seizures, and severe tremors. DTs last from 3 to 5 days and can be dangerous; medical intervention is required. Physical signs, particularly in cases of long-term alcohol dependence, are present in some individuals. They include hardening and scarring of the liver (cirrhosis), liver inflammation (hepatitis), inflammation of the pancreas (pancreatitis), and damage to the heart muscle (cardiomyopathy).

ABUSE VERSUS DEPENDENCE

In simple terms, alcohol abuse is drinking too much too often, while dependence refers to an inability to quit drinking. Alcohol abuse includes any pattern of drinking that makes it difficult or impossible for a person to fulfill family or work responsibilities or that results in physical danger to the person or others, such as driving a car under the influence of alcohol. Since alcohol abuse lacks the addiction that underlies alcohol dependence, it is easier to treat. Left untreated, however, it can develop into alcohol dependence.

CAUSES AND CONSEQUENCES

Recent studies indicate an inherited predisposition to alcohol dependence. People who come from a family with an alcohol-dependent parent are more likely to develop the disease than people who come from families without the disorder. A variety of environmental factors are

Impaired brain and nerve function; stroke

Permanent facial flushing

Hypertension, heart failure, rapid heart rate

Fatty liver, hepatitis, cirrhosis, liver cancer

Impaired immune function (spleen)

Pancreatitis (pancreas)

Gastritis; ulcers

Impotence; infertility

PHYSICAL EFFECTS OF ABUSING ALCOHOL
Long-term heavy drinking causes damage throughout the body and is a leading cause of death in the United States. A variety of serious health problems arise from drinking more than one drink a day for women or two drinks a day for men.

also thought to affect alcohol dependence.

Excessive alcohol consumption over a period of years has serious consequences, causing impaired health and premature death. Brain damage is common, beginning with blacking out while drinking. Short-term memory also suffers, and a severe brain impairment known as WERNICKE-KORSAKOFF SYNDROME, which involves partial paralysis and serious memory loss, can develop. Ulcers and other gastrointestinal problems, such as small bleeding tears in the lower esophagus are common, along with damage to the liver and pancreas. Large amounts of alcohol increase blood pressure and damage the heart muscle, leading to irregular heartbeat or heart failure. Alcohol dependence can cause sexual dysfunction in both men and women. It also increases the risk of cancer, particularly in the mouth, larynx, esophagus, stomach, liver, and pancreas. The pituitary and adrenal glands may also be affected. Poor nutrition and vitamin deficiencies are common in alcohol-dependent people since they often take in most of their calories in the form of alcohol and fail to eat a balanced diet.

Alcohol dependence has psychological and social consequences. Since depression often accompanies alcohol dependence, suicide is possible. Women who drink while pregnant may give birth to a baby with FETAL ALCOHOL SYNDROME, which causes a child to have mental retardation and a variety of serious physical problems. Alcohol dependence is associated with violence toward family members, including physical and sexual abuse and murder; an increase in accidents (for example, with firearms and motor vehicles); occupational or academic difficulties, such as trouble holding a job or staying in school; and legal troubles, particularly violations of drunk-driving laws.

TREATMENT
Since denial is a common element in alcohol dependence, the first step in treatment is getting the person to recognize the problem. In many cases, this requires a confrontation (sometimes called an "intervention"), often

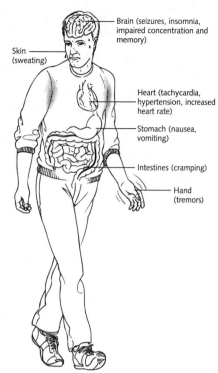

Skin (sweating)

Brain (seizures, insomnia, impaired concentration and memory)

Heart (tachycardia, hypertension, increased heart rate)

Stomach (nausea, vomiting)

Intestines (cramping)

Hand (tremors)

SYMPTOMS OF WITHDRAWAL
For an alcohol-dependent person, symptoms of withdrawal from alcohol start several hours after the last drink and may last from 3 to 7 days. The physical symptoms are sufficiently distressing to make "kicking the habit" very difficult.

as a result of a crisis, such as the diagnosis of an alcohol-related disease or an accident caused by alcohol abuse.

Once the problem is recognized, treatment can begin. The first step, called detoxification, involves the person's withdrawal from alcohol in a supervised setting that lasts from 4 to 7 days. Often the person is treated with tranquilizers and sedatives to ease the physical symptoms of withdrawal. Vitamins may be given to treat poor nutrition. Underlying psychological conditions such as depression are also treated, usually with medication.

The next step involves providing emotional and physical support to help the person remain abstinent from alcohol. Psychological support, counseling, and nursing and medical care are provided as needed. Drugs may also be prescribed.

Disulfiram (Antabuse) causes highly unpleasant symptoms, including rapid pulse and vomiting, if alcohol is consumed within 2 weeks of the time the drug is taken. Naltrexone, also used for recovery from heroin addiction, reduces the desire for alcohol and may be used during the first 3 months of recovery. Many people recovering from alcohol dependence rely on self-help peer groups, such as ALCOHOLICS ANONYMOUS (AA), which provides an effective model of sobriety and emotional support from fellow members.

Alcohol intoxication

The impaired mental or physical functioning that comes from the consumption of alcohol; also known as inebriation or drunkenness. Alcohol (known medically as ethanol, or EtOH) is a central nervous system depressant drug, one that slows the activity of the central nervous system, particularly the brain. Alcohol requires no digestion and is absorbed directly into the bloodstream. When alcohol is consumed, a portion enters the bloodstream through the mouth and throat, with the remainder entering through the stomach and intestines. Alcohol's effects are felt within 10 minutes and peak within 40 to 60 minutes.

The level of alcohol in the blood after drinking depends primarily on the amount consumed. Alcohol is metabolized largely in the liver, with some also expelled through the kidneys and lungs. Typically, an adult can metabolize approximately 1 ounce of alcohol per hour; that is the amount found in a 12-ounce can of beer, a 5-ounce glass of wine, or 1.5 ounces of whiskey, gin, vodka, or other distilled spirits. Drinking more alcohol than the body can absorb results in severe intoxication.

As the blood alcohol level rises, several stages of intoxication may occur. Initially, the person is talkative and sociable, with fewer inhibitions and some impairment of judgment. This occurs at a blood alcohol level of approximately 0.02 percent, which is less than the usual legal limit that defines DRUNK DRIVING. The person then becomes excited and

A

ALCOHOL INTOXICATION

Alcohol acts on a person's central nervous system as a sedative or tranquilizer would, slowing motor coordination and reaction time and impairing memory, reasoning, judgment, and self-control. A 5-ounce glass of wine, 12-ounce glass of beer, and 1.25 ounces of 80-proof liquor all have about the same amount of alcohol despite the difference in serving size. A 120-pound woman who drinks 2 bottles of beer (12 ounces each) can have a blood alcohol content (BAC) of 0.08 percent. A 140-pound man having 3 drinks would also have a BAC of 0.08 percent. Impairment begins, however, on as little as one drink and a BAC of 0.02 percent.

Women

NUMBER OF DRINKS*	BODY WEIGHT IN POUNDS									EFFECT
	90	100	120	140	160	180	200	220	240	
0	0.00	0.00	0.00	0.00	0.00	0.00	0.00	0.00	0.00	Only safe driving limit
1	0.05	0.05	0.04	0.03	0.03	0.03	0.02	0.02	0.02	Impairment begins
2	0.10	0.09	0.08	0.07	0.06	0.05	0.05	0.04	0.04	Driving skills significantly affected
3	0.15	0.14	0.11	0.10	0.09	0.08	0.07	0.06	0.06	Possible criminal penalties
4	0.20	0.18	0.15	0.13	0.11	0.10	0.09	0.08	0.08	
5	0.25	0.23	0.19	0.16	0.14	0.13	0.11	0.10	0.09	
6	0.30	0.27	0.23	0.19	0.17	0.15	0.14	0.12	0.11	Legally intoxicated
7	0.35	0.32	0.27	0.23	0.20	0.18	0.16	0.14	0.13	
8	0.40	0.36	0.30	0.26	0.23	0.20	0.18	0.17	0.15	
9	0.45	0.41	0.34	0.29	0.26	0.23	0.20	0.19	0.17	Criminal penalties
10	0.51	0.45	0.38	0.32	0.28	0.25	0.23	0.21	0.19	

Approximate Blood Alcohol Percentage†

Men

NUMBER OF DRINKS*	BODY WEIGHT IN POUNDS								EFFECT
	100	120	140	160	180	200	220	240	
0	0.00	0.00	0.00	0.00	0.00	0.00	0.00	0.00	Only safe driving limit
1	0.04	0.03	0.03	0.02	0.02	0.02	0.02	0.02	Impairment begins
2	0.08	0.06	0.05	0.05	0.04	0.04	0.03	0.03	Driving skills significantly affected
3	0.11	0.09	0.08	0.07	0.06	0.06	0.05	0.05	
4	0.15	0.12	0.11	0.09	0.08	0.08	0.07	0.06	Possible criminal penalties
5	0.19	0.16	0.13	0.12	0.11	0.09	0.09	0.08	
6	0.23	0.19	0.16	0.14	0.13	0.11	0.10	0.09	
7	0.26	0.22	0.19	0.16	0.15	0.13	0.12	0.11	Legally intoxicated
8	0.30	0.25	0.21	0.19	0.17	0.15	0.14	0.13	
9	0.34	0.28	0.24	0.21	0.19	0.17	0.15	0.14	Criminal penalties
10	0.38	0.31	0.27	0.23	0.21	0.19	0.17	0.16	

Approximate Blood Alcohol Percentage†

*One drink is 1.25 ounces of 80 proof liquor, 12 ounces of beer, or 5 ounces of table wine.   †Subtract 0.01 percent for each 40 minutes of drinking.

Data provided courtesy of the Pennsylvania Liquor Control Board.

erratic, with slowed reactions and poor judgment. The next step is some loss of control over talking and walking, with slurred speech, staggering, disorientation, double vision, and exaggerated mood. This occurs when the blood alcohol level reaches approximately 0.20 percent. With even more alcohol, the individual can walk only with assistance and may seem paralyzed. Vomiting and incontinence (loss of bladder control) are common. Unconsciousness follows, with slow reflexes and very slow, ineffective breathing. Death can occur, particularly at blood alcohol levels of 0.35 percent and higher.

A

Alcoholics Anonymous (AA)

A self-help group for men and women recovering from alcohol dependency that provides an effective model of total abstinence; commonly abbreviated to AA. Founded in 1935 on the principle that alcohol dependency is a disease and that each person's experience is unique, Alcoholics Anonymous follows the Twelve Steps (see TWELVE-STEP PROGRAM), which serve as practical suggestions to help people lead sober lives by accepting their powerlessness around alcohol and being honest about their past and present lives. AA is nonsectarian, although the organization espouses religious beliefs. There are no dues; the only membership requirement is a desire to stop drinking.

Alcoholism

A disorder involving addiction to alcohol and characterized by tolerance (the need to consume increasingly larger amounts of alcohol to feel its effects) to increasing amounts of alcohol, or by physical symptoms if alcohol is withdrawn, or both. See ALCOHOL DEPENDENCE.

Aldosterone

A hormone produced by the adrenal cortex (the outer layer of the adrenal glands). Aldosterone controls the levels of sodium and potassium in the blood to help regulate water balance, blood volume, and blood pressure. The production of aldosterone is stimulated by the hormone RENIN, which is produced by the kidneys.

Aldosteronism

A condition in which the adrenal cortex (the outer layer of the adrenal glands) secretes abnormally high levels of ALDOSTERONE, a hormone that regulates blood volume and the balance of sodium and potassium in the blood; also known as hyperaldosteronism. If aldosteronism results in a severe depletion of potassium, muscle weakness and even paralysis can result. Excessive water and sodium retention can abnormally elevate the blood pressure. Aldosteronism can also result in arrhythmias and other cardiac abnormalities.

Primary aldosteronism, also called Conn syndrome, may be caused by adrenal hyperplasia (see ADRENAL HYPERPLASIA, CONGENITAL), an enlargement of the adrenal gland caused by an abnormal increase in its cells, or by an adrenal tumor that secretes aldosterone. The secondary form of the condition is more common and is associated with congestive heart failure, cirrhosis, and kidney failure. In this form of the disease, alteration in renin secretion leads to an increased level of aldosterone. If a tumor, either benign (not cancerous) or malignant (cancerous), is causing excess aldosterone to be released, surgery may be considered. Spironolactone is a medication commonly used to treat the symptoms of a low potassium level that may result from aldosteronism.

Alendronate sodium

A bisphosphonate drug. Alendronate sodium (Fosamax) is prescribed for Paget disease of the bone and osteoporosis in postmenopausal women. Alendronate sodium helps to prevent loss of bone mass and can make bones stronger. The medication should be taken on an empty stomach with a full glass of water 30 minutes before eating.

Alexander technique

A method of improving posture and alleviating muscle tension through alignment of a person's head, neck, and back. The Alexander technique, a form of BODYWORK or MASSAGE THERAPY, was invented by Australian actor F. M. Alexander in 1904 as a vocal production technique, but he ultimately came to believe that his technique could solve many kinds of body problems, thereby eliminating back pain, excess tension, or lack of coordination. The basic idea behind the Alexander technique is that the relationship between the head and spine is of the utmost importance in determining the body's overall ease of movement and that through a person's awareness of posture, he or she can adopt new patterns to alleviate pain and improve function. Conditions that may respond to this therapy include scoliosis, asthma, and repetitive strain injuries.

Alexia

Loss of the ability to understand written language. Alexia is caused by brain damage associated with disorders such as stroke, dementia, or trauma to the head (in the visual cortex). This condition is diagnosed according to medical history, physical examination, neurological examination, and tests such as CT SCANNING (computed tomography scanning). Treatment depends on the nature of the problem and its underlying cause. Alexia is a more serious reading disorder than DYSLEXIA. Those with alexia without agraphia cannot read what they have written despite being able to write accurately.

Alienation

The feeling of being estranged from other people, society at large, or work. Alienation is thought to arise from a blocking of a person's feelings, leading him or her to be less effective in meeting the everyday demands of life. In psychiatry, alienation is the person's perception that his or her mental activities, actions, or body parts literally belong to someone else.

Alignment, dental

The positioning and spacing of teeth. The way the upper teeth relate to the lower teeth when the mouth closes is called OCCLUSION. Dental alignment is generally determined by heredity, but may also be affected by the premature loss of primary teeth and the subsequent effects on the development and eruption of permanent teeth. Problems with jaw growth can also affect tooth positioning. The proper alignment of teeth is important to appearance and the ability to chew. Improper alignment (MALOCCLUSION) makes the teeth difficult to clean and can lead to an increased risk of tooth decay and gum disease. Severe alignment problems may cause dental disease, difficulties with chewing food, and joint pain in the jaw. Problems with dental alignment are treated by an orthodontist.

Alimentary tract

Also known as the digestive or gastrointestinal (GI) tract, a series of joined and coiled tubes that extend from the mouth to the esophagus, stomach, small and large intestine, rectum, and anus. Food is propelled through the alimentary tract by a rhythmic series of muscular contractions called peristalsis. During digestion, enzymes, HYDROCHLORIC ACID (HCL), and BILE help break down food to promote its absorption into the body. Undigested matter is eventually expelled through the anus. See also DIGESTIVE SYSTEM.

Alitretinoin

A retinoid drug. Alitretinoin (Panretyn) is prescribed for skin lesions of KAPOSI SARCOMA (KS), a condition most commonly associated with HIV (human immunodeficiency virus). Alitretinoin is a vitamin A–related retinoid found naturally in the body that inhibits growth of KS cells; it works by activating retinoid receptors in normal human cells. Alitretinoin cannot prevent new KS lesions from forming. It is available as a gel and applied to individual lesions.

Alkali

A substance with basic properties; the hydroxide of an alkali metal. Akalis are usually bitter, caustic (burning), and able to neutralize acids by breaking them down into salts and water. An alkali will turn litmus paper blue. When found in soil or ground water, alkalis are harmful to agriculture. Most soaps and bleaches are made with mild alkali compounds.

Alkaloids

Organic compounds derived from plants that are made up of carbon, hydrogen, nitrogen, and often oxygen. Many alkaloids are poisonous but have medicinal properties when used in small quantities. Examples of such alkaloids include morphine and codeine, when used as pain relievers, and cocaine, when used as a local anesthetic. Other common alkaloids are nicotine, caffeine, quinine, LSD (lysergic acid diethylamide), lye, and strychnine (a rodent poison).

Allergen

Any foreign substance that is capable of causing an IMMUNE RESPONSE. Allergens produce what is called an allergic reaction. This occurs when the immune system mistakes allergens, which are normally nonharmful substances, for substances that are potentially harmful. A person may be exposed to an allergen by ingestion, inhalation, or physical contact. This exposure produces an allergic reaction if a person's immune system has become sensitized to the particular

allergen after repeated exposure, a process called SENSITIZATION.

The most common allergens are plant pollens, house dust mites, fungi spores, certain food items, medications such as penicillin, and the dander of domestic animals such as cats and dogs. The allergen in dogs that causes reactions is not the fur or hair itself, but rather a sticky substance produced by the animals' sebaceous glands. This substance clings to hair, fur, and skin cells and is distributed when this dander is shed by the dog. Every breed of dog produces this allergen, and cats, rabbits, hamsters, gerbils, rats, and horses produce a similar allergen that clings to their shed dander.

Allergens from cats produce particularly dramatic symptoms; male cats may produce more allergens than female cats, which may account for the variation in allergic symptoms when a person is exposed to different cats.

Studies have shown that even with thorough cleaning, it may take as long as 6 months for the cat allergen to completely disappear from the home.

Allergic reaction

A disorder caused by hypersensitivity to a substance, such as a medication. An allergic reaction occurs when the immune system attacks a substance that is normally harmless as if it were a disease-causing organism. The immune system produces antibodies that attach to mast cells, part of the immune system found in the skin, the stomach lining, the upper respiratory tract, and the

bronchial tubes (airways in the lungs). The immune system "remembers" the event and repeats it every time the substance enters the body, releasing powerful chemicals such as histamine that cause symptoms of an allergic reaction. Allergic reactions to medication can include hives, itching, wheezing, throat tightening, and rarely, shock, an intense reaction quickly leading to difficulty in breathing, low blood pressure, rapid pulse, sweating, and collapse.

Allergic reactions to medication are difficult to prevent, but symptoms can be treated with antihistamines, corticosteroids, or epinephrine. Medications are most likely to provoke allergic reactions when they are given by injection, because they enter the bloodstream directly. Drugs are less likely to cause an allergic reaction when they are taken in pill or capsule form because the digestive process breaks down some of the allergy-provoking substances.

The most common causes of medication allergies are aspirin and penicillin. People known to have allergic reactions to specific medications are urged to wear a medical alert bracelet.

Allergies

Abnormal and mistaken responses of the immune system that produce physical symptoms caused by contact with a substance that is normally harmless. Allergies occur when an ANTIBODY responds to a specific ANTIGEN. The substance producing the response is called an ALLERGEN. These antigens or allergens typically

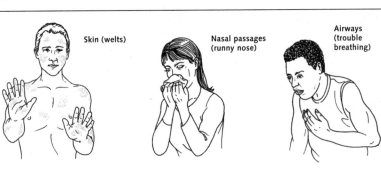

SITES OF ALLERGIC REACTION
The first step toward treating an allergy is to identify patterns of symptoms. Common sites of allergic reaction include the skin, which may develop raised, itchy welts; the nasal passages, which may produce a runny nose, itchy eyes, and sneezing; and the airways in the lungs, which may cause an asthmalike reaction with congestion, wheezing, and breathing difficulty.

do not produce a strong immune response in everyone exposed to them but can cause an immune rsponse in those who are allergic to the antigen.

Allergies occur when a person has a heightened sensitivity to an allergen that is ingested, breathed in, or touched. This sensitivity develops after the person has been repeatedly exposed to the allergen, a process called SENSITIZATION. Normally, the immune system can distinguish between the nonharmful substances that exist in the environment and the harmful substances, such as viruses and bacteria that cause illness. When exposure to these harmful substances occurs, the immune system reacts appropriately by producing antibodies that target them for destruction.

HOW ALLERGIES OCCUR
In some people, the immune system makes a mistake and responds to a harmless substance, such as house dust, pollen, mold, animal dander, certain foods, or certain medications. The resulting allergy is an altered reaction that occurs in the body's immune system. Allergic reactions occur when the immune system attacks what is perceived to be a hostile invader by producing antibodies to defend the body against the invader. The antibodies produced during an allergic reaction are in the IgE (immunoglobulin E) class of antibodies. The IgE antibody can be found on the surface of certain cells called mast cells and basophils. Allergens make contact with IgE antibodies, which triggers the allergy cells to release a series of chemicals called mediators. HISTAMINE, the best known of the mediators, may trigger an inflammatory response ranging from a mild runny nose and itchy, watery eyes to a severe life-threatening reaction called ANAPHYLAXIS.

The mediators respond very quickly, producing reactions immediately after a person has been exposed to an allergen.

WHY ALLERGIES OCCUR
A certain type of white blood cell is attracted to the site of the reaction and intensifies the reaction, causing swelling or inflammation in the affected area. If an allergen gets into the bloodstream, the effects may be more far-reaching. When this occurs, the allergen may cause symptoms in addition to those occurring at the site of the reaction. For example, a food allergen that is ingested may cause hives as well as gastrointestinal symptoms.

What makes people develop allergies to certain substances is not clearly understood. It is known that allergic reactions are initiated by repeated exposure to an allergen over time, ranging from a few weeks to several decades, in a process called sensitization. In some people, this involves production of memory cells that cause increased production of IgE antibodies on subsequent exposure. The immune system is then activated to attack the otherwise harmless substance each time exposure to the same allergen occurs.

SYMPTOMS, DIAGNOSIS, AND TREATMENT
Symptoms depend on the part of the body affected. If the allergic reaction occurs in the ears, nose, throat, or sinuses, the membranes lining these cavities become swollen as a result of the immune system's inflammatory response to the allergen. The person may have a stuffy or runny nose with frequent sneezing, coughing, and wheezing and an itchy sensation in the eyes, nose, throat, or roof of the mouth. If NASAL POLYPS have developed, the person may have difficulty breathing and a loss of the sense of smell. The allergy may be diagnosed after a doctor's evaluation of a complete history of symptoms including the time of day and the season in which the allergies occur. A skin SCRATCH TEST may be performed to determine the allergen responsible. Treatment is generally based on eliminating the person's exposure to the known allergen and on medications such as antihistamines and decongestants. A medical procedure known as immunotherapy, which is a series of injections to desensitize the system to specific allergens, may be tried.

Skin allergies may cause symptoms including a burning sensation in the eyes and mucous membranes and an itchy rash of small bumps, blisters, and general swelling of the skin's tissues. Welts on the skin that often itch and tend to appear and disappear intermittently may also occur. There may also be large welts below the surface of the skin, especially around the eyes and lips, but also on the hands and feet and possibly in the throat. Symptoms of skin allergies may occur as a result of exposure to heat, cold, sun, or rubbing. Diagnosis is generally made after the doctor physically examines the person's skin. The person may be asked to offer a detailed history of exposure to possible allergens, so the doctor can determine the substance responsible. Treatment may include antihistamines, in oral form or in preparations applied to the skin, avoidance measures if a trigger is identified, and sometimes adrenaline or corticosteroid medications if the allergic reaction is serious.

Food allergies can produce symptoms including abdominal pain, diarrhea, nausea, and vomiting. Nasal congestion may also occur, and the lips, eyes, face, tongue, and throat may become swollen. Hives and asthma may also develop from food allergies. The affected person may be required to follow a strict program, called an elimination diet, to determine the allergen causing the reaction. Skin scratch tests and specific blood tests may also be used in the diagnosis. The only treatment for food allergies is complete avoidance of the food. For some people, physical contact with the food allergen is to be avoided as strictly as ingestion of the allergens. People with serious food allergies must carry an emergency kit containing epinephrine at all times.

Allergies to medications can cause symptoms including wheezing and difficulty breathing, rash or hives, overall itching, and, in severe cases, shock or anaphylaxis. These allergies may be treated with adrenaline (epinephrine), antihistamines, or corticosteroid medications.

Allergies to insect stings may involve symptoms such as pain and severe itching at the site of the sting, hives, itchy eyes, and a constricted feeling in the throat and chest. Anaphylaxis can occur, causing severe swelling of the eyes, lips, or tongue and a swelling of the throat that makes it difficult to breathe. Anaphylaxis can involve obstruction of the airways and lungs and can even cause shock. Severe reactions can occur within 10 to 20 minutes of the insect bite and require emergency

A

THE ALLERGY RESPONSE

When the body's immune system is exposed to certain allergens, it becomes sensitized to them. Allergy symptoms usually occur when the body is again exposed to allergens it has become sensitized to.

STEP 1
When allergens enter the body, they are recognized by lymphocytes, a type of white blood cell.

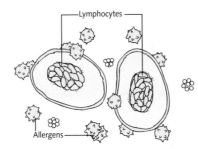

STEP 2
Lymphocytes create antibodies that are specific to the allergens.

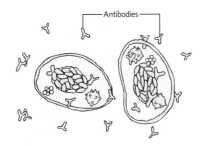

STEP 3
Antibodies attach to mast cells, which contain granules of histamine.

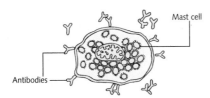

STEP 4
When allergens bind to antibodies on the surface of mast cells, histamine is released and allergy symptoms occur.

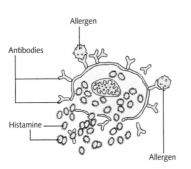

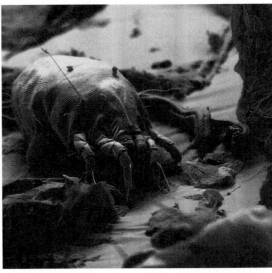

DUST MITE
Scanning electron micrograph shows a dust mite (enlarged 250 times) among scales of skin.

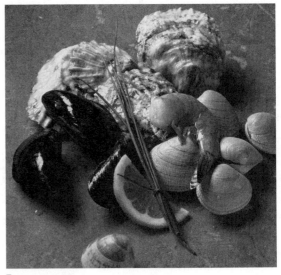

FOOD ALLERGEN
A common source of food allergy is shellfish.

medical attention, often an injection of epinephrine.

WHO IS AFFECTED

A large number of people living in the United States have allergies. Allergies tend to run in families, and heredity is known to be a risk factor. When both parents have an allergy, the offspring are at high risk for acquiring allergies themselves, although the reactions may not be produced by the same allergens.

A person may become sensitized in infancy, or the process may not begin until adulthood. Most allergies, particularly those caused by inhalation of an allergen, begin in childhood. Sometimes a child outgrows an allergy and another one develops. This rarely occurs in adulthood. It is uncommon for a new allergy to develop after the age of 40 years. Adult allergies tend to persist, although symptoms may become less severe with age.

It has been estimated that one in five Americans has a chronic allergy. One of the most common allergies is medically known as seasonal allergic rhinitis, which is also called HAY FEVER. This is usually caused by a reaction to airborne allergens, such as pollen, and occurs on a seasonal basis when the pollens are abundant in the outdoor environment. Another type of airborne allergy, called perennial allergic rhinitis, is a response to indoor allergens, including pet dander, dust mites, and household molds. As many as 6 to 10 million Americans have allergies related to cats, dogs, and other pets. About 50 million American people experience allergic reactions to poison ivy each year, and about 2 million have had allergic reactions to insect stings. Food allergies are less common; although many children younger than 6 years have symptoms of food allergies, only about half of this group have confirmed food allergies. A very small number of adults have allergies to food.

RISK FACTORS

While hereditary factors may predispose a person to allergies, environment is what tends to set allergic reactions in motion. An environment that supplies continual exposure to high levels of a particular allergen, especially inhaled allergens during infancy and childhood, seems to make a person more likely to acquire allergies at some point in life.

Allergist

A physician who specializes in IMMUNOLOGY and is specially trained in prevention, diagnosis, management, and treatment of allergies and asthma. An allergist has completed medical school, been awarded a medical degree, and been trained in internal medicine or pediatrics for 3 years. This training is followed by 2 years of study, called a fellowship, in an allergy/immunology training program. After completing this fellowship, the physician may become certified by the American Board of Allergy and Immunology by successfully passing the certifying examination.

Allograft

A surgical procedure in which tissue or an organ is taken from one person and transplanted into or implanted onto another individual.

In severe burns, for example, skin from donor cadavers is grafted onto the burn patient to cover the damaged area. Transplants of the cornea, heart, lung, liver, kidney, pancreas, and small intestine are also called allografts. See TRANSPLANT SURGERY.

Allopathy

A system of treating disease by inducing a second condition that is incompatible with or antagonistic to the disease being treated. This term was invented by homeopath Samuel Hahnemann to refer to traditional medicine (homeo means same; allo means order), which is practiced by all doctors with the medical degree MD.

Allopurinol

An antigout medication used to decrease the amount of uric acid in the body. Allopurinol (Zyloprim) is prescribed for various disorders including gout, gouty arthritis, leukemia, and tumors. Allopurinol acts on the enzyme system to reduce the amount of uric acid produced in the body, but it is not effective for an acute attack of gout.

Aloe

Dried juice of the leaves from various species of lilac plants. Aloe, or aloe vera, is chiefly used to ease the pain of sunburn, frostbite, and other skin irritations, but the natural medicine is not regulated by the Food and Drug Administration.

Alopecia

Baldness; absence of hair from areas where it normally is present. Alopecia can stem from genetic causes and is also associated with radiation therapy, chemotherapy, scarring, stress, endocrine disorders, certain drugs, and other factors. Male pattern baldness (androgenic alopecia), the most common type of baldness, is characterized by a progressive symmetrical loss of scalp hair in men in their 20s and 30s, starting at the front, eventually leaving only a peripheral ring of hair. It is an inherited condition that can also affect women, although somewhat later, with less severe loss of frontal hair. The trait seems to be aggravated by the presence of male sex hormones.

Alopecia areata is a loss of scalp and beard hair in patches, due to inflammation. It is usually reversible. Alopecia totalis is the entire loss of hair from the scalp due to alopecia

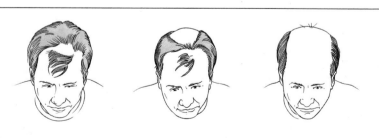

STAGES OF MALE PATTERN BALDNESS
Male pattern baldness occurs in varying degrees in a predictable pattern, advancing from the temples to the back and top of the head.

A

areata. In scarring alopecia, the hair loss is associated with inflammation and scarring of the hair follicles. Scarring alopecia is usually the result of a skin disorder, such as discoid lupus erythematosus, or infection by a fungus.

Alpha 1-antitrypsin deficiency

A common hereditary disorder characterized by a deficiency in levels of the blood protein alpha 1-antitrypsin (AAT). AAT is produced in the liver and inhibits the inflammatory response of the body. When AAT is deficient or absent, infection or inflammation can destroy tissue cells, a result seen most often in the lungs, particularly when they are exposed to cigarette smoke. Approximately 75 percent of adults with AAT deficiency who smoke will develop EMPHYSEMA, a serious respiratory disease, usually before age 40.

In one type of AAT deficiency, the liver produces an abnormal form of AAT that is not released from the liver into the blood. This form of AAT deficiency is called the Z variant. People with the Z variant may develop liver disease when excessive amounts of the protein build up in the liver.

AAT deficiency is a genetic disorder. It occurs when both parents pass on abnormal genes to the child. People with normal amounts of AAT have two normal genes. When a person inherits one normal gene and one abnormal gene, he or she is a carrier of the deficiency and can pass it on to his or her children. AAT deficiency occurs in one of about 10,000 people. Children with AAT deficiency have a 25 percent chance of developing CIRRHOSIS of the liver.

SYMPTOMS AND TREATMENT

Signs associated with AAT deficiency may include shortness of breath, unintended weight loss, wheezing, chronic cough, yellow skin (jaundice), barrel-shaped chest, accumulation of fluid in the tissues (edema), and abnormal liver test results.

Diagnosis is made on the basis of physical examination, chest X ray, and various tests, including tests of pulmonary function and arterial blood gases. A test to measure the AAT levels in the blood may also be done.

There is no proven treatment to reverse the deficiency itself. However, the disorders associated with it, such as emphysema, asthma, chronic bronchitis, and cirrhosis, can be treated. When the deficiency is detected before symptoms are present, treatment focuses on prevention, especially by avoiding smoking or stopping smoking. Nonsmokers with AAT deficiency rarely develop emphysema.

Researchers are currently investigating four different ways to correct AAT deficiency. In one approach, human AAT is administered intravenously every few weeks to people whose AAT is deficient. The replacement AAT is derived from human blood. In another, AAT is inhaled. A liver transplant can replace abnormal liver cells that produce the Z variant of AAT deficiency, thus correcting the deficiency. This method is primarily intended for children with severe AAT deficiency who develop cirrhosis. Gene therapy is being studied as well. In this experimental therapy, the normal gene for AAT is put into a noninfectious virus that is administered to the person. The virus invades tissue cells, causing production of normal AAT by the normal gene it contains. Results have been only partially successful, but the treatment is considered promising.

Alpha blockers

Drugs that help lower blood pressure by preventing blood vessels from constricting. Alpha blockers work by preventing stress hormones from stimulating receptors in the blood vessels, thereby preventing arteries and veins from constricting and raising blood pressure.

Alpha blockers represent a category of medications used to treat hypertension, usually in combination with other drugs. They are especially useful for people with high blood cholesterol levels, diabetes, an enlarged prostate gland (first line of treatment), and vascular disease.

Alpha blockers work in a specific, powerful way. They are associated with side effects including dizziness, headaches, heart palpitations, nausea, and mild fluid retention. The first dose of an alpha blocker may cause a person to feel faint from the rapid drop in blood pressure, but that unpleasant side effect can be avoided. A person taking the drug for the first time should talk to the doctor about taking a small dose just before going to bed for the night and then

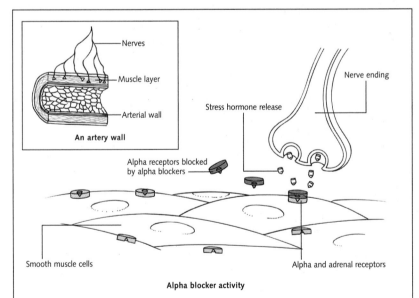

An artery wall

Alpha blocker activity

HOW ALPHA BLOCKERS WORK
By blocking the effects of stress hormones, alpha blockers help prevent the constricting of the smooth muscle layer of artery walls that leads to an increase in blood pressure. As a nerve ending releases the stress hormones norepinephrine and epinephrine, the drug blocks the receptors in the muscle wall, causing the muscle to relax.

gradually increasing subsequent doses. The person taking alpha blockers should learn not to make rapid changes in body position, such as jumping up from bed too fast upon waking.

Alpha-fetoprotein (AFP) test

See AFP TEST.

Alpha-tocopherol

Another name for VITAMIN E. Alpha-tocopherol protects cells from some kinds of damage and helps slow the cell damage that happens naturally as a person ages. Vitamin E is thought to interfere with the oxygen-controlled signals that make cancer cells grow, and it helps keep arteries from clogging by preventing the conversion of cholesterol into its most dangerous form. Vitamin E is found naturally in nuts, sunflower seeds, mayonnaise, cold-pressed vegetable oils, spinach, sweet potatoes, and yams.

Alprazolam

See BENZODIAZEPINES.

ALS

Amyotrophic lateral sclerosis, the most common form of MOTOR NEURON DISEASE, characterized by progressive muscle atrophy (shrinking) and the loss of muscle function. ALS is commonly referred to as Lou Gehrig disease (the only disease to be named after a patient), after the baseball player who died of the disease in 1939. ALS is a rare disorder in which the nerves that control muscle activity progressively degenerate within the brain and spinal cord. It specifically attacks specialized nerve cells called motor neurons. ALS causes upper motor neurons from the brain and spinal cord and lower motor neurons that exit the spinal cord to gradually disintegrate. This results in the characteristic muscle wasting and weakness. The cause of ALS is unknown. About one in ten people with ALS have a family history of the disorder.

SYMPTOMS

The onset of ALS generally occurs after age 50 years. This progressive disease affects the body's voluntary or skeletal muscles. There is initially no pain associated with ALS, and the involuntary muscles and the volun-

tary muscles that control the eyes are not affected. In limb-onset ALS, weakness is first experienced in the arms or legs, making it difficult to walk or perform tasks that require manual dexterity. Bulbar-onset ALS first involves problems with speaking or swallowing.

In ALS, muscle strength and coordination gradually decrease, while mental functioning remains unaffected. The eventual result is total paralysis. Upper motor neuron damage causes weakness, spasticity (muscle stiffness), and exaggerated reflexes. The damage to lower motor neurons leads to muscle wasting and twitching (fasciculations). When lower motor neurons in the bulbar region at the bottom of the brain are affected, the muscles responsible for speech and swallowing weaken. At the point

where the lower motor neurons in the spinal cord become involved, muscle function is lost in the limbs, neck, and trunk.

As the loss of muscle control continues to progress, and more muscle groups become involved, the person becomes more disabled. Eventually all four limbs become involved. Deterioration finally results in speech impairment, difficulty swallowing, and trouble breathing. Death results from paralysis of the respiratory muscles. This typically occurs in 3 to 5 years. However, exceptions occur, and some people have lived 20 years or more following diagnosis.

DIAGNOSIS

Accurate diagnosis of ALS can be difficult because it can be confused with a number of other neurological disorders that require different treatment.

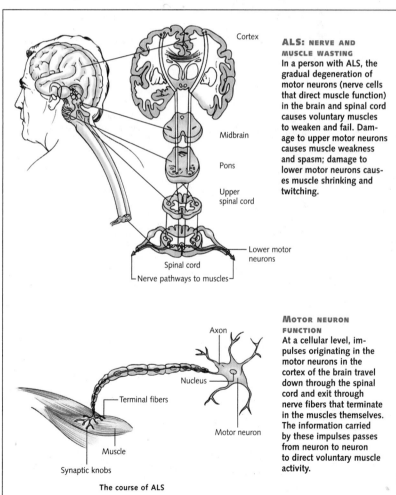

ALS: NERVE AND MUSCLE WASTING
In a person with ALS, the gradual degeneration of motor neurons (nerve cells that direct muscle function) in the brain and spinal cord causes voluntary muscles to weaken and fail. Damage to upper motor neurons causes muscle weakness and spasm; damage to lower motor neurons causes muscle shrinking and twitching.

Cortex
Midbrain
Pons
Upper spinal cord
Lower motor neurons
Spinal cord
Nerve pathways to muscles

MOTOR NEURON FUNCTION
At a cellular level, impulses originating in the motor neurons in the cortex of the brain travel down through the spinal cord and exit through nerve fibers that terminate in the muscles themselves. The information carried by these impulses passes from neuron to neuron to direct voluntary muscle activity.

Axon
Nucleus
Terminal fibers
Motor neuron
Muscle
Synaptic knobs

The course of ALS

Diagnosis of ALS is made through neuromuscular examination that indicates muscle weakness without loss of sensation. Weakness often begins in a single limb or in the shoulders or hips. Examination may also reveal tremors, spasms, contractions, and atrophy. There may be abnormal reflexes and a clumsy gait (walk). Tests to confirm diagnosis and rule out other causes include electromyography (measurement of muscle electrical activity). This test entails inserting electrodes into muscles and measuring the electrical signals. Other tests may include blood studies, CT (computed tomography) scanning, and MRI (magnetic resonance imaging), which help to rule out other causes of muscle weakness. At times, a muscle biopsy is necessary. Genetic testing may be recommended if there is a family history of ALS.

TREATMENT

Because there is no cure for ALS, the goal of treatment is to control symptoms. Medication may be prescribed to manage spasms and the ability to swallow. Since there is a progressive loss of the ability to care for oneself, helpful measures include physical therapy, rehabilitation, and orthopedic appliances (such as a wheelchair). To prevent choking, a tube may need to be placed into the person's stomach for feeding. Because mental functioning remains intact, emotional support is vital for coping with this disorder.

Alteplase

A drug that dissolves blood clots. Alteplase (Activase) is used to treat heart attack, stroke, or pulmonary embolism (clot in the artery of the lungs.) Alteplase, which is also known as t-PA, or tissue-type plasminogen activator, is one of several promising drugs to dissolve blockages rather than create detours around them, such as in artery bypass surgery. Alteplase can be used to open clogged arteries during and after an acute heart attack, unlike bypass surgery, which can only prevent one. Alteplase may be effective for strokes, but only if it is given within 3 hours of the first symptoms.

Alteplase is the first cardiac medication to have been genetically engineered. It was created by splicing genes together and is derived from human cells rather than bacteria, which can trigger an immune response in the body.

Side effects associated with alteplase include nausea and dizziness. More serious reactions include bloody urine, bloody bowel movements, bloody vomit, coughing up blood, nosebleeds, and heavy vaginal bleeding. People who are taking alteplase should alert their doctors at once if they experience any bleeding problems.

Alternative medicine

Techniques, methods, and practices of health care used as alternatives to conventional medicine. Interest in alternative medicine stems from the idea that conventional Western medicine has its limitations, and it reflects a desire on the part of some to take an active role in promoting their own health and well-being. Examples of alternative medicine include ancient healing traditions such as ACUPUNCTURE and HERBAL MEDICINE, in addition

---

A LOOK AT ALTERNATIVE MEDICINE

Every year, more than 40 percent of Americans use some form of alternative medicine, whether it be acupuncture for pain relief, meditation to help with life's stresses, or over-the-counter nutritional supplements to stay well.

There are several fields of practice under the large umbrella of alternative therapies. Mind-body or lifestyle practices include biofeedback, hypnotherapy, guided imagery, meditation, and yoga, while alternative systems include traditional Chinese medicine (such as acupuncture) and homeopathy. Alternative therapies also include what is called manual manipulation, such as chiropractic, acupressure, and massage therapy, while biologic treatments include areas such as aromatherapy and herbal medicines.

The National Institutes of Health, which now houses the National Center for Complementary and Alternative Medicine, estimates that Americans spend more than $27 billion a year on these treatments, also known as unconventional medicine.

Much of what is known about the effectiveness and safety of alternative therapies is based on anecdotal evidence, that is, the personal testimonials, theories, beliefs, and opinions of those who have experienced positive outcomes. Scientific research continues to expand as the field of alternative medicine becomes increasingly popular and the treatments more widely used, but only some therapies have been validated by clinical research thus far.

Still, alternative medical practice is considered to be outside the mainstream of currently established medical protocol. Regulation of alternative practitioners varies from state to state. Regulatory agencies can be contacted to verify the credentials of a person offering alternative treatments.

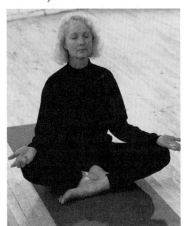

YOGA FOR GOOD HEALTH
Adults of any age can benefit from yoga, an ancient art enjoying a surge in popularity. Yoga is a gentle form of exercise that may give a person more energy while reducing stress.

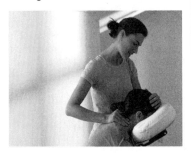

MASSAGING AWAY TENSION
Portable massage chairs allow a person to enjoy a quick massage that eases tension in the back, neck, shoulders, and arms while sitting up and fully clothed.

to newer methods, such as CHIROPRAC-TIC, and megavitamin therapy. Most techniques of alternative medicine have not been widely taught in medical schools, although many are increasingly recognized and considered effective by doctors. At the same time, however, many doctors are calling for more clinical research on alternative therapies to verify whether they work and are safe.

NATURAL HEALING
An idea key to all forms of alternative medicine is that health is more than simply the absence of disease. All forms of alternative medicine also assume that health care involves more than just the physical body. Alternative medicine generally focuses on the whole person and takes into account his or her physical, emotional, spiritual, nutritional, and social needs. One goal of alternative medicine is for people to take personal responsibility for their own balance and well-being.

Natural healing usually refers to the use of noninvasive, nonpharmaceutical techniques that help heal the person. These may include MASSAGE THERAPY, chiropractic, BODYWORK, and other techniques.

COMPLEMENTARY MEDICINE
Complementary medicine includes techniques often used by conventional medical practitioners together with traditional methods such as surgery and medication. The conventional technique is viewed as the primary tool, while the complementary technique is secondary. Massage therapy, bodywork, and MEDITATION are examples of techniques that may be used as complementary medicine; for example, a doctor may recommend meditation to help prepare for major surgery.

LIFESTYLE
Most methods of alternative medicine emphasize the importance of addressing the person's whole lifestyle as part of his or her therapy. Alternative medicine focuses on the whole person, not simply his or her symptoms, before selecting any remedy. While the various forms of alternative medicine differ from one another in many ways, they all subscribe to the importance of restoring inner balance or harmony to the whole person as an essential part of any successful therapy. Examples of lifestyle therapies include yoga and ayurveda, an ancient system of healing and health care that includes meditation, yoga, and herbal remedies.

Altitude sickness
A disorder caused by a lack of oxygen at high altitudes. Altitude sickness affects hikers and mountain climbers who climb too rapidly above 8,000 feet. The disorder occurs because as altitude increases, both atmospheric pressure and the amount of oxygen available in the atmosphere decrease. Initial symptoms, often referred to as acute mountain sickness, include headache, sleep disturbance, fatigue, shortness of breath, dizziness, and nausea, any of which may occur in 20 percent of people who ascend higher than 8,000 feet in a single day. Drinking extra water is recommended to compensate for excess water loss associated with acute mountain sickness, which wears off within 24 to 48 hours, as the body adapts to the higher altitude.

More serious symptoms can develop above 9,000 feet, causing high-altitude pulmonary edema and high-altitude cerebral edema, both of which can be fatal. High-altitude pulmonary edema is characterized by strong coughing that produces frothy, blood-tinged sputum, while high-altitude cerebral edema is associated with staggering, hallucinations, confusion, and coma.

Altitude sickness can usually be prevented by a slow ascent. It is thought that the symptoms occur because insufficient oxygen indirectly causes excess water to enter the cells of the body, which can lead to dangerous swelling in the lungs and around the brain. Symptoms of altitude sickness can usually be avoided by pausing for 1 day at 7,000 feet and by ascending no more than 2,000 feet per day above 7,000 feet. Hikers should avoid drinking alcohol and carbonated beverages and smoking cigarettes.

Aluminum
A silvery-white metallic element found in abundance in the Earth's crust. Aluminum is never found in a pure form but as a constituent of many minerals, such as bauxite, mica, and feldspar. It is used to form many alloys (metal combinations) that are lightweight but hard and resistant to corrosion. Aluminum foil is used as a wrapping material, and aluminum powder is used in paints for buildings. Aluminum is the main ingredient in some antacids. Too much aluminum in the body can cause brain injury, resulting in dementia.

Alveolectomy
Dental surgery to trim or remove the bone or gum tissue in the jawbone that holds the roots of the teeth. The procedure is usually performed along with tooth extractions. The purpose of alveolectomy is to eliminate protrusions or sharp surfaces in the dental ridge and to prepare the area for the placement of dentures. This procedure will also promote a quicker healing of the ridge, the soft tissue covering after tooth removal.

The person is usually given a general anesthetic before an incision is made in the gum. The surgeon exposes the uneven bone, which is reshaped. The gum is then sutured back together. The person can expect swelling and bruising, with the gum healing in about 2 weeks.

Alveoli
Microscopic air sacs within the lungs and the site of gas exchange. The alveoli are clustered together like grapes at the end of a bronchiole (small air tube). Each alveolus is made of connective tissue surrounded by very small blood vessels called capillaries. Air that is inhaled travels through the successively finer air passageways of the RESPIRATORY SYSTEM to the alveoli. The thin walls of the alveoli absorb the oxygen molecules from the air, which then pass through the capillary walls into the bloodstream to oxygenate the blood (which then circulates to body tissues). At the same time, the waste product carbon dioxide passes from the blood through the walls of the capillaries and into the alveoli and is expelled from the lungs in exhaled air. The exchange takes place at this cellular level because oxygen in the alveolus is at higher pressure than in the capillaries, and carbon dioxide is at higher pressure in the capillaries than in the alveolus. This gas exchange is called true respiration.

Alveolitis

A lung disease that results from an inflammation of the alveoli, which are the tiny round air sacs found at the ends of the bronchioles in the lungs. The alveoli are the terminal ends of the bronchioles, which are tiny airways that form after many divisions of the bronchi, the two airways that branch off from the windpipe, or trachea. There are millions of alveoli in each lung. Each alveolus is surrounded by a dense system of capillaries. When they function normally, the alveoli's very thin walls permit an exchange of oxygen and carbon dioxide between the alveoli and the blood in the capillaries.

CAUSES AND SYMPTOMS

Allergic alveolitis (also called hypersensitivity pneumonitis) is caused by an allergic response in those who are sensitive to organic dusts. Contact with organic dusts often occurs in the workplace, and the different forms of alveolitis are often named according to the manner in which they were acquired. The two most common of these are FARMER'S LUNG, which is generally caused by continual inhalation of spores from moldy hay, and BYSSINOSIS, which occurs in workers who produce cotton, flax, jute, and hemp for yarn or rope. Other forms of alveolitis include the following: humidifier lung, which is caused by a fungus that has contaminated a household humidifier, heating system, or air conditioner; BAGASSOSIS, which is caused by fungi that are found in sugar cane fiber mold; suberosis, which is caused by the inhalation of moldy cork dust; and sequoiosis, which is the result of exposure to moldy redwood sawdust. Additional forms of alveolitis include mushroom picker's disease, which is caused by inhalation of dust from moldy compost; maple bark stripper's disease, which occurs from exposure to rotting maple tree logs and bark; bird fancier's lung, or bird breeder's lung, which results from the inhalation of protein dust particles from bird droppings and feathers; malt worker's lung, which is caused by inhalation of malt dust; and detergent worker's lung, which results from the inhalation of dust that contains spores from enzyme additives to commercial laundry detergents.

In people who are sensitive to any of these specific dusts, exposure can cause symptoms, generally from 6 hours to days after exposure. The symptoms include a persistent cough, a sensation of tightness in the chest, wheezing, shortness of breath, and decreased lung function. There may also be recurrent episodes of fever, chills, dry coughing, and very labored breathing.

DIAGNOSIS AND TREATMENT

Diagnosis is based on characteristic symptoms and a history of environmental exposure and may be confirmed with the results of PULMONARY FUNCTION TESTS, X rays, and blood tests. Avoiding exposure to the dust that irritates the alveoli generally relieves symptoms. Proper cleansing of humidifiers, air conditioners, and heating systems is also recommended. In some cases, a corticosteroid may be prescribed to open airways and ease breathing.

People who smoke cigarettes or cigars are more susceptible to alveolitis, have more serious symptoms, and are advised to quit smoking.

Alveoloplasty

A surgical procedure usually performed after teeth are extracted to recontour the jawbone and increase the ridge size in preparation for dentures. If teeth need to be removed because of advanced PERIODONTAL DISEASE, severe decay, or fracture, the ridge of the jawbone that surrounded and held the roots of the teeth may need to be flattened. In this state, the bone and gum tissue cannot support dentures and must be reshaped or reconstructed, possibly with the use of grafting. If bone or skin grafts are used, the procedure may require hospitalization. Procedures using artificial bone grafts may be performed in a dental office. In addition to providing support for dentures, alveoloplasty helps to reduce the risk of jawbone fracture and may help to prevent the severe pain or facial numbness that can be caused by lower dentures pressing on facial nerves.

Alzheimer's disease

An irreversible brain disease, usually in older people, that causes a progressive decline in mental function. Alzheimer's disease (AD) is the most common cause of dementia, a syndrome characterized by a gradual loss of memory and other intellectual functions. (AD is also known as dementia of the Alzheimer type, or DAT.) Typically in AD, brain cells die and the connections between them deteriorate. About 5 percent of people age 65 are affected, with the incidence increasing as people age. Fifty percent of people over age 85 may have AD. Researchers suspect AD may be caused either by a deficiency in a brain chemical or a genetic defect. Early on, AD affects cells in the hippocampus, a brain area related to memory. Later, it targets the cerebral cortex, where language and reasoning originate. In addition to memory loss, a person with AD eventually loses the abilities to reason and communicate. Early signs of AD, such as forgetfulness and a loss of concentration, are subtle. But an affected person gradually worsens and at last becomes incapacitated. The course of the disease varies greatly among individuals. On average, people live from 8 to 10 years after diagnosis but can live as long as 20 years.

Anatomic hallmarks of the disease are the distinct pathologic abnormalities called plaques and tangles, which have been detected in the brain tissue of people who have AD. Plaques are dense protein deposits found around the brain's nerve cells. Tangles are twisted protein fibers that appear inside the nerve cells. Both are associated with AD, but their precise role in the disease is not clear.

SYMPTOMS AND DIAGNOSIS

Alzheimer's disease is uncommon before age 65, although it can occur anytime from age 40 on. Characteristically, it develops slowly and gradually progresses in a steady manner. At first a person may have difficulty remembering recent events or names of familiar people and objects. More noticeable symptoms of AD set in over a period of 4 to 8 or more years and grow increasingly severe. Cognitive abilities, such as reasoning, judgment, and

DAILY ASSISTANCE
When a person reaches the later stages of Alzheimer's disease, a spouse or other family member may have to assist with everyday functions such as eating. A healthy diet is particularly important because nutritional deficiencies can worsen the symptoms of the disease.

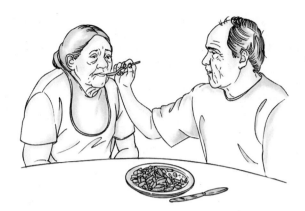

understanding, become impaired. Ordinary forgetfulness is not a sign of the disorder, but memory loss that interferes with function is. It is very common to forget where the car keys are; it is cause for concern to forget what the car keys are for. Affected individuals eventually can develop problems speaking, reading, writing, and doing simple math calculations. They may no longer remember the year or the city where they live. Personality may also change. Loss of interest in familiar activities and mood swings often occur. Individuals may become apathetic and indifferent or angry, frustrated, and aggressive. People with AD may wander and can get lost in once familiar surroundings. Eventually, they may not recognize loved ones and may forget how to perform basic activities of daily living such as dressing, washing, eating a meal, or using the toilet.

Other than a brain biopsy demonstrating the characteristic changes in brain tissue, no physical, psychological, or laboratory test provides a definitive diagnosis of AD. However, based on medical observation, the accuracy rate of AD diagnosis by experienced clinicians is high; autopsies bear out clinical AD diagnoses from 85 to 95 percent of the time.

Diagnosis is determined through a complete physical examination, personal and family medical histories, and tests. An important part of evaluating people for AD is ruling out possible causes of symptoms that may be reversible. For example, treatable conditions such as depression, hypothyroidism, or a vitamin B12

deficiency can all cause forgetfulness and confusion. Vision or hearing loss, alcohol use, or side effects of medications can be responsible for other Alzheimer-like symptoms. Unlike AD, these causes are treatable.

Tests may include basic analyses of blood and urine; a mental status examination; and neuropsychological tests of memory, problem solving, and language. Imaging studies of the brain, such as CT (computed tomography) scanning or MRI (magnetic resonance imaging) frequently are

SIMPLE REMINDERS
A person in the early stages of Alzheimer's disease may benefit from minor adjustments in the home environment. For example, labels on kitchen cabinets or dresser drawers may help the person remember where to find items he or she uses every day. While short-term memory is impaired, long-term memory may be all right in the beginning stages of the disease.

used to rule out other causes of dementia. Alzheimer's disease can be very difficult to distinguish from other forms of dementia. Alzheimer's disease is often confused with VASCULAR DEMENTIA (which is caused by strokes); it is possible for an older person to have both of these types of dementia at once. Because treatments and programs may vary for different types of dementia, correctly identifying the type is important.

TREATMENT
Medications called cholinesterase inhibitors can be taken to slow the progression of cognitive symptoms in the early to middle stages of the disease. The first medication marketed for this, tacrine, required careful monitoring. Later, donepezil became available; its side effects are mild, primarily occasional nausea or diarrhea. Donepezil inhibits the breakdown of a key NEUROTRANSMITTER (a type of messenger cell in the brain) and helps cognitive functions. People's responses to these medications can vary, and the risks and benefits of the medications require careful evaluation.

Behavioral approaches sometimes improve the control of symptoms

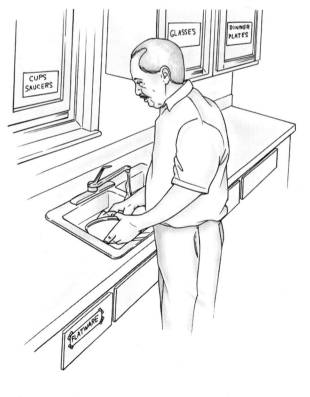

GLASSES

DINNER PLATES

CUPS SAUCERS

FLATWARE

A

such as depression, frustration, agitation, and anger. Such approaches include creating a more tolerant home environment and avoiding circumstances that are likely to provoke outbursts. Medications can help control symptoms such as sleeplessness, agitation, wandering, anxiety, and depression. Medica-tions are prescribed conservatively because possible side effects such as sedation and confusion can exaggerate the problems of older people who have AD.

Community resources are useful for dealing with the behavior of people with AD. Family caregivers often find support through groups of fellow caregivers who share strategies for coping with AD behavior and the difficulties associated with coping. State or AREA AGENCIES ON AGING are sources for information on available services such as transportation, home-delivered meals, home health services, and adult day care programs (see DAY CARE, ADULT). Most people with AD will eventually require the skilled and constant care of a LONG-TERM CARE FACILITY such as a nursing home.

RISK FACTORS AND OUTLOOK

Being genetically linked to a relative who has or had the disease is a risk factor for AD, as is being older than 65; the risk of developing AD doubles each decade after age 65. Researchers also have noted a possible link of AD to a history of head injury. There is neither a known way to prevent AD nor a cure. As life expectancy increases, the number of people with AD will grow. While researchers do not fully understand the causes of the disease, they know that complex changes in the brain, triggered by different variables, appear to precede the disease. Looking to improve treatments and disease prevention, researchers continue to explore the genetic and nongenetic factors that have a role in the disease. Other diseases, such as PICK DISEASE and LEWY BODY DEMENTIA, can cause memory loss and symptoms similar to AD. Although they have some distinct features, these diseases are less common than AD, and, frequently, doctors have difficulty identifying the exact disease that is causing the dementia.

Amalgam, dental

Silver-colored filling material used by dentists to fill a tooth that has been treated for the removal of TOOTH DECAY. Dental amalgam is a mixture of mercury and an alloy of silver, tin, and copper. It is considered to be one of the safest, most durable, and least expensive materials used to fill a dental cavity. Amalgam fillings cannot cause a person to have metal poisoning. The dentist mixes the amalgam, places it in the filling, and allows it to set, usually in a few minutes. It takes about 24 hours for the filling to harden completely, so some dentists advise avoiding chewing on the affected side.

Amaurosis fugax

Loss of vision in one eye that lasts for seconds to minutes and may last for up to 24 hours. Visual loss is often described as if a curtain is coming down from above or across the field of vision. The usual cause is a spasm or blockage in a small blood vessel leading to a lack of blood in the retina (the light-sensitive layer in the back of the eye). The condition can be a sign that a person is at increased risk for stroke. The name comes from a Greek word (amaurosis) meaning "darkening" and a Latin word (fugax) meaning "fleeting."

Ambidexterity

The ability to use either hand with equal skill. Ambidexterity is characterized by the ability to write with either hand, rather than being exclusively left-handed or right-handed. Ambidexterity also includes the ability to use either hand to perform a variety of other tasks, such as holding a tennis racket or using keys.

Amblyopia

Poor vision in one eye resulting from a failure to develop normal sight during childhood; commonly known as "lazy eye." Amblyopia results from functional and structural abnormalities after birth. The brain's center of vision usually develops from birth to age 6 or 7 years. If the brain's visual center has not developed by then, vision may be permanently impaired. A newborn can see, but must learn to focus and to coordinate images from both eyes into a single, three-dimensional image. If vision in one eye is distorted, nerve connections between that eye and the brain fail to develop properly. The brain learns to ignore the distorted image and relies only on the better eye. The result is amblyopia or a failure to develop normal vision in the affected eye.

Amblyopia can be caused by any disease that prevents clear focusing.

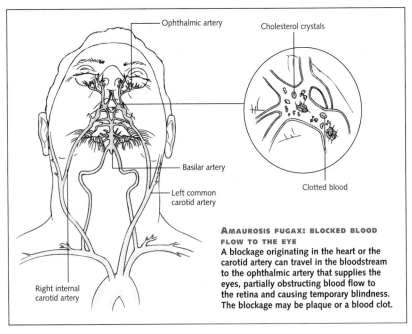

Ophthalmic artery

Cholesterol crystals

Basilar artery

Left common carotid artery

Clotted blood

Right internal carotid artery

AMAUROSIS FUGAX: BLOCKED BLOOD FLOW TO THE EYE
A blockage originating in the heart or the carotid artery can travel in the bloodstream to the ophthalmic artery that supplies the eyes, partially obstructing blood flow to the retina and causing temporary blindness. The blockage may be plaque or a blood clot.

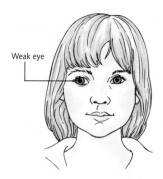

Weak eye

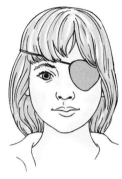

TREATING "LAZY EYE"
A common cause of amblyopia is strabismus, or a misaligned eye. The child with such a condition learns to "turn off" the vision in the misaligned eye, resulting in a loss of vision. Treatment involves patching the stronger eye, which trains the child to use the weaker eye.

The most common cause is STRABISMUS, known commonly as "crossed eyes." Other causes include farsightedness, nearsightedness, or astigmatism that is more severe in one eye than the other. In rare instances, amblyopia is caused by a cataract (clouding of the lens of the eye).

Except in obvious cases of strabismus, amblyopia can be difficult to detect. Physicians check for the condition by watching how well a child can follow objects with one eye covered. If amblyopia is present, covering the good eye will lead the child to try to remove the cover or to fuss and cry. Further examinations are then performed to determine the cause of the vision difference between the two eyes.

Amblyopia does not usually improve after the age of 9 years, making it very important to detect and treat it before then to ensure the development of normal vision. If not treated, irreversible serious visual defects can occur in the affected eye. Individuals with amblyopia have poor depth perception, and if a child should lose vision in the good eye from disease or injury, he or she may be left with permanently impaired eyesight.

Treatment is usually successful, particularly in younger children. Treatment relies on inducing the child to use the weak eye. Often this is accomplished by placing a patch over the good eye, requiring the child to rely on vision from the amblyopic eye for an extended period. In some cases, drops that blur vision in the good eye are used instead of a patch, but this approach is usually less effective. Strabismus usually requires corrective surgery to bring the eyes into alignment. Correcting vision with glasses or contact lenses may also be prescribed.

Ambulance

A vehicle designed to transport sick or injured people. Ambulances contain cots to keep the person stationary and are equipped with devices for administering oxygen, intravenous fluids, cardiac care, and other life-saving interventions. Ambulances are built for speed and smooth riding and have room for one or two sick or injured people plus medical personnel. Military ambulances are larger and designed for sturdiness rather than speed; they are built to carry four to six injured people to field hospitals.

Ambulatory surgery

Any surgical procedure in which the patient is not admitted to a hospital; the person returns home on the same day the surgery is performed. Also known as outpatient or same-day surgery, ambulatory surgery can be performed in a surgery clinic, within a hospital setting, or in a day surgery center.

Preparation for and recovery from ambulatory surgery varies, depending on the type of operation being performed. Since the patient will receive an anesthetic, food and drink are usually not allowed for 8 to 10 hours beforehand. When the person arrives at the surgery center (sometimes called a surgicenter), he or she is prepared for the procedure. A thin tube called an intravenous catheter is inserted into a vein in the hand or lower arm for presurgical medications. Blood pressure and heart rate are checked, and the area to be operated on is usually cleaned and shaved. After the procedure is performed and the recovery period is complete, the patient can be taken home by a friend or relative. Because of the lingering effects of anesthetics and other medications, the person should not drive or operate machinery for at least 24 hours. Once home, the person may need help with eating and bathing for a few days.

Ambulatory surgery, which now accounts for more than half of all surgical procedures in the United States, helps cut health care costs. Same-day procedures cost 30 to 60 percent less than surgical operations that require an overnight hospital stay. Many people prefer ambulatory surgery because they can recover in their familiar home setting rather than in a hospital.

Many different types of surgery can be performed as same-day procedures, including biopsies, removal of cysts, cataract surgery, gallbladder removal, laparoscopic surgery, vasectomy, hernia and hemorrhoid repair, tubal ligation, tonsil and adenoid removal, and arthroscopic surgery of the joints.

Amebiasis

An infectious intestinal disease caused by a microscopic, one-celled parasite. Amebiasis in its most severe form is called AMEBIC DYSENTERY. A small percentage of the people infected with the parasite actually become

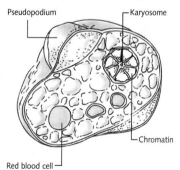

Pseudopodium

Karyosome

Chromatin

Red blood cell

ONE-CELLED PARASITE
An intestinal parasite (*Entamoeba histolytica*) causes amebic dysentery (or amebiasis). This parasite feeds on red blood cells and moves by means of a pseudopodium, an extrusion of part of the outer membrane. The nucleus of the organism contains genetic material (chromatin and karyosomes).

A

PREVENTING AMEBIASIS WHEN TRAVELING

Amebiasis is more common in developing countries where hygiene and water purification standards may be less rigorous than those of the United States. To avoid the disease, a traveller should:

- Adhere strictly to rules of personal hygiene, washing the hands carefully after use of the toilet and before handling food.
- Drink only bottled water or carbonated drinks in cans and bottles.
- Boil other drinking water for at least 1 minute, or water should be filtered through an "absolute 1 micron or less" filter (available at camping supply stores) and treated by dissolving iodine tablets in the filtered water.
- Avoid drinks with ice cubes and fountain drinks.
- Peel fresh fruit and vegetables just before eating; fruits and vegetables served peeled should be avoided.
- Avoid milk, cheese, and other dairy products that have not been pasteurized.
- Avoid food or beverages sold by street vendors.

ill, and in those who do get sick, symptoms are often mild. They include diarrhea, abdominal pain and cramping, nausea, weight loss, and sometimes fever. Symptoms of amebic dysentery include stomach pain, bloody mucous stools, and fever. In rare cases, the parasite may spread to the liver and form an abscess, and in even rarer cases, the parasite may invade other parts of the body, including the lungs or brain.

CAUSES

Infected people are the only source of the parasite that causes amebiasis, and it is spread by contact with fecal material from people who carry the parasite. Eating or drinking contaminated food or water can cause the infection. If a person touches a surface contaminated with the cysts of the parasite and the hands come in contact with the mouth, amebiasis may result. Oral-anal contact may also produce amebiasis. People who may develop

severe amebiasis when infected include pregnant women, malnourished individuals, infants, and persons receiving corticosteroid therapy. Symptoms usually occur within 2 to 4 weeks of exposure, but may appear within a few days to a few months. A person with amebiasis can carry the parasite for several weeks to several years, often with no symptoms.

The infection is most common in environments where poor sanitary conditions exist. People living in or traveling to developing countries and those residing in poorly maintained institutions may become infected.

DIAGNOSIS AND TREATMENT

Amebiasis is diagnosed by examining a person's stool sample under a microscope. It is not easily diagnosed because other cells and more common parasites look similar when seen through a microscope. Several stool samples are sometimes obtained on several different days because the parasite is not always found in every sample. A blood test may be recommended if there is the suspicion that the infection has spread to the wall of the intestines or to the liver. The blood test may be positive in a person who has had amebiasis in the past but is no longer infected.

The infection is treated with specific antibiotics. Once treated, a person will no longer carry the parasite in the intestinal tract and in most cases is unlikely to become reinfected.

Amebic dysentery

Inflammation of the colon caused by infection with an ameba (a single-celled parasite), causing bloody DIARRHEA, excess mucus secretion, and abdominal cramps. Amebic dysentery is most common in countries with poor sanitation and is caused by consuming water or food that is contaminated with particles of feces that contain amebae.

Diagnosis of amebic dysentery can be made by analyzing stool samples, by blood tests, or by SIGMOIDOSCOPY (visual examination of the sigmoid colon and rectum through a lighted tube called a sigmoidoscope). Anti-amebic drugs, such as metronidazole, are usually effective in treating the disease. After treatment, follow-up stool samples are required for 2 to 3

months to ensure that no parasites remain. Untreated amebic dysentery can cause an abscess in the liver (see LIVER ABSCESS) to develop. A liver abscess is a serious complication that can be detected by using ultrasound scanning. To prevent amebic dysentery, doctors recommend that travelers use bottled water, avoid fresh fruits, and eat only thoroughly cooked foods.

Amelogenesis imperfecta

An inherited condition that affects the enamel of the teeth. Amelogenesis imperfecta may cause the teeth to be varied in color, ranging from white to yellow or brown. The condition causes the tooth enamel surface to be abnormally thin and chalky, making the tooth more prone to decay. The condition can also cause the teeth to be sensitive to sweets and to heat. When parts of the teeth are missing or when there are aesthetic problems, the placement of dental crowns is often recommended.

Amenorrhea

The absence of menstruation either in a woman who has never menstruated or in a woman whose regular menstrual cycle has ceased temporarily or permanently. See MENSTRUATION, DISORDERS OF.

American Medical Association (AMA)

The largest physician organization in the United States. Founded more than 150 years ago, the AMA is committed to education, research, and service. It develops and promotes standards in medical practice, ethics, and research and promotes excellence in medical education and practice. In addition, the AMA serves as an advocate on behalf of physicians and patients in the legislative and judicial arenas, and it provides timely information on health matters through a wide range of sources, including accreditation and education activities, scientific journals, the AMA Web site (http://www.ama-assn.org), and physician and consumer book publishing divisions.

AMA policy is developed through a democratic process that gathers informed viewpoints on issues of importance to physicians and their patients. Its House of Delegates is the seat of policymaking. Its state, local, and specialty society representatives set policy through a consensus-building process.

Americans with Disabilities Act (ADA)

A civil rights law enacted in 1990 to eliminate discrimination against individuals with disabilities and to provide disabled Americans with a system of legal redress. The Americans with Disabilities Act (ADA) prohibits discrimination by private and public services in many areas, including employment, housing, public accommodations, education, transportation, communications, and health services, on the basis of disabilities.

The term "disability" is defined by the ADA to include a functional physical or mental impairment that substantially limits one or more major life activities. An individual with a history of an impairment, such as having had cancer or being treated for bipolar disorder, is protected by the ADA. Also protected under the ADA are people who are perceived by others as having an impairment.

Physical impairment generally refers to a physiological disorder or condition, a disfigurement, or an anatomical loss. Mental impairment refers to mental or psychological disorders such as mental retardation, emotional illness, and learning disabilities. Generally, a person with an acute, short-term condition (such as the flu or a broken bone) would not be covered. The ADA has certain specific exceptions to the definition of disability such as compulsive gambling and kleptomania (an obsessive impulse to steal). People with alcoholism are protected by the ADA from discrimination by an employer but applicants and employees who use illegal drugs are not.

The ADA prohibits discrimination in employment against any qualified person with a disability in matters such as recruitment, advertising, job applications, and hiring; training,

Terms in small capital letters—for example, PHYSICAL THERAPY or PAGET DISEASE—indicate a cross-reference to another entry with more information.

advancement, compensation, and fringe benefits; leaves, layoffs, and firings; and tenure and retirement. Reasonable accommodations that do not cause "undue hardship" must be made to a workplace by an employer.

The ADA has helped individuals with disabilities to gain access to public places such as schools, theaters, hotels, restaurants, museums, libraries, health care offices and facilities, and parks and expanded access to auxiliary aids and services such as listening devices, interpreters, and large-print material. The ADA facilitates telephone and other communication means for deaf and hearing-impaired people and enables those in the disabled community to participate more fully in society. In every case, however, the ADA does not override federal and state health and safety laws.

Amino acids

Organic compounds that make up all proteins. Amino acids are found in both plants and animals. The human body can synthesize some amino acids, while the essential amino acids must be obtained from protein consumed in the diet. Following the digestion of protein in food, amino acids are released from the intestines into the bloodstream, which carries them to various cells of the body, where they are used for growth, maintenance, and repair.

Aminoglycosides

Antibacterial antibiotics used to treat infections caused by aerobic, gram-negative bacteria. Aminoglycosides work by preventing proper protein synthesis in disease-causing bacteria. Among the bacteria that are vulnerable to aminoglycosides are *Pseudomonas, Klebsiella, Escherichia coli* (see E. COLI), *Staphylococcus aureus,* and *Mycobacterium tuberculosis.*

Aminoglycosides are available as nebulizer solutions, capsules, and eye ointments and by injection. Aminoglycosides are chiefly used for bacterial "blood poisoning" (septicemia), although they may be used to treat urinary tract infections. Neomycin, streptomycin, and kanamycin are used to treat active tuberculosis. Adverse and potentially serious side effects include kidney dysfunction, equilibrium disturbances, deafness, and muscle paralysis.

Amiodarone hydrochloride

An antiarrhythmic drug. Amiodarone (Cordarone, Pacerone) is used to treat arrhythmias, or irregular heartbeat. Amiodarone works by decreasing the sensitivity of heart tissue to nerve impulses. It is usually prescribed only when other medications do not improve a person's condition or when the abnormal heart rhythm is so severe as to be life-threatening.

Amitriptyline

An antidepressant drug. Amitriptyline (Elavil) is one of a class of antidepressants called tricyclic antidepressants (TCAs). TCAs work by blocking the passage of two neurotransmitters, serotonin and norepinephrine, into and out of nerve endings, thereby causing a sedative effect. Amitriptyline is usually prescribed to treat depression; sometimes it is used to control chronic pain due to migraine, tension headache, diabetic nerve pain, tic douloureux (SEE TRIGEMINAL NEURALGIA), pain associated with cancer, herpes lesions, and arthritis; to treat eating disorders including bulimia; and to treat a pathological weeping and laughing disorder associated with multiple sclerosis.

Amitriptyline must be taken regularly for several weeks before it becomes completely effective. It is associated with a number of side effects, including mild drowsiness, dry mouth, headache, nausea, restlessness, sleep disturbances, and cardiac arrhythmias. Amitriptyline makes the skin more sensitive to sunlight; people who are taking it should wear protective clothing and use a sun block with a sun protection factor (SPF) of 15 or higher. The drug can be lethal in overdoses.

Ammonia

A colorless alkaline gas with a strong, penetrating odor. Ammonia in solution with water is also called volatile alkali. Ammonia solutions are used to clean, bleach, and deodorize; to etch aluminum; and in the manufacture of chemicals. The ammonia used for household cleaning is a water solution of ammonium hydroxide that should be used with caution because it can harm the skin and the eyes. Ammonia solutions should never be mixed with bleach because a poisonous gas called chloramine can be generated, resulting in severe lung damage. Prolonged exposure to and breathing in of ammonia vapors can also cause lung damage.

Amnesia

The loss of memory. (See also MEMORY, LOSS OF.) Amnesia can be the result of brain damage or of severe emotional trauma. Depending on its cause, memory loss may be temporary or permanent and may come on slowly or suddenly. Common causes of amnesia include alcoholism, general anesthetics, brain surgery, drug reactions, ECT (electroconvulsive therapy), head trauma or injury, hysteria, and migraine. Although aging is associated with increased difficulty mastering new material or recalling previously learned facts, unless disease is involved it does not cause memory loss.

TYPES OF AMNESIA

There are three major forms of amnesia: anterograde, retrograde, and transient global amnesia. Anterograde amnesia is caused by brain trauma. It is characterized by an inability to form new memories or remember newly learned material. Although short-term memory disappears, a person with anterograde amnesia can clearly remember events before the trauma.

Retrograde amnesia, also the result of trauma, is in many ways the opposite of anterograde amnesia. In this form of memory loss, a person can recall only the events that occurred after the trauma. He or she can no longer recall past events and information.

In transient global amnesia, there is a sudden loss of memory and a transient inability to recall new information. An affected person is disoriented and confused, but his or her behavior is otherwise normal. The exact cause of transient global amnesia remains unknown. However, most attacks follow periods of emotional stress, intense physical activity, or exposure to extreme temperatures; there is no association with recent head trauma or seizures. Although unsettling and alarming, most attacks of transient global amnesia resolve within several hours.

DIAGNOSIS AND TREATMENT

It is essential to identify the underlying cause of memory loss. To that end, doctors usually conduct thorough physical and neurological examinations and take a detailed medical history. Tests that may be used include cerebral angiography, MRI (magnetic resonance imaging) or CT (computed tomography) scanning of the head, electroencephalogram (EEG), blood tests, and psychometric or cognitive tests. Treatment of amnesia depends on its underlying cause. Home care measures include family support and providing familiar objects or photographs to keep the person oriented. When memory loss compromises safety, doctors recommend placement in a long-term care facility, such as a nursing home.

Amnio infusion

A procedure used during labor in which saline (a salt solution that has the same concentration as body fluids) is instilled into the uterus at a constant rate. During the procedure, a catheter (a hollow needle) is placed in the uterine cavity through the cervix, and then saline is introduced through the catheter. The objectives of this treatment include flushing out thick waste-stained fluid and reversal of abnormal fetal heart rate patterns, which may be related to umbilical cord compression.

Amniocentesis

A test commonly performed between weeks 14 and 16 of pregnancy to diagnose hereditary diseases and congenital defects in a fetus. Amniocentesis involves removing some of the amniotic fluid that surrounds a fetus in the uterus. The test is performed in women thought to have an increased risk of bearing a child with a genetic disorder or other detectable birth defects. Those at risk include women older than 35 years, those identified by maternal blood tests, or those who have a family history of a genetic disorder. Special counseling about amniocentesis is available.

During the procedure, a very fine needle is passed through the abdominal wall into the uterine cavity to withdraw about an ounce of amniotic fluid for analysis. Fetal cells obtained from the amniotic fluid are then grown in a laboratory and analyzed to detect abnormalities in chromosomes or genes, such as the chromosomal abnormality that results in Down syndrome. Other disorders can be detected by biochemical assays, which are measurements of the amount of certain chemicals present in amniotic fluid. Amniocentesis is sometimes used to diagnose other congenital defects, such as spina bifida (a neural tube defect). In addition, amniocentesis may be performed to assess the maturity of the baby's lungs, for suspected infection, or occasionally to drain off excess amniotic fluid. The risk for a miscarriage or spontaneous abortion increases slightly for women who undergo amniocentesis early in pregnancy.

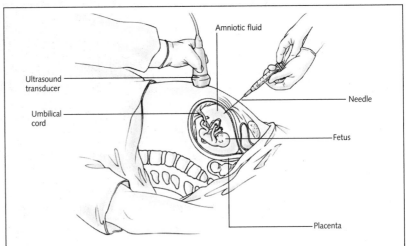

Amniotic fluid

Ultrasound transducer

Umbilical cord

Needle

Fetus

Placenta

HOW AMNIOCENTESIS IS PERFORMED
The woman is given a local anesthetic. Then a needle will be inserted into the uterus to withdraw amniotic fluid (the liquid that surrounds the fetus). The position of the fetus, placenta, and umbilical cord are monitored using ultrasound imaging.

THE PROCEDURE

In amniocentesis, a local anesthetic is injected into the abdominal wall to numb the site where the needle will be inserted to draw the amniotic fluid. An ultrasound is used to locate the positions of the fetus, placenta, and umbilical cord and to guide the insertion of the needle and withdrawal of amniotic fluid. Following the procedure, most women resume normal activities; a few require bed rest. Mild cramping, light bleeding, or leaking of amniotic fluid are commonly reported after the procedure. These reactions do not necessarily indicate a problem; however, a woman who experiences any of them should contact her doctor.

Amniotic fluid

The clear, watery fluid that surrounds and protects a fetus in the uterus (the organ in which the baby grows). The amniotic fluid is contained in a membrane called the amniotic sac. The fluid cushions the fetus from the pressure of the woman's internal organs and protects it from injury. Maintaining the proper amount of fluid is important to the health of the fetus. At each prenatal visit, the physician indirectly checks the amount of amniotic fluid by measuring and feeling the woman's abdomen. An ultrasound test may be used to assess the volume of the fluid more accurately for suspected abnormalities. POLYHYDRAMNIOS is a condition in which excess amniotic fluid is detected; it occurs once in about 250 pregnancies. OLIGOHYDRAMNIOS is an extremely rare condition in which an abnormally small amount of amniotic fluid is produced.

Amniotomy

A procedure used to start or speed up labor. The membranes of the amniotic sac surrounding the baby are broken and the AMNIOTIC FLUID is released, leading to stronger and more frequent contractions of the uterus. A painless procedure, amniotomy allows the doctor to place monitors in the uterus to monitor the labor and the baby's condition. See LABOR.

Amoxicillin

See PENICILLINS.

Amphotericin B

An antifungal drug. Amphotericin B (Abelcet, Fungizone) is used to treat severe infections caused by fungi. Amphotericin B is given by intravenous infusion, which lasts more than 1 hour and can cause the person to have fever, chills, loss of appetite, and headache. Most people receiving the drug will experience side effects and should be closely monitored.

Ampicillin

See PENICILLINS.

Amprenavir

A protease inhibitor. Amprenavir (Agenerase) is prescribed for HIV (human immunodeficiency virus) infection. When combined with other drugs, protease inhibitors reduce the amount of HIV in the bloodstream to levels that are virtually undetectable, although the drug cannot eradicate HIV or AIDS (acquired immunodeficiency syndrome).

Amputation, surgical

Surgical removal of a limb or appendage, such as a finger, hand, arm, toe, or leg. An amputation is necessary when a limb is irretrievably damaged in an accident or irreversibly infected by bacteria or when its blood supply is disrupted by diabetes, severe artery disease, frostbite, or gangrene (death of tissue).

An amputation is a major operation performed with the patient under general anesthesia. An incision is made around the limb to be amputated; then, the muscles, tendons, nerves, and bones are severed. The end of the bone is filed down smoothly and capped with the remaining healthy tissue. Large sutures (stitches) are used to close the muscle, and smaller sutures or staples are used to close the skin. Tubes are often left in the wound to allow drainage during the early healing period and then removed later. An amputation requires a hospital stay of 2 to 7 days and an at-home recovery period of about 6 weeks.

A person who has lost an arm or a leg is fitted with an artificial limb, or PROSTHESIS. Although the prosthesis is never as strong or agile as the original limb, it can help in handling the tasks of ordinary life. Usually a temporary limb is fitted soon after surgery to help the person get used to it. After the stump has healed, a permanent limb is designed to fit the need of the person. Physical therapy is often needed to help a person who has lost a leg, for example, relearn how to walk and drive.

Although an amputation is not usually life-threatening, the psychological consequences of the surgery can be difficult. Some people experience pain in the stump (PHANTOM LIMB PAIN, which is the sometimes painful feeling that the missing limb is still attached to the body). Counseling may help the person cope with self-esteem and image issues that arise after losing a limb.

A replantation of an arm just above the elbow may be an option after a traumatic amputation, for example, but the surgical procedure must take place within 12 hours. The limb should be placed in a plastic bag that contains saline solution, and the plastic bag should be placed on ice. A patient needs to be in good general health and younger than 60 years to be a replantation candidate. After the surgery, the patient must keep his or her arm elevated to prevent swelling. The major complications following a replantation include infection and clotting.

Amsler grid

A chart used to detect a type of age-related change in central vision known as MACULAR DEGENERATION. The chart looks like a piece of paper with dark lines forming a square grid around a dot in the center. The grid is held at a comfortable reading distance with one eye covered while the person focuses on the center dot; the test is then repeated with the other eye covered. Blurring of the grid or distortion of its lines into wavy, fuzzy, or missing areas of vision can indicate damage to the macula, most commonly from macular degeneration. See also VISION TESTS.

Amyloidosis

An uncommon disease caused by the abnormal protein amyloid being deposited in tissues or organs of the body, most frequently in the heart, kidneys, nervous system, or gastrointestinal tract. The associated disease may be inflammatory or cancerous.

Antibodies that cannot be broken down and recycled by the body lead to amyloidosis. When these antibodies accumulate in the bloodstream, they may be deposited in other areas of the body as amyloid. Depending on the affected organs, amyloidosis may present no symptoms, or the symptoms may be wide-ranging and include swollen legs and ankles, weakness, weight loss, shortness of breath, dizziness, diarrhea, severe fatigue, an enlarged tongue, and numbness or tingling in the extremities. The cause of amyloidosis is not known, but it is not believed to be contagious or related to stress or occupation. There may be a hereditary link. The majority of people affected are older than 40. Some people who have the form of bone marrow cancer called MULTIPLE MYELOMA may develop amyloidosis.

Amyotrophic lateral sclerosis

See ALS.

Amyotrophy

ATROPHY or wasting of the muscles. Amyotrophy is a common symptom of motor neuron diseases, such as ALS, but it is also seen in many other conditions, including diabetes, syphilis, and cancer.

Anabolic steroids

Synthetic male sex hormones (androgens). Anabolic steroids promote the growth of skeletal muscle (anabolic effects) and the development of male sexual characteristics (androgenic effects). They were originally developed to treat a condition called hypogonadism, in which the testes do not produce enough testosterone for normal growth and sexual functioning. Some athletes, especially bodybuilders, abuse steroids to increase muscle size and to decrease body fat. Anabolic steroids can cause liver failure, abnormal hair distribution, oily skin, and, in women, masculine characteristics.

Anaerobic

Lacking or needing no oxygen to survive; oxygen-deficient. Anaerobic is used to describe life forms, such as certain types of bacteria, that do not require oxygen for metabolism. Anaerobic life forms are able to live in the complete absence of oxygen and are called anaerobes.

Anaerobic respiration can occur during heavy exercise, leading to an oxygen deficit in the blood. When this happens, pyruvic acid interacts with hydrogen in such a way that lactic acid builds up in the tissues, causing muscle pain.

Anal dilation

The widening of the anal sphincter muscle to treat hemorrhoids or to repair an ANAL FISSURE, a tear or ulcer in the lining of the anal canal. It is

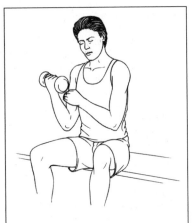

ONE FORM OF ANAEROBIC EXERCISE
Anaerobic exercise involves short, intense intervals of activity that oxygen cannot fuel alone; partial breakdown of carbohydrates is required to bring energy to muscles quickly. The partial breakdown leads to a buildup of lactic acid as a by-product, so anaerobic activities can be sustained for only a short time.

also performed if there is a narrowing of the anal canal that interferes with the normal passage of stools. The procedure can stop the pain, spasms, and bleeding associated with anal fissures, and healing is relatively quick. However, impaired continence can occur as a result of dilation. Anal dilation is performed under general anesthesia with the use of a mechanical dilator.

Anal discharge

Secretion of substances, such as blood, mucus, or pus, from the anus. Anal discharge is often the result of a relatively minor problem, such as hemorrhoids or an anal fissure (a tear or ulcer in the lining of the anal canal). However, in some cases, a discharge may be the sign of a more serious disorder, such as CROHN DISEASE, COLITIS, or colon cancer (see COLON, CANCER OF THE). For this reason, doctors recommend that individuals who experience an anal discharge seek medical attention as soon as possible. This is critically important in cases of a bloody discharge.

Anal fissure

A tear or ulcer in the lining of the anal canal that extends inside the canal from the anal opening. Fairly common, anal fissures may be linked to constipation and diarrhea, although their

SIDE EFFECTS OF ANABOLIC STEROIDS IN MEN
Overdoses of anabolic steroids cause severe hormonal disruptions; musculoskeletal growth problems; behavioral changes; and diseases of the skin, liver, kidney, and heart (in both men and women). Abusers often believe that they can manipulate dosages to prevent the side effects, but these practices (called stacking or pyramiding) are not proven.

Balding — Hallucinations, followed by depression
Acne
Permanent breast enlargement
High cholesterol, atherosclerosis, high blood pressure, heart damage
Liver disease and cancer
Kidney disease
Stunted bone growth
Shrinking of testicles, impotence, low sperm count

exact cause remains unknown. The first symptom of an anal fissure is usually rectal pain and occasional bleeding. The pain may be sharp and burning and increases during defecation. Pain may cause people to avoid defecation, which worsens the situation. Other symptoms include spasm of the anal muscles and anal discharge.

An anal fissure is usually diagnosed by physical examination. In most cases, topical ointments and stool softeners are prescribed. Doctors also recommend a high-fiber diet, adequate fluids, and warm baths after painful bowel movements to reduce spasms. With these measures, many anal fissures resolve spontaneously. In other cases, minor surgery is necessary. See ANAL DILATION and SPHINCTEROTOMY.

Anal fistula
Formation of an abnormal channel between the anal canal and the skin surrounding the anus. The continual discharge of watery pus from the fistula can irritate the skin and result in itching, discomfort, and pain. Most anal fistulas are caused by abscesses (pus-filled sacs) that spread from inside of the anus to the outer surface of the skin. Sometimes, a fistula may result from CROHN DISEASE, COLITIS, or colon cancer (see COLON, CANCER OF THE). The doctor will perform tests, such as X rays and a SIGMOIDOSCOPY (visual examination of the sigmoid colon and rectum with a lighted tube called a sigmoidoscope) to detect the underlying cause of the problem, which is then treated accordingly.

When an abscess is present, minor surgery is performed to remove the fistula and drain the abscess. Most fistulas persist until they are surgically removed. Depending on the severity of the fistula, this procedure may be done in the doctor's office under local anesthesia or at a hospital under general anesthesia. Afterward, stool softeners, antibiotics, and rest are usually prescribed.

Anal sex
Sexual stimulation of the rectal area for either sex, usually by penetration with the penis. Unprotected anal intercourse puts people at a high risk for sexually transmitted diseases (STDs), such as warts, or HIV (human immunodeficiency virus); use of latex condoms for anal sex helps prevent STDs.

Anal stenosis
Narrowing of the anus, which is also known as anal stricture. In this condition, the anal opening is too small to permit the normal passage of feces. Symptoms of anal stenosis include constipation and pain during defecation. In many cases, anal stenosis is present from birth. Sometimes, it is the result of INFLAMMATORY BOWEL DISEASE (IBD). The chronic inflammation characteristic of IBD causes scarring in the anus that can eventually lead to stenosis.

Diagnosis of anal stenosis is made by physical examination, X rays, and SIGMOIDOSCOPY (visual examination of the rectum and sigmoid colon using a lighted tube called a sigmoidoscope). Treatment with daily digital dilation may successfully widen the anal opening in infants. Sometimes, surgery is necessary to correct the condition.

Anal stricture
See ANAL STENOSIS.

Analgesia, patient-controlled
A method of diminishing pain, most commonly after surgery, in which the patient chooses, within limits set by the physician, how often to receive medication needed to overcome discomfort. Patient-controlled analgesia or PCA (pain control without loss of consciousness) is replacing periodic painkiller (analgesic) injections. Injections may produce highly variable pain control, working well soon after a medication is injected, but then losing effectiveness over several hours. Patient-controlled analgesia allows for a more even administration of medication, generally resulting in improved pain control. The medication is placed in an electronic pump and attached to a thin tube (catheter) that is inserted into a vein, usually in the patient's hand or lower arm. When the person feels discomfort, he or she presses a button that causes the pump to release a predetermined dose of medication. Limits set by the attending physician are programmed into the pump so that overdosing is unlikely. Patients controlling their own medication actually may use less medication than those receiving periodic injections of painkillers.

Patient-controlled analgesia has

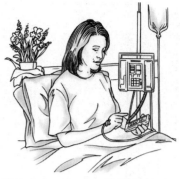

SELF-CONTROL OF PAIN MEDICATION
Patient-controlled analgesia (PCA) is delivered through an intravenous line connected to a bedside pump that also delivers fluids to prevent dehydration. The system is programmed to deliver a dosage of the drug based on the person's input and response to previous doses.

also been adapted for home care after surgery and for some cancer patients. The same type of device is used, except that the tube may be placed in a vial under the skin, rather than in a vein, before the patient leaves the hospital.

Analgesics
Painkillers. An analgesic is any drug used to relieve pain without loss of consciousness. Painkillers usually have only a temporary effect. Analgesic drugs range from nonnarcotics such as aspirin, acetaminophen, and ibuprofen, to narcotics such as codeine and morphine. There are more than 100 different analgesics on the US market. They are divided into two main classes: nonnarcotics and narcotics.

NONNARCOTIC PAINKILLERS
Nonnarcotics include acetaminophen and nonsteroidal anti-inflammatory drugs (NSAIDs), such as aspirin and ibuprofen.
■ **NSAIDs** The NSAIDs work by blocking the production of prostaglandins, naturally occurring substances present in many tissues that stimulate nerve endings, which are sensitive to pain. Prostaglandins help cause inflammation (redness, swelling, and pain), so by blocking their production, NSAIDs have anti-inflammatory properties. NSAIDs are particularly useful for muscle, joint, and menstrual pain.

NSAIDs have no effect on the condition or disease causing the pain,

A

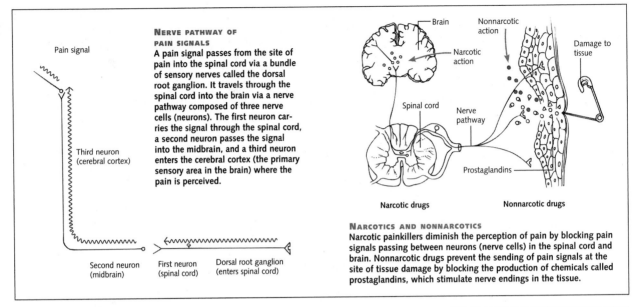

NERVE PATHWAY OF PAIN SIGNALS
A pain signal passes from the site of pain into the spinal cord via a bundle of sensory nerves called the dorsal root ganglion. It travels through the spinal cord into the brain via a nerve pathway composed of three nerve cells (neurons). The first neuron carries the signal through the spinal cord, a second neuron passes the signal into the midbrain, and a third neuron enters the cerebral cortex (the primary sensory area in the brain) where the pain is perceived.

Pain signal

Third neuron (cerebral cortex)

Second neuron (midbrain)   First neuron (spinal cord)   Dorsal root ganglion (enters spinal cord)

Brain
Nonnarcotic action
Narcotic action
Damage to tissue
Spinal cord
Nerve pathway
Prostaglandins

Narcotic drugs   Nonnarcotic drugs

NARCOTICS AND NONNARCOTICS
Narcotic painkillers diminish the perception of pain by blocking pain signals passing between neurons (nerve cells) in the spinal cord and brain. Nonnarcotic drugs prevent the sending of pain signals at the site of tissue damage by blocking the production of chemicals called prostaglandins, which stimulate nerve endings in the tissue.

but they can relieve the symptoms. Dosage varies from once a day to two to four times a day. Toxic effects of NSAIDs include stomach or kidney problems. COX-2 inhibitors are NSAID agents that are much less likely to cause stomach problems.

■ *Acetaminophen* Acetaminophen works by blocking the production of prostaglandins in the brain, but the drug has no ability to block production in the rest of the body so it cannot reduce inflammation. Acetaminophen is useful for common aches and pains such as a toothache or headache.

NARCOTIC PAINKILLERS

Narcotic analgesics combine with pain receptors in brain cells to block the transmission of pain signals within the brain and spinal cord. The most effective narcotic analgesics are the opioids, such as morphine, which are used to treat severe pain associated with diseases such as bone cancer. Milder narcotic analgesics, such as codeine, are less powerful than morphine and are used for moderately severe pain, such as after dental surgery. Any narcotic painkiller can impair a person's ability to drive and must be used with care. Synthetic drugs with morphinelike action include meperidine (Demerol), propoxyphene (Darvon), and tramadol (Ultram).

Narcotic analgesics are usually given under medical supervision to prevent addiction and abuse. Overdose can cause breathing distress, coma, and death.

Analysis, scientific

Determination of the identity of a substance or of the constituent parts of a compound. Qualitative analysis is the identification of the elements present in a substance; quantitative analysis is the determination of the amount or concentration of each element in a substance.

Anaphylactic reaction

A rapid allergic reaction that can be life-threatening. Anaphylaxis is an acute systemic type of allergic reaction, one that affects the entire body. An anaphylactic reaction is one in which the immune system has been triggered to recognize a substance as a threat to the body and react to its presence suddenly and aggressively. During the anaphylactic reaction, the immune system releases antibodies and the tissues release substances such as histamine, which causes the airways to narrow, resulting in wheezing and labored breathing. Histamine causes the blood vessels to dilate, or widen, which leads to a drop in blood pressure, resulting in shock. Hives often occur, and irregular heartbeats (arrhythmias) can occur during prolonged reactions.

Anaphylactic reactions occur infre-

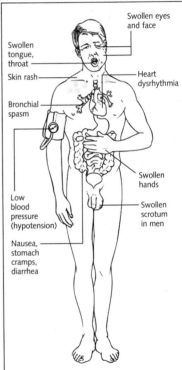

Swollen eyes and face
Swollen tongue, throat
Skin rash
Heart dysrhythmia
Bronchial spasm
Low blood pressure (hypotension)
Nausea, stomach cramps, diarrhea
Swollen hands
Swollen scrotum in men

EFFECTS OF ANAPHYLACTIC REACTION
Anaphylactic reactions are swift and severe, causing sudden release of histamines throughout the body. Swelling and spasm in the airways and abnormally low blood pressure (caused by swollen blood vessels) are the most dangerous symptoms. Effects on the heart may be a result of the low blood pressure.

quently but are considered life-threatening. They can occur in response to any allergen, or allergy-producing substance, but are commonly associated with insect bites or stings, horse serum used in certain vaccines, food allergies, and drug allergies. Pollen and other inhaled environmental allergens rarely cause anaphylactic reactions.

Anaphylactoid purpura

An allergic reaction of unknown origin that causes a skin rash and other potentially serious symptoms (see HENOCH-SCHÖNLEIN PURPURA).

Anaphylaxis

A severe, potentially life-threatening allergic reaction that is characterized by swelling of the throat, difficulty breathing, and a sudden fall in blood pressure. Anaphylaxis, which is also called anaphylactic shock, is an infrequent but very serious allergic reaction and an example of immediate HYPERSENSITIVITY. It usually occurs within seconds or minutes of exposure to minute amounts of an ALLERGEN (allergy-causing substance) to which a person is highly sensitized. The body's IMMUNE RESPONSE to the allergen involves the release of histamine and other body chemicals. These immune chemicals produce hives and swelling of the skin and severe breathing problems caused by swelling tissues in the throat and a narrowing of the airways. The blood vessels swell and become wider, which results in a dramatic drop in blood pressure. These symptoms are a medical emergency, and immediate medical attention can be lifesaving.

CAUSES AND SYMPTOMS

The specific allergens capable of triggering anaphylaxis vary from one individual to another. There are several substances that tend to be more commonly associated with this severe allergic reaction. In the case of food allergies, anaphylactic shock may be caused by eggs, seafood, nuts, grains, milk, or peanuts. Medications, particularly antibiotics from the penicillin and cephalosporin groups, and vaccinations can produce the reaction in sensitized individuals. In some people, insect stings cause anaphylaxis; the insects most often involved are bees, yellow jackets,

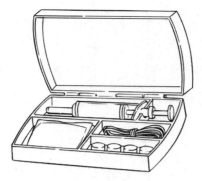

ANAPHYLACTIC KIT AND PEN
People with severe allergies should carry an emergency kit with them and be prepared to use it. An anaphylaxis kit includes premeasured doses of epinephrine or other drugs, equipment to administer it, and thorough instructions. Epinephrine is also available in easy-to-use hypodermic "pens" that can be included in any kit.

paper wasps, hornets, and South American fire ants. This severe allergic reaction may occur when analgesics, such as aspirin or nonsteroidal anti-inflammatory drugs, are injected intravenously. Latex and rubber products, including the latex gloves worn by health care workers, can cause allergic reactions that may escalate to anaphylaxis. Sometimes the cause of anaphylaxis may not be determined.

Symptoms appear immediately after the offending allergen has been ingested or physically contacted. Milder episodes can involve skin symptoms primarily, while more severe anaphylaxis causes severe breathing difficulties. The drop in blood pressure causes symptoms such as a rapid pulse, dizziness, wheezing, sweating, weakness, coughing, a sensation of tightness in the chest, and fainting or unconsciousness. The skin may turn a pale or bluish color. Intensely itching hives may affect large areas of swollen skin, and the lips, tongue, or eyes may become very swollen. Gastrointestinal symptoms may include nausea, abdominal cramps, vomiting, and diarrhea. Cardiac collapse may occur. The throat may feel constricted and swollen, and there may be hoarseness. An obstructed airflow makes it difficult to breathe. Once these symptoms have started, a person may die within minutes to hours if treatment is not started.

DIAGNOSIS, TREATMENT, AND PREVENTION

Anaphylaxis is recognized immediately by the characteristic symptoms. Since the affected person may not be able to provide a doctor information about the possible allergen, a companion may have to provide this information.

Treatment consists of an immediate injection of adrenaline (epinephrine) to open airways and reduce swelling, as well as rapid injection of intravenous fluids. CARDIOPULMONARY RESUSCITATION (CPR) to assist in breathing and to restore the person's heartbeat may be necessary. Sometimes an emergency tracheotomy to open the main airway and restart breathing may need to be performed. Subsequently, oxygen therapy and mechanical VENTILATION may be required to help the person breathe. Additional medications may be given, including ANTIHISTAMINES to block the effect of histamine or CORTICOSTEROIDS to halt inflammation and swelling. With proper medical treatment, a person who has undergone anaphylaxis can recover completely. However, a person who has had this reaction remains at risk for future episodes following ingestion of or contact with the causative allergen.

It is a good idea for a person who has experienced anaphylactic shock and determined the cause to wear a medical-alert bracelet or necklace that identifies the problem and its source. Allergens that trigger the symptoms must be strictly avoided. When food allergies are the cause, ingredients listed on packaged food labels should be scrutinized to make sure no amount of the allergen is contained in the food. Servers at restaurants should be asked about the ingredients in dishes before they are ordered. Allergies to insect stings may be prevented by avoiding outdoor activities that might result in exposure to insects, such as gardening and mowing the lawn. Scented personal products including perfumes, lotions, and hair care products should be avoided when outdoors, and the person should always wear shoes outside to avoid stepping on a bee and getting stung.

If it is not possible to avoid all situations that may cause exposure to the allergen that causes anaphylactic shock, a doctor may recommend that a person have available a preloaded syringe of epinephrine to be injected at the first sign of symptoms. These injections should be considered only as interim measures when anaphylactic shock occurs, and emergency medical attention should always be sought. Immunotherapy, which involves a series of allergy shots to gradually desensitize a person to the allergen, may be necessary for some people to prevent future severe reactions.

Anastomosis

A natural or artificial connection, usually by surgery, of two tubular channels that may or may not normally be joined. An anastomosis can involve the intestines, arteries, or veins. Most commonly, a natural anastomosis takes the form of two blood vessels converging. Surgical anastomosis is performed to treat various disorders. For example, it is often used to treat intestinal obstruction. In this procedure, the diseased part of the intestine is removed and the remaining healthy sections are joined together.

Anastrozole

An anticancer drug. Anastrozole (Arimidex) is used to treat advanced breast cancer in postmenopausal women. Anastrozole works by reducing the amount of the hormone estradiol produced in the body. Side effects may mimic menopause.

Anatomy

Physical structure of living things; scientific study of physical structure. Anatomy is concerned with the internal and external physical structures of animals, plants, and other organisms. Gross anatomy refers to structures that are visible to the naked eye, while microscopic anatomy, or histology, involves structures that can only be seen under the microscope.

Androgen hormones

The group of male SEX HORMONES that stimulate the development of the male sex organs and other male characteristics. Androgen hormones are produced by the testicles (see TESTICLE) and the adrenal cortex (the outer layer of the adrenal glands). Testosterone, the most powerful of

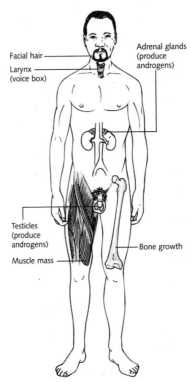

EFFECTS OF MALE SEX HORMONES
Androgen hormones, including testosterone, are absorbed by many different types of cells all over the body. They stimulate growth of facial hair; enlargement of the larynx, which deepens the voice; development of greater muscle mass; development of the penis and testicles; and bone growth.

the male hormones, is produced by the testicles. Small quantities of weaker androgen hormones, as well as small amounts of testosterone, are produced in the adrenal glands and ovaries of women.

Synthetic forms of these hormones may be prescribed as medications for various disorders and diseases. They may be taken orally, injected, applied as a topical skin patch, or implanted in muscle tissue, generally to replace the hormones when the body is unable to produce enough on its own. In women, in rare instances they are used to treat breast cancer and LICHEN SCLEROSUS, a skin problem of the vulva. In men, androgen hormones can correct hormone deficiencies associated with the pituitary gland or disorders of the testicles. The most common use of testosterone is to improve sexual function in men with low levels of

the hormone due to testicular or pituitary gland dysfunction or declining levels due to aging. Androgens may be prescribed to stimulate the beginning of puberty in boys who are late entering this phase of development. They may also be used to treat underdevelopment of the penis. Androgen is also used as a muscle-building and appetite-stimulating agent in people with HIV (human immunodeficiency virus). (Occasionally, athletes abuse androgens to enhance muscle mass and athletic performance, but there is no evidence that the weak androgens that can be obtained over-the-counter have muscle-strengthening properties.)

Side effects of synthetic androgens include edema, weight gain, acne, weakness, loss of appetite, irritability, and nausea. In women, high doses may cause an increased sex drive, absent menstrual periods, an enlarged clitoris, deepening of the voice, decreased breast size, male-pattern hair growth on the body, or male-pattern hair loss. In men, high doses of androgens may temporarily interfere with the production of sperm or cause breast enlargement or atrophy of the testicles.

People with disorders of the liver, people with diabetes, men with enlarged prostates or prostate cancer, and women with breast cancer usually cannot take androgens.

Androgens

Male sex hormones. Testosterone is the principal male steroid hormone, produced in the testes in men and in small amounts in the ovaries and adrenal glands in women. Testosterone is responsible for the growth and development of male sex organs as well as for some physical characteristics in men, such as beard, body hair, and a lowered voice. Androgen hormone replacement is prescribed to replace testosterone in men who have low levels of it in their blood or who have lost testicular function. Women may receive testosterone to treat metastatic cancer (cancer that has spread from one area of the body to another).

Andrology

The study of the male reproductive system and the diseases that affect it.

A

Anemia

A condition marked by the presence of an abnormally low number of red blood cells or hemoglobin molecules, the iron-containing compound in red blood cells that transports oxygen. There are many different types of anemia, each one with its own cause. As a group, anemias are the most common diseases affecting the blood.

In the healthy person, red blood cells are produced in the bone marrow and have a life span of approximately 120 days, at which point new red blood cells replace them. In healthy individuals, the formation of new red blood cells balances the destruction of old cells, and the amount of hemoglobin remains steady within the normal range. Anemia can result if red blood cells are destroyed prematurely, if the bone marrow loses the ability to make a sufficient number of new red blood cells, or if a person experiences blood loss from bleeding. The net result is a deficiency in red blood cells or hemoglobin. This loss in the body's ability to transport oxygen produces the symptoms of anemia.

SYMPTOMS

Most anemias start with mild symptoms that may hardly be noticed. Symptoms worsen as the disease progresses. A person with anemia may feel fatigued and appear paler than usual. The pallor is more apparent in the nail beds of the fingers and toes, the insides of the lips and eyelids, and the palms, where the creases may become as pale as the skin surrounding them. The heart rate often increases as the heart works harder to pump blood throughout the body in an effort to compensate for the oxygen deficit. Shortness of breath when exercising may also occur.

TYPES

The most common cause of anemia is iron deficiency (see ANEMIA, IRON-DEFICIENCY). Since iron is an essential component of hemoglobin, an iron deficiency leaves the body unable to produce enough hemoglobin to meet its needs. The usual causes of iron-deficiency anemia are inadequate diet, poor absorption of iron from food, and blood loss. In the United States, blood loss is the most common cause of iron deficiency in adults, which may be caused by conditions such as ulcers, colon polyps, or colon cancer or by the use of nonsteroidal anti-inflammatory drugs (NSAIDs).

Insufficient vitamin B12 causes pernicious anemia (see ANEMIA, PERNICIOUS). Insufficient folic acid (also known as folate) produces a folic acid deficiency anemia. Since vitamin B12 and folate are important building blocks for red blood cells, insufficient vitamin B12 or folic acid results in an inability of the bone marrow to produce enough new red blood cells to replace old ones.

Hemolytic anemias (see ANEMIA, HEMOLYTIC) involve disease processes in which red blood cells break down faster than bone marrow can produce them. The most common cause of hemolytic anemia is an acquired immunity to one's own red blood cells. Antibodies attack the cells as if they are foreign to the body and subsequently destroy them. Hemolytic anemia can also develop as a result of taking certain medications and from an inherited defect in enzymes such as glucose-6-phosphate dehydrogenase (G6PD).

In the aplastic anemias (see ANEMIA, APLASTIC), the bone marrow fails to properly develop all types of blood cells, including red blood cells.

Certain inherited anemias involve genetic abnormalities that cause the body to manufacture defective hemoglobin. Examples include SICKLE CELL ANEMIA and the thalassemias (see THALASSEMIA).

Many infections and chronic diseases occur in conjunction with anemia. Anemias that occur along with a chronic disease are relatively common and probably result from a combination of factors, including a decrease in the ability of the bone marrow to produce red blood cells, a shortened red blood cell life span, and impaired iron utilization. Examples of causative diseases include endocarditis (inflammation of the lining of the heart that usually involves the heart valves), osteomyelitis (inflammation of the bones), juvenile rheumatoid arthritis, rheumatic fever, Crohn disease, and ulcerative colitis.

Anemia, aplastic

A disease in which the bone marrow fails to produce all types of mature blood cells in sufficient numbers. "Aplastic" means "anatomically undeveloped." Symptoms develop as a result of the insufficient number of fully developed blood cells. ANEMIA (low red blood cell count) causes fatigue, weakness, shortness of breath, and rapid pulse. Leukopenia (low white blood cell count) increases the risk of infection. Thrombocytopenia (low platelet count) results in bleeding from the skin and the mucous membranes, such as those of the nose and gums, and causes easy bruising. Aplastic anemia may be acute or chronic, and it is always progressive, becoming worse over time. Left untreated, the disease leads to rapid death.

The bone marrow in a person with aplastic anemia contains very few stem cells, the cells from which

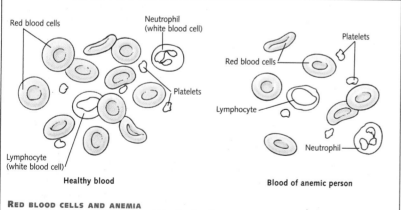

RED BLOOD CELLS AND ANEMIA
In healthy blood, there are enough red blood cells—the oxygen-carrying cells in the blood—to carry an adequate supply of oxygen to tissue cells throughout the body. In a person with anemia, the number of red blood cells in the blood is reduced and oxygen supply to cells is insufficient to fuel body activity.

mature bone marrow cells are derived. In some cases, aplastic anemia is thought to develop from an autoimmune disorder, in which a person develops antibodies against his or her own cells. Aplastic anemia can also be caused by exposure to toxins (such as organic solvents, cleaners, and paint removers), chemotherapy, radiation therapy, certain medications and illegal drugs, pregnancy, infections, and systemic lupus erythematosus. In many cases, no clear cause is identified.

Mild cases of aplastic anemia are treated with supportive care, such as blood transfusions and platelet transfusions to raise the number of blood cells to normal and antibiotics to fight infections. If the disease is severe and life-threatening, bone marrow transplant (see BONE MARROW TRANSPLANT, ALLOGENEIC) is the most effective treatment for people younger than 30. People who are older than 40 or who lack a matching bone marrow donor are treated with antithymocyte globulin, a serum that suppresses the immune system. Other immunity-suppressing drugs, such as cyclosporine, may also be used.

Anemia, Cooley

An inherited disease in which there is abnormal production of part of the hemoglobin molecule, resulting in the production of abnormal hemoglobin. Cooley anemia is also known as beta-thalassemia major, because it affects both genes that code for the beta chain of hemoglobin. If the defective gene is inherited from only one parent, the ANEMIA is mild and often symptom-free, and the person can live a normal, full life (thalassemia minor). If both parents contribute the gene, however, the disease is severe (thalassemia major; see THALASSEMIA). As a result of this molecular abnormality, the body produces too few red bloods cells, which have an unusually short survival time and do not have enough normal hemoglobin to transport oxygen effectively.

Infants with the severe form of Cooley anemia are healthy at birth, but a pronounced anemia (insufficient number of red blood cells) appears during the first year of life.

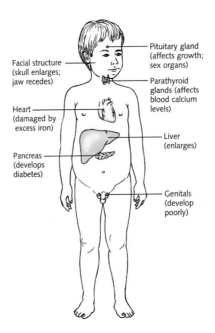

Facial structure (skull enlarges; jaw recedes)

Pituitary gland (affects growth; sex organs)

Parathyroid glands (affects blood calcium levels)

Heart (damaged by excess iron)

Liver (enlarges)

Pancreas (develops diabetes)

Genitals (develop poorly)

DAMAGE TO ORGANS
If Cooley anemia is untreated, bone marrow expansion causes skeletal deformities. Excessive absorption of dietary iron and the iron from transfusions to treat the anemia lead to a build up of iron in the tissues. The effects on the person vary with the location and extent of the damage.

Because the bone marrow expands to compensate for the impaired production of red blood cells, the skeleton becomes deformed. The cheek bones and upper jaw protrude, the ribs and spine are misshapen, and the long bones (for example, the thigh and upper arm) break easily. The intestinal system absorbs too much iron, which is deposited throughout the body. As a result, the heart and spleen grow abnormally large, the liver fails, and growth and sexual development are retarded. Without treatment, death occurs by the early 20s.

Cooley anemia is treated with transfusions of red blood cells. When treatment begins early, facial and skeletal deformities can be prevented. Excess iron accumulation is treated with medication that eliminates iron from the body.

Thalassemia is sometimes called Mediterranean anemia, because it is common in that part of the world. The disease is also prevalent among Chinese, other Asians, and Africans.

Anemia, Fanconi

A rare inherited disease that causes abnormally low numbers of certain blood cells accompanied by underdeveloped or missing thumbs, short stature, and mental and sexual retardation. A child with Fanconi anemia displays symptoms between 18 months and 10 years of age. An abnormally low number of platelets makes the child bruise easily and bleed from the skin and the mucous membranes, such as those of the nose and the gums. Red and white blood cell counts are also low, making the child pale, fatigued, and subject to infection. Patches of the skin may turn brown and discolored from deposits of the skin pigment melanin.

Anemia, hemolytic

A group of diseases in which red blood cells are destroyed faster than they are produced, resulting in ANEMIA (an abnormally low number of red blood cells). The word "hemolytic" comes from two Greek roots meaning "blood destroyer." Symptoms include fatigue, pallid skin, breathlessness, rapid heartbeat (particularly on exertion), jaundice, dark urine, and enlarged spleen. Hemolytic anemias are sometimes difficult to treat, but they are rarely fatal.

Some hemolytic anemias are inherited; others are acquired. An example of a hereditary form is a deficiency in the enzyme glucose-6-phosphate dehydrogenase (G6PD). Since the gene that causes this deficiency resides on the X chromosome, it is found almost entirely among men. The disease is particularly common among black men, affecting one or more of every ten, and it is also found among people of Mediterranean ancestry. Under normal circumstances, people with this disease are not anemic and show no symptoms. The anemia may develop during an infection or after exposure to certain chemicals, such as mothballs, and specific drugs, such as antimalarial agents, sulfonamide antibiotics, aspirin, nonsteroidal anti-inflammatory drugs (NSAIDs, such as ibuprofen), and quinine. This type of hemolytic anemia can be prevented by avoiding medications that may bring on a crisis.

An acquired form of the disease is idiopathic autoimmune hemolytic anemia. For unknown reasons, a person forms antibodies against his or her own red blood cells. The disease may begin very suddenly and severely. This hemolytic anemia is treated with prednisone, which slows the immune response. Since the spleen is the organ that removes red blood cells from the bloodstream, it is sometimes surgically removed. Drugs that suppress the immune system may also be prescribed.

Anemia, iron-deficiency

A decrease in the number of red blood cells caused by inadequate stores of iron in the body. Iron is the central component of hemoglobin, the pigment in red blood cells that transports oxygen through the body. When the iron supply in the body is inadequate, hemoglobin production falls and ANEMIA results.

CAUSES

Iron deficiency is the most common cause of anemia. It is estimated to occur in one of five nonpregnant women of childbearing age, in one of two pregnant women, and in 3 of 100 men. The principal causes of the disease are inadequate iron in the diet, insufficient iron absorption during digestion, and abnormal blood loss. Women are particularly prone to developing the disease because of blood loss during menstruation. Pregnancy is also associated with iron deficiency since the mother is producing blood cells for the fetus as well as for herself, thus increasing the demand for iron. Lactation also increases the need for iron, which is a component of breast milk. In women after menopause and in men, the most likely cause of iron-deficiency anemia is blood loss in the digestive tract from conditions such as ulcers, colon polyps, or colon cancer or the use of aspirin or other nonsteroidal anti-inflammatory drugs (NSAIDs), such as ibuprofen. In children, lead poisoning can interfere with iron utilization and cause anemia. Children and adolescents sometimes become iron-deficient during periods of accelerated growth, when demand for iron exceeds intake. Vegetarians who eat no animal products (vegans) for a period of several years have an increased likelihood of developing iron-deficiency anemia.

SYMPTOMS AND DIAGNOSIS

Mild iron-deficiency anemia often produces no symptoms. If the disease progresses, symptoms appear, which include pallid skin, fatigue, irritability, weakness, shortness of breath, postural hypotension (low blood pressure on standing up), brittle nails, headache, and sore tongue. Some people develop cravings for nonfood items such as clay, soil, and ice, a condition called PICA. Children are likely to experience decreased appetite.

Iron-deficiency anemia is diagnosed by blood tests that measure the amount of hemoglobin and iron in the blood. If the iron deficiency is thought to be the result of digestive tract bleeding, other tests may be performed to identify the bleeding site.

TREATMENT AND PREVENTION

Iron-deficiency anemia is treated by increasing dietary iron intake and by taking supplemental iron, typically in the form of ferrous sulfate. Iron-rich foods include red meat, raisins, fish, egg yolks, liver, poultry, legumes (peas and beans), potatoes, and whole grains. Occasionally people with iron-deficiency anemia are given supplemental iron by injection; in severe cases, blood transfusions may be given until the bone marrow can replace the blood that has been lost. In most cases, the iron level in the blood comes up to normal in 2 months. Therapy is continued for another 6 to 12 months to rebuild the stores of iron in the bone marrow. If bleeding from the digestive tract causes the anemia, the underlying condition needs to be treated to prevent continued blood loss.

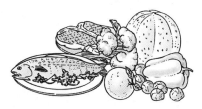

IRON AND VITAMIN C
Eating a well-balanced diet that includes iron-rich foods helps prevent anemia. Good sources of iron include red meat and liver, fish, and nuts. Vitamin C, which helps the body absorb iron, is plentiful in citrus fruits and cantaloupe, green peppers, and many other green vegetables.

Iron-deficiency anemia can be prevented by eating a healthy diet and taking iron supplements when at increased risk for the disease. Those at risk include menstruating women, pregnant women, children and adolescents, and vegans.

Anemia, megaloblastic

A blood disorder characterized by larger than normal red blood cells. Abnormal precursors of red blood cells called megaloblasts (from Greek roots meaning "big cell buds") occur in the bone marrow and give this anemia its name. Megaloblastic anemia commonly results from deficiency in vitamin B12 or folic acid (also known as folate). It can also be caused by leukemia, multiple myeloma, certain hereditary disorders, and some chemotherapy agents. The most common type of megaloblastic anemia is pernicious anemia (see ANEMIA and ANEMIA, PERNICIOUS).

Anemia, pernicious

A blood disorder characterized by abnormally low numbers of red blood cells and caused by an inability to absorb vitamin B12. To absorb vitamin B12, the cells lining a portion of the stomach make a substance called intrinsic factor that binds to vitamin B12 found in food. Only when combined with intrinsic factor can vitamin B12 be absorbed into the bloodstream from the intestine. People with pernicious anemia cannot produce intrinsic factor and become deficient in vitamin B12, which is needed for red blood cell production.

Pernicious anemia gets its name from the fact that, in the days before its cause was understood and effective treatment developed, it led to gradual, progressive deterioration and eventual death. Early symptoms include a sore tongue, a rapid heartbeat, limited endurance, weakness, abdominal discomfort, and weight loss due to poor appetite. The disease also affects the nerves, causing paresthesia (tingling or numbness) in the hands or feet, difficulty walking, clumsiness, slow thought processes, and impaired memory. Rarely there are psychiatric symptoms such as hallucinations or paranoia.

Pernicious anemia is usually diag-

A

nosed with blood tests that measure the level of vitamin B12 in the bloodstream. In some cases a biopsy sample of bone marrow is taken. Pernicious anemia is a megaloblastic ANEMIA, which is characterized by the presence of abnormal red blood cell precursors (megaloblasts) in the bone marrow.

Once pernicious anemia is diagnosed, it is treated with regular injections of vitamin B12. Treatment usually reduces symptoms in 48 to 72 hours. People with pernicious anemia require injections every month or two for the remainder of their lives. Treatment should begin as soon as the disease is diagnosed, since delay can result in permanent damage to the nervous and digestive systems. If treatment is started early, most people with pernicious anemia live a normal life.

Pernicious anemia usually does not appear before age 30, although there is an uncommon form of the disease that arises in children by age 3. Pernicious anemia is thought to be caused by an unidentified inherited characteristic and is most common in people of northern European descent, particularly those with fair hair. Pernicious anemia also is associated with autoimmune diseases involving the hormone-producing glands, such as type 1 diabetes mellitus, Addison disease, and Graves disease.

Anemia, sickle cell

See SICKLE CELL ANEMIA.

Anemia, sideroblastic

A group of blood diseases in which the red blood cells contain too much iron and hemoglobin production is defective. Sideroblastic anemia can be inherited. Other forms of the disease are acquired as a result of exposure to toxins (such as alcohol or lead), certain cancers (such as leukemia, lymphoma, or myeloma), or inflammatory disease (such as rheumatoid arthritis). In some cases, no cause can be identified. Symptoms include fatigue, shortness of breath, weakness, pallid skin, and an enlarged liver and spleen. Removing the toxin or treating the underlying disease often reverses the ANEMIA. Some people with sideroblastic

anemia respond to high doses of vitamin B6 (pyridoxine) or androgens to stimulate the bone marrow. In addition, blood transfusions may be required, and medication may be needed to rid the body of excess iron from multiple transfusions.

Anencephaly

A severe NEURAL TUBE DEFECT in which an infant's brain and spinal cord fail to develop in utero (within the uterus). Anencephaly occurs when the top portion of an embryo's neural tube fails to close in the early stage of pregnancy. As a result, the infant is born without a forebrain (the part of the brain responsible for thinking and coordination). Remaining brain tissue is often left exposed, uncovered by skin or bone. Although reflex actions such as breathing may occur, an affected infant is usually blind, deaf, unconscious, and unable to experience sensations, such as pain. The lack of a functioning cerebrum means that the infant cannot gain consciousness. When the infant is not stillborn, death usually occurs within hours or days after birth.

Some cases of anencephaly may be detected by checking the mother's alpha-fetoprotein level early in the pregnancy. The abnormality can often be confirmed on ultrasound examination before delivery. The risk for

anencephaly and other neural tube defects can be decreased if the mother takes a daily multivitamin containing 400 micrograms of folic acid as a part of regular prenatal care.

Anesthesia

A method, including medication, to cause the temporary absence of all sensation. Anesthesia makes surgery possible by eliminating the pain that a procedure would otherwise cause. Various forms and routes of pain suppression are available, depending on the person's medical history, preferences, age, and emotional makeup and on the type and duration of surgery performed.

There are two types of anesthesia used in surgical procedures. Under local or regional anesthesia, the person is conscious and sensation is temporarily deadened in only part of the body. An injection of drugs into the surgical site interrupts the nerve supply, preventing any pain sensation.

In general anesthesia, the person is injected with drugs that cause an unconscious state; this affects all parts of the body but particularly the brain and spinal cord so that the person has no discomfort during surgery. It is this kind of medication that renders a patient temporarily unconscious, most often referred to as

---

DIFFERENT TYPES OF ANESTHESIA

Anesthetics are drugs that block the sensation of pain in a part of the body or make a person temporarily unconscious—preventing any awareness of pain. Major types include:

- Local anesthesia, which stops sensation only in the area being treated, and is usually administered by injection, spray, or ointment. A common example is an injection of "novocaine" before a tooth is drilled and filled. Local anesthetics wear off quickly. The person is awake and alert while being treated but feels no pain.
- General anesthesia, in which the person is given medication that induces a loss of consciousness for major surgery. It requires that the patient not eat or drink for several hours before the procedure. The stomach needs to be empty because anesthesia can cause a person to vomit while unconscious, which can be dangerous if material is inhaled into the lungs.
- Regional anesthesia, which stops sensation in an entire region of the body, such as an arm, leg, or from the waist down. One of the most common regional anesthetics is called an epidural, which is given as an injection in the back.
- Patient-controlled analgesia, which is a method of diminishing pain, usually after surgery, in which the patient chooses, within physician controls, how often to receive medication needed to control any discomfort. The medication is placed in an electronic pump and attached to a thin tube or catheter, which is inserted into a vein of the person's arm or hand. The patient presses a button that releases a predetermined dose of medication, with limits set by the doctor.

"being asleep," as the anesthesiologist gives combinations of drugs by injection, inhalation, or both.

Anesthesia, ambulatory

A method to cause loss of sensation and consciousness to prevent pain during AMBULATORY SURGERY, when the patient is discharged the same day that the operation is performed.

A number of anesthetic methods are available, depending on the patient's medical history, preferences, age, and emotional makeup and on the type of surgery to be performed. Local anesthesia (see ANESTHESIA, LOCAL), which numbs the area to be operated on, can be used alone or in combination with CONSCIOUS SEDATION, which leaves the patient drowsy, relaxed, and insensitive to pain. Regional anesthesia (see ANESTHESIA, REGIONAL) numbs a portion or region of the body, such as the legs, while the patient remains awake. Conscious sedation may be combined with regional anesthesia. General anesthesia (see ANESTHESIA, GENERAL) causes the person to temporarily lose consciousness and sensation and suppresses pain over the whole body.

People undergoing ambulatory anesthesia must not eat or drink anything for 8 to 10 hours before the surgery. This precaution is taken to avoid the risk of vomiting during surgery and inhaling the vomit into the lungs, which may cause serious complications. After the surgery, the patient recovers in a special room (called postoperative recovery) until the anesthetic wears off. Heart and lung functions are monitored to watch for any side effects or surgical complica-

tions. Once the patient has recovered and can walk unassisted, drink fluids, and urinate, he or she is released to recover completely at home. Except in cases where local anesthesia is used alone—as, for example, in most dental work—the patient may not drive for the first 24 hours and should have someone designated to assist at home during the same period. Alcohol and herbal and nonprescription medications should also be avoided for the first day or longer, depending on the medications that the person may be taking.

Side effects from ambulatory anesthesia are usually minor and temporary, lasting for only a day or two after the procedure. They consist of drowsiness, nausea, and headache. If general anesthesia was used, an ENDOTRACHEAL TUBE inserted in the throat to provide airway access during surgery may leave the throat feeling mildly sore for several days.

Anesthesia, dental

The application or injection of medication to eliminate pain during dental treatment or surgery. Topical anesthesia is used by dentists to numb tissues in an area of the mouth in preparation for injecting a local anesthetic. A local anesthetic is injected to stop pain in a specific area of the mouth for a short period, usually about an hour. This form of dental anesthesia is most commonly used prior to potentially painful treatments, including repairing cavities, preparing the teeth for dental crowns, and minor surgical procedures.

CONSCIOUS SEDATION may be given, in combination with a local anesthetic for pain, to help the dental patient relax during a procedure. The dentist may administer an anesthetic agent, such as nitrous oxide, or a sedative by mouth, inhalation, or injection. A person under conscious sedation remains rational and responsive to the verbal commands of the dentist. General anesthesia, which puts a patient into an unresponsive, sleep-like state, is used when complex procedures are required or when the patient is extremely anxious.

Anesthesia, epidural

A method of anesthetizing the lower half of the body by administering medication into the epidural space (a narrow area around the spinal cord) in the lower back. Typically used in labor or surgery, the procedure is also called an epidural block or a lumbar epidural block. In epidural anesthe-

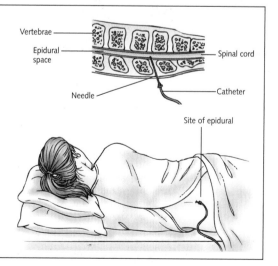

RECEIVING EPIDURAL ANESTHESIA
To administer an epidural anesthetic, the doctor inserts a hollow needle between the vertebrae in the lower part of the spine and threads a catheter (tube) through the needle. The regional anesthetic, which numbs the person from the waist down, is injected through the catheter into the epidural space—the region surrounding the spinal cord (see inset). The person receiving the anesthetic does not feel pain, but remains fully conscious and can still move the lower body, making the epidural a useful form of medication for a pregnant woman in labor.

Vertebrae

Epidural space

Spinal cord

Needle

Catheter

Site of epidural

sia, a hollow needle is inserted into the epidural space. A thin plastic tube (catheter) is threaded through the needle, and a local anesthetic (numbing agent) is injected through the catheter into the epidural space, numbing the body from the waist down.

In labor, epidural anesthesia is relatively safe for both the mother and the baby, since it does not enter the baby's bloodstream or make the mother drowsy. The catheter remains in place throughout labor and delivery, enabling the administration of more pain medication if needed. Most women experience complete pain relief with epidural anesthesia. However, it may slow labor and inhibit the ability to push. For that reason, the medication is often given during the earlier, more painful stages of labor and allowed to wear off for pushing. Often, epidural anesthesia affects the ability to urinate, and a catheter must be inserted into the bladder to drain it. See also PUDENDAL BLOCK.

Anesthesia, general

A method of preventing pain and discomfort during surgery that makes the patient temporarily unconscious. Under general anesthesia, patients respond minimally, if at all, to intense stimulation, including pain. Breathing, heart function, and protective reflexes, such as coughing, continue but are slowed.

General anesthesia is used for surgery in the chest, abdomen, limbs, neck, and head and for almost all types of laparoscopic surgery, in which the abdomen is inflated with gas to allow the insertion of instruments through small incisions. For general anesthesia, the person inhales anesthetic gases, and intravenous medication is given.

METHODS

After a surgical patient is placed on the operating table, a number of monitoring sensors are attached to his or her body to allow monitoring of heart rate, blood pressure, and blood oxygen levels. A breathing mask is placed over the face to allow the patient to breathe pure oxygen for several minutes before the anesthesia is given. This creates an oxygen reservoir in the lungs of the patient

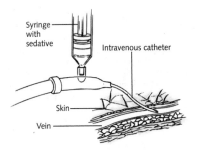

INDUCING UNCONSCIOUSNESS
To give a general anesthetic, a sedative is first administered to cause the person to lose consciousness immediately. This medication is usually injected through a catheter inserted into a vein in the hand or arm.

and increases the time available to the operating room team to handle any possible emergency.

Putting the patient in an anesthetic sleep is called induction. In adults, induction is usually brought on by medications that are placed in an intravenous line (catheter) in the arm or hand of the patient. In children (see ANESTHESIA, PEDIATRIC), inhaled gases may be used.

Once general anesthesia has started, an ENDOTRACHEAL TUBE is inserted through the mouth of the person and down the throat past the LARYNX (voice box). This flexible tube prevents stomach contents from entering the lungs (aspiration), and it protects the patient by providing an open and secure airway during the procedure. During surgery, a pump connected to the endotracheal tube helps inflate and deflate the lungs at a rate that maintains the appropriate levels of oxygen and carbon dioxide in the bloodstream. Anesthetic gases, or inhalation anesthetics, can also be given through the tube to maintain the loss of consciousness and insensitivity to pain. Additional medications may be given through the intravenous line in response to changes in blood pressure or heart rate. When the surgery has been completed, the patient is brought back to a state of consciousness by stopping each anesthetic agent at the appropriate time. The order and timing vary with the medications and type of surgery performed. Anesthetic gases stop working as soon as they are no longer pumped into the lungs of the person. Some intravenous medications need to be

reversed by administering reversal drugs that act as "blockers" or antagonists. As the anesthesia ends, pain medication is often given intravenously to control discomfort while the patient wakes up in the recovery room. The endotracheal tube is removed after the patient is breathing normally and before he or she returns to consciousness.

During recovery from general anesthesia, patients feel sleepy and fatigued. The time these effects last depends on the depth and length of the anesthesia and the reaction to the medication. Nausea is possible; vomiting is less common. Both conditions are temporary and can be diminished

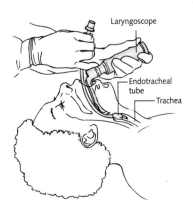

Inserting the tube

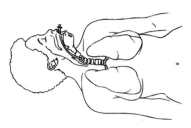

Position of tube

ADMINISTERING GENERAL ANESTHESIA
After the person is completely unconscious, an endotracheal tube is inserted through his or her mouth and into the trachea (windpipe). The doctor may use an instrument called a laryngoscope to guide the insertion of the tube. The endotracheal tube is connected to a ventilator that carefully regulates the amount of oxygen the person receives during the operation. Anesthetic drugs that can be inhaled are also given through this tube to keep the person unconscious and pain-free. The endotracheal tube remains in place throughout the operation.

by medication. Insertion and removal of the endotracheal tube sometimes causes a minor sore throat for a few days.

POSSIBLE COMPLICATIONS

Breathing difficulties can arise during general anesthesia because intermediate levels of anesthetic medications make the airways more irritable. This is most likely to occur at the beginning or end of anesthesia, and it poses the greatest risk to children, smokers, and people with asthma or other airway diseases.

Since general anesthetic agents depress heart function or cause blood vessels to relax, blood pressure drops. Blood loss and the evaporation of fluid from tissues exposed during surgery increase this effect. Medication may be needed to counteract the drop in blood pressure. The volume of blood loss can be corrected by giving the patient intravenous fluids and blood transfusions during surgery. Some anesthetic agents can cause an irregular heartbeat, but this is usually not dangerous.

Only very rarely is a patient who is under general anesthesia aware of pain or other sensations during surgery. Also rare is the allergic reaction called malignant hyperthermia (see HYPERTHERMIA, MALIGNANT), a genetically caused reaction to anesthetic gases that causes widespread metabolic disturbance and raises body temperature rapidly to as high as 108°F. Seizures, fast heart rate, high blood pressure, and abnormal heart rhythms can also occur. If not treated promptly, malignant hyperthermia can be fatal. Patients with immediate family members who have experienced malignant hyperthermia should make all of their physicians aware of this when deciding upon surgery.

Anesthesia, inhalation

A method of giving medication that is inhaled into the lungs as an anesthetic gas to suppress pain. Nitrous oxide, known as "laughing gas," is an odorless, colorless gas that was one of the first effective anesthetics discovered and is still the most widely used inhaled anesthetic agent, especially for dental procedures. It is very safe, with little effect on the circulatory and respiratory systems, and its effects stop as soon as the gas is dis-

continued. Nitrous oxide, however, is a relatively weak anesthetic and is not generally used alone. It is commonly administered with intravenous anesthetics or other medications to decrease anxiety, relax the patient, and enhance the effectiveness of the other intravenous medications.

Nitrous oxide may be given with halothane, another inhalation agent and a powerful anesthetic that suppresses pain very effectively. Halothane works quickly, and the anesthetic effect is reversed as soon as the gas is withdrawn. The disadvantage to halothane is that it depresses the circulatory system, leading to abnormally low blood pressure, and it can induce an irregular heartbeat (see ARRHYTHMIA, CARDIAC). Combining halothane with nitrous oxide enhances the anesthetic effect, reduces the amount of halothane needed, and lowers the risk of circulatory complications during surgery. ISOFLURANE, and the closely related and less widely used enflurane, are types of ether, the first inhaled anesthetic discovered. Isoflurane is well absorbed into the body and eliminated easily, putting few demands on the kidneys and liver.

Ether is obsolete in North America and Europe, but it is still used in poorer countries because it is cheap and relatively safe to use without sophisticated equipment. Recovery from ether is slow, however. Because the gas irritates the respiratory system, it carries a higher risk of lung complications after surgery.

Anesthesia, intravenous

A method that provides pain-suppressing medication through a small, flexible tube (intravenous catheter) inserted into a vein, usually in the hand or lower arm. Intravenous anesthesia can be used for general anesthesia (see ANESTHESIA, GENERAL), CONSCIOUS SEDATION, or regional anesthesia (see ANESTHESIA, REGIONAL).

Before surgery, the intravenous catheter is placed in the vein with a small needle that penetrates the skin and the vein. Once the catheter is in place, the needle is withdrawn and tape is applied to hold the catheter in position.

A number of different types of medication can be used as intra-

venous anesthetics. One group is the BARBITURATES, which work quickly and for a short time. Thiopental, known as "Sodium Pentothal," is used principally to induce anesthesia. Once the patient is asleep, the thiopental is withdrawn, and the anesthesia is maintained with inhaled anesthetics (see ANESTHESIA, INHALATION). Thiopental is also used to supplement nitrous oxide, which is a weak anesthetic by itself. The disadvantage to thiopental and other barbiturates is that they suppress the respiratory and circulatory systems, which can lead to breathing difficulties and an abnormally low blood pressure. The central nervous system and gastrointestinal tract may be affected, and other allergic reactions may occur with barbiturate use. The BENZODIAZEPINES reduce anxiety and induce relaxation. Diazepam (Valium) has been widely used. Midazolam (Versed) acts for a shorter period and is useful for anesthesia. Propofol is an agent that stops working as soon as it is withdrawn and produces mild side effects, such as nausea, headache, or vomiting. Like thiopental, it is used to put the patient to sleep and is also a useful agent for maintaining anesthesia during ambulatory surgery, when the surgical patient goes home on the same day. Narcotics (for example, MORPHINE SULFATE and FENTANYL) are used as medications before surgery, as supplements to weak anesthetics like nitrous oxide, and as regional anesthesia. The disadvantage of narcotics is that they suppress the respiratory system, which has to be properly controlled by the anesthesiologist. One of the HYPNOTIC DRUGS, ketamine, a relative of the illegal street drug called angel dust, is an excellent painkiller that works well for painful procedures on the surface of the body, such as skin grafts or changing dressings on severe burns. The disadvantage of ketamine is that it sometimes causes hallucinations or other psychological problems.

Anesthesia, local

A method used to give medication to induce loss of sensation to prevent pain in a surgical site. Most local anesthetics are given as injections, but ointments or sprays containing an

A

anesthetic agent can also be used. Local anesthetics block the nerve impulses that would otherwise communicate pain signals to the brain during diagnostic procedures, treatments, and surgery. They do not block all sensation; patients may still feel touch or pressure in the anesthetized area. Local anesthetics can be used alone or combined with CONSCIOUS SEDATION to keep the patient awake but relaxed, drowsy, and insensitive to pain.

For minor and same-day surgeries, such as stitching of small cuts or dental work, local anesthetics have a number of advantages over general anesthesia, which puts the patient in an induced sleep (see ANESTHESIA, GENERAL). Local anesthetics are generally safer because they have little or no effect on the respiratory or circulatory systems. Nausea and vomiting, which follow general anesthesia in some patients, are very rare with local anesthesia. For a short period, local anesthetics continue to have a painkilling effect after the surgery is complete; this can ease discomfort in the postoperative recovery period.

TYPES OF ANESTHESIA
Lidocaine is the most commonly used local anesthetic. It works for a relatively short time, which makes it suitable for minor surgeries, such as dental work or cleaning and suturing a bad cut. Mepivacaine and PROCAINE are similar to lidocaine. Ropivacaine and bupivacaine are longer lasting anesthetics that are also used for

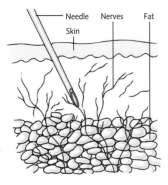

INJECTING A LOCAL ANESTHETIC
A local anesthetic, used before minor procedures, numbs the nerve endings in a limited area. The medication is usually injected under the skin in part of the body to be treated. It takes effect in a few minutes. In some areas such as the skin or eyes, local anesthetics can be applied as sprays or ointments.

regional anesthesia. Injected cocaine is used as a local anesthetic under certain circumstances. The local anesthetic may be mixed with other medications, such as EPINEPHRINE, which decreases bleeding, and sodium bicarbonate, which lowers the acidity in the medication and promotes faster absorption.

COMPLICATIONS
The most serious possible complication to local anesthesia is accidental injection of a large volume of medication into a vein. This can lead to seizures, an abnormal heart rhythm, and even cardiac arrest, which may prove fatal. As a safeguard during the injection of local anesthetic, the physician or nurse always injects slowly and pulls back on the syringe to look for blood to ensure that the medication is not being placed in a vein. See also ANESTHSIA, REGIONAL.

Anesthesia, pediatric
A method used to suppress pain in children undergoing a surgical operation. Anesthesia in children carries a greater risk than it does in adults. Since children have a higher metabolism than adults and require more oxygen, they suffer brain damage more quickly if a complication during anesthesia stops their breathing. The heart in a child lacks the flexibility of an adult heart and must work faster when required to pump more blood; this also increases the demand for oxygen. The respiratory muscles in children tire more easily, making breathing difficult when they are fatigued or stressed. The airway in children is weaker than in adults and more likely to collapse. Children often find hospital settings frightening, are extremely anxious about surgical procedures, and may struggle because of fear.

SEDATION, which makes the child relaxed and less anxious, is often used even before the child is taken to the operating room. The drugs can be given by mouth, by injection, or by rectal suppository. Children receiving general anesthesia are often put to sleep by breathing anesthetic gases before an intravenous catheter is placed in a vein. Pleasant smells, like bubble gum or strawberry, may be added to the mask to cover the smell of the gas, which some children find

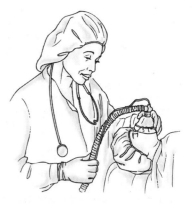

GIVING ANESTHETICS TO A CHILD
During surgery, every effort is made to make the child comfortable. A young person is often given a sedative (oral, injected, or in a rectal suppository) to relax even before going to the operating room. If the child is receiving a general anesthetic, the anesthesiologist may administer the drugs through a face mask. After the child is completely unconscious, an intravenous catheter can be placed in the arm.

unpleasant. This routine allows the child to be asleep and pain-free when an intravenous needle is placed in the hand or arm, which some children find frightening. If the intravenous catheter is to be placed while the child is still awake, an anesthetic cream rubbed into the skin an hour or so beforehand eliminates the pain and discomfort that might be caused by the intravenous catheter.

Regional anesthesia can be used during surgery in combination with CONSCIOUS SEDATION, which leaves the child awake, drowsy, and pain-free. This combination, with a spinal block as the regional anesthesia, is common for routine removal of the appendix. In other cases, a weak general anesthetic, such as nitrous oxide, may be combined with a regional anesthetic to allow the child to sleep through the procedure.

Children undergoing anesthesia are not allowed to eat or drink for a period beforehand, which varies with age. Newborns to infants 6 months old should have no solid food (including cereal mixed with formula) for 8 hours, formula for 6 hours, or clear liquids (breast milk, infant electrolyte solution, apple juice, and sugar water) for 3 hours. From age 6 months to 12 years, the solid food limit (including carbonated beverages, milk, orange juice, and chewing gum) is 8 hours, and for clear liquids,

A

it is 3 hours. If the child is older than 12 years, he or she should not have solid food after midnight, and clear liquids need to be discontinued 3 hours before the procedure. These guidelines may vary, so it is best to follow the orders detailed by the physician.

Anesthesia, regional

The use of medication to make a portion of the body unable to feel pain. Regional anesthesia works by blocking pain impulses from nerves located in the part of the body that is anesthetized. In some cases, regional anesthesia is combined with CONSCIOUS SEDATION, leaving the person awake, relaxed, and insensitive to pain. For many types of surgery, regional anesthesia is preferred to general anesthesia because it has no effect on the respiratory system and is safer for the patient.

The most common regional anesthesia for the arm is the brachial plexus block. This type of anesthesia involves the brachial plexus, a large bundle of nerves in which the branches control most of the arm and hand. The anesthetic medication is injected close to the nerve as it passes through the neck, under the collarbone or the armpit, depending on the surgery.

Another less common technique for anesthetizing the hand or lower arm is called intravenous regional anesthesia or the Bier block, named after Augustus Bier, the physician who developed spinal anesthesia. An intravenous catheter is placed in a vein in the hand; then, the blood is squeezed out the arm and back into the body by wrapping an elastic bandage up the arm. A tourniquet is placed around the upper extremity to keep the blood from flowing back into the arm. A local anesthetic is then pumped into the catheter to fill the veins of the arm and make the limb very numb. After surgery, the tourniquet is released and blood flow is restored to the arm. This is an effective technique for minor surgery on the hand and lower arm.

Anesthetic blocks of specific nerves are used less in the legs and feet than in the arms and hands because they are difficult to perform, require a number of injections rather than one, and produce small zones of numbness. Regional anesthesia in the lower part of the body is more commonly produced by injecting anesthetics into the spinal column; this procedure blocks pain impulses from nerves in the legs, groin, buttocks, and lower portion of the abdomen. This type of regional anesthesia is safer than general anesthesia, controls pain extremely well, and has a low risk of serious side effects. The procedure is commonly used in

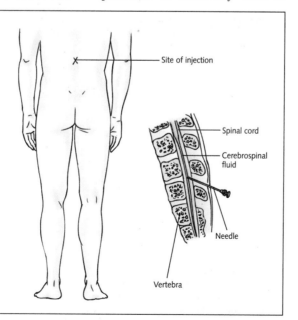

ANESTHETIZING THE ARM AND HAND
To numb the arm or hand before a surgical procedure, a regional anesthetic is most often injected into the brachial plexus, a large bundle of nerves that passes through the neck and branches down into the arm. The person remains fully conscious during the procedure.

epidural blocks for a woman having a baby. See also ANESTHESIA, SPINAL; ANESTHESIA, EPIDURAL; and CAUDAL BLOCK.

The medications used for regional anesthesia are the same as those available for local anesthesia. The choice of medication depends largely on the length of time that the surgical procedure requires.

Anesthesia, spinal

Making the lower part of the body insensitive to pain by injecting medications into the spinal column to block the nerves that lead to and from the legs, groin, buttocks, and lower region of the abdomen. Spinal anesthesia is also called a saddle block. Spinal anesthesia is used for repairing fractures in the legs and feet, hernia repair, removal of the appendix or uterus, surgery on blood vessels in the legs and lower part of the abdomen, lower back surgery, childbirth, and operations on the male and female urinary and reproductive systems. It produces excellent pain control without affecting the respiratory system.

HOW IT IS DONE

A local anesthetic is injected into the skin at the point where the spinal needle will be inserted. Next, a long, thin spinal needle is inserted through the skin into the space between two

ANESTHETIZING THE LOWER BODY
Regional anesthesia for the abdominal or pelvic areas or the legs is usually done by injecting the medication into the spinal column in the lower back. The needle is inserted between the vertebrae, into the cerebrospinal fluid within the spinal column (see inset). A single injection is commonly called a spinal; a continuous injection during surgery is called an epidural. The person remains fully awake but pain-free during the procedure. Regional anesthesia is somewhat safer than general anesthesia.

Site of injection

Spinal cord

Cerebrospinal fluid

Needle

Vertebra

RECEIVING SPINAL ANESTHESIA
A spinal anesthetic, sometimes called a saddle block, numbs and immobilizes the lower part of the body. To administer the anesthetic, a needle is inserted below the point where the spinal cord ends. A single injection delivers the medication between the vertebrae into the cerebrospinal fluid that surrounds the spinal cord (see inset). Because the medication blocks the nerves that conduct pain and also the nerves that control muscles, the person cannot move the affected area at all, making this form of anesthesia inappropriate for a woman undergoing vaginal childbirth.

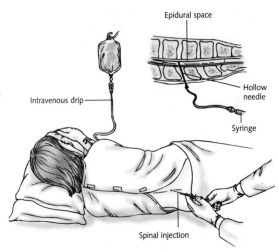

Epidural space

Intravenous drip

Hollow needle

Syringe

Spinal injection

vertebrae in the lower back and below the point where the spinal cord ends. The end of the needle penetrates the dura mater, the tough membrane that encloses the spinal column and is filled with a protective liquid called CEREBROSPINAL FLUID. The anesthetic is injected into the fluid, which transports it to the spinal nerves in the lower part of the body, and blocks sensitivity to pain. The needle itself does not touch or penetrate the spinal cord.

The medications used for spinal anesthesia are the same as those available for use in local anesthesia. The choice of medication depends largely on the length of time the surgical procedure requires.

Spinal anesthesia begins as a tingling sensation in the toes or the buttocks; then, it spreads across the entire lower part of the body. The medication blocks the nerves that control the muscles as well as the ones that convey pain, so that the patient cannot move the anesthetized area. The anesthesia may last from as little as an hour to as long as several hours. When it wears off, muscle control returns first and then feeling reappears. The possible complications of spinal anesthesia include abnormally low blood pressure (HYPOTENSION), severe headache during recovery from surgery, PARALYSIS, and MENINGITIS, an inflammation of the lining of the spinal cord that usually is due to infection. Hypotension is controlled by keeping the head of the patient lowered

during and after surgery. Severe headache is caused by continued leaking of cerebrospinal fluid through the puncture in the dura mater; it affects only one or two patients in every hundred who have spinal anesthesia. The pain can be controlled by medication until the dura mater heals and the leaking stops, usually within several days of surgery. Paralysis from needle damage or the use of the wrong anesthetic is very rare. Meningitis can be avoided with careful attention to a sterile environment in the operating room.

Anesthesiologist

A physician who specializes in anesthesiology, the practice of putting a person in an induced sleep to avoid pain during surgery. Anesthesiologists are medical school graduates who complete 4 years of advanced training, including a 1-year internship and 3 years in anesthesiology.

Before surgery, the anesthesiologist evaluates the person's medical condition and develops a plan based on the patient's physical status and the requirements of the surgical procedure. During surgery, the anesthesiologist manages the patient's anesthesia by administering appropriate medications and, with a variety of electronic devices, monitors the patient's vital functions, such as blood pressure, heart rate, and breathing. Following surgery, the anesthesiologist administers reversal medications that return the patient to full consciousness. The

anesthesiologist helps to manage pain control during recovery and monitors vital signs as needed.

Anesthesiologists also play key roles in emergency medicine and critical care, providing medical diagnosis and assessment of patients, supporting their respiratory and circulatory functions, and controlling pain. Because of their expertise in pain control, anesthesiologists help to manage chronic pain caused by injury or disease.

Anesthesiology

The medical specialty that focuses on relieving pain and providing medical care to surgical patients before, during, and after surgery. See also ANESTHESIOLOGIST.

Anesthetics

Drugs that cause a loss of sensation, including pain. Anesthetics may be general, which is when a temporary loss of consciousness is induced in a patient, or local, when specific nerves are targeted to produce numbness (and a loss of sensation) in only that part of the body.

GENERAL ANESTHETICS

General anesthesia involves the deliberate loss of consciousness, usually to relieve the pain of surgery. The first general anesthetics used were ether and chloroform. These early anesthetics had unpleasant side effects, such as vomiting during recovery, and they were administered in ways that permitted little or no dosage control.

Modern general anesthetics, such as trichloroethylene and halothane, are administered as gases from machines that mix the drugs with oxygen and nitrous oxide. The flow and composition of the gas mixture can be controlled, and the person's breathing can be maintained during chest surgery, for example, when complete muscle relaxation is required.

Short operations usually involve general anesthetics such as sodium thiopental (Pentothal) that can be injected into a vein in the hand or upper arm. Unconsciousness occurs within 10 or 15 seconds after starting the injection. This method is also used as a preliminary anesthetic before the anesthesiologist administers a gas mixture for a lengthier surgical procedure.

LOCAL ANESTHETICS

Local anesthetics work by blocking the passage of impulses along nerves. Many local anesthetics are synthetic cocainelike drugs. Painless childbirth can be achieved with an epidural block, a method that involves the injection of an anesthetic into the space surrounding the membrane that covers the lower end of the spinal cord, thereby numbing the nerves that serve the pelvic organs. Similarly, operations on the lower half of the body can involve local anesthetics that are injected into the space between the spinal cord and its outer membrane, in a method known as spinal anesthesia. A dentist may give a person a local injection of anesthetic into the gums before starting dental work.

Aneurysm

An abnormal widening or ballooning of a portion of a blood vessel. Common risk factors for aneurysms include HYPERTENSION (high blood pressure), ATHEROSCLEROSIS (narrowing of the arteries), and smoking. There are many different types of aneurysms. Two of the most common and serious types are cerebral aneurysms and aortic aneurysms.

CEREBRAL ANEURYSM

Aneurysms in the brain occur when there is a weakened wall in a blood vessel. They may be congenital or develop later in life. An aneurysm generally does not cause symptoms until it either ruptures or leaks blood. A cerebral aneurysm that has ruptured or burst is the most common cause of a subarachnoid hemorrhage (see HEMORRHAGE, SUBARACHNOID), or bleeding into the space between the brain and the arachnoid membrane (the middle membrane covering the brain). This is a life-threatening condition that can lead to STROKE, SEIZURE, BRAIN DAMAGE, or death. Permanent brain damage is a result of ischemia (loss of blood flow) or of bleeding into the brain tissue.

The primary symptom of a ruptured cerebral aneurysm and subarachnoid hemorrhage is the sudden onset of a severe headache and a stiff neck. This may be accompanied by nausea, vomiting, fainting, an altered level of consciousness, breathing problems, difficulty with speaking, trouble swallowing, confusion, irritability, vision

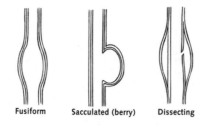

TYPES OF ANEURYSMS
An aneurysm is a bulging in the wall of a blood vessel that can occur in different ways. The entire wall can bulge uniformly (fusiform); a weak spot can cause the wall to yield on one side (sacculated, or berry); or the inner layer of the vessel wall can deteriorate, so that blood seeps between the layers (dissecting).

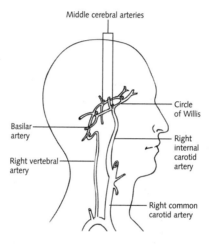

COMMON SITES OF BERRY ANEURYSMS
Berry (sacculated) aneurysms occur at various typical spots (see color) in the circulatory system in the head and neck. An individual is likely to have an aneurysm at only one site. The design of the system maximizes blood flow to the brain, even if small blockages are present.

problems, loss of movement or sensation, muscle aches, or seizure.

A suspected cerebral aneurysm requires immediate medical attention. Diagnostic evaluation includes a neuromuscular examination, CT (computed tomography) scanning, MRI (magnetic resonance imaging), and angiography. (See BRAIN IMAGING.) A spinal tap will reveal the presence of blood in cerebrospinal fluid. Treatment varies but usually includes lifesaving interventions and supportive measures. Surgery is usually required to remove large hematomas (collections of blood) and repair the damaged blood vessel. Analgesics and antianxiety drugs are

prescribed to relieve headache. Other possible medications include antihypertensives to control high blood pressure, anticonvulsants to control seizures, and calcium channel blockers to prevent cerebral vasospasm. In cerebral vasospasm, blood vessels in the brain narrow from a contraction of the smooth muscle in the blood vessel wall, creating a greater risk of tissue damage and death. Outcomes of subarachnoid hemorrhages vary widely. Even with prompt treatment, the death rate approaches 50 percent. Survivors may recover completely or have permanent brain damage.

AORTIC ANEURYSM

An abdominal aortic aneurysm is an abnormal widening of the abdominal part of the aorta (the major artery of the body). A common complication is rupture. This is a life-threatening medical emergency that can cause profuse bleeding. It is most often seen in men between age 40 and 70 years.

Symptoms of an aortic aneurysm include an abdominal hernia or pulsatile mass, abdominal pain and tenderness, rigidity, lower back pain, rapid pulse, paleness, nausea, vomiting, anxiety, fatigue, clammy skin, thirst, sweating, and fainting. Diagnosis is based on physical examination of the abdomen, blood tests, and radiographic tests such as X rays, ultrasound, MRI, CT scanning, and angiography.

If the aneurysm is unruptured, treatment depends on the size of the aneurysm and the general health of the person. Smaller aneurysms involve periodic evaluation to monitor the aneurysm's size. Medications may be prescribed for related conditions such as high blood pressure. Larger aneurysms are at greater risk for rupture, and surgical repair is often recommended. Once an aneurysm ruptures, it is a life-threatening event, and fewer than half of those who experience a ruptured abdominal aortic aneurysm survive. Emergency treatment includes supportive care and surgery to repair the damaged blood vessel.

Angina

A diffuse pain or discomfort in the chest that is often described as a tightness or heaviness; the cause is insufficient blood flow to the heart. Angina is also known as angina pectoris, which is Latin for "choking pain of the chest." In most cases, attacks of angina last only a few minutes and are brought on by physical exertion or emotional stress. Angina itself is not a disease, but a symptom of heart disease.

Not all pain in the chest is caused by angina. For more information on the various types, see CHEST PAIN.

SYMPTOMS AND CAUSE

People experience angina in different ways, but in a given individual the pattern is usually consistent. The pain is often described as dull rather than sharp, and it typically occurs over a wide area rather than a sharply defined spot. Asked to describe the location of the pain, many people place the whole hand or a clenched fist on the chest instead of pointing to a specific point. Mild cases of angina may be mistaken for indigestion. The discomfort is often felt under the breastbone (sternum) but may radiate out into the back, neck, shoulders, and arms, particularly on the left side. In some cases, pain occurs only in the arm or jaw. Pain and discomfort may be accompanied by nausea, sweating, shortness of breath, and light-headedness.

Angina results from conditions that reduce the flow of oxygen-rich blood to the heart. The most common cause is atherosclerosis, or fat deposits that narrow the coronary arteries (see CORONARY ARTERY DISEASE), which provide the heart with its blood supply. In some instances, the cause can be malfunction of the aortic valve, one of the four valves that control blood flow inside the heart, or a problem in the heart muscle itself.

Risk factors for angina include male gender, cigarette smoking, high cholesterol levels, hypertension (high blood pressure), diabetes mellitus, a family history of heart disease before age 55, lack of exercise, and obesity (being more than 30 percent over ideal body weight). Brief bouts of angina usually do no damage to the heart, but prolonged episodes may precede a heart attack.

TYPES

Stable angina arises during or just after situations in which the heart must work harder and needs increased oxygen. Examples include

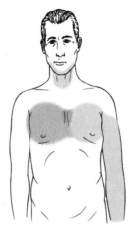

PRESSING OR SQUEEZING PAIN
Angina, a sensation of pain or pressure usually in the chest, occurs when the heart muscle is not getting enough oxygen from the blood. Usually felt under the breastbone, the pain of angina may also occur in the shoulders, arms, neck, jaws, or back. An episode of angina does not cause permanent heart damage.

cigarette smoking, eating a heavy meal, physical exertion (for example, climbing stairs, exercising, sexual activity), strong emotions such as anger or frustration, or exposure to cold temperatures or high altitude. An attack of stable angina usually lasts from 1 to 15 minutes, subsides with rest, and tends to occur more commonly between 6 AM and noon. Angina attacks lasting longer than 30 minutes are rare and merit emergency evaluation.

If stable angina worsens in frequency or severity of attacks or occurs at rest, it is called unstable angina. Such attacks may occur at any time, whether the person is moving or at rest, including during sleep. Unstable angina is a serious condition that indicates an increased risk for a myocardial infarction (heart attack). It is less common than stable angina and may require hospitalization.

Variant, or Prinzmetal, angina is also distinguished by attacks that occur when the person is at rest. This type of angina is not caused by fat deposits in the coronary arteries but by spasm of the arteries. Variant angina is often accompanied by abnormal heart rhythms, such as VENTRICULAR FIBRILLATION or ventricular tachycardia (see TACHYCARDIA, VENTRICULAR), which increase the risk of sudden death.

Another type of angina is known as

microvascular angina, because it seems to result from poor circulation in the capillaries (the tiniest blood vessels) in the heart. The capillaries are constricted, reducing blood flow, but the constrictions are too small to be detected by standard diagnostic tests.

DIAGNOSIS, TREATMENT, AND PREVENTION

In many cases, a doctor can decide whether angina is present from the way a person describes an attack. A variety of tests may be performed to identify the underlying cause of the symptoms and to determine the extent of coronary artery disease and any damage to the heart. These tests include exercise stress testing (monitoring the heart while exercising on a treadmill or a stationary bicycle), nuclear imaging (injecting a radioactive substance into the blood to produce images of the heart), echocardiogram (an ultrasound image of the heart), cardiac catheterization (inserting a thin tube through a blood vessel into the heart to locate artery blockages), and CT (computed tomography) scanning.

Once the severity and extent of the underlying condition have been determined, the best course of treatment can be chosen. Most people with mild stable angina are treated with a combination of lifestyle changes and medication. Typical lifestyle changes include a heart-healthy diet that is rich in fruits and vegetables and low in fats and oils, good control of diabetes and hypertension, regular exercise, quitting smoking, and avoiding secondhand smoke. A number of medications can be used to increase the flow of oxygen into the heart or to reduce the heart's need for oxygen. These include nitrates, such as nitroglycerin, which widen blood vessels; beta blockers, which slow heart rate and reduce the force of the heart's contraction; calcium channel blockers, which widen the coronary arteries and increase blood flow and are used to treat both variant and stable angina; antiplatelet medications, such as aspirin, which inhibit the formation of blood clots and reduce the risk of heart attack; and anticoagulants, which likewise inhibit blood clotting.

Persons with unstable or severe stable angina are often treated with an invasive catheter or surgical procedure. In BALLOON ANGIOPLASTY, an inflated balloon on the end of a catheter is used to compress the fat deposits narrowing a coronary artery. A STENT, a small tube of thin wire mesh, is often placed in the widened artery via a catheter to hold it open. Balloon angioplasty and stenting are commonly performed under local anesthesia on an outpatient basis and allow fast recovery. A minimally invasive procedure, sometimes referred to as keyhole surgery, which does not require the use of a heart-lung machine or splitting the sternum to expose the heart, can be used in some people with fewer than three blockages. BYPASS SURGERY is a major surgical procedure that entails using sections of the person's own blood vessels to detour around coronary artery blockages.

The same lifestyle changes advised for treatment of mild angina may also help prevent the condition, particularly in people whose family history places them at increased risk of coronary artery disease. A heart-healthy diet, avoiding tobacco, moderate alcohol intake, regular exercise, and maintaining an ideal body weight are prudent measures for preventing angina.

Angioedema

An allergic reaction in the skin and underlying tissue marked by swelling and red blotches. Angioedema is characterized by large welts below the surface of the skin, especially around the eyes and lips, and less frequently on the hands and feet and in the throat. It is caused by the release into the bloodstream of HISTAMINE and other chemicals related to the immune system.

There is known to be a hereditary component to the development of angioedema, but the specific cause of the reaction is often unknown. Foods, pollen, animal dander, medications, latex, insect stings, infections, illness, cold, heat, light, and emotional distress are common culprits. Among the foods that are known to cause angioedema in sensitized people are eggs, milk, peanuts, fish, shellfish, berries, and soy. Penicillin and aspirin are other possible causes, and inhalant allergens, such as pollen and animal dander, are sometimes responsible.

Diagnosis of angioedema is sometimes difficult because of the wide range of possible allergens or irritants that may cause it and because emotional conditions may intensify the reaction. A physical examination of the skin manifestations and a detailed history of exposure to possible irritants during the preceding 2 to 4 weeks may help a doctor determine a possible cause.

Treatment is generally centered on avoidance of the causative agent and may sometimes include medications such as adrenaline (epinephrine), antihistamines, and, occasionally, an oral corticosteroid.

Hereditary or recurrent angiodema is a rare form of the disorder that can be dangerous. It involves an abnormality in a blood protein in the immune system and may require specialized treatment. This form of angiodema usually includes swelling that does not itch and is sometimes accompanied by abdominal cramps and diarrhea. If hereditary angiodema affects the throat or tongue, the swelling can obstruct the air passage and be life-threatening. A physician should be informed of any possible family history of this disorder so it can be properly diagnosed and treated.

Angiogenesis

The growth of new blood vessels. Chemicals produced by cancers may stimulate angiogenesis. Some evidence suggests that angiogenesis may be necessary for cancers to grow or spread. Researchers are investigating new cancer therapies using angiogenesis inhibitors to prevent the formation of new blood vessels in cancerous tumors.

Angiogram

Also known as an angiograph; an X-ray film of blood vessels (either arteries or veins) after they have been filled with a CONTRAST MEDIUM. See also ANGIOGRAPHY.

Angiography

An X-ray procedure used to visualize blood vessels (both arteries and veins) after they have been injected with a CONTRAST MEDIUM. Blood vessels cannot be seen on X-ray film unless they have been injected with a radiographic contrast medium. When an angiogram is used to examine arteries, it is known as an arteriogram. In studies of the arteries, the contrast medium is most commonly injected through a catheter inserted into an accessible artery (such as one in an arm or a leg) and then threaded into the artery to be studied. For example, in a coronary angiogram, a catheter may be inserted into the femoral artery of the leg and threaded upward into the coronary artery. When an angiogram is used to examine the veins, it is called a venogram. Venograms generally involve the veins deep in the lower legs.

WHY IT IS PERFORMED
Angiography is generally used to detect abnormalities of the blood vessels or to evaluate the blood supply to various organs. The procedure may yield information about blood flow, the formation of an aneurysm (an abnormal ballooning of a weakened area in a wall of an artery), vascular anomalies, tumors, and hemorrhage. Deep leg veins may be examined by angiography to confirm the presence of deep-vein thrombosis, identify causes of edema, and assess vascular health after surgery.

Cardiac catheterization is a type of angiography that involves threading a catheter through a blood vessel until the catheter reaches the heart. The procedure is done so that the coronary arteries and other structures can be visualized. Catheterization can also be used to visualize the blood vessels of the legs, brain, liver, spleen, kidneys, and intestines.

Because angiography carries the risk of complications and is costly, it is generally used when other types of examinations have failed to provide information a physician needs to know. In some cases, angiography may be the only procedure that can yield the necessary information.

HOW IT IS PERFORMED
Angiography can be performed as an outpatient procedure in a hospital. The person being examined lies on a movable table and is given intravenous sedatives to relax him or her. Heart rate and oxygen levels are monitored throughout the procedure. A local anesthetic is applied to the area, a needle is inserted into an accessible blood vessel, and a guide wire is threaded through the needle. A very thin, flexible tube called a catheter is inserted over the guide wire and passed directly into the artery or vein. The catheter is then manipulated until it is in the desired location. Contrast medium is injected into the

CLOSE-UP ON ANGIOGRAPHY

Angiography is a an X-ray procedure that can identify narrowed, blocked, or abnormally wide arteries or veins. A radiologist inserts a catheter into a blood vessel and manipulates it until it reaches the artery or vein to be examined. Then a contrast medium, usually iodine dye, is injected into the artery or vein. Once the contrast medium passes through the blood vessel, a series of X rays is taken.

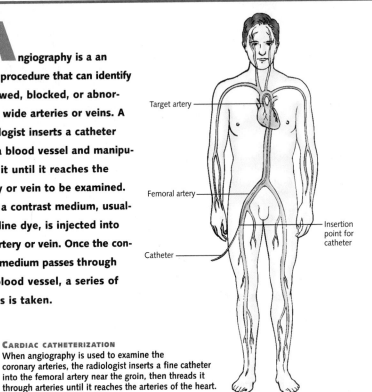

Target artery

Femoral artery

Catheter

Insertion point for catheter

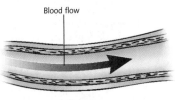

Blood flow

Healthy artery

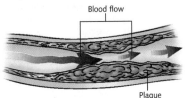

Blood flow

Blocked artery

Plaque

HEALTHY AND BLOCKED ARTERIES
In a healthy artery, the flow of blood is not obstructed. When plaque builds up on the artery walls, blood flow slows.

CARDIAC CATHETERIZATION
When angiography is used to examine the coronary arteries, the radiologist inserts a fine catheter into the femoral artery near the groin, then threads it through arteries until it reaches the arteries of the heart.

catheter, causing a mild sensation of warmth. The normal flow of blood carries the contrast medium to the selected blood vessels. As the contrast medium moves through the blood vessels, X-ray images are taken rapidly. The entire procedure usually takes between 1 and 2 hours.

The catheter is removed, and pressure is applied over the puncture site for 10 to 15 minutes. The person who has undergone angiography must remain in bed for up to 6 hours after the procedure to allow the puncture site to heal to prevent bleeding. Normal activity must be limited for 24 hours, and vigorous activity must be avoided for up to 72 hours.

RISKS
Because angiography is an invasive procedure, there are risks involved. The risks include bleeding at the puncture site, injury to a blood vessel, allergy or other reaction to the contrast medium or other medica-

tions, and infection. Very rarely, a heart attack or stroke may occur during or after angiography. See also DIGITAL SUBTRACTION ANGIOGRAPHY.

Angioma
A benign (not cancerous) growth on the skin consisting of blood vessels. Some examples include CHERRY ANGIOMAS (small, bright red, domelike spots on the skin caused by dilated blood vessels) and capillary hemangioma (a reddish purple birthmark caused by an abnormal distribution of blood vessels).

Angioplasty, balloon
See BALLOON ANGIOPLASTY.

Angiotensin
A hormone that causes blood vessels to constrict and raises blood pressure. Medications that prevent the forma-

tion of angiotensin, known as angiotensin-converting enzyme (ACE) inhibitors, lower blood pressure and reduce the workload on the heart. They are commonly used in the treatment of congestive heart failure (see HEART FAILURE, CONGESTIVE) and high blood pressure (see HYPERTENSION). Another class of medications, the angiotensin-receptor blocking agents, block the effect of angiotensin and have effects similar to those of ACE inhibitors.

Angiotensin-converting enzyme inhibitors
See ANTIHYPERTENSIVES.

Anhidrosis
An abnormal lack of SWEATING in response to heat. Sweating is the body's way of cooling itself, and its absence can result in potentially life-threatening overheating. Anhidrosis

can be seen in people who have a severe neck injury, diabetes mellitus, dehydration, or a heat illness. Treatment of anhidrosis is with drugs to stimulate sweating.

Animal experimentation

The use of animals in medical laboratory studies. Animal experimentation is a well-established standard in the process of pursuing solutions to human health problems and is considered essential by many medical scientists to find cures for life-threatening diseases and conditions. Most laboratory animals are rodents that are specifically bred for research because of the similarities between the physiological systems of humans and certain species.

There are numerous animal activist organizations and individuals who are opposed to this use of animals. Some activists believe that all animals have rights and deserve consideration and that society should not deny animals the same rights that protect people from being sacrificed for the common good.

Society and the medical community hold that the use of animals for medical research is beneficial for making sure that treatments are safe for humans and has proved, in some cases, to be essential for sustaining human life. Guidelines already exist to ensure that animals used in research are treated compassionately. Several relevant federal laws regulate the protection of animals involved in medical research.

In recent years, computer simulators, in-depth cadaver studies, and advances in research using living volunteers have been used to supplement and sometimes replace animal testing studies.

Animals, diseases from

Infections that may be transmitted from animals to humans under natural conditions. Diseases from animals are also referred to by the medical term zoonosis, or zoonotic disease.

WHO IS AT RISK

People who come in contact with infected animals or with disease vectors (carriers of disease that spread the infection from an infected animal to an uninfected person or animal) are at risk of becoming infected. Infants and small children who are exposed to animals may be at greater risk due to several factors; they are more likely to handle animals and put their hands in their mouths without washing them, and their immune systems are not fully developed, which makes them less resistant to infection.

A woman who is pregnant may be more susceptible, and her fetus may be at greater risk. Older people whose immune systems may be impaired and people who are being treated for cancer or who have HIV (human immunodeficiency virus) or AIDS (acquired immunodeficiency syndrome) have a greater risk for acquiring diseases from animals. Animal health care workers, including veterinarians, agricultural workers, zoo workers, and wildlife and primate researchers, have greater exposure to animals that may carry infections. Frequent hand washing is extremely effective in preventing infection, and hand-to-mouth activity (eating, smoking) should not occur when a person is exposed to animals. See also the following specific diseases from animals: ANTHRAX, BRUCELLOSIS, CAT-SCRATCH DISEASE, HANTAVIRUS INFECTION, LEPTOSPIROSIS, MENINGITIS, PLAGUE, RABIES, TICKS AND DISEASE, TULAREMIA, and WEIL DISEASE.

Anisometropia

A large difference in the refractive power of the two eyes. An individual who is farsighted in one eye and nearsighted in the other has anisometropia.

Ankyloglossia

See TONGUE-TIE.

Ankylosing spondylitis

An inflammatory disease of the joints in the spinal column and back of the pelvis that tends to progress to the shoulder, hip, and knee joints. Ankylosing spondylitis is a form of RHEUMATOID ARTHRITIS that generally develops in late adolescence or early adulthood, affecting young males predominantly. When it develops before the age of 17, it is termed juvenile ankylosing spondylitis. The disease

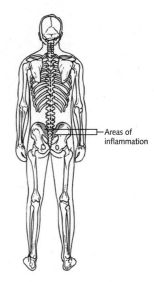

INFLAMMATION OF THE LOWER SPINE
Ankylosing spondylitis generally starts in the region of the sacroiliac joint between the flaring bones of the hip (ileum) and the bone at the base of the spinal column (sacrum). It causes episodes of back pain and increasing back stiffness.

can lead to extreme rigidity, deformity, and a fusion of the bones involved.

Symptoms include morning back pain with aching and stiffness that tends to improve in 1 or 2 hours. Movement tends to minimize this pain, which often returns when the body is stationary for long periods. Over a period of several months, the pain and inflexibility tend to become more severe, moving up the spine. Other spinal components, such as ligaments and muscles, become affected, causing severe muscle spasms. These spasms produce a forward flexing of the spinal column, which causes a rounded curvature of the back. The disks, joints, and ligaments of the spinal column and eventually the hip, knee, and shoulder joints become inflamed and hardened. In severe cases, the neck may be stiff, preventing the person from being able to lift his or her head. Sites other than the spinal column can be involved, such as the eyes, heart, aorta, and lungs.

The cause of ankylosing spondylitis is unknown, but the presence of the inherited gene HLA-B27, though not a cause, seems to increase susceptibility in some cases. It is also possible that common infections of the intestinal, genital, or urinary tract may activate the disease.

The diagnosis of ankylosing spondylitis is based on a clinical history, an evaluation of lower back stiffness and joint and tissue inflammation, and the results of laboratory tests and procedures, such as X rays and other imaging techniques. A person with this condition should sleep on a firm mattress with thin pillows to prevent muscle spasms of the back. Treatment may include physical and occupational therapy, nonsteroidal anti-inflammatory drugs (NSAIDs), and in rare severe cases, surgery to realign the spine and to replace destroyed joints in order to restore function and eliminate debilitating pain. See also SPONDYLITIS.

Ankylosis

Immobility and consolidation of a joint or joints caused by disease or injury. Ankylosis refers to the condition in which bones and other components of a joint are stiff or fixated, causing severe or complete loss of the joint's movement. It is also the term for a surgical procedure known as cervical spine fusion, which is performed to stabilize a joint, commonly in the neck or back.

Anodontia

A total or partial absence of teeth, usually due to heredity. Total anodontia is a rare condition in which the primary teeth or the permanent teeth fail to develop. In this case, some teeth may be present but they are cone-shaped or malformed. Partial anodontia is a more common condition that involves the lack of one or several permanent teeth, often the third molars. Primary teeth are usually not affected. The condition is sometimes referred to as hypoplasia of the DENTITION. Possible causes, in addition to heredity, include nutritional disturbances during the mother's pregnancy or the child's infancy, endocrine disorders, and diseases such as RICKETS and SCARLET FEVER. When permanent teeth do not appear after the primary teeth have come out, the most

> 📖 Terms in small capital letters— for example, PHYSICAL THERAPY or PAGET DISEASE—indicate a cross-reference to another entry with more information.

frequent causes are accidents that have damaged the gums or bone, or early TOOTH DECAY. The molars and premolars have natural grooves that tend to trap the bacteria that cause decay. In some instances, the permanent teeth simply fail to develop or, due to dental impaction (see IMPACTION, DENTAL), cannot grow through the gum tissue. Any missing teeth can eventually cause problems and should be evaluated by a dentist, who will probably recommend a bridge or denture.

Anomaly

A marked deviation from the norm or standard, particularly as a result of congenital or hereditary defects. Some anomalies are developmental, meaning that they stem from an imperfect development of the embryo. Other anomalies are caused by genetic defects.

Anorexia

See ANOREXIA NERVOSA.

Anorexia nervosa

A mental illness in which a person refuses to maintain normal body weight, is extremely afraid of gaining weight, and has a distorted image of his or her body, such as describing it as obese even when it is extremely thin. People with anorexia usually lose weight by restricting the amount and type of food they eat. In one type of anorexia similar to BULIMIA, some people engage in binge eating, or they purge themselves with self-induced vomiting, laxatives, diuretics, or enemas. People with anorexia may also exercise excessively. Even though the word anorexia comes from Greek roots meaning "lack of appetite," people with anorexia desire food but refuse to eat. The disease primarily affects females, particularly during adolescence, but it also affects women at other ages, and, rarely, men.

SYMPTOMS AND CONSEQUENCES

People with anorexia nervosa are preoccupied with weight, yet deny that they are too thin. They may develop extreme rituals around meals, such as eating only certain items (usually low-calorie), cutting their food in small pieces, hoarding food, or refusing to eat in the presence of others. Anorexia nervosa is

often accompanied by other mental diseases, such as depression, manic-depressive illness, self-mutilation, and obsessive-compulsive disorder. As their weight drops below normal, those with anorexia often experience low moods, withdraw from social contact, have trouble sleeping, exhibit irritability, and lose interest in sex. Physical symptoms include sensitivity to cold, yellowing skin, brittle nails, low blood pressure, lack of menstrual periods, slow heartbeat (bradycardia), and, if the person is inducing vomiting, damage to tooth enamel from stomach acid. Long, fine hair may develop on the body as a way of conserving heat. Anorexia nervosa can have serious medical consequences, including heart disease, anemia, kidney disease, dental problems, and brittle bones (osteoporosis). Death from heart failure is a major risk. In severe cases, hospitalization may be necessary.

CAUSES AND TREATMENT

The onset of anorexia nervosa often follows a stressful life event, such as leaving for college. The disease is more likely in societies where food is abundant and cultural norms favor thin body shapes; in the United States it is most prevalent in middle- and upper-class whites. Anorexia nervosa tends to run in families; women with a parent or sibling who

---

SIGNS OF ANOREXIA NERVOSA

People with anorexia do not usually think of themselves as sick; the disease is often detected by family or friends. The following are common symptoms:

- **Preoccupation with eating, food, weight, and calories**
- **Excessive exercise**
- **Repeatedly talking about being fat, especially if the person is thin**
- **Baggy clothes**
- **Irregular or absent menstruation**
- **Symptoms of self-induced vomiting, including retreating to the bathroom after meals, vomit odors in the bathroom, frequent "showers," swollen glands ("chipmunk face"), bloodshot eyes after a trip to the bathroom, and paleness, dizziness, or light-headedness**

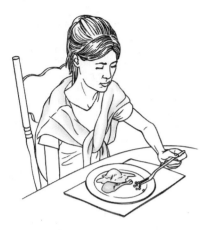

PREOCCUPATION WITH WEIGHT
A person with anorexia nervosa is engaged in self-starvation. In order to reduce body weight, he or she often devotes enormous energy to the avoidance of eating, becoming extremely picky about the type or preparation of food to be consumed. The rituals surrounding meals replace the meals themselves.

has the disease are more likely to develop it. Personality traits common in people with anorexia are low self-esteem, social isolation, and a perfectionist attitude; they are often good students and athletes.

Treatment consists of increasing the person's weight into the normal range by stabilizing eating patterns coupled with psychotherapy, especially family group therapy, aimed at understanding the emotional conflicts that underlie the disorder. In some cases, medication may be used to treat accompanying depression or anxiety. In extreme cases, the person will need nutrition through intravenous therapy. Prognosis is generally good, although relapses are common.

Anorgasmia
See ORGASM, LACK OF.

Anosmia
The loss of the sense of smell. Temporary anosmia is most commonly due to nasal congestion associated with colds or allergies. However, in some cases it is the result of more serious problems, such as neurological disorders or nasal polyps. Several medications and poisons can cause anosmia, as can a facial or skull fracture. Treatment of the underlying disorder may cure the problem. The sense of smell also tends to lessen as

a person ages, a condition that is not treatable.

Anovulation
See OVULATION, LACK OF.

Anoxia
An abnormal condition caused by a lack of OXYGEN. There are various types of anoxia, which can be local or system-wide. In anemic anoxia, the person's blood is unable to carry oxygen to tissues. In cerebral anoxia, circulatory failure causes a life-threatening lack of oxygen in the brain.

Antacids
Drugs used to relieve the symptoms of indigestion and heartburn. Antacids, which are available in over-the-counter preparations, neutralize stomach acid and effectively relieve symptoms. Most antacids contain one or more of the following active ingredients: sodium bicarbonate, calcium carbonate, magnesium hydroxide, and aluminum

hydroxide. Antacids are available as pills, powders that dissolve in water, chewable tablets, and liquids.

The use of antacids can mask the symptoms of more serious disorders, and the excessive or prolonged use of antacids can cause bloating or serious disorders of the kidneys or bones. A person who experiences indigestion, heartburn, or stomach pain for longer than 2 weeks should seek medical attention.

Antagonist
A drug that binds to a cell receptor without eliciting a biological response. Antagonist drugs are substances that tend to cancel out the action of active substances.

Antepartum hemorrhage
Any vaginal bleeding after the 20th week of pregnancy. Antepartum hemorrhage may have several causes, including damage to the cervix, sepa-

---

UNDERSTANDING ANTACIDS

Two distinct types of antacids are available to treat heartburn, stomach upset, or indigestion. It is important to understand which type of antacid is best suited for a person's condition because the drugs can differ in side effects and interactions with other medications. The first type, called non–histamine$_2$ (H$_2$) antagonists, neutralizes the gastric acid secreted from the stomach. This type contains at least one of the following ingredients: calcium carbonate, sodium bicarbonate, aluminum salts, or magnesium salts, which are available over-the-counter as chewable tablets or liquids.

The chemical compounds in non–H$_2$ antagonists each have different properties. Calcium carbonate, for example, is very potent in neutralizing acids but should not be taken for long-term therapy. Sodium bicarbonate–based antacids provide almost immediate relief. However, people on a salt-restricted diet or who have congestive heart failure, high blood pressure, cirrhosis, edema, or kidney failure, should consult with a doctor before taking antacids. Aluminum salts can cause constipation, and use is not advisable for people with kidney disease.

The second type of antacid, called an H$_2$ antagonist, blocks the formation of hydrochloric acid in the stomach. This type of antacid takes longer to give relief, especially if an abundance of stomach acid is already present. Certain conditions, such as hyperacidic stomach and duodenal ulcers, benefit from this type of antacid, which is sold over-the-counter as cimetidine (Tagamet), ranitidine (Zantac), and famotidine (Pepcid).

Antacid tablet

KEY

⬭ Antacid   ⬬ Stomach acid

⬰ Base-acid combination

TRADITIONAL ANTACIDS
A traditional antacid medication (nonhistamine antagonist) neutralizes stomach acid by introducing a chemical compound called a base. Newer antacids (histamine antagonists, or acid blockers) prevent the formation of hydrochloric acid in the stomach.

ration of the placenta from the uterine wall, or PLACENTA PREVIA, in which the placenta lies over the cervix. Most antepartum bleeding is mild and harmless. However, hemorrhage caused by placental separation, placental bleeding, and placenta previa can threaten both the mother and baby. Any bleeding during pregnancy should be reported to the doctor as soon as possible. Blood tests and ultrasound scanning can help identify the source of the hemorrhage. In the case of severe antepartum hemorrhage, hospitalization may be required. A blood transfusion may be needed, and the baby may need to be delivered as soon as possible, either by cesarean section or by induction of labor.

Antepartum testing

See PRENATAL TESTING.

Anterior

The front of something. In describing anatomy, anterior refers to surfaces, organs, and structures that are near the front of the body or the front of a particular body part. For example, the anterior surface of the heart faces the breastbone.

Anthrax

An infectious disease of farm animals that is occasionally spread to people. Anthrax is found in goats, cattle, sheep, horses, and exotic wildlife such as hippos, elephants, and the Cape buffalo. The disease is unusual in humans and generally occurs in developing countries in which exposure to infected animals and their products is not adequately prevented.

CAUSES AND SYMPTOMS

Anthrax is caused by a bacterial spore that is highly resistant and can remain viable in soil and in animals for decades. People may become infected with cutaneous anthrax by handling materials from animals that have died of anthrax (the bacteria enter via a scratch or sore when contaminated animal material is handled) or from eating contaminated meat. Pulmonary anthrax (sometimes called inhalation anthrax) may occur if a person with an acute respiratory infection inhales spores of the organism that causes anthrax. Anthrax has been used in BIOTERRORISM.

Symptoms of cutaneous anthrax include an enlarging skin eruption,

malaise, body aches, headache, fever, nausea, and vomiting. Pulmonary anthrax symptoms resemble those of the flu and may progress rapidly to severe respiratory distress, shock, coma, or even death.

DIAGNOSIS AND TREATMENT

Anthrax is suspected when there is a history detailing exposure to animals or their products, which may have transmitted the disease. Animal handlers, agriculture workers, butchers, wool sorters, and weavers are at risk. Cultures of skin lesions may be taken to identify the bacteria in cutaneous anthrax, and throat swabs and sputum samples may be evaluated if pulmonary anthrax is suspected.

The cutaneous form is treated with penicillin, tetracycline, or another antibiotic to prevent the bacteria from spreading through the body and to heal the open sore on the skin. Anthrax is not contagious from person to person. Pulmonary anthrax is usually fatal if not treated early with continuous intravenous penicillin and, possibly, corticosteroids.

Anthroposophical medicine

A holistic medical approach based on an integration of spiritual and physical factors in pursuit of good health. Founded by Rudolf Steiner, an Austrian physician in the 19th century, anthroposophical medicine seeks to meld conventional medical knowledge with its view of spiritual factors. Some important herbal remedies have come from the anthroposophical tradition.

Antiaging therapies

Treatments claimed to improve and maintain optimal health for people as they age. Antiaging therapy involves stimulation and addition of substances thought to help the body repair and regenerate itself as it ages. The elusive goal of antiaging therapy has been to help the body perform as well in old age as it did in youth. Antiaging therapies include the use of vitamins, minerals, hormones, and some drugs of unproven benefit.

AGING AND ANTIAGING

Aging is the disorganization, deterioration, dissolution, and wear and tear that gradually breaks the body down over time, making people look older in the process. How the aging process

happens is not entirely understood, though scientists have determined that it takes place at the molecular, cellular, and anatomic levels. The effects of aging are most visible at the anatomic level, although breakdown at the cellular level shows up as wrinkled skin, loss of muscle tissue, hair loss, and other familiar signs of aging.

At the molecular level, aging affects DNA and protein molecules, breaking them down by various means, including free radicals (atoms carrying unpaired electrons introduced to the body by smoking, pollution, and radiation and thought to have a role in promoting disease).

The antiaging process is part of life at every age. The body spontaneously repairs damage caused by aging, partly by constantly replacing molecules and cells. Antiaging therapies are intended to reverse the aging process by stimulating the body's natural antiaging mechanisms. There is no evidence that external therapies can reverse or retard the aging process.

HUMAN GROWTH HORMONE

Human growth hormone is assumed to promote antiaging. Growth hormone is present in the body in greatest quantity during adolescence, when people go through their final growth spurt. After adolescence, levels of human growth hormone decline as people age, especially after the age of 60. Decline in human growth hormone is associated with the wrinkled, sagging skin of older people, as well as with an overall decline in energy. Some antiaging therapies promote the use of synthetic growth hormones in an attempt to supplement the body's diminished supply and improve mental functioning and skin quality as well as increase muscle mass. No scientific evidence exists prove this can be done.

One fact that limits exploration of the use of human growth hormone to reverse the aging process is that it has many dangerous side effects. Too much growth hormone can lead to chronic diseases such as DIABETES MELLITUS, TYPE 2; ARTHRITIS; and CARPAL TUNNEL SYNDROME. It can also cause high blood pressure and fluid retention. Its prolonged use might increase the risk of cancer. Daily injections of human growth hormone, the minimum necessary to derive any benefits, cost between $10,000 and $35,000 per year.

OTHER ANTIAGING THERAPIES

Several chemicals found in the body are associated with aging, and antiaging therapies seek to limit their effects.

■ *Antioxidants* Antioxidants are natural substances that may counter the harmful effects of free radicals. Vitamins C and E and beta-carotene, related to vitamin A, are antioxidants found in many foods, as is the mineral selenium. Eating at least five servings of fruits and vegetables per day is recommended to obtain these and other natural antioxidants. Some researchers suspect that antioxidants in fruits and vegetables may slow the aging of the brain.

■ *DNA and RNA* As people age, more and more of the damage done to DNA in the cells of the body is not repaired. Some antiaging therapies promote the use of pills containing DNA or RNA to help the body repair its DNA. No evidence exists to demonstrate that this remedy is effective or that oral intake is plausible.

■ *DHEA* Because the hormone DHEA has boosted the immune systems of mice and has been shown to prevent cancer in some animals, products are being sold in health food stores that are labeled as containing DHEA. These products claim to extend life by boosting the immune system, although no research has been done to support such claims.

■ *Estrogen and testosterone* Some antiaging therapies recommend large doses of hormones, such as estrogen and testosterone, to reverse the aging process. No evidence exists to demonstrate that this remedy is effective, and large doses of hormones produce serious side effects and may cause cancer.

■ *Live cell therapy* Another form of antiaging therapy involves the injection of healthy live cells from animal embryos into the muscles of a person to supposedly "wake up" the person's own corresponding cells, creating new connective tissue in the process. LIVE CELL THERAPY is controversial and has not been approved for use in the United States by the Food and Drug Administration. Toxic reactions may include fever, lethargy, pain at the injection site, arthritis, and severe allergic reactions.

Antianxiety drugs

Antianxiety drugs, also known as anxiolytics, do not cure anxiety disorders but can effectively relieve unpleasant symptoms. Most antianxiety drugs are called BENZODIAZEPINES, which work by enhancing the function of a neurochemical called GABA (gamma-aminobutyric acid). Benzodiazepines are fast-acting but can be associated with addiction, abuse, and the impaired ability to drive.

Some antianxiety drugs are BETA BLOCKERS, which reduce the effects of adrenaline. Also fast-acting, these drugs are not habit-forming. Other drugs used to treat the symptoms of anxiety include ANTIDEPRESSANTS, many of which work by enhancing or regulating the activity of serotonin, a chemical in the brain known to affect a person's mood.

Antiarrhythmics

Drugs that correct an irregular heartbeat by restoring normal rhythm. Antiarrhythmics can also help the heart work more efficiently by slowing it down when it beats too fast. The pace at which the heart beats is controlled by electrical signals that start in one part of the heart and spread throughout the entire organ. Arrhythmias develop when this control mechanism is disrupted.

Antiarrhythmics are available only by prescription and come in different classes that differ in the way they work to control a person's heartbeat. They are available as capsules, tablets, and injections.

Antibiotics

Drugs used to treat bacterial infections. Originally, antibiotics were defined as substances produced by one microorganism that selectively inhibit the growth of another microorganism, but that strict definition is not always accurate because synthetic antibiotics are also available.

The first antibiotic to be used to treat disease was penicillin (see PENICILLINS), discovered by Alexander Fleming in 1926 and first used during World War II. Before that, doctors had no effective medicines to treat serious infections. There are now more than 100 antibiotics available to treat bacterial disease.

HOW ANTIBIOTICS WORK

Antibiotics were originally made

DNA strand
Drugs interfere with DNA and RNA metabolism
Example: Rifampin

Ribosomes
Drugs produce abnormal polypeptides and inhibit protein synthesis
Examples: Tetracycline, chloramphenicol

Cell wall
Drugs disrupt formation
Examples: Penicillins, cycloserine, cephalosporins

Plasma membrane
Drugs disrupt structure
Examples: Some antifungals

Cytosol
Drugs block metabolism by affecting production or breakdown of needed components
Examples: Isoniazid, sulfonamides

HOW ANTIBIOTICS DISABLE BACTERIA Various antibiotics interfere with cell activity in different parts of the bacterium in order to destroy it.

from molds and fungi, but now some of these drugs are made synthetically in laboratories.

The bacteria and fungi used to create antibiotics are known to kill harmful bacteria that cause infection and disease. When a person takes an antibiotic, it overpowers and kills the bacteria causing the infection, or it prevents the bacteria from multiplying. Doctors always recommend that a person finish the entire course of antibiotics. If a person feels better and stops taking the medication, the surviving bacteria, which have the highest resistance, will start to grow and multiply and the person can have a relapse that will be more difficult to treat.

USES OF ANTIBIOTICS

When organisms invade the body, they reproduce and multiply rapidly. At the same time, they compete with the body's natural metabolism, in some cases by producing poisons that injure cells. Bacterial infections can be extremely serious and even fatal. The extent to which an infected person is ill depends on the type and number of the invading organisms, as well as on the person's general health. There are several types of bacterial infection for which antibiotics are prescribed.

■ *Staphylococcal infections* Staphylococcal bacteria are responsible for a wide range of diseases. They cause skin infections, blood poisoning (bacteremia), food poisoning, osteomyelitis (infection of the bone), staphylococcal pneumonia, and toxic shock syndrome.

■ *Streptococcal infections*
Altogether, 21 species of streptococcal bacteria have been identified, of which three classes are responsible for most infections. These include strep throat (streptococcal pharyngitis), scarlet fever, and skin infections such as impetigo, erysipelas, and lymphadenitis. Other infections caused by streptococcal bacteria include pneumonia, otitis media (inflammation of the middle ear), endocarditis (inflammation of the interior lining of the heart), and meningitis (inflammation of the membrane surrounding the spinal cord or the brain.)

■ **E. coli** *infections* Escherichia coli (see E. COLI) and other bacteria that live in human intestines cause a great deal of the diarrhea seen in children. Travelers to Mexico, South America, and Southeast Asia are also at risk of developing diarrhea as a result of bacterial infection from contaminated food, especially salads.

■ *Others* Other bacterial infections that are usually treated with antibiotics include salmonella (an extremely common infection), typhoid fever, Lyme disease, botulism, diphtheria, dysentery, cholera, and tuberculosis.

LIMITATIONS OF ANTIBIOTICS
Antibiotics generally are only useful in the treatment of bacterial infection. Not all fevers are caused by infection, and not all infections are caused by bacteria. Many infections are caused by viruses, and antibiotics cannot treat viral infections. Colds and flu, for example, are respiratory infections caused by viruses.

Sometimes viral infections such as colds and flu can lead to secondary infections that are caused by bacteria.

Secondary bacterial infections, such as ear or sinus infections, can be treated with antibiotics. However, not all bacterial infections need to be treated with antibiotics. Many bacterial infections improve on their own; minor skin infections may be treated with local topical antiseptics, creams, or sprays.

Antibiotics are not useful for certain people. The very young and the very old, for example, tend to be vulnerable to the adverse effects of antibiotics. An older person is more likely to suffer from kidney damage or allergic reactions, while a newborn's immune system may be too immature to metabolize or excrete antibiotics. Pregnant women should not take antibiotics indiscriminately because some antibiotics can have adverse effects on fetal development.

RESISTANCE TO ANTIBIOTICS
Because over time antibiotics have been overused and used inappropriately, tough new strains of bacteria have developed that are resistant to antibiotics. As bacteria reproduce, they change their cellular makeup to protect themselves from future attack, including the attacks made on them by drugs. People who have taken a lot of antibiotics or who have not taken them as prescribed are especially vulnerable to resistant bacteria, as are people with immune systems weakened by age, illness, or long-term hospitalization.

Bacteria, whether normal or mutant, reproduce at incredible rates. While antibiotics can easily destroy most normal bacteria, mutant strains have developed that permit some strains to survive an antibiotic attack. Many bacteria have adapted and become invulnerable to antibiotics. As a result, the number of deaths from infectious diseases has risen, in part because many bacteria have acquired resistance against antibiotics.

Antibody

An effective tool for fighting infection within the body; a soluble protein that is produced in the body by B cells and reacts to antigens in a number of ways. An antibody recognizes a specific ANTIGEN and binds to it or coats it to inactivate or destroy the antigen. Antibodies are secreted into the body's fluids by B cells, which are a type of white blood cell called a lymphocyte.

Antibodies are able to interact with antigens in the body, but they cannot penetrate living cells. Each B cell makes a specific antibody to combat a specific antigen. For example, one B cell is programmed to make an antibody to block the virus that causes the common cold, while another antibody can stave off the *Streptococcus* bacterium that results in strep throat.

Antibodies interact with antigens the way a key fits a lock. Sometimes the fit is precise, and at other times it is less exact. In varying degrees, antibodies are able to interlock with antigens and mark them for destruction. Each Y-shaped antibody molecule is composed of two identical long polypeptides and two identical short polypeptides. The antibody molecules bind to an antigen at the ends of the Y-shape, forming an antigen-antibody complex. When this occurs, many large plasma cells are produced. Each of these cells acts as a factory by manufacturing more antibody molecules identical to the original one, and these molecules are poured into the bloodstream.

Antibodies consist of a large protein molecule that belongs in the group known as immunoglobulins, which can perform their functions in several different ways that vary with the nature of the antigen with which they are interacting. The most common of these is the release by the antibody-antigen complex of a group of serum enzymes that are lethal to the antigen. An antibody might also interlock with the toxins produced by certain bacteria and directly disable the toxic material; these antibodies are known as antitoxins. Other antibodies coat invading bacteria, making the bacterial microbes vulnerable to scavenger cells that can engulf and destroy them. Antigen cells that are coated by antibodies via a different process are primed for destruction by certain white blood cells. Another kind of antibody function blocks viruses from entering the body's cells, a function that is used in making vaccines.

Antibody, monoclonal

An ANTIBODY produced in large quantities by a single cell for use against a specific antigen. Monoclonal antibodies are currently developed as a method for identifying the myriad cells involved in the immune response and as diagnostic tools for cancer and other diseases.

The antibodies normally found in the body are generally polyclonal, which means they are produced by more than one cell. A specialized laboratory technique enables many monoclonal antibodies to be created in animals. When an animal is immunized with the desired antibody and begins to produce that antibody, the spleen is removed so that a suspension of cells can be prepared. Some of these cells produce the desired antibody. These are fused with a line of myeloma cells (cancerous cells produced in the bone marrow of people with multiple myeloma) that does not produce antibodies. The fusion of these two produces the desired monoclonal antibody, which is isolated, grown in tissue culture, and reinjected into the membrane lining the animal's abdominal cavity. Excess fluid in the abdomen that contains the monoclonal antibody in high concentrations is removed, and fermentation laboratories then produce commercial preparations of the monoclonal antibodies.

Preparations of monoclonal antibodies are currently used for a wide variety of medical goals. They can be used to measure proteins, medications, and other substances in the blood. They may be involved in typing tissue and blood and in identifying infectious agents. They are also used to treat allograft rejection in organ transplant recipients. In the diagnosis and treatment of leukemias and lymphomas, they may be used to identify cluster designations (abbreviated CD and used with a number, such as CD3; the CDs are used as markers in identification of tumors) for classification and follow-up. Monoclonal antibodies are useful for identifying tumor antibodies and autoantibodies in a variety of diseases.

Anticardiolipin antibodies

Antibodies directed against cardiolipin (see ANTIBODY). The presence of anticardiolipin antibodies is associated with systemic lupus erythematosus and with a syndrome characterized by an increased risk of blood clots, or thrombi, within the cardiovascular system.

Anticholinergic agents

Drugs used to treat various spastic conditions. Anticholinergics are used to treat Parkinson disease, muscle rigidity, and muscle spasms caused by psychoactive medications. Anticholinergics work by blocking acetylcholine receptors in the brain and other tissues, reducing the effects of acetylcholine and restoring balance with dopamine. Anticholinergics can be used to treat peptic ulcer disease and other gastrointestinal disorders by reducing acid secretion, but newer and more effective antiulcer drugs have been developed. Some anticholinergics are also used to prevent nausea and vomiting caused by motion sickness and to treat asthma.

Examples of anticholinergics include belladonna alkaloids, which contain naturally occurring anticholinergics that have been used for centuries, and benztropine (Cogentin).

Anticoagulants

Drugs that prevent clotting of blood; also called "blood thinners." Anticoagulants are used to maintain normal blood flow in people who are at risk for excessive clot formation, such as people who are bedridden. Anticoagulants prevent new clots or the enlargement of existing clots; they do not dissolve existing clots.

Anticoagulants are prescribed for people who have had recurrent heart attacks or stroke. They are also given to people who have transient ischemic attacks (TIAs), an arterial embolism, or a pulmonary embolism and to people at risk for developing blood clots, such as those with irregular heart rates. Anticoagulants are usually taken for at least 6 months, although people with artificial heart valves may have to take them indefinitely. Anticoagulants include ardeparin (Normiflo), dalteparin (Fragmin), danaparoid (Orgaran), enoxaparin (Lovenox), heparin, and warfarin (Coumadin). Heparin and warfarin use may require frequent blood monitoring.

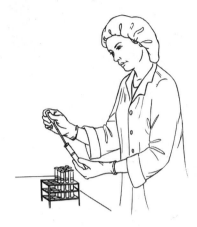

MONITORING BLOOD THINNERS
Persons taking some types of anticoagulants (blood thinners) will need to have blood samples taken every few weeks to ensure that the drug is working properly. Dosages can be adjusted as necessary.

Anticonvulsants

Drugs used to control seizures. Anticonvulsants are used to treat EPILEPSY and other SEIZURE disorders, such as a seizure following neurosurgery and a seizure associated with brain tumors. Anticonvulsants act on the central nervous system by inhibiting activity in the part of the brain responsible for grand mal or generalized seizures in which the entire body shakes uncontrollably. A doctor will choose a particular anticonvulsant based on the type of seizure being treated.

GRAND MAL SEIZURES
Among the many anticonvulsants available to treat grand mal seizures, also called tonic-clonic seizures, there are three commonly prescribed drugs: carbamazepine (Tegretol), phenytoin (Dilantin), and valproic acid (Depakene). Phenobarbital (Luminal, Solfoton), usually used in combination with phenytoin, has been used to control epileptic seizures. Newer antiepileptic drugs, including gabapentin (Neurontin), lamotrigine (Lamictal), and topiramate (Topamax), are also effective in combination with other drugs to control partial seizures.

Most people with a single type of seizure can be treated with a single anticonvulsant. People with different types of seizures frequently need to take more than one drug.

ABSENCE (PETIT MAL) SEIZURES

Anticonvulsants used to treat absence seizures (a condition in which a child will stare uncontrollably for several minutes) include ethosuximide (Zarontin), valproic acid (Depakene), and sometimes clonazepam (Klonopin).

MYOCLONIC SEIZURES

Myoclonic seizures, which affect a specific part of the body, are usually treated with clonazepam (Klonopin) or valproic acid (Depakene).

OTHER USES FOR ANTICONVULSANTS

Some anticonvulsants are used to treat various psychiatric conditions, including bipolar disorder, acute mania, schizoaffective disorder, and panic disorder. Some anticonvulsants are also used to treat neurological disorders, including trigeminal neuralgia and pain due to other neuropathies.

Antidepressants

Drugs used to treat DEPRESSION and other conditions associated with reduced levels of two neurotransmitters: norepinephrine and serotonin. Antidepressants work by raising the levels of norepinephrine and serotonin in the brain or by preventing their inactivation in the brain. Under normal circumstances, the neurotransmitters stimulate the brain when they are released and are reabsorbed by brain cells, then broken down by an enzyme called monoamine oxidase (MAO). When levels of these neurotransmitters are low, the brain is understimulated.

TRICYCLIC ANTIDEPRESSANTS

This class of antidepressants is named for its chemical structure. Tricyclics increase the levels of both serotonin and norepinephrine by blocking their reabsorption into nerve cell endings. Tricyclics are very effective at treating symptoms of depression, but they are associated with many troublesome side effects, such as drowsiness, dry mouth, and constipation. In overdose, they are deadly.

Examples of tricyclic antidepressants include amitriptyline (Elavil), desipramine (Norpramin), and nortriptyline.

MAO INHIBITORS

This class of antidepressants is named for its action. By inhibiting mono-

amine oxidase, the levels of neurotransmitters in the brain are increased. MAO inhibitors are very effective at reducing symptoms of depression, but MAO is also involved in the metabolism of tyramine, an amino acid. People who take MAO inhibitors must be very careful not to eat or drink certain foods or beverages, such as sour cream, aged cheese, pizza, sauerkraut, pea pods, avocados, red wine, beer, and champagne, among others. These foods contain large amounts of tyramine and can cause the person to have a dangerous increase in blood pressure. MAO inhibitors include phenelzine (Nardil) and tranylcypromine (Parnate).

SSRIs

Selective serotonin reuptake inhibitors (SSRIs) make up the newest class of antidepressants. They are less likely to cause side effects than either tricyclics or MAO inhibitors. They work by blocking the reabsorption of serotonin in the brain, thereby increasing the available supply and enhancing a person's mood. SSRIs are associated with some side effects, but they are usually mild. Some people taking SSRIs experience sexual difficulties, including lack of interest in sex and difficulties in having orgasm.

Examples of SSRIs include citalopram (Celexa), fluoxetine (Prozac), paroxetine (Paxil), and sertraline (Zoloft).

OTHER ANTIDEPRESSANTS

Several drugs have antidepressant activity but are not classified as antidepressants. These include bupropion (Wellbutrin), a dopamine inhibitor; mirtazepine (Remeron), a tetracyclic similar to a tricyclic but with fewer cardiac side effects; nefazodone (Serzone), a serotonin receptor antagonist; trazodone (Desyrel), similar to a tricyclic; and venlafaxine (Effexor), a serotonin and norepinephrine inhibitor.

Antidiuretic hormone

See ADH.

Antidote

Any drug or other remedy that counteracts the effects of a poison. Antidotes work in different ways. Antidotes may bind (or chelate) a metal toxin, thus helping its elimination from the body. They may also

protect certain organs from the adverse effects of a poison.

The key to the choice of antidote is knowing what the poison is. About 78 percent of poisoning cases can be handled in the home after telephone consultation with a local specialist at a POISON CENTER.

Antiemetics

Drugs used to prevent or relieve nausea and vomiting, usually from motion sickness, gastroenteritis, morning sickness, and cancer. Four kinds of drugs are prescribed for nausea and vomiting: phenothiazines, antihistamines, anticholinergics, and selective serotonin antagonists. Phenothiazines work by depressing the central nervous system; antihistamines have a depressant effect on nerve pathways; anticholinergics inhibit nerve impulse transmissions; and serotonin antagonists block the stimulation that causes vomiting. The latter type of drug is often used to treat nausea and vomiting due to cancer chemotherapy. All are powerful drugs that act at one or more of the places in the body responsible for causing nausea and vomiting, and they must be taken with care.

Some antiemetics are available without prescription. Many nonprescription antiemetics contain an antihistamine (see ANTIHISTAMINES) and may cause drowsiness. Most are also useful for motion sickness. The herbal agent ginger may also be useful as a mild antiemetic; it is sometimes used to treat motion sickness and morning sickness in pregnancy. Women who are pregnant should talk to their doctors before taking any medication.

Antiepileptic agents

See ANTICONVULSANTS.

Antifreeze poisoning

Poisoning following the consumption of motor vehicle antifreeze. Antifreeze is made up almost entirely of ethylene glycol, a clear, colorless, odorless liquid with a sweet taste. Antifreeze poisoning chiefly occurs when children accidentally drink antifreeze, which they sometimes consume in large amounts because it tastes sweet. Alcoholics also sometimes drink antifreeze as a substitute for ethanol, the intoxicating ingredient in liquor.

A

By itself, ethylene glycol is not particularly toxic, but metabolism in the body breaks it down into substances that are extremely poisonous. Even small amounts of antifreeze can cause kidney damage, especially to children, and death may occur within 24 hours. Anyone who suspects antifreeze has been ingested should call a POISON CENTER immediately or seek emergency medical attention.

Antifungal drugs

Drugs used to treat infections caused by fungi. Fungi are single-cell life forms that survive by invading and living off other living things. They thrive in moist, dark places, including some parts of the human body. Fungal infections on the skin can usually be treated with creams, ointments, or powders. But infections occurring inside the body may need to be treated with drugs taken in the form of a tablet, capsule, liquid, or vaginal suppository or by injection. Examples of such infections include candidiasis (also known as thrush or yeast infection), histoplasmosis, and aspergillosis.

Examples of antifungal drugs used to treat infections inside the body include fluconazole (Diflucan), itraconazole (Sporanox), and ketoconazole (Nizoral). All of these drugs are available by prescription only. Antifungal products applied to the skin, however, are usually available without a prescription and are sold as creams, ointments, liquids, powders, aerosol sprays, and vaginal suppositories. They are used to treat common fungal infections such as athlete's foot, jock itch, ringworm, and vaginal yeast infections.

Antigen

A substance that, on entering the body, is recognized as foreign and responded to by the person's immune system. An antigen is a molecule that can produce a specific IMMUNE RESPONSE when it is introduced into the bloodstream. A specific configuration on the surface of certain large molecules makes a particular molecule an antigen that attracts a specific ANTIBODY. Different types of antibodies recognize the different configurations as sites that they can combine with. The combining sites of the antibody and antigen emit powerful attracting forces that make them

interlock tightly at surface sites that match like pieces of a jigsaw puzzle.

Antigens are substances that can be recognized by B and T cells. Antigens can be divided into three types: immunogens, haptens, and tolerogens. An immunogen is a substance that can stimulate an immune response and serve as a target of that immune response. A hapten is a substance that cannot initiate an immune response by itself; however, when combined with a larger molecule called a carrier, it can stimulate an immune response. A tolerogen is a substance that inhibits responses against itself when exposed to the immune system.

Antihistamines

Any drug used to counteract histamine, a chemical released within the body during an allergic reaction. Antihistamines do not alter the cause of the reaction but suppress the symptoms associated with histamine, such as swelling, irritation, and

watery discharge from the eyes and nose. Antihistamines work by blocking histamine receptors.

ANTIHISTAMINES AND HAY FEVER
Antihistamines are most often used to suppress the symptoms of hay fever and related allergies. The allergic reaction is triggered when pollen is inhaled, irritating the lining of the nose and releasing histamine. Histamine acts on receptors in the nose to widen the blood vessels that supply blood to the mucous membrane, which leads to swelling (congestion) and a runny nose. Antihistamines help to block that inflammatory effect, thus reducing swelling, irritation, and mucus discharge.

Antihistamines are sometimes found in cough or cold remedies because they reduce nasal secretions. They are not effective for treating colds, however, and may actually make them worse by preventing or delaying clearance of the bronchial or nasal passages by drying them up.

HOW ANTIHISTAMINES WORK

People may misunderstand the purposes of antihistamines and decongestants because both types of drugs are frequently recommended for colds, allergies, and rashes. But the medications are markedly different in how they work to treat a person's symptoms. Decongestants relieve nasal congestion by narrowing blood vessels in the nasal membranes and by reducing mucus and swelling in the nasal lining.

Antihistamines have a broader effect than decongestants and work by blocking a chemical the body creates (called histamine) in response to an allergic reaction. Histamine causes small blood vessels in the eyes and skin to widen, causing redness and swelling. Too much histamine in the body can also cause sneezing, runny nose, itching, hives, and rashes; an antihistamine relieves these symptoms.

Antihistamines can have adverse side effects. If used for too long they can worsen nasal congestion. They are not recommended for people who have high blood pressure, glaucoma, thyroid disease, or heart disease or for some people who have asthma or diabetes. A person taking a sedative should not take antihistamines, since both types of drugs can cause drowsiness and impair a person's ability to drive.

ANTIHISTAMINES COUNTERACT HISTAMINES
Histamines are body chemicals produced in an allergic reaction. At a cellular level, they act through specialized histamine receptors on the walls of microscopic blood vessels to cause swelling, itching, and release of fluids. Antihistamines are similarly specialized to occupy the receptor sites to interfere with the actions of the histamines.

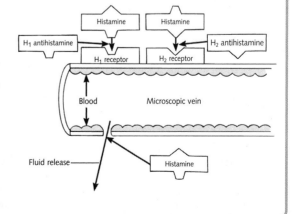

OTHER USES FOR ANTIHISTAMINES

Antihistamines are available in topical form as creams and ointments to reduce skin inflammation and itching caused by allergic reactions. Antihistamines may also be purchased over-the-counter without a prescription as sleep aids. They may be prescribed to help treat ear infections. Some over-the-counter antihistamines can cause drowsiness, resulting in an impaired ability to drive. Nonsedating antihistamines are available by prescription only.

Antihypertensives

Drugs that help lower blood pressure. Blood pressure measures the force with which blood moves through the blood vessels. While blood pressure normally varies throughout the day, rising during exercise and falling during sleep, in some people the blood pressure stays high all the time. Some cases of high blood pressure (hypertension) can be treated with lifestyle changes—losing weight, lowering salt intake, exercising more, stopping smoking—but in most cases, hypertension is treated with medication to help control the condition. There are five classes of medication used to treat hypertension.

DIURETICS

These drugs work by making it difficult for the kidneys to retain water and salt. By increasing the amount of urine, the amount of fluid in the bloodstream is reduced, which reduces pressure on the artery walls of the blood vessels. Examples of diuretics include bumetanide (Bumex), chlorothiazide (Diuril), chlorthalidone (Hygroton), furosemide (Lasix), hydrochlorothiazide (Esidrix, HydroDIURIL), metolazone (Zaroxolyn), and spironolactone (Aldactone).

BETA BLOCKERS

Beta blockers reduce high blood pressure by slowing the force and speed of the action of the heart, including the rate at which it contracts. The medication may also reduce blood pressure by directly affecting the central nervous system, altering the body's response to certain nerve impulses. Examples of beta blockers are atenolol (Tenormin), bisoprolol (Zebeta), carvedilol (Coreg), metoprolol (Lopressor), and propranolol (Inderal). Some beta blockers can cause drowsiness and possibly impair a person's ability to drive.

ACE INHIBITORS

Angiotensin-converting enzyme (ACE) inhibitors lower blood pressure by blocking production of angiotensin II, a chemical the body produces to raise blood pressure. Normally, angiotensin maintains blood pressure by tightening the arteries and causing the retention of sodium (salt) and water. ACE inhibitors reduce blood pressure very quickly. Examples include benazepril (Lotensin), captopril (Capoten), enalapril (Vasotec), fosinopril (Monopril), lisinopril (Prinivil, Zestril), moexipril (Univasc), quinapril (Accupril), ramipril (Altace), and trandolapril (Mavik).

ANGIOTENSIN II RECEPTOR ANTAGONISTS

Angiotensin II receptor antagonists lower blood pressure by blocking angiotensin from binding to receptor sites in the smooth muscles of the blood vessels. This stops the angiotensin from tightening the arteries and raising the blood pressure. Examples include candesartan (Atacand), irbesartan (Avapro), losartan potassium (Cozaar), and valsartan (Diovan).

CALCIUM CHANNEL BLOCKERS

Calcium channel blockers reduce blood pressure by dilating the arteries, thereby reducing resistance to blood flow. They include amlodipine (Norvasc), bepridil (Vascor), diltiazem (Cardizem, Dilacor XR, Tiazac), felodipine (Plendil), isradipine (DynaCirc), nicardipine (Cardene), nimodipine (Nimotop), nisoldipine (Sular), and verapamil (Calan, Covera-HS, Isoptin, Verelan).

OTHER DRUGS THAT CAN LOWER BLOOD PRESSURE

Several drugs relax the muscles in the walls of the arteries or veins, thus reducing blood pressure. These drugs are sometimes considered to be nerve blockers. They include clonidine (Catapres), guanfacine (Tenex), hydralazine (Apresoline), methyldopa (Aldomet), minoxidil (Loniten), and prazosin (Minipress).

A few drugs combine a calcium channel blocker with an ACE inhibitor in a single pill. The doctor decides which combination works best for various symptoms.

Antimicrobial agents

A general term referring to several categories of drugs, including antibiotics, antifungals, antiprotozoals, and antivirals. The most important characteristic of an antimicrobial agent is that it acts to inhibit or kill a target pathogen, or disease-causing entity, but has no toxic effect on the host. Antimicrobials affect the biochemical processes of microbes, but not those of humans or other animals.

Antineoplastons

Substances occurring naturally in the blood said to defend against cancer cells. Antineoplastons are small proteins, peptides, and amino acid derivatives found naturally in human blood and thought to work against cancer cells by "reprogramming" them and turning them back into normal cells. People with cancer have very low levels of antineoplastons in their blood—as low as 2 percent of those found in healthy people's blood. Some experiments have been

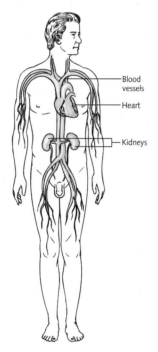

Blood vessels

Heart

Kidneys

SITES OF ANTIHYPERTENSIVE DRUG ACTION
Various types of antihypertensive medications work in different areas of the body to lower blood pressure. ACE inhibitors, angiotensin II receptor antagonists, and calcium channel blockers affect the blood vessels. Beta blockers slow the action of the heart. Diuretics act in the kidneys to increase the amount of urine, thereby decreasing the amount of fluid in the blood.

performed with synthetic antineoplastons to determine whether they can help cure cancer, but results have been inconclusive. The use of antineoplastons has not been endorsed by the Food and Drug Administration in the United States.

Antioxidants

Substances able to neutralize OXYGEN FREE RADICALS produced in the body during metabolism. Antioxidants act by interrupting a process called OXIDATION, in which free radicals (molecules with unpaired electrons) react with other molecules in a series of chain reactions. Free radicals are produced normally by the body, as are antioxidants, to help body systems maintain a healthy balance. Stress, aging, and pollution can add to the number of free radicals in the body, thereby disrupting the delicate balance by damaging DNA within body cells.

Because antioxidants prevent or slow oxidation by free radicals, they are assumed to provide a protective effect and are thought to be able to reduce the risk of cancer, heart disease, and stroke, among other diseases associated with aging. Antioxidants such as beta-carotene and VITAMIN E (alpha-tocopherol) are found naturally in fresh fruits and vegetables and are thought to protect cell membranes. Vitamin C, or ascorbic acid, which is also an antioxidant, removes free radicals from within cells. People who eat 5 to 8 servings of fruits and vegetables each day as part of a balanced diet are most likely consuming adequate amounts of foods containing antioxidants.

Although some people believe that adding antioxidants to the diet by consuming dietary supplements is desirable, this view is controversial and not medically proven. Some scientists think that regular consumption of dietary supplements may interfere with the body's natural production of antioxidants.

Anti-Parkinson drugs

Drugs that address an imbalance of the primary neurotransmitters dopamine and acetylcholine. Parkinson disease is caused by an imbalance of the two neurotransmitters responsible for transmitting nerve impulses from the brain to the muscles. One group of anti-Parkinson drugs works by stimulating production of dopamine in the brain, supplying the substance from which it is formed (levodopa) to be converted to dopamine in the brain. Dopamine levels can also be increased by reducing the breakdown of dopamine in the brain or by stimulating its release.

Another group of drugs, called anticholinergic drugs, restores the balance between the two neurotransmitters by blocking the action of acetylcholine.

Antipsychotic drugs

Drugs that reduce psychotic symptoms. Antipsychotic drugs do not cure schizophrenia or other psychotic disorders, but they do make it possible for people with those diseases to function more effectively. The condition of most people with psychotic disorders, including schizophrenia, improves when treated with antipsychotic drugs, although some people with psychotic illness are not helped much by medication. Antipsychotic drugs have been known by various names since they first became available in the 1950s, including psychotropics, neuroleptics, phenothiazines, major tranquilizers, and atypical antipsychotics.

HOW ANTIPSYCHOTIC DRUGS WORK

It is thought that in psychotic disorders, the brain cells release too much dopamine, which causes overstimulation of brain activity. Antipsychotic drugs block the stimulatory actions of dopamine. They are chiefly used to treat the hallucinations and delusions associated with schizophrenia and other psychotic disorders. Antipsychotic drugs are less able to modify symptoms such as reduced motivation or the absence of emotion.

NEUROLEPTICS

Older antipsychotic drugs are known as neuroleptics, major tranquilizers, or phenothiazines. Examples include chlorpromazine (Thorazine) and haloperidol (Haldol), which have been available since the mid-1950s. These drugs have been associated with significant side effects that have limited their usefulness, including drowsiness, restlessness, muscle spasms, tremor, dry mouth, and blurred vision. Most of these side effects can be limited by lowering the dose or by taking other medications.

Neuroleptics are associated with a serious disorder that represents a long-term side effect of their use called tardive dyskinesia (TD). This irreversible disorder is characterized by involuntary movements of the mouth, lips, and tongue. TD occurs in about 15 to 20 percent of people who have been taking neuroleptics for many years, although it can develop in people who have taken the drugs for shorter periods. Some of these agents can cause an impaired ability to drive.

ATYPICAL ANTIPSYCHOTIC DRUGS

Newer antipsychotic drugs available since 1990 are often more effective and cause fewer side effects than neuroleptics. Examples include clozapine (Clozaril), olanzapine (Zyprexa), and risperidone (Risperdal). Although the atypical antipsychotic drugs are rarely associated with the kind of side effects that characterize treatment with neuroleptics (including TD), they do have side effects. Weight gain, for example, is associated with taking these drugs. Clozapine has sometimes caused agranulocytosis, a condition in which the number of white blood cells that fight infection is greatly reduced. As a result, people taking clozapine must have their blood tested every 2 weeks.

Antipyretic drugs

Drugs that reduce FEVER. Fever can be reduced by drugs representing three different classes. Many of them are available without a prescription. The three types of antipyretics are salicylates, including aspirin; acetaminophen, sometimes called nonaspirin pain relievers; and nonsteroidal anti-inflammatory drugs (NSAIDs), such as ibuprofen, naproxen, and ketoprofen. Aspirin should not be taken by children because of its involvement in causing Reye syndrome, a rare disorder that can cause brain and liver damage. In children, the most commonly used antipyretic drugs are acetaminophen and ibuprofen.

Antireflux surgery

An operation to repair an abnormal condition (gastroesophageal reflux) in which stomach acids back up into the esophagus, damaging its lining and causing pain. The procedure involves tightening of the lower esophageal sphincter (valve) so that stomach juices cannot flow up into the esophagus, causing a person to have chronic heartburn. Gastroesophageal reflux disease (GERD; see ESOPHAGEAL REFLUX) may be caused by an abnormality of the lower esophageal sphincter, which may be too weak to prevent leaking from the stomach into the esophagus. Some people with gastroesophageal reflux disease have a hiatal hernia, a condition in which a portion of stomach protrudes abnormally through the diaphragm.

Most people with gastroesophageal reflux disease can control the disease with an improved diet, over-the-counter antacids, or prescription medications that decrease acid production in the stomach. In a small number of cases, the symptoms become extremely severe. The surgical procedure is recommended for a person whose symptoms are intolerable; who cannot eat because of inflammation of the esophagus; who has repeatedly suffered from asthma, laryngitis, or pneumonia caused by regurgitated stomach contents; or who has bleeding ulcers in the esophagus.

HOW IT IS DONE
To determine whether a patient is a candidate for antireflux surgery, the surgeon is likely to examine the lower portion of the esophagus and upper part of the stomach with an endoscope (a lighted viewing instrument) to assess for damage to the esophagus. Through a thin tube placed in the esophagus, the physician is able to monitor the acid reflux level for 24 hours and check on the strength of the lower esophageal sphincter at the same time.

Antireflux surgery can be performed either as an open procedure or with a laparoscope (a type of viewing tube.) Although the open procedure requires a larger incision and a longer recovery period than LAPAROSCOPIC SURGERY, it may be necessary in people who are obese, who have a large amount of dense scar tissue from prior abdominal surgeries, or who are likely to bleed abnormally during the operation.

Laparoscopic antireflux surgery is performed by making small (¼ to ½ inch) incisions in the abdomen and inserting narrow instruments connected to a tiny video camera. The camera gives the surgeon a magnified view of the esophagus on a television screen and allows the surgeon to manipulate surgical instruments to perform the repair. The surgeon wraps a portion of the upper end of the stomach around the base of the esophagus and attaches it tightly with sutures. If a hiatal hernia is present, the surgeon repairs it at the same time.

Laparoscopic antireflux surgery is preferred over the open procedure because of reduced postoperative pain, a shorter recovery period, and smaller scars.

OUTCOME AND COMPLICATIONS
Antireflux surgery is performed with a patient under general anesthesia, so a person should not consume any food or water after midnight on the day before surgery. The operation can take several hours to complete, and most patients stay in the hospital for at least one night or even longer, depending on the speed of recovery. Some patients need a liquid diet for a time after surgery, and solid foods are gradually reintroduced.

Pain following laparoscopic antireflux surgery is generally mild, and recovery takes from a few days to about 2 weeks. The open procedure causes more discomfort and requires 6 weeks of recovery. Once recovered, the patient should experience no difficulty with daily tasks, such as walking, lifting, playing sports, and driving. Antireflux surgery is highly effective; almost nine out of ten people no longer need medication. Long-term side effects and complications, such as feelings of stomach bloating and a reduced ability to belch, can occur but are uncommon.

Antiseptics

Substances that destroy or inhibit the growth of bacteria and other microorganisms. Antiseptics are used topically to treat wounds and infections, to sterilize surfaces and medical instruments, to promote general hygiene, to preserve foods, and to purify sewage. Common antiseptic chemicals include iodine, alcohol, hydrogen peroxide, and boric acid, each of which works differently. Iodine, for instance, can kill bacteria within 30 seconds, while other antiseptics work more slowly.

Antiseptics include germicides, which kill bacteria directly, but they do not include drugs such as antibiotics that destroy microorganisms internally. Disinfectants used to kill microorganisms on nonliving surfaces are antiseptics that are too harsh to apply to body tissue and are chiefly used to clean kitchen counters, bathrooms, or cutting boards, for example. The most effective antiseptics are physical rather than chemical, destroying microorganisms by sterilizing objects with heat by boiling, flaming, or burning.

Antiserum

A serum containing antibodies used to provide temporary immunity from a specific disease. Antiserum may be obtained from an animal that has been immunized against the disease in question, or it may be transmitted through infection with microorganisms containing specific antigens. Antiserum may be specific for a single antigen or specific against more than one antigen.

Antisocial personality disorder

See PERSONALITY DISORDERS.

Antitoxin

A specific type of ANTIBODY that combines with the toxins produced by certain bacterial microorganisms that enter the body and inactivate the toxins. Antitoxins are proteins that exist naturally in the body or develop in response to the presence of toxins in the bloodstream. Toxins known as exotoxins are produced by the bacteria that cause botulism, diphtheria, and tetanus and are among those that are inactivated by antitoxins.

Antituberculosis drugs

Drugs used to cure tuberculosis infection. Pulmonary tuberculosis is caused by a bacterium called *Mycobacterium tuberculosis* and is treated with daily oral doses of antibiotics for at least 1 year. In some cases, the bacteria that cause tuberculosis have developed immunity to specific antituberculosis drugs, so most people with the disease take three or four drugs, including isoniazid, rifampin, pyrazinamide, and ethambutol. Antituberculosis drugs are available by prescription. They are all associated with some side effects. Rifampin, for example, can turn urine and tears orange or brown. Isoniazid and rifampin can cause noninfectious hepatitis.

Antivenin

A substance containing purified antibodies used to neutralize the venom of a poisonous animal. Antivenin is a type of antiserum that comes from the serum of an animal that has been deliberately immunized against a particular venom. Antivenin is available to counteract animal bites from poisonous snakes, spiders, and scorpions.

Anuria

Serious kidney malfunction that results in little or no urine production. Failure to pass urine is an indication of a serious problem in the urinary tract. In patients with only one kidney, anuria is often caused by a stone. In patients with both kidneys, the condition may be caused by a tumor blocking the kidneys, kidney disease, or abnormally low blood pressure caused by shock. Treatment is urgent and depends on the cause of the condition. Dialysis may be used to rid the body of wastes until the kidneys are again able to function normally. Left untreated, anuria leads to uremia (excess waste products in the blood) and death.

Anus

The opening at the lower end of the DIGESTIVE SYSTEM through which the feces, or stool, passes out of the body. About 1 to 2 inches long, the anus comprises two circular muscles. The internal anal sphincter muscle is a smooth, involuntary muscle; the external anal sphincter is a voluntary, striated muscle that can be relaxed at will to allow a bowel movement. The two muscles work together to open and close the anus.

Anus, cancer of

An uncommon cancer that develops in the inch-long muscular tube where the rectum opens. Anal cancer is a form of colon cancer (see COLON, CANCER OF THE) that is highly treatable and potentially curable. The earliest sign of anal cancer usually is bleeding and is often mistaken as a sign of hemorrhoids. Other common symptoms include pain or itching in the anal area, straining during bowel movements, or a discharge from the anus. Less common symptoms may include swollen lymph nodes in the groin or anal area and changes either in bowel habits or in the size of the stool.

Anal cancer is often discovered during a rectal examination, in which the doctor inserts a gloved finger into the anus, feeling for lumps or growths. If a mass is found, other tests, including blood tests and a biopsy, may be ordered; CT (computed tomography) scanning, MRI (magnetic resonance imaging), and ultrasound scanning may be used to assess the extent of the cancer. A sigmoidoscope, a fiberoptic tube with a light at one end, may be used to examine the inside of the colon. Treatment usually consists of radiation and chemotherapy. If the tumor is not eradicated, surgery may be needed.

Anal cancer is somewhat rare. About 3,500 people in the United States develop the disease and about 500 die of it annually. Women are slightly more likely than men to get anal cancer; most people who have it are older than 50. Anal cancer is associated with HUMAN PAPILLO-MAVIRUS (HPV), smoking, and having anal sex.

Anus, imperforate

A birth defect in which an infant is born without a fully developed anus. (See also BIRTH DEFECTS.) The anus is the external opening of the rectum through which stools pass. When a baby is born with an imperforate, or closed, anus, there are two possible causes. The anus may be covered with skin, or, more rarely and seriously, the anal canal fails to develop before birth.

The main symptom is the failure of a newborn to pass any stools. To diagnose an imperforate anus, a finger or catheter is inserted into the rectum until it encounters an obstruction, the end of the rectum. Surgery is necessary to correct an imperforate anus. If the anus is simply covered, the surgeon will remove the skin. If the anal canal did not develop, more complicated reconstructive surgery is required. Most children recover completely. Eight of ten children born with an imperforate anus are toilet-trained by age 4.

Anxiety

A general feeling of uneasiness, dread, uncertainty, and fear in response to or in anticipation of a real or imagined threat. The physical symptoms of anxiety can include racing heart, palpitations, light-headedness, hyperventilation, appetite loss, diarrhea, urinary frequency, hesitancy or indecision, sweating, enlarged pupils, tremors, poor attention span, headache, sexual difficulty, sweating, irritability, sleeplessness (insomnia), fatigue, nightmares, dry mouth, diarrhea, or difficulty swallowing.

CAUSES

Anxiety can have a number of causes, including the threat itself; general physical and emotional stress, which is worsened by fatigue and overwork; grief over, for example, the death of a loved one or the loss of a job; a number of drugs, including caffeine, decongestants, asthma inhalers (bronchodilators), and thyroid supplements; withdrawal from addictive drugs; poor diet; or an overactive thyroid gland (hyperthyroidism), stroke, Parkinson disease, heart disease, or emphysema.

From time to time people may experience mild anxiety, a normal response to stress that resolves when the stress is removed. Anxiety becomes a medical problem requiring treatment if it consistently interferes with a person's day-to-day functioning.

TREATMENT

People who are experiencing anxiety should avoid caffeine, stimulants, alcohol, and other mood-altering drugs. Techniques such as biofeedback and relaxation therapy, which can help the person relax in times of stress, can help alleviate anxiety. Psychotherapy or counseling to understand and deal with underlying emotional conflicts, sometimes accompanied by antianxiety medication to relieve symptoms, is used when anxiety becomes severe and debilitating. See ANXIETY DISORDERS.

Anxiety disorders

A group of mental illnesses characterized by overpowering and long-lasting fear, dread, unease, apprehension, obsessions, compulsions, and unpleasant physical symptoms, such as sweating, elevated heartbeat, shaking, or trembling. Anxiety disorders

A

interfere with day-to-day functioning and may make it difficult or impossible for an individual to hold a job or enjoy a family or social life. They are the most common mental illnesses in the United States and are thought to affect approximately one in nine Americans a year. Anxiety disorders often accompany other mental illnesses, such as mood and eating disorders.

TYPES OF ANXIETY DISORDERS

■ *Generalized anxiety disorder (GAD)* The most prevalent type of anxiety disorder, GAD is characterized by excessive, constant anxiety and worry about a number of life problems, such as marriage and money, for a period of 6 or more months. GAD may begin in a person's 20s or 30s or as a childhood overanxious disorder. Men and women are affected equally, and the disorder tends to be chronic.

■ *Panic disorder* This disease is distinguished by unpredictable bouts of extreme anxiety that seem to start suddenly and peak quickly, usually within 10 minutes. Unpleasant physical symptoms can include elevated blood pressure and heartbeat, disorientation, dizziness, numbness, a looming sense of danger, choking sensations, and a strong desire to escape. People with panic disorder worry steadily about having another attack and may change their behavior to avoid situations they think trigger the bouts of panic. Panic disorder is sometimes accompanied by a serious fear of public spaces (agoraphobia). The disease is more common in women than men, and it usually begins between adolescence and age 35. See PANIC DISORDER.

■ *Phobia* An exaggerated, extreme, and irrational fear of specific situations or objects. The feared situation or object varies with the individual. Typical phobias include objects such as needles, knives, or animals, particularly snakes, dogs, or spiders (simple phobia); social situations (social phobia); and public spaces such as churches and stadiums (agoraphobia). These fears are common in children and are not a sign of a psychiatric disorder. See PHOBIA.

■ *Obsessive-compulsive disorder (OCD)* OCD is distinguished by persistent, intrusive, and distressing thoughts, images, or impulses that occupy the mind (obsessions) and by repetitive actions the individual thinks he or she must perform (compulsions). Typical obsessions include fear of contamination by dirt, germs, or viruses; extreme need for objects to be in an exact order; heightened vigilance, such as keeping all windows and doors locked at all times; and fear of unlucky numbers. Typical compulsions include washing the hands repeatedly, checking door and window locks again and again, and hoarding supplies against unlikely disasters. OCD is equally common in males and females. See OBSESSIVE-COMPULSIVE DISORDER.

■ *Posttraumatic stress disorder (PTSD)* The immediate or delayed response to a traumatic event that evokes intense fear, helplessness, and horror through flashbacks, or nightmares coupled with avoidance of all things associated with the event and increased vigilance and arousal, such as extreme alertness and difficulty sleeping. PTSD can arise after accidents involving maiming or death, natural disasters, war, physical abuse, assault, rape, and torture. It usually develops within 3 months of the trauma but can begin years later. See POSTTRAUMATIC STRESS DISORDER.

CAUSES

A number of factors contribute to anxiety disorders. Since these diseases tend to run in families, inherited brain chemistry probably has a role. The pattern of a person's life experiences and his or her overall personality are also factors. In some cases, the use of stimulants such as caffeine, decongestants, and cocaine contributes to the disease.

TREATMENT AND OUTCOME

Anxiety disorders are typically treated with a combination of medications to improve the person's physical and emotional symptoms and psychotherapy aimed at teaching the individual how to handle anxiety-provoking situations. A number of medications are available, including sedatives, antihistamines, tranquilizers, benzodiazepines, and antidepressants. People with anxiety disorders should avoid alcohol and stimulants, including caffeine. Therapy usually consists of training in relaxation and desensitization—that is, leading the person step by step through the anxiety-provoking situation and teaching him or her how to stay relaxed throughout the process. Anxiety disorders are difficult to eliminate entirely, but treatment (sometimes including hypnosis) offers significant improvement in almost all cases.

Anxiolytics
See ANTIANXIETY DRUGS.

Aorta
The largest artery in the body. All other arteries branch out from the aorta to carry oxygen-rich blood from the heart to the rest of the body tissues. The aorta, which is about an inch wide, begins in the lower left chamber, or left ventricle, of the heart. When the heart beats, the aortic valve opens to allow oxygen-rich blood to flow from the ventricle into the aorta. When the beat ends, the valve closes to prevent blood from flowing back into the ventricle. Arteries branching off the aorta carry blood into the upper body, arms, neck, and head. In the lower abdomen the descending aorta divides into two smaller arteries, which supply blood to the legs and the organs in the abdomen, including the stomach, kidneys, intestines, spleen, and reproductive organs. See CARDIOVASCULAR SYSTEM; HEART.

Aortic insufficiency
Leakage in the valve between the heart and the aorta (main artery of the body); also known as aortic regurgitation. Aortic insufficiency allows blood to leak back from the aorta into the heart, decreasing blood flow into the body and forcing the heart to pump harder to compensate. Over time, the heart chamber known as the left ventricle, where the aortic valve is located, may enlarge and weaken, causing congestive heart failure (see HEART FAILURE, CONGESTIVE).

The symptoms of aortic insufficiency include shortness of breath during exercise, difficulty breathing when lying down at night, weakness on exertion, swelling in the ankles, angina (chest pain), night sweats, fainting spells, and irregular heartbeat. The disease can be caused by degeneration of the aortic valve with aging, infection (associated with endocarditis or rheumatic fever), or congenital abnormality. Severity of the disease varies from mild to life-threatening.

Aortic insufficiency is diagnosed in a variety of ways. A doctor listening to the heart through a stethoscope may detect the characteristic sounds of a valve defect even before symptoms appear. An electrocardiogram can be used to measure the heart's electrical activity and detect enlargement of the left ventricle. A chest X ray can also detect enlargement. An echocardiogram can directly visualize the valve and quantify the amount of leakage. In some cases, the person may undergo cardiac catheterization, a procedure in which a thin tube is threaded into the heart through a blood vessel and contrasting dye is injected to allow visualization of the heart and quantification of the leakage.

A person with aortic insufficiency needs to take antibiotics before dental or invasive surgical procedures to prevent infection of the valve. A valve infection (such as that associated with ENDOCARDITIS, inflammation of the lining of the heart that usually affects the valves) is a life-threatening condition that worsens the disease. Other medications may be used to treat the symptoms of aortic insufficiency, such as angiotensin-converting enzyme (ACE) inhibitors and calcium channel blockers, which lower blood pressure and decrease the workload of the heart; anticoagulants, which inhibit the formation of blood clots; and diuretics, which eliminate excess salt and fluid from the body. In cases of severe aortic insufficiency, surgery to repair or replace the valve can offer the most effective treatment.

Aortic stenosis

Narrowing of the valve connecting the heart to the body's main artery (aorta). Because the narrowing partially blocks the aortic valve, blood flow to the body is reduced, and the heart must work harder to compensate. The greater workload can enlarge the heart chamber known as the left ventricle, where the aortic valve is located. Over time, the left

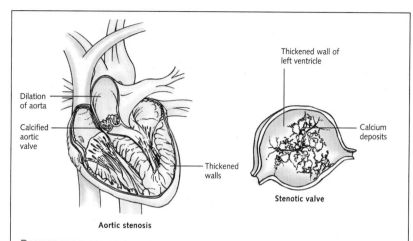

Thickened wall of left ventricle

Dilation of aorta

Calcified aortic valve

Thickened walls

Calcium deposits

Stenotic valve

Aortic stenosis

DAMAGE FROM AORTIC STENOSIS
A calcium buildup on the aortic valve, usually the result of aging, obstructs blood flow from the left ventricle into the aorta. Pressure builds in the ventricle (the heart's main pumping chamber) and, over time, its walls thicken. The aorta dilates (widens) in an effort to keep blood pumping adequately to the rest of the body.

ventricle thickens and enlarges, a condition known as ventricular hypertrophy. Congestive heart failure (see HEART FAILURE, CONGESTIVE), which is life-threatening, can result. Aortic stenosis is more severe if the coronary arteries are narrowed by fat deposits because the enlarged heart is deprived of the blood supply it needs.

Aortic stenosis may exist in a mild form for years before symptoms appear. Symptoms include fatigue, fainting spells, shortness of breath with exercise, difficulty breathing while lying down at night, angina (chest pain), and swelling in the ankles. The disease may be caused by damage to the heart from rheumatic fever, valve defects present at birth (congenital), or the buildup of calcium deposits on the aortic valve because of aging. The condition can appear at any age, but it is most common among those between 50 and 80 years old. Aortic stenosis is four times more likely to occur in men than in women.

Aortic stenosis is diagnosed in a variety of ways. A doctor listening to the heart through a stethoscope may detect the characteristic sounds of a valve defect even before symptoms appear. An electrocardiogram can be used to measure the electrical activity of the heart and to detect enlargement of the left ventricle. Chest X rays and echocardiograms can also

detect enlargement. An echocardiogram can allow doctors to see the size of the valve opening and quantify the severity of the narrowing and blood flow impairment. In some cases, the person may undergo cardiac catheterization, a procedure in which a catheter (thin tube) is threaded into the heart through a blood vessel and contrasting dye is injected to allow visualization of the heart. During this procedure, measurements are also made to accurately assess the degree of narrowing of the valve.

A person with aortic stenosis needs to take antibiotics before dental, medical, or surgical procedures to prevent infection of the valve, which worsens the disease. Other medications may be used to treat the symptoms of aortic stenosis, such as angiotensin-converting enzyme (ACE) inhibitors, which lower blood pressure and decrease the workload of the heart; anticoagulants, which inhibit the formation of blood clots; and diuretics, which help remove excess body fluid. Once symptoms of aortic stenosis become severe, surgery to repair or replace the valve is the preferred treatment. The long-term prognosis is poor for those who do not undergo surgery. If the person also has coronary artery disease, valve replacement surgery may be combined with coronary bypass surgery in a single procedure.

A

Aortitis

Inflammation of the aorta, the main artery leading from the heart into the body. Aortitis is commonly caused by advanced syphilis or rheumatoid arthritis.

Aortography

An X ray of the aorta, the large artery leading from the heart into the body. Before the X ray is taken, a contrast dye is injected to allow better visualization of the aorta.

Apert-Crouzon disease

See CRANIOFACIAL DYSOSTOSIS.

Apgar score

A scoring system used by doctors to assess the need for resuscitation and care of a baby at 1 minute after birth and again at 5 minutes after birth. To arrive at the Apgar score, the doctor evaluates five signs of the baby's condition: heart rate, breathing and crying, skin color, muscle tone, and reflexes. In the case of babies who are not white-skinned, skin color is scored by examining the soles of the feet, the palms of the hands, the whites of the eyes, and the insides of the mouth and lips. Each of the five signs is given a score from 0 to 2, and the scores are added up to make the baby's total Apgar score. The total score ranges from 0 to 10. Babies who have endured a long or difficult delivery may have low Apgar scores and may require medical attention right after birth. Apgar scores alone are of limited value in predicting long-term outcomes.

Aphakia

Absence of the natural lens of the eye. In the normal eye, the lens is a clear, crystalline structure located behind the iris (the colored part of the eye) that focuses light coming into the eye. The cause of aphakia can be a congenital abnormality (lacking lenses at birth), an injury that destroys the lens, or surgical removal. Surgical removal of the lens is standard treatment for cataract, a disease in which

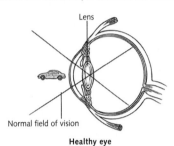

Normal field of vision

Healthy eye

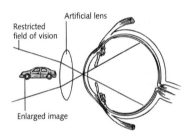

Artificial lens

Restricted field of vision

Enlarged image

Eye with aphakia

AN EYE WITHOUT A LENS
In a healthy eye, the lens focuses incoming light to produce an image within a large field of vision. In an eye with aphakia, the lens is absent and the ability to focus is severely restricted. The field of vision is greatly reduced, and the object of focus looks larger than it really is.

the lens becomes cloudy or opaque. Aphakia causes extreme farsightedness, which can be treated with glasses or contact lenses or by surgery to insert a plastic lens implant in the eye. In contemporary CATARACT SURGERY, a lens implant is used to replace the diseased lens. Aphakia can result in other complications, such as glaucoma (abnormally high pressure within the eye that may lead to blindness) or retinal detachment.

Aphasia

Language problems caused by injury to the brain. People with aphasia have problems with speaking, understanding, reading, or writing. Aphasia is sometimes confused with DYSARTHRIA, which is trouble speaking or forming words because of an impairment in the function of the muscles required for speech.

CAUSES
The brain controls the complex series of events required to speak and understand language. This is why brain injury, such as that resulting from the interrupted blood flow during a STROKE, can cause problems with communication. Depending on the location and extent of brain damage, the resulting difficulties can range from mild to severe. Other causes of aphasia include brain trauma and BRAIN TUMOR. The location of the brain injury determines the type of language problem. Lesions in the front part of the brain lead to problems with expression (Broca aphasia), while problems in the back of the brain lead to comprehension problems (Wernicke aphasia).

SYMPTOMS
The symptoms of aphasia vary widely from person to person. Problems range from trouble finding the right word to a complete inability to speak. Many affected persons have trouble understanding other people's speech. Their own words may be slurred or garbled, or they may say the wrong word or make sounds that are not real words. People with aphasia often have even more difficulty with reading and writing than with spoken words. However, although they have trouble putting their thoughts into words, people with aphasia generally continue to think clearly.

APGAR SCORE			
SIGN	**SCORE**		
	0	**1**	**2**
Heart rate	None	Fewer than 100 beats per minute	More than 100 beats per minute
Breathing and crying	None	Irregular breathing, weak crying	Regular breathing, strong crying
Skin color	Blue or pale	Pink body with blue hands and feet	Pink all over
Muscle tone	Limp	Some bending of arms and legs	Active bending of arms and legs
Reflex response	None	Grimaces	Cries

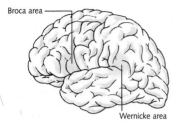

LANGUAGE CENTERS IN THE BRAIN
Aphasia results from an injury to a part of the brain that involves language. Damage to the Wernicke area, where the brain recognizes and understands spoken words, may cause problems with comprehension. Damage to the Broca area, where the brain plans spoken words and controls speech production, may result in an inability to express thought via speech.

DIAGNOSIS AND TREATMENT

A person who has experienced a brain injury is usually hospitalized under the care of a neurologist. After his or her condition has stabilized, most doctors recommend a thorough speech and language evaluation. This is usually conducted by a speech-language pathologist (or speech therapist), a professional who is trained at the master's or doctoral level to evaluate speech disorders and prepare plans to improve speech. A complete evaluation includes the testing of speaking, understanding, reading, and writing.

People who experience speech problems at any age can benefit from SPEECH THERAPY. Speech therapy can be helpful for people who are having trouble either speaking or expressing their thoughts. Speech therapists also work with those who have trouble swallowing. The therapist can help family members and friends devise a plan to make communication easier. Helpful techniques generally include asking short questions and making short requests; providing aids, such as glasses and hearing aids; and remembering that a person with aphasia has not lost his or her intelligence or common sense.

Apheresis

A special type of BLOOD DONATION in which only certain components of a donor's blood are collected. Apheresis is performed to collect plasma, platelets, or white blood cells. In contrast with whole blood donation, which takes 6 to 8 minutes, apheresis donation requires approximately 1½ hours. In this procedure, blood is drawn from one arm and passed through an instrument that separates and collects the desired blood components. The remaining components are returned to the donor through the other arm. The body normally replaces the removed blood component within 24 to 48 hours. Because apheresis donors give only part of their blood, they can donate more frequently.

Aphonia

Loss of the ability to produce the vocal sounds of normal speech. (Dysphonia is a difficulty in producing sounds; in spastic dysphonia, a person cannot speak because of spasmodic contraction of throat muscles.) Aphonia has a number of different causes. It may be caused by overuse of the vocal cords, disorders affecting the parts of the respiratory system needed to vocalize or produce speech, underlying disease, paralysis (aphonia paralytica), or psychological disorders (hysteric aphonia or aphonia paranoica). Speech therapy is useful in the treatment of some cases of aphonia. Sometimes botulinum toxin type A (Botox) injected in the vocal cords will relieve vocal cord spasms.

Aphrodisiac

A drug or food thought to arouse sexual desire. Aphrodisiacs are named after Aphrodite, the ancient Greek goddess of physical love. Many substances are reported to be aphrodisiacs, but almost all have no such effect. Certain foods are reputed to be aphrodisiacs, such as asparagus, eggs, chilies, curries, and ginseng. Some substances with a supposed aphrodisiac effect actually change mood rather than increase desire and may, therefore, make a person less inhibited and more open to sexual stimulation. Alcohol and certain amphetamine-like drugs are examples. One reputed aphrodisiac, known as Spanish fly or cantharidis, is a poison that burns the mouth and throat and can lead to serious infection of the urinary tract and even death. In some individuals, aphrodisiacs may appear to work simply because the person believes strongly that the substance has power. In recent years, injectable and oral medications have become available that produce erections in men who have had problems (see ERECTILE DYSFUNCTION). These drugs are not actually aphrodisiacs, however, because they do not increase sexual desire; rather they overcome the physical problems that block erections.

Apicoectomy

The surgical removal of the tip of the root in the tooth and the infected tissue surrounding it. This procedure is performed by an endodontist, a dentist specially trained to treat the nerves and pulp in teeth and gum tissue, usually as part of ROOT CANAL TREATMENT or to eliminate an area of infection. There are several reasons why an apicoectomy may be needed, and in some cases, this surgery may be the only alternative to a tooth extraction. Chronic pain after a root canal indicates the need for X rays, which can reveal a cyst or evidence of damage to the root of the treated tooth. An apicoectomy may also become necessary if the root of the tooth has not been filled adequately or if a post has been placed in the root of the tooth canal to anchor a crown, thus preventing further treatment.

WHAT TO EXPECT

The specialist administers local anesthesia to prevent pain during the procedure. He or she then opens the gum tissue near the tip of the root in the tooth, raising a flap to expose the outer layer of underlying bone. Sometimes, a small hole must be drilled to expose the tip of the root. A small, spoon-shaped instrument is used to remove the infected tissue or

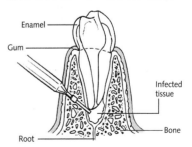

REMOVING THE TIP OF THE TOOTH ROOT
To complete an apicoectomy (removal of the tip of the root of a tooth), the root tip and infected tissue surrounding it are removed with a dental drill. The space is filled to seal the end of the root canal.

cyst. The tip of the root is removed with a dental drill. A small hole is drilled into the remaining root tip and a filling, usually of silver amalgam (see AMALGAM, DENTAL), is placed in the hole to seal the root canal. Most people can return to their normal routine within a day.

Apitherapy

See BEE VENOM AND BEE PRODUCTS, THERAPEUTIC.

Aplasia

The absence of an organ or tissue due to developmental failure. In aplastic anemia (see ANEMIA, APLASTIC), there is a failure in the normal generation and development of blood cells.

Apnea

A total cessation of breathing, either momentarily or for a prolonged period. Prolonged apnea, which can be life-threatening, may occur as a result of a stroke or transient ischemic attack (a brief interruption in blood supply to the brain, resulting in temporarily impaired sensation, movement, vision, or speech); as an effect of certain drugs; or as a result of airway obstruction. Loud snoring accompanied by pauses in breathing while sleeping is a symptom of potentially life-threatening SLEEP APNEA SYNDROME. Other symptoms of sleep apnea include daytime sleepiness, fatigue, and headache. Sleep apnea is most common in overweight people, as excessive body fat puts pressure on breathing passages. In CHEYNE-STOKES respiration, alternating periods of apnea and deep, rapid breathing occur. Common causes of Cheyne-Stokes breathing include congestive heart failure, respiratory diseases, and neurological diseases, such as stroke.

Treatment of apnea depends on its severity and underlying cause. For example, remedies for mild sleep apnea include weight reduction; exercise; avoidance of alcohol, tranquilizers, and sleeping pills; sleeping on the side or abdomen rather than the back; and the use of medications prescribed or recommended by the physician. More serious cases can require medication, the administration of oxygen using a mask during sleep, or surgery. Untreated sleep apnea can lead to hypertension, heart disease, and stroke.

Apolipoprotein

The protein component of lipoprotein complexes. See LIPID-LIPOPROTEIN METABOLISM.

Aponeurosis

A membrane connecting muscles. An aponeurosis is a broad, dense sheet of fibrous tissue that either joins muscles to one another or connects them to bone.

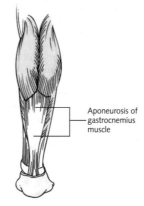

Aponeurosis of gastrocnemius muscle

CONNECTING MEMBRANE
The aponeurosis is tissue that is, in effect, an extension of a tendon, primarily attaching a muscle to the structure that it moves.

Apoptosis

The programming of cells in the body to age and die at a certain time. Also called programmed cell death, apoptosis is the process by which a cell kills itself. Normal cell growth is a balance between the proliferation of new cells and the death of old ones. Programmed cell death is regulated by specific genes that ensure that adequate numbers of healthy cells replace the dying cells. Abnormalities in apoptosis are thought to enable cancer cells to multiply while normal cells die. People with defects in the proteins that cause apoptosis, such as the suppressor protein p53, may develop multiple types of cancer. Certain chemotherapy drugs are designed to cause apoptosis in tumor cells by reprogramming them to die.

Appendectomy

Surgical removal of the appendix, a small finger-shaped pouch that branches off from the large intestine.

An appendectomy is performed to treat APPENDICITIS (an acute inflammation of the appendix) and is a simple operation associated with few risks. An appendectomy has traditionally been performed through an abdominal incision several inches long. In the absence of PERITONITIS, surgeons now remove the appendix through a tiny incision, using a laparoscope (a viewing instrument that both transmits images to the surgeon on a screen and cuts away the appendix). See also LAPAROSCOPY.

Recovery depends on the type of procedure performed. Generally, it is possible to begin to drink fluids 24 hours after a laparoscopy. After both traditional and laparoscopic surgery, the person leaves the hospital within a few days. Recovery time for laparoscopic surgery is generally shorter than for traditional surgery.

Appendicitis

Acute inflammation of the appendix (a small finger-shaped pouch that branches off from the large intestine in the lower right part of the abdomen). The appendix can become inflamed and fill with pus when a small piece of stool or debris blocks its opening. To avoid serious complications, an APPENDECTOMY (surgical removal of the appendix) is usually required.

SYMPTOMS AND DIAGNOSIS
The first symptom of appendicitis is usually vague pain and discomfort around the navel. Within a few hours, the pain moves to the lower right part of the abdomen and becomes more intense. In some cases, a day or two of constipation precedes the onset of pain. Other symptoms can vary and may include loss of appetite, nausea, vomiting, and fever.

Diagnosis is based on a physical examination of the abdomen by a doctor. Applying pressure to the spot where an inflamed appendix is located causes increased pain. If the diagnosis is uncertain, the doctor may order blood and imaging tests, such as abdominal X rays, a CT (computed tomography) scan, or ultrasound scanning. An exploratory operation called a laparotomy may be performed. See LAPAROTOMY, EXPLORATORY.

TREATMENT
An inflamed appendix must be removed as early as possible to prevent serious complications. Possible com-

plications include GANGRENE, an ABSCESS, or rupture of the appendix that can lead to PERITONITIS (a life-threatening inflammation of the peritoneum, the membrane that lines the abdominal cavity). Although removing an appendix is a simple operation, the risk of complications increases greatly if the appendix ruptures. If imaging tests or a laparotomy reveal that an abscess has formed around the appendix, removal of the appendix may be delayed in order to drain the abscess and administer antibiotics. Once the abscess subsides, an appendectomy can be performed.

Appendix

A small organ hanging down from the upper part of the large intestine (cecum) into the abdomen. Medically known as the vermiform, the appendix is an organ of the IMMUNE SYSTEM. The appendix contains abundant lymphatic tissue and apparently serves to destroy disease-causing microorganisms that might enter the body or multiply

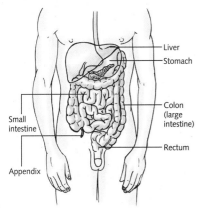

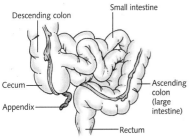

LOCATION OF APPENDIX
The appendix is a narrow tube, closed at one end, that extends down from the front portion (cecum) of the large intestine into the lower abdomen. It secretes mucus that flows into the cecum.

rapidly through the digestive system (although its role is not entirely clear). The most common disorder is APPENDICITIS, an inflammation of the appendix, which is treated by surgical removal of the appendix.

Appetite

A desire for food. Appetite is regulated by the hypothalamus and the cerebral cortex in the brain. A healthy appetite is a sign of well-being, while a change in appetite can be a symptom of physical or emotional problems. Signs of appetite problems include significant weight loss or gain, a lack of energy, and an alteration in bowel habits. Older people or people with chronic illnesses often experience a loss of appetite. People who experience a significant change in appetite are advised to consult their physician.

Appetite stimulants

Drugs used to stimulate feelings of hunger. These drugs are often used to help in the treatment of people with cancer and AIDS (acquired immunodeficiency syndrome). Appetite stimulants seem to be most effective if they are introduced during the early stages of weight loss.

Appetite suppressants

Drugs that are intended to reduce feelings of hunger. No convincing evidence is available showing that any product available over-the-counter can help people lose weight. Appetite suppressants can be dangerous if they are taken by people with high blood pressure, heart disease, glaucoma, diabetes, thyroid disease, or kidney problems.

Appetite, loss of

A decreased desire to eat even when there is a physical need for food. Loss of appetite can have a variety of causes, such as emotional upset, anxiety, loneliness, depression, school or work stress, fatigue, and acute infection or illness, such as the flu. Appetite can also be affected by drugs and medications, including amphetamines, chemotherapy drugs, antibiotics, cough and cold preparations, codeine, morphine, meperidine, and digitalis. Constant snacking during the day, which decreases the appetite

at mealtime; diseases of the digestive system, including cancer; and an eating disorder (see ANOREXIA NERVOSA) can also be culprits.

Treatment depends on the cause. If a disease of the digestive system is suspected, a detailed examination of the digestive system will be made, including X rays, CT (computed tomography) scans, and tests of liver, thyroid, and kidney function. If medication decreases appetite, the medication may be changed, or measures can be taken to make meals more appealing (such as using different spices) and to increase the number of calories consumed by serving higher calorie foods. If a mental disease or emotional difficulty is the cause, treatment is directed at that condition. In the case of acute disease or infection, appetite usually returns to normal after the sickness is over.

Appetite, loss of in older people

A gradual decline or loss of interest in eating and drinking that commonly occurs in older people. Because the organs of older people do not function with the same efficiency as those of younger people, consequences of loss of appetite can be serious. Older people need to follow a sensible and varied diet. Poor nutrition can result in fatigue, lack of stamina, confusion, and a wide array of other health problems.

A loss of appetite can be due to numerous factors. Illness, depression, and alcohol abuse can lead to a general lack of interest in food. Dental problems can make chewing food painful or awkward. Taste grows less acute over the years, making food less appealing. (See also TASTE, LOSS OF IN OLDER PEOPLE.) Medications commonly taken by older people may cause stomach discomfort, dry mouth, and nausea that interfere with eating. Individuals in a confused state may forget to eat altogether. Confusion can be either the side effect of a medication or a symptom of dementia, which requires medical attention.

STIMULATING APPETITE
When food tastes and smells less appetizing than it formerly did, increasing seasonings used in cooking may bring back some taste. Food can be diced or even ground to reduce the effort of chewing. In a

A

healthy but sedentary older adult, exercise may increase appetite. If an older person is taking medications that interfere with appetite, adjustments in dosage or type of medication often help. Underlying problems, such as illness, depression, or alcohol abuse, require consultation with a physician. Loss of appetite and weight can sometimes signal a serious disease, such as cancer, and may lead the doctor to search for an underlying cause.

Following dietary restrictions and recommendations is sometimes a source of stress for caregivers. For example, trying to force-feed a patient with a terminal illness may help maintain nutrition but can cause stress and arguments that interfere with quality of life. Also, prescribing a restricted low-fat diet may not make as much sense for a person at the end of life. Doctors suggest that regular mealtimes should be scheduled for older people with loss of appetite, especially for those who are ill or confused. Visits by home health aides can be arranged to help with shopping and cooking. Meals-on-Wheels can deliver meals, and many adult day care centers serve hot, nourishing food.

Applied kinesiology

A diagnostic and therapeutic approach to health care that focuses on neuromuscular problems. Kinesiology is the study of human movement, and applied kinesiology is a relatively new form of HOLISTIC MEDICINE derived from that study. Applied kinesiology is based on CHIROPRACTIC principles and assumes that muscles are associated with internal organs and glands in such a way that weakness in a muscle, for example, indicates a problem in the associated organ. Manual manipulation of the spine, extremities, and bones of the skull is associated with applied kinesiology. The goals of applied kinesiology are to restore postural balance, improve normal neuromuscular function, achieve balance among internal bodily functions, and prevent degenerative muscle diseases. However, there are no clinical studies yet verifying that applied kinesiology is effective or safe.

Apraxia

A loss of the ability to carry out previously learned skills or gestures despite normal muscle power and coordination. Apraxia is caused by brain damage associated with problems such as ALZHEIMER'S DISEASE, STROKE, brain tumor, or head injury. Symptoms can include difficulty using an arm or leg or even making purposeful facial movements on command.

Arachnoiditis

An inflammation of the arachnoid membrane that covers the brain and spinal cord (usually involving the lumbar spine). Arachnoiditis may be caused by infection (such as bacterial infections, syphilis, or tubular meningitis) or trauma (such as from surgery, a lumbar puncture, spinal anesthesia, or myelography). This debilitating condition is characterized by intractable pain and neurological deficits. As arachnoiditis progresses, symptoms increase. Few people with this condition are able to continue working; some develop progressive PARAPLEGIA (paralysis of the legs). There is no cure for arachnoiditis. Treatment is focused on pain management and is intended to help the affected person resume a functional role in society. Neurosurgery to release nerve roots can be helpful.

Arcus senilis

A gray or white, bow- or arch-shaped ring that commonly appears at the edge of the clear outer covering (cornea) of the eye in people older than 50 years. Arcus senilis (which means "old man's arch" in Latin) results from deposits of cholesterol and in people younger than 40 years can be a sign of high cholesterol levels in the blood. See HYPERLIPIDEMIAS.

Area Agencies on Aging

Also known as AAAs, a network of local offices of the Federal Administration on Aging that provides assistance to older people across the country. Agencies are funded by the Older Americans Act, which allocates federal money to states. States in turn distribute money to local AAAs to operate programs for people age 60 and older. Area Agencies on Aging do not charge for services. Area Agencies on Aging coordinate existing community services for older people and help them gain access to them. The types of assistance vary considerably from place to place, but may include transportation, home-delivered meals, home health aide services, and adult day care programs. (See also CAREGIVING FOR OLDER PEOPLE and DAY CARE, ADULT.) The AAA branch serving an area is usually listed in the government section of the telephone directory under "aging services" or "elder services." The Eldercare Locator, also federally funded, is a nationwide telephone service designed to help older people and their caregivers find local resources.

Arm, fractured

FOR FIRST AID
see Fractures (broken bones), page 1323

A break in one or several of the bones in the arm, generally caused by physical trauma, undue pressure, or other injury to the arm. A fractured arm is usually painful and may cause numbness and tingling. Immediately following the event that produces the fracture, there may be acute pain, localized tenderness to the touch, muscle spasms, and greater pain or numbness with movement or use of the arm, followed by numbness, tingling, weakness, or paralysis. A fractured arm is generally diagnosed by the presence of deformity and an evaluation of X rays. Treatment may depend on a person's age, the type of fracture, and the bone or bones involved. Generally, the broken bones are aligned into an immo-

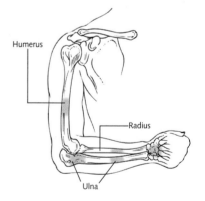

COMMON SITES OF FRACTURES
The parts of the arm that break frequently include the humerus (the long bone of the upper arm), the tip of the ulna at the elbow, and the shafts of the radius and ulna (bones of the forearm). Casting, splinting, or surgery is required, depending on the position and nature of the break.

A

bile position, usually with a cast or splint for a specified time. During the healing period, a sling may be used to support the arm and hold it stationary against the body. In more complex fractures, traction and surgical repair may become necessary. See also FRACTURE.

Aromatherapy

The use of plant oils for psychological and physical well-being. The plant oils are inhaled, rubbed onto the skin, or swallowed. (Only a few oils—for example, lavender and lemon—can be swallowed safely. Aromatherapy is a version of herbal medicine that features the use of fragrant substances to alter mood or improve health. Aromatherapy is said to help relieve stress, enhance the immune system, and unlock buried emotions.

Aromatherapy uses more than 100 essential plant oils, not perfume oils, which contain unnatural chemicals that do not provide therapeutic benefits. Essential oils come from flowers, fruits, grasses, leaves, roots, and wood resins. Aromatherapy is based on the idea that drawing essential oils into the body by smell stimulates the brain in positive ways. Oils believed to have a spiritual dimension are also used in massage and in bath water to help restore balance and harmony to the body and life in general.

Arousal

The mental state in which an individual responds to stimulation of the senses.

Arrhenoblastoma

A rare, benign tumor of the ovary that usually produces the male hormone testosterone and causes masculinization (male characteristics, such as facial hair). These tumors generally do not appear in girls before puberty.

Arrhythmia, cardiac

A disturbance or abnormality in the rhythm of the heartbeat. Cardiac arrhythmias vary in severity from annoying to life-threatening.

The heartbeat is controlled by electrical impulses that begin in a group of cells called the sinus node, which is located in the right atrium (upper right chamber) of the heart (see HEART for anatomical detail). The electrical signal moves across the two atria (upper chambers) of the heart, then to another group of cells called the atrioventricular (AV) node. The AV node connects to specialized fibers in the lower chambers (ventricles) of the heart that conduct the electrical signal into the ventricles and cause them to contract.

Cardiac arrhythmias result from some abnormality in this conduction system. The sinus node may initiate an abnormal rhythm, the normal conduction pathway can be disrupted, or some other part of the heart takes over the sinus node's role as pacemaker.

TYPES AND SYMPTOMS

The least serious and most common cardiac arrhythmia is the ectopic heartbeat, or extrasystole. This is a simple variation in a normal heartbeat, possibly the source of the phrase "my heart skipped a beat." An occasional extrasystole is harmless and requires no treatment. The most likely cause is stress, lack of sleep, or the use of caffeine, alcohol, or tobacco. Over-the-counter decongestants and weight-loss medications are also common causes of skipped heartbeats.

An arrhythmia that causes the heart to beat too slowly is called BRADYCARDIA. Since the heart may not pump fast enough to keep the body supplied with the oxygen-rich blood it needs, symptoms such as fatigue, dizziness, light-

---

THE HEARTBEAT

KEY
⇨ Electrical signal ➡ Blood flow

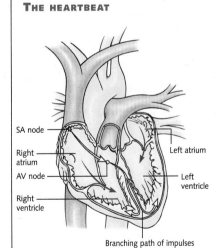

HEALTHY HEARTBEAT
An electrical impulse triggers each heartbeat. The impulse starts in a group of cells in the sinoatrial (SA) node—the heart's pacemaker—and travels through the atria, causing them to contract.

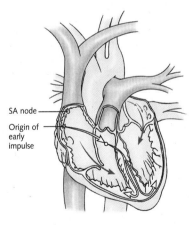

LESS BLOOD PUMPED
In one type of arrhythmia, the electrical impulse originates in a different place in the heart and occurs too early. The atria contract too soon and pump less blood through the heart and into the body.

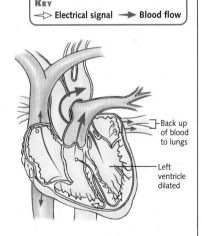

BACKING UP OF BLOOD
Some arrhythmias make the contraction of the atria irregular and ineffective. This can lead to a back up of blood in the lungs, causing congestive heart failure.

headedness, or fainting can occur in people with bradycardia.

An arrhythmia that causes the heart to beat too rapidly is known as TACHYCARDIA or tachyarrhythmia. Symptoms can include palpitations (the sensation of an unusually fast or irregular heartbeat), chest pain, dizziness, light-headedness, or fainting. If the atria are beating too rapidly, the condition is known as supraventricular tachycardia (SVT); if the beat of the atria is irregular, it is known as ATRIAL FIBRILLATION. Both SVT and atrial fibrillation tend to occur in episodes, with periodic attacks separated by periods of normal heart rhythm. They may become chronic or persistent over time. Atrial fibrillation and some types of SVT, such as atrial flutter, increase the risk of stroke, since blood pooling in the atria may clot, enter the circulatory system, and lodge in the brain. Anticoagulants may be prescribed to reduce the risk of stroke.

Paroxysmal supraventricular tachycardia (PSVT) (see TACHYCARDIA, PAROXYSMAL SUPRAVENTRICULAR) causes sudden attacks in which the heart races suddenly at between 140 and 240 beats a minute (versus the normal 60 to 100). PSVT is not usually life-threatening, but repeated attacks increase the risk of developing congestive heart failure.

In ventricular tachycardia (see TACHYCARDIA, VENTRICULAR), the ventricles contract too rapidly. Ventricular tachycardia, usually associated with heart disease, is a common complication during the first several days after a heart attack. In the more serious condition known as VENTRICULAR FIBRILLATION, the ventricles contract in such a weak and uncontrolled way that the heart essentially ceases to pump. If a normal rhythm cannot be reestablished within a few minutes, death can result.

DIAGNOSIS AND TREATMENT
Accurate, early diagnosis of a cardiac arrhythmia is important in order to begin treatment. Persons with symptoms suggesting arrhythmia may wear a HOLTER MONITOR, which is a portable device that records and analyzes the electrical activity of the heart. Depending on the person's symptoms and medical history, tests may include an electrocardiogram, which measures the electrical activity of the heart at rest or during exercise; an echocardiogram, which uses ultrasound waves to check the structure and function of the heart; and cardiac catheterization, in which a thin tube is threaded into the heart through a blood vessel and contrasting dye is injected to visualize the heart.

Treatment depends on the type of arrhythmia and its severity. Some arrhythmias can be controlled with lifestyle changes, such as avoiding caffeine and tobacco, reducing alcohol consumption, quitting smoking, avoiding certain medications (such as decongestants, which speed up the heart), and reducing stress. Medications that control or change heartbeat may also be prescribed. Examples include beta blockers, which slow heartbeat and reduce the workload of the heart; calcium channel blockers, which also reduce blood pressure; and digoxin, which increases the force of heart contractions and slows conduction of the heartbeat. For people with bradycardia, a PACEMAKER can be surgically implanted in the chest to accelerate the heart via electrical impulses whenever it beats too slowly. For people with ventricular tachycardia, a device called an implantable cardioverter DEFIBRILLATOR can be placed surgically in the chest. The defibrillator monitors heartbeat and corrects it if it becomes abnormally fast. Radiofrequency ablation (see ABLATION THERAPY), which uses radiofrequency energy emitted through a catheter threaded into the heart to destroy very small areas of tissue, can be used to change the conduction pattern of the heart and make it normal. This technique is most commonly used to treat atrial arrhythmias.

Arsenic

A poisonous chemical element used in dyes and agriculture. Arsenic is a gray metallic element that can cause nausea, vomiting, diarrhea, cramps, numbness, seizures, coma, and death when consumed in large quantities. Arsenic was used widely as rat and ant poison and on flypaper in the 19th century when it was used for deliberate poisoning more often than any other deadly poison. At that time, it was difficult to detect arsenic in the body.

Art therapy

This form of therapy uses creativity and images to allow insight into a person's experience of life and health and provides an avenue for emotional expression. It is most often used with children, including those with POSTTRAUMATIC STRESS DISORDER and ATTENTION DEFICIT/HYPERACTIVITY DISORDER, as well as with adults recovering from serious illness. Art therapists are professionally trained in both art and therapy; board certification by the American Art Therapy Association is granted after graduate level education and postgraduate supervised experience.

Arteries

Vessels that carry blood away from the heart to the rest of the body. The walls of the arteries have an elastic, muscular structure. The inner layer is a smooth lining, the middle layer is composed of elastic membranes and muscle, and the outer walls are tough, fibrous tissues. This structure enables the arteries to withstand the great force of blood being pumped rapidly from the heart. The elastic membranes stretch as the blood flows through, and then the muscular layer contracts; the arteries help pump the blood along and smooth out its flow. All arteries except the pulmonary artery (which carries blood from the right side of the heart to the lungs to receive oxygen) pump oxygen-rich blood. As arteries travel through the body, they branch into smaller vessels. Large arteries, such as the aorta or the carotid arteries in the neck, are about as thick as a finger. Medium arteries, such as the brachial artery that carries blood into the arm, are pencil-thin. Smaller branches are called arterioles (see ARTERIOLE), and the finest arterial vessels are known as capillaries (see CAPILLARY). As the vessels

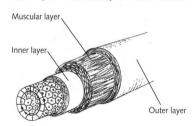

Muscular layer
Inner layer
Outer layer

STRUCTURE OF AN ARTERY
The layers of an artery wall help even out the pulsing of blood so that the pressure is fairly constant as blood circulates through the body.

become smaller and more delicate, the pressure of the blood flow decreases and evens out. See CARDIOVASCULAR SYSTEM.

Arteriole

A thickly muscled vessel that branches out from a larger artery and connects to minute capillaries. Arterioles are part of the system that carries oxygen-rich blood pumped out of the heart into body tissue. The nerves that supply an arteriole are finely tuned to regulate blood flow to tissues, depending on their specific requirements. Those requirements are greater in muscles or organs that are engaged in activity, or in times of stress.

Arteriosclerosis

Thickening and loss of elasticity in the walls of the arteries; also known

---

HARDENING OF THE ARTERIES

When an artery is diseased, calcium and cholesterol deposits narrow the opening and harden the arterial walls, and blood flow is affected. Gangrene may occur if the blood supply to the extremities is reduced, a heart attack may occur if the blood supply to the heart is reduced, and a stroke may occur if the blood supply to the brain is cut off.

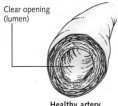

Clear opening (lumen)

Healthy artery

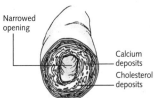

Narrowed opening

Calcium deposits

Cholesterol deposits

Evidence of atherosclerosis

INSIDE THE ARTERY
In a healthy artery, the opening (lumen) is clear and unobstructed. In an artery with arteriosclerosis, the lumen has narrowed because of an accumulation of calcium and cholesterol deposits along the arterial walls.

---

as hardening of the arteries. The most common type of arteriosclerosis is ATHEROSCLEROSIS, in which fat deposits build up in the arteries. Other types of arteriosclerosis include arteriolosclerosis (thickening of the walls of the arterioles or small arteries) and Mönckeberg arteriosclerosis (extensive deposits of calcium form on the media, or middle layer, of the arteries).

Arteriovenous fistula

An abnormal direct connection between an artery and vein. Blood flows from the artery into the vein through the fistula, bypassing the bed of capillaries (very small blood vessels) that normally lie between them. If a fistula is large, a substantial proportion of oxygen-rich blood bypasses the capillary bed, forcing the heart to work harder to supply the affected part of the body with blood and oxygen. Oxygen deprivation can result.

Arteriovenous fistulas are most commonly caused by accident or trauma, such as a deep wound that punctures an artery and vein that lie close together. When the wound heals, a passageway from the artery to the vein may remain. The condition may also be present at birth. One such congenital arteriovenous fistula occurs in the lungs. Symptoms include blue skin, enlargement of the fingertips, and a heart murmur. An arteriovenous fistula can be repaired with a surgical procedure or by clotting the blood in the passageway to close it.

Arteriovenous malformation

A tangled mass of small arteries intertwined with small veins that is present at birth; commonly abbreviated as AVM. Blood flows directly from the arteries into the veins, not through the bed of capillaries (very small blood vessels) that normally lie between them. An AVM is most serious when it occurs in the brain; this condition is called cerebral AVM. Since the vessels are fragile and lack normal support, they often bleed and cause hemorrhages.

Symptoms of a ruptured or leaky cerebral AVM include headache, blurred vision, slurred speech, vomit-

ing, stiff neck, muscle weakness and loss of sensation in a part of the body, fainting, drooping eyelid, altered vision, facial paralysis, or change in mood. A ruptured cerebral AVM can be fatal. Treatment usually consists of surgery to remove the malformation.

Arteritis

Inflammation of an artery or arteries. The inflammation can block the artery, reducing blood flow to the affected area and possibly swelling the artery into a balloonlike form called an aneurysm. Arteritis is usually treated with anti-inflammatory medications, such as corticosteroids. In some cases, surgery is needed to remove the blockage and restore normal blood flow.

Arteritis, giant cell

Chronic inflammation of large and medium arteries, usually in the head and neck, less commonly throughout the body; also known as temporal or cranial arteritis. The disease takes its name from the extremely large cells that develop in the inflamed blood vessels. Symptoms resulting from the inflammation include fever, headache, scalp tenderness, jaw pain, double vision or blindness, weakness, loss of appetite and weight, muscle aches, and excessive sweating. The cause of giant cell arteritis is unknown, but it is thought to result from a disorder of the immune system. About 50 percent of people with giant cell arteritis have polymyalgia rheumatica (a syndrome occurring primarily among older people that is characterized by muscle and joint pain and an elevated erythrocyte sedimentation rate). It occurs almost exclusively in people older than 50, and it is more common in women than in men and less common in blacks than in other ethnic groups. Treatment consists of anti-inflammatory medications, such as aspirin and corticosteroids.

Arthralgia

Pain experienced in a joint as a symptom of a disease or condition. Arthralgia is the medical term used when there is pain in a joint with no signs of localized inflammation or ARTHRITIS. Arthritis refers to a condition that involves inflammation and swelling in the joint in addition to pain; arthralgia refers to the isolated symptom of joint pain. This symptom may be present for several years before there are signs of arthritis. Or, arthritis may never develop. The pain is most commonly treated with acetaminophen or with anti-inflammatory drugs, such as aspirin or ibuprofen.

Arthritis

FOR SYMPTOM CHARTS
see Ankle or foot problems, page 18
see Hip pain, page 42
see Knee pain, page 44

The inflammation of a joint, which causes localized pain, swelling, and stiffness. There are several different types of arthritis. The most common type is OSTEOARTHRITIS, or degenerative arthritis, which involves changes in the joint cartilage as a result of aging and use. As the cartilage deteriorates, the bones of the joint thicken and become distorted. The affected joint may become swollen. Because movement of the joint is restricted and painful, the associated muscles begin to shrink from lack of use.

Osteoarthritis generally affects the large, weight-bearing joints, such as the spine, hips, and knees, but the finger joints may also be affected. The pain and discomfort of osteoarthritis may be lessened with aspirin, ibuprofen, or other nonsteroidal anti-inflammatory drugs (NSAIDs). When pain is intolerable, injections of corticosteroid drugs into the affected joint may be given on a limited basis. PHYSICAL THERAPY, such as exercise, massage, and heat treatments, may also be prescribed. When joints are severely damaged by osteoarthritis, producing chronic pain and preventing normal movement of limbs, they may be surgically replaced with artificial joints made of metal or metal combined with plastic or porcelain. (See JOINT REPLACEMENT.) Hip and knee joints are often successfully replaced. (See also JOINT REPLACEMENT, HIP; JOINT REPLACEMENT, KNEE.) Self-help treatments for osteoarthritis include losing weight, using a cane to relieve pressure on a joint, applying heat to ease pain, and exercising regularly to strengthen muscles surrounding the affected joints. Although many joints may be affected by osteoarthritis, the inflammation does not involve other organ systems.

Other types of arthritis include

EXERCISE MAY HELP ARTHRITIS

There are more than 100 types of arthritis, which cause varying degrees of pain and restricted movement, but in most cases, doctors agree that exercise can help lessen pain, increase range of movement, and help a person with arthritis feel better.

A person with arthritis should start by seeing his or her doctor, physical therapist, or specially trained health professional to learn range-of-motion exercises and strengthening exercises that are good for arthritis. But here are some other exercise ideas:

- Walking is the ideal exercise for most people because it burns calories, strengthens muscles, and builds denser bones without jarring fragile joints.
- Stretching is another simple way to keep joints and muscles flexible. Stretching relieves stress and can help a person maintain normal daily activities.
- Exercising in the water can build strength and increase range-of-motion while the buoyancy of the water reduces wear and tear on sore joints.
- Country line dancing, ballroom dancing, swimming, yoga, and T'ai chi are good for most people with arthritis and are fun exercises that take the work out of working out.

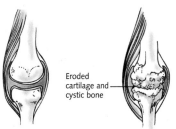

Eroded cartilage and cystic bone

Healthy joint   Osteoarthritic joint

EFFECTS OF ARTHRITIS
In a healthy, nonarthritic joint, a layer of cartilage at the ends of the bones helps the bones slide smoothly over each other. In a joint with osteoarthritis, the cartilage breaks down and the underlying bone is exposed. Cysts called osteophytes develop on the bone and make joint movement difficult.

gouty arthritis, which is caused by urate crystals forming in the joints (see GOUT), and a temporary form of arthritis that may accompany acute rheumatic fever. Infectious diseases, including hepatitis B and C and rubella (or German measles), can cause temporary arthritis, which is an uncommon side effect of the rubella vaccination. In these cases, as in the case of temporary arthritis with acute rheumatic fever, the joints are not permanently damaged or deformed.

Rheumatoid arthritis, an autoimmune disease, is a more serious, systemic form of arthritis, which may affect the heart, lungs, and eyes, as well as the joints. The suspected cause is an unidentified virus that stimulates the immune system. Disease-fighting cells that are subsequently released by the immune system inflame the joints. See also RHEUMATOID ARTHRITIS.

Arthrodesis

The surgical fusion or immobilization of the bones in a damaged joint for the purpose of supporting the joint and relieving pain. The procedure, often performed on the foot or ankle, involves removing the weight-bearing surfaces of the joint. A fixation device is then implanted to hold the bones together during the healing process. As they heal, the bones grow together until they are united.

Arthrogram

An image, taken by X ray, CT (computed tomography), or MRI (magnetic resonance imaging) of a joint that has been injected with a contrast dye to outline the internal anatomy of the joint. Arthrograms are generally taken of the knee, ankle, elbow, hip, wrist, or shoulder joint as part of an evaluation of joint injuries, possible damaged cartilage, and other suspected abnormalities. The images are used to determine the course of treatment and may also be used as a visual aid during corrective surgery. See ARTHROGRAPHY.

Arthrography

A diagnostic procedure performed with the use of CT (computed tomography), fluoroscopy, or MRI (magnetic resonance imaging) to create an image, called an ARTHROGRAM, of the inside of a joint. Arthrography with a CT scan reveals a three-dimensional view of the bones and soft tissues, such as cartilage, of the joint being observed. Fluoroscopy passes X rays through the body and onto an X-ray sensitive, fluorescent screen so that the interior structures of a joint can be viewed. MRI, a more expensive technique, uses magnetic fields and radio waves to produce images of the joint, thus avoiding exposure to radiation.

The procedure is performed to evaluate possible damage to or an abnormality of the joints at the ankle, elbow, hip, knee, shoulder, wrist, and other areas. Arthrography is usually performed by a radiologist on an outpatient basis or in a hospital. A local anesthetic is given at the site to be scanned. Fluid may be withdrawn from the affected joint, followed by the injection of a contrast dye and a small amount of air into the joint space to create a clearer X-ray image. A CT scanner or fluoroscope then records multiple images of the joint, which are evaluated by a radiologist with expertise in musculoskeletal imaging. Arthrography generally takes between 1 and 2 hours. Following the procedure, the area is bandaged, and the person is instructed to avoid wearing tight clothing to constrict the area and to rest the joint for 24 hours.

Arthroplasty

See JOINT REPLACEMENT.

Arthroscopic surgery

Joint surgery performed using a technique called arthroscopy, which involves the use of a specialized viewing instrument to observe the interior of a joint. An arthroscope is a small, tubular instrument containing an optical system of magnifying lenses, a fiberoptic light source, and a video camera. Tiny surgical instruments are used with the arthroscope to allow a surgeon to perform surgery on a joint, including the removal of unattached pieces of cartilage, the repair or removal of torn knee cartilage, and obtaining a biopsy specimen. Biopsy specimens from the joint area may be evaluated to diagnose infections, rheumatoid arthritis, gout, or disorders of the connective tissue. Repair or replacement of torn ligaments in the knee can be performed with the arthroscopic technique.

The conditions that may be treated with arthroscopic surgery include knee problems such as arthritis. It may also be used to repair tears in

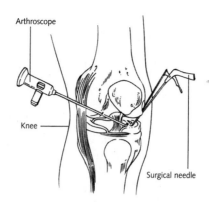

A COMMON ORTHOPEDIC PROCEDURE
Once inserted into a joint through small incision, an arthroscope transmits an image of the joint to a monitor, allowing the surgeon to see the area of operation, to insert surgical instruments, and to remove or repair damaged tissue.

the cartilage, tendons, or ligaments of the knee joint. Loose bodies or growths in the joints of the elbow, called osteophytes, or in the ankle, called osteochrondral lesions, may be removed or repaired by this surgical technique. It may be performed to repair tears in the rotator cuff of the shoulder joint and to reattach torn tissue in the shoulder joint. If there is arthritis or damage to the cartilage in the shoulder or wrist, the surgery may be done to smooth worn cartilage and remove loose cartilage fragments. Arthroscopic surgery may also be used to shave off bony fragments and smooth the joint area for the correction of damage to the cartilage in the wrist joint.

Arthroscopic surgery offers several advantages over what is medically termed an "open procedure," which involves a larger incision. The surgeon can gain access to a joint through one or several small incisions, each about the size of a small buttonhole, thus reducing the time the person would need to recover from one large incision. In addition, the use of arthroscopy in joint surgery allows the procedure to be performed in an outpatient setting, often in a special procedures room. Local anesthesia can often be used, but general anesthesia and a sedative may also be given before the procedure. Arthroscopic surgery causes less trauma to the body, minimizes pain and scarring, and allows a faster recovery than open-joint surgery.

Arthroscopy

See ARTHROSCOPIC SURGERY.

Artificial insemination

The placement of sperm inside the female reproductive tract by artificial means rather than sexual intercourse. During this procedure, a man's semen, which carries the sperm, is introduced either into the woman's cervical canal or into her vagina. A physician may place the semen in her cervical canal by using a syringe, or the woman can place the semen into her vagina herself. If a man's sperm count is low or when the woman's cervical secretions produce antibodies and repel sperm, the sperm can be separated from the semen and concentrated before they are introduced. A physician typically uses a syringe and catheter to introduce the sperm directly into the uterus.

Artificial insemination is used when the man has difficulty having natural intercourse or has a very low sperm count or semen volume. It is also often used when the woman's ovulation is being controlled with fertility drugs and timed so that the maximum number of sperm will reach the egg when it is released. (See also ASSISTED REPRODUCTIVE TECHNOLOGY; INFERTILITY.) Artificial insemination using donor sperm can be used for single women desiring pregnancy. It is also used when the male partner has no sperm or has a genetic disease that he does not want to transmit to his offspring.

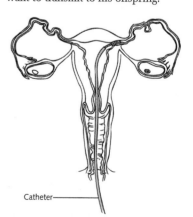

INSERTING SPERM INTO THE UTERUS
Artificial insemination places sperm directly into a woman's uterus just before ovulation. The procedure is generally done with a syringe and catheter. The sperm may come from a male partner or from a healthy donor.

A

Artificial kidney

Popular name for the machine that cleans and filters the blood by removing waste products and fluid. See DIALYSIS MACHINE.

Artificial respiration

The forcing of air into and out of the lungs of one person by another or by mechanical means. Artificial respiration, also called rescue breathing, is usually performed when natural breathing stops because of disease, trauma, overdose of drugs, or by suffocation caused by drowning or other means. If the brain is deprived of oxygen for even 5 minutes, permanent damage can result, and after a few more minutes, death is likely to occur. Because of the danger of going for even short periods without breathing, artificial respiration should always be started as soon as possible. Respiratory first aid called CARDIOPULMONARY RESUSCITATION (CPR) combines artificial respiration with chest compressions to keep blood moving throughout the body.

Methods of artificial respiration include rescue breathing, or mouth-to-mouth resuscitation, in which one person breathes into the mouth of an unconscious person once every 5 seconds until the person revives or help arrives. When a person stops breathing because of choking, the abdominal thrust, or HEIMLICH MANEUVER, is recommended. In this method, air from the lungs is used to dislodge the obstruction, by one person applying sharp pressure to the abdomen of the person in need.

Artificial respiration is also performed by mechanical devices, such as a portable resuscitator used by police and fire departments or by ventilators used to pump air into the lungs of people with respiratory failure from many different causes. Heart-lung machines are used to keep the blood oxygenated during open-heart surgery.

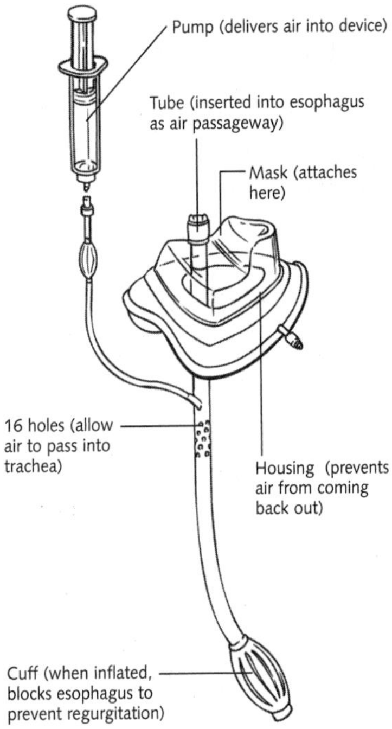
Pump (delivers air into device)
Tube (inserted into esophagus as air passageway)
Mask (attaches here)
16 holes (allow air to pass into trachea)
Housing (prevents air from coming back out)
Cuff (when inflated, blocks esophagus to prevent regurgitation)

PORTABLE RESUSCITATOR
For artificial respiration delivered by emergency personnel, a tube can be inserted directly into a person's trachea (windpipe) to deliver air (endotracheal intubation). If this procedure is not possible, a device that inserts into the person's esophagus can be used instead. Air is delivered to the person's trachea through holes in the tube at the level of the person's throat.

Artificial sweeteners

Low-calorie or no-calorie substitutes for sugar. Candy, chewing gum, jams, jellies, baked goods, and frozen desserts may all contain artificial sweeteners. There are two types of artificial sweeteners: nutritive and nonnutritive.

Polyols, or sugar alcohols, are considered nutritive sweeteners (as is sugar) because they provide energy. They provide a sweet taste and offer less energy and fewer calories than sugar. In addition, they are useful for preventing tooth decay and controlling blood glucose levels. Polyols such as sorbitol, mannitol, and xylitol occur naturally in fruits and berries, but these nutritive sweeteners are commercially synthesized rather than extracted from natural sources. Nutritive sweeteners are absorbed slowly and incompletely from the intestine and are generally safe; however, excess ingestion of polyols can cause diarrhea.

The Food and Drug Administration (FDA) has currently approved four nonnutritive sweeteners: SACCHARIN, ASPARTAME, acesulfame potassium (acesulfame-K), and sucralose. Nonnutritive sweeteners add sweetness to food without providing energy or calories. They are beneficial in weight management, prevention of dental caries, and control of blood glucose.

Although the United States leads the world in the consumption of nonnutritive sweeteners, some controversy has always surrounded their use. For instance, cyclamate was banned in the United States in 1969 because it caused cancer in laboratory mice. However, it continues to be used elsewhere and is under review by the FDA for approval. Although saccharin remains on the market, its label includes the information that it causes cancer in laboratory animals. Because saccharin can cross the placenta, women should consult an obstetrician about the safety of using this sweetener during pregnancy.

Asbestos

A tough, nearly indestructible fiber composed of mineral silicates. There are four types of asbestos: crocidolite, amosite, chrysotile, and tremolite. Asbestos exists in thousands of materials, including cement products, floor tiles, roofing, fireproofing material, and insulation. Inhalation of asbestos fiber particles can result in the fibers settling deep within the lungs and producing scars on the lung tissue. This produces a form of the lung disease PULMONARY FIBROSIS that is called ASBESTOSIS.

There are currently strict US government standards to prevent lung diseases that may be caused by exposure to asbestos. Products and materials that contain asbestos must be manufactured so that the fibers cannot release particles into the air where they may be inhaled. Current danger from asbestos exposure exists in the form of products and materials manufactured before the government guidelines were in place. Structures and buildings still exist that include asbestos-containing materials and may present the risk of asbestos particle inhalation. The removal or destruction of these materials must be undertaken with special procedures and extreme caution.

Asbestosis

A form of the lung disease PULMONARY FIBROSIS that is caused by breathing ASBESTOS dust particles and results in extensive scarring of the lung tissue. Asbestosis can also cause thickening of the membrane layer, called the pleura, that covers the lungs. The risk of developing asbetosis is greater among people who have ongoing exposure to asbestos, such as demolition workers who work on old buildings that are insulated with material containing asbestos. The greater and longer the exposure to asbestos-containing materials, the higher the risk becomes. Asbestosis also greatly increases the risk of LUNG CANCER in cigarette smokers, especially those who smoke more than one pack of cigarettes a day and experience prolonged exposure to asbestos.

SYMPTOMS AND DIAGNOSIS

Symptoms may not be evident until many scars have formed in the lung tissue and make the lungs less elastic. Initial symptoms include mild shortness of breath and a reduced capacity for strenuous activity. Coughing and wheezing are common among people who smoke heavily or have chronic bronchitis in addition to asbestosis. Over time, breathing becomes increasingly difficult. In severe cases, people with asbestosis develop severe shortness of breath and respiratory failure.

In some cases, the condition causes inflammation in the pleural space, the space between the two membranes that surround the lungs. In rare cases, exposure to asbestos can lead to fluid accumulation or to a malignant tumor called MESOTHELIOMA.

Diagnosis of asbestosis is based on a clinical history that includes prolonged exposure to asbestos combined with characteristic chest X-ray findings and the detection with a stethoscope of abnormal lung sounds called "crackles," which are typical of asbestosis and pulmonary fibrosis.

TREATMENT AND PREVENTION

Treatment (oxygen therapy, eliminating future asbestos exposure, and a procedure to drain fluid from around the lungs if present) is aimed at easing symptoms. Smoking cessation in those who smoke is essential to treating the condition. In severe cases, lung transplantation may be the only effective treatment.

Prevention of asbestosis focuses on minimizing or eliminating asbestos dust and fibers in the workplace. Asbestos must be removed from schools and homes by skilled workers who have been trained in safe removal techniques.

Ascariasis

An infection caused by a parasitic roundworm. Ascariasis occurs when food or drink contaminated with roundworm eggs is ingested. When the eggs hatch, the roundworm's larvae are released into the intestine. These larvae migrate through the intestinal wall into the bloodstream to the lungs, where they travel up the respiratory system and are swallowed. This returns the larvae to the intestines where they mature into adult roundworms. The mature roundworms live in the intestine and lay eggs that are expelled with the stool.

CAUSES AND SYMPTOMS

Ascariasis occurs in association with poor personal hygiene and poor sanitation. It is common in warm areas where human feces are used to fertilize food crops.

Illness may be caused by the migration of the larvae through the lungs and by the presence of the adult worm in the intestine. If many worms gather in the intestine, the infected person may experience poor absorption of food nutrients.

Symptoms of ascariasis may include the passing of roundworms in the stool, in vomiting, or through the nose or mouth. Other possible symptoms include fever, cough, bloody sputum, wheezing, shortness of breath, skin rash, and abdominal pain and cramps.

DIAGNOSIS AND TREATMENT

Ascariasis is diagnosed by an examination of stool samples for parasites and eggs and by abdominal X ray. The infection is treated with medication that destroys intestinal parasitic worms. The condition is usually cured with prescribed medication and may improve without treatment. Complications can occur with heavy infestation of the adult worms and their migration to the liver where they may cause an obstruction, a perforation, or an abscess. Obstruction of the intestines may also occur when large numbers of adult roundworms are present. In some cases, the larvae's migration through the lungs can cause pneumonia.

Ascites

A swollen abdomen that results from an abnormal collection of fluid inside the abdominal cavity. Ascites can be a symptom of cancer, infection, cir-rhosis (a severe liver disease), portal hypertension (increased blood pressure in the portal vein, which carries blood from the intestines to the liver), or heart or kidney disease. The underlying condition should be identified before the ascites is treated. Ascites itself can be treated with diuretic drugs and by restricting sodium intake. If this fails to reduce the amount of fluid, or if breathing becomes impaired, draining the ascitic fluid is required. A needle is inserted through the abdominal wall and can remove up to 5 quarts of fluid, which can be analyzed to find out what is causing the ascites.

Ascorbic acid

See VITAMIN C.

Aseptic technique

Any health care procedure in which strict precautions are observed to avoid contamination by microorganisms. For example, health care workers follow aseptic technique when drawing blood and preparing it for analysis. They use sterile gloves and instruments and make sure that the blood sample is not contaminated by organisms on the skin. The aseptic technique is used with any medical procedure that involves entering a person's body.

Aspartame

One of the nonnutritive ARTIFICIAL SWEETENERS. Nonnutritive sweeteners are beneficial in weight management, prevention of dental caries, and control of blood glucose levels. Aspartame, which is nearly 200 times sweeter than sugar, is used to sweeten a variety of foods and beverages. It is also used as a substitute for table sugar. A combination of the amino acids aspartic acid and phenylalanine, aspartame also contains a small amount of methanol.

Laboratory tests on animals have raised questions about the safety of aspartame. However, aspartame was given a thorough scientific review and approved by the Food and Drug Administration in 1981. Doctors have concluded that aspartame is safe for the general public, including children, women who are pregnant or breast-feeding, and people with diabetes. Individuals who are sensitive to phenylalanine, because they lack the enzyme to metabolize it, should avoid aspartame.

Asperger disorder

Asperger disorder is a pervasive developmental disorder (see DEVELOPMENTAL DISORDER, PERVASIVE) that is probably related to autism but is not associated with delays in language development. Unlike autism, coexisting mental retardation is very rare in Asperger disorder. Treatment is generally directed at symptoms, such as poor relationships with peers or family members or the inability to adapt to school or work. Methods of treatment may include family therapy, group social skills training, and individual coaching. Medication may be necessary to treat coexisting psychiatric disorders, such as depression, anxiety disorders, and obsessive compulsive disorder. Psychological evaluation for specific learning disorders and appropriate educational remediation is usually needed for people with Asperger disorder.

Aspergillosis

An opportunistic infection of the lungs and sinuses caused by a common environmental mold called *Aspergillus*. The mold that causes aspergillosis is found in compost heaps and other sites of decaying vegetation, on insulating materials, in air conditioning or heating vents, in hospital rooms and on hospital implements, and in airborne dust. Aspergillosis occurs when the mold's spores are inhaled or, more rarely, when the spores come in contact with broken skin.

The infection occurs most commonly among people with weakened immune systems, including people receiving chemotherapy and people receiving immunosuppressive therapy for organ transplants. It may also occur in people who are HIV-positive (they have the human immunodeficiency virus) and can be a late-stage manifestation of AIDS (acquired immunodeficiency syndrome). Factors that predispose a person to developing aspergillosis include long-term high-dose corticosteroid use, marijuana use, hereditary disorders, and previous lung disease.

Symptoms include cough, chest pain, labored breathing, fever, night sweats, sinus pain, and facial swelling.

Diagnosis is made by examining the fluid of the lung or sinus involved and by a sputum culture. For mild to moderate aspergillosis, the treatment is the oral antifungal medication ITRACONAZOLE. When the infection is invasive, intravenous AMPHOTERICIN B is the standard treatment.

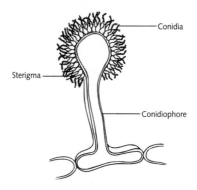

Conidia

Sterigma

Conidiophore

ENVIRONMENTAL MOLD
Under a microscope, the *Aspergillus* mold or fungus that causes aspergillosis has a stalk with a bulbous head covered with beady structures.

Asphyxia

Suffocation; interruption of breathing. Asphyxia is suffocation caused by a blocked airway or the breathing in of toxic gases. Asphyxia is the direct result of a lack of oxygen and an excess of carbon dioxide in the body, which leads to unconsciousness; if untreated, asphyxia may lead to death.

Aspiration

Drawing in or out with suction. Aspiration can also refer to normal breathing, the accidental inhalation of a foreign object or body fluids, the removal of harmful substances (such as bone fragments or body fluids), and the extraction of tissue samples for testing (as in a fine-needle aspiration of the breast).

Aspirin

Acetyl salicylate; a drug used to reduce pain, fever, and inflammation. Also known as acetylsalicylic acid, aspirin reduces pain by acting on the hypothalamus and by blocking pain impulses in muscles. The fever-reducing activity in aspirin involves the heat-regulating center in the hypothalamus: aspirin increases sweating, which leads to cooling of the body by evaporation.

At low doses, aspirin reduces blood clotting by preventing formation of a substance needed for clotting of platelets. Aspirin is used by doctors to treat people who have transient ischemic attacks (TIAs), thromboembolic disorders, and unstable angina, as well as to prevent heart attack. Ordinarily aspirin is useful for headaches, muscle ache from overexertion, and mild to moderate pain. But a person should not use aspirin for more than 3 days without consulting a doctor.

Although aspirin is widely available without prescription, it should be used with caution. Aspirin is associated with allergic reactions and is implicated in the development of REYE SYNDROME in children. Aspirin may also worsen an asthma attack. It can upset a person's stomach, so it is best if taken with food or after meals.

Assault

In law, the attempt or threat to use violence to harm another person; if actual violent contact is made with the other person's body, BATTERY has been committed in addition to assault. Assault is a crime of attempt that requires intent to harm; threatening words or intentions alone do not constitute assault. Criminal statutes differentiate among various degrees of assault, including simple assault; assault with a deadly weapon; and aggravated assault, which is defined as assault involving the intent to commit robbery or rape. See also ABUSE, PARTNER.

Assault, sexual

FOR FIRST AID
see Rape, page 1327

Forced sexual activity or contact without consent; also called rape. Sexual assault is a gender-neutral term currently in use in many states instead of "rape," which has traditionally been defined as forced vaginal penetration of women by men. Sexual assault is now recognized as a crime committed against males and females of all ages, from infants to elderly people. Sexual assault includes rape by strangers, acquaintances, and spouses. In 80 percent of all instances of sexual assault against women, the assailant is known to the victim (called DATE RAPE). About 5 percent of reported sexual assaults are committed against men.

Sexual assault is the most rapidly growing violent crime in the United States. In an average year, more than 700,000 females are sexually assaulted, and 61 percent of them are younger than 18. Experts believe that fewer than half of all cases of sexual assault are reported to authorities, and some experts suspect the percentage is as low as 10 percent. Sexual assault usually takes place in connection with the abuser's use of alcohol or drugs; sometimes the abuser gives drugs to the victim without that person's knowledge, to facilitate the assault. See also ABUSE, SEXUAL.

Assay
A test that measures the amount, purity, or effectiveness of drugs or other biologic substances.

Assisted living facility
Residential facilities for older people who no longer can manage all of their daily needs. Residents live in their own apartments and typically have meals in a common dining area. Fees usually include meals, housekeeping, and an agreed-upon amount of personal assistance with daily activities such as bathing, grooming, dressing, or bathroom use. Nursing care is usually not offered. See also LONG-TERM CARE FACILITY.

Assisted reproductive technology
Generally, infertility treatments using advanced technology to treat a variety of conditions associated with infertility. The most common form of assisted reproductive technology

(ART) is IN VITRO FERTILIZATION (IVF) for treating female infertility. Other ART techniques include gamete (the female egg and male sperm) intrafallopian transfer (GIFT), zygote intrafallopian transfer (ZIFT), and intracytoplasmic sperm injection (ICSI). Sperm for these procedures can be obtained by electroejaculation for men who are unable to ejaculate because of paralysis or neurological diseases. Sperm can also be obtained from men who have no sperm in their ejaculate (or who have had a vasectomy) by aspirating the sperm with a needle from their testicles or epididymis. ART may involve the use of donor sperm, eggs, or embryos. Embryos that have been frozen and stored can be used to achieve a future pregnancy by frozen EMBRYO TRANSFER. See also INFERTILITY.

Assistive listening devices
Equipment designed to help people who are hearing-impaired (see HEARING AIDS). The devices may be used

with hearing aids or as an alternative to hearing aids. They generally fall into three main categories: amplifying, alerting, and decoding devices.

Amplifying devices enhance sound from a television, radio, or stereo to headphones, allowing the user to adjust volume and pitch without affecting the sound from the speaker. Small amplifiers that can be attached to a telephone are also available. Some telephones are sold with amplifiers built into the receiver. Small personal amplifiers are available at many theaters and churches.

Alerting devices are systems that can be wired to a doorbell or telephone to alert a person by means of loud noises, flashing lights, or a vibrator attached to the user's wrist or bed. Advanced alerting systems can be used with alarm clocks, smoke detectors, and the timers on ovens and clothes dryers. These systems can be programmed to produce individualized alerts for specific sounds.

Decoding devices convert the sound of voices into written text on televisions. Televisions may be purchased with built-in, closed-captioned decoders. Decoders to attach to an existing television are also available. Closed-captioned service is currently offered by all news and prime time programs, as well as syndicated programming and many feature videos. Decoding devices can also convert voice to text via a specialized telephone system called a telephone teletypewriter (TTY).

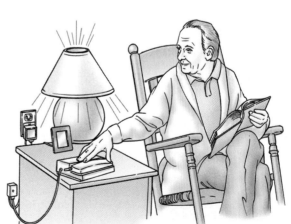

ALERTING DEVICES
An alerting device can be wired to a telephone so a light turns on or flashes when the telephone rings. The light plugs into an alerting unit that plugs into an electrical outlet; another cord connects the alerting unit to a telephone jack. Doorbells, smoke detectors, ovens, and other household appliances can be connected. Signals include lights, vibrations, or amplified sounds.

A

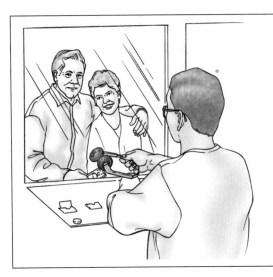

AMPLIFYING DEVICES
A small amplifier is often enough to bring ordinary sounds into an audible range for a person with a hearing impairment. Theaters, churches, and day-care centers may offer such devices. Special headphones permit users to adjust the volume without making their transmissions louder.

These systems convert voice into written text and allow the user to speak or type a response.

Astereognosis

A brain disorder characterized by an inability to identify objects by the sense of touch, even when there is no defect of sensation in the fingers or any difficulty holding the object (for example, an individual is unable to identify common objects, such as a coin or safety pin, placed in his or her hands). Astereognosis can occur on the left or right side. It is caused by brain damage to the part of the cerebrum that controls touch.

Asthma

An immunological condition that causes inflammation, excessive mucus secretion, and reversible constriction of the smooth muscle in the lung's airway. Asthma can produce wheezing, coughing, and shortness of breath; these symptoms may vary in severity. An asthma attack may be triggered by a person's sensitivity to certain substances, exercise, dusts, viral infections, and other conditions that produce inflammation of the airways.

SYMPTOMS

A dry cough at night or during physical activity may be the only symptom of asthma. The initial symptoms of an asthma attack are generally shortness of breath, coughing, or chest tightness. In children, an itching sensation on the chest or neck may be the first hint of an approaching attack.

The attacks sometimes have a sudden onset that can rapidly progress to pronounced wheezing and shortness of breath. In other instances, the attack starts slowly and symptoms gradually increase in intensity. An asthma attack may last for several minutes, for several hours, or even for days at a time.

Anxiety may accompany an asthma attack, especially if breathing becomes difficult. In very severe attacks, speaking is difficult and little air moves in or out of the lungs. If a person's air supply becomes seriously restricted, confusion and lethargy can occur, and the skin may turn blue. Emergency medical treatment is essential if these symptoms are present. Patients rarely die, even in cases of severe asthma attacks, if proper treatment is obtained early in the course of the attack.

CAUSES

The airway inflammation associated with asthma may be triggered by contact with an allergen to which a person is sensitive, by a viral infection, or by strenuous exercise.

In some people with defined allergies, asthma may be triggered by an abnormal reaction of the airways to specific stimuli. These stimuli may include pollens, dust mites, or animal dander, which certain cells in the airway recognize as allergens. The result is an immune response that causes certain cells to release substances such as HISTAMINE and leukotrienes that stimulate the smooth muscles in the airways to contract. Mucus secretion increases;

white blood cells, which secrete chemicals that cause an inflammation response, are transported to the area; and the tissues lining the airways become swollen and inflamed. This produces a narrowing of the airways, a condition that is called bronchoconstriction. Bronchoconstriction, which can impede air movement and make breathing difficult, can vary in frequency, duration, and severity.

Asthma may also occur in people who do not have defined allergies. Smoke, cold air, vigorous activity, stress, anxiety, a viral infection of the upper respiratory system, or any combination of these environmental conditions and events may produce similar changes that cause the narrowing of the airways in certain people. The resulting asthma attacks also vary in severity, frequency, and duration.

DIAGNOSIS

Asthma can be initially diagnosed on the basis of a description of characteristic symptoms. If a person has narrowed airways at the time he or she visits a doctor, the doctor may hear wheezing, in which case SPIROMETRY, a test that measures air movement in and out of the lungs, may confirm bronchoconstriction. Spirometry may also be used to determine the extent of airway obstruction and to monitor asthma treatment.

If the diagnosis of asthma seems likely and spirometry results are normal, the doctor may recommend a trial of bronchodilators. If the symptoms resolve, then asthma is the probable diagnosis. In rare cases in which the diagnosis is uncertain, the doctor may give a small amount of a bronchoconstrictor to inhale. Inhalation at this dosage does not produce narrowing of the airways in a healthy person, but does result in bronchoconstriction in a person with asthma.

Identifying and avoiding asthma triggers is the first line of defense against asthma attacks. In cases in which it is vital to identify the substance that triggers asthma attacks, allergy skin testing may be done. To diagnose exercise-induced asthma, a person is given spirometry tests before and following exercise on a treadmill or stationary bicycle.

TREATMENT

The most commonly used medications to relieve asthma symptoms are

FOCUS ON ASTHMA

Tobacco smoke, cold air, cat dander, and grass are common irritants that can irritate the airways and help trigger an asthma attack. If a person is hyperresponsive and hyperreactive to these irritants—that is, if one's body overreacts to irritants and the airways become inflamed and filled with mucus in a manner that restricts airflow and affects breathing—an asthma attack results. Asthma attacks may also be triggered by viral infections or strenuous exercise.

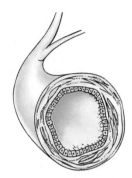

NORMAL BRONCHIOLE
A bronchiole unaffected by irritants is open and clear of obstruction.

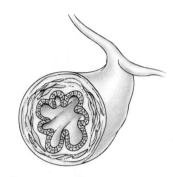

NARROWED BRONCHIOLE
During an asthmatic spasm, the bronchiole narrows and is obstructed by mucus.

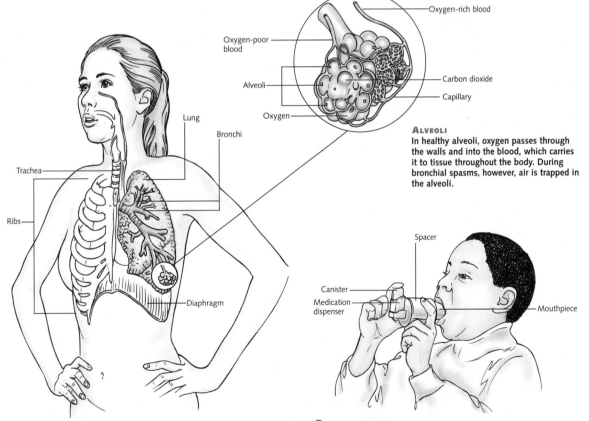

Oxygen-rich blood

Oxygen-poor blood

Alveoli

Carbon dioxide

Oxygen

Capillary

ALVEOLI
In healthy alveoli, oxygen passes through the walls and into the blood, which carries it to tissue throughout the body. During bronchial spasms, however, air is trapped in the alveoli.

Lung

Bronchi

Trachea

Ribs

Diaphragm

HEALTHY RESPIRATORY SYSTEM
Inhaled air enters through the trachea (windpipe), passes through the bronchi, and moves to the alveoli (the air sacs) in the lungs.

Spacer

Canister

Medication dispenser

Mouthpiece

BRONCHODILATORS
Drugs called bronchodilators relax the smooth muscle of the bronchi and reopen the airway during an asthma attack.

A

BRONCHODILATORS, which stimulate certain receptors in the airway to relax the smooth muscle and dilate (widen) the airways. Bronchodilators may be taken by mouth, by injection, or by inhalation. Inhaling devices deposit the medication directly into the airways during an attack and immediately dilate the airways, but in cases of severe bronchoconstriction they may not transport the medication to all the affected airways. Oral bronchodilators can reach all the obstructed airways but act more slowly than inhaled forms and usually have more side effects than inhaled bronchodilators; oral agents must be taken on a regular basis to prevent asthma attacks. They may be taken orally via short-acting tablets, sustained-release capsules, or in syrup form. Bronchodilators can be given by injection, but these are usually used to treat severe asthma attacks.

Inhaled, oral, or injected CORTICO-STEROIDS can counteract the inflammatory response and are very effective at controlling symptoms. Inhaled corticosteroids are used most often in those with moderate or severe asthma. When taken over time, these medications gradually act to prevent attacks by reducing inflammation and blocking the sensitivity of the airways to allergens and other stimuli. When severe asthma does not respond to other treatments, long-term oral corticosteroids may be prescribed to control symptoms. Long-term use of oral corticosteroids is limited to the most severely affected people because of the potential for serious side effects, including inhibited wound healing, weakening of the bones, slowed growth in children, bleeding from the stomach, cataracts, increased blood sugar level, weight gain, and mental disturbances. Inhaled corticosteroids used over the long-term do not have these same side effects.

Other medications that may be prescribed to prevent or control asthma include CROMOLYN SODIUM and nedocromil, which inhibit the release of inflammatory substances and help prevent airway constriction. The

Terms in small capital letters—for example, PHYSICAL THERAPY or PAGET DISEASE—indicate a cross-reference to another entry with more information.

ASTHMA ATTACK PREVENTION

Asthma attacks may be prevented by taking several precautions.

- Eliminating exposure to indoor allergens including dust mites, feathers, cockroaches, and animal dander can reduce the frequency and severity of asthma attacks.
- Exposure to dust mites present inside the home may be controlled by lowering indoor relative humidity and removing carpeting that tends to harbor them. Specialized coverings for pillows, mattresses, and comforters can reduce exposure to mites, as can the use of air conditioning in hot weather.
- Animal dander should be eliminated by removing household pets from living quarters.
- Secondhand cigarette smoke and other irritating environmental fumes should be avoided.
- In some people, certain substances may trigger attacks and should be avoided. These substances include the yellow coloring agent tartrazine, which is used in some tablet coatings and processed foods, and sulfites, a common preservative used in some salad bar food items and in beer and wine. Ingredients listed on the labels of these beverages should be checked.
- Certain people, particularly those who have nasal polyps, may be sensitive to aspirin and other nonsteroidal anti-inflammatory medications (NSAIDs), which can trigger asthma attacks when taken.

---

newest medications used to control asthma are leukotriene modifiers (for example, montelukast, zafirlukast, and zileuton), which prevent the action of chemicals that cause the inflammation associated with asthma attacks.

Persons diagnosed with asthma are generally prescribed a handheld, metered-dose inhaler that uses pressurized gas to propel the bronchodilator medication, which is inhaled through the mouth into the airways. Inhaled bronchodilators work rapidly to relieve shortness of breath and wheezing by relaxing the smooth muscles of the airways. For people with frequent asthma attacks (more than two to three asthma attacks a week), cromolyn or inhaled corticosteroids may be added as daily medications. Another group of oral medications called leukotriene receptor antagonists is also used to control symptoms. Oral THEOPHYLLINE is prescribed less commonly but can be useful for treating persistent symptoms, particularly nighttime symptoms.

An acute asthma attack should be treated immediately using additional medications or higher doses or different forms of the medications used on an ongoing basis to control or prevent asthma. A handheld inhaler may be used by a person during an asthma attack, or a NEBU-LIZER may be used to direct pressur-

ized air through a solution of the medication. The nebulizer produces a continuous mist that can be inhaled. Intravenous asthma medications, including EPINEPHRINE or corticosteriods, are sometimes used to treat severe asthma attacks. Oxygen and intravenous fluids may also need to be given, and antibiotics may be necessary if an underlying infection is present.

Asthma, cardiac

Wheezing that results from the pooling of fluid in the lungs because of heart failure (see HEART FAILURE, CONGESTIVE). Similar symptoms can arise from other diseases, including PANIC DISORDER, COR PULMONALE, and SLEEP APNEA SYNDROME. Cardiac asthma often occurs in association with paroxysmal nocturnal dyspnea (a sudden, severe shortness of breath that occurs at night). A person with paroxysmal nocturnal dyspnea awakens abruptly from sleep, feels a need to sit up, and may open a window in an attempt to get more air. The episode can include coughing, wheezing, or a smothering sensation. To get relief, the person must sit upright and sometimes must resort to sleeping in a chair.

Astigmatism

A defect in vision caused by uneven curvature of the eye's clear outer covering (cornea). The normal

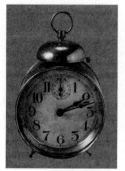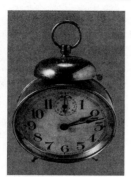

HOW ASTIGMATISM AFFECTS VISION
A person with severe astigmatism that is corrected with glasses or contact lenses may see a somewhat tilted or distorted image compared with the normal image of the face of a stopwatch. The corrective lenses must provide more power to one section of the eye than another, and the fit is difficult to achieve.

Normal image   Image for person with severe, corrected astigmatism

cornea is round, curving equally from top to bottom and side to side. In astigmatism, the cornea curves more in one direction than the other, making it asymmetrical. Astigmatism is usually present at birth and often increases through childhood. A minor degree of astigmatism is very common and considered normal and often requires no correction. More pronounced astigmatism changes little during school years. It can lead to blurred near and distance vision. Glasses or contact lenses specially designed to counteract the astigmatism are used to correct the condition; the correction provided by glasses or contact lenses for greater degrees of astigmatism can lead to tilting and distortion effects. Astigmatism can occur with other vision defects such as nearsightedness or farsightedness.

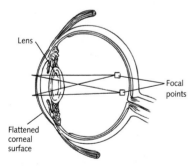

Lens

Focal points

Flattened corneal surface

TWO FOCAL POINTS
A person with astigmatism has a cornea that is flatter and elliptical, like a football, rather than spherical. The curvature of the corneal surface is greater in some areas and flatter in others, creating two points of focus in the eye. One focal point may lie at or near the retina, while the other falls in front of or behind it.

Aston-patterning

Form of BODYWORK that relieves muscle pain and fatigue by improving faulty patterns of body movement. Developed by dancer Jane Aston in the 1970s, Aston-patterning changes habitual patterns of body usage to improve energy, stability, mobility, and balance. Massage is generally used to release tension and make it possible to learn new patterns of movement. See ROLFING.

Astringents

Agents that cause contraction after they are applied to the skin. Examples include calamine lotion, used to dry minor skin irritations associated with poison ivy, mild sunburn, and insect bites; and witch hazel, used to cool and soothe superficial skin irritations such as hemorrhoids or diaper rash.

Astrocytoma

A type of brain tumor that develops from glial (supportive) brain tissue. Astrocytomas can be benign or malignant and account for about 10 percent of all brain tumors. Astrocytomas are usually slow-growing in adults but can be fast-growing in children. Symptoms in children can include movement disorders, while in adults, symptoms are usually vague and can go undiagnosed for years. A diagnostic workup, or evaluation, may include CT (computed tomography) scanning or MRI (magnetic resonance imaging), followed by a tissue biopsy. Treatment generally includes surgical removal, followed by radiation therapy.

Asymptomatic

A term that describes a person who does not have symptoms or any indications of sickness or disease. When a person has a condition but exhibits no recognizable signs of it, he or she is said to be asymptomatic. See also SYMPTOM.

Asystole

The absence of a heartbeat. See also CARDIAC ARREST.

Ataxia

Lack of coordination caused by nerve or brain damage. Ataxia may impair balance, gait, movement, or speech. The term "ataxia" is often used in a general way to refer to symptoms associated with dysfunction of the cerebellum (the part of the brain that helps control balance) and brain stem but can also occur with sensory loss (sensory ataxia). Ataxia can be caused by intoxication with medications or alcohol, infections, strokes, tumors, or chronic hereditary degenerative syndromes, such as FRIEDREICH ATAXIA or olivopontocerebellar atrophy. Slow or clumsy movement in the early stages of these diseases can eventually become so pronounced that a person requires a wheelchair. Hereditary ataxias may also affect speech and swallowing. These progressive diseases do not always result in total disability. However, they may shorten a person's life span as a result of complications such as heart disease and respiratory difficulties. The treatment of ataxia is based on the cause. Physical and occupational therapy can be helpful when the ataxia cannot be cured by treating the cause.

Atelectasis

A chronic or acute condition that arises when a portion of the lung collapses, usually caused by obstruction of a bronchial tube. As a result, the collapsed tissue is unable to properly exchange oxygen. The condition may be caused by mucous plugs or obstruction of the airway by a tumor or foreign bodies lodged in the bronchi. Abnormalities in the bronchial structures or external compression of an airway from an enlarged lymph node or tumor may also produce this condition in the

A

lung. Other causes of atelectasis include compression of the lungs caused by the abnormal presence of fluids or gases.

Atelectasis is a common complication of surgery performed in the upper abdomen, on the lungs, or on the heart. These types of surgeries can cause pain that makes it difficult to take deep breaths that open the airways and, therefore, can impair a person's ability to cough up mucus that can plug the airway. Chronic cases may be caused by a collapsed lobe of the lung, which is produced by compression from structures and organs outside the lung, or by an infection that causes bronchial obstruction.

SYMPTOMS, DIAGNOSIS, AND TREATMENT
Atelectasis may cause few symptoms or may cause chest pain, cough, and shortness of breath. If a person's oxygen supply is affected, there may be a blue discoloration of the skin, a drop in blood pressure, an irregular heartbeat, and an elevated temperature. Chronic atelectasis may have no symptoms or may result in severe, dry coughing. Acute pneumonia may develop from the chronic form.

Atelectasis is diagnosed on the basis of a physical examination and X-ray findings that reveal a decrease in lung size and an opaque, airless area within the lung. A CT (computed tomography) scan may be used to view the chest, and a fiberoptic bronchoscope may be used to detect the cause of obstruction.

Treatment is generally aimed at the cause of the condition. If a bronchial obstruction is determined, suctioning or respiratory and physical therapy are used. A plug or foreign body may be removed through a bronchoscope, which will allow air into the lung so that it can inflate. Chronic atelectasis is treated with appropriate physical therapy, including forced coughing and deep breathing, possibly with the aid of an incentive spirometer (see SPIROMETRY). Antibiotics are used to treat underlying infections.

In some chronic cases, surgery may be recommended. If a tumor is producing the obstruction, it may be treated with surgery, radiation therapy, or chemotherapy. Laser therapy may be effective in removing some tumors located inside a bronchial tube.

Atenolol
See BETA BLOCKERS.

Atherectomy
See BALLOON ANGIOPLASTY.

Atheroma
An abnormal growth of fatty tissue in or on the walls of a major artery. The term comes from the Greek word for "porridge," which refers to the soft, lumpy appearance of atheromas. Atheromas have a central role in the disease ATHEROSCLEROSIS.

Atherosclerosis
A disease in which deposits of fat and other materials accumulate in and on the inner walls of the arteries, narrowing them and causing them to lose their elasticity, strength, and flexibility. The fatty deposits are often called atheromas or plaques. Atherosclerosis comes from two Greek roots: "ather," which means "porridge" and refers to the soft, lumpy appearance of the fatty deposits; and "sclerosis," which means "hardening." Atherosclerosis is often referred to popularly as hardening of the arteries.

DISEASE PROCESS AND SYMPTOMS
Atherosclerosis is thought to begin when an injury stimulus (for example, elevated levels of cholesterol, high blood pressure, or tobacco use) damages the smooth lining of the arterial walls. White blood cells are then attracted to the injury sites; at the same time, the damaged walls allow more fats to accumulate, which stimulates the smooth muscle cells of the arteries to proliferate. Clot-producing platelets collect over the site, trapping even more white blood cells and fat particles. As the plaque builds, it may develop a thick covering of calcium, which causes the characteristic hardening of the artery. In addition, the growing plaque narrows the opening in the artery and restricts blood flow. If the plaque ruptures, a clot can form at the site and obstruct the blood flow, which prevents tissues from receiving enough oxygen and can

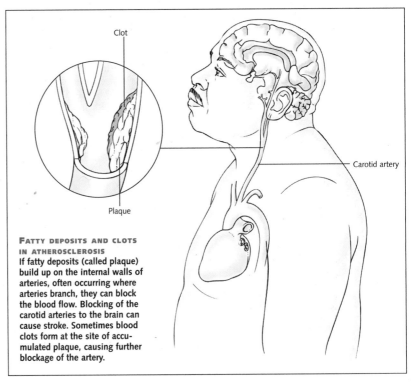

Clot

Carotid artery

Plaque

FATTY DEPOSITS AND CLOTS IN ATHEROSCLEROSIS
If fatty deposits (called plaque) build up on the internal walls of arteries, often occurring where arteries branch, they can block the blood flow. Blocking of the carotid arteries to the brain can cause stroke. Sometimes blood clots form at the site of accumulated plaque, causing further blockage of the artery.

result in myocardial infarction. Alternatively, a piece of the plaque can break free and travel through the bloodstream, where it can lodge in a smaller artery and block it, resulting in an EMBOLISM.

The coronary arteries, which surround the heart and supply it with blood, are a common site of atherosclerosis. If the blood flow is restricted to the extent that there is an imbalance of oxygen supply to oxygen demand, the chest pain known as ANGINA often results. Complete blockage of one of the coronary arteries by atherosclerotic plaque is a principal cause of heart attack, and it can lead to sudden death.

Atherosclerosis in the arteries that supply blood to the brain (the carotid and cerebral arteries) is one cause of STROKE. Severe plaque in the arteries providing blood to the lower limbs (see CLAUDICATION) may cause poor circulation, sores, and gangrene, and amputation may be necessary.

DIAGNOSIS

Sometimes a doctor suspects atherosclerosis during a routine physical examination. Through a stethoscope applied to the neck, groin, or abdomen, the doctor may be able to hear the characteristic bruit (blowing sound) caused by turbulent blood flow that results from atherosclerotic narrowing. Also, a weak pulse in the wrists, legs, or feet may indicate partially obstructed blood flow.

When atherosclerosis is suspected, a number of noninvasive tests can be used to identify and assess the disease. One is the electrocardiogram (ECG). This test measures the electrical activity of the heart and shows any damage or irregularity limiting blood flow into the heart. An ECG can be performed while a person is immobile or exercising (CARDIAC STRESS TESTING), typically on a treadmill or a stationary bicycle. In a nuclear stress test, the person being tested is injected with a very small dose of a radioactive substance; then his or her heart is photographed with a radiation-sensitive gamma camera both at rest and while exercising. In echocardiography, the heart is visualized with ultrasound waves, and an image of the beating heart plays on a video screen, where the doctor can check the thickness, size, and function of the heart. Ultrafast CT (computed tomography) scanning takes multiple views of the heart and is useful in determining the amount of calcification in the artery. A doctor may also detect narrowing in the blood vessels of the legs by comparing the blood pressure in the vessels around the ankle and on top of the foot with the blood pressure in the arm.

When atherosclerosis is advanced, an invasive test called an angiogram is often performed. To assess atherosclerosis in the coronary arteries, a thin tube called a catheter is inserted into a blood vessel, usually in the thigh, and threaded into the heart. Contrast dye is injected through the catheter, and X rays are taken of the heart. A similar test is performed to diagnose atherosclerosis in the arteries leading into the brain or the lower extremities.

RISK FACTORS

Certain factors are known to increase the risk of atherosclerosis. Some can be controlled by individual choice; others cannot.

The uncontrollable risk factors include age, sex, and heredity. Growing older does not of itself cause atherosclerosis, but the risk of heart disease increases with age. When younger than 60, men are more likely than women to suffer heart attacks caused by atherosclerosis. After that age, the risk for both men and women is more or less equal. Atherosclerosis tends to run in families. People with a parent who suffered a heart attack because of atherosclerosis at a relatively young age are at greater risk for the disease.

A principal controllable risk factor for atherosclerosis is smoking. Tobacco use increases the risk for depositing fatty materials in the arteries and increases the likelihood of heart attack and sudden death. Hypertension (high blood pressure) also contributes to the hardening of arteries and damages the heart. Hypertension is particularly dangerous in people who smoke. Diabetes mellitus also raises the risk of atherosclerosis. Men with diabetes mellitus have double the normal risk of coronary artery disease, while women with diabetes mellitus have five times the normal risk. High blood cholesterol and a diet rich in fats and oils can contribute to atherosclerosis. Obesity (being 20 percent heavier than ideal body weight) typically increases cholesterol levels and blood pressure and contributes to a sedentary lifestyle, which is another risk factor.

TREATMENT

The best treatment for atherosclerosis is preventing the disease in the first place, by eliminating or reducing the controllable risk factors for the disease. Stopping tobacco use, controlling diabetes and hypertension with medication and diet, reducing fats and oils in the diet, maintaining a healthy weight, and exercising moderately to vigorously several times a week lower the chances of developing atherosclerosis. If the disease does develop, the preventive precautions can slow its advance or even reverse the disease process.

A number of medications are useful in treating atherosclerosis. Aspirin inhibits the formation of blood clots and may help prevent a damaged blood vessel from becoming blocked. ANTIHYPERTENSIVES such as beta blockers reduce the workload on the heart. Nitrates relax the heart and blood vessels, increasing the flow of oxygen-rich blood to heart. The angiotensin-converting enzyme (ACE) inhibitors have a similar effect. Drugs to lower blood cholesterol levels may be prescribed for people with elevated blood fat levels. Certain vitamins may also be helpful, particularly folic acid, one of the B vitamins.

Invasive procedures are used for advanced disease, particularly when an artery has been blocked. In BALLOON ANGIOPLASTY, a balloon-tipped catheter is threaded through a blood vessel into the coronary artery and inflated to press the plaque down and widen the opening. A STENT is a wire-mesh sleeve inserted into a widened artery by catheter to further stretch and support it. Surgical procedures to bypass a blocked artery may be used to help those with severe blockage that cannot be controlled with medications or less invasive methods.

CAROTID ENDARTERECTOMY, a procedure to correct a narrowing in the carotid artery that supplies blood to the brain, is performed to reduce the risk of stroke. In coronary artery bypass surgery, veins harvested from the legs are grafted to the coronary arteries to bypass blockage.

Athetosis

An involuntary movement disorder characterized by slow, writhing, continuous movements of the extremities. Athetosis most commonly affects the head, face, neck, and limbs. There may also be facial grimacing. Athetosis is caused by damage to the basal ganglia (clusters of nerve cells deep in the brain) and is associated with medical disorders such as CEREBRAL PALSY and HUNTINGTON CHOREA. It is often difficult to distinguish from chorea (a more rapid involuntary movement disorder) and is sometimes called choreoathetosis.

Athlete's foot

A common infection of the skin between the toes, which leads to itching and soreness; also known as tinea pedis. Athlete's foot is a form of TINEA (a group of related skin infections caused by different species of fungi). Fungi thrive in moist, warm areas. Athlete's foot seldom affects children younger than age 12.

The rash may spread to other parts of the foot; in some people, it may manifest as redness and scaling on the soles and sides of the feet. Infection may spread to the toenails (onychomycosis), causing scaling, crumbling, and thickening of the nails. Possible complications of athlete's foot include secondary bacterial infections.

SYMPTOMS AND DIAGNOSIS

Athlete's foot is usually characterized by a red, scaly, cracked rash between the toes. Often the rash itches and burns. If blisters develop and break, exposed areas of tissue cause pain and swelling. When the rash is scratched, it can become raw and ooze. There is often an unpleasant odor. Athlete's foot is diagnosed by the characteristic appearance of the skin and by examining pieces of skin, obtained through scraping, under a microscope, or cultured in special

media to detect fungus growth. To obtain proper treatment, it is important to distinguish athlete's foot from other skin problems such as dermatitis or psoriasis.

TREATMENT

Simple cases of athlete's foot respond well to treatment with antifungal creams. The skin should be kept clean and dry. If there are blisters, sometimes doctors recommend soaking the feet before applying creams. Severe infections require stronger oral antifungal medications that may cause side effects. To control or prevent athlete's foot, it is important to wash feet daily and dry them thoroughly, especially between the toes; wear cotton socks and change them frequently; wear sandals in warm, humid weather; avoid tight shoes; go barefoot when at home; and use antifungal powder.

Atony

A loss of muscle tone (the normal degree of resistance a relaxed muscle gives to passive movement) resulting in weakness of the body or of a muscle or organ. Atony is a symptom of many diseases, including MULTIPLE SCLEROSIS, MUSCULAR DYSTROPHY, MYASTHENIA GRAVIS, and STROKE. The cause of weakness is diagnosed according to its location, quality, progression, and accompanying symptoms. The doctor will also investigate factors that aggravate or relieve atony.

ATP

Adenosine triphosphate. ATP is a molecule that serves as the principal immediate source of usable energy for the metabolism of cells. ATP is composed of adenine, ribose, and three phosphate units. The conversion of ATP to adenosine diphosphate (ADP) provides the fuel to drive nerve signal transmission, muscle movement, protein synthesis, and cell division.

Atresia

From birth, the absence of a normal body opening or the abnormal closure of an opening. Examples of atresia include a closed anus, the absence or closure of the outer ear canal, and narrowing of certain blood vessels.

Atrial fibrillation

A rapid, highly irregular heartbeat caused by abnormalities in the electrical signals generated by the atria (upper chambers) of the heart. In the normal heart, the heartbeat begins in the sinus node, which is located in the upper portion of the heart. The sinus node usually generates the impulse for a heartbeat between 60 and 100 times a minute, which then spreads across the rest of the heart. In atrial fibrillation, rapid firing of electrical impulses from the atrium increases the heart rate to 100 to 175 beats per minute, with irregular inter-

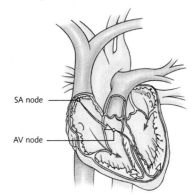

SA node

AV node

Normal electrical signals

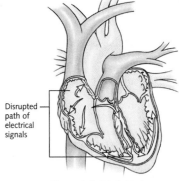

Disrupted path of electrical signals

Abnormal electrical signals

KEY
⟹ Electrical signal ⟶ Blood flow

ELECTRICAL SIGNALS IN THE HEART
In the healthy heart, electrical signals originate in the sinoatrial (SA) node, and the atrioventricular (AV) node conducts the electrical signals throughout the heart. When electrical signals travel through the atria in a disorganized way, the coordination of atrial contraction is disrupted and an irregular heart rhythm results.

vals between the beats. Instead of contracting correctly, the atria quiver. The ventricles (lower chambers) of the heart beat irregularly and rapidly in response to this abnormal rhythm, making the heart less effective and efficient.

At first, atrial fibrillation tends to occur in episodes lasting minutes or hours, with long periods of normal heart rhythm separating the attacks. When atrial fibrillation occurs, it is likely to cause palpitations (the physical sensation of rapid heartbeat). If the attack is severe, chest pain, shortness of breath, light-headedness, fainting, or fatigue can also result. Over time, atrial fibrillation can become chronic.

The principal risk posed by atrial fibrillation is stroke. Since the atria are not contracting properly, blood may pool and clot. If a clot dislodges, travels in the bloodstream to the brain, and lodges in an artery (see EMBOLISM), a stroke results. An embolism can also affect other organs, particularly the lungs, kidneys, and lower extremities. Atrial fibrillation also increases the risk of heart failure (see HEART FAILURE, CONGESTIVE), CARDIOMYOPATHY (impaired heart muscle function), and HEART ATTACK.

Atrial fibrillation is the most common type of sustained abnormal heart rhythm (see ARRHYTHMIA, CARDIAC, for information on how atrial fibrillation compares with other heartbeat disorders). The disease is estimated to affect 2 million Americans.

RISK FACTORS

The risk of atrial fibrillation increases with age. Among people 50 years old or younger, the disease affects fewer than 1 in every 100; among those older than 80, it affects 10 of every 100. Atrial fibrillation affects both men and women equally. It is more common in people with hypertension (high blood pressure), coronary artery disease, congenital (present at birth) heart disease, thyroid disease, pericarditis (inflammation of the membrane covering the heart), congestive heart failure, chronic lung diseases (such as asthma or chronic obstructive lung disease), abuse of alcohol or drugs (particularly cocaine), excessive use of caffeine or decongestants, and heart valve disease.

DIAGNOSIS

The episodic nature of atrial fibrillation makes diagnosis difficult in some cases. A doctor using a stethoscope can listen for heart rhythms that indicate atrial fibrillation, usually an irregular, rapid pulse. An electrocardiogram (ECG) measures the electrical activity of the heart and reveals irregularities in rhythm. The Holter monitor uses a portable ECG device that is worn by the person as he or she goes through normal activities for 1 or 2 days. An event recorder, which is usually kept at home for up to a month, is particularly good for detecting occasional or sporadic episodes of cardiac arrhythmia. The stress test is another type of ECG, in which readings are taken while the person exercises, typically on a treadmill or a stationary bicycle. In echocardiography, the heart is visualized with ultrasound waves, and an image of the beating heart is displayed on a video screen, which helps the doctor assess the thickness, size, and function of the heart. This test may also be used to detect blood clots in the atria.

Transesophageal echocardiography uses a small transducer attached to an endoscope (flexible tube) that is inserted through the mouth and throat and into the esophagus to provide a clear, detailed picture of the function of the heart. This test is useful for detecting clots in the atria and for examining the mitral valve for narrowing that may be causing atrial fibrillation. In an electrophysiology study, a catheter is inserted in a blood vessel and threaded through the circulatory system to the heart. Electrical activity of the heart is recorded to identify any abnormality.

TREATMENT

Treatment depends on the severity of the atrial fibrillation. Any underlying condition, such as hypertension or coronary artery disease, must be treated as well.

A number of medications are useful in the treatment of atrial fibrillation. Beta blockers, calcium channel blockers, and digoxin slow the ventricular heart rate, reduce the work load on the heart, and lower blood pressure. Anticoagulants, such as aspirin and warfarin, are used to prevent clots and lower the risk of stroke. Antiarrhythmic medications stabilize heart rhythm. The use of anticoagulant and antiarrhythmic drugs, however, requires careful monitoring since side effects can be dangerous.

More invasive treatments are available if needed. CARDIOVERSION uses drugs or electrical shock to return the heart to a normal rhythm. A device called an implantable cardioverter DEFIBRILLATOR (ICD) can be placed surgically in the chest. The ICD monitors heartbeat and corrects it if it becomes abnormally fast. Radiofrequency ablation (see ABLATION THERAPY), which uses radiofrequency energy emitted through a catheter threaded through the blood vessels into the heart to destroy very small areas of tissue to change the conduction pattern of the heart, is a newer procedure that has been developed for the treatment of atrial fibrillation. In the Maze procedure, which requires surgical opening of the chest, the surgeon makes small cuts in the atrial wall to create a new pattern of electrical pathways and prevent atrial fibrillation.

Atrial flutter

A rapid but relatively regular heartbeat caused by abnormalities in the electrical signals generated by the atria (upper chambers) of the heart. Atrial flutter is a common type of cardiac arrhythmia, or abnormal heartbeat.

In the healthy heart, the beat begins in the sinus node, which is located in the atria, then spreads across the rest of the heart, usually at a rate of 60 to 100 times a minute. In atrial flutter, rapid firing of abnormal tissue, usually in the lower right atrium, causes the atria to contract approximately 300 times a minute. The ventricles (lower chambers of the heart) beat in response to every second, third, or fourth atrial contraction, so that the overall heartbeat varies between 75 and 150 beats per minute. Atrial flutter causes the heart to pump less effectively, reducing the amount of blood being pumped throughout the body. The condition is often associated with heart attack or surgery on the heart or lungs.

Atrial flutter tends to occur in episodes lasting minutes or hours, with periods of normal heart rhythm separating the attacks. When an

A

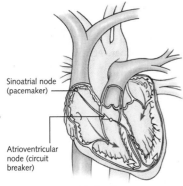

Sinoatrial node (pacemaker)

Atrioventricular node (circuit breaker)

Healthy heartbeat

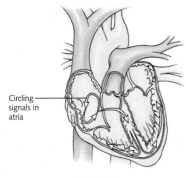

Circling signals in atria

Atrial flutter

KEY
⟹ Electrical signal ⟶ Blood flow

QUICKENED HEARTBEAT
If electrical problems in the heart cause the atria to beat too quickly, but evenly, the result is atrial flutter. Impulses travel in circles in the atria, causing the atria to beat far too rapidly. Some signals make it into the ventricles, which also beat too quickly.

attack occurs, it is likely to cause palpitations (the physical sensation of rapid heartbeat). If the attack is severe, chest pain, shortness of breath, lightheadedness, fainting, or fatigue can result.

The episodic nature of atrial flutter makes diagnosis difficult in some cases. A doctor using a stethoscope can listen for heart rhythms that indicate atrial flutter, usually suggested by the presence of a regular rapid pulse of approximately 150 beats per minute. An electrocardiogram (ECG) measures the electrical activity of the heart and can reveal an abnormal rhythm. The Holter monitor, which records a person's heartbeat, can be worn as he or she goes through nor-

mal activities for 1 or 2 days. An event recorder is particularly good for detecting occasional or sporadic episodes of atrial flutter and is typically worn by a person who can trigger the device to record when he or she experiences symptoms, such as palpitations and dizziness. The stress test is another type of ECG, in which readings are taken while the person exercises, typically on a treadmill or a stationary bicycle. In echocardiography, the heart is visualized with sound waves, and an image of the beating heart is displayed on a video screen, where the doctor can assess the thickness, size, and function of the heart.

A number of medications are useful for treating atrial flutter. Beta blockers, calcium channel blockers, and digoxin slow the overall heart rate, reduce the workload on the heart, and lower blood pressure. CARDIOVERSION uses drugs or electrical shock to return the heart to a normal rhythm.

Atrial natriuretic peptide
A hormone (chemical messenger) that is produced by the atria (upper chambers) of the heart to regulate blood pressure and fluid balance by its action on the kidneys. The name "atrial" comes from the hormone's origin in the cells of the atria and "natriuretic" refers to its role in excreting sodium in the urine.

Atrial septal defect
See SEPTAL DEFECT, ATRIAL.

Atrium
Either of the two upper chambers of the heart. The right atrium receives oxygen-depleted blood from the body and moves it into the right ventricle, where the blood is pumped into the lungs to dispose of waste products (carbon dioxide) and receive oxygen. The oxygen-rich blood then returns to the left atrium, passes into the left ventricle, and is pumped through the aorta into the rest of the body. The tricuspid valve divides the right atrium from the right ventricle, letting blood flow from the one into the other and preventing backwash. The mitral valve performs the same function between the left atrium and the left ventricle. See HEART.

Atrophy
Wasting or diminution in size or activity of a part of the body. Atrophy is caused by factors such as disease, aging, nutrition, immobility, and lack of exercise. For example, in a person who has polio, affected muscles decrease in size, or atrophy. As people age, the brain decreases in size, although this does not directly correlate with a decrease in intelligence or brain activity.

Atropine
A drug used to relax muscles by inhibiting nerve responses. Atropine is given by injection, as eye drops, or in oral form. It is used in emergency cardiac situations to speed up the heart rate. See ANTICHOLINERGIC AGENTS.

Attending physician
The physician in charge of a person's overall care in the hospital. The term is also used to refer to full-fledged members of a hospital medical staff. An attending physician may be a primary care doctor, a doctor on the hospital staff, or a specialist. In a teaching hospital, an attending physician also teaches and directs staff composed of medical students, residents (doctors who recently graduated from medical school and training in a specialty), and fellows (doctors have completed residency and are receiving training in a subspecialty).

Attention deficit disorder
See ATTENTION DEFICIT/HYPERACTIVITY DISORDER.

Attention deficit disorder, in adults
See ATTENTION DEFICIT/HYPERACTIVITY DISORDER.

Attention deficit/hyperactivity disorder
A mental illness characterized by difficulty paying attention and a high degree of restlessness and impulsive behavior; the name of the disorder is commonly abbreviated as ADHD. Symptoms begin before age 7, last for at least 6 months, and cause the child substantial difficulty in at least two settings, usually family and school.

HYPERACTIVITY OR INATTENTION
Attention deficit/hyperactivity disorder, or ADHD, may cause behavior that is inattentive, hyperactive, or a combination of both. A child whose behavior is impulsive or hyperactive may frequently interrupt or intrude on the activities of others, have difficulty playing quietly, or be unable to take turns.

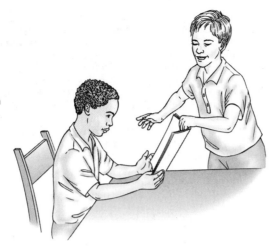

In some cases, the disorder resolves during adolescence. More often, it lasts into adulthood and becomes a lifelong condition, although the symptoms may be less pronounced than they were in childhood. ADHD is more common in males than in females.

TYPES AND SYMPTOMS
Psychiatrists distinguish among three types of ADHD, based on the relative amount of attention deficit versus hyperactivity. In the predominantly inattentive type, the individual fails to pay attention to details or makes careless mistakes, finds it difficult to attend to tasks or leisure activities, dislikes tasks requiring sustained concentration, fails to follow through on instructions, is forgetful, or is easily distracted. In the predominantly impulsive type, the individual fidgets or squirms when seated, leaves his or her seat at inappropriate times, moves restlessly, blurts out answers, talks excessively, interrupts or intrudes on others, and has difficulty waiting in line or for his or her turn. In the combined type, which is the most common, the individual exhibits symptoms of both attention deficit and hyperactivity. The combined type is found principally among elementary school boys; the inattentive type, among adolescent girls.

ADHD is often accompanied by other disorders. Approximately half of the children with the disorder are hostile and negative in their behavior, and a smaller number engage in aggressive behavior toward people or animals, vandalism, or breaking important rules. Anxiety and depression may also affect children and adults with ADHD. Untreated ADHD increases the risk of substance abuse, academic and vocational problems, marital discord, and emotional distress. There is also a connection between ADHD and TOURETTE SYNDROME, a disease of the nervous system that causes repeated involuntary movements called tics. Only a small number of people with ADHD have Tourette syndrome, but approximately half of those with Tourette have ADHD.

CAUSE
Studies show that ADHD is not caused by bad parenting, emotional problems in the family, excessive television viewing, food allergies, or too much sugar. Certain food additives may be responsible for a very small number of cases. Likewise, brain injuries account for only a small percentage of cases of ADHD.

Recent research points to the likelihood that ADHD is most often caused by biological factors that affect the chemical activity of the brain. Scientific studies that allow the researcher to view the brain as it works show a connection between an individual's ability to pay attention and brain activity. In people with ADHD, the areas of the brain that control impulsive behavior and focus attention are less active than in people without the disorder. It is believed this lower level of activity, which is thought to be related to abnormal activity of the brain chemical dopamine, leads to ADHD.

The reason for the altered activity of dopamine is uncertain. Some theories suggest that exposure of the fetus to cigarettes, drugs, or alcohol may be the cause. Since ADHD tends to run in families, it also appears that this pattern of brain activity is inherited. Children born into a family in which a parent or sibling has ADHD are much more likely to develop the disorder.

TREATMENT
ADHD is usually treated with a combination of medications to stabilize brain activity and counseling or therapy to help the individual learn how to cope with the disorder. The most commonly used medications are stimulants, such as methylphenidate (Ritalin), amphetamine, and pemoline (Cylert). All these medications increase the activity of dopamine and thus may help raise the level of activity in areas of the brain that control attention and impulse control. Antidepressants are also used, sometimes in combination with stimulants. Tranquilizers along with clonidine (Catapres), a medication to treat high blood pressure, have also proved useful.

Children with ADHD respond well to behavior therapy that rewards them for controlling impulses and learning how to focus. They also need patience and understanding from parents and teachers, and they benefit from classroom environments adapted to fit their needs and from individualized education plans developed in cooperation with the school district. For adults, coaching in skills that help them cope with problem behaviors, such as disorganization or having a lack of concentration, is often helpful. Support groups for parents of children with ADHD and for adults with the disorder can provide a social network that helps overcome feelings of isolation.

Treatments that have not been shown scientifically to work on people with ADHD include chiropractic adjustment, large doses of vitamins, biofeedback, special diets, allergy treatments, and wearing glasses with colored lenses.

Audiologist

A specialized health care professional who holds a master's or doctoral degree from an accredited university graduate program and is trained to identify, evaluate, and rehabilitate hearing loss, balance disorders, and related problems. Audiologists recommend and fit hearing aids and other rehabilitative devices. They may also provide and fit protective hearing devices and offer consultation on the effects of noise on hearing. Audiologists may also be involved in research related to hearing loss and balance disorders. Since audiologists are not physicians, they cannot treat infections or prescribe medication.

Audiology

The study of hearing. This branch of scientific study deals with the identification, assessment, and nonmedical management of auditory (hearing-related) and balance disorders.

Audiometry

Measurement of hearing ability using specific tests. The hearing tests are performed with specialized equipment in a doctor's office, in a free-standing facility, or in a hospital audiology department's soundproof testing room. The purpose of the tests is to diagnose hearing problems, including HEARING LOSS from any cause. The tests are painless, accurate, and take 30 to 45 minutes.

The first part of a typical test measures how well a person hears sounds that are conducted through air. The person being tested wears earphones and listens with one ear at a time to sound frequencies ranging from low tones to high tones. The second part of the test measures a person's ability to hear sounds conducted through the bones of the head. The person being tested may wear a special headband or earphones that vibrate against the head. In both parts of the test, the person raises a hand or presses a button to indicate which tones are heard. The level of sound increases from an inaudible level to a level that can just barely be heard. This level is known as that person's threshold for that frequency. A person's thresholds in both parts of the test are recorded on a graph called an audiogram, which displays the results in grid form. Hearing is evaluated by determining how well sound is transmitted through air compared with how well it is conducted through bone. This comparison helps to specify which part of the hearing mechanism is responsible for hearing loss.

Aura

An unusual sensation that is often a warning of an impending MIGRAINE headache or a SEIZURE, a sudden episode of uncontrolled electrical activity in the brain, causing a series of involuntary muscle transactions or a temporary lapse in consciousness. An aura may consist of a strange feeling, abnormal perceptions, or visual disturbances such as seeing stars or flashes. For example, preceding the onset of migraine pain, a person may experience a tingling sensation or see zigzagging lights. When it precedes a seizure, an aura may help identify the seizure's focal point in the brain. It is important to diagnose and treat the underlying disorder that is causing auras.

Auranofin

A drug used to treat rheumatoid arthritis. Auranofin (Ridaura) is taken orally as an anti-inflammatory agent and is thought to work by altering the immune system. It usually has fewer side effects than some other drugs used to treat rheumatoid arthritis.

Auricular therapy

See ACUPUNCTURE, EAR.

Autism

A nervous system disorder beginning in early childhood and characterized by impaired social interaction, problems with communication and imagination, and unusual or limited activities or interests. Doctors classify autism as one of the pervasive developmental disorders (see DEVELOPMENTAL DISORDER, PERVASIVE). It affects from 2 to 4 people in 10,000 and varies widely in its severity and symptoms. Some individuals are only mildly affected, while others exhibit extremely repetitive, unusual, aggressive, or self-injurious behavior. Autism is found in all races and social classes but is four times more common in males than in females. Some degree of mental retardation occurs in 75 percent of those affected. However, in some people, an inability to communicate and other symptoms conceal a considerable intelligence. Some individuals who have autism possess unique aptitudes that are often quite remarkable, such as musical ability.

SYMPTOMS

The symptoms of autism may be obvious from early infancy or may gradually become apparent in a child's first 2 to 3 years. Symptoms vary widely. Sometimes, parents mistake autism for deafness. Autistic infants may be quiet and passive or they can be agitated and cry a great deal. Some crawl and walk early for

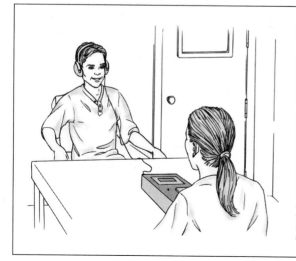

MEASURING SOUND RECEPTION
A typical hearing test is performed in a soundproof room, and the person wears earphones that emit tones or speech at varying volume levels. The listener indicates hearing tones with hand signals or words by repeating them. The person can take the test without special preparation; he or she can take usual medications—including decongestants or nasal sprays. A person who uses a hearing aid should bring it to the test center.

their age, while others experience considerable delay. Nearly always, there is a delay in the development of spoken language, particularly in conversational language.

Impaired social interaction is the hallmark symptom of autism. Many babies with autism avoid eye contact and fail to bond with parents. They may resist physical contact by stiffening or going limp when parents pick them up and try to cuddle them. Children with autism often have overly sensitive responses to touch, sounds, and other stimulation. As autistic children grow older, they have trouble interpreting the tones of voice and facial expressions of their peers. Making friends is difficult for them. Autistic children may avoid eye contact. They do not pick up on or use nonverbal cues about appropriate behavior. They seem unaware of the emotions of others. In severe cases, children appear oblivious to the presence of other people or to the effects their behavior has on others. Some children with autism engage in repetitive behaviors such as rocking and hand gestures, but those behaviors are also seen in children who do not have autism. Often, children with autism may have trouble sleeping and eating. Some appear to be excessively active.

Individuals with autism often repeat words or phrases over and over again in a singsong fashion. They typically have a narrow and unusual range of interests. Many dwell conversationally on their favorite topics with little or no regard for the interest of listeners. They can also be inflexibly wedded to specific rituals and routines. When those patterns are disturbed, they may become extremely upset. Some engage in self-injurious activities such as biting and head banging. Although they may hurt themselves, many people with autism have a reduced sensitivity to pain.

DIAGNOSIS AND TREATMENT

The exact cause of autism remains unknown. Researchers believe that a combination of genetic and environmental factors contribute to its development. Earlier theories suggesting that parental practices were responsible have been disproved. There is no specific medical test to diagnose autism. Children are diagnosed according to their symptoms and results of psychological testing. Because hearing problems can be confused with autism, children who experience delayed speech development also should have their hearing checked. An evaluation by a speech and language pathologist is important.

Treatment is designed to meet the individual needs of each child. Educational and behavioral interventions can help children to develop social and language skills. Therapists offer highly structured, skill-oriented training that is most effective when begun at a very young age. Child and adolescent psychiatrists or other physicians with special training in autism may prescribe medication to ameliorate symptoms, such as aggressive behavior. These drugs are thought to influence the balance of serotonin and other chemical messengers in the brain. Other medications are prescribed to control associated problems such as EPILEPSY or symptoms of overactivity or poor attention (see ATTENTION DEFICIT/ HYPERACTIVITY DISORDER). Because raising an autistic child is stressful and challenging, parents may find it beneficial to join a support group with other parents of autistic children. Counseling may also be helpful.

Outlook is often related to intellectual ability. Symptoms change over time, requiring different needs to be met. For example, adolescence may bring difficulties such as depression or increased behavior problems. Meanwhile, other symptoms may improve with treatment or as children mature. Only one of six children with autism grow up to be functionally independent adults. Some children with autism are able to live at home with their parents and follow largely normal lives. Severely autistic individuals may need to live in residential facilities or group homes.

Autoclave

The apparatus used to sterilize objects by steam under pressure. Autoclaves are used to destroy microorganisms on medical equipment to prevent infection and the spread of disease. The autoclave

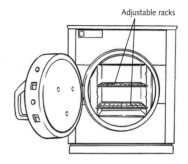

Adjustable racks

STERILIZING UNIT
An autoclave sterilizes surgical instruments with hot steam at temperatures of 250°F. The instruments are placed on perforated racks in the unit and undergo a 15-minute steam cycle and a 10-minute drying cycle.

works in the same way a pressure cooker does, allowing steam to flow around all objects placed in the chamber. The steam is able to penetrate cloth or paper packaging to sterilize the contents.

Autoimmune disorders

Disorders that occur as a result of a mistaken IMMUNE RESPONSE to the body's tissues. Autoimmune disorders develop when a HYPERSENSITIVITY reaction causes the immune system to respond inappropriately, excessively, or inadequately. Normally, the immune system defends the body against potentially harmful agents, called antigens, including microorganisms such as bacteria that can cause illness, in addition to toxins, cancer cells, blood, and transplanted tissue donated by another person. The introduction of these agents into the body causes the immune system to attack the foreign substances.

Usually, the immune system can differentiate between antigens that enter the body and a person's own body tissues. But when the immune system attacks naturally existing body tissues, an autoimmune disorder results. This occurs when a normal control process within the immune system malfunctions for unknown reasons. It is possible that certain microorganisms or medications trigger the malfunction, especially in people who have inherited a susceptibility to autoimmune disorders. This disruption in the immune system's normal controls

A

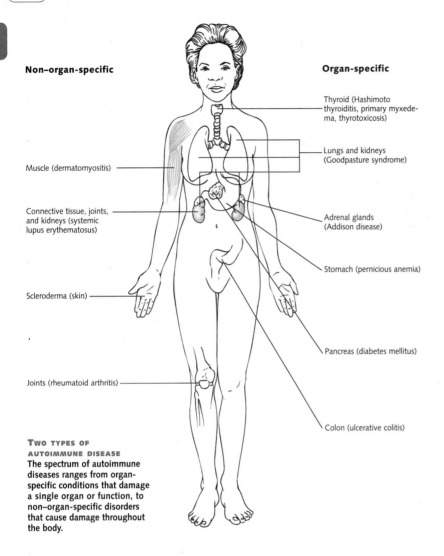

Non–organ-specific

Organ-specific

Thyroid (Hashimoto thyroiditis, primary myxedema, thyrotoxicosis)

Muscle (dermatomyositis)

Lungs and kidneys (Goodpasture syndrome)

Connective tissue, joints, and kidneys (systemic lupus erythematosus)

Adrenal glands (Addison disease)

Stomach (pernicious anemia)

Scleroderma (skin)

Joints (rheumatoid arthritis)

Pancreas (diabetes mellitus)

Colon (ulcerative colitis)

TWO TYPES OF AUTOIMMUNE DISEASE
The spectrum of autoimmune diseases ranges from organ-specific conditions that damage a single organ or function, to non–organ-specific disorders that cause damage throughout the body.

can prompt some lymphocytes to become sensitized to the body's own tissues. Or sometimes, the mistaken response may occur when normal body tissue undergoes changes that interfere with the immune system's ability to recognize it as a natural part of the body.

Autoimmune disorders can destroy one or more organs or types of body tissues. The resulting destruction of tissue can cause abnormal growth of an organ or changes in the organ's function. Tissues of the muscles, joints, and skin are commonly affected. Blood components, including red blood cells and blood vessels, can also be destroyed by autoimmune disorders, as can connective tissues and endocrine glands, including the thyroid and the pancreas. Kidney disease can also occur.

Autoimmune responses can occur in several ways. There may be an interaction between the body's molecules and another reactive agent, such as a reactive chemical or infectious agent. The result may be an altered body molecule that is subject to attack by the immune system. Autoimmune responses can also occur when an antigen that is normally hidden by the immune system suddenly becomes visible. Having never been seen by the immune system, it is recognized as foreign and subsequently attacked. Another way autoimmune responses can occur is through a process called reactive antigens. For example, rheumatic fever may result from cross-reactivity between bacterial *Streptococcus* antigens and heart tissue.

SIGNS, SYMPTOMS, AND DIAGNOSIS
Signs and symptoms of autoimmune disorders are related to the specific disease or condition that results and the tissues or organs affected. These include RHEUMATOID ARTHRITIS, systemic lupus erythematosus (see LUPUS ERYTHEMATOSUS, SYSTEMIC), ADDISON DISEASE, diabetes mellitus (see DIABETES MELLITUS, TYPE 1; DIABETES MELLITUS, TYPE 2), HASHIMOTO THYROIDITIS, MULTIPLE SCLEROSIS, REITER SYNDROME, SJÖGREN SYNDROME, and GRAVES DISEASE.

Nonspecific symptoms are frequently associated with all disorders related to autoimmunity. These include a tendency to tire quickly or be easily fatigued, dizziness, general malaise, weight loss, and a low-grade fever. Autoimmune disorders may be diagnosed with a specialized blood test that may reveal increased amounts of white blood cells and elevated levels of certain proteins called complements, as well as specific immunoglobulins or antigens.

TREATMENT
Symptoms and deficiencies related to specific disorders are treated accordingly. If the disorder results in insufficient hormones or other substances essential to normal body functions, vitamins, thyroid supplements, insulin, or other medications can be taken or administered to compensate for the deficiency. If components of the blood are affected, blood transfusions may become necessary. If the bones, joints, or muscles are affected, therapies and equipment to aid in the performance of everyday activities can become part of treatment.

Most autoimmune disorders are chronic, but they can be managed with proper medical treatment of specific symptoms and of the underlying disorder. Treatment of autoimmunity strives to control the autoimmune process and maintain the body's ability to defend itself against disease. This involves controlling immunity by means of a balanced suppression of the immune system: the immune response against normal body tissue needs to be reduced, and the immune response to potentially harmful antigens or abnormal tissues needs to be preserved. Controlling the immune response may be accomplished with corticosteroids and immunosuppressants, such as cyclophosphamide and azathioprine. Side effects to these medications can sometimes be severe and must be weighed against beneficial effects.

Autologous blood donation

Donation of one's own blood to oneself. Autologous blood donation may be used by people with a scheduled surgical procedure to ensure that any blood they may require during the surgery will be their own. The blood is drawn and stored before surgery in sufficient time to allow the body to replace the red blood cells. Blood may be stored for up to 42 days from the day of donation. The advantage of autologous blood donation is that it is the safest blood available.

Autologous bone marrow transplant

See BONE MARROW TRANSPLANT, AUTOLOGOUS.

Automatism

A condition in which a person performs or acts without awareness of what he or she is doing and without any memory of the acts afterward; also known as automatic behavior. Sleepwalking is an example. Other examples of automatism include lip smacking, swallowing, chewing, pacing, humming, or mumbling. These symptoms usually last only about a minute. As with other instances of automatism, a sleepwalking person may appear to function normally, but he or she shows no signs of personality. Automatism may represent a trance following severe trauma, and it can also be a sign of certain forms of EPILEPSY, migraine, and some mental diseases.

Autonomic nervous system

The part of the NERVOUS SYSTEM that controls involuntary activities, such as blood pressure and heartbeat. The autonomic nervous system consists of a network of nerves divided into two parts: the parasympathetic nervous system and the sympathetic nervous system. The two systems act together and normally balance each other. The parasympathetic nervous system predominates during times of relaxation, acting to conserve and restore energy. The sympathetic nervous system prepares the body to cope during times of stress. It quickens the heartbeat and the breathing rate as if it were preparing for a FIGHT-OR-FLIGHT RESPONSE.

Autopsy

Examination of a body after death. An autopsy, a legal and medical procedure also called a postmortem examination, is performed by a medical examiner or by a pathologist to establish the cause of a death or to detect

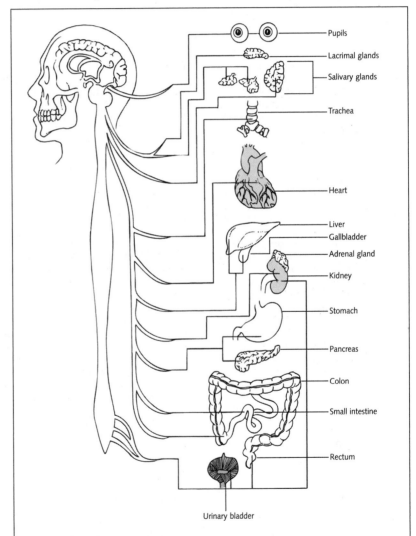

Pupils
Lacrimal glands
Salivary glands
Trachea
Heart
Liver
Gallbladder
Adrenal gland
Kidney
Stomach
Pancreas
Colon
Small intestine
Rectum
Urinary bladder

FUNCTION OF AUTONOMIC NERVOUS SYSTEM
The autonomic nervous system controls the involuntary action of various organs or body parts when the body is at rest and also when it is under stress. Various nerves control various parts of the body as shown.

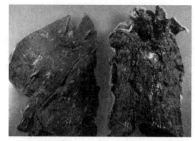

Normal lung   Smoker's lung

POSTMORTEM EXAMINATION
An autopsy can plainly establish the presence and extent of disease. The healthy lung contrasts with that removed from the body of a smoker.

the presence or absence of disease or injury. Injury can be the result of physical trauma or medical procedures. An autopsy involves a detailed dissection of a body, using surgical procedures to conduct a systematic external and internal examination. Chemical analyses of body fluids for medical information and detection of the presence of drugs and poisons are usually part of an autopsy. Various laboratory tests may be undertaken, and X rays may be done; organs may be examined for evidence of infection.

When a death has occurred as the result of a suspected crime, an autopsy may be ordered by legal authorities to gather evidence for use in judicial proceedings. An autopsy is also used to investigate contagious diseases and industrial hazards that may threaten public health. With the approval of the next of kin, an autopsy can be used to remove corneas and internal organs for transplant and to help educate physicians and improve care by providing feedback on treatment and diagnosis. An autopsy can help to establish a family's risk for developing certain diseases. It may also provide important information to family members when a death has been unexplained. However, an insurance company may not agree to pay for it.

Autosomal dominant traits

Hereditary traits carried by genes that are more likely to be expressed than those of other genes. A dominant trait expresses itself regardless of the function of its corresponding gene. For example, a person who inherits the genes for brown eyes and blue eyes will have brown eyes because that is the dominant trait. An individual needs only one copy of the dominant gene to be affected. This means that if one parent carries the trait, offspring have a 50 percent chance of inheriting it. A dominant gene may be inherited, or it may occur due to a spontaneous mutation that causes dominance of a particular gene.

Autosomal recessive traits

Hereditary traits carried by genes that are expressed only when an individual has two copies of the gene. A child needs to inherit the affected gene from both parents for the genetic trait to be expressed. When a disease is inherited as an autosomal recessive trait, the parents do not usually have the disease themselves but are symptomless carriers. Examples of autosomal recessive disorders include Tay-Sachs disease, sickle cell anemia, and albinism. See also AUTOSOMAL DOMINANT TRAITS.

Avascular necrosis of femoral head

A hip disorder in children. Avascular necrosis causes pain and stiffness in the affected thigh and limited range of motion in the hip joint. A child with this condition may limp. The condition is caused by the death of bone cells at the top of the thighbone due to a poor blood supply. It can result from an injury to the blood vessels that supply the femur. Taking a corticosteroid drug (see CORTICOSTEROIDS) for an extended period or having sickle cell anemia increases the risk for developing avascular necrosis.

DIAGNOSIS AND TREATMENT

Avascular necrosis is diagnosed by creating images of the thighbone, using radionuclide scanning, MRI (magnetic resonance imaging), or X rays, that will show abnormalities in the bone. Medication can reduce the pain and swelling, while physical therapy may help maintain the full range of motion in the hip. In some children, surgery is necessary to repair avascular necrosis. In the early stages, a surgeon can remove dying bone and replace it with new bone. In the advanced stages, the entire hip joint may need replacement. In a form of avascular necrosis called Legg disease (also called Legg-Calvé-Perthes disease; see OSTEOCHONDROSIS), the problem resolves itself as blood supply to the femur is restored on its own.

Aversion therapy

A technique used to stop or alter an unwanted behavior by coupling that behavior with an unpleasant or painful experience. Aversion therapy has been used, for example, to help a person stop smoking by giving an electrical shock or a nausea-producing drug when the person smokes a cigarette. Repeated over time, the pairing of the desire for tobacco with the shock or nausea produces a disagreeable emotional reaction to cigarettes that eventually leads the person to avoid smoking. Aversion therapy has also been used to eliminate self-mutilation in autistic children, and to reduce or eliminate sexual deviant behavior. Nausea-producing drugs have also been used as aversion therapy to treat alcoholism. These drugs interfere with the metabolism of alcohol and produce extremely unpleasant side effects. Nausea and vomiting, for example, occur if even a small amount of alcohol is ingested within 2 weeks of taking the drugs. (Aversion therapy for alcoholism is often used in conjunction with counseling.)

Aviation medicine

The branch of medicine that focuses on the special health and medical problems associated with flight, such as HYPOXIA (reduced oxygen concentration in blood and tissues), JET LAG, BAROTRAUMA, dehydration, restricted body movement, blood clots, and ear pain. Aviation medicine also encompasses the assessment of the fitness of crew members and passengers to fly, the management of medical emergencies in the air, and the investigation of aircraft accidents.

AVM

See ARTERIOVENOUS MALFORMATION.

Avoidant personality disorder

See PERSONALITY DISORDERS.

Avulsed tooth

A tooth that has been completely dislodged from its socket by excessive pressure or accidental trauma. Sometimes called traumatic avulsion, a tooth that has been knocked out requires immediate treatment by a dentist. If the person is bleeding, a clean piece of gauze or tissue should be folded into a pad and placed over the tooth wound. The tooth should be placed in a cup of milk to be taken to the dentist. If milk is unavailable, the tooth may be placed in cool water or saline (salt) solution or wrapped in clean wet cloth or gauze. It should not be placed in tap water because the minerals in the water can harm the tooth.

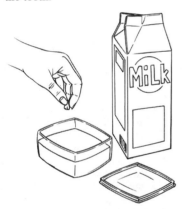

PRESERVING A KNOCKED-OUT TOOTH
If a person's tooth is knocked out, the tooth should be carefully preserved to keep it alive until a dentist can treat the person. If possible, the tooth should be placed in cold, whole milk, in a container with a tight-fitting lid. The milk (whole, not skim) contains nutrients that help keep the tooth alive.

Getting to the dentist quickly can make the difference between saving the tooth and losing it. The tooth must be replaced in the mouth before a blood clot forms in the socket, usually within 2 hours. When the person arrives at the dentist's office, the tooth will be disinfected and placed back in its socket. Often, the tooth will be attached to its adjacent teeth for a couple of weeks, until it tightens. Periodic checkups will be necessary to check for nerve damage.

Axilla

Underarm; armpit. The axilla is the cavity underneath the area where the arm joins the body.

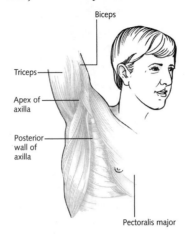

Biceps

Triceps

Apex of axilla

Posterior wall of axilla

Pectoralis major

MUSCULAR ARMPIT
The armpit, or axilla, is the hollow created between the major muscles of the arm, shoulder, and chest, including the biceps and triceps, the latissimus dorsi, and the pectoralis major.

Axillary lymph node dissection

Removal of some or all of the LYMPH NODES in the underarm area, typically as part of breast cancer surgery (see MASTECTOMY; LUMPECTOMY). Axilla is the medical name for the armpit. Since cancer cells spread from their point of origin through the LYMPHATIC SYSTEM, testing of the removed nodes can determine whether the cancer has traveled beyond the breast.

A patient who has undergone an axillary lymph node dissection experiences temporary soreness, numbness, or a combination of the two along the length of the arm to the wrist. Sometimes, the pain is confined to the triceps area. Very brief but intense pain may flow down the arm and into the hand for months after surgery. Small pillows should be placed under the arm during rest or sleep to elevate it. It is important to use the arm as soon as possible after surgery and to follow any prescribed exercise regimen to regain full range of motion. Occasionally, axillary node dissection causes lymphedema, a condition in which the arm swells with lymphatic fluid because it is not draining normally. Cuts, scrapes, and other injuries to the affected arm should be avoided, and any sign of infection—redness, additional swelling, numbness, pain, warmth—requires immediate medical attention.

Ayurveda

Ancient system of healing and health care that includes yoga, meditation, and herbal remedies. Ayurveda origi-

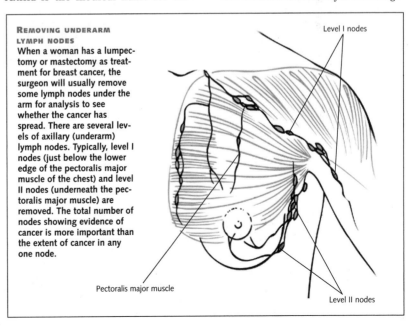

REMOVING UNDERARM LYMPH NODES
When a woman has a lumpectomy or mastectomy as treatment for breast cancer, the surgeon will usually remove some lymph nodes under the arm for analysis to see whether the cancer has spread. There are several levels of axillary (underarm) lymph nodes. Typically, level I nodes (just below the lower edge of the pectoralis major muscle of the chest) and level II nodes (underneath the pectoralis major muscle) are removed. The total number of nodes showing evidence of cancer is more important than the extent of cancer in any one node.

Level I nodes

Pectoralis major muscle

Level II nodes

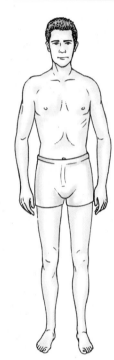

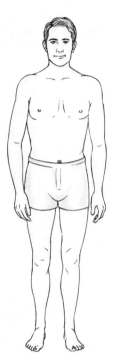

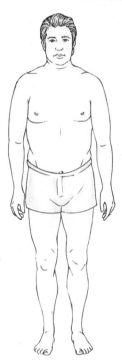

AYURVEDA: COMBINATIONS OF ELEMENTS
Ayurveda beliefs describe three doshas, or combinations of elements, that tend to indicate a person's general body type, personal qualities, and predisposition to certain health problems. Any one person may be made up of more than one dosha, although one predominates. The three doshas are evaluated by taking the pulse at the radial artery, a technique known as nadi vigyan. It is by this technique that an ayurvedic practitioner is able to determine which herbs and other ayurvedic therapies should be administered to treat a person's ailments.

Vatha (thin, dark skin, highly creative, often constipated)

Pitta (medium build, fair-skinned passionate, large appetite)

Kapha (large, overweight, good memory, sweats copiously)

ELEMENTS OF AYURVEDA

To restore and maintain a healthy balance, the practitioner of ayurveda will likely follow a health plan that consists of the following:

- Yoga postures and yoga breathing exercises
- Meditation used to quiet the mind and listen to the inner body
- Dietary practices intended to bring the person into balance and harmony, including the use of HERBAL MEDICINE and the practice of occasional fasting to detoxify the body
- Massages and baths with or without herbal oils

nated in India 3,500 years ago and is a complex science made up of physical, psychological, and spiritual components. Ayurveda is chiefly devoted to the promotion of good health, the prevention of disease, and personal growth, although ayurvedic practices are used to treat health problems as well. Ayurveda is a word from Sanskrit that means "the science of life"; the method is practiced by more than 300,000 doctors worldwide.

Ayurveda is based on the idea that a person's lifestyle is the source of disease. The goal of ayurveda is to restore and maintain the person's balance, which is a function of diet, environment, climate, thought patterns, and emotions.

Azithromycin

An antibiotic used to treat chlamydial and bacterial infections of the skin and respiratory tract. Azithromycin (Zithromax) is a derivative of erythromycin. It is associated with several side effects, including nausea, diarrhea, dizziness, sensitivity to sunlight, and vaginal candidiasis (yeast infection).

Azoospermia

The absence of sperm cells in a man's semen, the thick white liquid expelled from the penis at sexual climax. Azoospermia results in infertility. The condition is generally due to a disorder of the testicles or an obstruction in the passageways leading from the testicles. These disorders include hormonal imbalances; cystic fibrosis, which in many cases prevents development of vas deferens, the tube that transports sperm cells from the testicles; and exposure to certain chemicals and medications, X rays, or radioactive materials. An obstruction can be caused by a disease that inflames and scars the reproductive tract, such as mumps in adolescent or adult men, or it can be a complication of surgery.

Treatment depends on the cause of the condition. Some types of hormonal imbalances can be treated with medication, and in certain cases, obstructions must be repaired surgically.

AZT

See ZIDOVUDINE.

B

B cell

A type of white blood cell; B lympho-cyte. B cells are formed in the bone marrow and circulate in the blood and lymphatic system. They have an essen-tial role in immunology. Many B cells mature into plasma cells, which manu-facture antibodies, proteins necessary to fight infections. Other B cells mature into memory B cells that "remember" the antigen that originally stimulated them to mature. This allows the body to recognize the antigen as a foreign body if it reencounters it in the future and to make antibodies to destroy it. For example, if a person is exposed to a particular bacterium, antibodies are formed to coat it. This coating then allows other white blood cells to destroy the bacteria and prevents an infection from developing. Once anti-bodies are formed, whenever the body is reexposed to the same bacteria the body recognizes the infectious organ-ism and starts making antibodies to combat it.

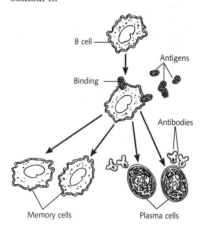

SMART CELLS
During invasion by a disease organism, certain B cells identify the specific invader (antigen) and bind to it. Then they multiply quickly, becoming either memory cells, which develop antibodies to stop future infections by the same antigen, or plasma cells, which develop antibodies that seek out that antigen in the body and destroy it.

Babesiosis

A rare disease caused by a parasite that is transmitted to people who are bitten by infected ticks. The parasite attacks the red blood cells. Babesiosis is rare in humans, but potentially fatal. Common in animals, the infec-tion is similar to LYME DISEASE in that it is spread by deer ticks, which are generally carried on deer, meadow moles, and mice. A person can be infected with both babesiosis and Lyme disease at the same time.

Most people who become infected have no symptoms, but people who are older or ill with other conditions may experience the symptoms of babesio-sis. These may first appear within 1 month to 1 year after exposure and include fatigue and loss of appetite. As the infection grows more severe, symp-toms may include fever, chills, drench-ing sweats, muscle aches, jaundice, and headache. The infection is diag-nosed by laboratory analysis of a blood test that identifies the parasite in the red blood cells. Babesiosis is treated with a combination of antiparasite medications. There is no vaccine avail-able against the infection.

RISK FACTORS

The symptoms of babesiosis may appear earlier and be more pro-nounced in older people, those with weakened immune systems, and espe-cially people who have had their spleens removed, for whom complica-tions and death are more likely. People who do not have these risk factors tend to have a milder illness, often without symptoms and often improving with-out treatment. Complications of the infection may include very low blood pressure, liver problems, severe ane-mia, and kidney failure.

Babesiosis occurs principally in the spring, summer, and fall, in coastal areas of the United States, especially on the offshore islands of New York and Massachusetts, but cases of babesiosis have been reported in Georgia, California, and Wisconsin, as well as in some countries of Europe. Babesiosis is currently con-sidered a health threat throughout the United States, as cases of the infec-tion and deaths have occurred in areas where the risk of infection was not believed to exist previously.

Babinski reflex

An abnormal reflex response to stimu-lation of the plantar (bottom) surface of the foot indicating upper MOTOR NEU-RON DISEASE (damage to the brain or spinal cord). During a neurological examination, people demonstrating a Babinski reflex will extend and point their great toe up in response to irritat-ing stimulation along the bottom of the foot, which indicates an abnormality in the brain or spinal cord (central nervous system).

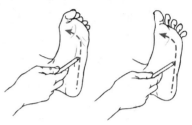

Healthy response   Babinski reflex

TESTING A REFLEX
Doctors check for the Babinski reflex to test motor nerve function. In a healthy person, stroking the side of the sole of the foot caus-es the toes to curl downward. A person with some nerve damage in the brain or spinal cord will respond with the Babinski reflex: the big toe bends up, and the smaller toes fan out.

Baby bottle tooth decay

TOOTH DECAY in children younger than 3 years caused by sugar-contain-ing liquids. The main cause of bottle caries is the practice of allowing a child to suck on a bottle of milk, for-mula, fruit juice, or other sweet drinks throughout the day or while in bed. These liquids cling to the teeth for hours, especially while the child is sleeping, since saliva flow and swallowing are reduced then. The bacteria in the mouth interact with the natural or refined sugars in the liquid, forming acids that can dis-solve the tooth enamel and decay the teeth. Ultimately, the decayed teeth may be lost. Usually the upper front teeth (the incisors and canines) and the lower back teeth (the molars) are most affected.

Decay can begin in the PRIMARY TEETH when a child is as young as 8 months old. These teeth are impor-tant to the appearance of a child, as well as to his or her ability to learn to speak and to chew properly. The pri-mary teeth hold spaces in the mouth and jaw for the development of the PERMANENT TEETH. When they are lost too early, the adjacent teeth may shift position, blocking the correct align-

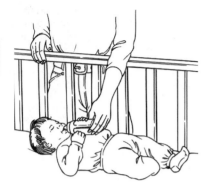

PROTECTING BABY TEETH
Baby bottle tooth decay may develop in a child who is allowed to suck on a bottle of milk, formula, or juice while in bed. The liquids cling to the teeth and cause decay, and the problem is worse when a child is sleeping because he or she is not producing as much saliva or swallowing as much as during waking hours. Parents can help prevent this form of tooth decay by taking the bottle away altogether at bedtime.

ment of the emerging permanent teeth. This can cause crowding, MAL-OCCLUSION (improper bite), or both, requiring treatment by a dentist who specializes in ORTHODONTICS.

PREVENTION
Children should not be permitted to fall asleep with a bottle of milk, formula, fruit juice, or any other sweet liquid, nor should they continually suck on a bottle of these drinks. Cool water in a bottle can be given for comfort at nap time and at night. A clean pacifier recommended by a physician or dentist may also be given; pacifiers should never be dipped in sweet liquids, sugar, jelly, or honey. After feedings, the gums of the child can be wiped clean with a damp washcloth or moistened gauze. As soon as the first tooth appears, it should be brushed gently with the use of a soft, small toothbrush. When most or all of the baby teeth have appeared, flossing should be added to the brushing routine. Children who are 1½ years old should be drinking primarily from a cup; it is suggested that a child be taught to use a cup as he or she approaches the first birthday. Any red or swollen area in the mouth or dark spots on the teeth of a child should be evaluated by a dentist. Regular dental visits should be started by a child's first birthday.

Baby teeth
See PRIMARY TEETH.

Bach flower remedies
Homeopathic remedies derived from plants and flowers intended to treat the emotions. The 38 Bach flower remedies are thought to work by balancing the emotions and helping people to feel better about themselves and their lives. Developed by British doctor Edward Bach in the 1930s, the Bach flower remedies reflect their inventor's belief that physical illness stems from an unhealthy mental state. Each remedy is designed to address a particular disturbing mood or attitude—the remedy for doubt or discouragement, for example, is gentian.

Bacilli
Rod-shaped BACTERIA, some of which cause disease by infecting the body. Bacilli can cause anthrax, a potentially lethal germ disease, as well as dysentery, tetanus, diphtheria, and tuberculosis.

Bacitracin zinc
An antibiotic available as a cream, spray, or ointment used to treat infections from minor cuts, scrapes, or burns. Bacitracin is widely available without a prescription, both as a brand name and a generic product. It treats or prevents infections caused by many bacteria, including various types of *Staphylococcus* and *Streptococcus* organisms.

Back pain

FOR SYMPTOM CHART
see Backache, page 20

Discomfort, ranging from mild and intermittent aches to constant and severe pain, at any point along the spine. Back pain is common, with eight of ten people experiencing it at some point in their lives. Back pain occurs most commonly in the lower region of the spine, which bears the majority of the body's weight. Lower back pain is sometimes called lumbago. The medical terms describing the different types of back pain are acute, subacute, and chronic. Acute back pain is a mild to severe, short-lived discomfort, possibly caused by an accident or injury, and usually lasting from 1 to 7 days. Subacute refers to pain that

is not related to other illnesses or conditions; it is usually mild, though sometimes severe, and lasts from a week to several months. Chronic back pain may be mild to severe; it either lasts a long time or occurs frequently, generally over a period of 3 months or more, and may be related to other illnesses or conditions.

CAUSES
Back pain is a common health problem in the United States, although its specific cause is often not clear. The source of back pain is often the result of a spasm of the muscles with pressure on the nerves in the back. A minor injury or a change in any single component of the spine's carefully balanced structure can produce pain with movement. This pain, due to spinal imbalance, may be the result of overuse, fatigue, or injury of related muscles and joints. Poor posture, lack of muscle tone in the abdomen, or the back, lack of exercise, and obesity (particularly extra weight in the abdominal area) can cause or aggravate an aching back. Emotional stress may be involved in back pain and is known to slow the rate of recovery.

Back pain is often the result of injuries caused by sudden or unexpected movements of the back, which produce muscle strain. These injuries may result in severely painful muscle spasms that usually last from 2 to 3 days, after which the pain subsides and lingers for a few more days or weeks. Mild back injuries may take up to 4 weeks to heal completely; if muscle strain is severe or if ligaments have been strained, recovery may take up to 12 weeks. Stresses or injuries to the back may result in inflamed joints along the spine or strained, stretched, or torn muscles, tendons, or ligaments along the backbone, all of which produce pain.

TYPES OF BACK PAIN
OSTEOARTHRITIS produces bony spurs on the vertebrae of the spine and narrows the disks that cushion them. This can put pressure on nerves exiting the spinal canal and produce back pain. Osteoarthritis is a result of degenerating cartilage in the vertebrae, as well as degeneration of the disks, and is considered a common component of aging.

Polymyalgia rheumatica is a joint disorder that can cause pain in the lower back lasting several months or

BACK PAIN EXERCISES

Regular exercise can help strengthen and stretch your back. Try doing this series of exercises for at least 15 minutes. If you have back pain or other health problems such as osteoporosis, talk to your doctor before exercising your back.

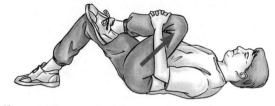

KNEE TO SHOULDER STRETCH
Lie on your back on a firm surface with knees bent and feet flat. Pull your right knee toward your chest with both hands. Hold that position for 15 to 30 seconds. Return to the starting position and repeat the exercise with the left knee. Repeat with each leg three to four times.

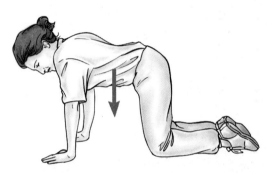

"CAT" STRETCH, STEP 1
Get down on your hands and knees, with hands and arms spread apart the width of your body. Let your back and abdomen sag toward the floor.

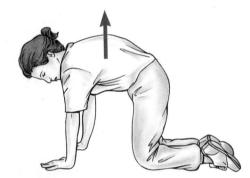

"CAT" STRETCH, STEP 2
Slowly round or arch your back away from the floor. Hold for several seconds and repeat the movement three to four times.

HALF SIT-UP
Lie on your back on a firm surface with your feet flat and knees bent. Stretch your arms toward your knees until your shoulder blades lift off the ground. Do not hold your knees, but keep the reaching position for a few seconds before returning slowly to starting position. Repeat several times.

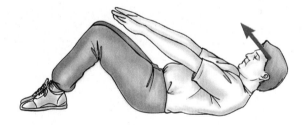

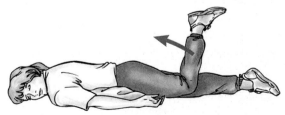

LEG LIFT 1
Lie face down on a firm surface with a large pillow under your hips and lower abdomen. Keep one leg flat to the ground, but raise the other knee until it is bent with the bottom of the foot facing upward. Hold the position for about 5 seconds and repeat on each leg several times.

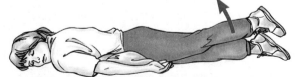

LEG LIFT 2
With the pillow still tucked under your hips and lower abdomen, raise one leg slightly just a foot or so off the ground and hold the position for about 5 seconds. Switch to the other leg and repeat the exercise for each leg several times.

B

One way to prevent back pain may be as simple as learning how to lift properly. Many back injuries are caused when a person tries to lift an object much too heavy or when an individual uses an improper technique. Here are some strategies for correct lifting:

- First, test the load before lifting. A person should push the object lightly with his or her hands or feet to see how easily it moves. If it is too heavy, get help or try breaking the package down, if possible, into smaller loads.
- Do not arch the back when lifting over the head.
- Take care to keep the load close to the body and bend from the hips and knees, not the back.
- Use slow and smooth movements.
- Keep the body facing the object before trying to lift it.
- Only "lift with the legs" if it is possible to straddle the load. To lift with the legs, bend the knees to pick up the load, not the back. Keep the back straight.
- Try to carry the load close to the body in the space between the shoulder and the waist; this puts less strain on back muscles.

years. (See MYALGIA.) FIBROMYALGIA produces pain and stiffness in muscles and tendons, especially in the neck and upper back. Back pain is sometimes but not always a symptom of PAGET DISEASE, a disorder of uneven calcium distribution in the bone.

A ruptured intervertebral disk (see DISK, INTERVERTEBRAL) is a painful condition sometimes called a herniated or SLIPPED DISK. An injury, simple bending and lifting, or no apparent trauma may precede the pain of a slipped disk. When a disk moves out of place and bulges into the spinal canal, it presses on nerve endings, irritating them and causing severe pain. If the disk compresses the roots of spinal nerves, back pain, muscle spasms, and SCIATICA result. Sciatic pain, as well as numbness, radiates into the hip, down the leg, and sometimes into the foot. This pain is often worsened by coughing or sneezing. This kind of pain warrants medical attention because the disk's continuing pressure on the spinal nerve may damage the nerve and weaken surrounding muscles.

SPINAL STENOSIS, the narrowing of the spinal canal, is another factor in back pain caused by compression of the spinal nerves, which results in numbness and weakness in the legs in addition to pain. ANKYLOSING SPONDYLITIS is a form of arthritis that causes the joints in the spine to become stiff, producing back pain.

Back pain may also be caused by OSTEOPOROSIS, which produces small fractures of the spine's vertebrae, usually in postmenopausal women. REITER SYNDROME produces arthritis

and back pain, generally in adult men. SPONDYLOLISTHESIS causes back pain as a result of the forward shifting of one vertebra onto another, which puts pressure on nerves. Infection of the spinal fluid is a cause of back pain that is sometimes confused with a ruptured disk because the symptoms are similar. It is diagnosed by withdrawal and analysis of a sample of spinal fluid. Back pain can also be a symptom of spinal tumors, which are generally detected by MRI (magnetic resonance imaging).

DIAGNOSIS

Back pain is rarely a symptom of a serious illness or disorder. The exception to that is if a child has back pain that awakens him or her while sleeping; an immediate evaluation should be sought by a doctor because the pain may be due to an infection or a tumor. If a person of any age develops serious back pain after a fall or other physical trauma to the spine, a doctor should be contacted immediately. Timely medical attention should also be sought if one or both legs feel weak or numb or if bladder or bowel problems occur.

A physician or orthopedist can diagnose back pain by physically examining the back and possibly the abdomen, the rectum, and the pelvis. The doctor may also evaluate general muscle tone, deep tendon reflexes, and posture. X rays, as well as CT (computed tomography) and MRI examinations, may be performed, especially if a disk problem is suspected. In addition, a diskogram, in which the intervertebral disk itself is injected with a contrast material and

then visualized, may also be done. In some cases, a myelogram (X ray involving the injection of a contrast solution into the spine; see MYELOGRAPHY) may be necessary to produce a clear image of the affected disk. Bone scans, involving the injection of a small amount of radioactive liquid that is concentrated in the bones for a short time, can reveal damage to spinal bones or tumors in the spine. Electrodiagnostic studies can confirm the presence of nerve compression at the spine. Blood tests can determine the presence of an illness such as rheumatoid arthritis.

TREATMENT

If back pain is mild to moderate, the prescribed course of treatment may be a few days of bed rest with the use of medications, including over-the-counter aspirin or acetaminophen, prescription nonsteroidal anti-inflammatory drugs (NSAIDs), or muscle relaxants. Injections of corticosteroids may be given in some cases. Physical therapy treatments may be prescribed, including alternating applications of heat and cold, gentle massage, and exercises designed to improve flexibility, strengthen the muscles of the back and abdomen, and improve posture. A physical therapist may also be instructed to use a procedure called transcutaneous electrical nerve stimulation (TENS), which involves the placement of electrodes on the skin near the painful area to block nerve signals from traveling to the brain. TRACTION treatment in a hospital setting may be used to relieve pressure on spinal nerves. In some cases, orthopedic braces (see BRACE, ORTHOPEDIC) that support the back may be prescribed for short periods on occasions when there is undue stress on the spine. A physician may refer a person who suffers from back pain to a program in back education, sometimes called a back school, which is available in some communities. The course teaches the anatomy and function of the spine, offers practice sessions on how to protect the back in common situations, and demonstrates techniques for managing pain and preventing the recurrence of problems.

Surgery may be a last resort in the treatment of back pain, usually only becoming an option when there is constant pain with increasing muscle weakness from compression of a spinal nerve. Surgical procedures for back pain include the following: A herniated disk may be surgically removed. LAMINECTOMY is a surgical procedure for the purpose of relieving leg pain, rather than back pain, and involves the removal of bone spurs or disk fragments. This can often be performed through a small keyhole-like incision using a microscope. Fusion is a surgical technique, which may involve the use of metal implants, with the goal of eliminating pain caused by the movement of vertebrae by joining two vertebrae together. Fusion is generally considered as a treatment in cases of an unstable spine or following a laminectomy when there is degenerative SPONDYLOLISTHESIS. Sometimes, the spine is fused in both the front and back. Injections into intervertebral disks, as well as electrocautery (electric heat), are alternatives to surgery in the treatment of ruptured disks.

PREVENTION

Measures to protect the back and prevent future incidents of back pain or the exacerbation of existing pain may be learned from a physician or orthopedist, from a physical therapist, or from a program of back education. Elements of good posture, healthy body weight, proper rest and sleep positions, correct positions for lifting, and exercises to strengthen back muscles are all essential to preventing back pain.

Baclofen

A skeletal muscle relaxant. Baclofen (Lioresal) is a drug used to treat muscle spasms in multiple sclerosis and other disorders involving the spinal cord. It can cause impaired ability to drive.

Bacteremia

A bacterial infection in the blood; often called blood poisoning (sepsis). The infection begins in one area, such as a tooth abscess or urinary tract infection, and then spreads. Once infectious bacteria reach the bloodstream, they can travel throughout the body. Symptoms include sudden fever, chills, rapid heartbeat with a drop in blood pressure (septic shock), flushed skin, red streaks leading from a wound, confusion, and mental impairment. Left untreated, bacteremia causes shock and can result in death. A blood culture test is used to diagnose bacteremia. When diagnosed promptly, bacteremia can be treated successfully with intravenous antibiotics and other supportive therapy.

Bacteria

A large group of single-celled microorganisms, some of which cause disease in humans. Bacteria, commonly known as "germs," are one of the six principal types of infectious organisms, with the others being viruses, protozoa, rickettsia, fungi, and parasites. Infectious bacteria can enter the body in food, drink, or air; through a wound or opening in the skin; or through a natural opening in the body. Bacteria multiply by cell division; one bacterium becomes two, then four, then eight, and so on. As a result, bacteria multiply rapidly under favorable conditions. Bacteria are simple organisms that lack a true cell nucleus. Some bacteria have long, whiplike filaments called flagella that allow them to move easily in the body. Others have short filaments (pili) that do not move but help in attaching the bacteria to tissue surfaces, such as the lining of the intestine, and colonizing them. Many bacteria are surrounded by a protective capsule that prevents them from being destroyed by the special white blood cells that attack invading microorganisms. Certain bacteria can

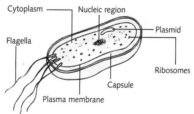

STRUCTURE OF BACTERIA
Some bacteria are encased in an outer protective structure called a capsule. Within the capsule, the cell has a rigid cell wall for protection and an inner flexible membrane called the plasma membrane surrounding the fluid interior. All metabolic processes take place in the fluid content, which is called the cytoplasm. In the cytoplasm, the cell's nucleic region carries the genetic information (DNA) needed for the cell to copy itself. Plasmids also carry additional helpful genetic material. Bodies called ribosomes form proteins that are essential to the cell's reproduction. Tails, or flagella, on the bacterium give it mobility.

produce spores, dormant forms that survive difficult environmental conditions and grow into bacteria when those conditions improve.

TYPES

Since bacteria normally have no color, they have to be stained to be seen under a microscope. Bacteria that absorb the dye known as GRAM STAIN appear blue under a microscope and are called gram-positive. Those that do not absorb it are gram-negative. The distinction is important because gram-positive bacteria can be treated with penicillin and similar antibiotics, while gram-negative bacteria are usually resistant to these medications.

Bacteria come in a number of basic shapes. Rods are bacilli, one of which is the bacterium that causes anthrax;

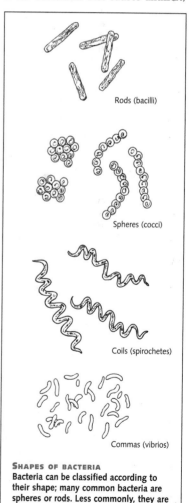

Rods (bacilli)

Spheres (cocci)

Coils (spirochetes)

Commas (vibrios)

SHAPES OF BACTERIA
Bacteria can be classified according to their shape; many common bacteria are spheres or rods. Less commonly, they are shaped like spirals or commas.

B

UNDERSTANDING BACTERIA AND INFECTIONS

Bacteria comprise a numerous group of microscopic, single-celled organisms, some of which cause disease in humans. Most bacteria, abundant in the air, soil, and water, are harmless to humans. Some bacteria are actually helpful, residing on the skin or in the gastrointestinal tract to fight off other bacteria and build up resistance against other more virulent strains of bacteria that can cause disease. However, harmful organisms actively reproduce and cause disease directly by damage to cells or indirectly by toxins they release.

Infection is the invasion of the body by disease-producing organisms that can enter the body through air that is breathed, in ingested food or liquid, directly through the skin, or from another part of the body. Beyond hand washing and good hygiene, the best defense the body has against viruses and bacteria is keeping the skin clean and promptly treating any cuts or sores, along with maintaining a healthy immune system.

---

spheres, also called cocci, include *Streptococcus,* which causes strep throat; coils, or spirochetes, are bacteria that cause diseases such as syphilis and Lyme disease; and commas are known as vibrios or the cholera bacterium. Bacteria differ in their ability to live with oxygen. Certain kinds can live only in the presence of oxygen and are known as obligate aerobic bacteria. Anaerobic bacteria live only where there is no free oxygen. An example is the tetanus (lockjaw) bacterium, which lives in the soil below the air but can grow in the body only if introduced through a puncture wound. Facultative anaerobes, such as the *Staphylococcus* that can cause severe infections of the skin and underlying tissues, prefer an environment with oxygen but can survive without it.

ROLE IN DISEASE

When infectious bacteria invade the body and multiply into large numbers, they release poisons (toxins) that cause disease. Symptoms depend on the type of bacterium and the toxins it releases. Bacterial toxins from organisms that cause cholera and food poisoning can cause diarrhea, paralysis (from tetanus and botulism), rash, fever, tissue destruction, and organ failure. The extent of the infection also determines the severity of the disease. Bacterial infection may remain localized in a single area, such as an abscess, or it can enter the blood, spread throughout the body, and cause septic shock, a severe life-threatening condition in which the heart, lungs, kidneys, and liver fail. Most types of infectious bacteria can be weakened or destroyed with antibiotics. These medications pre-

vent the infection from growing larger or destroy it directly.

Bacteria, flesh eating

The common name for a severe but rare destructive infection of the skin and underlying tissues that rapidly advances into shock. Known medically as necrotizing FASCIITIS, it can cause death if left untreated.

The bacterium that causes the infection is called streptococcus group A, which is the same microorganism responsible for STREP THROAT. Strep throat, however, is not the usual cause of necrotizing fasciitis. A particularly virulent strain of the bacterium gets under the skin, probably through a minor scrape or cut, and grows rapidly. The skin becomes extremely painful, red, hot, and swollen; then, it takes on a violet color and blisters as tissue under the skin dies. Fever follows, along with

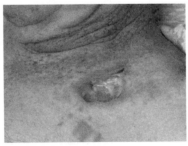

AFTER SURGERY
A rare form of *Streptococcal bacteria* can infect a relatively minor wound and destroy surrounding tissue. If left untreated, the condition can be fatal. In an infected wound, the skin becomes extremely painful, swollen, and inflamed. As the tissue under the skin dies, the area turns violet and blisters. Immediate treatment with antibiotics is critical, and surgery or even amputation is necessary in some cases.

low blood pressure and a rapid heartbeat. The infection proceeds very rapidly, often in a matter of hours.

Treatment includes antibiotics, along with surgery to remove diseased tissue (DEBRIDEMENT). Such operations may have to be repeated daily until all diseased tissue has been removed. If a large amount of tissue is involved, the limb may need to be amputated. RECONSTRUCTIVE SURGERY is usually needed after the infection has been stopped.

Bacterial vaginosis

See VAGINOSIS, BACTERIAL.

Bacteriology

The branch of biological and medical science that studies BACTERIA, one of the principal causes of infectious disease.

Bacteriuria

The presence of bacteria in the urine. Bacteriuria is usually a sign of an infection in the urinary tract. The bacteria are identified by placing a small sample of urine on a slide and viewing it through a microscope. In some cases, the bacteria are also grown (cultured) to determine their exact identification and concentration, which will determine the medications likely to eliminate them. In most cases, antibiotics are used to eliminate the infection.

Bad breath

Unpleasant mouth odor, sometimes called halitosis. Bad breath is usually caused by certain foods or beverages, tobacco use, poor oral hygiene, TOOTH DECAY, a DRY MOUTH, PERIODONTAL DISEASE (disease of the gums), an infection, or a medical disorder. When strong-flavored food—garlic and onions, for example—is eaten or when coffee or alcohol is consumed, they are absorbed into the bloodstream and transferred to the lungs where their odors are expelled during breathing. These odors persist in the breath until the food is eliminated from the body. When small particles of food collect between the teeth, on dentures, and on the tongue and other tissues of the mouth, they decompose and collect bacteria, which produce an offensive odor. The bacteria can also cause tooth decay, which contributes to bad breath. Removing these particles by regular flossing and brushing the teeth helps to prevent tooth decay and bad breath. Brushing the tongue and cleaning dentures will also help to prevent bad breath.

Halitosis may be caused by dry mouth (xerostomia), a decrease in the flow of saliva, which serves to clean the mouth and dislodge the food particles that cause mouth odors. Gum disease may cause persistent bad breath or a bad taste in the mouth. Smoking or chewing tobacco produces odors in the mouth and also contributes to other causes of bad breath, including gum disease. When a dentist cannot determine the cause of chronic mouth odor, a physician should be consulted. Bad breath may be a symptom of respiratory tract infections, sinusitis, postnasal drip, and bronchitis, as well as diseases of the kidneys, liver, or gastrointestinal tract.

PREVENTION AND SELF-HELP

Regular dental visits, including treatment of gum disease and professional cleanings, are the first line of defense against bad breath. The teeth should be brushed twice daily with a FLUORIDE toothpaste to remove food particles and plaque; the tongue should also be brushed and dental floss or interdental cleaners should be used daily. Mouthwashes do not correct bad breath for any length of time. Antimicrobial or fluoride mouth rinses may be recommended by a dentist to help control conditions such as gum disease and tooth decay that contribute to bad breath. Rinsing the mouth with water and chewing sugarless gum can stimulate saliva flow, which keeps the mouth clean and reduces odors by helping to dislodge food particles and wash away bacteria. A dentist can provide recommendations to help correct a dry mouth.

Avoiding odor-producing foods, beverages, and tobacco can prevent bad breath. If bad breath persists despite increased attention to oral hygiene, a dentist should be consulted.

Bagassosis

A lung disease characterized by inflammation of the alveoli in the lungs. Bagassosis is caused by exposure to a certain mold found on sugar cane and sugar beets and their products. The disease is a form of allergic ALVEOLITIS.

Baker cyst

An inflamed and swollen membrane-lined sac, called a bursa, which is located behind the knee. A Baker cyst can be very painful and may involve extensive swelling that spreads down the back of the leg into the calf and ankle. In its normal state, a bursa is flat and contains very little fluid; it functions as a cushion between bones and soft tissues, such as muscles, tendons, ligaments, and skin. A Baker cyst, which is caused by inflammation of the main muscle in the calf and the knee joint, may be due to overuse, injury, infection, or arthritis.

It is important to seek early medical attention if a Baker cyst is suspected because the cyst can rupture and cause symptoms that could be confused with blood clots in the deep veins of the leg. The condition is readily diagnosed by a physical examination of the swollen area and confirmed with ultrasound scanning. Treatment generally includes applying local heat, immobilizing and elevating the affected leg, the use of nonsteroidal anti-inflammatory drugs (NSAIDs) such as aspirin and ibuprofen, possibly drawing fluid out through aspiration, or the injection of a local corticosteroid. Physical therapy may be prescribed to help regain mobility of the knee joint. The physical therapy may include exercises designed to restore strength in associated muscles that have been weakened by the condition. In some cases, the fluid inside the cyst may be infected and require removal by fine-needle aspiration, in addition to a course of oral or intravenous antibiotics.

Balance

The ability to remain upright, maintain a position, or move without falling over. Balance depends on the complex interaction of body systems and organs, such as the ears, eyes, muscles, heart, brain, and nervous system. Information about balance is processed by the brain, which enables various parts of the body to perform the changes needed to maintain balance.

Various disorders can disrupt balance. These include disorders of the inner ear, such as LABYRINTHITIS and MENIERE DISEASE. Rarely, OTITIS MEDIA (inflammation of the middle ear) disturbs balance. Other causes of balance problems include stroke, brain tumor, spinal cord tumor or injury, diseases of the cerebellum or basal ganglia (clusters of nerve cells deep within the brain), nerve degeneration, muscular diseases, and vascular disorders.

Balanitis

Inflammation of the foreskin and head (glans) of the penis in an uncircumcised male. The usual cause is bacterial infection from inadequate cleaning under the foreskin. Symptoms can include pain, redness, and swelling of the glans and the foreskin; foul-smelling discharge; a burning sensation on urination; chills and fever; and enlarged lymph nodes in the groin. Ulceration and spread of the infection to deeper tissues of the penis are possible complications. Balanitis is treated with corticosteroid creams to control swelling, antibiotics to fight the infection, and medications to stop pain and fever. If balanitis recurs despite good hygiene, circumcision (removal of the foreskin of the penis; see CIRCUMCISION, MALE) may be the best treatment.

Ballismus

The abnormal swinging, flinging, and jerking movements that are sometimes seen in HUNTINGTON CHOREA (a progressive disorder involving degeneration of nerve cells in the cerebrum) or other diseases affecting the basal ganglia (clusters of nerve cells deep within the brain). Ballistic movements are involuntary and uncontrollable. They are caused by irregular muscle contractions and most commonly affect the arms and legs as a result of inappropriate signals from the brain. The most common cause of hemiballismus (ballistic movement affecting one half of the body) is a stroke in a deep area of the brain called the subthalamic nucleus.

Balloon angioplasty

A minimally invasive procedure to open arteries narrowed or blocked by fatty deposits, a disease known as ATHEROSCLEROSIS. Atherectomy is another type of balloon angioplasty (see next page). The technical name for balloon angioplasty is percutaneous transluminal coronary angio-

B

RESTORING BLOOD FLOW

Depending on the type of arterial blockage, a balloon angioplasty or a rotational burr angioplasty (atherectomy) may be performed. If the blockage is relatively soft, a balloon angioplasty can widen arteries and restore circulation. If the blockage is calcified, a rotational burr (surgical drill) can be used to bore a hole through the plaque. If restenosis occurs (plaque rebuilds within the artery) within 6 months, angioplasty may be repeated or coronary artery bypass may be performed.

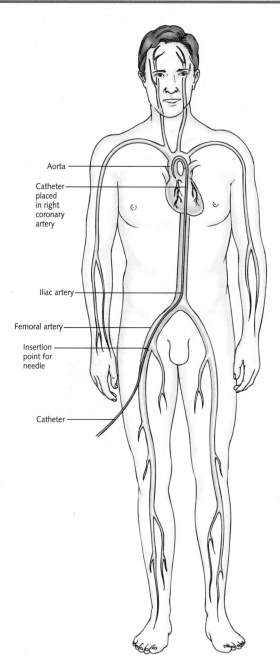

Aorta

Catheter placed in right coronary artery

Iliac artery

Femoral artery

Insertion point for needle

Catheter

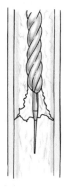

PTCA (STEP 1)
In percutaneous transluminal coronary angioplasty, or PTCA, the deflated balloon is threaded into the obstructed coronary artery and positioned so that it crosses the site of the blockage.

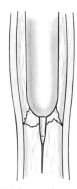

PTCA (STEP 2)
The balloon is inflated and deflated several times, creating a wider opening and pressing the plaque against the vessel wall. The balloon is then deflated, and the catheter and guide wire are removed.

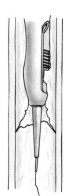

ATHERECTOMY
In atherectomy, a catheter with a rotational burr is used along with the balloon. A balloon is inflated to position the atherectomy burr on the plaque deposit. Then the burr shears the plaque off the artery wall. The shavings are collected in the catheter tip and are removed as the catheter is withdrawn.

INSERTING A BALLOON CATHETER
A hollow needle is inserted into the femoral artery, usually at a point in the groin. Then a long guide wire is threaded through the iliac artery and the right coronary artery into the heart. A 2-millimeter catheter with a sausage-shaped balloon attached to its tip is threaded over the guide wire into the blocked artery.

plasty (PTCA), which means that the procedure is performed through the skin (percutaneous) and inside an artery (transluminal) that feeds the heart (coronary), for the purpose of reshaping that artery (angioplasty). Variations of the procedure are also used to treat narrowed or blocked arteries in areas other than the heart, such as the neck or leg.

Balloon angioplasty has become increasingly popular in recent years as an alternative to coronary BYPASS SURGERY. Bypass surgery involves opening the chest by cutting through the breastbone to expose the heart, requires the use of a heart-lung machine, and entails several months of recovery. Balloon angioplasty, which can be very effective, involves only a small incision and allows recovery in days or weeks.

Balloon angioplasty is performed for those who have angina (chest pain) during exercise or have had a heart attack. It is usually most effective when only one coronary artery is narrowed or blocked.

THE PROCEDURE

Balloon angioplasty is performed under conscious sedation; the person undergoing the procedure is conscious but relaxed, drowsy, and insensitive to pain. Local anesthetic is injected before a small incision is made to expose an artery. Usually this is done in the groin, but sometimes the arm or wrist is used. A short tube called a sheath is inserted into the artery, and a hollow, flexible tube called a catheter is threaded through the sheath and down the artery. The guide catheter is passed through until it reaches the heart; the surgical team watches its progress through a televised X ray. Small amounts of dye are injected through the catheter to allow visualization of the diseased artery. Once the catheter is in place, a smaller catheter with a deflated balloon at its tip is passed through the catheter and positioned at the point of narrowing or blockage. The balloon is then inflated, usually for 30 seconds to 2 minutes, to compress the fatty deposit, stretch the artery wall, and increase the artery's diameter. In some people, inflation of the balloon causes pain since blood flow to a portion of the heart is cut off temporarily. The pain ends when the balloon is deflated. The balloon is typically inflated and deflated several times, then more dye is injected to assess the effectiveness of the procedure. In many cases, a wire-mesh sleeve called a stent is positioned in the artery to keep it open and provide support. The catheters are then withdrawn.

The sheath is left in place for 4 to 24 hours after the angioplasty is performed. Anticoagulant drugs are given to prevent clotting in the sheath, and the person's condition is monitored continuously to ensure normal heart function. If the sheath is in the leg or groin, the person is kept in bed until it is removed; if the sheath is in the arm, the person can move about immediately after the procedure. Most people go home within 24 to 48 hours and return to work in approximately 7 days. Various medications are commonly prescribed during the first few weeks, including nitroglycerin to relax the coronary arteries, calcium channel blockers to prevent coronary artery spasms, and platelet inhibitors, such as aspirin, to lower the risk of blood clots. Pain and bruising around the incision usually heal within a few days.

RESULTS AND COMPLICATIONS

The principal complication of balloon angioplasty is a sudden, complete closure of the treated artery, which typically happens within 24 hours of the procedure. However, this complication is rare, and the use of a stent makes it even less likely. Should the artery close, emergency bypass surgery may need to be performed.

In 20 to 40 percent of those who undergo balloon angioplasty, the repaired artery closes again within 6 months of the procedure, in which case the balloon angioplasty is repeated or bypass surgery is performed.

Since balloon angioplasty does not resolve the underlying atherosclerosis that caused the narrowing or blockage of the artery, other treatments may be needed. These include lifestyle changes, such as quitting smoking, reducing fat in the diet, and taking medications to keep the coronary arteries relaxed, lower blood pressure, reduce the workload on the heart, and lower cholesterol levels.

Balloon catheter

A thin, hollow tube with an inflatable balloon at its tip. A balloon catheter is inserted into an artery that is narrowed or blocked by fatty deposits. Then the balloon is inflated to compress the deposits, widen the artery, and restore normal blood flow. (For more information, see BALLOON ANGIOPLASTY.) A balloon catheter may also be used to open narrowed heart valves in the procedure known as VALVULOPLASTY.

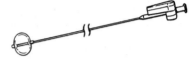

LESS INVASIVE TOOL
Balloon catheters vary in design, and different types can be used for monitoring, diagnosis, or treatment. The device can be threaded through a blood vessel or inserted through an incision in a vessel. It does not interfere with blood flow, requires a relatively small incision, and reduces the length of time required to perform many procedures.

Balloon valvuloplasty

See VALVULOPLASTY.

Bandage

A piece of material used to bind a diseased or injured part of the body. Bandages may be in the form of a pad or a strip. Bandages are used to stop the flow of blood, to absorb drainage from a wound, to cushion the injured area, to prevent contamination or infection, to hold a medicated dressing in place, to immobilize an injured part of the body, and to speed healing.

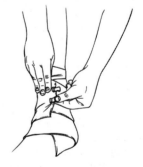

ELASTIC BANDAGES
An elastic bandage is used to decrease bleeding or support a joint or group of muscles. Applied properly, it is very effective, but if wrapped too tightly, it can cut off circulation, particularly if swelling occurs, a significant danger with elastic bandages.

B

Barbiturates

Central nervous system (CNS) depressant drugs. Barbiturates, such as phenobarbital (Luminal), secobarbital (Seconal), and pentobarbital (Nembutal), among others, act on the brain and CNS to induce drowsiness. Barbiturates can be used to control seizures in diseases such as epilepsy, and they are sometimes used to treat insomnia for short periods. Some short-acting barbiturates are used as general anesthetics.

For many years, barbiturates were used as sedatives, but they have been replaced by the BENZODIAZEPINES. Barbiturates can become addicting if used for long periods, and they are associated with severe side effects when taken in overdose or when abruptly stopped. They should not be used to relieve the anxiety or tension of everyday life. Barbiturate use can cause an impaired ability to drive.

Bariatric surgery

An operation to aid an obese person in losing weight by controlling appetite and the ability to absorb food. The word "bariatric" means "management of weight" in Greek. Bariatric surgery is not cosmetic; it involves a procedure that should only be used to eliminate the serious, and sometimes fatal, medical problems caused by obesity. A common procedure involves stapling across the upper part of the stomach to reduce the amount of food that a person can consume.

COMPLICATIONS OF OBESITY

A person who weighs 100 pounds above his or her ideal body weight is classified as morbidly obese. An individual whose weight is 200 percent over his or her ideal weight (or twice as much as it should be) is considered to be superobese. Obese people are subject to medical problems such as diabetes mellitus, hypertension, heart disease, sleep apnea syndrome, degenerative arthritis, an elevated blood cholesterol level, and an increased incidence of certain cancers, such as colon and rectum, prostate, uterus, and possibly breast. As a result, the death rate for obese people is much higher than for individuals of normal weight.

Bariatric surgery is a possible treatment option for people who are severely obese or who have been unable to lose sufficient weight through carefully managed diet regimens. A person thinking about this procedure needs to be well informed and motivated about improving his or her condition and healthy enough to undergo the procedure. In all cases, the decision to undergo surgery involves weighing the risks and benefits in close consultation with a physician. A person who abuses drugs or alcohol, who has certain psychiatric disorders, or who may not follow medical care instructions is not considered a good candidate for bariatric surgery.

THE PROCEDURES

Bariatric surgery reduces the amount of food that can be held in the stomach before it passes into the small intestine. Two procedures are currently in use.

A gastroplasty (also called a gastric partitioning) involves the creation of a small pouch in the top of the stomach—large enough to hold only 1 ounce of food—and restricts the passage of the food through the stomach by stapling a band of synthetic mesh across the bottom of the pouch. Newer gastric-partitioning procedures involve the use of an adjustable gastric band that is insert-ed through the use of a laparoscope (a small viewing tube). Patients feel full after eating only a small amount of food and retain the full feeling longer than they did before surgery. Overeating causes nausea and possibly vomiting.

In the second procedure, a gastric bypass, the surgeon constructs a small stomach pouch and then connects this pouch directly to the intestine. With this procedure, food bypasses the remainder of the stomach after it has traveled through the surgically constructed pouch. A gastric bypass can also limit the kinds of food that can be eaten. Possible side effects include low absorption of iron because the gastric bypass eliminates most acid content, which iron needs for absorption.

Both procedures have the effect of reducing the amount of food that a person can eat at a given meal. In the unaltered stomach, the passage of food into the intestine is regulated by a valve at the bottom of the stomach. When it functions normally, the valve releases high-calorie concentrated sweets into the intestine more slowly than it does more digestible foods. Since this mechanism no longer functions after a gastric bypass, eating sweets causes unpleasant bloating

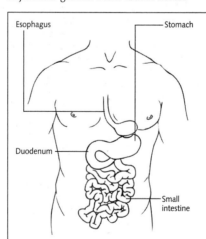

GASTROPLASTY
Gastroplasty is a procedure in which the surgeon partitions off the upper part of the stomach with a band of silicone mesh to create a small pouch, leaving only a narrow outlet into the rest of the stomach. The new pouch holds only about 1 ounce of food, so the person feels full after eating very small meals.

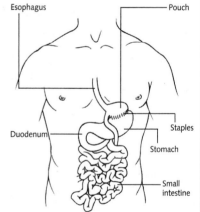

GASTRIC BYPASS
In a gastric bypass, a small pouch is created in the upper portion of the stomach. This pouch has no outlet into the remainder of the stomach. To allow passage of food into the intestine, a piece of the intestine is brought up and attached to the pouch. As a result, food bypasses part of the intestine where some digestive processes take place.

and cramping as the food passes swiftly into the intestine.

WHAT TO EXPECT

Both types of bariatric procedures are major surgeries. The intestine must be emptied with enemas or laxatives the night before the procedure, and the patient must fast after midnight. The procedure, which takes 2 to 3 hours, is performed through an incision that runs from under the sternum (breastbone) and reaches to the navel. A tube is run through the nose and into the stomach to drain fluids during healing. In some cases, another tube connected to the stomach is left in place after the procedure to help control distension of the stomach during the early stages of healing. The tube is removed approximately 4 weeks later in a simple ambulatory surgical procedure.

After surgery, the patient usually spends 4 to 9 days in the hospital. The patient cannot eat or drink immediately after surgery. After the tube is removed, first liquids, and then solid foods, are reintroduced to the diet. Full recovery takes 4 to 6 weeks.

On average, most people who undergo bariatric surgery lose 50 to 60 percent of their excess weight, with a maximum weight loss reached at 18 to 24 months after the procedure. Some weight-related complications, such as type 2 diabetes mellitus, hypertension, and obstructive sleep apnea, may also be resolved following the weight loss. Patients must continue on a carefully controlled diet, often with vitamin and mineral supplements to ensure proper nutrition, and stay in regular contact with their physician.

Barium enema

Also known as a lower gastrointestinal tract series; an X-ray procedure that uses barium sulfate and sometimes air to outline the lining of the colon and rectum. Barium sulfate, a CONTRAST MEDIUM, is administered rectally and held briefly inside the intestine while a series of X rays is taken. The barium is not penetrated by the X rays and appears white on an X-ray image, allowing abnormalities to show up as dark shapes along the intestinal lining. In an air-contrast, or double-contrast examination, air may also be pumped into the

TWO TYPES OF BARIUM ENEMA
A single-contrast barium infusion involves injecting barium sulfate solution into the colon to detect blockages or prominent abnormalities. In a double-contrast barium infusion, air is blown into the colon in addition to the solution for a better view of the interior.

Barium infusion—single contrast (shows blockages and prominent abnormalities)

Barium infusion—double contrast (shows smaller abnormalities, such as diverticula)

intestine to sharpen the outline of the intestinal wall.

WHY IT IS PERFORMED

A barium enema is ordered to check for abnormalities such as tumors, ulcers, obstructions, or polyps of the colon and rectum and to diagnose diverticulosis (the presence of small sacs in the gastrointestinal wall). It is also sometimes recommended as a screening test for colorectal cancer instead of a COLONOSCOPY. In such cases, it may be performed once every 5 to 10 years, starting at age 50 years.

HOW IT IS PERFORMED

To provide the best X-ray images, the colon and rectum must be emptied before a barium enema. In preparation for the procedure, the doctor may tell the person to modify his or her diet, for example, by drinking only clear liquids for 24 hours before the test. The person undergoing the procedure may be asked to drink extra fluids to ensure adequate hydration before and during the procedure. To empty the colon completely, he or she may be instructed to take a laxative and administer suppositories at home, or a laxative and suppositories may be administered just before the procedure.

As the person lies on his or her side, a lubricated enema tube is inserted into the rectum, and the barium sulfate fluid flows through the tube and into the colon. The introduction of the fluid may produce a small amount of discomfort such as a feeling of pressure, an urge to move the bowels, and cramping pains. A small balloon at the tip of the enema tube may be inflated

to help keep the barium inside. The person will be instructed to maintain a tight contraction of the anal sphincter against the enema tube. While the barium is held inside the intestines, a series of X-ray pictures is taken. The person being tested is asked to hold his or her breath and to remain still as the X rays are taken. At other times, he or she is asked to move into different positions, and the table is rotated and tipped slightly to allow the barium fluid to flow into different areas of the colon to offer different views. The flow of the barium solution is monitored on a fluoroscope, a device that is equipped with a fluorescent screen.

After the X rays have been taken, the enema tube is removed. The person is assisted to a toilet to expel as much of the barium as possible from the intestines. Some X rays may be taken after the barium has been expelled.

When an air-contrast examination is performed, air is gently introduced into the colon after the barium is administered, and more X rays are taken. The air and the thin film of barium that adheres to the intestinal lining enhance the images of the intestine. The enema tube is removed, and the colon is emptied.

To help clear the remaining barium from the intestines, which may take several days, the person will be told to drink water, take laxatives, and use an enema. The stool may be an

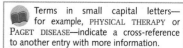
Terms in small capital letters—for example, PHYSICAL THERAPY or PAGET DISEASE—indicate a cross-reference to another entry with more information.

B

B

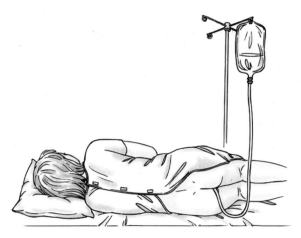

HOW AN ENEMA IS DONE
For a barium enema, the person lies on his or her side and a lubricated tube is gently inserted into the rectum. The barium solution is in a hanging bag, and the fluid flows through the tube into the colon. The person will be asked to hold the solution in the colon while X rays are taken. The flow of the solution is monitored on a screen.

unusually light color for a day or two after a barium enema.

RISKS

Barium enema is considered a safe procedure. There is a minimal risk of intestinal blockage if the barium fluid is not entirely cleared from the colon. The physician's recommendations for cleansing the intestine should be followed carefully to prevent blockage. The doctor should be notified if, after a barium enema, a person experiences severe abdominal or shoulder pain, nausea, vomiting, or blood in the stools, as this may indicate that a perforation occurred. If the person has difficulty moving the bowels or if the stool is extremely narrow or does not return to its normal color, medical attention may be required.

Barium swallow

Also known as an esophagogram or barium meal; an X-ray procedure that uses barium sulfate to outline the pharynx and esophagus. A flavored solution containing barium sulfate, a CONTRAST MEDIUM, is swallowed, and a series of X rays is taken. The barium coats the pharynx and esophagus and appears white on X-ray film, allowing structural and functional abnormalities to show up as dark shapes.

WHY IT IS PERFORMED

A barium swallow is usually ordered to evaluate the function of the pharynx and the esophagus and to detect abnormalities such as a tumor or a stricture (narrowing) in the esophagus that may be causing difficulty swallowing. It is also used to check for ulcers or other inflammatory conditions in the lining of the esophagus.

HOW IT IS PERFORMED

The person having the examination should modify his or her diet by having only a light, liquid meal the evening before testing and not eating or drinking anything after midnight the night before testing. He or she may be instructed not to take any antacid medications. If the person undergoing the test takes medication, the doctor will advise the person whether he or she should take the medication before the test. The procedure is performed by a radiologist in a doctor's office, X-ray

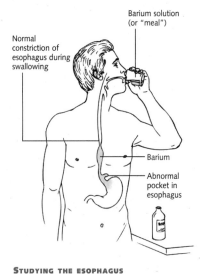

STUDYING THE ESOPHAGUS
When a person swallows a barium solution, a technician (using a device called a fluoroscope) can follow the path of the liquid as it flows down the esophagus and into the stomach. The barium shows the configuration of the esophagus and makes a condition such as an abnormal pocket clearly visible.

facility, or radiology department of a hospital.

The person is given a barium preparation to drink. The barium solution is the consistency of a milkshake and has a chalky taste. During the test, the person will drink about 12 to 14 ounces of the barium solution. The person must remain totally still while the X rays are being taken. The flow of the barium solution is monitored on a fluoroscope, a device that is equipped with a fluorescent screen.

After the test, the person may be given a laxative to help eliminate the barium. The stool may be an unusually light color for a day or two after a barium swallow.

Barotrauma

Injury to the middle ear caused by a change in air pressure. The conditions inside the pressurized cabin of an airplane during takeoff and especially during landing are typically responsible for barotrauma. Scuba divers and high-altitude pilots face similar risks. When air pressure is greater on the outer surface of the eardrum than on its inner surface, the eardrum is pushed inward. Middle ear infections, sinusitis, or allergies may increase a person's susceptibility by producing congestion that blocks the eustachian tube (the tube connecting the middle ear to the back of the nasal cavity). This blockage prevents the normal flow of air that equalizes pressure in the middle ear. If the eustachian tube is completely blocked, pressure changes within the middle ear may be severe enough to rupture the eardrum or cause bleeding into the middle ear, either of which may cause a temporary, mild hearing loss.

SYMPTOMS

The symptoms of barotrauma include mild to considerable ear pain, some degree of hearing loss, a plugged feeling in the ear, and possibly dizziness, as well as TINNITUS (ringing, buzzing, or roaring in the ears). These symptoms usually clear up within 3 to 5 hours.

TREATMENT

If symptoms for air travelers do not improve within a few hours of landing, consultation with a doctor is recommended. A physician may perforate the eardrum and remove fluid

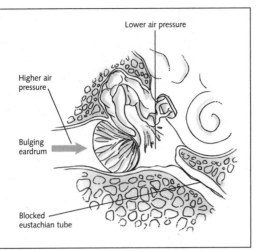

Lower air pressure

Higher air pressure

Bulging eardrum

Blocked eustachian tube

from the middle ear to equalize air pressure inside the ear. The eardrum generally heals on its own within 1 to 2 weeks. If the eardrum has been ruptured, the doctor may prescribe an antibiotic and place a temporary paper patch over the eardrum. A week-long course of a corticosteroid drug (see CORTICOSTEROIDS) may also be used to treat the hearing effects of barotrauma. If there is a small persistent perforation in the eardrum, the physician may close it by performing a procedure in his or her office.

PREVENTION OF BAROTRAUMA

When a person with a congested nose must travel by air, taking a decongestant medication, with or without an antihistamine, an hour before departure may be beneficial. On long flights, taking the medication an hour before landing may help prevent symptoms. Swallowing, yawning, or chewing gum will help open the eustachian tube, reducing pressure in the middle ear. Infants may be given a bottle or pacifier to suck on during an airplane's ascent and descent to prevent discomfort. The Valsalva maneuver (blocking the nostrils with thumb and index finger and exhaling gently with the mouth closed) may be a helpful technique to try at the first signs of ear discomfort. People who have recently had surgery involving the inner or middle ear are especially vulnerable to pressure changes and should not fly without first consulting their doctor.

Bartholin abscess

See BARTHOLIN GLANDS, DISEASES OF.

Bartholin cyst

See BARTHOLIN GLANDS, DISEASES OF.

Bartholin glands, diseases of

Disorders affecting the two Bartholin glands, located on either side of the vaginal entrance, that secrete lubricating fluid during sexual arousal. The gland openings can become blocked from infection or injury. As a result, a Bartholin cyst may form, usually causing no symptoms. However, if the cyst (a fluid-filled sac) becomes infected and an ABSCESS appears (Bartholin abscess), the woman may feel pain and tenderness just inside

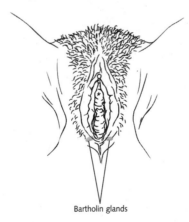

Bartholin glands

LOCATION OF BARTHOLIN GLANDS
Bartholin glands are under the skin on either side of a woman's vaginal opening. They release lubricating fluid as a part of sexual arousal and activity. If they become blocked by infection or injury, they may develop a small cyst or a painful abscess. Either condition can be treated in a doctor's office.

the vagina, where there will be a warm, swollen lump. Treatment includes an antibiotic for the infection. If the abscess does not respond to antibiotics, the doctor may lance and drain it. About 1 percent of all cancers of the vulva are carcinomas of the Bartholin glands. A tumor of the Bartholin glands or duct may resemble a benign Bartholin cyst.

Bartonellosis

See CAT-SCRATCH DISEASE.

Basal body temperature (BBT)

The temperature of the body, taken immediately after awakening in the morning and before getting out of bed. Typically, the BBT is used by women to identify the days during the menstrual cycle when OVULATION (the release of an egg from the ovary) takes place. A woman's temperature often falls by a few tenths of a degree during the 12 to 24 hours before ovulation; then, it rises for several days after ovulation. By measuring the BBT with a thermometer that is able to detect slight changes and by recording the temperature on a chart every day for several months, an ovulation pattern can be detected. A woman is most likely to become pregnant if she has sex on the days just before, after, or on the day of ovulation. Tracking of the BBT can be used by women who are trying to become pregnant or by women who want to avoid becoming pregnant. See CONTRACEPTION, OTHER METHODS.

Basal cell carcinoma

The most common form of SKIN CANCER. Skin cancer is the most common type of cancer in the United States, and basal cell carcinoma accounts for three of four cases. Its principal risk factor is sun exposure. The two other common types of skin cancer are SQUAMOUS CELL CARCINOMA and malignant melanoma (see MELANOMA, MALIGNANT). Of the three, basal cell carcinoma has the best prognosis, with a cure rate of more than 95 percent. Basal cell carcinoma rarely spreads to other parts of the body. However, early diagnosis and treatment are important because, without treatment, basal cell carcinoma can eventually extend below the skin and invade nearby structures.

B

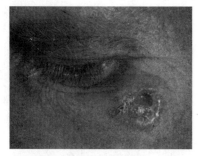

A SORE THAT DOES NOT HEAL
Basal cell carcinoma, the most common form of skin cancer, often appears on the face, neck, or head where the skin has been exposed to the sun. The lesion looks like a small sore that does not heal, sometimes bleeding and scabbing, or that recurs regularly in the same place.

SYMPTOMS AND DIAGNOSIS

Basal cell carcinoma most often develops on areas of the body that are frequently exposed to the sun's ultraviolet rays such as the head, neck, hands, and chest. Basal cell carcinoma tumors can appear as small, shiny, fleshy nodules (solid masses of tissue) or bumps or as flat, scaly, red areas. They vary from white to light pink to brown. Sometimes blood vessels are visible in the lesions themselves or in the surrounding skin. These tumors grow very slowly and can take months or years to expand to a diameter of half an inch. Basal cell carcinoma tumors bleed easily after a minor injury. Left untreated, they bleed and crust over repeatedly.

For the early detection of skin cancer, doctors recommend regular skin self-examination. It is important to know the regular pattern of freckles, moles, and other marks on skin. It is necessary to get medical attention for a new skin growth; changes in the surface or color of a mole; a spot or bump that is getting larger, scaling, oozing, or bleeding; a sore that does not heal within 3 months; or itchiness or pain in a lesion. In cases of suspected skin cancer, complete personal and family medical histories are taken, and the history of the lesion such as when it first appeared or changed in size or appearance is considered. The lesion is examined for size, shape, color, and texture, and the rest of the body is checked for other lesions. Diagnosis of skin cancer is made by a skin biopsy (taking a small sample from the lesion and examining it under a microscope).

TREATMENT

Most basal cell carcinoma tumors can be cured through minor surgery. The type of treatment depends on factors such as the size, type, depth, and location of the cancer. Surgical options include EXCISION (cutting out the tumor), CURETTAGE (scraping), electrodesiccation (burning with an electric current delivered through a probe), and MOHS SURGERY (microscopically controlled surgery removing one layer of skin at a time). Radiation may be helpful for tumors that are difficult to treat surgically and for people unable to tolerate surgery. Less frequently, CRYOSURGERY (freezing with liquid nitrogen) may be used. In most cases, surgery is performed on an outpatient basis using a local anesthetic. In the removal of large cancers, skin grafting and reconstructive surgery may be necessary.

RISK FACTORS AND PREVENTION

Basal cell carcinoma occurs primarily in middle-aged and older people. However, it is beginning to appear more often in young people, particularly those who frequent tanning salons or sun bathe. This type of cancer is most common in fair-skinned people with blond or red hair and blue or green eyes. Whites are at greater risk than other groups. Men are two to three times more likely than women to develop basal cell carcinoma, probably because of more sun exposure due to outdoor occupations. Other risk factors are a family or personal history of skin cancer; a tendency to burn or freckle easily when exposed to the sun; having spent a lot of time outdoors; overexposure to X rays or other forms of radiation; and exposure to arsenic, coal, industrial tar, paraffin, and certain types of heavy oils.

It is not uncommon for people who have had a basal cell carcinoma tumor to get another (in the same site or in a new location) within 5 years. Consequently, doctors recommend both monthly self-examinations and regular examinations by a health care provider every 6 to 12 months.

The most effective way to prevent basal cell carcinoma is to avoid harmful radiation from the sun. Doctors recommend applying a sunscreen with a sun protection factor (SPF) of at least 15 before going outdoors; using a broad-spectrum sunscreen that provides UVA and UVB protection; reapplying sunscreen every 2 hours (more often if swimming or sweating); avoiding exposure to the sun between the hours of 10 AM and 4 PM when rays are at their most intense; wearing a broad-brimmed hat, sunglasses, and protective clothing that covers most of the body; and, when possible, staying in the shade.

Basal ganglia

A motor control area of the brain. The basal ganglia are clusters of nerve cells (neurons) deep within the brain that help control voluntary movement. In movement disorders such as HUNTINGTON CHOREA (a progressive disorder involving degeneration of nerve cells in the cerebrum), there is an untimely deterioration of nerve cells in the basal ganglia. Parkinson disease is caused by degeneration of dopamine-producing cells in the basal ganglia. Dopamine is an important neurotransmitter that stimulates the nerves in the basal ganglia. When the basal ganglia nerve cells do not function properly, symptoms of Parkinson disease occur, which include muscle stiffness, tremor, slowness, and imbalance.

Baseball elbow

An overuse injury common among adolescent pitchers. Similar to tennis elbow, baseball elbow is caused by repeated stress to the elbow as it flexes and extends during overhead throwing. The medial, or inside, portion of the elbow may be injured by the throwing motion made in baseball, while the lateral, or outside, structures of the elbow are compressed by this movement. Baseball elbow is seldom severe, but in the worst cases, the cartilage of the elbow joint may be permanently damaged. A child who plays baseball, especially as a pitcher, and complains of persistent elbow pain should be examined by a doctor. The elbow joint should be rested, and physical therapy may be considered to teach the child appropriate stretching and strengthening exercises. Adjustments in throwing technique are sometimes recommended before resuming participation in the sport.

Baseball finger

An injury resulting from the fingertip being jammed or struck by a thrown ball. Baseball finger, which is sometimes called "mallet finger," causes pain and sometimes discoloration in the joint of the finger closest to the tip. The injury may make it difficult or impossible to fully straighten the finger. X rays are necessary for a diagnosis as they may reveal an avulsion fracture, which is a bone that breaks as a result of a tendon separating from the bone. Baseball finger is generally treated with a finger splint that must be worn continuously for 1 to 6 weeks, after which a follow-up of orthopedic care is recommended. If proper healing has not occurred, an additional 4 weeks of splinting may be needed. The doctor may suggest appropriate pain medication to relieve discomfort. If healing is not complete within that amount of time, surgical repair may become necessary. There are several kinds of finger splints available for purchase, but one can also be made at home by wrapping a paper clip in tape, positioning it under the injured joint, and wrapping it firmly with gauze strips to hold it in place.

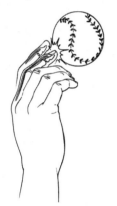

INJURY TO THE FINGERTIP
A blow to the end of the finger may tear a tendon at the first joint, causing pain and making movement of the finger difficult. A splint may be the recommended treatment.

Battery

By law, the illegal application of physical force to another person. Battery need not include force; a mere touch is sufficient. A person can commit battery indirectly, by striking the property of another, by administering poison or drugs to another, or by deliberately communicating a disease to another person. Battery is a crime that is related to but different from assault, which is a crime of attempted or threatened battery. See ASSAULT, SEXUAL; INCEST; VIOLENCE, FAMILY; VIOLENCE, SCHOOL; and VIOLENCE, STREET.

BCG vaccination

Bacille Calmette-Guérin vaccination; a live vaccine derived from a strain of *Mycobacterium bovis*, a form of bacteria that causes TUBERCULOSIS (TB). BCG vaccination is used to immunize against strains of tuberculosis that are resistant to the medications isoniazid and rifampin. Once BCG vaccine is administered, it reduces the ability of tuberculin skin tests to detect TB infection. Therefore, BCG vaccine is not recommended for an adult who is at high risk for contracting TB. Health care workers who have a negative PPD (purified protein derivative) result and are not immunodeficient may be considered for vaccination with BCG if they have a continued risk of exposure to TB. Children and infants may be candidates for BCG vaccination if they have close contact with people who have active, ineffectively treated, or drug-resistant TB and cannot take preventive treatment (isoniazid) or if they live in areas in which there are high rates of new TB infection that is unresponsive to treatment.

Becaplermin

A human growth factor drug. Becaplermin (Regranex) is produced in a laboratory and is used to stimulate wounded tissue to heal faster, such as in person who has diabetes and ulcers on the lower limbs and feet. Becaplermin is available by prescription as a gel and is applied to the wound in a thin layer to promote healing.

Beclomethasone

See CORTICOSTEROIDS.

Bed bath

The bathing of a person in bed; also called a sponge bath. A complete bed bath is used for the thorough washing of a person who is completely unable to clean himself or herself, such as an individual who is unconscious. A partial bed bath can be given by the bedridden person himself or herself, using a basin, soap, and water.

Bed rest

Staying in bed to rest when ill. Bed rest is used to help someone who has been sick to recover by resting completely. In the past, doctors often prescribed bed rest. However, prolonged bed rest has many possible harmful side effects (for example, PRESSURE SORES), and most doctors now recommend limiting its use.

Bedpan

A shallow toilet pan used by persons confined to their beds. Bedpans can be used by both men and women to urinate and defecate; men may also use a URINAL. A bedpan should always be emptied and cleaned immediately after it is used.

Bedridden

Confined to bed because of illness or injury. A person who is bedridden is one who is forced to stay in bed all the time because of illness, injury, or weakness.

Bedsores

See PRESSURE SORES.

Bed-wetting

Involuntary urination during sleep; also known as nocturnal enuresis. Bed-wetting is common and normal among preschool children, with more than a third of 3-year-olds wetting the bed at night. By age 5, most children are able to control their bladders while sleeping. Bed-wetting is more common in boys than girls. Primary enuresis means the child has never been dry at night. Secondary enuresis refers to the child who has been consistently dry for a number of months before wetting the bed again.

A child usually wets the bed for one of two reasons. His or her bladder may not be sufficiently developed to hold urine through the night, or during sleep the child fails to recognize the need to urinate and sleeps through the impulse. Bed-wetting tends to run in families. A school-aged child who has not achieved nighttime bladder control usually has a parent who experienced the same problem. Bed-wetting may also be related to drinking caffeinated or carbonated beverages, citrus juice, or a

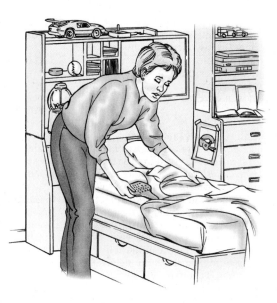

BED-WETTING ALARM SYSTEM
Many doctors recommend a bed-wetting alarm system to help a child awaken in time to go to the bathroom. A moisture-sensitive pad attached to the child's underpants is connected to a signaling device clipped to the child's pajama top. At the first signs of dampness on the pad, a buzzer sounds near the child's ear so that he or she can wake up and get to the bathroom. The system helps train the child to wake up on his or her own in response to the urge to urinate. The child will need 2 or 3 months to learn to get up without the alarm.

great deal of water. A child who has been dry at night and suddenly starts wetting the bed again is probably responding to stress. Factors such as a new sibling, a death, or a divorce in the family may be responsible. Enuresis also may be the result of abuse or an underlying disease such as a urinary tract infection. Bed-wetting in a formerly dry child should be evaluated by a pediatrician or family physician. (See also ABUSE, CHILD.)

DIAGNOSIS AND TREATMENT
The physician will conduct a thorough physical examination and ask questions about a child's bed-wetting problem. In the vast majority of children, bed-wetting is not due to a serious underlying medical problem. However, about 1 percent of cases are related to diseases or disorders such as diabetes mellitus, a urinary tract infection, or a structural abnormality. (See also DIABETES MELLITUS, TYPE 1; DIABETES MELLITUS, TYPE 2; and URINARY TRACT INFECTIONS.) To determine whether bed-wetting is the sign of a more serious problem, the doctor will test the urine for signs of infection. In rare cases, X rays or ultrasound scanning of the kidneys and bladder may be ordered. If imaging tests detect a structural abnormality, the child will be referred to a urologist (a doctor who specializes in disorders of the urinary tract). Treatments can be prescribed for infections and structural problems.

If there are no underlying causes for bed-wetting, a pediatrician can recommend techniques and habits to control bed-wetting. For example, children should use the toilet before bedtime and avoid drinking too many liquids in the evening. Keeping a plastic cover on the mattress and a fresh supply of clean linens and pajamas near the bed can reduce the stress created by bed-wetting. Children need reassurances that bed-wetting is not their fault. They should be praised for staying dry. Children should never be punished, pressured, or criticized for the problem.

For a child of 7 or 8 who is still wetting the bed, the physician may recommend a special pad with an alarm system. Urine on the pad triggers an alarm to wake the child to go to the bathroom. Bladder stretching exercises are sometimes recommended to increase bladder capacity. During the day, the child gradually increases the time between urinating. Medications can be prescribed to manage bed-wetting. Pills and nasal sprays can concentrate urine to make urination less frequent. Other pills strengthen the sphincter tone and inhibit bladder contractions. Doctors generally do not prescribe medications to treat bed-wetting for children younger than age 7. Older children who are troubled by bed-wetting may benefit from seeing a mental health professional.

Bee pollen

A combination of pollens and nectar collected by bees and mixed with bee saliva. Bee pollen is a natural substance thought by some people to enhance the performance of an athlete or to cure hay fever. Bee pollen has been studied as a promising alternative medical treatment, but there is insufficient evidence to back up these claims. Bee pollen can trigger serious allergic reactions in some people, so it should be used with care.

Bee stings

Painful injuries caused when stinging insects inject venom into the skin. Stinging insects include female bees, wasps, and ants. A bee sting begins as a sharp pain lasting a few minutes, after which it becomes a dull ache and is likely to itch. The sting site will become red and swollen as the body flushes venom from the area. Most bee stings in the United States involve honeybees, whose stingers usually remain in the skin after the bee stings. It is important to remove the stinger immediately, because venom continues to enter the skin from the stinger for 45 to 60 seconds after the sting. If removed within 15 seconds of the sting, the severity of the reaction is reduced.

In addition to removing the stinger, first aid for bee stings involves washing the wound and applying hydrocortisone cream or calamine lotion to reduce the itching and swelling. An oral antihistamine may help relieve symptoms. A small number of people—one or two out of every thousand—are allergic to bee stings. Allergic reactions to bee stings can include hives, nausea, vomiting, and headaches. Life-threatening allergic reactions such as anaphylactic shock (see SHOCK, ANAPHYLACTIC), dizziness, unconsciousness, and difficulty breathing may also occur immediately after the sting or up to 30 minutes later and may last for hours.

People who are aware that they are allergic to stings should carry sting kits and wear medical identification bracelets or necklaces to inform others about their allergy. Bee stings can be avoided by wearing light-colored clothing that covers as much of the body as possible, choosing unscented soaps and cosmetics, and avoiding flowering plants.

Bee venom and bee products, therapeutic

The medicinal use of honeybee products; apitherapy. Bee products, including honey, pollen, royal jelly, beeswax, and venom, have been used to treat medical conditions since ancient times. Bee venom has been studied extensively by scientists, who have identified at least 18 active substances in it. Bee venom is used by apitherapists to treat arthritis and other inflammatory conditions; acute and chronic injuries such as bursitis or tendonitis; scar tissue; and multiple sclerosis. Bee venom is administered by deliberately provoking a bee to sting in order to mobilize the body's self-healing ability. Apitherapists also use bee products to treat skin disorders, infections, viruses, high blood pressure, asthma, arthritis, depression, menstrual cramps, and allergies. Bee pollen contains 50 percent sugar, as well as other substances, which should be noted by people with either form of diabetes mellitus. Some people, however, are allergic to bee pollen and may develop a life-threatening ANAPHYLACTIC REACTION; ANAPHYLAXIS.

Behavior therapy

A method of treating psychological and psychiatric conditions that focuses on changing outward behavior rather than uncovering emotional conflicts that may help explain that behavior.

Behavior therapy holds that many psychiatric and psychological conditions thought to be illnesses are actually a collection of abnormal behaviors that cause problems in daily life. Since these behaviors are learned just as normal behaviors are, behavior therapy focuses on helping the individual learn new ways of behaving that eliminate or reduce difficulties. Behavior therapy is often combined with techniques aimed at changing thought patterns (see COGNITIVE-BEHAVIORAL THERAPY). Behavior therapy has been shown to be effective for treating specific problems such as abnormal fears (phobias), depression, sexual dysfunction, panic and anxiety attacks, and childhood behavior problems. It can also be effective in weight reduction. It is not effective for treating acute psychotic reactions, such as schizophrenia.

Behavior therapists use a wide variety of techniques in their work, adjusting these tools to the needs of the person being treated. Typically, the therapist helps the individual break the problem behavior down into its component parts and then creates a program for that individual to learn a new and more adaptive way to behave. These techniques can include guided imagery, role-playing, recording of physiological responses (such as panic symptoms) as the person is observed in the problematic situation, as well as BIOFEEDBACK and homework assignments requiring the person to try a new behavior and pay attention to what happens.

Behavior therapy is based on the theory of operant conditioning (see LEARNING), which holds that people will increase behavior that rewards them (positive reinforcement). Thus, children may be given sweets when they perform the desired behavior, such as sitting still in a chair for a certain number of minutes. Behavior therapy also uses techniques that increase a behavior as a way of avoiding an unpleasant consequence (negative reinforcement), to help the individual learn that the same behavior in different settings may have different consequences (discriminant learning), and to encourage a desired behavior in settings other than the one in which it was learned (generalization).

Belching

The expulsion of air from the digestive tract through the mouth. Many people unconsciously swallow air while eating, chewing gum, or smoking. STRESS or poorly fitted DENTURES may also cause too much air to be swallowed. Swallowing air leads to upper intestinal gas, which can also be produced by drinking carbonated beverages. Although much gas is passed into and absorbed by the small intestine, some may be belched out. Belching alone is usually not caused by a disease. However, belching that is accompanied by a sour or bitter fluid, or is more common when lying down, may be a symptom of ESOPHAGEAL REFLUX (the backward flow of acid from the stomach up into the esophagus). Belching after meals may be a sign of indigestion or gallbladder disease.

Management of belching depends

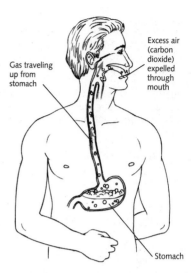

BELCHING EXCESS AIR
A person often swallows air with food, in carbonated beverages, or with inhaled smoke. Much of this air passes into the intestine and is absorbed, but some air from the upper digestive tract may be expelled back through the mouth. Belching is usually a normal phenomenon.

on its cause. Doctors may recommend that people avoid carbonated beverages or chewing gum, eat slowly, quit smoking, make sure that dentures fit properly, avoid lying down immediately after eating, or practice stress management. If belching is excessive or accompanied by other symptoms, the doctor will conduct a variety of tests to determine its underlying cause. Medications are usually not effective in reducing belching.

Bell palsy

An abnormal neurological condition characterized by weakness or paralysis of muscles on one side of the face. People with Bell palsy cannot move one side of the mouth, close the eye, or furrow the brow on the affected side. Other possible symptoms of Bell palsy include changes in the production of tears and saliva and altered senses of taste and hearing. This condition is caused by damage to or dysfunction of the facial nerve. Nerve inflammation is sometimes the result of a virus, such as the one that causes cold sores and fever blisters. Possible causes of facial nerve damage that mimic Bell palsy include strokes, tumors, and infections (such as shingles or Lyme disease). Any case of facial weakness or paralysis requires prompt and careful evaluation by a physician. Most cases of Bell palsy resolve without treatment. However, treatment options include corticosteroids, antiviral medications, and facial massage. Artificial tears or a patch may be necessary to protect the eye from damage. In rare cases, surgery may be recommended.

Benazepril hydrochloride
See ANTIHYPERTENSIVES.

Bends
See DECOMPRESSION SICKNESS.

Benign
A term that describes a condition that is not malignant (cancerous), invasive, or recurrent and does not metastasize (or spread.) A benign tumor is one that is not cancerous.

Benign familial tremor
A neurological disorder characterized by shaking. (See also TREMOR.) Benign familial tremors tend to run in families and are usually harmless. Although they can develop at any age, these tremors are more common in older people. They may manifest themselves as head nodding, difficulty holding small objects, or a quivering voice. Over time other parts of the upper body (such as the eyelids or arms) may be affected, but the lower body is usually not involved. Benign familial tremors generally worsen during periods of activity, purposeful movement, or emotional stress. Diagnosis is made on the basis of physical examination and personal and family medical history. Sometimes tests such as CT (computed tomography) scanning and MRI (magnetic resonance imaging) are ordered to rule out other causes of tremors. Treatment is often not necessary. Although they affect movement or speech, benign familial tremors seldom cause any other problems. However, if tremors are severe and interfere with one's ability to perform daily activities, the doctor can order medications such as anticonvulsants, beta blockers, or tranquilizers. It is also helpful to avoid caffeine and other stimulants.

Benign prostatic hyperplasia
See PROSTATE, ENLARGED.

Benzodiazepines
Synthetically produced sedative-hypnotic drugs. Benzodiazepines have replaced barbiturates as the treatment of choice for anxiety and convulsive disorders and to provide sedation, because they cause less drowsiness and are less likely to be fatal if taken alone in an accidental overdose.

Most benzodiazepines, often referred to as minor tranquilizers, are used to treat anxiety and tension. Three benzodiazepines—diazepam, midazolam, and lorazepam—are used as surgical drugs to sedate patients and prevent them from remembering details of the surgery. Diazepam is also used to treat neurologic conditions involving muscle spasm. Four types of benzodiazepines—diazepam, clonazepam, clorrazepate, and lorazepam—are used as anticonvulsants.

Benzodiazepines should not be taken for long periods, because they can cause physical dependency and withdrawal symptoms when stopped. All types of benzodiazepines can cause an impaired ability to drive. Drinking alcohol increases the sedative effect, so alcohol intake should be limited.

Benzoyl peroxide
An antiacne medication. Benzoyl peroxide is the active ingredient in many lotions and creams available without prescription to spread on infected skin. Benzoyl peroxide works by causing skin to shed cells more quickly than usual, thus preventing pores from closing around the built-up oily secretion associated with acne infection.

Bereavement
Intense sorrow that results from the death of a loved one. Bereavement is characterized by many symptoms of depression, including loss of appetite and insomnia. However, bereaved persons do not feel ill and usually do not seek psychiatric care. Intense mourning typically lasts about 3 to 4 months, with lingering feelings for up to a year. Abnormal bereavement is a clinical or major depression with the loss of a loved one, the trigger pushing the person over some threshold into illness. See GRIEVING.

Beriberi
A disease caused by a deficiency in thiamin. Thiamin (vitamin B1) is essential for energy production from carbohydrates and for nerve and muscle function. It is found in foods such as pork, liver, leafy green vegetables, whole grains, and enriched breads and cereals. Beriberi frequently occurs in Asia, where it is caused by a diet limited to white rice. Rare occurrences in the United States are usually associated with stress-related conditions such as infection, hypothyroidism, alcoholism, pregnancy, or breast-feeding.

Symptoms of beriberi include diarrhea, fatigue, heart failure, and weight loss. Impaired nerve function leads to muscle weakness, wasting of the limbs, impaired sensation, and confusion. Administration of thiamin cures and prevents most cases of beriberi. Types of beriberi include alcoholic beriberi, atrophic beriberi, cardiac beriberi, and cerebral beriberi.

Berylliosis
An environmental, chronic, inflammatory disorder of the lungs caused by the inhalation of beryllium dust. Materials that contain beryllium may be found in the aerospace, electronic, and nuclear weapon industries. The symptoms of berylliosis may not develop until several years after exposure. They include chest pain, shortness of breath on exertion, a dry cough, and, occasionally, fever and chills. Berylliosis is often treated with CORTICOSTEROIDS.

Beta blockers
Antihypertensive drugs. Beta blockers are very effective drugs that lower blood pressure by blocking the effects of norepinephrine, thereby easing the heart's pumping action and indirectly widening blood vessels. Current research demonstrates that beta blockers reduce the risk for heart attacks and other cardiovascular events. Beta blockers are inexpensive, safe, and effective for most people with hypertension and no complicating health problems. People with asthma should never use beta blockers because they can narrow

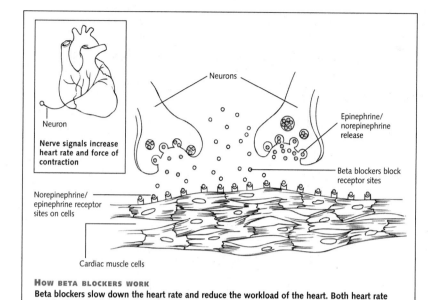

HOW BETA BLOCKERS WORK
Beta blockers slow down the heart rate and reduce the workload of the heart. Both heart rate and the force of heart muscle contractions are controlled by neurons extending into the heart. At a cellular level, the hormones norepinephrine and epinephrine stimulate cardiac muscle cells by locking onto receptor sites on heart muscle cells. Beta blockers occupy the receptor sites and block the effect of the hormones, thereby lowering the heart rate.

bronchial airways. Beta blockers can also be useful for people with angina to slow heart rates; they can also be used as eyedrops for glaucoma.

Examples of beta blockers include acebutolol (Sectral), atenolol (Tenormin), betaxolol (Kerlone), carteolol (Cartrol), carvedilol (Coreg), metoprolol (Lopressor), nadolol (Corgard), penbutolol (Levatol), pindolol (Visken), propranolol (Inderal), and (Blocadren). Beta blockers may differ in their effects and benefits as well as in their side effects; some can cause an impaired ability to drive.

Beta-carotene
A form of CAROTENE, a substance found in plants that is converted to VITAMIN A by the intestines, lungs, and liver.

Bezoar
A ball of indigestible material in the stomach. Bezoars can be composed of hair, fiber, or other indigestible material. Although they are most common in children, bezoars can also occur in adults following partial GASTRECTOMY (surgical removal of part of the stomach). People with diabetes are also more likely to develop bezoars. Trichobezoars are bezoars made of hair only; they develop in children

who chew on their hair or pull it out and swallow it. This type of bezoar may also occur in emotionally disturbed adults who eat their hair. A bezoar may produce loss of appetite, nausea, vomiting, and abdominal pain. Treatment usually requires breaking up the bezoar, using a gastroscope. If this is not successful, surgical removal is required. Thereafter, medications can sometimes prevent their recurrence.

BIA
See BIOELECTRIC IMPEDANCE ANALYSIS.

Bifocal
In optics, eyeglasses made up of two portions, one for seeing near and the other for far distance vision. Bifocals are eyeglasses in which each lens is made up of two sections with different strengths. The upper part is usually used for distant vision, while the lower part is for reading or other close work. Bifocals are generally prescribed for older adults, whose eyes gradually lose the ability to see clearly at close range (called PRESBYOPIA).

Bigeminy
A double heartbeat, in which a normal beat is coupled with an abnormal

beat. Bigeminy is typically experienced as a missed beat or flip-flop in the chest. Occasional bigeminy is harmless, but repeated episodes can be a sign of a heart rhythm problem. See ARRHYTHMIA, CARDIAC.

Biguanides
Oral hypoglycemic agents; medications for the treatment of type 2 (non–insulin-independent or adult-onset) diabetes. Biguanides make up one of five classes of oral medications used to treat diabetes. Oral hypoglycemic agents are not oral insulin but are designed to help reduce blood sugar levels when diet and exercise alone are not enough. Oral medications are effective only if the pancreas is still producing some insulin, as is generally the case with middle-aged and older people with diabetes. People with type 1 diabetes do not secrete enough insulin for the oral medications to be effective.

Only one biguanide is currently available in the United States: metformin (Glucophage). Biguanides increase the sensitivity of the liver and muscle to insulin, thereby helping to lower blood sugar.

Bilateral
Having two sides. Bilateral kidney disease, for example, affects both the right and left kidneys.

Bile
A yellow-green liquid that aids digestion. Bile is secreted by the liver and concentrated and stored in the gallbladder. The liver produces about 3 cups of bile each day. When a hormone released by the small intestine causes the gallbladder to contract, bile is released through the bile ducts into the small intestine. The substances in the bile, including bile salts and lecithin, make fats soluble so that they can be absorbed by the intestine and pass into the bloodstream.

Another important function of bile is to carry BILIRUBIN (a normal by-product of the breakdown of hemoglobin from aging red blood cells) from the liver to the gallbladder and into the small intestine. The bilirubin is broken down by intestinal bacteria and eventually excreted in the stools. If this process of bilirubin metabolism is interrupted, excess bilirubin

B

accumulates in the bloodstream and causes JAUNDICE (a yellowing of the skin and the whites of the eyes). Jaundice is a symptom of many different liver disorders.

Another component of bile is CHOLESTEROL, a fatlike substance that is excreted by the liver. Serum cholesterol is an important constituent of cells; however, high levels of cholesterol increase the risk of ARTERIOSCLEROSIS, a disease in which the walls of arteries become inflamed and thickened with plaque. Excess cholesterol can also lead to the formation of GALLSTONES, solid masses that can form in the gallbladder.

Bile duct

One of several tubes that carry bile from the LIVER to the gallbladder and then to the first section of the small intestine (duodenum). Bile is a greenish watery liquid, produced in the liver and stored in the gallbladder, that contains salts and pigments necessary for digestion. A system of bile ducts (the biliary system) starts in liver tissue, in units called lobules, and channels bile into successively larger ducts. Two large tubes, the hepatic ducts, leave the liver and join to form the common hepatic duct. From the common hepatic duct, bile flows either into the gallbladder for

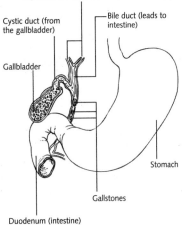

Right and left hepatic ducts (from the liver)

Cystic duct (from the gallbladder)

Bile duct (leads to intestine)

Gallbladder

Stomach

Gallstones

Duodenum (intestine)

BLOCKED BILE DUCTS
As bile passes from the liver and gallbladder into the intestine, it travels through a series of ducts. Its passage can be blocked by gallstones, scar tissue, or cancer. Gallstones are hardened masses of cholesterol or salts that can form in the gallbladder or bile ducts and are a common cause of obstruction.

storage or into the common bile duct to be carried toward the small intestine. The common bile duct joins a duct from the pancreas, and they form a single opening into the small intestine, through which digestive secretions from both organs flow.

Bile duct cancer

Cancer in the ducts that carry BILE, a necessary fluid in digestion, from the liver to the gallbladder and small intestine. Bile duct cancer occurs most frequently between ages 50 and 70. People who have a history of colitis or gallstones are more likely to develop the disease. JAUNDICE, a yellowing of the skin and the whites of the eyes, is the primary symptom of bile duct cancer. Symptoms may also include itching, weight loss, abdominal pain, nausea, vomiting, and an enlarged liver. Diagnosis is made by physical examination, blood tests, and imaging studies.

Treatment consists of surgery to remove the cancer. Often, the tumor spreads to the liver, from which the tumor may be difficult or impossible to remove. If bile ducts become blocked, they can be treated by inserting tubes through the blockage by using ERCP (endoscopic retrograde cholangiopancreatography), a procedure that utilizes X rays for guidance and a special viewing tube that can perform some surgical procedures. When surgery is successful, periodic CT (computed tomography) scanning is necessary to detect cancer should it recur. Doctors may also recommend CHEMOTHERAPY or RADIATION THERAPY. See also BILE DUCT OBSTRUCTION.

Bile duct obstruction

A condition in which BILE is blocked from entering the intestines, creating pressure in the bile ducts, the system that drains bile from the gallbladder and liver into the intestine. Bile duct obstruction may be due to scar tissue from inflammation, GALLSTONES (hard masses that can form in the gallbladder), BILE DUCT CANCER, or pancreatic tumors (see PANCREAS, CANCER OF THE).

The primary symptoms of bile duct obstruction are JAUNDICE (a yellowing of the skin and the whites of the eyes), itching, and BILIARY COLIC (severe pain in the upper abdomen). The pain may also radiate to the back

and is often accompanied by nausea and vomiting.

DIAGNOSIS AND TREATMENT
Bile duct obstruction is diagnosed by ultrasound examination, CT (computed tomography) scanning, or ERCP (endoscopic retrograde cholangiopancreatography), the most invasive procedure. ERCP can usually identify the cause and site of the blockage and can be used to treat some types of obstruction. In ERCP, a sedative is given and the throat is anesthetized locally. Then, a flexible, lighted tube called an endoscope is inserted through the mouth and guided down to where the bile system drains into the small intestine. A contrast dye is injected through the endoscope to make the bile ducts and surrounding organs visible on X rays. If the test reveals a gallstone or narrowing (also known as stricture) of the ducts, additional instruments can be inserted to remove or work around the obstruction. Balloons can be inserted to dilate strictures. A sample of the tissue (see BIOPSY) may also be taken for analysis. The procedure lasts from 30 minutes to 2 hours. Further treatment varies according to the underlying cause of obstruction.

Bilharziasis

See SCHISTOSOMIASIS.

Biliary atresia

A potentially fatal disorder in newborns, in which the bile ducts inside or outside the liver fail to develop or develop abnormally. Biliary atresia causes JAUNDICE (a yellowing of the skin and the whites of the eyes) and CIRRHOSIS (a severe liver disease). The symptoms of biliary atresia appear from 2 to 6 weeks after birth. Jaundice is the primary symptom. An infant may also experience pale stools, dark urine, an enlarged and hardened liver, and a swollen abdomen. Some babies develop an intense, uncomfortable itching that can make them very irritable. The cause of biliary atresia is not known.

DIAGNOSIS AND TREATMENT
Several tests are performed to diagnose biliary atresia definitively because many liver diseases also cause similar symptoms. Diagnostic procedures may include blood and urine tests, LIVER FUNCTION TESTS, a test for blood-clotting function, ultra-

sound scanning, X rays, and a liver BIOPSY.

When ducts are completely obstructed, surgery is necessary to drain bile from the liver. In an operation called the Kasai procedure, the surgeon removes damaged ducts outside the liver and replaces them with healthy tissue from the baby's intestine. The goal is to permit excretion of bile from the liver to the intestine. In babies who respond to the surgery, bile starts to flow several days following surgery. This surgery is not effective when obstructed bile ducts are inside the liver.

Complications frequently occur after surgery. CHOLANGITIS (inflammation of the bile ducts) and continuing liver damage are common. ESOPHAGEAL VARICES (large, swollen, varicose veins in the lower portion of the esophagus) can develop when cirrhosis is present; infection, excessive sleepiness, and retention of body fluid also may occur. If the Kasai procedure is not successful and complications of cirrhosis become life-threatening, a liver transplant may be considered.

Biliary cirrhosis

An uncommon type of cirrhosis that causes gradual, progressive destruction of bile ducts in the liver. Because its normal excretion is interrupted, bile accumulates in the liver and can damage liver cells. This chronic liver disease is classified as either primary biliary cirrhosis (PBC) or secondary biliary cirrhosis.

PRIMARY BILIARY CIRRHOSIS
The major problem in the initial stages of PBC is liver inflammation. As time goes on, continuing inflammation around damaged bile ducts leads to severe scarring and eventually life-threatening CIRRHOSIS; PBC may exhibit no symptoms for many years. Often, the first symptom is intense itching. Eventually, such signs as JAUNDICE (a yellowing of the skin and the whites of the eyes), fatigue, cholesterol deposits in the skin, fluid accumulation, and darkening of the skin arise. Related disorders include impaired function of the salivary glands (that causes dry mouth) and of the eyes, arthritis, thyroid problems, and thinning of the bones that can lead to fractures.

Doctors believe that the cause of PBC has a genetic component. While not inherited, PBC occurs more frequently in families in which a previous member has already been affected. The disease may be caused by a disturbance in the immune system. PBC more commonly affects women than men and usually occurs between the ages of 40 and 60. Because initially there are few symptoms, abnormal laboratory test results (such as liver function tests) are often the first indication of PBC. A number of additional tests must be performed to rule out other possible causes (such as bile duct obstruction). Treatment begins with the elimination of potentially harmful foods or drugs. Specific symptoms also are addressed. For example, salt restriction or diuretics can reduce fluid buildup. Other medications relieve severe itching. Doctors are also investigating the use of medications, such as colchicine and methotrexate, to slow the course of PBC. In severe cases, a liver transplant may be considered.

SECONDARY BILIARY CIRRHOSIS
This form of the disease is also characterized by accumulation of bile in the liver (cholestasis). Secondary biliary cirrhosis results from long-term BILE DUCT OBSTRUCTION or from BILIARY ATRESIA, a congenital condition in which the bile ducts are abnormal or fail to develop. Symptoms include intense abdominal pain, enlarged liver, fever and chills, and some blood abnormalities. Treatment is as for bile duct obstruction or biliary atresia.

Biliary colic

Severe, constant pain in the upper abdomen. Pain may radiate to the right shoulder and the back and can mimic the pain of a heart attack. Biliary colic is often accompanied by nausea and vomiting. Attacks occur intermittently and generally last for hours. GALLSTONES (solid masses that form in the gallbladder) are the most common cause of biliary colic. At times, a stone leaves the gallbladder and becomes lodged in the bile duct. Colic occurs as the gallbladder and bile duct muscle clamp down in an attempt to expel the stone into the intestines. CHOLECYSTITIS (inflammation of the gallbladder) may also develop.

Ultrasound scanning is usually used to find out the cause of the pain. CHOLECYSTOGRAPHY (an X ray of the gallbladder and common bile duct after they have been filled with a contrast dye) is sometimes recommended when ultrasound scanning fails to provide a diagnosis. ERCP (endoscopic retrograde cholangiopancreatography), another type of imaging procedure, may be done when initial tests are negative, but symptoms persist. In ERCP, a slim tube called an endoscope is inserted through the mouth and guided down to the bile ducts. A contrast dye is injected through the endoscope to make the ducts and surrounding organs show clearly on X rays. If the ERCP reveals gallstones, they are usually removed. In people with recurrent biliary colic or severe symptoms, removal of the gallbladder is usually recommended. See CHOLECYSTECTOMY.

Biliary system
The organs in which bile is formed, concentrated, stored, and transported to the small intestine. The biliary system removes waste products from the liver and carries bile to the intestine. The biliary system is composed of the bile ducts, gallbladder, bile, and various other structures. The gallbladder, a small pouch that lies under the liver, stores and concentrates BILE, which flows through the bile ducts from the liver into and out of the gallbladder. A hormone released by the small intestine causes the gallbladder to contract and release bile into the small intestine, where it helps neutralize stomach acid and make fats soluble to permit their digestion. See also BILE DUCT.

Bilirubin
A breakdown product of hemoglobin, the blood pigment that transports oxygen. When red blood cells are destroyed, the bilirubin that results from the breakdown of hemoglobin is transported to the liver and excreted as part of the bile into the gallbladder and small intestine. A small amount of the bilirubin reenters the bloodstream after it is taken up by the small intestine; later it is excreted in the urine. By measuring the amount of bilirubin in the blood and urine, a physician can tell whether the liver and gallbladder are functioning nor-

mally. If an obstruction is blocking the bile ducts or gallbladder, the level of bilirubin in the blood increases. Abnormally high levels of bilirubin can cause jaundice, a yellowish discoloration of the skin and the sclera (whites of the eyes), that can be a sign of liver or gallbladder disease. In addition to liver and gallbladder disease, hemolytic anemia, in which there is an increased destruction of red blood cells, can cause bilirubin levels to rise.

Billroth operation

A type of partial GASTRECTOMY (surgical removal of all or part of the stomach). The Billroth operation was developed by the Austrian surgeon Christian Billroth in the 19th century and became the first successful operation on the stomach. It is still used today in the treatment of some types of peptic ulcers and for gastric cancer.

Binet test

Also known as the Binet-Simon Scale; the first intelligence test designed to measure intelligence and cognitive functions. It was created by Alfred Binet and Theodor Simon in 1905. The modern Stanford-Binet Scale is a direct descendant of the original test; it assesses intelligence across four major areas: verbal reasoning, quantitative reasoning, abstract/visual reasoning, and short-term memory. See also INTELLIGENCE TESTS.

Bioavailability

The degree to which a drug or other substance is absorbed; the fraction of the oral drug that reaches central blood circulation. Bioavailability measures the extent to which a drug or dietary supplement becomes available to work on the body tissue after it is taken.

Biochemistry

The study of chemistry involving biological processes. Biochemistry is the scientific study of substances found in living organisms, as well as the chemical reactions involved in life processes. Biochemists use the tools and concepts of chemistry to understand and explain living systems. A particular focus of biochemistry is the living cell and the various chemical reactions that allow it to grow, store energy, maintain itself, and reproduce.

Biochemists are also interested in

biomolecules, compounds that contain carbon and make up various parts of the living cell. Examples of biomolecules include proteins, carbohydrates, lipids, and nucleic acids, such as DNA (deoxyribonucleic acid) and RNA (ribonucleic acid). Biochemists also study the chemistry of vitamins and the chemistry of the immune response.

Bioelectric impedance analysis

A tool used in the assessment of human body composition. Bioelectric impedance analysis (BIA) determines a person's percentage of body fat. In this method, electrodes are placed on the foot and hand to measure the body's resistance to electricity. The greater the resistance, the higher the percentage of body fat. Body fat measurements are useful because excess body fat puts people at a higher risk of health problems such as cardiovascular disease, cancer, diabetes, and stroke. The accuracy of BIA depends on the state of hydration, the amount of fluid retained by cells. Dehydration causes an overestimation of body fat, while fluid retention (bloating) causes an underestimation.

Like BODY MASS INDEX (BMI), BIA is safe, easily used, and noninvasive. Tools such as these are important because weight alone is not an accurate assessment of body fat. The percentage of body fat varies from person to person, depending on age, fitness, and genetic makeup. Other factors such as the distribution of weight are likewise important. (See WAIST-TO-HIP RATIO.) BIA must not be used by people who have pacemakers.

Biofeedback

A technique in which sight or sound signals allow a person to become aware of and control specific bodily functions that are not normally controlled voluntarily, such as heart rate, blood pressure, muscle tension, and brain wave activity. In a typical biofeedback session for a person wanting to lower blood pressure, a blinking light or beeper is activated every time a sensor detects that blood pressure is rising. As the individual learns to associate sensations in the body with the light or beeper, he or she can become conscious of the physical changes

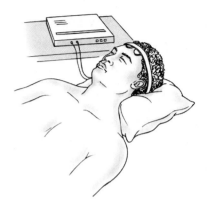

TRAINING TO CONTROL BODY FUNCTIONS Biofeedback equipment emits a light or sound signal to make a person conscious of changes in an involuntary function such as blood pressure, heartbeat, or urine excretion. With training, the person becomes able to recognize the signs of these changes and control the function voluntarily.

associated with rising blood pressure and learn to bring them under control. After a number of training sessions, the individual learns how to keep blood pressure from rising even when the light or beeper is not used. Biofeedback has been used successfully to treat a wide variety of conditions, diseases, and symptoms, including migraine and tension headaches; chronic pain; high blood pressure (hypertension); digestive disorders; irregular heartbeat (cardiac arrhythmia); attention deficit/hyperactivity disorder; Raynaud phenomenon, a circulatory condition that causes uncomfortably cold hands; epileptic seizures; mood changes before menstruation (premenstrual syndrome); difficulty holding urine in adults (incontinence); bed-wetting in children; and movement disorders, such as paralysis from spinal injury.

Biomechanical engineering

The application of mechanical laws and engineering principles to explain the function of the human body and to treat disorders. For example, biomechanical engineering may involve the examination of the range of motion around a joint or the reaction of bones to stress. Its practical applications are varied, ranging from the design of exercise programs for people with arthritis to the creation of braces or artificial joints.

Biopsy

A diagnostic test in which a specimen of tissue is removed for microscopic examination or testing. The doctor may use imaging techniques such as CT (computed tomography) or ultrasound scanning to direct the procedure. Methods of tissue removal vary from biopsy to biopsy. For example, in a NEEDLE BIOPSY, a needle is inserted through the skin to remove tissue that may be diseased; in a punch biopsy, a small cylinder of skin is removed. During a bone marrow biopsy, a needle is placed in a pelvic bone to remove and analyze the bone marrow. Biopsy is used to diagnose cancer or certain infections.

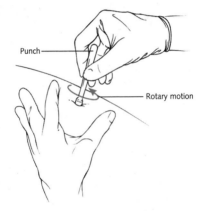

PUNCH SKIN BIOPSY
Punch biopsies are usually done to obtain a sample of skin rash, moles, or lumps. The doctor gives a local anesthetic, then twirls a small punch into the skin. The cylindrical sample is cut out from the bottom with scissors, and the opening is stitched shut. Scarring is minimal.

Biorhythms

Natural physical cycles. Examples of biorhythms include the sleep-wake cycle and the reproductive cycle. Biorhythms are thought by some people to affect behavior and mood physically, emotionally, and intellectually. According to this view, biorhythms can help explain why people have good days and bad days.

The theory behind the study of biorhythms is that each person has an internal clock that correlates with susceptibility to disease and the likelihood of having accidents. Despite considerable research into the validity of this theory, it remains controversial and unproven.

Bioterrorism

The intentional use of chemical or germ (infectious biological) agents on a population as a weapon. Health care workers are usually the first to recognize when such an outbreak has occurred. The infectious agents are usually invisible, odorless, colorless, and tasteless, but are highly potent and capable of doing great harm.

Chemical agents, such as cyanide or nerve gas, usually cause symptoms within minutes of exposure, while bacterial and viral agents may not cause disease until 24 hours or more after being inhaled or ingested. All of these agents are dependent on atmospheric temperature, weather, and geography in relationship to their disease-causing ability and persistence in the environment. Most bacterial and viral agents, such as anthrax and smallpox, need to be inhaled or ingested to cause disease, while chemical agents usually can cause disease through inhalation or by entering through the skin.

Response to such outbreaks is usually coordinated through the military, the Centers for Disease Control and Prevention (CDC), and local departments of public health. See chart on next page.

Biotherapeutic agents

Medically useful drugs whose manufacture involves microorganisms or enzymes produced by microorganisms. Most biotherapeutic agents are produced by genetic engineering, or bioengineering. Because biotherapeutic agents are either identical or similar to proteins produced naturally in the body, they are expected to have less potential to cause side effects than traditional drugs. This is particularly important in cancer therapy.

Some dietary supplements are biotherapeutic agents, among them acidophilus and *Saccharomyces cerevisiae* (brewer's yeast). Acidophilus is a species of bacteria naturally found in the body. Used as a supplement, acidophilus is intended to treat or prevent yeast infections of the mouth or vagina, urinary tract infections, and diarrhea related to antibiotic use. Brewer's yeast is a fungus used as a supplement to help treat acne and acute diarrhea and to relieve premenstrual symptoms.

Biotin

Vitamin H. A vitamin found in a variety of foods, including liver, salmon, bananas, carrots, cereals, and peanuts. Biotin aids the action of various enzymes in cells. Its functions include helping to form proteins from amino acids, breaking down fats, and forming new fatty acids and glucose.

Bipolar disorder

FOR SYMPTOM CHART
see Depression, page 32

A mental illness characterized by swings in mood from extreme elation and energy (mania) to abnormal sadness and lethargy (depression). The swings may be brief (minutes) or long (years). Bipolar disorder is also known as manic-depressive illness. Since a person with manic-depressive illness loses contact with reality, the disease is considered a PSYCHOSIS.

MANIA AND DEPRESSION
Both mania and depression affect sleep pattern, level and amount of daily activity, physical energy, appetite, mood, self-esteem, sex drive, and relationships. Mania is characterized by a persistently euphoric mood, decreased need for sleep, high physical energy, increased sexual activity, rapid speech, agitation, loss of self-control and judgment, unrealistic beliefs in one's powers and abilities, racing thoughts, and disturbed appetite. Drug abuse, particularly of alcohol, cocaine, or sleeping medications, is common. Some people with bipolar disorder experience a less severe mood disturbance known as hypomania, an abnormally expansive, elevated, highly energized, or irritable mood that comes on quickly. People with hypomania can function well in family, school, and job settings, but those with mania are faced with considerable difficulty in their social roles.

Depression is characterized by sadness, melancholy, crying, slowed mental processes, and changes in such physical patterns as eating and sleeping. People with depression sometimes have thoughts about suicide and may attempt to kill themselves. Medically, depression is defined as the daily presence for 2 weeks of at least five of the following nine symptoms: melancholy mood or

B

TREATING BIOTERRORISM

These bacterial, viral, and biological agents are being tracked and investigated by the Centers for Disease Control and Prevention. The incubation period is the time between exposure to the agent and the appearance of symptoms.

AGENT	TYPE	INCUBATION PERIOD	SYMPTOMS	TREATMENT
Anthrax: cutaneous, gastrointestinal, inhalational	Bacterial	1 to 60 days (usually 1 to 5)	Skin lesions, nausea, vomiting, abdominal pain, bloody diarrhea, infection, flulike symptoms	Antibiotics; corticosteroids for skin lesions
Botulinum toxin (botulism)	Biological	12 hours to 5 days (usually 12 to 36 hours)	Blurred vision, dry mouth, fatigue, double vision; if not treated, paralysis, respiratory distress, and death	Supportive care, ventilator, and and appropriate antitoxins
Brucellosis	Bacterial	5 to 60 days (usually 30 to 60)	Flulike symptoms: fever, headache, weakness, fatigue, nausea, vomiting	Antibiotics
Enterotoxin B	Biological	3 to 12 hours	Sudden fever, chills, headache, cough	Fever control, intravenous fluids, blood pressure control
Inhalational (pneumonia) tularemia	Bacterial	1 to 21 days (usually 3 to 5)	Sudden weakness, chills, headache, body aches, dry cough, chest pain	Antibiotics
Pneumonic plague	Bacterial	1 to 10 days (usually 2 to 3)	Sudden flulike symptoms: chest discomfort, cough, respiratory distress	Antibiotics
Q fever	Bacterial	2 to 40 days (usually 2 to 14)	Chills, cough, weakness, fatigue, chest pain; possible pneumonia	Antibiotics
Ricin toxin	Biological	4 to 24 hours	Weakness, chest tightness, fever, cough, respiratory failure, circulatory collapse	Fever control, intravenous fluids, blood pressure control, ventilator
Smallpox	Viral	7 to 17 days	High fever, headache, vomiting, delirium followed by rash and scabs in 2 to 3 days	Fever control, intravenous fluids, blood pressure control
T-2 mycotoxins	Biological	Minutes to hours	Airway irritation; pain in skin, eyes, and gastrointestinal tract	Clinical support; soap and water washing within 1 hour may eliminate toxic effects; washing 4 to 6 hours after exposure reduces toxic effects to skin
Viral encephalitis	Viral	2 to 14 days	Spiking fever, fatigue, headache, seizures	Fever control; anticonvulsants as needed
Viral hemorrhagic fever	Viral	4 to 21 days	Fever, malaise, headache, vomiting, diarrhea	Fever control, intravenous fluids, blood pressure control

Adapted from American Medical Association's *Quick Reference Guide to Biological Weapons* (November 2001).

sadness (sometimes experienced as apathy or irritability) for most of the day; loss of pleasure in practically all activities, particularly ones the person previously enjoyed; disturbed appetite or either weight gain or loss; disturbed sleep, particularly the inability to sleep through the night (insomnia); slowed or agitated physical activity; fatigue or very low energy, often leading to a diminished or nonexistent sex drive; feelings of worthlessness, low self-esteem, or inappropriate guilt; difficulty concentrating and thinking; and morbid or suicidal thoughts or actions.

COURSE AND CAUSES

Bipolar disorder tends to follow one of two patterns. In some people, the episodes of mania or hypomania and depression may follow each other closely. In others, periods of normal mood may occur between the manic and depressive episodes or following them. As a person with the disease ages, the time between mood changes decreases.

Bipolar disorder is equally common in men and women. In men, the disease usually begins with a hypomanic or manic episode. In women, depression is usually the first symptom. Typically, women with the disease are likely to have an episode soon after the birth of a child. Ongoing episodes of mania, hypomania, or depression tend to worsen in the few days before a woman with the disease begins her menstrual period. In both men and women, changes in the sleep-wake schedule, such as air travel across time zones or sleep deprivation, may precipitate an episode or exacerbate an ongoing period of depression, mania, or hypomania.

The precise cause of bipolar disorder remains undetermined. Evidence suggests that genetic inheritance has a role. A person who has a parent or sibling with the disease is more likely to suffer from it than a person who lacks a close relative with the disorder. Studies of twins and adopted children also point to a pattern of inheritance.

TREATMENT AND OUTCOME

Untreated bipolar disorder usually leads to repeated bouts of illness, with hospitalization likely. Most patients with bipolar disorder respond well to medication for the disease. Supportive therapy for patients and their families is also helpful.

The drug most commonly used for bipolar disorder is LITHIUM, a drug that has been prescribed since the 1950s. Lithium stabilizes mood, is not sedating, and prevents the extremes of both mania and depression. The length of time that a patient uses lithium after an episode of depression or mania depends on individual factors. Since lithium can cause harm to a developing fetus, it should not be taken by a woman who is pregnant or planning to become pregnant.

In about one half of individuals, lithium alone is not effective. Particularly in the early stages of mania, lithium is sometimes initially combined with major tranquilizers or benzodiazepines (see SEDATIVES). Lithium can also be combined with carbamazepine, an antiepilepsy medication. Other drugs for epilepsy can be used as alternatives for people whose disease does not respond well to lithium. ANTIDEPRESSANTS are prescribed for some people with bipolar disorder whose episodes of mania and depression cycle rapidly.

Birth

The process in which a baby is delivered from the mother. In an uncomplicated vaginal delivery, the baby is pushed out of the uterus and through the vaginal passage known as the BIRTH CANAL by involuntary contractions (see DELIVERY, VAGINAL). Usually, the baby is delivered head first, but sometimes babies are born buttocks first (BREECH DELIVERY) or feet first (footling breech delivery). Under certain conditions, the doctor may perform a surgical operation called a CESAREAN SECTION (or C-section), in which the baby is delivered through an incision in the mother's abdomen. A cesarean section may be needed when the baby is in a BREECH PRESENTATION or in serious distress; the labor is not progressing or is abnormally long; there is a dangerous infection; the birth canal is not large enough for the baby's passage; or in another situation in which a cesarean is thought to be safer for the mother or baby. See also CHILDBIRTH; LABOR; and NATURAL CHILDBIRTH.

Birth canal

The passage from the cervix to the vaginal opening through which a baby moves during CHILDBIRTH. When the cervix is fully dilated (open), the baby's head enters the birth canal, at the top of the vagina, and continues down and out of the body through the vaginal opening. See also REPRODUCTIVE SYSTEM, FEMALE.

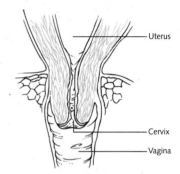

Birth canal in nonpregnant woman

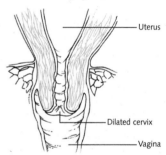

Birth canal of woman in early childbirth

AN EXPANDABLE PASSAGEWAY
The birth canal is that part of a woman's reproductive system between the cervix (the neck of the uterus) and the vaginal opening. Usually the cervix, which is a muscular ring, is contracted. During labor and childbirth, the cervix opens (dilates) to allow the passage of the baby's head and body.

Birth control

See CONTRACEPTION.

Birth control pill

See CONTRACEPTION, HORMONAL METHODS.

Birth defects

Physical problems or abnormalities present in a baby at birth. Birth defects, also known as congenital anomalies, can affect the baby's appearance or how his or her brain or other organs function. The cause of

B

most birth defects is unknown. However, some birth defects are inherited from the baby's parents; others may be acquired prenatally, for example, when a woman contracts a specific infection (such as rubella, toxoplasmosis, cytomegalovirus, or syphilis), or if the fetus is exposed to a chemical substance (such as drugs or alcohol) during pregnancy. Birth defects may also be acquired during labor and delivery.

When a birth defect is inherited from the parents, it is called a genetic disorder because the problem involves genes, the basic units of heredity. Genes are carried by chromosomes, tiny structures that are present in every human cell. Birth defects may result from problems with the number or structure of chromosomes. In the birth defect known as DOWN SYNDROME, for example, there is an extra copy of the 21st chromosome. Babies born with Down syndrome can have mental retardation, abnormal facial features, and medical problems. When planning a family, a couple concerned about birth defects can get GENETIC COUNSELING to learn their risks.

SCREENING FOR BIRTH DEFECTS

To assess the risk of a baby having certain genetic problems, such as Down syndrome, or structural defects, such as SPINA BIFIDA, maternal serum screening tests, such as an alpha-fetoprotein (AFP) test, are performed. If the AFP test shows abnormal levels of AFP or other indications suggesting fetal problems, the doctor may conduct more tests. Further investigations may include ultrasound imaging (see ULTRASOUND, OBSTETRICAL); AMNIOCENTESIS, in which the amniotic fluid surrounding the fetus is analyzed; or CHORIONIC VILLUS SAMPLING (CVS), in which a sample of tissue from the placenta is analyzed.

Birth rate

The number of live births within a population in 1 year divided by the average or midyear number of people in that population. If total population (that is, males and females of all ages) is used, the result is called the crude birth rate. If population is restricted to females of childbearing age, the so-called true birth rate is the result. Birth rate is a key statistic in deter-

---

CRUDE BIRTH RATES

Crude birth rates, the annual number of male and female births per 1,000 total population, vary greatly from one continent to another.

©2000 Population Reference Bureau

---

mining whether a population is growing, remaining steady, or declining in size.

Birth weight

The weight of a baby immediately after birth. Newborns usually weigh between 5½ and 9 pounds. The average full-term infant birth weight in the United States is 7½ pounds. Newborns weighing from 3⅓ to 5½ pounds are considered to be low-birth-weight babies, and those weighing less than 3⅓ pounds at birth are very low-birth-weight babies. See also PREMATURE BIRTH.

Birthing centers

Facilities that provide a broad range of care at a single location for pregnant women who are at low risk for having complications in labor. Traditionally operated by nurse-midwives or physicians in freestanding locations, birthing centers typically offer prenatal education and care, a site for labor and delivery, and postnatal care in a single location, with access to acute care as needed. The birthing center approach has been adopted by many hospitals. Women

with heart disease, diabetes, multiple fetuses, or other conditions that increase the risk of complications for the mother or the baby should not deliver outside a traditional hospital.

Birthing centers provide a natural, homelike setting and typically utilize the pain management techniques of NATURAL CHILDBIRTH. Family participation is often encouraged. Midwives often work in consultation with doctors, but if complications arise while a woman is in a freestanding birthing center, she may be transferred to a hospital.

Birthmark

An area of discolored skin that is present from birth or appears during the first few weeks of life. Vascular (relating to blood vessels) birthmarks are common and usually benign (not cancerous). They are composed of blood vessels bunched together in the skin. They can be brown, pink, tan, blue, or red, and they can be flat or raised. The most common types are capillary and cavernous HEMANGIOMA and PORT-WINE STAIN, both of which are reddish purple birthmarks caused by an abnormal distribution or malformation of blood vessels.

Births, multiple

See TWINS; MULTIPLE BIRTHS.

Bisacodyl

A stimulant laxative. Bisacodyl has a direct stimulant effect on the colon, speeding up peristalsis (the smooth muscular contractions that move food through the digestive tract) and bowel movements. Bisacodyl is available without prescription under many brand names.

Bisexuality

The condition of being erotically attracted to individuals of both sexes. The exact line dividing homosexuality (desire for the same sex) and heterosexuality (desire for the opposite sex) from bisexuality is unclear. Some people who have had sexual relations with people of both sexes do not describe themselves as bisexual, while others who have had sexual contact with only one sex consider themselves bisexual based on sexual desire and fantasy. Bisexuality does not imply that a person has partners of different sexes at the same time. Over the course of his or her life, a bisexual person may spend some time with partners of one sex and some time with partners of the other.

Bismuth

An element of bismuth subsalicylate, which is commonly used to treat mild diarrhea. Bismuth subsalicylate is the active ingredient in such commonly used products as Pepto-Bismol and Bismatrol. It is available without prescription in tablets, chewable tablets, and liquid. It can cause dark stools and discoloration of the tongue.

Bisoprolol

See BETA BLOCKERS.

Bisphosphonates

A class of nonhormonal drugs used to treat bone and calcium metabolism diseases. Bisphosphonates are used to prevent and treat osteoporosis and to treat Paget disease of bone as well as certain bone cancers. The drugs work by inhibiting bone resorption, preventing a loss of bone density. Bisphosphonates can lead to an increase in bone mass.

Examples of bisphosphonates include alendronate (Fosamax), etidronate (Didronel), pamidronate (Aredia), and risedronate (Actonel).

Bite

The relationship between the upper and lower teeth that determines the way the teeth meet when the mouth closes. When the teeth are properly aligned, the top front teeth extend slightly over the lower front teeth, and the top and bottom molars meet evenly on both sides of the mouth when the mouth closes.

A person's bite (OCCLUSION) is generally determined by his or her heredity. Few people have perfectly aligned teeth. Bite problems may be caused by habits such as tongue thrust (when a child pushes his or her tongue forward) or sucking the thumb, fingers, or lower lip, all of which apply pressure to the teeth. Top teeth that are too far forward and bottom teeth that are too far back are typically called an OVERBITE. Lower teeth that are too far forward and upper teeth that are too far back are

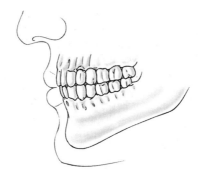

ALIGNMENT OF TEETH
The way in which the upper and lower teeth and jaws meet is called bite (or occlusion). In a person with a well-aligned bite, the top front teeth extend slightly over the lower front teeth, and the top and bottom molars fit together when the mouth is closed. A misaligned bite can cause dental problems.

referred to as an UNDERBITE. A CROSS-BITE refers to some of the upper teeth closing inside or outside some of the lower teeth. An improper bite is called a MALOCCLUSION. Bite problems can also be created by the premature loss of primary teeth or permanent teeth. Bite problems that are cosmetically unacceptable or causing dental disorders are treated by an ORTHODONTIST.

Bites and stings

FOR FIRST AID
see Bites and stings, page 1314

Wounds delivered to people through contact with humans, animals, and insects. Potentially dangerous bites and stings can be delivered by pets, wild animals, snakes, spiders, scorpions, ticks, bees, wasps, jellyfish, and humans. Bites and stings can be minor or serious. Minor bites are those in which the skin is broken but not torn, with limited bleeding, while serious bites can result in deep puncture wounds, badly torn skin, and persistent bleeding. Both minor and serious bites may become infected, causing swelling, redness, pain, and pus draining from the wound. Certain diseases such as RABIES can be transmitted through bites and scratches, causing such symptoms as fever, headache, and flulike symptoms and can progress to coma and death.

Mild insect bites, such as BEE STINGS, can usually be handled with first aid,

unless the person who has been stung is allergic. Poisonous bites can occur with some kinds of spiders or scorpions and will require emergency medical attention. Other insect bites (see BITES, INSECT) can transmit serious diseases such as Lyme disease, which is the result of tick bites (see BITES, TICK). Most reptile bites (see BITES, REPTILE) are mild, except in the case of poisonous snakes. Certain forms of marine life, even after they are dead, can inject venom through their tentacles into the skin of swimmers; examples include jellyfish and Portuguese men-of-war. The chief symptoms of marine stings are pain and stinging that cause redness and swelling on the skin, although if a great deal of venom is transmitted, symptoms can include muscle cramps, fainting, coughing, vomiting, and difficulty in breathing.

Bites, animal

FOR FIRST AID
see Bites and stings: animal bites, page 1314

Puncture wounds occurring when a person's flesh is caught between the upper and lower teeth of an animal. Animal bites are usually puncture wounds and are most often from pets, particularly dogs. Cat bites are more

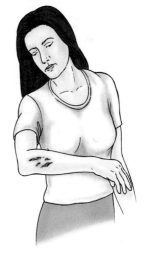

WHEN TO GET MEDICAL HELP
Any animal bite should be washed and bandaged. Most bites should be checked by a doctor, particularly if any of these symptoms is present: redness, swelling, pus, increasing pain, sensation of warmth around the bite, red streaks leading away from the bite, or fever.

serious than dog bites, because they are deeper and thus much more likely to become infected. Animal bites may cause superficial skin breaks with no bleeding, puncture wounds, major lacerations, or crushing injuries. Medical treatment should be sought if the person bitten has not had a tetanus shot within 10 years; if there is swelling, redness, pus, or pain present after the bite; or if the wound needs stitches.

Bites from wild animals are potentially more serious than those caused by pets because of the risk of rabies infection transmitted by the animal's saliva. Rabies is a rare but potentially fatal disease carried primarily by raccoons, bats, skunks, and foxes. Although there is no cure for rabies once symptoms develop, people can be vaccinated after having been exposed to the disease, thereby becoming immune. Any person bitten by an unknown or wild animal should seek immediate emergency medical assistance.

Bites, human

An injury resulting when a person's flesh is caught between the upper and lower teeth of another human being. Human bites usually cause puncture wounds and pose a high risk of infection because of the many types of bacteria and viruses found in the human mouth. Human bites may also cause injury to tendons and joints, especially if the wound extends below the skin. Human bites may be deliberate, or they may happen accidently, as when someone injures his or her knuckles on another person's teeth during a fight.

FIRST AID FOR HUMAN BITES

Human bites can be more dangerous than most animal bites and should never be ignored. If a person receives a human bite that breaks the skin, the following first aid measures should be followed. The person should:

- Stop the bleeding by applying pressure.
- Flush the wound for several minutes under running water.
- Wash the wound thoroughly with soap and water.
- Apply a clean bandage.
- Get emergency medical care, including a tetanus shot if needed.

Bites, insect

FOR FIRST AID
see Bites and stings: insect bites and stings, page 1314

A sting or bite from an insect. Insect bites involve the injection of venom or other agent into the skin, which triggers an allergic reaction. Most reactions are mild, involving only an annoying itching or stinging sensation and mild swelling. Delayed reactions can occur, including fever, painful joints, hives, and swollen glands. A small percentage of people develop severe allergic reactions to insect venom, and many have difficulty breathing, faintness, rapid heartbeat, confusion, or swelling of the lips or throat. A severe reaction must be considered a medical emergency.

The most troublesome insect bites are those caused by bees, hornets, wasps, yellow jackets, and fire ants. Mosquitoes, ticks, biting flies, and most spiders generally cause only mild bites. Mild bites are usually treated by removing the stinger, applying ice or a cold pack to the bite area to reduce pain and swelling, applying hydrocortisone cream to the area, and taking an oral dose of a mild antihistamine. The most serious insect bites are those caused by poisonous spiders, which should be treated at a hospital. Tick bites can cause ROCKY MOUNTAIN SPOTTED FEVER or LYME DISEASE, and any person bitten by a tick should observe the site carefully for the development of a rash.

Bites, reptile

Injuries caused when a person's flesh is pierced by the fangs of a reptile. Most reptiles, such as turtles and snakes, are not poisonous, and their bites can be treated with first aid, including thorough washing of the area, applying antibiotic cream or ointment, and bandaging. The best way to reduce the risk of being bitten by a reptile is not to handle them. Only people with proper training in the handling of reptiles should pick them up.

The first thing to do in the event of a reptile bite is to determine if the reptile is poisonous. If the skin in the area of the bite changes color, swells, or is painful, the reptile is probably poisonous. Poisonous snakes in the

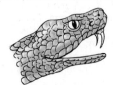

Pit viper (venomous)

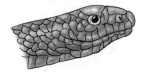

Rear-fanged snake (venomous)

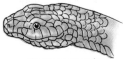

Nonvenomous snake

SNAKES WITH FANGS
Generally, snakes with fangs are poisonous and leave fairly obvious fang marks on the skin when they bite. A pit viper has a short jaw with long, prominent fangs in the front. Another type of snake has short fangs at the rear of its long jaw bone. A nonvenomous snake may have teeth but no fangs.

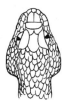

Poisonous snake

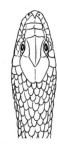

Nonpoisonous snake

IDENTIFYING POISONOUS SNAKES
In general, a poisonous snake can be identified by its head. Most poisonous snakes have triangular heads, oval or slit-like eyes, deep pits (poison sacs) between their nostrils and eyes, and fangs. The head of a nonpoisonous snake is round, with round eyes, no pits between the eyes and nostrils, and no fangs.

B

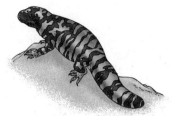

Gila monster

POISONOUS LIZARDS
There are only two poisonous lizards in North America—the gila monster and the Mexican beaded lizard. Both of these lizards are more than a foot long and heavy-bodied, with round, thick tails. Although poisonous, their bites are rarely fatal. The gila monster hangs on tightly after it bites.

United States include the cottonmouth (water moccasin), copperhead, coral snake, and rattlesnake. In this case, the person should lie down quietly, taking care to keep the bite area lower than the heart, to limit circulation of the venom. If the bite is on an arm or leg, that limb should be bandaged tightly above the bite, between it and the heart, to slow the spread of the venom. Emergency medical care should be sought, either at a hospital or on the scene of the injury if the person cannot be moved. See also SNAKEBITE.

Bites, spider

FOR FIRST AID
see Bites and stings: spider bites, page 1314

Stings or bites from a spider. Only a few spiders in North America are poisonous to humans; these include the black widow spider and the brown recluse spider. Both prefer warm climates and dark, dry places where flies are plentiful; they often live in outdoor toilets, wood, rock, and brush piles or in dark garages and attics. Bites usually occur on the arms or hands of people who reach into woodpiles or who rummage in attics or garages. Often, the person does not realize he or she has been bitten until a swelling or bite mark is noticed.

The black widow spider can be recognized by a red hourglass marking on its belly. The symptoms of its bite include intense pain and stiffness within a few hours, with or without nausea, fever, severe abdominal pain, and chills. The brown recluse spider has a violin-shaped marking on its

back. Its bite causes intense pain within 8 hours and a fluid-filled blister that forms at the site of the bite and then falls off, leaving a deep, growing ulcer. Mild fever and nausea may occur. First aid measures to be taken in the case of a bite from either spider include placing a snug bandage above the bite to slow the spread of the venom, applying a cold compress or ice bag to the bite, and obtaining emergency medical aid.

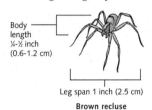

Body length ¼-½ inch (0.6-1.2 cm)

Leg span 1 inch (2.5 cm)

Brown recluse

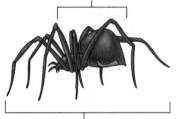

Body length 1 inch (2.5 cm)

Leg span 2-3 inches (5.1-7.6 cm)

Black widow

POISONOUS SPIDERS
Of the few poisonous North American spiders, the brown recluse and the black widow are the best known. The body of the brown recluse is soft and yellow-tan to dark brown. Its long, delicate legs are covered with short, dark hairs. A distinctive violin-shaped marking lies just behind the head. The black widow has a shiny black, round body. A reddish hourglass-shaped marking appears on the underside.

Bites, tick

FOR FIRST AID
see Bites and stings: tick bites, page 1315

Bites caused by a small insect called a tick. All ticks attach themselves to any warm-blooded animal that brushes by them, including humans. Some ticks transmit organisms that cause serious illnesses, including LYME DISEASE and ROCKY MOUNTAIN SPOTTED FEVER. The risk of receiving such a bite depends on the area of the United States in which a person lives, whether he or she spends much time in wooded areas, and pre-

PREVENTING TICK BITES

The easiest way to prevent getting bitten by a tick is to dress appropriately. The person should:

- When outdoors, wear long sleeves, long pants tucked into socks, and a hat with hair tucked inside.
- Use insecticides that repel or kill ticks, but be aware that they are not 100 percent protective; repellents containing DEET may be used on exposed skin (except on the face); insecticides containing permethrin may be used on clothing, but not on skin.
- After time spent outdoors, check for ticks, especially in areas where they tend to become attached including behind knees, between fingers and toes, under the arms, in and behind the ears, on the neck, around the hairline, and on top of the head.
- Remove a tick before it has been lodged in the skin for 24 hours, which will greatly reduce the risk of infection; remove a tick with tweezers, grabbing the head as close to the skin as possible; do not squeeze, coat with petroleum jelly, or burn ticks with a match while they are attached to skin.

ventive measures taken to avoid tick bites.

Ticks are often very tiny and hard to see; the deer tick that causes Lyme disease, for instance, is about the size of a grape seed. Nevertheless, if a person is bitten by a tick, the first thing to do is to remove it promptly and carefully, using tweezers while wearing protective rubber gloves, if possible, to grasp it by its head and gently pull it out. Once the tick has been removed, the area should be washed with soap and water, and antibiotic ointment or an antiseptic should be applied. The person handling the tick should wash his or her hands. If part of the tick stays in the skin, or if the person develops a rash or flulike symptoms, medical help should be sought. The symptoms of infection caused by a tick bite may not appear until days or weeks after the bite. To be effective, Lyme disease is best treated early as treatment is slower and less effective in the later stages of the infection.

The deer tick associated with Lyme

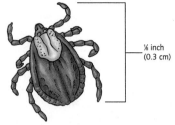

Rocky Mountain wood tick

⅛ inch
(0.3 cm)

IN CASE OF A TICK BITE
A person bitten by a tick should remove it and
seal it in a plastic bag if possible. In case medical help is required, it is useful to take the tick
to the doctor's office for identification. A person who has been bitten should see a doctor if
symptoms such as rash, fever, muscle aches,
or joint pain develop.

disease is found in more than 40
states. It is found around beaches and
in wooded and grassy areas. Tick bites
can occur throughout the year, but in
northern areas of the United States the
risk is greatest from May through
August, when ticks are most active.
Preventive measures that should be
taken by people in areas likely to have
deer ticks include wearing long-
sleeved shirts, long pants, socks, and
shoes and applying insect repellent at
the recommended dose.

Bitolterol

A bronchodilator prescribed for the
treatment of asthma and bronchospasm. Bitolterol (Tornalate)
works by relaxing bronchial smooth
muscle, relieving bronchospasm and
reducing airway resistance.

Black cohosh

An herbal remedy used for premenstrual discomfort and menopausal
disorders. Black cohosh is derived
from the root of the cohosh plant,
which is also known as black snake
root, bugbane, bugwort, rattle root,
richweed, and squaw root. It has an
effect similar to that of the female hormone estrogen and was widely used
by early American colonists and native
Americans for the relief of menstrual
cramps and for rattlesnake bites.

Black hairy tongue

Dark discoloration of the tongue
accompanied by an overgrowth of
papillae (tiny, circular bumps) on the
upper surface of the tongue. The condition is not considered medically

serious and may be caused by any one
of several factors. Antibiotic treatment, especially tetracycline, can
cause the bacteria normally present in
the mouth to multiply and accumulate
in the creases of the tongue. This gives
the tongue a darkened appearance and
causes the papillae to become extended and appear hairlike. Black hairy
tongue may also be related to a fungal
infection of the mouth or to using
over-the-counter antacid medications
containing bismuth. Some people's
tongues have very deep crevices and
cracks that trap food, drink, and other
substances. For these people, drinking
tea or coffee, chewing tobacco, or
smoking may cause black or dark
brown discoloration of the tongue.

Blackhead

A pimple that has darkened at the top
due to exposure to the air. Blackheads
typically develop as the plug of greasy
material (keratin) blocking a sebaceous gland (see SEBACEOUS GLANDS) is
exposed over time to oxygen in the air.
Blackheads are often a characteristic
of acne and usually appear on the face,
chest, shoulders, and back.

Blackout

A temporary loss of CONSCIOUSNESS or
vision. When a blackout occurs, a
doctor should be consulted to determine the cause.

Bladder

The sac that holds urine produced in
the kidneys until it is expelled from
the body. The bladder, one of the

organs in the urinary tract, is located
inside the pelvis. Two tubes called
ureters lead from the kidneys into
the back of the bladder. At the base
of the bladder, a circular muscle
forms a sphincter that can be opened
to allow urine to flow into a tube
called the urethra, which exits the
body in the genital area. The walls of
the bladder are muscular and can
stretch or expand to hold as much as
a pint of urine and then contract to
expel it.

In an infant, bladder function is
entirely reflexive. Sensory signals
originate in the bladder, indicating
that the bladder walls are stretching.
Those sensations are received in the
spinal cord, which sends motor signals to open the sphincter muscle
and allow the bladder to empty. But
as the child grows, the function
becomes conscious, so that the urge
to urinate is under voluntary control.

Bladder and bowel management

The control of urination and the passage of feces. Many factors, ranging
from diet to muscle and nerve coordination, contribute to proper bladder
and bowel management. People who
experience problems such as fecal or
urinary incontinence need to see a
doctor for medical evaluation and
treatment.

Bladder cancer

Abnormal growth and cell division of
the tissues of the bladder, the hollow
organ that holds urine. Most bladder

ANATOMY OF THE BLADDER
Urine (waste liquid fil-
tered out of the blood
by the kidneys) flows
into the bladder through
the ureters. The muscu-
lar walls of the bladder
expand to hold as much
as 2 cups of urine and
contract to expel it.
Sphincter muscles at
the base of the bladder
control the release of
urine into the urethra,
the tube that carries
the urine outside the
body.

Ureters

Openings from
ureters into
bladder

Muscular wall

Sphincter muscles

Urethra

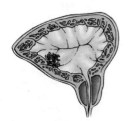
Stage A: Inner lining only

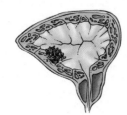
Stage B-1: Less than one half of muscle thickness

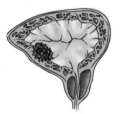
Stage B-2: More than one half of muscle thickness

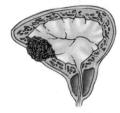
Stage C: Penetration of bladder wall

STAGES OF BLADDER CANCER
To plan treatment for bladder cancer, a doctor needs to know the extent of the growth of the cancer cells. At an early stage (A), cancer cells are present only in the inner lining (mucosa) of the bladder. At stage B-1, the cancer has invaded the muscular wall of the bladder, but has penetrated less than half of the thickness. At stage B-2, more than one half of muscle thickness is involved. At stage C, the cancer cells have penetrated the bladder wall.

cancers are transitional cell carcinomas, which are cancers that begin within the layers of the cells lining the inner wall of the bladder. When bladder cancer is confined to the surface layer it is called superficial bladder cancer. If superficial bladder cancer metastasizes, or spreads, through the lining of the bladder and invades the muscular wall of the bladder, it is called invasive bladder cancer. Invasive bladder cancer may spread to nearby organs.

If bladder cancer reaches the lymph nodes surrounding the bladder, it may eventually spread to other organs such as the lungs or bones. The affected organs will have the same kind of abnormal cells that constitute the tumor that originated in the bladder.

SYMPTOMS
Visible blood in the urine or blood in the urine that can be detected only through urinalysis is one symptom of bladder cancer. Pain during urination, difficulty urinating, or the urge to urinate frequently are other symptoms of bladder cancer and may result from irritation caused by tumor growth. A medical evaluation should

be sought if these symptoms persist longer than 2 weeks. However, bloody urine and urination problems are also symptoms of less serious conditions such as bacterial infections and kidney stones.

DIAGNOSIS AND TREATMENT
Initially, a doctor may suspect a person has bladder cancer based on the person's symptoms. Very rarely, a doctor may be able to feel a bladder tumor through the vagina or rectum. Urine samples may be examined for the presence of blood and cancer cells. After the person is given either a local or a general anesthetic, a physician may observe the bladder directly through a specialized instrument called a cystoscope. During a CYS-TOSCOPY, a biopsy sample may be taken to definitively diagnose bladder cancer. In some cases, the entire tumor may be removed at the time of biopsy.

After the stage of bladder cancer has been determined, treatment may include surgery, radiation therapy, chemotherapy, and biological therapy.

CAUSES AND RISK FACTORS
The causes of bladder cancer are not fully understood. There may be a genetic factor involved. This cancer

tends to occur after the age of 55 but may also develop in younger people. In the United States, whites are more susceptible to bladder cancer than African Americans, and men are more susceptible than women.

Smoking cigarettes is known to be a major risk factor for bladder cancer, as it is for other cancers. Stopping smoking reduces this risk. Exposure to carcinogens in the workplace can be a risk factor for workers in jobs involving the treatment and manufacturing of rubber, dyes, chemicals, and leather. Hairdressers, machinists, metal workers, printers, painters, textile workers, and truck drivers may also be at greater risk.

Bladder tumors

Tumors occurring in bladder tissue. Bladder tumors may be benign (noncancerous) or malignant (cancerous; see BLADDER CANCER). Examples of a benign bladder tumor include transitional cell papilloma, which is very rare and occurs in the lining of the bladder, and nephrogenic ADENOMA, which is a rare, tumorlike lesion of the bladder.

Blastomycosis

A chronic infection caused by a fungus inhaled into the lungs and transported by the bloodstream to other organs, principally the skin and bones. The fungus that causes blastomycosis is found in the soil, primarily in the southeastern United States and the Mississippi Valley. The infection is common in dogs, but it is not known to be transmitted from animals to humans. It occurs mostly in middle-aged men.

Blastomycosis often has no symptoms and improves on its own. When the infection first occurs in the lungs, the symptoms may be similar to those of a mild cold. It may eventually affect the lungs and the skin, causing symptoms that may include cough, weight loss, chest pain, skin lesions, localized swelling, and coughing up blood. The skin lesions are most common on the exposed skin of the face, hands, wrists, and lower legs. If the infection spreads throughout the body's system, it may affect the urinary tract, skin, liver, spleen, bone, lymph nodes, heart, adrenal glands, gastrointestinal tract, and pancreas.

DIAGNOSIS, TREATMENT, AND RISK FACTORS

Because the symptoms tend to vary, blastomycosis is difficult to diagnose. Diagnostic procedures may include direct culture, special stains, and antibody measurement. Blastomycosis is usually treated with antifungal medications. The infection is generally eliminated with early medical treatment. The success of treatment is less predictable if the disease has spread throughout a person's system. If the skeletal bones become involved, OSTEOMYELITIS and ARTHRITIS may occur.

Bleaching, dental

A cosmetic process to whiten teeth that have become discolored. Dental bleaching is considered safe for the teeth and gums when supervised by a dentist, who can determine whether a person's teeth can be lightened and what type of bleaching system is appropriate. The most immediate results involve applying a bleach solution to the teeth, followed by exposure to a high-intensity heat lamp for 5 minutes, and then applying a fluoride gel to reduce sensitivity. Laser bleaching can also be performed by a dentist in his or her office. Some people choose to buy a whitening system that can be used at home; this is often the least expensive and most common form of dental bleaching. It is effective for people

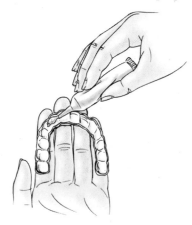

BLEACHING THE TEETH AT HOME
Commercial products are available to bleach or whiten the enamel on the teeth at home. One of these products features a tray that can be filled with a bleaching gel and fitted over the teeth. Bleaching works best on teeth that are yellowed from age or from drinking beverages containing caffeine.

who have healthy, unrestored teeth that have become darkened due to age or from drinking tea or coffee. Yellowish shades of teeth tend to respond best to dental bleaching. If the teeth are gray-shaded, which may be caused by FLUOROSIS (excessive fluoride), smoking, or taking tetracycline, dental bleaching may not help, or the change may be negligible.

WHAT TO EXPECT

A dentist or a dental hygienist first makes an impression of the teeth, which is used to custom-make a thin, lightweight, mouth-guard tray. The tray is designed to be comfortably worn during waking hours (it does not interfere with speaking), or while a person sleeps. Dental bleaching involves placing a bleaching gel in the tray before it is positioned over the teeth. Most bleaching gels contain carbamide peroxide, which is broken down by the moisture in the mouth to release hydrogen peroxide to lighten the enamel of the teeth. Possible side effects include irritation of the gum tissue, tooth sensitivity, or gastrointestinal discomfort; the treatment should be discontinued if these occur. The best results of dental bleaching provide lightening of the teeth two shades lighter as measured on a dental-shading guide. The whitening can last from 1 to 5 years; smoking and drinking coffee or tea will shorten the lasting effects. The treatment may need to be repeated.

Bleeding

Loss of blood from blood vessels. Bleeding can occur internally or externally through a natural opening, such as the nose or vagina, or through a break in the skin. The amount of bleeding is not necessarily a good indicator of how serious an injury is, because some relatively minor injuries, such as scalp wounds, bleed profusely. Some very serious injuries do not bleed much at all, such as puncture wounds, which are dangerous because of the risk of infection, including tetanus. Internal bleeding may not be noticeable externally, but it can cause physiological shock, in which the skin becomes clammy and the blood pressure drops severely.

First aid measures to be taken depend on whether the bleeding is

mild or severe. Most bleeding usually stops by itself within a few minutes, and direct pressure applied to a wound will stop most external bleeding. For severe bleeding, it may be necessary to apply pressure to the vein or artery above the bleeding point in such a way that the vessel is pressed against the bone behind it. Emergency medical assistance should always be sought for severe bleeding and whenever internal bleeding is suspected.

Bleeding disorders

Diseases involving malfunction of the blood's clotting system or other problems that result in prolonged bleeding. Bleeding may result from problems with clotting, the platelets, or fragile blood vessels. Some bleeding disorders are congenital (present at birth), and others develop during illness or are acquired as a result of medical treatment.

In normal blood, clotting, or coagulation, is a complex process that involves the blood cells known as platelets and as many as 20 proteins (coagulation factors) found in the plasma (the liquid portion of the blood). In a bleeding disorder, something goes wrong with the platelets or with one or more of the coagulation factors. The resulting bleeding can range from mild to severe. Symptoms may include easy and extensive bruising, excessive bleeding after injury, uncontrolled bleeding inside the body, heavy and repeated nosebleeds, and abnormally copious menstrual bleeding.

HEMOPHILIA

HEMOPHILIA is an example of an inherited bleeding disorder. Since the gene that causes hemophilia is sex-linked (that is, carried on the X chromosome), it appears almost exclusively in males and is carried by females. Boys and men with hemophilia lack a specific clotting factor and are prone to episodes of serious bleeding.

VON WILLEBRAND DISEASE

A deficiency in the clotting protein known as von Willebrand causes VON WILLEBRAND DISEASE, which is named after the Finnish physician who first described it. An inherited disorder, von Willebrand disease affects males and females equally. It has varying degrees of severity, with the more severe forms being the most rare.

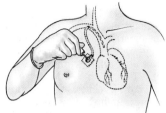

SELF-CARE FOR HEMOPHILIA
A child with hemophilia can have an infusion device implanted under the skin on the chest so that he or she can administer clotting factor at home. It is important that the child learn sterile technique, including sterilizing the site of injection and the needle, and proper disposal of the needle.

DISSEMINATED INTRAVASCULAR COAGULATION

The key symptom in disseminated intravascular coagulation (DIC; also known as intravascular coagulation) is severe bleeding that can be caused by an injury or following surgery. DIC results from excessive, inappropriate clotting in small blood vessels throughout the body, which uses up most of the supply of coagulation factors and allows bleeding to continue unabated at the site of the wound. DIC is a rare, life-threatening disorder and occurs primarily as a complication of other diseases, such as cancer, severe infections, and snakebites.

THROMBOCYTOPENIA

Taken from Greek roots meaning "a poverty of clotting cells," THROMBOCYTOPENIA results from a shortage of platelets. Thrombocytopenia can result from the production of antibodies to platelets, which destroy them, and an inability of the bone marrow to make a sufficient number of platelets.

DEFECTS IN THE BLOOD VESSEL

Certain diseases cause defects in the blood vessel wall. These vessels are more fragile and more prone to bleed than normal blood vessels. Causes include aging, vitamin C (ascorbic acid) deficiency, hereditary abnormalities, and some drugs.

Bleeding gums

See PERIODONTAL DISEASE.

Blepharitis

Inflammation of the edges of the eyelids. The eyelids look sticky, crusty, and reddened, with scales that cling to the bases of the lashes. The eye may feel gritty when blinking and

itch or burn. Eyelashes can fall out. Blepharitis has a number of possible causes, including bacterial infection, lice in the eyelashes, or a skin condition known as SEBORRHEIC DERMATITIS, which causes scaling and yellow crusty patches and appears on other parts of the body besides the eyelids, particularly the scalp. The lining of the eye may also become infected, resulting in CONJUNCTIVITIS (pinkeye). In rare instances of severe infection, the clear outer covering of the eye (cornea) can ulcerate. In most cases, blepharitis does not threaten sight. Crusts are removed by cleaning the eyelids with a clean cloth soaked in warm water; mild baby shampoo can also be used. Antibiotic or corticosteroid ointments may also be prescribed to fight infection and reduce swelling. If lice are present, they can be eradicated by placing petroleum jelly on the base of the eyelashes.

Blepharoplasty

See EYELID SURGERY.

Blepharoptosis

Drooping of one or both upper eyelids; also called ptosis. The cause is usually weakness in the muscle that raises the lid. In mild cases, the upper range of vision is blocked; in severe cases, the person can see little or nothing out of the eye without raising the eyelid by hand or tilting the head back. In children who are born with blepharoptosis, usually only one eye is affected. The condition also appears as people age, usually as a result of overall loss in muscle tone. Less often, blepharoptosis is a result of injury or such diseases as diabetes

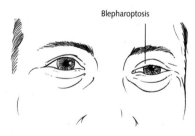

Blepharoptosis

DROOPING LIDS
Normally, the eyelid falls over only a small portion of the iris and does not cover any part of the pupil. In a person with blepharoptosis, the drooping lid makes the eye look smaller and diminishes the crease above the eyeball. Often the person tries to compensate by raising the eyebrows or lifting the head slightly.

mellitus, type 1 and type 2; myasthenia gravis; or cancer in locations that affects nerve and muscle responses (for example, the base of the neck).

Children born with blepharoptosis are treated surgically since the drooping eyelid limits normal use of the covered eye and can hamper development of normal vision (see AMBLYOPIA, or "lazy eye"). The age at which surgery is performed depends on the severity of the blepharoptosis. Mild cases are treated between ages 3 and 5 years; severe cases are treated earlier. Surgery usually involves suspending the weak eyelid by using artificial tissues attached to a normally functioning muscle in the forehead.

In adults, treatment of blepharoptosis depends on cause. If an underlying disease is causing the eyelids to droop, treatment of that disease may remedy the condition. Blepharoptosis from aging can be treated surgically, either for cosmetic reasons or to improve vision. This surgery involves repairing the weakened muscle and removing pockets of fat or loose tissue that give the eyelids a baggy appearance (see EYELID SURGERY).

Blepharospasm

Repeated, involuntary twitching or quivering of the eyelid. Usually the upper eyelid is affected. Once these spasms begin, they may continue for one or more days. Although annoying, temporary blepharospasms cease on their own without treatment. The condition is very common, affecting almost everyone at one time or another. The usual causes are stress and fatigue. Rest and gentle message often help relieve the condition.

Severe, persistent blepharospasm may also be caused by certain eye diseases, such as GLAUCOMA, inflammation of the eyelids (blepharitis), dry eyes, infection, or inflammation within the eye. Treatment of the underlying disease often alleviates the spasm.

Less common is a condition known as essential blepharospasm, which causes progressively more severe spasms of the eyelids and may also involve other muscles of the face and neck. Essential blepharospasm usually begins after age 50 years and is more common in women than men. The cause is uncertain, but it is thought to arise from miscommunica-

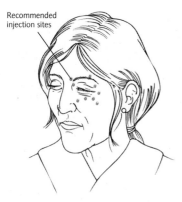

Recommended injection sites

SITES OF INJECTION FOR BLEPHAROSPASM
Injections of botulinum toxin, administered about every 3 months in carefully adjusted doses, can block the nervous transmissions that result in blepharospasm. The injections are done at specific sites around the eye to block nerve pathways.

tion in parts of the brain responsible for muscle control. Essential blepharospasm typically begins with increased blinking or squinting and progresses to repeated strong closing of the eyelids followed by difficulty in opening them. The person may be effectively blind because the eyelids cannot be kept open. Stress, fatigue, bright lights, watching television, driving, and social interactions often worsen the condition. Treatment by injecting medication into the eyelid is successful in some cases. Surgery to remove the involved muscles is also used.

Blind loop syndrome

A condition resulting from alterations in the structure of the intestine. In blind loop syndrome, one or more nonfunctioning segments of intestine are created either inadvertently or purposely by a surgical procedure. For example, a blind loop occurs following a partial removal of the stomach. A new opening is made into the small intestine, bypassing the first part of the intestine, which becomes a blind loop or dead end. Blind loop syndrome can also be present at birth.

Blind loop syndrome can lead to bacterial overgrowth and to complications, such as an intestinal obstruction, MALABSORPTION SYNDROME (impaired absorption of nutrients through the small intestine), or necrosis (death of tissue cells). Symptoms may include foul-smelling diarrhea, fatigue, and weight loss. Treatment with antibiotics may succeed, but if the condition persists, diseased segments of the intestine must be surgically removed and healthy segments rejoined.

Blind spot

The area on the retina (the light-sensitive layer at the back of the eye) from which the optic nerve emerges; also known as the optic disc. Since this part of the retina lacks light receptors, the optic disc is insensitive to light. In normal vision with both eyes, the blind spot is not perceived since the blind spot of one eye is covered by a seeing area of the other eye. The term "blind spot" is also sometimes used to refer to apparent holes (scotomas) in the visual field in which nothing can be seen. These scotomas are often a result of retinal disease or glaucoma.

Blindness

Total or partial loss of sight caused by a disease or disorder of the eye, optic nerve, or brain. In most cases, blindness refers to a loss of vision that cannot be corrected with glasses or contact lenses. Blindness does not always refer to a total loss of sight. Some people who are legally blind can perceive slow-moving objects or colors. The term "low vision" is used for people who have moderately impaired vision but are not classified as blind. Color blindness is not actually a form of blindness, since it refers only to a lack of perception of certain colors and not to a loss of vision.

ASSESSMENT

Physicians assess vision with two measurements. Visual acuity measures the ability to see details. Normal vision is defined as 20/20. Any loss of visual acuity raises the second number. For example, a person with 20/200 vision must stand 20 feet away from an object to see details that a person with normal vision can perceive at 200 feet. The second measurement is visual field, which refers to the size of the area around the center of vision. A normal visual field is 180 degrees, or half a circle. In the United States, blindness is defined legally as acuity of 20/200, even with glasses or contacts, or a visual field of 20 degrees or less.

CAUSES

■ *Glaucoma* This disease often results from abnormally high pressure within the eye and leads to progressive deterioration of vision from irreversible destruction of the optic nerve. It is the leading cause of preventable blindness in the United States and the principal cause of blindness among African Americans. Since the absence of symptoms makes glaucoma difficult to detect in the early stages, the disease may go untreated and lead to blindness. If detected before damage is severe, glaucoma can be treated and blindness prevented in most cases. See GLAUCOMA.

■ *Cataract* Cloudiness of the normally clear lens of the eye, usually as a result of aging, can lead to loss of sight. The disease is treated surgically, by removing the lens and replacing it with an artificial lens implant. If a lens implant is not used, contact lenses or very thick glasses must be worn. See CATARACT; CATARACT SURGERY.

■ *Diabetic retinopathy* Diabetes mellitus, type 1 and type 2, can cause disease in the small vessels that supply blood to the retina (the light-sensitive layer at the back of the eye), resulting in visual impairment. Laser treatment may be effective in treating the disease at certain stages. In some cases, when there is a hemorrhage inside the eye, lost vision can be restored by surgically removing the normally clear gel in the center of the eye and replacing it with a salt solution, a procedure known as VITRECTOMY. See RETINOPATHY, DIABETIC.

■ *Injury* Physical damage to the eye or the optic nerve may lead to partial or total loss of sight. Injury to an area of the brain that controls vision, as in a fall or a stroke, is another cause of blindness.

■ *Trachoma and river blindness* Rare in North America and Europe, trachoma is a common disease in Africa, the Middle East, South and Southeast Asia, and parts of Latin America. Trachoma results from infection with the *Chlamydia trachomatis* bacterium, which is spread easily by eye-hand contact, certain flies, and contaminated articles such as towels. Trachoma affects the mucous lining (conjunctiva) and the clear outer covering (cornea) of the eye and can be

Visual Impairment Aids

Many assistive devices are currently available for people with visual impairment, enlisting the other senses to help the person see.

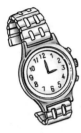

Talking watch
With the press of a button, the time of day is announced electronically. Watches for people with visual impairment usually also feature oversized numbers and hands and the use of color on the face or hands to make the watch more useful to people who are partially sighted.

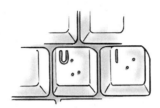

Braille computer keytops
Raised bumps representing the Braille alphabet are stamped onto transparent keytops that, once snapped in place, permit the original key legends to show through. Large print and large print/Braille combination keytops are also available for people with varying degrees of visual impairment.

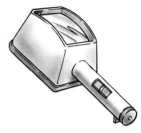

Magnifying glass
For people with poor or impaired vision, magnifiers are available with LED (light-emitting diode) and halogen lighting, interchangeable lenses, and color filters. Although larger than an ordinary magnifying glass, these enhanced magnifiers are still portable.

treated effectively with antibiotics and other medications. River blindness is known technically as onchocerciasis, and it is the second leading infectious cause of blindness worldwide, surpassed only by trachoma. The cause is a nematode worm spread by biting flies, which are most prevalent along rivers in sub-Saharan Africa.

■ *Nutritional deficiency* A diet deficient in vitamin A (beta carotene), usually associated with malnutrition, can lead to visual impairment as a result of severe drying of the conjunctiva that leads to deterioration and ulceration of the cornea. Although completely preventable, vitamin A deficiency is the major cause of childhood blindness in developing countries and widely prevalent in Asia, the Middle East, Africa, and South America.

■ *Other causes* Macular degeneration produces a blind or empty spot in the center of vision and is a leading cause of vision loss in the United States among people older than 65 years. Sickle cell anemia can cause blindness by blocking and damaging small blood vessels leading to the retina. Other diseases that destroy or

impair the eye, such as tumors or severe infections, may also lead to vision loss or blindness.

TREATMENT
Blindness caused by cataracts can often be reversed by surgery to remove and replace the cloudy lens. In loss of sight from most other causes, blindness can be prevented only by early detection and treatment of the underlying condition. If blindness does result, it is generally permanent.

Treatment for blindness consists of teaching the affected person how to adapt to a lack of sight. People who have some remaining vision can use vision aids, such as eyeglasses equipped with a telescopic lens, handheld lighted magnifiers, and specially tinted glasses. More and more high-tech aids are becoming available as well: sonar and radar devices that tell the user about objects in the vicinity, computers that translate printed text into synthetic speech and print dictation as text, computer-driven closed-circuit TV systems that read and magnify text, and typewriters and word processors that use Braille, a tactile alphabet used by the blind.

Blister
A small swelling of the skin filled with fluid; also known as a vesicle or bulla. Blisters can develop anywhere that the skin experiences friction and frequently occur on the feet. Groups of blisters or blisters involving more than one body location should be evaluated by a doctor for proper treatment. Although they are common and, in most cases, minor injuries, blisters require attention to prevent infection. They must be covered with an adhesive bandage or gauze pad and should not be punctured unless they are painful or prevent a person from performing essential activities such

INFECTED BLISTERS
It is essential to check blisters for signs of infection such as redness or pus. If a blister becomes infected, the person should see a doctor. Often a short course of antibiotics can quickly remedy the problem. In people who have diabetes or poor circulation, it is especially important to observe blisters carefully to prevent serious complications.

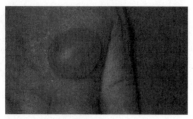

PROTECTIVE SWELLING
A blister is a fluid-filled sac that forms to shield the skin from friction or burning. An intact blister protects the underlying tissues from bacteria and decreases the risk of infection, so the best treatment is to cover the blister to prevent it from breaking.

as walking. Large blisters should only be punctured by a dermatologist. To puncture a blister, wash hands and the blister area with soap and warm water. Puncture the blister in several places around the perimeter with a sterile needle and let the fluid drain. Leave the skin covering the blister intact. Again wash hands and the blister area with soap and warm water. Cover the blister with an antibiotic ointment and gauze.

Blocking
Interruption of a train of speech before a thought or idea has been completed. After a period of silence, which may last from a few seconds to minutes, the person indicates that he or she cannot recall the topic of conversation. Blocking may or may not be a sign of a mental illness.

Blood
The red fluid that circulates in veins and arteries throughout the body. The blood transports oxygen, nutrients, and other chemicals throughout the body to every tissue and carries away waste materials. It also defends the body against infections. Because blood loss could be so damaging, blood has the capability to help seal damaged blood vessels, create clots at the sites of injuries to stop bleeding, and help repair damaged tissue. The heart pumps the body's blood supply in a continuous cycle through the arteries to the lungs and all other organs and tissues and then back to the heart through the veins. (See CARDIOVASCULAR SYSTEM.) A typical adult's body contains about 10 pints of blood. At rest, the heart pumps about 10 pints

of blood per minute. About 55 percent of the blood's volume is made up of a fluid called plasma, which transports blood cells, proteins, minerals, and nutrients to the body's tissues. The blood cells—including red blood cells, white blood cells, and platelets—account for the remaining blood volume.

BLOOD CELLS
The three major types of cells each have specialized functions. Red blood cells (erythrocytes) carry oxygen to body tissues and exchange it at a cellular level for the waste product carbon dioxide. White blood cells fight infection by roaming the body, detecting invading microorganisms and fighting them. Platelets help the blood to clot to stop bleeding from sites of injury and repair damaged blood vessels. Most blood cells are manufactured in the bone marrow by a series of cell divisions beginning with a single cell called a stem cell. About 99 percent of the blood is composed of red blood cells. Together, platelets and white blood cells make up the remaining 1 percent.

■ *Red blood cells* By using an iron-based chemical component called HEMOGLOBIN, red blood cells (also known as red corpuscles or erythrocytes) carry oxygen from the lungs to the tissues and then carry carbon dioxide waste back to the lungs where it is exhaled (see RESPIRATION). The relatively large surface area of the doughnut-shaped blood cells allows them to absorb and release oxygen molecules efficiently. They also have the flexibility to maneuver through tiny blood vessels. Differing structural characteristics among red blood cells distinguish the various blood type groups, such as A, B, AB, or O (see BLOOD GROUPS).

Each red blood cell contains large quantities of hemoglobin, an iron-rich protein that can transport oxygen, as well as enzymes, minerals, and sugar, which give energy and structure to the blood cell. When hemoglobin combines with oxygen, as it does very effectively in the lungs where the oxygen level is high, a substance called oxyhemoglobin is formed, accounting for the bright red color of oxygen-rich blood. In the tissues, where oxygen levels are lower, the hemoglobin just

as effectively releases oxygen, and the oxygen-depleted blood that flows back through the veins is considerably darker.

It takes about 5 days for red blood cells to be formed in the bone marrow. The rate at which they are produced depends on the supply of nutrients and a hormone produced in the kidneys. Red blood cells circulate in the blood for about 4 months before they age and wear out. As red blood cells die, they lodge in small blood vessels and the spleen until they are destroyed by macrophages, cells derived from white blood cells that eat other cells and microorganisms.

■ *White blood cells* White blood cells (also called leukocytes or white corpuscles) are larger than red blood cells but less numerous. There are three main types of white blood cells—granulocytes, monocytes, and lymphocytes. Each of the three types of white blood cells has a different role in defending the body against infectious organisms and other foreign materials.

Granulocytes are further divided into three types called neutrophils, basophils, and eosinophils. The most important type, making up 60 percent of all white blood cells, is the neutrophil, which isolates and kills invading bacteria. Neutrophils stay in the blood for only about 6 to 9 hours before moving through the blood vessels and into the tissues, where they live for a few days. Basophils can dilate or constrict small blood vessels and influence the nervous system. Eosinophils have a role in allergic reactions and increase in numbers to fight certain infections.

Monocytes circulate in the blood for 6 to 9 days, consuming microorganisms to defend the body against infection. Lymphocytes, white blood cells that are usually formed in the lymph glands, have an important role in the immune system. T-type lymphocytes are involved in allergies, and B-type lymphocytes form the antibodies that protect against second attacks of certain diseases. Lymphocytes survive in the blood anywhere from 3 months to 10 years.

■ *Platelets (thrombocytes)* The smallest type of blood cells, platelets, are colorless cells that repair injured

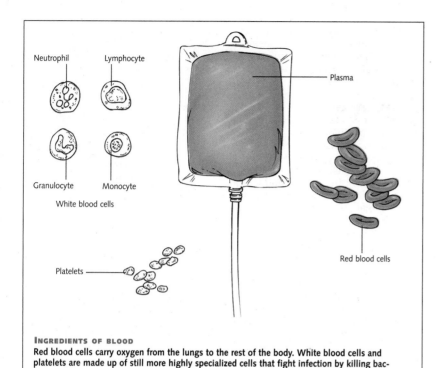

Neutrophil Lymphocyte

Plasma

Granulocyte Monocyte

White blood cells

Red blood cells

Platelets

INGREDIENTS OF BLOOD
Red blood cells carry oxygen from the lungs to the rest of the body. White blood cells and platelets are made up of still more highly specialized cells that fight infection by killing bacteria and forming antibodies. Platelets help heal damaged blood vessel walls and clot blood. Plasma (about 55 percent) is the liquid part of blood, composed of water and nutrients.

Blood cell count, complete

See BLOOD COUNT; CBC (COMPLETE BLOOD CELL COUNT).

Blood cells

The three major types of cells carried in plasma, the liquid portion of the BLOOD. They have specialized functions. Generally, red blood cells (erythrocytes) carry oxygen to the body; white blood cells (leukocytes) defend against invasions by bacteria, viruses, fungi, and other foreign material; and platelets (thrombocytes) help the blood to clot and repair damaged blood vessels. Most blood cells are manufactured in the bone marrow, and all three types are generated by a series of cell divisions beginning with a single cell called a stem cell. Red blood cells make up about 99 percent of blood cells, while white blood cells and platelets make up about 1 percent.

Blood clotting

The process by which blood turns from a liquid into a semisolid mass to stop bleeding. It begins when an injury to a blood vessel exposes the blood to cells in the blood vessel's lining. The blood cells known as platelets aggregate (adhere to one another) at the site of the injury. As the platelets aggregate, they trigger a cascade of reactions among various proteins known as coagulation factors, which results in the formation of a clot. The clot that seals the point of bleeding is made up of both the aggregated platelets and fibrin. When the wound heals, other proteins help dissolve the clot.

Blood count

A common blood test that provides information on the number and types of cells in the blood; also known as complete blood cell count or CBC. The term "count" refers to the numerical counting of each blood cell type. To do the test, a small quantity of blood is drawn from a vein into a syringe through a needle. Then the number of red blood cells, the number and kind of white blood cells, and the number of platelets in a given volume of the blood are determined. The test also provides data on the total amount

blood vessels, stemming blood loss. They live up to 9 days. When a blood vessel is damaged, platelets gather to plug the site of the injury, the first process in clot formation or coagulation. Proteins circulating in the blood, called clotting factors, complete the process (see PLATELETS; BLOOD CLOTTING; and BLOOD COUNT).

PLASMA
Plasma, the basic component of blood, is a yellow liquid, made up largely of water, proteins, acids, and salt. Plasma is the transport system and medium for nutrients, waste products, and blood cells, and it helps maintain blood pressure, distributes heat evenly throughout the body, and maintains a steady acid-base balance in the bloodstream. Measurement of the levels of the dissolved constituents within plasma helps doctors diagnose diseases. The primary chemical components of plasma include waste products, nutrients, proteins, and hormones.

■ *Waste products* Urea and BILIRUBIN are the major waste products in plasma. Urea is the main product of tissue metabolism and is transported in the

plasma to the kidneys. The waste product from the destruction of hemoglobin is bilirubin, a yellow pigment that is removed from the plasma by the liver and turned into bile. In a person with liver disease or anemia, bilirubin levels become abnormally high, causing the skin and eyes to turn yellow.

■ *Nutrients, proteins, and hormones* Sugars, fats, and amino acids that cells need to make proteins, vitamins, and minerals are transported to the tissues in the plasma from the intestinal tract or after release from storage organs such as the liver. Some blood proteins are involved in blood clotting and coagulation, while others decrease coagulation. The main plasma protein is albumin, a small molecule that maintains the water content in the bloodstream. The organs of the endocrine system secrete hormones directly into the bloodstream. Hormones work as chemical messengers that regulate the body's rates of metabolism of the cells, growth, and sexual development and the body's response to stress or illness.

B

of hemoglobin (the oxygen-carrying pigment) in the blood and hematocrit (the fraction of the blood composed of red blood cells).

A blood count is useful for diagnosing and managing many diseases. It can show problems resulting from loss of blood volume (for example, as the result of internal bleeding), abnormalities in blood cells, chronic or acute infection, allergies, and abnormal clotting.

Blood donation

The collection of whole blood or its components from a person. Whole blood donation takes 6 to 8 minutes, while APHERESIS (in which components of a donor's blood are collected) requires approximately 1½ hours. Blood collection is strictly regulated by the Food and Drug Administration (FDA). The process is very safe because all collection equipment is used only one time for each donor. Donated blood is used for persons undergoing bone marrow transplant, organ transplant, heart surgery, burn treatment, and treatment after motor vehicle accidents or other trauma. In autologous transfusion, a person donates blood in advance for his or her own use. In directed donation, family and friends donate the blood for a person's transfusion. See also BLOOD TRANSFUSION.

Blood gases

A laboratory test that measures the amounts of oxygen and carbon dioxide in the blood and determines the acidity; also known as arterial blood gas analysis. A sample for blood gases is taken from an artery, usually in the wrist, the groin, or the arm. The site is cleaned and disinfected, then a local anesthetic is injected. Once the area is numb, a needle is inserted into the artery and a sample of blood is withdrawn into a special syringe that prevents contamination by outside air. After the sample is drawn, pressure must be applied to the site for 5 to 15 minutes to prevent bleeding.

Blood gas analysis is useful for evaluating diseases that affect breathing, such as pneumonia, chronic obstructive pulmonary disease, and tuberculosis. It also provides information about the effectiveness of oxygen

therapy. Information about the acidity of the blood provides a measure of kidney function and can also provide information that can be used to assess the body's metabolism.

Blood groups

A system that classifies blood by the proteins contained in its red blood cells; also known as blood types. Blood group is important in determining the safety of blood transfusions. If blood from one blood group is transfused into a person with a different blood group, antibodies in the recipient's blood will attack the donated blood as a foreign substance. Transfusions between people of the same blood group almost always succeed.

There are four principal blood groups: A, B, AB, and O. The blood groups are further divided by the presence or absence of the Rh factor (see RH INCOMPATIBILITY). Blood with the Rh factor is Rh-positive (+); blood without it is Rh-negative (–). The most common blood group among Americans is O+, followed in order by A+, B+, O–, A–, AB+, B–, and AB–.

Blood groups are inherited in a predictable manner. This makes blood group data useful for identifying the father of a child whose paternity is in dispute.

Blood loss

BLEEDING, or loss of blood from blood vessels, that can occur internally or externally. Direct pressure halts most external bleeding. If bleeding is severe, or if internal bleeding or shock is suspected, emergency assistance should be sought.

Blood poisoning

The popular name for bacterial infection spreading through the blood. See SEPTICEMIA.

Blood pressure

A measurement of the force exerted by the blood against the walls of the arteries. Blood pressure results from two forces. One is the force of the heart as it contracts; the other is the resistance of the arteries to blood flow, which is a function of their flexibility and size. In general, the more blood the heart pumps with each beat and the narrower and less flexible the

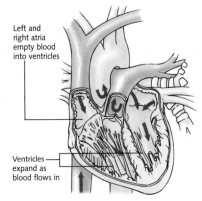

Left and right atria empty blood into ventricles

Ventricles expand as blood flows in

Diastolic pressure

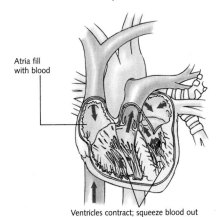

Atria fill with blood

Ventricles contract; squeeze blood out

Systolic pressure

FILLING AND PUMPING
Diastolic (dilating) pressure occurs as the heart relaxes and blood flows from the holding chambers (atria) into the pumping chambers (ventricles). Systolic (squeezing) pressure occurs as the ventricles contract and pump blood out of the heart. Blood flows from the right ventricle to the lungs; from the left ventricle to the rest of the body. The atria start to fill with blood again while the ventricles are contracting.

blood vessels, the higher the blood pressure.

Blood pressure is measured in millimeters of mercury (mm Hg) and given as two numbers written like a fraction, such as 125/75. The first, larger number represents the blood pressure when the heart is contracting, or the systolic pressure. The second, smaller number represents the pressure between beats when the heart is relaxed, or the diastolic pressure.

Blood pressure lower than 120/80 is considered optimal for cardiovascular health. Blood pressure of 120 to 139 over 80 to 89 indicates that

MEASURING YOUR OWN BLOOD PRESSURE

If your blood pressure is too high or too low, monitoring it at home can be an important part of managing the condition. Blood pressure is measured with a device called a sphygmomanometer, which consists of a central unit connected to a cuff that fits around the arm. Some models need to be used with a hand bulb and a stethoscope, while others work automatically.

Before taking a blood pressure reading, a person should rest quietly for at least 5 minutes. Blood pressure should not be taken if the bladder is full or if one has recently drunk a cup of coffee or smoked a cigarette, since all three raise blood pressure.

The basic procedure is as follows:
- The arm should be positioned at heart level by resting it on a table or the arm of a chair.
- The cuff should be slipped over the bare upper arm. The fit should be snug, with the lower edge of the cuff about 1 inch above the elbow.
- If an automated device is being used, the start button should be pushed. The cuff will inflate, then slowly deflate, and display the reading. Some models provide the pulse rate as well.
- If a stethoscope is used, its disk should be placed between the elbow and the edge of the cuff.
- The hand bulb should be squeezed until the pressure is 30 mm Hg above the expected systolic pressure, at which point no pulse sound will be heard in the stethoscope.
- The cuff should then be deflated slowly while listening for the pulse sound. The pressure when the pulse is first heard should be noted. This is the systolic pressure.
- As the cuff continues to deflate, the reading when the pulse sound disappears should be noted. This is the diastolic pressure.
- To ensure an accurate reading, the procedure should be repeated after a few minutes have passed.

the person has PREHYPERTENSION. Readings that are consistently over 140/90 indicate the presence of HYPERTENSION (high blood pressure). Untreated hypertension can lead to damage to the heart, kidneys, and eyes and is a contributing factor to heart attack and stroke. HYPOTENSION (low blood pressure) may cause fainting or dizzy spells. Hypotension is one symptom of shock following serious injury and blood loss, and it may also result from chronic disease or pregnancy.

Blood pressure is never constant. It rises and falls during the day in response to a number of variables, including emotions, fatigue, stress, and physical exertion. As a result, blood pressure readings should be taken in a relaxed setting with the person sitting and at rest. Any abnormal reading should be confirmed with additional measurements taken over the subsequent days and weeks.

Blood pressure cuff

The inflatable band placed around the upper arm to measure blood pressure. The blood pressure cuff is part of an instrument called a SPHYGMOMANOMETER, the most accurate method of measuring blood pressure. A sphygmomanometer consists of a pressure gauge, an inflater bulb or pressure pump, and the blood pressure cuff, which is connected by way of a rubber tube to a measurement panel.

Blood pressure is measured by inflating the blood pressure cuff after it has been wrapped around the person's upper arm. Once inflated, the blood pressure cuff exerts pressure on a large artery until the blood flow stops. That pressure is released slowly and gradually, permitting a nurse or doctor to listen to the pulse through a stethoscope. The health care worker can determine both the systolic and diastolic blood pressures, which can be read on a graduated scale on the measurement panel or electronically.

Blood products

The forms in which blood donations are stored before a transfusion. Blood products include whole blood and various blood components, each of which is used for different purposes.

Whole blood is used to replace blood lost during surgery or following a severe injury, but it can only be stored for 3 to 4 weeks after donation.

Packed red blood cells are prepared by removing some of the blood plasma to produce a concentrate useful for treating some kinds of chronic anemia that do not respond to medication. Packed red blood cells restore hemoglobin levels without overwhelming the person with excess fluid, and they can be frozen for long-term storage.

White blood cells (granulocytes)

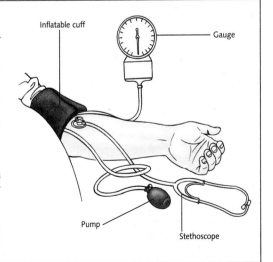

MEASUREMENT OF BLOOD PRESSURE
When a person has a blood pressure check, the cuff around the arm is inflated so that the pressure in the cuff is higher than the systolic (pumping) pressure of the heart and the heartbeat is inaudible. As the doctor deflates the cuff, he or she measures the systolic pressure by checking the gauge at the moment that the heartbeat suddenly becomes audible again—meaning that cuff pressure is the same as the systolic pressure in the artery. As the cuff deflates further, the doctor measures the diastolic (resting) pressure at the moment the sound of the heartbeat disappears again—which occurs when the cuff pressure goes below the diastolic pressure in the artery.

Inflatable cuff
Gauge
Pump
Stethoscope

can be separated from normal blood or taken from the blood of people who have too many such cells, and given to people who have life-threatening infections or abnormally low levels of granulocytes.

Platelets are used to treat people with blood disorders involving clotting. Plasma is used shortly after collection to correct bleeding and clotting disorders. Shock caused by severe blood loss can be temporarily treated with plasma protein solutions until whole blood is available.

Concentrated clotting factors VIII and IX can be collected and used to treat HEMOPHILIA, although the concentrate must be heat-treated to reduce the spread of HEPATITIS and AIDS (acquired immunodeficiency syndrome).

Immunoglobulins (antibodies), can be concentrated from the plasma of people recovering from viral diseases such as rubella and hepatitis B and from the plasma of people who have recently been immunized against diseases such as tetanus. Such a concentrate can be used to protect people who are unable to produce their own antibodies or who have just been exposed to a viral disease.

Blood smear

A laboratory test that provides information about the number, type, and shape of blood cells; also known as a peripheral smear or differential stain. A small amount of blood is drawn from a vein, usually in the elbow or on the back of the hand, and examined under a microscope. The number of white and red blood cells relative to other types of blood cells is counted, any abnormalities in cell shape are noted, and the total number of white blood cells and platelets is roughly estimated. A blood smear also allows doctors to classify the blood by its color and by the shape and size of the cells. A blood smear may be performed as part of a routine health examination or when diagnosing an illness, particularly one that involves abnormally shaped blood cells.

Blood tests

A series of laboratory studies of blood samples used to screen for or to diagnose diseases. Some tests require only a drop or two of blood, and the sample is usually taken from the tip of the finger. When the test requires a larger sample, it is normally taken by needle from a vein in the elbow or on the back of the hand; the blood is collected in a sterile syringe or vacuum tube. Blood tests are usually painless, and complications are minor and rare.

There are hundreds of available blood tests. The ones listed here are the most common.

BLOOD COUNT

This common blood test provides information on the number and types of cells in the blood; also known as complete blood cell count or CBC. The term "count" refers to the numerical counting of each blood cell type. To perform the test, a small quantity of blood is drawn from a vein through a needle. Then the number of red blood cells, the number and kind of white blood cells, and the number of platelets in a given volume of the blood are determined. The test also provides data on the total amount of hemoglobin (the oxygen-carrying pigment) in the blood and hematocrit (the fraction of the blood composed of red blood cells).

The blood count is useful for diagnosing and managing many diseases. It can show problems resulting from loss of blood volume (for example, as a result of internal bleeding), abnormalities in blood cells, chronic or acute infection, allergies, and abnormal clotting.

BLOOD SMEAR

This test provides information about the number and shape of blood cells; it is also known as a peripheral smear or differential stain. A small amount of blood is drawn from a vein, usually in the elbow or on the back of the hand, and examined under a microscope. The number of white blood cells relative to other types of blood cells is counted, any abnormalities in cell shape are noted, and the total number of white blood cells and platelets is roughly estimated. A blood smear may be performed as part of a routine health examination or when diagnosing an illness, particularly one that involves abnormally shaped blood cells.

BLOOD CHEMISTRY

This group of tests provides information as to how well major organs are functioning. Blood chemistry tests generally identify the levels of electrolytes (sodium, potassium, chloride, and phosphorus) in the blood; the level of glucose, or blood sugar, which is important for detecting diabetes mellitus; liver function tests (including bilirubin levels); and kidney function tests (including blood urea nitrogen and creatinine levels). Additional tests may be added to the group if a doctor deems them necessary.

LIPIDS

This test measures the blood levels of total cholesterol, high-density lipoproteins, low-density lipoproteins, and triglycerides, all of which have a role in the development of heart disease. (See CHOLESTEROL for more information on blood fats.)

SEDIMENTATION TEST

This test determines how long it takes for red blood cells to sediment (settle) to the bottom of a liquid-filled test tube. A faster than normal rate suggests anemia (low red blood cell count), infection, inflammation, rheumatoid arthritis, or certain cancers. (See ESR.)

BLOOD GASES

The blood gases test measures the amounts of oxygen and carbon dioxide in the blood and determines the acidity of the blood; it is also known as arterial blood gas analysis. Unlike most other blood tests, for which samples are drawn from a vein, the blood gases sample is taken from an artery, usually in the wrist, groin, or arm. The site is cleaned and disinfected, then a local anesthetic is injected. Once the area is numb, a needle is inserted into the artery and a sample of blood withdrawn into a special syringe that prevents contamination by outside air. After the sample is drawn, pressure must be applied to the site for 5 to 15 minutes to prevent bleeding.

Measurement of blood gases is useful for evaluating diseases that affect breathing, such as pneumonia, chronic obstructive pulmonary disease, and tuberculosis. It also provides information about the effectiveness of oxygen therapy. Information about the acidity of the blood provides a measure of kidney function and information that can be used to assess the body's metabolism.

CROSSMATCHING

This laboratory test is used to determine a person's blood group by identifying the proteins on the red blood cells; it is also known as blood typing and ABO typing. Crossmatching is important for determining the safety

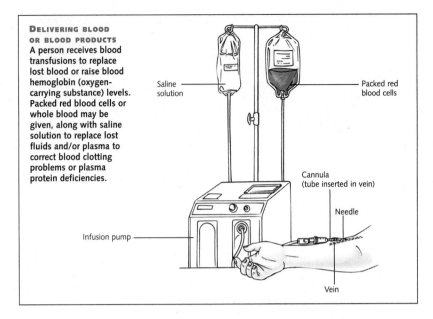

DELIVERING BLOOD OR BLOOD PRODUCTS
A person receives blood transfusions to replace lost blood or raise blood hemoglobin (oxygen-carrying substance) levels. Packed red blood cells or whole blood may be given, along with saline solution to replace lost fluids and/or plasma to correct blood clotting problems or plasma protein deficiencies.

Saline solution

Packed red blood cells

Cannula (tube inserted in vein)

Needle

Infusion pump

Vein

Blood-brain barrier

A double layer of cells that inhibits substances from crossing from the bloodstream into brain tissues. It protects the brain by slowing or stopping the passage of certain chemical compounds, including some drugs, and disease-causing organisms (such as viruses) from the bloodstream into the brain.

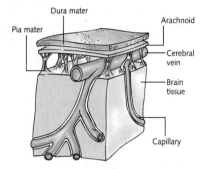

Dura mater

Pia mater

Arachnoid

Cerebral vein

Brain tissue

Capillary

BRAIN TISSUE
A cross-section of brain tissue reveals the protective layers over the brain: the tough dura mater, the weblike arachnoid layer containing blood vessels, and the pia mater that adheres to the brain surface. Capillaries, which penetrate the tissue, are lined with endothelial cells that form the blood-brain barrier.

of blood transfusions. If blood from one blood group is transfused into a person with a different blood group, antibodies in the recipient's blood will attack the donated blood. Transfusions between people of the same blood group almost always succeed.

The four principal blood groups, A, B, AB, and O, are further divided by the presence or absence of the Rh factor (for rhesus, the name of the species of monkey in which the factor was discovered). Blood with the Rh factor is Rh-positive (+); blood without it is Rh-negative (–). The most common blood group among Americans is O+, followed by A+, B+, O–, A–, AB+, B–, and AB–.

Crossmatching is performed by mixing a sample of blood with anti-A serum (one that has antibodies against type A blood), then with anti-B serum. If the blood is type A, it clots in the anti-A serum, not in the anti-B serum. If it is type B, it clots in the anti-B serum, but not in the anti-A serum. If it is type AB, it clots in both; if type O, it clots in neither. The same serum test is then repeated with a serum sample (that is, blood from which all cells have been removed) to ensure accuracy. Rh type is determined similarly with an anti-Rh serum. Clotting means the blood is Rh-positive; no clotting means the blood is Rh-negative.

Crossmatching is a particularly im-

portant test for a person receiving a blood TRANSFUSION and for women during pregnancy (see RH INCOMPATIBILITY).

Blood transfusion

The infusion of whole blood or its components directly into the bloodstream to replace blood loss from surgery, injury, or disease. A blood transfusion may also be needed to improve clotting or to enhance the body's ability to transport oxygen to tissues. In a transfusion, a nurse administers the blood intravenously. Before it is transfused, donor blood is carefully screened to make certain it is free from infectious disease organisms and is compatible with the recipient's blood. Incompatibility can provoke serious transfusion reactions such as chills, fever, hives, wheezing, shock, and kidney failure. In autologous transfusion, a person donates blood in advance for his or her own use. In directed donation, family and friends donate the blood for a person's transfusion. See BLOOD DONATION; TRANSFUSION.

Blood urea nitrogen

See KIDNEY FUNCTION TESTS.

Blood vessels

The tubes that carry blood from the heart to the body and back again; a general term for arteries, veins, and capillaries that are structures of the CARDIOVASCULAR SYSTEM.

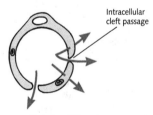

Intracellular cleft passage

Typical capillary

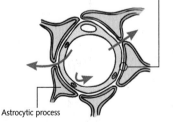

Tight junctions (cell connections)

Astrocytic process

Brain capillary

SPECIALIZED BRAIN CAPILLARIES
A typical capillary allows transport of substances into surrounding tissue, via openings in the wall (for example, intracellular cleft passages) and structures that allow passage through the wall itself. A brain capillary is almost completely surrounded by structures called astrocytic processes that fit tightly to the wall, restricting transport through the walls.

Bloodless surgical techniques

Techniques that minimize the amount of blood lost during a surgical procedure and make blood transfusions from outside donors unnecessary. Bloodless surgery was developed to meet religious objections to transfusions and to address concerns about the safety of the blood supply following the spread of AIDS (acquired immunodeficiency syndrome) and hepatitis. Bloodless techniques are used in many different types of surgical procedures.

A number of technologies are used to make bloodless surgery possible. Meticulous dissection techniques reduce bleeding by cutting less tissue, and an advanced cell-saver system conserves and recirculates blood that would otherwise be lost. Electrical surgical instruments use heat to seal off cut blood vessels during surgery and also to help the blood to clot, to prevent or limit bleeding. Patients can be given intravenous fluids that water down the blood and decrease the number of red blood cells lost. A medication given before surgery called synthetic ERYTHROPOIETIN, a hormone that stimulates the bone marrow to produce more red blood cells, helps to reduce the effects of blood loss.

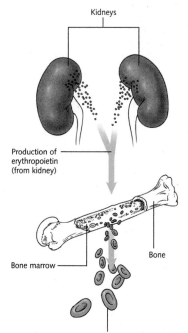

HORMONES AND RED BLOOD CELL PRODUCTION
The kidneys produce the hormone erythropoietin, which stimulates the bone marrow to produce more red blood cells as necessary. A person having surgery can be given a synthetic form of the hormone so that blood lost during surgery is quickly replenished.

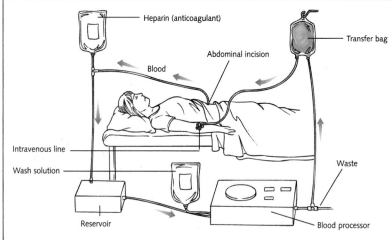

SURGERY WITHOUT TRANSFUSIONS
The cell-saver system collects the patient's own blood, washes it, and returns it into circulation. Blood is withdrawn from the patient's abdomen and mixed with heparin, a drug that prevents the blood from clotting. The blood is pooled in a reservoir and then disinfected in a processing unit. Waste products are channeled off, and the cleaned blood moves into a transfer bag where it is held before being introduced back into the person's body through an intravenous line.

Blow-out fracture

A break in the floor of the bony socket (orbit) surrounding the eye. The usual cause is a hard blow from a nonpenetrating blunt object, such as a fist, a ball, or a car's dashboard during an automobile collision. The fracture may entrap some of the muscles that move the eye, causing double vision, especially when the person looks up. Other symptoms include bruising around the eye, protrusion of the eyeball, and numbness in the cheek or upper teeth. Tests, including a CT (computed tomography) scan, are performed to determine whether eye muscles are involved in the fracture. A blow-out fracture involving muscles requires surgical repair, which is usually performed within 14 days of the injury. If no muscles are involved, if there is no persistent diplopia (double vision), or if no serious cosmetic defect is present, the fracture is allowed to heal on its own.

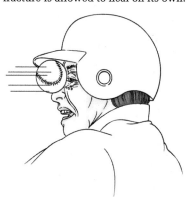

BLOW TO THE FRONT OF THE EYE
A blow to the front of the eye (as with a ball or fist) may leave the rim of the eye socket intact, but cause a break in the paper-thin floor of the socket. Portions of the eye muscles may be trapped in the break, causing abnormal eye movement and double vision.

Blurred vision

A lack of sharpness when viewing an object, resulting in unclear visual details. Blurred vision can have a number of causes, including farsightedness, nearsightedness, astigmatism (distortion caused by asymmetry in the eyeball), cataract (clouding of the lens of the eye, usually caused by aging), deterioration of the light-sensitive layer (retina) of the eye (because of macular degeneration or diabetic retinopathy, for example), glaucoma (a disease that results in damage to the optic nerve), infection in or injury to the eye, extreme fatigue, exposure to the elements (such as snow blindness), and drugs and medications (such as alcohol and antihistamines). Blurred vision that persists should be evaluated professionally. Treatment depends on cause. Refraction problems such as farsightedness and nearsightedness can be treated with glasses or contact lenses. Surgery may be necessary for cataracts, certain kinds of retina problems, or injury. Glaucoma can be treated with medication, laser surgery, and traditional surgery (see TRABECULECTOMY). If a drug is the cause of blurring, abstaining or changing to a different medication may resolve the vision problem; talking to the doctor about a change in medication is the first step.

Blushing

Temporary and involuntary reddening of the skin. Blushing can be brought on by excitement, exercise, fever, or embarrassment. Blushing occurs when the nervous system causes the capillaries of the skin of the cheeks and neck to widen, thus increasing blood flow that causes reddening.

BMI

See BODY MASS INDEX.

Body image

The subjective picture of one's physical attributes, including attitudes about oneself and physical experience of the world, carried in the mind. Distortions in body image are associated with ANOREXIA NERVOSA and BULIMIA, disorders in which thin persons perceive themselves as fat and alter their eating patterns to lose excessive amounts of weight.

Distortion of body image can also occur in the brain as parietal lobe disease or be caused by hallucinogen use. Phantom limb disorder, schizophrenia, and migraine headache can also affect a person's body image.

Body mass index

Also called BMI; a measurement of body weight relative to height. The BMI is closely associated with body fat percentage, an important factor that can be difficult to measure. Body weight is more sensitive to fluctuations in muscle mass and water reten-

BODY MASS INDEX TABLE

Generally, a BMI of 27 is considered overweight, and 30 or above is severely overweight. However, figures vary with height. Below is a partial table of BMIs for people of different weights and heights.

WEIGHT (pounds)	HEIGHT (feet, inches)					
	5'0"	5'3"	5'6"	5'9"	6'0"	6'3"
110	21	19	18	16	15	14
120	23	21	19	18	16	15
130	25	23	21	19	18	16
140	27	25	23	21	19	18
150	29	27	24	22	20	19
160	31	28	26	24	22	20
170	33	30	27	25	23	21
180	35	32	29	27	25	23
190	37	34	31	28	26	24
200	39	35	32	30	27	25
210	41	37	34	31	28	26
220	43	39	36	33	30	27
230	45	41	37	34	31	29
240	47	43	39	35	33	30
250	49	44	40	37	34	31

Adapted with permission of the American Dietetic Association.

tion than is BMI and, therefore, does not reflect body fat changes as accurately.

Standard BMI tables, which show weight-to-height ratios, are useful tools for examining the relative healthiness of a person's weight. When a BMI is above the normal range, a person is considered OVERWEIGHT or obese. The higher the BMI, the more overweight an individual is. A BMI of 25 to 27 generally means that a person is overweight. Exceptions are people such as athletes, who have a high BMI because of excess muscle rather than fat. A BMI of 27 to 30 or higher is a sign of OBESITY, which is an even more serious health threat than being overweight. A diagnosis of obesity means that an individual weighs 20 percent or more than the average for his or her height. When the BMI is above 40, a person is carrying approximately 100 pounds of excess weight.

To determine BMI, an individual's weight in pounds is multiplied by 700, divided by the person's height in inches, and divided by the height again. Because this is a rather intimidating calculation that individuals may be discouraged from undertaking on their own, standard BMI tables are readily available. BMI is easily determined on the accompanying table by finding one's weight in the left-hand column and one's height at the top of the table. The BMI for that weight and height is found where the columns corresponding to these two numbers intersect within the table.

WEIGHT-RELATED HEALTH CONSIDERATIONS

An individual who is overweight or obese has a higher than average percentage of body fat and, consequently, faces increased risks for health problems. A high BMI is associated with serious problems such as high blood pressure, a high cholesterol level, cardiovascular disease, diabetes, stroke, and cancer. Obesity has been linked with colon cancer and prostate cancer in men and with cancer of the breast, uterus, and endometrium in women. Other concerns include back pain, sleep apnea (a potentially life-threatening condition in which individuals stop breathing for short periods during sleep), gallstones, osteoarthritis, heartburn, gout, and varicose veins. Studies have shown that heavier people generally have a shorter life expectancy. Excess weight has been associated with increased emotional and psychological problems.

WEIGHT MANAGEMENT

Overweight and obese individuals should see a doctor or a registered dietician (RD) to discuss nutritional needs and a WEIGHT LOSS plan. Effective weight loss programs emphasize slow, gradual loss based on healthful eating and exercise. For people with an extremely high body mass index (above 40), surgery may be an option. An operation may also be considered for people with a BMI between 35 and 40 who have obesity-related, life-threatening health problems such as heart disease or diabetes.

Body piercing

The practice of creating holes in body parts for cosmetic purposes. Body piercing enables people to wear jewelry in such body parts as the earlobes, lips, nose, navel, eyebrows, nipples, and genitals. Body piercing has been practiced in almost every society, chiefly involving ears, nose, and mouth. Nontraditional body piercing has become increasingly popular in Western societies, such as the United States.

Navel piercing is associated with a high infection rate because the jewelry inserted in the navel tends to irritate the skin. Ears of infants and young children that have been pierced at home by their parents have been associated with severe bacterial infections, including TOXIC SHOCK SYNDROME and TETANUS. Other problems associated with body piercing include torn ear lobes and torn nipples, which may be caused by earrings or nipple rings being forcibly removed. Piercing in the mouth has caused airway obstruction, chipped or cracked teeth, and chewing problems. Body piercing is a potential route of transmission for HIV (human immunodeficiency virus) and other blood-borne diseases if instruments

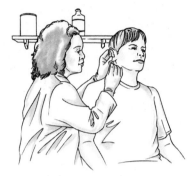

STERILE PROCEDURES
The major health risk associated with body piercing is infection from unsanitary piercing equipment. These infections can be painful and unsightly; more important, serious diseases such as hepatitis, tetanus, and HIV (human immunodeficiency virus) infection can be transmitted. Use of sterile gloves and sterilization of needles, body part, and jewelry are essential.

contaminated with blood are used between clients or improperly sterilized.

Some of the problems associated with body piercing can be avoided by careful selection of a piercing studio. Guidelines include making sure that the studio either uses sterilized disposable equipment or sterilizes its equipment in an AUTOCLAVE. Plastic ear-piercing guns should be avoided because they cannot be sterilized in an autoclave. Some people develop allergies to nickel as a result of body piercing; this can be prevented by wearing hypoallergenic, nickel-free jewelry.

Bodywork

Methods of therapeutic manipulation of the body to reduce pain and improve patterns of movement. Bodywork includes more than 80 different types of MASSAGE THERAPY, most of which are used to release muscle tension, improve blood flow, and reduce pain associated with muscle spasm. Other forms of bodywork seek to organize and integrate the body by correcting inappropriate patterns of movement, thereby bringing about more balanced use of the body. Several approaches to bodywork exist, including the ALEXANDER TECHNIQUE, the FELDENKRAIS METHOD, ROLFING, and the TRAGER APPROACH. Other forms of bodywork, such as THAI MASSAGE and REFLEXOLOGY, seek to restore balance or harmony to the

body by applying pressure to key points on the body thought to be associated with the flow of energy, or qi (pronounced "chee").

Boil

A tender, red, inflamed, pus-filled area of skin; also known as a furuncle. Most boils are caused by infection of a hair follicle with staphylococcal (staph) bacteria. Boils most commonly occur on the face, neck, armpits, buttocks, and thighs as painful, red lumps that gradually swell and fill with pus. A head forms with a yellow center, and pain increases until the boil finally bursts.

Boils should never be squeezed as this can cause the infection to spread. While most boils resolve without treatment within 2 weeks, it is helpful to apply warm compresses to the boil for 30 minutes several times a day. In the meantime, the boil and the surrounding area must be kept clean with antibacterial soap. Applying a sterile dressing prevents spread of draining material, and an antibiotic ointment prevents further infection. A cluster of boils affecting adjacent follicles is called a CARBUNCLE. Carbuncles and severe boils may require surgical draining. In some cases, oral antibiotics are prescribed. People with diabetes, atopic dermatitis, and weakened immune systems are more prone than others to boils, although poor hygiene can be a contributing factor.

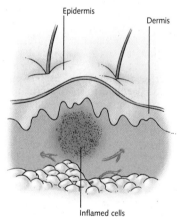

SKIN ABSCESS
A boil is an infection deep in the skin, in the underlying layer called the dermis. The dense accumulation of inflamed cells is most often caused by bacteria, but can also result from a clogged pore, inflammation of sweat glands, or in some cases, from prolonged pressure.

Bolus

A relatively large quantity of a substance, such as a dose of a drug; a chewed portion of food or other substance that is ready to be swallowed. An intravenous bolus is a relatively large volume of fluid or dose of a drug given rapidly and intravenously to speed up or magnify a response.

Bonding

The emotional attachment that forms between parent and child. Bonding begins before the child is born, and it is enhanced by close physical contact between mother and child in the hours after birth. Fathers who spend time with their children, especially while they are very small, form a similar attachment. When parents and child are separated immediately after birth (such as with premature infants who need intensive nursery care), bonding occurs when they are able to begin physical contact.

Bonding, dental

A process in which a tooth-colored resin material is attached to a tooth to repair it, improve its color, or reshape it. Dental bonding, also called dental composite bonding, has many uses: it can treat cavities or replace older, more obvious silver amalgam fillings, repair exposed roots, or close the spaces between teeth.

HOW IT WORKS

After preparing the tooth to be treated, the tooth surface is roughened so that a bonding agent will adhere to the tooth. The tooth is then ready for the composite, which is applied in layers and cured with a special light. The composite is then shaped to fit the tooth and polished to prevent staining and increase durability. The process can usually be completed in one office visit. Because dentists can blend shades to create a color close to the shade of the tooth to be repaired, the result is a natural, improved appearance. Dental bonding adheres to teeth and supports the remaining tooth structure when it is used to treat cavities. The bonding process may help to prevent breakage of a tooth and insulate it from uncomfortable temperature changes. Composite bonding generally lasts as long as silver fillings when used to treat cavities of average size; in larger restorations, it may be less durable than

silver amalgam. The composite resin material used in dental bonding is more brittle than the material of natural teeth and can chip more easily. It also stains more easily. The dentist can apply a clear plastic coating over the composite to prevent possible color changes. Beverages such as coffee, tea, and red wine will stain the bonded teeth.

Bone

The living tissue of which the skeleton is made. Bone is a form of connective tissue (tissue that supports or holds structures of the body together) that is uniquely hard and strong because of a high concentration of the mineral calcium.

STRUCTURE

A mature bone has several distinct layers. Covering the surface except at the ends is a membrane called the PERIOSTEUM, containing arteries, veins, and nerves that penetrate the underlying bone layers. Under the periosteum is a layer of hard (cortical) bone tissue. This dense material is composed of the structural protein collagen, arranged around microscopic channels called the haversian canals, through which the blood vessels and nerves pass. Within the hard bone lies a layer of spongy (cancellous) bone, composed of a mesh of cavities surrounded by hardened tissues. Adult bone contains about 65 percent calcium and other minerals and about 35 percent collagen. BONE MARROW lies in the cavities of spongy bone and also in the hollow core of long bones. There are two types of marrow—red marrow, in which blood cells are formed, and yellow marrow that is largely fatty tissue.

Bone tissue contains deposits of calcium and phosphorus that give bone its density and strength. The structure of spongy bone enables it to absorb stress, giving bone considerable resiliency.

FUNCTION

Overall, the bones of the skeleton form a framework that supports parts of the body and protects fragile internal organs and soft tissues. The muscles that are attached to the skeleton provide power for movement, and the bones act as levers. But beyond these physical functions, bone also is the site of the manufacture of blood cells, both red and white. Bone also ware-

houses its calcium and phosphorus and releases these minerals into the bloodstream as necessary.

DEVELOPMENT AND GROWTH

Bone tissue develops from cartilage, which hardens into bone in a process called ossification. In a newborn, many bones are still in the form of cartilage that will gradually ossify. This process continues until young adulthood, when bone reaches its peak density. In an infant or child, bone growth occurs at the end of the bone in an area called the epiphysis or growth plate. The ends of bones are composed mostly of spongy bone that hardens when bone growth (which is stimulated by hormonal activity) is complete in adolescence.

Bone is continually replacing itself throughout life, a process called rebuilding. Bone cells called osteoblasts build up bone by depositing calcium on the structural framework of the tissue, and other cells called osteoclasts break it down and reabsorb it. Until young adulthood, the rate of bone formation exceeds the rate of breakdown, and the density and strength of the bone tissue increases. Between the ages of about 20 and 35, the rate of bone formation starts to fall; after about age 35, the rate of breakdown exceeds the rate of formation, and bone density begins to decrease. See SKELETAL SYSTEM.

Bone abscess

A pus-filled pocket or cavity located on or in the bone and surrounded by inflamed tissue. A bone abscess is generally composed of white blood cells, bacteria, and dead tissue. The bacterial infection that most commonly gives rise to a bone abscess is caused by a staphylococcal infection. (See INFECTION.) Bone abscesses are rare and potentially fatal. They are treated with a surgical procedure to drain the abscess, as well as with appropriate antibiotics. See also OSTEOMYELITIS.

Bone cancer

Cancer that originates in bone tissue. Some cancers can spread to the bones and erroneously are called bone cancer. Also called primary bone cancer, cancer that first develops in bone tissue is uncommon and occurs chiefly in children and adolescents, ages 10 to 25. Cancer can affect any bone, but in adolescence, it typically appears in the long bones of the arms and legs. Bone cancer most often develops in the area around the knee joint. The most common symptom of bone cancer is pain, frequently accompanied by fatigue, fever, weight loss, and anemia. Swelling over a bone can be a sign of bone cancer, particularly if the swelling becomes progressively larger and more tender. Bone cancer can weaken bones and cause them to fracture.

The condition is assessed by blood tests and by using imaging tools, such as an X ray, a bone scan, CT (computed tomography) scan, or fluoroscopy. Diagnosis is confirmed by a bone biopsy, in which a small piece of the bone is removed and examined under a microscope. The most common type of primary bone cancer is osteosarcoma, which usually develops in bone areas with the greatest growth activity. A second type, Ewing sarcoma, begins in immature nerve tissue found in bone marrow. Another type, chondrosarcoma, develops in cartilage and is found more often in adults than in children or adolescents. Although the cause of primary bone cancer is not entirely clear, certain people are known to be at risk. Children and young adults who have had radiation or chemotherapy for other conditions have a greater risk for developing bone cancer. Adults with a noncancerous condition called PAGET DISEASE, which is characterized by the rapid turnover of bone tissue, also have an increased risk.

Treatment of bone cancer depends on the type, size, location, and stage of the cancer and the age and health of the individual. Surgery is often the primary treatment. Amputation of an affected arm or leg may be necessary, although sometimes surgeons can preserve part of the limb and remove only the cancerous section of a bone, replacing it with an artificial device or a bone graft. This is called limb-sparing surgery. Chemotherapy and radiation also are used alone or in combination.

> Terms in small capital letters—for example, PHYSICAL THERAPY or PAGET DISEASE—indicate a cross-reference to another entry with more information.

Bone cyst

An abnormal closed cavity or sac lined with tissue and filled with fluid that originates in the bone tissue and is usually noncancerous (benign). Bone cysts are rare and tend to occur in children between the ages of 5 and 15 years. They generally develop in long bones, such as the upper arm bone (humerus) or thighbone (femur), and make the affected bones more susceptible to fracture. A simple bone cyst has a well-defined border and may involve some degree of bone expansion and thinning of the cortex. Bone cysts may be diagnosed by means of X rays, including CT (computed tomography) scanning or MRI (magnetic resonance imaging). Surgery to remove bone cysts may be recommended to prevent fracture of the bone involved. Some bone cysts respond to being drained (which is called aspiration) and being injected with a corticosteroid.

Bone density testing

Tests done to evaluate the density of bones. Bone density testing is done to measure bone strength, predict fracture risk, and assess the degree of OSTEOPOROSIS, a condition that results in the bones slowly losing mass and deteriorating. A certain amount of bone loss is a normal consequence of aging in both men and women. Done periodically, bone density tests can help determine whether and how quickly the bones are losing calcium. Bone density testing should be considered if a woman is older than 40 years and has already experienced a bone fracture; has a close female relative who has had osteoporosis or a bone fracture; takes medication (such as corticosteroids or antiseizure medication) that accelerates bone loss; has a low body weight or a slight build; has a light complexion; or has a history of heavy drinking or smoking. Men are at less risk of osteoporosis than women but should be tested if they have a risk factor for osteoporosis such as taking corticosteroids.

The most accurate imaging technique to measure bone density is DUAL-ENERGY X-RAY ABSORPTIOMETRY (DEXA), which can detect extremely small degrees of bone loss. DEXA, using a low dose of radiation to detect bone loss, takes only a few minutes.

Bone graft

A surgical procedure to repair lost or damaged bone by replacing it with bone tissue taken from another part of the body or with a compatible synthetic material. Medical procedures that may involve bone grafts include fusion of the spine and of the arm and leg joints, closure of gaps in bones due to trauma or infection, oral or maxillofacial surgery, and the repair of certain bone fractures. Bone grafts are typically used to fill fracture defects in the growth plate at the end of the long bones in the arms and legs. Generally, the bone tissue or synthetic material is formed to fit into the area needing the graft, and rigid internal fixation is supplied by means of plates, pins, and screws, which hold the grafted, or implanted, material to the healthy bone tissue. Cells of the host bone regenerate on the porous framework of the bone graft, which provides support for the new bone tissue and related structures, stimulating their growth and enabling them to establish new connections between the separated segments of bone.

MATERIALS

Synthetic bone void fillers are artificial grafts that are sterile and can be sculpted to fit into a gap in fractured bones. Their use precludes the need for preliminary surgery to collect bone tissue for grafting. One synthetic bone graft material is composed of sea coral, which is chemically processed to create the same mineral content as human bone. The use of this synthetic material requires a 3-day hospital stay.

Autograft involves taking bone grafts from other bone tissue in a person's body; the bone is usually taken from the pelvis. This procedure requires two separate operations, one to obtain the needed bone and the other to implant it, but provides compatible living bone cells to repair the damaged bone tissue. The hospital stay for autograft procedures is generally a week.

An allograft surgical procedure involves using bone tissue from a cadaver, eliminating the need for two surgical procedures but introducing the risk of immune system rejection or viral contamination.

Bone imaging

Techniques that may use magnetic fields or radiation, often in combination with computers, to record and display images of bone structure. Bone imaging can reveal elements that are important to a complete diagnosis and are not provided by physical examination or laboratory tests. Conventional X RAYS, in which high-energy electromagnetic waves are passed through the body to produce images on film, are one kind of bone imaging. Because bone is dense, few X rays pass through bone structures, and bones appear white on the image, enabling a doctor to observe irregularities such as fractures.

Another approach to bone imaging, CT SCANNING (computed tomography scanning), sends many X-ray beams from different directions through the area to be observed. The CT scan records how much of each beam is absorbed by the bone and uses a computer to produce a series of vertical or horizontal, cross-sectional, three-dimensional images.

MRI (magnetic resonance imaging) is a form of bone imaging that uses a magnetic field in combination with radio waves to create signals that are analyzed by a computer, which then uses the information to construct an image. These images may be used to reveal tears in the tendons that attach muscle to bone or tumors that have infiltrated a bone. MRI requires that a person lie motionless inside a cylinder-shaped device (surrounded by a large magnet) for as long as an hour. An "open MRI" means the machine is not completely enclosed.

A radionuclide scan, sometimes called a BONE SCAN, involves the intravenous injection of a small amount of a radioactive substance, called a tracer or isotope, that travels through the body to the target organ. There, it produces small amounts of gamma rays that are detected by an instrument called a gamma camera. Malignant cells that have spread from a cancerous tumor to bone tissue may be revealed through radionuclide scanning. Abnormal sites of inflammation or a bone fracture line may also be highlighted by this type of scan. The rays emitted are analyzed by a computer, which images the organ. See also ARTHROSCOPIC SURGERY; DUAL-ENERGY X-RAY ABSORPTIOMETRY.

Bone loss

The decline in living bone tissue due to a combination of influences caused by aging that produce accelerated bone resorption (the normal dissolving phase of bone regeneration) and a decrease in the speed at which the bone is rebuilt. Bone loss is a complication of OSTEOPOROSIS, a disease that thins and weakens the bones, which then become porous and vulnerable to fracture. In postmenopausal women, a reduced amount of the hormone estrogen at menopause is associated with bone loss, since estrogen helps the bones retain calcium to keep them dense and strong. Insufficient intake of calcium and vitamin D, which aids in calcium absorption, may also have a role. Men and women may be affected by bone loss. With age, fat mass increases, while muscle mass and skeletal mass decline. Weight-bearing exercise and all activities that put stress on bones, including weight-lifting, are known to maintain bone density and may even increase it. Weight training also strengthens muscles, which protect the bones and joints, and may help slow bone loss.

Certain medications can contribute to bone loss over time by decreasing the body's ability to absorb ingested calcium or vitamin D from the intestines. These medications include glucocorticoids, or corticosteroid drugs; high doses of thyroid hormones; antiseizure medications such as phenytoin and phenobarbital; aluminum-containing antacids; gonadotropin-releasing hormones; and the cholesterol-lowering medication cholestyramine. Physicians may advise people who are taking such medications or who are at risk for bone loss to increase their calcium intake. Women may be prescribed hormone replacement therapy to stimulate greater calcium absorption.

Bone marrow

A soft, organic material rich in blood vessels, found in the cavities and the spongy bone layer of most bones; also known as myeloid tissue. There are two types of bone marrow. Red marrow is the primary production site for blood cells, particularly red blood cells (erythrocytes) and certain kinds of white blood cells (granular leukocytes). Red marrow contains little fat.

Yellow marrow gets its color from the large amount of fat it contains; it is usually found in the body's long bones. It produces some types of white blood cells.

In infants and young children, red marrow is found throughout the skeleton, but as a person ages, the marrow loses its blood cell–producing ability and becomes yellow marrow. In adults, red marrow is limited to the sternum, vertebrae, ribs, collarbone, hip, and skull.

Stimulated by hormones, cells called erythroblasts within the marrow divide rapidly to produce blood cells. The blood cells mature in the bone before entering the bloodstream through blood vessels that penetrate the outer layers of hard bone. Although the blood cells cannot repair or reproduce themselves, the marrow produces them so abundantly that the supply is maintained. If the blood supply is lost or damaged through injury or disease, the bone marrow steps up its production of blood cells to restore the supply.

Bone marrow biopsy

Microscopic examination of a piece of bone and bone marrow. The procedure can be performed in a doctor's office, using a local anesthetic. A hollow needle is guided into the back area of the pelvic bones or the breastbone (sternum); a core sample of bone with marrow inside is removed. Bone marrow biopsy is used to diagnose blood or bone marrow cancers, such as leukemia or multiple myeloma, or to determine if a malignant tumor from another organ of the body has spread to the bone marrow. It is also used to check for infections, to follow up on the effectiveness of treatment, or to find out how well the bone marrow would produce new blood cells if aggressive chemotherapy were to be used.

Bone marrow transplant, allogeneic

The replacement of an individual's defective bone marrow with the bone marrow or stem cells of a healthy donor. Stem cells (cells from which the different types of blood cells develop) are present in normal bone marrow and blood. They can be harvested by removing bone marrow

TRANSPLANTING BONE MARROW

For an autologous bone marrow transplant, bone marrow or blood cells are withdrawn from a person's own body. The stem cells are filtered out and frozen. Then the person is given massive doses of chemotherapy or radiation to destroy diseased cells. Finally, the frozen cells are thawed and injected back into the person's bloodstream. These healthy stem cells travel to the bone marrow and multiply. In an allogeneic transplant, the donor of the healthy cells is usually a relative whose blood is closely matched to that of the recipient. The healthy stem cells are similarly sorted, frozen, processed, and transfused into the person.

TRANSPLANT PREPARATION
Before an allogeneic bone marrow transplant, the recipient has chemotherapy, radiation, or sometimes both to kill bone marrow cells. If an autologous bone marrow transplant is being done, healthy cells are harvested first, and then chemotherapy, radiation, or both are used to kill diseased cells.

Radiation

Chemotherapy

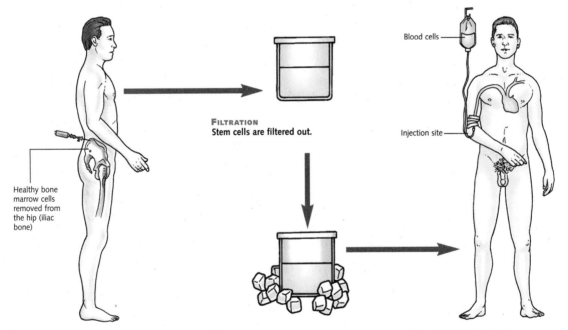

FILTRATION
Stem cells are filtered out.

Blood cells

Injection site

REMOVAL OF HEALTHY CELLS
Healthy bone marrow (or blood) cells are taken, either from the person who will be undergoing autologous bone marrow transplant or from a donor (allogeneic bone marrow transplant).

Healthy bone marrow cells removed from the hip (iliac bone)

PROCESSING CELLS
Stem cells are frozen in liquid nitrogen and processed.

TRANSPLANTING CELLS
Healthy blood cells are given intravenously into the recipient's bloodstream.

from a donor or by drawing the blood of a donor and using a blood pheresis machine, a device that separates blood into its different components. In an allogeneic transplant, the donor is usually a sibling, other relative, or a nonrelative whose marrow is closely matched to that of the recipient's. To find a match, scientists look at six genetic markers (HLA TYPES) found on white blood cells. The transplant is more likely to succeed if most or all of the markers of the donor and recipient match.

The purpose of a bone marrow transplant is to allow the administration of very large doses of chemotherapy or radiation, doses so large that they may completely destroy the bone marrow. Replacing the damaged bone marrow with new bone marrow helps destroy the cancer and helps the recipient fight off infections. Bone marrow transplant is considered an effective treatment of leukemia and lymphoma; it is being studied in several other cancers, including those of the brain, breast, and lung, and multiple myeloma. Recent studies suggest that bone marrow transplants are not effective for curing breast cancer that has spread throughout the body. The procedure has proved to be effective in the treatment of some noncancerous diseases, such as aplastic anemia.

Bone marrow transplant, autologous

A treatment in which an individual with cancer receives his or her own previously harvested healthy bone marrow or stem cells to replace bone marrow that has been damaged by chemotherapy or radiation. Autologous bone marrow transplant avoids the problems associated with using bone marrow from a donor whose cells may not be a good genetic match for the recipient. In cases of a poor genetic match, donor cells may be rejected by the recipient or may attack the recipient's cells in a "graft-versus-host" reaction (see GRAFT-VERSUS-HOST DISEASE).

The purpose of a bone marrow transplant is to make it possible to treat someone who has cancer with very high doses of radiation or chemotherapy that may otherwise be fatal. In the three-step procedure,

approximately a pint of bone marrow is removed from the hip bone, usually when the disease is in REMISSION or when cancer cells are not detectable. An anesthetic is usually required for this step, which involves 150 to 200 separate needle punctures.

Sometimes, instead of removing bone marrow, blood is drawn from the individual, and the stem cells are isolated by a blood pheresis machine. The harvested bone marrow or stem cells are then frozen in liquid nitrogen and stored. Next, the individual undergoes high-dose chemotherapy or radiation treatment, which kills all bone marrow cells, cancerous and healthy. Then, the stored healthy bone marrow or stem cells are reintroduced to the body, where they reproduce and replace the destroyed bone marrow. The body will not reject the bone marrow in this instance. However, the risk exists that some of the cells in the replacement bone marrow may turn out to be cancerous.

Bone scan

A NUCLEAR MEDICINE procedure that uses a radioactive isotope to make an image that identifies areas of bone in which cells are unusually active. The unusual activity could be caused by a tumor, infection, degenerative disorder, or a mending fracture.

WHY IT IS PERFORMED

Bone scans can be used to examine the skeleton for bone or joint infections and bone fractures. They help doctors locate abnormalities, but other techniques such as CT SCANNING (computed tomography scanning) and MRI (magnetic resonance imaging) are usually used to make a definite diagnosis. Bone scans are also commonly used to look for cancerous tumors that have originated in the bones or that have spread to the bones from other parts of the body. A bone scan may be ordered for any type of unusual bone pain, such as shin splints, or to evaluate the skeletal structure after a trauma.

HOW IT IS PERFORMED

A bone scan is generally done on an outpatient basis in a hospital or special testing facility. Before the procedure begins, the person being tested is usually instructed to drink several glasses of water. Drinking large quantities of water will help flush the

radioactive solution used in the procedure out of the body. There are no dietary restrictions before or after this procedure.

A small amount of a radioactive tracer called an isotope (one of two or more atoms having the same atomic number but of different masses) is mixed with a calciumlike material and is injected into a vein. Because bone absorbs calcium, the calciumlike substance and the isotope travel specifically to bone. For a 2-hour period after the injection, the isotope moves through the bloodstream and is taken up by bone tissue. The person can often leave the hospital or facility during this period.

After the 2 hours are up, and before the actual images are taken, the person will be asked to empty his or her bladder. He or she then lies down on a table and assumes various positions as a special camera scans the body from head to toe. In the bones, the isotope emits gamma rays, which are detected by the camera and analyzed by a computer to form an image of the bones. In areas where the bone cells are unusually active, the emitted rays are more intense and show up as hot spots. These hot spots occur because there is increased uptake of the isotope in areas where bone formation is occurring at a faster rate than that of surrounding bone. The scanning generally takes about an hour.

RISKS

The isotopes used in a bone scan are considered safe because the isotopes are quickly eliminated by the body through urination. Radiation levels are lower in bone scans than in some conventional X-ray procedures. Side effects from the isotope are very rare.

Booster

An additional dose of a vaccine administered at determined intervals to promote IMMUNIZATION against a specific disease or diseases and to advance the immune system's ability to defend the body against the disease or diseases. Booster shots for tetanus and diphtheria are commonly recommended for adults at 10-year intervals after the initial vaccination.

Borborygmi

Loud, rumbling, gurgling noises produced by the intestines. Borborygmi are sometimes referred to as a growling stomach. They occur during hyperactive intestinal peristalsis (the wavelike muscle movement that moves food through the digestive tract). This increased activity may be the result of GASTROENTERITIS, DIARRHEA, or hunger. When they are high-pitched and accompanied by other symptoms, such as vomiting, distension, and abdominal cramps, borborygmi may indicate an intestinal obstruction (see INTESTINE, OBSTRUCTION OF).

Borderline personality disorder

See PERSONALITY DISORDERS.

Bottle-feeding

Feeding of milk or formula to babies usually through sterilized bottles. Most formula is derived from cow's milk that has been fortified with vitamin D and other vitamins, in an effort to make it as much like human milk as possible. Specially prepared formulas are available for infants with milk allergy or specific digestive disorders. See FEEDING, INFANT.

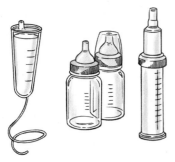

TYPES OF BABY BOTTLES
The right kind of bottle can make feeding time easier and more pleasant for both baby and parent. Some products for a baby with special needs allow the baby to pace the flow of the feeding. A typical bottle comes with a top for travel. For children with conditions that interfere with feeding, a specially designed bottle has an elongated nipple with a slit tip to keep the baby from swallowing air, a valve that adjusts the flow to suit the child, and a one-way valve that prevents flooding the child during feeding.

Botulinum toxin, type A

A neurotoxin produced by certain strains of the bacterium *Clostridium botulinum*, also known as botulism toxin. When consumed in food, botulinum toxin, type A can cause paralysis and death. The neurotoxins produced by *Clostridium botulinum* are among the most potent poisons known. In a purified form, botulinum toxin, type A (Oculinum and Botox) has been used to treat blepharospasm (involuntary contraction of the eyelid), strabismus (crossed eyes), and esophageal achalasia (dilated esophagus). When injected under the skin, Botox reduces the appearance of wrinkles for up to 6 months, but then additional Botox injections are needed.

Botulism

FOR FIRST AID
see Food poisoning: botulism, page 1322

A rare, potentially fatal, paralyzing illness caused by a nerve toxin that is formed by certain spores of a bacterium called *Clostridium botulinum*. The bacteria can multiply in low oxygen conditions and form spores that are found in food, most often in home-canned food, raw food, or improperly cooked food; the spores are also present in dust and soil.

There are three basic categories of botulism: Food-borne botulism is caused by eating food that contains the toxic bacteria. Wound botulism occurs when an open wound is infected with the bacteria. This form of botulism can be prevented by seeking prompt medical care for infected wounds and by avoiding the use of injected illicit drugs.

And finally, infant botulism is caused when children younger than 1 year of age consume food containing the spores of the bacteria, which then grow in the intestines and release toxins into the nervous system. It is believed that infants younger than 1 year of age have not yet developed sufficient beneficial digestive bacteria to control botulism spores. Infant botulism may be linked to some cases of SUDDEN INFANT DEATH SYNDROME (SIDS), because breathing is affected in severe cases.

Botulinum toxins may be cultivated by terrorists for use in BIOTERRORISM. Botulism could be spread in the food supply or water supply or sprayed in the air.

SYMPTOMS
The symptoms of food-borne and wound botulism may include double vision, blurred vision, drooping eyelids, slurred speech, difficulty swallowing, dry mouth, constipation, and

---

PREVENTING BOTULISM

Though rare, the illness known as botulism can cause a person to become seriously ill. But commonsense prevention can prevent people from becoming ill from the bacteria.

- Home-canned foods with low acid content—including asparagus, green beans, beets, and corn—are vulnerable to contamination with botulism. Persons who can foods at home should follow strict hygienic practices to reduce the risk. Home-canned foods should be boiled for 10 minutes before eating as the botulism toxin is destroyed by exposure to high temperatures.
- Dented, swollen, or leaking cans should not be used or purchased as they may also be a potential source of botulism.
- Other sources of botulism may include chopped garlic in oil, chili peppers, tomatoes, baked potatoes wrapped in aluminum foil, and home-canned or fermented fish. These foods should be carefully cleaned and handled and, when possible, boiled for at least 10 minutes.
- Honey is the main source of infant botulism and should not be given to children younger than 12 months.

---

muscle weakness. These symptoms generally occur within 18 to 36 hours of eating contaminated food, but may be experienced as soon as 6 hours or as long as 10 days after exposure. Infant botulism causes symptoms including lethargy, poor feeding, constipation, poor muscle tone, and weak crying or sucking. In adults and infants, the symptoms are considered a medical emergency because the illness can be fatal.

DIAGNOSIS AND TREATMENT
A clinical history and physical examination may suggest botulism, but medical tests are essential for ruling out other possible conditions with similar symptoms. The tests may include brain scans, spinal fluid examinations, and ELECTROMYOGRAPHY (EMG). Diagnosis is usually confirmed by testing for the particular bacteria in the stool.

When food-borne and wound botulism are diagnosed early, treatment may involve induced vomiting and the use of enemas to remove contaminated food from the stomach or intestines. The illness may also be treated in adults with an antitoxin that blocks the action of the toxin circulating in the bloodstream. This treatment can take many weeks. If respiratory failure and paralysis have occurred, treatment may include the use of a ventilator with full-time nursing care for an extended time. Paralysis slowly subsides after several weeks of treatment. Wound botulism may require surgery.

Supportive hospital care is a routine treatment for all forms of botulism. Fatigue and shortness of breath may persist for years after successful treatment of botulism poisoning and can require long-term therapy.

Bougie

A slender, cylindrical instrument inserted into tubular body passages. A bougie may be rigid or flexible, hollow or solid. Bougies are commonly used to dilate the urethra, to open constricted areas for examination, or to give a person medication.

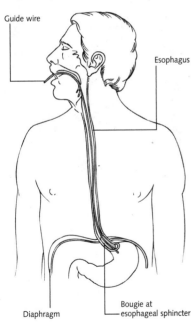

Guide wire

Esophagus

Diaphragm

Bougie at esophageal sphincter

EXPANDING A PASSAGE
To expand an esophagus narrowed by disease, a doctor may insert bougies (cylindrical rods with rounded tips) of increasing size down a guide wire into the passageway. The procedure, which gradually widens the esophagus, can be repeated as necessary and is generally effective and safe.

Bow legs

An outward curving of the bones in the legs. A normal part of development, bow legs are common in children younger than age 2. As a child grows, the curve normally straightens. Bow legs that persist beyond age 2 and into adolescence usually are an inherited trait. In rare cases, they are the result of a more serious underlying condition, such as RICKETS (a vitamin D deficiency that causes bones to soften), a fracture, infection, tumor, or JUVENILE RHEUMATOID ARTHRITIS.

In most cases, bow legs correct themselves over time and require no treatment. Providing shoes that fit correctly and ample opportunity to exercise are strongly advised. If bow legs persist after age 6, children are usually referred to a pediatric orthopedist for treatment. At this age, a corrective cast or brace (see BRACE, ORTHOPEDIC) may be required to correct the problem. In severe cases, corrective surgery may be necessary. In younger children, these measures are not recommended and may cause physical or emotional damage.

Bowel

Another name for the INTESTINE, that portion of the canal that extends from the stomach to the anus.

Bowel movements, abnormal

A sign of a disorder in the digestive system. Normal frequency of bowel movements can range from as many as three a day to as few as three a week. Although changes in bowel habits may be due to a harmless condition, a sudden and sustained change may be a symptom of an underlying disease.

Changes in bowel movements that last longer than a week require medical attention. Three or more loose movements a day are considered DIARRHEA. Persistent diarrhea can be a sign of an underlying disorder, such as COLITIS or CROHN DISEASE. In constipation, bowel movements become infrequent and feces are hard and dry. Infrequent or irregular bowel movements may be due to the overuse of LAXATIVES, a low-fiber diet, inadequate fluid intake, physical inactivity, the use of certain medications, ignoring the urge to defecate, or a disorder such as DEPRESSION. Constipa-

tion and pain with bowel movements can be due to HEMORRHOIDS or an ANAL FISSURE. Pain can lead to avoiding defecation, which only worsens the situation. Abnormal color in bowel movements is another sign of an underlying disorder (see also FECES, ABNORMAL). Pale stools may be a sign of a liver or gallbladder disorder. Sticky dark or black feces may indicate dangerous internal bleeding and are considered a medical emergency. The presence of blood or pus in the feces suggests colitis, Crohn disease, or cancer (see also FECES, BLOOD IN THE). The appearance of blood in stools requires immediate medical attention, which may include a FECAL-OCCULT BLOOD TEST that can identify traces of blood in the stool, and a rectal examination. Other tests that a doctor may order to determine the cause of abnormal bowel movements include a GASTROINTESTINAL (GI) SERIES, GASTROSCOPY, PROCTOSCOPY, SIGMOIDOSCOPY, and COLONOSCOPY.

Bowel sounds

Sounds produced by liquid and air moving through the digestive tract. Doctors use a stethoscope to assess bowel sounds. Normal bowel sounds include irregular, gurgling noises. Loud, rumbling, gurgling noises (BORBORYGMI) occur during hyperactive intestinal peristalsis (the wavelike muscle movement that moves food through the digestive tract). Hyperactivity may be the result of GASTROENTERITIS, DIARRHEA, or hunger. Rushed, high-pitched bowel sounds can be an early indication of an intestinal obstruction. The absence of bowel sounds can be a serious symptom of an obstruction. Soft, low, hypoactive sounds occur after surgery when the person has been given general anesthesia.

Bowen disease

The earliest form of SQUAMOUS CELL CARCINOMA, a type of skin cancer; also known as squamous cell carcinoma in situ. In Bowen disease, cancer cells are entirely within the epidermis (the outer layer of skin) and have not yet entered the dermis (the middle layer of skin). Skin cancer is the most common type of cancer in the United States. Its principal cause is long-term sun exposure. Light skin and a family or personal history of skin cancer are additional risk factors. When Bowen disease occurs on the anal or genital skin, it is often related to a sexually transmitted infection with the HUMAN PAPILLOMAVIRUS that causes genital warts.

Bowen disease is characterized by red, scaly, crusted patches on the skin. Patches are often larger than half an inch in diameter. Like other forms of skin cancer, Bowen disease is diagnosed through a biopsy. Early detection is critical. The cancer is removed by fairly minor surgery, which usually takes place on an outpatient basis using a local anesthetic. Surgical options include simple EXCISION (cutting), CURETTAGE (scraping), electrodesiccation (burning with an electric current delivered through a probe), MOHS SURGERY (microscopically controlled surgery removing one layer of skin at a time), and CRYOSURGERY (freezing with liquid nitrogen). The type of treatment chosen depends on factors such as the size and location of the cancer.

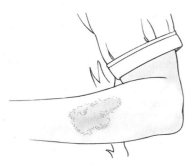

SEVERELY DAMAGED SKIN CELLS
Bowen disease is a very early form of skin cancer in which the cells are severely damaged or altered but are all in the outermost skin layer (epidermis). The lesion appears as a bright red or pink, scaly patch on skin, usually as the result of sun exposure.

Brace, orthopedic

An appliance that supports a bone or joint structure and its associated muscles, tendons, and ligaments to aid in repair following injury or surgery or that is worn to promote proper positioning of the spine or the extremities. Orthopedic braces may be prescribed for the treatment of instability in the shoulder or knee and to treat conditions including kyphosis (excessive backward curvature of the spine).

In growing children with adolescent SCOLIOSIS, the use of orthopedic braces during the years of active growth may prevent the curve from getting worse, although the braces cannot improve or cure scoliosis. The type of brace prescribed for scoliosis is generally an underarm, polypropylene "body jacket" type brace that is worn under clothing for 16 hours daily, for a period of 3 to 4 years. The more visible Milwaukee brace, a type of external back brace, may also be used. Extended orthopedic braces include some form of head and neck support attached to spinal support and may be used in cases of paralysis and following certain back surgeries.

Braces, dental

Metal or plastic appliances worn on the teeth that apply steady, gentle pressure over an extended period to move teeth into the proper position. See ORTHODONTICS.

Brachial plexus

A network of nerves in the upper part of the chest that controls muscles in the chest, shoulders, and arms. Nerve roots exit the spinal cord in the neck and combine to form three nerve trunks. The nerve trunks travel across the shoulder, giving off branches that are the nerves to the chest and shoulder. The trunks then rearrange into three nerve cords, which then provide branches that form the nerves of the arms.

Brachial plexus block

A method of anesthetizing the lower arm and hand for surgery by injecting medication into the bundle of nerves (brachial plexus) in which the branches control feeling in the arm. A brachial plexus block is a form of regional anesthesia (see ANESTHESIA, REGIONAL). The anesthetic medication is usually injected close to the nerve that passes through the armpit, a placement that numbs the hand and lower arm. For surgery on the upper arm, the injection can be made into the brachial plexus in the neck, or under the collarbone for shoulder surgery. In most cases, the injection into the area of the nerve is made with the person under CONSCIOUS SEDATION, a method of controlling pain that leaves the person awake but pain-free.

Surgery on the arm often requires a tourniquet to control bleeding, and a brachial plexus block stops the pain of the tourniquet. Another advantage to this nerve block is that it lasts for several hours after surgery is complete, controlling pain effectively at the time when it is often worst.

POSSIBLE COMPLICATIONS

The complications of brachial plexus block include damage to the nerve, which can cause temporary paralysis, and possibly muscle weakness, which can last up to several months. Injection of an anesthetic agent into a vein may lead to seizures and cardiac arrest. Injection into the shoulder has a small risk of penetrating the upper lobe of the lung, which lies close to the skin in this area. Injection in the neck is complicated by the proximity of the nerve that controls the diaphragm, the carotid artery, the jugular vein, and the spinal column.

Brachialgia

Neck or arm pain, including radiating pain from the shoulder or upper arm and difficulty moving the affected area. Brachialgia is caused by cervical disk syndrome, which may be due to trauma to the neck or disk abnormalities. Treatment generally consists of bed rest, traction, limiting physical activity for a period of 2 weeks, and the use of analgesics or muscle relaxants. PHYSICAL THERAPY may also be prescribed, and a cervical collar can be worn. If pain does not decrease or mobility is not restored following treatment, brachialgia may be suspected of being associated with other conditions, such as OSTEOPOROSIS or a malignant tumor. Inflammation from SCOLIOSIS may also cause brachialgia.

Brachytherapy

A type of internal radiation therapy used to treat cancer. In brachytherapy, also known as interstitial radiation therapy, a radioactive source is sealed in a container and placed on the surface of the body, near the affected area, or implanted directly into the tumor in the form of small radioactive "seeds" of gold or iodine. This procedure permits a very high but localized dose of radiation to be administered to a tumor without endangering surrounding tissue. Brachytherapy is most often used to treat tumors of the head, neck, prostate, cervix, and breast. It is generally used in combination with external radiation. The usual side effects include inflammation, redness, scarring, and discomfort.

Bradycardia

An unusually slow heartbeat, typically less than 50 beats per minute. One type of bradycardia, known as sinus bradycardia, occurs in well-trained athletes and during deep relaxation. It produces no symptoms and is considered normal. Other forms of bradycardia are abnormal and may require treatment, depending on type, severity, and symptoms.

When the heart beats too slowly, it fails to provide the body with enough blood to function properly. The usual symptoms of bradycardia are fatigue, shortness of breath, light-headedness or dizziness, or sudden fainting. Since these symptoms can result from conditions other than bradycardia, testing is required to isolate their cause.

There are three principal types of abnormal bradycardia. In SICK SINUS SYNDROME, the heart's natural pacemaker (the sinus node) malfunctions, producing an irregular heartbeat. In HEART BLOCK (also known as atrioventricular, or AV, block), the electrical impulse moving from the sinoatrial node to the ventricles (lower chambers) of the heart is delayed or even completely blocked. In its least severe form, heart block causes minor symptoms or no symptoms at all; however, if the blockage is complete, sudden death due to complete stoppage of the heart can result. In BUNDLE BRANCH BLOCK, electrical impulses are delayed or blocked along their normal pathway through the ventricles. This condition often produces no symptoms.

When bradycardia requires treatment, the person usually is instructed to stop taking any medication that may slow the heartbeat. In some cases, a PACEMAKER is implanted in the chest to maintain a normal heartbeat.

Bradykinesia

Abnormal slowness of voluntary movement and speech. Bradykinesia may occur as a side effect of medication, such as tranquilizers, or it can be caused by medical problems such as PARKINSON DISEASE (a progressive, degenerative disease of the nervous system characterized by muscle rigidity, weakness, and tremor).

Brain

The principal and most complex organ in the NERVOUS SYSTEM; the major control center for both basic body system maintenance and the highest levels of thought, emotion, and learning.

The brain and the spinal cord extending down from it together make up the CENTRAL NERVOUS SYSTEM. From the brain and spinal cord, a network of nerves branches out to connect the central nervous system to every part of the body. These nerve pathways are called the PERIPHERAL NERVOUS SYSTEM. Much like a computer, the brain receives sensory information from receptor sites throughout the body, sorts and analyzes it, and then sends information out to direct the body's response. The incoming and outgoing signals are in the form of electrochemical impulses traveling along nerve fibers made up of individual nerve cells called neurons (see NEURON). A large part of brain activity is largely directed toward regulating such basic, continuous, and vital body functions as breathing and heartbeat.

Because the brain operates continuously to ensure the body's survival, and to direct higher functions such as voluntary movements and conscious thought, it requires an enormous supply of blood. The brain weighs about 3 pounds, but 20 percent of the body's blood supply is channeled to the brain at any time. Blood flows to the brain through four arteries, two on either side of the neck called the carotid arteries, and two running along the spinal cord called the vertebral arteries. Arteries and veins branch throughout the wrinkled surface of the brain. A complex mechanism called the BLOOD-BRAIN BARRIER allows vital substances within the blood to penetrate the walls of the brain's capillaries, while preventing potentially harmful substances such as certain drugs from entering.

To protect the soft, gelatinous brain and its blood vessels, three layers of membranes called the MENINGES lie under the skull. (The meninges also cover the spinal cord.) The tough outer layer is called the dura mater.

Between the dura mater and the next membrane, called the arachnoid, is the subarachnoid space, which contains a cushioning fluid called the cerebrospinal fluid. The innermost membrane is the pia mater, which adheres to the surface of the brain.

The brain itself is composed of three main structures: the CEREBELLUM, the BRAIN STEM, and the forebrain, mostly occupied by the large CEREBRUM.

FOREBRAIN

The bulk of the brain is called the forebrain, and the cerebrum is by far the largest mass of the forebrain. The cerebrum is divided into two hemispheres, connected by a wall of nerve tissue known as the corpus callosum. The thin outer layer covering each of the hemispheres is called the cerebral cortex. It is composed of gray matter, which is rich in nerve cells, and it is the site of many of the brain's highest functions such as thinking and memory. The cerebral cortex is deeply wrinkled to allow the greatest possible surface area. The deepest wrinkles, called fissures or sulci, divide the cerebrum into four lobes, the names of which—frontal, parietal, occipital, and temporal—correspond to the bones of the skull that lie over them. Beneath the cerebral cortex, the inner mass of the cerebrum is made of white matter, which is entirely composed of nerve fibers connecting different parts of the cortex to each other and to other structures within the brain. Deep within the white matter in each of the hemispheres are bodies of gray matter (nerve cells) called basal ganglia. They are linked to the brain stem and cerebellum and are involved with the coordination of voluntary movement.

Of the two hemispheres of the brain, the left hemisphere is usually dominant, controlling such higher functions as language and mathematical skills. In right-handed people, the left hemisphere is always the dominant one; in left-handed people, the same is usually true. The right hemisphere regulates spatial orientation and balance and is also involved in some areas of creative thought and artistic ability. Many types of higher brain functions do not take place on one side of the brain or the other, but probably involve both hemispheres working together.

B

THE COMPLEX BRAIN

The brain is the primary control system of the body; different areas of the brain perform different functions.

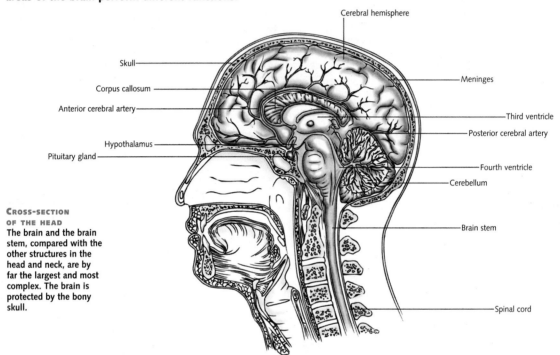

Cerebral hemisphere

Skull

Corpus callosum

Anterior cerebral artery

Hypothalamus

Pituitary gland

Meninges

Third ventricle

Posterior cerebral artery

Fourth ventricle

Cerebellum

Brain stem

Spinal cord

CROSS-SECTION OF THE HEAD
The brain and the brain stem, compared with the other structures in the head and neck, are by far the largest and most complex. The brain is protected by the bony skull.

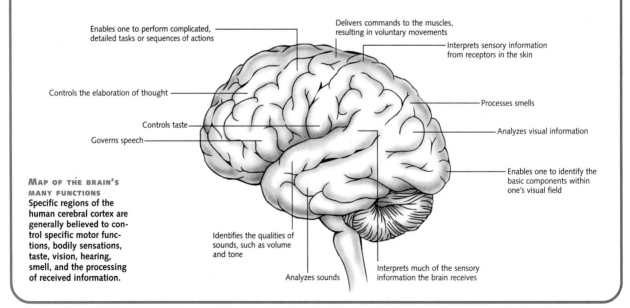

Enables one to perform complicated, detailed tasks or sequences of actions

Delivers commands to the muscles, resulting in voluntary movements

Interprets sensory information from receptors in the skin

Controls the elaboration of thought

Controls taste

Governs speech

Processes smells

Analyzes visual information

Enables one to identify the basic components within one's visual field

MAP OF THE BRAIN'S MANY FUNCTIONS
Specific regions of the human cerebral cortex are generally believed to control specific motor functions, bodily sensations, taste, vision, hearing, smell, and the processing of received information.

Identifies the qualities of sounds, such as volume and tone

Analyzes sounds

Interprets much of the sensory information the brain receives

Apart from the cerebrum, there are several other structures centered deep in the forebrain. The THALAMUS transmits information about body sensations to the cortex and may have a role in memory. The HYPOTHALAMUS, at the base of the brain, activates and regulates the AUTONOMIC NERVOUS SYSTEM (involved in many automatic, unconscious body functions), thirst and appetite, hormonal activity, body temperature, and sleep. The tiny PITUITARY GLAND is connected to the hypothalamus and produces some hormones that influence other glands in the body, and it is involved in growth and sexual development.

CEREBELLUM AND BRAIN STEM

The cerebellum, located at the back and underside of the brain, controls some unconscious and automatic functions involved with balance and coordinates some voluntary body movements. The brain stem, which includes structures called the pons and the medulla, extends from the middle and back part of the brain. It contains nerve tracts that connect the brain to the spinal cord and thereby to the rest of the body. The brain stem is concerned mainly with basic survival functions such as breathing, heartbeat, and consciousness. Both the cerebellum and brain stem function by unconscious REFLEX action, receiving sensory input from body organs and tissues and then signaling the body's automatic response.

Brain abscess

Also known as a cerebral abscess, a pus-filled cavity surrounded by inflamed tissue in the brain. A brain abscess is a life-threatening medical emergency. It may occur as a complication of other infections (such as chronic ear or sinus infection, mastoiditis, or epidural or lung abscess) or as a result of head injury. The inflammation of the abscess may cause swelling of the brain and create a mass effect that can put pressure on brain structures. Symptoms of a brain abscess include headache, muscle weakness, loss of sensation, vomiting, fever, and seizures. These may come on gradually or suddenly. Diagnosis is made through physical and neurological examination and tests such as a blood culture, chest X ray, electroencephalogram (EEG), CT (computed tomography) scanning, or MRI (magnetic resonance imaging). Treatment includes medications such as antimicrobials and antibiotics as well as diuretics and corticosteroids to reduce brain swelling. In some cases, surgery is necessary.

Brain damage

Injury, degeneration, or death of nerve cells within the brain. Damage can be wide and diffuse or localized and specific.

DIFFUSE DAMAGE

Diffuse brain damage can lead to severe mental or physical handicap. Its most significant cause is HYPOXIA, or an inadequate level of oxygen reaching the brain. Brain cells require a continuous supply of oxygen-rich blood. When cells are deprived of this nourishment, they die. Hypoxia may occur during birth or later in life as the result of problems such as CARDIAC ARREST (a sudden cessation of the heart's pumping action), RESPIRATORY ARREST (cessation of breathing), poisoning, drowning, STATUS EPILEPTICUS (prolonged seizures), genetic disorders, or environmental pollutants. Other causes of diffuse brain damage include ENCEPHALITIS and some degenerative disorders.

LOCALIZED DAMAGE

Localized brain damage can result in specific deficits of brain function that affect behaviors such as speech, balance, or coordination. Head trauma is a common cause of localized brain damage. Other causes include BRAIN TUMOR, BRAIN ABSCESS, and STROKE (a type of brain injury that occurs when blood supply to part of the brain is suddenly interrupted or when a blood vessel in the brain ruptures). ISCHEMIA is the term for the decreased blood supply to the cells. Brain cells die when they no longer receive oxygen and nutrients from the blood or when they are damaged by sudden bleeding into the brain.

SYMPTOMS AND TREATMENT

The symptoms of brain damage depend on the part of the brain that is affected and the nature and extent of the damage. People who have strokes, head trauma, or brain tumors have widely variable symptoms. CEREBRAL PALSY is an umbrella term used to describe a group of chronic disorders indicating brain damage in the first few years of life. Its broad range of symptoms includes seizures, muscle contractions, delayed development, mental retardation, spasticity, speech difficulties, vision problems, and hearing abnormalities.

Treatment of brain damage depends on the diagnosis of its underlying cause. Unfortunately, nerve cells do not recover their function after they have been destroyed. However, other parts of the brain can sometimes be trained to compensate for damaged areas. Rehabilitation is a very important part of any treatment plan for people with brain damage. Occupational therapy, physical therapy, and speech therapy are often helpful.

Brain death

Irreversible cessation of all functions of the entire brain, including the brain stem. This is the definition of death that was developed by Harvard Medical School in 1968. While brain death is diagnosed by a careful clinical examination, the diagnosis is confirmed by a variety of tests that determine an absence of reflexes, unresponsiveness to stimuli, a lack of spontaneous respiration or movement, and the absence of electrical activity of the brain as indicated by a flat ELECTROENCEPHALOGRAM (EEG). In addition, it must first be determined that nothing is suppressing the person's responses, such as hypothermia (cold body temperature) or drugs (for example, excessive phenobarbital levels can result in a coma and suppression of EEG activity). If after 24 hours there is no change in a person's status, he or she is declared dead. This definition of brain death allows for the certification of death even if the lungs and heart continue to function with machine assistance but electrical activity in the brain has ceased. After brain death has been determined, the person's organs can be donated.

Brain hemorrhage

See HEMORRHAGE, CEREBRAL; HEMORRHAGE, EPIDURAL; and HEMORRHAGE, SUBARACHNOID.

Brain imaging

The process of making pictures of the brain and its structures. Special imaging techniques developed in recent years have dramatically improved the diagnosis of brain injury and disease.

CLOSE-UP ON PET SCANNING

Whereas CT (computed tomography) scanning and X rays detail the structure of the brain, PET (positron emission tomography) scanning is one of the most effective ways of generating images of the working brain. PET scanning is a relatively new brain imaging technique, the uses of which are just beginning to be realized by medical researchers. For example, doctors use PET scanning to follow disease progression in Parkinson disease and Huntington disease and to study functional changes in the brain after injury, stroke, or other neurological diseases.

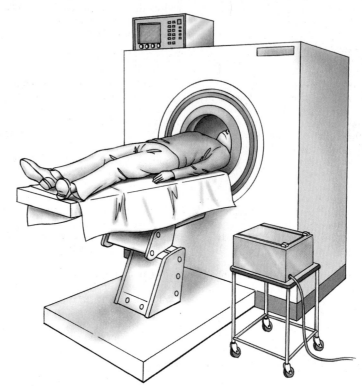

AN OPEN SCAN
During PET scanning, the person lies on a comfortable platform and holds his or her head very still within the round opening of the scanner.

PET IMAGING
During PET scanning, radionuclides, which are injected or swallowed, emit positrons. Positrons, a type of electron with a positive electrical charge, emit two beams of gamma rays when they collide with electrons. Since gamma radiation is symmetrical, a pair of detectors (coincidence detectors) positioned 180° from each other is needed to detect both emissions simultaneously and create a "living" image of brain tissue.

The most commonly used brain scans are CT SCANNING (computed tomography scanning), MRI (magnetic resonance imaging), and PET SCANNING (positron emission tomography scanning). CT scanning and MRI reveal the structure of the brain, which is useful in the diagnosis of brain tumors, cysts, and other structural abnormalities. PET and a special type of MRI known as a functional MRI are used to monitor the brain's activity and identify possible abnormalities. A relatively new brain scan called SPECT (single-photon emission computed tomography) may be used to locate problems such as the focus of a seizure in the brain. New techniques on the horizon include magnetic resonance spectroscopy (to detect abnormalities in the brain's biochemical processes) and near-infrared spectroscopy (to detect oxygen levels in brain tissue).

CT SCANNING

Also known as CAT scanning or computed axial tomography, CT scanning uses a sophisticated X-ray machine and a computer to create a detailed image of the brain's tissues and structures. CT scanning is readily available at most hospitals and produces images rapidly. It is also one of the safest ways to study the brain. It is particularly useful for identifying abnormal collections of blood in the brain. Radiopaque dye may sometimes be given intravenously to enhance blood vessels on a CT scan and improve the ability to detect certain diseases.

MRI

This technique uses a magnetic field and radio waves to create images of brain tissue. Unlike CT scanning, MRI does not use radiation. MRI provides images from various angles that allow physicians to put together a three-dimensional image of the brain. The images are much more detailed, and abnormalities are more readily seen. Special types of MRI are functional MRI and MRA (magnetic resonance angiography). Functional MRI monitors brain activity by using a magnet to pick up signals from oxygenated blood. MRA is used to map blood flow in order to detect problems such as narrowing or blockage of brain arteries. Gadolinium, a magnetically active dye, may be used to enhance the MRA's image of the brain's blood vessels.

PET SCANNING

Positron emission tomography provides an image of brain activity rather than brain structure. PET scanning uses glucose that has been labeled with a radioactive tracer and injected into the bloodstream. The brain uses glucose for energy. Detectors placed around a person's head detect the labeled glucose and its distribution around the brain. Since the brain uses glucose for energy, PET scanning creates images based on the metabolic activity of the nervous tissue. For example, malignant tissue absorbs more glucose than normal tissue, and this difference shows up on the scan. Degenerating neurons, as in Alzheimer's disease, use less glucose.

OTHER TYPES OF BRAIN IMAGING

Although no longer widely used for diagnosis, ANGIOGRAPHY still has an occasional role in the diagnosis of brain injury and disease. Angiography is an X-ray procedure that is used to visualize the inside of blood vessels after they have been injected with a contrast medium. The widespread use of CT scanning and MRI has supplanted the use of angiography for diagnosing most brain disorders. Plain X rays do not provide good images of brain tissue. However, they can be helpful in certain cases, such as when there are suspected abnormalities in the bones that make up the skull.

Brain stem

The lowest portion of the BRAIN, lying just above the spinal cord with nerve pathways that connect the spinal cord to other areas of the brain. Most of the activities carried on in the brain stem are unconscious functions such as breathing and heartbeat. The brain stem also contains the nerve endings of most of the cranial nerves, which send and receive sensory information from sense organs and structures.

STRUCTURE

The brain stem encompasses three structures: the midbrain, the pons, and the medulla. The midbrain lies at the top of the brain stem, just beneath the thalamus. The pons is under the midbrain, in the middle of the brain stem. The medulla lies in the lower portion of the brain stem, just above the spinal cord. Within the brain stem is the fourth ventricle (cavity) of the

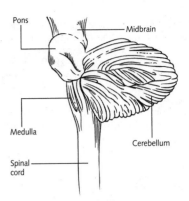

THREE-PART BRAIN STEM
The brain stem, which includes the midbrain, pons, and medulla, controls basic vital life functions such as breathing and heartbeat. It is in some ways the simplest part of the human brain, resembling the entire brain of lower animals. It links the rest of the brain to the spinal cord.

brain, containing cerebrospinal fluid to cushion and protect structures of the brain and spinal cord.

FUNCTION

The medulla contains the nerve cell bodies of the 9th to 12th cranial nerves, which send and receive sensory signals about taste from the tongue and some signals related to speech production. It also contains centers that regulate vital functions such as heart rate, blood pressure, and respiration. These centers are closely linked and function in concert. They involve both parasympathetic (resting) and sympathetic (responding to stress) brain activity.

The pons contains nerves that connect to the cerebellum, a separate structure that is attached to the brain stem and regulates some unconscious functions. The nerve cell bodies for the fifth to eighth cranial nerves lie in the pons, communicating sensory information from the ear about hearing and balance as well as signals from the face and teeth.

The midbrain holds the nerve cell bodies of the third and fourth cranial nerves; the midbrain controls some eye movements, the opening and closing of the pupil, and some limb movements. See CENTRAL NERVOUS SYSTEM.

Brain tumor

An abnormal growth of tissue found inside the skull.

TYPES OF BRAIN TUMORS

Tumors are classified as benign or

malignant (cancerous). In most parts of the body, benign tumors are not especially dangerous. However, any abnormal growth in the skull can put undue pressure on sensitive tissues and impair the function of the nerve tissue.

Tumors are further classified as primary (originating in the brain) or secondary (having traveled to the brain, or metastasized, from another location). Primary tumors rarely arise from neurons (nerve cells), because mature neurons no longer divide and multiply; instead, they usually develop from the connective tissues within the brain. The central nervous system (CNS) consists of the brain and spinal cord; brain tumors are more common than spinal cord tumors. Primary CNS tumors such as gliomas and meningiomas are named by their location, the type of cells they are made of, or both. (See also GLIOMA; MENINGIOMA.) The cause of most primary brain tumors remains unknown.

Metastatic brain tumors are secondary tumors caused by the spread, or metastasizing, of cancer cells from elsewhere in the body. Cancer cells travel through the bloodstream, pass through blood vessel walls, and may lodge in the brain, where they develop into cancerous growths. One in four people who have cancer that spreads within the body develops metastasis within the central nervous system.

SYMPTOMS

The symptoms of brain tumors vary according to their size, type, and location. In general, symptoms develop slowly and worsen over time. They commonly include headache, seizures, nausea, vomiting, vision or hearing problems, behavioral and cognitive symptoms, motor problems, and balance difficulties. Symptoms generally reflect the particular area of the brain that is damaged by the abnormal growth. For example, when tumors affect areas responsible for movement, they can cause weakness, paralysis, or lack of coordination.

DIAGNOSIS

When the medical history, symptoms, and the neurological examination suggest the possibility of a brain tumor, a number of tests can confirm the diagnosis. These include neurological examination, imaging studies, ELECTROENCEPHALOGRAM (EEG), LUMBAR PUNCTURE, and biopsy. Special imaging techniques developed in recent years have dramatically improved the diagnosis of brain tumors. The most commonly used brain scans are CT SCANNING (computed tomography scanning), MRI (magnetic resonance imaging), and PET SCANNING (positron emission tomography scanning). CT scanning and MRI reveal the structure of the brain, while PET and a special type of MRI known as a functional MRI are used to monitor the brain's activity and possible abnormalities in its function. A definitive diagnosis requires a biopsy. A biopsy involves removing a piece of the lesion from the brain through a small incision and having it analyzed by a pathologist to determine the type and grade (severity) of the tumor.

TREATMENT

Surgery, radiation, and chemotherapy are the three most commonly used treatments. Surgery to remove as much of the tumor as possible is usually the first line of treatment. New techniques such as MICROSURGERY and STEREOTACTIC SURGERY have made it possible to operate on many brain tumors that were once considered inaccessible. If the tumor is malignant, doctors usually recommend radiation or chemotherapy following surgery. When surgical removal is not possible, tumors are treated with radiation or chemotherapy. Chemotherapy can be given orally or intravenously, or it can be injected right into the tumor during either surgery or a biopsy procedure.

Bran

The skin or husk of cereal grains such as wheat, rye, and oats. Bran provides one of the most concentrated sources of dietary fiber (see FIBER, DIETARY). A diet high in bran and other fiber-rich foods helps maintain proper bowel function and prevent intestinal disorders ranging from constipation to irritable bowel syndrome. Additional benefits may include protection against cardiovascular disease, cancer, and diabetes.

Based on its capacity to dissolve in water, dietary fiber is considered either soluble or insoluble. One serving of bran flake cereal (¾ cup) contains 5½ grams of total fiber: 5 grams insoluble and ½ gram soluble. Insoluble fiber in bran does not mix well with liquid and passes through the digestive tract largely intact. It offers protection against a range of bowel disorders. When mixed with a liquid, soluble fiber forms a gel. In combination with a diet low in saturated fat and cholesterol, soluble fiber in bran can help lower total cholesterol levels and, thus, reduce the risk of heart disease. When it reaches the large intestines, soluble fiber is broken down by bacteria. This process contributes to the health benefits attributed to soluble fiber.

Doctors recommend that people consume 20 to 35 grams of fiber with one fourth of the total as soluble fiber each day. Eating a bowl of bran cereal for breakfast every day is an effective method to increase total fiber intake. However, fiber must be added to the diet gradually. A sudden increase in fiber intake can lead to flatulence (gas) and bloating. Drinking adequate water can help overcome these side effects. Because bran is high in valuable nutrients in addition to fiber, doctors recommend that people consume bran in natural products such as cereal and muffins rather than in dietary supplements.

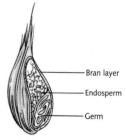

A CEREAL GRAIN
A grain is encased in a husk called the bran layer, which contains particularly fiber-rich carbohydrate, some B vitamins, and minerals such as iron. Underneath, the endosperm contains starch and protein used in refined flour. The germ contains protein, B vitamins, minerals, and carbohydrates.

Branchial cleft abnormalities

A group of abnormalities involving elongated openings located on the sides of the neck of a fetus in the embryo stage of development. Branchial cleft abnormalities are cysts or tubelike tracts produced by remnants of tissue from gill-like grooves on the fetus's neck. Surgical removal of the cyst or tract is the preferred treatment. When there is acute inflammation of the area, the cyst is usually drained and antibiotic treatment is given to clear up the infection before surgery is performed.

Braxton Hicks contractions

Mild contractions of the uterus during the final weeks of pregnancy. Braxton Hicks contractions, named for the doctor who first described them, are not true LABOR contractions, although they are often mistaken for them. Mild, irregular, and usually painless, Braxton Hicks contractions last from 30 seconds to 2 minutes. Also known as false labor, they do not indicate the start of true labor but are a sign that the body is preparing for it.

BRCA

Breast cancer genes. When present in a mutated form, these genes indicate that a woman has inherited a tendency to develop breast cancer. Their presence also increases a woman's risk for ovarian cancer. Two mutated genes, BRCA-1 and BRCA-2, are present in 85 to 90 percent of all cases of hereditary breast cancer. Some women born with BRCA-1 or BRCA-2 may never develop breast cancer, despite their increased risk for it. The mutated genes are inherited in certain families. Five to ten percent of all breast cancers occur in "breast cancer families."

Antioncogenes normally discourage tumor development. BRCA-1 and BRCA-2 are antioncogenes, genes that have mutated and become unable to keep abnormal cells from dividing. A woman's risk of developing breast cancer increases significantly if she is born without enough normal antioncogenes or if her antioncogenes mutate later in life. Genetic testing can be done to detect BRCA mutations, although the results cannot predict if or when cancer will develop, only that there is an increased risk. Experts recommend that women who have these altered genes should be monitored closely with frequent mammograms and breast examinations. Some women with the genes choose to reduce their risk of cancer by having their breasts and ovaries surgically removed. Surgery may not prevent breast cancer in every case, because the disease can develop in the tissue that remains.

Breakthrough bleeding

Bleeding (spotting or staining) between menstrual periods. In some women, breakthrough bleeding occurs as a normal part of ovulation. It is important for a woman to report breakthrough bleeding to her doctor, because it can occasionally be a sign of a reproductive system disorder, such as CERVICAL POLYPS, CERVICITIS, ENDOMETRIOSIS, or cancer. Breakthrough bleeding may also occur during the first few months after a woman begins taking birth control pills, as her body adjusts to the new levels of hormones. If the breakthrough bleeding continues beyond a few months, changing to another type of birth control pill with a different balance of hormones may eliminate the spotting. See MENSTRUATION.

Breast

One of the pair of organs attached to the chest consisting of milk-producing glands, blood vessels, fat, and connective tissue. In women, the foremost function of the breasts is to secrete milk to feed an infant. The breast is also sensitive to sexual stimulation.

STRUCTURE

Breast tissue is primarily composed of fat, which surrounds and protects milk glands and ducts and supportive fibrous tissue. The size and shape of the breast vary widely, depending in part on heredity and in part on body weight. At the center of the breast is the nipple, which contains 15 to 20 small holes that are openings to milk ducts or oil glands. The pigmented area surrounding the nipple is called the areola. Muscles under the areola enable the nipple to become erect when stimulated.

The underlying system of milk ducts radiates out from the nipple like the spokes of a wheel. When a woman becomes pregnant, a system of tiny glands called lobules secretes milk into the ducts. The glands and ducts are clustered into lobules, cushioned by fat and connective tissue. The breasts contain very little muscle, but a layer of muscle lies under the breast next to the chest wall.

BREAST DEVELOPMENT

At PUBERTY, between the ages of 8 and 15 years, a girl's breasts begin to grow, stimulated by the female hormone estrogen. So-called breast buds, slight swellings of the nipples, are often the first sign of puberty getting underway. During this time, some tenderness is normal. The duct system within begins to develop, and by age 18 or before, a girl's breasts have reached their mature size.

The breasts may go through various normal changes that correspond to the woman's menstrual cycle. They may enlarge slightly or become tender at about the midpoint of the cycle and may be uncomfortable and sensitive just before a woman's period.

After menopause, when a woman is no longer producing estrogen and progesterone, the proportion of fat in the breast tissue increases. As a result the breasts may begin to sag as the tissue becomes less dense.

FUNCTION

During pregnancy and while a woman is BREAST-FEEDING an infant, the breasts change considerably. The breasts grow larger, the veins become more visible from the outside, and the nipples and areola may darken and enlarge. Within the breast, the milk-producing cells multiply rapidly, and the system

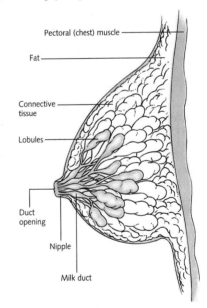

Pectoral (chest) muscle

Fat

Connective tissue

Lobules

Duct opening

Nipple

Milk duct

THE FEMALE BREAST
The female breast is specialized to produce milk. Lobules of glandular tissue are capable of secreting milk through a system of successively larger ducts that carry the milk toward the nipple. Fibrous connective tissue and fat protect and support the breast. In a pregnant woman, hormones stimulate the breast to begin milk production.

of milk ducts develops fully. Oil glands inside the breast enlarge and secrete an oily substance to help soften and lubricate the breast during breast-feeding. A few days after childbirth, the milk begins to flow. Breast milk, which contains a unique mixture of nutrients and proteins, is the healthiest food for an infant.

Breast abscess

An infected area of the breast that fills with pus and forms a lump. Symptoms of a breast abscess include swelling, tenderness, and redness and may include fever. An abscess typically occurs in women who are breast-feeding. It may be preceded by MASTITIS, an inflammation of the breast tissue caused when bacteria from the baby's mouth enter the breast tissue through cracks in the nipples. A woman who suspects she has a breast abscess or has a breast lump should see her doctor. For a breast abscess, the doctor may prescribe antibiotics to fight the infection and an anti-inflammatory medication, such as aspirin or ibuprofen, to reduce pain and fever. If antibiotic treatments do not eliminate the abscess, the pus may need to be removed by the doctor.

Breast cancer

FOR SYMPTOM CHART
see Breast pain or lumps, page 22

A disease in which cancer cells develop in the breast tissue and can spread to other organs. Breast cancer is the second most common cancer (after skin cancer) among women and the second most common cause of cancer death (after lung cancer) in women. Breast cancer also occurs in men. Women's breast tissue contains fat cells and glandular tissue that form milk-producing lobules. The lobules are separated by fibrous tissue and transport milk through thin tubes called ducts. Breast cancer most commonly develops as a lump in the fibrous tissue or in the ducts.

SYMPTOMS AND DIAGNOSIS
Frequently, a breast lump can be discovered during a monthly BREAST SELF-EXAMINATION or a doctor's annual breast examination. A MAMMOGRAM, a special X ray of a breast, can often detect breast cancers that are too

---

TESTING FOR BREAST CANCER

Recommendations by age are as follows:

- Self-examination – monthly, starting at menses
- Doctor examination – every 3 years, starting at menses
- Doctor examination – annually after age 40
- Establish baseline mammogram – age 40
- Mammogram every 2 years – age 40 to 50
- Mammogram annually – age 50 and over

---

small to feel, although some tumors cannot be detected by a mammogram. Also, mammography cannot differentiate a cancerous tumor from a benign one with certainty. Besides a lump, other signs of breast cancer include swelling, dimpled skin, and tenderness of the breast; or indentation or discharge from the nipple.

When a breast lump has been discovered, or the results of a mammogram are abnormal, the doctor usually will conduct other tests, such as a BIOPSY, aspiration, or ULTRASOUND SCANNING, to help diagnose or rule out cancer. Sometimes, breast cancer can be detected by mammogram when it is in its earliest stage, called carcinoma in situ (in situ means in place). At that stage, the cancer is confined to the cells lining the milk ducts. In a biopsy, the doctor removes the lump and then sends a sample of tissue from the lump to a pathologist to examine it for cancer cells. The pathologist can identify the type of cancer. Sometimes, a breast biopsy is done by inserting a needle into the breast lump and aspirating (drawing out) some of the tissue or fluid to examine it for cancer cells. Ultrasound is used to create images of breast tissue and can help ascertain whether the lump is solid or filled with fluid. If a biopsy shows that a breast lump contains cancer cells, the tissue sample will be tested to see if the cancer cells have receptors that can bind to the hormones estrogen and progesterone, which can stimulate cancerous cells to grow. This test, called a hormone-receptor test, is important in helping the doctor plan treatment and to determine what

---

chemotherapy is most likely to have the best effect. Part of the diagnosis involves assessing the stage of the cancer. Breast cancers are classified in stages, from carcinoma in situ at stage 0 to the most serious, stage IV, in which the cancer has spread to other organs in the body.

CAUSES AND RISK FACTORS
About 5 percent to 10 percent of women's breast cancers are genetically inherited. A woman whose mother, sister, or daughter has had breast cancer is at an increased risk of developing breast cancer herself, especially if her relative developed it at an early age or in both breasts. Other risk factors include age, obesity, and the woman's menstrual and pregnancy histories. A woman's risk for developing breast cancer increases with age. Eight of ten women with breast cancer are postmenopausal (past the onset of MENOPAUSE). Women who started menstruation early (before age 12) or went through menopause late (after age 55) have a slightly greater chance of getting breast cancer. Those who never had children or had their

---

BREAST CANCER RISK AND AGE

Risk for developing breast cancer increases with age. Family history of breast cancer increases one's risk beyond the following averages:

AGE	RISK
25	1 in 19,608
30	1 in 2,525
35	1 in 622
40	1 in 217
45	1 in 93
50	1 in 50
55	1 in 33
60	1 in 24
65	1 in 17
70	1 in 14
75	1 in 11
80	1 in 10
85	1 in 9
90	1 in 8
95	1 in 8

Adapted with permission of the National Cancer Institute.

BIOPSIES OF BREAST LUMPS

Any lump in a breast should be reported to a doctor for further evaluation. He or she may find a lump upon manual examination, or a mammogram may reveal a lump. In any case, a biopsy of the affected breast is often the next step. Biopsy samples of tissue can help determine for certain if a lump is cancerous.

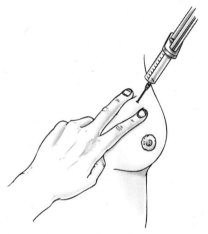

NEEDLE BIOPSY OF BREAST LUMP
The doctor steadies the lump between his or her forefinger and middle finger, inserts a thin needle, and withdraws fluid or tissue. The fluid or cells are then sent to a laboratory to be examined.

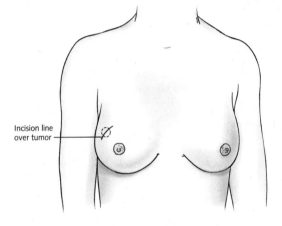

Incision line over tumor

INCISIONAL OR EXCISIONAL BIOPSY
In an incisional biopsy, only a portion of the lump is removed. Incisional biopsies are usually done only if removing the entire lump would involve an extensive operation. In an excisional biopsy (which is more common), the whole lump is removed.

first child after age 30 are also at risk, in theory, because they have been exposed to higher levels of the hormone ESTROGEN over the course of their lifetime. Estrogen replacement therapy (see HORMONE REPLACEMENT THERAPY) may also elevate the risk of developing breast cancer. (However, hormone replacement therapy may help prevent osteoporosis.) Women who have used oral contraceptives (birth control pills) seem not to have an increased risk for breast cancer. Other risk factors for breast cancer include exposure to ionizing radiation or chemicals such as pesticides; alcohol and smoking may play a role.

TREATMENT
Treatment options for breast cancer include surgery, radiation therapy, chemotherapy, and hormonal therapy.
■ *Surgery* Most women with breast

cancer have surgery to remove the cancer from the breast. Usually, some of the lymph nodes under the arm are also taken out and examined microscopically to see if they contain cancer cells. Two types of operations are performed to remove breast cancer: LUMPECTOMY and MASTECTOMY. Selection of the surgical procedure is based on the potential for disfigurement, side effects, the need for additional treatments (such as radiation therapy), and the emotional impact of each alternative.

A lumpectomy involves surgically removing the breast lump and some of the tissue around it. It is usually followed by radiation therapy to the breast and armpit to destroy any residual tumor. Most surgeons also remove some of the lymph nodes under the arm. Mastectomy is the surgical removal of the entire breast

and usually the lymph nodes under the arm. Mastectomy is often no more effective than removal of the lump alone. Therefore, it is usually used only when the woman's breast is small and the lump is so large that a lumpectomy would be more disfiguring than removing the whole breast; if the cancer cells have spread throughout the entire breast; or if the lump is simply very large (larger than 5 centimeters). A modified radical mastectomy consists of the removal of the breast, some chest muscles, and all of the lymph nodes under the arm. For many years, the modified radical mastectomy was the operation most used to treat breast cancer, but it is no longer considered necessary in the majority of cases. Radical mastectomies, removing all chest muscles and additional skin and fat from the chest, were per-

WARNING SIGNS OF BREAST CANCER

See your doctor if you have:

- **Any new lump**
- **A nipple discharge, particularly if the discharge is dark**
- **A nipple that draws inward or points in a new direction**
- **A dimpling of the skin of the breast**

formed in the 1960s and 1970s but are generally no longer done.

■ *Radiation therapy* High doses of X rays are sometimes used to kill cancer cells and shrink tumors. Radiation may come from a machine outside the body (external radiation therapy) or from introducing radioactive substances (radioisotopes) into the area where the cancer cells are found (internal radiation therapy). Radiation treatments last only a few minutes each time, but typically must be given 5 days a week for about 6 weeks. Radiation therapy is given following a lumpectomy to destroy any cancer cells that may remain in the woman's breast. It is sometimes used following a mastectomy to kill cancer cells that may remain in nearby tissues. Side effects of radiation therapy may include nausea or loss of appetite, swelling and redness of the breast, tiredness, muscle pain, and sensitivity to exposure to the sun.

■ *Chemotherapy* If tests show that cancer cells are present in the lymph nodes or have spread to other parts of the woman's body, drugs are used to kill the cancer cells. They are administered as pills or injections into a muscle or intravenously. Chemotherapy is most effective in younger (premenopausal) women whose lymph nodes show signs of cancer. Side effects of chemotherapy vary with the types of drugs used, but can include nausea, hair loss, and fatigue.

■ *Hormonal therapy* The presence of hormone receptors in breast cancer cells makes it more likely that the cancer cells will respond to hormonal therapy. Hormonal therapy can help stop hormones from stimulating cancer cells to grow. This is done by using drugs that block the hormones (particularly estrogen) or by surgical removal of organs that create hormones, such as the ovaries. Hormone therapy with the antiestrogen drug

called tamoxifen is often given to patients in the early stages of breast cancer, especially in postmenopausal women older than 50 years of age; it may be combined with other chemotherapy.

OUTLOOK

The chance of recovery and choice of teatment depend on the stage of the cancer (whether it is only in the breast or has spread to other organs), the type of breast cancer, specific characteristics of the cancer cells, and whether the cancer has been found in both breasts. A woman's age, weight, general health, desire for future pregnancy, and whether she is still having menstrual periods can all influence the prognosis and choice of treatment.

Breast cancer genes

See BRCA.

Breast enlargement

A surgical procedure to increase the size of the breasts by inserting a fluid or gel-filled implant between the breast tissue and the chest wall. Also called breast augmentation, breast enlargement is typically done on a woman who has lost most or all of a breast to cancer. Breast enlargement surgery is also performed on women who have one breast that is markedly smaller than the other and on women who choose, for cosmetic reasons, to enlarge their breasts.

THE PROCEDURE

Breast enlargement can be performed in a hospital, with the patient staying overnight. More commonly, it is done in an ambulatory surgery setting, with the patient returning home on the same day.

Anesthesia depends on the preferences of the plastic surgeon performing the enlargement and those of the patient herself. General anesthesia allows the patient to sleep through the operation, but it involves a greater risk of respiratory and heart problems and is more likely to cause side effects, such as nausea, vomiting, and a mild sore throat from the endotracheal tube used to assist breathing. Local anesthesia, combined with CONSCIOUS SEDATION, in which the patient is drowsy and insensitive to pain, has fewer complications; yet, it controls any discomfort. Nausea and vomiting are significantly less likely during

recovery, and an endotracheal tube is usually not used.

Once the patient is under anesthesia, the surgeon makes an incision to expose the internal breast tissues. Depending on the preference of the surgeon and the anatomy of the patient, the incision may be made in the areola (the dark tissue surrounding the nipple), in the crease where the breast joins the skin covering the chest, or in the armpit. Working through the incision, the surgeon lifts the breast tissue and skin away from the chest to make a pocket. The pocket may lie either behind the breast tissue (and over the muscles covering the chest wall) or under the muscles and the chest wall. The implant is then placed inside the pocket. The implant most commonly used today consists of a SILICONE shell, filled with saline solution or salt water, that has the consistency of natural breast tissue. For a woman who is having her breast reconstructed after cancer surgery (MASTECTOMY), the surgeon may use the tissues of the woman during the surgery (see BREAST RECONSTRUCTION). Once the implant is centered behind the nipple, the incision is closed. A gauze bandage and tape may be placed over the incision for support. Typically, the surgery takes 1 to 2 hours. The breast enlargement procedure may be combined with a BREAST LIFT to provide the best appearance.

WHAT TO EXPECT

Blood and urine laboratory studies may be required before and/or after surgery. As with any surgery involving anesthesia, the woman must have nothing to eat or drink after midnight on the night before. The surgeon may also provide instructions about medications or nutritional supplements to be avoided or added before surgery. Soreness and fatigue will last for several days after surgery, but patients are usually up and around within 24 to 48 hours. Ice packs on the surgical wounds and the pain medication, prescribed by the surgeon, help to control pain.

Gauze dressings over the incisions will be removed in a few days, according to the instructions of the surgeon. The stitches are removed in a week to 10 days, depending on the rate of healing; if dissolvable sutures have been used, they will disappear

BREAST ENLARGEMENT SURGERY

Surgery to enlarge the breasts involves making an incision in the breast and separating the breast tissue from the muscular chest wall to form a pocket for an implant. The implant can be positioned either under or on top of the chest muscles underlying the breast tissue. The surgery may include a breast lift to enhance the results.

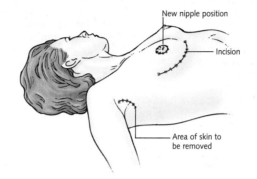

New nipple position
Incision
Area of skin to be removed

INCISION LINES FOR BREAST ENLARGEMENT
A breast enlargement requires an incision under the armpit, around the areola (the dark tissue surrounding the nipple), or under the bottom portion of the breast. The most common site for inserting the implant is the fold under the breast.

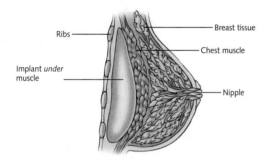

Ribs
Breast tissue
Chest muscle
Implant *under* muscle
Nipple

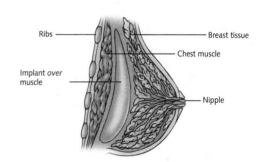

Ribs
Breast tissue
Chest muscle
Implant *over* muscle
Nipple

CHOICES FOR LOCATION OF IMPLANT
A breast implant can be inserted either under or over the chest muscle, centered under the nipple. An implant placed under the chest muscle makes it easier to detect tumors.

in the same period. Driving can be resumed in a week, and normal work schedules, depending on the degree of physical activity, can be resumed within a few days. Patients with small children should not lift them until the surgeon gives approval for that.

The breasts will be sensitive to the touch for 2 to 3 weeks, and direct physical contact should be avoided. A burning sensation in the nipples is common for the first 2 weeks. It normally subsides as healing progresses. Swelling of the breasts is normal after enlargement surgery. The swelling goes down as the breasts heal and usually disappears within 3 to 5 weeks.

After breast enlargement, mammograms should be continued at the regular intervals recommended by the physician. Breasts that have been surgically enlarged require a special mammogram technique; women should use a mammography facility that is familiar with it.

POSSIBLE COMPLICATIONS
The most common problem after breast enlargement is when the tissue surrounding the implant tightens around it and causes the entire breast to feel hard. This problem, called capsular contracture, may be reduced by massage and can be treated by the surgeon who removes the scar tissue. Sometimes, the implant has to be replaced or removed. On rare occasions, breast implants may break or leak, usually because of a penetrating injury. The body absorbs the harmless saline solution within a few hours after the implant deflates.

Surgery will be required to replace the implant.

If a break occurs in implants filled with silicone gel—which, because of concerns about safety, are now used only for women in government-approved clinical trials—the silicone may travel through the breast or even migrate to another part of the body. The implant must be replaced, and as much of the silicone gel as possible has to be removed.

Breast lift
A surgical procedure to restore a more youthful shape to breasts that have sagged due to aging, weight loss, pregnancy, or breast-feeding. A breast lift is also known as a mastopexy. In some cases, the procedure is combined with BREAST ENLARGEMENT to

add fullness and volume to the re-shaped breast.

Breast lifts are most successful in women who have relatively small breasts and do not plan to have any more children. The procedure works with breasts of any size, but its effect is likely to last a shorter time in a woman with large, heavy breasts. Likewise, pregnancy after a breast lift will shorten the effectiveness of the procedure by stretching the breast tissue and allowing sagging to occur again.

Typically a breast lift is done as AMBULATORY SURGERY, and the patient goes home on the same day. The procedure is usually performed with the patient under general anesthesia, although sometimes a surgeon may recommend a local anesthetic combined with conscious sedation, an intravenous medication that keeps the person relaxed, pain-free, and drowsy but awake.

Blood and urine laboratory tests may be required before or after surgery. As with any surgery that involves anesthesia, the woman must have nothing to eat or drink after midnight on the night before. The surgeon may also provide instruc-tions about medications or nutrition-al supplements to be added or avoid-ed in preparation for surgery.

WHAT TO EXPECT
In the most common breast-lift technique, the surgeon makes an incision along the natural contours of the breast. The surgeon removes excess skin and then raises the nipple and areola into the new, higher position. The incision is closed with sutures around the areola, in a line heading down from the nipple. The surgery takes from 1 to 3 hours.

Following surgery, an elastic bandage or surgical bra is worn over the gauze dressings that cover the sutured incisions. The breasts look bruised and swollen for several days, but pain is usually mild to moderate and well controlled with oral medications prescribed by the surgeon. In a few days, the surgical bra is replaced by a soft bra, which is worn for 3 to 4 weeks. Stitches are removed 1 to 2 weeks after surgery; if dissolvable sutures have been used, they will disappear in a couple of weeks.

OUTLOOK
Women can return to work in a week or two, depending on how they feel and the type of work. For 3 to 4 weeks after surgery, they should not lift heavy objects over the head. Some surgeons advise women to refrain from sexual activity for a week or more to avoid swelling in the breasts. Contact sports may be resumed after a month.

A breast lift does leave permanent scars. At first, the scars are red and lumpy, but they become less obvious with time and often fade to no more than thin, white lines. Usually the scars are placed so that they cannot be seen while the person is normally dressed. Excessive bleeding and infection of the surgical incision are possible but rare complications of a breast lift. Either condition can widen the scars that remain after the procedure.

Breast lump

A mass in the breast frequently detected by a woman during BREAST SELF-EXAMINATION or by a doctor during an annual examination. Breast lumps are common and usually are not cancerous. In addition to cancer, a breast lump may be a sign of FIBRO-CYSTIC BREASTS or FIBROADENOMA. In fibrocystic disease, cysts (small sacs filled with fluid) occur that vary in size with the woman's menstrual cycle. In some women with fibrocystic disease, pain and tenderness occur a week or two before the menstrual period; caffeine or similar stimulants may aggravate the symptoms. Fibroadenomas are solid, noncancerous lumps that occur most often in young women. Another possible cause of a breast lump is an infection, or BREAST ABSCESS. To diagnose or rule out cancer, a woman who has found a lump in her breast should see her doctor, who will perform a breast examination and recommend appropriate tests, which may include a MAMMOGRAM, ULTRASOUND SCANNING, an ASPIRATION, or a BIOPSY. See also BREAST CANCER.

Breast milk

Mother's milk. Beginning with the COLOSTRUM produced the first few days after childbirth, breast milk provides babies with the ideal balance of nutrients in forms readily available to the infant's immature digestive tract, plus valuable protection against disease. See also BREAST-FEEDING.

Incision line for skin removal

Nipple's higher position

Area of skin that is removed

Nipple and breast repositioned

STEPS IN A BREAST LIFT
A breast lift, also known as a mastopexy, begins with an incision that follows the natural contour of the breast and defines a new higher position for the nipple. Then excess skin under the incision line is removed, and the breast (including the nipple) is sutured into a higher position.

Breast pump

A device used to extract breast milk without nursing. Breast pumps can be rented or purchased and can be operated manually or electrically by battery or on house current.

Some mothers pump milk to be fed to their babies later in their absence. A pump can be used when an emergency separates a mother from her baby for a period of time. It is common for women who return to jobs after childbirth to continue BREAST-FEEDING by pumping their breasts at work and storing the milk. It can be refrigerated or frozen and given to the baby later when the mother is away. Similarly, premature babies who remain in the hospital after their mothers return home can also drink mother's milk. By pumping, a mother establishes her milk supply for when the baby comes home.

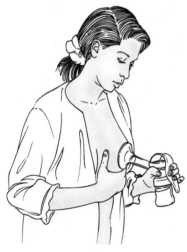

MANUAL BREAST PUMP
A breast pump is a simple convenience for a nursing mother who sometimes cannot be present at feeding time. To use a manual breast pump, a woman supports and positions her breast with one hand and uses the other hand to work the pump. She can then refrigerate or freeze the expressed milk so that another person can feed it to the baby when she is away.

Breast reconstruction

A surgical procedure to create a new breast to replace one that has been removed, usually because of cancer (see BREAST CANCER). Breast reconstruction can be performed when the breast is removed in a MASTECTOMY or at a later date. The surgery serves cosmetic and psychological purposes, allowing a woman who has lost a breast to disease to recover a sense of physical wholeness. It does not increase or decrease chances for further breast cancer.

Breast reconstruction requires more than one surgical procedure. Some women and their surgeons decide to begin the series of procedures at the same time that the mastectomy is performed. Others prefer to wait until after healing from the mastectomy is complete and then begin reconstruction.

OPTIONS

Two types of reconstruction are available. The choice between them depends on a number of factors, both medical and personal, and should be made by the woman and her surgeon.

■ *Skin expansion* The most common technique involves stretching the skin to accommodate a synthetic breast implant after mastectomy (removal of the breast). Following traditional mastectomy, the surgeon inserts a balloon expander under the skin of the chest where the breast and skin have been removed. A saltwater solution is added to the balloon through a small valve implanted beneath the skin, filling the balloon over a period of months and slowly stretching the skin. Some balloon implants are meant to be left in place. Others are replaced in a subsequent procedure with a breast implant of the same kind used in breast enlargement—a silicone shell filled with a saltwater or saline solution.

■ *Flap reconstruction* In this type of procedure, a new breast mound is fashioned from skin and underlying tissue taken from another part of the body, such as the back, abdomen, or buttocks. Flap surgery is performed in two ways. In the first, a flap of tissue is removed from one site and transplanted in the breast area. The surgeon uses a microscope to connect the blood vessels in the flap to blood vessels in the chest. In the other method, the flap, usually taken from the back of the woman, is tunneled under the skin to the transplant site on the chest while remaining connected to its original blood supply.

Flap reconstruction is more complex than skin expansion, but the results may be more natural, and the possibility of leaking or ruptured implants is avoided.

■ *Follow-up procedures* Once the breast reconstruction is complete, the nipple and the areola (the dark surrounding tissue) are reconstructed. Since the surgeon cannot create a new breast to identically match the other breast, surgery on the healthy breast may be recommended to achieve a symmetrical appearance. See BREAST ENLARGEMENT; BREAST LIFT; AND BREAST REDUCTION.

THE PROCEDURE

Blood and urine laboratory studies are usually required before and after surgery, and the woman is screened for undetected conditions that may affect safety and outcome, such as high blood pressure or diabetes. As with any surgery that involves anesthesia, the woman must have nothing to eat or drink after midnight on the night before. The surgeon may also provide instructions about medications or nutritional supplements to be added or avoided.

The initial procedure is almost always performed in a hospital, with the patient asleep under general anesthesia and pain-free. The usual stay in the hospital depends on the procedure performed, but it averages 2 to 5 days. Depending on their extent and complexity, follow-up procedures may be done with a local anesthetic, coupled with conscious sedation, an intravenous medication that leaves the patient awake but drowsy and pain-free.

Following the initial reconstructive surgery, women generally feel sore and tired for 1 to 2 weeks. Pain is usually well controlled by oral medications prescribed by the surgeon. In many surgeries, a drain is placed in the incision to remove excess fluid. The drain is normally taken out within a week to 10 days. Sutures are removed in a week to 10 days. If dissolvable sutures have been used, they will disappear within the same period.

The time required for full recovery depends on the extent of surgery as well as the general health of the woman. If a mastectomy is combined with flap reconstruction, 6 weeks of recovery is typical. Less time may be required with skin expansion, particularly if it is performed after complete healing from the mastectomy.

B

RECONSTRUCTING A BREAST

When all or part of a breast has been removed, usually because of cancer, many women choose to have a surgical procedure to reconstruct the breast. A new breast may be formed from tissue from the woman's back or abdomen. More commonly, an implant is put in place. All the procedures are done with the patient asleep under general anesthesia.

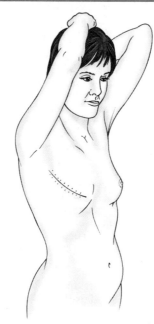

BEFORE
The right breast has been removed in a mastectomy for treatment of cancer.

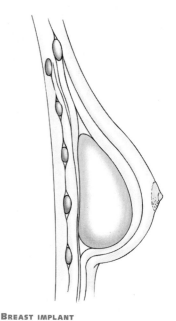

BREAST IMPLANT
One option is to insert a saline implant under the pectoral muscle. For a larger breast, the skin is first stretched over a period of months.

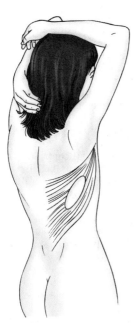

FLAP RECONSTRUCTION USING TISSUE FROM THE BACK
A second option is using a flap of skin, muscle, fat, and attached blood vessels from the back. The tissue flap is tunneled under the skin and attached to the chest.

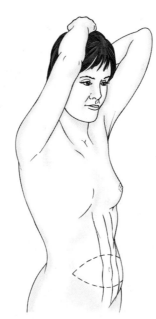

FLAP RECONSTUCTION USING TISSUE FROM THE ABDOMEN
A third option is to use tissue from the abdomen to reconstruct the breast. The tissue is tunneled under the skin to the breast site.

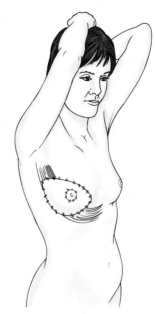

AFTER
In a later procedure, a nipple can be created using tissue from the thigh and some tissue from the remaining breast. The woman now has a breast and nipple that look reasonably natural.

The recovery period involves some restrictions. Most surgeons advise refraining from overhead lifting, strenuous sports, and sexual activity for 3 to 6 weeks. Special stretching exercises may be advised to restore flexibility and muscle tone to the chest area.

A reconstructed breast does not deliver the same sensations as a normal breast, but in time, it may develop some feeling. The scars left by the procedure are permanent but they often fade over time to no more than thin, white lines.

POSSIBLE COMPLICATIONS

As with any surgery, breast reconstruction can cause bleeding, infection, or the collection of blood under the skin (hematoma). These conditions may widen the scars that remain after the procedure. If an implant is used, the most common complication is capsular contracture, when tissue surrounding the implant tightens and causes the entire breast to feel hard. This problem can be treated by removing or scoring the scar tissue; sometimes, the implant has to be replaced or removed.

On rare occasions, breast implants may break or leak because of an injury or as a result of normal body movement. The body absorbs the harmless saline solution within a few hours after the implant deflates. Surgery is required to replace the implant.

If a break occurs in implants filled with silicone gel—which, because of concerns about safety, are now used only for women in government-approved clinical trials—the silicone may travel through the breast or even migrate to another part of the body. The implant must be replaced, and as much of the silicone gel as possible has to be removed as well.

Breast reduction

The surgical removal of skin, fat, and underlying tissue to make the breast smaller. Breast reduction is performed most often to solve the problems faced by women with very large, heavy breasts. The excessive weight can cause neck and back pain, skeletal deformities in the skin, bra strap indentations in the skin, skin irritation, and even breathing problems. Overly large breasts may create a high degree of self-consciousness.

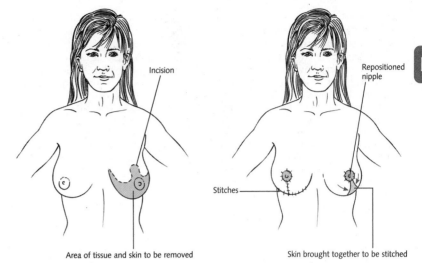

Incision

Repositioned nipple

Stitches

Area of tissue and skin to be removed

Skin brought together to be stitched

REDUCING BREAST SIZE
To do a breast reduction, the surgeon makes an incision across the breast and above the nipple that outlines where the nipple will be repositioned and the area of skin and underlying tissue that will be removed. Excess skin, breast tissue, and fat are removed, and the nipple is moved up. Then the skin is brought together under the now smaller breast and stitched in a vertical line down from the nipple and along the crease under the breast.

The procedure is also performed in women who have had a BREAST RECONSTRUCTION following the surgical removal of a breast because of cancer. In this case, the reduction serves to make the remaining natural breast more similar in appearance to the reconstructed breast.

THE PROCEDURE
In almost all cases, breast reduction is performed in a hospital with the patient asleep under general anesthesia. The entire procedure takes from 3 to 5 hours, occasionally longer.

First, the surgeon marks the area where the nipple and areola (the dark surrounding area) will appear after surgery. Then, in the most common procedure, an incision is made that encircles the areola and follows the curve of the crease below the breast. The surgeon then removes excess skin, glandular tissue, and fat and moves the nipple and areola into a new, higher position. Depending on the size of the original areola, some of it may be removed so that its size matches the dimensions of the new breast. The skin from the sides of the breast is then drawn down to create the new contour of the breast. In some cases, the surgeon may use LIPOSUCTION to remove excess fat, especially from under the armpit.

In most breast reductions, the nip-

ple and areola remain attached to their original nerves and blood vessels and usually retain some sensation after surgery. If the breasts are particularly large, however, the nipple and areola may have to be removed and grafted into their new position. In this case, normal sensation is lost.

The incisions are closed with stitches around the areola, down to the crease of the breast, and along the crease. Gauze bandages are placed over the incisions, and the breasts are wrapped in an elastic bandage. Sometimes, the patient is able to wear a surgical bra soon after the operation.

BEFORE AND AFTER SURGERY
Blood and urine laboratory studies are usually required before surgery, as well as after, and the woman is screened for undetected conditions that may affect safety and outcome, such as high blood pressure or diabetes. As with any surgery that involves general anesthesia, the woman must have nothing to eat or drink after midnight on the night before. The surgeon may also provide instructions about medications or nutritional supplements to be avoided in preparation for surgery.

The usual hospital stay after breast reduction is overnight, and patients are typically up and around in a day or two. The bandages are removed 1 or 2 days after surgery, and stitches are taken out in 1 to 3 weeks. If dissolvable sutures have been used, they will disappear in the same period. A surgical bra needs to be worn 24 hours a day for several weeks until bruising and swelling subside. Thereafter, a soft sports bra is advised until healing is complete.

Medication prescribed by the surgeon should control the pain and discomfort that are to be expected during the first week after surgery. Aching may continue for up to 6 weeks, and shooting pains in the breasts sometimes occur over a period of several months. Swelling of the breasts during the first menstrual period after surgery may also cause pain. After breast reduction, women should avoid heavy lifting for 6 weeks and driving for a month. Most surgeons advise women to refrain from sexual activity for a week or more to keep the incisions from swelling.

Some loss of feeling in the nipple following surgery is normal. Sensation usually returns within 6 weeks, although a year may pass before the breast feels normal. Scars are red and raised at first. Usually the scars fade considerably within the first year, but they are permanent and will not disappear completely. Breast-feeding after breast reduction will not be possible because the milk ducts are removed during surgery.

Possible complications include bleeding, infection, the collection of blood under the skin (hematoma), and permanent loss of sensation in the breast or nipple. The nipple and areola may not graft properly because of a disrupted blood supply; they can be reconstructed with a skin graft in a follow-up procedure.

Breast self-examination

FOR SYMPTOM CHART
see Breast pain or lumps, page 22

A visual and physical examination of one's own breasts in order to detect breast lumps. Monthly self-examination is recommended. During a self-examination, a woman checks for visual changes in the breasts, including alterations in texture, color, shape

and size. Fingertips are used gently to feel for lumps in the breast tissue. A woman who menstruates should do the examination a few days after her period ends or on the day she begins a new pack of oral contraceptives. Women who do not menstruate should pick a day and do the exam on that day each month. The detection of a new lump requires a visit to the doctor for further evaluation. See BREAST LUMP; BREAST CANCER; and MAMMOGRAM.

Breast-feeding

Nourishing an infant with milk from a woman's breast. Breast-feeding, also called nursing, is the medically preferred way to feed a baby; it is inexpensive, nurturing, and convenient and benefits both the mother and child. Breast-feeding traditionally has been thought to provide protection against pregnancy. Although breast-feeding inhibits ovulation and reduces the risk of pregnancy, it is not a reliable means of birth control.

Breast milk provides all the nutrients, hormones, and proteins that an infant needs in the first few months of life. It also contains antibodies that protect babies from illness. Breast-fed babies have fewer infections of the ears and digestive and respiratory tracts than bottle-fed infants; they have a significantly reduced risk for many acute and chronic diseases, develop fewer food allergies, and are less likely to become constipated. Breast-feeding may promote cognitive development. Nutritionally, commercial formulas are nearly identical to breast milk; however, they lack the protective antibodies and hormones of breast milk. Most pediatricians recommend that breast-feeding be continued at least throughout the first year of an infant's life. If weaning becomes necessary, doctors recommend formula over cow's milk.

Most women can breast-feed. However, prior surgery, medications, or an illness may reduce a woman's milk supply. Breast-feeding may not be appropriate for women who are undergoing chemotherapy, who are HIV-positive (HIV is the human immunodeficiency virus that causes acquired immunodeficiency syndrome, or AIDS), or who have hepatitis B (a viral disease that damages the liver). Medications and some types of

infection can pass from the mother into breast milk. A woman should consult her doctor about the advisability of breast-feeding if she is taking medications, has an illness, or has special concerns about it.

THE NURSING WOMAN
During pregnancy, the breasts undergo many changes in preparation for breast-feeding. As early as 6 to 8 weeks into a pregnancy, the fat layer in the breasts thickens and the number of milk glands increases. The nipples may protrude more, and the areolas (the skin surrounding the nipples) grow larger and darken. In the fourth or fifth month of pregnancy, a small amount of colostrum may leak from the breasts. Colostrum is a thin, yellowish, milky liquid that is secreted shortly after childbirth. It is rich in maternal antibodies, which protect the baby from infection, and it contains all the nutrition that a newborn needs in the first few days of life. A woman's milk usually does not flow until 2 to 5 days after delivery.

When a baby starts to nurse, nerves in the nipple signal the brain to secrete the hormones oxytocin and prolactin. Oxytocin tells the breasts to let the milk flow, and prolactin stimulates glands in the breasts to produce more milk and release it through the milk ducts. Pressure from the baby's sucking forces milk out through the nipple. The longer and more frequently a woman breast-feeds, the more milk her breasts will produce. The infant's cry can stimulate a woman's brain to release oxytocin, but not prolactin. In addition to causing milk to flow, oxytocin also helps shrink the uterus back to its prepregnancy size.

Women who breast-feed their infants need an adequate supply of fluids and nutritious food. To produce milk, a woman who is breast-feeding needs about 600 more calories per day than she did before she became pregnant. A well-balanced diet helps ensure that the extra calories consumed provide the nutrients specifically needed for breast-feeding. Particularly, women who are breast-feeding need about 1,200 milligrams of calcium (the same as for pregnancy). Salmon, broccoli, and dairy products, such as milk, yogurt, and cheese, are rich in calcium. Women who do not ingest enough calcium while they

BREAST SELF-EXAMINATION

Most breast lumps are found by women themselves during regular breast self-examination. Every woman should examine her breasts each month. Detecting any new lump or anything else unusual requires an immediate visit to the doctor for further evaluation.

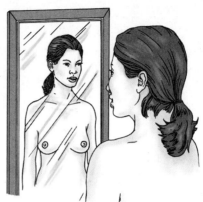

STEP 1
In a mirror, inspect each breast from all angles for changes such as puckering, dimpling, or redness of the skin.

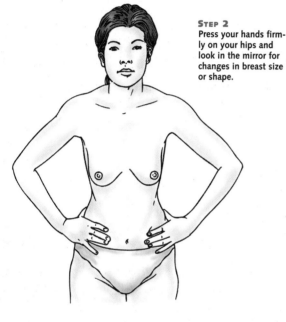

STEP 2
Press your hands firmly on your hips and look in the mirror for changes in breast size or shape.

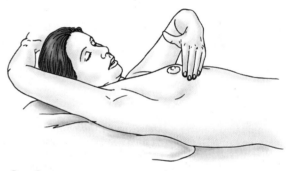

STEP 3
Lie flat on your back with a pillow under your right shoulder and right arm over your head. You will use your left hand to examine your right breast.

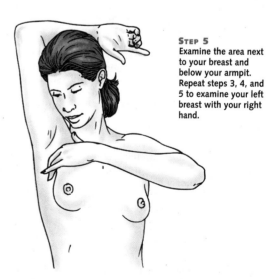

STEP 5
Examine the area next to your breast and below your armpit. Repeat steps 3, 4, and 5 to examine your left breast with your right hand.

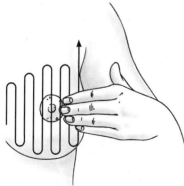

STEP 4
Examine the entire right breast in an up-and-down pattern as shown. Feel the breast with the pads of your index and middle fingers. Compress gently, feeling for lumps. Then, circle the nipple to examine that area; also look for any discharge.

B

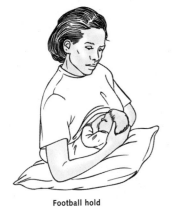 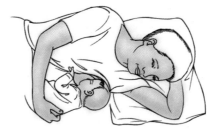

Football hold   Lying down

VARYING POSITIONS FOR BREAST-FEEDING
Changing breast-feeding positions from one feeding to another helps prevent breast soreness for a nursing mother. The so-called football hold, in which the mother holds the baby close to her side, is a good position for a very small baby. Both mother and baby may find the lying-down position comfortable. In any nursing position, the baby's entire body should be facing the mother, and the baby's head may need support from a hand or arm as shown in the football hold.

are breast-feeding risk losing calcium from their bones. To meet daily requirements for vitamins and minerals, many doctors recommend that women who breast-feed continue to take prenatal vitamins. Drinking several glasses of skim milk each day can help a woman meet her body's needs for fluids and calcium. Women who breast-feed lose the weight gained in pregnancy sooner because producing milk burns calories.

HOW TO BREAST-FEED
There are two ways to breast-feed. A baby may be fed directly from the breast, or milk may be expressed (pumped) from the breast and given to a baby later in a bottle. Many working women breast-feed while they are on maternity leave from work. After returning to work, they may manually express milk or use a breast pump (a device for removing milk from the breast) to provide a supply of milk for the baby while the mother is away.

A baby can begin sucking at the breast as early as 1 hour after birth. At first, some babies have difficulty attaching to the nipple, but soon become adept. To signal hunger, a baby may cry, suck, or nuzzle against his or her mother's breast. A baby who is finished nursing will let go of the breast. Most newborns nurse for about 10 to 20 minutes on each breast, although each baby sets his or her own pattern. The amount of milk the infant consumes cannot be measured; however, monitoring the baby's growth can indicate whether the food intake is adequate. Babies who are well fed typically soil six or more diapers a day, sleep well, and steadily gain weight. For any persistent nursing problems, a doctor, nurse, or lactation specialist should be contacted. La Leche League, an international volunteer group, provides reliable information and support for women who are breast-feeding.

A woman can breast-feed for as long as is practical, although breast milk should be supplemented with other foods after the infant is about 6 months of age. It is best to wean (stop breast-feeding) slowly. Lactation experts recommend starting the weaning process by substituting a bottle or cup at the child's least favorite feeding time and increasing the number of substitute feedings gradually. Women who gradually diminish breast-feeding begin to produce less milk and often experience less discomfort from engorgement (the breasts being too full).

BREAST-FEEDING PROBLEMS
Once the baby and mother have established a routine, serious breast-feeding problems are rare. There are several common difficulties that can be easily treated.

■ *Engorgement* When a woman's milk comes in, her breasts may be overfull and tender, and she may have a low fever. Breast-feeding usually relieves this condition. To further relieve the discomfort of engorgement, a woman may massage her breasts, take a hot shower, or place hot packs on her breasts.

■ *Sore nipples* Soreness usually diminishes as the breasts become accustomed to the baby's sucking. Sore nipples can also result from not properly drying the nipples between feedings or from not breaking the suction of the baby's mouth before taking the baby off the breast. Harsh soaps, creams, or lotions can irritate the skin of the nipples and can be bad for the baby, who is likely to ingest anything that is applied to the nipple. A doctor or midwife can suggest safe products.

■ *Blocked ducts* A tender lump in the breast of a woman who is breast-feeding may be a sign of a blocked milk duct. A woman can help clear a blocked duct by massaging the breast, taking warm showers, applying heat to the breast, and nursing longer and more frequently.

■ *Mastitis* An inflammation of the milk ducts, mastitis occurs when bacteria, usually from the baby's mouth,

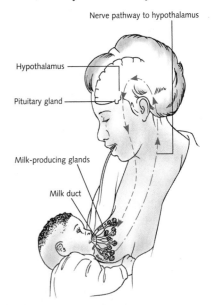

HOW BREAST-FEEDING WORKS
When a baby sucks on the mother's breast, he or she triggers the let-down reflex. The baby's sucking action stimulates nerve endings in the areola (the pigmented area surrounding the nipple) of the breast. Nerve impulses carry a message to the hypothalamus (a structure at the base of the brain) via the pituitary gland (a gland in the brain that produces and stimulates many hormones) to cause the production of oxytocin. Oxytocin contracts muscles in the alveoli to release milk through the milk ducts in the breast.

enter the breast through the nipple. Mastitis can lead to the formation of a BREAST ABSCESS, a hard, pus-filled lump in the breast. Symptoms of mastitis can include fever and chills, pain, swelling, hardness, redness, and a hot feeling of the breasts. A woman who has these symptoms should contact her doctor immediately. Mastitis is treated with antibiotics and, often, an anti-inflammatory drug to reduce pain and inflammation. Most doctors recommend discontinuing breast-feeding until the infection resolves.

■ **Breast lumps** While most breast lumps in nursing women are due to blocked ducts or abscesses, any lump that does not resolve with treatment within a week or two needs to be evaluated, since breast cancer can occur, although rarely.

Breath, shortness of

The sensation of having difficulty breathing comfortably. Shortness of breath is also referred to as DYSPNEA and is commonly associated with exercise or physical exertion. A person experiencing shortness of breath may feel that he or she has an insufficient supply of air and is unable to inhale and exhale fast enough or deeply enough. This may be accompanied by an increased exertion of the chest muscles, which may produce a sensation of tightness in the chest. There may be anxiety because of the urgency sensed in not getting enough air.

Strenuous physical activity causes the body to create more CARBON DIOXIDE and require more OXYGEN. Breathing becomes rapid during exertion to compensate for the extra carbon dioxide in the body, which must be expelled, and the increased need for oxygen, which must be inhaled. The heart and lungs must be operating adequately to compensate for this acceleration in exhaling carbon dioxide and breathing in oxygen. Shortness of breath with strenuous activity is normal, but in disorders affecting the heart and lungs, shortness of breath may occur

> Terms in small capital letters—for example, PHYSICAL THERAPY or PAGET DISEASE—indicate a cross-reference to another entry with more information.

with only slight physical exertion and, in some cases, when a person is at rest.

Shortness of breath that occurs during a slight increase in physical activity may be caused by structural conditions that limit the ability of the lungs to exchange air normally. A pulmonary function test can identify abnormal lung function. A narrowing of the airways, associated with asthma or infections of the upper respiratory system, can obstruct airflow and produce shortness of breath. Fluid may accumulate in the lungs as a result of abnormal heart function and cause shortness of breath and sensations of heaviness in the chest or smothering. Fluid in the lungs can also lead to spasm of the smooth muscles in the airways, resulting in a narrowing that can cause severe shortness of breath and wheezing and can produce cardiac asthma (see ASTHMA, CARDIAC).

Congestive heart failure (see HEART FAILURE, CONGESTIVE) may cause shortness of breath that first occurs only when a person lies down and is relieved when the person sits or stands upright. Sudden attacks of shortness of breath during sleep that prompt a person to awaken gasping for air may be a sign of heart failure. Severe blood loss or anemia may prevent the blood from carrying sufficient oxygen to the tissues and can cause a form of shortness of breath that produces rapid deep breathing in an attempt to take in more oxygen.

Anxiety may cause shortness of breath and produce the sensation that the air supply is inadequate. The sensation is unpleasant and frightening and may be heightened if a person believes that the cause is a serious physical problem, such as a heart attack. The person may breathe more rapidly and hyperventilate, causing an unpleasant sensation created by reduced carbon dioxide levels in the blood, which exacerbates shortness of breath. Tingling in the extremities and face and a sensation of distance from one's surroundings are signs of HYPERVENTILATION.

When shortness of breath occurs at rest, it is generally a symptom of heart or lung abnormalities or of psychological problems that may require professional treatment.

Breathing

The process of taking air into the lungs and letting it out again. In breathing, air is inhaled into the lungs through the nose or mouth as a result of muscle contractions, and it is exhaled as a result of muscle relaxation.

Breathing exercises

Exercises intended to promote deep, slow, calm breathing to maximize the amount of oxygen in the blood. Breathing exercises enable the breather to use the lungs to their full capacity by emphasizing "abdominal" or "diaphragmatic" breathing, in which the diaphragm (the muscle separating the chest from the abdominal cavity) is used to its full potential. Breathing exercises may be used to learn how to breathe correctly while lying down, sitting, and walking. Also, many people use breathing exercises to manage stress.

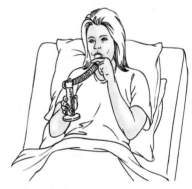

RESPIRATORY THERAPY
A person whose lung function has been impaired may be encouraged to do breathing exercises using a device called a spirometer, which measures the amount of air inhaled and exhaled. Using a spirometer regularly can help a person gradually improve his or her lung function.

Breathing problems

Difficulties with normal respiration that may be caused by structural irregularities in the respiratory system, acid-base irregularities, or infections that affect the organs involved in breathing. Breathing problems occur when normal breathing function is disrupted. During normal breathing, air is taken in through the nose and propelled to the back of the throat and the larynx, or voice box. The air passes through the windpipe and enters the bronchi, or airways, which distribute the inhaled air to the air sacs of the lungs, where oxygen and carbon dioxide are exchanged. Any inflammation, abnormality, or obstruction in these structures can inhibit the flow of air and produce breathing problems.

Movements of the diaphragm, the ribs, and the muscles between the ribs allow the chest to expand during this process. Abnormalities that inhibit these movements can decrease the flow of air and result in breathing problems.

Normal breathing is controlled by the respiratory center in the brain, which is located in the medulla, near the top of the spinal cord. Breathing in and out through the nose occurs automatically at a pace set by this area of the brain. When nasal passages are blocked by inflammation or obstructions, people breathe deliberately through the mouth. This can dry the tissues of the mouth, tongue, and upper throat and make breathing uncomfortable.

Breathing problems can be a symptom of an underlying medical condition. WHEEZING, the high-pitched whistling or purring sound that occurs on exhalation, may be caused by a respiratory infection (such as the common cold [see COLD, COMMON]), allergies, ASTHMA, exposure to toxic fumes, an obstruction in the airways, PNEUMONIA, or a genetic abnormality of the lungs. Wheezing, particularly in children, should be evaluated medically.

Whooping cough (PERTUSSIS) and CROUP can cause breathing problems, especially in young children. Breathing problems in children that are accompanied by drooling, an inability to swallow, or cyanosis (blue discoloration of the skin and mucous membranes) require emergency medical treatment.

Breathlessness

See DYSPNEA.

Breech delivery

A birth in which the baby proceeds through the cervix in a BREECH PRESENTATION, buttocks-first or feetfirst. At birth, most babies are in a head-down position, facing the mother's spine; about 3 or 4 percent of babies are born in a breech position. A breech baby can be delivered vagi-

nally, but a CESAREAN SECTION is often performed if labor does not progress, the woman's pelvis is too narrow for the baby to pass through it, or the baby shows signs of distress. The decision may also depend on the physician's level of experience in breech delivery.

Because a baby's position may shift before birth, confirming whether a baby has settled into a breech position can be difficult. When a breech position is suspected, the doctor feels for the baby through the mother's abdomen and uterus to find out where the baby's head is. An ultrasound can confirm the diagnosis. Less commonly, X rays can be used to confirm the baby's position and also to measure the size of the mother's pelvis. Prior to delivery, the doctor may try to turn the baby through external VERSION, a procedure in which the doctor manually attempts to gently reposition the baby into the headfirst position. External version usually is performed in a labor and delivery unit because, occasionally, the umbilical cord becomes pinched, requiring a prompt cesarean section. A baby who has been turned by external version may shift back into a breech presentation. If a doctor decides that it is safe, a breech baby may be delivered vaginally.

THE PROCEDURE

During a typical delivery, the largest part of the baby, the head, molds a passage through the birth canal, and the body follows. In a breech delivery, the head is delivered last. The primary problem of a breech delivery is that the buttocks or feet may not force the cervix to open wide enough for the baby's head. Forceps (a grasping tool) delivery is often necessary to ease the head through the birth canal. Electronic FETAL MONITORING of the heart is usually used to assess the condition of the baby. An EPISIOTOMY, a surgical incision in a woman's vagina, may be needed to enlarge the vaginal opening to ease delivery. A breech baby is at an increased risk of injury during delivery and of receiving an insufficient supply of oxygen as a result of cord prolapse, a serious situation in which the umbilical cord drops through the cervix into the vagina. In this position, the cord can become compressed, and a baby's oxygen

supply can be reduced or cut off. To prevent further compression of the umbilical cord after a cord prolapse, the mother may be asked to get on her hands and knees, with her head lower than her hips. The doctor then manually pushes the baby's head up and off of the umbilical cord.

If labor fails to progress, or if the baby shows signs of distress, the baby will be delivered by cesarean section. In deciding whether to deliver a breech baby vaginally, a doctor will consider a variety of factors, such as the size of the mother's pelvis and the specific position and location of the baby in the birth canal. The baby should weigh less than 8 pounds, and his or her gestational age should be at least 36 weeks. Very premature babies are fragile and have head sizes that are much larger than their bodies, making delivery of the head through a less dilated cervix dangerous. Women who have had prior uncomplicated births of similar or higher birth weight babies are more likely to deliver a breech baby safely and quickly through the vagina.

Breech presentation

A condition in pregnancy or labor in which, instead of the head, the baby's buttocks, foot, or feet, are positioned against the mother's cervix. In most deliveries, the baby moves into a head-down, facing-back position. But about 3 to 4 percent of babies are in a breech presentation at delivery. A breech presentation is more likely in pregnancies with a small fetus, more than one fetus, or too much or too little amniotic fluid. Women who have had several children are also at greater risk for a breech presentation because the muscles of the abdomen and uterus are more relaxed and permit the fetus to move more easily into a breech position.

Three types of breech presentation occur. In a frank breech position, the baby's buttocks present with the hips bent and legs extended. In a complete breech, the buttocks present with the hips and knees flexed. In a single- or double-footling breech, one or both of the baby's feet present before the buttocks. See also BREECH DELIVERY.

COMMON BREECH POSITIONS

Late in pregnancy, the fetus is usually head down, with its face toward the mother's back. If a fetus is in the breech position instead, its buttocks are resting on the mother's cervix. The three most common breech positions are the frank breech, footling breech, and complete breech. A doctor may be able to manually turn the fetus in the uterus, delivery via the vagina may proceed despite the breech, or a cesarean delivery may be necessary.

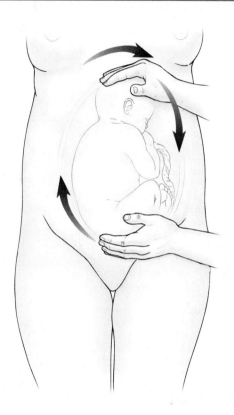

TURNING THE BABY TO NORMAL BIRTH POSITION
Sometimes it is possible for the doctor assisting the delivery to reposition the fetus while it is still in the uterus (known as external version). With the woman lying on her back, the doctor gently manipulates the fetus from outside the mother's abdomen and tries to rotate it into a more normal position.

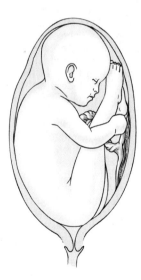

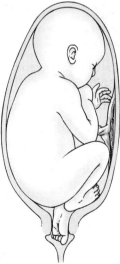

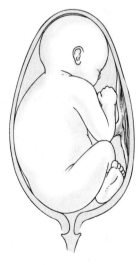

FRANK BREECH
The fetus's hips are bent, and its legs are extended up toward the head. A vaginal birth is usually possible.

FOOTLING BREECH
One (or both) of the fetus's feet sticks out or covers the woman's cervix. The baby is usually delivered by cesarean.

COMPLETE BREECH
Both hips and knees are bent. A vaginal birth is sometimes possible.

B

B

Bridge, dental

A dental appliance of false teeth that is attached to natural teeth on either side. A fixed bridge is attached to the teeth that have been filed down in order to be fitted with crowns (see CROWN, DENTAL). Fixed dental bridges are more commonly used than removable, partial denture bridges, except in cases in which there are several adjacent teeth missing or the span of empty space is relatively wide. Unlike partial dentures, fixed dental bridges cannot be taken out by the person wearing them.

The fixed bridge is usually made up of two crowns that are permanently cemented to the remaining teeth with a pontic, which is a device attached to the two crowns to fill in the space where a tooth has been removed. A resin-bonded bridge is commonly used on the front teeth when the teeth are healthy. In this style of bridge, the pontic is fused to metal bands, which are bonded to the back of the teeth with cement so they cannot be seen. When there are healthy, natural teeth on only one side of the space where a tooth is missing, a bridge may be installed. This dental bridge anchors the pontic to one or more adjacent teeth on one side of the space.

Dental bridges fill the cosmetic function of replacing missing teeth so that the surrounding facial features are supported and the appearance of the mouth is improved. They also improve the overall function of the teeth and oral hygiene. A fixed bridge corrects the bite in the area where a tooth is missing and restores the ability of the person to chew and speak normally. The space left by a missing tooth can cause the surrounding teeth to loosen and/or shift out of their proper position. This can create conditions in the mouth that lead to gum disease and tooth decay, both of which may lead to a further loss of teeth.

WHAT TO EXPECT

Placement of a fixed dental bridge can usually be accomplished in two or more dental appointments, sometimes with a specialist in PROSTHODONTICS, who replaces missing teeth. The procedure may take 2 weeks or longer, depending on the complexity of the appliance and the time required to match the crowns and pontic to the natural shade of teeth.

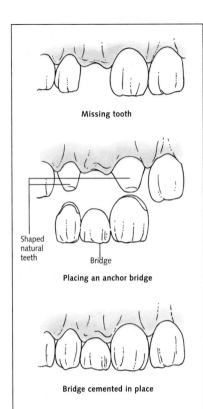

Missing tooth

Shaped natural teeth

Bridge

Placing an anchor bridge

Bridge cemented in place

FITTING A BRIDGE
A fixed dental bridge provides an artificial tooth (called a pontic), attached to natural teeth on either side, to replace a missing tooth. The natural tooth is removed, and the two teeth on either side are shaped to be fitted with crowns that are permanently cemented to the new artificial tooth. When the bridge is in place, the new tooth looks and functions like the lost tooth.

At the first appointment, the dentist uses a drill to file down the teeth that will anchor and support the pontic. The dentist or hygienist makes a dental impression of the area (see IMPRESSION, DENTAL), and a temporary bridge is fitted to be worn until the permanent bridge is ready. A metal framework for the crowns and pontic is made from the impression; then, it is coated with a ceramic material that resembles the natural surface, texture, and shade of teeth. The final bridge is then fitted over the teeth, adjusted for fit and color, and permanently cemented onto the teeth.

Good oral hygiene, including regular brushing, flossing, and dental checkups, is essential to maintaining a dental bridge. The dentist may recommend and instruct the person

wearing a bridge in the use of floss threaders to remove food debris, plaque, and bacteria from the spaces between the bridge and adjacent teeth and gums. Proper care can prevent infections, which could lead to loss of the bridge. A fixed dental bridge can last up to 10 years.

Brimonidine

An alpha agonist drug used to treat open-angle glaucoma and ocular hypertension (high pressure inside the eye). Brimonidine (Alphagan) reduces the amount of the liquid produced inside the eyeball (aqueous humor) and increases the rate at which fluid flows out of the eyeball. It is given as eye drops.

Brittle bones

A genetic disorder, also known as osteogenesis imperfecta, that is characterized by bones that break easily, often with a minimum or total absence of physical trauma. The range in severity of this disorder is extreme; some affected individuals have a few broken bones, and others have experienced as many as several hundred fractures over the course of a lifetime. Brittle bones are caused by a genetic defect affecting the amount or quality of the person's COLLAGEN. The defective amount or type of collagen results in weak bones that break easily. When there is insufficient collagen, the person may experience fractures before puberty and have a tendency toward spinal curvature and brittle teeth. In the most severe form of osteogenesis imperfecta in which collagen is not properly formed in a newborn, the infant could die because the condition causes severe respiratory problems. Other types of osteogenesis imperfecta related to improper collagen formation may produce symptoms present at birth, including a blue or gray tint to the whites of the eyes, bone deformity, loose joints, poor muscle development in arms and legs, spinal curvature, a barrel-shaped rib cage, triangular face, and hearing loss.

This disorder may be diagnosed during a physical examination or with laboratory or DNA tests. There is no cure, but treatment is aimed at managing symptoms and developing optimal bone mass and muscle strength. Physical therapy may be beneficial. A type of surgery called rodding, which implants metal rods into the central canals of the long bones, can buttress the bones, preventing or correcting deformity.

Broken blood vessels

Damage to blood vessels that may lead to internal or external BLEEDING. When trauma breaks small blood vessels near the surface of the skin, it causes a BRUISE.

Broken tooth

A tooth that has lost part of its structure, usually because of physical trauma that has chipped or split off a piece of it. When a tooth is broken, a dentist should be seen as soon as possible. In the interim, warm water rinses will help to keep the mouth clean, and cold compresses applied to the outside of the cheek next to the injured tooth will help to reduce swelling in the area. Chewing on the tooth should be avoided. An aspirin substitute can help to reduce pain in the area. Repair of the tooth may require treatment by a dentist specializing in tooth replacement or by an oral surgeon. Small chips can often be smoothed down without the need for a restoration. Larger breaks may need a filling or crown. If the fracture goes below the gum line, then the tooth might be lost.

Bronchiectasis

A condition that refers to the dilation (widening) of portions of the airways, called the bronchi, that branch off the lower part of the windpipe. Bronchiectasis occurs as a result of damage to tissue of the bronchial wall. The tissue becomes chronically inflamed, thickened, and flaccid. Parts of the tissue are damaged or destroyed, the firm tone of the bronchial wall is diminished, and excess mucus is produced, which promotes the growth of bacteria in the area. Infected secretions from the bacterial infection may pool and further damage the tissue of the airway wall. Tiny, balloonlike sacs may develop and protrude into the lungs. The inflammation can spread to the lung tissue and result in BRONCHO-PNEUMONIA, and the obstruction of airways can result in dangerously low levels of oxygen in the blood.

SYMPTOMS AND CAUSES

The process that leads to bronchiectasis generally originates in early childhood but may develop later in life. Symptoms sometimes do not appear until after the condition is well established. In some instances, there are no symptoms. When symptoms appear, they tend to start gradually, most commonly following a respiratory tract infection. These symptoms tend to worsen over the years. A chronic cough with mucus may be the first and only symptom. Coughing up blood may also occur. Coughing spells commonly occur early in the morning and late in the day. Wheezing and shortness of breath (see BREATH, SHORTNESS OF) are symptoms of widespread bronchiectasis. Severe disease that causes heart strain may cause swelling in the feet and legs, an accumulation of fluid in the abdomen, and labored breathing in the prone position.

Causes of bronchiectasis also include respiratory infections, airway obstructions, inhalation of toxic substances, aspiration of stomach acid or food particles, certain genetic conditions such as CYSTIC FIBROSIS, and abnormalities in immune function.

DIAGNOSIS AND TREATMENT

Bronchiectasis is diagnosed on the basis of characteristic symptoms and indications of associated conditions such as chronic bronchitis, emphysema, and asthma. Chest X rays can identify the location of tissue damage and evaluate the extent of the condition. Because chest X rays do not always reveal the lung abnormalities that indicate bronchiectasis, CT (computed tomography) scans are generally required to confirm a diagnosis.

Once the diagnosis is confirmed, additional tests may help identify underlying conditions or obstructions. The tests may include blood tests, cultures of nasal and bronchial secretions, and sputum specimens. A specialized diagnostic tool that allows the doctor to observe the inside of the airways, a fiberoptic bronchoscope, can determine if there is a bronchial obstruction leading to bronchiectasis.

Underlying infections are generally treated with antibiotics, often prescribed for long-term use to prevent recurrent infections. Anti-inflammatory medications, including corticosteroids, may be prescribed, as may

medications that thin the pus and mucus to help drain the accumulated fluid. Oxygen therapy may be given if the blood oxygen concentration is low, and diuretics may be used to control swelling associated with heart failure. Bronchodilator medications often prove helpful in alleviating shortness of breath and wheezing. In rare cases, when the condition is resistant to treatment or when excessive amounts of blood are lost in coughing, surgical removal of affected tissue may be required. A surgical procedure to control bleeding may also be considered.

Bronchioles

Small airways in the lungs that branch off the bronchi (large tubes) within the lung. The bronchioles terminate in clusters of air sacs called alveoli, deep within LUNG tissue.

Bronchiolitis

Inflammation of the bronchioles, usually due to a viral lung infection. Bronchiolitis is most commonly caused by respiratory synctial virus (RSV). It generally occurs in children younger than 2 years who usually contract the infection during the winter and early spring. Older people, people with heart or lung disease, and people who have immune deficiency disorders may also be susceptible. The virus is contracted when infectious material comes in contact with mucous membranes of the eyes, mouth, or nose. It is spread by the respiratory secretions of infected persons, either by contact with airborne droplets from their coughs or sneezes or by contact with contaminated surfaces and objects. The virus can be destroyed by washing the hands with soap and water and by using disinfectants on contaminated surfaces.

SYMPTOMS, DIAGNOSIS, AND TREATMENT

Initial symptoms of bronchiolitis include excess nasal mucus and a low fever for 2 to 3 days. This is followed by coughing, labored breathing, and wheezing for the next 2 to 3 days. Symptoms last for about 7 to 15 days, and most children completely recover. Some young children may require hospitalization, particularly infants younger than 6 months.

The infection is diagnosed by tests to confirm the presence of viral antigens or an increased level of antibodies. A chest X ray may also be done to rule out pneumonia. The most common approach to treatment of mild infections in children is alleviating symptoms; acetaminophen is generally given to reduce fever, increased liquids are given to relieve dehydration, a mild cough syrup is given to decrease cough, a steam-filled bathroom from hot running water in a shower or tub may also quiet coughing, and a cool-mist vaporizer may be used in the bedroom during sleep to keep airways moist. When more severe disease is present, intravenous fluids, bronchodilators, oxygen therapy, and, in severe cases, mechanical ventilation may be required. Doctors may prescribe ribivarin, a nebulized form of antiviral therapy to treat RSV infection. No vaccine against the virus is currently available.

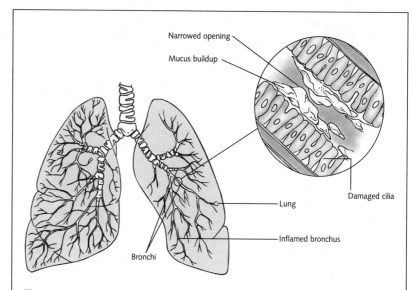

NARROWED, CLOGGED AIRWAYS
Bronchitis affects the mucous membranes lining the bronchi that branch into the lungs. The walls of the tubes become swollen and inflamed, and excess mucus clogs the passage. The cilia (tiny hairs) lining the tubes, which help pass mucus up and out of the lungs, may be damaged, allowing infection to spread.

Bronchitis

FOR SYMPTOM CHART
see Coughing, page 28

An illness caused by inflammation of the mucous lining of the airways, called bronchi. Bronchitis occurs when the bronchial tubes become irritated. The irritation may be caused by cigarette smoking or by bacterial or viral respiratory infections. The viral infections responsible for the common cold (see COLD, COMMON) are the most frequent cause of bronchitis, which occurs when the virus spreads to the airways. The walls of the airways respond to the irritation by secreting copious, thick mucus, which clogs the inflamed, swollen airways and obstructs the flow of air through them.

Air pollution and inhalation of industrial particles are also associated with bronchitis. Workers exposed to dust, such as coal miners, grain handlers, and metal workers, tend to have higher than normal rates of a form of the illness that may be referred to as industrial bronchitis.

SYMPTOMS
Bronchitis may be acute or chronic. In the acute form, bronchitis is a common infection that usually occurs at the same time as or following a chest cold and has as its primary symptom a productive cough. There may also be a sensation of tightness and generalized pain in the

area of the chest, chills, a low fever, feelings of malaise, and a wheezing sound during breathing. Acute bronchitis is caused by a virus in 90 percent of cases, and typically the condition is not helped by antibiotics. Acute bronchitis almost always clears up in less than a week without lasting effects, although a cough may persist for 4 to 6 weeks.

Chronic bronchitis is defined by a persistent cough that produces mucus and recurs on most days for 3 months of the year over a period of 2 successive years without another identifiable underlying disease. This disease is most common among those who smoke cigarettes, especially those older than 35. Being overweight is a risk factor for chronic bronchitis.

A cough that produces yellowish gray phlegm is the most common symptom of both forms of bronchitis. The illness generally follows a characteristic pattern of development in which the initial symptoms are similar to those of acute bronchitis. Those symptoms may resolve, but the distinguishing productive cough of bronchitis may last for several weeks afterward. In chronic bronchitis, as the disease progresses, the cough lasts throughout the year. There is often severe coughing that brings up

yellow or green phlegm upon awakening in the morning. The cough associated with chronic bronchitis is distinctive in that it sounds loud, deep, and wet. Bouts of coughing may last several minutes, and shortness of breath is often experienced at the same time as or directly following an episode of coughing. In the United States, chronic bronchitis is almost always associated with smoking.

DIAGNOSIS AND TREATMENT
The short-lived symptoms of acute bronchitis following a cold generally do not merit a doctor's attention unless chronic heart or lung problems are present, including asthma, emphysema, and congestive heart failure. When medical consultation is sought, the diagnosis is generally based on the discolored sputum that is produced by coughing. If the phlegm is yellow, gray, or green, an antibiotic may be prescribed. In some cases, one of the BRONCHODILATORS may be prescribed to open the narrowed airways. Otherwise, treatment is generally based on self-help strategies, including aspirin for fever (do not use aspirin for children), bed rest, and increased fluids. Over-the-counter cough medicine may be helpful if coughing interferes with sleep. Avoiding inhaled irritants, especially

B

cigarette smoking and secondhand smoke, is essential. The use of a vaporizer may be beneficial because warm, humid air helps ease the irritated airways.

Chronic bronchitis is diagnosed by the characteristic cough and its ongoing occurrence over several years. The diagnosis may be confirmed by a medical history, a physical examination, and an evaluation of lung function test results and chest X rays. If detected early and if the person who has chronic bronchitis does not smoke, he or she may expect a good survival rate. However, survival rates are low for people with severe forms of this illness that go untreated.

The first line of treatment is to stop smoking. Care must be taken to avoid respiratory infections that will exacerbate chronic bronchitis by limiting exposure to people who have colds or

other infections and by being vaccinated for pneumonococcal pneumonia. Annual flu shots are recommended for people who have chronic bronchitis. Aggravating factors to avoid include dust, cold air, inhalation of noxious fumes including paint fumes, automobile exhaust, and, in some cases, common household cooking odors and perfumes. Increased fluid intake can help thin the thick mucus so that it is coughed up more easily.

If the sputum of a person with chronic bronchitis abruptly changes in color, quantity, or density, a broad-spectrum antibiotic, such as tetracycline or ampicillin, may be prescribed for 7 to 10 days. If wheezing is present or reversible bronchial constriction is detected on lung function tests, a bronchodilator may be prescribed. Chronic bronchitis may

impede the body's ability to get oxygen from the lungs; if this occurs, oxygen therapy may become necessary either in a hospital setting or via oxygen delivery devices suitable for home or portable use.

Bronchodilators

Drugs that enlarge the airways to allow unrestricted passage of air. Bronchodilators are prescribed for people with asthma who have wheezing or breathing difficulties. Examples of oral bronchodilators include aminophylline and theophylline. All of these bronchodilators relieve coughing, wheezing, shortness of breath, and troubled breathing. They are available in liquid, tablet, and capsule forms for the treatment of acute attacks and in extended-release form for long-term treatment.

TAKING BRONCHODILATORS

Bronchodilators are the first line of medication for asthma. These drugs relax the muscular walls of the airways to help prevent muscle spasms that constrict the air passages (bronchospasms). The drugs act most quickly and efficiently if they are inhaled in aerosol form, using a device called an inhaler. A doctor can teach people with asthma, including small children, how to use an inhaler.

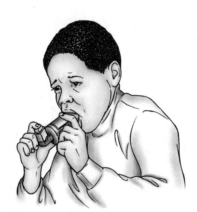

FORMING A SEAL
A person using an inhaler learns to form a tight seal around the device with his or her lips. Pressing a button delivers a dose of the drug into the canister of the inhaler.

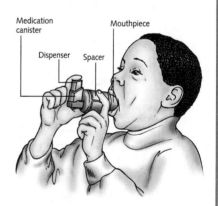

INHALING
With the head back, the user takes a slow, deep breath to fill the lungs and then holds the breath for as long as 10 seconds.

NARROWED AIRWAYS
In a person with asthma, the airways in the lungs are narrowed by inflamed and swollen membranes and accumulation of excess mucus. When a muscular spasm in the airway walls (a bronchospasm) constricts the diameter of the airway, the passage of air is further restricted or blocked.

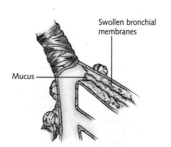

Swollen bronchial membranes

Mucus

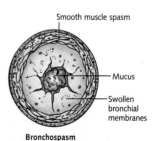

Smooth muscle spasm

Mucus

Swollen bronchial membranes

Bronchospasm

B

Bronchopneumonia

An infection of the tissues of the lungs that occurs principally in the smaller branches, called bronchioles, of the airways, or bronchial tubes. Bronchopneumonia, which is also called bronchial pneumonia, may be caused by bacteria such as pneumococci, staphylococci, and streptococci or by viruses such as the influenza virus. The disease may develop as a complication of a common cold (see COLD, COMMON) or influenza. Some forms of bronchopneumonia are contagious.

The disease occurs when infection produces pus and mucus, which clog and inflame the air sacs and bronchioles. The resulting symptoms may initially seem to be those of a serious cold, especially in younger people in good health. Symptoms can intensify rapidly in people with heart or lung ailments, in older people, and in people with weakened immune systems. Symptoms can include a cough that produces blood-streaked sputum, chest pain, fever, chills, and difficulty breathing. In severe cases when insufficient oxygen is delivered to the body, the skin may acquire a bluish tinge and mental confusion can occur. Death may occur within 24 hours to those who are particularly susceptible and have severe infection.

DIAGNOSIS AND TREATMENT

Bronchopneumonia may be initially suspected in those with a cough and fever when abnormal breath sounds are detected by listening to the chest with a stethoscope. Chest X rays are generally used to confirm the presence of an infection and determine its severity. Sputum and blood samples may be tested to identify the infectious agent. Analysis of blood oxygen levels is helpful to assess severity.

People who contract bronchopneumonia require medical attention and monitoring. Hospitalization is sometimes necessary. If bacteria are the cause of disease, antibiotic medications are prescribed. Fluoroquinolones are the first-line agents used to treat older people and those with severe symptoms. Macrolides (such as erythromycin, azithromycin, and clarithromycin) and doxycycline can be used to treat younger persons and those who are less severely ill. Oxygen therapy may be required.

Pneumococcal vaccination is considered effective against some of the organisms that cause pneumonia and is recommended for healthy people older than 65 and for people with chronic heart or lung disease, compromised immune systems, or alcoholism. The vaccine is also recommended for those who have had their spleens removed.

Bronchopulmonary dysplasia

A chronic lung disease in newborns marked by inflammation of the airways. Bronchopulmonary dysplasia is caused by use of intensive oxygen therapy and/or breathing assistance with a mechanical VENTILATOR (also called a respirator or life-support machine). Most commonly, it occurs in newborns being treated for RESPIRATORY DISTRESS SYNDROME, a life-threatening disorder caused by the lack of a necessary chemical (SURFACTANT) in the lung lining. Infants with respiratory distress syndrome usually require mechanical ventilation to provide enough oxygen for survival and to prevent tissue damage. A ventilator controls their rate of breathing and amount of oxygen intake. Bronchopulmonary dysplasia occurs when the infant's lungs and airways are damaged by protracted exposure to oxygen and the pressure of the ventilator. An affected infant may experience shrill wheezing and noisy, rapid, labored breathing. The skin may turn blue from lack of oxygen. The baby may experience lung infections, impeded growth, and problems with feeding.

DIAGNOSIS AND TREATMENT

Bronchopulmonary dysplasia is diagnosed when chest X rays reveal damage to the lungs. An infant with this condition continues to need oxygen therapy, often with a ventilator, in order to breathe (see OXYGEN, SUPPLEMENTAL). With good nutritional support, such as feeding the baby intravenously or with a tube that passes through the nose or mouth into the stomach, the baby's lungs will begin to heal. The oxygen levels and pressure can be slowly decreased as the baby recovers, usually over many months. When the infant no longer needs the ventilator, oxygen may be administered through a removable mask or a tube in the nose. Depending on the infant's condition, therapy may continue for weeks or months. Treatment may also include medications to open airways or prevent fluid buildup in the lungs. During this period, the baby may need to be fed through a tube inserted through the abdominal wall into the stomach or a nasogastric tube that is directed into the stomach from the nose or mouth. After recovery, a child may have an increased risk of asthma and respiratory infections.

Bronchoscopy

A technique that uses a rigid or flexible fiberoptic instrument for the visual examination of the airways, or bronchial tubes. Bronchoscopy involves the use of a narrow tube, called a bronchoscope, that can be passed deep into the multiple branches of the bronchial tubes. A fluoroscope, which is a guiding X ray,

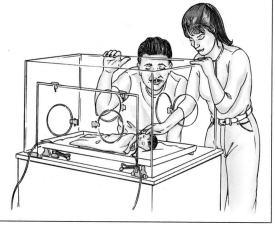

MECHANICAL VENTILATORS FOR INFANTS
An infant born with respiratory distress syndrome or other heart or lung disorders may require oxygen therapy and a mechanical ventilator to breathe. High concentrations of oxygen and the pressure of the ventilator may cause bronchopulmonary dysplasia, a serious lung disease. An infant with this disease will still need continued oxygen therapy and the ventilator, but the oxygen levels can be slowly decreased.

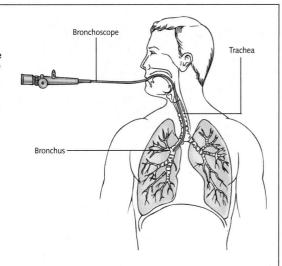

Bronchoscope

Trachea

Bronchus

enables a doctor to direct the instrument to the proper area of the lung. An inner channel of the instrument permits the insertion and movement of wire instruments and can be used to suction secretions or remove foreign bodies obstructing the airways. The procedure can be used to obtain samples of tissue from the bronchial tubes and air sacs of the lungs. Color video bronchoscopy is used when photographic records are needed, particularly of lesions in the bronchi, and to enhance visualization.

Bronchoscopy may be used diagnostically to detect disease or abnormalities and therapeutically to correct disorders. Flexible bronchoscopy may be performed without sedation or with minimal sedative medication as an outpatient procedure. Rigid bronchoscopy, which may be used when large airways are obstructed and is more commonly used in children, usually requires general anesthesia, but may be performed with local anesthesia and sedation. Premedication to decrease secretions and suppress coughing is generally given.

Bronchospasm

A narrowing and constriction of the muscles surrounding the airways, or bronchi, reducing the flow of air. Bronchospasm may be associated with ASTHMA, inflammation caused by infection, chronic BRONCHITIS, or exercise. Bronchospasm caused by exercise is called exercise-induced

bronchospasm and tends to occur within a few minutes of completing strenuous physical activity. The episode tends to peak within 5 to 10 minutes and may persist for an additional 20 to 30 minutes. Bronchospasm is generally treated with one of the BRONCHODILATORS, which relaxes smooth muscle and opens the airways to permit normal breathing.

Bronchus

A tube that is an airway from the trachea (windpipe) into each LUNG. The main bronchus branches in the lung into smaller passages called segmental bronchi, which in turn branch further into smaller tubes called bronchioles.

Brucellosis

A rare disease that primarily affects dogs and may affect farm animals. While humans are resistant to the illness, there have been cases of human infection, which have generally occurred as a result of direct contact with infected animals. Brucellosis is most commonly transmitted by contact of infectious secretions with cuts or abrasions in the skin, inhaling the organisms from the vaginal discharge or aborted material of female animals, or by ingestion of unpasteurized dairy products.

The disease develops within 2 to 4 weeks of exposure. The symptoms of brucellosis include fever, sweats, malaise, loss of appetite, and back

pain. Diagnosis is confirmed by culture of the organism from blood or tissue. A diagnosis can be made on the basis of high or rising specific antibodies. Antibiotic therapy is generally prescribed for 6 weeks.

Bruise

A collection of blood in unbroken tissue; also known as a contusion. Bruises are usually the result of an injury that causes blood vessels to break, causing bleeding into tissues beneath the skin. Most fade slowly within 10 to 14 days. As a bruise fades, the changing colors represent chemical changes in the hemoglobin of red blood cells as they are broken down and reabsorbed into the bloodstream. Bruises do not require a bandage. If bruises do not fade, if they appear for no reason, or if they are accompanied by persistent pain or headache, medical attention is needed.

Bruit

An abnormal sound heard when a stethoscope is placed over an artery. A bruit is a sign of partial obstruction of the artery by fatty deposits and can be a sign of increased risk for heart disease and stroke (see ATHEROSCLEROSIS). "Bruit" (pronounced "brwe" or "broot") is a French word meaning noise.

Bruxism, dental

The medical term for involuntary clenching or grinding of the teeth, especially at night during sleep. Over time, dental bruxism can cause sensitivity and may also force the jaw to move out of proper balance. Bruxism may be due to nervous tension, emotional stress, MALOCCLUSION (improper BITE), and possibly sleep disorders. Some antidepressants and antipsychotic drugs can actually cause bruxism.

SYMPTOMS AND TREATMENT

The symptoms of dental bruxism may not be apparent until the condition has persisted for some time. It is helpful to recognize the behavior before the teeth are seriously damaged. Early symptoms can be a tired jaw and headache first thing in the morning. Other symptoms may include a flattening of the biting surfaces of the teeth, indentations in the tongue, and transient tooth pain. In addition to pain in the jaw, tense facial muscles, and headaches, bruxism can cause facial pain associated with temporomandibular joint disorder (TMJ) or CLICKING JAW A clicking or popping sound in the jaw, caused by TMJ, may also be felt. If the teeth are worn down and the enamel begins to rub off, the DENTIN inside the tooth may become exposed and sensitive to hot, cold, and sweets.

A dentist can evaluate bruxism and may recommend a course of therapy to teach a person with bruxism how to relax the tongue, teeth, and lips. The dentist may suggest a plastic mouth appliance, called a night guard or MOUTH GUARD, which is made to be worn during sleep. The night guard absorbs the pressure of biting, and it can help to prevent future damage to the teeth, as well as to change the behavior. In some cases, a specialist in oral surgery may be consulted for treatment. If tension or stress is a factor, treatment by a psychologist may help. A mild sedative may be prescribed for treating bruxism. BIOFEEDBACK therapy may help people who clench and grind their teeth during waking hours; the therapy can teach them how to reduce muscle activity consciously.

Bubonic plague

An acute, infectious disease caused by a bacterial organism found in wild rodents and transmitted to humans by fleabites or the ingestion of flea feces. Bubonic plague, also called plague, can be transmitted from one infected person to another by the spread of infected droplets from coughing, which is produced when the infected person contracts PNEUMONIA. When this occurs, it is referred to as pneumonic plague. If the infection spreads from the lungs to other sites in the body, the blood becomes infected, and the disease is called septicemic plague.

SYMPTOMS

Initial symptoms of bubonic plague are headache, nausea, vomiting, aching joints, and general malaise. Lymph nodes of the groin, armpit, or neck become painful and swollen. Body temperature, pulse rate, and respiration rate are increased. Death can occur within 4 days. In nonfatal cases, the infection can improve within 2 weeks.

In pneumonic plague, there is blood in the person's saliva, which may flow freely and become bright red. Death may occur within 3 days of the first appearance of symptoms. A sudden, high fever and a deep purple coloration of the skin are the symptoms of septicemic plague, which can cause death within 24 hours.

DIAGNOSIS, TREATMENT, AND PREVENTION

Tests that may indicate a plague infection include culturing the lymph nodes, sputum, and blood. Immediate treatment with antibiotics such as streptomycin, chloramphenicol, or tetracycline is essential to prevent death. Oxygen, intravenous fluids, and respiratory support may be necessary. Infected persons must be isolated and may be given sedatives to control pain and delirium.

Bubonic plague can be prevented by maintaining good standards of sanitation, eliminating rats, and preventing the transport of rats that arrive in ships from ports where the disease is endemic. Famine reduces resistance to the disease and contributes to the spread of it. Plague is rare in developed countries.

Budd-Chiari syndrome

A rare disorder in which the veins that drain blood from the liver become blocked or narrowed. Budd-Chiari syndrome leads to a swollen liver, portal hypertension (increased blood pressure in the portal vein, which carries blood from the intestines to the liver), and liver failure. Blockage of the veins may be due to a blood clot, pressure from a tumor, or a congenital abnormality. If left untreated, this syndrome is often fatal.

Buerger disease

A severe form of inflammation and obstruction of the blood vessels in the extremities, usually the feet and less often the hands; also known as thromboangiitis obliterans. Normal blood flow is restricted or blocked, causing severe pain or a burning sensation, particularly in the arch of the foot, and eventually destroying the tissues. Pain worsens with exercise, and the hands or feet may look pale or blue and feel cold to the touch. The superficial blood vessels may

appear red and inflamed. Infection and gangrene often result, necessitating amputation.

Buerger disease occurs almost exclusively in men younger than 30 who smoke or chew tobacco. While the disease cannot be cured, it may be slowed or reversed by stopping all tobacco use and avoiding cold temperatures and other factors that reduce circulation to the extremities. Warmth and gentle exercise may be used to increase circulation. If pain is persistent and intolerable, surgery may be required to cut the nerves to the affected area.

Bulimia

A mental illness characterized by recurrent episodes of binge eating and extreme countermeasures to reduce the effect of the food, often by self-induced vomiting. Binges consist of eating abnormally large amounts, typically high-calorie sweets such as ice cream or cake, in a relatively short period. During the binge, the person feels out of control, as if he or she is incapable of stopping until all the food has been consumed. Following the binge, the person tries to eliminate the calories by self-induced vomiting, by purging (using diuretics or laxatives), or by excessive exercise or fasting.

To be classified as bulimia, binges and countermeasures have to occur an average of twice weekly over a period of 3 months. Unlike people with anorexia, most people with bulimia have body weights within or near the normal weight range, but they perceive themselves as fat and put extreme emphasis on body image. The disorder usually begins in late adolescence or early adulthood.

SYMPTOMS AND CONSEQUENCES

Most people with bulimia are aware that their eating is abnormal and are secretive about their behavior. The illness is often associated with symptoms of depression (such as low self-esteem and bouts of crying), heightened anxiety, and substance abuse, particularly of alcohol or stimulants. PERSONALITY DISORDERS also occur, but the person exhibits normal sexual activity. Typically, people with bulimia who purge show more psychological symptoms than those who do not purge. Purging behavior can produce a variety of physical symptoms, such as imbalances in metabolism, abnormal heart rhythm, significant and permanent loss of tooth enamel from acid in the vomit, an increase in dental cavities, swelling of the salivary glands (causing "chipmunk face"), irregular or absent menstruation, abdominal pain and bloating, scars or calluses on the back of the hand from forcing it down the throat, and dependence on laxatives. In a small number of cases, hospitalization is required. Death from bulimia is rare.

CAUSES AND TREATMENT

Bulimia occurs with the same frequency in the United States as in the other industrialized nations (Canada, Europe, South Africa, Japan, New Zealand, and Australia). People with bulimia are typically white, but the disorder appears in other ethnic groups as well. About nine in every ten people with bulimia are female. The exact cause of bulimia is unknown. Contributing factors may include cultural overemphasis on physical appearance, family problems, emotional conflicts, and depression.

Since the person with bulimia is aware that his or her eating behavior is abnormal, treatment focuses on breaking the pattern of binge eating. Treatment may include behavior therapy (in which the person monitors eating and is rewarded for normal behavior), family therapy (involving relevant members of the bulimic person's family), individual counseling, and group therapy. If the person has depression, antidepressant medications may be used. Another medication (naltrexone hydrochloride), which affects the pleasure centers of the brain and is used to treat alcoholism, is also used with some success to treat bulimia. Lithium, another drug, and electroconvulsive therapy are also used. See also EATING DISORDERS.

Bulla

See BLISTER.

Bumetanide

A diuretic used to treat edema (excess fluid) associated with congestive heart failure, kidney and liver disease, cancer, and premenstrual syndrome. Bumetanide (Bumex) works in the kidneys by promoting the excretion of sodium, water, magnesium, chloride, and potassium.

BUN

Blood urea nitrogen. See KIDNEY FUNCTION TESTS.

Bundle branch block

A delay or obstruction in the passage of electrical impulses through the ventricles (lower chambers) of the heart. In the healthy heart, the electrical signal that begins the heartbeat starts in the sinus node, located in the upper region of the heart, then travels to the atrioventricular node and through the bundle of His. There the signal branches, following the right bundle branch to the right ventricle and the left bundle branch to the left ventricle and coordinating the heartbeat in the lower chambers with that in the upper chambers (atria). In bundle branch block, damage to a bundle delays the signal in its passage to either the right or left ventricle. The delayed signal makes a detour around the damaged area, so that the affected ventricle still beats but slightly slower than its counterpart. Bundle branch block may have the effect of slowing the heartbeat (see BRADYCARDIA).

Bundle branch block is a common abnormality. It is often present at birth or develops later in life for no known reason. In some people, bundle branch block is caused by aging, hypertension (high blood pressure), past heart attack, viral infection, disease of the heart valves, heart failure, or chronic obstructive pulmonary disease.

In many cases, bundle branch block produces no symptoms and does not require treatment. The condition is usually detected with an electrocardiogram (ECG), which measures the electrical activity of the heart. If the blockage is severe and the heartbeat very slow, the individual may experience periods of fainting or near-fainting. Surgical implantation of a PACEMAKER, a device that speeds up the heartbeat if it falls below a certain rate and thereby overrides the faulty electrical impulse, usually remedies the problem. In addition, any underlying disease needs to be treated. Persons with bundle branch block that produces no symptoms should be examined regularly by a doctor to check for any unexpected changes in heart function.

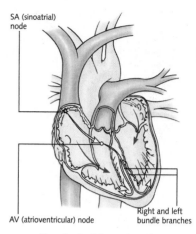

SA (sinoatrial) node

AV (atrioventricular) node

Right and left bundle branches

Normal path of electrical impulse

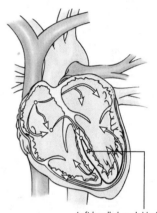

Left bundle branch block

Bundle branch block

KEY
⇨ Electrical signal   ➡ Blood flow

BLOCKED ELECTRICAL IMPULSES
In a healthy heart, a heartbeat begins with an electrical impulse that is transmitted from the atria via a nerve bundle, which then branches off to the left and right ventricles. If coronary artery disease or another disorder blocks the impulse in one branch, the impulse must take a longer, slower route, and one ventricle contracts a fraction of a second later than the other.

Bunion

A painful, inflamed, bony protrusion at the base of the big toe. A bunion is caused by an abnormal enlargement of the joint of the big toe, which is forced inward against the other toes and may overlap the toe next to it. This irregularity in the position of the big toe, called hallux valgus, is what pushes the bony base of the big toe outward to form the protrusion known as a bunion. The cause tends to be hereditary and is more common in females, but may also be related to flat feet and the wearing of narrow shoes with high heels and a constricted toe box. Symptoms may include swelling, soreness, and redness near the toe joint, an inflamed bursa and calluses at the affected area, and persistent or intermittent pain. Self-help treatment for bunions emphasizes wearing extra-wide, soft leather, flat-heeled shoes to relieve pressure on the inflamed bump by the big toe. A bunion splint may be applied. In severe cases, an orthopedic surgeon or podiatrist can correct the condition with a surgical procedure.

Buphthalmos

An abnormal enlargement of the eye. The outer layers of the eye are over-sized and distended. Buphthalmos, which comes from two Greek roots meaning "ox eye," is also known as infantile glaucoma or megophthalmos (Greek, meaning "big eye").

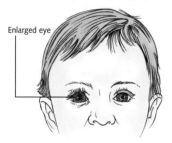

Enlarged eye

INFANTILE GLAUCOMA
Buphthalmos is a rare, inherited condition in which the eye's drainage system does not develop properly. Pressure builds up in the eye and damages the optic nerve, causing enlargement of the eye, cloudy vision, and sensitivity to light. Medication and surgery can usually correct the problems.

Buprenorphine

A narcotic painkiller used before and during surgery, dental surgery, and labor and delivery. Buprenorphine (Buprenex and others) acts in the central nervous system to relieve moderate to severe pain, but it can cause breathing problems. This drug can cause an impaired ability to drive.

Bupropion

An antidepressant; also used to help people stop smoking. Bupropion (Wellbutrin for depression; Zyban for smoking cessation) seems to work by blocking the uptake of the neuro-transmitter dopamine. Bupropion is generally prescribed only when other antidepressants have failed because it may cause seizures in some people.

Burkitt lymphoma

A malignancy of the lymph glands, often in the jaw or the abdomen. In Burkitt lymphoma, tumors grow rapidly within the jaw, displacing nearby teeth, or within the abdomen, where massive tumors can appear. Burkitt lymphoma is a fast-growing cancer that can eventually invade the central nervous system and the bone marrow.

Burkitt lymphoma was first discovered in Africa, where it is very common. It chiefly affects children in areas of tropical Africa and New Guinea and is currently thought to be associated with the Epstein-Barr virus. Burkitt lymphoma is rare in the United States, except as an AIDS-related cancer.

Burning tongue, idiopathic

A condition characterized by a severe, recurrent burning or aching sensation in the back of the mouth, the throat, and the ear. There may be brief episodes of very severe pain in the tongue or elsewhere in the mouth, lasting several seconds or minutes. Talking or swallowing can trigger these episodes, but the cause of this condition is unknown. Burning tongue is a form of neuralgia (pain caused by nerve irritation or damage). Over-the-counter pain relievers may sometimes alleviate discomfort. Under medical supervision, prescription drugs are often helpful. Duration of treatment varies widely because symptoms of the condition may diminish or disappear.

Burns, chemical

Injury to the skin caused by corrosive chemicals. Chemical burns are reactions that occur when a person's skin comes in contact with acids, alkalis, or other corrosive agents, in which chemical energy is converted into heat. Chemicals will usually continue to burn the skin as long as they are in contact. The stronger the chemical and the longer the contact, the worse the burn. Examples of chemicals that can burn the skin include cleaning agents, garden chemicals, and paint removers. Many can be found in the workplace or the home.

Chemical burns should always prompt a person to seek emergency medical care, because the depth of injury may be difficult to assess. First aid measures that may be started include brushing off any powdered chemicals and flushing the area with large amounts of cool, running water. Jewelry and clothes that might hold chemicals next to the skin should be removed. For burns affecting a person's eye, it is important when flushing that eye with cool water to make sure that the water does not run into the unaffected eye. If possible, the person should cover the burn with a cool, wet cloth. Ointments are not recommended.

Burns, electrical

FOR FIRST AID
see Burns, electrical, page 1316

Injury caused by contact with electricity. Sources of electricity that can cause burns when an unprotected portion of a person's body comes in contact with them include power lines, lightning, defective household electrical equipment, and unprotected electrical outlets. As electrical current goes into the body, it is converted to heat that can cause extensive damage to blood vessels, nerves, bone, and muscle. The severity of an electrical burn depends on how long the body is in contact with the source of electricity, the type and strength of the electrical current involved, and the direction the electricity takes through the body.

TYPES OF BURNS
Three types of burns are associated with electricity.

■ ***Contact burn injuries*** This is a true electrical injury in which the current passes through the body and leaves two burns—one where the electrical current entered the body and the other where it exited. Even if the entrance and exit wounds look minor, the tissues underneath may be severely damaged.

■ ***Electrical flash burn*** This type of burn is an electrothermal (heat generated by electricity) injury caused by the arcing of the current.

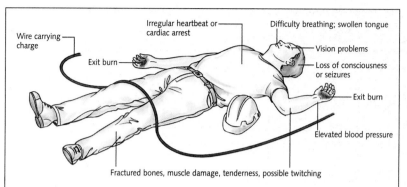

INJURIES FROM ELECTRIC SHOCK
In a person who has received a large electric shock, the burns are not the major problem. Respiratory and cardiac arrest are immediate possibilities. The first priority is to ensure that the person has an open airway and to provide cardiac life support. Care for injuries, burns, and medical shock is also necessary.

■ *Flame burn* This type of burn occurs when electricity ignites clothing or surrounding material.

Any person with an electrical burn should receive emergency medical care. It is never wise to approach a person injured by electricity unless the power source has been turned off.

Burns, heat

Injury caused by exposure to dry heat sufficient to damage the skin. Heat burns, also called thermal burns, can have many causes, including contact with an open flame, hot objects, explosions, and the sun. Heat burns are classified according to degree of severity. About 2 million people in the United States receive burns each year; 300,000 of them are serious injuries. Burns are the third largest

cause of accidental death in the United States.

The goals of first aid for burns are to remove the person from smoke or fumes, to reduce the effect of heat on the skin, to relieve pain, to prevent fluid loss, to prevent infection, and to summon emergency medical help when necessary. Correct first aid can be important in hastening recovery. In the case of small burns, cool water will lessen pain and stop tissue damage. The person should remove any constricting jewelry and cover the burn area with a dry, sterile bandage or clean cloth. For burns covering a large surface area, the person may be in shock and should lie flat, if injuries permit, with feet elevated, until medical help arrives. See also Classifying burn injuries, next page.

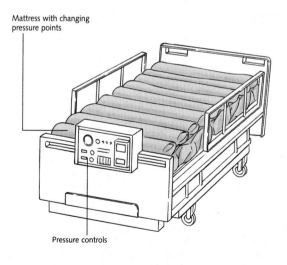

SPECIAL BURN BED
This special mattress overlay changes pressure points over the body every 5 minutes and circulates air in a wavelike motion throughout the mattress. The features help prevent pressure ulcers and help stimulate the person's circulation.

Mattress with changing pressure points

Pressure controls

Burns, scald
See SCALDS.

Burping
See BELCHING.

Burr hole

A small, circular opening made in the skull to remove blood clots in or on the brain, which usually form after an injury or accident. The special drill with a rounded tip used to make the hole is called a burr. During an emergency, a burr hole may be made in the skull of a person with a severe head injury to relieve pressure on the brain. Burr holes can also be made to permit a biopsy of the brain, to drain an abscess or cyst, or to inject gas or medication.

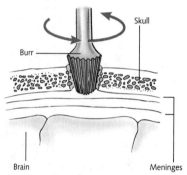

Skull

Burr

Brain

Meninges

RELIEVING PRESSURE ON THE BRAIN
A small precision drill called a burr is used to drill through the skull to remove blood clots on the brain. The hole (burr hole) that is created penetrates the bone, and the protective membranes that cover the brain (meninges) are drawn up through the hole and snipped to make an opening. Through this opening, a surgeon can pass instruments into the brain itself to vacuum out blood, pus, and dead brain tissue.

Bursa

A fluid-filled, enclosed sac of connective tissue designed to reduce friction between moving body parts. Bursae are located between the skin and bone and between tendons and bones, muscles and bones, and ligaments and bones to cushion the movements of one body part over the other.

Bursitis

An inflammation of a bursa, the fluid-filled sac that serves to reduce friction against moving bones. Bursitis most commonly affects bursae of the shoulder, the elbow, the hip, and

B

CLASSIFYING BURN INJURIES

When the skin is exposed to a temperature of 120°F or higher for even a short time, skin cells are damaged. Burns are classified by depth and extent.

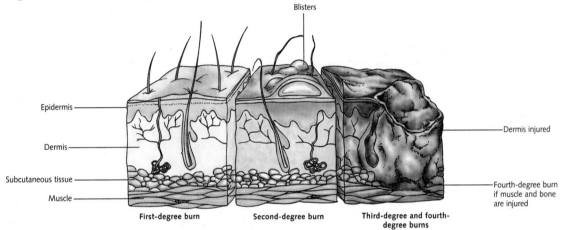

Blisters

Epidermis

Dermis

Subcutaneous tissue

Muscle

Dermis injured

Fourth-degree burn if muscle and bone are injured

First-degree burn

Second-degree burn

Third-degree and fourth-degree burns

DEPTH OF BURNS
In a first-degree burn, damage is limited to the outer skin layer, including redness, warmth, occasional blisters, and tenderness. In a second-degree burn, damage goes through the outer layer and into deeper layers of skin, causing blisters. In a third-degree burn, the skin is totally destroyed, exposing seared, charred tissue. In a fourth-degree burn, the muscle and bone are also injured.

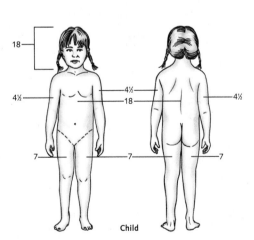

Child

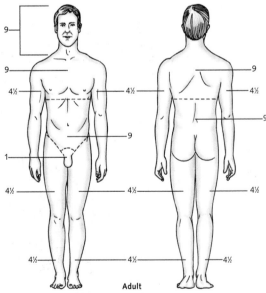

Adult

RULES OF NINES
The "rule of nines" is used to calculate the extent of body surface burned by dividing the total surface into sections of about 9 percent, or fractions or multiples of 9 percent. The percentages for children and adults differ slightly because of the differences in body proportions.

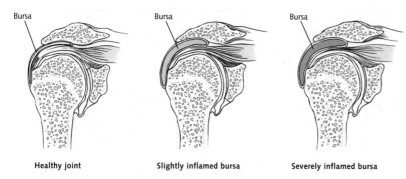

Bursa   Bursa   Bursa

Healthy joint   Slightly inflamed bursa   Severely inflamed bursa

SWOLLEN BURSA
In a healthy shoulder joint, the fluid-filled bursa cushions the tendons, muscles, and bones and lubricates the motion of the joint. When the bursa becomes inflamed and swollen, it puts pressure on the surrounding tissues, causing pain and limiting movement.

areas directly above and below the knee. Repeated movement can cause persistent friction between a bursa and the muscles and bones surrounding it. The ongoing friction causes irritation and swelling. This friction, or less commonly minor trauma or infection, results in inflammation of the bursa, which becomes enlarged and puts pressure on nearby tissues. Movement increases the pressure, causing more pain. Joint movement near the inflammation is limited by the pain. The entire area affected by bursitis eventually becomes painful. The pain may radiate to nearby muscles and tendons. The site may also feel hot to the touch and become red and swollen. When bursitis persists, the bursa can become calcified, and deposits may form, limiting movement of the tendons.

DIAGNOSIS AND TREATMENT
Bursitis is diagnosed by physical examination and the use of imaging, which can reveal the enlarged bursa and possible calcified deposits. The condition can be managed by avoiding activities, such as kneeling, ball-throwing, and repeated raising of the arms above the head, that put pressure on or irritate the bursa.

Self-help techniques include applications of ice to treat pain and swelling, wrapping to control swelling and provide support, and range-of-motion exercises to aid in regaining motion. Medical treatments may include acetaminophen for pain and anti-inflammatory drugs, such as aspirin and ibuprofen, to ease discomfort from inflammation. Corticosteroids may be injected into the bursal area, and if infection is present, antibiotics may be prescribed. The fluid inside the bursal sac can be drawn out with a fine needle (aspirated) to help relieve the swelling. In severe cases, arthroscopic surgery may be recommended.

Buspirone

A tranquilizer; an antianxiety drug. Buspirone (Buspar) is used to treat chronic anxiety and has been used to treat anxiety with depression and premenstrual syndrome. Unlike other antianxiety drugs, such as the benzodiazepines, buspirone seems less likely to be habit-forming or to cause drowsiness.

Butalbital compound

A barbiturate. Butalbital is one ingredient among several in a number of combination drugs containing a barbiturate, an analgesic (painkiller), and sometimes a narcotic and caffeine. One example is Fiorinal with codeine, which contains butalbital, aspirin, caffeine, and codeine; another example is Fioricet, which contains butalbital, acetaminophen, and caffeine. Both combinations are prescribed for migraine and tension headaches. Butalbital can cause an impaired ability to drive.

Bypass surgery

A procedure to detour around obstructions in the arteries providing blood to the heart. Bypass surgery, known technically as coronary artery bypass grafting (CABG), is used to treat ATHEROSCLEROSIS, a disease in which deposits of fat and other mate-

rials clog the arteries, causing angina (chest pain) and often leading to heart attack. Bypass surgery is the treatment of choice when a simpler approach to treating atherosclerosis, such as medication or BALLOON ANGIOPLASTY, is insufficient. Bypass surgery is often recommended for people with debilitating angina, blockage of the left main coronary artery, impaired function of the left ventricle (the heart's main pump), or multiple blockages.

THE OPERATION
Bypass surgery is a major procedure performed under general anesthesia that takes 3 to 6 hours to complete, depending on the complexity of the case. The chest is opened by cutting through the skin and splitting the breastbone to expose the heart. The person is then connected to a heart-lung machine, a device that circulates and oxygenates the blood and performs the work of the heart and lungs. The heart itself is stopped to make it easier for the surgeon to work. Studies of off-pump surgery have been promising, in which the heart is not stopped; however, long term effects of off-pump surgery are not known.

Two methods of creating the bypass are commonly used. In one, a section is taken from the saphenous vein in the leg. One end of the vein graft is stitched into the aorta (the artery that carries oxygenated blood from the heart to the body), and the other end is stitched into the blocked coronary artery downstream from the blockage. If there is more than one blockage, additional sections of saphenous vein are stitched around them in the same way. The second method uses one or both of two arteries known as the internal mammary arteries, which arise from the subclavian arteries and lead to the inside of the chest well. The surgeon frees the lower end of the internal mammary artery from the chest wall and stitches it to a blocked coronary artery below the blockage, rerouting its blood supply. Because artery grafts tend to stay open longer than vein grafts following surgery, many heart surgeons prefer to use them in bypass surgery; radial artery grafts from the forearm are now being used more frequently for this procedure.

REPAIRING HEART BLOCKAGE

Although alternatives to surgery exist for those with coronary artery disease, bypass surgery is preferable for certain people: those with more than 50 percent blockage in the left main artery, those with a long section of diseased artery, and those with three or more blocked arteries. Bypass surgery is also considered to be the preferred treatment for people who have both coronary artery disease and diabetes mellitus.

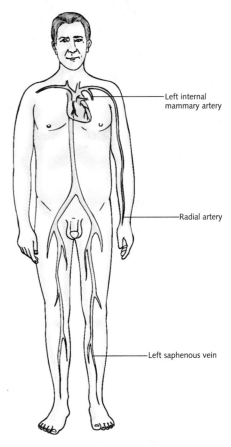

- Left internal mammary artery
- Radial artery
- Left saphenous vein

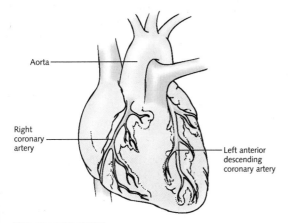

Aorta

Right coronary artery

Left anterior descending coronary artery

THE HEALTHY HEART
No blockage obstructs the arteries, and blood flow throughout the heart is normal.

BYPASS GRAFTS
Arterial bypass grafts are commonly taken from a site in the chest, arm, or leg.

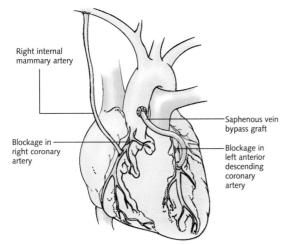

Right internal mammary artery

Saphenous vein bypass graft

Blockage in right coronary artery

Blockage in left anterior descending coronary artery

BLOCKAGES CORRECTED
Transplanted arteries channel blood around sites of arterial blockage.

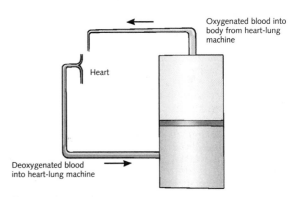

Oxygenated blood into body from heart-lung machine

Heart

Deoxygenated blood into heart-lung machine

HEART-LUNG MACHINE
During the procedure, blood is diverted from the vena cavae (veins bringing blood into the heart) to a heart-lung machine, which oxygenates the blood and returns it to the body via the aorta.

After the bypasses are completed, the heart is restarted with an electric shock. Once the heart is beating normally, the heart-lung machine is disconnected, and the incision is closed.

MINIMALLY INVASIVE BYPASS SURGERY

In recent years a procedure known as minimally invasive direct coronary artery bypass surgery has been developed as an alternative to the standard bypass operation. Instead of making a large incision through the breastbone, the surgeon creates a small opening between the ribs and creates the bypass with an internal mammary artery. No heart-lung machine is used, although the heart is slowed during surgery. Minimally invasive direct coronary artery bypass surgery causes less trauma and postoperative pain and requires less medication than standard bypass surgery; however, it seems to carry a greater risk of heart attack or stroke. In addition, it cannot be used for people with multiple blockages or, in most cases, with blockages on the right side of the heart.

RECOVERY AND RESULTS

Following surgery, the person spends 24 to 48 hours in a special cardiac care unit, where heart functions are carefully monitored. In most cases, a person who has undergone bypass surgery uses a ventilator for breathing during this period. Once the ventilator is removed and breathing occurs normally, another 4 to 7 days in the hospital is usually required. Full recovery at home can take up to several months, but those with nonphysical jobs can usually return to work in 4 to 6 weeks. Physical activities, such as driving or lifting heavy objects, are restricted until the incision is fully healed.

Since bypass surgery increases blood flow to the heart, results are often pronounced and immediate. The pain, pressure, and breathlessness of angina disappear almost immediately.

Fewer than 1 percent of those undergoing bypass surgery die of heart attack or stroke during or shortly after the procedure. The risk is highest for older people, people with diabetes mellitus, those with other major health problems, and people undergoing a second bypass procedure. Other complications, such as high blood pressure or irregular heart rhythm, can result but are often temporary or can be controlled with medication. In some cases, the bypass grafts clog over time, and the surgery has to be repeated. See also ANGIOGRAM; CARDIAC STRESS TESTING; CHEST PAIN; CORONARY ARTERY DISEASE; and ECG (electrocardiogram).

Byssinosis

A narrowing of the airways, or bronchi, produced by the inhalation of cotton, flax, or hemp particles. Byssinosis occurs almost exclusively among people who work with these materials. Susceptible workers exposed to bales of raw cotton and the initial stages of cotton production are most affected. Symptoms include tightness of the chest and wheezing, occurring most commonly on the first day of the workweek when renewed exposure to the material follows a period away from it. Cotton workers often experience diminished symptoms with ongoing exposure throughout the workweek, but when there has been continuous exposure over many years, chest tightness may persist for as long as a person is exposed to cotton dust.

Byssinosis is diagnosed with the use of lung function tests that reveal decreased lung capacity. The reduced lung capacity is usually most pronounced on the first day of the workweek. Treatment is based on controlling dust from certain materials in the workplace. Episodes may be treated with asthma medications—BRONCHODILATORS, such as ALBUTEROL SULFATE, delivered by inhalation devices, or orally in tablet form, such as THEOPHYLLINE.

C-reactive protein

A protein produced in the liver and released into the bloodstream when INFLAMMATION is present in the body. Levels of C-reactive protein (CRP) can be detected by a blood test. An increased level of CRP may indicate an increased risk of heart disease and stroke in some people. Inflammation is part of the disease process in ATHEROSCLEROSIS and other diseases. As an artery becomes inflamed with plaque, the level of CRP increases in the blood. In a person with elevated levels of CRP who has other risk factors for heart disease, a doctor will recommend the same treatments that help prevent heart disease to also help reduce the level of CRP. See also HEART DISEASE, ISCHEMIC.

CA-125 test

A blood test used in the diagnosis of cancer of the ovary (see OVARY, CANCER OF). Elevated levels of the protein CA-125 are suggestive of ovarian cancer, although not definitive, and doctors must use other tests and procedures to diagnose the disease. The test is also used to follow the progress of ovarian cancer while it is being treated or has gone into remission.

A blood test is used to measure a woman's CA-125 level, which is expressed numerically. Most women (99 percent) have a CA-125 level that is below 35. The higher the level above 35, the more likely the result is indicative of ovarian cancer.

CA-125 has been found at elevated levels in women with several noncancerous conditions such as fibroid tumors, liver disease, endometriosis, and pelvic infections. Also, some types of ovarian cancer do not produce elevated levels of CA-125. However, CA-125 levels can be elevated in the presence of other cancers, including those of the liver, lung, cervix, breast, stomach, and colon. Because benign conditions commonly diagnosed in younger women, including pregnancy, are sometimes associated with an elevated CA-125 level, the test is considered to be of limited value for women before menopause.

Cachexia

General ill health marked by extreme weight loss and a wasted appearance. Cachexia is associated with chronic infections and malignant conditions, such as cancer and AIDS. Drugs such as megestrol acetate and somatropin are often used to stimulate appetite.

Cadaver

Dead human body; corpse. Cadavers are used by physicians and other scientists to study anatomy and disease. Autopsies performed on cadavers allow doctors to identify disease sites, to help determine causes of death, and to provide tissue to repair defects in living human bodies. All medical students dissect cadavers as part of their medical education.

Cadmium poisoning

Poisoning that is caused by the inhalation or ingestion of cadmium. Cadmium may be accidentally inhaled in fumes from melting, welding, or other industrial processes that involve soldering. Ingestion or breathing in of the cadmium used in photography or engraving causes serious symptoms, such as vomiting, difficulty breathing, and headache. Kidney disease and liver damage are also possible. Treatment of acute cadmium poisoning includes decontamination, CHELATION THERAPY, and intravenous fluids.

Café au lait spots

Benign (not cancerous), light-colored to brown spots found on the skin; the color is produced by melanin. (The name is French for coffee with milk.) Café au lait spots are flat and uniform in color and may be half an inch to several inches in diameter. Spots are present at birth or develop in childhood. In some cases, café au lait spots are a sign of the inherited disorder NEUROFIBROMATOSIS. Although most people with these spots have no disease, any new or changing lesion should be examined by a doctor.

Calciferol

Vitamin D2. A fat-soluble, crystalline unsaturated alcohol. Calciferol occurs naturally as cholecalciferol in milk and fish liver oils and as ergocalciferol in plant foods such as spinach, broccoli, soybeans, and other dried beans. Calciferol helps the body use calcium and is used in the treatment of osteomalacia, osteoporosis, rickets, and hypocalcemic disorders. See also VITAMIN D.

Calcification

The buildup of calcium salts that occurs normally in bone development. Calcification may also refer to the accumulation of calcium salts that cause calcium deposits in a person with persistent BURSITIS, a painful inflammation affecting the shoulder, elbow, hip, or knee area. A calcium deposit may be detected by X rays. If the calcification is enlarged, the deposit may be removed by arthroscopic surgery.

Calcification, dental

A natural stage in which calcium crystals build up on the outer layer of the developing teeth. This layer calcifies into hardened tissue that covers the crowns, or top of the tooth, forming a hard covering called enamel. Dental calcification is a normal stage of development in the tooth bud, which begins in the human embryo. Any interruption to this process can cause enamel defects.

Calcinosis

Calcification of the skin and other soft tissues, which particularly affects the skin of the hands. Calcinosis is characterized by swollen hands, pinpicks of red coloration on the skin of the hands, thickened nails, and sores on the fingers. Calcinosis is one of five elements in a form of scleroderma called CREST SYNDROME. The "C" in the acronym CREST stands for calcinosis.

Calcitonin

A peptide hormone drug prescribed for osteoporosis and Paget disease of the bone. Calcitonin (Calcimar, Miacalcin, Osteocalcin, Salmonine) is a synthetic hormone that is virtually identical to the normal calcitonin found in humans, a hormone secreted by the thyroid gland. The drug slows down the process by which bone is naturally broken down. The calcitonin used in this drug is more potent than human calcitonin and is based on the calcitonin found in salmon.

Calcitonin maintains bone density to reduce the risk of vertebrae fractures associated with back pain, which is characteristic of osteoporosis in postmenopausal women. Calcitonin is available as an injection and as a nasal spray.

Calcium

An element found in food that is essential for neurotransmission, muscle contraction, bone formation, and proper heart function. Imbalances of calcium can lead to many health problems, and an excess of calcium in nerve cells can cause their death. Calcium supplements are available for people who are unable to ensure an adequate intake through diet, particularly during periods of bone growth in childhood and adolescence, as well as during pregnancy and breast-feeding. The bones serve the body as a storage site for calcium, continuously giving it up to the bloodstream and replacing it from food as the needs in the body change from day to day. When there is not enough calcium in the blood, calcium is taken from the bones.

A diet low in calcium throughout the younger adult years may add to the risk of developing OSTEOPOROSIS, a disease characterized by deteriorating bone, which is why many doctors recommend that menstruating women receive 1,200 milligrams of calcium per day.

Postmenopausal women may need calcium supplements to prevent osteoporosis. Most women get about 500 milligrams of calcium through their daily diets, but after menopause, their doctors may recommend calcium supplements to increase the daily total. Men and women ages 31 through 50 are urged to get 1,000 milligrams of calcium per day; men and women 51 through 70 years old should receive 1,200 milligrams a day.

Calcium channel blockers

A class of drugs used to treat hypertension (high blood pressure), chronic angina pectoris (chest pain), and cardiac arrhythmias and to prevent migraine headaches. Calcium channel blockers lower blood pressure by decreasing contractions of the heart and widening blood vessels. Calcium channel blockers work by preventing or slowing the influx of calcium ions into the smooth muscle cells of the heart and the blood vessels, relaxing arteries, and increasing the supply of blood and oxygen to the heart.

Calcium channel blockers are available by prescription, including some sustained-release preparations. Examples of calcium channel blockers include amlodipine (Norvasc), diltiazem (Cardizem, Dilacor), felodipine (Plendil), isradipine (DynaCirc), lercanidipine (Zanidip), nicardipine (Cardene), nifedipine (Adalat, Procardia), nisoldipine (Sular), and verapamil (Calan, Isoptin, Verelan).

Calculus, dental

A mineralized, porous deposit that hardens and adheres to the crowns and roots of the teeth. Dental calculus, also called TARTAR, is caused by the accumulation of plaque (see PLAQUE, DENTAL). Once calculus has formed, it traps more plaque. The bacteria in the plaque produce toxins that irritate the gums and can cause the destruction of fibers that anchor the teeth to the gums. When this occurs, gingival pockets (see POCKET, GINGIVAL) are formed between the tooth and gum, which leads to PERIODONTAL DISEASE. The pockets may extend deeper and eventually involve the bone that holds the tooth in place, which can lead to tooth loss.

Bacterial plaque is constantly forming on the teeth and must be removed by regular daily brushing and flossing to prevent the formation of calculus and gum disease. A dentist can remove calculus by using probelike instruments or ultrasonic units to scale the surfaces of the teeth. The surfaces are then smoothed and polished to prevent further deposits of calculus. If the calculus is present deep in the gum pockets, then a procedure called a root planing or deep scaling is performed. A dentist may use local anesthesia to perform more rigorous scaling to remove both the

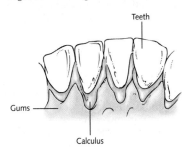

Teeth

Gums

Calculus

A MINERAL BUILDUP ON THE TEETH
Dental calculus is a yellowish or black mineral deposit that forms around the teeth and tooth roots when calcium and other minerals in saliva combine with existing plaque. Calculus traps more plaque, and the resulting buildup can only be removed by a dentist. Left untreated, calculus can cause gum disease and tooth loss.

calculus and any dead tissue in the periodontal pockets.

Calculus, urinary tract

A stone that forms in the organs that produce and transport urine, including the kidneys, ureters (tubes connecting the kidneys and bladder), and the bladder. These stones form from crystalline materials normally present in the urine. They begin most often in the kidney and are commonly known as kidney stones; the rarer bladder calculi are called bladder stones and are found almost exclusively in men. Calculi can partially or completely block the passage of urine from the kidney affected, causing serious symptoms and side effects. (See URINARY TRACT, MALE; URINARY TRACT, FEMALE.)

SYMPTOMS

Urinary tract calculi usually cause no symptoms until the stones obstruct and irritate the urinary tract. The first symptoms are often severe pain, inflammation, and swelling. The pain usually begins suddenly, ranges from dull to sharp, and can be severe enough to wake the person from sleep. Location of the pain depends on the position of the calculus. Discomfort can appear in the side, the back, or the groin, pelvis, and genitals.

Blood in the urine is also common. In some cases, the blood is seen in the toilet; in others, it can be detected only with a laboratory test. There may also be an urgent need to urinate, with a burning sensation upon urination. Nausea and vomiting often accompany calculi in the kidney and upper ureter. Infection with fever and chills may also be present; the combination of urinary tract calculi with fever is a medical emergency.

DIAGNOSIS AND TREATMENT

Since the pain caused by urinary tract calculi can mimic that of other diseases, the presence of calculi must be established by direct physical examination, analysis and testing of the urine, or X rays.

Most small stones pass out of the urinary tract without medical intervention, usually within 6 weeks after symptoms begin. Patients are advised to drink large amounts of water to increase the amount of urine and to help flush the calculi out. Medications are sometimes used to dissolve the calculus or make it small enough

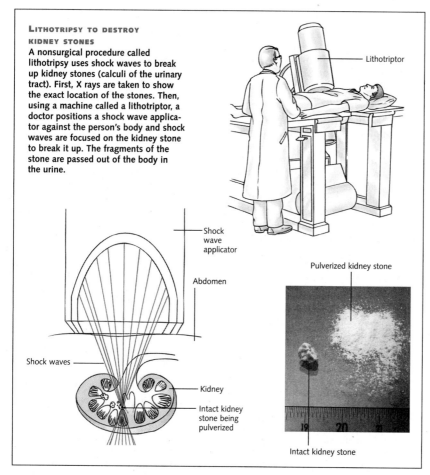

LITHOTRIPSY TO DESTROY KIDNEY STONES
A nonsurgical procedure called lithotripsy uses shock waves to break up kidney stones (calculi of the urinary tract). First, X rays are taken to show the exact location of the stones. Then, using a machine called a lithotriptor, a doctor positions a shock wave applicator against the person's body and shock waves are focused on the kidney stone to break it up. The fragments of the stone are passed out of the body in the urine.

Lithotriptor

Shock wave applicator

Abdomen

Shock waves

Kidney

Intact kidney stone being pulverized

Pulverized kidney stone

Intact kidney stone

to pass out. Some calculi can be removed with shock waves that break the stone into smaller pieces, which are easier to pass, in a procedure known as LITHOTRIPSY. High-frequency sound waves are focused on the calculus from outside the body until the calculus crumbles, usually in about 45 minutes.

If these approaches do not succeed, or if the calculus completely blocks the flow of urine, the obstruction must be removed and any accumulated urine must be drained. Calculi in the bladder and the lower ureters may be removed by running a flexible viewing tube into the urinary tract to remove the calculus or to break it up with shock waves or an electrical spark. In some cases, the stone must be removed through an outpatient surgical procedure requiring general anesthesia. To drain the urine, a tube may be inserted through

the bladder into the kidney or through the skin into the kidney. Patients may resume normal activities within several days.

OUTLOOK AND PREVENTION
Urinary tract calculi usually form as the result of a combination of factors. Infection of the kidney and bladder, high concentrations of crystal-forming salts in the urine, a physical condition that slows the normal flow of urine (such as an enlarged prostate), obesity, and a family history of calculi can play a role. Calculi are more common in affluent countries; among white-collar workers rather than manual laborers; in people who eat diets high in fat, protein, and salt; and in hot climates.

People who have developed a urinary tract calculus have a 50 percent likelihood of developing another stone within 5 years without follow-up preventive treatment. Prevention begins with evaluating the metabo-

lism of the person to determine which crystal-forming salts are overly concentrated in the urine. Diet can be modified and medications prescribed to decrease or eliminate the problem. People who have had stones are also advised to drink six to eight glasses of water a day to dilute urine and increase the number of urinations during the day.

Caliper splint
An orthopedic appliance made of plastic or metal used to support a weakened lower arm or leg.

Callus, bony
The newly formed soft bone that develops after a bone fracture and during the bone's healing process. Bony callus may also refer to a thickening of the surface layer of the skin over a bony prominence, usually on the feet, but also on the hands. Such a callus usually forms in response to pressure. Typically, a callus on the foot develops from the friction or compression of ill-fitting shoes. On the hands, a callus may be caused by frequent and long-term contact with hard, rough materials or from repetitive labor with hand tools. Symptoms include pain with pressure. With foot calluses, the pain is made worse when the foot is bearing weight, especially in thin-soled or high-heeled shoes. Resting and relieving pressure on the affected foot or hand relieves the pain. Such calluses rarely cause more than minor discomfort. On the feet, this can be readily remedied by wearing shoes that do not press against the site. On the hands, it is relieved by not using the rough materials or by avoiding rigorous labor activity that caused the callus. In most cases, these do not require medical attention, unless they become very painful or ulcerated. An emery board or pumice stone can be used to sand them down.

A person with diabetes mellitus needs to give special attention to a callus, since the disease can increase the risk of infection and prompt complications from poor circulation in the feet. In persistent cases, a foot specialist, such as an orthopedic surgeon or podiatrist, may find that the underlying bone is causing pressure and needs to be removed to relieve symptoms.

Callus, skin

An area of tough, thickened skin caused by pressure or friction. Calluses commonly develop on the palms, fingertips, and soles of the feet. They are similar to corns, which usually appear on the toes. Calluses are most often associated with specific types of work and sport. Tennis players and construction workers, for example, tend to develop calluses on their hands, violinists and guitarists on their fingertips, and runners on the soles of their feet. In some cases, it is beneficial to have calluses because they prevent blisters. However, calluses can also cause tenderness or pain under the skin. Self-treatment of calluses includes using a file, pumice stone, or towel to rub away excess skin when the skin is damp, such as after showering or bathing, or applying a salicylic acid plaster or other over-the-counter medicated preparation to soften the skin. Medical treatment by a dermatologist, foot doctor, or orthopedic surgeon includes paring the thickened skin with a scalpel. In some cases it may be necessary to wear protective pads or orthopedic shoes or to have surgery to correct deformities that cause calluses to develop.

Caloric test

A procedure used to determine whether abnormalities or disease are present in the ear of a person experiencing dizziness, balance problems, or hearing loss. The test is usually part of a group of diagnostic methods called electronystagmography (ENG) that evaluates the function of the vestibular system (inner ear nerve system essential to balance) and associated areas of the brain. Caloric tests are performed by a doctor in his or her office or in a diagnostic clinic. The physician infuses water of varying temperatures into the external ear canal and monitors reflex flickering of the eyes. These involuntary eye movements are recorded and interpreted to detect abnormalities in the inner ear, the vestibular system, and the nerves that connect the vestibular system to the brain and the muscles of the eye. Those taking the test are instructed to avoid sedatives and tranquilizers for 2 to 3 days before the test, to abstain from consuming caffeine and alcohol for 24 to 48 hours before testing, and to avoid eating for 4 hours before taking the test. Caloric testing takes about an hour. It is not painful but may cause nausea.

Calorie

A measurement of energy provided by food for use by the body. A difference exists in how the term is used popularly and in the scientific community. Scientifically, a calorie is 1/1,000 of a kilocalorie. Popularly, however, the term calorie is used sometimes interchangeably with the scientific term kilocalorie. Scientifically, a kilocalorie is a measure of the amount of heat required to raise the temperature of 1 kilogram of water 1 degree Celsius (centigrade). This measurement is used because it can be determined readily.

Most of the energy consumed in food is released as heat to maintain body temperature. The three basic components of the diet—proteins, carbohydrates, and fats—produce different amounts of energy or calories. Alcohol and soluble fiber can also provide energy. Excess calories are stored as body fat. Mildly active adults need about 25 calories (kilocalories) per kilogram of body weight per day to meet their basic energy needs. Another way to estimate daily calorie needs by weight in pounds is to multiply the body weight by 10. That equals basic caloric needs. For less active individuals, add on a sum that is 3 times their weight. For the mildly active, add on 5 times the weight, for the extremely active, 10 times. Hence, the formula for a less active person who weighs 160 pounds is: 160 lb $\times$ 10 + 480, totaling approximately 2,100 calories. To lose weight, an adult needs to consume fewer calories daily than this total.

Calorie requirements

The amount of energy required by the body for normal function, growth, repair, and physical activity. Daily calorie requirements vary from person to person and depend largely on how active an individual is. To maintain health, sedentary women and older people must take in about 1,600 calories a day. Active women, children, teenage girls, and sedentary men require approximately 2,200 calories. Very active women, teenage boys, and active men need about 2,800 calories daily. However, because individual needs vary, individuals are encouraged to consult their physicians to determine their own calorie requirements.

A calorie is a measurement of energy. The three basic components of the diet—proteins, carbohydrates, and fats—provide different amounts of energy or calories, as do alcohol and soluble fiber. Carbohydrates and fats are the body's main sources of energy. Every gram of fat contains more than double the number of calories in a gram of protein or carbohydrate. In the average, healthful daily diet, 50 to 60 percent of calories should derive from carbohydrates, no more than 30 percent (and preferably less) from fat, and 10 to 20 percent from protein. However, the typical diet consumed by the average American has a much higher percentage of calories derived from fats.

CALORIES AND BODY WEIGHT

Excess calories are stored as body fat. To shed pounds, doctors recommend that people who are OVERWEIGHT (weighing 10 to 20 percent more than average) consume 500 calories a day less than the amount needed to maintain their weight. Those who are obese (more than 20 percent overweight) should consume 750 calories less than required. (See also OBESITY.) However, it is important to monitor calories from fat as well as calorie intake, because a low-calorie diet is not necessarily low in fat. High fat intakes make weight loss more difficult and contribute to health risks. Portion size is also important because large servings of even low-calorie

---

CALORIC ENERGY IN FOOD

Most food provides some energy; the higher the number of calories, the more energy available to be used or stored as fat. Listed below are the number of calories per gram in:

- Fat   9
- Protein   4
- Carbohydrate   4
- Alcohol   7
- Soluble fiber   2

foods can undermine weight loss. Exercise is another essential element of weight loss. Weight loss takes place when calorie intake is less than calories burned for energy. For example, if an older person gradually becomes less active, maintaining the same amount of calories consumed in youth may lead to weight gain.

Before embarking on a weight-loss plan, individuals should consult a physician. Doctors advise that the safest weight loss plan is one based on a balanced, nutritious diet and regular exercise. Long-term, slow weight loss is also most likely to be enduring.

Certain people require more, not fewer, calories. A high-calorie diet is one that provides 1,000 or more calories beyond the normal recommendation. Doctors sometimes prescribe such diets for women who are in the later stages of pregnancy or breast-feeding, people who have severe weight loss due to illness, and people such as athletes who have high energy requirements or metabolic rates.

Calorimetry

Measurement of the amount of heat energy produced by an individual. Calorimetry is used by dieticians to determine the energy needs of people who are very ill. It can be conducted either directly or indirectly. Direct calorimetry involves putting a person in a device called a calorimeter and measuring how much heat he or she gives off. This method is expensive and impractical, so indirect calorimetry is usually preferred. Indirect calorimetry uses a device that measures oxygen consumption and carbon dioxide production to calculate energy expenditure and respiration rate. This calculation is used to devise a nutrition care plan for critically ill patients (for example, those who require mechanical ventilation).

Calvé-Perthes disease

See OSTEOCHONDROSIS.

Campylobacter

A type of bacteria that is the most frequent cause of bacterial DIARRHEA in the United States. Stomach cramps and fever are additional symptoms of *Campylobacter* infection. Infection is usually caused by eating foods, such as undercooked chicken, that have been contaminated by *Campylobacter.*

Normally, the symptoms of *Campylobacter* infection are relatively mild. The problem may resolve on its own, or a doctor may prescribe an antibiotic to speed recovery. However, a growing problem in recent years has been a strain of *Campylobacter* that is resistant to antibiotics. This is thought to result from the practice of adding antibiotics to the feed of chickens. Symptoms last longer in people who are infected with the resistant strain. *Campylobacter* can be a serious problem for older people, young children, and people who have compromised immune systems.

Cancer

Any of a group of diseases characterized by an uncontrolled, abnormal growth of cells that can spread throughout the body. The terms malignancy and neoplasia are often used interchangeably with cancer. Cancer is thought to develop from a single cell or a small set of cells after changes have occurred in their DNA, the genetic material that instructs cells how to behave. Some cancers result from inherited genetic abnormalities, and others are triggered by carcinogens, environmental agents capable of causing

---

SIGNS OF CANCER

Different cancers have different symptoms. Any of these seven basic warning signs may signal the presence of cancer. However, they also can be signs of noncancerous conditions. A doctor can conduct tests to identify the problem:

1 **Change in bowel or bladder habits**
2 **A sore that does not heal within 2 weeks**
3 **Unusual bleeding or discharge**
4 **A lump that does not go away**
5 **Indigestion or difficulty in swallowing**
6 **A change in a wart or mole**
7 **Persistent hoarseness or cough**

Source: American Cancer Society.

---

genetic mutations (see CARCINOGEN). Sometimes, viruses interact with genes in cells and make them more likely to become cancerous. Often, the reason that a cell becomes cancerous is unknown.

Cancer cells cause harm in several different ways. They can deprive normal cells of nourishment or space; they can form a mass, or TUMOR, that may eventually invade and destroy normal tissue; and they can metastasize (spread) by traveling through the bloodstream or the lymphatic system to other parts of the body. Most cancers take years to develop; cancer that is detected and treated before it has invaded adjacent organs or spread throughout the body has the best chance of being cured.

Cancer is classified into five major groups. From 80 to 90 percent of cancer cases are carcinomas. A CARCINOMA is a tumor that originates in the surface tissue of an organ. A SARCOMA is a tumor that originates in the bone, cartilage, muscle, connective tissues, or fatty tissues. Myeloma originates in the plasma cells of the bone marrow. LYMPHOMA originates in the lymph system, and LEUKEMIA originates in the blood-forming cells of the bone marrow.

A number of investigations or workups can be done to help identify cancer. However, a tissue biopsy, which involves taking a sample of affected cells for analysis under a microscope, is the only absolutely accurate method of diagnosing cancer.

There are four general types of treatment for cancer: surgery, RADIATION THERAPY, CHEMOTHERAPY with anti-cancer drugs, and biological therapy, which helps the body's own immune system to fight the cancer. Many people with cancer will receive treatments that combine some or all of the available therapies. Different types of cancer vary in their rates of growth, patterns of spreading, and responses to treatment. People with cancer need treatment that is tailored to their particular disease.

Half of all men and a third of all women in the United States will develop cancer at some time. Cancer can affect individuals of any age or ethnic background. Today, millions of people are living with cancer or have been cured of the disease. Based on normal life expectancy, the chance

A CLOSE-UP ON CANCER

Each year, more than half a million people die of various forms of cancer. Researchers study how tumors grow to develop treatments for them. Cancers start with changes in oncogenes, cells that control cell growth.

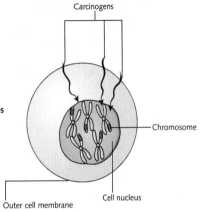

STEP ONE IN THE DAMAGE THAT RESULTS IN CANCER
Carcinogens penetrate the cells and cause damage to the oncogenes on the chromosomes. Oncogenes regulate important processes, including cell division. The oncogenes try to repair themselves.

Carcinogens

Chromosome

Cell nucleus

Outer cell membrane

GENETIC CHANGES CONTINUE
Damage to the oncogenes continues. Some oncogenes are able to repair themselves, but other chromosomes are permanently damaged.

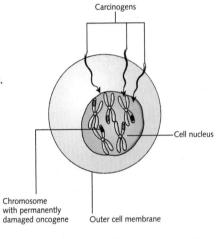

Carcinogens

Cell nucleus

Chromosome with permanently damaged oncogene

Outer cell membrane

GENETIC DAMAGE RESULTS IN CANCER
As too great a percentage of the oncogenes become permanently damaged, the cell becomes unable to perform key functions. Eventually, the cells no longer function and become cancerous.

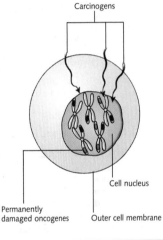

Carcinogens

Cell nucleus

Permanently damaged oncogenes

Outer cell membrane

HOW CANCER SPREADS IN THE BLOOD: STEP ONE
The cancerous cells multiply out of control, forming a large tumor. The growing tumor ruptures the surrounding blood vessels, and the cancerous cells go into general circulation in the bloodstream.

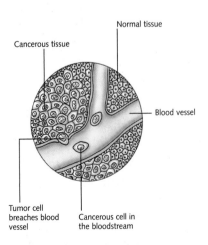

Normal tissue

Cancerous tissue

Blood vessel

Tumor cell breaches blood vessel

Cancerous cell in the bloodstream

HOW CANCER SPREADS IN THE BLOOD: STEP TWO
Cancerous cells float in the bloodstream and become lodged in a capillary far from the original site. A secondary tumor is formed.

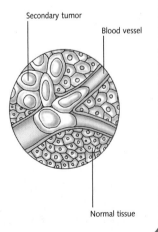

Secondary tumor

Blood vessel

Normal tissue

C

CANCER STATISTICS

THE INCIDENCE OF CANCER IN US MEN IN 2002

197,700	Genital system cancers, including prostate cancer
100,700	Respiratory system cancers, including lung cancer
130,300	Digestive system cancers
62,200	Urinary system cancers
31,900	Lymphoma
32,500	Skin excluding basal and squamous cancers*
18,900	Oral cavity and pharynx cancers
17,600	Leukemia
14,000	Other and unspecified primary site cancers
9,600	Brain and other nervous system cancers
7,800	Multiple myeloma
6,000	Endocrine system cancers, including thyroid cancer
4,400	Soft tissue cancers, including heart
1,300	Bone and joint cancers
1,500	Breast cancers
1,100	Eye and eye orbit cancers

THE INCIDENCE OF CANCER IN US WOMEN IN 2002

203,500	Breast cancers
120,300	Digestive system cancers
81,400	Genital system cancers, including ovarian cancers
82,500	Respiratory system cancers, including lung cancer
28,500	Urinary system cancers
29,000	Lymphoma
25,800	Skin excluding basal and squamous cancers*
16,200	Other and unspecified primary site cancers
16,700	Endocrine system cancers, including thyroid cancer
13,200	Leukemia
10,000	Oral cavity and pharynx cancers
7,400	Brain and nervous system cancers
6,800	Multiple myeloma
3,900	Soft tissue cancers, including heart
1,100	Bone and joint cancers
1,100	Eye and eye orbit cancers

*Note: Figures exclude basal and squamous cell skin cancers and in situ carcinomas, except urinary bladder cancers.

ESTIMATED TOTAL DEATHS FROM CANCER IN BOTH SEXES IN THE UNITED STATES IN 2002

161,400	Respiratory system cancers, including lung cancer	13,100	Brain and other nervous system cancers
132,300	Digestive system cancers	10,800	Multiple myeloma
40,000	Breast cancer	9,600	Skin, excluding basal and squamous cancers*
30,800	Male genital system cancers, including prostate cancer	7,400	Oral cavity and pharynx cancers
43,700	Other and unspecified primary site cancers	3,900	Soft tissue cancers, including heart
83,300	Female genital system cancers, including ovarian cancers	2,300	Endocrine system cancers, including thyroid cancer
25,800	Lymphoma	1,300	Bone and joint cancers
24,900	Urinary system cancers	200	Eye and eye orbit cancers
21,700	Leukemia		

*Note: Figures exclude basal and squamous cell skin cancers and in situ carcinomas, except urinary bladder cancers.
Adapted with permission of American Cancer Society.

SMOKING AND CANCER

Deaths from many different types of cancer are attributed to smoking cigarettes, in varying percentages.

TYPE	SEX	% DEATHS
Lung	M	90
	F	79
Larynx	M	81
	F	87
Oral cavity	M	92
	F	61
Esophagus	M	78
	F	75
Pancreas	M	29
	F	34
Bladder	M	47
	F	37
Kidney	M	48
	F	12
Stomach	M	17
	F	25
Leukemia	M	20
	F	20
Cervix	F	31

Source: Newcombe PA, Carbone PP. The health consequences of smoking: cancer. *Medical Clinics of North America* 1992; 76: 305-331.

of surviving for at least 5 years with cancer is 50 percent.

Quitting smoking significantly reduces the risk of developing cancer. Cancers that have been associated with smoking include LEUKEMIA, urinary bladder cancer, and cancers of the cervix, esophagus, larynx, lung, kidney, oropharynx, pancreas, and stomach. Eating a diet rich in nutrients and exercising regularly can also help reduce the risk of cancer. For information about specific types of cancer, see the entry for the site of cancer—for example, BREAST CANCER or COLON, CANCER OF THE.

Cancer screening

Tests performed on people without symptoms to identify possible cancer at an early stage. Screening tests have been used effectively for cancers of the breast, cervix, gastrointestinal tract, and prostate gland. Screening for lung cancer is not yet successful.

A PAP SMEAR can detect precancerous conditions in the cells of the cervix and is recommended for all women who are sexually active or who are age 18 or older. In women at low risk for cervical cancer, Pap smears are generally performed annually or, in low-risk individuals, every 3 years after having three tests with normal results. New cases of cancer of the cervix in the United States decreased by half after the Pap smear was introduced in 1945.

Breast cancer can be detected by a MAMMOGRAM, an X ray of the breasts. Experts differ on whether women between the ages of 40 and 49 should have mammograms every year or every 2 years. However, most agree women older than age 50 should have an annual mammogram. Mammography cannot definitively diagnose cancer, but it can highlight an area where cancer may exist, often before a lump is felt. Such a finding requires further investigation and a biopsy. When a woman has a palpable breast mass, it should be evaluated with a biopsy even if the mammogram result is normal.

A simple test for colon and rectal cancer is the digital rectal examination, which is recommended once a year for men and women older than age 40. This examination can also detect cancer of the prostate at an early stage. A FECAL-OCCULT BLOOD TEST, which checks for colon and rectal cancer, is recommended annually for all people age 50 or older and for those at high risk for developing those cancers. This test can detect small amounts of blood that are present but not visible in the stool. Another screening test for colon and rectal cancer is SIGMOIDOSCOPY, in which the rectum and lower (sigmoid) colon are examined directly by means of a flexible tube with a light at one end.

Cancer, hereditary risk factors for

An increased risk for certain kinds of cancer due to inheriting mutated genes. Some cancers, such as those of the cervix, lung, or bladder, are rarely inherited. Others, including cancers of the breast, colon, and ovary, sometimes occur repeatedly in families because of an inherited genetic defect. When a particular cancer has occurred more than once in a family, and in a person of younger-than-average age for that cancer, family members should be screened for it.

Cancer researchers believe that normal cells are transformed into cancer cells as a result of changes in the cells' genetic material (DNA). When the DNA, which spells out the genetic code, has been altered, cells may begin to function and divide in abnormal ways, which may lead to cancer. An individual who inherits an altered gene has an increased risk for cancer, which may develop when the altered genes are exposed to internal or external carcinogenic influences, such as hormones, cancer-causing chemicals, or radiation.

A single defective gene can make people susceptible to certain types of cancer. These inherited cancers include NEUROFIBROMATOSIS, in which tumors and patches of brownish pigment appear on the skin; familial polyposis, a disorder characterized by abnormal growths called polyps inside the large intestine (see POLYPOSIS, FAMILIAL); and TUBEROUS SCLEROSIS, in which abnormal growths appear on the skin and in the brain, stomach, and heart. People with neurofibromatosis and tuberous sclerosis are usually identified by age 10, while carriers of familial polyposis can be identified by DNA analysis of a blood sample.

People with strong family histories of specific cancers may have inherited the tendency to develop those cancers, even though the abnormal gene in question has not yet been identified. People with family histories of cancer should therefore be examined regularly for early signs of the disease; the earlier cancer is detected, the more effective treatment is likely to be. Cancer screening is recommended particularly for people with family histories of colon cancers, such as hereditary nonpolyposis colon cancer (HNPCC); breast cancer, which can be caused by specific genes (BRCA-1, BRCA-2); or cancer of the ovaries, which is known to occur in families.

Candidiasis

See YEAST INFECTIONS.

Canker sore

A small, painful sore or ulcer that occurs inside the mouth. It is usually surrounded by an area of redness less than 2 inches in diameter. Canker sores commonly first appear when a person is in his or her 20s or 30s. The sores tend to disappear in 1 to 2 weeks. Recurrences are common and may be induced by trauma, eating spicy or citrus foods, and menstru-ation.

Women get canker sores more frequently than men do, and the sores appear to run in families. Sometimes they are believed to be associated with immune system disorders or conditions, nutritional deficiencies, or gastrointestinal problems. There is no cure for canker sores. Doctors recommend avoiding eating acidic, abrasive, or spicy foods and brushing teeth gently. In severe cases, a doctor or dentist can prescribe a local anesthetic to control pain and oral and topical medications to manage inflammation. See also COLD SORE.

Cannabis

Marijuana. See DRONABINOL.

Cannula

A hollow tube that can be inserted into a body cavity, such as a blood vessel or the bladder. A cannula usually contains a sharp, pointed, solid core called a trocar that eases insertion. Cannulas are used to draw off fluid (or fat, in the case of liposuction) or to give medication.

Cap, dental

See CROWN, DENTAL.

Capecitabine

An antimetabolite drug prescribed for breast cancer that has metastasized (spread to other parts of the body). Capecitabine (Xeloda) is used to treat breast and colorectal cancer that has spread despite previous therapy. Capecitabine can be taken by mouth and has fewer side effects than other cancer drugs. It works by interfering with the growth of cancer cells.

Capgras syndrome

A specific delusional belief in which the person is convinced that some important person, commonly the spouse, has been replaced by an identical-appearing impostor. This occurs commonly in schizophrenia, bipolar disorder, delusional disorder, and postpartum psychosis. It can also occur in neurological disorders such as cerebral hemorrhage, epilepsy, Parkinson disease, and Alzheimer's disease or after the person has had brain surgery.

Capillary

A microscopic blood vessel that connects the smallest arteries (arterioles) and the smallest veins (venules) to complete the circulation of blood at a cellular level. A network of capillaries is present in all body tissues. The capillary walls are membranes through which nutrients and oxygen pass from the blood into body cells, while waste such as carbon dioxide passes out. See also HEART.

Capitation

A method of payment for health care services. In capitation, a fixed payment is made for a specific period (monthly or annually) for each person assigned to a physician, hospital, or other health care provider, regardless of the number and nature of services provided.

Caplet

A solid, capsule-shaped tablet coated with a water-soluble shell. People who have trouble swallowing tablets may find caplets easier to take.

Capsaicin

A pain-relieving cream, gel, lotion, or roll-on. Capsaicin (Capsagel, Dolorac, Salonpas-Hot, Zostrix) is a natural chemical used on top of the skin to relieve the pain of arthritis, shingles, or diabetic neuropathy. Pain relief will be only temporary. Capsaicin is available without a prescription.

Capsule

A form in which certain drugs are prepared. A capsule is a shell made of gelatin that contains the drug in powdered form, liquid, or tiny slow-release particles.

Capsulitis, adhesive

See FROZEN SHOULDER.

Captopril

See ANTIHYPERTENSIVES.

Car restraints

Safety devices used in motor vehicles to minimize the risk of injury or death during accidents. Car restraints include lap and shoulder safety belts, CHILD SAFETY SEATS, and AIR BAGS. Safety restraints are designed to prevent injuries that can result from colliding with any part of the car's interior in a crash or sudden stop. The most effective safety protection is provided by the use of all three forms of restraint. Safety belt laws have been enacted in virtually all states within the United States.

SAFETY BELTS

The use of lap and shoulder seat belts provides the greatest possible protection against being thrown out of a vehicle during an accident. The lap belt keeps passengers and drivers from being thrown out of their seats during a crash. The lap belt should be worn snugly over the lower part of the pelvis, not across the stomach, where it might cause internal injury during a crash. If the lap belt is worn too loosely, the person may slide under it during a crash. Sitting up straight prevents the lap belt from riding up.

The shoulder harness is intended to prevent the upper body from being thrown forward during a crash. It should be positioned over the top part of the shoulder and across the chest. To maximize protection, there should never be more than 1 inch of slack between the body and the shoulder belt. The shoulder belt should never be tucked under the arm, where it can put pressure on the ribs and possibly break them in an accident. In some models of cars, the shoulder belt is automatically positioned when the car is turned on.

The use of lap and shoulder seat belts reduces the risk of fatal injury to front-seat occupants of cars by 45 percent and the risk of moderate to critical injury by 50 percent. In light trucks, the use of safety belts reduces the risk of fatal injury by 60 percent and the risk of moderate to severe critical injury by 65 percent. Between 1975 and 2001, an estimated 147,246 lives were saved by the use of seat belts, and more than 2 million moderate to critical injuries were prevented.

AIR BAGS

Air bags, which are designed to work together with lap and shoulder seat belts, provide supplemental protection. Together, air bags and safety belts provide the most effective safety protection possible. Air bags are designed to inflate in moderate to severe crashes, not those that occur at lower speeds. They provide an additional 10 percent reduction in the risk of fatal injury.

CHILD SAFETY SEATS

Child safety seats range in size according to the age and weight of the child and are equipped with shoulder harness clips designed to keep the lap and shoulder belts in the correct positions. Child safety seats must be selected to accommodate the type of seat belt restraint provided in the model and make of motor vehicle in which the seat will be used. Most children younger than 10 years should use a booster seat to ride safely. Lap and shoulder belts usually do not fit properly until a child is at least 4 feet, 10 inches tall and weighs 80 pounds.

The use of child safety seats has reduced fatal injuries in infants by 69 percent and in toddlers by 47 percent. However, at least half the child car seats in use in the United States are incorrectly installed. Because

methods of installation can vary considerably, it is important to read the labels and follow the instructions carefully.

Carbamazepine

A drug used to treat seizure disorders and trigeminal neuralgia, a painful nerve disorder. Unlabeled use (meaning it does not have Food and Drug Administration approval but is used by a physician for that purpose) of carbamazepine (Tegretol, Carbatrol) includes treatment of bipolar disorder, intermittent explosive disorder, restless leg syndrome, chorea in children older than age 6, posttraumatic stress disorder, and schizophrenia that is resistant to treatment.

Carbamide peroxide

An antiseptic. Carbamide peroxide, which is available as a solution, gel, or ear drops without a prescription under many brand names, has many uses. It is used as a disinfectant for minor mouth irritations such as canker sores, and it has a deodorant effect as a result of its ability to inhibit bacteria that cause odor. Carbamide peroxide is found in products that remove ear wax from the ear canal, and it is used as a bleach in hair products. When carbamide peroxide comes in contact with bacteria, a chemical reaction occurs in which oxygen and hydrogen are released in bubbles (fizzing). Once the fizzing stops, the product is no longer effective.

Carbohydrates

Essential nutrients that are the body's main source of energy. There are two primary types of carbohydrates: simple (SUGAR) and complex (starch). Starches and sugars in fruits, vegetables, and grains are all examples of carbohydrates. Although both kinds of carbohydrates contain the same amount of calories, the complex carbohydrates found in foods such as whole-grain breads and baked potatoes are preferred to the simple sugars in cookies, candy, and cakes. The more refined or processed the source of the carbohydrate, the more likely that significant amounts of its nutritional value have been removed. Both simple and complex carbohydrates may be refined; sources of these carbohydrates are said to have "empty

calories" because they contribute no nutritional value other than energy.

SIMPLE CARBOHYDRATES (SUGARS)

Sugars are found in many forms beyond sucrose, the simple white table form that is spooned into coffee. Natural sugars, such as fructose, glucose, and lactose, occur in fruit and milk. Although sugars provide energy, they possess little or no additional nutritional value. Excess sugar in the diet may also lead to cavities in the teeth. Sugars are often used in desserts that are rich in fat and calories, which can contribute to weight gain. The US Department of Agriculture FOOD GUIDE PYRAMID advises consumers to derive the smallest proportion of their diet from fats, oils, and refined sugars.

COMPLEX CARBOHYDRATES (STARCHES)

Complex carbohydrates provide more lasting sources of energy than simple carbohydrates because they are absorbed more slowly. The foods that are rich in complex carbohydrates—starches such as potatoes, pasta, rice, and beans—are often rich in vitamins, minerals, and fiber. For highest nutritional value, it is best to eat complex carbohydrates in

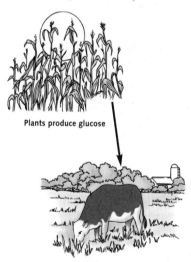

Plants produce glucose

Animals consume complex carbohydrates

CARBOHYDRATES: FUEL FOR THE BODY
Plants produce glucose, the most simple carbohydrate, and string the molecules together to form complex carbohydrates called starches. Animals and people consume complex carbohydrates from plants, and their digestive systems break down the carbohydrates into glucose molecules that can enter the bloodstream.

C

unrefined forms, such as brown rice rather than white rice and bread made from whole wheat rather than white flour.

CARBOHYDRATES AND ENERGY
Carbohydrates are the body's main source of fuel. Doctors advise that 50 to 60 percent of a person's total calorie intake come from carbohydrates. While fats also provide energy, they contain more than double the amount of calories per gram as carbohydrates, and excess fat in the diet is associated with increased health risks. See also FATS AND OILS.

Because complex carbohydrates are more healthful choices overall, the most carbohydrate intake should be from food sources of complex rather than simple carbohydrates. Simple sugars such as sucrose are rapidly broken down by the body and take only minutes to reach the bloodstream as glucose. Complex carbohydrates generally take more time to be converted into glucose. Carbohydrates that are not used for energy are stored in the body as glycogen, or, if consumed in amounts well in excess of energy requirements, they are stored as body fat.

Carbon dioxide

A colorless, odorless, tasteless gas formed from carbon and oxygen. Carbon dioxide is found in nature, both as part of the atmosphere and in combination with other elements as carbonates. Natural mineral waters contain bubbles of excess carbon dioxide that cause them to sparkle, or effervesce; this same effect is created artificially in the production of carbonated soft drinks. Carbon dioxide causes bread dough to rise and is used in fire extinguishers, among many other uses. Carbon dioxide is a product of the burning of fuels that contain carbon, such as coal, oil, gasoline, and natural gas, and its presence in the atmosphere has been growing steadily, thus upsetting the natural balance of the ecosystem and leading to the GREENHOUSE EFFECT and GLOBAL WARMING. It can accumulate in indoor areas that have poor ventilation. Too much carbon dioxide in these areas can cause headaches, difficulty concentrating, and shortness of breath. Carbon dioxide may also be a cause of SICK BUILDING SYNDROME.

Carbon tetrachloride

A heavy, colorless, poisonous chemical compound. Carbon tetrachloride is toxic when inhaled or absorbed through the skin. It is used commercially in dry cleaning and to extinguish fires. Carbon tetrachloride should never be used in the home as a spot remover because of its poisonous qualities. It can cause liver problems, along with headaches.

Carbuncle

A cluster of painful, pus-filled boils (see BOIL) on the skin. A boil results when a hair follicle becomes infected with staphylococcal (staph) bacteria. In a carbuncle, boils in adjacent follicles expand and join to form a mass with multiple drainage points. Although they can develop anywhere, carbuncles are most common on the back and the buttocks. They are usually the size of a pea but may grow as large as a golf ball.

Good hygiene is essential to treat a carbuncle. Both the carbuncle and the area surrounding it must be kept clean with antibacterial soap. A sterile dressing prevents spread of draining material, and an antibiotic ointment prevents further infection. Clothing and bedding that have come in contact with infected areas must be laundered. Carbuncles must never be squeezed because this can spread the staph infection. Many carbuncles resolve by applying warm compresses for 30 minutes several times a day for about 2 weeks and keeping the area scrupulously clean. This helps decrease inflammation. Some carbun-

---

CARBUNCLE DANGER

Serious complications can result from carbuncle infections, including the spread of the infection; formation of abscesses (pus-filled sacs); or SEPSIS, a potentially fatal condition. A doctor should be contacted if:

- **Carbuncles persist for more than 2 weeks**
- **Fever is present**
- **Red streaks extend from the carbuncle**
- **Fluid collects around the carbuncle**
- **Pain worsens**
- **New symptoms appear**

---

cles are deep in the skin and cannot drain on their own; they require surgical drainage and sometimes treatment with oral antibiotics. People with diabetes mellitus, atopic dermatitis, and weakened immune systems are more prone than others to carbuncles, although poor hygiene can be a contributing factor.

Carcinogen

An agent capable of causing or promoting cancer. Carcinogens, such as cigarette smoke, can be created by humans, or they may exist naturally in the environment (for example, ultraviolet radiation from the sun). Smoke, sunlight, X rays, and viruses are all known carcinogens, as are asbestos, air pollution, fatty foods, and certain chemicals used to preserve food. Carcinogens cause cancer in different ways. Some change normal cells into cancer cells, while others create conditions that enable other factors to cause cancer.

Carcinogenesis

The origin or development of cancer in previously healthy cells. Carcinogenesis is a multistep process, beginning with a series of changes in the genetic material (DNA) of a single cell. Cells are routinely exposed to substances that can alter their genes, but usually, natural processes of cell repair prevent such alterations. However, when the cell is unable to prevent alterations, its DNA can be permanently changed. When the cell reproduces itself, the new changes in the DNA are reproduced, too. In this way, a single cancer cell can give rise to a family of cells that are not controlled by normal cell repair processes. Unregulated, the new cells will divide rapidly and eventually invade surrounding tissues to form a tumor. Eventually, new cells may break off and move to distant parts of the body, where they can form colonies of cancer cells, called metastases.

The likelihood that a person will begin to develop cancer increases with age, because cancer is a slowly progressing, multistep disease. All forms of cancer are thought to originate from a single cell.

Carcinoid syndrome

A disorder associated with carcinoid tumors of the lung and small intestine that secrete the hormone sero-tonin into the bloodstream. Excess quantities of the hormone can trigger symptoms that include flushed skin, watery diarrhea, and asthmalike wheezing. The syndrome occurs in about 10 percent of people who have carcinoid tumors that have spread to the liver. Treatment with drugs that block the effects of the serotonin can reduce symptoms. In rare cases, the carcinoid tumor is removed surgically from the lung, intestine, or liver.

Carcinoma

A cancerous tumor arising from cells in surface tissues or the linings of organs. Carcinoma is one of the five basic kinds of CANCER and the most common form, accounting for about 80 to 90 percent of all cancers. Carcinoma develops from epithelial tissues of the skin and mucous membranes, which line surfaces and cavities within the body. Carcinomas tend to invade nearby tissues and metastasize (spread). Cancers of the lungs, skin, breast, cervix, and prostate gland are usually carcinomas.

Several types of carcinoma have been identified, including those affecting squamous cells, basal cells, transitional cells, and glandular epithelium (tissues lining the glands). Because carcinoma is the most common form of cancer, the word "carcinoma" is frequently used as a synonym for cancer.

Carcinomatosis

A condition in which CARCINOMA spreads to multiple sites in the body. Carcinoma may grow extensively in the organ where it originates, damaging both the organ and surrounding tissue. In carcinomatosis, it spreads to numerous other organs.

Cardiac arrest

FOR FIRST AID
see Resuscitation (CPR), page 1328

A sudden and immediate cessation of the heartbeat. Breathing stops, and, since blood flow to the brain is cut off, the person loses consciousness. Unless a normal heart rhythm is reestablished within 4 to 6 minutes, the person will die of irreversible brain damage.

Cardiac arrest almost always occurs in a heart affected by underlying heart disease (see HEART DISEASE, CONGENITAL; HEART DISEASE, ISCHEMIC), such as coronary artery disease, or by damage to the heart muscle, which is often the result of a previous HEART ATTACK. Cardiac arrest is commonly preceded by VENTRICULAR FIBRILLATION, a condition in which the lower chambers of the heart beat so fast that the heart tires and stops completely. Ventricular fibrillation can result from a previous or current heart attack, disease affecting the heart muscle (for example, cardiomyopathy), congenital defects, heart valve disease, cardiac arrhythmias (abnormal heart rhythms), and a number of other diseases and syndromes. Recreational drug use can also cause cardiac arrest.

Cardiac arrest is a medical emergency requiring immediate response. CARDIOPULMONARY RESUSCITATION (CPR) can help maintain blood flow to the brain until adequate medical help arrives. A device called a DEFIBRILLATOR is often used to restart the heart with an electrical shock. A person who has survived cardiac arrest is at increased risk of another. Therefore, it is important to identify and treat any underlying disease.

The risk for cardiac arrest can be reduced by preventing the underlying heart disease that can trigger such an event. This includes reducing blood cholesterol levels, managing stress, avoiding tobacco, and controlling hypertension (high blood pressure) and diabetes mellitus.

Cardiac output

The amount of blood the heart pumps per minute. Cardiac output is reduced in people with heart failure or those who have had a heart attack that injured the heart muscle. In critical situations, cardiac output can be measured by inserting a thin tube called a pulmonary artery catheter, or Swan-Ganz catheter, into a vein and threading the tube into the heart and pulmonary artery. Cardiac output gives doctors a sensitive indicator of changes in the heart's functioning efficiency and provides an early warning of developing problems. The presence of weakness, fatigue, dizziness, hypotension (low blood pressure), and cold extremities caused by poor blood flow can lead doctors to suspect poor cardiac output, in which case an echocardiogram can measure the pumping action of the heart and can indirectly assess cardiac output.

Cardiac rehabilitation

A medically supervised program designed to speed recovery and improve mental and physical functioning in people with heart conditions. Cardiac rehabilitation is commonly recommended after a heart attack, heart surgery (such as balloon angioplasty or bypass surgery), or diagnosis of heart disease (for example, congestive heart failure, hypertension, or congenital heart disease). Cardiac rehabilitation programs are usually based in hospital or community settings and are tailored to meet the needs of each person.

In a typical cardiac rehabilitation program, a person is prescribed medications to treat the disease, such as beta blockers to lower blood pressure and drugs to reduce blood cholesterol levels. Psychological counseling is included as a component of cardiac rehabilitation because heart disease often causes depression and other mental health problems. Lifestyle changes involve quitting tobacco use, learning stress management techniques to deal with day-to-day pressures, changing diet to reduce cholesterol and fat intake, reducing weight, and exercising. Most cardiac rehabilitation programs take 3 months to complete.

Research has shown that cardiac rehabilitation is highly successful. Benefits include decreased risk of a subsequent heart attack, lower blood pressure, improved blood cholesterol levels, improved heart functioning, less need for medication, lower weight, slowed or reversed atherosclerosis (buildup of fatty plaques in the arteries), and greater psychological well-being.

Cardiac stress testing

Procedures that measure and compare heart function at rest and during exercise. Faster heart rates make it easier to detect impaired blood flow to the heart or abnormal heart rhythms. Cardiac stress testing is performed to diagnose a heart condition,

TESTING THE HEART

During exercise, the body needs more oxygen and the heart needs to circulate more blood. Tests measuring cardiac stress, which may be triggered by exercise or medications, reveal whether blood supply is reduced in the arteries that supply the heart. Cardiac stress testing can also help determine the type and degree of exercise that is appropriate for a person. There are two types of cardiac stress testing available. Whether one is more appropriate than the other is determined by a person's physical fitness and activity level.

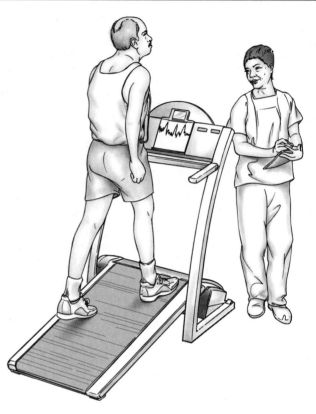

EXERCISE STRESS TEST IN ACTION
For those able to exercise, the heart rate is monitored with electrode leads attached to the chest while the person walks or runs on an elevated treadmill. Alternatively, a stationary bicycle may be used.

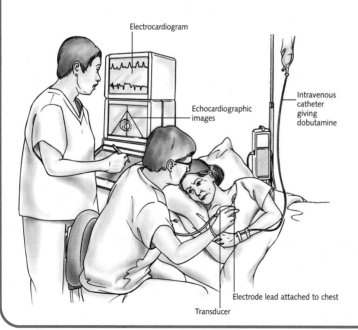

Electrocardiogram

Echocardiographic images

Intravenous catheter giving dobutamine

Electrode lead attached to chest

Transducer

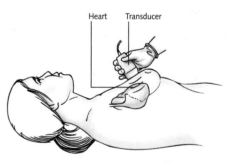

Heart   Transducer

TRANSDUCER PLACEMENT
The echocardiogram transducer, when placed on the chest, emits painless sound waves that are translated into images of the heart.

DOBUTAMINE STRESS ECHOCARDIOGRAM
For those unable to exercise, echocardiographic images are taken using a transducer, and the heart rate is monitored using electrode leads attached to the chest while a drug called dobutamine is administered intravenously to make the heart beat faster.

monitor progress in those who have had a heart attack or have undergone heart surgery, and determine safe exercise levels for people who have heart disease or are at risk for developing it. Cardiac stress testing is safe, quick, and noninvasive.

STRESS ECG

The stress ECG is a variation of the standard electrocardiogram (see ECG), which measures the electrical activity of the heart while at rest. In the stress ECG, 12 electrodes are attached to the upper body, arms, and legs, and an electrocardiogram is taken. Blood pressure is also monitored continuously. Next, heart rate is raised as the person exercises on a treadmill or a stationary bicycle. The level of exertion is increased gradually by raising the slope or speed of the treadmill or the resistance of the bicycle pedals. The test continues until the heart rate hits a predetermined upper limit or until the person being tested can no longer continue because of fatigue, angina (chest pain), or breathlessness. ECGs are taken throughout the exertion and during the 10- or 15-minute period afterward, at which time the person cools down and recovers from the exertion. Changes in heart function before, during, and after exertion can reveal underlying heart disease and allow a doctor to assess its type and severity.

PHARMACOLOGICAL STRESS TEST

Also known as the chemical stress test, this method is used for those who cannot perform a physical activity like walking on a treadmill or riding a bicycle. The person to be tested is injected with a drug such as dobutamine or adenosine, which causes the heart rate to speed up even though the person is actually resting. An ECG is administered before the drug is given and then again after the drug takes effect. This information allows diagnosis and assessment of the function of the heart, much like a standard stress ECG.

STRESS ECHOCARDIOGRAM

In echocardiography, a small device called a transducer, which emits ultrasound waves and captures the returning echoes, is placed against the chest. A machine then turns the echoes into an image of the heart. Echocardiography allows doctors to visualize the heart as it is moving and to observe its main pumping cham-

bers, the shape and thickness of the chamber walls, the valves, and the outer covering and major vessels of the heart. It is also possible to determine the volume and direction of blood flow through the heart. For a stress echocardiogram, echocardiography is performed before, during, and after exertion on a treadmill or bicycle. The echocardiogram can then detect changes in the motion of the heart muscle after exercise, suggesting underlying heart disease.

NUCLEAR STRESS TEST

This type of cardiac stress testing is valuable for determining which parts of the heart muscle have good blood flow and which do not. The person is injected with an extremely small amount of a radionuclide (radioactive substance), usually thallium. The thallium, which travels through the bloodstream, can be detected by a gamma camera. Areas of the heart with good blood supply appear dark on the gamma camera because of the presence of the thallium, while areas with reduced or absent blood flow appear gray or white. By taking gamma camera pictures of the heart before, during, and after exercise, doctors can determine whether areas of heart muscle have been damaged and whether normal blood flow is blocked or obstructed. A nuclear stress test is safe because the amount of radioactivity is minuscule and because the thallium loses its radioactivity in a matter of hours.

Cardiologist

A physician who specializes in preventing, diagnosing, and treating heart disease.

Cardiology

The branch of medicine that specializes in studying the structure and function of the heart and the diseases that affect it.

Cardiomegaly

Enlargement of the heart. The heart can increase in size as a result of disease that places extra workload on it, such as hypertension (high blood pressure), congestive heart failure, or excessive alcohol use. This condition is known as pathological cardiomegaly. For some, cardiomegaly arises from no known cause, in which case it is said to be idiopathic.

Cardiomegaly can cause a number of symptoms, such as edema (swelling) in the lower extremities, shortness of breath, weakness, dizziness, cardiac arrhythmias (irregular heart rhythms), and palpitations (fast, irregular heartbeat). Treatment consists of treating the causative condition and making necessary lifestyle changes, such as abstaining from alcohol.

Cardiomegaly can also result from intense athletic training, a condition commonly known as athlete's heart. Cardiomegaly in athletes is usually not dangerous, produces no symptoms, and does not require treatment.

Cardiomyopathy

A type of heart disease in which the heart muscle is abnormally enlarged, thickened, or stiffened, reducing its ability to pump effectively. The word cardiomyopathy combines three Greek roots meaning heart (cardio-) muscle (myo) disease (-pathy).

There are two basic types of cardiomyopathy: ischemic (resulting from a lack of oxygen to the heart muscle) and nonischemic (not resulting from a lack of oxygen). Ischemic cardiomyopathy is caused by CORONARY ARTERY DISEASE, in which deposits of fat and other materials block blood flow into the arteries supplying oxygen to the heart muscle. The heart enlarges as a result of working without sufficient oxygen. Ischemic cardiomyopathy tends to develop in older adults. Nonischemic cardiomyopathy is less common than ischemic cardiomyopathy. It is a progressive disease and often occurs in young adults and even children. People with nonischemic cardiomyopathy often require heart transplantation.

TYPES, SYMPTOMS, AND CAUSES

There are three principal varieties of nonischemic cardiomyopathy.

■ *Dilated cardiomyopathy* This type refers to overall dilation (enlargement) of the heart, particularly the ventricles (lower chambers), which do most of the work of pumping blood into the lungs and the body. As the heart weakens, it pumps out a smaller portion of the blood in its chambers. In

> Terms in small capital letters— for example, PHYSICAL THERAPY or PAGET DISEASE—indicate a cross-reference to another entry with more information.

order to move the needed amount of blood into the body, the heart enlarges, creating a larger volume to make up for decreased pumping power. Eventually, this compensatory mechanism cannot keep up, and the heart weakens. Heart failure sets in, and fluid accumulates in the legs, abdomen, and lungs. Shortness of breath caused by fluid accumulation in the lungs is a common symptom. Swelling in the liver often causes pain in the abdomen. Blood clots can form in the enlarged heart chambers, break loose, travel through the bloodstream, and block arteries, particularly in the legs, lungs, kidneys, or brain.

Dilated cardiomyopathy has a number of possible causes, including excessive alcohol consumption over a period of years, particularly when combined with a poor diet; toxins, including certain chemotherapy drugs used to treat cancer; inflammation of the heart muscle, usually because of viral infection; certain disorders of the blood (such as HEMOCHROMATOSIS, which leads to abnormal iron deposits in the heart muscle) or the nervous system; hypertension (high blood pressure); current or recent pregnancy; and genetic tendency. In some cases, dilated cardiomyopathy occurs without any clear cause. This form of the disease is most common in middle-aged people, primarily men, but it has been diagnosed in individuals of all ages, including children.

■ *Hypertrophic cardiomyopathy* This type results from abnormal thickening of the heart wall, most often the septum (wall) between the ventricles. It can also affect just the tips of the ventricles or the entirety of one or both ventricles. The thickening decreases the amount of blood the heart can pump with each beat, leading to an inadequate supply of oxygen-rich blood to the body. In advanced disease, the thickening may actually block the aorta (the main artery leaving the heart), so that little or no blood actually reaches the body.

The major symptoms of hypertrophic cardiomyopathy are shortness of breath; angina (chest pain), which is often long-lasting and occurs after rather than during exercise; and loss of consciousness or light-headedness with exertion. Heart rhythm may also be affected, producing palpitations (uncomfortably fast, irregular heartbeat). Sudden death due to cardiac arrest can occur as a result but is rare.

Hypertrophic cardiomyopathy can result from heart valve problems or a history of uncontrolled hypertension. The disease can also be hereditary. The inherited form of the disease usually starts in the teens or 20s, with symptoms developing by age 35. It is more common in men than in women and in blacks than in whites.

■ *Restrictive cardiomyopathy* This is the least common type of cardiomyopathy. The heart muscle becomes so stiff that during the relaxation phase between heartbeats little blood enters the ventricles. Since the heart can only pump the blood it actually receives, the flow of blood into the lungs and the body decreases. A person with restrictive cardiomyopathy is likely to complain of fatigue, have swollen hands and feet, and experience difficulty breathing during exertion. Pain in the upper right abdomen, nausea, bloating, and loss of appetite are also common. Angina may occur as well. Congestive heart failure (see HEART FAILURE, CONGESTIVE) and cardiac arrhythmias (heart rhythm problems) can result.

Restrictive cardiomyopathy can result from any condition that causes extensive scarring of the heart muscle. The heart can scar in reaction to radiation or drug treatment for cancer or in reaction to the cancer itself. Diseases that affect connective tissue throughout the body (for example, SCLERODERMA) can scar the heart. Restrictive cardiomyopathy can also result from diseases that cause deposits of abnormal materials, such as amyloidosis, in which certain blood cells produce protein that accumulates in the heart, kidneys, liver, skin, blood vessels, and intestinal tract.

DIAGNOSIS AND TREATMENT
Depending on symptoms, a number of tests may be needed to determine whether cardiomyopathy is present and, if so, in which form. A chest X ray can show the size of the heart and reveal the presence of pulmonary congestion. An ECG (electrocardiogram) is useful for determining the electrical patterns of the heart, which are often disturbed by cardiomyopa-thy. In echocardiography, a transducer transmits ultrasound waves that bounce off the heart and into a machine that translates the echoes into an image of the heart. This image allows doctors to visualize the heart while it is beating and to determine the volume and direction of blood flow through the heart. If infection is suspected, the doctor may perform a biopsy of heart tissue for examination.

Treatment of cardiomyopathy depends on the type and severity of disease and its symptoms. A number of medications are useful. Diuretics, which increase urine production and rid the body of excess fluid and salt, help in the treatment of edema, bloating, and shortness of breath. Beta blockers neutralize the effect of adrenaline, which can have a role in enlargement of the heart. Medications called vasodilators, which cause the arteries to dilate (widen), reduce the workload on the heart. Diuretics, beta blockers, and vasodilators all reduce blood pressure, which may also improve the symptoms of cardiomyopathy. In some people, medications that increase the pumping power of the heart, such as digitalis, are prescribed. Anticoagulants, which reduce the blood's ability to clot, are appropriate for those in whom slowed blood flow may increase the risk of stroke. If cardiomyopathy has resulted from excessive use of alcohol, abstinence from drinking alcohol will often stop and possibly even reverse the disorder. For people in whom the cardiomyopathy is caused by myocarditis (inflammation of the heart muscle), treatment of the infection may resolve the inflammation and reverse the heart muscle disease.

For some cardiomyopathies, surgery is a treatment option. The most common surgical procedure is removal of part of the thickened septum in hypertrophic cardiomyopathy, a procedure called a myectomy (literally, "muscle removal"). A PACEMAKER is often implanted in people whose cardiomyopathy causes irregularities in heart rhythm. If cardiomyopathy cannot be halted or reversed and the disease progresses despite the use of medications, a HEART TRANSPLANT offers the best chance for continued survival.

Cardiopulmonary resuscitation (CPR)

Lifesaving techniques used to maintain oxygen and blood flow to people who are unconscious and have stopped breathing. CPR is a combination of rescue breathing, used to maintain oxygen flow to the lungs, and chest compressions, used to maintain blood circulation while awaiting emergency medical assistance.

CPR is performed in emergencies involving cardiac arrest, choking, drowning, or when the person is unconscious and has stopped breathing. Death can occur in 8 to 10 minutes when a person has stopped breathing, and brain death can occur in only 4 to 6 minutes. CPR should be given only by people who have been trained in CPR.

CARDIOPULMONARY ARREST

Cardiopulmonary arrest is a combination of two life-threatening conditions, the absence of breathing and the absence of a pulse, the sign of a beating heart. CPR is given only if the person is unresponsive and has stopped breathing. CPR keeps oxygenated blood flowing to the brain and other organs until medical treatment is available to restore normal heart function.

The key techniques involved in CPR are rescue breathing and chest compression. The airway is opened to ensure that there is nothing blocking the windpipe; mouth-to-mouth rescue breathing is necessary to get oxygen to the person's lungs; and chest compressions replace the missing heartbeat to maintain blood flow to the brain and other organs.

■ *Airway* In CPR, the first action is to open the airway, which may be obstructed by the person's tongue. The person is placed flat on his or her back, on a firm surface, with the neck extended. To open the mouth and airway, the person's chin is lifted forward. A careful check is made to see if the person is breathing. If the person is not breathing, rescue breathing should be started.

■ *Rescue breathing* Once it has been determined that the person is not breathing, mouth-to-mouth breathing will involve closing the person's nostrils with one hand and breathing into his or her mouth once every 5 seconds. If the person's chest does not rise as a result of mouth-to-mouth breathing, the airway may be blocked and must be opened by repositioning the head followed by a chin lift or with the HEIMLICH MANEUVER, pressing upward on the abdomen sharply to dislodge the obstruction.

■ *Chest compression* If an unresponsive person is not moving or breathing, chest compressions can keep the blood flowing until help arrives. By placing the hands over the chest, with elbows straight and weight centered above the person's chest, the person performing CPR can push on the person's chest at a rate of 80 to 100 times per minute. After 15 chest compressions, two rescue breaths should be given; and the person's pulse and breathing should be checked after every four cycles of 15 compressions and two breaths.

CPR FOR INFANTS AND CHILDREN UNDER 8

When CPR is performed on an infant younger than 1 year, the same techniques already described are used, with the following exceptions. Mouth-to-mouth rescue breathing should be performed while covering the baby's mouth and nose tightly with the rescuer's mouth. Chest compression should be performed on an infant by encircling the chest with the rescuer's hands and compressing with two thumbs or by placing two fingers over the lower breastbone. This is performed in a cycle of five compressions followed by one rescue breath. Pulse and breathing should be reassessed after every 10 cycles.

For children aged 1 to 8, chest compressions should be given with the heel of one hand in a cycle of five compressions followed by one rescue breath. Pulse and breathing should be reassessed after every 10 cycles.

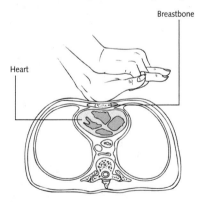

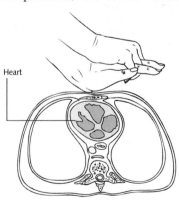

Breastbone

Heart

Heart

Compression stage

Release stage

PROVIDING PUMPING ACTION
When a person administers CPR, the compression stage physically forces blood out of the heart and into the lungs and the rest of the body. When the pressure is released and the chest wall returns to its normal position, blood is drawn back into the heart from the lungs and the rest of the body.

Cardiorespiratory fitness

The capacity of the heart and lungs to function during physical activity. Cardiorespiratory fitness is measured using equipment that records a person's heart rate, blood pressure, and respiration. The testing is called pulmonary exercise testing, incremental exercise testing, CARDIAC STRESS TESTING, or (more informally) exercise stress testing.

The person being tested is attached to devices that measure and analyze the heart rate, blood pressure, and oxygen in the blood while he or she cycles, walks, or runs on exercise equipment in a hospital, doctor's office, or pulmonary function laboratory. Electrocardiogram (ECG) electrodes may be attached to the chest, a blood pressure cuff is positioned on the arm, and a pulse oximeter is placed on the finger, ear, or nose. A nose clip may be used to prevent exhaled air from escaping through the nostrils, allowing the air to be exhaled through the mouth and collected for analysis.

The exercise begins at a given rate, and the intensity is increased every 2 to 3 minutes until the person being tested reaches his or her point of maximum exercise capacity within 8 to 12 minutes. This point of maximum capacity is calculated based on the person's medical history, height, weight, and sex. The exercise may be stopped if the person being tested cannot reach maximum capacity because of exhaustion or because the test shows signs of medical problems or ECG abnormalities. The test's measurements reveal the heart rate, respiratory rate, oxygen uptake by the lungs, and concentration of oxygen and carbon dioxide in the exhaled air. The analysis of these measurements can establish the cause of limitations in a person's cardiorespiratory fitness, or ability to exercise.

Cardiothoracic surgery

Any procedure used to treat a disease, abnormality, or injury in the chest (thorax), particularly in or around the heart. This includes coronary artery bypass and valve surgery of the heart; removal of lung tumors and abscesses; and repair of injuries to the heart, lungs, and chest walls.

Cardiovascular

Pertaining to the heart and blood vessels.

Cardiovascular fitness

The ability of the heart to sustain exertion without undue stress. Cardiovascular fitness is promoted by regular exercise—at a minimum, 20 to 30 minutes a session, 3 times a week—that strengthens the heart and lungs. Cardiovascular fitness activities include walking, jogging, bicycling, jumping rope, racket sports, cross-country skiing, swimming, rowing, and dancing.

Cardiovascular surgeon

A physician who specializes in operating on the heart and blood vessels. Cardiovascular surgeons earn a medical degree (MD or DO), then complete 5 to 6 years of general surgery training, followed by an additional 2 to 3 years of cardiovascular surgical training. They perform such procedures as bypass surgery, heart valve repair, and removal of aortic aneurysms (abnormal widening or ballooning of the aorta).

Cardiovascular system

The HEART and the BLOOD VESSELS, also called the circulatory system, which transports the BLOOD that carries oxygen, carbon dioxide, nutrients, antibodies, enzymes, and waste materials throughout the body. This vast system is vital to maintaining life.

THE HEART

The heart is the center of the cardiovascular system, the 1-pound muscular organ that keeps blood circulating throughout the body. The heart functions as two side-by-side pumps, each of which sends the blood through a different system of circulation. The left side of the heart controls the systemic circulation, which pumps oxygen-rich blood to all tissues in the body. The right side of the heart controls the pulmonary circulation to the lungs, where exhausted blood is rejuvenated with fresh oxygen.

Systemic circulation begins in the left atrium, the upper left chamber of the heart, which receives oxygen-rich blood from the pulmonary circulation. The blood travels into the left ventricle, the lower left chamber of the heart, which forcefully pumps it out into the aorta, the main artery of the body. Arteries branching off from the aorta carry blood to different parts of the body and into smaller arteries called arterioles that reach various organs. Arterioles branch into smaller, finer blood vessels called capillaries. Through the microscopic walls of the capillaries, oxygen and other nutrients pass from the blood into body tissues at a cellular level.

Pulmonary circulation begins when the oxygen-depleted blood flows from the capillaries into small veins called venules, carrying with it carbon dioxide and other waste products of the chemical activities in body tissues. The venules combine to form veins, which carry the blood back to the right side of the heart. The blood travels from the right atrium into the right ventricle, which pumps it through the pulmonary artery to the lungs. In the lungs, carbon dioxide is exchanged for oxygen (which has entered the lungs from the air). The newly oxygenated blood then flows back into the heart's left atrium to reenter the systemic circulation.

BLOOD VESSELS

Blood vessels include both arteries and veins; the functional difference between the two is the direction the blood is flowing. Arteries carry blood away from the heart, while veins carry blood toward the heart. Both veins and arteries are made up of three layers of tissue, but arteries are thicker, more muscular, and more elastic than veins because the blood moving through them is under higher pressure. Arterial blood moves not only because of the heart's pumping action, but also because of the muscular contraction, or pulse, passing through the artery walls. This pulse can be felt easily in places like the wrist or alongside the neck in the large artery called the carotid artery. Veins do not have a pulse, but the movement of muscles surrounding the veins helps push the blood through them. In many parts of the body, such as the arms and legs, arteries and veins travel alongside one another, so that the pulse of the artery also helps propel the venous blood toward the heart. The veins of the arms and legs have one-way valves that keep the blood moving against gravity and in the direction of the heart. There are no valves in the veins of the head, neck, and torso.

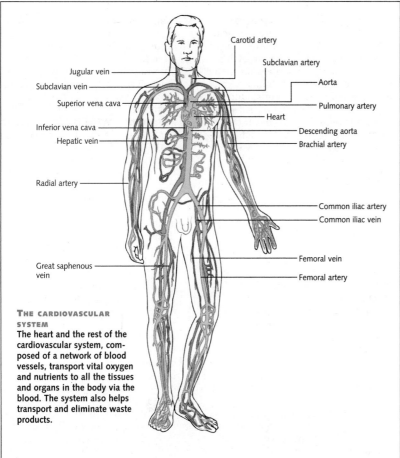

Carotid artery
Subclavian artery
Jugular vein
Subclavian vein
Aorta
Superior vena cava
Pulmonary artery
Inferior vena cava
Heart
Hepatic vein
Descending aorta
Brachial artery
Radial artery
Common iliac artery
Common iliac vein
Femoral vein
Femoral artery
Great saphenous
vein

**THE CARDIOVASCULAR
SYSTEM**
The heart and the rest of the
cardiovascular system, composed of a network of blood
vessels, transport vital oxygen
and nutrients to all the tissues
and organs in the body via the
blood. The system also helps
transport and eliminate waste
products.

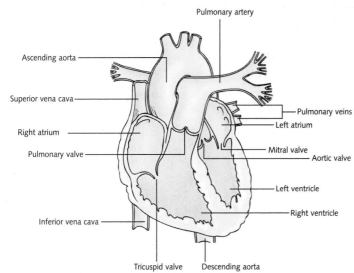

Pulmonary artery
Ascending aorta
Superior vena cava
Pulmonary veins
Left atrium
Right atrium
Mitral valve
Pulmonary valve
Aortic valve
Left ventricle
Right ventricle
Inferior vena cava
Tricuspid valve   Descending aorta

THE HEART
The heart is a muscular organ that pumps blood throughout the body. The right side receives
blood from the body and sends it to the lungs, where it picks up fresh oxygen. The oxygen-rich
blood then flows to the left side of the heart, which pumps it back out to the rest of the body.

FUNCTIONS
The cardiovascular system has key
roles in several fundamental body
processes. In addition to supplying
the oxygen that the body's cells need
to survive and function, the cardiovascular system also carries nutrients
throughout the body as a function of
the systemic circulation. Blood is
diverted into the liver (via portal circulation) where capillaries carrying
proteins, fats, carbohydrates, minerals, and other nutrients from the
stomach and other digestive organs
pass these nutrients into the liver to
be processed for use or to be stored.
Blood from the liver then travels back
into the systemic circulation.

The cardiovascular system also participates in the function of the IMMUNE
SYSTEM, which protects the body from
infection. White blood cells, which
help guard the body against invading
viruses, bacteria, and other microorganisms, are transported in the blood
into the LYMPHATIC SYSTEM, a complex
system of nodes and vessels that carry
fluids throughout the body. White
blood cells patrol the body, circulating
through the blood and the lymphatic
vessels to detect germs and remove
damaged cells.

Cardioversion

A procedure in which an electrical
shock is administered to the heart in
an attempt to restore an abnormal
heart rhythm to normal. Cardioversion is similar to the emergency procedure known as DEFIBRILLATION,
except that it uses a smaller amount
of electricity, is rarely used in an
emergency, and is applied most often
to cardiac arrhythmias (heartbeat
abnormalities) that are not immediately life-threatening. Cardioversion
is a standard treatment for ATRIAL FIB-
RILLATION (the upper chambers of the
heart quiver rather than contract,
causing an abnormally fast and rapid
heartbeat) and ventricular tachycardia (a fast heartbeat that begins in the
lower heart chambers rather than the
upper; see TACHYCARDIA, VENTRICULAR).
In chemical cardioversion, medications are used in place of electric
shock to produce the same effect on
an abnormal heartbeat.

THE PROCEDURE
In preparation for cardioversion, anticoagulant medications are prescribed
for some people for 3 weeks before

C

the procedure and 4 weeks after the procedure to decrease the risk of blood clots. All persons undergoing cardioversion are instructed to refrain from eating or drink anything for 8 to 12 hours before the procedure. The person is connected to a heart monitor and given medications intravenously to aid in relaxation. Large sticky patches containing electrodes are attached to the chest and connected by wires to a defibrillator, which the doctor has calibrated to deliver the appropriate amount of electrical shock at the correct time. Before the shock, the person undergoing the procedure is given a strong sedative or a quick-acting general anesthetic, so that he or she is insensitive to pain. The shock lasts only 1 second; in many cases, subsequent shocks are given at incrementally higher doses. Once the heart rhythm returns to normal, the anesthetic or sedative is withdrawn and the person returns to waking consciousness. A typical cardioversion takes approximately 30 minutes, and the person is unconscious for only 2 or 3 minutes of that time. Following the procedure, the person's condition is monitored for several hours to ensure a stable heart rhythm and normal blood pressure. Driving should be avoided for 24 hours after cardioversion to ensure full recovery from the anesthetic and sedatives.

OUTCOMES AND COMPLICATIONS
Most persons who undergo cardioversion achieve a normal heart rhythm immediately. Antiarrhythmic medications are prescribed for many of these people to maintain a normal heartbeat following the procedure. In some cases, cardioversion has to be repeated periodically, or a device (implantable cardioverter defibrillator) must be placed in the chest surgically to monitor the heart and maintain a normal heartbeat.

The principal risk of cardioversion is dislodging a blood clot in the heart, which can then travel through the bloodstream and lodge in an artery, usually in the lungs, brain, kidneys, or legs. Anticoagulant medications reduce this risk.

Caregiving for older people

Assistance to older adults, ranging from minor help to constant care. Most caregivers are unpaid family members. About three fourths of them are women, and about one fourth of all family-member caregivers are in their 50s and 60s. Infirm older people may require professional care or nursing services. More than half the older people who receive assistance from a caregiver live independently. Caregivers enable them to avoid the expense of a nursing home or other LONG-TERM CARE FACILITY.

Many older people prefer to preserve their independence and remain among familiar surroundings and friends for as long as possible. Nursing homes, while providing extensive care, are expensive and, in most cases, are not covered by Medicare.

ASSISTANCE WITH DAILY ACTIVITIES
Caregiving can involve personal help with dressing and bathing or assistance with grocery shopping, cooking, and money management. When recovering from an injury or surgery, an older individual may temporarily need constant help. Those who have a chronic health problem such as dementia (a progressive brain disorder that causes increasing memory loss and confusion) require much more attention. ALZHEIMER'S DISEASE is the most common cause of dementia, and most people who have this condition eventually need around-the-clock care.

PROFESSIONAL SERVICES
Older people who are homebound or bed-bound may need professional home care. In such cases, the physician can arrange for allied health professionals to visit the home. For example, a nurse may come to give injections or manage a catheter. After hip surgery, a physical therapist can make regular visits to help an older person regain muscle strength and flexibility. People who have had a stroke may need speech therapy to relearn how to speak or how to swallow without choking. An occupational therapist might visit the home to suggest better ways to perform daily tasks such as bathing. He or she may also recommend home modifications to make houses and apartments safer and easier to get around in, preventing accidents such as falls. See also FALLS, IN OLDER PEOPLE.

SUPPORT FOR CAREGIVERS
Despite the personal rewards of caregiving, most family-member caregivers experience depression or high levels of stress at some time. Tending to the needs of older people is often physically and emotionally demanding. For example, an older person may need physical assistance getting in and out of bed or may experience periods of anxiety and forgetfulness. Such conditions require considerable patience on the caregiver's part. Caregivers commonly experience

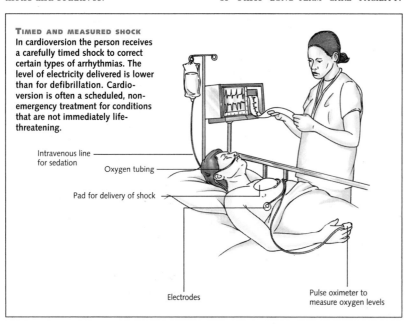

TIMED AND MEASURED SHOCK
In cardioversion the person receives a carefully timed shock to correct certain types of arrhythmias. The level of electricity delivered is lower than for defibrillation. Cardioversion is often a scheduled, non-emergency treatment for conditions that are not immediately life-threatening.

Intravenous line for sedation

Oxygen tubing

Pad for delivery of shock

Electrodes

Pulse oximeter to measure oxygen levels

CHANGING THE SHEETS

One of the tasks involved in providing home care for someone who is immobile or bedridden is changing the bed sheets regularly. Sheets must be changed whenever they are soiled, and at least every 4 or 5 days. Sheets made of 100-percent cotton are best because they absorb perspiration.

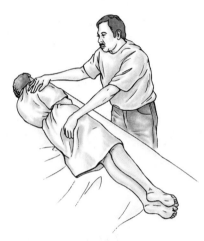

CHANGING THE BED: STEP ONE
It is possible to replace the bottom sheet with a clean sheet safely when a person is unable to get out of bed. After determining the person is not in pain or distress, the caregiver loosens the bottom sheet and gently rolls him or her onto one side.

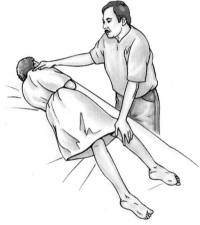

STEP TWO
Next, the caregiver moves the person toward himself or herself—near the edge of the bed—making sure that the person's position is stable. In this way, a fall can be prevented.

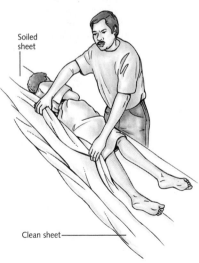

Soiled sheet

Clean sheet

STEP THREE
Next the caregiver rolls half of the soiled bottom sheet lengthwise against the person's back. Then the caregiver rolls half the clean sheet lengthwise and places it on the bed as shown.

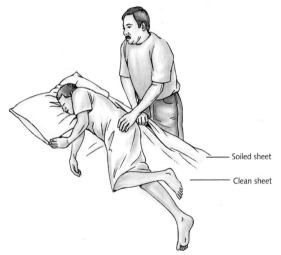

Soiled sheet

Clean sheet

STEP FOUR
The person is rolled carefully onto the flat clean sheet, and the dirty sheet is removed. The caregiver then unrolls the remainder of the clean sheet, smoothing out the wrinkles and tucks it in at the corners.

C

C

MOVING A PERSON

People who provide home care for someone who is weak or bedridden need to learn how to move the person safely. A caregiver must use proper technique in order to avoid injuring his or her back and also avoid injuring the patient. Use of a transfer belt—a special device placed around the person's waist—may be helpful.

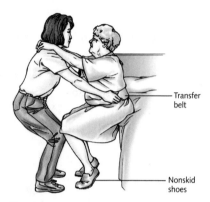

Transfer belt

Nonskid shoes

TRANSFERRING FROM BED TO CHAIR: STEP ONE
The caregiver and the patient should both wear shoes or slippers with nonskid soles. A transfer belt makes it easier to grip the person who needs help and provides leverage. Step 1 is to guide the person to a sitting position on the side of the bed, with feet flat on the floor. The caregiver can brace the peson against his or her knees.

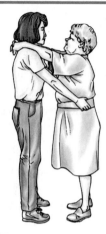

STEP TWO
After pausing to make sure the person does not feel dizzy, the caregiver helps the person to a standing position. At that point the caregiver can safely guide the patient to a chair.

family conflicts and feelings of guilt as they struggle to balance the needs of aging parents with the care of their own children, the demands of a job, and other responsibilities. As a consequence, many caregivers suffer insomnia, fatigue, or other physical or emotional problems.

The strains of caregiving can be alleviated with emotional and community support, counseling, training in how to provide home care, and RESPITE CARE. Respite care provides a temporary break for the caregiver. It is available from services that offer home health care, adult day care (see DAY CARE, ADULT), and temporary, short-term institutional care. Nursing homes and board-and-care facilities will often accept a resident for a short period of time. Home health agencies can arrange for care in the home, or an older person can spend part of each day in an adult day care program. These arrangements may allow a caregiver to go on vacation or spend more time with other family members. State or AREA AGENCIES ON AGING can provide information about training for caregivers and respite care. Community support services

may include transportation, home-delivered meals, home health services, and adult day care programs.

Caries, bottle
See BABY BOTTLE TOOTH DECAY.

Caries, dental
See CAVITY, DENTAL.

Carisoprodol
A muscle relaxant used to relieve the pain of specific muscle injuries. Carisoprodol (Soma) is prescribed for the pain and discomfort associated with sprains, spasms, strains, and other muscle injuries. The medication does not relax muscles directly, but relieves discomfort through a sedative effect that can cause drowsiness and impair a person's ability to drive.

Carotene
An orange pigment found in plants that is converted to VITAMIN A by the liver, lungs, and intestines. Orange fruits and vegetables such as cantaloupe, papaya, carrots, sweet potatoes, and pumpkin are rich in carotene. This substance is also found in dark green, leafy vegetables

such as spinach and kale. Vitamin A is essential for growth and development and helps maintain healthy eyes, skin, and mucous membranes and normal bone structure. Carotene is an antioxidant chemical that may prevent damaging changes in cells. Studies are ongoing to find out whether antioxidants help reduce the risk of heart disease and certain types of cancer.

Carotid artery
One of four major blood vessels of the neck and head. In the lower neck, there are two common carotid arteries (left and right), with two branches (internal and external). The left common cartoid artery leads from the aorta and runs up the neck on the left side of the trachea (windpipe). Just above the larynx (voice box) it divides in two, forming the left internal carotid and the left external carotid arteries. The right common carotid artery leads out from the subclavian artery, itself a branch of the aorta, and then divides in a similar fashion on the right side of the neck.

The external carotid arteries subdivide to supply the face and scalp,

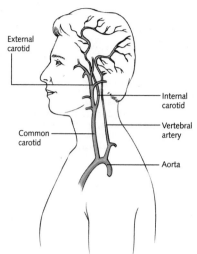

MAJOR BLOOD VESSEL
The carotid arteries arise from parts of the aorta, then branch out into the internal and external carotids in the neck. The external carotids supply blood to most of the face, scalp, mouth, and jaws. The internal carotids supply the brain and eyes.

while the internal carotid arteries form a network to supply the eyes and the brain. At the base of the brain, the internal carotids and another artery (the basilar artery) form a major ring of blood vessels called the circle of Willis.

Carotid endarterectomy

A surgical procedure used to remove the buildup of fat and cholesterol in the principal artery supplying blood to the brain, restore normal blood flow, and lower the risk of STROKE. Fat and cholesterol deposits (plaques) form as a result of ATHEROSCLEROSIS. Plaque buildup in the carotid artery is most common at the point where it divides into its two branches: the internal, which supplies the eye and the brain, and the external, which supplies the remainder of the head. Plaque is stripped away during carotid endarterectomy, widening the opening in the artery and increasing blood supply to the brain.

Carotid endarterectomy is usually performed in those who have already had a stroke or a temporary strokelike event (see TRANSIENT ISCHEMIC ATTACK) and who have at least a 50 percent blockage in the carotid artery. The procedure is sometimes used to treat persons who have not experienced a

stroke or transient ischemic attack but who have 80 percent or greater blockage in the carotid artery.

Carotid endarterectomy is done with the person asleep under general anesthesia or sedated and numbed with a local anesthetic in the surgical area. The surgeon makes an incision in the neck to expose the carotid artery. Either the artery is clamped above and below the blockage, or a bypass tube is installed to route the blood past the blockage during surgery. The surgeon then opens the artery, removes the plaque and the internal artery lining, and closes the artery, often using a patch of synthetic or natural material to add strength. The neck incision is closed after removal of the clamps or bypass tube.

The procedure typically requires a hospital stay of 1 to 2 days. During this period the person needs to lie flat and turn the head as little as possible. Aching or soreness in the neck persists for approximately 2 weeks after surgery.

Carotid endarterectomy is effective in reducing the risk of future stroke or transient ischemic attacks. Possible complications include infection of the incision, hypotension (low blood pressure) after surgery, and heart attack, stroke, or sudden death during surgery. In some cases, hyperperfu-

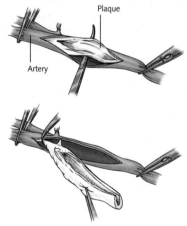

CLEANING ARTERIAL WALLS
To remove accumulated cholesterol and debris (plaque) from the wall of an artery , the surgeon closes off a section of the artery, opens the wall, and lifts the plaque from the wall lining. He or she snips off the plaque, taking care to make a clean endpoint so that the interior wall of the artery is smooth.

sion syndrome results, in which the brain adapts poorly to the increased blood supply, leading to headache, seizure, or stroke.

Carpal tunnel syndrome

Compression of the median nerve that causes numbness, tingling, weakness, or pain in the hand or wrist. Carpal tunnel syndrome is an example of a nerve entrapment syndrome and is by far the most common compression syndrome. See also COMPRESSION SYNDROME; NERVE ENTRAPMENT; and PINCHED NERVE.

CAUSES

The median nerve supplies sensation and movement to the hand. Carpal tunnel syndrome is caused by pressure on or compression of the median nerve as it passes between the bones and a ligament at the front of the wrist. In some individuals, carpal tunnel syndrome is the result of a REPETITIVE STRAIN INJURY, which is caused by activities such as uninterrupted computer keyboard use. Other conditions associated with carpal tunnel syndrome include pregnancy; diabetes mellitus, type 2; obesity; arthritis; hypothyroidism; and trauma. However, in many people, the cause of this condition is unknown.

SYMPTOMS

A trapped or compressed median nerve causes symptoms such as numbness, tingling, weakness, and pain. People with carpal tunnel syndrome initially experience numbness and tingling of the hand in the areas supplied by the median nerve, including the thumb and index, middle, and part of the fourth fingers. These sensations are often more pronounced at night and may cause wakening. As the disease progresses, there may be burning, cramping, and weakness of the hand. Decreased hand grip can cause dropping of objects. Sometimes shooting pains are experienced in the forearm. Chronic carpal tunnel syndrome can eventually lead to wasting or atrophy of hand muscles.

DIAGNOSIS

Physical examination usually reveals a weak hand grip and decreased sensation in the palm, index finger, thumb, middle finger, and thumbside of the ring finger. When the doc-

PROTECTING THE WRISTS

When the median nerve of the hand is damaged or the ligaments of the wrist press against the nerve, numbness, tingling, burning, or aching of fingers and thumb may result. These symptoms can be treated with a splint to immobilize the wrist or with nonsteroidal anti-inflammatory drugs to reduce swelling near the nerve. If symptoms are more severe, surgery may be recommended. Some simple habits can help prevent the problem known as carpal tunnel syndrome.

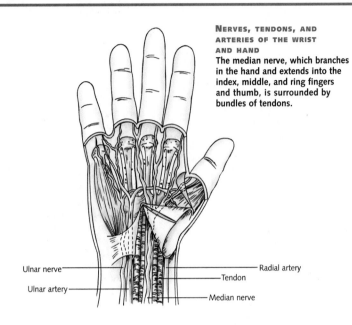

NERVES, TENDONS, AND ARTERIES OF THE WRIST AND HAND
The median nerve, which branches in the hand and extends into the index, middle, and ring fingers and thumb, is surrounded by bundles of tendons.

Ulnar nerve

Ulnar artery

Radial artery

Tendon

Median nerve

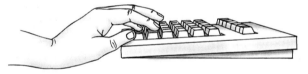

CORRECT WRIST POSITION
Wrist joints should be held parallel to the floor when working at a keyboard to prevent carpal tunnel syndrome.

INCORRECT WRIST POSITION
Letting the wrist joint bend for extended periods can lead to carpal tunnel syndrome.

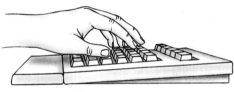

WRIST PRESS EXERCISE
People who use their hands extensively for their jobs should do a 5-minute warm-up before starting work.

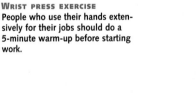

BALL SQUEEZE EXERCISE
Squeezing a ball is an example of a strengthening exercise that can help prevent carpal tunnel syndrome.

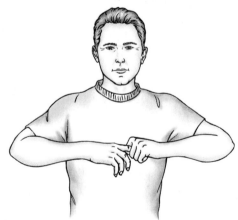

FINGER PULL EXERCISE
Periodic stretching exercises are recommended to prevent carpal tunnel syndrome.

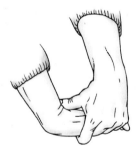

tor taps the median nerve at the front of the wrist, it may cause sensations of tingling (Tinel sign). Bending the wrist forward increases the compression on the nerve and may also reproduce symptoms (Phalen maneuver). The doctor may order a nerve conduction study to determine the severity of pressure on the median nerve. Wrist X rays and electromyography may provide additional useful information.

TREATMENT

Most cases of carpal tunnel syndrome can be treated with braces or splints. These are worn to relieve or minimize pressure on nerves. It is also important to identify and avoid or control the activity (such as repetitive, uninterrupted work at a computer keyboard) that contributes to the problem. In some cases, nonsteroidal anti-inflammatory drugs (NSAIDs) are prescribed to reduce inflammation and swelling. If splints and NSAIDs fail to control an individual's symptoms, a corticosteroid injection may prove beneficial. A corticosteroid injection may reduce inflammation and swelling, which in turn lessens the nerve compression. A small number of people require surgery. This entails opening the wrist and cutting the fibrous tissue across the wrist to relieve the pressure.

Carrier

A person in whom the specific organisms of a disease reside, but who does not show any apparent symptoms of the disease. A carrier is capable of transmitting the infection to another person. In genetics, a carrier is a person who has a recessive gene and therefore displays no trait from it but can still transmit the trait to offspring.

Cartilage

A smooth, fibrous, and dense connective tissue that is an important component of the skeleton. It is not as hard as bone, but is composed of the same material, a structural protein called collagen. Cells in cartilage also secrete a gelatinous substance that gives cartilage some of its flexibility. There are three types of cartilage in the human skeleton: hyaline, elastic, and fibrocartilage. Hyaline cartilage is strong and smooth, covering the ends of bones in free-moving joints such as the shoulder, elbow, and knee. It also is found in the nose, trachea, and bronchi. Elastic cartilage is also flexible and soft and is found in the outer ear and the epiglottis. The third type, fibrocartilage, is very dense and highly resistant to impact and twisting. It is found in the disks that join the vertebrae in the spinal column, and in the knee. Cartilage lacks its own blood supply, which is why it heals slowly when torn or damaged in a sports injury or trauma. Slower, wear-and-tear damage to cartilage in joints will also gradually repair itself.

The skeleton of a developing fetus is composed of cartilage that gradually hardens into bone—a process called ossification. Throughout childhood, the ends of the long bones contain growth plates at either end composed of cartilage cells that continually form new layers of bone tissue. Once these cells stop dividing, the growth plates harden into bone, and bone growth is complete.

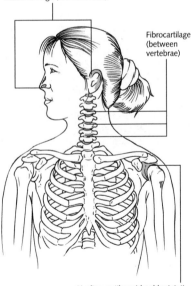

Elastic cartilage (nose and ears)

Fibrocartilage (between vertebrae)

Hyaline cartilage (shoulder joint)

THREE TYPES OF CARTILAGE
Specialized cartilage is found on different areas of the skeleton. Elastic cartilage (ear, nose, larynx) provides flexibility even as it helps support and maintain the shape of organs, Fibrocartilage (between vertebrae, in pelvis, hip, shoulder) absorbs shock, provides sturdiness, and lines sockets. Hyaline cartilage (shoulders, breastbone, ends of bones) reduces friction at joints and allows movement.

Case manager

A professional who is trained to assess, plan, implement, coordinate, and monitor the options and services necessary to meet a person's health care needs. Case managers work in a variety of situations, including hospitals, health care plans, physicians' practices, skilled nursing facilities, and assisted living centers.

Case-control studies

A design for human research that involves matching a group of people (known as the case patients) who have a particular disease, chronic condition, or injury with another group of people (known as the controls) who lack the disease, condition, or injury in order to detect the differences between them. Although case-control studies are considered statistically crude, they are often the most practical method for studying harmful outcomes, such as cancer caused by exposure to an environmental pollutant or industrial chemical.

Cast

A firm splinting device used to enclose and immobilize injured bones and soft tissues in the limbs or torso so that healing can occur. By keeping broken bones and injured soft tissues covered and compressed, a cast maintains a bone in place so that it can heal properly and prevents movement that might cause further injury. See FRACTURE.

A cast may be used to provide stability to an unstable fracture and to provide rest and relieve the pain of certain injuries. Casts may also be used to aid in joint stability and in the realignment of deformed or improperly positioned tissues, such as those occurring with club foot, congenital hip dislocation, or dysplasia. Casts are made of plaster or synthetic material, most commonly fiberglass. Plaster, which requires 24 hours to dry entirely, is generally preferred for its strength, plasticity, and close fit. Synthetic casts are more lightweight and water resistant. The length of time necessary for a cast to be worn depends on the type of condition being treated and the individual progress of healing.

Complications connected with the use of casts are rare but include pres-

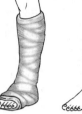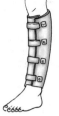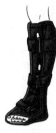

Plaster cast   Fiberglass cast   Air splint

TYPES OF CASTS
A plaster cast is the strongest, most rigid, and most tightly fitting type of immobilization for a broken bone. A fiberglass cast is lighter and more durable and provides for clearer X-ray examination of the fracture as it heals. An air splint, or half cast, provides less support but can be adjusted as the injury heals; it may be used for sprains and minor fractures or late in recovery.

sure ulcerations, compression of the nerves and blood vessels, skin infection, and COMPARTMENT SYNDROME. Casts are removed with a cast cutter (a specialized, small vibrating saw) that cuts through the plaster from one end of the cast to the other but should not injure underlying skin if properly used. A pair of blunt-end scissors is used to cut through the protective skin coverings, which may be stockinette, sheet wadding, or spandex. After a cast is removed, there may be swelling, stiffness, soreness or weakness of muscles surrounding the injured bone and increased tenderness with pain.

Castration

Surgical removal of the testicles in a man or the ovaries in a woman; most often performed as part of cancer surgery. Castration may be used in the treatment of some breast and prostate cancers since estrogen stimulates the growth of some breast cancers and testosterone stimulates the growth of prostate cancer. See ORCHIECTOMY for the male surgery and OOPHORECTOMY for the female.

Cat-scratch disease

An uncommon disease caused primarily by the *Bartonella* bacteria, which are transmitted among cats by fleas. Cat-scratch disease (CSD) is usually but not always associated with a history of a cat's scratch or bite. It may be contracted from environmental sources of *Bartonella* bacteria or from other animals, including dogs. Bartonellosis is a more comprehensive term for CSD, which is also referred to as cat-scratch fever or benign lymphoreticulosis.

The disease is generally mild and improves without treatment. It most frequently affects people younger than 17 years, especially children younger than 12 years. Often, many members of a family may be infected at once.

SYMPTOMS AND DIAGNOSIS

The symptoms of CSD typically include a small reddish lesion at the site of a cat scratch or bite on the skin, swollen lymph nodes, and sometimes a fever. Swelling in the lymph nodes (armpit, neck bone, and above the collarbone) may persist for months. Headaches, joint pain, and eye redness may occur. Diagnosis is typically made by blood tests and sometimes from cultured tissue samples.

RISK FACTORS AND PREVENTION

Treatment of CSD is not usually required, although associated problems rarely may include tonsillitis, encephalitis, hepatitis, pneumonia, and other serious diseases. People who have AIDS (acquired immunodeficiency syndrome), cancer, or other conditions involving compromised immune systems are most at risk for complications.

Because kittens are more likely to carry the bacteria than adult cats, people who have weakened immune systems are advised to avoid cats younger than 1 year of age. Infected cats appear to be in good health. Scratches or bites from cats should be cleaned immediately with soap and water; teasing or rough play with cats should be discouraged.

Catalepsy

A rare, abnormal state of trancelike consciousness accompanied by postural rigidity. Catalepsy may last for hours. During this time, a person's expression and body position remain the same, even if the position appears uncomfortable (such as an upraised arm). Efforts to change the person's position will be met with resistance. Catalepsy may be a symptom of epilepsy, hysteria, or schizophrenia. It can also occur during hypnosis or as a result of brain disease.

Cataplexy

A sudden loss of voluntary muscle control. Cataplexy is a classic symptom of NARCOLEPSY (a sleep disorder characterized by sudden and irresistible collapses into sleep). Signs of cataplexy include slight weakness, a nodding head, garbled speech, sagging facial muscles, buckling knees, and limp arm muscles. In some cases, there is a total collapse, during which a person appears unconscious but remains awake and alert. Attacks last from several seconds to 30 minutes. They are triggered by emotions such as anger, fear, laughter, and surprise. Stress and fatigue increase a person's susceptibility to cataplexy.

Cataract

A cloudiness or opacity in the normally clear lens of the eye. The lens is made of water and protein, which are arranged in a specific way to preserve the clarity of the lens. A cataract forms when alterations in the proteins occur and form a cloudy or opaque area in a portion of the lens. Over time, the cataract tends to grow and affect more and more of the lens. In most cases, cataracts affect both eyes, although the condition may be more advanced in one eye than the other.

Cataracts that are present at birth or develop shortly thereafter are known as congenital cataracts. Adult cataracts develop with advancing age, usually over an extended time, and are most likely to affect vision in people older than 60 years. Cataracts are very common, affecting approximately seven of every ten people older than 75 years.

SYMPTOMS

In the early stages, a cataract has little effect on vision. As the cataract grows, vision may become blurred or cloudy. Lights can look too bright, appear to be surrounded by halos, and may cause increased glare, an effect that often hampers the ability to drive at night. Colors may seem muted, and overall night vision often worsens. Vision can become double or multiple. In advanced cases, the pupil of the eye is visibly milky or white rather than black.

CAUSES

Congenital cataracts often develop because of genetic inheritance, intrauterine infections (for example, rubella), or an inherited metabolic condition, such as galactosemia. Some congenital cataracts are sporadic, or occur without any other associated systemic or genetic impairment. Adult cataracts can develop as the result of an injury to the lens or because of metabolic disease, particularly diabetes mellitus, type 1 and type 2. Most cataracts are age-related and caused by changes in the proteins of the lens. Risk factors for adult cataract include exposure to the ultraviolet (UV) light present in sunlight, radioactivity, smoking, abnormally low levels of calcium in the blood, corticosteroid drugs (used for long-term treatment of rheumatoid arthritis, for example), and a family history of cataracts.

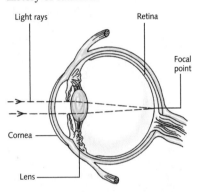

Healthy eye

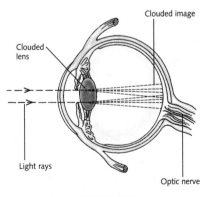

Eye with cataract

A CLOUDY LENS
A cataract is the result of chemical changes in the lens that create cloudy or opaque areas in the otherwise transparent structure. In healthy eyes, the lens focuses light on the retina to produce a clear image. A lens with a cataract blocks or alters the light transmission so that the image is blurred.

DETECTION, TREATMENT, AND PREVENTION

In most cases, cataracts are identified in the course of a professional eye examination, often before the individual has noticed any change in vision. In the early stages of the disease, glasses, magnifiers, and special lights may compensate for the vision change. The only lasting treatment is surgery, which involves removing the cloudy lens (see CATARACT SURGERY). The risk of getting cataracts may be reduced by protecting the eyes against UV light with UV-blocking sunglasses, avoiding tobacco, and treating diabetes and other metabolic diseases.

Cataract surgery

A procedure to restore vision lost because of cloudiness in the normally clear lens of the eye (see CATARACT for more information about this disease). The cloudy lens is removed and usually replaced with an artificial lens implant placed inside the eye. Rarely, when an implant cannot be placed, contact lenses or glasses with thick lenses are used.

Not everyone who has cataracts needs to have cataract surgery. In many cases, glasses, contact lenses, or improved lighting can compensate for the vision problems caused by cataracts. Surgery is indicated only when cataracts cause difficulty with reading, driving, and other basic visual tasks. Cataract surgery has become more common over the past decade because of its safety, ease, and excellent outcome.

In most cases, cataracts are present in both eyes. Surgery is performed first on one eye, then on the other, after the first eye has recovered.

THE PROCEDURE

In children with cataracts, surgery is performed with general anesthesia, usually in a hospital setting. In adults, the procedure is most often done under local anesthesia in a hospital or an outpatient surgical center. Conscious sedation is also frequently used—that is, the person is awake, but relaxed and insensitive to pain.

Before surgery, drops are placed in the eye to dilate the pupil, and the area around the eye is washed and cleaned. Working with a special microscope, the surgeon makes a small incision in the outer surface

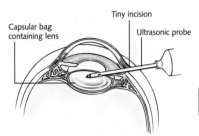

Inserting the probe

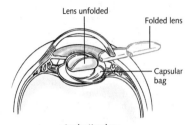

Implanting lens

REPLACEMENT OF DAMAGED LENS
Phacoemulsification is a type of cataract surgery that requires only a tiny, self-healing incision and an ultrasonic probe. The first step is to make the incision in the cornea and insert the probe to break up and suction out the old lens. The second step is to insert a new lens, folded to fit through the incision, and smooth it out into its proper position in the eye.

(cornea) of the eye. The lens is then removed, sometimes by cutting part of it away and suctioning out the remainder, sometimes by breaking the lens up with ultrasound waves and suctioning it out. In most cases, an intraocular lens implant is positioned inside the eye to replace the removed lens. The incision is so small it usually seals itself, but occasionally the incision needs extremely fine sutures to close it and a patch placed over the eye to protect it. The entire procedure lasts from 20 minutes to 1 hour. In most cases, people undergoing the procedure can be taken home soon after surgery.

RECOVERY AND OUTCOME

Following cataract surgery, itching and mild discomfort in the eye are normal. The eye may leak fluid and be sensitive to light and touch. If pain is present, a pain reliever every 4 to 6 hours is usually effective. In most cases, discomfort ends within 1 or 2 days of the surgery, although complete healing requires approximately 6 weeks. For a few days after surgery, drops to control pressure inside the eye may be prescribed. Most activity

C

is permitted during recovery, except bending and lifting, which raise pressure inside the eye.

Vision may be blurry soon after surgery, as the corrected eye learns to adjust to the other eye. Colors may also seem abnormally bright or blue-tinged. Color changes normally disappear within a few weeks.

People who have received a lens implant and who wear contact lenses or glasses typically need a new prescription a few weeks after surgery. If no intraocular lens has been placed in the eye, special contacts or glasses will be prescribed.

Complications from cataract surgery are not common. These include infection, bleeding, inflammation, loss of vision, light flashes, or retinal detachment. Prompt medical attention resolves most problems. In a few cases, a so-called after-cataract develops when a membrane from the original lens, which is intentionally left in the eye after surgery, becomes cloudy and blurs vision. After-cataract can be treated with a simple laser procedure in a doctor's office.

Catatonia

An extreme expression of physical activity in which the individual is either completely immobile or frantically overactive. A person immobilized by catatonia may hold a bizarre posture for hours or resist being moved; those who are hyperactive engage in frantic behavior that has no apparent purpose. Symptoms may also include resistance to all instructions, inability to talk (mutism), stupor, strange gestures or grimaces, unusual mannerisms, purposeless repetition of a word just spoken by someone else (echolalia), and repeated imitation of someone else's movements. People with catatonia may pose a risk to themselves or others and require supervision.

Catatonia has a number of possible causes. These include medical conditions that affect the function of the brain, such as brain cancer, inflammation of the brain (encephalitis), diseases of the brain's blood vessels, trauma, and certain metabolic abnormalities, as well as the adverse effects of some medications. Catatonia may also be a symptom of major DEPRESSION, BIPOLAR DISORDER, or SCHIZOPHRENIA. Patients are usually

treated in an inpatient psychiatric facility. Tranquilizers or electroconvulsive therapy may be used.

Catharsis

A sudden, often overpowering outpouring of repressed unconscious feelings surrounding an emotional conflict. This healthful or therapeutic release of ideas may occur through "talking out" conscious material during psychotherapy.

Cathartics

Agents that cause bowel movements by stimulating the movement of food through the digestive system. In the case of constipation, cathartics work by accelerating the passage of feces through the large intestine and elimination from the rectum.

Cathartics are sometimes given to people who have been poisoned because they decrease the available amount of the poison in the body by accelerating its expulsion from the digestive tract. Cathartics should never be given to a person who has been poisoned without the advice of a doctor or a specialist at a poison center.

Catheter

A flexible, hollow tube inserted into various body cavities. Catheters are commonly used to empty the bladder through the urethra (see CATHETERIZATION, URINARY) or to enter the heart

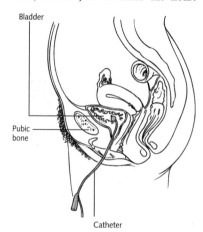

FLEXIBLE DRAINAGE TUBE
A urinary catheter is a common device used to drain urine from the bladder, often while a person recovers from surgery. The catheter, inserted into the urethra, carries the urine out of the body into a holding bag.

through a vein in the arm or leg for examination (see CATHETERIZATION, CARDIAC). Catheters are also used in PERITONEAL DIALYSIS for treatment of kidney failure.

Catheterization, cardiac

A minimally invasive procedure that involves threading a catheter (thin tube) through a blood vessel into the heart to obtain diagnostic information about the heart, coronary arteries (the arteries on the surface of the heart), and the aorta (the main artery leaving the heart). The doctor tracks the passage of the catheter through the circulatory system to the heart on a fluoroscope, an X-ray device that displays its image on a monitor. By injecting a special dye through the catheter, the doctor can take accurate X-ray pictures of the heart and its arteries.

INDICATIONS
Cardiac catheterization is performed primarily for three reasons. The first is to help make a diagnosis in cases in which symptoms, such as breathlessness or chest pain during exercise, suggest heart disease and preliminary test results are inconclusive. The second reason for cardiac catheterization is to assess the need for surgery. Once a disease has been diagnosed, cardiac catheterization may be used to get a detailed picture of the problem and to determine whether a person is a good candidate for surgery and whether any other defects that might complicate the surgery are present. The third reason cardiac catheterization is performed is for treatment (for example, BALLOON ANGIOPLASTY and STENT placement).

THE PROCEDURE
Depending on circumstances and the health of the person, cardiac catheterization can be performed as either an outpatient or inpatient procedure. The test is done in a catheterization laboratory, which resembles an operating room equipped with a wide variety of X-ray cameras, video displays, and monitoring equipment. The person to be tested lies on a table. An intravenous line is inserted into a blood vessel in the wrist or arm, and a mild sedative and other medications, such as anticoagulants, are injected into the bloodstream. The sedative relaxes the person

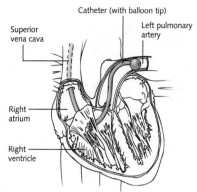

MEASURING HEART FUNCTION
One type of cardiac catheter is threaded through a blood vessel (often in the groin or elbow) into the heart and into the pulmonary artery (to the lungs). It is used to measure cardiac function and blood pressure. It is often placed in a person in an intensive care unit, when precise monitoring is necessary.

undergoing the procedure, but he or she remains aware and conscious during the test. The anticoagulants prevent blood clots. Monitoring devices are taped to the body to monitor heart rate and rhythm.

Many cardiologists use the groin or upper thigh to insert the catheter, but some prefer the elbow or wrist. The insertion site first is cleaned, shaved, swabbed with a disinfectant, and numbed with a local anesthetic. There are two ways to place the catheter. In the first, a needle is inserted into an artery, and a very thin guide wire is threaded through it. A device called a sheath is then pushed over the wire into the artery, and the catheter is inserted through the sheath, which is equipped with a one-way valve to prevent leaking. In the second method, the cardiologist makes a small incision to expose the artery, and the sheath is inserted through another small incision in the artery wall.

As the catheter is threaded through the artery to the heart, the cardiologist observes its progress on a monitor displaying a real-time X-ray image. In some cases, more than one catheter is inserted. This part of the procedure may cause discomfort, but it is not painful. Once the catheter or catheters are in position, the cardiologist begins testing.

A number of specific tests can be performed, depending on a person's symptoms. One is the left ventriculogram. A catheter is placed in the left ventricle (lower left chamber of the heart), which is the main pump for propelling blood into the body. A special dye or contrast medium is injected through the catheter, and X rays are taken to give a picture of the structure and to assess the function of that portion of the heart. The coronary arteries, which surround the heart and supply it with blood, are tested in a similar manner, by injecting contrast medium into them as X rays are taken. This part of the procedure is called a coronary angiogram. Blood pressure and blood oxygen measurements may be taken at different locations in the heart and in the pulmonary arteries, which carry blood into the lungs. In some cases, X rays of the aorta (the main artery carrying blood from the heart into the body) are taken with contrast medium. Blood samples can also be obtained. If infection of the heart is suspected, a small sample (biopsy) of heart tissue may be removed through the catheter.

During the testing portion of cardiac catheterization, particularly when contrast medium is used, the person may experience a flush through the entire body, queasiness or nausea, headache, and palpitations (the sensation of an unusually fast heartbeat). These sensations are common and short-lived.

When testing is complete, the cardiologist removes the catheter or catheters. The sheath may be left in place for 4 to 6 hours while the anticoagulants wear off. Then it is removed, and pressure is applied to the insertion site for a short time to prevent bleeding. Alternatively, the sheath is removed immediately after the catheter, and the wound is sealed with a tool called a vascular closure, or hemostatic, device. Stitches are used if an incision was made.

Cardiac catheterization usually takes from 30 to 60 minutes. The recovery period depends on where the catheter was inserted. If the arm was used, the person may be able to go home in as little as 2 hours after removal of the sheath, once the sedative has worn off. Insertion in the groin or upper thigh requires 6 to 8 hours of recovery before the person can get out of bed and stand or walk. Exercise and sexual activity can usually be resumed 24 hours after the catheterization. Bruising and soreness around the insertion point last for a few days and usually heal completely within 10 days to 2 weeks.

OUTCOMES AND COMPLICATIONS
Cardiac catheterization provides a great deal of information about the heart and is extremely useful for diagnosing disease, assessing the severity of disease, determining the value of surgery for a given individual, and planning that surgery. The test is relatively safe; major complications occur rarely but include bleeding around the insertion site, infection, embolism (a blood clot that can travel to other sites of the body and lodge there), cardiac arrhythmia (abnormal heartbeat), allergic reaction to the contrast medium, perforation or other damage to a blood vessel, heart attack, or stroke.

Catheterization, urinary

Insertion of a thin, flexible tube (catheter) into the bladder to drain urine. Catheters may be used temporarily, such as during surgery and recovery, or continuously in people who cannot retain urine normally or empty their bladder (see INCONTINENCE, URINARY). Typically, the catheter has a balloon tip that is inflated with air or sterile liquid to hold it in place after it is inserted. The balloon is then deflated to remove the catheter. The urine

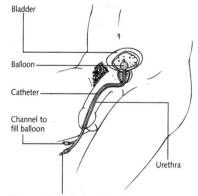

DRAINING URINE MECHANICALLY
The catheter usually has a balloon tip that is inflated inside the bladder to hold the tube in place, then deflated before the tube is removed. A catheter is often inserted before a surgical procedure to take care of urination during and immediately after surgery. A catheter can be placed permanently in someone who has lost bladder function entirely.

drains into a bag that is emptied periodically.

Complications of urinary catheterization include infection of the urinary tract, injury to the urethra (the tube that carries urine from the bladder out of the body), bladder stones, blood in the urine, and, rarely, bladder cancer, but only after many years of catheterization.

Catheter-related infections

Infectious complications associated with the use of catheters. Catheter-related infections are considered NOSOCOMIAL INFECTIONS, which means they are acquired while a person is hospitalized. When a catheter is inserted into the body to drain fluids or perform other medical procedures, microbes present on the catheter may be introduced into the body, producing an infection. Treatment consists of antibiotics and removing the catheter.

Cauda equina

A group of nerve roots with a common covering at the lower end of the spinal cord. Nerve roots in the cauda equina provide motor and sensory function to the legs and bladder.

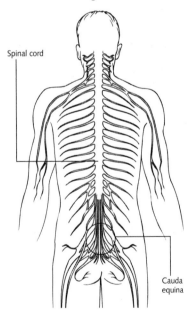

Spinal cord

Cauda equina

DESCENDING NERVE ENDS
The spinal cord ends between the first and second lumbar vertebrae, and from that point on, a cascade of nerve roots called the cauda equina descends through the remaining (sacral) vertebrae.

Cauda equina syndrome

A rare but severe neurologic disorder caused by compression of the cauda equina (a group of nerve roots at the end of the spinal cord). Possible causes could include a herniated disk, tumor, or a blood clot that compresses the spinal cord. Compression of the nerves can lead to incontinence, paralysis, and lack of sensation in the legs if left untreated.

Caudal

A term that usually refers to a position toward the end of the spine; literally means "of the tail."

Caudal block

A type of nerve block in which a local anesthetic is injected into the lowest portion of the spinal canal. Obstetric and gynecological surgical procedures often benefit from this type of anesthesia.

A needle is inserted into the skin between the upper part of the buttocks and the coccyx (the bone at the spine's base) until it penetrates the membrane in the spine called the dura mater. The anesthetic medication is injected beneath the dura mater. There, it mixes with the CEREBROSPINAL FLUID, which flows around the lower spinal nerves and renders those nerves insensitive to pain.

The caudal block is a variation of the epidural block (see ANESTHESIA, EPIDURAL). It requires more anesthetic medication to achieve the same level of numbing, but it carries almost no risk of nerve damage.

Causalgia

A sensation of severe, burning pain. Causalgia most often affects the extremities after nerve trauma. See also REFLEX SYMPATHETIC DYSTROPHY.

Caustic

Any strongly corrosive chemical substance. Caustic agents cause irritation and burning, and they destroy tissue. Examples of caustic agents include silver nitrate and caustic soda. While caustic agents are sometimes used to remove dead skin or warts, care must be taken to protect the surrounding skin.

Caustic ingestion

See POISONING, SWALLOWED CAUSTICS.

Cauterization

The use of a hot instrument, an electrical current, a corrosive chemical, or some other agent to destroy tissue or to stop bleeding. Cauterization can be used, for example, to seal blood vessels cut during surgery or to remove tonsils or other diseased tissue.

Cavernous sinus thrombosis

A potentially fatal condition caused when a blood clot in the cavernous sinus becomes infected with bacteria, which accumulate in the blood and produce toxins. Cavernous sinus thrombosis is usually a consequence of bacterial sinusitis. The infection may spread into other sinus areas through associated veins. Symptoms may include headache, a high fever, seizures, and loss of consciousness.

A person with cavernous sinus thrombosis may have a red, swollen, bulging eye with loss of movement. CT (computed tomography) scanning of the sinuses and brain may be performed to confirm the diagnosis. Treatment includes intravenous antibiotics, such as ceftriaxone (see CEPHALOSPORINS) at high doses, and surgical drainage of the infected sinuses. The prognosis is considered grave, even with prompt treatment.

Cavity, dental

A hole in a tooth caused by decay. A cavity is caused by the formation of dental plaque (see PLAQUE, DENTAL), which is made up of bacteria, food particles, and saliva. The bacteria interact with sugars in food particles that remain in the mouth and on the teeth to form acid, which dissolves the calcium and phosphate in the enamel of the tooth. This damage to the structure of the tooth is the first stage in the development of a dental cavity. If the cavity is not treated, it can reach the inner structures of the teeth, inflame the pulp (see PULP, DENTAL) of the tooth, and cause persistent pain, especially after eating or drinking foods or beverages that are sweet, hot, or cold. Dental cavities are treated by a dentist who removes the decayed tissue by using a dental drill. He or she then fills the prepared tooth with an amalgam or composite filling (see AMALGAM, DENTAL; BONDING, DEN-

TAL). If the cavity is advanced, it may require ROOT CANAL TREATMENT or even TOOTH EXTRACTION. See also TOOTH DECAY.

PREVENTION

Brushing the teeth daily with FLUORIDE toothpaste and the daily use of dental floss (see FLOSS, DENTAL) will help to prevent dental cavities. Foods that contain sugar should be eaten in moderation, and the teeth should be cleaned as soon as possible after eating. Fluoride can stop very early decay; it is available in toothpaste and mouthwash as well as in drinking water. Regular dental examinations and cleanings also help to prevent cavities. A dentist may recommend the use of a dental sealant (see SEALANTS, DENTAL), a plastic coating applied to the teeth to shield them from decay-causing bacteria. This coating is applied to the grooves on the chewing surface of the permanent molars, which are the most common spots for decay.

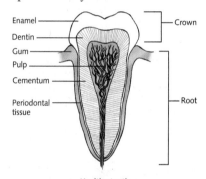

Healthy tooth

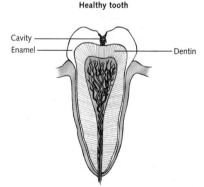

Decayed tooth

TOOTH DECAY

A dental cavity forms when bacteria interact with sugars in food debris to make an acid that eats through the protective enamel on the tooth. If the cavity is not treated, the acids and bacteria can penetrate the pulp of the tooth and cause considerable pain.

CBC (complete blood cell count)

The number of red blood cells, white blood cells, and platelets in one cubic millimeter of blood. This laboratory test is commonly used to diagnose disease, especially infections and anemia. The CBC may indicate a need for more tests of the kidneys or liver. It is also used to guide decisions about the TRANSFUSION of red blood cells and platelets.

CCU

See CORONARY CARE UNIT.

CD4 cell

A designation that refers to specific molecules present on the surface of immune cells called helper T lymphocytes, which are critical to effective immunity in a variety of infections. During HIV (human immunodeficiency virus) infection, the virus binds to the CD4 molecules on the helper T cells. This allows the virus to attack the helper T cell, making it incapable of activating other immune cells, which decreases the immune system's function and makes a person more susceptible to infection by other pathogens.

Infection with HIV is characterized by a significant decline in the number of CD4 cells and in their ability to function. When T-cell function is sufficiently impaired, the infection progresses to AIDS (acquired immunodeficiency syndrome).

CDC

See CENTERS FOR DISEASE CONTROL AND PREVENTION.

Cecum

The saclike first section of the large INTESTINE, located in the lower right abdomen. The small intestine ends at the cecum, and the appendix branches from it.

Cefaclor

A broad-spectrum cephalosporin antibiotic used to treat bacterial infections. Cefaclor (Ceclor) is prescribed for infections of the respiratory or urinary tract, for otitis media (inflammation of the middle ear), and for skin infections.

Cefadroxil

See CEPHALOSPORINS.

Cefixime

See CEPHALOSPORINS.

Cefpodoxime

See CEPHALOSPORINS.

Cefprozil

See CEPHALOSPORINS.

Ceftazidime

See CEPHALOSPORINS.

Ceftibuten

See CEPHALOSPORINS.

Ceftriaxone sodium

See CEPHALOSPORINS.

Cefuroxime

See CEPHALOSPORINS.

Celecoxib

A nonsteroidal anti-inflammatory drug (NSAID) used to treat arthritis. Celecoxib (Celebrex) relieves the pain and inflammation of osteoarthritis and rheumatoid arthritis. It was the first of a new subclass of NSAIDs called COX-2 inhibitors to come on the market for the treatment of arthritis. Celecoxib, like older NSAIDs such as Motrin (ibuprofen) and Naprosyn (naproxen), fights pain and inflammation by inhibiting the effect of a natural enzyme, COX-2. Unlike the older drugs, celecoxib does not also interfere with the enzyme COX-1, which protects the stomach lining. Celecoxib is less likely than the older drugs to cause gastrointestinal bleeding and stomach ulcers.

Although celecoxib is less likely than other NSAIDs to affect the stomach, it does present some risk to the digestive tract. People who have had stomach ulcers or gastrointestinal bleeding must take celecoxib with particular care.

Celiac disease

A disorder in which the lining of the small intestine is damaged by an immune reaction to gluten, a protein found in grains, such as wheat, rye, and barley. Celiac disease damages the tiny protrusions called villi on the small intestine's lining. This leads to MALABSORPTION (the impaired absorption of nutrients in the small intestine). Celiac disease is also known as gluten intolerance, gluten-sensitive enteropathy, and nontropical sprue.

C

Common symptoms include abdominal bloating and pain, weight loss, chronic diarrhea, and flatulence. Stools often are greasy, pale, bulky, and foul-smelling. In children, malnutrition may result, causing anemia, delayed growth, and FAILURE TO THRIVE. In some cases, the symptoms are not limited to the digestive system. They may also include fatigue, bone pain, behavioral changes, muscle cramps, joint pain, seizures, rash, numbness or tingling in the legs, sores in the mouth, tooth discoloration, and menstrual irregularity. In other cases, symptoms are virtually absent. There is an increased rate of intestinal cancer among individuals who have celiac disease.

Celiac disease is an autoimmune disorder (see AUTOIMMUNE DISORDERS), which means it is caused by a malfunction in the body's own immune system. It can be an inherited disorder, meaning that it runs in families. The disease can occur at any age and can be triggered by a stressful event, such as surgery, an infection, pregnancy or childbirth, or severe emotional stress. Breast-feeding appears to offer protection against the disease. In addition, the age at which an individual begins to eat foods that contain gluten (such as baby cereal) may also be a factor.

DIAGNOSIS AND TREATMENT
Because the symptoms mimic those of many other digestive disorders, establishing an accurate diagnosis can be difficult. To confirm a diagnosis, doctors test blood to measure the level of specific antibodies. A BIOPSY, in which a small piece of tissue is removed from the small intestine and analyzed, may be necessary to check for damage to villi.

The only effective treatment is a change in diet. Avoidance of all foods that contain gluten is prescribed. Eating even a small amount of gluten can damage the intestine. A gluten-free diet entails not only avoiding most grains, but also pasta, cereal, and many processed foods. Scientists continue to investigate whether it is also necessary to avoid oats and products made with oats. Left untreated, celiac disease can lead to complications, such as cancer, osteoporosis, miscarriage, congenital defects, short stature in children, or seizures.

Cell

The fundamental structural unit of all body tissue and all living things. The human body is composed of billions of cells, specialized to carry out specific roles in the vast system of processes that keep the body functioning.

Although different types of cells—bone cells, blood cells, and nerve cells, for example—vary dramatically in terms of what activity they perform, their basic structure is similar. Each microscopic cell has a nucleus that directs the activity of the cell; the nucleus is surrounded by a fluid called cytoplasm, and the cell is enclosed in an outer cell membrane. Every cell functions by manufacturing proteins, the complex chemicals that are the essential structural elements of life.

STRUCTURE
The cell centers on its nucleus, contained within the cytoplasm by a nuclear membrane. The nucleus directs the manufacture of cell proteins, and the type and quantity of proteins determine the structure and function of the cell. Amino acids are the chemical compounds that are the structural building blocks of proteins; the difference between various proteins is determined by the arrangement of the amino acids. The cell nucleus contains the master pattern for these amino acids, as well as the mechanism for reproducing the same pattern for a new cell.

The cytoplasm surrounding the nucleus is where most of the chemical activities of the cell take place. The cytoskeleton is the framework that supports it from within, gives the cell its shape, and enables it to move. A variety of structures in the cytoplasm are collectively called the organelles. The mitochondria, suspended within the cytoplasm, supply the cell with energy, depending on its requirements. A muscle cell, for instance, needs a great deal of energy to fuel its activities.

Smaller units called ribosomes make protein (a process called protein synthesis) either for use by the cell itself or for transport to other cells. Protein that is synthesized to be sent out of the cell moves through a structure called the endoplasmic reticulum for processing. The protein passes into another internal system, the Golgi apparatus, and moves to the cell's surface. Units of protein called vesicles fuse to the cell membrane and expel their contents. Specialized vesicles called lysosomes can digest bacteria entering the cell; others known as perisomes can detoxify harmful substances.

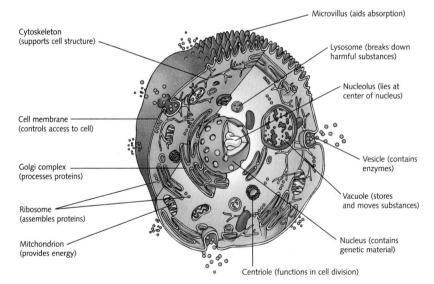

Cytoskeleton (supports cell structure)

Cell membrane (controls access to cell)

Golgi complex (processes proteins)

Ribosome (assembles proteins)

Mitchondrion (provides energy)

Microvillus (aids absorption)

Lysosome (breaks down harmful substances)

Nucleolus (lies at center of nucleus)

Vesicle (contains enzymes)

Vacuole (stores and moves substances)

Nucleus (contains genetic material)

Centriole (functions in cell division)

INTRICATE STRUCTURE OF A CELL
Within every cell, proteins are manufactured and processed to support the cell's specialized activity. The cell is also capable of replicating itself to form a new cell with the same function. An individual cell is microscopic and is composed of still smaller structures that work together to keep the cell functioning.

The cell's outer layer, the cell membrane, contains the cell's contents and controls the passage of substances into and out of the cell. The membrane must allow nutrients and oxygen to enter and waste materials to leave. The membrane also has the mechanism to allow the cell's products to cross out of the cell.

CELL REPLICATION

The genetic material of the cell, a chemical compound called DNA, is in the nucleus. The DNA is the chemical blueprint, or master plan, for the cell. The DNA is organized on string-like structures called chromosomes, and each chromosome contains smaller units known as genes. Each gene holds the instructions for making a specific protein, composed of a sequence of amino acids. The cell can divide and multiply, making exact copies of itself, because the chromosomes transmit the characteristics of the cell to the copy. The DNA (close to a particular gene on the chromosome) directs the formation of a related chemical called RNA, which carries an encoded message for the making of a specific protein. The RNA moves out of the nucleus into the cytoplasm and enters the ribosomes, where the protein is assembled according to the code of amino acids. In this manner, the cell is able to accurately and efficiently copy its own complex composition, passing along its unique characteristics to a new cell. See also CHROMOSOMES; GENE; and HEREDITY.

Cell division

A process by which a cell divides into two new cells. In cell division, the nucleus of the cell can divide in either of two ways—MITOSIS (in which identical cells are formed by division of the parent cell) or MEIOSIS (in which the new cells have half the number of chromosomes of the original cell). Once nuclear division is complete, the cytoplasm of the cell is divided in a process called cytokinesis. Cell division is the basis of all life forms.

Cellulitis

An acute, spreading infection of the skin. Cellulitis often follows trauma to the skin; it is usually caused by a staphylococcal or streptococcal infection in otherwise healthy individuals. Common symptoms include red-

COMPARING CELSIUS AND FAHRENHEIT		
EVENT	DEGREES CELSIUS	DEGREES FAHRENHEIT
Absolute zero	−273.15	−459.67
Freezing point of water	0	32
Normal body temperature	37	98.6
Boiling point of water	100	212

ness, warmth, and tenderness of the affected area, as well as fever, chills, and malaise. Cellulitis is a serious disease because infection can spread via the lymph system or the bloodstream. Cellulitis is diagnosed by appearance, and the organism responsible for causing the condition may be identified in some cases by cultures of the blood. Cellulitis is treated with antibiotics.

Celsius scale

A temperature scale based on the difference between the freezing and boiling points of water. In the Celsius scale, the freezing point of water is 0° (32° Fahrenheit), and the boiling point is 100° (212° Fahrenheit). Named for a Swedish astronomer, the Celsius scale is also known as the centigrade scale, because it is divided into 100 degrees. The Celsius scale is used to measure temperature throughout most of the world.

Cementum

A thin, bone-hard layer of tissue covering the surface of the root of the tooth. When excessive cementum (bonelike tissue) has formed on the roots of the teeth, the condition is known as hypercementosis, which is sometimes associated with tooth infections located at the tip of a root.

Centers for Disease Control and Prevention

Also known as the CDC, a federal agency based in Atlanta, Georgia. The mission of the CDC is to promote health and quality of life by preventing and controlling disease, injury, and disability. It seeks to accomplish this mission by working with foreign and domestic partners to monitor health, investigate health problems, advocate sound public

health policies, institute prevention strategies, promote healthy behavior, foster a safe environment, and train future leaders. The CDC has a critical role in controlling infectious diseases, such as AIDS (acquired immunodeficiency syndrome) and TUBERCULOSIS.

Central nervous system

The BRAIN and the SPINAL CORD, which together monitor and control all the body's functions, responses, and behaviors, both conscious and unconscious. The central nervous system (CNS) works together with the PERIPHERAL NERVOUS SYSTEM, composed of the nerves emanating out from the CNS to all parts of the body. See NERVOUS SYSTEM.

The sensitive structures of the CNS are armored in bone: the brain lies within the SKULL, and the spinal cord is encased inside the bones of the spine. The brain is the center for data collection, storage, and analysis. With the sensory information it

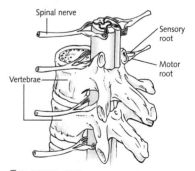

Spinal nerve

Sensory root

Motor root

Vertebrae

THE SPINAL CORD
The spinal cord, which links the brain to the rest of the body, is enclosed within the bony vertebral column for protection. Extending out from the spinal cord are the spinal nerves, including the sensory roots that convey information to the brain about body sensations and the motor roots that send information from the brain or spinal cord to muscles and organs.

C

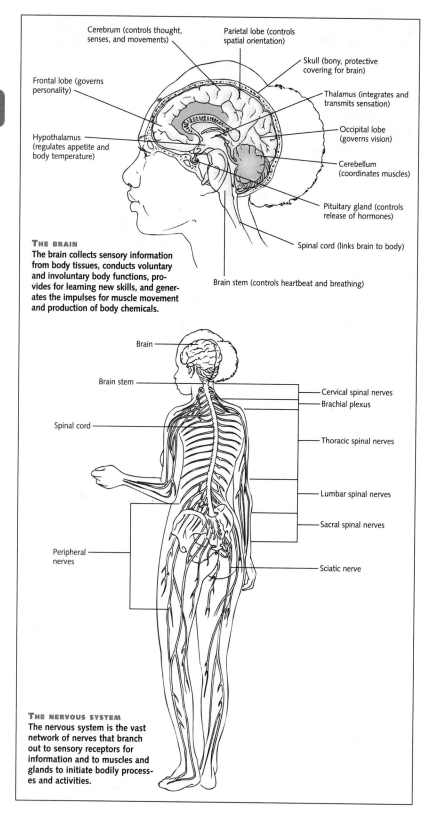

Cerebrum (controls thought, senses, and movements)

Parietal lobe (controls spatial orientation)

Skull (bony, protective covering for brain)

Frontal lobe (governs personality)

Thalamus (integrates and transmits sensation)

Hypothalamus (regulates appetite and body temperature)

Occipital lobe (governs vision)

Cerebellum (coordinates muscles)

Pituitary gland (controls release of hormones)

Spinal cord (links brain to body)

Brain stem (controls heartbeat and breathing)

THE BRAIN
The brain collects sensory information from body tissues, conducts voluntary and involuntary body functions, provides for learning new skills, and generates the impulses for muscle movement and production of body chemicals.

Brain

Brain stem

Spinal cord

Cervical spinal nerves

Brachial plexus

Thoracic spinal nerves

Lumbar spinal nerves

Sacral spinal nerves

Peripheral nerves

Sciatic nerve

THE NERVOUS SYSTEM
The nervous system is the vast network of nerves that branch out to sensory receptors for information and to muscles and glands to initiate bodily processes and activities.

receives about both internal body states and functions and external stimuli, it organizes and directs the body's response. The spinal cord, extending down the length of the body from the brain, contains bundles of nerve fibers that transmit information between the brain and the rest of the body. It can also receive some information and respond independently of the brain for some automatic functions.

The brain and spinal cord receive, process, and send information in the form of electrochemical impulses transmitted between individual nerve cells called neurons. The complex nerve pathways that make up the CNS are entirely composed of these specialized cells. See NERVE; NEURON.

Centrifuge

A device that uses centrifugal force to separate two or more substances of different density. A simple centrifuge is a container that is spun rapidly to speed the process of separation of substances that normally would separate slowly under the influence of gravity. The spin cycle of an automatic washer is an example of a centrifuge, one in which water is drained away from wet laundry. Another example is a centrifuge that separates blood cells from whole blood.

Cephalexin

An antibacterial drug; a cephalosporin antibiotic available in capsules, tablets, and liquid. Cephalexin (Keflex, Keftab) is a first-generation cephalosporin active against many gram-positive organisms, including staphylococcal organisms and organisms that cause pneumonia. It is also active against some gram-negative organisms, including *Escherichia coli* (see E. COLI), and it can be used to treat respiratory and urinary tract infections, as well as skin and middle ear infections. Cephalexin may also be used to treat infections of the bone and skin.

Cephalhematoma

A birth injury in which a hemorrhage forms underneath the periosteum, the membrane covering the baby's skull. Swelling is usually not visible until several hours after birth. Rarely, a cephalhematoma is a sign of an underlying skull fracture. Such fractures are usually the result of injuries caused by the stresses of birth, such as pressure applied with FORCEPS or VACUUM EXTRACTION. Depending on their size, most cephalhematomas are absorbed within 2 weeks to 3 months, though a few remain for some years as bumps on the skull. They generally require no treatment.

Cephalosporins

A class of antibiotic drugs used to treat infections caused by bacteria. Cephalosporins work by killing bacteria or preventing their growth. Cephalosporins are used to treat urinary tract infections, tonsillitis, celulitis, and respiratory tract infections such as pneumonia. Cefaclor (Ceclor) can be used to treat lower respiratory tract infections, including pneumonia. Cephalosporins will not work for colds, flu, or other viral infections.

Cephalosporins should be used with caution for people who are allergic to penicillin-type antibiotics; about 10 percent of people allergic to penicillins are also allergic to cephalosporins. Allergic reactions may include rash, itching, fever, and very rarely, a severe ANAPHYLACTIC REACTION.

Cerclage, cervical

A surgical procedure that places a stitch called a cerclage in the cervix to hold it closed during pregnancy. The cerclage is used to try to stop PRETERM LABOR or to make an INCOMPETENT CERVIX better able to resist the pressure of the growing pregnancy. In the most common approach, the cerclage draws the cervix closed like a drawstring. The procedure is usually performed between the 13th and 16th weeks of pregnancy; the stitch is removed at about the 37th week, allowing labor and delivery to proceed normally thereafter. It is not clear how effective the cerclage is in stopping preterm labor.

Cerebellum

A portion of the BRAIN, located in the lower back of the skull and connected to the brain stem. This two-hemisphere structure coordinates balance and muscular movement. The cerebellum is linked to the brain stem via a connection of thick nerve tracts. The nerve fibers from these nerve

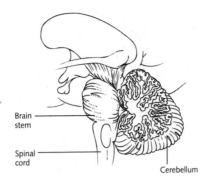

Brain stem

Spinal cord

Cerebellum

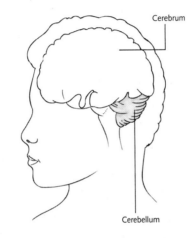

Cerebrum

Cerebellum

THE "LITTLE BRAIN"
The cerebellum is located under and behind the cerebrum and is involved with the coordination and control of voluntary movement. Like the cerebrum, it has two lobes and a convoluted surface. It integrates data about the body and past experience to learn, plan, and execute body movements.

tracts fan out toward the surface (cortex). The surface itself consists of gray matter (interconnected nerve cells) arranged in three layers. Via the brain stem, the cerebellum receives information from organs, such as the inner ear, concerning the body's posture and balance. From the muscles, joints, and tendons, it receives signals about movement. It also receives input about a motor plan for movement originating in the cerebral cortex, and it contains programs for previously learned movements. The cerebrum integrates this information and adjusts movement as it progresses. The cerebellum continually corrects the movement by adjusting signals to the motor nerve cells in the spinal cord and by updating the motor plan.

Cerebral contusion

Damage to the surface of the brain and its underlying tissues from an acute head injury, such as that sustained in a fall. This results in a bruise on the brain as opposed to a concussion, which results in an alteration in consciousness but no structural damage.

Cerebral hemorrhage

See HEMORRHAGE, CEREBRAL.

Cerebral palsy

An umbrella term for a group of chronic disorders that impair control of movement, appear in the first few years of life, and generally do not worsen over time. Cerebral palsy is characterized by a broad range of symptoms that may include seizures, muscle contractions, delayed development, mental retardation, gait (walking) abnormalities, spasticity, speech difficulties, vision problems, and hearing abnormalities.

CAUSES

Cerebral palsy is not a single disease with a single cause. It was once a commonly accepted belief that cerebral palsy was caused by a lack of oxygen during birth. Today doctors no longer believe this is true. Probably fewer than one in ten children have cerebral palsy as a result of oxygen deprivation. When doctors try to find the cause of cerebral palsy, they review the symptoms, the mother's and child's medical histories, and the onset of the disorder.

In the United States, 10 to 20 percent of children with cerebral palsy develop this condition after birth. Acquired cerebral palsy is usually the result of BRAIN DAMAGE from head injury or infection such as bacterial MENINGITIS. Congenital cerebral palsy is present at birth, although it may not be diagnosed until some months later. Causes of congenital cerebral palsy include infections during pregnancy, jaundice in a newborn infant, Rh incompatibility, and severe oxygen shortage in the brain or trauma to the head during labor and delivery. Additional risk factors include breech presentation, complicated delivery, low birth weight, premature birth, low Apgar score, multiple births, nervous system malformations, maternal bleeding late in pregnancy, maternal mental retardation or seizures, and seizures in the newborn.

SYMPTOMS

Symptoms of cerebral palsy include seizures, muscle contractions, delayed development, mental retardation, gait abnormalities, spasticity, speech difficulties, vision problems, and hearing abnormalities. The initial signs of cerebral palsy usually occur before age 3 years. Parents are often the first to notice that an infant is not developing on schedule. He or she may lag in developmental milestones such as rolling over, sitting, crawling, smiling, or walking. This is usually known as DEVELOPMENTAL DELAY.

Some children also have abnormal muscle tone. An affected baby may have HYPERTONIA, or increased muscle tone. Other babies may first be suspected of having cerebral palsy because they seem exceptionally floppy—like rag dolls. (See also FLOPPY INFANT.) Affected children may also have an unusual posture.

As time goes on, poor control of the muscles of the throat, mouth, and tongue can cause drooling. Difficulty with eating and swallowing may lead to a failure to thrive. Another common complication is incontinence in older children. About 50 to 70 percent of children with cerebral palsy have some intellectual impairment.

DIAGNOSIS

Diagnosis of cerebral palsy is based on medical history and the examination of a baby's motor skills. Doctors check for slow development, abnormal muscle tone, and unusual posture. The physician will also check reflexes and look for hand preference. Babies with cerebral palsy may show a hand preference in the first 12 months of life, which is unusual. It is also important to rule out other causes of symptoms, such as Down syndrome, Tay-Sachs disease, or muscular dystrophy. The doctor may order tests such as CT (computed tomography) scanning, MRI (magnetic resonance imaging), ultrasound, or electroencephalogram (EEG). Intelligence and vision tests are sometimes also recommended.

TREATMENT

There is no cure for cerebral palsy. However, proper management of neurological problems can enable people with cerebral palsy to lead close-to-normal lives. Each treatment plan must be carefully designed to meet an individual's unique needs. Usually cerebral palsy is managed by a team of health care professionals. General treatment measures include medication to control seizures and spasms; special braces to compensate for muscle imbalance; mechanical aids such as computers to overcome impairments; counseling for emotional and psychological needs; and physical, occupational, speech, and behavioral therapy. Surgery is sometimes recommended for contractures, conditions in which muscles become fixed in a rigid, abnormal position causing distortion or deformity.

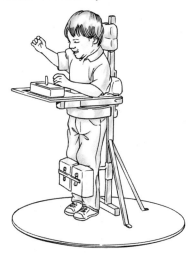

BRACING AND SUPPORT
To help a child with cerebral palsy reach his or her full potential for movement, a combination of physical therapy, braces, and surgery are customized to the child's needs. Braces and supports will help a child stand and walk safely and compensate to some extent for muscle weakness.

Cerebral thrombosis

A clot or thrombus that forms in and blocks an artery in the brain. When the clot completely blocks the artery, cutting off blood and oxygen to the brain, brain cells die and a STROKE occurs. This can cause permanent damage to that area of the brain or death. Stroke is the third leading cause of death in the United States.

CAUSES

The most important risk factor for a thrombotic stroke is ATHEROSCLEROSIS, or hardening of the arteries.

Thrombotic strokes are most common in older people. Clots rarely form in healthy arteries. However, in atherosclerosis, there is a thickening and loss of elasticity in artery walls. The arteries narrow and become lined with PLAQUE. Blood flow slows, and clots are more likely to form. When a clot becomes lodged in an artery in the brain, the result is a stroke. Most thrombotic strokes develop from clots that form in blood vessels. Another type of blood clot called a cerebral embolism results when a blood clot is formed elsewhere in the body, such as the heart, and is carried through the bloodstream until it lodges in an artery in the brain.

SYMPTOMS

Changes in brain function depend on the location and extent of injury to the brain. Common symptoms of a stroke are paralysis, weakness, numbness, tingling, decreased sensation, cognitive decline, impaired vision, AGNOSIA (inability to recognize or identify stimuli), problems with swallowing, loss of coordination, loss of memory, vertigo, personality changes, depression, changes in consciousness (such as sleepiness, apathy, stupor, or loss of consciousness), and lack of control over the bladder or bowels. Language difficulties, or APHASIA, following a stroke may include difficulty speaking or understanding speech, slurred speech, and problems with reading or writing. Symptoms most commonly affect only one side of the body.

DIAGNOSIS AND TREATMENT

Immediate medical attention is required to diagnose and treat cerebral thrombosis. Diagnostic tests may include MRI (magnetic resonance imaging), CT (computed tomography) scanning, angiography, ultrasound, functional MRI, and magnetic resonance angiography (MRA) (see BRAIN IMAGING). An electrocardiogram (ECG) or echocardiogram may be used to detect any heart involvement. Blood tests are also important, and examination may include neurological, sensory, and motor evaluation.

A stroke is a life-threatening condition for which immediate emergency

Terms in small capital letters— for example, PHYSICAL THERAPY or PAGET DISEASE—indicate a cross-reference to another entry with more information.

treatment is required. Hospitalization is necessary and usually includes lifesaving interventions and supportive measures. There is no cure for a stroke. The goal of treatment is to limit the damage to the brain, control symptoms, and maximize an affected person's ability to function. Rarely, surgery may be required to remove the blood clot or to repair damage. Possible medications include diuretics, anticonvulsants, and analgesics. Outcomes vary widely. Even with prompt treatment, death may occur. A person may also recover completely or suffer permanent BRAIN DAMAGE. People who experience brain damage may improve over time and with rehabilitation therapy.

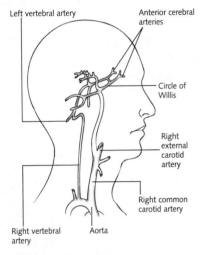

Arteries supplying brain

BLOCKED BLOOD FLOW TO THE BRAIN
Thrombosis is a disease process in which plaque in the blood accumulates, usually at branches and curves in the arteries. Cerebral thrombosis (often the result of aging) involves the blockage of arteries supplying blood to the brain. Shaded areas indicate where blockage often forms.

Cerebrospinal fluid

Also known as CSF, the clear, watery fluid that circulates inside and around the brain and spinal cord. Normal cerebrospinal fluid contains chemicals, such as glucose and proteins, and few if any white or red blood cells. The brain and spinal cord float in cerebrospinal fluid and are cushioned and nourished by it. In a diagnostic test called a LUMBAR PUNCTURE, a sample of CSF is removed for analysis in order to diagnose problems such as bacterial or viral meningitis, inflammation, tumors, hemorrhages, brain abscesses, and neurosyphilis.

Cerebrovascular accident

The sudden rupture or blockage of a blood vessel within the brain, leading to acute neurological damage; commonly referred to as STROKE. Cerebral infarctions, or thrombotic strokes, result from blockage caused by thrombosis (clot formation) or embolism (interruption of blood flow as a result of obstruction by a clot or plug of insoluble material carried in the bloodstream). An embolism usually results in a sudden onset of symptoms, while a thrombotic stroke usually begins more gradually. Hemorrhagic strokes are classified based on the pattern of bleeding. In a cerebral hemorrhage (see HEMORRHAGE, CEREBRAL), bleeding occurs within the brain. In a subarachnoid hemorrhage (see HEMORRHAGE, SUBARACHNOID), bleeding occurs around the brain. Despite their differences, hemorrhage, thrombosis, and embolism are also all commonly referred to as strokes when they occur in the brain.

Cerebral infarction, which results in the death of brain cells from inadequate blood supply, is the most common type of stroke. This may occur as a result of blockage of large arteries or smaller vessels (lacunar strokes) or from embolic stroke. Cerebral hemorrhages cause the death of brain cells because of the pressure caused by bleeding. As blood collects and clots, it can impair blood flow and cause damage to brain tissues. Subarachnoid hemorrhages cause stroke by irritating the blood vessels and causing them to spasm. The spasm of the smooth muscle in the blood vessel wall constricts the blood flow to that area of the brain and can lead to damage of the nerve tissue.

Cerebrovascular disease

Any disease affecting an artery within and supplying blood to the brain. The brain requires approximately 20 percent of the blood circulation in the body. Even a brief interruption in its supply of blood and oxygen can result in decreases in brain function (neurological deficit). The nature of changes in brain function depends on the location and extent of injury to the brain.

There are many different types of cerebrovascular disease. In ATHEROSCLEROSIS (narrowing of the arteries), there is a thickening and loss of elasticity in artery walls. The arteries narrow and become lined with PLAQUE. Blood flow slows, and clots (thrombi) are more likely to form. When a clot becomes lodged in an artery in the brain, the result is a stroke. Strokes are a group of brain disorders that are caused by an interruption of blood supply to the brain. They are the third leading cause of death in the United States. Risk factors for cerebrovascular disease include HYPERTENSION (high blood pressure), cigarette smoking, heart disease (see HEART DISEASE, ISCHEMIC; HEART DISEASE, CONGENITAL), warning signs or history of stroke, and diabetes (see DIABETES MELLITUS, TYPE 1; DIABETES MELLITUS, TYPE 2).

Cerebrum

The most developed, complex, and largest portion of the brain; the site of most conscious and intelligent activity. The cerebral cortex is the site of language, sensation, voluntary movement, memory, emotion, and imagination.

STRUCTURE

The cerebrum has two hemispheres (cerebral hemispheres) composed of white matter, covered by a thin, deeply wrinkled layer of gray matter (the cerebral cortex). The wrinkles and fissures of the cerebral cortex greatly enlarge its surface area. The two hemispheres are divided by the central fissure, but are connected by an underlying trunk called the corpus callosum. Within the two hemispheres are two of the ventricles of the brain, filled with cushioning cerebrospinal fluid. The surface areas of the cerebrum are divided into four lobes named for the bones of the skull that lie over them—frontal, temporal, parietal, and occipital.

The cerebral cortex is the site of thought, language, sensation, voluntary movement, memory, emotion, and imagination. Much of the cerebral cortex has been mapped according to what is known about the regions that serve certain functions. The prefrontal cortex involves concentration, long-

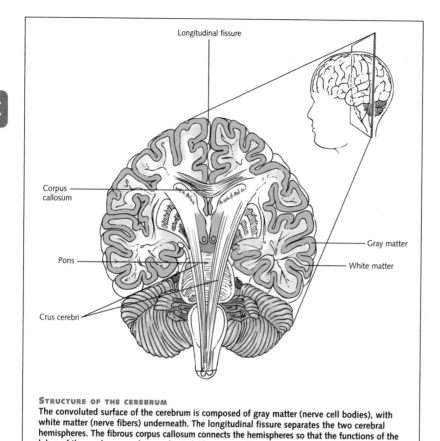

Longitudinal fissure

Corpus callosum

Pons

Crus cerebri

Gray matter

White matter

STRUCTURE OF THE CEREBRUM
The convoluted surface of the cerebrum is composed of gray matter (nerve cell bodies), with white matter (nerve fibers) underneath. The longitudinal fissure separates the two cerebral hemispheres. The fibrous corpus callosum connects the hemispheres so that the functions of the lobes of the cerebrum can be coordinated. The crus cerebri is a large bundle of nerve tracts.

range planning ability, and problem solving. The premotor cortex coordinates skilled movements such as athletic performance or playing a musical instrument. The motor cortex controls voluntary movements, from simple to complex. The primary somatic sensory cortex receives sensory signals from the skin and distinguishes sensations such as pain and pressure. The primary visual cortex interprets visual input about light and dark, shapes, and borders. The primary auditory cortex interprets input about sound, such as tone and volume. The Broca area plans and coordinates speech, and the Wernicke area integrates many types of sensory input and interprets the information into language.

Areas of the cortex near sites of known function are called association areas. These areas interpret input received from the primary areas of the cortex and develop voluntary or involuntary responses. The association areas also regulate many higher functions such as recognition and memory that are essential to learning and emotional response.

Some brain activity is localized in one hemisphere or the other. The so-called dominant hemisphere (left in most people) generally directs logical functions such as language and mathematical skills. The nondominant hemisphere regulates such activities as spatial orientation and relationships and some aspects of artistic and creative ability. As more is learned about brain function, it is becoming apparent that higher functions usually involve many areas of the brain and are not easily localized.

Certificate of need

Also known as a certificate of necessity, a written statement issued by a government agency affirming that the proposed construction or modification of a health care facility will be needed at the time of its completion. A certificate of need is given to the group or person seeking to construct or modify the facility. The intention of this measure is to help contain medical costs.

Certification, board

The process through which a physician's qualifications in a medical specialty are recognized by one of the specialties that make up the American Board of Medical Specialties (ABMS). Established in 1933, the ABMS is the umbrella organization for the 24 approved medical specialty boards in the United States. The governing body of each member board is composed of specialists qualified in the specialty represented by the board. Member boards evaluate physician candidates who voluntarily seek certification. To become certified in a specialty (for example, pediatrics or surgery), a physician must generally complete an approved residency training program and pass a comprehensive examination. Physicians who successfully receive certification are known as diplomates of their respective specialty board.

Cerumen

See EARWAX.

Cervical cap

A barrier method of birth control that keeps sperm from entering the cervix. A cervical cap is a firm rubber dome that fits over a woman's cervix and is held in place by suction and a flexible ring. A cervical cap must be fitted by a physician and is used with a spermicide. See CONTRACEPTION, BARRIER METHODS.

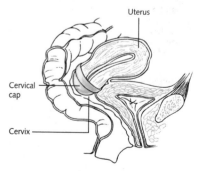

Uterus

Cervical cap

Cervix

PLACEMENT OF A CERVICAL CAP
A cervical cap fits tightly over the cervix to prevent sperm from entering. The cervical cap is similar to but smaller than a diaphragm and, therefore, is somewhat more difficult for a doctor to fit and for the woman to position.

Cervical dysplasia

The presence of abnormal cells on the surface of the cervix. They are not cancerous, but have characteristics similar to early cancer cells when viewed under a microscope. The abnormal cells can turn into cancer cells if cervical dysplasia is not detected and treated early. Usually, it produces no symptoms; however, symptoms can include bleeding from the vagina between menstrual periods (see BREAKTHROUGH BLEEDING), after having sex, or after menopause, or a heavy vaginal discharge. Cervical dysplasia is often linked to HUMAN PAPILLOMAVIRUS (HPV), a sexually transmitted disease that causes venereal warts; HPV occurs more commonly in women who have had many sexual partners or who began having sex before they were 18 years old.

Cervical dysplasia is usually detected during a routine PAP SMEAR, a screening test for abnormal cell growth on the cervix. When abnormal cells are present, the doctor usually performs a COLPOSCOPY (a greatly magnified visual inspection), and often a biopsy (removal of cells for examination under a microscope). Many mild cases of cervical dysplasia resolve on their own, while more severe cases usually require removal of the abnormal cells either surgically or by destroying the abnormal tissue with laser treatment or cryotherapy.

Cervical incompetence

See INCOMPETENT CERVIX.

Cervical intraepithelial neoplasia

See CIN.

Cervical osteoarthritis

See OSTEOARTHRITIS.

Cervical polyps

Grapelike growths of tissue that may protrude from the opening of the cervix. Cervical polyps are very common and can appear as either a single polyp or a cluster of polyps. Sometimes cervical polyps occur as a result of injury. As the cervical tissue heals, new tissue becomes overgrown, forming polyps. In some women, hormonal changes during

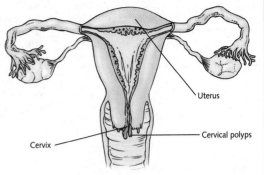

A COMMON GROWTH
Cervical polyps are benign lumps on the cervix (the neck of the uterus that leads into the vagina), caused by overgrowth of the cells that line the cervix. The polyps sometimes dangle down into the vagina, where they can be bumped easily (for example during intercourse) and cause bleeding. Cervical polyps usually can be removed in a minor procedure at a doctor's office.

Uterus

Cervical polyps

Cervix

pregnancy stimulate the growth of polyps, which can grow up to an inch in width. The usual symptoms of polyps are bleeding during and after intercourse and/or a bloody discharge from the vagina. Some women who have polyps have no symptoms at all, and the polyps are discovered during a routine pelvic examination.

While cervical polyps are usually harmless, a woman who has the symptoms of polyps should report them to her doctor because similar symptoms are produced by cancer of the cervix (see CERVIX, CANCER OF). The doctor will likely perform a PAP SMEAR and BIOPSY to rule out cancer. In rare cases, a polyp that is blocking the entrance to the cervix can interfere with a woman's ability to become pregnant. Most cervical polyps are easily removed in a brief, painless procedure that can usually be performed in a doctor's office under local anesthesia. Although cervical polyps are rarely cancerous, the removed polyp is sent to a pathologist for examination. If polyps recur, a D AND C (dilation and curettage) may be required.

Cervical rib

A small extra rib present at birth and occurring as an appendage to the seventh cervical vertebra in the lower neck. A cervical rib does not usually cause problems. In some cases, the rib may press against adjacent nerves and blood vessels, producing pain that radiates to the arm and hand. If pain or symptoms like those associated with RAYNAUD PHENOMENON (a circulatory condition featuring discoloration and coldness in the hands and feet) are present, the cervical rib is often removed.

Cervicitis

An inflammation of the CERVIX, the lower part of the uterus. Symptoms may include an abnormal vaginal discharge, pain during sexual intercourse, bleeding after sexual intercourse, aching in the lower abdomen, frequent or painful urination, burning, itching, or fever. To diagnose cervicitis, a doctor performs a pelvic examination, a Pap smear (to rule out the possibility of cervical cancer), and tests to culture for infectious organisms. The doctor may also perform a colposcopy (a magnified examination of the surface of the cervix).

Cervicitis is usually caused by a bacterial or viral infection, such as a sexually transmitted disease. However, cervicitis can also be caused by irritation of the cervix during childbirth or an abortion, or by an intrauterine device, a pessary (a device placed in the vagina to support a displaced uterus), or a forgotten tampon. If tests show that an infection is causing the cervicitis, antibiotics or other medications may be given. In cases in which a foreign object has caused the irritation, simply removing the object may be all that is needed. For severe cases of cervicitis, doctors sometimes perform cauterization (burning with an electrical probe), CRYOSURGERY (freezing), or laser treatment to eliminate the abnormal cells. A woman who suspects that she may have cervicitis should contact a doctor; untreated cervicitis can lead to PELVIC INFLAMMATORY DISEASE, fertility problems, or difficulty in delivering a healthy baby. A history of multiple sexual contacts, especially without using condoms, increases a woman's

C

chances of developing VAGINITIS (vaginal inflammation) and cervicitis. For women at high risk for cervicitis, a doctor may obtain cultures during an annual pelvic examination to screen for sexually transmitted diseases.

Cervix

A small, cylindrical organ made up of fibrous tissue and muscle located between the uterus and the vagina. An opening in the middle of the cervix connects the cavity of the uterus with the vagina. This passage is large enough to allow menstrual fluid to pass out of the vagina, but is too small to allow foreign objects to enter. Glands inside the cervix produce mucus that helps prevent microorganisms from entering the vagina. The cervix has a circular muscle that expands in size and shape during pregnancy and childbirth. During childbirth, the cervix can expand to about 4 inches wide. See also REPRODUCTIVE SYSTEM, FEMALE. After the baby is born, the muscles in the cervix contract, and the canal returns to its original size and shape.

Cervix, cancer of

A curable, slow-growing cancer that initially develops in the cervix and, if untreated, can spread to the other reproductive organs. Cancer of the cervix chiefly occurs in women between the ages of 30 and 55 and is nearly 100 percent curable when caught in the precancerous stage. It is one of the few cancers that has well-defined, recognizable precancerous stages. Before the cancer appears, abnormal changes occur in the cells on the surface of the cervix. The precancerous condition, CERVICAL DYSPLASIA, is categorized in various stages. The mildly abnormal cells may return to normal or may eventually develop into cancer. Severe dysplasia and early cancer can be treated and entirely cured.

TYPES OF CANCER

There are two main types of malignant cancer of the cervix. About 85 to 90 percent are squamous cell carcinomas. Most of the others are adenocarcinomas. Cancers that have aspects of both are called adenosquamous carcinomas.

■ *Squamous* The most common type of cancer of the cervix, the squamous

type, has been linked to sexual intercourse. Scientists believe that this cancer may result from a virus that is transmitted during sex. The human papillomavirus (HPV), usually introduced by a male sex partner with genital warts, may cause cervical dysplasia. One strain of the virus, HPV-16, has been implicated in 90 percent of squamous-type cervical cancers. Risk factors for developing squamous cell cancer of the cervix include having had sexually transmitted viral infections, such as genital warts or herpes; many sex partners; sex before age 18; or many pregnancies, beginning at an early age; and being a smoker.

■ *Adenocarcinoma* A much rarer form of cervical cancer, adenocarcinoma affects both women who are sexually active and those who have never had sexual intercourse. Its causes remain unclear.

SYMPTOMS AND DIAGNOSIS

The warning signs of cancer of the cervix may include vaginal bleeding after sexual intercourse or between periods, genital warts, an abnormal vaginal discharge, and pain during intercourse. However, the precancerous stage (dysplasia) usually exhibits no symptoms. Diagnosis of cancer of the cervix may involve a series of procedures. First, a Pap smear is performed. The Pap smear, also called a cervical smear test, is a procedure in which a small sample of cells from the cervix is removed for analysis. If dysplasia is detected, another Pap smear may be done, or a colposcopy (examination of the cervix under illuminated magnification) or biopsy (taking a tissue sample) may be performed. Sexually active women are advised to have a Pap smear done at age 18 or soon after their first sexual experience and, depending on their risk, every 1 to 3 years thereafter. The incidence of cancer of the cervix is

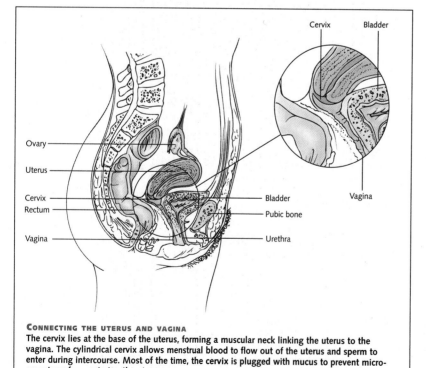

CONNECTING THE UTERUS AND VAGINA
The cervix lies at the base of the uterus, forming a muscular neck linking the uterus to the vagina. The cylindrical cervix allows menstrual blood to flow out of the uterus and sperm to enter during intercourse. Most of the time, the cervix is plugged with mucus to prevent microorganisms from entering the uterus.

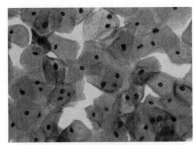

Normal cervical cells

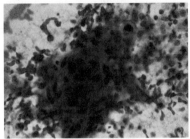

Cervical cells in carcinoma

**NORMAL VERSUS ABNORMAL
CERVICAL CELLS**
A micrograph (top photo enhanced by a microscope) shows cervical cells from a normal Pap
test. The nuclei in the cells (the dark ovals)
are small and regularly shaped. By contrast, the
bottom photo shows a cervical smear taken
from a woman diagnosed with a carcinoma.
The tumor cells have clumped together, and
the nuclei are misshapen and irregular.

increasing in the United States; however, fewer women die of it because
of early detection through extensive
Pap smear testing.

TREATMENT
If an area of abnormal cell growth
persists, or if early cancer is diagnosed through colposcopy or biopsy,
treatment is necessary. A local anesthetic will be given, and the doctor
will destroy the cells with laser
surgery, using extreme heat, or cryosurgery, using extreme cold. If cancer
has been diagnosed, several treatments may be considered. The affected tissue may be removed in a cone
biopsy. In more advanced cases, radiation may be used to kill or shrink the
cancer cells. Chemotherapy using
drugs that kill cancer cells may be
given either orally or intravenously,
or surgery may be performed.
    Several kinds of surgery are per-
formed for cancer of the cervix,
depending on how far the cancerous
cells have spread. If the cancer affects
only the cervix, the usual treatment is

a simple hysterectomy, in which the
uterus and cervix are removed. The
remaining tissues may be treated
with radiation. When the cancer has
spread beyond the cervix but remains
localized to the pelvis, more extensive surgery removing the surrounding tissue, such as the ovaries and
fallopian tubes, is performed. If the
cancer involves the colon, bladder,
and rectum, those organs can be surgically removed. Once cervical cancer has spread to the lungs, liver, and
other organs, only palliative therapy
(treatment that relieves the symptoms
but does not cure the disease) is available. After surgery for cervical cancer,
a woman will no longer be able to
become pregnant.
    Follow-up care is important after
treatment to detect the reappearance
of abnormal cells. Survival rates are
much higher when the cancer is identified in its early stages.

Cesarean section

A surgical procedure in which a baby
is delivered through incisions in the
mother's abdominal and uterine
walls. A cesarean delivery may be
planned before labor starts, or it may
be done unexpectedly as the result of
a complication during labor. It is performed in situations where it has
been judged the safest method of
CHILDBIRTH. A cesarean section may be
performed if labor fails to progress
(the contractions are not adequately
dilating the cervix); in a multiple
pregnancy; or if a baby is in distress,
in a BREECH PRESENTATION, or is too big

to pass safely through the mother's
birth canal. A cesarean section may
also be needed if the mother has a
serious medical condition, such as
diabetes, blood pressure problems,
ECLAMPSIA, or active genital herpes.
    A complete cesarean section takes
approximately 40 to 60 minutes,
although an obstetrician can remove a
fetus much more quickly in an emergency. The procedure is typically done
using regional or general anesthesia
(see sidebar, ANESTHESIA) in a hospital
operating room. The doctor usually
makes a horizontal (Pfannenstiel) incision in the abdomen and another in
the uterus; after rupturing the amniotic sac, the doctor gently pulls the baby
out. The placenta and other materials
are removed, and the incisions are
sutured closed.

AFTER A CESAREAN SECTION
A woman for whom regional anesthesia is used can usually hold her baby
as soon as a physician ascertains that
he or she is healthy and has a good
heartbeat and respiration. The mother's pulse, blood pressure, breathing
rate, and abdomen are regularly
checked, and she will be given intravenous fluids for 1 to 2 days. The
hospital stay is usually 3 to 4 days.
After returning home, a woman may
need to limit her activity while her
abdomen heals. If she has older children, she should refrain from lifting
them. She may experience side
effects, such as mild cramping, bleeding or discharge, and passing blood
clots from her vagina. Pain in the area
of the incisions can be treated with

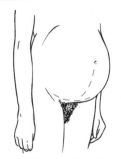

Two options for skin incision

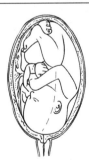

Vertical incision

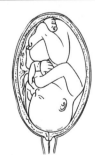

Bikini-line incision

INCISIONS FOR CESAREAN DELIVERY
The most common incision for a cesarean birth is the so-called bikini-line incision, a horizontal
cut in the skin just above the pubic hairline. Sometimes a vertical incision is done, extending
from the navel down to the public hairline. Under the incision in the skin, a second incision is
made in the wall of the uterus. This incision is usually horizontal. The broken lines indicate the
location of the incisions relative to the fetus.

C

medication. Pain that worsens or is accompanied by a fever requires a doctor's attention.

A woman who has had a cesarean section may deliver vaginally in a future pregnancy. However, there is some risk of rupturing the uterus at the site of the scar. The risk is least with a horizontal scar on the uterus. Because the direction of the uterine incision may have been different from that of the abdominal scar, the doctor reviews prior surgical records before determining the safest approach to each birth.

Cetirizine

See ANTIHISTAMINES.

Chagas disease

A potentially fatal infection caused by a parasite called *Trypanosoma cruzi*. Chagas disease, also called American trypanosomiasis, is most common in low-income, rural areas of South and Central America. It has been reported in Texas in humans and domestic dogs. It is transmitted to humans by reduviid insects, which are also called "kissing bugs" or "assassin bugs." These insects live in cracks and holes in substandard housing, especially thatch, mud, or adobe houses, and become carriers of the infection upon biting an animal or person who has Chagas disease. The infection is then spread to humans when an infected insect deposits feces on a person's skin. The feces may be accidentally rubbed into the wound formed by the insect's bite or into an open cut, the eyes, or the mouth. The disease may also be transmitted from an infected pregnant woman to her fetus during pregnancy, at delivery, or when breastfeeding. It is sometimes contracted via blood transfusion or organ transplant or by ingesting uncooked food contaminated with the feces of infected insects.

SYMPTOMS, DIAGNOSIS, AND TREATMENT

The early stage of Chagas disease may produce symptoms within several days to a few weeks of contracting the infection. Acute symptoms are rare and include swelling of the eye that has been infected, fatigue, fever, enlarged liver or spleen, diarrhea, vomiting, and swollen lymph glands. Swelling of the brain can develop in

very young children and infants and may cause death.

Chronic symptoms sometimes do not develop for 10 to 20 years and may include an enlarged heart, irregular heart rate, heart failure, or cardiac arrest. Enlargement of parts of the digestive system may occur and produce severe constipation or swallowing problems. The infection can destroy nerve cells of the colon causing a condition called megacolon. Chronic Chagas disease decreases life expectancy by an average of 9 years.

Diagnosis is made by blood tests, which reveal the presence of the parasite or antibodies that the body has created to help fight the parasite. Medication may be prescribed to treat acute Chagas disease, but there is no effective medication to treat the infection once it has progressed. In the chronic stage, the disease is treated by managing the symptoms.

Chakra balancing

A method of self-healing based on the belief that life-force energy transmitted by energy centers called chakras can be harnessed through visualization, meditation, and controlled breathing. The word "chakra" comes from Sanskrit and means "wheel of light." Chakra balancing depends on seven main chakras thought to be connected to, or part of, the body. Each chakra transmits and receives life-force energy, also called prana. When a person is sick, his or her chakras are assumed to be distorted, stagnant, blocked, or unbalanced, a situation that is thought to prevent life-force energy from flowing in and out of the body freely. Chakra balancing may use colors, crystals, light, sound, aromatherapy, or meditation and visualization to achieve its goal of self-realization and well-being. It is used for relieving anxiety, headaches, and stress.

Chalazion

An inflamed, tender lump on the eyelid caused by the blockage of a small gland that has a role in producing the oil layer of tears. A chalazion appears some distance from the edge of the eyelid, unlike a stye, which occurs close to the eyelashes. A chalazion may cause discomfort in the eye, sensitivity to light, and increased tearing. Over time a chalazion forms a

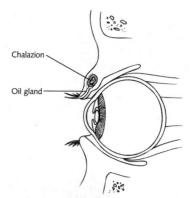

Chalazion

Oil gland

INFLAMED OIL GLAND
A chalazion differs from a stye in that it does not contain an active bacterial infection. It forms when debris blocks the natural drainage of oils from glands in the eyelid. A chalazion tends to be less painful than a stye but often is more long-lasting, taking a month or more to diminish.

cystlike swelling, which may put pressure on the eyeball and distort vision (astigmatism) or become infected. In many cases, chalazions resolve on their own within a few months. Applying warm compresses (a clean cloth soaked in hot water and wrung out) for 10 minutes four times a day may speed healing. If swelling continues, a chalazion can be drained surgically under local anesthesia in the doctor's office.

Chancre

A painless, ulcerated lesion that may be produced by an inflammatory reaction that occurs 10 to 60 days after exposure to SYPHILIS. Chancres are usually located on the genitals and tend to heal spontaneously, although the syphilis infection persists.

Chancroid

A sexually transmitted disease (STD) caused by the bacterium *Haemophilus ducreyi* when it enters the body through a scrape, sore, or crack on the surface skin of the genitals. Chancroid is spread via direct contact with a chancroid sore during sexual contact, including vaginal, anal, or oral sex.

Generally, within 2 to 5 days of sexual contact, the initial symptom of chancroid appears in the genital area as one or more small, painful, open, red sores, which may bleed when touched. The sores may produce pus and a bad odor and can spread to the thighs and abdomen. If they become infected, they may cause the lymph nodes in the groin to become painful and swollen.

Untreated, the infection can produce ongoing ulcers on the genitals; the sores may persist for months. Chancroid is successfully treated with antibiotics. The associated open lesions usually heal within 2 weeks. Warm compresses along with saline washes four times a day on the sores can help heal the chancroids. The infection can recur at any time after it has been cured, including immediately following treatment.

Chancroid is contagious for as long as a person has open sores. Because the open sores contain bacteria, any contact with them can transmit the infection. This can be prevented by following safer sex practices, including the use of a condom, and by limiting the number of sex partners. If a person suspects that he or she has chancroid, medical care should be sought immediately, and sexual contact should be avoided until the infection has been cured and all sores have completely disappeared.

Charcoal

A substance obtained by partly burning organic material; almost pure carbon. Charcoal is produced by heating wood or other organic substances in an enclosed space, without air. Charcoal is used as a fuel and an absorbent, in the melting of metals, in explosives, and by artists for drawing. Activated charcoal, which is charcoal that has been treated with oxygen to create pores among carbon atoms, is used to absorb certain poisons that have been ingested.

Charcoal, activated

A substance used to treat diarrhea and gastrointestinal gas; also a treatment for many drug overdoses. Activated charcoal is used to relieve painful pressure caused by excess gas in the digestive tract. Its use as a poison treatment is based on its ability to help prevent the poison from being absorbed from the stomach into the body. It is not effective against all poisons; for example, it does not work on lye, boric acid, lithium, cleaning fluid, iron, gasoline, kerosene, or alcohol. Charcoal

is available without a prescription, but it should not be used as a poison treatment without first consulting with a doctor or specialist at a poison center.

Charcot joint

The chronic degeneration of a joint that may pass unnoticed because of a neuropathy (loss of sensation) affecting the joint. Charcot joint is usually caused by neurological disorders, such as diabetic neuropathy (see DIABETES MELLITUS, TYPE 2), leprosy, and syphilis. It is characterized by swelling, hemorrhage, heat, instability, and atrophy of joints, such as the knee. Early diagnosis and treatment can sometimes prevent further damage. However, in severe cases, joint replacement may become necessary.

Charcot-Marie-Tooth disease

A group of inherited neuromuscular disorders characterized by weakness and loss of muscle tissue in the lower legs, feet, and hands. Charcot-Marie-Tooth disease (CMT) occurs when the insulating tissue surrounding peripheral nerve fibers or the nerve fibers themselves degenerate. The disease is named for the three French doctors who first identified it. The peripheral nerves carry signals from the brain and spinal cord to control voluntary muscles; they also send sensory signals in response to pain and pressure back to the brain and spinal cord. CMT chiefly affects muscular and sensory function in the limbs. About 1 of 2,500 people has a form of CMT, which is one of the most common hereditary neurologic disorders. Around 100,000 to 125,000 people in the United States have the disease. CMT is generally inherited as an autosomal dominant gene trait. This means that if one parent has the disease, offspring have a 50 percent chance of getting it. The genetic abnormality leading to the most common forms of CMT has been identified, and genetic testing is available.

SYMPTOMS

Individuals with CMT slowly lose normal use of their hands, feet, arms, and legs as the nerves to the extremities degenerate. CMT is also associated with foot deformities, such as high arches or flexed toes. Often, a high-arched foot is the first sign of the dis-

order. Mild loss of sensation can often occur. Symptoms develop slowly and usually become obvious between mid-childhood and age 30.

CMT varies in severity, even among members of the same family. Most individuals have difficulty participating in sports and often sprain ankles or fracture the bones of the lower leg and foot. The leg and foot problems are rarely so disabling as to require a wheelchair, however. When the muscles of the hand are affected, help may be needed to open screw caps, write, fasten buttons, and turn doorknobs. Neither intellect nor life expectancy is affected by Charcot-Marie-Tooth disease, and most people with the disease live full, active lives.

DIAGNOSIS AND TREATMENT

A doctor experienced with the disease will suspect CMT based on a characteristic pattern of foot, leg, and hand weakness. A family history and tests will be used to confirm the diagnosis. Tests may include an ELECTROMYOGRAM (EMG), which records the electrical activity of muscle cells; a nerve conduction velocity test, which measures the speed at which nerve impulses travel along the nerves; and DNA studies. The nerve impulses of people with CMT are slower than normal; therefore, the damage to their peripheral nerves shows up in a characteristic pattern of electrical activity on an EMG.

Treatment may involve physical therapy, lightweight lower leg braces, shoe inserts, and sometimes surgery to correct foot deformities. There is no cure for CMT.

Checkup

A thorough examination of a person's health. One of the main objectives of regular checkups is the early detection or prevention of disease. In some cases, early diagnosis makes the difference between cure and serious illness or death. A primary care doctor will advise people how often they need checkups, depending on age and health history. See also EXAMINATION, PHYSICAL.

Cheilitis

Inflammation of the skin on and around the lips. Cheilitis can result from atopic dermatitis, oral retinoid therapy, sun exposure, vitamin deficiency, or habitual lip licking.

C

Irritating substances in lipstick, mouthwash, and toothpaste may be factors. Actinic, or solar, cheilitis is a sun-induced inflammation of the lips.

Chelating agents

Substances that can bond strongly to metal ions. Medical applications of chelation came into use during the 1940s to combat poisoning with heavy metals, such as arsenic, lead, iron, mercury, copper, and aluminum. Chelation therapy involves the person receiving a series of these agents that will bind with the metals to help remove them from storage sites in the body, such as the liver or kidney, while promoting their excretion by the urine. Chelating agents may be given orally, by injection, or by intravenous infusion. Examples of chelating agents include penicillamine, dimercaprol (BAL), ethylenediaminetetraacetic acid (EDTA), and succimer (Chemet).

Chelation therapy

Traditional treatment for people poisoned with heavy metals; alternative medical therapy used for heart and arterial disease. Chelation is the process of removing undesirable metals from the body by administering substances that bind chemically to the metals in the blood. The metal and the chelating substance form a compound that can be excreted in the urine.

TRADITIONAL CHELATION THERAPY

Chelation therapy is a standard medical treatment for people poisoned with lead, iron, arsenic, mercury, copper, zinc, aluminum, manganese, and other metals. Its effectiveness in humans was discovered in 1948, when the US Navy began to use it for sailors who had absorbed lead from the paint used on ships.

Chelation therapy uses a synthetic amino acid called EDTA, or ethylenediaminetetraacetic acid, to remove minerals and metals from the body. When EDTA comes in contact with lead, iron, copper, zinc, magnesium, calcium, and other substances, it binds to them. In traditional chelation therapy, EDTA is given intravenously, a procedure that takes 3 to 4 hours.

ALTERNATIVE CHELATION THERAPY

Because EDTA binds to calcium, an ingredient in the plaque that forms on the walls of the arteries and causes atherosclerosis ("hardening of the arteries"), some doctors have speculated that EDTA might remove plaque-filled calcium from the arteries. Most doctors, however, have concluded that this speculation is baseless, chiefly because EDTA cannot pass through arterial cell membranes to reach calcium deposits, and the results of most studies have been negative.

Many alternative medical practitioners, however, continue to believe that chelation therapy is effective in the treatment of atherosclerosis and other chronic diseases of the circulatory system. They believe that chelation is able to remove enough calcium from the arteries to be able to smooth the artery walls, thereby improving blood flow and reducing the pain of angina (chest pain).

In an alternative medical treatment plan, chelation therapy may be combined with vitamin and mineral supplements, a low-fat diet, an exercise plan, smoking cessation, and limited alcohol and caffeine intake.

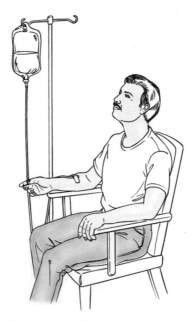

REMOVING METALS FROM THE BLOOD
Chelation therapy is traditionally used to treat metal poisoning by administering a chemical called EDTA that binds with metals so that they can be separated from the blood and excreted. For a severe case of metal poisoning, as many as 20 to 40 treatments may be required initially.

Chemical peel

The use of a caustic agent, usually an acid, to remove the damaged, outer layers of the skin and to improve and smooth its texture. Chemical peels are used for people with wrinkles caused by sun exposure, aging, blemishes, acne scars, and uneven pigmentation. A chemical peel can be applied to the entire face or to specific areas.

A number of different agents can be used for chemical peels, depending on the type of treatment the patient needs. Beta-hydroxy acid, a chemical peel agent, and the alpha-hydroxy acids, a group that includes glycolic acid, are the mildest. Both produce a light peel suitable for fine lines and wrinkles. Trichloroacetic acid (TCA) yields a medium peel. It is used for pigmentation problems and superficial blemishes, as well as for lines and wrinkles. Phenol, the strongest solution, removes coarse wrinkles, blotchy skin, or precancerous skin growths. Since phenol can lighten the color of the treated area, it may be unsuitable for people with dark skin. Phenol can also pose a risk for people with heart disease because of its associated side effects.

The mild beta-hydroxy and alpha-hydroxy peels can be used on a one-time basis or in a series of treatments. The agent may cause a slight stinging or burning sensation, but no anesthetic is needed. After treatment, the skin may flake or scale and turn red and dry; these effects disappear as the skin heals.

A TCA peel may also cause some stinging as the chemical is applied, but the sensation passes quickly and no anesthesia is required during the procedure. A crust or scab forms over the treated area, and there may be substantial swelling and some discomfort during healing. This usually lasts no more than a week, and new, bright-pink skin growth becomes apparent within a week to 10 days. Two or more peels spaced over a period of several months may be required to achieve the desired effect.

With phenol, only one treatment is usually needed, but it takes longer—1 to 2 hours versus 15 minutes for TCA, beta-hydroxy acid, or alpha-hydroxy acid. Adhesive tape or petroleum jelly may be applied over the treated

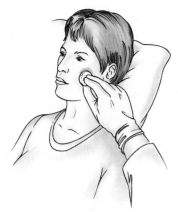

CHEMICAL SKIN TREATMENT
To remove damaged skin, a doctor can apply several different types of caustic chemicals, depending on the condition being treated. The chemical agent can be applied to the entire face or to a specific area to treat wrinkles caused by sun exposure, blemishes, acne scars, blotchy pigmentation, and precancerous growths.

area. Swelling can be substantial over the first 2 or 3 days and may require the patient to eat a liquid diet and avoid talking. The treated area scabs over, and new skin appears in a week to 10 days. The new skin is red at first and then lightens to a pinkish color during the following weeks and months.

After all types of chemical peels, the new skin must be protected against exposure to the sun to prevent damage and blotching. Patients should shade the face with a hat or visor and use a sunblock with a sun protection factor (SPF) of 30 or higher.

Chemonucleolysis

A procedure used in the treatment of herniated disks. In chemonucleolysis, a chemolytic agent, such as the enzyme chymopapain, is injected into a disk to dissolve the nucleus pulposus at the center of the disk. Chemonucleolysis has fallen out of favor because of inconsistent results and side effects.

Chemotherapy

Treatment with drugs, especially for cancer. Cancer chemotherapy includes any and all medications used to treat cancer, whether the drugs are antineoplastic (anticancer) or cytotoxic (cell-killing). Chemotherapy is often the first choice of

cancer therapy because it reaches throughout the entire body rather than a localized treatment, such as surgery and radiation, which target a specific area. Chemotherapy can treat cancer cells that have spread beyond the original site of the disease to other parts of the body. More than 100 drugs are available for cancer chemotherapy.

HOW CHEMOTHERAPY WORKS

Cancer chemotherapy takes advantage of the normal life cycle of a cell. All living tissue is made up of cells and is maintained by the process of cell growth and reproduction. Cells lost through injury or normal wear and tear are replaced. The cell cycle consists of five steps, which can last a number of hours or, in the case of the resting phase, years. The cycle is important to oncologists (cancer specialists), because many cytotoxic drugs work only on actively reproducing cells and are ineffective on cells in the resting phase.

When chemotherapy drugs attack reproducing cells, they cannot differentiate between normal tissues that are replacing worn-out cells and the targeted cancer cells. The normal cells will be damaged by chemotherapy along with the cancer cells, which results in side effects. Each time a person is treated with chemotherapy for cancer, the doctor must achieve a balance between

THE HICKMAN CATHETER
The Hickman catheter is a device for the delivery of cancer drugs. While the person is anesthetized, the thin, flexible tube is inserted in the chest through a small incision (entry site) in the jugular vein and slid under the skin between the neck and shoulder to another incision on the chest or stomach (exit site).

destroying cancer cells to cure or control disease and sparing normal cells to minimize side effects.

GOALS OF CHEMOTHERAPY

The first goal of chemotherapy is to destroy the cancer in order to treat it and prevent it from returning. When the cancer cannot be treated, the goal of chemotherapy is to prevent the disease from growing and spreading to maintain the best possible quality of life for the person. Chemotherapy is often used to help relieve symptoms caused by the cancer to enhance a person's quality of life, even when it is no longer possible to extend life.

Chemotherapy is often combined with other therapies, such as radiation or surgery. Chemotherapy may be given before surgery to shrink a large tumor so it can be removed. It may also be given after surgery to destroy stray cells that may have been left behind after a tumor has been removed.

TYPES OF DRUGS USED IN CHEMOTHERAPY

Oncologists select drugs to use in chemotherapy based on the type of cancer and its stage (how far it has spread). Many factors are considered in choosing anticancer or cytotoxic drugs, including the person's age, general health, and medical history. The regimen may include one drug or, more likely, a combination of several drugs.

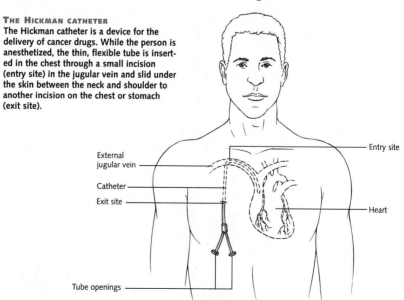

External jugular vein

Catheter

Exit site

Tube openings

Entry site

Heart

Chemotherapy drugs are divided into several categories based on how they affect chemicals in cancer cells, the specific cellular processes the drug interferes with, and the phase of the cell cycle the drug affects.

■ *Alkylating agents* These drugs work directly on DNA to prevent the cancer cell from reproducing. The agents work in all phases of the cell cycle. They are used to treat chronic leukemia, non-Hodgkin lymphoma, multiple myeloma, and some cancers of the breast, ovary, and lung. Examples include busulfan, cisplatin, cyclophosphamide, dacarbazine, ifosfamide, mustargen, and melphalan.

■ *Nitrosoureas* Nitrosoureas inhibit enzymes needed for DNA repair. Because these drugs can travel to the brain, they are used to treat brain tumors. They also are used to treat non-Hodgkin lymphomas, multiple myeloma, and malignant melanoma. Examples include carmustine and lomustine.

■ *Antimetabolites* These drugs interfere with the growth of RNA and DNA. They are used to treat chronic leukemias and tumors of the breast, ovary, and gastrointestinal tract. Examples include cytarabine, fludarabine, gemcitabine, methotrexate, and 5-fluorouracil.

■ *Antitumor antibiotics* These drugs have both antimicrobial and cytotoxic activity. They also interfere with DNA by inhibiting certain cellular activities, and they work in all phases of the cell cycle. Examples include bleomycin, dactinomycin, daunorubicin, doxorubicin, and idarubicin.

■ *Mitotic inhibitors* These drugs can inhibit cell division (mitosis) or interfere with other parts of cell reproduction. Mitotic inhibitors include natural products and plant alkaloids. Examples include docetaxel, etoposide, paclitaxel, vinblastine, vincristine, and vinorelbine.

■ *Other cancer drugs* Other drugs used to treat cancer that do not fit into any of these categories include amsacrine and asparaginase.

Corticosteroids, sex hormones, and immunotherapy drugs are also given to people who have cancer. Sometimes these drugs are used to kill cancer cells or to slow their growth, but at other times they are used to increase the effectiveness of chemotherapy. Immunotherapy drugs are intended to stimulate the immune system so that the person's system can recognize and attack cancer cells.

Cherry angiomas

Harmless, small, bright red, domelike spots on the skin caused by dilated blood vessels (see ANGIOMA). Also known as De Morgan spots. Cherry angiomas develop mostly on the torsos of older people but can be found anywhere on the body. They can be removed by a dermatologist.

Chest pain

FOR SYMPTOM CHART
see Chest pain, page 24

Any pressure, squeezing, or general discomfort in the chest, which includes the heart, breast, and neck areas. Depending on its cause, chest pain can be mild or severe, dull or sharp, long-lasting or temporary, or frequent or occasional. It may occur randomly or only in association with certain activities, such as during exercise or immediately after a meal. Chest pain is not a condition in itself but a symptom of an underlying cause that can be serious, such as heart attack, or trivial, such as indigestion or a strained muscle.

HEART-RELATED CHEST PAIN
The most common type of chest pain related to the heart is ANGINA, a diffuse pain often described as a feeling of tightness or heaviness in the chest. Angina is caused by insufficient blood flow to the heart. In most cases, attacks of angina last from 1 to 15 minutes and are brought on by physical exertion or emotional stress. Angina is a symptom of heart disease. Examples of other heart-related causes of chest pain include malfunction of the heart's mitral valve (MITRAL VALVE PROLAPSE [MVP]) or aortic valve (AORTIC STENOSIS), inflammation of the tissue surrounding the heart (PERICARDITIS), and inflammation of the heart muscle itself (MYOCARDITIS).

CHEST PAIN FROM OTHER CAUSES
About one in five people who see a doctor for chest pain are experiencing difficulty with the esophagus, the tube that leads from the throat to the stomach. The most common disease of the esophagus that causes chest pain is HEARTBURN, which can be a symptom of ESOPHAGEAL REFLUX (acidic stomach contents entering the esophagus) or HIATAL HERNIA (a portion of the stomach protrudes through the diaphragm muscle). Chest pain can also result from an ULCER in the stomach or upper portion of the small intestine (see STOMACH ULCER; DUODENAL ULCER). Ulcer pain worsens when the stomach is empty and improves after eating. Gallbladder disease (see CHOLECYSTITIS) can also cause chest pain.

Injury or disease in the chest itself can also cause chest pain. A severe

---

SIDE EFFECTS OF CHEMOTHERAPY

While the purpose of cancer chemotherapy is to kill cancer cells, it can also damage normal cells. Cells that divide rapidly under normal conditions, such as blood cells, cells of hair follicles, and cells in the reproductive and digestive tracts, are most likely to be damaged by chemotherapy. Damage to such cells accounts for many of the side effects of chemotherapy. Examples of such side effects include the following:

- Myelosuppression, or bone marrow suppression, which can lead to abnormally low numbers of red blood cells, white blood cells, and platelets
- Leukopenia, or low white blood cell count, which can limit the ability of the body to defend itself against infection
- Anemia, or low red blood cell count, which can produce symptoms such as dizziness and fatigue. (Serious cases may require blood transfusions.)
- Thrombocytopenia, or low platelet count, which can cause serious blood loss from injury or bleeding and can damage internal organs
- Hair loss, which is almost always temporary
- Appetite and weight loss, which are usually temporary
- Nausea and vomiting
- Fatigue
- Heart damage
- Damage to reproductive tissues, which can lead to temporary sterility, irregular menstrual periods, and painful intercourse

CHEST PAIN AND HEART ATTACK

In popular thinking, the key symptom of heart attack is pain in the chest. However, not all chest pain signals a heart attack, nor does every heart attack cause chest pain. The key is knowing the type of pain and accompanying symptoms that are most likely to indicate a heart attack.

According to the American Heart Association, there are three classic warning signs of heart attack. One or more of the following is likely to occur if a heart attack is taking place:

- Uncomfortable pressure, fullness, squeezing, or pain in the center of the chest that lasts more than a few minutes. The pain may also go away and then return.
- Pain radiating from the chest to the shoulders, neck, or arm (usually the left). In women particularly, it may affect the jaw.
- Chest pain accompanied by light-headedness, fainting, nausea, or shortness of breath.

A number of other symptoms occur less commonly but may also indicate heart attack:

- Unusual pain in the chest, abdomen, or stomach
- Nausea or dizziness without chest pain
- Shortness of breath or difficulty breathing without chest pain
- Anxiety, fatigue, or weakness lacking apparent cause
- Cold sweating, palpitations, or pallor

If a heart attack is suspected, medical attention should be sought immediately.

blow to the chest, such as hitting the steering wheel or dashboard in an automobile collision, may produce persistent pain, even after the injury has apparently healed. Chest pain may also be caused by an infection (for example, pneumonia), inflammation (such as bronchitis or pleurisy), a disorder in the lungs (such as asthma), or any condition that produces persistent heavy coughing. Severe anxiety, particularly in the form of PANIC DISORDER, can also result in chest pain and is typically accompanied by palpitations (uncomfortably rapid heartbeat).

DIAGNOSIS AND TREATMENT

Since chest pain is not a condition but a symptom, treatment depends on the source of the problem. The principal diagnostic objective is to determine whether the pain originates in the heart or in another organ. Further testing, such as an ECHOCARDIOGRAM or CARDIAC STRESS TESTING, may be ordered. On the other hand, if the doctor suspects heartburn, a medication to reduce stomach acid may be prescribed. Resolution of the chest pain while taking medications to reduce stomach acid suggests a gastrointestinal problem rather than a cardiac problem. Medications, angioplasty, and

surgery are all potential options to treat angina. The choice depends on a person's health status, a person's preferences, and the type of vessel narrowing that is causing the problem.

Chest tube

A medical instrument used to drain accumulations of fluid in the pleural space, a condition called PLEURAL EFFUSION. A chest tube is inserted through a small incision in the chest wall. The tube is then connected to a suction device to aid in draining the fluid and reexpanding the lungs. When bleeding occurs in the pleural space between the chest wall and the lungs, a condition called HEMOTHORAX, a chest tube may be inserted through the chest wall to drain the blood. The tube is left in place after the draining to aid the lung in expanding again. Chest tubes may also be inserted to drain pus that may accumulate in the pleural space as the result of severe pneumonia.

Chest X ray

The most common diagnostic tool for producing images of the structures, organs, and tissues inside the chest. X rays can be used to screen, diagnose, and evaluate conditions of the chest. X rays are high-energy electromagnetic waves with a shorter wavelength

than visible light. When X-ray beams are passed through the chest, dense structures such as bone do not allow many X rays to pass through them. For this reason, structures such as the rib cage appear white on an X-ray image. Hollow structures such as the lungs allow most of the X rays to pass through and appear black on the X-ray image. Tubular structures such as the blood vessels in the chest are outlined more clearly on X-ray film if they are filled with a CONTRAST MEDIUM. Chest X rays may be used to diagnose lung diseases such as cancer or pneumonia or to help identify conditions such as an enlarged heart, congestive heart failure, and other consequences of heart disease.

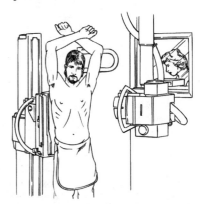

SIMPLE X-RAY PROCEDURE
For a chest X ray, the technician will probably take a side and a front view. For a side view, the person stands with one shoulder on the plate containing the film and arms overhead; for a front view, the person's chest is against the plate. The person is asked to hold his or her breath during the filming.

Chewing tobacco

Tobacco that has been pressed together for chewing rather than smoking; also called smokeless tobacco. Chewing tobacco contains nicotine, and the hazards of addiction to smokeless tobacco compare to those of smoking. Chewing tobacco wears away tooth enamel, erodes the gums, and contributes to bone loss, thus loosening the teeth. Because sugar is added to chewing tobacco to improve its taste, people who chew tobacco are at increased risk of tooth decay. All forms of smokeless tobacco contain high concentrations of cancer-causing agents, and users are at risk of developing oral cancers and cancer of the pharynx, larynx, and esophagus.

Cheyne-Stokes

An abnormal respiratory pattern characterized by alternating episodes of APNEA (in this case, a temporary cessation of breathing) and deep, rapid breathing. Each cycle lasts from 45 seconds to 3 minutes and includes a 10- to 20-second period of apnea. Causes of Cheyne-Stokes respiration include cerebrovascular disease, brain tumors, metabolic disturbances affecting the brain, and head trauma. In older people, the problem is frequently caused by congestive heart failure or respiratory diseases, such as pneumonia. Cheyne-Stokes can also affect younger, healthy people when they hyperventilate or are exposed to high altitudes. This breathing pattern occurs most commonly during sleep. See also SLEEP DISORDERS.

Chickenpox

An acute, highly contagious illness caused by the varicella-zoster virus, which also causes SHINGLES, a later reactivation of the virus. Chickenpox is transmitted by direct contact with a person who has the illness or by respiratory exposure to infected droplets. It occurs most commonly in late winter and spring. The incubation period is 14 to 16 days, and it can be transmitted within 10 to 21 days following exposure. To prevent transmission to another person, the individual who has chickenpox should be isolated until all the skin lesions have crusted over.

SYMPTOMS

An itchy rash of red-outlined, fluid-filled bumps is the first symptom of chickenpox. Moderate fever, mild headache, and general malaise may also be present. The bumps form clear fluid blisters that become dry and crusty and then scab over in 4 to 5 days. This progression may take place at different intervals on different sites of the body. Generally, no new lesions appear by the fifth day, most have become crusted by the sixth day, and most of the crusted lesions have disappeared by the 20th day. The mouth, throat, eyes, upper respiratory tract, and mucous membranes of the vagina and rectum may

also be involved. When the lesions appear on the scalp, there may be swelling and pain in the lymph nodes of the neck.

DIAGNOSIS AND TREATMENT

Diagnosis may be made on the basis of a physical examination and medical history and confirmed by detection of viral antigens in the lesions or blood.

In mild cases, only the symptoms of chickenpox are usually treated. Wet compresses may be applied to control itching and scratching. To prevent infection of the lesions, frequent bathing with soap and water and frequent changes of underclothing are recommended. In severe cases, oral antihistamines or pain relievers are sometimes given. The risk of severe, even fatal, disease is higher in adults and in persons with depressed T-cell immunity (for example, those with AIDS [acquired immunodeficiency syndrome]) or people taking corticosteroids or receiving chemotherapy. Oral acyclovir, which has been found to decrease somewhat the length and severity of chickenpox, can be given to those at risk within 24 hours after the rash first appears.

A vaccine is recommended for all healthy children who have not had chickenpox, beginning at the age of 12 to 18 months, or between 19 months and 13 years of age. Healthy adolescents and young adults may be immunized if they have no history of varicella infection. The vaccination is highly effective at preventing severe disease.

Once a person has had chickenpox, the person is considered immune from contracting it again. A blood test can determine immunity in a person who is uncertain of his or her medical history.

Chilblains

See PERNIO.

Child abuse

See ABUSE, CHILD.

Child development

The predictable stages children pass through as they achieve physical, intellectual, and emotional maturity. Mental growth follows a definite pattern through childhood and adolescence. As a child develops, new intellectual and emotional abilities

emerge and become part of the personality. Typically, this pattern of development is complete by late adolescence. In the work of important psychological theorists, such as Sigmund Freud, childhood development is central to adult personality and to emotional problems that appear later in life.

DEVELOPMENTAL STAGES

Children develop as a result of the complex interaction between what they have inherited and what they learn from their environment. Since each individual is unique, the pattern of development varies somewhat from child to child.

■ *Infant (from birth to 1 year)* In the first months of life, behaviors and emotions are governed largely by reflex. Examples are the rooting and sucking reflexes. When the baby's lips or cheeks are stroked, the baby turns toward the sensation and roots for the nipple. As soon as the nipple enters the mouth, the baby begins to suck. These particular reflexes usually disappear by about the fourth month, but they may arise in a sleeping infant as old as 7 months. In the hand-grasp reflex, stroking the palm causes the baby to close the fingers strongly over the stroking object. Although most infant reflexes cease after the first few months, the baby's brain stores information learned during reflexive movements and uses the information later.

Most babies can smile at other people by about 8 weeks. In the fifth month, babies can clearly distinguish parents from strangers and may express fear of strangers. At 8 months, infants are highly attached to the parent providing most of their care, and they may express fear (SEPARATION ANXIETY) when that parent leaves the room. Other fears, such as of vacuum cleaners, loud noises, or baths, may develop at this age; usually they last only a short time. Typically, infants of 11 and 12 months start saying "no" and may begin to have tantrums.

■ *Toddler (1 through 3 years)* Toddlers seek independence, and their desire to go off on their own challenges parental discipline. Toddlers need to learn in a consistent manner what behavior is appropriate. They often start activities they are not yet skilled enough to complete and

DEVELOPMENTAL MILESTONES

Although children learn and grow at their own pace, they typically acquire physical, mental, and social skills at predictable ages, as their nervous system matures.

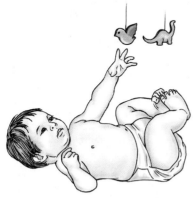

INFANT INTERACTION

Babies love to reach for and touch brightly colored objects, such as an overhead mobile attached to the crib. A child 9 months or older enjoys toys with moving parts, levers, and wheels.

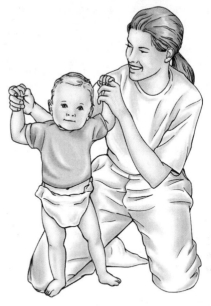

BABY STEPS

By 11 or 12 months, many infants will want to try to stand or walk with assistance. Children also enjoy taking steps while holding onto furniture or their parent's hands. This activity, called cruising, is a good activity to learn before walking.

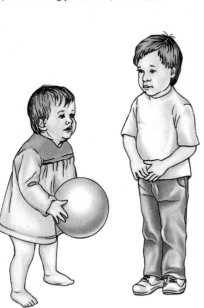

LEARNING TO PLAY AND SHARE

Toddlers use a lot of energy in play. Parents should encourage and supervise play with other children, but they should not expect a child younger than 3 to share his or her toys. Children at this age often play side by side, not together.

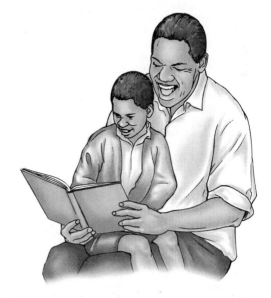

READING TOGETHER

Reading aloud to a child is one of the most important things a parent can do to stimulate development. Children of all ages enjoy being read to by their parents, grandparents, and baby-sitters. Many parents make reading a daily habit.

C

exhibit a high degree of frustration and anger as a result. Temper tantrums, crying, screaming, and breath holding are common. Throughout this period, children use language more and more complexly. They first try words at 12 to 15 months, and by age 3 may be arranging events in chronological order and telling stories.

■ *Early childhood (4 through 5 years)* Four- and 5-year-olds are highly social, with vivid imaginations that are expressed in complex make-believe play. They can now think about language and speak in ways that are understood by people outside their own families. Children learn to count small numbers of objects, can draw simple objects, play games that involve taking turns and following rules, and may begin to write the alphabet and read a few words.

■ *School age (6 through 12 years)* Acceptance by peers is extremely important at this stage of life. Friendships tend to be with members of the same sex. In early school age, many children denounce or condemn members of the opposite sex, a behavior that lessens as the child approaches adolescence. Many children try lying, cheating, and stealing as they learn to negotiate the various and conflicting rules of school, family, and friends; appropriate responses from parents and teachers help children learn acceptable social behavior. As school-aged children grow older, their capacity to pay attention increases, typically from approximately 15 minutes in a 6-year-old to 1 hour in a 12-year-old.

■ *Adolescence (13 through 18 years)* Adolescents are painfully self-conscious, constantly comparing themselves with their peers. Sexuality is very important, as girls begin their first menstrual periods (menarche) and boys start experiencing wet dreams (nocturnal emissions of semen). Adolescents pull away from parents to establish their own identities. At first, they associate largely with members of their own sex, then the peer group widens to include members of the other sex. Dating, sexual experimentation, and the desire to establish sexual relationships are issues of overriding importance. Adolescents tend to think of themselves as indestructible and immortal, believing that unfortunate events like unwanted pregnancy or an auto accident while under the influence of drugs or alcohol cannot happen to them.

THEORIES OF NORMAL AND ABNORMAL DEVELOPMENT

■ *Sigmund Freud (1856–1932)* Freud believed that the essential adult personality forms during the first 5 or 6 years of life. In addition, he saw the pattern of childhood changes in sexual terms, which are often referred to as the psychosexual stages of development. According to Freud, disruption of a given stage would cause an individual to focus exclusively (fixate) on the issues of that stage for the rest of his or her life.

In the first, or oral, stage (birth to 18 months), the child derives erotic pleasure from the mouth, lips, and tongue. Trauma at this stage produces so-called oral personalities, typified by people who smoke or drink excessively. Between 18 months and 3 years, children are in the anal stage, the period in which they learn bowel and bladder control. Fixation at this point produces an anal personality, which is orderly, stubborn, or generous. During the phallic stage, which lasts from ages 3 through 6, the penis or clitoris becomes the most important erogenous zone. The child forms a strong erotic desire for the parent of the opposite sex, a formation Freud called the Oedipal complex (after the Greek tragic hero Oedipus, who unknowingly killed his father and married his mother). These desires are repressed by the time the child enters the latency period, which lasts until puberty. During latency boys and girls are uninterested in each other and restrict their friendships to same-sex groups. Puberty begins the genital stage, when sexual desire returns and adolescents seek out members of the opposite sex. The genital stage continues throughout the rest of the person's life.

■ *Harry Stack Sullivan (1892–1949)* Sullivan agreed with Freud on the importance of childhood, but he argued that development continued well past the early years. He divided development into seven developmental epochs, and he focused strongly on the child's relationship with his or her mother and on the need for healthy interpersonal relationships during the teenage years. Most important, Sullivan divided adolescence into three distinct epochs, each with its own demands. In preadolescence (ages 9 to 12), the child needs an intimate relationship with a close friend of the same sex. During early adolescence (ages 13 to 17), the child enters puberty and begins to desire relationships with the opposite sex. In late adolescence (18 to early 20s), the individual seeks out a long-term sexual relationship and focuses more on finances and occupation.

■ *Erik Erikson (1902–1994)* Erikson divided life into eight stages, of which the first five occur during childhood and adolescence. Each stage is marked by a crisis, which is less a cataclysmic event than a turning point when both potential and vulnerability increase. If the passage from one stage to another is made successfully, the person enjoys enhanced function, while an unsuccessful transition produces maladjustment. The stages are related; the manner in which an individual resolves one crisis affects the next.

The first stage, called trust versus mistrust, occurs in the first year of life. If the child is consistently nurtured and cared for by the parents, he or she learns to regard the world with trust. Failure to nurture and care produces distrust. The second stage, autonomy versus shame and doubt, occurs in the second year. As the child develops and seeks independence and self-control, he or she learns autonomy from success and shame and doubt from failure. Success in this stage yields a balance of willfulness and self-restraint; failure leads to either strict obedience or constant defiance.

The third stage, initiative versus guilt, happens during the third or fourth year, as children try out social roles in family and peer groups and develop a conscience. Success leads to a balance between initiative and conscience, while a stifling of healthy initiative produces paralyzing guilt. The fourth stage is industry versus inferiority, and it covers school age until adolescence. Children discover the importance of working and applying themselves. They also learn that overwork at the expense of playfulness and imagination is dangerous. Success delivers a feeling of competence that carries over into adulthood, while failure leads to a lingering sense of inferiority. The final stage, identity versus role confusion, lasts through adolescence, as the individual tries to establish a feeling of inner sameness. Success leads to the ability to be true to oneself; an individual who fails to find inner sameness may never understand who he or she is. Adolescents often band together in a desire to define themselves and exclude others, an impulse that in the extreme can be cruel to outsiders and may lead to criminal behavior.

■ *Jean Piaget (1896–1980)* Piaget focused on the development of cognitive power, or intelligence, in children. In the sensorimotor period (birth to approximately 2 years) the child begins with simple reflexes and develops basic mental schemes to deal with the world. The preoperational period lasts from ages 2 to 7 years, as the child develops language and symbols (such as the alphabet and numbers), begins to think internally, can search for hidden objects, and understands past, present, and future. In the concrete operational period (approximately 7-11 years), the child can add, subtract, classify, and put objects in order, and he or she is more socially oriented than self-centered. With the formal operations period, beginning at approximately age 11 or 12, the child can think abstractly, reason deductively, develop and test hypotheses, and decide whether answers solve problems.

Child safety seats

Safety seats designed to protect infants and children in a motor vehicle accident. The use of child safety seats is required by law throughout the United States, and most hospitals will not permit a parent to take a newborn baby home unless the car is equipped with a safety seat. The safety seat is designed to diffuse the forces in a crash over the child's entire body and to keep the child from being thrown out of the car or from striking anything within the car during a crash. An infant's chance of surviving

a crash is greatly improved by the proper use of a child safety seat.

The infant safety seat is designed for a baby weighing less than 20 pounds. It should be installed in the center of the rear seat of the car so the baby faces the back of the car. Some infant safety seats can be converted to an upright, forward-facing seat when the baby is about a year old and weighs about 20 pounds. Such a seat will protect a baby until he or she weighs about 40 pounds, at which point a belt-positioning booster seat should be used, together with both lap and shoulder seat belts. Children age 12 and younger should always ride in the back seat of any vehicle. See CAR RESTRAINTS and Types of child safety seats, next page.

Childbirth

FOR FIRST AID
see Childbirth, page 1317

The process of giving birth to a child, involving the three stages of LABOR. Childbirth can take place safely at a hospital, a birthing center (see BIRTHING CENTERS), or at home, with proper preparation. Usually, babies are delivered with the help of a medical caregiver. Medical professionals trained to handle childbirth include doctors, such as family practitioners and obstetrician/gynecologists, and certified nurse-midwives and licensed midwives (see MIDWIFE). Doulas are trained to assist with nonmedical pain management, providing emotional support, and birth education, but cannot help deliver a baby. Some women cannot deliver their babies by vaginal delivery (see DELIVERY, VAGINAL) and must have them by CESAREAN SECTION (C-section), a surgical procedure in a hospital in which the baby is born through an incision in the abdomen.

Childbirth, emergency

FOR FIRST AID
see Childbirth, page 1317

Delivery of a baby when no medical help is available. Emergency childbirth is sometimes needed when access to medical help is blocked, or when the labor is proceeding faster than expected. Childbirth is a natural process that should normally proceed

without interference, and bystanders should intervene only when necessary. It is never advisable to try to delay delivery. Simple first aid measures that can assist a mother who is delivering a baby without medical assistance include calling 911, making the woman comfortable, and keeping her calm.

To assist a woman in an emergency situation, it is essential for the person helping to wash his or her hands well with soap and water and to wear rubber gloves, if possible. The pregnant woman should lie on her back on top of clean sheets, if possible, with knees bent and spread apart. She should be encouraged to breathe slowly between contractions. The baby will need to be supported gently as he or she emerges, and the umbilical cord should be gently moved if it is wrapped around the baby's neck. Rubbing the back while holding the baby so its head is lower than its feet should help him or her start to breathe. The baby should be dried with a towel and wrapped in a clean towel; the white material on the baby's skin should be left intact. A string should be tied around the umbilical cord at least 4 inches from the baby's navel. A second string should be tied with a tight square knot about 6 to 8 inches from the baby or 2 to 4 inches from the first knot. About 1 minute after birth, the cord should be cut between the two ties, using a sterilized knife or clean scissors. The placenta should be expelled by the mother within 30 minutes and should be saved for the medical personnel to inspect when they arrive. Until that happens, the mother and baby should be kept warm.

There are only three situations in which a person might require emergency childbirth: when no transportation to a hospital is available, when the delivery is expected within 5 minutes, or when the doctor or hospital cannot be reached because of a natural disaster or other catastrophe.

Chinese medicine

Ancient form of HOLISTIC MEDICINE based on herbology, nutrition, acupuncture, massage, exercise, and the idea that health involves a state of balance of body, mind, and spirit. In

TYPES OF CHILD SAFETY SEATS

Child safety seats are required in most states and are proven to save lives and young children from serious injury. The best type of seat depends on the age and weight of the child.

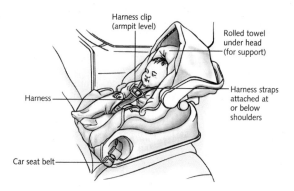

Harness clip (armpit level)

Rolled towel under head (for support)

Harness

Harness straps attached at or below shoulders

Car seat belt

INFANT-ONLY SEAT
An infant who weighs 20 pounds or less should be placed in the infant-only car seat facing the rear of the car in the middle of the back seat. It is important to make sure the car seat belt firmly buckles and secures the infant seat so that it does not move easily.

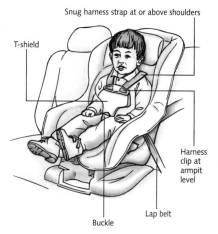

Snug harness strap at or above shoulders

T-shield

Harness clip at armpit level

Buckle

Lap belt

T-SHIELD SEAT (20 TO 40 POUNDS)
A child who weighs 20 to 40 pounds should be placed in the back seat of the car in a T-shield–type car seat, which gets its name from the shape of the restraint that is placed over the chest of the child and locked in place between the child's legs.

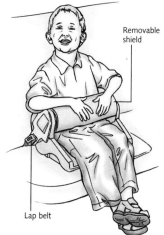

Removable shield

Lap belt

REMOVABLE SHIELD BOOSTER
A child who is 5 or 6 years old may be seated in a removable shield-type booster, which is secured in place with a lap belt and with a padded armrest that locks the child snugly in place.

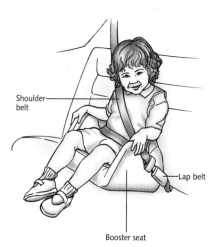

Shoulder belt

Lap belt

Booster seat

BOOSTER SEAT WITH BELT ADJUSTMENT SLOT
The safest type of seat for a child who weighs 30 pounds or more but no more than 100 pounds is a booster seat with a seat belt–type harness that secures a seat belt–across the child's lap and has a restraining belt that crosses over the child's chest.

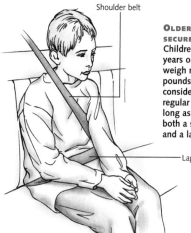

Shoulder belt

Lap belt

OLDER CHILD IN SECURE SEAT BELT
Children who are 10 years or older and weigh more than 80 pounds are usually considered safe in a regular seat belt, as long as the belt has both a shoulder belt and a lap belt.

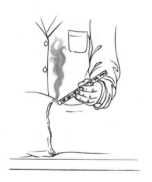

Applying the moxa stick

MOXIBUSTION
Moxibustion treatments involve burning an herb called moxa and applying the heat to specific acupoints on the body. The burning moxa stick does not touch the skin and is removed if the person becomes uncomfortable.

Chinese medicine, body, mind, and spirit are not viewed as separate entities, and the person is looked at as a whole.

CAUSES OF DISEASE
Chinese medicine is based on the idea that health is a state of balance and illness a sign of imbalance. Chinese medicine holds that disease can have both external and internal causes. External causes of disease include poor diet, climate, congenital abnormalities, injury, lack of exercise, and exhaustion.

Internal causes are emotional and affect the mind and the spirit. Once the mind or spirit is troubled, the person's energy is reduced through imbalance, and chronic physical disease develops. The core belief of the Chinese system of medicine is the realization that imbalance of a person's emotions inevitably leads to imbalance of his or her physical functioning. Avoiding extremes, or following the "Middle Way," is a practice fundamental to the Chinese medicine view of promoting longevity by avoiding illness.

DIAGNOSIS
In Chinese medicine, diagnosis is based on observation, questioning, listening, smelling, and physical examination. The aim of diagnosis is to identify the "pattern of disharmony" that is disrupting the person's state of balance. The aim of treatment is to restore harmony and balance to the body or mind, rather than to eliminate disease. When

balance is restored, Chinese medicine holds that signs and symptoms usually disappear. Health is defined as the absence of disharmony or imbalance.

THERAPIES
A characteristic attitude reflected in Chinese medicine is that "illness is good." This means that being sick tells a person that he or she is out of balance in body and mind and must stop, rest, and take steps to recover and regain balance. By the same token, health is a constantly changing flow of energy, or qi ("chee"). According to traditional Chinese medicine, imbalances in qi result in illness.

Therapies in Chinese medicine are directed at restoring balance to qi. ACUPUNCTURE uses the insertion of needles to adjust qi, while herbology uses herbal remedies to normalize qi in the blood and other organs. Particular foods are selected to balance qi and other fundamental substances in the body, and exercise is designed to move qi. Tui-Naor Chinese massage therapy, balances qi

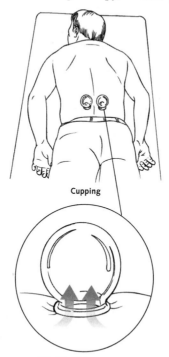

Cupping

Skin lifted into a vacuum

CUPPING
In a treatment called cupping, moxa may also be placed in a metal cup, lit, and applied in a similar manner.

in the body by applying pressure to the body with the hands. Qi is stimulated externally in various ways, including ACUPRESSURE (pressing points on the body); CUPPING (applying pressure created by vacuums in special cups); and MOXIBUSTION (burning herbs to heat acupuncture points.)

Chinese restaurant syndrome

Symptoms such as headache, nausea, diarrhea, sweating, chest tightness, and a burning sensation at the back of the neck that occur as a reaction to MSG (monosodium glutamate) in food. Because MSG is best known for its role in some Asian cooking, the reaction to it has been called Chinese restaurant syndrome. MSG is used to enhance flavor in a variety of restaurants and in many processed foods.

Chiropractic

The practice of physical manipulation to diagnose, treat, and rehabilitate disorders of the neuromusculoskeletal system. The word "chiropractic" literally means "doing by hand." Chiropractic is based on the ideas that the human body has an innate self-healing ability and that it seeks balance. Chiropractors believe that small internal misalignments, called vertebral subluxations, interfere with proper functioning of the nervous system and the body's ability to maintain a healthy balance. Chiropractic seeks to bring a misaligned body back into balance through the manual manipulation of the spine, joints, and muscles.

Techniques used by chiropractors include manipulation of joints in ways that are similar to cracking the knuckles—pressure is applied to a joint to return it to its proper position. Other techniques include soft tissue manipulation, deep tissue massage, and ultrasound to stimulate circulation. About 90 percent of chiropractors use X rays to identify dislocations.

The manual manipulation of the spine practiced by chiropractors is widely considered to be effective for the relief of acute lower back pain. Chiropractic can also ease pain in areas such as the neck, the joints, or the middle of the back. It is some-

C

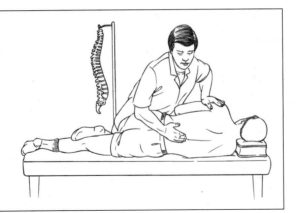

SPINAL REALIGNMENT
A typical chiropractic manipulation involves realigning the spine by massaging specific vertebrae to release tension and then applying a rapid thrust to move them into their proper position. Treatments may last from 15 minutes to an hour and may be repeated as frequently as several times a week.

times used to relieve the pain of headaches, muscle spasms, and nerve inflammation. Chiropractic has not been found to be successful in studies as a treatment for asthma, high blood pressure, or neurological pain.

Chiropractic, network

A holistic approach to chiropractic in which physical adjustments are intended to promote the body's self-healing potential. Network chiropractic was developed by practitioners who believed that chiropractic had become overly mechanical and had abandoned its original holistic approach to health and wellness. Network chiropractors believe they follow the original intent of chiropractic, which is that physical adjustments are performed to release the interference that enables the body to heal itself.

Chlamydia

The most common bacterial sexually transmitted disease (STD; see SEXUALLY TRANSMITTED DISEASES) in the United States. Chlamydia is caused by the bacterium *Chlamydia trachomatis* and is usually transmitted by sexual activity. The bacteria that cause the infection are carried in the blood, semen, or vaginal fluid of an infected person, entering the body via contact with these fluids.

SYMPTOMS AND RISK FACTORS

In men, chlamydia can cause nonspecific urethritis (NSU), with symptoms including a discharge from the penis and pain when urinating. In about one fourth of infected men, there are no symptoms. Chlamydia may also cause a swelling of the testes, which

can lead to sterility, although this complication is rare.

Women often have no symptoms of chlamydia. If symptoms occur, they may include a yellow-green vaginal discharge, pain during urination, persistent lower abdominal pain, pain during sexual intercourse, spotting between menstrual periods, and possibly nausea and fever.

Without treatment, chlamydia may persist for as long as 15 months, during which time it is communicable to sexual partners. The infection can eventually spread to the upper reproductive tract in women and result in serious complications, including inflammation of the fallopian tubes (SALPINGITIS) or the cervix (CERVICITIS) and PELVIC INFLAMMATORY DISEASE (PID). These conditions can cause INFERTILITY. Chlamydia also raises the risk of ectopic pregnancy in women in whom the infection has not been treated. In pregnant women, the bacteria can be passed to the fetus, causing eye infections, pneumonia, and persistent respiratory disease.

A person can have chlamydia for weeks or even months, with symptoms that come and go over time. Medical care should be sought in the presence of any symptoms or if a sexual partner has been infected.

DIAGNOSIS AND TREATMENT

Chlamydia may be diagnosed by culturing cells, which takes 3 to 7 days for results. Newer and more efficient methods are available for diagnosing chlamydia, and results can be determined within a few hours. Both methods require a sample of a man's urine or a swab from a woman's cervix or urethra. A 7-day course of oral antibiotics, such as tetracycline

or erythromycin, is generally prescribed to treat chlamydia.

Chloasma

Temporary discoloration of facial skin during pregnancy or while taking hormonal contraceptives (see CONTRACEPTION, HORMONAL METHODS). Hormonal changes cause darkening of patches of the skin over the forehead on the bridge of the nose and on the cheekbones, generally after 16 weeks of pregnancy. The discoloration is intensified by exposure to sunlight and is most marked on women with dark complexions.

Chlorpheniramine maleate

An antihistamine. Chlorpheniramine maleate is used to relieve symptoms due to the common cold or allergies such as hives, rash, watery eyes, runny nose, itching, and sneezing. It is also used as a sleep aid for insomnia and to treat motion sickness and anxiety. Common brand names include Chlor-Trimeton and Teldrin.

Choking

FOR FIRST AID
see Choking (Heimlich maneuver), page 1318

A breathing emergency caused by an airway that has been blocked by food or another object. Choking is a common emergency, usually the result of inadequately chewed food that has become lodged in the throat or windpipe. This often happens when a person has been talking while chewing a piece of meat. Choking also may happen when a person who wears dentures chews his or her food inadequately; this can occur because dentures exert less pressure on food than teeth. Choking can also occur when a person runs, walks, or plays with food or other objects in the mouth.

Choking is usually accompanied by panic, with a visible expression of terror on the person's face. He or she may turn purple, the eyes may bulge, and the person may wheeze or gasp. If the person can cough freely, has normal skin color, and can speak, he or she is not choking; coughing will probably resolve the problem. However, if the cough sounds more like a gasp and the person is turning blue, he or she is most likely choking. If in

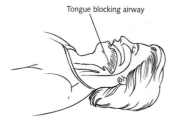

Tongue blocking airway

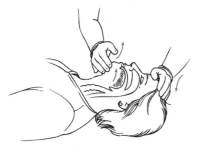

Head-tilt technique

OPENING THE AIRWAY
Many choking situations occur because the person's tongue slides into the airway. If the person is unconscious, the danger of choking is greater because the jaw muscles relax. The rescuer can reposition the person's tongue by pressing the head back and down and closing the lower jaw.

doubt, ask the person if he or she can speak. A person who is choking will only be able to communicate through gestures, and the universal sign for choking is a hand clutching the throat, with fingers extended. The HEIMLICH MANEUVER may be used by trained persons to dislodge the obstruction. Even if the blockage is removed and the person's breathing restored, emergency medical assistance should always be sought, because complications can arise from both the emergency and the first aid measures taken.

Cholangiocarcinoma

A cancer of the bile ducts, the tubes that carry bile from the liver and gallbladder to the small intestine. This uncommon cancer occurs most frequently in men and women in their 50s. Symptoms include jaundice (yellowing of the skin), pale stools, and dark urine, often accompanied by weight loss and fatigue. Individuals with gallstones or gallbladder inflammation, chronic inflammation of the large intestine, or infection by a certain type of parasite found in Asia have an increased risk for developing

this cancer. No effective treatments have been developed, and the prognosis is usually poor. Complete surgical removal of the affected duct is sometimes attempted if the cancer is small and localized.

Cholangiopancreato-graphy

A diagnostic procedure performed to evaluate diseases of the bile ducts of the liver such as stones or narrowing. In conventional ERCP (endoscopic retrograde cholangiopancreatography), a CONTRAST MEDIUM is injected directly into the bile ducts. In magnetic resonance cholangiopancreatography (see MRI), the bile ducts are visualized without the use of a contrast medium during an abdominal magnetic resonance examination.

Cholangitis

Inflammation of the bile ducts, the channels that carry bile from the liver to the gallbladder and to the intestines. (See BILARY SYSTEM.) Cholangitis is most commonly the result of obstruction of bile flow and consequent bacterial infection. The most common symptoms of cholangitis are abdominal pain, fever, and jaundice (a yellowing of the skin and the whites of the eyes). In some cases, abdominal symptoms are minimal, but chills and fever are present.

Cholangitis is usually caused by a bacterial infection that is triggered when a gallstone blocks the bile ducts. Gallstones are solid masses, primarily of cholesterol, that form in the gallbladder. Bile duct blockage may also be due to strictures (narrowing of part of the ducts from injury or accumulation of scar tissue). When the passage of bile is obstructed, trapped bacteria rapidly multiply. Less commonly, bile duct inflammation is caused by primary sclerosing cholangitis, an autoimmune disorder, which means that it is caused by a malfunction in the body's own immune system that causes it to attack itself. Primary sclerosing cholangitis is frequently associated with ulcerative COLITIS and sometimes with Crohn disease, and can gradually destroy the bile ducts in the liver.

DIAGNOSIS AND TREATMENT
When the symptoms suggest cholangitis, it is important to discover the underlying cause and location of

obstruction to avoid recurrence. Cholangitis is diagnosed by ultrasound and CT (computed tomography) scanning or ERCP (endoscopic retrograde cholangiopancreatography). In ERCP, a slim, flexible, lighted tube called an endoscope is inserted through the mouth and guided down to the bile ducts. A contrast dye is injected through the endoscope to make the bile ducts and surrounding organs show clearly on X rays. If the test reveals a gallstone or narrowing of the ducts, additional instruments can be inserted to remove or work around the obstruction. Balloons can be inserted to open up blockages. A sample of tissue may also be taken for analysis. Further treatment varies with the cause of the obstruction.

Cholecystectomy

Surgical removal of the gallbladder. A cholecystectomy is performed in severe cases of CHOLECYSTITIS, or inflammation of the gallbladder. Cholecystitis is usually the result of gallstones (solid masses, primarily of cholesterol, formed in the gallbladder). Cholecystectomy is also indicated for patients with recurrent symptoms due to gallstones.

Today, laparoscopic cholecystectomy is the preferred surgical treatment of symptomatic gallstones. It has largely replaced open cholecystectomy, which requires a long abdominal incision. In a laparoscopic cholecystectomy, the gallbladder is removed with a fiberoptic viewing instrument called a laparoscope. After this procedure, there is less postoperative pain and disability, a shorter hospital stay, and a more rapid recovery than for the open method.

Throughout the operation, the surgeon views the abdominal cavity on a monitor. First, a needle is inserted through a small keyhole incision near the navel. Carbon dioxide is pumped through the needle to distend the abdomen. Three additional tubes are inserted in the right side of the abdomen. Tiny instruments are passed down the laparoscope through the incisions to remove or crush gallstones and free the gallbladder. Air and bile are removed from the gallbladder, the organ is extracted, and the cystic duct is tied off and cut.

C

C

LAPAROSCOPIC CHOLECYSTECTOMY

A cholecystectomy is the surgical removal of the gallbladder. Up until the development of laparoscopic surgery, gallbladders were usually removed with abdominal cholecystectomies—making a large incision (about 6 inches long) in the abdomen. This type of cholecystectomy is still the preferred method if there are gallstones in the common bile duct or if acute cholecystitis or certain other conditions exist. In other cases, however, the surgeon may use the laparoscopic cholecystectomy technique shown here, which reduces the length of the hospital stay and recovery time.

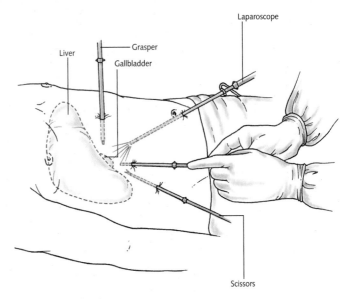

MAKING THE SMALL INCISIONS
The surgeon creates four punctures, or ports, through which the laparoscope (viewing tube) and the tiny surgical instruments are inserted.

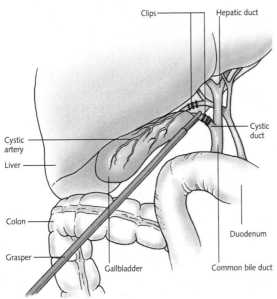

CLOSING OFF THE CYSTIC DUCT AND THE CYSTIC ARTERY
First, the surgeon pushes the gallbladder away from the small intestine and colon. Then, the surgeon uses clips to close off the cystic duct from the common bile duct and to close off the cystic artery.

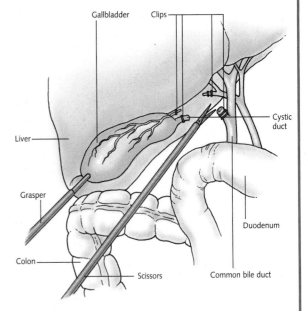

REMOVING THE GALLBLADDER
After the cystic duct and the cystic artery are severed, the surgeon seals off the blood vessels to the gallbladder, removes the bile, and pulls the gallbladder out through a port. Finally, the ports are stitched closed with one or two sutures.

A laparoscopic cholecystectomy is done in a hospital under general anesthesia. The procedure lasts less than an hour, and patients usually return home later on the same day or the next day. After surgery, a small dressing covers the incisions. Eventually, only minor scars remain.

Cholecystitis

Inflammation of the GALLBLADDER. Cholecystitis is usually the result of GALLSTONES (solid masses, primarily of cholesterol, which form in the gallbladder). When a gallstone in the cystic duct blocks the flow of bile from the gallbladder to the intestine, acute cholecystitis occurs and requires immediate treatment. Very often, surgical removal of the gallbladder (CHOLECYSTECTOMY) is necessary.

A stone that lodges in the cystic duct can cause extreme cramping pain in the upper abdomen. The pain may radiate to the right shoulder and the back and can be mistaken for a heart attack. As the gallbladder becomes increasingly inflamed, nausea and vomiting occur. Left untreated, jaundice (a yellowing of the skin and the whites of the eyes) and CHOLANGITIS (inflammation of the bile ducts) may develop. A rare but extremely serious complication of cholecystitis can be rupture of the gallbladder. This causes a severe form of peritonitis (inflammation of the peritoneum, the membrane that lines the abdominal cavity). A life-threatening emergency, peritonitis requires immediate medical treatment.

Gallstones are the most common cause of the inflammation. Of those affected, 75 percent have experienced previous gallbladder problems. Repeated attacks of acute cholecystitis lead to chronic cholecystitis. In this condition, the gallbladder shrinks, its walls thicken, and it eventually ceases to function. Less commonly, cholecystitis is due to an accident (trauma), surgical injury, or an infection that spreads into the gallbladder from the intestine. When acute inflammation of the gallbladder develops and no gallstones are present, the condition is called acalculous cholecystitis.

DIAGNOSIS AND TREATMENT

Imaging tests, such as ultrasound scanning and ERCP (endoscopic retrograde cholangiopancreatography), are administered to detect the presence of gallstones or bile duct blockage. CHOLECYSTOGRAPHY (an X ray of the gallbladder and common bile duct after they have been filled with a contrast dye) may be recommended when ULTRASOUND SCANNING fails to provide a definite diagnosis. However, today this procedure is performed much less frequently than in the past. In ERCP, a slim, flexible, lighted tube called an endoscope is inserted through the mouth and guided down to the gallbladder and bile ducts. A contrast dye is injected through the endoscope to make organs show clearly on X rays. If the test reveals gallstones in the duct, an additional instrument can be inserted to remove stones caught in the common bile duct. When there are no gallstones present, as in acalculous cholecystitis, the diagnosis is more difficult to make.

In some cases, a stone that obstructs the bile duct may pass on its own into the duodenum or fall back into the gallbladder. However, in most cases, gallstones must be removed by using an endoscope or by surgery. Very often, especially when there is a history of recurrent gallbladder problems, doctors recommend surgical removal of the gallbladder. If inflammation and infection are severe, a course of antibiotics may be ordered before surgery.

Cholecystography

An X-ray procedure for examining the gallbladder and common bile duct, which cannot be seen in a normal X ray. In cholecystography, a contrast dye that can make the organs visible in an X ray is administered either orally or intravenously. The dye can reveal the presence of gallstones or blockages; failure of the dye to become concentrated in the gallbladder may indicate a diseased gallbladder. Cholecystography can help to diagnose problems such as CHOLECYSTITIS (inflammation of the gallbladder that is most often caused by GALLSTONES) and BILIARY COLIC. Cholecystography has been replaced by ultrasound scanning as the first choice for imaging the gallbladder. It is now used when ultrasound scanning fails to provide a definite diagnosis.

Twelve hours before oral cholecys-tography is done, the individual has a fat-free meal and takes tablets that contain an iodine-based contrast material (dye) that is opaque to X rays. Alternatively, the contrast material may be administered intravenously. The dye is excreted by the liver into the gallbladder after 12 hours. X rays are then taken, and the individual is given a fatty meal or cholecystokinin (a substance that causes the gallbladder to expel bile and iodine into the bile duct). More X rays are taken about an hour later.

Cholera

An acute intestinal infection that occurs in developing countries of Africa and Asia and in parts of Latin America, where basic sanitation is lacking because of poverty. Cholera is caused by the bacterium *Vibrio cholerae*. In epidemics, the organism is spread by water contaminated directly or indirectly with feces or vomit from people who are infected. The organism that causes cholera is able to grow well in some foods, including rice, but it cannot grow or survive in acidic foods, including carbonated beverages, and is killed by heat. Large epidemics are usually associated with fecal contamination of a water supply and street food. It can also be contracted by eating raw or undercooked shellfish that have been contaminated by sewage.

People infected with cholera may have only mild diarrhea or no symptoms at all. In severe cases, death may occur within hours of becoming infected. Profuse watery diarrhea and vomiting cause a rapid, life-threatening loss of vital fluids and salts, with the possibility of circulatory collapse and shock. Cholera can be fatal if it is not diagnosed and treated promptly.

DIAGNOSIS AND TREATMENT

Cholera is diagnosed by laboratory tests that isolate the toxin-producing organism in the stool or vomit sample. Blood tests are also used to diagnose the infection.

For milder cases, treatment is generally based on having the person drink an oral rehydration solution or, in more severe cases, administration of intravenous solutions until the person is able to ingest fluids. Antibiotics such as tetracycline or doxycycline can decrease the length of the illness. The medication can

C

also lessen the excretion of the live cholera bacteria and the volume of fluids lost, but it is not considered essential for a successful cure.

At present, there is no recommended vaccine against cholera available in the United States, nor are there any cholera vaccination requirements for entry or exit in any country in the world. Adequate sanitation helps prevent cholera outbreaks.

Cholescintigraphy

A nuclear imaging study used to visualize the gallbladder and bile ducts. A small amount of radioactive substance is administered intravenously and is concentrated by the gallbladder. A special scanner is used to make a screen image of the gallbladder and bile ducts from the concentrated radioactive material. Cholescintigraphy is useful for diagnosing acute cholecystitis and detecting blockages in the bile duct system.

Cholestasis

Diminished bile flow from the liver. Cholestasis leads to jaundice (a yellowing of the skin and the whites of the eyes) and liver damage. It may be detected in a physical examination, in which the physician can detect jaundice by sight and can determine from tapping and feeling the abdomen whether the liver is tender or enlarged. Other investigations may include blood tests, ultrasound scanning, and a liver biopsy. To prevent liver damage, diagnosis and treatment of the underlying cause of cholestasis is essential.

Cholesteatoma

A benign mass or tumorlike growth formed by an accumulation of dead cells in the middle ear and/or mastoid (the prominent bone behind the ear). The condition is caused by repeated or chronic middle ear infections and inflammation and is usually associated with poor eustachian tube function. Cholesteatomas are formed when the skin of the eardrum grows into the middle ear. This skin forms a ball-shaped pocket that fills up with dead cells shed by the eardrum. The pocket erodes the bone that lines the middle ear cavity, often damages the delicate bones of hearing in the middle ear, and may become infected.

SYMPTOMS

Mild to moderately severe hearing loss and a recurring discharge from the ear are usually the symptoms of cholesteatoma. The discharge may consist of pus or other unpleasant-smelling fluids from the ear. Headache, earache, weakness of the facial muscles, and dizziness are less common symptoms that may precede serious complications.

DIAGNOSIS

People who experience any of the symptoms of cholesteatoma, and especially those with a history of ear infections, should see their doctor, who will probably refer them to an otolaryngologist (ear, nose, and throat specialist) for an examination and hearing test. A surgical microscope is often necessary to properly inspect the ear canal. If a cholesteatoma is detected, CT SCANNING (computed tomography scanning) may be ordered to determine how much the growth has spread and how severely the bones of hearing have been eroded.

TREATMENT

The first phase of medical treatment for cholesteatoma with drainage concentrates on drying the fluid that is causing the infection within the ear. Antibiotics may be prescribed to be taken orally or as drops to be applied in the ear. In some cases, intravenous antibiotics are necessary. Antibiotic treatment combined with weekly cleanings of the ear using a surgical microscope can sometimes clear up the infection. If there are polyps (growths of inflamed tissue) in the ear canal, they may have to be surgically removed before the infection will clear up. In children, removal of these polyps may have to be done in a hospital under general anesthesia. Once the infection has cleared up and the ear is dry, MICROSURGERY and complete removal of the cholesteatoma by an ear surgeon are usually recommended. If the growth is small or at an early stage, it may be possible to remove it entirely and thoroughly clean out the middle ear cavity. If the cholesteatoma is large, removal is more complicated, and the operation may involve rebuilding hearing structures and repairing a broken eardrum. Because the condition can recur, annual examinations by an otolaryngologist are essential. If the person's hearing is badly damaged, a hearing aid (see HEARING AIDS) may be necessary.

RISK FACTORS

Cholesteatomas contain enzymes that erode bone. The mastoid bone (bone located behind the outer ear and connected to the middle ear) may become involved. In time, a cholesteatoma can erode the bone leading into the inner ear and the thin plate of bone that separates the roof of the middle ear from the brain. This erosion of bone can cause profoundly impaired hearing, severe imbalance, and facial nerve paralysis. In extreme cases, it can lead to severe complications such as epidural abscess (accumulation of pus in the space between the skull and the outermost membrane covering the brain), brain abscess, and MENINGITIS (inflammation of the membranes that cover the brain and spinal cord).

Cholesterol

A chemical that is an essential component of cells and is a building block for many hormones. Cholesterol, a sterol, is a form of lipid (see LIPIDS). A certain amount of cholesterol is required by the body. Elevated levels of this waxy, fatlike substance are associated with an increased risk of ATHEROSCLEROSIS, a condition in which blood vessels are narrowed by fat deposits, which can compromise the blood flow to vital organs. Eventually, there may be sufficient blockage of an artery to cause a HEART ATTACK or STROKE. Eating too much fat, especially saturated fat, can raise blood cholesterol levels. See also FATS AND OILS.

CHOLESTEROL AND HEALTH

Many experts recommend checking blood cholesterol levels in one's 20s, particularly in individuals with a family history of heart disease or high blood cholesterol levels. If the results are normal, the test should be repeated every 5 to 10 years. If the results are abnormal, the blood cholesterol level should be monitored more closely; treatment may be required. A person's cholesterol levels are determined by a combination of genes and lifestyle. When blood cholesterol is high, lifestyle changes, such as diet and exercise modification, may bring it under control. A diet high in animal fat is likely to dramatically raise cholesterol levels. Regular exercise may

CHOLESTEROL LEVELS

Doctors assess an individual's cholesterol levels with a simple blood test that measures LDL (bad), HDL (good), and total cholesterol levels.

A total blood cholesterol level of:
- Less than 200 is ideal
- 200 to 239 is borderline high
- 240 or above is high

A low-density lipoprotein (LDL) level of:
- Less than 100 is ideal
- 100 to 129 is slightly elevated
- 130 to 159 is borderline high
- 160 or above is high

A high-density lipoprotein (HDL) level of:
- 60 or above is healthy
- 40 to 59 is slightly low
- Less than 40 is too low

Adapted from American Heart Association guidelines.

help control weight and cholesterol levels. If diet and exercise cannot reduce the cholesterol to an acceptable level, medication is advised.

When the total blood cholesterol level is elevated, additional tests can detect the levels of the different types of blood cholesterol. Cholesterol does not float freely in the bloodstream, but is attached to special carriers called lipoproteins. The two most important carriers are low-density lipoprotein (LDL) and high-density lipoprotein (HDL). The levels of LDL and HDL have opposite effects on the heart. High levels of LDL, referred to as "the bad cholesterol," are associated with a buildup of plaque (fat deposits) in the arteries, leading to atherosclerosis and heart disease. High levels of HDL, "the good cholesterol," reduce the risk of disease.

CHOLESTEROL IN FOODS

Because the liver can manufacture all the cholesterol needed by the body, there is no need for cholesterol in the adult diet. However, dietary cholesterol is present in all animal products (meat, poultry, dairy products, eggs, cheese, butter, and fish). Red meats (beef, pork, and lamb) contain the most LDL cholesterol. Fish and poultry generally contain lesser amounts. There is no cholesterol in any plant product or the oils made from them.

Although not a fat itself, cholesterol is closely related to fats. The amount of saturated fat in the diet can be even more damaging to blood cholesterol levels than cholesterol in foods such as egg yolks or red meat. Saturated fat from both animal and plant products is a major factor in raising blood cholesterol levels. Animal products contain considerably more saturated fat than most plant products. Large amounts of dietary cholesterol consumed with large amounts of saturated fat increase blood cholesterol levels more than large amounts of cholesterol alone. Saturated fats come from meats, poultry, dairy products, certain tropical vegetable oils (palm, palm kernel, coconut), and solid vegetable fats that are hard at room temperature. These are the fats most responsible for high blood cholesterol levels and an increased risk of heart disease.

Like saturated fats, trans-fatty acids (also known as trans fats) raise levels of harmful LDL cholesterol, promote clogged arteries, and increase the risk of heart disease. Trans-fatty acids are made through the hydrogenation process that solidifies liquid oils for use in food products. They may be present in stick margarine, crackers, cookies, and deep-fried foods.

UNSATURATED FATS

Unsaturated fats such as fish oils and pure vegetable oils are healthier choices than saturated fats and hydrogenated oils. Some unsaturated fats even lower cholesterol levels and may reduce the risk of cardiovascular disease. As a result, doctors advise consumers to avoid saturated fats and trans-fatty acids and instead incorporate unsaturated fats into their diets. Unsaturated fats are divided into two groups: monounsaturated and polyunsaturated.

Canola oil and avocado oil are good sources of monounsaturated fats, as are a variety of nuts: almonds, hazelnuts, macadamias, pecans, and pistachios. Monounsaturated fatty acids lower levels of harmful LDL cholesterol and have no negative effect on the helpful HDL variety. Polyunsaturated fats are found in corn, safflower, soybean, and sunflower oils. Omega-3 fatty acids, another type of polyunsaturated fats, are found in fish. Polyunsaturated fats lower the total blood cholesterol

level even more than monounsaturated fats. However, the non–omega-3 types do so by lowering helpful, heart-protective HDL as well as harmful LDL cholesterol levels.

Cholesterol-lowering drugs

Drugs used to lower cholesterol levels and reduce the risk of heart disease. Most people with high cholesterol levels are able to reduce their levels with improved diet and increased exercise, but for some, these measures are not enough, and cholesterol-lowering drugs must be prescribed. There are four types of drugs used to lower cholesterol levels.

STATINS

These drugs, also called HMG-CoA reductase inhibitors, lower levels of total cholesterol and LDL (low-density lipoprotein) cholesterol ("bad" cholesterol). They also lower levels of lipids, such as the triglycerides. Statins work by interfering with the manufacture of cholesterol in the body, blocking an enzyme called HMG-CoA reductase that is needed by the body to create cholesterol. Less cholesterol in the body encourages the liver to remove LDL cholesterol from the bloodstream, thus lowering the risk of clogged blood vessels and heart disease.

Statins work quickly, lowering cholesterol levels within 1 to 2 weeks, but many people will need to continue to take them for a long time. Common side effects include rash and upset stomach.

Examples include atorvastatin (Lipitor), fluvastatin (Lescol), lovastatin (Mevacor), pravastatin (Pravachol), and simva-statin (Zocor).

BILE ACID SEQUESTRANTS

Bile acid sequestrants, sometimes called bile acid resins, are synthetic substances that lower overall and LDL cholesterol levels. The body does not absorb these drugs, so they are relatively free of serious side effects. They work by preventing bile acids from recycling repeatedly through the liver and the intestines, by binding to the acids and causing their elimination in the stool. With fewer bile acids in circulation, the liver is forced to convert cholesterol into bile acids, thereby removing LDL from the blood.

Bile acid sequestrants have draw-

> **BRINGING DOWN CHOLESTEROL LEVELS**
>
> When high cholesterol levels are detected, the first recommended step is typically dietary change. A diet that limits all foods high in saturated fat and cholesterol—for example, red meat, butter, and other foods with a high fat content—is recommended. Foods such as fruits, vegetables, and whole grains, which are high in fiber and complex-carbohydrates and low in fat, are better for people with high cholesterol levels.
>
> Exercising at least three times a week for 30 minutes a day can raise the HDL (high-density lipoprotein) cholesterol or "good" cholesterol level. A higher HDL cholesterol level protects against atherosclerosis by removing cholesterol from the interior lining of the arteries.
>
> When dietary changes and exercise fail to lower a person's cholesterol level sufficiently, cholesterol-lowering drugs may be prescribed. A doctor may also recommend medication if a person has other risk factors such as a family history of coronary heart disease, high blood pressure, or a low HDL cholesterol level or if the person smokes or lives with a smoker.
>
> Some common side effects of cholesterol-lowering medication include constipation, abdominal pain, and abdominal cramping.

backs, including constipation, gas, bloating, nausea, and heartburn. The constipation associated with this therapy tends to diminish over time. It can be treated with laxatives, stool softeners, or increased fluid and fiber intake. In general, eating low-fat foods will help the medications to be more effective.

Bile acid sequestrants are often given in combination with statins or niacin. Examples include the lipid-lowering agent cholestyramine (Questran) and colestipol hydrochloride (Colestid).

NIACIN (NICOTINIC ACID)

Niacin is the B vitamin needed for carbohydrate metabolism. When taken in very large quantities, niacin becomes an effective, versatile, low-cost drug that lowers LDL cholesterol and triglyceride levels while raising HDL (high-density lipoprotein) cholesterol ("good" cholesterol) levels. When combined with a bile acid sequestrant, niacin can reduce LDL cholesterol levels by as much as 40 to 60 percent.

There are disadvantages to niacin. Some forms of it must be taken three times a day, and the sustained-release form can have toxic effects on the liver. Because niacin can make the body resistant to the effects of insulin, people with diabetes should not take it.

Niacin comes in two forms: sustained release and immediate release. With the exception of the prescription drug Niaspan, which is taken only once a day, the sustained release form is particularly associated with toxic effects on the liver. Niacin comes in tablets, capsules, and liquids. All forms should be taken with or following a meal to avoid stomach upset.

FIBRIC ACID DERIVATIVES

Fibric acid derivatives lower the levels of triglycerides and very low-density lipoproteins. Although fibric acid derivatives raise HDL cholesterol levels, they do not lower LDL cholesterol levels as effectively as other drugs. These drugs are chiefly used to treat people with exceptionally high levels of triglycerides. They work by reducing the production of triglycerides in the liver or by preventing their synthesis.

Fibric acid derivatives can cause dizziness, drowsiness, blurred vision, chest pain, flulike symptoms, and liver disorders, among many other side effects. For this reason, as well as their inability to reduce LDL cholesterol levels, fibric acid derivatives are not used to reduce cholesterol levels as much as they once were. Examples include gemfibrozil (Lopid), clofibrate (Atromid-S), and fenofibrate (Tricor).

Cholestyramine resin

A cholesterol-lowering agent; a bile acid sequestrant; a lipid-lowering agent. Cholestyramine resin (Questran) is used in combination with other drugs to treat high cholesterol levels.

Chondritis

Inflammation of the cartilage that covers the surfaces of the bone ends, such as the joints in the arms and legs or the ends of the ribs in the chest. Chondritis causes pain in the affected area, especially with movement of the joint. The inflammation of cartilage is commonly due to mechanical pressure, stress, injury, or local inflammation.

Chondrocalcinosis

Deposits of calcium in the cartilage of a joint surface. An X ray reveals chondrocalcinosis in a joint. A release of calcium pyrophosphate dihydrate (CPPD) crystals into the joint causes the form of arthritis called PSEUDOGOUT.

Chondromalacia

The progressive softening and erosion of cartilage, most commonly appearing in the undersurface of the kneecap (patella). When it affects the cartilage of the knee joint, the condition is known as chondromalacia patella. Chondromalacia causes this cartilage, which is normally smooth and glossy, to appear rough and frayed when observed with MRI (magnetic resonance imaging) or with arthroscopic diagnostic techniques. The principal symptom of the condition is tenderness or pain behind and around the kneecap(s). Activities that involve repeated or prolonged bending of the knee, such as walking on an incline, climbing and descending stairs, squatting, or sitting for a long time, intensify the pain. Athletic adolescents and young adults are most often affected. A previous traumatic injury is frequently associated with chondromalacia, and the knee joint may be misaligned.

Treatment provided by a physician specializing in sports medicine generally includes applying heat and taking anti-inflammatory medication, such as aspirin, ibuprofen, or other nonsteroidal anti-inflammatory drugs (NSAIDs). A doctor or physical therapist may also recommend a series of special exercises to strengthen the muscle and support the knee joint. Avoiding heavy lifting, squatting, and stair climbing should also be considered. A knee sleeve or other appliance that supports the kneecap may relieve pain, as may an injection of a corticosteroid. Cases not responding to traditional therapy may require arthroscopic surgery and a realignment of the kneecap.

Chondromatosis

A condition in which benign cartilage masses or tumors covering a movable joint become detached and remain in the joint space. These free bodies are sometimes called "joint mice." Chondromatosis most commonly affects the knee joint. The symptoms include limited range of motion in the affected joint, and, if the condition persists over time, there is a risk of degenerative joint disease. The cause is unknown. Chondromatosis is more common in men and usually occurs after the age of 40.

Chondrosarcoma

A rare malignant tumor of cartilage tissue. Chondrosarcoma usually affects the thighbone, upper arm bone, ribs, collarbone, or pelvis. Symptoms depend on the location and stage of the tumor. Severe pain may indicate a fast-growing tumor; moderate discomfort and swelling may point to a slower-growing tumor. When chondrosarcoma affects the pelvic bone, there may be urinary frequency or obstruction, and the tumor may be felt as a pull in the groin muscle. X rays, CT (computed tomography), and biopsy are the diagnostic tools used to identify chondrosarcoma. MRI (magnetic resonance imaging) is an essential tool for surgical planning. Treatment of chondrosarcoma is surgical removal of the tumor and wide margins of tissue around the tumor, sometimes followed by limited use of chemotherapy or radiation treatment. The location, size, grade, and stage of the cancerous growth determine survival rates. The survival rate is excellent when chondrosarcomas are found early and removed.

Chordee

An abnormal downward bowing of the erect male penis, which prevents sexual intercourse. Chordee results from abnormal development because of infection or trauma. Treatment options depend on the severity of the disease, but may include surgery.

Chorea

A condition of involuntary, purposeless, rapid, jerking movements, as if the person affected is "dancing." See HUNTINGTON CHOREA.

Choreoathetosis

Involuntary movements that are irregular and writhing, creating an appearance of restlessness. Choreoathetosis can involve the face, neck, arms, legs, trunk, and respiratory muscles. Movements range from subtle to wild and ballistic. They can be a side effect of the drug levodopa (used to treat PARKINSON DISEASE) and an effect of Huntington disease.

Chorioamnionitis

In pregnancy, inflammation of the amniotic membranes typically after their rupture. The cause is an infection by bacteria that reach the uterus through the vagina. Chorioamnionitis occurs in about 2 percent of all pregnancies. Symptoms in the mother include fever, abdominal pain and cramping, a drop in blood pressure, and tenderness of the uterus. Symptoms in the fetus include a higher than normal heart rate.

Chorioamnionitis generally occurs at the end of a pregnancy, when more than 24 hours have elapsed between rupture of the membranes and delivery, permitting bacteria to multiply. To avoid the risk of infection, doctors will choose to induce labor if it has not begun spontaneously within 12 to 36 hours of membrane rupture. In rare instances, an infection occurs when there has been no obvious rupture of the membranes and sometimes may cause PRETERM LABOR. AMNIOCENTESIS may be used to confirm the presence of an infection.

Chorioamnionitis is treated in a hospital with antibiotics given intravenously. Because the antibiotics cannot penetrate the placenta to treat the fetus, immediate delivery is recommended. If the baby is born with an infection, antibiotics may be given intravenously.

Choriocarcinoma

A highly malignant tumor that invades the walls of the uterus. Choriocarcinoma usually appears months after a MOLAR PREGNANCY, an ECTOPIC PREGNANCY, or a miscarriage, although in about 15 percent of cases, it accompanies or follows normal pregnancies. Some choriocarcinomas develop from placental cells left behind after an abortion or pregnancy. Symptoms include vaginal bleeding and excessive nausea. Pelvic examination may show that the uterus is larger than expected. Urine and blood tests will show higher than normal levels of the hormone HUMAN CHORIONIC GONADOTROPIN (HCG).

Treatment includes removing the contents of the uterus during a D AND C. HYSTERECTOMY is sometimes recommended, particularly if the woman no longer wishes to bear children. CHEMOTHERAPY almost always cures choriocarcinoma, even when it has spread to other organs. Blood tests are used to monitor the level of HCG until it returns to normal.

Chorionic villi

During pregnancy, tiny fingerlike projections attached to a membrane that eventually becomes the part of the PLACENTA closest to the baby. The fetal blood vessels project into the villi, which are surrounded by the mother's blood.

Chorionic villus sampling

A prenatal test that detects genetic abnormalities in a fetus. In chorionic villus sampling (CVS), a small sample of chorionic villi (projections in the placenta that absorb nutrients from the mother's blood) is taken from the placenta. Guided by ultrasound, the doctor inserts either a catheter through the cervix or a needle through the mother's abdominal wall, removing a sample of cells from the villi. The sample is sent to a laboratory, where the cells will be grown and studied for genetic abnormalities. The test can identify conditions, such as Down syndrome and Tay-Sachs disease, some inherited conditions, and sex.

Chorionic villus sampling can detect most of the same defects as AMNIOCENTESIS, but it can be performed earlier. The test is usually performed in a hospital, between the 9th and 12th weeks of the pregnancy, with results available in about 10 days. If results indicate an abnormality in the fetus, the pregnancy can be terminated, either late in the first trimester or at the beginning of the second, when abortion is safest. Such

---

Terms in small capital letters—for example, PHYSICAL THERAPY or PAGET DISEASE—indicate a cross-reference to another entry with more information.

C

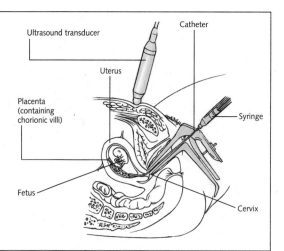

PRENATAL TESTING
For chorionic villus sampling (CVS), the doctor inserts a catheter into the uterus via the vagina and, guided by ultrasound, extracts cells from a part of the placenta called the chorionic villi. (Less commonly, a needle is inserted into the lower abdomen.) The extracted cells contain the same genetic material as the cells of the fetus, so the sample can be tested to check for genetic abnormalities such as Down syndrome.

Ultrasound transducer

Catheter

Uterus

Syringe

Placenta (containing chorionic villi)

Fetus

Cervix

early diagnosis allows parents to choose whether to terminate the pregnancy privately, before it is apparent to others. After the test, a woman may feel tired; she may experience some bleeding. Chorionic villus sampling is not without risk, including the risk of injury or infection of the cervix. The risk of miscarriage is greater with CVS (1 in 100) than with amniocentesis (1 in 200). Rarely, the test causes harm, such as limb deformities to the fetus, especially when performed before the 10th week of pregnancy.

Choroidal melanoma
See EYE TUMORS.

Christian Science
A religion based on religious teachings that promote the belief that healing comes from God through "heartfelt, yet disciplined prayer." Christian Scientists turn to prayer rather than conventional medicine to heal illness.

Christian Scientists maintain that a transformation or spiritualization of a sick person's thoughts will change his or her condition rather than medication and other traditional methods used to treat disease. Christian Science holds that the origin of evil, including physical illness, is to be found in the mind's ignorance of true reality, and healing of the sick is believed to come about through the transforming action of religious belief. Those involved in the religion refuse blood and blood product transfusions and forbid drinking alcohol and smoking.

Chromium
A gray, metallic element essential for energy in the human diet. In its active form, chromium helps insulin to remove glucose, or blood sugar, from the bloodstream to the cells. A diet that is low in chromium can affect the ability of insulin to process carbohydrates, proteins, and fats. As many as 90 percent of American diets may be low in chromium because chromium is lost during the process of refining processed foods. Elderly people, people with diabetes mellitus, and children who do not eat enough protein are at particular risk for chromium deficiency. The best dietary source for chromium is brewer's yeast grown in chromium-rich soil. Cooking in stainless steel cookware increases the chromium content of food.

Chromium picolinate
A complex mineral important for converting carbohydrates and fat into energy and maintaining normal blood sugar levels. Chromium picolinate is naturally present in whole grains, brewer's yeast, nuts, and dried beans. Only trace amounts are required by the body. Supplements of chromium picolinate have become popular in recent years for weight loss and for managing glucose levels.

Chromosomal abnormalities
Variations from normal in the number or structure of chromosomes, which may or may not cause genetic defects. Chromosomes carry genes, which determine an individual's char-

acteristics. About one in 500 newborns has a chromosomal abnormality. Abnormalities generally occur while egg and sperm cells are forming.

Egg and sperm cells are formed through a process called MEIOSIS. The process begins with cells that have the normal number of chromosomes, 46, and ends with four sex (sperm or egg) cells, each having only 23 chromosomes. At conception one of the egg cells that has 23 chromosomes joins with a sperm cell that has 23 chromosomes to form an embryo that has 46 chromosomes. This enables each individual to have two types of each chromosome and gene, one from the mother and one from the father.

Sometimes the process of meiosis is disrupted unexpectedly. A particular egg or sperm cell may be formed with an abnormal number of chromosomes. If the abnormal sex cell then participates in the process of fertilization, the resulting embryo will have an abnormal number of chromosomes, represented by a specific chromosome abnormality.

Chromosomal abnormalities are diagnosed through KARYOTYPING, a process for analyzing chromosomes through a blood, skin, bone marrow, or other tissue sample. The chromosomes are examined under a microscope where they are counted and structural defects are identified. Prenatal testing is available to diagnose a chromosomal abnormality in a fetus when there is a high risk or the suspicion of a problem.

TYPES OF ABNORMALITIES
Chromosomal abnormalities can range from very severe and leading to early death, to disorders that involve mental retardation, to relatively mild disorders, depending on which chromosomes are involved. Some pregnancies are at higher risk than others for abnormalities. Influential factors include a family history of genetic disorders and the mother being older than age 35. About half of miscarriages are due to chromosomal abnormalities that are so severe that prenatal development cannot proceed.

One error that can occur during meiosis is an irregular number of chromosomes. Sometimes a fetus can inherit the wrong number of chromosomes, and instead of receiving the normal 46 (23 from each parent), it

DOWN SYNDROME
The karotype (a photograph of chromosomes arranged in pairs) of a person with Down syndrome has an extra chromosome in pair 21, which usually results from the failure of a pair of chromosomes to separate early in the process of cell division in an egg or sperm. Down syndrome is the most common chromosome abnormality

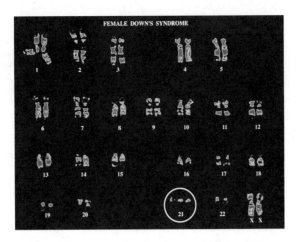

FEMALE DOWN'S SYNDROME

will receive an extra set, for a total of 69 chromosomes. Sometimes a fetus inherits a single extra chromosome from a parent or may be missing a chromosome. Various conditions, such as DOWN SYNDROME (trisomy 21 syndrome), TRISOMY 18 SYNDROME, and TRISOMY 13 SYNDROME, involve having an abnormal number of chromosomes. Abnormalities can also occur due to structural changes within chromosomes. Sometimes a chromosome breaks in one place, only to reunite the broken parts at a different location on the same chromosome or even on a different chromosome. Sometimes genetic material is lost. These types of changes can result in mental retardation and other birth defects. It is unknown why such breaks occur.

BIRTH DEFECTS
Birth defects associated with chromosomal abnormalities can be divided into two categories: those that occur in sex chromosomes and those that occur in other chromosomes. Most human chromosomal abnormalities occur in the autosomes, the 22 pairs of chromosomes that are the same in males and females. Chromosomal abnormalities associated with sex chromosomes, however, are only slightly less common than autosomal abnormalities, and they are usually less severe. Both autosomal and sex chromosomal abnormalities usually can be diagnosed before birth by AMNIOCENTESIS and CHORIONIC VILLUS SAMPLING.

■ *Autosomal abnormalities* The most common serious autosomal abnormality is Down syndrome. People with Down syndrome have an extra copy of the autosomal chromosome 21, making pair 21 a triad instead of a

pair. However, in 3 to 5 percent of cases, the third copy of chromosome 21 has been relocated to another chromosome, most commonly, chromosome 14 or 15.

Down syndrome occurs in one of every 800 births, and older mothers have a greater risk of having a baby with the condition. Women who have already had a baby with Down syndrome are at slightly higher risk for having other children with the condition; and women who have Down syndrome themselves are also at higher risk. Amniocentesis or chorionic villus sampling is routinely offered to all pregnant women who are 35 or older to identify fetuses with Down syndrome.

■ *Sex chromosome abnormalities*
Sex chromosomes include the female chromosome X and the male chromosome Y; both appear in chromosome 23 in males. Males with a normal genetic makeup inherit an X and a Y chromosome, while females with a normal genetic makeup inherit two Xs. A single Y chromosome produces maleness, and its absence is necessary for femaleness. Sex chromosome abnormalities in females are caused by variations in the number or structure of X chromosomes; abnormalities in males are the result of irregular numbers or structure of the X or the Y chromosome or both.

TURNER SYNDROME is a female sex chromosome abnormality. In this disorder, females inherit only one X chromosome instead of two. The condition is rare, affecting an estimated one in 2,000 to 3,000 female infants. It typically results in short stature and infertility. Females with three X chro-

mosomes, called triple-X females, are usually taller than average with unusually long legs and slender torsos. Unlike females with Turner syndrome, they are not sterile, although they are usually in the low normal range of intelligence and may have slight learning difficulties. This chromosomal abnormality is uncommon, affecting one in 1,000 female infants, and little is known about it.

Like triple-X females, males with XYY syndrome, who carry an extra Y chromosome, are usually taller than average, generally appearing and acting normal. They are able to reproduce. The frequency of the syndrome is not certain; estimates range from one in 900 male births to one in 2,000.

Males with KLINEFELTER SYNDROME have inherited one or more extra X chromosomes, resulting in a GENOTYPE such as XXY, XXXY, XXXXY, or XY/XXY mosaicism. This syndrome is one of the most common chromosomal abnormalities, occurring in as many as one in 500 male births. Males with Down syndrome in rare cases also have Klinefelter syndrome, which typically is associated with infertility and increased incidence of learning disabilities.

Chromosome analysis
See KARYOTYPING.

Chromosomes
Genetic material in the nucleus of cells where genes are located. Chromosomes consist of highly compacted threads of deoxyribonucleic acid (DNA) and associated proteins. Each species normally has a characteristic number of chromosomes in each cell; 46 chromosomes are found in human cells, including two that determine the sex of the individual.

Chromotherapy
See COLOR THERAPY.

Chronic
Long-lasting; long-term; always present. In medicine, a chronic condition is one lasting 3 months or more.

Chronic care facility (CCF)
A residential facility that provides medical and nursing care for people with CHRONIC diseases or conditions.

A chronic care facility cares for people with disorders that persist for a long time. This is in contrast to a hospital, which is geared toward the treatment of people with acute health problems such as heart attacks or strokes.

Chronic fatigue syndrome

A serious, often disabling illness characterized by persistent, unrelenting, and severe exhaustion, as well as muscle pain and cognitive disorders that are sometimes referred to as "brain fog." Chronic fatigue syndrome (CFS) is not associated with significant muscle weakness, psychological disorders, or physical illness. The condition affects women three times more often than men. Adolescents may be affected, but less frequently than adults.

CFS is also referred to as chronic fatigue and immune dysfunction syndrome (CFIDS) and myalgic encephalomyelitis (ME). The syndrome can be confused with LYME DISEASE, FIBROMYALGIA, or other diseases that cause chronic fatigue. CFS was once thought to be chronic EPSTEIN-BARR VIRUS (EBV) infection because high levels of EBV antibodies were found in many people with CFS. Researchers found, however, that equally high levels of EBV antibodies could occur in healthy people as well as those with CFS. In addition, it was discovered that some people without EBV antibodies experienced symptoms of chronic fatigue syndrome.

The cause is unknown, and the disease is something of a mystery. Ongoing research involves investigations into possible causes related to cardiology, immunology, virology, and endocrinology. It is believed that genetic and environmental factors may have a role in the development or persistence of chronic fatigue syndrome.

People who are affected by CFS may become bedridden or may be able to work or attend school only on a part-time basis. Disability insurance benefits are often denied because sometimes the condition is not viewed as a serious illness, but rather as a mental health issue with no objective, laboratory-confirmed abnormalities.

SYMPTOMS

The earliest symptom of CFS may be a strong, noticeable feeling of exhaustion that comes on suddenly and persists or continually comes and goes. A good night's sleep does not alleviate the feeling of tiredness. The person may have symptoms of a viral infection, including swollen glands, severe fatigue, fever, and upper respiratory distress.

The intense fatigue, either ongoing or intermittent, generally lasts for 6 months or more and interferes with daily activity and function. It is often made worse by exertion. Other stresses, including exercise, may worsen the condition. Swollen, tender lymph glands, sore throat, headache, aching joints, abdominal pain, muscle pain, low-grade fever, short-term memory impairment, and difficulty concentrating and sleeping are other symptoms.

For many people, the onset of CFS follows an illness such as the common cold, bronchitis, hepatitis, or an intestinal infection. For others, symptoms of chronic fatigue syndrome appear after infectious mononucleosis or a period of high stress. Other people may develop CFS gradually with no previous illness involved.

DIAGNOSIS AND TREATMENT

Two criteria are used in the medical diagnosis of chronic fatigue syndrome: the person diagnosed must have experienced severe and chronic fatigue for 6 months or longer without other known medical conditions that have been clinically diagnosed. In addition to the severe chronic fatigue, the person must have four or more of a set of specific symptoms at the same time, including substantial impairment in short-term memory or concentration, sore throat, tender lymph nodes, muscle pain, multijoint pain without redness or swelling, headaches different from those previously experienced, unrefreshing sleep, and malaise lasting more than 24 hours following exercise.

Further diagnostic evaluation for chronic fatigue syndrome is usually based on the exclusion of other possible illnesses. An initial assessment may include routine blood tests and tests for thyroid-stimulating hormone. Other tests may include a chest X ray, blood tests, and antibody tests for Lyme disease, hepatitis, and HIV (human immunodeficiency virus). A diagnosis of obvious depression or severe anxiety can rule out the diagnosis of CFS.

Treatment of CFS is aimed at relieving symptoms. Many people suffering from chronic fatigue syndrome report an improvement with antidepressant therapy, as long as the specific medication chosen does not increase feelings of fatigue. Psychotherapy on an individual or group basis may help some people. High-dose vitamins are sometimes recommended, but their effectiveness has not been proven.

Some people experience significant improvement within the first 5 years of illness; a larger number improve over a 10-year period. Many people continue to experience some symptoms even after generally recovering.

Chronic obstructive lung disease

See CHRONIC OBSTRUCTIVE PULMONARY DISEASE.

Chronic obstructive pulmonary disease

An obstruction of the airways that progressively limits the ability to breathe. Chronic obstructive pulmonary disease, or COPD, is caused by chronic BRONCHITIS or EMPHYSEMA or a combination of the two. Emphysema is characterized by destruction of the tissue that makes up the walls of the air sacs, or alveoli, which results in overinflation of the air sacs. Chronic bronchitis is characterized by a daily cough and sputum production for 3 months or longer. Habitual cigarette smoking is the primary cause of COPD; COPD is irreversible. The disease is most common among people who are middle-aged or older, occurring primarily among those between 55 and 65 years of age.

SYMPTOMS

Symptoms of COPD may appear within as little as 5 years of habitual smoking and generally begin with a cough that produces mucus and usually occurs upon awakening in the morning. The associated cough tends to be mild and may be dismissed as a "smoker's cough." When a person who has COPD acquires a common cold (see COLD, COMMON), the infection tends to progress quickly to the chest area. Frequently, the mucus coughed up during chest colds is yellow or green as a result of pus in the sputum. Chest infections, which sometimes produce wheezing, may occur more frequently in a person with COPD.

If COPD progresses, shortness of breath (see BREATH, SHORTNESS OF), which becomes more pronounced over time, usually occurs with physical exertion. This symptom may eventually restrict everyday activities, such as getting dressed and preparing food, and may increase in severity after eating. Leg swelling can occur as a result of related heart failure (see HEART FAILURE, CONGESTIVE). Ultimately, COPD can produce shortness of breath with minimal activity or even when a person is at rest.

CAUSES

Factors including heredity and environment contribute to developing COPD, but the major cause is smoking tobacco. Cigarette smoking can produce three types of lung injuries: the overproduction of mucus and an associated cough to bring up sputum, the narrowing of airways with a reduction of the ability to exhale, and the destruction of the walls of the air sacs in the lungs.

The process by which irritants such as cigarette smoke result in COPD begins with the inflammation of the air sacs in the lungs. When this inflammation becomes established, permanent damage of the air sacs may result. White blood cells collect in the inflamed air sacs and release enzymes that damage connective tissue in their walls. Continued smoking damages the cilia (tiny hairlike cells lining the airways), causing further impairment of lung function. Under normal conditions, the cilia transport mucus toward the mouth and help the body expel toxins. This function is severely compromised by the damage caused by smoking.

A rare hereditary condition can result in the underproduction of a protein, alpha 1-antitrypsin, that protects the air sacs of the lungs. This promotes the development of emphysema, especially in those who smoke at an early age.

Once well established, COPD causes air to become trapped in the lungs and decreases the amount of capillaries in the walls of the air sacs. This inhibits the oxygen–carbon dioxide exchange between the air sacs and the blood. At first, blood oxygen levels are reduced, with carbon dioxide levels remaining constant. In time, the carbon dioxide levels become elevated as the oxygen levels continue to decrease.

DIAGNOSIS

People with advanced COPD may demonstrate labored breathing even at rest. Mild or early cases of COPD, however, are sometimes difficult to diagnose. In the early stages of COPD, chest X rays are usually normal; in advanced stages of COPD, they may demonstrate characteristic changes. SPIROMETRY, a test that reveals reduced airflow with a forceful exhalation, can indicate that the airflow is obstructed and will confirm the diagnosis. Analysis of arterial blood gases can determine oxygen and carbon dioxide levels in the bloodstream. When COPD is suspected in younger people, the blood level of a certain protein may be measured to determine the presence of a hereditary condition called alpha 1-antitrypsin deficiency that predisposes a person to the condition.

TREATMENT

There is no cure for the condition, but several strategies may be helpful. Smoking cessation is the first and most important approach. Although many of the effects of COPD are irreversible, giving up cigarettes generally provides some benefits regardless of the point in the disease process at which smoking is stopped. For example, quitting smoking at a mild or moderate stage in the illness may prevent or delay disabling symptoms. Avoidance of exposure to all airborne irritants is also generally helpful.

Because bouts of INFLUENZA or PNEUMONIA can intensify the symptoms of COPD and because a person who has the condition may be more susceptible to these infections, annual influenza vaccinations and a pneu-

mococcal vaccination every 6 years are recommended. When bacterial infections occur, antibiotics may be prescribed early to help control the intensified COPD symptoms these infections can cause.

Some of the conditions produced by COPD, including bronchospasm, wheezing from spasm of the muscles lining the airway, inflammation, and excessive secretions, can be improved. BRONCHODILATORS in metered-dose inhalers or oral medications can relax constricted bronchial airways and help relieve wheezing. In some people with COPD, CORTICOSTEROIDS may decrease inflammation. Increased fluid intake is helpful for thinning secretions so they may be expelled more efficiently, and RESPIRATORY THERAPY is sometimes used to loosen chest secretions in people who have severe COPD.

Very low oxygen levels in the blood associated with extreme disease may be treated with long-term oxygen therapy (see OXYGEN, SUPPLEMENTAL) used continually throughout the day. This therapy may prolong the life of a person with a low blood oxygen level. Oxygen therapy can improve mental functions and may also help control shortness of breath on exertion and reduce the risk of heart failure.

Exercise therapy is often recommended to increase movement and enhance the quality of life by improving the ability for daily activities, including cooking, self-care, and sexual activity. This can be helpful in establishing greater independence. However, prescribed programs of exercise do not improve lung function and must be maintained on a reg-

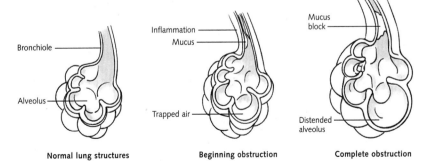

Bronchiole

Alveolus

Inflammation

Mucus

Trapped air

Mucus block

Distended alveolus

Normal lung structures   Beginning obstruction   Complete obstruction

PERMANENTLY DAMAGED LUNGS
Chronic obstruction pulmonary disease permanently harms delicate lung structures. The bronchioles are narrowed by inflammation and congested with excess mucus. Air that reaches the alveoli is trapped, and the tiny alveoli distend. The affected person has increasing difficulty exhaling.

ular basis to provide benefits. Exercise programs can decrease the number of hospital stays and shorten their duration. Oxygen therapy may be recommended for use during exercise sessions.

Although surgery to reduce lung volume is a complex procedure, it may be an option for people with severe COPD. Candidates for the procedure must stop smoking for 6 months before the operation and adhere faithfully to a strenuous training program. Lung volume reduction surgery is effective in improving lung function and exercise capacity in some people, but it is not known how long these benefits last. LUNG TRANSPLANTATION is considered for some people younger than 50. People whose disease is caused by a hereditary condition involving a missing protein can receive replacement treatments, involving costly, weekly intravenous infusions of the protein.

OUTLOOK

When airway obstruction is mild and treatment strategies, including smoking cessation, are adhered to, the prognosis can be favorable. When the obstruction is moderate to severe, the risk of death becomes greater, but with proper care and appropriate lifestyle changes, good survival rates can be achieved. COPD also involves an increased risk of fatal LUNG CANCER. Death associated with COPD may also result from respiratory failure, pneumonia, leakage of air into the pleural space surrounding the lungs, abnormalities in heart rhythm, or obstruction of the arteries that lead to the lungs.

Cidofovir

A drug used to treat an eye infection caused by cytomegalovirus (CMV). Cidofovir (Vistide) is chiefly used in persons infected with HIV (human immunodeficiency virus) who contract a CMV infection in the eye. The infection may or may not improve with this treatment.

Cilia

Microscopic hairlike extensions reaching out from the surface of a cell. Cilia have a wave motion in the lining of the inner ear and the lungs, for example, that help move fluids or mucus and other surface material.

Cilostazol

A drug used to reduce symptoms caused by blood flow disorders. Cilostazol (Pletal) is given to people with blood disorders, such as peripheral vascular disease, and those with insufficient blood flow to the leg muscles that causes leg pain while walking.

Cimetidine

A drug used to treat benign stomach and duodenal ulcers and other disorders. Cimetidine (Tagamet) works by blocking the secretion of acid from the stomach. Oversecretion of gastric acids and stress have long been considered contributing factors in the creation of stomach ulcers. Cimetidine is usually prescribed in addition to antibiotics to treat benign stomach ulcers.

Cimetidine is also used to treat gastroesophageal reflux disease (GERD), heartburn, and sour stomach. It is available both with and without prescription. Since it is metabolized in the liver, it can interact adversely with other drugs. A person should talk to his or her doctor before taking cimetidine.

CIN

Cervical intraepithelial neoplasia. Abnormal cells on or near the CERVIX; also, one of four classification systems used to categorize abnormal PAP SMEAR results. CIN is a precancerous condition without symptoms that is detected by Pap smear. In CIN, abnormal cells are found in the cell layers of the surface of the cervix. The extent of the abnormal cells is classified according to the CIN system along a continuum. At one end, all cells are normal, while at the other end is invasive cancer. The points in between represent mild, moderate, and severe states of abnormal cell growth, called CIN 1, CIN 2, and CIN 3. In some women, the abnormal cells will develop into cancerous conditions, while in others, they will return to normal. Because there is no way to predict what will happen, it is essential that all cases of CIN be treated or watched closely, with repeated Pap smears and other diagnostic tests.

When a woman receives an abnormal result indicating CIN from a Pap smear, her doctor may perform COL-POSCOPY. If an abnormality is identified, the doctor may perform a BIOPSY. Pap smears and colposcopies can be repeated as part of watching CIN closely to see if and how it develops. Treatments for CIN range from the very mild to the serious. The mildest treatment is the "wait and see" approach, including Pap smears and colposcopies. More serious treatments include destruction of abnormal cells by CRYOTHERAPY (freezing), LASER, or other technologies.

Ciprofloxacin

See FLUOROQUINOLONES.

Circadian rhythm

The occurrence of biological processes in cycles of about 24 hours. Circadian rhythm is determined by a "biological clock" that is set to coincide with recurring daily cycles of light and darkness. Biological processes that occur according to circadian rhythm include hormone secretion, sleeping, eating, and sensitivity to drugs and stimuli. See also BIORHYTHMS.

Circulatory system

See CARDIOVASCULAR SYSTEM.

Circumcision, male

Surgical removal of the foreskin (prepuce) of the penis. Circumcision is performed routinely on many newborn males for social or cultural reasons. There is no medical reason for routine circumcision of infants. In later life, conditions may develop in uncircumcised males that require circumcision. These include inability to pull the foreskin back from the head of the penis, inability to return the retracted foreskin to its normal position, and repeated infections of the foreskin and glans (BALANITIS). These conditions usually develop because of poor hygiene.

In newborns, circumcision is performed by the surgeon placing a bell-shaped piece of plastic or metal over the glans and then cutting off the foreskin and removing the device. The wound should be protected with petroleum jelly at each diaper change until it heals. In older boys and adults, the foreskin is cut away and the wound is closed with stitches. To relieve pain, ice packs can be applied to the surgical site for the first 24

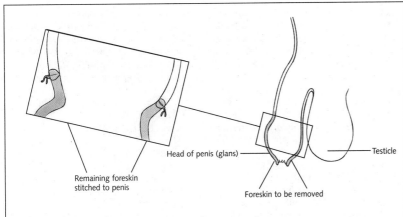

REMOVING THE FORESKIN
To perform a circumcision, the doctor removes the foreskin, the skin and underlying mucous membrane that covers the head of the penis. The remaining rim of the foreskin is stitched to the skin covering the shaft of the penis, just behind the head.

Labels: Head of penis (glans) — Testicle — Remaining foreskin stitched to penis — Foreskin to be removed

hours. Oral pain medications may also be prescribed.

Complications of circumcision can include excessive bleeding and infection. In rare instances, the glans or the urinary opening may be damaged and require surgical repair.

Cirrhosis

A chronic disease that causes degeneration of healthy, functioning liver cells that are gradually replaced by scar tissue. The scarring destroys the normal structure of the liver. As scar tissue replaces healthy tissue, the liver is less able to remove toxins from the bloodstream and carry out its normal functions. Eventually, if enough liver cells are damaged, liver failure and death result. The scarring can also cause portal hypertension (an increase in the pressure of the blood system of the liver). Portal hypertension can cause ESOPHAGEAL VARICES (the dilation of the veins of the esophagus), a potentially life-threatening condition in which the veins are prone to bleeding. Cirrhosis also increases the risk for liver cancer.

SYMPTOMS AND CAUSES

The early stages of cirrhosis cause few symptoms. Eventual symptoms may include loss of appetite, weight loss, indigestion, weakness, and fatigue. Spidery red lines called angiomas may appear on the face, arms, and upper trunk. In many people, there is a general loss of a sense of well-being. In the late stages of cir-

rhosis, as the tissue damage becomes severe, there are signs such as ascites (an abnormal accumulation of fluid in the abdominal cavity), bleeding in the digestive tract, and, sometimes, jaundice (the yellowing of the skin and the whites of the eyes). There may also be a loss of interest in sex, development of breasts in men, a cessation of menstrual periods in women, general swelling, irritability, confusion, impaired memory, and an inability to concentrate.

Alcoholism, fatty liver, and hepatitis C (a viral infection) are the most common causes of cirrhosis in the United States. Alcoholic cirrhosis usually occurs only in people who consume large amounts of alcohol for 5 or more consecutive years. Women are more susceptible than men to liver damage from alcohol because of their smaller size and their lack of certain enzymes that break down alcohol. Although daily heavy drink-

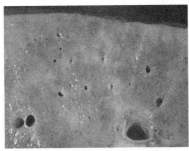

LIVER DAMAGE IN CIRRHOSIS
Scar tissue is evident on the liver of a person who was chronically dependent on alcohol.

ing is more likely to cause liver damage, even intermittent use of alcohol can harm the liver. Other causes of cirrhosis include viral infection, autoimmune disease, MALNUTRITION, parasites, drug reactions, toxic chemicals, metabolic defects, and congestive heart failure (see HEART FAILURE, CONGESTIVE). Sometimes, the cause cannot be identified.

DIAGNOSIS AND TREATMENT

Because many liver diseases cause similar symptoms, a number of tests must be performed to make a definitive diagnosis of cirrhosis. In addition to conducting a physical examination and taking a medical history, the doctor may order tests, such as blood and urine tests, liver function tests, ultrasound scanning, X rays, and a liver biopsy. The physician must also be made aware of the person's history of alcohol consumption.

In the early stages of cirrhosis caused by alcohol, it is often possible to halt the progression of cirrhosis by completely avoiding alcohol. Alcohol consumption causes all forms of cirrhosis to worsen. As cirrhosis progresses, medications can be prescribed to treat symptoms. For example, diuretics relieve fluid retention and antacids ease abdominal discomfort. Hospitalization is required in severe cases of gastrointestinal bleeding, vomiting blood, or excessive fluid accumulation. In some cases, a transfusion is necessary.

A liver transplant may be recommended for people with advanced disease who have BILIARY CIRRHOSIS or whose disease is caused by hepatitis, fatty liver, or toxins. If cirrhosis caused by alcohol is accompanied by the deterioration of additional organs (such as the heart and brain), a liver transplant is less likely to be recommended. However, for people who permanently stop drinking and are otherwise healthy, a liver transplant is an option.

Cisapride

A drug formerly used to treat heartburn caused by gastroesophageal reflux disease. In 2000 the manufacturer removed cisapride (Propulsid) from the US market because of potentially serious cardiac side effects. Cisapride is available only for patients who meet specific criteria.

Cisplatin

A drug used in cancer chemotherapy. Cisplatin (Platinol) is one of a group of chemotherapy drugs known as alkylating agents, used to slow or stop the growth of cancer cells. Cisplatin is used to treat several cancers, including small cell carcinoma of the lung and cancers of the testicles, ovaries, bladder, head, and neck, among others.

Cisplatin is usually prescribed in combination with other anticancer drugs. It is most often given intravenously.

Citalopram

An antidepressant drug. Citalopram (Celexa, and others) is one of a group of selective serotonin reuptake inhibitors (SSRIs) that are thought to work by raising levels of serotonin in the brain, which helps to elevate a person's mood. Side effects include nausea, constipation, and dry mouth.

Clarithromycin

Antibiotic used to treat bacterial infections. Clarithromycin (Biaxin) is used to treat a wide variety of infections, including those of the skin and respiratory tract, as well as duodenal ulcers.

Claudication

Pain or cramping in the limbs, usually the feet and legs, caused by ATHEROSCLEROSIS (narrowing or blockage of the arteries by deposits of fat and other materials). Symptoms result from insufficient blood flow to the limbs and depend on the severity of the claudication. In the early stages, pain appears only during exercise, usually in the calves or feet, and disappears after a period of rest. Some people feel little pain and instead experience fatigue, aching, cramping, numbness, or weakness. In later stages, pain occurs even at rest, and the affected limbs become cold, pale, and painful. People with severe claudication may have to use a cane, walker, or wheelchair and are at increased risk of developing gangrene, for which amputation may be required.

Other possible signs of claudication include cold or numb feet, loss of hair on toes or legs, impotence (erectile dysfunction) in men, cyanosis (bluish skin) or paleness, sores on feet or legs that do not heal, and thickened toenails. Since similar symptoms can arise from other conditions (for example, a pinched nerve in the spine), tests such as X-ray examination of the arteries after injection of a special dye are usually required for accurate diagnosis. Risk factors for claudication include arteriosclerosis, hypertension (high blood pressure), high blood cholesterol levels, high blood homocysteine levels, diabetes mellitus, smoking, obesity, lack of exercise, and being age 60 or older.

Lifestyle changes are important in the treatment of claudication. These include regular exercise, particularly walking, which develops the leg muscles and encourages the growth of new blood vessels around the site of the narrowing. In addition, wearing comfortable shoes, eating a heart-healthy diet low in cholesterol and fat, avoiding tobacco, and increasing the intake of B vitamins and folic acid to reduce homocysteine levels are important. Medications may also be used to treat claudication. Aspirin or other antiplatelet drugs lower the risk of developing blood clots. Cholesterol-reducing drugs can slow the buildup of fats in the arteries, and vasodilators widen blood vessels to increase blood flow. Other medications may be used if a person has hypertension or diabetes mellitus. If blockage in a major artery is severe, a catheter (a long, thin tube) fitted with a balloon can be inserted into the artery and inflated to compress the fat deposits and increase blood flow (see BALLOON ANGIOPLASTY). Alternatively, a graft around the blocked artery may be created with a section of vein taken from elsewhere in the body or with synthetic material.

Claudication can be prevented or slowed by the same measures used to prevent atherosclerotic heart disease. These involve abstaining from tobacco use, controlling hypertension and diabetes mellitus, eating a low-fat diet, exercising regularly, maintaining a healthy weight, and reducing blood cholesterol levels. Reducing blood homocysteine levels by taking folic acid supplements may also be of benefit.

Claustrophobia

A fear of confined areas or enclosed spaces that can lead to extreme anxiety or panic. Often part of PANIC DISORDER, claustrophobia may be treated with therapy and the use of a mild tranquilizer.

Clavicle

See COLLARBONE.

Clawhand

Also known as main en griffe, an abnormal condition of the hand in which the fingers are in extreme flexion. This is often seen in an ulnar neuropathy (compression of the ulnar nerve at the elbow), in which the muscles innervated by the ulnar nerve are weakened by nerve damage.

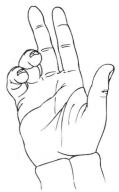

PARTIAL PARALYSIS
Damage (from disease or injury) to nerves in the arm and hand can cause paralysis of muscles in the hand. Most commonly, the index and third fingers are extended and the ring and little fingers are excessively flexed, creating the "clawhand" appearance.

Cleft lip and palate

Birth defects in which the lip or the roof of the mouth fail to close. Cleft lip and palate can occur in combination or separately. A baby born with a cleft lip has an elongated opening where parts of the upper lip have not fused. This opening can vary from a small notch at the top of the lip to a complete separation extending all the way to the nose. Cleft lip, with or without cleft palate, is both more common and more likely to be an inherited defect than is cleft palate alone. One of 1,000 babies is born with a cleft lip, with or without a cleft palate; only one of 2,500 babies is born with a cleft palate alone.

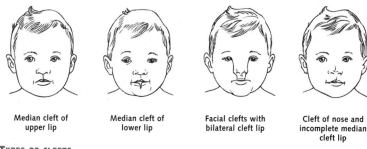

Median cleft of upper lip

Median cleft of lower lip

Facial clefts with bilateral cleft lip

Cleft of nose and incomplete median cleft lip

TYPES OF CLEFTS
When the two sides of the lips or palate do not meet and fuse properly, the resulting cleft, or split, can take various forms. In a cleft lip, either the upper or lower lip can be affected, both sides of the lip and the nostrils may be split, or the nose and upper lip may be involved.

Cleft lip and palate may be caused by genetic factors or by a TERATOGEN (an agent such as a drug or a chemical that causes abnormalities in developing fetuses) or by a combination of genetic and environmental factors. Risk factors include a family history of cleft lip or palate. Babies born with a cleft lip or palate sometimes have other birth defects. There is no known way to prevent cleft lip or palate.

TREATMENT AND COMPLICATIONS
Babies born with cleft lip or palate have immediate problems with feeding. A special device, called an obturator, can be fitted over the palate so the baby can be fed. It must be replaced every few weeks to keep up with the baby's rapid growth. A cleft palate may interfere in normal speech development, even with corrective surgery. Cleft lip and palate in children are associated with recurring ear infections, hearing loss, excessive dental caries (cavities), and displaced teeth. Orthodontia (braces) is often required.

Cleft lip is usually closed surgically at 1 or 2 months of age. Because cleft lip is sometimes associated with widening of the nose, another operation may be required during adolescence to complete the repair. A cleft palate is generally closed surgically during the first year of life to allow the baby to develop speech. If the operation is not done within the first 3 years of life, the child may require a special device to learn to speak intelligibly.

For affected individuals or those with a family history of cleft lip and palate, a genetic counselor can help identify the chance of recurrence in offspring. Ultrasound scanning during pregnancy can detect the defect.

Clicking jaw

A symptom of temporomandibular joint or TMJ syndrome, which involves an irregular functional relationship between the jaw joints and the supporting muscles and ligaments. Other possible symptoms of TMJ syndrome include limited jaw movement, headache, and facial pain.

Clinical trial

A test or study of a medical treatment to determine whether it is safe and effective. Clinical trials are research studies designed to measure the effectiveness of a drug or medical device in people who volunteer to participate in the research. Clinical drug trials are undertaken only after the drug has been studied intensively in laboratory animals.

All drug trials take place under very strict rules. In the United States, the Food and Drug Administration (FDA) monitors all clinical trials very closely. The trials are carried out in a series of phases, with each new phase building on the information accumulated in the previous ones.

Phase 1 studies are intended to find the best way to safely give a new treatment to a small group of healthy volunteers who are given small doses of the drug; doses are slowly raised to see whether the drug causes any side effects.

Phase 2 studies are designed to see whether the new drug actually works and is effective against the disease it is intended to treat. Slightly larger

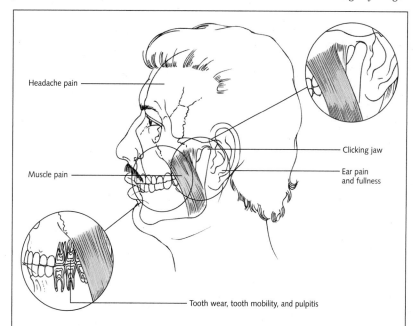

Headache pain

Clicking jaw

Ear pain and fullness

Muscle pain

Tooth wear, tooth mobility, and pulpitis

SYMPTOMS OF TMJ
The symptoms of temporomandibular joint (TMJ) syndrome go far beyond the clicking jaw. Other symptoms include muscular pain in the sliding joint between the skull and the lower jaw, especially when chewing; tooth wear from grinding of the teeth, movement of teeth, and inflammation of the inner pulp of the teeth (pulpitis); ear pain and ringing in the ears; headache in the temples and the back of the head; and sensitivity to light and blurred vision.

C

groups of volunteers with the disease participate.

Phase 3 studies compare standard treatments with the new one. These studies require large numbers of volunteers, who are assigned at random to one of the drugs being compared. The results are compared to see whether the new drug is at least as effective and safe as the standard therapy. In addition, less common side effects are identified.

Clitoridectomy

Removal of the CLITORIS. Clitoridectomy has been used for centuries in many countries, but is currently only used as part of ritual female circumcision (see FEMALE GENITAL MUTILATION) in some African countries and in parts of Asia. Although clitoridectomy was used in some Western countries as a brutal and ineffective remedy for masturbation and promiscuity in the 19th century, it is not performed in the West today except in cases of cancer of the vulva.

Clitoris

A small, rounded, highly sensitive structure that is part of a woman's external sexual organs (see REPRODUCTIVE SYSTEM, FEMALE). The clitoris, which is richly supplied with nerves and blood vessels, is above the opening to the vagina, where the labia majora join. The clitoris becomes swollen with blood during sexual arousal, and the structure has a central role in a woman's erotic sensations.

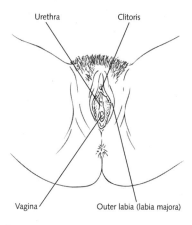

LOCATION OF CLITORIS
The clitoris is a very small mound of erectile tissue located just below the pubic bone, where the two outer labia meet.

Clomiphene citrate

A fertility drug. Clomiphene citrate (Clomid, Serophene) is used to treat women who have ovulation problems and want to become pregnant. Clomiphene citrate induces ovulation by stimulating the production of certain hormones related to pregnancy. The drug is associated with multiple ovulations and increased probability of multiple births.

Clonazepam

See BENZODIAZEPINES.

Clone

A group of genetically identical cells or organisms derived from a single original cell or organism by asexual reproductive methods. In medicine, a clone refers to an exact replica of an original parent cell. Plants have been cloned for centuries by obtaining cuttings of their leaves, stems, or roots. The body cells of animals, including humans, can be cloned in the laboratory. Because they are genetically uniform, clones are useful in biological research.

Clonidine

An antihypertensive drug used to treat mild to moderate high blood pressure. Clonidine (Catapres) works by relaxing and dilating blood vessels through actions in the brain stem. It is also used to treat nicotine withdrawal, ulcerative colitis, Tourette syndrome, neuralgia, opiate withdrawal, and symptoms of menopause.

Clonus

An abnormal muscle response, in which stretching sets off a series of quick muscle contractions. Clonus is usually the sign of a central nervous system disease and is associated with brisk reflexes and spasticity.

Clopidogrel bisulfate

A drug used to prevent heart attacks, strokes, and other circulatory problems. Clopidogrel (Plavix) is used to treat vascular diseases caused by narrowed blood vessels ("hardening of the arteries"). It works by inhibiting the formation of blood clots, which can impair blood flow to the brain, heart, and body.

Clostridium difficile

An organism that causes an acute inflammation of the colon. *Clostridium difficile (C. difficile)* is one of several forms of the common bacilli clostridia, which are normally found in dust, soil, vegetation, and the gastrointestinal tracts of humans and animals. Clostridia are usually harmless, but some forms, including a pathogenic strain of *C. difficile*, produce toxins that cause diarrhea and colitis, often after antibiotic treatment.

Infection may occur via heat-resistant spores of *C. difficile*, which can persist for long periods in the environment, including at hospitals and nursing homes.

Antibiotic therapy, which may produce an imbalance in the normal flora of the intestines, is usually the cause of the overgrowth of *C. difficile* in the colon. Many antibiotics can produce this alteration in the normal colonic flora, but clindamycin, ampicillin, amoxicillin, and the cephalosporins are most often implicated. Older people tend to be more susceptible, but young adults and children may be affected. People who are hospitalized and taking antibiotics are at particularly high risk because of the prevalence of the spores or this organism in a hospital environment.

SYMPTOMS, DIAGNOSIS, AND TREATMENT

Antibiotics inhibit the growth of many bacteria but permit certain bacteria, including *C. difficile*, to flourish in the intestines, which may lead to antibiotic-associated colitis. Symptoms include diarrhea, abdominal cramps, and low-grade fever.

The symptom of diarrhea generally begins within 4 to 10 days of starting antibiotic treatment, but sometimes develops after the medication has been discontinued. Symptoms usually stop when antibiotic therapy is discontinued.

Diagnosis is made by performing tests on a stool sample for the presence of a toxin produced by *C. difficile*. Endoscopy of the colon may also show visual evidence of pseudomembranous colitis, the most serious form of antibiotic-induced diarrhea, and this can be confirmed by a biopsy of the colon.

Treatment is based on stopping the antibiotic treatment that may be causing the diarrhea. Many people do well after discontinuing antibiotics.

CLONING DOLLY

The cloning of Dolly, a Scottish sheep, is noteworthy because it proves that cells from adult animals are not too specialized to create a new organism, as scientists once believed. Before Dolly was cloned, scientists thought that adult cells that had differentiated into specialized cells—like muscle or liver cells, for example—could never be altered into their original, undifferentiated state, from which they can develop into a whole new animal. To clone an animal, scientists had to find a way to remove the genetic material from an adult cell, without destroying the cell in the process.

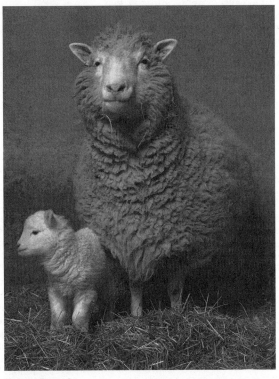

HELLO, DOLLY!
When Dolly was born healthy, scientists could prove that her DNA was the same as that of another cell from the sheep who had contributed the nucleus. None of her genes were the same as those of the sheep who had provided the egg or the sheep who had been her surrogate mother. Dolly aged rapidly and died at an early age.

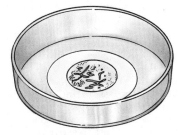

ISOLATING DONOR CELLS
The breakthrough method used to clone Dolly began with an egg cell removed from a ewe and isolated in a laboratory. Donor cells were placed in a medium that causes all genes to become inactive.

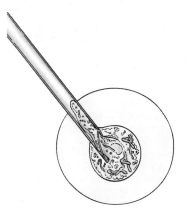

REMOVING THE NUCLEUS
The nucleus of the egg was sucked out, creating an egg with no genes at all.

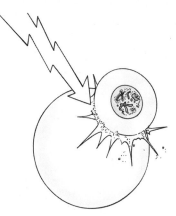

INSERTING A NEW NUCLEUS
The nucleus of a cell from another sheep was inserted in the egg and fused with an electrical impulse.

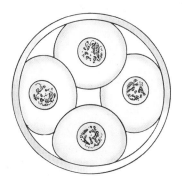

FORMATION OF AN EMBRYO
The egg began cell division to form a new embryo, which was implanted in another ewe.

Relapses may occur and require further courses of medication. Others can become seriously ill with persistent diarrhea and dehydration. In some cases, antibiotic-associated colitis caused by *C. difficile* may become life-threatening. The more severe symptoms may be treated with oral vancomycin or metronidazole.

Clotrimazole

An antifungal drug used to treat athlete's foot, oral thrush, and other fungal infections. Clotrimazole is available as oral lozenges (Mycelex) to treat thrush, as a cream to treat athlete's foot and ringworm (Lotrisone), and as a cream to treat vaginal yeast infections (FemCare, Gyne-Lotrimin, Mycelex-7).

Clubbing

A condition often caused by chronic lung disease in which the tips of the fingers or toes become enlarged and the area where the nail emerges from the nail bed becomes rounded. Clubbing may be caused by diseases other than lung disease. The condition is sometimes unrelated to disease and is hereditary.

Clubfoot

See TALIPES.

Coarctation of the aorta

A birth defect in which the aorta, the main artery leading from the heart into the body, is severely narrowed. Usually the narrowing occurs just past the point where the subclavian artery, which supplies the upper body, branches off the aorta. This narrowing causes a discrepancy in blood pressure between the upper body (which will have higher blood pressure) and the lower body (which will have lower blood pressure). Other complications include hypertension (high blood pressure), congestive heart failure (see HEART FAILURE, CONGESTIVE), enlarged heart, kidney failure, premature development of blockages in the coronary arteries surrounding the heart, aneurysm (ballooning) and possible rupture of the aorta, stroke, or heart attack. Left untreated, coarctation of the aorta usually results in death before age 40.

In most cases, coarctation of the aorta is discovered during early childhood,

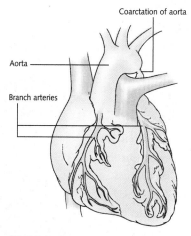

Coarctation of aorta

Aorta

Branch arteries

CONSTRICTED AORTA
Narrowing of the aorta, either from the inside or from structural underdevelopment, obstructs blood flow from the left ventricle (pumping chamber) through the aorta and its branching arteries. The constriction makes the ventricle work harder and causes pressure to increase in the arteries between the heart and the constricted area.

but occasionally it escapes detection until adolescence. Signs of the disease include cyanosis (a bluish tint to the skin) in the lower body, high blood pressure in the arms but not the legs, and a weak pulse in the groin along with a strong pulse in the carotid arteries. Symptoms can include dizziness, headache, cramps in the legs with exercise, fainting, and nosebleeds.

Surgery is the usual treatment. The procedure may be performed as soon as the condition is detected or, if diagnosed in infancy, delayed until childhood. The surgery involves removing the narrowed portion of the aorta and sewing the two free ends back together, sometimes with a patch of synthetic material or a flap of tissue from a nearby blood vessel. A hospital stay of 3 to 4 days is typically needed after surgery. In some cases, BALLOON ANGIO-PLASTY is used in place of surgery. Although angioplasty or surgery is successful in most cases, follow-up and medical management are required. For example, antibiotics may need to be taken before dental, medical, or surgical procedures to lower the risk of infection in the aorta or heart.

COBRA-EMTALA

Consolidated Omnibus Budget Reconciliation Act (COBRA)–Emergency Medical Treatment and Active Labor

Act (EMTALA). COBRA addresses the issue of continuation of health insurance coverage after termination of employment. EMTALA covers the requirement of hospital emergency departments to provide care for individuals who come to the emergency department for treatment.

COBRA requires employers with 20 or more employees to offer continuing group health insurance coverage to certain former employees, retirees, spouses, and dependent children. The length of time the coverage continues depends on the specific occurrence (for example, if the person quits a job or is fired) that caused the discontinuation of group health insurance coverage of a covered employee and his or her spouse and dependent children. A spouse and dependent children of a covered employee can also qualify after a divorce or legal separation from, or death of, the covered employee. The covered employee may be required to pay the insurance premium in addition to a surcharge of up to 2 percent to cover administrative costs.

EMTALA requires hospital emergency departments to provide services to individuals who come to an emergency department for care of an emergency condition or women who are in active labor, regardless of their ability to pay or lack of insurance coverage. EMTALA also established standards for transferring patients to other emergency departments.

Cocaine

See CRACK COCAINE.

Coccidioidomycosis

A potentially fatal fungal infection caused by *Coccidioides immitis*, a fungus that lives in the semiarid, sandy soil common to the southwestern United States, Mexico, and Argentina. Coccidioidomycosis is caused by inhaling an airborne form of the fungus at a certain stage in the organism's life cycle. The risk is increased following human disturbance of soil or after natural disasters, including windstorms, dust storms, and earthquakes. Construction and agricultural workers, as well as archeologists in endemic areas, are particularly vulnerable.

Coccidioidomycosis most commonly affects the lungs, but may progress to involve the kidneys, spleen, lymph nodes, brain, and thyroid gland.

SYMPTOMS, DIAGNOSIS, AND TREATMENT

The symptoms of coccidioidomycosis include flulike malaise with fever, fatigue, cough, headaches, rash, muscle aches, and weight loss. Symptoms may also begin as acute pneumonia or, rarely, as chronic pneumonia. One form may affect the skin, bone, and meninges, which are the membranes lining the brain and spinal cord. In people infected with HIV (human immunodeficiency virus), severe pulmonary disease may develop.

Diagnosis is made by discovering the fungus in a person's saliva or from a culture made from the main airways of the lungs. Skin testing is no longer considered an accurate diagnostic measure.

Long-term treatment with the medication FLUCONAZOLE may be effective in curing coccidioidomycosis if treatment begins early and there are no complications. Even with treatment, the mortality rate is high, especially for people with weakened immune systems. Meningitis, the most serious complication of the infection, is usually fatal if untreated.

Developing an effective vaccine is currently seen as the most promising approach to controlling coccidioidomycosis because surviving an infection provides lifelong immunity.

Coccydynia

A continuous aching pain in the area of the coccyx, the structure formed by the small, fused bones at the base of the spine. Coccydynia may also be called coccygodynia. The condition is associated with a musculoskeletal abnormality in the area of the spine. Coccydynia may be caused by injury to the coccyx, possibly related to a heavy backward fall. It may occur after childbirth.

Medical treatments may include repeated injections of a local anesthetic at the painful site or the injection of a corticosteroid and a local anesthetic into the tissues around the coccyx area, combined with physical manipulation of the coccyx for a short period following the injections. With the use of fluoroscopic X rays, the anti-inflammatory corticosteroid may be injected directly into the affected joint. Repairing associated

ligaments by injecting them with an irritant, a treatment called prolotherapy, acts by causing inflammation that ultimately shortens and strengthens the ligaments and may be effective in relieving the pain of coccydynia. In some cases, surgical removal of the coccyx may be recommended.

Coccygodynia

See COCCYDYNIA.

Cochlea

The fluid-filled, snail-shaped structure in the inner EAR that translates sounds into electrical impulses and relays them to the brain. Sound waves that reach the inner ear vibrate a membrane called the oval window, which transmits the sound waves into the fluid environment within the cochlea. In the cochlea is a structure called the organ of Corti, which contains millions of tiny hair cells and acts as an analyzer of the frequency of sound waves. The movement of the fluid stimulates the hair cells. Higher pitched tones maximally stimulate the hair cells at the base of the cochlea, and lower pitched sounds stimulate the hair cells at the farther end. The bending of the hair cells converts pitch and volume information into nerve impulses that are transmitted via the eighth cranial nerve to the auditory cortex, the area of the brain where sound is perceived and interpreted.

Cochlear implant

An electronic device designed to restore partial hearing to children and adults who are severely hearing impaired due to damage to the COCHLEA (inner ear) and are unable to benefit from HEARING AIDS. Cochlear implants involve several components, including a surgically implanted transmitter, which is activated by a device worn outside the ear. Cochlear implants differ from hearing aids in that they do not enhance sound to make it louder or clearer. Instead, the cochlear implant bypasses damaged parts of the hearing system, converts speech and environmental sounds into electrical signals, and directly stimulates the hearing nerve.

Cochlear implant surgery involves positioning a special receiver/stimulator under the skin in a shallow inci-

sion made in the bone behind the ear. Electrodes (very thin wires) are inserted about 1 inch into the inner ear to stimulate the auditory nerve (nerve responsible for hearing). Other components are worn outside the body. A transmitting coil, a ring about 1 inch wide, is held in place over the implanted receiver behind the ear by small magnets in both the coil and the receiver. A microphone is worn behind the ear, as a person might wear a hearing aid. A signal processor, about the size of a pocket calculator, is generally worn on a belt or in a pocket. Two small cables, which can be worn under clothing, connect the three external components.

Cochlear implant is the only medical treatment currently available for profound sensorineural hearing loss (a form of total hearing loss in which sounds reach the inner ear but are not passed on to the brain by the auditory nerves). Sensorineural hearing loss is usually caused by damage to the inner ear or the hearing nerve. The damage may occur as a result of aging. It can also be caused by exposure to loud music, machinery noise, viral infections, or side effects from certain medications. Heredity may have a role, and some infants are born with this form of hearing loss. Cochlear implant surgery may safely be performed on children aged 2 years and older and possibly even on younger children in the future. The auditory nerve must be intact for these implants to be of sufficient benefit to provide a hearing-impaired person with increased hearing ability. Implants that stimulate the brain stem directly are being developed.

HOW IT WORKS

The microphone worn behind the ear captures incoming sound and transmits the sound to the signal processor. The processor converts the sound into electrical impulses, or signals, which travel up one of the cables to the transmitting coil behind the ear. The coil transfers the signals to the implanted receiver and the electrodes inside the inner ear. The electrodes directly stimulate the auditory nerve fibers to transmit the signals, sound-generated nerve impulses, to the brain's hearing center. The brain translates the impulses into meaningful speech and environmental sound.

The implant surgery is performed

under general anesthesia by an ear surgeon. The operation may be performed on an outpatient basis or may require a hospital stay of several days, depending on the device used and the anatomy of the inner ear. One month after surgery, the microphone, transmitting coil, and signal processor are positioned and adjusted. The person who has received the implant is then taught how to listen to sound through the implant. Regular follow-up visits to readjust the system are usually needed.

Results of using cochlear implants vary from one person to another, and the benefits for those who receive the implants are improving continually. Most individuals who are profoundly hearing impaired find they are better able to receive some sound with the implants. They may find their ability to lip-read is improved and overall communication enhanced. Normal hearing is not entirely restored, but many implant recipients can successfully talk on the phone. Results with infants and children are very promising. The degree of benefit may depend on how long a person has been hearing impaired, the amount of surviving auditory nerve fibers he or she has, and the person's motivation to learn to hear.

Codeine

A narcotic pain reliever. Codeine is used to relieve mild to moderate pain associated with dental surgery, bone fracture, headache, burns, shingles, and childbirth. It also suppresses coughing. Codeine, like other narcotics, is habit-forming and, therefore, is not recommended for long-term use.

Codeine is often prescribed as part of a combination drug, such as aspirin with codeine (Empirin with Codeine, Emcodeine) or acetaminophen with codeine (Tylenol with Codeine, Phenaphen with Codeine, Pyregesic-C), to relieve pain. Other drugs involving codeine are a combination of a barbiturate, aspirin, and codeine, to treat headaches and other pain; a combination of muscle relaxant (carisoprodol), aspirin, and codeine, to treat muscle pain and stiffness; and some combinations of antihistamine, decongestant, and antitussive, used to treat hay fever, colds, and flu and to suppress cough.

Codependence

A pattern of behavior found in a person who enables someone addicted to alcohol, drugs, or compulsive gambling to maintain his or her ADDICTION. The behavior is usually unwitting. The codependent person honestly wishes to help but does so in ways that prevent the person who is addicted from recognizing the addiction for what it is. For example, a codependent person may shield the person addicted by inventing excuses for absences from work due to drinking or drugs or may take on family responsibilities the person cannot fulfill because of the addiction. Codependence is found principally in the spouses, children, friends, and coworkers of the person with the addiction and in the clergy. It has been suggested that people who exhibit codependence have low self-esteem and consider themselves of value only when they are helping others. Some experts in the field consider codependence a disease, much as drug addiction or alcohol dependency. Treatment consists of helping the codependent person recognize the pattern of enabling behavior and take steps to change it.

Coffee enemas

A method used to relieve pain by administering enemas containing caffeine from coffee. The method was invented accidentally by a field nurse in World War I, who administered enemas to several badly wounded soldiers because she had run out of painkillers. Coffee enemas have been used by some alternative practitioners to treat people with cancer on the

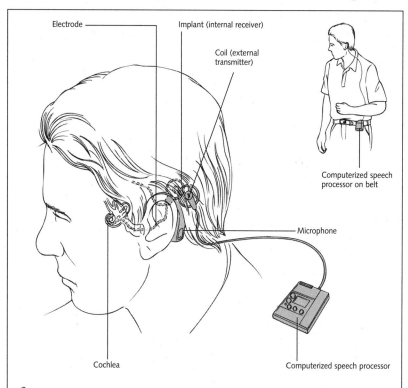

Electrode — Implant (internal receiver)

Coil (external transmitter)

Computerized speech processor on belt

Microphone

Cochlea

Computerized speech processor

COMPONENTS OF A COCHLEAR IMPLANT
A cochlear implant helps a person with sensorineural hearing loss (nerve deafness) more clearly distinguish speech and other sounds. A microphone worn behind the ear picks up sounds, which are sent to a small computerized processor (often worn under the clothing) that converts the sounds to electric impulses. These signals travel via wires up to an external transmitting coil worn behind the ear. The coil sends the signals to an electrode receiver implanted in the inner ear. The signals go to the cochlea (part of the inner ear that changes sound vibrations into nerve impulses). Electrodes directly stimulate auditory nerve fibers, bypassing damaged hair cells that have caused the hearing loss. The nerve impulses carry sound information to the brain's hearing center, which interprets it as meaningful sounds.

principle that caffeine taken rectally stimulates the action of the liver, increases the flow of bile, and opens the bile ducts, thereby emptying the liver of toxic products of tumor breakdown and substances that cause pain. This form of DETOXIFICATION is used as often as needed to remove toxins, including those believed to come from the use of conventional pain-relieving drugs. The effects claimed for coffee enemas cannot be obtained by drinking coffee; to be effective, the caffeine must enter the liver without first passing through the digestive tract. However, coffee enemas are clinically unproven and may, in fact, cause chemical imbalances in the blood along with severe diarrhea and dehydration.

Cognitive-behavioral therapy

An approach to resolving emotional conflicts and mental illnesses that emphasizes techniques focused on current thinking (cognition) and direct experience (behavior). Different varieties of cognitive-behavioral therapy are known as rational-emotive therapy, reality therapy, and transactional analysis. Cognitive-behavioral therapy is typically used for a period of weeks rather than an extended time. It is effective for specific emotional issues, mild depression, anxiety, and problems with anger.

BASIC CONCEPTS

Cognitive-behavioral therapy is based on the theory that personality is determined largely by how a person thinks and behaves. Unlike traditional psychoanalysis, which seeks to uncover childhood emotional conflicts buried in the subconscious, cognitive-behavioral therapy focuses on dysfunctional thinking in the present. The therapist and the person work together as a collaborative team to test the person's thinking against reality and to determine which beliefs help the person adapt and which ones cause distress and need to be changed in a more positive direction.

Cognitive-behavioral therapists maintain that specific attitudes, known as schemas, predispose people to behave or react in distressful ways. Schemas are structures of fundamental beliefs that develop in childhood, are reinforced by events, and are carried forward into adult life. Therapy consists of testing schemas against reality as a way of making the person aware of them and highlighting the need to change beliefs that are not logical. Correcting these cognitive errors can alleviate emotional distress.

For example, research has shown that people with depression have characteristic misbeliefs. These include relating negative events to oneself even when there is no basis to do so (personalization); seeing choices as only black or white (dichotomous thinking); focusing on the most negative aspects of a situation (selective abstraction); and distorting the importance of events, such as making small problems into major obstacles (magnification-minimization). Cognitive-behavioral therapy seeks to create awareness of such schemas and help the person think in ways that are more conducive to coping and that offset depressive feelings.

TECHNIQUES

Cognitive-behavioral therapy centers on examining illogical beliefs and testing them against reality. A number of methods are commonly used. At the beginning of therapy, the person may be asked to keep a detailed log of all activities, which the individual then shares with the therapist. Next, the therapist and the person may develop a schedule of weekly activities to ensure that the person is making positive efforts toward therapy goals. An example would be planned social outings for someone who is isolated because of depression. Role-playing is commonly used to help the individual work through the feelings surrounding difficult tasks, such as shyness in starting a conversation. Pretending to be strangers, the therapist and the individual can practice ways of initiating a social interaction. In some cases, the therapist may accompany the person in problematic situations to observe how he or she behaves and then help create new ways of dealing with those circumstances. A system of rewards for behaving in a desired way may be used, a technique known as behavior modification.

Cohort study

A design for human research that involves observing a group, or cohort, of people free of disease, over time to determine what diseases occur in people with particular characteristics or exposures. For example, observing a group of people who had been exposed on the job to a particular industrial chemical would allow the researcher to determine how many of the overall group developed cancer, high blood pressure, or heart disease after exposure and whether the disease rate in this subgroup was higher than the unexposed subgroup. The advantage of cohort studies is that they provide a good measure of disease risk. The disadvantage is that accuracy requires a large number of people in the cohort, which makes such studies particularly expensive and difficult to use.

Coinsurance

Also called a copayment; the percentage of health care costs that people must pay themselves after paying their DEDUCTIBLE (the dollar amount that is paid for health care each year before health plans begin to pay). For example, if a person owes a 20 percent coinsurance payment and makes an office visit that costs $100, he or she is responsible for a copayment of $20 for that visit.

Coitus

The sexual union of two people of the opposite sex, in which the man's penis enters the woman's vagina. See SEXUAL INTERCOURSE.

Coitus interruptus

A birth control method commonly known as withdrawal. Coitus interruptus relies on a man withdrawing his penis before he ejaculates into a woman's vagina. Coitus interruptus is extremely unreliable because semen containing sperm can be released before a man has an orgasm and ejaculates. Pregnancy can occur after a drop or two of semen enter the vagina. See CONTRACEPTION, OTHER METHODS.

Colchicine

A drug used to treat gout attacks and gouty arthritis. Colchicine relieves the pain and swelling of gout and helps to prevent further attacks. It is also used to treat other diseases affecting joints, skin, and internal organs and is available as a pill and by injection.

C

Cold injury

An abnormal and potentially serious physical condition that is caused by exposure to cold temperatures. Cold injuries range from FROSTBITE to HYPOTHERMIA. Frostbite occurs when tissue freezes. Blood vessels are deprived of oxygen, leading to edema (swelling) and necrosis (tissue death). Treatment is with gentle warming, such as immersion into warm bath water. Affected body parts should not be rubbed. Chilblains (see PERNIO), a condition in which there is constriction of small blood vessels because of cold weather, causes burning, itching, and ulceration similar to that caused by burns; treatment is the same as for frostbite.

Hypothermia occurs when the core body temperature drops below 94°F. Symptoms of hypothermia include shivering; slurred speech; slow breathing; cold, pale skin; poor coordination; fatigue; and lethargy. Children and older people are especially susceptible to hypothermia, and need emergency attention for it.

The best course of action is preventing cold injuries. The head, face, and neck should be covered because much of a person's body heat is lost there first because of the large blood supply in those areas. Multiple layers of waterproof clothing work best to preserve body heat. Sweating should be avoided because it causes the body to lose even more heat; it is important to stay as dry as possible.

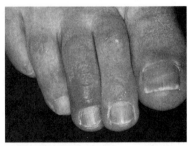

COLD INJURY ON THE TOES
Pernios or chilblains on the foot of a woman seem especially severe on the middle toe.

Cold remedies

Prescription or nonprescription medications that relieve some of the symptoms of the common cold. Cold remedies cannot prevent or cure the viral infections that cause the cold, but they can sometimes make the per-

son who has a cold feel more comfortable. These cold remedies fall into several general categories: ANTIHISTAMINES, DECONGESTANT DRUGS, nose sprays, COUGH REMEDIES, pain relievers, and multisymptom or combination "cold and flu" preparations.

ANTIHISTAMINES

Antihistamines are drugs that block the action of histamines, which are body chemicals that stimulate blood vessels to expand in the membranes of the nose. Histamines are responsible for several cold symptoms, including a runny or stuffy nose, sneezing, itchy eyes, and nasal congestion. Antihistamines may alleviate some or most of these symptoms but have some side effects. Some people experience an uncomfortably dry mouth and nose. The main side effect for most people is drowsiness, which is usually most noticeable after the initial dose is taken. Because of this side effect, it is recommended that antihistamines be taken at bedtime. In fact, it may be dangerous to take antihistamines during the day, especially when driving. Antihistamine remedies may temporarily make breathing easier by clearing nasal passages, but they achieve this by shrinking and drying up tissues inside the nose, a process that can thicken nasal mucus and make it potentially harder to drain from the nose. Antihistamines should be taken for no more than a few days.

DECONGESTANTS

Decongestants are cold remedies that cause constriction or tightening of the blood vessels in the membranes of the nose and air passages. Viral infections involved in the common cold often cause these blood vessels to expand or dilate, producing congestion in the nose, sinuses, and chest. Decongestants constrict the blood flow so that the nasal tissues shrink, and the air passages open up. Taking a decongestant may also help promote nasal secretions, relieve obstruction, and provide relief from the discomfort of a stuffy nose. Topical decongestants should not be taken for more than a few days. The active ingredients in decongestant remedies are chemically related to EPINEPHRINE (adrenaline), a natural decongestant and a type of stimulant. The possible side effects include jittery feelings and nervousness, insom-

nia, elevated blood pressure and pulse rate, difficulty urinating, and upset stomach. Cold remedies containing decongestant ingredients should not be used by anyone who has high blood pressure, an irregular heart rhythm, heart disease, glaucoma, diabetes mellitus, or prostate or thyroid problems.

Over-the-counter nose sprays are decongestants directly applied to the inside of the nose. They constrict blood vessels in the nasal passages. Nasal sprays tend to give faster and greater relief from congestion because of the direct application of the decongestant to the membranes in the nose. These nasal sprays can also impair circulation in the nose somewhat, and after a few hours, the vessels dilate or expand again as a "rebound" effect. The result may be increased mucus production and intensified congestion. A person may respond by using the spray more and more, which continues the cycle. The rebound effect from nasal sprays can cause rhinitis (inflammation of the membrane lining the nose) within a few days. People who have overused nose sprays may need to take a decongestant by mouth to break the cycle. When medical attention is sought, a corticosteroid drug (synthetic drugs sometimes used to treat inflammatory disorders; see CORTICOSTEROIDS) may be prescribed.

Topical decongestants should not be used in infants, and their use should be avoided in children.

Decongestant nose sprays should not be used for more than 3 days. A safer alternative to decongestant nose sprays, saline drops or spray, may help soothe and clear a stuffed nose. Mix ½ teaspoon of table salt in 6 ounces of water and apply 3 drops in each nostril. Also, laying a hot, wet cloth over the nose may help loosen and drain mucus from the nose.

COUGH REMEDIES

Over-the-counter cough remedies containing cough suppressants may offer minimal help for reducing the frequency of coughs. In general, nonprescription cough suppressant lozenges are best at soothing the throat. When coughing is so severe that it interferes with sleeping or with everyday conversation, a doctor should be consulted. Prescription medications containing dextromethorphan or CODEINE can help control dry, unproductive coughing. EXPECTORANTS help a person cough up phlegm; they release and expel infected mucus from the throat and may be more beneficial when coughing is a bothersome symptom of an uncomplicated common cold. Popular cough remedy preparations combining an expectorant, which promotes coughing, with a cough suppressant, intended to prevent coughing, do not make sense. For sore throats, sucking on hard candy or cough drops may be soothing and help alleviate pain. Ingredients such as honey, glycerin, and menthol can help ease throat irritation.

RISKS

Adults with cold symptoms, including headache, body aches, and fever, may find aspirin or acetaminophen helps relieve these symptoms, but these painkillers may intensify a cold's symptoms. Researchers have found that aspirin and acetaminophen may sometimes suppress certain immune responses (see IMMUNE RESPONSE) and actually increase nasal congestion in adults. Doctors recommend that children and teens with a cold take acetaminophen or ibuprofen rather than aspirin, if necessary to relieve pain and fever. Aspirin use carries the risk of REYE SYNDROME, a very rare and potentially fatal condition that occurs in children with viral illness, especially if they have taken aspirin.

Multisymptom cold and flu preparations often contain medications for a wide variety of symptoms. A person with a cold who uses these products may end up treating symptoms he or she does not have. Multisymptom remedies in liquid or pill form may combine antihistamines, decongestants, drying agents, both cough suppressants and expectorants, plus pain relievers. It is recommended that a person choose a remedy with specific ingredients targeted to his or her specific symptoms. If a product label does not specify the functions of individual ingredients, a pharmacist can help. Cold remedies labeled "extra-strength," "maximum strength," and "long-acting" are potentially more effective than their standard counterparts, but higher doses increase the risk of side effects and their severity.

VITAMINS AND HERBAL REMEDIES

Scientific study has not revealed conclusive results in the testing of vitamins and herbal remedies for the treatment of viral infections associated with colds or for the treatment of symptoms of these infections. The best approach to the use of vitamins and herbal preparations is to consult with a physician. The doctor should be reminded of all prescription and nonprescription medication currently being taken because some combinations can be harmful.

Cold sore

A small blister around the mouth caused by the herpes simplex virus (see HERPES, OROLABIAL); also known as a fever blister. Although most people carry this virus, it is usually dormant. Many factors, such as stress, sun exposure, fever, injury, colds, or other illness, can trigger an outbreak. Cold sores frequently affect adolescents and young adults. Blisters tend to recur at the same site and usually appear on the lips but may also develop on the cheeks, chin, nostrils, or gums.

A cold sore begins with a tingling or burning sensation, followed in 2 days by the appearance of a small blister filled with clear, yellow liquid. Both the blister and the red, raised skin around it are tender and painful. In some cases, a number of small blisters merge to form one large sore. Blisters eventually break, ooze, and crust over.

There is no known cure for the virus that causes cold sores. They generally resolve without treatment in 7 to 14 days, but doctors can prescribe oral antiviral agents such as acyclovir and famciclovir to shorten the duration. Treatment should start when the tingling begins. Self-care measures for

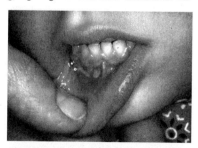

COLD SORES NEAR THE GUM LINE
The herpes simplex virus caused the cold sores in this child's mouth. The virus can be spread by sharing towels or eating utensils.

cold sores include using topical over-the-counter and prescription ointments, avoiding irritants such as spicy foods, and not picking at the blisters. Cold sores are highly contagious and are usually spread by direct skin contact. Kissing and other skin contact should be avoided when a person has a cold sore. People who are prone to cold sores should regularly use sunblock on their lips to protect their lips from the sun.

Cold, common

FOR SYMPTOM CHART
see Coughing, page 28

Infection of the respiratory tract, caused by any one of more than 200 different viruses. Sometimes called a head cold, the infection causes inflammation of the mucous membranes lining the nose and throat. Nasal congestion, sore throat, and sometimes other symptoms, usually confined to the nose and throat, are produced by the inflammation. The larynx (organ in the throat that contains vocal cords) may also become involved, causing laryngitis.

SYMPTOMS

The symptoms of the common cold usually begin 2 to 4 days after the person has become infected. Colds sometimes seem to come on quickly because viruses can multiply rapidly in the body. The major symptoms usually include nasal congestion and nasal discharge. At first the nasal discharge may be thin and watery, later becoming thick and greenish yellow. Sneezing, watering eyes, sore throat, hoarseness, coughing, a congested feeling in the head and chest, and headache are other common symptoms. Sometimes a person with a cold experiences achiness, mild fatigue, and fever. Fever associated with the common cold is usually slight, but can be as high as 102°F in infants and young children. The fever may cause shivering and chills. In adults, higher temperatures with more severe body aches are more likely to be symptoms of INFLUENZA, or flu.

The length of the symptoms may depend on which virus is causing the cold. A common cold generally lasts from 7 to 13 days. Most cold sufferers recover within a week. Symptoms lasting much longer than 2 weeks

C

WHERE A COLD VIRUS STRIKES
A cold can affect any part of the respiratory tract. Most commonly, the linings of the nose and throat become inflamed, causing a runny nose and sneezing. The infection may also irritate the larynx and trachea, causing a hoarse voice, sore throat, and coughing. If the infection spreads to the lungs, a more serious condition such as pneumonia may result.

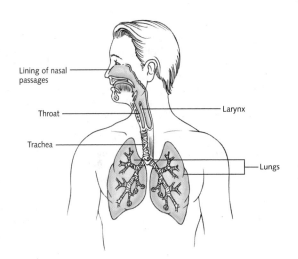

Lining of nasal passages

Throat

Trachea

Larynx

Lungs

may be the result of an allergy rather than a cold, or they may be caused by a secondary infection brought on by bacteria. A physician should be consulted if the symptoms of a cold persist for more than 10 days. Specific symptoms that require a doctor's attention include earache, pain in the face or forehead, or a fever lasting longer than 4 days or going above 102°F. A combination of symptoms including persistent hoarseness or sore throat, shortness of breath and wheezing, and a dry, painful coughs may indicate PNEUMONIA and require immediate medical attention.

CAUSES
Almost everyone gets colds occasionally, regardless of their age or sex. Children are extremely susceptible to the nasal viral infections that cause cold symptoms when they are 1 or 2 years old. In this age range, they can have as many as six to ten colds a year. Adults average about two to five colds a year. Women (especially young mothers) aged 20 to 30 have more colds than men, possibly because they have more contact with young children. As they grow older, children may gradually become immune to many of the common viruses that cause colds. Frequency of infection may increase again during the early school years because there are types of viruses to which children have not been previously exposed in the school environment. Also, children may be more careless about covering their mouths when they sneeze and cough. Most people acquire greater immunity to colds

with age and catch fewer and less severe colds as they grow older.

The major way to catch a cold seems to be through hand-to-hand contact. Typically, an infected person will touch a moist surface such as the eye, nose, or mouth and then touch the hand of an uninfected person. If this person touches a similar surface within 10 to 15 minutes, the cold may be transmitted. Coughing may spread a related illness, and a hearty sneeze may transport a cold virus as far as 12 feet through the air. Relatively large particles of infected respiratory secretions can be transported briefly in the air, while smaller infectious particles may remain suspended in the air for long periods. Breathing in these particles can give a person a cold.

No one is exactly sure how all colds are spread, but some popularly held beliefs about how people catch colds are known to be untrue. Colds are not caused by exposure to drafts or cold weather. Nor are they caused by getting chilled or overheated. Factors such as exercise and diet or enlarged tonsils or adenoids are not believed to be related to susceptibility. Research suggests, however, that psychological stress, allergies affecting the nasal passages or the throat, and a woman's menstrual cycles may have an impact on susceptibility to a cold.

In the United States, most colds occur during fall and winter, beginning in late August or early September. The incidence of colds increases slowly and remains high until March or April when it begins to decline. These seasonal variations may be

related to school openings in the fall. Also, colder winter weather may result in more time spent indoors where the chances are increased that viruses will spread from one person to another. Seasonal changes in relative humidity may also affect the prevalence of colds. Many common cold–causing viruses survive better when humidity is low as it is during the colder months of the year. Cold weather also dries out the lining of the throat and nasal passages, making them more vulnerable to viral infection.

TREATMENT
There is no effective prescription drug treatment for the common cold. The antiviral agents are usually most effective for influenza and not the common cold. A physician will not usually prescribe antibiotics for a person with a cold because the virus causing the cold does not respond to antibiotic medication. However, people who have recurrent bouts of SINUSITIS or BRONCHITIS or frequent ear infections should see a physician at the first sign of a cold since these conditions may present complications. A doctor can explain how a cold affects the specific situation and recommend appropriate treatment, which may include antibiotics or other prescription medication.

While there is no medical treatment for the virus causing the common cold, the symptoms of the infection can be relieved to decrease the discomfort of the person who has a cold. Among the treatments doctors recommend are bed rest, drinking plenty of fluids, gargling with warm salt water for sore throats (½ teaspoon in 6 ounces of warm water), and applying petroleum jelly to soothe a raw nose. Nasal sprays may reduce sneezing and nasal congestion if given within 1 day of symptom onset.

No conclusive scientific study has definitively proven that the use of vitamins or herbal medicine can cure or prevent colds or alleviate the symptoms of the infection. There are over-the-counter remedies that may help alleviate some of the symptoms.

When a person has symptoms of a cold, he or she should stay at home to avoid giving the infection to others, as well as for his or her own rest and recuperation. Self-help techniques that may prove beneficial for alleviating cold symptoms at home include keeping the room temperature warm but not overheated and increasing the humidity in the air with a central or room humidifier, especially when indoor heating systems are on. Taking a hot shower and inhaling steam can also be helpful. Breathing in humid air helps prevent nasal passages from drying out and allows the mucus to drain, or be gently blown out, more easily. Blowing the nose properly is important. It should be done by lightly blowing into a disposable tissue, clearing the nostrils one at a time by pressing on one side of the nose while blowing easily through the other nostril. Pressing both nostrils while blowing should be avoided as this prevents a thorough clearing of mucus from the nose and may spread the infection into the ears.

Drinking extra fluids will help thin the mucus blocking nasal passages and may ease congestion. Taking in ample liquids can help replace fluids lost through perspiration and nasal discharge and also keep body tissues well hydrated to help protect them against further infection. Hot soup and other hot beverages have been shown to relieve some of the respiratory symptoms of colds. Hot liquids can also help relieve a sore throat.

PREVENTION

Doctors recommend frequent hand washing during cold season as possibly the simplest and most effective

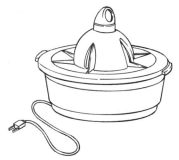

BREATHING MOIST AIR
A cool vaporizer sprays a fine mist of water particles into the air to increase humidity in the room. For a person with a cold, breathing warm, humid air prevents irritated nasal passages from drying out and helps mucus drain out more smoothly. It is best to keep the room temperature warm and use a cool-water vaporizer, to avoid the fire and scalding risks of a steam vaporizer.

way to keep from getting a cold. Avoiding touching the nose or eyes is another preventive measure. Cleaning environmental surfaces with a virus-killing disinfectant may also help prevent spread of infection. Also, close, prolonged exposure to people with colds should be avoided.

Colectomy

The surgical removal of all or part of the colon. A colectomy is performed to treat serious diseases, such as colon cancer (see COLON, CANCER OF THE), DIVERTICULAR DISEASE, and severe COLITIS. A light or liquid diet is prescribed for several days before a scheduled procedure. Antibiotics and bowel-cleansing enemas may also be given to rid the intestine of stool and bacteria. A colectomy may also be performed on an emergency basis if there is an imminent risk of perforation or an obstruction.

A colectomy is done in a hospital under general anesthesia. The surgeon begins by making an incision in the abdominal wall. Next, the tumor or diseased part of the colon is removed. When possible, only part of the colon is excised, allowing the healthy remaining sections to be joined together to maintain a passageway for stools. Usually the operation involves a large incision and scar.

When this is not possible, an opening called a STOMA is made in the abdominal wall. This allows the discharge of feces into a bag attached to the skin. A COLOSTOMY is a procedure in which an opening from the colon is made through a stoma. The procedure in which the ileum (the lower part of the small intestine) opens through a stoma is an ILEOSTOMY. Both procedures can be temporary or permanent.

After a colectomy, nutrients are given intravenously while fluid is drained from the abdomen. In 2 to 3 days, a special diet is prescribed and waste begins to pass into the colostomy bag. When colostomies and ileostomies are temporary, another procedure will be scheduled to close the stoma once the intestine has recovered from the initial surgery. Doctors may also recommend chemotherapy, radiation, or both after a colectomy for colon cancer.

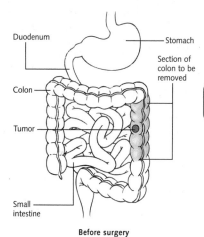

Before surgery

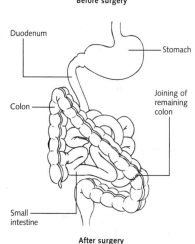

After surgery

REMOVING PART OF THE COLON
A partial colectomy is done to remove a section of the colon that is diseased, usually with cancer. The two ends of the remaining healthy colon are then joined to form a shorter but continuous passage.

Colestipol hydrochloride

A drug used to lower serum cholesterol levels. Colestipol hydrochloride (Colestid) is used to lower cholesterol levels in order to prevent heart disease. It is available as a tablet, taken orally, or in granule form to mix with water, another liquid, or food.

Colic

Gastrointestinal pain experienced by infants. Many doctors believe that colic is the result of an immature digestive system, although its exact cause remains unknown. Colic occurs in both breast-fed and bottle-

C

fed babies. The condition is harmless. Continual, intense crying, along with fussiness and irritability, are the hallmarks of colic. During colicky spells, the baby's abdomen may be distended or hard. Infants may clench their hands and draw their knees up toward the abdomen. An attack ends when a baby has a bowel movement, passes gas, or eventually falls asleep from exhaustion.

Episodes of colic are most common in the late afternoon and early evening. Almost all affected infants will have the onset of symptoms by 3 weeks of age. Colic usually occurs at least three times a week and lasts for 3 hours or more. It rarely lasts beyond the first 3 months of an infant's life. Colic can be a sign of a more severe medical problem. A colicky baby who is vomiting or whose bowel movements contain blood or mucus needs to be seen by a pediatrician or family physician. The doctor will examine the child to exclude a more serious problem, such as an intestinal obstruction. See also CRYING IN INFANTS.

TREATMENT

Colicky symptoms generally improve as the child matures. The pediatrician can suggest a number of calming techniques. For example, many babies feel better when they are soothed by continuous motions or sounds. Because colic is common, parents have found an array of activities that may comfort a colicky baby. They range from rocking and patting to running the vacuum cleaner or clothes dryer. Many babies find relief when held in the "football" position (face down along the length of an adult's arm, with the head and neck carefully supported on the hand). The gentle pressure on the baby's abdomen helps alleviate pain. Laying an infant face down across the knees and massaging his or her back also can relieve pressure. In some cases, a physician may recommend an antigas medication, although it may provide no more than a placebo effect.

Researchers believe that food sensitivity may have a role in some cases of colic (see food intolerance). Although formula changes are probably of limited usefulness for treating colic, many parents and doctors will try a formula change. For example, if bottle-feeding, a soy formula may be a better choice than one based on

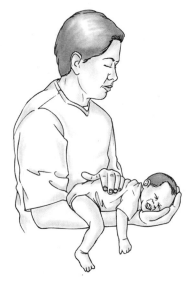

COMFORTING A COLICKY CHILD
The "football hold" may bring some comfort and relief to a colicky baby. When a baby is held face down along the length of an adult's arm, with hand support for the neck and head, the gentle pressure along the length of the abdomen sometimes helps ease his or her pain. A light touch or massage on the back may also be soothing.

cow's milk, on the chance that the symptoms are related to milk allergies. Breast-feeding mothers often try eliminating potentially irritating foods from their diet. Typical offenders may be dairy products, caffeine, chocolate, onions, spicy dishes, and gas-producing foods such as cabbage, broccoli, and beans.

Parents of colicky babies may become frustrated, exhausted, or angry. They may think, wrongly, that they have caused the colic. To avoid serious stress, doctors say, parents should let a caretaker watch the child for a short while and take some time off.

Colitis

Inflammation of the lining of the colon. Colitis may affect the entire colon or only parts of it. One type of colitis is caused by bacterial infection. Sometimes, this form of the disease occurs after treatment with antibiotics and is treated with another type of antibiotic. A more serious type of colitis, ulcerative colitis, shares many similarities with CROHN DISEASE, and both diseases are considered types of INFLAMMATORY BOWEL DISEASE.

The most common symptom of colitis is blood in the feces (see FECES, BLOOD IN THE). An attack of diarrhea that contains blood and pus is a typical sign of colitis. Other symptoms may include abdominal pain, persistent diarrhea, fever, and weight loss. An anal fissure (a tear or ulcer in the lining of the anal canal), an anal fistula (an abnormal channel between the anal canal and a hole in the skin surrounding the anus), or an abscess in the anal canal can also develop.

DIAGNOSIS

Colitis is diagnosed by a complete physical examination and tests, such as stool analysis, blood tests, a lower GASTROINTESTINAL (GI) SERIES (an X-ray procedure also called a barium enema), SIGMOIDOSCOPY, and COLONOSCOPY. In sigmoidoscopy and colonoscopy, the colon and rectum are examined by using a slim, flexible, lighted tube inserted through the anus. The colonoscopy (ENDOSCOPY of the entire colon) is a more extensive procedure than the sigmoidoscopy (an endoscopy of the rectum and sigmoid colon). A biopsy (analysis of a tissue sample) can confirm the presence of ulcerative colitis.

ULCERATIVE COLITIS

Shallow and widespread bleeding ulcers are typical of ulcerative colitis. The inflammation usually occurs in the rectum and lower part of the colon, but may affect the entire colon. Constant healing and scarring may lead to the formation of inflammatory polyps. In some cases, cancerous cell changes are associated with ulcerative colitis. It is sometimes difficult to differentiate between ulcerative colitis and Crohn disease. Both cause recurrent bouts of colon inflammation, damage the digestive tract, and can be associated with cancerous cell changes and complications in other parts of the body. However, there are also significant differences. For example, ulcerative colitis usually occurs only in the colon, while Crohn disease can affect any part of the digestive tract; ulcerative colitis affects the lining of the colon, while all layers of the intestine are involved in Crohn disease; and the inflammation of the bowel is patchy in Crohn disease, while it is continuous in ulcerative colitis. Ulcerative colitis is slightly more common than Crohn disease in the United States.

The first episode of ulcerative colitis often occurs in late adolescence and may be severe. Remission is possible, but it can continue throughout an individual's life. The exact cause of the disease remains unknown. However, doctors believe that an agent, such as a virus or bacterium, alters the body's immune system, triggering inflammation of the intestinal wall. Other contributing factors may include genetic predisposition, diet, and stress. Ulcerative colitis may have an autoimmune component, suggested by the fact that complications of the disease occur in parts of the body other than the intestine. These include SACROILIITIS (inflammation of the sacroiliac joint at the base of the back), SPONDYLITIS (a painful type of arthritis that affects primarily the joints of vertebrae in the back), ERYTHEMA NODOSUM (a skin condition in which red areas of swelling appear on the legs), and iritis (inflammation of the iris in the eye). When the symptoms of colitis subside, these conditions also generally improve.

TREATMENT

Anti-inflammatory drugs are the main treatment for ulcerative colitis. The goal of both aspirin-based anti-inflammatory drugs, such as sulfasalazine, and corticosteroids, such as prednisone, is to suppress the inflammatory response so the body can heal itself. Powerful corticosteroids more successfully control stubborn cases of inflammation, but they also have many unwanted side effects. These include bloating, weight gain, brittle bones, nervousness, and insomnia. In selected cases,

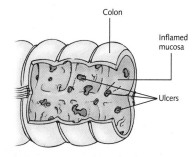

INFLAMMATION OF THE COLON LINING
In a person with ulcerative colitis, the innermost lining (mucosa) of the colon becomes inflamed and small ulcers form. The most common symptom of the disease is blood in the stool, or bloody diarrhea.

anti-inflammatory drugs may be administered as enemas to deliver the medication to the site of the inflammation and reduce side effects. Other drugs that may be prescribed to manage colitis include immunosuppressants and antibiotics. Severe attacks of colitis generally require hospitalization and intravenous administration of medication. If a great deal of blood has been lost, a transfusion may be required.

In some cases, surgical removal of all or part of the colon (a COLECTOMY) becomes necessary. When possible, only part of the colon is excised, allowing the healthy remaining sections to be joined together. This maintains a passageway for stools. When this is not possible, an opening called a STOMA is made in the abdominal wall to allow the discharge of feces into a bag attached to the skin.

Colitis, antibiotic associated

See CLOSTRIDIUM DIFFICILE.

Collagen

A strong, fibrous protein that is the major component of connective tissue. Connective tissue, which includes tendons, ligaments, organ walls, blood vessels, cartilage, and the soft inner material of the bone, requires collagen for strength and elasticity. Collagen is also the component of scar tissue that holds a wound together to promote healing and prevent infection. Vitamin C is important in the production of collagen.

Collagen diseases

Disease of the connective tissue, which is an essential part of every structure in the body. Collagen diseases are sometimes referred to as connective tissue diseases, immunologic rheumatic diseases, or AUTOIMMUNE DISORDERS. The characteristic symptom of all the disorders in this group is the inflammation that damages the connective tissues of the body, many of which are composed of collagen. Collagen is a fibrous protein and the main component of connective tissues, like those that make up tendons. Collagen diseases share certain elements, but each of the diseases also has a distinctive set of symptoms. All diseases in this group are caused by alterations in the immune system.

With collagen diseases, the body's antibodies begin to attack the affected person's own body cells and their components, instead of attacking bacteria, viruses, and other invaders as antibodies normally do.

All the body's systems may be affected. The soft tissue or joints are often involved, but there is often little damage to the affected bone and cartilage. For some people, the symptoms appear and disappear at intervals. For others, the disease ends independently and never recurs. Many people lead active lives despite their disorder; others are profoundly affected and do not regain full health. There is no cure. Certain medication, including corticosteroids, may be used to treat the symptoms and delay the progression of the condition. See CONNECTIVE TISSUE DISEASE, MIXED. Also see specific collagen diseases: LUPUS ERYTHEMATOSUS, SYSTEMIC; SCLERODERMA; SJÖGREN SYNDROME; POLYMYOSITIS; DERMATOMYOSITIS; POLYCHONDRITIS, RELAPSING; and POLYMYALGIA RHEUMATICA.

Collagen injections

Placing a natural protein substance under the skin to fill in the wrinkles, creases, furrows, and other changes in the skin caused by aging or sun damage. Collagen injections can also be used to add fullness to lips and cheeks or to fill in shallow areas, including certain kinds of scars. They may be used alone or along with some other cosmetic procedure, such as a FACE-LIFT.

Collagen is a naturally occurring protein found in skin, bone, and ligaments. The material is extracted from cattle or humans. Since the body metabolizes collagen placed in the tissues, the injections have a temporary effect that can last from a few weeks to an indefinite period of months or even years. The exact factors that control the longevity of collagen injections remain unknown.

When given alone, collagen injections are administered in the office of a physician. The collagen is mixed with lidocaine, a local anesthetic. Additional painkillers, such as topical cream anesthetic or a Freon spray to numb the area to be injected, may be used to treat patients who are particularly sensitive. The collagen is injected with a thin needle placed at several points along the site to be

C

Collagen, a naturally occurring body protein, can be injected under the skin to smooth wrinkles and other skin irregularities caused by sun damage or aging. The collagen, along with a local anesthetic, is injected at several points along the area of skin being treated. Because the body metabolizes collagen, the results of the injections are temporary—anywhere from a few weeks to a year or more.

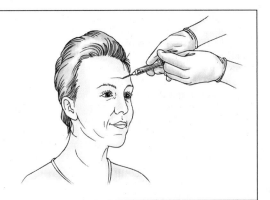

filled. Some minor stinging or a burning sensation may accompany the injections.

After treatment, the area will look overfilled. The collagen mixture contains salt water, which is soon absorbed by the body, decreasing the amount of fill. In some cases, the injected area may swell or appear to be bruised, but these effects pass soon, as do sensations of stinging or throbbing. Redness is normally gone within 24 hours, but may last up to a week in fair-skinned people. Small scabs sometimes appear where the needle was inserted, and these, too, disappear within a week. No bandages are needed, and makeup with sunblock can be worn over the injected area.

The principal risk in collagen injections is an allergic reaction. To determine whether a patient may be allergic, the surgeon will administer a skin test about a month before the injection procedure. Any redness, swelling, or itching should be reported to the surgeon.

Collagen injections are not suitable during pregnancy, in people who are allergic to beef or to lidocaine, and in people with autoimmune disorders.

Collar, orthopedic

A therapeutic device worn around the neck to provide support to the cervical vertebrae, or bones of the neck. An orthopedic collar may be made of rigid plastic for firm support during daily activities. During sleep, a softer, more comfortable, cotton collar may be worn. Orthopedic collars may be the first line of treatment for cervical osteoarthritis when there is persistent pain. The collar may also be a component of ongoing treatment

for OSTEOARTHRITIS, as well as for a prolapsed disk in the neck portion of the spinal column. A sudden and forceful jolt to the neck (such as that caused by a motor vehicle collision) may cause neck pain (WHIPLASH) that can be treated by wearing an orthopedic collar for rest and support for 1 to 2 days. The wearing time can be decreased as symptoms improve.

Collarbone

The bone that spans the top of the chest from the upper sternum (breastbone) to an extension of the shoulder blade (scapula). Because the collarbone (also called the clavicle) functions as a strut that forces the shoulder blade out and back to form the shoulder, it is subject to stress and fracture.

Colles fracture

A transverse break in the two bones of the forearm, called the radius and ulna. A Colles fracture is generally caused when a person's outstretched hand bears the brunt of the body's full weight in a forward fall. The two bones buckle near their ends just above the wrist, displacing the hand so that it is positioned backward and upward by about an inch in relation to the wrist. Colles fracture is diagnosed by X ray, which generally shows an irregularity in the surface of the bone. If the fracture is severe, the X ray will show a break through the bones. This kind of fracture may be treated with a splint or cast and sling for 5 to 8 weeks to immobilize the bones and allow repair. Surgery involving internal fixation appliances is sometimes indicated for severe fractures. In some cases with people who are older, complete mobility of

the wrist joint may be lost, even after treatment. If the ligaments are injured, chronic pain may result. Later complications of Colles fracture include carpal tunnel syndrome.

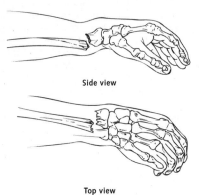

Side view

Top view

A COMMON FRACTURE OF THE ARM
A Colles fracture usually occurs when a person extends his or her hand to break a fall. Women whose bones are weakened by osteoporosis are particularly at risk.

Colon

The largest portion of the large INTESTINE extending from the end of the small intestine to the rectum. The colon loops around the small intestine and has four sections. The ascending colon, starting with a saclike structure called the cecum, starts on the lower right side of the abdomen and curves left below the liver. The transverse colon extends across the abdomen and curves upward next to the stomach on the left side of the body. The descending colon drops down the left side to the level of the pelvis, where it curves under the small intestine. The final portion, the sigmoid colon, is an S-shaped section that connects to the rectum.

The colon receives waste products of digestion from the small intestine in liquid form. The colon absorbs the water through the colon wall, forming the waste material (fecal matter) into a solid. There are no digestive enzymes in the fecal matter, but there are high concentrations of harmless bacteria. Some of the bacteria consume nutrient traces that are later reabsorbed, particularly if the body is nutritionally deficient. Other bacteria ferment some foods and produce gas, which is expelled from the body.

The colon functions as a storage

area for solid wastes before they are passed out of the body in a bowel movement. The feces moves slowly through the colon to allow for absorption of liquids, and the body usually requires only about one bowel movement a day. After each meal, a reflex stimulates the colon and part of the feces is pushed down into the sigmoid colon toward the rectum. When the feces reaches the rectum, it stretches the walls of the rectum and instigates the need to defecate, a reflex that can be allowed to continue or voluntarily controlled. If the action is allowed to go forward, the sigmoid colon continues to move the feces along and the bowel movement passes through the rectum and out of the body. See DIGESTIVE SYSTEM.

Colon and rectal surgeon

A surgeon who has received special training in the diseases, repair, and removal of the colon and rectum. Colon and rectal surgery, also called colorectal surgery, may involve removal of hemorrhoids, polyps, and parts of the intestine and other surgical interventions.

Colon cancer, hereditary nonpolyposis

A form of colon cancer that does not develop from polyps and arises in individuals who have an inherited susceptibility to it. Hereditary nonpolyposis colon cancer (HNPCC) is also known as Lynch syndrome. Individuals who have at least three relatives in two generations who have had colon cancer, with one having had it before age 50, are considered to be at significant risk—two to three times the average risk—for HNPCC. It usually develops at a relatively young age, and women with HNPCC also have an increased risk for developing cancer of the endometrium (lining of the uterus).

Hereditary nonpolyposis colon cancer occurs in two forms. HNPCC type 1 is characterized by the development of carcinomas in only the colon and the rectum, while HNPCC type 2 develops in other locations in addition to the colon and the rectum, including the stomach, larynx, bladder, ovary, and bile ducts. The genetic defect in HNPCC has been discov-

ered. The defect occurs in a special type of repair gene; consequently, errors that occur in DNA replication are not corrected. The accumulation of cells with errors in the DNA leads to cancer.

Colon cleansing

A controversial procedure intended to flush toxic substances from the bowel. Colon cleansing, which is also called colonic irrigation, is a method of DETOXIFICATION based on the idea that impacted fecal material can stick to the lining of the colon instead of being excreted in the normal manner. Colon cleansing is accomplished by administering through a rubber tube an enema of 20 gallons or more of warm water, coffee, herbs, or enzymes intended to promote healing. Advocates of this procedure believe that toxic waste products in the fecal material are reabsorbed by the colon and cause a variety of symptoms, including bad breath, headaches, allergies, and digestive disorders. Most doctors object to the procedure on the grounds that irrigation removes essential protective bacteria that naturally occur in the intestines. Critics of colon cleansing also point out that eating a healthy, high-fiber diet is a better way to prevent constipation and fecal impaction and warn that serious infections can be introduced in the colon.

Colon, cancer of the

Cancer of the large intestine, which is made up of the colon and rectum. Colon and rectal cancers are often grouped together as colorectal cancer (see also RECTUM, CANCER OF THE). Colon cancer is the second most common cause of cancer death in the United States. With early detection and removal of polyps, this cancer has a very high cure rate. Men and women are equally susceptible to the disease, which is most common after age 40.

SYMPTOMS AND CAUSES

Warning signs include blood in the stool and a sudden change in bowel habits. A rapid onset of persistent, inexplicable constipation or diarrhea after years of regularity is cause for concern. Blood in the stool with a change in bowel habits merits prompt medical attention. Other possible symptoms include frequent gas pains, a change in the diameter of

bowel movements, and a feeling that the bowel has not emptied completely after a bowel movement. There may also be tenderness or a mass in the abdomen. In some cases, bloating, discomfort, rumbling, and gurgling occur. Sometimes, there are no symptoms until the intestine ruptures or the cancer causes an intestinal obstruction See INTESTINE, OBSTRUCTION OF.

Colon cancer usually arises from polyps, abnormal growths on the colon walls that over time can become cancerous. Polyps may develop as a result of inflammatory diseases of the bowel, such as ulcerative COLITIS and CROHN DISEASE. As cancer cells multiply, a visible growth can develop in the intestinal lining that enlarges and may become bloody and ulcerated and constrict bowel movements. Left untreated, the cancer can spread to nearby organs. While the underlying cause has not yet been identified, this disease is more common in countries where a diet low in fiber and high in refined foods is common.

DIAGNOSIS AND TREATMENT

When polyps in the colon are identified at an early stage, they can be removed before they become cancerous. Diagnostic tests may include a

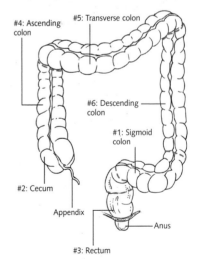

#4: Ascending colon
#5: Transverse colon
#6: Descending colon
#1: Sigmoid colon
#2: Cecum
Appendix
Anus
#3: Rectum

FREQUENCY OF COLON CANCER
Cancer of the colon (large intestine) occurs with greater frequency in some parts of the colon than others (see numbers). Most cancers occur in the front portion that leads from the small intestine up the right side of the abdomen (ascending colon) or, even more frequently, in the latter portion (sigmoid colon) leading down the left side of the abdomen toward the anus.

FECAL-OCCULT BLOOD TEST (a test for traces of blood in the stool), a rectal examination, blood tests, and stool sample analysis. Tests commonly used to identify causes of polyps include a lower GASTROINTESTINAL (GI) SERIES, SIGMOIDOSCOPY, and COLONOSCOPY. A lower GI series or barium enema uses the chemical barium sulfate, which is visible on X rays, to enable doctors to see the inside of the colon and rectum. In sigmoidoscopy and colonoscopy, the rectum and colon are examined by using a flexible viewing tube passed through the anus. A CT (computed tomography) scan of the abdomen is also used to see the colon and surrounding organs.

Surgery is the best treatment of

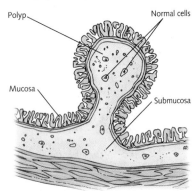

Polyp — Normal cells
Mucosa — Submucosa

Noncancerous polyp

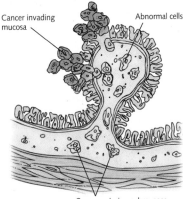

Cancer invading mucosa — Abnormal cells
Cancer entering submucosa

Cancerous polyp

CANCER ARISING FROM POLYPS
Most colon cancer develops from polyps, which are growths in the mucosa (inner lining) of the colon. Most polyps are benign, but an adenomatous polyp, or adenoma, can become cancerous. Its cells begin to multiply, and they invade the mucosa and then the deeper layers of the colon lining. Left untreated, they can grow through the outer colon wall.

> **SIGNS OF COLON CANCER**
>
> Signs resemble those of other colon problems and require a doctor's attention:
> - **Bleeding from the rectum**
> - **Blood in the stool**
> - **Any changes in bowel movements—persistent diarrhea or constipation, narrow stool, a feeling that the bowel does not empty entirely**
> - **Abdominal pain (below your stomach or on either side)**
> - **Unexplained weight loss**
> - **Severe anemia (which may indicate internal bleeding)**

colon cancer. In a procedure known as a COLECTOMY, tumors are removed and the healthy remaining sections of the colon are joined together. This maintains a passageway for stools. In other cases, a temporary or permanent opening called a STOMA is made in the abdominal wall. This allows the discharge of feces into a bag attached to the skin. A procedure called a COLOSTOMY is done so that the colon opens through a stoma. The procedure to open the lower part of the small intestine, or ileum, through a stoma is known as an ILEOSTOMY.

RISK FACTORS AND PREVENTION
Because most colon cancers develop and spread slowly, early detection saves as many as nine out of ten lives. Regular screening tests greatly reduce the incidence and severity of colon cancer. The American Cancer Society recommends an annual fecal-occult blood test and a sigmoidoscopy every 5 years after age 50. Colonoscopy is recommended for those at high risk because of prior colon cancer, a family history of the disease, or a history of chronic digestive problems.

Colon, irritable

See IRRITABLE BOWEL SYNDROME.

Colon, spastic

See IRRITABLE BOWEL SYNDROME.

Colonoscopy

A diagnostic examination of the inside of the colon through a long, flexible instrument called a colonoscope. A colonoscope is a type of ENDOSCOPE used specifically to examine the colon and has attachments such as lenses, a light, and a small video camera. Many

---

colonoscopes contain small video computer chips that can scan the inside of the colon and transmit images to a video screen. Instruments passed through or attached to a colonoscope may be used to take a biopsy sample or to remove polyps. Colonoscopy differs from sigmoidoscopy in that the entire colon is examined in a colonoscopy but only the lower third in a sigmoidoscopy.

WHY IT IS PERFORMED
Colonoscopy is used to check for inflammation, abnormalities, and other problems of the colon. For example, it can locate bleeding sites, ulcers, polyps, and colorectal cancer (see COLON, CANCER OF THE and RECTUM, CANCER OF THE). It may be recommended to confirm a preliminary diagnosis of colitis in a person who has symptoms. Because colorectal cancer has a very high cure rate, colonoscopy is also used as a screening test for people who are at high risk of colon cancer such as individuals who have had colon cancer, chronic colitis, or a strong family history of colon cancer.

HOW IT IS PERFORMED
Because the intestine needs to be as empty as possible during a colonoscopy, the person undergoing the procedure may be instructed to follow a liquid diet for a day or two before the procedure and take a laxative or give himself or herself an enema the night before. The procedure is performed in a doctor's office or the ambulatory suite of a hospital and can take up to an hour. A sedative or pain medication is given to relax the person and to minimize discomfort.

The person undergoing the procedure lies on his or her left side on an examining table. The colonoscope is gently inserted into the rectum and slowly threaded all the way up the colon. The doctor may inflate the colon with air, which dilates (widens) the colon and can make maneuvering the colonoscope easier.

While slowly withdrawing the tube, the doctor examines the inside of the colon directly through the scope or on a video monitor. Inflamed tissue, abnormal growths, bleeding, ulcers, and even muscle spasms can be seen.

RISKS
Although uncommon, it is possible for the colon to be punctured or otherwise injured during the procedure.

CLOSE-UP ON COLONOSCOPY

Colonoscopy is a procedure in which the inside of the colon is examined using a fiberoptic colonoscope, an elongated flexible viewing tube that transmits images to a monitor. Bleeding sites, inflamed tissue, ulcers, polyps, and colorectal cancer can be easily visualized and identified using colonoscopy.

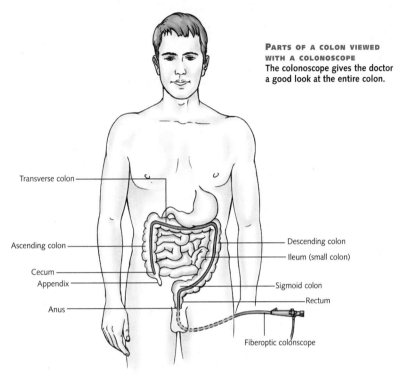

PARTS OF A COLON VIEWED WITH A COLONOSCOPE
The colonoscope gives the doctor a good look at the entire colon.

Transverse colon

Ascending colon

Cecum

Appendix

Anus

Descending colon

Ileum (small colon)

Sigmoid colon

Rectum

Fiberoptic colonscope

POSITIONING OF THE PERSON DURING COLONOSCOPY
The person lies on his or her left side. The flexible viewing tube is threaded through the entire colon. Examination of the colon lining occurs as the doctor slowly withdraws the tube.

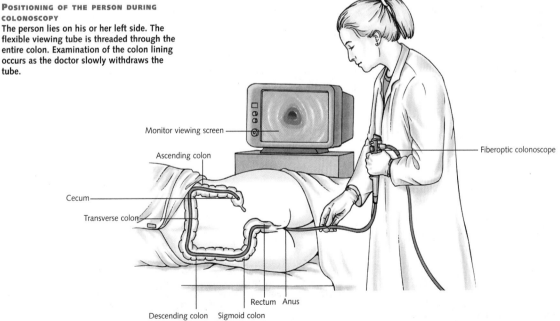

Monitor viewing screen

Ascending colon

Cecum

Transverse colon

Fiberoptic colonoscope

Descending colon   Sigmoid colon   Rectum   Anus

C

Color blindness

The inability to perceive colors normally. The level of defect varies from mild to severe. Affected people cannot distinguish between certain shades of color, most commonly red and green. Only rarely do people who are color blind see the world only in various shades of gray.

CAUSES

Specialized cells called cones in the light-sensitive layer (retina) at the back of the eye contain chemicals that are maximally sensitive to red, green, and blue wavelengths. The cone cells transform light stimuli into nerve impulses that are conducted to the brain. The brain then translates these impulses into the many hues the human eye can perceive. Color blindness arises from a deficiency in one or more of the light-sensitive chemicals. As a result, the eye fails to perceive that color. The severity of the defect depends on the proportion of missing chemical.

In most cases, color blindness is passed from mother to son. Because women and girls usually carry a gene that counterbalances color blindness, the condition affects females much less often than males. By various estimates, from 30 to 120 boys in every 1,000 are born with color blindness, but fewer than 3 girls in 1,000 have it. Inherited color blindness is usually red-green.

Less commonly, color blindness is acquired as a result of eye disease. Disorders of the optic nerve, inadequate vitamin A (beta-carotene) in the diet, inflammation of the eye, and cataracts can all impair color vision. Acquired color blindness is usually blue-yellow.

TREATMENT

Inherited color vision deficiencies cannot be cured. In some cases, tinted eyeglasses can be worn to increase contrast between colors. Color vision loss caused by eye disease may be improved with treatment of the disease.

Color therapy

A method of restoring health by applying colors to the body; chromotherapy. Color therapy is based on the idea that colors, derived from light, represent energy states that can be delivered to the body. In color therapy, sick bodies are considered deficient in one or more of the color types, and balance is restored by applying certain colors to the body. Tools used in color therapy include gemstones, flowers, candles, prisms, wands, colored fabrics, and bath treatments containing essential oils and waters. Color therapists have identified specific colors that they believe to be associated with certain emotions and body parts. An example of how conventional medicine uses light therapy is the use of ultraviolet light for the treatment of psoriasis. However, there is no scientific proof for color therapy in general.

Color vision

The ability to perceive colors. Specialized cells called cones in the light-sensitive layer (retina) at the back of the eye contain chemicals that are maximally sensitive to red, green, and blue wavelengths. When stimulated by light, the cone cells transmit impulses to the brain. These impulses are then blended in the brain to produce the many hues the human eye can perceive. A defect in color perception is known as COLOR BLINDNESS.

Colorado tick fever

FOR SYMPTOM CHART
see Rashes, page 50; 52

FOR FIRST AID
see Bites and stings: tick bites, page 1315

A viral infection transmitted by the bite of a wood tick. Colorado tick fever is endemic to areas with elevations above 4,000 feet in the western states of the United States and Canada. It is rare in other areas. There is a seasonal peak for infections lasting from late May through early July.

Symptoms generally begin within 4 to 5 days of the tick bite, but may not appear for as long as 20 days following a bite. General malaise with high fever and a fine, red rash are the usual symptoms. Recovery is usually within a week to 10 days, but the virus can live in the red blood cells for several months. Accordingly, people who have been infected cannot donate blood for 6 months following infection.

Cases of Colorado tick fever affecting the liver or central nervous system have been reported. Hallucinations and memory loss may occur with

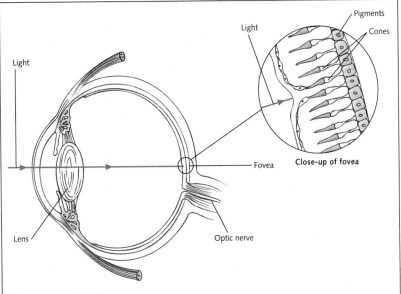

SENSITIVITY TO COLOR
The perception of color starts in tiny structures in the retina called cones. The cones are photoreceptors (sensitive to light) and contain pigments that are sensitive to wavelengths in the visible color spectrum. The cones connect to nerve fibers that carry the sensory impulses through the optic nerve to the brain, where they are interpreted as colors.

severe infection. Rarely, the infection causes pathological changes in the heart, brain, and lungs and can be fatal. Some deaths due to Colorado tick fever are suspected to have been ascribed to Rocky Mountain spotted fever, which carries a higher risk of fatality.

There is no vaccine for Colorado tick fever. Preventive steps can be taken, however, to avoid getting wood tick bites, including tucking long pants into socks to protect the legs while hiking through tick-infested areas and wearing shoes and long-sleeved shirts. Immediate treatment usually involves fully removing the tick from the skin and taking a pain reliever, if necessary. If complications develop, medical treatment will focus on controlling the symptoms.

Colostomy

A surgical procedure in which a STOMA, an artificial opening, is created in the abdominal wall to allow the discharge of feces into a bag attached to the skin. Colostomy is similar to ILEOSTOMY, in which the lower part of the small intestine, or ileum, opens through a stoma. A colostomy is sometimes necessary to treat serious digestive diseases, such as ulcerative colitis, DIVERTICULAR DISEASE, and colon cancer. Surgeons sometimes perform a colostomy as part of COLECTOMY, an operation in which all or part of the colon is removed. Through an incision in the abdominal wall, the tumor or diseased part of the intestine is removed. If the remaining healthy sections cannot be rejoined, a stoma is created to allow the feces to pass from the body.

A colostomy can be temporary or permanent. If it is temporary, the stoma will be closed in a second procedure once the intestine has recovered from initial surgery. A permanent colostomy requires keeping the stoma clean and regularly emptying the bag that collects the waste. People who have colostomies usually return to a normal bowel routine. Often, bowel movements are so regular that only a small pad is worn over the stoma for most of the day. The most frequent problem is skin irritation around the stoma, caused by leakage of digestive fluids. See Colostomy step by step, next page.

Colostrum

The first breast milk produced after childbirth. Low in fat and carbohydrates and high in protein, colostrum is easy to digest and is rich in antibodies that defend the newborn against infection. Colostrum has a laxative action and is the ideal first food for the newborn. After 3 to 5 days, colostrum is replaced by mature milk. See BREAST-FEEDING.

Colposcopic biopsy

Removal of tissue from one or more sites on the CERVIX during COLPOSCOPY in order to examine it for abnormal cells. Colposcopy may be done on an outpatient basis, without the use of anesthesia. Most women experience some cramping during the biopsy and spotty bleeding thereafter.

Colposcopy

A procedure to examine the surfaces of the vaginal walls and the cervix for abnormal cells, using a colposcope, a lighted magnifying instrument. The examining physician may apply a diluted solution of acetic acid to the cervix and vaginal wall to help identify areas of abnormal cells. The acid discolors the abnormal areas, which can then be checked for cancer by doing a biopsy (a microscopic examination of a small sample of the abnormal tissue). A colposcopy is performed in a doctor's office and takes about 15 minutes. It usually is not painful, although some discomfort may result from the SPECULUM that props the vagina open throughout the procedure. If a biopsy is performed, the woman may feel pain similar to menstrual cramping.

Coma

A profound or deep state of unconsciousness. A coma may occur as an outcome of an underlying illness, or it may be caused by trauma. A person in a coma lacks both wakefulness and awareness. In addition to providing treatment to reverse the coma, medical care includes providing nutrition and preventing infection (especially pneumonia) and pressure sores. Physical therapy may be used to prevent permanent muscular contractions and orthopedic deformities.

Comas rarely last longer than 2 to 4 weeks. The prognosis for a person in a coma depends on its cause and the nature of neurological damage. In some cases, a prolonged coma is followed by a persistent VEGETATIVE STATE, in which a person has lost cognitive neurological function and awareness of the environment, yet retains noncognitive function and a sleep-wake cycle. Other times, people emerge from comas with a variety of physical, intellectual, and psychological difficulties. These require special attention and close medical supervision. Recovery is gradual, and degrees of recovery vary. However, many people eventually regain full awareness.

Commensal

A normally harmless organism or bacterium that lives in or on the body. Commensals may cause disease, but usually only in people with impaired immune systems.

Commode

A chair with a toiletlike attachment under the bottom, which can be removed for cleaning. A commode is used to help people who are partially bed-bound and for whom a trip to the bathroom is difficult. A commode is like a child's potty chair, but large enough for adults.

Common cold

See COLD, COMMON.

Communicable disease

A disease that is transmitted from an infected person, insect, or animal. Communicable diseases include the forms of infection transferred from one person to another by direct contact with the infected person or that person's bodily discharges, whether it be blood, saliva, urine, or feces, as well as diseases conveyed indirectly via an organism, such as an insect that transmits a pathogen.

Community health

See PUBLIC HEALTH.

Compartment syndrome

An acute or chronic condition caused by exercise or injury and characterized by pain and swollen muscle tissue. Also called exertional compart-

C

COLOSTOMY STEP BY STEP

A colostomy is a procedure in which a stoma, or opening, is created in the abdominal wall to remove solid waste from the body. Colostomies may be either temporary or permanent. These illustrations show the steps in a permanent colostomy, performed because the rectum and the anus must be removed. Reasons for performing colostomies include cancer of the colon, obstructive tumors, and diverticulitis.

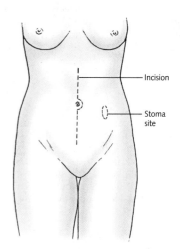

INCISION SITE AND STOMA SITE
This diagram shows the usual incision line and stoma site on a person who is undergoing a colostomy. The exact positions of these incisions vary from person to person. The surgeon makes an 8- to 10-inch incision to remove the rectum and the anus and to close off the colon with a clamp.

Incision

Stoma site

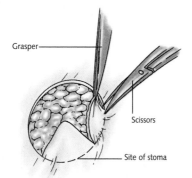

Grasper

Scissors

Site of stoma

AREA OF SKIN REMOVED ON STOMA SITE
The surgeon removes a circular area of skin and fat from the stoma site. He or she then cuts through the abdominal muscles to the colon and pulls the colon out through the stoma.

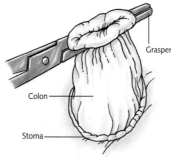

Grasper

Colon

Stoma

PULLING COLON THROUGH STOMA SITE
The surgeon uses a grasper to pull the colon out through the stoma site. After this step in the procedure, he or she is able to close the main incision on the stomach.

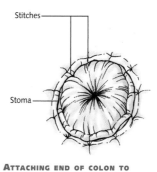

Stitches

Stoma

ATTACHING END OF COLON TO EXTERIOR SKIN
This diagram shows how the surgeon attaches the end of the colon to the skin using absorbable sutures. The result is an opening, to which a stoma appliance is attached.

A PERSON WITH A PERMANENT COLOSTOMY
The person with a permanent colostomy wears a disposable bag, which attaches to the stoma appliance. This bag collects the semisolid waste from his or her body. Having a colostomy necessitates some dietary changes. Also, the stoma site must be carefully cleaned.

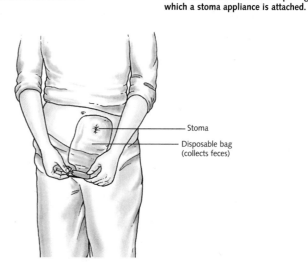

Stoma

Disposable bag (collects feces)

ment syndrome (ECS), the swelling is produced by increased pressure of the fluids within the closed muscle compartment. This increased pressure occurs normally during exercise and diminishes soon after the activity is stopped. With compartment syndrome, the built-up pressure persists after the exercise session is over. The condition most commonly occurs in the leg, especially in the front of the lower leg, but may also affect the forearm, thigh, and buttocks.

SYMPTOMS AND DIAGNOSIS

The symptoms include severe pain and swelling when a person stretches. Symptoms may also include numbness, motor loss, or weakness in the affected muscle. Many people experience a gradual onset of aching and a sensation of fullness in the affected muscle or muscles after starting to exercise or after reaching a certain level of intensity. The pain may occur on one side of the body or both, sometimes with more severe pain on one side.

The symptoms of compartment syndrome are generally relieved when a person stops exercising or rests. Compartment syndrome may be acute (coming on suddenly) or chronic (persistent for a long time). The more common chronic form usually occurs in conditioned athletes younger than the age of 40. The acute form tends to occur in people of this group who already have chronic ECS and then dramatically increase their training level. Chronic compartment syndrome also occurs in relatively sedentary people who begin a strenuous exercise program.

ECS is diagnosed by physical examination and clinical history. X rays may be taken to rule out other possible causes of the pain, such as stress fractures. MRI (magnetic resonance imaging) may aid in evaluating any possible abnormality in the muscle. To confirm a diagnosis, intracompartmental pressure must be measured.

TREATMENT

Treatment may include exercising on a different surface, changing footwear, and adjusting a person's train-

---

Terms in small capital letters—for example, PHYSICAL THERAPY or PAGET DISEASE—indicate a cross-reference to another entry with more information.

---

ing intensity. The use of orthotics, special shoe inserts designed to provide extra support, as well as strengthening and stretching exercises, may be recommended. In severe and persistent cases of compartment syndrome, a surgical procedure called fasciotomy, which relieves the pressure on muscles, may be recommended.

Complementary medicine

Alternative health care; medical practices not currently part of conventional medicine but often used as a complement to it. Most alternative medical systems are based on theories and practices that have been developed independent of conventional biochemical medicine. Many systems are practiced in Asian, Native American, Aboriginal, African, Middle-Eastern, Tibetan and Central and South American cultures.

Complementary medicine usually depends on comprehensive systems incorporating body, mind, and spirit, giving equal emphasis to each component. Traditional Indian medicine, for example, treats disease with combinations of diet, exercise, meditation, herbs, massage, sunlight, and controlled breathing. Another system, homeopathy, is based on the belief that "like cures like," meaning that the same substance that in large quantities produces disease can cure it in very small doses. Homeopaths use small doses of plant extracts and minerals to stimulate the body's own healing mechanisms to treat disease.

Other systems of complementary medicine include herbal remedies, plant-derived materials that are recognized as dietary supplements by the Food and Drug Administration (FDA), and vitamins, which are also recognized by the FDA as over-the-counter medications. Other systems of complementary medicine include substances such as bee pollen and shark cartilage to treat disease.

Complex

An idea or group of ideas that is repressed into the subconscious yet continues to generate a powerful emotional charge. An example is the OEDIPUS COMPLEX, which is the name given by Sigmund Freud for the sexual

love a son has for his mother. The female counterpart of a daughter's love for her father is the ELECTRA COMPLEX.

Compliance

A person's adherence to a physician's prescribed course of medical treatment. For example, it is important to comply with a doctor's instructions to take the complete course of antibiotics prescribed for a bacterial infection, even after symptoms have disappeared. Otherwise, the infection may recur—possibly in a more severe form. Compliance is a key aspect of controlling or curing disease. Compliance may be difficult in patients with chronic illnesses that require complicated treatment regimens.

Complication

In medicine, a disease or problem arising in addition to the original condition or following surgery. For example, surgical complications include postoperative infections that may or may not be related to the disease being treated.

Composite, dental

See BONDING, DENTAL.

Compress

A pad of cloth or other material that is pressed firmly against a body part for a period of time as part of therapy. Compresses may be dry or wet, and they may be cold, lukewarm, or hot. Wet compresses may contain medications and are used chiefly to relieve inflammation. Dry compresses are often used to stop bleeding.

Compression fracture

A break in a vertebra, or bone of the spine, caused by a collapse of the bone tissue in one or more vertebrae. A compression fracture may also be called a vertebral compression fracture. The symptoms of a compression fracture depend on the area of the back affected. If the fracture occurs in the lower back, walking may make the pain worse. Most compression fractures do not affect the nerves. However, if the fracture puts pressure on the nerves or spinal cord, symptoms may include numbness, tingling, or weakness. The causes of compression fractures include OSTEOPOROSIS,

SPINAL INJURY, and malignant growths, such as tumors. The treatment depends on the underlying cause. When there are multiple compression fractures, the spine may curve forward forming a hump on the upper back, a condition called KYPHOSIS.

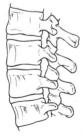 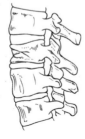

Healthy vertebrae   Compression fracture

COLLAPSED VERTEBRA
A compression fracture usually occurs as the result of the bone-thinning disease osteoporosis. The fracture is very painful at first and may weaken the spine. The collapsed vertebra cannot be reconstructed in any way.

Compression syndrome

A collection of symptoms caused by pressure on a nerve or nerves that supply the muscles and carry sensations from a particular area of the body. Symptoms of a compression syndrome include weakness, numbness, tingling, and pain. CARPAL TUNNEL SYNDROME (compression of the median nerve at the wrist) is by far the most common compression syndrome. Possible treatments for a compression syndrome include identifying and avoiding the activity that contributes to the problem and wearing a splint. Nonsteroidal anti-inflammatory drugs (NSAIDs) are often recommended to reduce inflammation. If the damage is severe, surgery may be needed to relieve the pressure on the nerve.

Compulsive behavior

An action repeated again and again as a way of warding off anxiety or distress, not for the purpose of creating pleasure or satisfaction. In many cases the person feels driven to perform the action to stave off a dreadful event. Failure to perform the compulsive behavior produces a high level of distress or anxiety. Compulsions are either excessive and exaggerated or not related realistically to the

event they are supposed to prevent. A person worried about bacterial contamination, for example, may wash the hands so often that the skin is red and raw; another person concerned about security may check every lock in the house multiple times an hour; a compulsive gambler cannot stop wagering even after all the money is used up. Compulsive behavior can be a sign of OBSESSIVE-COMPULSIVE DISORDER.

Computed tomography scanning

See CT SCANNING.

Concentration

The mental capacity to focus attention and effort on a particular task.

Conception

The fertilization of an egg by a sperm that initiates pregnancy. During sexual intercourse, 300 million or so sperm are ejaculated into the vagina. About 3 million of them penetrate the cervix to get to the uterus; the rest are killed by vaginal secretions or are excreted from the body. The sperm that reach the egg secrete an enzyme that breaks down the outer covering of the egg. Once a single sperm has penetrated the egg, the outer covering immediately changes, to prevent other sperm from entering. The nucleus in the head of the sperm and the nucleus of the egg fuse to form a fertilized egg, also called a ZYGOTE. The zygote is made up of a unique combination of genes, half of which come from the man's sperm and half from the woman's egg.

Conception depends largely upon timing. A woman in her childbearing years is most likely to conceive if she has sex in the period between 2 days before and 1 day after OVULATION each month. An egg is capable of being fertilized up to 24 hours after ovulation. Sperm are capable of fertilization for up to 48 hours, and it takes most of them 4 to 7 hours after ejaculation to reach the fallopian tubes (see FALLOPIAN TUBE), where fertilization occurs.

A woman is most fertile in her 20s, and her ability to conceive diminishes gradually as she ages, ending completely at MENOPAUSE. Men can be fertile well into old age. See also How conception occurs, facing page.

Concussion

A brief loss of consciousness following a head injury. A concussion may result from a fall in which the head strikes an object, or it may happen when a flying object hits a person's head. The length of time the person is unconscious may relate to the severity of the concussion. People frequently have no memory of events immediately preceding or following the injury and loss of consciousness. A concussion may be accompanied by headache, faintness, nausea or vomiting, slightly blurred vision, and difficulty concentrating.

As a general rule, concussion is a minor, temporary injury that does not cause permanent damage to the brain. However, any head injury is potentially serious, so any head injury that results in a person losing consciousness should receive medical attention. About one third of all people with concussion may experience symptoms after the event, including insomnia, irritability, restlessness, depression, moodiness, or the inability to concentrate. Concussion is usually self-healing, although the doctor may prescribe a pain reliever other than aspirin for any headache.

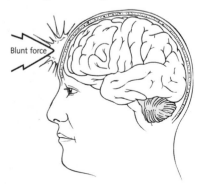

Blunt force

MILD HEAD INJURY
A concussion occurs when an impact on the head causes it to accelerate or decelerate abruptly, and the brain shifts within the head. Symptoms can range from a brief loss of concentration to a loss of consciousness for more than a minute. The injury is generally mild, but medical attention is recommended.

Conditioning

A type of learning that connects an event in the environment or a stimulus with a physical, emotional, or behavioral response in the individual. There are two types of conditioning. In classical or Pavlovian conditioning,

How conception occurs

This is the process involved in fertilizing an egg.

1. Just before conception, a mature egg and some nourishing cells are released from one of a woman's ovaries and travel up the nearest fallopian tube toward the uterus with the aid of tubelike projections called fimbriae.
2. During intercourse, millions of sperm in ejaculated semen move up the woman's uterus and into the fallopian tubes from the opposite direction.
3. One of the sperm penetrates the egg, usually in a fallopian tube, mixing their genetic material.
4. The cells of the fertilized egg start to divide again and again while the fertilized egg continues toward the uterus.
5. Within 2 to 7 days, this mass of cells (now an embryo) embeds itself within the inner lining (endometrium) of the wall of the uterus.

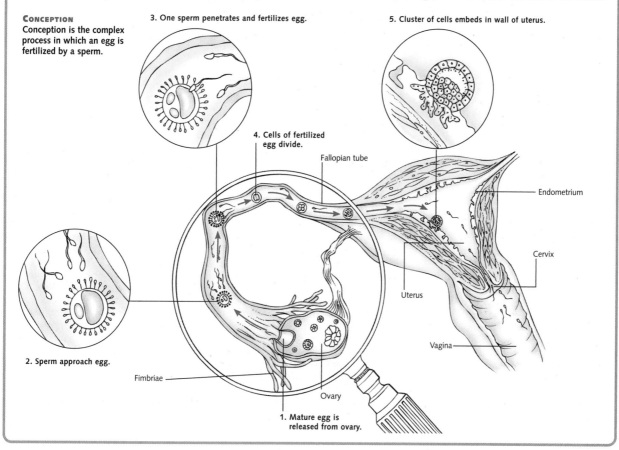

CONCEPTION
Conception is the complex process in which an egg is fertilized by a sperm.

3. One sperm penetrates and fertilizes egg.

5. Cluster of cells embeds in wall of uterus.

4. Cells of fertilized egg divide.

Fallopian tube

Endometrium

Cervix

Uterus

Vagina

2. Sperm approach egg.

Fimbriae

Ovary

1. Mature egg is released from ovary.

---

an unconscious or automatic response is connected with a stimulus not associated physiologically with that response. Classical conditioning creates a new connection between the stimulus and the response. It occurs independent of rewards and punishments and of the action of the individual. In operant conditioning, a behavior increases in frequency when it is followed by a reward (reinforcement) and decreases when it is followed by a punishment. The word "operant" refers to the fact that the individual has to perform a behavior, or operate,

before receiving the reinforcement or punishment. See LEARNING.

Condom

A thin sheath placed over a man's erect penis to prevent sperm from entering a woman's uterus, helping to prevent pregnancy; latex condoms also help prevent spread of disease through sexual intercourse. Other names for a condom include rubber and prophylactic. A polyurethane female condom that lines the vagina is also sold. See CONTRACEPTION, BARRIER METHODS.

Condyloma

See HUMAN PAPILLOMAVIRUS.

Condyloma acuminatum

A sexually transmitted viral infection that is caused by the HUMAN PAPILLOMAVIRUS (HPV) and produces genital warts (also known as venereal warts). Condyloma acuminatum is currently one of the most common sexually transmitted diseases among men and women living in the United States. The wart virus is transferred during vaginal sexual intercourse, oral sex, and anal sex. All sexually active people are susceptible, but those with more than one sexual partner and people who have had other sexually transmitted diseases are at greater risk for infection.

Once a person is infected, the warts may appear within 2 weeks, within several months, or even within several years. In women, the warts appear in the vagina, around the opening of the vagina, on the cervix, and in or around the anus. The infection may also cause itching and a vaginal discharge. In men, the warts are located on the penis and are usually too small to be observed by visual examination. The warts may cause itching, irritation, or bleeding. They may be hard and flesh-colored or dark pink to red. There may be one or two small warts or clusters of tiny eruptions.

DIAGNOSIS AND TREATMENT

A PAP SMEAR will reveal the presence of the wart virus in women. A COLPOSCOPY to examine the vagina and cervix through a magnifying lens may also be used in the diagnosis of condyloma acuminatum in women. Men may be diagnosed by applying a weak solution of acetic acid to the penis and looking for warts with the aid of magnification.

Some warts improve without treatment. Other treatment procedures to remove warts can be performed in a doctor's office. These include using liquid nitrogen to destroy the warts by freezing the tissue or applying one of the topical chemicals bichloroacetic acid (BCA), trichloroacetic acid (TCA), or podophyllin, which is later washed off. Other treatments include laser treatments or burning off the warts with an electrical instrument. Destroying visible warts may not destroy the virus, which may remain in the tissue and produce new warts. Repeated treatments, as often as weekly, may be required for complete recovery.

RISK FACTORS

Early diagnosis and treatment are important for both men and women. Genital warts are linked to changes in a woman's cervical tissue that may become precancerous if untreated. These changes can be noted in a Pap smear and are easily treated if diagnosed early. There is recent evidence that men with condyloma acuminatum may be at increased risk for penile and other cancers if not promptly diagnosed and treated.

Other complications involve bleeding due to flat warts located inside a man's penile urethra and obstruction of the urethra in women. Untreated wart lesions may cause disfigurement of affected areas.

It is important that an infected person advise his or her sexual partners so they can be examined and treated if necessary. Condoms should be used until the virus is completely cured, and in general, the use of condoms can help prevent the spread of condyloma acuminatum.

Condyloma latum

A secondary eruption; the second stage of SYPHILIS. The warts are painless, moist, gray-white to red, and found under breasts, in armpits, fingers, toes, and the genital area. Condyloma latum is highly contagious; it is treated with antibiotics.

Cone biopsy

A procedure in which a cone-shaped or cylindrical section of tissue is removed from a woman's cervix for diagnosis or treatment of cervical dysplasia or localized cancer of the cervix. It is performed when a woman has had a PAP SMEAR that is more than moderately abnormal. When used for diagnosis, the removed tissue is preserved and then examined microscopically by a pathologist. When a cone biopsy is used therapeutically, a pathologist checks to see that all the abnormal cells have been removed or are surrounded by a margin of normal tissue. A cone biopsy is performed with a scalpel or a laser, and it may be done with the patient under local anesthesia or general anesthesia. Some bleeding is likely to occur after the procedure.

Confabulation

The concoction of detailed, realistic stories about situations or experiences to compensate for gaps in memory. This type of fabrication can be a symptom of a brain disorder known as KORSAKOFF PSYCHOSIS.

Confidentiality

The protected privacy of identifiable personal health information. The medical profession generally extends the promise of confidentiality to people who seek medical care. The patient-physician relationship depends on an assurance of confidentiality to encourage full disclosure of pertinent health and lifestyle information that may affect a person's medical diagnosis and treatment.

LIMITED ACCESS TO MEDICAL RECORDS

The need for privacy among people receiving medical care and the release of personally identifiable information must be weighed against the benefits that the availability of medical data can offer in certain situations. Having access to the medical records of people who are unconscious and have been brought into hospital emergency departments may save lives. Similar access may also help pharmacists prevent lethal combinations of prescription medications. Public health authorities may use computerized records to track and manage epidemics of infectious diseases. Databases also provide researchers with valuable information about the causes of illness. Medical record information also serves as the basis for health insurance coverage.

State law requires that certain medical information be reported to state and local governments. This information is maintained in databases and includes the reporting of sexually transmitted diseases to public health agencies, informing child-welfare agencies of child abuse, and advising law-enforcement agencies of injuries caused by firearms.

Confidentiality may also be breached if there is a potential for harm to a third party. For example, a psychiatrist has a duty to warn authorities about a patient's homicidal tendencies.

POTENTIAL ABUSE OF ACCESS TO MEDICAL RECORDS

Release of confidential medical information is not always prohibited by law. In some states, pharmacies may sell prescription records to pharmaceutical companies to be used for marketing purposes. Breaches of confidentiality in the past have included, for example, unauthorized release to the press of the medical records of political candidates, the sale of medical records to malpractice lawyers seeking clients, and unauthorized disclosure of a person's HIV (human immunodeficiency virus) status to the media.

The Health Insurance Portability and Accountability Act (HIPAA) further protects medical record information. The HIPAA regulations will require that this information not be released by health care personnel, providers, or payers for medical services (such as insurance companies and public agencies) without the authorization of the person receiving medical care.

Confusion in older people

Disorientation regarding time, places, people, or situations that is more commonly experienced by people over age 65 than by younger individuals. It sometimes results from lifestyle-related causes and may pass quickly when the underlying problem is corrected. In other cases, confusion stems from a more serious disorder, such as ALZHEIMER'S DISEASE. Confusion over time that changes a person's level of functioning requires a doctor's evaluation.

CAUSES

Prolonged confusion in older people can be due to underlying causes ranging from depression to Alzheimer's disease. Contributing factors may include medications, acute illness, exhaustion, alcohol use, and poor nutrition. Often confusion is a sign of delirium, dementia, or depression.

Delirium is a temporary state of acute confusion, agitation, and disorientation usually caused by an underlying disorder such as metabolic changes, infection, stress, or exhaustion. It may also be a side effect of medication.

Dementia, a more chronic brain disorder, causes progressive memory loss and confusion. Unlike delirium, dementia is usually permanent. Its early signs may be mistaken as delirium. As time goes on, dementia leads to a decline in normal function and eventually to incapacitation. Not a normal part of aging, dementia is a result of progressive, degenerative disease. The chief causes of dementia are Alzheimer's disease and vascular disease. Potentially reversible causes of dementia include thyroid dysfunction and vitamin deficiencies.

Depression is a common disorder in older people that can lead to confu-

sion. The individual might complain of aches and pains or fatigue. Other symptoms include loss of interest and pleasure in normal activities, feelings of guilt or worthlessness, persistent sadness, difficulty with concentration and memory, insomnia, and irritability. Depressive symptoms lasting for more than 2 weeks require a physician's care. (See also DEPRESSION, IN OLDER PEOPLE.)

DIAGNOSIS AND TREATMENT

Diagnosis is based on a detailed medical history, a complete physical examination, and, usually, diagnostic tests. In the history, a doctor will look for changes in mental status. Confusion that comes on abruptly indicates delirium or depression. More gradual symptoms suggest dementia. A physician will also review all medications that the individual is taking to determine whether drug reactions are the cause. A physical examination can help detect the underlying causes of confusion.

Medical tests used to diagnose cases of confusion may include the basic tests of blood and urine cultures to detect infection; neuropsychological tests of memory, problem solving, and language; and imaging studies of the brain, such as CT (computed tomography) scanning or MRI (magnetic resonance imaging). Sometimes a lumbar puncture, or spinal tap, is needed to rule out an infection of the central nervous system.

Depending on the diagnosis, treatment is directed at the underlying problem. It may involve, for example, discontinuing a new medication that coincides with the onset of symptoms or administering antibiotics for infections. Depression typically responds well to psychotherapy and medication. Reversible causes of dementia, such as thyroid disorders, can also be treated. Although Alzheimer's disease is an irreversible form of dementia, medications can control some of its symptoms and slow the disease's progression.

Congenital

Any condition existing at birth. Congenital conditions usually exist before birth and may or may not be inherited. A congenital abnormality is a structural abnormality present at birth.

Congenital hypothyroidism

A condition present at birth in which the thyroid gland is absent or produces too little thyroid hormone. Congenital hypothyroidism is usually caused by developmental defects of the thyroid gland. Females are twice as likely to have congenital hypothyroidism as males, and it is much more common among white than among black infants.

If any portion of the thyroid gland system fails to form or to function correctly, a baby may develop hypothyroidism. Delayed diagnosis or inadequate treatment of hypothyroidism can lead to failure to grow properly or to irreversible mental retardation. If hypothyroidism is diagnosed and appropriate treatment begun within the first 4 weeks of life, however, the baby may develop normally. Congenital hypothyroidism can be difficult to diagnose because symptoms are usually subtle and vague. In the United States, a universal screening system ensures that all babies are checked for congenital hypothyroidism soon after birth, usually by measuring the amount of the thyroid hormone, T4, in the baby's blood. Once the condition is diagnosed, treatment with a daily dose of thyroid hormone can proceed. Most babies who are treated for congenital hypothyroidism grow and develop normally.

Congestive heart failure

See HEART FAILURE, CONGESTIVE.

Conjunctiva

The thin mucous membrane that lines the inside of the eyelids and covers the white, exposed surface (sclera) of the EYE. Cells in the conjunctiva produce a fluid similar to tears that lubricates the lids and the cornea to keep the eye moist.

Conjunctivitis

Inflammation of the membrane lining the eyelids and the exposed outer surface of the eye (conjunctiva). Popularly known as pinkeye, conjunctivitis is the most common eye disease in the Western hemisphere. The disease's severity ranges from mild to severe. Symptoms can include redness, irritation and pain, excessive tearing, itching, blurred vision, a grainy or gritty feeling in the eye, increased sensitivity to light, and crusts that form on the eyelids overnight.

CAUSES

Conjunctivitis can result from a number of different causes. Viral infection is the most common. Various kinds of bacteria can also cause the disease. Typically, the overnight formation of crusts on the eyelids that create the sensation that the eye is glued shut is a sign of bacterial infection. Other causes of conjunctivitis include allergies (usually to pollen, house dust, or pet dander), exposure to chemicals (including swimming pool chlorine), and certain systemic diseases. Wearing contact lenses, particularly extended-wear lenses, increases the risk of conjunctivitis.

Conjunctivitis can also arise in newborns as a result of exposure to bacteria during passage through the birth canal. If the inflammation comes from the bacterium that causes gonorrhea (see SEXUALLY TRANSMITTED DISEASES), it can result in blindness. Prompt treatment is required. In most states, drops are placed in a newborn's eye shortly after birth to prevent this infection.

PREVENTION AND TREATMENT

Viral conjunctivitis is highly contagious and can cause local epidemics, particularly among young children. Spread of the disease can be stopped or slowed with good hygiene, such as frequent hand washing; keeping the hands away from the eyes; changing pillowcases frequently; replacing eye cosmetics regularly; not sharing eye cosmetics, towels, or handkerchiefs; and cleaning and using contact lenses properly. Conjunctivitis caused by exposure to pollen, other allergens, and chemicals can be prevented by avoiding the irritating substance.

Treatment of conjunctivitis depends on the cause. Viral conjunctivitis clears up on its own; antibiotics are of no use. Bacterial conjunctivitis is treated with antibiotic drops or ointments. Discomfort from both viral and bacterial conjunctivitis can be relieved by applying warm compresses (a clean cloth soaked in warm water and wrung out) to the eyes several times a day. Allergic conjunctivitis can be treated with eye drops containing antihistamines (which

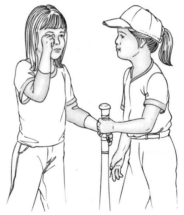

A CONTAGIOUS INFECTION
Conjunctivitis is inflammation caused by a viral infection that can be easily passed along when the infected person rubs his or her eyes and then makes contact with someone else. Washing hands frequently can help prevent spreading the infection to others.

counteract histamine, the chemical that causes allergy symptoms), systemic antihistamine medications (such as over-the-counter or prescription allergy drugs), or immunotherapy (so-called allergy shots, which desensitize the body to the irritating substance).

A type of conjunctivitis known as giant papillary conjunctivitis is common among soft contact lens wearers who are prone to allergy. Giant papillary conjunctivitis may also be caused by exposed sutures and ocular prostheses. Symptoms usually develop gradually. They include decreased comfort during lens wear, mild itching, excessive lens movement, and excess mucus production. Treatment usually consists of changing contact lens brands, changing contact lens solutions, switching to glasses for a time to allow the eyes to heal, replacing the contact lenses with a clean pair, using a scrupulous cleansing regimen, or increasing enzyme use and using antihistamine drops.

Connective tissue

Any tissue that connects, binds, or supports a structure of the body. Different connective tissues are derived from different combinations of cells, fibers, and substances found in bones, arteries, and veins. Loose connective tissue is so called for its irregularly arranged fibers. The fibrous support in this tissue comes

from collagen, a strong, linked protein, and from elastic fibers made of the protein elastin. This kind of connective tissue is found, for example, in the lower layers of the skin. Adipose tissue is made of fat cells supplied with lymph and blood. Besides serving as a source of fuel, adipose tissue, such as the buttocks and breasts, helps insulate and pad body organs. In dense, regular connective tissue, masses of fibers lie in a tight parallel arrangement. Able to stretch, yet strongly resistant to twisting forces, this kind of connective tissue forms tendons and ligaments. Dense, irregular connective tissue contains loosely arranged fibers and few cells. It envelops muscle tissue and certain internal organs, forms joint capsules, and makes up the dermis, the thick, inner layer of the skin. This type of connective tissue resists impact well even though it receives only a minimal blood supply.

Connective tissue disease, mixed

A chronic inflammatory autoimmune disease. Mixed connective tissue disease is a term used to describe overlapping groups of collagen diseases that cannot be individually categorized as one of the specific disorders. The diagnosis of mixed connective tissue disease (MCTD) may be similar to that of RHEUMATOID ARTHRITIS or systemic lupus erythematosus (see LUPUS ERYTHEMATOSUS, SYSTEMIC). MCTD is characterized by symptoms including muscle weakness and pain in the joints. There may be other symptoms relating to disorders of the heart, lungs, and skin. Kidney disease and a dysfunction of the esophagus, including swallowing problems, may be associated with the abnormalities in the body. See also COLLAGEN DISEASES.

Conscious sedation

A method of controlling discomfort during surgery in which the patient is awake but drowsy and insensitive to pain. Conscious sedation is sometimes used alone for minor procedures. It can also be combined with regional or local anesthesia to provide additional pain control for more extensive surgery.

The medication is given through a line or tube that is inserted into a vein in the hand or arm of the patient.

A variety of medications may be used, depending on the condition of the person and the pain-control requirements that the procedure may demand. The medications are given in small, continuous doses or pumped automatically into the bloodstream. The medications currently used are very short-acting so that the sedation can be increased or decreased as needed, permitting faster recovery to full consciousness when the surgery is complete.

Most people who undergo conscious sedation do not have pain during surgery, and they have no memory of anything that happened in the operating room during the procedure. Recovery with conscious sedation is faster than with general anesthesia, and nausea and vomiting are much less likely. During surgery, conscious sedation causes less suppression of the respiratory system. Patients can breathe without the assistance required during general anesthesia. If the person vomits during surgery, he or she is able to clear the throat. As a result, the risk of inhaling regurgitated material into the lungs (aspiration) is very small.

Complications with conscious sedation can arise if either too much or too little medication is given. If the dose is too low, the patient will have no memory of pain but may move on the operating table in response to pain. If the dose is too high, the breathing rate may fall abnormally low and the patient could have trouble breathing. This problem can be resolved by placing a mask on the patient to allow inhalation of pure oxygen.

Consciousness

The knowledge or awareness of what is happening around oneself. A person in a state of consciousness is cognizant of external stimuli, sensations (especially visual and auditory), and feelings. A conscious individual is awake, is able to feel and think, and knows what he or she is doing and intends to do. The spinal cord is the first relay point for sensory information en route to brain centers. Conscious thought and memory depend on the proper functioning of the brain, especially the cerebral cortex. A host of circumstances, from injury to disease, can lead to a dis-

turbance of consciousness. Symptoms of this include impaired attention, concentration, and understanding. If the level of consciousness continues to deteriorate, a person may pass into a state of STUPOR and then COMA.

Consensual sex

Sexual contact between two consenting adults. In contrast, nonconsensual sex refers to sexual contact without mutual consent or agreement. It may range from forced touching or fondling to RAPE.

Constipation

FOR SYMPTOM CHART
see Constipation, page 26

Infrequent or irregular bowel movements in which feces are hard and dry. Although most people have one bowel movement a day, as many as three movements a day or as few as three a week are considered normal. Regularity and ease of defecation are more important than frequency. Doctors recommend that anyone who experiences constipation after years of regularity seek medical help. This is especially important when constipation is accompanied by other symptoms, such as weight loss, abdominal pain, or rectal bleeding (see feces, blood in the).

Constipation occurs when colon muscles fail to contract and propel stools forward as usual. The colon continues to absorb water from stools, making them hard and dry and more difficult to pass. Primary causes usually include not eating enough fiber or drinking enough fluids. Repeatedly ignoring the urge to defecate can also be a factor. Other causes include the overuse of LAXATIVES,

physical inactivity, the use of certain medications (such as antacids, iron, or codeine), HEMORRHOIDS, an ANAL FISSURE, IRRITABLE BOWEL SYNDROME, DIVERTICULAR DISEASE, or HYPOTHYROIDISM. In some cases, the abrupt onset of constipation is a symptom of colon cancer (see COLON, CANCER OF THE).

DIAGNOSIS AND TREATMENT
Diagnostic tests to determine the cause of constipation include a lower GASTROINTESTINAL (GI) SERIES (an X-ray procedure also called a barium enema) and SIGMOIDOSCOPY or COLONOSCOPY (examinations of the rectum and colon using flexible viewing tubes passed through the anus). Blood tests may be helpful in identifying an electrolyte deficiency that may impair colonic function.

Treatment depends on the cause. Doctors generally recommend adding fiber-rich vegetables, fruits, and bran to the diet, drinking adequate fluids, and responding promptly to the urge to defecate. Because constipation is a side effect of many medications, the doctor will review all medications that a person is taking and adjust them as necessary. Laxatives should be used cautiously and infrequently, since long-term use may damage the colon. An enema is used to treat severe constipation, but should not be used regularly. Painful conditions, such as hemorrhoids, may cause some people to avoid defecation, which worsens constipation. When the cause is an underlying problem, such as hemorrhoids or irritable bowel syndrome, the person should see a doctor.

Contact dermatitis

A skin reaction caused by exposure to an external agent. In allergic contact dermatitis (see also SKIN ALLERGY),

---

PREVENTING CONSTIPATION

Laxatives are generally not needed to maintain regular bowel movements. The following measures may prevent or relieve constipation. Constipation that persists despite these practices requires medical attention:

- Drinking eight to ten (8-oz.) glasses of water or fluid daily
- Consuming 25 to 30 grams of fiber daily in the forms of grains and fruits and vegetables (an orange has 3.1 grams of fiber; two slices of whole wheat bread, 3.9)
- Responding promptly to the urge to defecate
- Walking briskly for at least 15 minutes daily
- Taking a psyllium-based fiber supplement with water (when combined with water, psyllium softens stools)

there may be no apparent inflammation the first time a person is exposed to the substance. But on subsequent occasions, after the skin has become sensitive or allergic to the substance, exposure produces a skin eruption. Allergic contact dermatitis differs from irritant contact dermatitis. Irritant contact dermatitis is a rash caused by contact with any substance, such as strong soaps or detergents, that produces skin inflammation in most people. Many substances can be both irritants and allergens.

Symptoms of contact dermatitis vary from person to person but may include redness, itching, inflammation, blistering, crusting, scabbing, scaling, thickening, and pigment (color) changes. It may be difficult to distinguish contact dermatitis from other forms of dermatitis. A doctor will ask about any exposure to irritants or a history of ALLERGIES. Diagnosis is based on skin examination and PATCH TEST results that indicate sensitivity to commonly encountered substances. In patch testing, small amounts of possible allergens are applied to the skin for a short time. Some materials—such as latex, nickel, perfumes, cosmetics, hair dyes, feminine deodorants, poison ivy, wool, soaps, and detergents—are

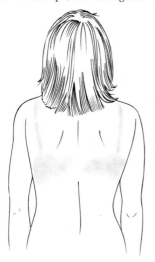

EXTERNAL AGENT OF SKIN IRRITATION
Contact dermatitis may look and feel like other forms of dermatitis, with redness, blistering, and itching. However, the symptoms of contact dermatitis are confined to the area of skin that was exposed to an irritating agent or allergen—such as the rubber in a bra (above), poison ivy, or detergents.

more likely than others to produce contact dermatitis. People with contact dermatitis should avoid the allergens or irritants that cause their reactions. A dermatologist can help identify products that do not cause reactions. Treatments to control symptoms may include corticosteroids and antihistamines. Scratching should be avoided. To control itching, doctors recommend applying cold compresses and soothing lotions, taking oatmeal baths, avoiding excessive heat and humidity, and wearing loose clothing.

Contact lenses

Small, thin, plastic disks shaped to correct visual defects and designed to be worn on the surface of the cornea (the clear outer covering on the front of the eye) over the iris and pupil. Contact lenses float on the thin layer of liquid that lubricates the cornea. They are particularly useful for people who suffer from pronounced refraction errors, such as severe nearsightedness, farsightedness, or astigmatism (a lack of symmetry in the cornea); possess a cone-shaped cornea (keratoconus); or have undergone CATARACT SURGERY. Since contact lenses require manual dexterity to insert and remove, they are not suitable for small children or for people with diseases that limit mobility of the hands, such as arthritis or Parkinson disease. They are also unsuitable for people with frequent eye infections, dry eyes, or severe allergies or for people who work in dusty or dirty environments.

TYPES

There are two basic types of contact lenses. Hard lenses are made from a relatively rigid plastic. Modern hard lenses are fitted with grooves that make it easier for oxygen to pass to the cornea; such lenses are called gaspermeable. Soft lenses use a plastic with a higher water content, which makes them more flexible and also allows oxygen to reach the cornea. Oxygen is important for preserving the health of the cornea lying under the contact lens.

Daily-wear contact lenses are designed to be replaced daily. Extended-wear lenses can be worn for longer periods without removal and cleaning; in the United States, Food and Drug Administration rules

limit this period to 7 days. Extended-wear contact lenses that can be worn for up to 30 days are available in Canada and Europe.

Hard lenses offer the advantage of sturdiness; they are less likely to tear or scratch. They also require less maintenance than soft lenses, and they provide sharper vision. Hard lenses are more likely to develop a buildup of proteins that can cause blurred vision. Most people find hard lenses less comfortable than soft, because they are more difficult to keep in position on the eye and because they cause more friction with the eyelid. In corneal refractive therapy, hard lenses are worn at night (on a prescribed basis) to reshape the cornea, treating nearsightedness.

Many soft lenses are disposable. They are worn for a set period, which varies from 1 day to 2 weeks, and then replaced with a fresh set of lenses. So-called frequent-replacement lenses are worn for a longer period, usually from 1 to 3 months, before replacement. Disposable and frequent-replacement lenses reduce cleaning problems and the risk of infection.

Contact lenses can be made with a single-vision correction, or they can be designed as bifocals, with one part of the lens for distance vision and another for close. Some people find bifocal contact lenses difficult to use and choose monovision instead—that is, one eye is corrected for distance vision, and the other for near vision. Monovision requires more adjustment of head position and causes some loss of depth perception.

Astigmatism is corrected with toric contact lenses, which are usually hard. Toric lenses compensate for the asymmetry in the cornea and remove or reduce the resulting distortion in vision.

RISKS AND COMPLICATIONS

Contact lenses raise the risk of eye infection, particularly if the lenses are not removed and cleaned regularly and properly. In rare cases, infection with a bacterium or a fungus can cause an ulcer on the cornea (see CORNEAL ULCER). This condition is serious, and it may threaten sight. The risk of infection is higher with extended-wear lenses than with daily-wear lenses.

Giant papillary conjunctivitis is a

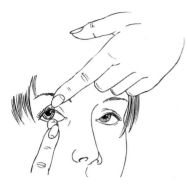

RIGID CONTACT LENSES
Rigid, gas-permeable contact lenses usually provide sharper vision than soft lenses. They are longer-lasting and require less maintenance than do soft lenses. They may feel less comfortable on the eye at first, but after the wearer has adapted to them, they are comfortable and resistant to infection.

common reaction among soft-lens wearers who are prone to allergy. It is believed that lipid deposits on the lens cause the membrane (conjunctiva) of the upper eyelid to become bumpy and inflamed. Symptoms usually develop gradually. They include decreased comfort during lens wear, mild itching, excessive lens movement, and excess mucus production. Treatment usually consists of switching to glasses for a time to allow the eyes to heal, replacing the contact lenses with a clean pair, a scrupulous cleansing regimen, and increasing enzyme use and using antihistamine drops.

If too little oxygen penetrates the contact lens, problems can arise in the cornea. In corneal vascularization, tiny blood vessels grow into the normally vessel-free cornea. In extreme cases, the new blood vessels cloud vision. Switching to another type of contact lens or to eyeglasses usually resolves the problem. In corneal warpage, the cornea changes shape because of oxygen deficiency. Again, changing lens type or switching to glasses resolves the problem.

Contact tracing

A measure that allows public health officials to locate people who have come in contact with individuals diagnosed with a serious INFECTIOUS DISEASE. People who have been exposed to these diseases may be infected themselves. Contact tracing, usually coordinated by local public health agencies, involves the process of finding and informing people who have had contact with an infected person. This procedure can help limit the spread of infectious diseases by offering diagnostic testing and treatment to people who may not know they have been exposed, as is often the case with sexually transmitted diseases.

Contagious

An infection or disease that is communicable by contact. A contagious disease is one that is transmitted by contact with a person infected with it, with that person's bodily fluids, or with objects and surfaces touched by the infected person.

Continuing care retirement communities

See LONG-TERM CARE FACILITY.

Contraception

Also called birth control. The deliberate prevention of pregnancy or conception by various means. Common methods of contraception include barrier and hormonal methods, intrauterine devices (IUDs), coitus interruptus (withdrawal), natural family planning, spermicides, and sterilization. Various methods of contraception have been in use for thousands of years. Honey douches and a spermicide made from crocodile dung were used by ancient Egyptians. Condoms made of animal intestines first appeared in Europe in the late 16th century, and the first rubber condom surfaced in 1842. Hormonal contraception in the form of birth control pills came out in 1960. Each method of birth control has benefits and drawbacks. For example, some barrier methods protect against sexually transmitted diseases but are not as effective at contraception as birth control pills.

Contraception, barrier methods

Methods of contraception that prevent pregnancy by keeping sperm from entering a woman's uterus. There are several types of barrier contraceptives, including condoms (both male and female), diaphragms, and cervical caps. A doctor can provide information on the advantages and disadvantages of contraceptive methods. (See also CONTRACEPTIVE.)

TYPES OF BARRIER METHODS

All barrier methods of contraception should generally be used with a spermicide. Spermicides kill sperm on contact. Some barrier methods also offer protection from sexually transmitted diseases (STDs). Barrier methods are not as effective as some other contraceptives, such as hormonal methods (see CONTRACEPTION, HORMONAL METHODS) and intrauterine devices (IUD; see IUD). Lifestyle, health history, and level of comfort should be considered when selecting a barrier method of contraception.

■ *Condom* A condom is thin sheath placed over a man's erect penis to contain the semen and prevent sperm from entering a woman's vagina. Condoms provide the fullest possible protection against the spread of STDs. Also called rubbers, prophylactics, and sheaths, condoms usually are made of latex and often are pretreated with spermicide. Condoms are inexpensive, easy to use, and widely available without a prescription. In use, a rolled-up condom is placed over the tip of a man's erect penis and unrolled down. After a man ejaculates, he withdraws his penis while he or his partner holds the condom at its rim to prevent semen from leaking out. A water-based lubricant may be used to avoid discomfort. Petroleum jelly is not recommended because petroleum weakens latex. Used condoms should always be discarded.

■ *The female condom* A polyurethane sleeve that lines the vagina, the female condom shields the vagina and cervix from semen. At the upper end, the sleeve has a round cap, braced by a light ring; a much larger ring opens the sheath for penile penetration at the vaginal entrance. To insert the condom, the inner ring is squeezed and pushed up into the vagina until it is just behind the pubic bone. About an inch of the open end will remain outside of the woman's body. Both oil- and water-based lubricants may be used with the female condom because the lubricants do not degrade polyurethane, as opposed to latex. To remove the condom after ejaculation, the outer ring is squeezed, twisted, and gently pulled from the vagina for disposal.

C

USING BARRIER CONTRACEPTIVES

Barrier methods of contraception are more effective when used correctly. Each device must be used with a jelly or cream spermicide, which kills sperm on contact.

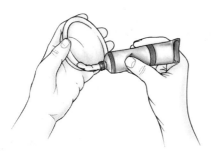

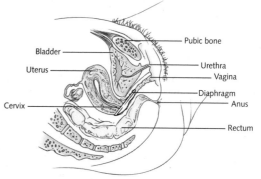

BEFORE INSERTING A DIAPHRAGM
Place about a tablespoon of spermidical cream or jelly inside the diaphragm, then apply some around the rim.

CORRECT POSITION OF A DIAPHRAGM
The diaphragm has to cover the entire cervix.

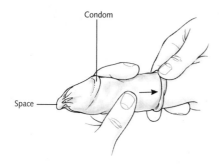

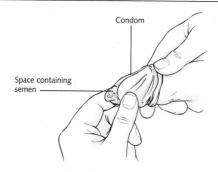

PUTTING ON A MALE CONDOM
Always leave a space at the tip of the condom to hold the semen. Squeeze the space at the tip to make sure there is no air inside, then roll the condom all the way down to the base of the penis.

REMOVING A MALE CONDOM
Remove the male condom immediately after ejaculation and withdrawal, while holding the base firmly to prevent semen from escaping. Never reuse a condom.

CORRECT POSITION OF A FEMALE CONDOM
A female condom has a small inner ring that is inserted inside the woman's vagina up against the cervix and a larger outer ring that fits outside the body against the outer genitals.

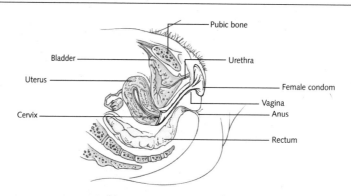

■ *Diaphragm* A flexible rubber dome that is propped against the pubic bone to cover the cervix and part of the uterus. To obtain a diaphragm, a woman must see a doctor to determine proper fit and to get a prescription for the device and spermicide to use with it. The diaphragm must hold the spermicide firmly against the cervix. Diaphragms may be inserted just before or up to 6 hours before intercourse; if inserted earlier, additional spermicide should be inserted into the vagina with an applicator just before intercourse. If intercourse is repeated, the position of the diaphragm should first be checked and new spermicide should be added. Oil-based lubricants that contain petroleum should not be used because they can damage the latex. After intercourse, a diaphragm must be left in place for 6 hours before it can be removed and cleaned. A woman whose diaphragm slips or who has had pelvic surgery, been pregnant, or gained or lost a significant amount of weight should have a doctor check the fit of her diaphragm. Diaphragm users have a higher risk of urinary tract infections and, therefore, should drink extra fluids and urinate after intercourse.

■ *Cervical cap* A firm rubber dome that fits snugly over a woman's cervix. Like a diaphragm, a cervical cap can only be obtained by prescription and requires a doctor's examination to determine the correct size. Similarly, a cervical cap must always be used with a spermicide and should not be used with oil-based lubricants. Cervical caps require less spermicide than diaphragms, but can be difficult to put into place. The position of the cap must be checked before each act of intercourse. After intercourse, the cap must stay in place for at least 6 hours; it can remain inserted for up to 36 hours.

■ *Contraceptive sponge* Made of absorbent polyurethane foam that has been impregnated with a spermicide, the round sponge has a dimple in the middle of one side and a polyester loop for removal on the other. It works by bracing spermicide against the cervix while blocking the cervical opening. The sponge is moistened with water to activate the spermicide and is placed high in the vagina, with the dimple-side up and the loop fac-

ing down. It continuously releases spermicide, and no additional applications of spermicide are necessary. Sponges can be inserted up to 24 hours before intercourse and must stay in place for 6 hours after intercourse. The sponge is available without a prescription. Its failure rate is relatively high, because it can be easily displaced inside the vagina. On average, 24 percent of the women who use the sponge become pregnant in 1 year. The failure rate for women who have borne children is higher than for others.

Contraception, emergency postcoital

Birth control that a woman may use after having unprotected sex or having been the victim of sexual assault. Two common methods are used, either oral medication or insertion of an intrauterine device (IUD). Both require a visit to a doctor or clinic.

Morning-after pills are usually a series of birth control pills containing estrogen and progestin, which inhibit the growth of the lining of the uterus (endometrium), making it impossible for a fertilized egg to grow there. Two pills are taken as soon (up to 72 hours) after intercourse as possible, followed by two more pills 12 hours later. Another morning-after pill, mifepristone (not widely available), when taken within 72 hours after having sex, can cause changes in the lining of the uterus that block a fertilized egg from implanting there. Taking a morning-after pill does not guarantee that a woman will not become pregnant. Morning-after pills are not as effective as daily forms of hormonal birth control, and their higher dosages typically cause nausea. Since the hormones are either identical or similar to those found in birth control pills, the contraindications for the morning-after pill are similar to those for birth control pills. See CONTRACEPTION, HORMONAL METHODS.

Another method of emergency contraception is the insertion of a copper-releasing IUD within 5 days after having sex. In normal use, IUDs prevent fertilization. When used as emergency contraception, IUDs are thought primarily to prevent implantation of a fertilized egg in the uterus.

Contraception, hormonal methods

Methods of preventing pregnancy by changing the levels of female hormones in a woman's body. Hormonal birth control methods include birth control pills, hormone implants or injections, an intrauterine device (see IUD) impregnated with hormones, and morning-after pills. Hormonal birth control methods are easy to use, highly effective, and relatively inexpensive. Hormonal methods work by preventing ovulation. They also cause changes in a woman's cervical mucus and uterus that help prevent pregnancy. Hormonal birth control methods are relatively safe, but not every woman may be able to use them. Women with certain health conditions, such as high blood pressure or an inherited tendency to develop blood clots, may not be good candidates for using hormonal contraception. Hormonal methods do not protect against sexually transmitted diseases; they should be used in combination with condoms in a nonmonogamous relationship.

BIRTH CONTROL PILLS

Birth control pills are the most widely used hormonal birth control method. Obtained only by prescription, they can work in several ways. They prevent ovulation, thicken the mucus lining of the cervix, change the lining of the uterus, and inhibit the smooth muscles that transport eggs down the fallopian tubes. There

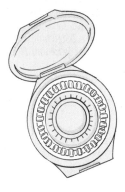

BIRTH CONTROL PILLS
Birth control pills, available only with a prescription, provide a daily dose of female hormones. The widely used combined pill contains both estrogen and progestin. The minipill contains only small amounts of progestin, without the estrogen. Both types are highly effective for preventing pregnancy when taken as prescribed.

C

are several types of birth control pills. Most contain the hormones estrogen and progestin and are called combination pills. Others, called minipills, contain only progestin. Progestin-only pills are slightly less effective than combination pills in preventing pregnancy.

Birth control pills are safe and effective when taken daily, as prescribed. The failure rate for birth control pills rises if a woman misses taking pills. If that happens, a back-up form of birth control should be used for the remaining part of the monthly cycle. Some antibiotics and anticonvulsants also may compromise the pill's effectiveness.

Some women, such as those who smoke, have an increased risk for complications from using birth control pills. Conditions that rule out using the pill include pregnancy, any disease or condition associated with blood clotting, hepatitis or other liver diseases, abnormal genital bleeding, cancer of the breast or reproductive organs, or being a smoker who is age 35 or older. A doctor can help a woman judge whether birth control pills are a safe choice, based on her medical history, age, and lifestyle.

OTHER HORMONAL METHODS

Hormonal implants are a safe and very effective form of birth control. Available only by prescription, implants are small, soft-plastic capsules that are placed beneath the skin usually in a woman's upper arm. They release a steady but low-dosage stream of hormones. Before the insertion of implants, a woman is given an injection of a local anesthetic at the site of the implantation. A small incision is made, and the implants are put in place. After insertion, no further steps need to be taken to prevent pregnancy. Each implantation lasts about 5 years and eliminates the possibility of user error. At the end of 5 years, the old implants can be replaced with new ones. If a woman wishes to stop using them at any time, implants can easily be removed. The hormones in implants may make a woman's periods irregular, and spotting sometimes occurs.

Hormonal injections are another safe and effective form of birth control, available only from a doctor. The intramuscular injections work primarily by preventing ovulation. Each

---

WHO SHOULD NOT TAKE ORAL CONTRACEPTIVES?

Women who:

- **Smoke cigarettes and are over age 35**
- **Think they may be pregnant**
- **Have had blood clots in the veins of their legs, eyes, or lungs during pregnancy or while taking oral contraceptives in the past**
- **Have certain types of heart disease or who have had a heart attack**
- **Have high blood pressure**
- **Have breast cancer**
- **Are experiencing vaginal bleeding of an unknown cause**
- **Have active liver disease, such as hepatitis or cirrhosis**
- **Have advanced diabetes**

---

injection provides birth control for 3 months, although contraceptive protection appears to extend somewhat past the deadline for the next shot. While the injection is in effect, a woman does not need to take any further steps to prevent pregnancy. By using shots, the possibility of user error is nearly eliminated, although the user must return for another injection every 3 months to maintain protection. Women who have hormonal injections may have irregular periods.

A woman who has had sex without using any birth control method or who has been the victim of a sexual assault may be able to use the morning-after pill. This type of hormonal birth control involves taking high doses of certain kinds of birth control pills within 72 hours after having sex. A doctor should be consulted immediately if a woman believes that she may need this form of birth control. See CONTRACEPTION, EMERGENCY POST-COITAL.

Contraception, other methods

In addition to barrier methods and hormonal methods of contraception, some other methods include the Rhythm Method (natural family planning), spermicides, coitus interruptus (the withdrawal method), intrauterine devices (IUDs), and sterilization. Each method works in a different way to prevent pregnancy.

Some are often used in combination with other methods. For example, the rhythm method is based on the assumption that pregnancy can be avoided by not having intercourse around the days a woman ovulates, the time of the month when she is most fertile. This method is not reliable; it works best when women have regular cycles and ovulate predictably and when it is used with a spermicide or a barrier method of birth control.

Spermicides contain a chemical that kills sperm or makes them unable to fertilize an egg. Inexpensive and easy to use, spermicides are widely available without a prescription. Available as creams, gels, foams, suppositories, and films, spermicides are inserted into the vagina near the cervix before intercourse. Instructions provided with the spermicide must be followed closely for the best results. Spermicides are most effective at preventing pregnancy when used with a barrier method, such as a diaphragm, condom, or cervical cap. Using a spermicide may offer some protection against some sexually transmitted diseases, including chlamydia and gonorrhea.

Coitus interruptus, more commonly known as the withdrawal method of birth control, relies on a man withdrawing his penis before he ejaculates into a woman's vagina. This

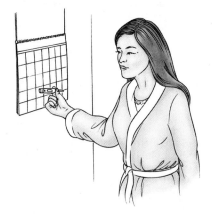

TEMPERATURE METHOD
The temperature method of family planning requires a woman to take her temperature daily to watch for fluctuations that signal ovulation. Body temperature rises slightly (less than 1°F) before, during, or right after ovulation. The woman must meticulously take her temperature with a specialized thermometer at exactly the same time each day.

EFFECTIVENESS OF CONTRACEPTIVES

Of 100 women using each contraceptive method for 1 year, this many become pregnant. "Used perfectly" means the method was used correctly 100 percent of the time. "Used typically" shows the effectiveness in groups of typical users, including those who may use the method incorrectly. If no contraceptive is used, 85 of 100 women become pregnant.

METHOD	USED PERFECTLY	USED TYPICALLY
Birth control pill (all types)	Less than 1	5
Condom, female	5	21
Condom, male	3	14
Spermicidal products	6	26
Sponge (previous birth)	9	20
Sponge (no previous birth)	20	40
Diaphragm with spermicide	6	20
Implant	0.05	0.05
Intrauterine device (all types)	0.1 to 1.5	0.1 to 2
Withdrawal	4	19
Sterilization, female	0.5	0.5
Sterilization, male	0.10	0.15

Contraceptive Technology, (Contraceptive Technology Communications, Inc).

behavior method of contraception is ineffective because sperm can be released before a man ejaculates.

Sterilization is another option. It involves surgical procedures for both women and men. Sterilization should be considered a permanent method of birth control because attempts to reverse it are complicated, costly, and not always successful. Sterilization should only be chosen as a form of birth control when a woman or man is certain that she or he will not want to have children in the future. Sterilization does not impair sexual functioning. Sterilizing women involves a procedure called a TUBAL LIGATION, commonly called tying the tubes. In a tubal ligation, the fallopian tubes are clipped or banded closed, cut and tied off, or burned (cauterized) with an electric current and cut. For men, sterilization is done with a VASECTOMY, in which the two vas deferens (the tubes that carry sperm from the testicles to the penis) are cut to prevent sperm from being ejaculated by the penis.

Intrauterine devices are small devices containing copper or hormones that are placed in the uterus to interfere with ovulation and conception. A hormonal IUD must be replaced every year; the copper ver-sion can be kept in place for up to 12 years. Women who have multiple sex partners are at an increased risk for pelvic infection; they should probably use another form of birth control, because IUDs tend to make pelvic infections worse and therefore can render a woman infertile or at risk for ectopic pregnancy. See IUD.

Contraceptive

A device or agent used to prevent conception, the fertilization and implantation of an egg in the uterus. Various contraceptives accomplish this is different ways. Contraceptive choices include barrier methods, such as the condom, diaphragm, cervical cap, and sponge; spermicides, such as jellies and foams; the intrauterine device (see IUD); hormonal methods, such as birth control pills, implants, and injections; and other methods, including natural family planning (the rhythm method); withdrawal (coitus interruptus); and sterilization. See CONTRACEPTION, BARRIER METHODS; CONTRACEPTION, HORMONAL METHODS; and CONTRACEPTION, OTHER METHODS.

CHOOSING A CONTRACEPTIVE

A common cause of contraceptive failure is using the method incorrectly. Because contraceptives must be used properly to be effective, it is important that the user select a method that he or she is likely to use properly. Some issues involved in choosing a contraceptive are convenience, price, reliability, comfort, personal health, and lifestyle. For some people, a contraceptive that requires interruption of FOREPLAY is not convenient. The cost of another method may be prohibitive. For example, the initial cost of some contraceptives, such as IUDs and implants, is high compared with other methods. However, the cost for these methods is actually lower over time, because of the duration of their effectiveness. Reliability is a concern for everyone and must be factored into every decision. Rates of effectiveness vary from 99 percent for some birth control pills to 74 percent for spermicides alone. People also need to feel comfortable using a chosen method. If they feel awkward, they are not likely to use it often. Personal health considerations can rule out some choices. Women older than 35 years who are smokers, for example, are not good candidates for birth control pills because of their increased risk for heart attack and stroke. The method must fit the person's lifestyle, too. For example, single people who may have multiple sex partners should use condoms to prevent sexually transmitted diseases, in addition to another form of birth control.

Contraceptive foam and jelly

Products that are used, usually in combination with a barrier method of contraception, to kill sperm in the vagina as a means of birth control. They can be purchased without a prescription. To be effective, they must be applied no earlier than 30 minutes before intercourse and reapplied if intercourse is repeated. See CONTRACEPTION, OTHER METHODS.

Contraceptive implant

A form of hormonal birth control, administered through soft-plastic tubes that are implanted in a woman's upper arm. Contraceptive implants provide birth control for up to 5 years after insertion. See CONTRACEPTION, HORMONAL METHODS.

C

Contraction stress test

In pregnancy, a test in which contractions (see CONTRACTIONS, UTERINE) are induced in the mother's uterus, and the heart rate of the fetus is monitored electronically to measure the fetal response to the contractions. Monitoring the baby's heartbeat assesses the baby's health and can help the doctor decide whether to let the pregnancy proceed or to induce labor. Two methods can be used to conduct the contraction stress test. In the first, the woman's nipples are stimulated, causing her brain to secrete oxytocin, a hormone that induces uterine contractions. The second method is the OXYTOCIN CHALLENGE TEST (OCT), in which a small amount of synthetic oxytocin (Pitocin) is introduced intravenously to stimulate contractions.

Contractions, uterine

The strong, rhythmic tightening of the muscles of the uterus, increasing in intensity, frequency, and duration, that accompanies labor. Uterine contractions cause the cervix to dilate (widen) so that the baby can pass into the vagina. At first, the contractions may be mild, irregular, and infrequent. Early contractions can feel like gas pains, menstrual cramps, or a backache. As labor progresses, the contractions become stronger and more regular. Relaxation between contractions helps reduce pain and conserve energy for the next contraction. Preceding labor, particularly in the last month or two of pregnancy, sporadic, mild contractions called BRAXTON HICKS CONTRACTIONS may occur. They are not associated with the progressive opening of the cervix or the pain seen with labor contractions. See also LABOR.

Contracture

A deformed or distorted joint caused by abnormal shortening of muscles and tendons surrounding the joint or by the shrinking of scars in the connective tissue capsule or skin associated with the joint. Shortened muscles and tendons are caused by a lack of regular use and movement of a joint. The hip, knee, shoulder, and hand joints of older people who are not active are often affected by joint contracture.

Contraindication

A factor in a person's condition that makes it inadvisable to participate in a particular treatment, such as taking a certain medication or undergoing surgery. For example, pregnancy is a contraindication for the administration of many drugs, and an allergy to penicillin is a contraindication for using a penicillin type of antibiotic.

Contrast medium

A substance used in RADIOGRAPHY to increase the contrast of an image. The contrast medium can be introduced either in or around the structure. Because of the difference in the way that X rays are absorbed by the contrast medium and the surrounding tissues, the structure can be visualized. Usually, a contrast medium is a substance through which X rays cannot pass, such as barium. However, air can also be used as a contrast medium. Other commonly used agents are iodine-based mediums for INTRAVENOUS PYELOGRAPHY, CT SCANNING (computed tomography scanning), and ANGIOGRAPHY and gadolinium for MRI (magnetic resonance imaging).

Controlled substance

A substance regulated by US federal law to prevent abuse. Controlled substances are divided into five schedules, based on their medicinal value, harmfulness, and potential for abuse or addiction. The term "controlled substance" comes from the Controlled Substance Act of 1970, which regulates the prescribing and dispensing of dangerous drugs.

Schedule I includes the most dangerous drugs, such as heroin, LSD (lysergic acid diethylamide), mescaline, and some amphetamines, all with high potential for abuse and no accepted medical use in the United States.

Schedule II includes certain drugs extracted from substances of vegetable origin, such as morphine, opium, and methadone, that have a high potential for abuse but have currently accepted but restricted medical uses in the United States.

Schedule III includes drugs with some potential for abuse and currently accepted medical uses in the United States, such as certain barbiturates and anabolic steroids.

Schedule IV includes drugs with low potential for abuse relative to schedule III and that have currently accepted medical uses in the United States, such as phenobarbital and diazepam (Valium).

Schedule V includes drugs with less potential for abuse than those in schedule IV and that have currently accepted medical uses in the United States, such as drugs containing small amounts of codeine and opium.

Contusion

See BRUISE.

Convalescence

The process of recovery after an injury, illness, or surgery. During convalescence, a person gradually regains strength before resuming normal activities. The period of convalescence may be a matter of days (as after a viral infection) or a number of weeks (as after major surgery).

Conversion disorder

A mental illness that is not due to any physical cause, but in which a distressed person develops physical symptoms that mimic a disease of the nervous system or a general medical condition. The symptoms are due to a psychological conflict and are not faked. Typically, they occur at the same time as or soon after a troubling event. The symptoms are severe enough to significantly impair the person's ability to function in family life or work and can include difficulty walking, paralysis or localized weakness, inability to speak, difficulty swallowing ("lump-in-the-throat" feeling), inability to urinate, loss of sense of pain or touch, blindness, double vision, deafness, hallucinations, and seizures. In most cases, symptoms are inconsistent and do not fit with the actual structure or function of the body. For example, a person with an arm paralyzed by conversion disorder may unknowingly move the limb while dressing, or an individual who has a hard time swallowing may experience equal difficulty with solids and liquids, when solids should pose more of a challenge.

The term "conversion" comes from the idea that the symptoms represent a symbolic solution to an emotional crisis. For example, an individual who has seen a traumatic event may become blind to avoid the distress of being an eyewitness to future trauma. Conversion disorder can occur alone, or it may be associated with other disorders such as depression or a personality disorder.

Conversion disorder usually begins between ages 19 and 35. In most cases, symptoms arise suddenly; less often they develop gradually. Usually the symptoms last only a short time. Recurrence is common; people who have had the disorder once are at increased risk of having it again.

Treatment consists of a physical examination by a doctor to rule out any underlying disease, followed by psychiatric treatment to help the person understand the emotional basis of the disorder. Conversion disorder is not life-threatening, but it can result in damage such as muscle wasting caused by lack of exercise in a paralyzed limb. Hypnosis can aid as a stress management tool in treating this disorder.

Convulsion

Involuntary jerking movements, now called a SEIZURE.

Cooley anemia

See ANEMIA, COOLEY.

COPD

See CHRONIC OBSTRUCTIVE PULMONARY DISEASE.

Copper

A mineral that is essential for manufacturing collagen (a protein that is a major component of connective tissue) and for enabling oxygen to bind to hemoglobin, an oxygen-carrying protein in red blood cells. Copper deficiency causes an anemia that resembles iron deficiency anemia. Copper is also necessary for healthy functioning of the heart, efficient energy production, and absorption of iron from the digestive tract. Dietary copper is found in whole grains, nuts, liver, and oysters.

Cor pulmonale

Enlargement of the right ventricle (lower right chamber of the heart) because of disease in the lungs. Cor pulmonale is a Latin phrase meaning "lung-affected heart." The right side of the heart pumps blood into the lungs, where it takes on oxygen for transport into the rest of the body. In a healthy person, little pressure is required to pump blood into the lungs. As a result, the muscle of the right ventricle is not as strong as the left, which pumps blood into the body. However, if the lungs are impaired by diseases such as EMPHYSEMA or PULMONARY FIBROSIS, the heart must work much harder to deliver blood. The right ventricle enlarges to accommodate this overload. At first the heart can compensate, but over time it fails.

Cor pulmonale is a serious disease that can shorten a person's life. In some cases, it is acute and reversible; more often than not, it is chronic. In addition to treating the underlying respiratory disease, the doctor may recommend using supplemental oxygen, restricting salt and water intake, and taking diuretic medications to reduce fluid accumulation in the lungs and lessen the heart's workload.

Cordotomy

An operation performed to divide bundles of nerve fibers within the spinal cord. Cordotomy is done to relieve persistent pain that has failed to respond to other measures, such as strong analgesic medication or TENS (transcutaneous electrical nerve stimulation). It is most often performed for severe, unremitting pain associated with cancer in the lower trunk and legs.

Cornea

The transparent, curved structure forming the front of the eyeball. Covered by the conjunctiva (the lining on the surface of the eye and inside the eyelids), the cornea contains five layers of clear tissue that help to focus light onto the retina. It joins the sclera (white of the eye) at its outer rim, and the black pupil and colored iris lie under it. The cornea itself is difficult to see because of its transparency.

The cornea helps focus light rays onto the retina at the back of the eye and protects the front of the eye. The top layer of the cornea is extremely sensitive to the slightest scratch, in order to protect the structures beneath it. An inner layer of cells continually moves fluid out of the eye to keep the cornea clear. The cornea is kept moist by the fluid-producing cells in the conjunctiva and the tears coming from the lacrimal gland.

The front of the cornea is curved outward, much like the lens of a camera. As light enters the eye, the convex cornea bends the light rays, which will be further bent by the lens inside the eye. The cornea needs more help from the lens to focus on close objects. The eye continually changes shape to achieve good focus, rounding to focus on near objects and flattening to focus on distant ones.

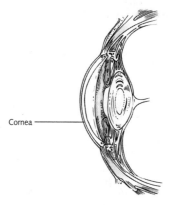

Cornea

FOCUSING LIGHT INTO THE EYE
The cornea is the stronger focusing structure in the eye (stronger than the lens), and it continually changes shape to adjust the focus of entering light rays. It also serves as a protective "windshield." Fluid moves over it constantly to keep it clear and to wash away foreign particles and microorganisms.

Corneal abrasion

An injury to the thin skin (epithelium) overlying the transparent covering (cornea) of the eye. Corneal abrasion can be caused by a speck of sand or other small object, a fingernail, or a contact lens that is worn too long. Symptoms may include severe pain in the eye, sensation of a foreign body in the eye, abnormal vision, sensitivity to light, redness, and swollen eyelids. Treatment consists of removing any foreign body that may be present, lubrication with artificial tears or ointment, and antibiotic drops or ointment in the eye if infection poses a risk. Most doctors recommend covering the eye with a patch to allow healing and relief of pain. Corneal injuries heal quickly with treatment, and the eye typically returns to normal within 24 to 48 hours.

Corneal transplant

See KERATOPLASTY, PENETRATING.

Corneal ulcer

An open sore on the transparent outer covering of the eye (cornea). Signs and symptoms include impaired vision, severe pain, redness, a visible white patch on the cornea, sensitivity to light, and increased tearing. Corneal ulcers usually arise from infection by bacteria, often through contamination of an injury to the cornea. Fungi and protozoa (amoebas) can also cause corneal ulcers. Wearing contact lenses overnight increases the risk of corneal ulcer, as do dry eyes, severe allergies, inflammatory disorders, and immunosuppression (with medications, such as corticosteroids, or through HIV [human immunodeficiency virus] infection, for example).

Corneal ulcers are serious and can lead to vision loss if left untreated. A medical examination is conducted, and laboratory tests of tissue from the ulcer are performed to determine the cause of the infection. If a corneal ulcer is present, then the appropriate antibacterial, antiviral, or antifungal agent is prescribed, usually in the form of eye drops. If the ulcer erodes through the cornea, surgery is required. In cases of severe scarring of the cornea, a corneal transplant (see KERATOPLASTY, PENETRATING) may be needed to restore vision.

Coronary artery bypass

See BYPASS SURGERY.

Coronary artery disease

Narrowing or blockage of the arteries that nourish the heart by deposits of cholesterol, calcium, and other materials; also known as coronary heart disease. Even though blood flows through the heart, the heart takes the oxygen it needs from the coronary arteries, which branch off from the base of the aorta (the main artery carrying oxygen-rich blood out of the heart). The coronary arteries travel over the surface of the heart, encircle the top, and branch out toward the bottom, forming the pattern of a crown (corona means "crown" in Latin).

In the United States, coronary artery disease is the leading cause of heart attacks and of death in both men and women.

DISEASE PROCESS AND SYMPTOMS

Coronary artery disease results from ATHEROSCLEROSIS, in which deposits (plaques) of fat and other materials accumulate in and on the inner walls of the arteries, narrowing them and reducing their elasticity, strength, and flexibility. Atherosclerosis is known popularly as hardening of the arteries. Narrowed or blocked coronary arteries restrict blood flow; as a result, the heart may receive less oxygen than it needs. The symptoms and complications of coronary artery disease are caused by this deficiency in oxygen supply, which is medically known as cardiac ischemia.

The symptoms of coronary artery disease vary from one person to another. The most common is ANGINA, diffuse chest discomfort or pain often described as a feeling of tightness or heaviness that is brought on by exertion but relieved by rest. Critical vessel narrowing may cause pain even when resting. Other symptoms can include shortness of breath, especially after stress or exercise; cardiac arrhythmia (irregular heartbeat); nausea or upset stomach; severe sweating; weakness or fatigue; and (in women) breast pain or a feeling in the upper abdomen that is comparable to indigestion. When coronary artery disease produces no symptoms, it is said to be silent.

Coronary artery disease, with or without angina, can result in a HEART ATTACK when a blood clot forms in a narrowed artery and blocks it completely. The section of heart muscle downstream from the blockage is subsequently damaged by the lack of oxygen. In most cases, a heart attack is painful, but pain-free attacks occur and are known as silent heart attacks.

Coronary artery disease can lead to congestive heart failure (see HEART FAILURE, CONGESTIVE). The weakening heart falls behind the body's demand for blood, and fluid accumulates in the heart and lungs. Congestive heart failure, like heart attack, can result in disability and death.

A less common form of coronary artery disease is coronary artery spasm, the temporary contraction of an artery that results in a reduction of blood flow to the heart. While coronary artery spasms can take place in healthy arteries, they occur most often in arteries narrowed by plaque. The abrupt onset of angina (chest pain) associated with coronary artery spasm usually happens when a person is at rest, most frequently between midnight and 8 AM. Coronary artery spasms are temporary and usually halt spontaneously, with the artery resuming its normal function and appearance. Smoking tobacco, cocaine use, and genetic factors are thought to be contributing causes of coronary artery spasms. A severe or prolonged coronary artery spasm may result in permanent muscle damage or a heart attack. If symptoms fail to improve on their own, coronary artery spasms can be treated with medication, such as nitroglycerin.

RISK FACTORS

The chances of developing coronary artery disease vary with a number of inherited and lifestyle risk factors. They include a family history of early-onset coronary artery disease (younger than age 55 in men and younger than age 65 in women), low levels of high-density lipoprotein (HDL) cholesterol and high levels of low-density lipoprotein (LDL) cholesterol in the blood (see CHOLESTEROL for a discussion of cholesterol types and their role in disease), uncontrolled HYPERTENSION (high blood pressure), a high-fat diet, smoking, lack of exercise, being overweight or obese, uncontrolled diabetes mellitus, and high blood levels of homocysteine (an amino acid produced by the metabolism of meat). Some research points to a link between chronic stress and depression and coronary artery disease. Chronic bacterial infections may also be involved; research on this connection and other emerging risk factors is being explored. By gathering information on each of these factors, doctors can assess a person's risk profile for coronary artery disease.

DIAGNOSIS

If coronary artery disease is suspected, either because of the presence of symptoms or because of a person's risk profile, one or more of several tests may be used to check for abnormality. A resting ECG (electrocardiogram) records the electrical activity of the heart and can help detect irregular heart rhythms and other changes

UNDERSTANDING HEART DISEASE

Family history of heart disease, high blood pressure, smoking, high cholesterol levels, obesity, lack of exercise, and diabetes are all factors that increase the risk of developing coronary artery disease. Fortunately, many of these risk factors are controllable. Medications are available to reduce high blood pressure and lower high cholesterol levels, while lifestyle changes, such as maintaining a healthy weight, regular exercise, eating a low-fat diet, and not smoking can greatly reduce the risk of developing heart disease.

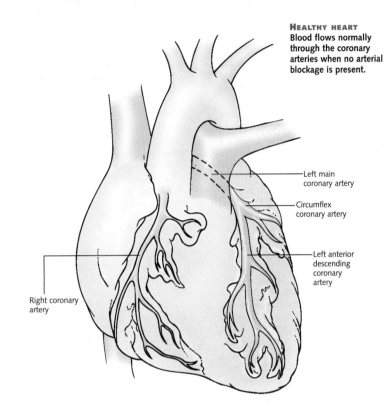

HEALTHY HEART
Blood flows normally through the coronary arteries when no arterial blockage is present.

Left main coronary artery

Circumflex coronary artery

Left anterior descending coronary artery

Right coronary artery

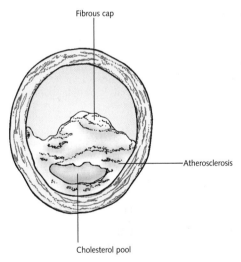

Fibrous cap

Atherosclerosis

Cholesterol pool

ATHEROSCLEROSIS
Partial blockage of a coronary artery can reduce blood flow in the heart and lead to angina (chest pain).

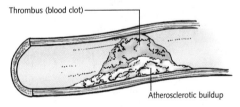

Thrombus (blood clot)

Atherosclerotic buildup

ATHEROSCLEROSIS WITH THROMBUS
A coronary artery with atherosclerotic buildup and thrombus (blood clot) causes total blockage and results in myocardial infarction (heart attack).

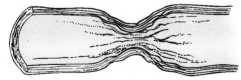

CORONARY ARTERY SPASM
Blood flow is temporarily interrupted by coronary spasm.

caused by coronary artery disease. The ECG may also be performed while the person exercises on a stationary bicycle or a treadmill (see CARDIAC STRESS TESTING) to measure the performance of the heart during exertion and to detect changes brought about by exercise. The ECHOCARDIOGRAM uses ultrasound waves to visualize the structure and function of the heart and the major arteries. In myocardial perfusion imaging, the person is injected with a small amount of a mildly radioactive substance that shows up on a special camera and allows doctors to observe the pattern of blood flowing through the coronary arteries.

If the results of any of these tests are abnormal, the person who has been tested is likely to undergo a minimally invasive procedure known as cardiac catheterization (see CATHETERIZATION, CARDIAC), in which a catheter (thin tube) is threaded through a blood vessel into the heart to obtain diagnostic information about the heart, the coronary arteries, and the aorta. The passage of the catheter is tracked through the circulatory system to the heart with a fluoroscope, an X-ray device that displays images on a monitor. By injecting a special dye through the catheter, accurate X-ray pictures of the heart and its arteries can be obtained. Cardiac catheterization allows doctors to pinpoint the location of plaques narrowing the coronary arteries and helps determine their severity.

TREATMENT AND PREVENTION
Treatment of coronary artery disease depends on the severity of the disease, the location of the narrowed arteries, the symptoms, and a person's overall health. The doctor treating the person with coronary artery disease has a number of options, including recommending lifestyle changes, prescribing medication, and performing surgery or less invasive interventional techniques.

Typical lifestyle changes include following a heart-healthy diet rich in fruits and vegetables and low in fats and oils; good control of diabetes and hypertension (high blood pressure) with diet and exercise, plus medication as needed; regular exercise; and quitting smoking and avoiding the intake of secondhand smoke. A number of medications can be used to increase the flow of oxygen into the heart or to reduce the heart's need for oxygen. These include nitrates such as nitroglycerin, which widen blood vessels and increase blood flow to the heart; beta blockers, which slow heart rate and reduce the force of the heart's contraction; calcium channel blockers, which widen the coronary arteries and increase blood flow to the heart muscle; antiplatelet medications such as aspirin, which inhibit the formation of blood clots and reduce the risk of heart attack; and statins, which lower cholesterol levels in the blood and may reduce plaque buildup in the coronary arteries.

In cases of severe narrowing or blockage, the interventional technique known as BALLOON ANGIOPLASTY is commonly used. Similar to cardiac catheterization, a catheter with an inflatable, balloonlike tip is threaded into a coronary artery and inflated to compress the fat deposits narrowing it. A stent (a small tube of thin wire mesh) is often placed in a widened artery via catheter to hold the artery open and provide support. Balloon angioplasty and stenting are commonly performed on an outpatient basis with the person under local anesthesia and, compared with BYPASS SURGERY, require a relatively short recovery period. Bypass surgery is a major surgical procedure that entails using sections of the person's blood vessels to detour around coronary artery blockages.

Coronary care unit

A part of the hospital dedicated to treating people with serious acute heart disease; commonly abbreviated as CCU. A cardiologist (heart specialist) heads the CCU, and a resident physician may also be present at all times. The CCU combines specialized equipment for constant electronic monitoring of heart function with highly trained personnel who can detect the signs and symptoms of heart problems and intervene as needed.

When a person is admitted to the CCU, cardiac monitor electrodes are attached to his or her skin. The cardiac monitor keeps constant track of heart rhythm and rate and is often equipped with an automatic alarm to signal a serious problem. Another monitoring device may also be insert- ed through a vein and into the pulmonary artery to measure the amount of blood the heart pumps per minute (cardiac output). Blood pressure is also monitored closely. An intravenous needle provides medications and fluids. Supplemental oxygen may also be provided.

If the condition or function of the heart deteriorates, if a heart attack occurs, or if the heart stops beating (cardiac arrest), CCU staff are equipped to respond quickly. Electroshock equipment (such as a defibrillator) and medications are readily available.

Once the condition of a person in the CCU improves, either less extensive monitoring or transfer to another unit is the first step toward rehabilitation.

Coronary heart disease

See CORONARY ARTERY DISEASE.

Coronary thrombosis

Partial or complete blockage by a blood clot of one of the arteries that nourish the heart. Since the surface arteries (coronary arteries) provides the heart with oxygen-rich blood, the clot cuts off the oxygen supply to the heart muscle downstream. The result is myocardial infarction, or heart attack.

Under normal circumstances, blood clots form when blood flow is sluggish or when a blood vessel is injured. Clotting can occur in the coronary arteries if they are narrowed by deposits of fats and other materials that form plaque on the inside of the artery and stiffen the artery wall, a disease process called ATHEROSCLEROSIS. If atherosclerotic plaque fractures, it triggers a cascade of events that can cause a clot to form and block the artery. Coronary thrombosis is more likely in people who smoke, are overweight, do not exercise regularly, have high blood pressure, take oral contraceptives, have high cholesterol levels, are of advanced age, or have an inherited tendency toward easy clotting.

Medications called thrombolytic agents, which can dissolve the clot when administered a short time after it has formed, can be used to treat coronary thrombosis. These medications may be given through a vein in the hand, arm, or leg, or they may be introduced to the site of the clot through a catheter (thin tube) threaded through a vein. Catheter treatment allows a stronger dose of medication over a shorter time. Anticoagulant medication is used as a follow-up treatment to prevent the formation of subsequent blood clots.

The risk of coronary thrombosis is lessened by avoiding tobacco use, exercising regularly, and maintaining a healthy body weight. Anticoagulant medication may also be prescribed for people with a history of blood clots. Lowering cholesterol levels and treating hypertension (high blood pressure) also lower the risk of coronary thrombosis.

Coroner

A public official who inquires into the cause of a person's death when the cause of death is not known or is suspected to have been a result of foul play or violence. A coroner may be elected or appointed and does not have to be a doctor in some jurisdictions.

Corpus luteum cyst

An ovarian cyst in which a fluid-filled sac develops from a persistent corpus luteum, the yellow pouch that remains after an egg has been released from a follicle (egg sac) in the ovary. If the egg is not fertilized, the body normally resorbs the corpus luteum. Corpeus luteum cysts usually go away in a few weeks but can grow as large as 4 or more inches in diameter and can cause pain in the woman's lower abdomen, usually on only one side. A corpus luteum cyst may cause delayed menstrual periods or bleeding between menstrual periods. Corpus luteum cysts may also cause symptoms that are similar to more serious conditions such as cancer of the ovary. If a woman develops symptoms of a corpus luteum cyst, her doctor will usually perform a PELVIC EXAMINATION and may order tests such as ULTRASOUND SCANNING, to rule out conditions such as cancer, ECTOPIC PREGNANCY, or other noncancerous ovarian growths.

Corpuscle

Most often refers to two types of blood cells. Red blood corpuscles, or erythrocytes, are iron-rich cells that transport oxygen through the bloodstream. White blood corpuscles, or leukocytes, have key roles in defending the body against invasion by viruses, bacteria, and fungi.

Corset

A cloth and elastic back support brace worn to relieve strain by restricting motion in the lower back when a person is in a seated or standing position. Corsets can offer comfort and warmth, as well as support, to the back. Corsets are obtained by prescription or over-the-counter at medical supply stores and some pharmacies. They are typically worn by people who have back injuries and whose work involves lifting; their use should be limited to this purpose. It has never been demonstrated that lumbar corsets prevent back pain. A corset eventually weakens the back muscles if used too frequently or worn for prolonged periods, during which support of the back is provided mostly by the brace and not the muscles.

Corticosteroid hormones

The group of three types of hormones produced by the adrenal cortex (the outer layer of the adrenal glands). The steroid group of hormones includes androgens and estrogens, the two SEX HORMONES that affect sexual development and reproduction; glucocorticoids, which maintain glucose (sugar) regulation, suppress the immune and inflammation responses, and secrete CORTISOL in response to stress; and mineralocorticoids, which include ALDOSTERONE, a hormone that regulates sodium and potassium balance, controls sodium levels in the urine, and maintains blood volume and blood pressure. Corticosteroid hormones are essential to life. They are produced in response to stimulation by corticotropin hormones, which are produced by the pituitary gland in response to CRH (corticotropin-releasing hormone) produced by the hypothalamus. Synthetic corticosteroids are used in topical creams to treat various skin disorders such as dermatitis, eczema, and hives. Cortico-steroid inhalants may be prescribed for chronic bronchitis, asthma, postnasal drip, and nasal polyps. Oral corticosteroids are used to treat asthma, arthritis, autoimmune disorders, and inflammatory bowel disease. They are also used after kidney transplantation. See also CORTICOSTEROIDS.

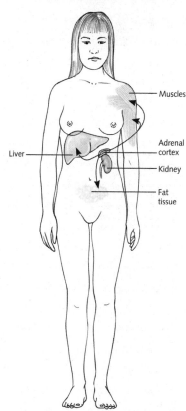

HORMONES FROM THE ADRENAL CORTEX
The adrenal cortex, or the outer layer of the adrenal glands, produces a large group of important hormones called corticosteroids. They regulate metabolism of carbohydrates, fat, and protein and influence the balance of water and electrolytes in the body.

Corticosteroids

Steroids produced by the adrenal glands in response to the release of adrenocorticotropic hormone (ACTH) by the pituitary gland. Corticosteroids are used for hormonal replacement therapy, for suppression of ACTH secretion by the pituitary gland, to suppress the immune response, and as anticancer, antiallergy, and anti-inflammatory agents.

Corticosteroids have many uses and forms. In paste form, they are used by dentists to relieve the discomfort of some mouth and gum conditions.

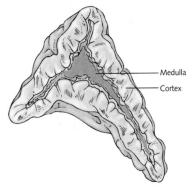

SYNTHETIC CORTICOSTEROIDS
Corticosteroid drugs are synthetic forms of the body's own corticosteroid hormones produced in the adrenal glands (located on top of the kidneys). Some steroids are produced in the outer layer, called the cortex, and others are produced in the inner portion, called the medulla. These hormones work together to control blood pressure, the immune system, and the body's response to stress.

Corticosteroids, such as triamcinolone, are inhaled to help prevent the symptoms of asthma. As a nasal spray, corticosteroids such as beclomethasone are used to treat the symptoms of allergy.

As eye drops, corticosteroids such as hydrocortisone are used to treat certain eye diseases and to relieve discomfort, redness, and irritation of the eye. Corticosteroids are used to treat ulcerative colitis, hemorrhoids, and other rectal problems. As a skin cream, corticosteroids are used to relieve redness, swelling, itching, and discomfort of many skin problems. Corticosteroids called glucocorticoids, including methylprednisolone, affect the immune system. They are important for treatment or prevention of asthma, rheumatoid arthritis, and organ and tissue transplant rejection.

Side effects from prolonged use include weight gain, susceptibility to infections, easy bruising, and muscle weakness. When corticosteroids are used for more than 2 weeks, the medication should be discontinued on a gradual or tapered basis, according to the doctor's instructions.

Corticotropin

See ACTH.

Corticotropin-releasing hormone

See CRH.

Cortisol

A glucocorticoid hormone produced in the adrenal cortex (the outer layer of the adrenal glands); also known as hydrocortisone. Glucocorticoids affect almost every organ and tissue in the body. Cortisol is a potent hormone that regulates the metabolism of glucose (sugar), other carbohydrates, proteins, and fats. By stimulating the release of glucose that is stored in cells, cortisol increases the blood sugar level. Cortisol also helps maintain blood pressure and cardiovascular function, helps balance the effects of insulin in breaking down sugar for energy, and helps slow the inflammatory response produced by the immune system when diseases or injuries occur.

The release of cortisol is one feature in a complex system. The adrenal cortex is stimulated to produce cortisol by the production of ACTH (adrenocorticotropic hormone), which is produced by the pituitary gland. The pituitary gland produces ACTH in response to stimulation by CRH (corticotropin-releasing hormone), which is produced by the hypothalamus in the brain. As cortisol levels increase in the blood, further production of CRH and ACTH is curtailed.

CORTISOL LEVELS

Because cortisol has a part in so many vital functions within the body, the amount produced and released is precisely balanced. In healthy people, cortisol secretion is increased during the hours before a person awakens and reaches a peak in the early waking hours. The hormone tends to fall to very low levels in the evening and during the first phases of sleep. The normal daily fluctuations of cortisol secretion may be impaired by infection, injury, exertion, severe illness, and a person's exposure to intense levels of heat or cold. Emotional stress may influence the release of cortisol in an otherwise healthy person.

Increased levels of cortisol may be associated with physical stress, HYPERTHYROIDISM (overactivity of the thyroid gland), obesity, ACTH-producing tumors, and certain medications such as estrogen, oral contraceptives, cortisone, and spironolactone. CUSHING SYNDROME is caused by excessive production and release of cortisol and may be diagnosed by a lack of normal fluctuation in cortisol levels at different times of the day.

The failure to produce normal levels of cortisol is called adrenal insufficiency. When the problem is caused by a disorder of the adrenal glands, it is known as primary adrenal insufficiency. When the lack of cortisol is the result of inadequate secretion of ACTH by the pituitary gland, it is called secondary adrenal insufficiency. Decreased cortisol levels may also be related to low thyroid conditions, hypopituitarism, tuberculosis, fungal infections of the adrenal glands, adrenal hemorrhage, and certain medications such as lithium, danazol, levodopa, androgens, and other corticosteroid medications. ADDISON DISEASE is caused by a deficiency of cortisol.

Tests to determine the amount of cortisol in the blood and urine are used to diagnose malfunctions in the adrenal glands, including Cushing syndrome and Addison disease.

Cortisone

See CORTICOSTEROIDS.

Cosmetic dentistry

Treatments to improve the appearance of the teeth. There are several dental techniques that can make the teeth look better by improving their color or shape. When discolorations of a tooth are superficial, a dentist or a dental hygienist can use a rotary polisher with polishing paste to remove the discoloration. If this process is not sufficiently effective, the teeth can be whitened, a common procedure provided by dentists. (SEE BLEACHING, DENTAL.) Com-

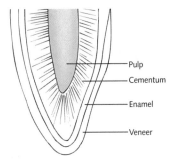

TOOTH VENEER
Dental veneer is a porcelain or acrylic laminate, applied in thin layers, that adheres to the surface of the tooth to form a coating over the natural enamel. The veneer can alter the color, texture, and shape of the tooth. Results last from 3 to 12 years.

C

COSMETIC IMPROVEMENT OF TEETH

Several options are available to improve the appearance of darkened or stained teeth:

- **Bleaching**: Lightens teeth that have darkened from tobacco, food stains, or age. This painless procedure can be performed by a dentist. The dentist paints the teeth with a bleaching solution and then uses heat or light to activate the whitening process. The dentist may apply the bleaching solution by painting it on the teeth or by using a mouthpiece. The treatment lasts at least 1 year, but its effects can be prolonged with home kits.
- **Bonding**: Involves applying a coating to teeth to help cover stains, fill gaps, or disguise cracks. The dentist applies a resin material onto the tooth and hardens it with a special curing light. Repairs last for up to 5 years.
- **Veneers**: Are thin shells that are attached to the surface of a tooth to correct uneven, stained, or chipped enamel. The veneer is applied with a soft plastic powder; the tooth is then shaped and polished. The procedure is painless, and results last from 3 to 12 years.

---

posite bonding may also be used to achieve the desired results. See BONDING, DENTAL.

Dental veneers (see VENEERS, DENTAL) can change the shape and texture of the tooth as well as its color. This procedure involves bonding a thin layer of porcelain or composite over the surface of a tooth to create an improved appearance. Veneering can correct irregularities in tooth enamel that has become stained, pitted, or worn. It may be recommended when there are overly wide, natural spaces between teeth or for irregularly spaced or crooked front teeth. Veneers can be used only on the surface that is not involved with chewing, such as the front teeth. The materials used can be blended to a shade that very closely matches the color of the surrounding teeth. Composite resin can be applied to the tooth or teeth in a series of very thin layers, which adhere to the enamel of the tooth. This procedure can be done in one visit. The porcelain veneer is a two-step process in which the front and top of the tooth are smoothed down and an impression is taken and sent to a dental laboratory. On the second appointment, the porcelain veneer is bonded onto the front of the tooth with a thin resin. The porcelain veneer is strong and resists staining.

Cosmetic surgery

Any procedure to enhance the appearance or beauty of a person rather than to resolve a medical problem. Common examples are FACE-LIFT, CHEMICAL PEEL, and EYELID SURGERY. Cosmetic surgery, considered a form of plastic surgery, involves procedures that primarily improve the appearance of an otherwise healthy person.

CONSIDERING COSMETIC SURGERY

Since cosmetic surgery is elective (nonessential), it is important to consider possible risks or complications as well as to acknowledge the benefits of a particular procedure. The decision to have cosmetic surgery is a personal one. The person considering the surgery needs to make sure that he or she is electing to have the surgery for the right reasons—and not to please someone else or as a way to find a mate or earn a job promotion.

The person should talk to the doctor about what kind of realistic results are achievable. Someone considering having a face-lift, for example, should realize that cosmetic surgery is still surgery and the body needs time to heal. It is important to talk to the doctor beforehand about how long it will be before bruising and swelling subside and positive results will become noticeable. People considering cosmetic surgery should also ask about the risks and side effects of the anesthesia that will be used.

Costochondritis

An inflammation of the cartilage attaching the front of the ribs to the breastbone, causing localized pain and tenderness. The area affected is generally the second or third rib attachment. The pain, which may be severe, tends to become more intense with movement or exercise. Pressure applied directly to the site can make the pain worse. Redness and swelling are not usually present. When there is swelling in the tender area, the condition is called Tietze syndrome. If the cause is not associated with physical injury to the rib cage, it may be difficult to determine the exact cause, which is often unknown. Because the onset of costochondritis yields sudden and intense chest pain, the condition may be mistaken for a heart attack. Diagnosis is by a process of elimination, including tests that exclude other possible causes. These tests may include chest X rays, electrocardiograms, and certain blood tests. Costochondritis is primarily treated with medication to relieve the associated discomfort, such as aspirin, ibuprofen, and other nonsteroidal anti-inflammatory drugs (NSAIDs). If the pain persists, a corticosteroid, such as cortisone, may be injected into the area to reduce the inflammation.

Co-trimoxazole

An antibiotic; a sulfonamide or sulfa drug. Co-trimoxazole, a trimethoprim-sulfamethoxazole combination drug (Bactrim, Septra), is used to treat several bacterial infections, including urinary tract infections, ear infections in children, *Pneumocystis carinii* pneumonia, other types of pneumonia, chronic bronchitis, and traveler's diarrhea.

Cough

FOR SYMPTOM CHART
see Coughing, page 28

A reflex that produces a sudden burst of air through the airways. Coughs clear material from the airways and help expel material from the lungs, including inhaled particles and sputum. Sputum, which is also called phlegm, is composed of a mixture of mucus, debris, and cells that have been shed from the lungs. Dry coughs do not produce sputum, but a productive cough indicates sputum production. Sputum that is yellow, green, or brown indicates a bacterial infection. When it is white, clear, or watery, a virus, allergy, or irritant is generally the cause. When sputum is examined microscopically, the presence of bacteria and white blood cells can confirm the diagnosis of an infection. Sputum can also be sent to a laboratory for culturing and special tests to identify the underlying disease.

A cough is a symptom that may be accompanied by other symptoms such as chest pain, shortness of breath, breathlessness, hoarseness, sore throat, and dizziness. In evaluating a cough, a doctor may need to know the length of time it has been present, the time of day it occurs, the presence of accompanying symptoms, the amount of sputum if any is produced, and the appearance or color of sputum. It may also be helpful to know whether factors such as cold air, body posture, talking, eating, or drinking may aggravate coughing.

Coughs may be related to several conditions, including infection, allergy, or fluid in the lungs. Treatment is usually directed at the underlying cause rather than at suppression of the cough, especially if large amounts of sputum are produced. Bringing up sputum and clearing the airways are important functions that should not be inhibited in some cases. Suppressing coughs with medication is appropriate when there is a nonproductive dry cough and the cough interferes with normal activities or sleep. Cough medications may also be used, even if sputum is produced, if coughing prevents sleep and causes exhaustion.

There are two types of cough medications, antitussives and expectorants. Antitussives suppress the cough reflex, and expectorants thin bronchial secretions and help loosen mucus so it is easier to bring up and expel. Antitussive medications include codeine, a narcotic painkiller that suppresses the cough center in the brain and must be prescribed by a doctor; dextromethorphan, an ingredient available in over-the-counter cough medications that suppresses the brain's cough center; demulcents, usually in lozenges and syrups to coat the irritated lining of the airways; and local anesthetics, cough reflex inhibitors that may be administered by a doctor to prevent coughing during examinations. Steam inhalation from a vaporizer and moisture inhalation from a cool-mist humidifier are techniques that reduce irritation in the pharynx and airways and loosen secretions so they are easier to expel.

Expectorants include iodides, guaifenesin, and terpin hydrate, which are common ingredients in over-the-counter cough products.

Cough remedies

Products available without prescription to help alleviate a cough. Coughing is a useful process in which secretions (mucus) are cleared from the throat and the lungs (a "productive" cough); productive coughs should never be suppressed, since they serve a valuable purpose. Sometimes, however, dry or unproductive coughing hurts the throat or interferes with sleep, and in those cases a cough remedy may be helpful. In all, there are more than 800 products on sale in the United States to help people cope with symptoms of colds, including cough.

Cough remedies are divided into three categories. Cough suppressants help to control a dry cough, usually in the early stage of a cold. Dry cough can irritate the throat, which leads to more coughing. Expectorants can help by loosening mucus congesting the lungs in order to cough it up. Cough-cold combinations are chiefly useful for relieving the cough associated with colds, flu, or hay fever. These combination drugs may also contain antihistamines, decongestants, and pain relievers.

Cough, chronic

FOR SYMPTOM CHART
see Coughing, page 28

A noisy expulsion of air from the lungs, usually sudden and involuntary, that is recurrent and may either produce a dry, hacking sound or bring up phlegm. Coughing is a protective reflex, generally activated when membranes lining the respiratory tract secrete excessive mucus or phlegm. These secretions help to protect the airways by accumulating and trapping viruses, bacteria, and foreign particles. By expelling this accumulation, coughing helps keep breathing passages open. Coughing may also prevent infectious mucus from coming in contact with the lungs and bronchial tubes, where it could lead to serious illnesses like PNEUMONIA or BRONCHITIS. When a cough recurs and is persistent for more than 3 weeks, it is termed a chronic cough.

CAUSES
The most common cause of coughing is an infection of the upper respiratory tract or a common cold. Usually within 2 weeks, when the infection clears up, the cough also disappears. Three medical conditions account for the majority of instances of chronic cough: POSTNASAL DRIP syndrome (inflammation of sinuses or lining of the nose causing a discharge that flows into the throat), ASTHMA, and chronic heartburn. In a smaller number of incidences, whooping cough, also called PERTUSSIS, may cause a persistent, unexplained cough; there is an effective vaccine available. Smokers or ex-smokers also may develop persistent coughs, which may be caused by chronic bronchitis, EMPHYSEMA, and CANCER of the lung and throat. Congestive heart failure (see HEART FAILURE, CONGESTIVE) may also cause coughing.

A physician should be consulted when a cough continues to get worse after about a week. This prolonged duration of coughing, together with other possible symptoms, may indicate the presence of a serious medical problem. Laboratory tests or imaging studies may be necessary to diagnose the underlying cause.

Cough, smoker's

A noisy expulsion of air from the lungs that is associated with cigarette or cigar smoking. See also COUGH; COUGH, CHRONIC.

Coughing up blood

Expelling sputum that contains blood. Coughing up blood, also called hemoptysis, occurs somewhat frequently, and, while it may be alarming, it is not usually serious if there is not a large quantity of blood. The presence of blood flecks in sputum may indicate acute or chronic BRONCHITIS. When large amounts of blood are coughed up, however, a prompt medical evaluation is necessary.

CAUSES
Tumors of the respiratory tract, particularly lung tumors, may result in coughing up blood. In people who smoke and are older than 40, the presence of blood in the sputum requires an evaluation to rule out cancer.

Another cause of this symptom is blockage of an artery supplying blood to the tissue of the lungs, a condition called PULMONARY EMBOLISM, which occurs when a blood clot lodges in the artery. When this condition causes lung tissue to die, a condition called PULMONARY INFARCTION, the person may cough up bloody sputum.

Heart failure, lung infections, and bronchiectasis can also cause the coughing up of blood. Also, blood vessels of the lungs may be damaged inadvertently during a medical procedure to measure blood pressure in the heart and lungs. This procedure involves inserting a CATHETER into an artery or vein of the lungs. If damage occurs, there may be severe bleeding with coughing.

DIAGNOSIS AND TREATMENT
Diagnosing the underlying cause when a person coughs up blood is crucial. The first step is a chest X ray, which may help identify the underlying cause. Often an examination called BRONCHOSCOPY uses a viewing instrument to observe the bronchial tubes to locate the area of bleeding. A perfusion scan, which uses a radioactive marker, can reveal the blockage of a lung artery, which is usually a sign of a pulmonary embolism. When sputum contains only a few blood streaks that are determined to be caused by an infection, treatment may not be necessary; alternatively, antibiotics may be prescribed to clear up the infection causing the blood-streaked sputum.

If the bleeding occurs in a major blood vessel and a large amount of blood is coughed up, treatment to stop the bleeding is usually necessary. Bronchial artery embolization may be used to close off the bleeding vessel. This procedure involves the use of X rays to guide a catheter into the affected vessel where a chemical that closes the vessel is injected. Bleeding caused by heart failure or pneumonia generally subsides when the condition is medically treated.

If the blood in the respiratory system produces clots large enough to block the airways and inhibit breathing, it is important to avoid suppressing the cough. In some cases, RESPIRATORY THERAPY is required to aid in this process. If the clot is large and located in a major bronchial tube, it can be removed with the use of a bronchoscope.

Surgery may be required to remove a diseased area of the lung if this is causing coughed up blood. If a tumor is discovered that is inoperable, treatment with radiation and chemotherapy should be considered. Conditions that cause clotting abnormalities may contribute to coughing up blood and can be treated with transfusions of plasma, clotting factors, or platelets to promote clotting.

Counseling, psychological

A relationship in which a trained professional helps another person understand and resolve his or her emotional problems. In most types of psychological counseling, the individual talks about his or her problems with the counselor or therapist. The counselor tries to understand the problems troubling the person, raises the individual's awareness, and helps him or her deal with thoughts, feelings, or behaviors that cause distress.

Sometimes the word "counseling" refers to the treatment of people with mild problems, and "psychotherapy" describes the treatment of severe disturbance. However, the words are often used interchangeably. Psychological counseling is also known as talk therapy.

Psychological counseling can be effective for dealing with problems such as alcohol or drug abuse, anxiety, or depression that cannot be resolved by talking with family or friends. Counseling can also be helpful with issues that are particularly uncomfortable, such as sexual abuse. In many cases, simply talking about the problem with a professional can help alleviate distress. Depending on the problem, psychological counseling may be combined with other forms of treatment, such as prescribed medication.

The methods used in psychological counseling vary with the training of the particular counselor. See BEHAVIOR THERAPY; COGNITIVE-BEHAVIORAL THERAPY; and PSYCHOANALYSIS.

Couples therapy

Counseling or psychotherapy that focuses on the interactions between two people in a long-term relationship. Also known as marital therapy or marriage therapy, couples therapy is used for married couples, homosexual partners, and unmarried heterosexual couples. Common reasons for entering into couples therapy include feelings of being unloved, criticized, constantly belittled, or neglected in the relationship. Concern about incompatibility and complaints about sex are also common. Couples therapy is sometimes used when a family problem, such as an emotional disturbance in a child, can be traced to emotional upset between the adult partners.

HOW IT IS DONE
A number of approaches and techniques are used. Behavioral couples therapy emphasizes replacing troubling behaviors with beneficial ones by creating ways for the couple to discuss problems, develop solutions, and come to agreements. Integrative behavioral therapy adds techniques designed to help each partner accept the other's personal differences as a necessary and desirable part of their relationship.

Research shows that when the problem bringing the couple to therapy is a relationship issue, therapy with both partners together is more effective than individual therapy. To date, no one therapeutic approach has been shown to be superior to any other.

Coxa vara

A congenital deformity of the hip joint in which the neck of the thighbone bends downward.

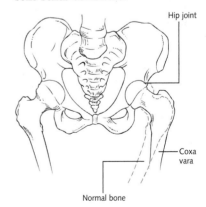

A HIP DEFORMITY
Coxa vara causes a difference in the way the two hip joints bear weight, usually resulting in a shortened leg and a limp.

Coxsackievirus

Any of a group of viruses that cause a variety of infectious diseases, including a mild form of MENINGITIS and HAND-FOOT-AND-MOUTH DISEASE. Coxsackie-viruses are always present in the environment in forms that change from one year to the next, mostly occurring in the summer months. The infection from one form of the virus may not cause symptoms, while other forms of the virus can cause a variety of symptoms. The most common symptoms of an infection include flulike malaise, fever, and muscle aches. There may also be coughing, nasal congestion, diarrhea, and vomiting.

Coxsackieviruses can cause a mild form of meningitis, called aseptic meningitis, and, rarely, transient paralysis. The symptoms of aseptic meningitis include pain and stiffness in the neck and back, muscular aches, fever, malaise, loss of appetite, and vomiting. The symptoms may disappear within a week, but fatigue and irritability may persist for a month or longer.

When the virus causes hand-foot-and-mouth disease, most commonly in infants and children, a skin rash develops on the face, neck, and chest. Fever may develop, and the infection may progress to aseptic meningitis.

Inflammation of the heart muscle (MYOCARDITIS) and inflammation of the membranous sac that encloses the heart (PERICARDITIS) may also be caused by a coxsackievirus. Myocarditis in newborns produces symptoms including a sudden fever and feeding difficulties. It can be fatal to infants. In adults, the symptom is chest pain, but complete recovery is common.

CAUSE AND DIAGNOSIS

Infections with coxsackieviruses occur by exposure to an infected person via inhalation of that person's respiratory droplets or by exposure to fecal discharges. One group of these viruses is identified in sewage, suggesting that contact with contaminated water may transmit the infection. Like all viruses, coxsackieviruses can replicate themselves only in living host cells, so the viruses do not increase in number while in water.

Coxsackievirus infections are diagnosed by isolating the virus from the throat or stool specimens. Because it is a virus, medical options are limited and treatment is directed toward managing symptoms.

Crab lice

Small, crablike organisms that attach themselves to human hairs. Crab lice usually live in pubic hair, but may also become attached to eyelashes, eyebrows, and hair in the armpits or on the face. The lice, also called pubic lice or pediculosis pubis, can survive outside the human body for up to 48 hours and may be transmitted by contact with an infested person's bed linens, towels, or clothes. Infestations are transmitted by direct physical contact with a person who has crab lice, especially of the genital areas during sexual activity. They are not generally transferred from furniture or toilet seats as the lice rarely survive falling from a host. Also, they do not jump from one person to another in everyday contact and are not transmitted to or from animals.

Infestations of crab lice occur when the adults lay their white, shiny eggs, which are called nits, on the hair shafts close to the skin. The nits hatch within 7 to 10 days. The nits are the size of a pinhead and difficult to see; they may resemble dandruff. The hatched crab lice are grayish-white or brown and may blend with skin tones. The brown lice can be mistaken for small moles.

SYMPTOMS AND TREATMENT

There may be no symptoms of infestation, or symptoms may appear immediately or may take several

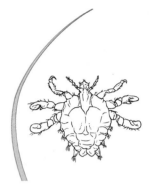

HATCHED LICE
A hatched crab louse is about the size of a pinhead (here it is magnified in size and compared to a human hair) and is gray or brown. The lice cling tightly to the skin and are easy to overlook. They may even appear to be tiny moles. Itching is the most noticeable symptom.

weeks to become noticeable if the eggs have not hatched. In most instances, the lice cause itching, which becomes worse at night. A bluish rash is sometimes observed at the site of the bites. If lice are in the eyelashes or eyebrows, the eyes may become inflamed.

When an infestation of crab lice is suspected, medical attention should be sought. The nits cannot be banished by soap and water washing as they cling tightly to the hair shafts. Destroying them requires an over-the-counter medication, usually lindane or pyrethrin solution. Instructions for use must be followed precisely.

People with dense body hair should

PREVENTING LICE REINFESTATION

Because crab lice are so highly contagious, it is essential to clean every item that may have come in contact with the lice, including bed linen, clothing, undergarments, and even the bathroom and bedroom where the person with the lice has been. To prevent reinfestation, the person should:

- Machine wash in very hot water all items that have come into contact with the skin since symptoms started, including all undergarments, clothing, towels, bed sheets, and pillowcases. "Dry clean only" items can be sealed in plastic bags for 30 days or dry-cleaned.
- Wear only clean undergarments and clothing following treatment.
- Clean the bathroom, shower, and bedroom thoroughly. In the bathroom, a 70 percent alcohol solution, bleach, or bathroom cleanser should be used. Spray products are available for sanitizing mattresses, upholstery, and carpeting.
- Set aside all items that cannot be thoroughly cleaned and avoid all contact with them for 2 weeks to allow lice eggs to hatch and die before transferring to a human.
- Advise sexual partners to seek a medical examination for crab lice, and abstain from sexual contact until infestation has been completely resolved.
- Discard infected combs and hats.

apply the medication to the trunk, thighs, armpits, and all other areas where infestation may have occurred. Nits may not be destroyed by the medication and can be removed with a fine-toothed comb for this purpose that can be purchased at a pharmacy. It may be necessary to reapply the medication 1 week later.

Itching may persist after treatment. If the areas affected by crab lice show signs of redness, swelling, tenderness, or drainage following treatment, medical attention should be sought. Once medical treatment is completed, it is important to take measures to prevent recurrence.

Crack cocaine

A particularly addictive form of the drug cocaine that can be smoked to produce an intense, short-lasting state of euphoria or "high." The most potent stimulant of natural origin, cocaine comes from the leaves of the coca plant (*Erythroxylon coca*), which is found in the Andean highlands of South America. The leaves are cooked into a coca paste, which is then processed into a powder form, usually cocaine hydrochloride. Processing cocaine hydrochloride with ammonia or baking soda (sodium bicarbonate) and water, then heating the mixture to remove the hydrochloride yields crack cocaine. The end product is a form of cocaine that can be smoked. Crack cocaine, so named because of the cracking sound made by the baking soda when the drug is heated, is also called rock cocaine because of its stonelike appearance.

Cocaine is highly addictive, particularly when smoked. Smoking delivers the drug to the bloodstream as quickly as an injection, and it affects the person's brain almost immediately, causing euphoria, reduced fatigue, and decreased mental clarity that lasts 5 to 10 minutes. Crack cocaine can also produce aggressively paranoid behavior, which may cause the person to explode into violent actions. Speech may be slurred, and the user may feel confused and anxious. In most cases, the high diminishes with repeated use of the drug, and the user may increase the dose to recapture the lost pleasure. Addiction can come from as little as one use. People who stop using crack cocaine often experience depression

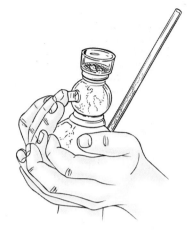

SMOKING CRACK COCAINE
Crack cocaine is a highly purified form of cocaine that has been chemically altered so that it can be smoked in a pipe or injected (unlike powdered cocaine, which is usually sniffed). Either smoking or injection delivers the drug to the bloodstream rapidly and efficiently, which is why crack cocaine is especially dangerous.

and may return to the drug to raise their mood.

Crack cocaine carries considerable physical risk. Cocaine can sharply raise body temperature, heart rate, and blood pressure. Its use can lead to seizures and sudden death from respiratory failure, stroke, cerebral hemorrhage (bleeding in the brain), or heart failure. Lung trauma and bleeding can cause coughing, severe chest pain, and shortness of breath.

Mental health is also affected. Crack cocaine addiction may cause violent or erratic behavior, hallucinations (for example, the sensation that bugs are crawling over the person's skin), confusion, anxiety, depression, and loss of interest in food, sex, friends, sports, hobbies, and other pleasurable pursuits. When crack cocaine is simultaneously used along with alcohol, the liver combines them into a third substance, cocaethylene, which intensifies the cocaine euphoria but also may increase the risk of sudden death from cardiac causes.

Cradle cap

A condition in babies in which thick, yellow scales form in patches over the scalp. Cradle cap is a form of SEBORRHEIC DERMATITIS. Cradle cap is common during the first 3 months of life

but infrequent after 1 year of age. However, episodes of seborrheic dermatitis may return in adolescence (when the sebaceous or oil-producing glands become more active) and persist throughout life. Cradle cap usually resolves on its own without any special treatment by age 12 months. Remedies include using over-the-counter medicated shampoos, massaging mineral oil into the scalp, and using a soft toothbrush to remove scales. If cradle cap is causing discomfort, parents should consult a pediatrician. If over-the-counter shampoos fail to cure cradle cap, a doctor can prescribe a more potent shampoo.

Cramp

A sudden, painful spasm in a muscle due to an excessive and prolonged contraction of the muscle fibers. Common causes include overuse, muscle stress, and dehydration. Exercise-related cramps usually occur during or immediately after workouts, due to muscle fiber damage and a buildup of chemicals such as lactic acid. Less common causes of cramps include overuse, as in writer's cramp (see CRAMP, WRITER'S); an inadequate blood supply, which may be due to ARTERIOSCLEROSIS (narrowing of the arteries); compression of nerves in the spine; potassium loss (possibly due to diuretic medications); and pregnancy.

Muscle cramps most often affect the leg muscles. Nighttime leg cramps may be caused by poor circulation. Measures to relieve cramps include drinking plenty of fluids to avoid

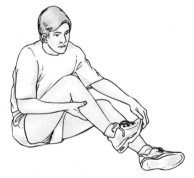

RELIEVING A CRAMP
When a leg muscle cramps, gently flexing the foot upward often helps. Massage or walking around briefly may also give relief. Cramps are not usually a sign of a serious medical problem.

dehydration, stretching before and after exercise, massage, application of heat and cold packs, and over-the-counter medications such as analgesics. Any unexplained cramp that is not relieved by simple self-care measures should be evaluated by a doctor.

Cramp, writer's

Painful spasms in the muscles of the hand that make it difficult to write. A simple and transient case of writer's cramp affects the thumb and first two fingers of the writing hand; it is caused by using the same muscles for long periods. A more serious form of writer's cramp is believed to be caused by abnormal functioning of the brain. This is a separate problem from overuse conditions and may require treatment with oral medications, botulinum toxin injections, or surgery.

Cranberry

A natural substance used to treat urinary tract infections. Components of cranberry prevent bacteria from adhering to the lining of the bladder. Cranberry is available in pill form as well as in sweetened juice products.

Cranial nerves

Twelve pairs of nerves originating in the brain that control most of the functions in the head and face, including the sense organs. Most of the cranial nerves originate in the brain stem, but two (the olfactory and optic nerves) connect to the cerebrum. Nerve pathways may also relay information from the cranial nerves to higher areas of the brain. Some of the cranial nerves carry only sensory signals from the sense organs, others carry motor messages to move the muscles of the organs and structures of the head, and some carry autonomic (involuntary) messages for functions such as heartbeat. Some of the cranial nerves have all three capabilities.

The first cranial nerve, called the olfactory nerve, controls the sense of smell. The second cranial nerve is the optic nerve, which controls sight. The third, fourth, and sixth cranial nerves (oculomotor, trochlear, and abducent) direct eye movements. The fifth, the trigeminal nerve, is concerned with facial sensations and jaw movements. The seventh, the facial

nerve, directs facial expressions and taste. The eighth, the acoustic (or vestibulocochlear) controls hearing and balance. The ninth, the glossopharyngeal nerve, controls movement and sensation from the back of the tongue to the throat, the secretion of saliva, and some branches of the facial nerves responsible for taste. The tenth cranial nerve, also called the vagus nerve, is concerned with the vital functions of breathing, circulation, and digestion. The 11th, the spinal accessory nerve, directs movements of the neck and back, and the 12th cranial nerve, the hypoglossal nerve, regulates the movements of the tongue. See How cranial nerves function, page 417.

Craniofacial dysostosis

A birth defect comprising a characteristic group of deformities that involve an abnormal fusion, or joining, between some of the bones of the skull and face (see BIRTH DEFECTS). The fusion does not allow the craniofacial bones (bones of the skull and face) to grow normally, which affects the shape of the head and the appearance of the face as well as the positioning of the teeth. Sometimes called Apert-Crouzon syndrome, or Crouzon disease, after the doctor who first observed the birth defect, craniofacial dysostosis is caused by an abnormal-

ity in the genes. If neither parent shows signs of the syndrome, the abnormality may be the result of a change in the genetic material at the time of conception; the exact cause of this change is not known.

Craniofacial dysostosis varies in severity. The major associated problem is an underdevelopment of the upper jaw, causing a facial deformity characterized by bulging eyes and a sunken middle portion of the face. An abnormal relationship between the upper and lower jaws, called MAL-OCCLUSION, is also a feature of the syndrome. Dental and plastic surgery specialists can monitor facial growth and sometimes correct such deformities. Mental retardation is not usually a feature of the syndrome. Individuals born with it may have ear problems, including ear disease and hearing loss, as well as eye problems such as crossed eyes, excessive tearing, or dry eyes. It is recommended that parents of an infant born with craniofacial dysostosis contact a craniofacial center for a complete evaluation of the child, as well as for treatment planning and comprehensive related services.

Craniopharyngioma

A slow-growing, calcified, cystic tumor of the brain that is usually benign (not cancerous), develops near the pituitary gland, and usually

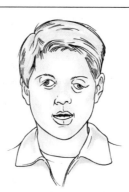

DYSOSTOSIS
A child born with craniofacial dysostosis (Crouzon syndrome) may have an unusually shaped head, receded cheekbones or jaw, bulging or prominent eyes, crossed eyes, or irregular teeth because of abnormal growth and joining of the bones of the skull and face. He or she may also have some vision or hearing problems. Mental capacity is usually normal.

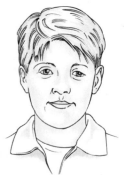

AFTER SURGERY
Dental and facial surgery can correct many characteristics of craniofacial dysostosis. In the child's first year, the rigid joints between the bones of the skull may be released to permit brain growth. For best results surgery is generally performed in several stages as the child grows. With surgical and other treatment, many affected children can be active and have a normal appearance.

HOW CRANIAL NERVES FUNCTION

Each of the 12 pairs of cranial nerves has a different job. Some deliver sensory information from organs, such as the eyes, ears, and nose, to the brain. Others transmit the messages that move the facial muscles and tongue or that stimulate the salivary glands. A few of the nerves have both sensory and motor functions.

THE 12 CRANIAL NERVES
All but two of the cranial nerves connect in the brain stem; the other two, the olfactory and optic nerves, link directly with parts of the cerebrum.

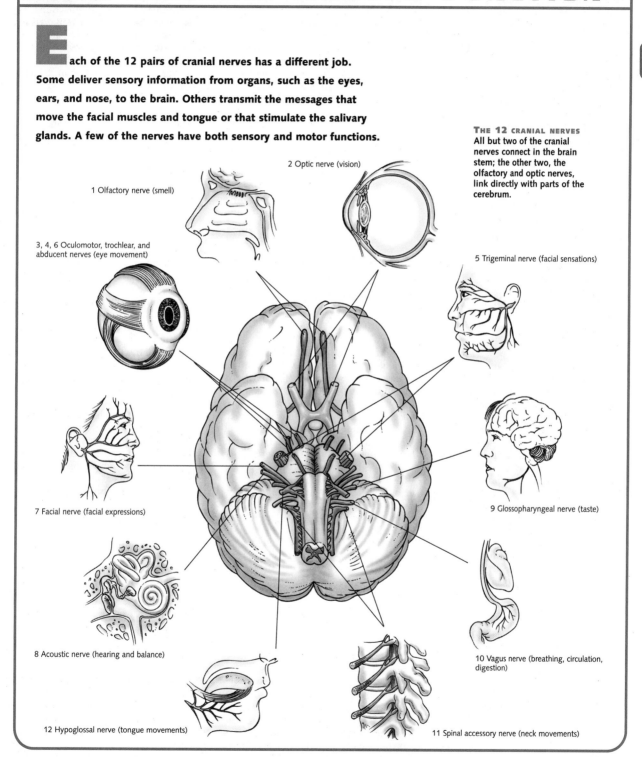

1 Olfactory nerve (smell)

2 Optic nerve (vision)

3, 4, 6 Oculomotor, trochlear, and abducent nerves (eye movement)

5 Trigeminal nerve (facial sensations)

7 Facial nerve (facial expressions)

9 Glossopharyngeal nerve (taste)

8 Acoustic nerve (hearing and balance)

10 Vagus nerve (breathing, circulation, digestion)

12 Hypoglossal nerve (tongue movements)

11 Spinal accessory nerve (neck movements)

affects children or older adults. A craniopharyngioma may be associated with increased pressure within the cranium. The tumor usually develops in the pituitary stalk and projects into the hypothalamus. In rare instances, it may develop in or migrate to the opening between the nose and throat or extend into the cervical spine.

In children, a craniopharyngioma generally consists of cells that have been derived from the membrane that lines the inside of the embryonic craniopharyngeal canal (the duct between a part of the brain and the mouth and throat in a fetus). This passageway narrows and closes by the end of the second month of gestation. Craniopharyngioma may originate in the fetus from remnant cells from this activity. In adults, the tumor generally originates from an overgrowth of cells at the front of the pituitary gland.

SYMPTOMS

Craniopharyngiomas are generally considered nonfunctioning tumors, meaning that they do not produce excess levels of hormones that are released into the bloodstream. Although the tumors are almost always benign, they can invade surrounding structures. Symptoms, if any, may not become evident for several years because the tumor grows so slowly.

There may be no symptoms of these tumors. If there are symptoms, they are the result of the pressure the tumor applies to tissues surrounding the pituitary gland. A common symptom is a slowly progressive, dull, and localized headache. Other symptoms include weight gain, fatigue, constipation, intolerance to cold, hypoglycemia (low blood sugar), cardiac arrhythmia, lethargy, confusion, loss of appetite, nausea, vomiting, excessive thirst and urination, and, in men, decreased sexual drive and erectile dysfunction. Children with a craniopharyngioma may fail to grow at a normal rate, and puberty may be delayed. Vision problems may occur if there is pressure on the optic nerve from the tumor. Other symptoms may

---

> Terms in small capital letters—for example, PHYSICAL THERAPY or PAGET DISEASE—indicate a cross-reference to another entry with more information.

---

include obesity, muscular movement disturbances, emotional immaturity, loss of short-term memory, and incontinence.

DIAGNOSIS AND TREATMENT

A craniopharyngioma is diagnosed by general physical examination, a neurologic evaluation, and MRI (magnetic resonance imaging). Other tests may include those for pituitary function.

If a craniopharyngioma causes excessive pressure on the brain or other conditions that are considered serious and possibly life-threatening, surgical removal of the tumor may become necessary, followed by radiation therapy. If the tumor adheres to surrounding blood vessels, it may be impossible to remove it entirely. Craniopharyngiomas have a tendency to recur at their original site. Survival rates are excellent for children and people younger than 20 years but are poor for those older than 65 years.

Craniosacral technique

See VISUALIZATION.

Craniosynostosis

Premature or early closure of one or more of the openings in the skull of a newborn. Babies are normally born with the seven bones of the skull separated by fibrous borders (sutures). The soft spot where sutures intersect is called a FONTANELLE. The fact that the bones of the skull are not solidly fused at birth enables the shape of the infant's head to mold as it passes through the birth canal and later permits the skull to expand as the brain grows in early infancy. In craniosynostosis, the sutures close too early. A deformed skull, pressure on the brain, and vision problems can result. The cause is not always known, although some types of craniosynostosis are inherited. In some cases, it occurs because the brain is not growing properly. Craniosynostosis is sometimes accompanied by another birth defect, polydactyly, the presence of extra fingers and toes at birth.

Craniosynostosis takes two forms. Isolated craniosynostosis usually involves only one cranial suture and is not an inherited condition. Craniosynostosis syndromes, by contrast, usually involve the premature

---

closure of several sutures and may be associated with facial deformities. This type of craniosynostosis is usually inherited, and genetic counseling is recommended to parents with a family history of the problem.

DIAGNOSIS AND TREATMENT

Craniosynostosis is usually first suspected by a pediatrician, family physician, or geneticist, who may refer the child to a pediatric neurosurgeon or a craniofacial surgeon. The suture ridges and fontanelles are examined. The child's face and head are measured, and CT (computed tomography) or photographic images of the brain may be used to identify places where the bones of the skull have fused.

The fusion of a single suture may not need treatment. However, the treatment of more extensive craniosynostosis requires procedures performed by teams that specialize in craniofacial surgery. The type of surgery depends on the location of the prematurely fused bones. The extent of the fusion determines how soon after birth surgery is required. When all the sutures are fused, for example, the baby should be operated on as soon after birth as possible to permit the brain to grow normally and to relieve the pressure on the eyes and brain. Most surgery for craniosynostosis is done between 3 and 6 months of age, when the bones of the skull are comparatively easy to manipulate. Because the growing brain continues to reshape the skull and face after the surgery, a second operation is sometimes required when the child is 4 or 5 years old.

Craniotomy

A procedure to remove a section, or flap, of the skull to expose and operate on the tissues underneath, usually the brain. A craniotomy is used to repair aneurysms and ruptured blood vessels, remove tumors of the brain, fix malformed arteries and veins, and treat blockages in the flow of cerebrospinal fluid (a condition called HYDROCEPHALUS).

In a craniotomy, small burr holes (see BURR HOLE) are first drilled into the skull; then, a saw is used to cut between the holes and free the flap so it can be removed. After the surgery is

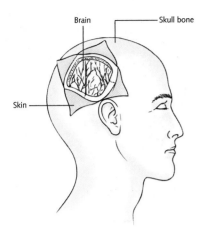

OPERATING ON BRAIN TISSUE
In order to operate on the brain—to remove a tumor or repair an injured blood vessel, for example—a surgeon must remove a section of the skull. To perform a craniotomy, the surgeon drills small holes in the bone and then saws between the holes. The section of bone is removed to operate on the brain, and then the bone is replaced and attached with wire sutures or titanium screws.

complete, the flap is put back in place with wire sutures or titanium screws. If the opening was made in an area such as the forehead where it affects appearance, small titanium plates are placed over the burr holes to erase indentations in the skin.

Cranium
The part of the SKULL that encloses the brain; sometimes used to refer to all the bones of the skull.

Creatinine
See KIDNEY FUNCTION TESTS.

Creatinine clearance
See KIDNEY FUNCTION TESTS.

Creative visualization
See VISUALIZATION.

Cremation
An alternative to burial in which a dead body is disposed of by burning it to ashes. The ashes can be kept by the family or discarded by the crematorium. A physician must examine a body if it is to be cremated in order to prevent destruction of any possible evidence to a crime.

Crepitus
An abnormal sound, such as the grating of fractured bones when moved or a rattling in the lungs that indicates a diseased condition. Gas or air trapped within the tissues of the skin leads to rapid swelling and creates a crackly sensation or noise when the swollen area is pressed with fingers. This type of crepitus is associated with gas GANGRENE, a rare but severe form of tissue death that follows an infection by *Clostridium* bacteria, usually at the site of trauma or a recent surgical wound.

CREST syndrome
A form of the disease SCLERODERMA, an autoimmune disorder in which the body's immune system attacks its own tissues.

CREST is an acronym that includes the following syndromes: calcinosis, which is a calcification in the skin; Raynaud phenomenon, which causes a sequence of color changes in the fingers and toes in response to cold; esophageal dysfunction, which may be gastroesophageal reflux or difficulty swallowing; sclerodactyly, which is a narrowing and hardening of the skin of the fingers or toes; and telangiectasia, which is a dilation of the tiny blood vessels, especially those in the skin.

Scleroderma, the disease responsible for CREST syndrome, may be caused by a malfunction of the immune system and an inflammation in the connective tissue surrounding the capillaries. The inflammation causes internal scarring as it heals, and this shrinks and stiffens the tissues involved. Usually the skin and the esophagus are affected. The lungs and kidneys may be affected as well. It usually begins between the ages of 20 and 40 and is more common in women than in men.

Creutzfeldt-Jakob disease
A rare, fatal condition characterized by a rapidly progressive mental deterioration and muscle wasting. An abnormal cellular protein causes degeneration of nerves and glial (connective) tissue in the brain causing vacuoles (holes) within the brain called spongiform encephalopathy. People with Creutzfeldt-Jakob disease

develop seizures and involuntary movements, as well as weakness, imbalance, and confusion. These changes ultimately lead to death. See MAD COW DISEASE.

CRH
Corticotropin-releasing hormone. A hormone produced by the hypothalamus that stimulates the pituitary gland to release ACTH (adrenocorticotropic hormone).

Cricothyroidotomy
An emergency intervention to provide an open breathing passage for an individual who cannot breathe or breathes only with great difficulty because of a blockage in the upper respiratory system. A needle is inserted into the TRACHEA (windpipe) through the skin and a membrane called the cricothyroid, which lies just below the prominent bulge of the LARYNX (voice box). A breathing device attached to the hollow needle then sends air in and out of the lungs.

A cricothyroidotomy is now generally preferred to a TRACHEOSTOMY, in which an opening for breathing is

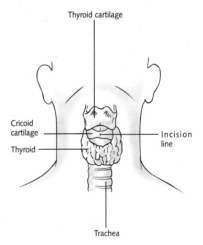

AN EMERGENCY AIRWAY
For a person whose breathing is obstructed (for instance, when someone is choking on an inhaled object), a doctor can perform an emergency procedure to open an airway. The doctor makes an incision in the neck between two pieces of throat cartilage—the cricoid and thyroid cartilages. The incision is just below the Adam's apple (thyroid cartilage). A hollow needle is inserted through the incision into the trachea (windpipe). A tube attached to the needle keeps air moving in and out until the obstruction is removed.

made in the trachea below the larynx. A tracheostomy involves a greater risk of bleeding because large blood vessels in the area can be cut accidentally. No such vessels are found in the cricothyroid area, making this procedure safer.

Crisis intervention

Providing immediate care or advice to people with acute physical or psychological problems. In psychiatry, crisis intervention constitutes a form of intense, short-term therapy that centers on the event that triggered an emotional trauma.

Critical

Pertaining to a period of crisis in a person with a life-threatening medical condition. In critical or intensive care, doctors use technologically sophisticated equipment to treat and monitor the conditions of people who are recovering from surgery or who have experienced life-threatening problems such as heart attacks or severe injuries or burns.

Less acute medical conditions are commonly described as serious (when vital signs are unstable and not within normal limits), fair (when vital signs are stable and within normal limits and the person is conscious but may be experiencing some degree of discomfort), or good (when vital signs are within normal limits and the person is conscious and comfortable). When a person's medical condition does not get worse or improve, it is typically described as stable.

Critical care

Assessing and treating the health of a person at immediate risk of dying. A patient who may die is referred to as being in critical condition. Critical care, also known as intensive care, covers the whole process of treating seriously ill patients.

The INTENSIVE CARE UNIT of the hospital provides state-of-the-art, 24-hour care by doctors and nurses who are trained to take aggressive and immediate action to intervene, whenever necessary, to save the life of a patient. Critical care staff keep a constant watch on their patients by monitoring blood pressure, blood gases, kidney and lung function, brain activity, body temperature, and urine

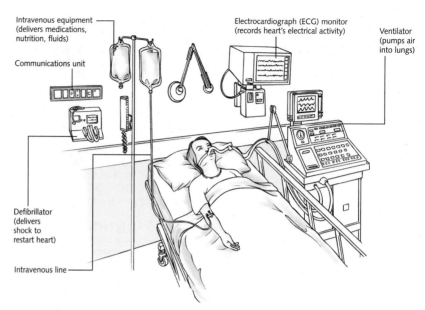

CRITICAL OR INTENSIVE CARE UNIT
The sophisticated equipment in the critical care unit is designed for immediate treatment of life-threatening developments in a person's condition. The specialized critical care staff closely monitors a person's vital signs and body functions so that they can intervene at the first signs of difficulty.

output. Critical care also involves grief counseling and support for relatives and close friends if the person who is being cared for dies.

Crohn disease

Chronic inflammatory disease of the digestive tract. Crohn disease is also known as enteritis, ileitis, and regional enteritis. Although it can occur anywhere in the digestive tract, from the mouth to the anus, this disease most frequently affects the colon (large intestine) and the ileum (small intestine) where they join. Crohn disease shares many similarities with ulcerative COLITIS, and the two are considered types of INFLAMMATORY BOWEL DISEASE.

SYMPTOMS AND CAUSES

Abdominal pain and diarrhea are the most common symptoms of Crohn disease. Frequently, these problems follow a meal. Other signs include fever, joint pains, loss of appetite, and weight loss. Inflammation of the lining of the intestine, anal fissure (a tear or ulcer in the lining of the anal canal), anal fistula (an abnormal channel formed between the anal canal and a tiny hole in the skin surrounding the anus), or an ABSCESS may also develop. The disease usually first develops between ages 20 and

30. Although remission is possible, the disease often continues intermittently throughout a person's life.

The cause is unknown. However, doctors believe that an agent, such as a virus or bacterium, alters the body's immune system, triggering inflammation in the intestinal wall. Contributing factors may include genetic predisposition, diet, and stress. Several complications occur far from the intestine, supporting the theory that there is an autoimmune component to this disease (see AUTOIMMUNE DISORDERS). Such complications may include sacroiliitis (inflammation of the sacroiliac joint at the base of the back), spondylitis (a painful type of arthritis that affects primarily the joints of vertebrae in the back), erythema nodosum (a skin condition in which red areas of swelling appear on the legs), and iritis (inflammation of the iris in the eye). When the symptoms of Crohn disease subside, these conditions also generally improve.

DIAGNOSIS

Diagnosis is based on a complete physical examination and tests, such as stool analysis, blood tests, a lower GASTROINTESTINAL (GI) SERIES (an X-ray procedure also known as a barium enema), and SIGMOIDOSCOPY or COLON-

OSCOPY (examinations of the rectum and colon using flexible viewing tubes passed through the anus). It can be difficult to differentiate between Crohn disease and ulcerative colitis. Crohn disease is slightly less common than ulcerative colitis in the United States.

TREATMENT
Treatment is with anti-inflammatory drugs. The goal of both aspirin-based anti-inflammatory drugs, such as sulfasalazine, and corticosteroids, such as prednisone, is to suppress the inflammatory response so the body can heal itself. Powerful corticosteroids more successfully control stubborn cases of inflammation, but they also have many unwanted side effects. These include bloating, weight gain, brittle bones, nervousness, and insomnia. Immunosuppressants and antibiotics may also be prescribed. Severe attacks generally require hospitalization and intravenous administration of medication. If a great deal of blood has been lost, a transfusion may be required.

When medication cannot control the symptoms or a complication develops, a colectomy (surgical removal of all or part of the colon) becomes necessary. When only part of the colon is removed, the healthy remaining sections are joined to maintain a passageway for stool. When this is not possible, a colostomy is performed, in which an opening called a STOMA is made in the abdominal wall to allow discharge of feces into an external bag. A similar procedure on the small intestine, or ileum, is known as an ILEOSTOMY. Colostomies and ileostomies can be temporary or permanent.

Cromolyn sodium

An antiasthma drug. Cromolyn (Intal) is prescribed as an inhalant to prevent asthma, especially exercise-induced asthma attacks. Cromolyn (Nasalcrom) is available as nose drops to treat a stuffy or runny nose caused by hay fever, sinusitis, or other allergies. Cromolyn (Gastro-crom) is a liquid medicine used to treat food allergy reactions, inflammatory bowel disease, and symptoms of systemic mastocytosis (abnormal proliferation of mast cells in various tissues).

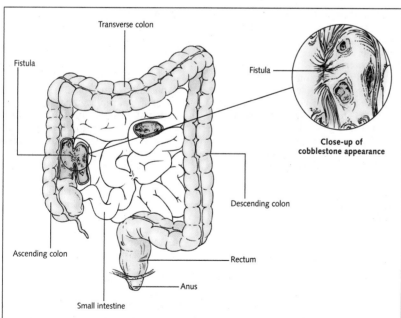

INFLAMMATION OF THE INTESTINE
A person with Crohn disease experiences chronic inflammation of the intestine. The disease can occur anywhere in the digestive tract, but most commonly affects the area close to the junction of the large and small intestines. The swelling and inflammation cause the inner intestinal wall to have a cobblestone appearance. Ulceration from the disease can create fistulas (abnormal channels between organs or parts of organs).

Crossbite

A form of irregular alignment (MALOCCLUSION) that involves the way the teeth meet when a person bites down. Some of the upper teeth tend to close inside or outside the lower teeth. A crossbite may sometimes be referred to as a deep bite. As with all bite irregularities, the problem may be cosmetic and may also involve problems with increased tooth decay because the teeth are harder to clean. In some cases, a crossbite may result in problems with the other teeth, which do not meet properly. Jaw problems and pain in the jaw sometimes occur. A crossbite may be due to heredity, to improper jaw growth, to habits such as sucking on the fingers and lips, or to tongue thrust, when a person unknowingly thrusts his or her tongue forward and puts pressure on the teeth. A dentist specializing in ORTHODONTICS can correct a person's crossbite with dental braces (see BRACES, DENTAL).

Crossed eyes

See STRABISMUS.

Crossmatching

A laboratory test to determine a person's blood group by identifying the proteins on the red blood cells; also known as blood typing and ABO typing. Crossmatching is important for determining the safety of blood transfusions. If blood from one blood group is transfused into a person with a different blood group, antibodies in the recipient's blood will attack the donated blood. Transfusions between people of the same blood group almost always succeed.

There are four principal blood groups: A, B, AB, and O. The blood groups are further divided by the presence or absence of the Rh factor (for rhesus, the name of the species of monkey in which the factor was discovered). Blood with the Rh factor is Rh-positive (+); blood without it is Rh negative (–). The most common blood group among Americans is O+, followed by A+, B+, O–, A–, AB+, B–, and AB–.

Crossmatching is performed by mixing a sample of blood with anti-A serum (one that has antibodies against type A blood), then with anti-B serum. If the blood is type A, it clots in the anti-A serum, not in the anti-B serum. If it is type B, it clots in the anti-B serum, but not in the anti-A serum. If it is type AB, it clots in both; if type O, it clots in neither. The same serum test is then repeated with a serum sample (that is, blood from which all cells have been removed) to ensure accuracy. Rh type is determined similarly with an anti-Rh serum. Clotting means the blood is Rh positive; no clotting means it is Rh negative.

Crossmatching is particularly important for people receiving transfusions (see TRANSFUSION) and for women during pregnancy (see RH INCOMPATIBILITY).

Cross-tolerance

Resistance to the effects of a drug that develops through the repeated use of another, similar drug. Usually cross-tolerance arises with drugs that are chemically similar and have similar effects. For example, a person tolerant to heroin is usually tolerant to morphine and methadone as well.

Croup

FOR SYMPTOM CHART
see Coughing, page 28

An acute viral inflammation of the voice box and windpipe that narrows the airway just below the vocal cords, causing difficult and noisy breathing. Croup is a common illness in young children, especially those aged 6 months to 3 years. After the age of 3, the windpipe is more developed and swelling is less likely to interfere with breathing. Croup occurs most frequently between October and March.

When it is caused by influenza, croup tends to be severe and can affect a wider range of ages in children. The infection is spread via the air or by direct contact with infected secretions. The illness usually lasts 3 to 4 days and may seem improved by day, then worsen at night.

There are two types of croup; both often begin with a common cold (see COLD, COMMON). Spasmodic croup is caused by mild upper respiratory infection or allergy and begins suddenly, often at night. The symptoms include gasping for breath, hoarseness, and a distinctive barking cough. Usually there is not a fever with spasmodic croup, and it can reoccur.

Viral croup usually develops from a

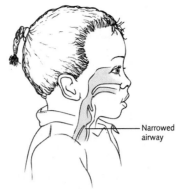

SWOLLEN TRACHEA
In a child with croup, the trachea (windpipe) is swollen, causing a narrowing of the airway. The characteristic harsh breathing noises, called stridor, result from difficulty drawing air in through the swollen passage. The vocal cords may also swell, causing the child's voice to become hoarse.

cold and progresses to a barking cough. It is caused by a viral infection in the voice box and windpipe. The child's airway swells and more fluid is secreted, causing labored, noisy breathing, a condition called STRIDOR. If stridor occurs when a child is resting and not crying or moving, it may indicate severe croup. Low fever often accompanies symptoms of viral croup, but the child's temperature may get as high as 104°F.

TREATMENT
The danger of croup in young children is that the inflammation may cause progressive swelling and obstruct breathing. A pediatrician should be called if there is a suspicion of croup, and emergency medical services should be sought if any of the following symptoms develop: extremely labored breathing, a whistling sound with breathing that increases in volume with each breath, inability to speak for lack of breath, difficulty inhaling, pallor with blue coloration at the mouth and fingertips, wheezing when inhaling during rest, and drooling, with great difficulty swallowing saliva.

Severe cases of croup are rare. When they occur, a child may need to be admitted to the hospital to receive oxygen, intravenous feeding, and medication. Sometimes a tube is inserted through the nose or mouth and into the windpipe to bypass the inflammation in the larynx and trachea.

For milder cases of croup, home

treatment is often effective. Sitting in a steamy bathroom for 15 to 20 minutes often helps restore normal breathing. (The shower should be turned on to be as safe and hot as possible and the bathroom door closed to create enough steam in the room.) Following this steam treatment, using a cold water vaporizer or humidifier in a child's room while he or she sleeps can help. Inhaling cool, moist night air during a croup attack is also sometimes helpful.

If these home treatments are not helpful in dealing with croup, a pediatrician may prescribe a corticosteroid medication, which will reduce the inflammation in the throat and shorten the illness. Because antibiotics are helpful only in treating bacterial infections, they are not useful in treating croup, which is almost always due to a virus or allergy. Cough syrups are also ineffective because they do not affect the larynx or trachea where the infection and inflammation are located.

Crouzon disease
See CRANIOFACIAL DYSOSTOSIS.

Crowding, dental
See OVERCROWDING, DENTAL.

Crown, dental
The visible part of the tooth that normally protrudes above the gum line. A dental crown is also the name for the artificial replacement placed over a dental implant or the remaining structure of a natural tooth, most often because of a fracture or tooth decay. Dental crowns are sometimes called caps; they restore the structure, size, shape, function, and appearance of a normal tooth. A crown is required when there is not enough tooth structure remaining to hold onto a filling or when a weak tooth needs additional support. If there is insufficient tooth structure to hold a crown, typically after root canal treatment, a post may be cemented into the root to provide sufficient structure to hold the crown. Crowns may also be used when a tooth is cracked to hold the tooth together and seal the cracks. Other uses of a crown include the need to attach a dental bridge (see BRIDGE, DENTAL), to guard against cracking when teeth are weakened, or as a cos-

CROWNING A TOOTH
If a tooth is severely decayed, broken, or fragile, the dentist may construct an artificial crown. First, the dentist removes any decay and files the natural tooth down to make room for the crown. An impression is made of the stub and surrounding teeth to guide the sculpting of the crown. The new crown is cemented in place and filed to duplicate the bite of the original tooth.

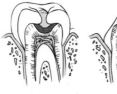

Decayed tooth

Tooth filed to a stub

Crown fitted over stub

metic solution when teeth are misshapen or discolored. The purpose of a crown is to replace the structure of a tooth, to improve the appearance of a tooth or teeth, or to replace missing teeth with a dental bridge, including a pontic (a false tooth attached to one or more crowns).

HOW CROWNS ARE PLACED
Most dentists are skilled at placing crowns. Dentists with a specialty in PROSTHODONTICS, who have extra training in placing crowns, may be recommended when the problem is complex. Placing a dental crown is usually accomplished in two visits to a dental office. On the first visit, and after local anesthesia, the dentist prepares a tooth for a crown by using a dental drill to reduce the structure of the tooth so the crown can fit over it. A dental impression (see IMPRESSION, DENTAL) of the reduced and reshaped tooth, as well as the surrounding teeth, is then made. The impression is sent to a dental laboratory where the crown will be created, with specifications regarding the color as well as the bite, shape, and length of the tooth or teeth being made. Crowns are generally made of porcelain, gold, or a combination of the two materials. The crown is designed to look as much as possible like the natural teeth of the person.

The dentist uses a temporary crown, usually plastic, to cover the prepared tooth while the permanent crown is being made. This usually takes 1 to 2 weeks. During the second visit, the temporary crown is removed, the permanent crown is cemented onto the tooth, and the BITE is adjusted as needed.

SELF-CARE OF CROWNS
In general, care should be taken to avoid biting on hard or sticky foods to prevent cracking or losing the crown. Teeth grinding (see BRUXISM, DENTAL) should be treated because it can dam-

age crowns. Twice daily brushing is very important to keep crowns clean, and regular cleaning between the teeth with dental floss or interdental cleaners (small brushes designed for this task) is essential to proper care of crowns. To prevent decay of the tooth structure under the crown and to prevent gum disease, plaque (see PLAQUE, DENTAL) must be removed from the surfaces where the gum meets the crown. In some cases, special floss threaders may be necessary to floss in hard-to-reach areas and under bridges.

Cruciferous vegetables

Nutrient-rich vegetables from the cabbage family. Cruciferous vegetables are named for their four-petaled flowers that look like a crucifer or cross. Cabbage, bok choy, broccoli, brussels sprouts, cauliflower, collard greens, kale, kohlrabi, mustard greens, radishes, rutabagas, turnips, and watercress are all cruciferous vegetables. Studies suggest that a diet high in cruciferous vegetables offers protection against colon cancer and rectal cancer. Some experts believe that substances found in cruciferous vegetables such as beta-carotene, vitamin C, fiber, and indoles (plant chemicals that influence metab-

olism of the hormone estrogen) have cancer-fighting abilities. Cruciferous vegetables are rich in valuable nutrients and phytochemicals and are fat-free. They appear to contain indoles, which affect the way the body metabolizes estrogen, a hormone with a metabolism that has been associated with breast cancer.

Crush syndrome

The consequence of prolonged continuous pressure on the limbs, which decreases the blood supply to skeletal muscles and may damage muscle tissue. The damaged muscle can release breakdown products such as myoglobin into the bloodstream, which can be toxic to the kidneys. See also RHABDOMYOLYSIS.

Crutch palsy

A condition producing paralysis in the arm because of pressure in the underarm area from improper or overuse of crutches as support and walking aids. This commonly occurs when a person leans his or her entire body weight on the shoulder pads at the tops of the crutches, causing excess pressure on the axillary, or armpit area. A sensation of numbness and tingling down the arm and into the thumb is often the first sign of crutch palsy. Properly distributing body weight on the elbows, shoulders, hands, wrists, and working leg, rather than solely on the muscles located under the arms, helps prevent this condition. Crutches that include a back-of-the-shoulder extension to stabilize the crutch behind the user may help reduce the risk of the axillary nerve damage that causes crutch palsy, which usually improves without therapy.

VEGETABLES IN THE CABBAGE FAMILY
Eating cruciferous vegetables may be particularly beneficial in helping to prevent breast, colon and rectal, and prostate cancer. Plant geneticists are studying different species of these vegetables to develop hybrids that offer the most cancer protection.

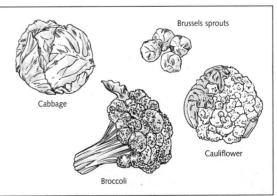

Brussels sprouts

Cabbage

Cauliflower

Broccoli

C

Crying in infants

Crying is a baby's way of communicating his or her needs. Babies normally cry a lot in the first year of life. Many newborns cry loudly whenever they are awake, frequently for no obvious reason. As babies grow older, wakefulness without crying is more common, and parents become more adept at interpreting the cause of tears. Physical factors that prompt babies to cry may include hunger, a wet or dirty diaper, sleepiness, gas, or pain. Babies also cry when they feel insecure or frightened or need attention. Infants who cry excessively and cannot be comforted may have COLIC, an intense pain that seems to have gastrointestinal origins. For a baby 6 months of age or older, crying can be a symptom of teething. Harsh or persistent crying can be a sign of illness.

The first response to an infant's crying is to satisfy the need that he or she may be communicating. Picking up and holding the baby, providing a feeding or a dry diaper, or removing a blanket may help quiet the child. Continuous rhythmic motions (patting or rocking) or sounds such as a vacuum cleaner or washing machine may comfort colicky infants. Burping a baby—holding him or her upright against the shoulder and gently rubbing or patting the back—can help relieve gas. Teething rings, pacifiers, and cold, wet washcloths reduce teething pain. A baby whose crying consistently is not stopped by such measures needs to be seen by a doctor.

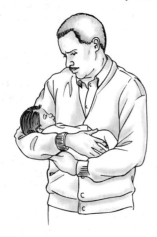

ROCKING AND WALKING
The rhythmic motions of gentle rocking and walking, in addition to the comfort of being held, may help soothe a crying baby.

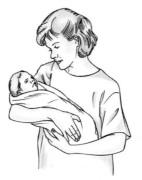

SWADDLING
Swaddling a child, which simply means wrapping in a blanket or shawl, provides warmth and security that may make a crying newborn feel more secure. A swaddled child should not be laid down for napping because he or she needs to be able to move.

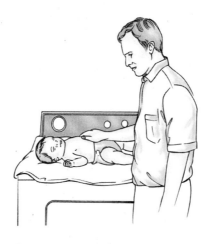

RESTING ON A DRYER
Some crying infants are lulled by the warmth and gentle vibrations of a clothes dryer in operation. The baby needs a soft blanket to lie on, and an adult must be present with a hand resting on the child, for both safety and reassurance.

Excessive high-pitched crying or weak and infrequent crying can be a sign of illness. The doctor should be consulted if crying is accompanied by other symptoms such as a fever, runny nose, diarrhea, a cough, or vomiting, all possible signs of a disease or infection.

A consequence of a baby's excessive crying is that parents become tired, irritable, or impatient. To protect the safety of the infant, professionals urge stressed parents to seek relief. They suggest leaving the room of the crying baby for a few moments.

Resting at the same time the baby rests can help a parent catch up on lost sleep. Tasks such as housework and cooking should take second place to caring for the baby. Anxious parents can relieve stress by asking a qualified friend to baby-sit and simply get away from the baby for a short time.

Cryopreservation

The use of extremely low temperatures to preserve sperm or embryos for use at a later time. Frozen sperm can be thawed and used for ARTIFICIAL INSEMINATION or ASSISTED REPRODUCTIVE TECHNOLOGY procedures. Frozen embryos can be thawed for EMBRYO TRANSFER after a failed fresh embryo transfer or for a subsequent pregnancy after a successful pregnancy. Techniques for successfully freezing human eggs have not yet been developed.

Cryosurgery

Using a temperature below freezing to remove abnormal or diseased tissue. Cryosurgery is used to remove lesions, such as warts, from the skin and to treat cancer or precancerous conditions of the CERVIX. The freezing agent used is typically liquid nitrogen, which has a temperature of approximately $-256°F$.

For lesions of the skin, both cancerous and noncancerous, a dermatologist applies the liquid nitrogen with a cotton-tipped applicator. In most cases, no anesthesia is required. After freezing, the skin stings briefly and then reddens and swells into a blister over the next 2 or 3 days. The blister ruptures on its own within about 2 weeks and forms a scab. When the area heals completely and the scab falls away, little or no scar remains. This type of cryosurgery is performed as an outpatient procedure.

Cryosurgery of the cervix, which is generally performed after administration of a local anesthetic, involves the doctor using a metal probe containing liquid nitrogen or another freezing agent that is inserted into the vagina to reach the cervix. The procedure may cause slight cramping. The woman can resume most normal activities almost immediately after the procedure, but the surgeon may recommend avoiding sexual intercourse for several weeks. After the surgery, a watery fluid containing the

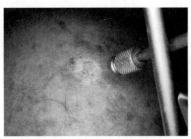

CRYOSURGERY USED ON A MOLE
Dermatologists often use cryosurgery to remove moles. Liquid nitrogen is sprayed on the mole. The nitrogen freezes the lesion, causing it to shrivel and drop off after the skin warms up.

cervical tissue discharges from the vagina. This flow gradually slows, with healing complete in about 2 or 3 weeks.

Another form of cryosurgery (called cryoblation of liver tumors) involves a general anesthetic and a surgical procedure in which an incision is made into the abdomen to gain access to the liver. Multiple metal probes containing liquid nitrogen are inserted into the tumors to freeze and kill the tumor cells. The liver heals by regeneration and scarring.

Cryotherapy

Also known as CRYOSURGERY; the use of very low temperatures to destroy tissue by freezing. Cryotherapy is used to control pain or bleeding, reduce the size of brain lesions, remove lesions of the uterine cervix, and treat malignant and benign tumors and common skin conditions (such as skin tags and warts). In this procedure, cold is given through a probe that has liquid nitrogen flowing through it. The tissue must be cooled to −20°C (−4°F) through the use of liquid nitrogen. Blistering, followed by necrosis (death of tissue cells) follows. The tissue sloughs off when it thaws. If necessary, the procedure is repeated.

Cryptococcosis

An infection that is contracted when soil contaminated with a specific yeast, often from pigeon droppings, is inhaled. Cryptococcosis infections may be limited to the lungs, or they may spread to the meninges (the membrane surrounding the brain), the skin, the bones, or other areas of the body. The risks are greatest for

people with weakened immune systems, including those with AIDS (acquired immunodeficiency syndrome), Hodgkin lymphoma, diabetes, mellitus, or cirrhosis and people undergoing long-term corticosteroid therapy. In these people, the infection can progress to PNEUMONIA or MENINGITIS. In others, cryptococcosis generally remains confined to small areas of the lungs, heals spontaneously without antifungal therapy, and may not require medical treatment.

Diagnosis of cryptococcosis is made by identifying the yeast in sputum, urine, blood, cerebrospinal fluid, or other body secretions. If treatment becomes necessary, antifungal therapy is usually prescribed.

Cryptorchidism

See TESTICLE, UNDESCENDED.

Cryptosporidiosis

A parasitic infection transmitted by eating or drinking food or water that is fecally contaminated. Cryptosporidiosis may be contracted by swallowing contaminated water while swimming, by exposure to surfaces contaminated with fecal matter, and by the fecal-oral route, especially during sexual activity.

The symptoms generally begin within 2 to 14 days of exposure and last between 2 and 14 days. They often include profuse watery diarrhea, abdominal cramps, nausea, and a moderate fever. The gallbladder may also be infected. Sometimes, the infection may not cause symptoms and improve on its own, but in people with weakened immune systems,

cryptosporidiosis can be severe and even fatal.

Unpasteurized apple cider and apple juice (contaminated by fallen apples lying in manure) have been associated with outbreaks of cryptosporidiosis. People who visit or live in developing countries are at greatest risk in the rural areas of those countries. Eating or drinking in areas where sanitation is poor increases the risk of contracting cryptosporidiosis. Chlorine treatment alone cannot adequately disinfect water contaminated with the parasite that causes the infection. There is no vaccine currently available, and no antiparasitic drug has been discovered to treat cryptosporidiosis.

Cryptosporidium

A microscopic parasite that lives in the intestines of humans and animals and causes CRYPTOSPORIDIOSIS. *Cryptosporidium* is carried in animals without symptoms, particularly in cattle, deer, and sheep. The parasite can survive outside the body in feces for prolonged periods. It causes infection when it contaminates food and water. *Cryptosporidium* is resistant to chlorine disinfection.

Crystal therapy

A method of healing by placing stones on the body over the chakra points. Crystal, or gem therapy, is an ancient art in which the chakras, or energy centers (see CHAKRA BALANCING), are thought to promote the body to heal itself by resonating to the colors or energy states of specific gems, stones, and crystals. Gems and crys-

---

PREVENTING CRYPTOSPORIDIOSIS

In areas of a country where hygiene and sanitation are below acceptable standards, the following precautions should be observed:

- Only canned or bottled carbonated beverages, including bottled carbonated water, should be used.
- Any wet surface that comes in contact with the mouth, such as the opening of a bottle and the rim of a can, should be thoroughly dried before the container is opened.
- Ice should be considered contaminated and not used in beverages.
- Drinking water should be boiled vigorously for 1 minute and allowed to cool without the addition of ice before drinking.
- If water is chemically disinfected with iodine, it must be allowed to sit for 15 hours to kill any parasites before drinking.
- Raw food, including salads, uncooked vegetables, and unpasteurized milk and milk products, should be avoided. Fruit should be peeled, and cooked food should be eaten when hot.

tals, and particularly quartz, are said to emit vibrations that can affect the energy flow within the body. Crystal therapy is unproven by any scientific research.

C-section

See CESAREAN SECTION.

CT scanning

Computed tomography scanning; formerly known as CAT (computerized axial tomography) scanning. A diagnostic imaging technique in which multiple projections of X rays (passed through the body from several angles) are analyzed by a computer to produce cross-sectional images of structures. The digital images obtained through CT scanning are more detailed than the images obtained through standard X rays. CT scanning combines RADIOGRAPHY with comput-

er analysis of tissue density. The procedure is a painless, noninvasive method of visualizing detailed views of internal organs and structures; in many cases, it can eliminate the need for more invasive procedures.

CT scanning reveals bone and also shows soft tissues such as organs, muscles, and tumors. Light and dark tones of the images can be adjusted to highlight tissues of similar density. By using graphics software, the computer data from multiple cross-sections can be assembled into three-dimensional images.

WHY IT IS PERFORMED

CT scanning was originally designed to image the brain, but it is now also used to diagnose disorders of the body cavity and bones. It may be used to detect organ damage, tumors, bleeding, and other abnormalities that cannot be visualized on standard

X rays. CT scanning can aid in surgery and in the diagnosis of many different conditions. It may be used in association with treatments such as radiation therapy, in which knowing the precise density, size, and location of a tumor is essential to providing the correct dosage of radiation. CT scans of the blood vessels can be performed to locate and detail precisely the nature of conditions such as an aneurysm (abnormal ballooning of a weakened area in the wall of an artery).

HOW IT WORKS

As the scanner moves, a computer calculates the amount of X-ray penetration through the specific planes of the body parts being examined. Each amount is given a numerical value, called the density coefficient. This numerical information is supplied to a computer, which translates the val-

CLOSE-UP ON CT SCANNING

A rotating X-ray tube within the CT scanning mechanism directs X rays through the body, allowing image data to be obtained from various angles. Special computer equipment is used to compile the information from the images. The result is a detailed, cross-sectional view of all types of organs and tissues.

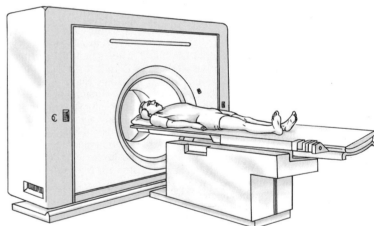

TYPICAL CT SCANNING EQUIPMENT
The person undergoing a CT scan of the head lies on a movable table that slides into the cylindrical scanner.

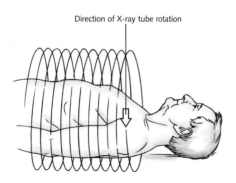

Direction of X-ray tube rotation

SPIRAL CT
Spiral, or helical, CT is a new vascular imaging technique that is 8 to 10 times faster than regular CT. There are no gaps between images, and exposure to radiation is lower.

ues into different shades of gray. The images produced by the computer are displayed on a monitor and photographed, creating a series of images that depict a cross-section of the parts being examined.

Ultrafast CT scanning is a type of CT scanning that involves the use of an electron beam for examining calcifications of the coronary arteries. Coronary artery calcifications are related to the level of atherosclerosis found in the blood vessels of the heart.

HOW IT IS PERFORMED

CT scanning is performed in a hospital radiology unit or outpatient diagnostic clinic. The equipment includes a tube-shaped, X-ray scanner, a computer, and a monitor.

The person being scanned lies on a narrow table that slides into a tube-shaped scanner. The scanner then takes multiple X-ray images. In helical, or spiral CT scanning, there is continuous scanning as the examination table slides through the unit. Spiral scanning reduces the amount of time needed for scanning the entire body, enhances the contrast if a contrast medium is used, and improves the reconstruction and manipulation of the images.

WHAT TO EXPECT

Beforehand, the person performing the procedure usually explains what is involved in the scanning process. For some CT scans, an intravenous contrast medium containing iodine may be administered to make the blood vessels show up more clearly, or a flavored barium drink may be given to provide contrast to internal structures.

The person being scanned lies on a narrow table that slides into the scanner. The table moves continuously in spiral scanning or may stop and start several times, depending on the part of the body being scanned, to obtain scans at different angles. A small area, several sections, or the whole length of the body may be scanned.

After the scan, there will be special instructions if a contrast medium was used. For example, the person may be instructed to drink large amounts of water to help flush the contrast medium through the system. A radiologist will then interpret the results of the scan and provide a report to the referring physician.

Culture

The process of taking a sample of material from the body, encouraging the growth of microorganisms it may contain, and identifying them.

Microorganisms are collected and cultivated so that the doctor can accurately diagnose an infection. Cultivation produces large numbers of microorganisms that can be tested further if need be. The type of specimen depends on the suspected site of infection in the patient. A throat swab is made if a STREP THROAT is suspected; a urine specimen is collected if the doctor suspects a urinary tract infection; a sputum sample is taken if a respiratory infection is suspected; or a stool, or feces, sample is obtained if a gastrointestinal infection is suspected. A blood sample can be cultured if the bloodstream is thought to be infected.

HOW IT IS DONE

The sample of material is collected in a sterile container and is incubated in a special liquid or solid used for culturing various types of bacteria. The culture is incubated for about 2 or 3 days under conditions of temperature and humidity that promote the growth of microorganisms. Any bacteria present will multiply to form visible colonies. Microorganisms causing infection are then viewed under a microscope and identified. A culture is often used to determine the

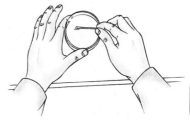

Sample placed in dish

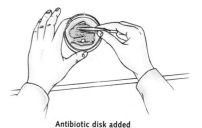

Antibiotic disk added

GROWING MICROORGANISMS
In a laboratory, a doctor or technician can place a sample of body fluid or tissue into a sterile dish and encourage the microorganisms in the sample to grow. When the bacteria or other organisms have multiplied, they can be identified and tested further. A technician then places a disk of antibiotic into a colony of bacteria to test its effectiveness.

cause of a suspected infection and to select the correct medication to treat it. In a person with a severe sore throat, a culture is used to diagnose strep throat, which is caused by the *Streptococcus* bacterium and can be treated with antibiotics. The sample

---

DIFFERENT TYPES OF CULTURES

Culture is the procedure for growing microorganisms artificially in a laboratory so that once an organism is identified, appropriate antibiotic therapy can begin. There are 10 different types of cultures that can be grown in a laboratory after a tiny sample of blood, urine, mucus, or other body fluid is obtained. Here are the types of cultures and what they check for:

- **Throat culture:** Usually checks for strep throat
- **Sputum culture:** Checks for respiratory diseases, such as bronchitis, tuberculosis, lung abscess, and pneumonia
- **Nasopharyngeal (mucus removed from nose) culture:** Checks for upper respiratory tract diseases, such as meningitis and whooping cough
- **Blood culture:** Checks for infection in the bloodstream (sepsis) and identifies cause
- **Urine culture:** Checks for urinary tract infections
- **Duodenal-contents culture:** Checks for bacterial infection of the biliary tract and duodenum (first part of the small intestine)
- **Wound culture:** Checks for a wound infection
- **Stool culture:** Checks to identify bacteria causing intestinal infections
- **Gastric culture:** Checks gastric fluid obtained from the stomach to confirm a diagnosis of tuberculosis; also helps to identify the cause of bacterial infections in the bloodstream of newborns
- **Urethral or cervical culture:** Checks for sexually transmitted diseases, such as gonorrhea or chlamydia

C

for a throat culture is taken by wiping a special cotton-tipped swab across the back of the throat to collect a small amount of mucus, which is then incubated and tested for growth of microorganisms causing infection. A throat culture can also be used when other diseases, such as diphtheria, thrush, or whooping cough, are suspected. Secretions from the lower respiratory tract can be cultured to look for pneumonia and tuberculosis; urine is cultured to diagnose bladder and urinary tract infections. Cultures can be done of the blood to check for infections of the heart, brucellosis, or blood poisoning; the stomach and intestinal tract for bacterial, fungal, or parasitic infections or in dysentery; and fluid and pus to check for infection from an infected wound. Once the microorganism causing the infection is identified, the physician can prescribe a medication known to be effective against it.

Cunnilingus

Oral stimulation of a woman's clitoris and vagina with a partner's mouth and tongue. See ORAL SEX.

Cupping

Technique used in CHINESE MEDICINE to increase the flow of qi ("chee") or energy within the body. Small rounded cups made of glass or bamboo are placed over the person's acupoints for 5 to 10 minutes to draw blood and qi toward them. A lighted taper is placed inside the cup briefly, then removed; the cup is then placed on the skin, usually on the back. Because the flame has consumed the oxygen in the cup and a vacuum has been created, the cup will stick tightly to the skin, drawing up the skin as the cup cools. This is thought to increase the flow of blood and qi. Cupping is used to treat back or shoulder pain, influenza, the common cold, and other diseases.

Cure

The restoration to health of a person who has a disease or disorder.

Curet

A sharp surgical instrument that is tipped with a ring, loop, or scoop and used to scrape the walls of a body cavity. A procedure performed with a

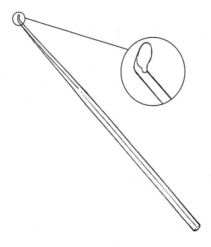

THE VERSATILE CURET
A curet may be tipped with a ring, blade, or spoon to scrape body tissues or surfaces. Different types of curets are used in many diagnostic and treatment procedures.

curet is known as CURETTAGE. A curet is used for many surgical purposes, such as removing adenoids or tissue remaining in the uterus after a miscarriage, or cutting away inflamed gum tissue in the cavity surrounding a tooth.

Curettage

A procedure in which a thin layer of the lining (endometrium) of the UTERUS is removed by scraping the inside with a metal loop, called a CURET. Curettage is used either to remove tissue or to obtain a sample of it for microscopic analysis. The procedure is part of a D AND C.

Curettage, dental

The deep scaling (see SCALING, DENTAL) on the surface of the root of the tooth below the gum line to remove calculus (see CALCULUS, DENTAL) and diseased gum tissue. Dental curettage is sometimes called root planing; it may also be used to remove bacteria and diseased tissue from the socket of the tooth after a tooth extraction. Dental curettage is generally performed by a dentist who specializes in PERIODONTICS using a small instrument called a curet or scaler. The instrument is inserted into the space between the gum and teeth at the base of the gum pocket to scrape away materials that adversely affect the health of the gums and to smooth the

root surface. The gums usually bleed during the procedure, and a local anesthetic may be given to prevent discomfort.

Cushing syndrome

A rare hormonal disorder produced by the extended exposure of tissues in the body to increased levels of the hormone CORTISOL in the bloodstream; also known as hypercortisolism. Cushing syndrome tends to affect adults between the ages of 20 and 50 years.

SYMPTOMS
Cushing syndrome has varying symptoms. The disorder is generally characterized by the wasting of muscles, thinning of skin, severe fatigue, high blood pressure, hyperglycemia (high blood sugar), and weakened bones. In most cases, there tends to be upper body obesity, rounding of the face, and an increase in fat tissue in the neck area. This is offset by thin arms and legs. The skin bruises easily and heals poorly. There may be dark pink or purple stretch marks on the abdomen, thighs, buttocks, arms, and breasts. Weakened bones may interfere with routine movements; lifting objects, bending down, or simply getting up from a chair can cause backaches or fractures of the ribs or spine. An affected person may experience anxiety, depression, and irritability.

In children, Cushing syndrome may produce general obesity and slowed growth rates. Women may experience irregular or absent menstrual periods along with excess hair growth on the face, neck, chest, abdomen, and thighs. Men may have a diminished sex drive, and their fertility may be decreased.

CAUSES
Cushing syndrome occurs when excessive levels of cortisol in the bloodstream expose tissues to abnormal amounts of this hormone for extended periods. Glucocorticoid hormone medications—including prednisone taken for asthma, rheumatoid arthritis, lupus, or other inflammatory diseases—may cause excess cortisol in the bloodstream and produce symptoms of Cushing syndrome.

This hormonal imbalance may also be caused by a breakdown in the normal interaction among the hypothalamus, pituitary gland, and adrenal glands, which signal each other to produce and release varying amounts of precisely balanced hormones. A problem at any level of this delicate progression may ultimately stimulate the adrenal glands to release excessive amounts of cortisol.

A pituitary ADENOMA, which is a benign (not cancerous) tumor of the pituitary gland, is a common cause of Cushing disease, a form of Cushing syndrome that tends to affect women more often than men. Another cause of Cushing syndrome is when tumors, which may be benign but are usually malignant (cancerous), grow outside the pituitary gland and secrete ACTH (adrenocorticotropic hormone). This stimulates the adrenal glands to release cortisol. Called ectopic ACTH syndrome, this condition is seen most commonly in some types of lung cancer. Abnormalities of the adrenal glands, especially benign adrenal tumors called adrenal adenomas, may be responsible for releasing excessive amounts of cortisol into the blood. Rarely, adrenal cancers may be involved in causing Cushing syndrome.

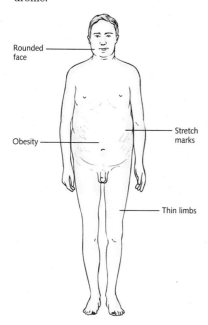

SYMPTOMS OF CUSHING SYNDROME
Overproduction of corticosteroid hormones by the adrenal glands results in the characteristic symptoms of Cushing syndrome: rounding of the face, stretch marks on the side and abdomen, obesity, and thin arms and legs (a result of muscle wasting). Other symptoms include high blood pressure, fatigue, and diabetes mellitus.

DIAGNOSIS AND TREATMENT

Cushing syndrome is diagnosed on the basis of medical history, physical examination, and laboratory tests. The main screening test for Cushing syndrome is the 24-hour urinary free cortisol level test, in which a person's urine is collected for a 24-hour period and the cortisol level is measured. If the level is abnormal, the dexamethasone suppression urine test will help distinguish a pituitary adenoma from an ectopic ACTH-producing tumor, and the corticotropin-releasing hormone stimulation blood test will differentiate ectopic ACTH syndrome from an adrenal tumor.

CT (computed tomography) scanning and MRI (magnetic resonance imaging) of the pituitary gland offer direct visualization of tumors and may be used after Cushing syndrome has been diagnosed, to determine if a pituitary adenoma is the cause.

Treatment of Cushing syndrome is related to the cause of excess cortisol production and may include surgery, radiation, chemotherapy (if the disorder is due to cancer), and the use of cortisol-inhibiting drugs. A pituitary adenoma may be surgically removed, and then a synthetic cortisol medication in the form of either hydrocortisone or prednisone may be taken. The medication is usually taken for less than a year after the surgery. When surgery is not successful or cannot be performed, radiation therapy in combination with a course of cortisol-suppressing medication may be an effective treatment for tumors of the pituitary gland. In some cases, surgical removal of the adrenal glands becomes necessary.

Cusps, dental

The raised, rounded points on the surface of the upper and lower back teeth. Cusps serve to tear and chew food. The teeth that have dental cusps include the following: the cuspids (the pointed teeth next to the incisors, called canines or eye teeth); the bicuspids (the teeth located between the canines and molars, called premolars); and the molars (the large teeth at the back of the mouth).

Cutaneous

Pertaining to the skin.

Cutdown

An incision through the skin to identify a vein and insert a catheter for intravenous infusion. A cutdown is performed when an infusion cannot be begun by VENIPUNCTURE (piercing of a vein with a needle). Following the procedure, the incision is sutured and a sterile dressing is applied.

Cutting and burning

See SELF-MUTILATION.

CVS

See CHORIONIC VILLUS SAMPLING.

Cyanide

A poisonous, colorless liquid with the odor of bitter almonds. Cyanide is used in the making of plastics, in the recovery of gold and silver from ores, and in the electroplating of metals such as silver, gold, copper, and platinum. However, because only a few milligrams of cyanide can be rapidly fatal to humans, it is chiefly known as a deadly poison. Cyanide prevents the use of oxygen by body tissues, and if a large dose is consumed, death will occur almost immediately.

The treatment for cyanide poisoning varies, depending on the nature of the compound in question. Cyanide may be swallowed as a liquid or inhaled as a gas. As with any suspected poisoning, the first thing a person should do is call a POISON CENTER and follow the instructions or go to the nearest hospital emergency department.

Cyanocobalamin

Vitamin B12 (see VITAMIN B). Cyanocobalamin is involved in the metabolism of folic acid and some fatty acids.

Cyanosis

A bluish cast to the skin or mucous membranes caused by a lack of oxygen in the blood. Mild cyanosis, particularly in dark-skinned people, is most obvious in the mucous membranes (such as the inside of the nose and mouth) and the nail beds. It may also appear on the ears, nose, and feet. In advanced cases, the bluish color may spread over the entire surface of the body, as in babies who are born with certain heart defects, a condition commonly known as blue baby. Cyanosis has many other possi-

C

ble causes, including asthma, high altitude, exposure to cold temperatures, suffocation, severe pneumonia, pulmonary edema (fluid in the lungs), heart disease, seizure, drug overdose, and shock. Treatment for cyanosis depends on the cause.

Cyclobenzaprine

A drug that treats pain and stiffness caused by muscle spasms. Cyclobenzaprine (Flexeril) relaxes muscles, relieving pain and discomfort of strains, sprains, spasms, and other muscle injuries. It may cause drowsiness and should be used with care.

Cycloplegia

Paralysis of the ciliary muscles surrounding the lens of the eye. Since these muscles are central to reshaping the lens for focusing on near objects (see ACCOMMODATION), the eye loses its ability to focus on objects close to the eye. Drops that dilate the eye often cause temporary cycloplegia.

Cyclosporine

A drug prescribed to prevent rejection of organ transplants. Cyclosporine is currently available in two slightly different formulations. One of these, Sandimmune, is also given to treat alopecia areata (localized areas of hair loss), aplastic anemia (shortages of red and white blood cells and platelets), Crohn disease (chronic inflammation of the digestive tract), and kidney disease. Sandimmune is always given with a corticosteroid and is available as a capsule, a liquid, and by injection.

A newer formulation of cyclosporine (Neoral) is used to treat certain severe cases of psoriasis and rheumatoid arthritis. It also is prescribed to prevent organ rejection.

Cyclothymia

A psychological disorder characterized by chronic mood swings between mild depression and excitement (hypomania) over a period of at least 2 years. The mood changes are abrupt and unpredictable and cause considerable distress. Cyclothymia is similar to BIPOLAR DISORDER except that the moods are less extreme. In some cases, the disorder progresses into persistent depression or bipolar disorder. Long-term treatment with mood-

stabilizing medication, such as lithium, and psychotherapy is helpful.

Cyst

A small, closed sac filled with liquid, semisolid, or solid material. A cyst can become inflamed, infected, and painful. If cysts become infected or are otherwise troublesome, they can be removed through draining or EXCISION (cutting). See also DERMOID CYST and EPIDERMAL CYST.

Cystectomy

Surgical removal of the bladder. BLADDER CANCER, which invades the muscular bladder wall, is the most common reason for cystectomy. If the cancer is restricted to one site, only part of the bladder is removed (partial cystectomy), but that is rarely performed today. More often, the cancer occurs in more than one site, and the entire bladder is removed along with associated structures (radical cystectomy). In men, the prostate gland and seminal vesicles are also removed; in women, the urethra, uterus, cervix, and the front wall of the vagina are removed. Lymph nodes in the area are also removed and checked for cancer. To replace the role of the bladder in storing urine, a new reservoir is created surgically from a portion of the small or large intestine. Depending on the surgery, a person who has undergone radical cystectomy either must wear a urine collection bag at all times or can drain the internal reservoir periodically. In some cases, a section of intestine may be brought down to the urethra, allowing the patient to urinate normally. Radical cystectomy is an effective treatment for bladder cancer.

Cystic fibrosis

An inherited disease characterized by thick, sticky mucus in the lungs and other organs and increased salt content in sweat. Cystic fibrosis (CF) affects the respiratory and digestive systems and is the most common fatal hereditary disease in white children in the United States. Boys and girls have an equal chance of being born with the disease. CF occurs in one in every 2,500 babies born in the United States. It occurs mostly in whites whose ancestors came from northern Europe. CF is less commonly seen in blacks, Native Americans, and

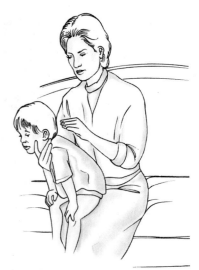

LOOSENING MUCUS
In a child with cystic fibrosis, mucus builds up in the lungs and obstructs the airways. Clapping on the child's back and chest will help dislodge the mucus.

Asians, although it is seen in all races and ethnic groups. Since CF is a recessive genetic disorder, a person must inherit an abnormal copy of the CF gene from each parent in order to be affected. About 4 percent of whites are carriers of the gene. A blood DNA test can detect whether an individual carries the gene.

The CF gene was identified in 1989, leading to a better understanding of how the disease occurs. It is caused by a defect in the gene responsible for manufacturing the protein cystic fibrosis transmembrane conductance regulator (CFTR). In healthy people, CFTR permits chloride ions to enter and leave the cells that line the lungs, pancreas, sweat glands, and small intestine. In people with CF, CFTR either malfunctions or is entirely absent, which prevents chloride from entering or leaving cells, leading to production of the thick, sticky mucus that clogs the internal organs. Mucus blocking the airways in the lungs makes it hard for the body to fight infections and leads to the destruction of lung tissue. Thickened mucus clogs the pancreatic ducts, preventing the enzymes needed to digest fats and proteins from reaching the intestines. Faulty CFTR also prevents the normal process by which most people reabsorb the chloride in their own sweat, allowing excessive amounts of salt to escape in the sweat of people with cystic fibrosis.

SYMPTOMS AND TREATMENT

The first sign of CF in an infant may be intestinal blockage. Some babies with CF may have bulky stools, poor weight gain, or slow growth, all the result of low levels of digestive enzymes in the intestines. Children with CF may also have chronic coughs, wheezing, or respiratory tract infections. People with CF tend to become dehydrated because they lose too much salt in their sweat. Often parents of children with CF report that their infants taste salty when they kiss them. Chronic lung infections associated with the disease gradually destroy lung tissue, eventually leading to death. The average life expectancy for people with CF is 20 to 30 years.

Even though CF remains incurable, various treatments can relieve discomfort and slow the deterioration of tissue. Intestinal blockage in newborns can be removed surgically. Malabsorption can be improved by giving pancreatic enzymes with meals. To compensate for their inadequate digestive system, most people with CF must eat a high-calorie diet that includes higher than normal amounts of fat, in addition to adequate protein and vitamin supplements. Respiratory infections are treated with antibiotics and bronchodilators, which are inhaled to fight infection and open the airways. Caretakers may provide chest therapy, in which they apply force to the person's back and chest to dislodge mucus that obstructs the airways. Some people with CF may require lung transplants.

Cystitis

FOR SYMPTOM CHART

see Urination in woman, painful or
frequent, page 57

Inflammation of the interior lining of the bladder; the most common urinary tract infection in women. Cystitis occurs when bacteria from the colon that live on the skin near the rectum or in the vagina enter the urinary tract through the urethra. The bacteria travel up the urethra, infecting the bladder. Sexual intercourse can precipitate cystitis in women, because bacteria can be massaged into the urethra by the movements of the penis. Symptoms can include more frequent urination, a burning sensation while urinating, and blood in the urine. Even though the urge to urinate may be strong, only small amounts of urine are released, and it may have a strong smell. Fever and soreness in the lower abdomen or back may also occur.

Cystitis is very common; it can be prevented by drinking plenty of fluids, wiping from front to back after urination or a bowel movement (in women), and by emptying the bladder immediately before and after sexual intercourse. Drinking about 2 quarts of water or other fluids for a day may relieve symptoms. Cranberry juice is sometimes thought to help prevent cystitis. A physician should be consulted when symptoms persist or are severe. Antibiotics or other drugs may be prescribed.

Cystocele

A protrusion of the bladder into the vagina. A cystocele, which is sometimes called a fallen or dropped bladder, is caused by the stretching and weakening of the pelvic muscles and most often occurs after childbirth. Women who have had large babies, many pregnancies, or long and difficult labors are particularly likely to develop cystoceles. Although many women experience no problems, symptoms can include pressure or aching in the vagina, difficulty in urinating, and problems with penetration during sexual intercourse. Stress incontinence, in which urine leaks out when a woman laughs or coughs, is also common. Some women with cystoceles are predisposed to developing urinary tract infections. Problems may not arise until after menopause, when the loss of estrogen weakens pelvic muscles even further.

A doctor can easily detect a cystocele during a routine pelvic examination. In mild cases, symptoms may be relieved with regular practice of KEGEL EXERCISES. Postmenopausal women may find that HORMONE REPLACEMENT THERAPY will reverse some of the weakening of the pelvic muscles. Insertion of a vaginal PESSARY may provide temporary support of the bladder and urethra and improve urinary control. If symptoms are severe or interfere with daily activities, a surgical procedure can correct a cystocele by pushing the bladder upward and sewing it into position. Another surgical procedure alters the bladder opening through an abdominal incision. Both surgeries can be painful and may require lengthy recoveries.

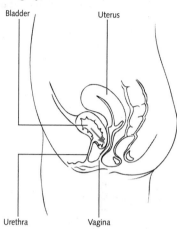

Bladder   Uterus

Urethra   Vagina

A DROPPED BLADDER
In a woman whose pelvic muscles have been weakened, most often by childbirth, the base of the bladder may drop against the vagina—a condition called a cystocele (arrow indicates area of pressure). In some cases, the fallen bladder pulls the urethra into an angle that makes urination difficult.

Cystography, voiding

A detailed X-ray study of the bladder. The test may be performed when an infection, tumor, bladder stones, or reflux of urine into the kidneys is suspected. The patient first empties his or her bladder by normal urination. Then, a thin, flexible tube (catheter) coated with anesthetic jelly is inserted through the urinary tract. The bladder is filled with dye through the catheter, and X rays are taken with the patient in different positions. The patient voids the dye by urinating, and another X ray is taken. Voiding cystography is not painful, but it can be uncomfortable. After the test, the patient may experience tenderness in the urinary tract for 24 hours. There is a small risk of infection marked by chills, fever, and burning during urination after the first 24 hours.

Cystometrogram

A test to help determine the cause of abnormal bladder emptying found in certain diseases, such as diabetes mellitus. First, the patient urinates normally, and the amount of urine, length of time during urination, and any amount of straining or dribbling are recorded. Then a thin, flexible tube (catheter) coated with anesthetic jelly is inserted through the urinary tract into the bladder; the amount of urine remaining in the bladder is drained and measured. Next, saline solution at room temperature is pumped into the bladder through the catheter, and the patient reports any sensation. After the saline solution is drained, a device that measures bladder pressure (cystometer) is connected to the catheter. Water, or in some cases carbon dioxide gas, is slowly pumped into the bladder. The amount of water or gas and its pressure are recorded as the patient reports first the need to urinate, then a sense of fullness, and finally the point at which urination begins. The data gathered in a cystometrogram, often combined with other test results, can help a physician diagnose the cause of abnormal bladder function.

A cystometrogram causes discomfort and may produce pain, flushing, sweating, nausea, and an unpleasant urge to urinate. There is a slight risk of infection and blood in the urine.

Cystoscopy

Visual examination of the inside of the lower urinary tract and bladder through a special viewing instrument tipped with a light (cystoscope). Long, thin instruments can also be inserted into the bladder through the cystoscope to crush stones, take tissue samples, remove tumors, or repair defects. Cystoscopy is performed for a number of reasons, including blood in the

urine, inability to control urination (incontinence), infection, congenital abnormalities, calculi, and tumors. The cystoscope is lubricated and inserted through the urinary opening into the urethra and the bladder. The amount of urine remaining in the bladder is measured, and a sample is taken. Fluid is pumped into the bladder to inflate it and allow inspection of the entire bladder wall. Tissue is sampled, tumors are treated, and stones are crushed as needed. Dye may be injected into the tubes connecting the bladder and kidneys (ureters), and X rays of the upper urinary tract are taken. The cystoscope is then removed.

Cystoscopy is often performed in the office of the doctor, but if a biopsy is performed or a stone is treated, it will be performed in the hospital. Nonprescription painkillers usually control discomfort. Sexual relations can be resumed as soon as the surgeon determines that healing is complete. Vigorous exercise should be avoided for 2 weeks. Complications include infection and, rarely, damage to the urinary tract or bladder and injury to the penis.

Cystotomy

A surgical incision made into the bladder, usually to inspect or repair the bladder or for placement of a tube to aid in urination.

Cystourethrocele

A condition in which the tissues supporting the bladder and urethra are weakened in women. The weakness can cause stress incontinence, in which urine leaks out when the woman sneezes, coughs, jumps, or lifts heavy objects. Most women with cystourethroceles develop them as a result of childbirth, which can weaken the

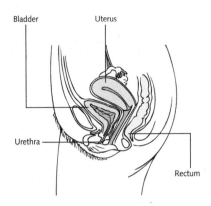

Normal bladder

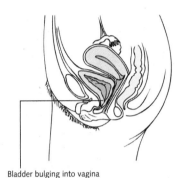

Bladder bulging into vagina

Weakened bladder

LOSS OF BLADDER SUPPORT
A cystourethrocele, a weakening of the tissues supporting the bladder and the urethra, causes the neck of the bladder, where it connects with the urethra, to bulge into the vagina. The condition can cause stress incontinence, lower back pain, or a sensation of uncomfortable pressure.

surrounding pelvic muscles. Symptoms may not appear until after menopause, when the lack of estrogen weakens the pelvic muscles even further. In addition to stress incontinence, some women also experience lower back pain, a feeling of pelvic pressure, or discomfort in the vaginal area.

A doctor can detect a cystourethrocele during a routine pelvic examination. When a woman has stress incontinence, the doctor may perform other tests, such as a CYSTOSCOPY, an examination of the inside of the urethra and bladder, to determine the extent of the problem. Treatment can include KEGEL EXERCISES in mild cases, medications that increase the tone of the muscles around the urethra, hormone replacement therapy in women who are past menopause, or surgery.

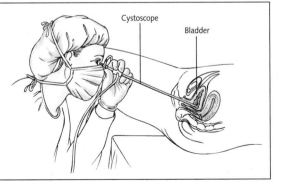

EXAMINING THE BLADDER
During a cystoscopy, a doctor inserts a hollow, lighted tube (cystoscope) through the urethral opening and into the bladder to examine the length of the urethra and the interior of the bladder. Instruments can also be inserted through the cystoscope to take tissue samples, crush stones, or even remove tumors. The cystoscope can be either rigid (shown here) or flexible.

C

Cytokines

A generic term for hormonelike peptides produced by various types of cells of the human body in response to an inflammatory stimulus. They are important in the immune response. Examples include INTERLEUKINS and INTERFERONS.

Cytologist

A person who specializes in cytology, the branch of biology that focuses on the formation, origin, structure, function, activities, and pathology of cells. For example, a cytologist may perform a microscopic evaluation of cells on a slide made during a Pap smear to check for signs of a malignant tumor.

Cytology

The branch of biology that is concerned with the formation, origin, structure, function, activities, and pathology of cells.

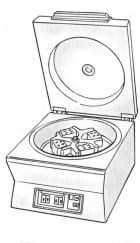

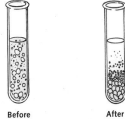

Before   After

HOW A CENTRIFUGE WORKS
Cytologists sometimes use a machine called a centrifuge to separate out certain types of cells for examination. A sample of body fluid is placed in the centrifuge, which whirls it around to create centrifugal force. The more dense cells sink to the bottom, and the lighter fluid elements rise to the top.

Cytomegalic viral retinitis

Infection of the light-sensitive layer (retina) at the back of the eye with CYTOMEGALOVIRUS (CMV). CMV infection usually produces no symptoms, except in people with compromised immune systems, such as people with AIDS (acquired immunodeficiency syndrome) or those who have undergone bone marrow or organ transplants or are receiving chemotherapy for cancer. Cytomegalic viral retinitis (also called cytomegalovirus retinitis) occurs in approximately one of every four people with AIDS and may lead to blindness. Symptoms include floaters (small, moving shapes in the visual field), impaired vision, blind spots, and loss of vision to the sides. Treatment is difficult, since antiviral medications stop the virus from reproducing but do not destroy it. In addition, the medications have many side effects and may be difficult to take. Recently, intraocular injections and implants with antiviral drugs have shown great benefit without the side effects of systemic drugs. Isolation of persons undergoing immunosuppression or chemotherapy can be an effective measure to prevent CMV infection at the time of greatest vulnerability.

Cytomegalovirus

A member of the herpesvirus group, which also includes herpes simplex virus types 1 and 2, varicella-zoster virus (the virus that causes chickenpox), and EPSTEIN-BARR VIRUS (the virus that causes infectious mononucleosis; see MONONUCLEOSIS, INFECTIOUS). Cyto-megalovirus (CMV) can survive in the body in a dormant state for months to years after a person has been infected. Once infected, a person retains the living virus within his or her body for life. However, the disease rarely recurs in healthy people.

The virus exists throughout the world at all socioeconomic levels, although CMV infection is more widespread in developing countries and in lower socioeconomic groups. A large percentage of adults in the United States have been infected by the age of 40 years. CMV is the most common virus transmitted to a fetus before birth.

SYMPTOMS

After an initial infection, the majority of adults and children who contract cytomegalovirus have few or no symptoms and no long-term health consequences. A prolonged infection follows, during which time a person does not experience clinical illness and is generally unaware of the presence of the virus. Factors that may influence the dormant or latent stage of the infection and its reactivation are not completely understood, but it is known that impairment of the body's immune system from therapeutic treatments (such as chemotherapy) or from disease, such as AIDS (acquired immunodeficiency syndrome), consistently reactivates the virus causing recurrent infection with CMV.

When reactivated, the virus may or may not produce symptoms. If there are symptoms, they may include a mononucleosislike syndrome with prolonged fever, sore throat, fatigue, and swollen glands. Mild HEPATITIS may be experienced. People with weakened immune systems can develop eye infections, pneumonia, colitis, and encephalitis.

CAUSES

Cytomegalovirus is spread via bodily secretions, including saliva, urine, feces, blood, tears, breast milk, semen, and cervical secretions. Close or intimate contact among people, including kissing and sexual activities, can transmit the infection from one person to another. The virus may also be passed from a pregnant mother to her developing fetus, and the newborn may become infected during delivery or during breast-feeding if the mother has CMV. It can also be contracted in the process of receiving a blood transfusion or an organ transplant.

CMV is not considered highly contagious, but has been shown to spread in households among family members and other residents and among children and adult workers in day care centers. It is most often transmitted in these environments via infected body fluids. When a person's hands come in contact with these fluids and the hands then touch the mouth, nose, or eyes, the virus that is latent in these fluids is absorbed into the susceptible person's body. Frequent hand washing is effective in killing the virus. Education and effective hygiene are recommended for those who live or work with young children, especially those who are in contact with oral secretions or soiled diapers.

DIAGNOSIS AND TREATMENT

Because CMV is so common and rarely produces symptoms, most infections are not diagnosed. Screening is not considered valuable for healthy children or adults who may carry the virus. The protocol for deciding to test for CMV infection is generally based on a person having symptoms of infectious mononucleosis with negative test results for that virus, or the Epstein-Barr virus, or showing signs of hepatitis A, B, or C, with negative test results for these infections. A woman who is pregnant who develops mononucleosis-like symptoms during pregnancy should be evaluated for CMV infection. In such cases, laboratory tests, including blood tests and urine or throat swab cultures, may be performed to discover the virus or antibodies to it.

To measure antibodies in the blood, the enzyme-linked immunosorbent assay, or ELISA test, is most commonly used. Since a person who has been infected with CMV develops antibodies that persist in the person's body for a lifetime, antibody blood tests may indicate a previous infection with CMV, rather than a current one. Antibody blood tests may be performed on an initial suspicion of the infection and again 2 weeks later to determine an active infection. In combination with positive test results from urine or throat specimens, a diagnosis of an active CMV infection can be made.

There is no treatment for CMV infection in an otherwise healthy person at this time. Several antiviral medications are available for infants and persons with weakened immune systems

who develop serious infections. Vaccines are also being researched, but they may be many years from development and widespread use.

The very small percentage of women who contract CMV for the first time during pregnancy are at risk of having a baby who has symptoms at birth or who may develop disabilities at a later time. CMV remains the most significant cause of congenital viral infection in the United States. Infants who are infected by their mothers before birth may have a generalized infection with symptoms that are apparent at birth. These may range from jaundice caused by moderate enlargement of the liver and spleen to fatal disease. Up to 90 percent of these infected infants may have complications within the first few years of life. These complications can include a small head, hearing loss, vision impairment, developmental delays (see DEVELOPMENTAL DELAY), and varying degrees of mental retardation.

People using organ transplant equipment and those receiving chemotherapy or other medication can become more seriously ill if they contract CMV. Those who have immune deficiency diseases, such as AIDS, are also at risk of developing more severe illness with CMV infection.

Cytopathologist

A physician who specializes in CYTOPATHOLOGY, the study of disease-related changes within cells. Cytopathologists are usually trained in anatomical pathology (the study of the effects of disease on the structure of the body), and they focus on disease at the cellular level.

Cytopathology

A branch of pathology is concerned with the manifestations of disease in

cells. Cytopathology is particularly useful in the diagnosis of precancerous and cancerous diseases.

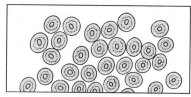

Well-differentiated cells

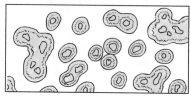

Moderately differentiated cells

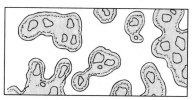

Poorly differentiated cells

CYTOPATHOLOGY IN CANCER DETECTION
A cytopathologist examines cells taken from samples of body tissue or fluid under a microscope to help diagnose disease. The appearance of cells in a tumor of the prostate show the advance of cancer. At a very early stage in the tumor's growth, the cells are still small, uniform, and very tightly packed—the cytopathologist calls these cells well differentiated. As the tumor grows, the cells become more irregularly shaped and dissimilar; they begin to disperse, and some of the cells fuse together. These cells are moderately differentiated. At an advanced stage of the cancer, the cells are fused into highly irregular masses that have invaded the connective tissue of the prostate; the cells are now poorly differentiated.

D and C

Dilation and curettage. A procedure in which the ENDOMETRIUM (the lining of a woman's uterus) is scraped away with a spoon-shaped instrument called a curet. A D and C may be done as a diagnostic or therapeutic procedure to treat a variety of disorders, such as excessive bleeding during menstrual periods. A D and C is also commonly performed after a woman has a miscarriage or for an abortion. In this outpatient procedure, a local anesthetic is given to numb the cervix; a sedative may be given for relaxation. A SPECULUM is used to expand the vagina, and then the cervix is gradually opened with a series of plastic or metal wedges called dilators. The doctor inserts a curet through the cervix into the uterus to remove the surface of the endometrium. The scrapings are then examined under a microscope for abnormalities, such as cancer or polyps.

A woman usually rests for a few hours and then returns home. Most women experience mild cramping and light bleeding after this procedure. Complications, although rare, may include perforated tissue, excessive bleeding, or infection. Until the cervix contracts to its normal size, a woman is at increased risk for bacterial infection. For this reason, it is important not to use a tampon or have sexual intercourse after the procedure. A doctor will usually advise that a woman refrain from intercourse or using tampons until she has healed, generally in about 4 weeks. She may continue most of her regular activities after a day or two of rest. As a new lining begins to form in the uterus, the woman's next period may not occur at the regular time. A follow-up appointment with her doctor is needed to confirm that she is healing properly.

D and E

Dilation and evacuation. A procedure in which a woman's cervix is dilated and the contents of the uterus are removed by suctioning. Almost always an outpatient procedure, D and E is typically performed as part of an abortion procedure or after a miscarriage. When performed during the first trimester of pregnancy, the procedure may be referred to as vacuum aspiration, vacuum curettage, suction curettage, or suction D and C.

Before the procedure, a sedative may be given, as well as a local anesthetic to numb the area around the cervix. In some cases, general anesthesia may be used. Laminaria (long slender rods that expand on contact with moisture) may be used hours before the procedure is begun to help the cervix dilate (open). A woman may experience a cramping pain as her cervix dilates. Once the cervix is sufficiently dilated, the doctor will insert a metal or plastic tube called a cannula into the woman's uterus. The outer end of the cannula is attached to a pump that will remove the contents of the uterus, causing it to contract. Some women experience mild pain as this occurs, but others feel intense menstrual-type cramps. The procedure lasts from 5 to 15 minutes. The aftermath of the D and E is medically similar to that for a dilation and curettage (see D AND C). A potential for infection exists for about 4 weeks, so a woman should refrain from sexual intercourse and the use of tampons until then.

Dacryocystitis

Inflammation of the tear sac and the tear duct leading from the eye to the nose. The cause is usually bacterial, but viruses or fungi may be the cause. Symptoms include warm, painful swelling of the lower eyelid close to the nose, oozing of pus from the eye when pressure is applied to the swollen area, and fever. Since tears normally drain from the eye through the tear duct into the nose, blockage of the duct from dacryocystitis may cause tears to stream from the eye. The condition is most common in infants and in adults older than 40 years. Infection may be acute (come on suddenly) or chronic (persist over time). In some cases, an abscess may form and rupture through the skin.

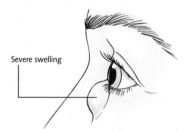

Severe swelling

BLOCKED TEAR DUCT
Any blockage in the tear duct (caused by malformation, disease, injury, or the effects of aging) can result in a buildup of bacteria in the duct called dacryocystitis. The tears that normally drain into the nose flow from the eye instead. Symptoms include pain, redness, swelling, excessive tearing, discharge, and fever.

Applying a warm compress (a clean cloth soaked in very warm water and then wrung out) can help relieve pain and promote drainage. In infants, gentle massage of the tear duct four times a day for up to 9 months can help drain the blockage and create normal flow. Antibiotic ointments or oral medications can be used against infection. In some cases, a tiny tube is inserted into the tear duct and the duct is flushed with a sterile saltwater solution. If these treatments fail, surgery to open and drain the tear duct is performed; on rare occasions,

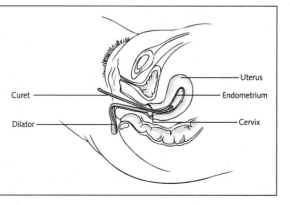

SCRAPING THE UTERINE LINING
In a D and C procedure, the vagina is expanded with a speculum. The cervix is gradually dilated (opened) by inserting a series of successively larger rods called dilators. Then the doctor uses a curet to scrape the lining of the uterus (the endometrium). The procedure is done using a local anesthetic.

Curet

Dilator

Uterus

Endometrium

Cervix

the tear sac is removed to prevent further infection. Abscesses resulting from dacryocystitis are also drained surgically.

Danazol

A synthetic androgen (male hormone). Danazol (Danocrine) is prescribed to treat endometriosis, fibrocystic breast disease, and hereditary angioedema, which is swelling of different parts of the body. Danazol should not be taken by a woman who is pregnant.

Dandruff

Excessive shedding of skin from the scalp. The body normally sheds a certain amount of dead skin from the body surface. Dandruff results in itching and noticeable loose flakes of skin. To control itching and flaking, doctors recommend over-the-counter dandruff shampoos that contain ingredients such as coal tar, salicylic acid, selenium sulfide, sulfur, and zinc pyrithione. Medicated shampoos can be harsh on the hair and scalp and may require use of a conditioner afterward.

If the scalp is red, irritated, or severely itchy or scaly, it is important to see a doctor to rule out other causes such as SEBORRHEIC DERMATITIS and PSORIASIS. Topical medications can be prescribed to control the problem.

Dapsone

An antibiotic used to treat leprosy. Dapsone (Avlosulfon) is an antibiotic that is effective against the bacterium *Mycobacterium leprae*, which causes leprosy. Dapsone is also used to treat dermatitis herpetiformis (a skin disease), pemphigus, malaria, and AIDS (acquired immunodeficiency syndrome)–related pneumonia.

Date rape

FOR FIRST AID

see Rape/sexual assault, page 1327

Sexual contact that is forced on a person who is acquainted with the rapist. Date rape, also known as acquaintance RAPE, is most common among women between the ages of 16 and 24 years. The use of alcohol and drugs also can be a factor, especially when the man puts drugs in a woman's drink or food without her knowledge.

Day care, adult

Assistance, ranging from health care to social programs, for older people who continue to live in their homes. Services may include health assessment; physical, occupational, or speech therapy; and hot, nourishing meals. Day care centers provide older adults opportunities for companionship with peers and recreational activities. They also provide respite for caregivers (see RESPITE CARE). Centers usually operate on weekdays during business hours. Often, transportation is provided. Many adult day care centers are subsidized by voluntary or public organizations, such as civic or religious groups, hospitals, and senior centers. Services are often provided free or on a sliding scale. When full fees are charged, community organizations often sponsor those who cannot afford to pay. Medicaid may cover a portion of the costs in some states, depending on a person's eligibility. See also CAREGIVING FOR OLDER PEOPLE.

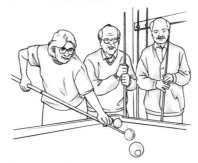

ADULT DAY CARE CENTERS
Older people may benefit from the services offered at a daytime care center. The benefit may be as simple as a place to socialize, play games, or eat meals with friends. Many centers offer more comprehensive services including various types of therapy and light nursing care. A day care center also provides temporary time off for the caregiver.

Day treatment program

Extended psychotherapy, counseling, and education in a nonresidential setting. Day treatment programs are used for a wide variety of emotional, psychological, and neurological problems, such as alcohol and substance abuse, anxiety disorders, and stroke. Day treatment may also be recommended for people with attention deficit/hyperactivity disorder (ADHD), traumatic brain injury, Alzheimer's

disease, Parkinson disease, seizure disorders, mood disorders (such as depression, manic-depressive illness, and dysthymia), physical and sexual abuse, and eating disorders. Most day treatment programs focus on helping people learn self-management and develop independent living skills. These programs also involve families in treatment and teach them to serve as advocates for family members in need of care.

De Morgan spots

See CHERRY ANGIOMAS.

de Quervain disease

A painful inflammation of the sheath surrounding the tendon that is attached to the bone at the outside of the wrist. It is seen in individuals who use their thumbs and hands in a repetitive manner. The sheath is enclosed in a narrow tunnel, and the tendon becomes compressed when the sheath is swollen. This puts excessive pressure on the tendon, which causes the severe wrist pain commonly produced by de Quervain disease. Pressure on the nerve can cause numbness and tingling over the thumb and index finger. X rays may be recommended to rule out a fracture.

Treatment may include limitation of activities involving movements of the wrist and the use of a thumb brace to rest and support the area. Ice and nonsteroidal anti-inflammatory drugs (NSAIDs) may be recommended for pain management. A thumb splint may also be used for 3 weeks. A cortisone or anesthetic injection in the area is sometimes helpful. If the pain persists, outpatient surgery performed with a local anesthetic may become necessary. The surgical technique requires making a small incision at the wrist and opening the sheath to relieve pressure on the tendon. de Quervain disease is also called chronic tendovaginitis.

Deafness

An inability to hear, which may affect any age group, with consequences ranging from minor to severe. A small proportion of hearing-impaired persons in the United States are considered profoundly deaf, meaning their hearing loss is so severe they cannot benefit from hearing aids or other forms of mechanical sound amplification. A much larger proportion of people who are hearing impaired can benefit, in varying degrees, from the use of amplification devices.

CAUSES

Deafness is usually caused by illness or accidents. It may also run in families and be inherited. Certain conditions such as rubella (German measles) during a woman's pregnancy create a risk that her baby will be born deaf. A person's environment may contribute to loss of hearing if there is ongoing exposure to noise levels that result in progressive hearing loss.

There are four general categories of hearing loss: conductive hearing loss, sensorineural hearing loss, mixed hearing loss, and central hearing loss. The cause of a person's loss of hearing is what determines the type and, in most cases, how the loss will be treated. Conductive hearing loss is caused by diseases or obstruction in the outer or middle ear; this condition is not generally severe and can be helped by a hearing aid, by performing surgery on the eardrum or middle ear, or simply by cleaning earwax or other obstructions from the ear canal. Sensorineural hearing loss results from damage to the sensory nerves or hair cells in the inner ear and ranges in severity from mild to profound. Because this type of hearing loss affects certain sound frequencies more severely than others, a person with sensorineural hearing loss perceives distortions in sound, even when the sound is amplified. In such cases, hearing aids may not help a person with sensorineural hearing loss. Mixed hearing loss is caused by problems in the outer or middle ear, as well as in the inner ear. Central hearing loss is caused by damage to or impairment of centers or connections in the brain.

DIAGNOSIS AND TREATMENT

An evaluation of the degree and type of hearing loss is made with the help of hearing tests (see AUDIOMETRY). The results of these tests determine the course of treatment. A person with hearing loss will be evaluated and fitted with various kinds of hearing aids and other mechanical sound amplifiers, including ASSISTIVE LISTENING DEVICES. A surgical procedure may be required to restore or improve hearing ability.

Communication systems are frequently used to benefit people who are deaf. These systems, generally taught to deaf children in special schools and classes, encourage the combined use of certain methods of communicating that are suitable to the child or adult who cannot hear. The goal is to establish or enhance the ability of a person who is deaf to transmit thoughts and ideas to other people. American Sign Language (ASL) is a language system formed by making distinctive shapes and movements with one or both hands. Individual hand signs are related in both concrete and abstract meaning to English words. The grammar of ASL is created by facial expressions and movements of the body, as well as the spacing of the hands and the directions they face. Finger spelling is a system based on forming shapes with the hands that correspond to the letters of the alphabet. Words are literally spelled out by means of these letter shapes made by the hands. Cued speech supplements lip-reading with the use of eight different hand movements to communicate the pronunciation of spoken syllables. Oral communication is a system taught to deaf children using speech as an expressive skill for articulating thoughts to another person. Lip-reading is used along with oral communication as a means of understanding another person. Other communication systems for helping deaf individuals include manually coded English, art, electronic media, mime, gesture, and reading and writing.

Death

The end of life. By medical definition, death generally occurs when a person has sustained irreversible cessation of circulatory and respiratory functions. When a person's heartbeat and respiration are being maintained mechanically, death occurs when there is an irreversible cessation of all functions of the entire brain, including the brain stem. This definition of death was proposed in 1981 by the President's Commission for the Study of Ethical Problems in Medicine and is a modification of a definition developed at Harvard Medical School

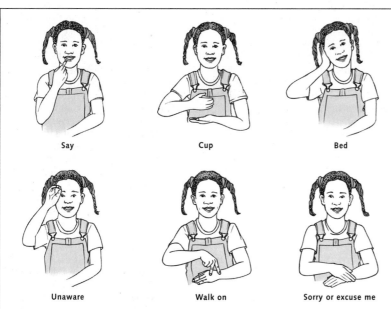

Say   Cup   Bed

Unaware   Walk on   Sorry or excuse me

AMERICAN SIGN LANGUAGE
American Sign Language (ASL) is a communication system that teaches the hearing-impaired person how to make hand gestures to convey words. The hand gestures are further differentiated and enhanced by facial expression and body posturing. The girl pictured is expressing six words—including different parts of speech and some abstract concepts. By assigning a single gesture for a whole word, ASL differs from finger spelling, which assigns a gesture to a letter.

in 1968. The Harvard definition described death as brain death verified by tests that detect a total unawareness of stimuli, an absence of spontaneous muscle movement or respiration, an absence of reflexes, and the cessation of electrical activity in the brain as indicated by a flat line on an electroencephalogram. Because of advances in medical technology, death can no longer be defined as it once was, the cessation of heartbeat and respiration, since these bodily functions may be artificially prolonged for a considerable time by medical technology.

WHY DEATH MUST BE MEDICALLY DEFINED

The measure for when death has occurred is fluid because it is influenced by changes in medical science, social thought, and the legal system. To address the necessary issues, it is important to have a medical, and generally accepted, definition of death for the protection of patients and people in the medical profession.

There are practical medical implications, and patient care reasons for needing a precise definition of death. When death occurs, all medical care may be stopped, and personnel and resources, such as limited space in an intensive care unit, may be made available for other patients. A determination of death also helps indicate when vital organs may be removed to maximize the success of a transplantation procedure to another patient.

Death certificate

An official and legal document stating that a person is dead and identifying the cause of death. Only a licensed physician can fill out and sign a death certificate, which is needed before burial or disposal of the person's remains. A death certificate is also necessary for collecting insurance benefits and for tax purposes and other financial transactions.

Death rate

The number of deaths within a group of people in 1 year divided by the average or midyear population of that group. If total population is used, the result is called the crude death rate. Death rate can also be calculated for the population within certain age groups; the result is the age-specific death rate. Death rate may be meas-

ured in people with a specific disease or condition, such as a gunshot wound (homicide rate), heart disease, or a type of cancer.

Debility

Generalized weakness, feebleness, or loss of strength and energy. Debility may be caused by a physical disease or a psychological disorder.

Debridement

Surgical removal of foreign material or damaged, dead, or contaminated tissue from a severe wound or injury. Surgical debridement usually requires an anesthetic because it involves cutting away the damaged tissue with sharp instruments or a laser. Debridement helps promote healthy healing of badly damaged skin, tissue, muscle, and bone.

In autolytic debridement, special dressings are used to keep the wound fluid in contact with damaged tissue. Over time, the defense mechanisms in the body soften and liquefy dead cells so that the cells can slough away. Autolytic debridement is virtually painless, but it is slower than the surgical alternative and poses a higher risk of wound infection.

Enzymatic debridement uses fast-acting enzymes, some of which work only on dead tissue and others that work on any tissue that they come into contact with. This method is expensive, can be painful or uncomfortable, and requires a doctor who is skilled in the procedure.

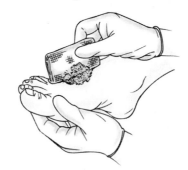

CLEANING A WOUND
Debridement, or cleansing, of a wound may involve removing material such as sand, glass, or dead or contaminated tissue. Some chemical agents soften or liquefy damaged cells so that the body can slough them off naturally (a process called autolytic debridement). Other agents use enzymes (proteins) that destroy the cells altogether (enzymatic debridement).

Decalcification, dental

The loss of calcium from the hard enamel covering the teeth. The enamel is made up almost entirely of calcified material. The result of dental decalcification is the loss of the hard, smooth tooth surface, which becomes chalky and porous as the enamel dissolves. This makes the tooth more susceptible to decay. The condition is common in young children who habitually suck on baby bottles filled with sweet liquids. (See BABY BOTTLE TOOTH DECAY). It is also seen on teeth after braces are removed, because of food impinging on the wires. The teeth cannot naturally replace enamel destroyed by decalcification. A dentist should be consulted to treat the condition. Bonding may be needed to restore the tooth to its original condition.

Decerebrate

The state of being without a functioning cerebrum (the main controlling part of the brain). This condition occurs when the brain stem is damaged. When in response to stimulation the arms of a comatose person are extended and internally rotated, he or she is said to be in decerebrate posture. See also COMA.

Deciduous teeth

The first teeth to appear in the mouth of an infant, usually at the age of about 6 months. Sometimes called baby or primary teeth, deciduous teeth are so named because they shed or fall out at the end of a growth period, much like a tree that annually sheds its leaves. Deciduous teeth typically shed between the ages of 4 and 12 years to make room for the 32 permanent teeth. There are normally 20 deciduous teeth. See PRIMARY TEETH.

Decompression sickness

The health problems caused by nitrogen bubbles in a scuba diver's bloodstream, which can block the flow of blood. Decompression sickness, also called "the bends," usually results from an ascent to the surface of the water that is too rapid to allow the release of excess nitrogen absorbed with oxygen during the descent into the water. During a diver's descent, the increasing pressure of the deep water causes his or her body to absorb an increased amount of air made up of nitrogen and oxygen. The extra oxygen is quickly metabolized by the body. Nitrogen, which is an inert gas, is not metabolized by the body and may be especially retained in fatty tissue, which means that in overweight individuals, the nitrogen may be released more slowly. All of it must be released from the body through exhalation. This is particularly important when a diver ascends; as the pressure surrounding the diver decreases, he or she must release the excess nitrogen. When the ascent is too rapid, the nitrogen can escape, and this can result in nitrogen bubbles forming in the diver's blood, preventing normal blood flow. The side effects of this blockage may range from discomforts such as headaches, to more severe impairment including confusion and paralysis, to dire outcomes, such as coma and death. The treatment for decompression sickness is hyperbaric oxygen therapy. See DIVING MEDICINE.

Decompression, spinal cord

A surgical procedure to relieve pressure on the spinal cord or on a nerve root emerging from the cord. Spinal cord decompression is performed to treat conditions such as disk prolapse (a ruptured disk; see SLIPPED DISK), SPINAL STENOSIS (narrowing of the spinal canal), a tumor, or a vertebral fracture. Surgery is usually indicated when the problem becomes disabling or interferes with walking or bladder or bowel control.

In a decompression LAMINECTOMY, the surgeon removes bone, fluid, or tissue that presses on the spinal cord. Fractured vertebrae may be stabilized by fusion of the bones or the insertion of hardware. Bed rest is required after surgery to allow the spine to heal, and physical or occupational therapy may be necessary. The success rate of surgery varies from person to person.

Decongestant drugs

Drugs used to relieve nasal congestion. Decongestants are widely available in many forms to treat a congested (stuffy) nose typical of colds and allergies. Decongestants relieve only

HOW DECONGESTANTS WORK
The mucus-producing cells that line the nasal passages are supplied with blood by vessels that widen when a person has an infection or allergy. The enlarged vessels increase the flow of fluid into the cells of the mucous membrane, which swells and produces more mucus. Decongestants promote chemical action that narrows the blood vessels, diminishing both the swelling and the production of mucus.

Engorged cells of mucous membrane — Mucus buildup — Enlarged blood vessels

Untreated congestion of nasal membrane

Reduced mucus production — Decreased swelling

Contracted blood vessels

After decongestant treatment

a stuffy nose and are not effective against other symptoms of colds or allergies. Decongestants cannot cure colds.

HOW DECONGESTANTS WORK

Nasal congestion occurs when membranes lining the nose become swollen. Decongestants narrow the blood vessels that supply the nose, thus reducing blood supply to the swollen membranes, which makes them shrink.

Because decongestants are chemically related to epinephrine, a natural decongestant and stimulant, they should not be used by people who have irregular pulse, high blood pressure, heart disease, or glaucoma.

FORMS OF DECONGESTANTS

Decongestants are sold in many forms: tablets, capsules, caplets, gelcaps, liquids, nasal sprays, and nose drops. Some decongestants are available only by prescription, while others are available over-the-counter.

PRECAUTIONS

Even though decongestants are widely available without prescription, they are drugs that can cause problems. Nasal sprays and nose drops, for example, should never be used for longer than 3 days, because they can cause rebound congestion if used over several days. Rebound congestion is a condition in which the nose remains stuffy or gets worse with every dose. The only way to

stop this cycle is to stop using the drug altogether, in which case the stuffiness will go away in about a week.

Some decongestants can cause drowsiness and should not be used by people who are driving or operating machinery. Older people and children are more sensitive to the effects of decongestants and should take them only in very small amounts.

Decorticate

The state of being without a functioning cortex in the brain. When, with stimulation, the arms of a comatose person are rigidly flexed at the elbows and wrists, he or she is said to be in decorticate posture. See also COMA.

Decubitus ulcers

See PRESSURE SORES.

Deductible

The dollar amount people must pay themselves for health care before their health insurance plans begin to pay for services. See also COINSURANCE.

Defecation

The elimination of FECES or stool from the body in a bowel movement. Food is first broken down in the digestive tract. Toward the end of the tract, as waste passes through the colon, most of the remaining fluid is absorbed. The solid waste that remains is composed of a mixture of undigested and indigestible material, including vegetable fibers (roughage), bile pigments, mucus, bacteria, and dead cells.

When feces move from the colon into the rectum, the walls of the rectum are stretched. This stretching is perceived as the need to defecate. It triggers a reflex that can be either allowed to occur or overridden. If the reflex is heeded, the rectum contracts and the anal sphincters relax. Along with increased peristalsis (muscular contractions that propel food through the alimentary tract) in the sigmoid colon, this usually expels feces through the anus. At times, it is also necessary to bear down with voluntary contractions of the abdominal muscles. The defecation reflex is overridden by deliberately tightening the anal sphincters. Repeatedly ignoring the urge to defecate is a common reason for CONSTIPATION. Regularity and ease of defecation are considered more important than frequency. However, a change in the pattern of defecation can be the sign of a problem (see BOWEL MOVEMENTS, ABNORMAL).

Defense mechanisms

Automatic, unconscious psychological processes that protect a person against anxiety in response to stress and internal emotional conflict. Typically, defense mechanisms occur outside the person's awareness. Defense mechanisms are grouped by how well or how poorly they help the individual adapt to the reality of his or her situation. Some allow conscious awareness of ideas, feelings, and their consequences and aid the person in finding balance among conflicting motives. Examples are affiliation (turning to others for help), humor (emphasizing the amusing or ironic aspects of the situation), or altruism (dedicating oneself to meeting the needs of others). Some defense mechanisms drive potentially threatening ideas or emotions out of consciousness. Examples are displacement (transferring feelings about one individual, such as one's boss, to someone else, such as the person's spouse or child), repression (expelling the disturbing thoughts,

desires, or experiences from consciousness), and intellectualization (excessive use of abstract thinking or generalization to control or minimize feelings).

Other defense mechanisms keep unpleasant or unacceptable emotions, ideas, and impulses out of consciousness by misattributing them to external causes, such as projecting disturbing feelings onto other persons (projection) or denying their existence altogether (denial). Some defense mechanisms involve distortions of reality, such as omnipotence (acting as if one has special powers) or excessive daydreaming as a substitute for more effective behavior (autistic fantasy). Sometimes people use action (acting out) or apathetic withdrawal as a defense mechanism. If defense mechanisms fail to improve how the person reacts to stress reactions, the individual may suffer a complete break with reality, as happens in delusion.

Defibrillation

An emergency procedure used to stop an uncontrolled, rapid, and ineffective heartbeat by administering an electric shock to the heart. The machine used to provide the shock is known as a DEFIBRILLATOR. An uncontrolled, rapid, and ineffective heart-

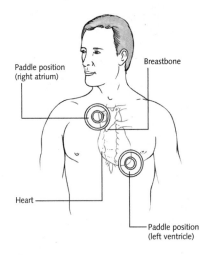

Paddle position (right atrium)

Breastbone

Heart

Paddle position (left ventricle)

PLACEMENT OF EXTERNAL PADDLES
An external defibrillator has paddles that are positioned on the chest to deliver one or more shocks to a person with sudden cardiac arrest. The person using the device can check the victim's heart function on a monitor after each shock. A person without a medical background can be trained to use a defibrillator.

beat (ventricular fibrillation) often follows a heart attack. If left untreated, it can lead to brain damage or sudden death. Defibrillation is thought to stop the heart briefly and allow a normal heartbeat to resume when the heart starts up again. The sooner defibrillation is given after ventricular fibrillation sets in, the more likely it is to be effective at preventing death or brain damage.

Defibrillator

A device used to administer an electric shock to the heart to stop an uncontrolled, rapid, and ineffective heartbeat. Such a heartbeat, which can develop after a heart attack, is known as ventricular fibrillation. Left untreated, it may lead to brain damage or sudden death. A defibrillator is thought to stop the heart briefly and allow a normal heartbeat to resume when the heart starts up again. The sooner a defibrillator is used after ventricular fibrillation sets in, the more likely it is to be effective in preventing brain damage or death.

There are three basic types of defibrillators. The manual defibrillator is used in a hospital setting to administer a high-energy electrical charge to a person experiencing ventricular fibrillation or cardiac arrest (no heartbeat). Handheld paddles are placed against the chest wall on both sides of the heart. The command "Clear!"—a fixture of television emergency-room dramas—is called out before the shock is given to prevent accidentally shocking anyone touching the person being treated. Manual defibrillators are also used for the nonemergency procedure known as CARDIOVERSION, which is used to regulate an abnormal but not immediately life-threatening heart rhythm.

An automatic defibrillator can be used by people who are not doctors, such as firefighters and emergency medical technicians. This device not only administers the electric shock but also reads and interprets the heart rhythm and determines the proper amount of electricity to provide.

The third type of defibrillator is the implantable cardioverter defibrillator (ICD), which is placed surgically in the chest to monitor the heartbeat and administer electric shock as needed to correct an abnormal heartbeat. The ICD contains an electronic memory of

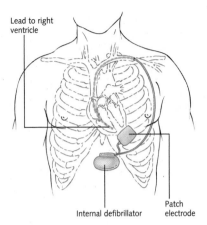

INTERNAL DEFIBRILLATOR
A defibrillator can be implanted under the skin to shock a heart that goes into certain kinds of arrhythmia. The device is slightly larger than a pacemaker and delivers a stronger shock. A wire threaded into the heart monitors the rhythm, a computer in the defibrillator determines the need for stimulus, and a patch electrode delivers the shock through the wire, if necessary.

adverse events that can be retrieved and analyzed. An ICD is similar to a PACEMAKER, but while pacemakers are generally used for people with bradycardia (abnormally slow heartbeat), ICDs are typically used for those with tachycardia (a tendency toward overly fast heart rhythms).

Defoliant poisoning
The effects of exposure to herbicide defoliant chemicals on animals and humans. Defoliant chemicals, which for years have been used routinely in agriculture to kill unwanted weeds, were widely used by US forces during the Vietnam War to expose enemy guerrilla forces in forested areas. Exposure to defoliants, especially AGENT ORANGE, has been linked to chemical acne, non-Hodgkin lymphoma, HODGKIN DISEASE, and soft-tissue SARCOMA.

To prevent defoliant poisoning among agricultural workers, US law requires that any persons handling defoliants wear protective clothing, face masks, and gloves. In addition, agricultural workers and others using defoliants must pass a course on the safe handling of such chemicals.

Deformity
Abnormal size or shape; permanent change from normal body structure.

A deformity may be present at birth (congenital), or it may develop after birth (acquired).

Degeneration
In medicine, a disease process causing deterioration in a body part with consequent loss of function. Degeneration also refers to deterioration in which cells are replaced by other cells, as in malignant tumors. Degeneration is also used in medicine to describe a general worsening of mental or physical qualities.

Degenerative joint disease
See OSTEOARTHRITIS.

Dehiscence
The splitting open of a partially healed surgical wound, usually because of infection. Dehiscence can be superficial, it can involve only a few layers of tissue, or it can be complete and involve the entire surgical wound. Dehiscence usually requires additional surgery and lengthens the hospital stay.

Dehydration
FOR FIRST AID
see Dehydration, page 1319

A decrease in the body's water level below that required for adequate circulation. Dehydration has many symptoms, including increased thirst, anxiety, weakness, confusion, and fainting. A decrease in urine output, dry and pale skin without the normal elasticity, sunken eyes, and decreased tears are also signs of dehydration. Dehydration can have several causes, including water loss, inadequate intake of fluids, or a combination of both. Excessive water can be lost through vomiting, diarrhea, excessive urine output, or sweating, particularly in hot weather. Dehydration in children is usually the result of a combination of factors, such as when the child refuses fluids and loses excessive fluid by sweating during fever.

Severe dehydration must be treated quickly to avoid cardiovascular collapse and death. A fluid loss of up to 5 percent of normal is considered mild; a loss of between 5 and 10 percent is considered moderate; and a loss of 10 to 15 percent is considered

severe. The best treatment for dehydration is prevention. Adequate fluids must be consumed at all times, particularly during illness. Infants and young children can be given special solutions, available over-the-counter in drug stores, that provide the correct balance of electrolytes when they are at risk of dehydration. Older people, children, and athletes are at greatest risk of dehydration.

Dehydro-epiandrosterone
See DHEA.

Déjà vu
A sense of familiarity when facing a situation or event one has not encountered before. The new situation is mistakenly viewed as a repetition of a previous event. Déjà vu is not usually a sign of a psychological disorder.

Deletion 22q syndrome
A condition in which part of chromosome 22 is missing or deleted. This deletion of genetic material can lead to a wide range of disorders and physical manifestations, including learning disabilities, abnormal facial features, malformations of the heart, abnormalities of the parathyroid and thymus glands, and cleft palate (a hole in the roof of the mouth). (See also CLEFT LIP AND PALATE.) Deletion 22q syndrome is estimated to occur in one of every 4,500 births.

Most cases of deletion 22q syndrome occur at random and represent an apparently spontaneous mutation on chromosome 22, rather than an inherited genetic condition. In some cases, however, the deletion is transmitted directly from parent to child. Newborns found to have deletion 22q syndrome should have an evaluation of areas that may be affected, including the heart; the palate; the ear, nose, and throat; and the endocrine, immune, and nervous systems.

Delirium
A state of mental confusion that develops over a few hours or days and tends to fluctuate, often rapidly. Delirium involves changes in consciousness, such as reduced awareness of the person's surroundings and a loss of attention or concentration,

and in impaired memory, disorientation to time or place, or impaired use of language, such as difficulty naming objects.

Delirium is caused by a disturbance in brain function and may be due to a general medical condition, such as a high temperature (fever), encephalitis, malaria, liver or kidney disease, or high blood pressure. Another cause may be certain chemical substances, including some toxins, certain medications, and recreational drugs such as cocaine, marijuana, hallucinogens, opium, and heroin. Alcoholism also may be a cause. In some cases, delirium is caused when a drug is withdrawn from a person addicted to it. Withdrawal from alcohol causes so-called delirium tremens (the "DTs"), for example. Treatment of delirium depends on the underlying cause and often involves hospitalization and medication (usually tranquilizers) to control mood or stabilize brain function. In most cases, delirium lasts approximately 1 week, although it may take several weeks or even months for cognitive function to return to normal. Full recovery depends on the cause and pre-existing medical and neurological conditions. If delirium occurs in older people, it may be a sign of a serious medical illness.

Delirium tremens

A disorder involving severe physical and psychological symptoms that can occur when alcohol is withdrawn from a person dependent on it (see ALCOHOL DEPENDENCE); commonly abbreviated to DTs. Individuals who drink the equivalent of 7 or 8 pints of beer, or 1 pint of distilled alcohol (for example, whisky or vodka), every day for several months or who have been alcohol-dependent for more than 10 years are most at risk for DTs.

The disorder usually begins within 72 hours of the last drink, but may not occur for 7 to 10 days. Physical symptoms include feeling shaky or nervous, irritability, depression, fatigue, sweating, pale skin, headache, nausea and vomiting, inability to sleep (insomnia), and loss of appetite. Psychological symptoms can include rapid mood changes, decreased attention span, confusion, disorientation, agitation, hallucinations (usually visual, such as snakes

or insects crawling on the walls or the person's body), stupor, and lethargy. The disorder is a medical emergency that may require life-support measures, antiseizure medications, tranquilizers, and antipsychotic drugs. Once the person survives the acute episode, treatment for alcohol dependency can begin.

Delivery, vaginal

FOR FIRST AID
see Childbirth, page 1317

The passage of a baby through the vagina, or birth canal, and out of the mother's body. Vaginal delivery is the most common type of birth. When a vaginal delivery is not considered safe or possible, a CESAREAN SECTION, in which the baby is removed through an abdominal incision, is performed. In a vaginal delivery, involuntary uterine contractions push the baby out of the uterus. As the baby's head enters the vagina, deliberate pushing by the mother can help deliver the baby. Most babies are delivered headfirst. See also BREECH DELIVERY.

BABY'S MOVEMENTS
Babies go through a classic sequence of eight movements to ease their way through the birth canal. In the first movement, the head reaches the top of the cervix. The second movement begins the baby's descent through the birth canal, caused at first by uterine contractions and later by the mother pushing. In the third movement, the head tips forward with the chin tucked tightly against the chest and the most narrow part of the head descends through the birth canal first. In the fourth movement, the head, which has been slightly sideways, rotates to face the maternal spine. In the fifth movement, the head tilts backward, and lifts the chin to accommodate a bend in the birth canal at the bottom. At this point, the baby's head can be seen through the vaginal opening. In the sixth movement, the head emerges from the vagina and turns slightly so that it is aligned with the shoulders. In the seventh movement, the shoulders turn within the birth canal in order to fit through the pelvis. In the eighth and final movement, the baby's body turns downward, and an upper shoulder emerges from under the

mother's pubic bone. Then the lower shoulder emerges from the bottom of the vagina. Following the passage of the shoulders, the rest of the body slides out quickly with no further turns by the baby and no particular effort by the mother.

BIRTHING ASSISTANCE
The doctor or MIDWIFE helps the baby's head emerge slowly from the vaginal opening, checking for the location of the UMBILICAL CORD. If the cord is looped around the baby's neck, as is the case about 25 percent of the time, the doctor slips it over the head or back over the shoulders. As the head emerges, the doctor wipes the AMNIOTIC FLUID off the baby's face and suctions fluid from its mouth and nose so that it does not inhale fluid when it starts breathing.

When the baby has fully emerged from the vagina, the doctor, midwife, or nurse clamps and cuts the umbilical cord, first usually waiting for it to stop pulsating. Two clamps are attached to the cord close to the baby's body, and the cut is made between them. The clamp closest to the baby is left on for 24 hours, and the remnant of the cord dries and eventually falls off naturally. Once the cord has been clamped, the newborn often is placed on the mother's abdomen. See also CHILDBIRTH and LABOR.

Delusion

A persistent, unshakable, and false belief that is held despite obvious evidence to the contrary. The belief that is held, however, is not shared by other family members, for example. Delusions can take many forms: persecution (that others are plotting against the individual); grandeur (that a person is a well-known figure); jealousy (that one's lover or spouse is unfaithful); somatic (that a person's body emits foul odors or is infested with insects); and erotomania (that a famous or powerful person is secretly in love with the individual). Arguing against the delusion or presenting contrary evidence is futile because the person tries to use the evidence to support the delusion. In some cases, delusion makes the person a threat to himself or others.

Delusions can be caused by the abuse of substances such as crack cocaine, a general medical condition such as Alzheimer's disease or systemic lupus erythematosus, or underlying mental illness, such as delusional disorder, manic-depressive illness severe depression, and schizophrenia. Treatment depends on the underlying cause.

Dementia

A syndrome marked by a progressive loss of memory and other intellectual functions. Although it can occur at any age, dementia is most common in older people. Its early signs may be as subtle as simple forgetfulness and confusion. However, an affected person gradually cannot function normally and eventually becomes incapacitated. Dementia is not a normal consequence of aging. More than half of all cases are caused by Alzheimer's disease and are irreversible. Among the potentially reversible causes of dementia are thyroid gland problems and vitamin deficiencies.

SYMPTOMS

Memory impairment, especially for recent events, is the hallmark of dementia. Other cognitive symptoms may include confusion, decreased judgment and understanding, disorientation, impaired speech, an inability to name objects, and difficulty concentrating. Emotional problems such as mood swings, personality changes, indifference, apathy, irritability, and depression may follow. Eventual symptoms may include agitation, anger, frustration, aggression, paranoia, restlessness, and wandering.

In the early stages of dementia, people may have trouble using the telephone, keeping track of finances, or remembering the names of familiar people, places, and objects. As the condition progresses, ability to reason and understand is increasingly impaired. An individual may lose interest in familiar activities. Over time, basic functions such as eating, dressing, washing, and using the toilet will be more difficult or impossible. This gradual mental and physical deterioration may take place over a period of 4 to 8 or more years. For some individuals, it may occur more rapidly or more gradually.

CAUSES AND DIAGNOSIS

Dementia results from diseases that damage normal brain cells. Damage to brain cells can occur from a variety of causes such as multiple

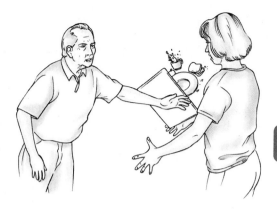

COPING WITH DEMENTIA
A person with dementia may exhibit uncharacteristic mood swings, anger, irritability, or other emotional symptoms. Caretakers may be able to help diminish some of these responses by providing a reliable routine, changing aspects of the care or surroundings that provoke repeated outbursts, or providing memory aids that help the person function as smoothly as possible.

strokes, Alzheimer's disease, HUNTINGTON CHOREA, PARKINSON DISEASE, LEWY BODY DEMENTIA, and PICK DISEASE. There is no known physical, psychological, or laboratory test that provides a definitive diagnosis. The diagnosis is based on a complete physical examination, medical history, and test results. These may include basic tests of blood and urine; neuropsychological tests of memory, problem solving, and language; and imaging studies of the brain, such as CT (computed tomography) scanning or MRI (magnetic resonance imaging).

An important part of the diagnosis is ruling out other possible causes of a person's symptoms. For instance, depression can cause pseudodementia, a syndrome that resembles dementia. Depression and thyroid gland problems, vitamin deficiencies, alcohol use, drug reactions, and brain tumors are potentially treatable problems that can bring on dementialike symptoms. See also ALCOHOL AND OLDER PEOPLE; DEPRESSION, IN OLDER PEOPLE.

TREATMENT

Most forms of dementia are irreversible. However, when symptoms are due to a potentially treatable underlying cause (such as thyroid problems or drug reactions) dementia may be treatable, and with appropriate management, symptoms of dementia usually lessen. Some form of daily supervision is necessary to ensure the comfort and safety of a person with dementia, even in its early stages. Those who have dementia may forget to eat or may wander off and become lost and distressed. Providing a regular mealtime schedule and memory aids, such as labels describing the contents of kitchen cabinets or bedroom drawers, may be necessary. There is no known cure for Alzheimer's disease, the leading cause of dementia. However, in its early to middle stages, medications such as donepezil can slow the progression of the disease and may lessen some of the cognitive symptoms.

The behavioral problems of dementia can be minimized. Modify-ing the home environment and avoiding situations that are likely to provoke outbursts can help. Medications can be used to control symptoms such as sleeplessness, agitation, wandering, anxiety, and depression. However, medications are usually prescribed only after other measures have been tried. Common drug side effects such as sedation and confusion can be troubling, especially to older people who have dementia. Often, the use of medications increases the risk of falls (see FALLS, IN OLDER PEOPLE) and fractured bones. Eventually, a person with dementia may require the skilled and constant care that is only available at a LONG-TERM CARE FACILITY, such as a nursing home or a specialized Alzheimer's center.

Demyelination

Breakdown of the fatty sheaths that surround and insulate nerve cells. See MULTIPLE SCLEROSIS.

Dendritic ulcer

See HERPES KERATITIS.

Dengue

An acute viral illness that is characterized by high fever and transmitted by the *Aedes aegypti* mosquito, usually found in tropical or subtropical regions and especially in urban areas.

People living in or traveling to these areas are at risk of contracting the illness. Dengue, also called dengue fever, has rare, but severe forms that may be fatal. These include dengue hemorrhagic fever and dengue shock syndrome.

SYMPTOMS AND DIAGNOSIS

In addition to a sudden fever, dengue symptoms include chills, severe frontal headache, pain behind the eyes, and muscle and joint aches. These symptoms may last for several days. After a brief absence of symptoms and seeming recovery, symptoms may reappear with fever, body aches, and a red rash that resembles measles.

Dengue hemorrhagic fever is characterized by extremely elevated body temperature and internal bleeding. Dengue shock syndrome includes those symptoms as well as very low blood pressure. Diagnosis is made on the basis of clinical history and examination and confirmed by blood tests.

OUTLOOK

Epidemics of dengue fever are currently larger and more frequent than they have been in the past. The increase in incidence of the illness is associated with increased urbanization in tropical regions and the rapid dispersal of the virus via air travel. The movement to control this health problem is based on educating the medical community in affected areas and developing community-based prevention programs aimed at controlling the mosquito population. Research priorities include developing improved, specific diagnostic tests and a vaccine.

Densitometry

The measurement of bone density using special X-ray techniques. Dual photon absorptiometry (DPA) and DUAL-ENERGY X-RAY ABSORPTIOMETRY (DEXA) are often ordered to measure the density of the vertebrae in the lower back and hip. A woman's bone density is generally checked at the beginning of menopause and again 6 months to 1 year later to evaluate bone density and identify changes that may indicate early signs of osteo-

> Terms in small capital letters—for example, PHYSICAL THERAPY or PAGET DISEASE—indicate a cross-reference to another entry with more information.

porosis and to monitor any response to treatment.

Density

The compactness of a substance, such as tissue. In radiology, density of tissue is determined by the amount of light or darkness seen in an area of a scan and is based on how dense the tissue is to radiation. Differences in tissue density are what allows CT (computed tomography) scans and MRI (magnetic resonance imaging) to create images of the body's organs and tissues.

Dental assistant

The person who assists a dentist with a variety of tasks and helps with patient care. The duties of a dental assistant may include preparing patients for treatments, sterilizing or disinfecting instruments, handing instruments to the dentist, developing X rays, offering postoperative instructions, and teaching at-home oral health care. Some dental assistants are also responsible for obtaining dental records, scheduling and confirming appointments, filing treatment records, billing, and ordering dental supplies. Dental assistants who do laboratory work may make casts of teeth from dental impressions (see IMPRESSION, DENTAL), clean and polish removable dental appliances, and make temporary crowns (see CROWN, DENTAL). Many dental assistants are trained and certified by accredited programs.

Dental dam

A barrier device commonly used in dental procedures that may also be used during oral sexual activity to prevent possible transmission of SEXUALLY TRANSMITTED DISEASES (STDs). The use of a dental dam is recommended by health professionals for use during oral-vaginal sex, oral-penile sex, or oral-anal sex. These devices help prevent the spread of STDs including AIDS (acquired immunodeficiency syndrome) from the anus or vagina to the mouth and from the mouth to the vagina or anus. The use of dental dams has not been clinically tested to prove their effectiveness, but their use is recommended as one component of safer sex.

Dental dams are generally 6-inch squares of latex, although hygienic

nonlatex dental dams are also available. They are available in various colors and in varying gauges from thin to extra heavy. There are scented and flavored dental dams.

Before use, the device must be rinsed to remove the powdery talc coating, then patted dry with a lint-free towel or air dried. Before oral-vaginal sex, the dam is spread over the entire vaginal opening and clitoris. The edges of the dam are held with the hands. Before oral-anal contact, the dam is used to cover the anus. A new dental dam should be used for each oral sexual activity, and only one side of the device should be used before discarding it. A dental dam used in the anal region should not be used for oral-vaginal activity, as organisms from the anus can be harmful to the vagina.

Plastic wrap may be used as a dental dam during oral sex, and nonspermicidal latex condoms may be cut to form a dental dam. Latex from a condom may be thinner and more susceptible to breakage than the latex used in conventional dental dams.

Dental examination

An exploration and analysis of the mouth, teeth, and gums by a dentist. A dental examination may be performed as a routine yearly checkup or to assess a complaint. Before the examination, the person answers questions regarding general health, current medications, prior dental treatments, special conditions (such as mitral valve prolapse and other heart conditions), diseases (such as diabetes), allergic reactions to medication, allergies, recent surgery, and pregnancy. These questions should be answered carefully because the information that they provide can be extremely important to the decisions made by the dentist regarding treatment.

WHAT TO EXPECT

During the examination, the dentist first looks at the overall condition of the entire mouth, to see if there are signs of disorders not related to the teeth, such as gum disease and diseases of the tissues lining the mouth and tongue. A cancer screening is usually done at this time. The dentist next examines the teeth, one by one, with a small, round mirror (for observing the backs of teeth), and a pointed probe, to determine if exist-

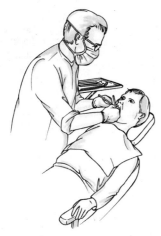

KEEPING MOUTH AND TEETH HEALTHY
Regular dental checkups and cleaning will help prevent serious problems such as gum disease and give the dentist an opportunity to check for signs of oral cancer or disorders of the jaw. A dentist will become familiar with a patient's medical history, talk to a patient about how to keep the teeth and mouth healthy before problems arise, and thoroughly discuss concerns about procedures before they are performed.

ing fillings (see FILLING, DENTAL) are sound and if there is new TOOTH DECAY. If the person being examined wears DENTURES, the dentures are examined for proper fit as well as for their effect on the gums and natural teeth. The gums and supporting structures are also checked at this appointment.

At the first dental examination and at 6-month intervals thereafter, dental X rays may be taken to look for conditions that cannot be observed visually, such as the status of wisdom teeth (see WISDOM TOOTH) or the effects of possible PERIODONTAL DISEASE on the bone supporting the teeth. Dental X rays enable the dentist to check for cavities between teeth and under existing fillings.

Dental examinations are generally followed by the scheduling of appointments for necessary treatments.

Dental hygienist

A dental professional trained to examine, clean, and scale the teeth; take and develop X rays; and offer instruction on proper dental care. The primary responsibility of the dental hygienist is professional cleaning of the teeth. Some dental hygienists also give local anesthesia, perform root-planing procedures, and place sealants. They are trained in specialized schools and have passed a state licensing examination in their field. Dental hygienists usually work as staff members with a dentist.

Dental implants

See IMPLANTS, DENTAL.

Dental laboratory technician

A highly trained professional who makes or repairs dental appliances. By using dental impressions taken from the patient by the dentist or dental hygienist, a dental laboratory technician (also called a denturist) constructs or repairs fixed and removable dental appliances, such as a crown or denture.

Dental X rays

See X RAYS, DENTAL.

Dentin

The main tissues located beneath the enamel of the surface of the tooth. Dentin, which is primarily composed of calcium, is less brittle than enamel and softer, which makes it more vulnerable to infection and TOOTH DECAY. If the enamel in a tooth is eroded or the gums recede to expose the roots of a tooth, the dentin loses its essential protective covering. When exposed, dentin is very sensitive to touch or pressure, heat, cold, foods that are either sweet or sour, and even airflow. For this reason, the condition commonly known as having sensitive teeth is medically termed dentin hypersensitivity. A person who experiences sensitivity in the teeth should consult his or her dentist. Treatment may include the use of a desensitizing toothpaste, the daily application of a prescription fluoride solution, or a dental procedure to cover the exposed surfaces with bonding materials (see BONDING, DENTAL).

Dentist

A person who has received specialized training in dentistry and has met the necessary legal qualifications to practice in the field. Dentists are educated at university-affiliated dental colleges and graduate with a DDS degree (doctor of dental surgery) or a DMD degree (doctor of dental medicine). After passing an examination, they are licensed by the state where they practice dentistry. Most dentists are general practitioners who provide comprehensive dental care including cleaning, filling, and extracting teeth; treating gum disease; correcting BITE irregularities; performing minor surgery on the mouth or jaw; and making and placing dental restorations and DENTURES.

All licensed dentists can practice any of the specialized areas within the field. Some dentists receive additional training to become specialists in one or more of the subdivisions in the profession. Board-certified dental specialists must satisfy training requirements and have mandated clinical experience in their area of expertise. Dental specialty programs require 2 to 3 years of postgraduate training, while an oral surgeon designation requires a minimum of 4 years of additional training. A dentist in general practice may refer a person to a specialist when circumstances indicate the need for more specialized care. Dentists who specialize include oral surgeons, orthodontists, prosthodontists, periodontists, endodontists, and pediatric dentists (see ORTHODONTIST; PERIODONTIST; and ENDODONTIST).

Dentistry

The medical profession concerned with the health of the teeth, gums, and tissues of the mouth. Dentistry involves preventing, diagnosing, and treating disorders in these structures; dentists are practitioners of this profession.

Dentition

The characteristics and position of the teeth in the upper and lower arches of the jaw. The term is sometimes used to describe incoming teeth. Mixed dentition refers to the presence of some PRIMARY TEETH and some PERMANENT TEETH in the mouth of a child at the same time. Permanent dentition refers to the 32 permanent teeth in the mouth of an adult.

Dentures

An artificial replacement for missing natural teeth and adjacent tissues in the upper jaw, the lower jaw, or both. Dentures are made of a strong acrylic resin, sometimes in combination with various metals. Partial dentures, either fixed or removable, are used to replace one or several missing PERMANENT TEETH (see BRIDGE, DENTAL). A full denture (false teeth) becomes necessary when a dentist or a specialist in PROSTHODONTICS determines that all the teeth—top, bottom, or both—must be removed (see TOOTH EXTRACTION). Saving the permanent teeth may be impossible if a person has serious PERIODONTAL DISEASE or severe TOOTH DECAY. Dentures may also be a solution if all or many teeth are lost in an accident or physical trauma. If there are a few strong, healthy natural teeth present in the mouth, they may be used to help anchor what is called an overdenture, a denture that fits over the remaining healthy teeth. The remaining teeth that will help support the overdenture may require ROOT CANAL TREATMENT and the placement of restorations, or dental crowns (see CROWN, DENTAL), before the overdenture can be fitted. Dental implants (see IMPLANTS, DENTAL) are another alternative to the replacement of permanent teeth; they may be used to support missing teeth, ranging from one tooth to all the teeth.

Full dentures must be carefully fitted by a dentist or prosthodontist so that they will rest comfortably on the gum ridges of the lower jaw and be

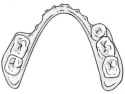

Partial denture

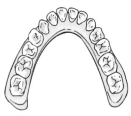

Full denture

REPLACING LOST TEETH
Dentures can replace all natural teeth and tissue in the upper or lower jaw or a single tooth or series of teeth. Dentures must be carefully fitted to be comfortable and secure. Food particles, saliva, and bacteria (plaque) can build up on dentures just as they do on natural teeth, so dentures require the same care and cleaning as the teeth they replace. The gums on which dentures rest also need lifelong care.

held securely in place by suction on the upper gum ridges. After the teeth are extracted, the gums and jaw are generally allowed to heal before the dentures are fitted. In some cases, the dentures may be prepared in advance and placed on the gum ridges immediately after the teeth have been extracted. The disadvantage to immediate placement of the dentures is that they may have to be relined after healing has taken place.

In preparation for the initial fitting of dentures, impressions (see IMPRESSION, DENTAL) are taken of the gums, and the natural BITE is measured and recorded. Decisions are made regarding the size and color of the dentures; the dentist may offer choices to the person being fitted. The dentist will set the teeth in wax and create preliminary dentures, which can be correctly fitted before being finished in acrylic.

POSSIBLE PROBLEMS
All dentures require proper cleaning as recommended by the dentist. Regularly scheduled, periodic fitting adjustments by the dentist are also essential to prevent the risks of mouth sores and bone loss. Full dentures on the lower jaw may be difficult to retain in place, even when they fit well, and may require the person wearing them to use surrounding muscles to keep them stable. Gum inflammation (gingivitis), mouth ulcers, and sores occur when dentures are not held firmly in place. Pain when chewing, red or swollen gums, or sore, white patches on the gums require the care of a dentist. Fungal infections of the gums may be treated with antifungal drugs. If the gums shrink due to bone loss, there are surgical treatments to correct the problem; the tissues of the gum and bone may be built up, or a metallic support may be implanted in the bone.

SELF-CARE
Avoiding certain hard foods that cause pain when chewing with dentures may help to prevent problems. Special preparation methods—removing corn from the cob, cutting firm fruits like apples into small pieces—may also be helpful. Daily cleaning of dentures, preferably after each meal, is important for removing food particles and plaque (see PLAQUE, DENTAL). Full, removable dentures should be taken out of the mouth at night to rest the gums and

prolong the longevity of the ridges. The gums should be cleaned daily with a soft brush or cloth, and massaged with clean fingers; the cleaning and stimulating of the gums are essential to ORAL HYGIENE and to the overall health of the mouth. Full dentures should be regularly soaked in a denture-cleaning agent that is mixed with water; dentures that are not placed in water during storage tend to warp and become ill-fitting. The dentist will probably recommend having an extra set of dentures for emergencies.

Deoxyribonucleic acid

Commonly known as DNA, the fundamental genetic component of all cellular organisms and some viruses. DNA is the chemical that forms the structure of genes. With the exception of identical twins, each person's DNA is unique. In any one individual, DNA is a component of each cell and is identical in every cell, whether a skin cell, bone cell, or other cell. DNA gives cells their specialized functions. Located on the chromosomes in the nucleus of each cell, DNA carries the information that instructs cells to produce the proteins by which they function. For example, DNA instructions enable nerve cells to produce the proteins that let them receive and send messages to the brain. DNA copies itself for each descendent cell, passing along the information needed for protein synthesis. DNA ensures that specialized cells, such as brain or liver cells, are produced at the right place in the right amount.

The DNA molecule is continuous, double-stranded, and shaped like a twisted ladder with the footholds representing nucleotide bases, the substances that form genes. Specific genetic instructions depend on the sequence (code) in which the nucleotide bases appear within a gene. DNA instructions are carried out by RIBONUCLEIC ACID (RNA), a chemical messenger that transports the DNA's orders into the part of the cell where proteins are made.

Dependence

A pervasive and excessive need to be taken care of when no physical reason makes such care necessary.

Dependence leads a person to become clingy, submissive, and fearful of separation. Dependent people have great difficulty making ordinary day-to-day decisions, such as which shirt or blouse to wear. They are so passive that they allow others, usually parents or a spouse, to make decisions for them, and they have great difficulty expressing disagreement with others, particularly people they depend on because they fear losing the relationship in the event of conflict. A dependent person shows little initiative and rarely does things on his or her own. The person may go to excessive lengths to win support and care. Since dependent people are preoccupied with fears of being left to care for themselves, they urgently seek a new relationship to provide support when a current relationship ends. Dependent people are typically pessimistic and self-doubting, belittling of their own abilities, and often refer to themselves as "stupid." They seek out protection and dominance from others because they lack faith in themselves. Dependent individuals may endure long-term physical or sexual abuse rather than end an abusive relationship out of fear of being left alone and independent.

Dependence can be a sign of a psychological disorder, such as panic disorder, agoraphobia, or depression. If the condition exists in the absence of another disorder or a general medical condition, it may mean the person has a dependent personality disorder. There is no known cure for this disorder, although psychotherapy can be helpful.

Dependence may also indicate addiction to a substance. See ALCOHOL DEPENDENCE; DRUG ADDICTION.

Depersonalization

The feeling that one's body is unreal, unfamiliar, floating, dead, changing in size, or being observed by the self from the outside. Isolated incidents of depersonalization are normal and no reason for concern. Depersonalization that continues for long periods or recurs often can be a sign of depression, schizophrenia, or panic disorder. Treatment is directed at the underlying disorder. Depersonalization differs from DEREALIZATION, in which the individual perceives the environment as unreal.

Depression

FOR SYMPTOM CHART

see Depression, page 32

An abnormal and persistent mood state characterized by sadness, melancholy, slowed mental processes, and changes in such physical patterns as eating and sleeping. While feelings of being blue or down usually improve on their own after a few days, depression continues. Medically, depression is defined as the daily presence for 2 weeks of at least five of nine symptoms. Those symptoms, of which one symptom must be either melancholy mood or loss of pleasure, include melancholy mood or sadness (sometimes experienced as apathy or irritability) for most of the day; loss of pleasure in practically all activities, particularly ones the person previously enjoyed; disturbed appetite or either weight gain or loss; and disturbed sleep, particularly the inability to sleep through the night (insomnia). Other symptoms include slowed or agitated physical activity; fatigue or very low energy, often leading to a diminished or nonexistent sex drive; feelings of worthlessness, low self-esteem, or inappropriate guilt; difficulty concentrating and thinking; and morbid or suicidal thoughts or actions.

In very severe cases, depressed people develop psychotic symptoms, such as hearing voices that tell them to kill themselves. Depression impairs a person's ability to function in family relationships, school, and job roles. Depression may alternate with periods of high excitement and energy (mania); in this case, the disease is BIPOLAR DISORDER. The most serious complication of depression is suicide.

COURSE AND CAUSES

Major depression is a common disorder. It usually begins in a person's 20s, although the disorder can appear in adolescents and children. In some cases, the first depressive episode is preceded by milder but chronic symptoms (DYSTHYMIA), which escalate into depression. Depression usually recurs. Depressive episodes are likely to come and go over periods of months or years. In some people, depression becomes chronic. Depression often occurs along with other disorders, such as anorexia nervosa, bulimia, obsessive-compulsive disorder, and substance abuse.

The precise cause of depression is unknown. The disorder is twice as common in women as in men. Most likely, this is due to differences in sex hormones since women are predisposed to two types of depression (premenstrual syndrome and postpartum depression), both of which are related to fluctuations in a woman's hormone levels. Imbalances in certain brain chemicals (neurotransmitters) also appear to be involved, since some of the most effective medications for depression affect the levels of these chemicals. Depression tends to run in families, indicating a genetic component. Life events, such as a history of childhood neglect or abuse; emotional stress, such as divorce, the death of a loved one, or financial difficulties; alcohol or drug abuse; and physical illness, such as cancer or stroke in certain parts of the brain, can also be causes. Older people are at increased risk of depression; it may be related to multiple medical problems and repeatedly losing close friends and loved ones.

Because depression may cause suicide, the disorder can be life-threatening. About one in seven people with untreated depression kill themselves. Rarely, depressed persons think of harming others or acting out those thoughts.

TREATMENT

Depression can be treated effectively

RISK FACTORS FOR SUICIDE

Women are three times more likely than men to attempt suicide, but men are three times more likely to complete suicide, usually by violent methods. The exact cause of suicide is unclear and often complex. Here are some known risk factors for those most likely to attempt to kill themselves:

- Male
- White or Native American
- Older (more than 60 years)
- Lack of social support
- Financial difficulties
- Recent humiliation
- Chronic or severe medical illness
- Family history of suicide
- Substance abuse

D

D

in almost all cases. The most common approaches are psychotherapy (also called counseling or talk therapy) and antidepressant medication, sometimes used alone or in combination with psychotherapy. Therapy for depression focuses on discovering and altering negative ways of thinking; teaching patients ways of coping with low moods; and, for people who have suffered stressful events like sexual abuse or the death of a spouse, dealing with the emotions connected to those events.

A variety of effective ANTIDEPRESSANTS are available, all of them effective. The choice of medication and the dosage depend upon the person's symptoms and any side effects caused by the particular drug. How long the medication is used is determined by the person's response to the drug and the course of his or her disorder.

In severe, chronic cases of depression that does not respond to medication, ECT (electroconvulsive therapy) is used. This consists of inducing a seizure by running a small electrical current through the brain. ECT is very effective, but it cannot prevent the recurrence of depression. People who have had ECT may have the treatment repeated. Sometimes, antidepressants are prescribed as a preventive measure.

Depression, in older people

Persistent feelings of sadness, accompanied by other symptoms such as insomnia, poor appetite, and weight loss. In older adults, disorientation, memory loss, and distractibility may be particularly prominent. Depressed older people may complain of aches and pains or fatigue, rather than sadness. They often complain of memory loss or inability to concentrate. Other traits typical of depression include irritability and excessive crying. See also DEPRESSION.

Older adults sometimes must cope with difficult issues that often cause grief. The loss of loved ones and friends, retirement, chronic illness, or moving into a long-term care facility can all temporarily result in sadness and a sense of loss. That is part of the normal grieving process and is not depression. However, feelings of sadness that persist for longer than 2 months may be a sign of depression. Other indications of depression may include suicidal thoughts, deep feelings of worthlessness, reduced physical activity, prolonged functional impairment (such as a lack of coordination), and hallucinations other than visits from a recently deceased person, which are not uncommon.

DIAGNOSIS AND TREATMENT

Depression in older people frequently is overlooked. The more obvious physical complications that accompany aging may overshadow the symptoms of depression. Often the signs of depression in older people are dismissed as grumpiness, crankiness, or part of the aging process. Sometimes, the inattention, lack of concentration, confusion, and disorientation caused by depression can be mistaken for DEMENTIA, a chronic brain disorder in which there is a progressive loss of memory and other intellectual functions. Depression can also accompany ALZHEIMER'S DISEASE (the most common form of dementia), particularly in its early stages.

A physician can determine whether there is an underlying physical cause for depression or whether it may be linked to prescription or over-the-counter drugs an older person is taking. Depression may also accompany other chronic diseases, such as PARKINSON DISEASE, STROKE, or hormonal disorders. If the doctor believes the symptoms are related to depression, he or she may initiate treatment.

Psychotherapy and medication are used to relieve depression in older people. Medications known as antidepressants can relieve depression. Some of the newer varieties, notably serotonin reuptake inhibitors, are associated with fewer side effects than older antidepressants. Severe cases of depression may require more intensive treatment, such as hospitalization in a psychiatric unit.

Support groups at senior centers may help many older people cope with major life changes. Talking with peers or a mental health professional can help combat feelings of being alone.

Derealization

The perception that the environment is unreal. The individual feels separated from the surroundings, as if he

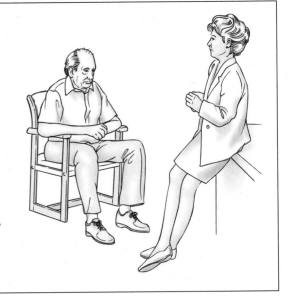

IDENTIFYING DEPRESSION
Depression in an older person can be difficult to identify. Medical problems, side effects of medications, or the effects of aging itself may mask symptoms of depression. An older person often experiences loss of friends or family, change in lifestyle, limited mobility, loneliness, or medical problems that could cause depression, and he or she needs extra attention to address these concerns. Friends and family can help by spending as much time as possible talking and listening to an older person. A physician can treat depression with therapy, antidepressant medications, or a combination of both.

or she were watching a movie. Derealization differs from DEPERSON-ALIZATION, in which the individual perceives himself or herself as unreal.

Dermabrasion

The removal of the surface layer of the skin by high-speed planing or sanding. Originally, dermabrasion was performed to improve the appearance of scars that resulted from injury or disease. It is now also used to treat acne scars, remove tattoos, and correct sun-related skin damage such as fine wrinkles and age spots.

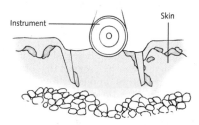

REMOVING OUTER SKIN LAYER
In dermabrasion surgical instruments are used to sand down or plane off the surface of the skin to smooth scars or wrinkles, or even remove tattoos. The procedure will remove superficial irregularities altogether, but deeper scarring or pigment can be improved only somewhat in appearance.

Dermabrasion is performed in an office or outpatient facility. Sedatives may be given to reduce anxiety, and topical anesthetics are used to reduce discomfort. During the procedure, a rotary abrasive instrument (a rapidly swirling wire brush, diamond cutting tool, or sandpaper) is used to remove or sand upper layers of the skin, removing irregularities. Afterward, soothing ointments and dressings are applied.

After dermabrasion, the sensation is similar to that of a severe sunburn. However, the doctor can prescribe medication to alleviate discomfort, and most people resume their normal activities within 7 to 10 days of the procedure. Good hygiene and the regular use of moisturizing lotions help speed healing. Eventually a new layer of skin forms, giving the skin a smoother appearance. At first, the newly formed skin tends to be lighter than the original skin tone. The pink or lighter skin gradually fades, and skin returns to normal color in 8 to 12 weeks. Makeup can be used to

hide redness in the meantime. Exposure to sunlight should be avoided for 3 to 6 months after dermabrasion; sunscreen must be used whenever going outdoors. Complications of this procedure are uncommon but may include pigment changes, thickened skin, and fever blisters in people prone to herpes infections.

Dermatitis

Inflammation of the skin; also known as eczema, which is the general term for noninfectious skin rashes. Dermatitis can be due to an allergen or irritant or a genetic predisposition. Symptoms vary from person to person but may include redness, itching, inflammation, blistering, crusting, scabbing, scaling, thickening, and pigment (color) changes. Dermatitis is often aggravated when intense itchiness causes a person to scratch, which worsens the itch.

Diagnosis of dermatitis is based on the appearance of the skin, patch test results, tissue biopsy, and personal and family medical history. The doctor will ask about any exposure to irritants or history of allergies. Often a person is referred to a dermatologist for further evaluation. Treatment depends on the underlying cause.

Doctors may prescribe medications such as corticosteroids and antihistamines. Some cases of dermatitis respond well to PHOTOTHERAPY (treatment with light). It is important to identify and avoid irritants, which may include substances such as synthetic fibers, perfumes, and soaps. To control itching, doctors recommend applying cold compresses and soothing nonfragrant lotions, taking oatmeal baths, avoiding excessive heat and humidity, and wearing loose clothing. People who are prone to atopic dermatitis (see sidebar below) should use a moisturizer frequently and take brief, lukewarm showers rather than long, hot baths.

Dermatitis artefacta

A type of DERMATITIS that is self-induced, such as by scratching; also known as factitial dermatitis.

Dermatitis, atopic

Inflammation of the skin. This form of DERMATITIS is closely linked with atopy, an inherited predisposition to become hypersensitive or allergic to substances such as pollen, ragweed, dust mites, molds, and animal scales or droppings. It is often associated with other atopic disorders such as

---

TYPES OF DERMATITIS

Dermatitis, or the general term eczema, includes the following:

- **Atopic dermatitis**: a chronic, noninfectious skin disease characterized by itchy, inflamed skin (people with atopic dermatitis usually also have asthma or hay fever)
- **Contact dermatitis**: a localized reaction that includes redness, itching, and burning due to contact with an allergy-causing substance such as nickel or nail polish or an irritant such as a cleaning agent or other chemical
- **Dyshidrotic eczema**: irritation of the skin on the palms of the hands and the soles of the feet that is characterized by clear, deep blisters that itch and burn
- **Hand dermatitis**: redness and inflammation of the hands usually due to irritants such as soaps, chemicals, or detergents
- **Neurodermatitis**: scaly patches of skin that are caused by a localized itch that becomes intensely irritated when scratched
- **Nummular eczema**: coin-shaped plaques (patches of thick, raised skin) of irritated skin—frequently on the arms, back, and lower legs—that may be itchy, crusted, and scaling

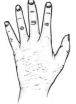

Neurodermatitis   Dyshidrotic eczema

TYPES OF DERMATITIS
The appearance of the skin is a good indication of various types of dermatitis. Affected skin on the back of the hands may be scaly and itchy, which is characteristic of neurodermatitis. Another type of dermatitis, called dyshidrotic eczema, causes deep blisters on the palms of the hands.

hay fever and asthma. Atopic dermatitis affects approximately one in ten infants and young children. Some outgrow it, although their skin usually remains dry and easily irritated. Environmental influences can bring on the symptoms of dermatitis.

SYMPTOMS

The symptoms and severity of dermatitis vary significantly from person to person. Severe itching is the primary sign. Very often there are also cracks behind the ears and rashes on the cheeks, arms, and legs. Other common symptoms include redness, inflammation, blistering, crusting, oozing, peeling, scabbing, scaling, thickening, and pigment (color) changes. Typical lesions include papules (small superficial bumps on the skin), plaques (patches of thick, raised skin), and scales and crusts (flaking, peeling layers of skin).

The symptoms most often begin in infancy and occur on and off throughout life. Episodes of atopic dermatitis may be set off by emotional stress. People with the disorder usually have very dry, sensitive skin. In adults, skin may become thick and leathery and develop painful cracks. People who have long-standing dermatitis also tend to get secondary bacterial infections.

DIAGNOSIS AND TREATMENT

There is no single test to diagnose dermatitis. Diagnosis is based on the appearance of the skin and a thorough medical history. The doctor will ask about any family or personal history of allergy, exposure to irritants, previous treatment for skin-related symptoms, and the impact of symptoms on lifestyle. Tests such as a PATCH TEST or a skin biopsy may be performed. It is important for the doctor to rule out other causes of symptoms. Often a person is referred to a dermatologist for further evaluation.

Treatment varies according to severity. The regular use of moisturizers on dry, atopic skin is helpful. Doctors also prescribe medications such as corticosteroids, antihistamines, drugs to control secondary infections, or immunosuppressant medications. Many people respond well to PHOTOTHERAPY (treatment with light). Ultraviolet (UV) B light is the preferred form of phototherapy for severe cases. PUVA (the drug psoralen plus UVA) is also used in some cases. Psoralen helps maximize the effects of ultraviolet light on the skin. People who tend to have atopic dermatitis should wear loose cotton fabrics and keep their homes free of potential irritants, such as dust, animal dander, and molds. To control itching, doctors recommend applying cold compresses and soothing creams and taking oatmeal baths. Irritants and excessive heat and humidity must be avoided. People who are prone to dermatitis should use a regular moisturizer and take brief, lukewarm showers rather than long, hot baths.

Dermatitis herpetiformis

An intensely itchy skin eruption that is associated with gluten-sensitive enteropathy (a disorder in which the lining of the small intestine is damaged by an allergic reaction to gluten, a protein found in grains such as wheat, rye, and barley). Dermatitis herpetiformis is a chronic skin disease characterized by clusters of papules (small, superficial bumps on the skin) or blisters that occur in a symmetrical pattern on the elbows, knees, buttocks, scalp, and shoulders. The itching, burning, and stinging of dermatitis herpetiformis are extremely uncomfortable. Consequent scratching leads to crusting and changes in skin color.

The severity of dermatitis herpetiformis varies. Although rashes may come and go, the disease is a lifelong condition. It typically begins when a person is in his or her 30s or 40s and affects more men than women. Although there are usually no gastrointestinal symptoms, treatment is with a gluten-free diet and medications such as dapsone. A gluten-free diet entails avoiding not only most grains but also pasta, cereal, and many processed foods. Proper diet is important to reduce symptoms, and it lowers the dosage of oral medication needed.

Dermatofibroma

A nodule (a solid mass of tissue) or small, round bump on the skin. Dermatofibromas may be pink or brown and are commonly found on the arms and legs of adults. They are believed to follow mild trauma or injury. Dermatofibromas are common, benign (not cancerous), and painless. However, they may persist indefinitely. A diagnosis is made through medical examination if the nodule dimples inward when the doctor squeezes it between his or her thumb and forefinger. No treatment is required, although surgical removal may be performed for cosmetic reasons.

Dermatographism

HIVES produced by rubbing, stroking, or friction on the skin; also known as dermographism. In dermatographism, histamine is released, causing capillaries (small blood vessels) to dilate, leading to redness and localized swelling. Dermatographism is a nonallergic cause of hives and is usually brought on by scratching. Long, raised, narrow, and itchy hives exactly follow the lines where stroking or scratching has occurred. Hives begin to appear on the skin immediately after the irritation and fade in less than an hour. Treatment is often unnecessary, but antihistamines are often prescribed if the hives cause extreme or persistent discomfort.

Dermatologist

A physician who specializes in the study of the skin, including its anatomical, physiological, and pathological characteristics. In addition to 4 years of medical school and 1 year of residency in general medicine, dermatologists have at least 3 more years of medical and surgical training in the diagnosis and treatment of skin, hair, and nail disorders.

Dermatology

The study of the skin, including its anatomical, physiological, and pathological characteristics. Dermatology encompasses the diagnosis and treatment of skin, hair, and nail disorders. Special concerns include diagnosing and preventing diseases of the skin; treating and preventing damage to the skin; and performing cosmetic procedures to improve the appearance of the skin due to injury, aging, sunlight, or disease. Dermatology may involve such procedures as CHEMICAL PEEL, DERMABRASION (removal of the surface layer of skin by high-speed sanding), LASER RESURFACING, LASER SURGERY, LIPOSUCTION (surgery in which fat is removed through suction), and surgical procedures to remove growths or unwanted varicose veins.

Dermatomycosis

A fungal infection of the skin. It usually affects moist areas of the body such as the groin (see also TINEA).

Dermatomyositis

A rare disease of the connective tissue characterized by skin rashes and inflammation and degeneration of muscles throughout the body. Although its exact cause remains unknown, doctors believe that dermatomyositis is caused by an autoimmune reaction (see AUTOIMMUNE DISORDERS) or a viral infection. Certain drugs or vaccines can cause this disease.

Early symptoms include a red rash and muscle weakness. The rash may appear on the upper eyelids, face, neck, shoulders, upper chest, and back. Muscle weakness, which either comes on suddenly or develops gradually over a period of weeks or months, can lead to problems with walking, standing, and climbing stairs. It may become difficult for the person to raise his or her arms over the head. As the disease progresses, joint pain and swelling, inflammation of the heart, and lung disease can develop. Complications may cause difficulty swallowing, shortness of breath, and carpal tunnel syndrome. In rare cases, malignant tumors are associated with this disorder.

Dermatomyositis is diagnosed by physical examination, electromyography, blood tests, and a muscle biopsy. Treatment is with corticosteroid medications and physical therapy. Immunosuppressant drugs may also be required, and associated tumors are removed whenever possible. Although it can strike at any age, dermatomyositis most commonly affects adults between the ages of 50 and 60 and children between 5 and 15. Women are affected twice as often as men. Children rarely have malignant tumors with this condition. See also POLYMYOSITIS, a similar condition but without the skin rashes.

Dermatophyte infections

Infections such as JOCK ITCH and ATHLETE'S FOOT caused by moldlike fungi (dermatophytes). See also TINEA.

Dermoid cyst

A cyst that is lined by skin. Dermoid cysts can contain a variety of tissues such as hair, sebaceous (oily) material, sweat glands, and, depending on where they occur in or on the body, even cartilage or bone. Dermoid cysts that occur in the ovary that develop from embryo cells can even grow teeth. Dermoid cysts are usually benign (not cancerous). The most common locations for dermoid cysts are the eyebrows, nose, and scalp.

DES

See DIETHYSTILBESTROL (DES).

Desensitization

A therapy for treating extreme fears (phobias) in which a person learns how to avoid anxiety and panic when facing the feared object or event. In the technique called systematic desensitization, the person is taught how to relax on cue, then presented with the feared situation in progressive steps, from least frightening to most, and trained to relax at each step. This technique works well with phobias such as fear of flying, heights, or insects such as spiders.

Desensitization, allergy

A therapy that involves repeatedly, and in a controlled manner, exposing a person's body to small amounts of extract from a substance (called an ALLERGEN) that causes allergies in the person, with the goal of eventually building up a tolerance to the allergy and reducing the allergic reaction in that person. Allergy desensitization may be called allergen immunotherapy, desensitization therapy, or, more commonly, allergy shots. The repeated introduction of an allergen in increasingly larger doses is intended to normalize the immune system's reaction to the harmless allergen so that the person will eventually be able to tolerate exposure to the antigen. The process is thought to occur by changing the response of the T lymphocytes of the immune system from allergy-provoking to allergy-protective.

Allergy shots are usually given once or twice a week initially and continued at those intervals in incremental doses until the concentration reaches a maintenance dosage level. When a maintenance level is reached, the injections may be spread out over intervals of once every 2 to 4 weeks. Eventually, there may be intervals of several years between treatments.

People who receive allergy desensitization usually benefit within 1 to 2 years of treatment, and most continue the therapy at longer intervals for the following 3 to 5 years.

Side effects are uncommon but can be severe. A rare, but extremely severe allergic response to this form of exposure to an allergen is anaphylactic shock, which is characterized by a swelling of body tissues including those in the throat, difficulty breathing, and a sudden fall in blood pressure. Because of this risk, allergy shots should be given only by a physician and a medical staff trained in immunology and the management of potential complications.

Designer drugs

Slang for drugs created by underground chemists to mimic illegal drugs. Designer drugs are usually created by changing the molecular structure of an existing drug to create a new substance, one that is not officially listed as a controlled substance. The best-known of the designer drugs, also known as club drugs, is MDMA, or Ecstasy, which resembles the stimulant methamphetamine and also has some psychedelic features. Use of Ecstasy is associated with "raves," all-night underground dance parties attended by teenagers and college students who are attracted to Ecstasy because it helps them to stay up all night.

Another type of designer drug (fentanyl analogue) is similar to heroin in that it blocks pain and causes euphoria. The fentanyl analogues have proved to be even more dangerous than heroin: two of them have been sold illegally under the names China White and New Heroin. China White has caused large numbers of fatal overdoses, while New Heroin can cause symptoms similar to those of Parkinson disease in its users.

Desipramine

An antidepressant drug. Desipramine (Norpramin) is prescribed to treat depression, obsessive-compulsive disorder, and bulimia nervosa, an eating disorder.

D

Desmoid tumor

An abnormal growth that is firm, fibrous, and rubbery. Desmoids most often occur in the abdominal wall, but may also develop in the head, neck, arm, or legs. In the abdomen, these tumors are most common in women who have had children. Growths may also develop at the site of old surgical incisions. Most desmoid tumors are local problems and do not spread or grow. Desmoid tumors usually require surgical removal. Sometimes, chemotherapy is an effective treatment.

Desogestrel

See ESTRADIOL.

Desoximetasone

See CORTICOSTEROIDS.

Detoxification

In holistic medicine, the practice of neutralizing toxins to render them more readily excreted. Colon cleansers (see COLON CLEANSING), blood purifiers, oxygen supplements, hydrogen peroxide, digestive and circulation aids, COFFEE ENEMAS, and CHELATION THERAPY are all used to help rid the body of so-called toxins. Many of the products used in body detoxification are herbal products. People who undertake body detoxification believe that poor elimination of waste products by the liver, kidneys, and colon is responsible for disease and lowered immunity.

Fasting is also used to detoxify the body. There are two types of fasts commonly used: the water fast and the juice fast. In the water fast, the person consumes a minimum of 1 and a maximum of 2 quarts of water for 24 to 36 hours, usually on weekends, until such symptoms as furry-feeling tongue and headaches have ended. In a juice fast, vegetable juices (carrot, celery, green bean, parsley, and watercress) are consumed exclusively for about 10 days. Sometimes a special bedtime drink of lemon and grapefruit juice, garlic, and olive oil is used to detoxify the liver. Juice fasting is not recommended on a regular basis.

Special detoxification diets are also followed. In these, large quantities of water, herbal teas, yogurt, and organic vegetables are consumed, although some diets restrict the dieter to a single food or only raw foods. Special detoxification diets can last for a few weeks or even years.

Detoxification programs

A medical process, usually in a hospital setting, in which a person addicted to alcohol or drugs is withdrawn from the addictive substance under the care of a physician. Detoxification is not a treatment for the addiction; rather, it is designed to manage the serious, even fatal physiological effects of stopping drug use, such as DELIRIUM TREMENS in alcohol-dependent people. Medications are available to help in detoxification from opiates (for example, heroin and morphine), nicotine (tobacco), benzodiazepines, alcohol, barbiturates, and other sedatives. A detoxification program normally lasts from 4 to 7 days and should be followed by a treatment program to address the psychological, social, and behavioral issues surrounding the person's addiction.

Developmental delay

The condition in which a child under age 5 has not attained the physical, intellectual, or social development considered normal for his or her age. In the first 5 years of life, children continually change, achieving skills in four areas: movement, language, intellect, and sociability. While individual children vary, defined developmental milestones exist within which normal children develop certain skills. For example, most children can walk by age 18 months. A child of that age who cannot walk may be experiencing developmental delay. Problems such as hearing or vision impairments can cause delay in language and intellectual development; once these impairments are treated, development can proceed. Babies who were born prematurely may lag behind other infants the same age but catch up fully by age 2.

The causes of developmental delay generally are categorized chronologically. Prenatal causes include chromosomal abnormalities or infections, such as RUBELLA, that occur during pregnancy. Perinatal causes refer to problems at birth such as oxygen deprivation. Postnatal causes are infections or injuries that occur after birth, such as MENINGITIS or severe head injuries.

TYPES OF DEVELOPMENTAL DELAY
Research has provided a refined understanding of how children proceed through the four areas of development. Based on this work, many screening and diagnostic tests have been designed to measure a child's development of skills and detect delays.

■ *Movement skills* The abilities to sit, crawl, walk, grasp and hold objects, and stack blocks are all movement or motor skills. Children usually master each of these skills by specific ages. Of all the developmental skills, motor skills are the least connected to intelligence. The cause of severe delay in motor skills is more likely to be a serious disease such as SPINA BIFIDA or CEREBRAL PALSY rather than a mental problem. Cerebral palsy primarily manifests itself as a motor abnormality.

■ *Language skills* Language development follows a predictable course. In stages, the child progresses from babbling to individual words, phrases, and full sentences. Deafness can cause language skill delays. Other causes are lack of verbal stimulation in the home, a family history of delayed speech, and damage to the organs and muscles used in speech.

■ *Intellectual skills* Normal intellectual skills include gestures such as smiling in response to learned cues at 4 months of age. Later skills may include searching for a hidden toy, matching similar objects, counting to 10, and by age 5, drawing stick figures. Delayed intellectual development is characteristic of chromosomal disorders such as FRAGILE X SYNDROME and DOWN SYNDROME. Exposure to infections before or after birth or injury in early childhood can also impair intellectual development.

■ *Social skills* Allowing for individual personalities, social development is predictable. Children usually smile by 3 months of age and laugh by 4 or 5 months. A child who does not establish eye contact, refuses to be comforted, is aggressive, or has no interest in other people may have a developmental delay. Sometimes the cause may be a lack of good interaction between parents and child. In other cases, the child may have a developmental disorder such as AUTISM.

2-year-old

3-year-old

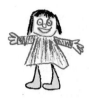
7-year-old

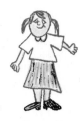
12-year-old

MILESTONES IN INTELLECTUAL SKILLS
To some extent, the way a child draws a person indicates his or her intellectual growth and development. As a child's perception of other people and hand-and-eye coordination develop, his or her drawings show a fairly typical progression. From left to right: a 2-year-old draws a person with a prominent head and face, indicating the importance of adult facial expressions at this stage; a 3-year-old draws a figure that includes a body in some form; a 7-year-old depicts a person with main features and body parts in place; a 12-year-old draws a person in reasonably lifelike proportion. The way in which a child depicts a human figure is only one of many milestones in intellectual development. Observation of these progressive skills may help identify developmental delay.

TREATMENT

Doctors routinely check development around 6 weeks, 6 months, and at 1, 2, and 3 years of age. Often, a developmental delay will be detected at an infant's or a child's regular examination. When a delay is found, the next step is finding its cause. Vision and hearing tests and a full developmental assessment will be conducted. Further investigation may involve a neurologist, psychologist, speech pathologist, occupational therapist, or physical therapist. Specific treatments may involve eyeglasses, hearing aids, regular therapy, or enrolling the child in a school or institution that has special facilities or programs appropriate to the child's disorder.

Developmental disorder, pervasive

Severe and extensive impairment in social interaction, language skills, and motor skills beginning in childhood. Children with pervasive developmental disorders typically have limited interests and activities and exhibit unusual behavior, such as repetitive hand movements and lack of eye contact. Often some degree of mental retardation accompanies these problems. The exact cause of the disorders is unknown. Often the term pervasive developmental disorder is mistakenly used interchangeably with AUTISM. However, it is a general term referring to autism and several other more rare disorders including RETT SYNDROME and the extremely uncommon ASPERGER DIS-ORDER. Autism is usually diagnosed within the first 3 years of life. It is characterized by impaired communication, mental retardation, and varying degrees of unusual, aggressive, or self-injurious behavior. In Rett syndrome, girl babies who at first appear normal gradually regress, becoming severely retarded. Asperger disorder is similar to autism except that it does not cause delays in language development. See also DEVELOPMENTAL DELAY.

DEXA

See DUAL-ENERGY X-RAY ABSORPTIOMETRY.

Dexamethasone

An anti-inflammatory drug; a corticosteroid. Dexamethasone (Decadron, NeoDecadron) reduces swelling and inflammation and is used in many disorders, including skin diseases such as hives and psoriasis; allergic conditions; cancer; anemia; digestive problems; eye disorders; and arthritis and bursitis. It is available as eye drops, tablets, injection, and an oral concentrate that must be taken with food.

Dextroamphetamine

A stimulant drug. Dextroamphetamine (Adderall, Dexedrine, DextroStat) is a prescription drug that stimulates nerve cells in the brain. It is used to treat narcolepsy, epilepsy, Parkinson disease, and hyperactivity in children. Dextroamphetamine is a drug that is easily abused and may cause many cardiovascular side effects.

Dextrocardia

An abnormal condition in which the heart lies on the right side of the chest rather than the left. The bottom of the heart points to the right instead of the left. In some cases, the abdominal organs also lie on opposite sides. In others, the organs remain in their normal positions. Dextrocardia is a congenital condition (present at birth), and, despite its abnormal position, the heart is able to function normally.

Dextromethorphan hydrobromide

A cough suppressant. Dextromethorphan is a nonprescription drug that suppresses a dry, unproductive cough without the addictive, sedative, and pain-relieving effects of codeine. It is available under many brand names as lozenges, syrups, and chewable tablets.

Dextrose

A type of sugar or glucose. Dextrose is added to processed foods to make them sweeter and as a preservative to prevent bacterial growth. A high proportion of sugar in the diet provides the body with few nutrients and unnecessary energy that may be stored as fat. Pharmaceutical preparations of dextrose are used in hospitals to provide nutrition via intravenous infusions.

DHEA

Dehydroepiandrosterone. A chemical naturally produced by the adrenal glands. DHEA is related structurally to the hormones ESTROGEN and TESTOSTERONE. After age 30, the body begins to make less DHEA. This has led manufacturers to produce and market DHEA supplements as antiaging remedies. Numerous claims have been made suggesting that DHEA supplements increase muscle, decrease fat, and boost immunity, energy, and strength. However, reliable evidence is lacking to support these claims, and liver damage may be a consequence of using them even for a short period.

Diabetes insipidus

A disease of the pituitary gland or kidneys characterized by the passage of large amounts of urine. It can be distinguished from diabetes mellitus (see DIABETES MELLITUS, TYPE 1 and DIABETES MELLITUS, TYPE 2) in two ways: it does not involve insulin production, and there is no excessive glucose (sugar) in the urine.

Diabetes insipidus is caused by an insufficient supply of ADH (antidiuretic hormone) or by the resistance of the kidneys to the effects of ADH. When an abnormally low level of ADH is produced by the hypothalamus, the disease is referred to as central diabetes insipidus. If a kidney disorder prevents the kidneys from responding to ADH in the bloodstream, the disorder is called nephrogenic diabetes insipidus. As a result of the malfunctioning mechanism that controls the output of urine, the output may be ten times greater than the normal urine output.

CAUSES AND TREATMENT

When diabetes insipidus is due to

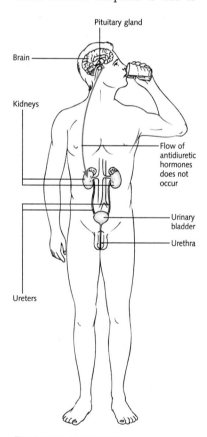

Pituitary gland

Brain

Kidneys

Flow of antidiuretic hormones does not occur

Urinary bladder

Urethra

Ureters

RARE FORM OF DIABETES
In a person with one type of diabetes insipidus, the pituitary gland is not producing adequate amounts of antidiuretic hormones that normally maintain water balance in body cells. Without the hormones, the kidneys lose excessive amounts of water, leading to dehydration. The person feels constantly thirsty.

insufficient ADH, the causes may include pituitary gland surgery, serious head injury that involves the hypothalamus or pituitary gland, or tumors of the pituitary gland or brain. Often the cause of inadequate ADH is not identifiable. When the disease is caused by a failure of the kidneys to respond to ADH in the blood, the underlying cause may be a genetic disorder, inadequate potassium in the blood, excess calcium in the blood, or certain medications.

The abnormal output of urine in central diabetes insipidus can be successfully reduced with a synthetic form of ADH called desmopressin, which is given orally. When excess urination is associated with nephrogenic diabetes insipidus, the condition may be treated by therapy aimed at correcting potassium or calcium levels in the blood. Drug-induced diabetes insipidus usually resolves when the medication that caused the disease is stopped. Treatment with NONSTEROIDAL ANTI-INFLAMMATORY DRUGS (NSAIDs) can help reduce excessive urine output in both the central and nephrogenic forms of the disease.

Diabetes mellitus, type 1

The less common of the two main groups of conditions characterized by an abnormally high glucose (sugar) level in the blood; formerly known as insulin-dependent diabetes or juvenile-onset diabetes. Type 1 diabetes mellitus, which accounts for 5 to 10 percent of all cases of diabetes, is due to little or no insulin production by the pancreas, the large endocrine gland behind the stomach where insulin is normally produced. People with type 1 diabetes require insulin injections to live. Type 1 diabetes most often occurs in children and young adults, but it can also develop in people older than 40 years. Parents of young people with type 1 diabetes play a major role in coping with the condition.

Glucose metabolism begins when intestinal enzymes break down carbohydrates into simpler sugars the body can absorb. One of these sugars is glucose, which circulates in the bloodstream and fuels the activities of important organs, including the brain. For the cells of organs to use glucose, the hormone insulin, which is made by the pancreas, must be

released into the bloodstream in proper amounts. Without insulin, the glucose cannot be properly metabolized, and the glucose level in the blood rises.

Because people with type 1 diabetes produce and release little or no insulin, glucose accumulates in the blood and is not made available to the vital organs. The excess glucose can no longer be reabsorbed by the kidneys during urine production, and excess glucose spills over into the urine without being used by the body for energy. The severe deficiency of insulin and the resulting buildup of glucose in the blood also cause a breakdown in the storage system of nutrients, resulting in an excess level of fatty acids in the bloodstream.

CAUSES

The cause of the inability of the pancreas to produce insulin is thought to be an autoimmune disorder. This disorder results when the infection-fighting mechanism in the body, the immune system, begins to destroy the insulin-producing beta cells in the pancreas. Why the immune system attacks and destroys these cells is unknown, but a number of factors may play a part. Exposure to certain viruses and other substances early in life, a person's diet, and genetic predisposition are among the possible contributing factors.

SYMPTOMS

Frequent urination (especially noticeable at night), excessive thirst, and weight loss are the classic symptoms of type 1 diabetes and relate to the elevation in blood sugar and the excess amount of sugar in the urine. The excess sugar in the urine draws water from the body, increasing urination. Excess sugar in the urine, in conjunction with the elevated blood sugar level, also causes increased thirst. The inability to use glucose as fuel causes the person to lose weight. To compensate for the inadequate fuel supply, the body tends to burn stored fat. This can cause a combination of unexplained weight loss and increased hunger. People with type 1 diabetes can lose weight despite eating more. The inability of the body to metabolize glucose can result in other symptoms, including fatigue. Blurred vision and slow healing are also symptoms that are often associated with type 1 diabetes.

Without available glucose to use as fuel, the body breaks down stored fats and proteins. The body converts the broken-down fats into waste products called ketones, which may build up in the blood and be released into the urine. Ketone levels in the blood can increase to produce a life-threatening condition called ketoacidosis, which requires emergency medical attention. The symptoms of ketoacidosis are abdominal pain, vomiting, rapid breathing, and extreme tiredness or drowsiness. Severe cases of ketoacidosis may cause mental confusion or even coma.

DIAGNOSIS

Because the complications of type 1 diabetes may begin before obvious symptoms develop, early diagnosis can be important. The fasting plasma glucose test is most commonly used to diagnose type 1 diabetes. The normal range for a fasting blood glucose level is between 70 and 100 milligrams per deciliter (mg/dL) of blood. If the glucose level is 126 mg/dL or higher on the results of two fasting plasma glucose tests, or very high (more than 200 mg/dL) on one test, a diagnosis of diabetes is usually made. The diagnosis may also be made if results of the fasting plasma glucose test reveal a high glucose level in combination with other symptoms of diabetes.

INSULIN TREATMENT

Daily insulin medication is essential for treating type 1 diabetes. Synthetic insulin, which is chemically identical to human insulin, is the lifesaving drug for people with type 1 diabetes. Before the availability of insulin, type 1 diabetes was a life-threatening disease.

Since insulin is destroyed by digestive enzymes and cannot be taken orally, it must be delivered directly into the tissues by one of several methods. Insulin injection is accomplished with the use of a needle and syringe, insulin pen, or jet injector. The insulin pen includes a replaceable insulin cartridge and a sterile, disposable needle. The pens eliminate the need for carrying extra syringes and insulin containers. Jet injectors use high pressure, instead of a needle, to propel insulin through the skin.

Insulin can also be delivered via an insulin pump. The pump is a device about the size of a pager that is worn externally on a belt or inside a pock-

---

A POSSIBLE CURE FOR TYPE 1 DIABETES MELLITUS

Pancreas gland transplants or transplantations of islet cells (the insulin-producing groups of cells inside the pancreas) have been successful in treating type 1 diabetes in many people. Pancreas gland and islet cell transplants are not appropriate treatment for everyone with type 1 diabetes for several reasons. Since the immune system tends to reject transplanted tissue, powerful and expensive medications must be taken to prevent rejection. These medications carry the risks of serious side effects and additional health problems.

Researchers have been exploring the development of less risky medications and improved transplant techniques that offer less possibility of rejection. Among this research is the exploration of an approach that would encapsulate the islet cells in a membrane that would protect them from an attack by the immune system. Other research includes inducing the immune system to tolerate the transplant by implanting the islet cells in the thymus gland and the use of bioengineering methods to produce artificial islet cells that can secrete insulin in response to a heightened blood sugar level.

---

et. This device delivers a constant flow of insulin through a flexible tube connected to a needle that is inserted just under the skin, usually in the abdomen. Using a pump requires frequent blood sugar monitoring so that insulin dosage can be adjusted. Extra insulin may be necessary, especially before meals, according to blood glucose levels and the foods to be eaten. The use of implantable pumps is currently being researched.

In the future, it may be possible to inhale insulin to treat diabetes.

Several different insulin preparations are available with different onset and duration of action. Rapid-acting insulin (regular insulin) has a shorter duration of action. It usually begins to lower blood sugar about 30 to 60 minutes after injection, peaks in about 2 hours, and lasts 6 to 8 hours. Intermediate-acting and long-acting insulins are available. Usually a combination of rapid-acting insulin and a longer-acting insulin is used to control the blood sugar level. Longer-acting insulins provide a baseline level of insulin, while rapid-acting insulin can be adjusted as needed for meals and exercise. Because exercise has a tendency to cause fluctuations in the levels of glucose in the blood, blood sugar levels should be checked before a person with type 1 diabetes exercises or begins a strenuous activity. If the blood sugar level is low, it may be necessary to eat a snack before the activity because exercise can reduce the blood sugar level even further. If the blood sugar level is high, extra insulin may need to be taken before the activity because the exercise may

cause the blood sugar level to go even higher. In some cases, a person may have to lower his or her insulin dose before a planned session of exercise or sports activity.

The amount of insulin required is determined by a doctor and is based on a number of factors, including the person's age, height, weight, food intake, and exercise level, as well as individual differences in the degree of difficulty controlling the blood sugar level. The doses must be balanced with meal times and activities. The required insulin dose may be affected by illness, stress, or unexpected events.

MONITORING THE BLOOD GLUCOSE LEVEL

Once a person has been diagnosed with type 1 diabetes, frequent self-monitoring of the blood glucose level helps maintain a near-normal blood sugar level (known as maintaining "tight control" of diabetes) and helps the person identify the causes of fluctuations. Insulin doses can then be adjusted accordingly.

Self-monitoring of the blood glucose level is a procedure that can be accomplished using a blood glucose meter. A drop of blood is taken (usually from a fingertip) and placed on a coated strip. In most home blood glucose meters, the strip is inserted into the meter, which gives a digital reading of the blood sugar level in about a minute. Glucose meters provide accurate measurement of blood sugar levels. The meters are small and lightweight, and some meters have memory functions that are capable of storing readings for up to several

D

LIVING WITH TYPE 1 DIABETES

In most people, insulin routinely moves blood sugar (glucose) into the cells, supplying the body with fuel. Type 1 diabetes, insulin-dependent diabetes mellitus, occurs when the pancreas does not pro-duce enough insulin. Half of those diagnosed with type 1 diabetes are younger than 20 years, and so this type of diabetes used to be called juvenile-onset diabetes.

HOW THE BODY IS AFFECTED BY TYPE 1 DIABETES

Type 1 diabetes must be kept under tight control in order to prevent serious complications in various parts of the body.

Brain People with diabetes are more likely to have strokes.

Eyes Elevated blood sugar levels slowly damage the eye blood vessels, leading to diabetic retinopathy or other eye problems.

Blood supply and heart A long-term complication of diabetes is increased fat deposits in the arteries.

Pancreas
The immune system decreases the ability of the pancreas to produce insulin.

Kidneys Diabetes causes the capillaries in the kidneys to become plugged and hinders the kidneys' filtering of wastes.

INSULIN INJECTIONS AT SCHOOL

The parents of children with type 1 diabetes should consult with the school nurse or a teacher before school starts. In many states, it is necessary for the parent to give written permission so that school personnel will be allowed to give insulin injections to the child.

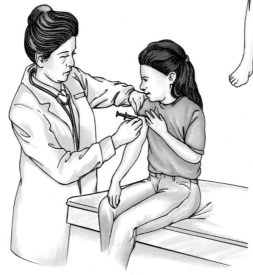

INJECTION ZONES FOR CHILDREN

Insulin injections should be given into a skin fold with some fatty tissue in order to prevent inadvertent injection into a muscle. Injection sites should be rotated to reduce possible tissue dam-age. Also, the child should be trained to inject straight in and apply some pressure to the site after the injection to minimize bruising.

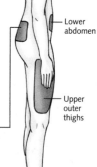

Upper outer arms

Lower abdomen

Upper outer thighs

Buttocks

HEALTHY SNACKS

Children with type 1 diabetes typi-cally follow a regimen in which they eat three meals a day, plus three healthy snacks, in order to keep their blood sugar levels steady. Possible snacks include a piece of fruit such as an apple, a low-fat muffin, a con-tainer of low-fat yogurt, or celery sticks—depending on the dietary requirements of the child.

weeks. The meter must be used correctly to obtain accurate results; a health care professional can offer instructions on how to operate and maintain the meter. Manufacturers' recommendations generally provide information on calibrating the meter for accuracy. In the absence of a meter, the strip can be evaluated by visual examination. The amount of sugar in the blood determines the color changes on the strip; a person who reads the strip visually compares the changed color with colors on a special chart to determine the blood sugar level.

Many factors—including diet, alcohol consumption, activity level, stress, illness, medications, and hormonal changes—can cause fluctuations in blood sugar levels. Informed daily decisions such as those regarding the timing of self-testing, insulin administration, diet, and exercise can help the person manage the blood sugar level successfully. A personal diabetes diary may be helpful for keeping track of the daily influences on blood sugar levels.

A person with type 1 diabetes should have his or her blood tested with the glycosylated hemoglobin test (hemoglobin A1c test) every 3 to 6 months. This test measures the amount of glucose attached to hemoglobin A, a protein found in red blood cells. The percentage of glucose attached to hemoglobin depends on the average glucose concentration and is a good measure of diabetic control for the preceding 3 to 4 months.

RISKS AND COMPLICATIONS

The two main risks for people with type 1 diabetes are hypoglycemia and hyperglycemia, both of which are caused by interference with the balance between insulin and the blood sugar level in the blood. If too much insulin is taken, the sugar in the blood may become depleted, causing hypoglycemia. When there is too little insulin in the blood, the glucose level may become too high, producing hyperglycemia. Each of these conditions carries the potential for serious medical emergencies. As a safety precaution, a person with diabetes should wear a medical identification bracelet or necklace that identifies him or her as having diabetes.

Hypoglycemia (low blood sugar) is referred to as insulin reaction (or shock). It may result from taking too much insulin, delaying meals, not eating enough food, exercising, or drinking alcohol. The symptoms of hypoglycemia include irritability, fatigue, excessive perspiration, increased appetite, confusion, and mild tremors.

A person who experiences hypoglycemia can usually correct his or her low blood sugar quickly by eating or drinking a sugar-containing food or drink or by taking glucose tablets. A medication that can raise the blood sugar level, GLUCAGON, is available by prescription; if the person with diabetes becomes so dazed that he or she cannot function, a relative or friend should inject glucagon immediately. Severe hypoglycemia can cause a person to lose consciousness or be unable to swallow, indicating the need for immediate emergency medical help.

People with type 1 diabetes should avoid the potential dangers of hypoglycemia by always testing blood sugar levels before exercise or driving. They must also always carry with them sugar-containing snacks and drinks or glucose products.

Hyperglycemia (high blood sugar) may be produced by taking an insufficient amount of insulin, eating excessive amounts of food, lack of exercise, illness, or stress. The symptoms of hyperglycemia include excessive thirst and urination, tiredness, blurred vision, vomiting, and weight loss. Over time, persistent hyperglycemia can affect vital functions. The large and small blood vessels can be damaged, leading to complications in different structures of the body, including the kidneys, eyes, gums, nerves, and heart. Recent studies show that maintaining tight control of the blood sugar level reduces other complications.

Damage to the large blood vessels results from an increased risk of atherosclerosis. Clinically, this causes a greater incidence of heart attack, stroke, and blockage of the blood supply to the legs and feet.

Diabetic nephropathy, kidney disease associated with type 1 diabetes, can be life-threatening. It develops when there is damage to the small blood vessels that filter waste products in the bloodstream. Ultimately, this may lead to kidney failure, requiring a kidney transplant or dialysis (a procedure that uses a machine to remove harmful substances from the blood).

Other diabetic complications include diabetic retinopathy (a disorder that causes bleeding of the blood vessels in the retina of the eye), leading to eye damage and vision loss. Eye disease caused by diabetes is the leading cause of adult blindness. Diabetic neuropathy (nerve damage) can produce numbness in the extremities, particularly the feet. People with type 1 diabetes must protect their feet from injury; open sores and infections of the feet heal poorly and can develop into a devastating infection that may eventually lead to loss of a foot or leg. Other forms of nerve damage may affect the heart, stomach, sexual organs, eyes, ears, facial muscles, and urinary tract. Infections of the gums and bones that hold the teeth in place can result in the teeth loosening and falling out.

It is important for women with type 1 diabetes who wish to become pregnant to make sure the blood sugar level is kept under tight control. This requires consultation with a doctor specializing in the care of pregnant women with diabetes. Controlling the blood sugar level at the time of conception and during the first 2 months of pregnancy is important for reducing the risks of major birth defects. For the remaining 7 months of the pregnancy, tight control of the blood sugar level is vital to the health of the developing fetus and can reduce the complications of premature delivery.

Diabetes mellitus, type 2

FOR SYMPTOM CHART
see Weight loss, page 62

The more common of the two main groups of conditions characterized by an abnormally high glucose (sugar) level in the blood; formerly known as non–insulin-dependent diabetes or adult-onset diabetes. Type 2 diabetes, which accounts for 90 to 95 percent of all people with diabetes, is characterized by INSULIN RESISTANCE that causes interference with the ability of the body to use glucose (sugar) for energy. Many people with type 2 diabetes do not require daily insulin therapy. Although diabetes usually begins in adults older than 40 years and is most common in people older than 55 years, it is becoming increasingly common in younger people, apparently due to obesity and reduced levels of physical activity. Type 2 diabetes is associated with the abnormal response in the body to the hormone insulin, which is produced by the pancreas, the large endocrine gland behind the stomach where insulin is normally produced. In this way, it differs from type 1 diabetes, which involves an inadequate supply of insulin produced and released by the pancreas. In fact, early in the course of the illness, many people with type 2 diabetes have high levels of circulating insulin as the pancreas attempts to compensate for the insulin resistance. An elevated blood sugar level develops as the beta cells (the insulin-producing cells of the pancreas) can no longer produce enough insulin to overcome the insulin resistance in the body. Over years, the beta cells can continue to lose more of their ability to produce insulin, and the insulin level may fall below normal.

Glucose is produced when carbohydrates or sugars are broken down by digestive enzymes. Once absorbed, glucose is carried throughout the body by the bloodstream, causing the blood glucose level to rise. Elevation in the blood sugar level stimulates the pancreas to release insulin. Insulin has an important role in allowing tissues such as muscle, liver, and fat cells to take up glucose. Under normal conditions, insulin accomplishes this task; the organs receive the energy they need to function, and the blood sugar level returns to normal. But, in people with type 2 diabetes, the sugar in the blood is not metabolized properly, and the glucose level in the blood is above normal.

CAUSES

Most people with type 2 diabetes have insulin resistance, along with an inability of the pancreas to secrete sufficient amounts of insulin to compensate for the resistance in the body. Two possible causes of insulin resistance have been identified. The first involves the receptors with which insulin must bind in order to function. People with type 2 diabetes may not have enough of these receptors or may have defects on the receptors. The second possible cause involves the inability of the cells to properly process insulin's signal to metabolize glucose; this may take place after the insulin has bonded with the receptor.

Obesity, particularly weight carried around the waist, is associated with insulin resistance and is thought to place an increased demand on the pancreas. A lack of physical fitness and a sedentary lifestyle are other associated factors.

Other risk factors for type 2 diabetes include heredity and ethnic background. A person is more likely to develop diabetes if family members have it. The condition commonly occurs among African Americans, Hispanics, Native Americans, and Native Hawaiians. The ethnic risk factor may be due to a combination of heredity and environmental influences such as diet. Sex is not a risk factor for type 2 diabetes except among African Americans; African American women are more likely than African American men to develop type 2 diabetes. Increased age is also a contributing factor. Certain medications—including diuretics used to treat high blood pressure and corticosteroids such as prednisone—can contribute to an elevated blood sugar level.

SYMPTOMS

Many people with type 2 diabetes do not have any symptoms at first. In time, they may develop symptoms such as recurrent infections, vision difficulties, or neuropathy (nerve damage). Other common complications include fatigue, a general ill feeling, sudden inexplicable weight loss, frequent urination (especially noticeable at night), and excessive thirst. These symptoms are the result of the excess sugar in the blood and the inability of the body to process and use glucose. The frequent urination is caused by the body trying to eliminate the extra glucose, which causes excessive thirst as the body tries to replace the lost fluid. Infections of the urinary tract may be slow to heal, and there may be genital itching in women. Slow-healing infections of the skin and gums, weakness, inability to concentrate, and loss of coordination may also be associated with type 2 diabetes. Rarely, loss of consciousness or coma from an extremely abnormal blood sugar level occurs.

DIAGNOSIS

The typical symptoms of extreme thirst and frequent urination will cause a doctor to check for the disease. Risk factors including being overweight, heredity, and ethnicity may also be taken into account, and the doctor may screen for diabetes even in individuals without symptoms. Type 2 diabetes may be diagnosed as a result of related health problems such as arteriosclerosis, ischemic heart disease, stroke, vision problems, numbness in the feet and legs, obesity, and slow-healing sores. Doctors examining a person with these problems are likely to check the person for type 2 diabetes.

Usually, a doctor diagnoses type 2 diabetes on the basis of a person's medical history, physical examination results, and blood glucose level. If the glucose level is 126 milligrams per deciliter (mg/dL) or higher on the results of two fasting plasma glucose tests, or very high (more than 200 mg/dL) 2 hours after a meal, a diagnosis of diabetes is usually made.

If diabetes is suspected, several types of blood tests may be administered to test the glucose level in the blood. The fasting blood glucose test is the simplest and most commonly used test to detect diabetes. A nonfasting or random glucose level of more than 200 mg/dL along with classic symptoms of diabetes usually also results in a diagnosis of diabetes. The oral glucose test, which is a blood test that measures the glucose level after a person has had a drink containing glucose and other sugars, can detect diabetes when other blood tests have not. In a person without diabetes, this drink causes the glucose level to rise quickly and then fall gradually as the body metabolizes the glucose. In a person with diabetes, the drink causes the blood sugar level to increase but, instead of gradually falling, the glucose level remains elevated. The test is used most commonly to diagnose gestational diabetes. Urine testing is no longer used to establish a diagnosis of diabetes.

TREATMENT

The goals are to normalize the blood sugar level, eliminate symptoms such as thirst and weakness, and prevent long-term complications such as

THE RISKS OF DRINKING ALCOHOL FOR PEOPLE WITH TYPE 2 DIABETES

People with type 2 diabetes should follow their doctor's guidelines on the safety of drinking alcoholic beverages. Here are some special considerations for people with type 2 diabetes:

- Drinking one or two alcoholic beverages on occasion is normally safe. However, alcohol is high in calories, and some drinks may be higher in sugar than others, which should be taken into account when planning daily food intake.
- Taken on an empty stomach, alcoholic beverages can produce hypoglycemia (low blood sugar), which is particularly risky for anyone taking oral hypoglycemics or insulin. A person may shake, feel dizzy, and pass out; onlookers may not provide necessary medical treatment because they think the person is intoxicated.
- Combining certain diabetes medications, including tolbutamide and chlorpropamide, with alcohol may cause dizziness, flushing of the face, and nausea.
- Over time, alcohol abuse causes liver damage. The blood glucose level becomes more difficult to control in a person with liver damage because the liver stores and releases glucose.
- Excess drinking can raise the levels of fats in the blood, which further increases the risk of heart disease.

heart disease and eye disease caused by diabetes. In treating type 2 diabetes, diet and weight loss are generally the first approaches to controlling the blood glucose level.

■ *Diet* Diet is the cornerstone of treatment for all people with diabetes. The doctor may recommend a diet or refer the person being treated to a nutritionist or dietician. Dieticians offer advice to ensure that the diet is healthful and easily followed. Careful control of food intake may help a person achieve and maintain a desirable weight and, in many cases, help control the blood glucose level. Because there is no known cure for type 2 diabetes, dietary approaches must be followed throughout a person's lifetime. For a person with type 2 diabetes, diet should help the person achieve and maintain an ideal weight, maintain a normal blood glucose level, and limit foods that may increase the already high risk of heart disease.

Most experts in the field of diabetes recommend that the daily diet consist of 50 to 60 percent of calories from carbohydrates, 10 to 20 percent of calories from protein, and 30 percent or less of calories from fat. Calories from saturated fats and cholesterol should be restricted and replaced with unsaturated and monounsaturated fats to help lower the blood cholesterol level. Lowering the cholesterol level to prevent heart disease is essential because people with diabetes have a higher risk for heart disease. Eating high-fiber foods, including fresh fruits and vegetables, legumes, and whole grains, has been shown to lower the blood glucose level. Scheduling smaller meals at regular intervals throughout the day also helps to maintain a normal blood glucose level. A doctor or dietician can offer help with these guidelines and individualize recommendations to a person's food preferences and lifestyle.

Exchange lists may help an individual with diabetes follow a healthful diet because the lists offer more choices than rigid diet plans. Exchange lists group together foods with similar nutrient and caloric values so that a person can plan the number of servings from each exchange to be eaten during the day.

It is known that foods high in carbohydrates, including whole grains, fruits, and vegetables, cause the blood glucose level to rise, but until recently it was unknown whether specific types of food within the carbohydrate category differed in their effects on the blood glucose level. Current research suggests that it is the total amount of high carbohydrate foods eaten at one time, rather than the specific type of food eaten, that affects the blood glucose level most significantly. Cooked foods raise the blood glucose level more than do raw foods eaten unpeeled.

■ *Exercise* People with type 2 diabetes derive many benefits from physical activity. Regular exercise in combination with the proper diet can help weight reduction efforts by burning extra calories. It can also improve the way the body responds to insulin (it decreases insulin resistance) and improve utilization of glucose in the body. Exercise can also help reduce the risks of heart disease by lowering fat and cholesterol levels, lowering blood pressure, and increasing production of high-density lipoprotein (HDL), the "good" cholesterol. Exercise also provides positive psychological effects that may help a person with diabetes avoid the stress that can cause fluctuations in the blood glucose level.

A doctor's guidance is important in planning the right exercise program for a person with type 2 diabetes. Factors such as the condition of the person's heart and circulatory system and overall level of fitness must be taken into account. For example, a person with high blood pressure or diabetic retinopathy (a disorder that causes bleeding of the blood vessels in the retina of the eye) must avoid exercises that involve straining such as lifting heavy weights. The goal is to establish an enjoyable exercise routine that suits a person's everyday life to encourage regular participation. Walking is often recommended. People who have problems with their feet must select footwear carefully and examine their feet regularly for sores that may become infected. Swimming or bicycling may be preferable for some people.

■ *Oral medications* Medications for people with type 2 diabetes do not replace diet and exercise programs but are used in combination with them when those elements of treatment alone are not sufficient to control the diabetes. People with type 2 diabetes who still produce some insulin may be treated with sulfonylureas. These agents are oral hypoglycemics and work by stimulating the pancreas to produce more insulin. They are most useful for people of normal weight who have never taken insulin or take less than 40 units a day, are younger than 40 years, and have had diabetes for less than 5 years. They are not known to be safe for pregnant women or nursing mothers.

The chemical names for the sulfonylureas currently in use in the United States include glyburide, glipizide, glimepiride, and chlor-propamide. In prescribing a specific medication, a doctor may take into account several factors such as the degree to which the blood glucose level must be lowered, other medications the person is taking, and the impact of the possible side effects of a medication. Side effects are unusual but, in rare instances, may include hypoglycemia (from reducing the sugar level too much), nausea, skin rashes, headache, sensitivity to sunlight, and either water retention or increased urination. A newer medication called repaglinide, which also stimulates insulin production, is now available.

Nonsulfonylureas are another group of medications used to treat diabetes. These are the insulin-sensitizing agents metformin, rosiglitazone, and pioglitazone. Metformin decreases the release of glucose stored in the liver and increases the sensitivity of the cells to insulin. Rosiglitazone and pioglitazone improve insulin action. Some of these medications carry a slight risk of injury to the liver or kidneys, and their use must be monitored in people with kidney, liver, or cardiac impairment. A doctor can determine the appropriate medication for a given individual.

Another class of agents, the glucosidase inhibitors, such as acarbose, work by inhibiting the breakdown of sugars by intestinal enzymes. As a result, they slow digestion and absorption of sugar, making these medications most useful for people experiencing marked elevations in the blood sugar level after eating.

A person who takes one of the oral

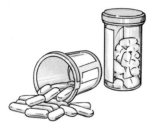

ORAL MEDICATIONS
Some people need medication to control diabetes. Different types of drugs may act to stimulate the pancreas to produce more insulin; limit the release of glucose from the liver and make cells more sensitive to the action of insulin; or slow down digestion and absorption of sugars to prevent problems after meals.

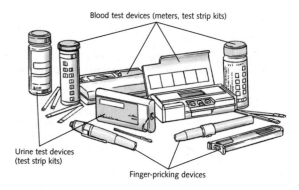

MONITORING DEVICES
Home monitoring of blood sugar levels is made easier with automatic finger-pricking devices. The blood sample is placed on a test strip that changes color to indicate blood sugar levels or can be read on a meter. Urine test kits also involve test strips that are placed in urine samples; color changes indicate blood sugar levels from several hours before the test.

Blood test devices (meters, test strip kits)

Urine test devices (test strip kits)

Finger-pricking devices

hypoglycemic medications must eat regularly and be aware of the effects of physical activity on lowering the blood glucose level. The symptoms of low blood sugar are headache, weakness, shakiness, and, in severe cases, physical collapse. Oral medications cannot control the blood sugar level in all people with type 2 diabetes; some may require insulin. In other people, over time, oral medications lose their effectiveness and insulin may be needed.

■ *Insulin* A synthetic or bioengineered form of injected insulin may be necessary for treating some people with type 2 diabetes, particularly those unable to control the glucose level with diet, exercise, and oral medication. Other considerations taken into account are the person's age, weight, and difficulty controlling the blood sugar level; history of side effects from oral hypoglycemics; or other health concerns that make the oral medications unsafe to use. Insulin may be used for people with type 2 diabetes who are pregnant or undergoing surgery. The doctor determines the correct type of insulin to be administered and offers instructions on its use. Weight control is still important for insulin to be most effective.

MONITORING THE BLOOD GLUCOSE LEVEL
Because controlling the blood sugar level is the single most important factor in preventing the possible long-term complications of type 2 diabetes, it is essential that a person keep track of his or her glucose level. The blood sugar level can fluctuate, making it useful for a person with this form of diabetes to learn self-monitoring techniques. At one time, home urine testing was used exten-

sively. But it is less accurate than blood testing and reflects the blood sugar level from several hours before the test. Also, certain medications and vitamins can affect the results.

Blood tests that can be done at home using special kits are more accurate and offer a more immediate reading. A drop of blood is drawn with a spring-operated device, and the blood is placed on a special strip that can be examined visually for color changes that indicate blood sugar level or inserted into a meter that gives a digital readout.

A doctor will recommend how often a person should test his or her blood sugar level. Several tests a day may be necessary. Self-testing offers a good indication of how a person's glucose level responds to food intake, exercise, stress, medication, and other events or treatments.

The glucose level of a person with diabetes is also regularly tested at visits to a doctor's office. The glycosylated hemoglobin test (hemoglobin A1c test) measures the amount of sugar that is attached to the red blood cells. Red blood cells remain in the bloodstream for about 3 months, enabling this laboratory test to reveal the average blood sugar level for the past 12 weeks. The results of this test are not affected by short-term fluctuations. The American Diabetes Association recommends that people who are using insulin treatment have this test every 3 to 4 months. People with diabetes who do not take insulin should be tested a minimum of twice yearly.

RISKS AND COMPLICATIONS
Hyperglycemia (high blood sugar) can occur in a person with this form of diabetes and produce symptoms that require urgent medical care. Stress, illness, hormone levels, and

other events and conditions may produce hyperglycemia. Hypoglycemia (low blood sugar) may be experienced when the effects of insulin or oral medicine are intensified by insufficient food intake, excessive activity, or drinking alcoholic beverages. For safety, a person with diabetes should wear a medical identification bracelet or necklace that identifies him or her as having diabetes.

The symptoms of hyperglycemia include extreme thirst and frequent urination. Untreated, hyperglycemia can result in dehydration, leaving a person weak, confused, and, if severe enough, unconscious with shallow breathing and a rapid pulse. Usually a person has signs of dehydration such as dry lips and tongue, and the hands and feet are cool to the touch. Medical attention should be sought immediately.

Hypoglycemia produces symptoms including nervousness and weakness. A person in this state may perspire profusely, feel extremely hungry, and have a headache. At the onset of these symptoms, a person with diabetes should eat or drink something that contains sugar. Suggested snacks include fruit juice, skim milk, raisins, honey, or sugar cubes. Hard candies and glucose tablets, available over-the-counter, will also help. It is recommended that a person with diabetes keep these provisions handy. When severe, hypoglycemia results in a loss of consciousness, which requires immediate medical care.

It is important that type 2 diabetes be diagnosed and treated as early as possible because it can cause severe health problems over time, in some cases before a person realizes that he or she has the disorder. Specifically, the heart, blood vessels, eyes, kidneys, and nerves are at risk from conditions produced by type 2 diabetes.

The risk of life-threatening heart disease that can lead to fatal heart attacks is often linked to diabetes. Associated risk factors include obesity, high blood pressure, high fat and cholesterol levels in the blood, and cigarette smoking. Treating diabetes and reducing these risk factors can help reduce the risk of heart disease.

Most people with diabetes do not develop kidney disease or damage, but individuals with diabetes are at much greater risk than the average

person. Treatment of diabetes and monitoring blood pressure reduces the risk.

Blurred vision associated with diabetes may result from a fluctuating glucose level affecting the balance of fluid in the lens of the eye. The function of the nerves that control eyesight may also be affected. People with diabetes are also at risk for developing retinopathy, a disease of the eye's light-sensitive tissue (the retina) in which the capillaries can bleed or leak, causing damage to the retina. High blood pressure and smoking cigarettes can worsen diabetic retinopathy, which is treatable. Cataract and glaucoma are two eye diseases that tend to occur more frequently in people with diabetes.

Any foot problems that develop must be medically treated early or they may lead to a life-threatening situation that requires amputation. The changes caused by diabetes in blood vessels and nerves in the legs and feet can cause peripheral vascular disease, a condition caused by fatty deposits narrowing the blood vessels, reducing the blood supply to the lower extremities. When nerves are affected, there may be a loss of sensation; sores on the feet and legs may not be noticed. If infection sets in, healing may be slow due to poor blood circulation. Proper care and cleansing of the feet on a daily basis and the use of special shoes or shoe inserts can help prevent problems. A form of nerve disease called diabetic neuropathy can dull the nerves and cause extreme pain and possibly psychological depression because of the pain. Diabetic neuropathy can also cause changes in the nerves that control functions including blood pressure and digestion; indigestion and diarrhea may result. Men may also experience erectile dysfunction.

Infections of the teeth and gums (including periodontal disease) and infections of vaginal tissue in women can develop more often in people with type 2 diabetes.

Diabetes, gestational

A condition of INSULIN RESISTANCE in pregnant women in which the effects of the hormone insulin, which is produced by the pancreas, are partially

blocked by other hormones produced by the placenta. These hormones—including estrogen, cortisol, and human placental lactogen—are essential for a healthy pregnancy. However, they induce a resistance to insulin, resulting in an increase in the insulin requirement. In most women, the pancreas has enough reserve to produce a sufficient amount of insulin to maintain normal glucose (blood sugar) levels. However, if the pancreas is incapable of making enough insulin to meet the increased requirement during pregnancy, gestational diabetes develops. Most cases of gestational diabetes develop during the latter half of pregnancy and resolve after childbirth, when the placenta is delivered and the hormone elevations associated with pregnancy drop. However, the impaired insulin reserve probably explains why these women are at risk of developing diabetes latter in life, when aging and weight gain induce insulin resistance.

RISK FACTORS AND SCREENING

Risk factors for developing gestational diabetes include obesity, family history of diabetes, an excess of amniotic fluid during pregnancy, a previous stillbirth, or a previous delivery of an extremely large infant or an infant with a birth defect.

There are several methods of screening for gestational diabetes. The most common is measurement of the glucose level after the ingestion of a glucose solution, usually administered between the 24th and the 28th weeks of pregnancy. A final diagnosis is usually dependent on an abnormal result of a 3-hour glucose tolerance test.

Maintaining a near-normal blood sugar level and monitoring fetal health during pregnancy and at delivery help ensure that the fetus's health is not compromised by the mother's gestational diabetes. Methods of monitoring fetal health include fetal movement records, fetal monitoring, nonstress testing, stress testing through the OXYTOCIN CHALLENGE TEST (OCT), and amniocentesis.

POSSIBLE COMPLICATIONS

Complications of gestational diabetes are usually prevented by early diagnosis of the condition and keeping the blood sugar level as near normal as possible for the remainder of the pregnancy. A pregnant woman can monitor her own blood sugar level by using a glucose meter at home.

A mild elevation in the blood sugar level is usually managed by a diet that provides adequate nutrition to the pregnant woman and the fetus while maintaining a healthy body weight for the pregnant woman. Dietary recommendations that help maintain proper pregnancy weight and a normal blood sugar level include avoiding sugar and sugar-containing foods, eating complex carbohydrates and foods high in dietary fiber, and restricting dietary fats.

Moderate levels of exercise during pregnancy may also help regulate insulin in the body and help control weight. In some cases, insulin injections may be necessary to manage gestational diabetes.

A common complication associated with gestational diabetes is thought to be related to the high level of glucose in the pregnant woman's blood, resulting in excess insulin production by the fetus. The excess insulin affects fetal tissue and causes the fetus to grow excessively large. The increased size of the fetus may preclude a normal vaginal delivery and necessitate a CESAREAN SECTION. The size of the fetus is determined by physical examination and often by DIAGNOSTIC IMAGING such as an ultrasound test, which uses sound waves to produce images and does not expose the fetus to radiation.

A baby born to a mother with gestational diabetes may have hypoglycemia (low blood sugar) immediately after delivery if the mother's increased blood sugar level raised the fetus's insulin level. Hypoglycemia is generally treated by giving the newborn intravenous glucose to restore the glucose level to normal. At birth, the infant may have other treatable chemical imbalances, including low levels of calcium and magnesium in the blood.

Jaundice may develop in the infant of a mother who had gestational diabetes. This most commonly occurs when extra red blood cells are destroyed, and bilirubin, a pigment that produces a yellow discoloration of the skin, is released. Many infants are born with minor jaundice. When

it is problematic, the baby is placed under special lights that clear away the pigment. Rarely, in severe cases, blood transfusions are necessary.

Gestational diabetes may increase the chances of the pregnant woman's developing PREECLAMPSIA, a complication characterized by high blood pressure, protein in the urine, and swelling of the face and extremities. Preeclampsia, which occurs infrequently, can impair the function of the nervous system and lead to seizures, stroke, or other serious complications. Early delivery may be recommended if preeclampsia develops.

Diabetes, insulin-dependent

See DIABETES MELLITUS, TYPE 1.

Diabetes, non-insulin-dependent

See DIABETES MELLITUS, TYPE 2.

Diabetic coma

FOR FIRST AID
see Diabetic coma, page 1319

A complication of type 2 diabetes mellitus that results in extremely high glucose (blood sugar) levels without the presence of ketones, a by-product of fat metabolism. Diabetic ketoacidosis, high blood sugar with ketones in the urine, may also be a cause of diabetic coma. Diabetic coma, which is also known as nonketotic hyperglycemic coma (NKHC), is characterized by decreased consciousness,

extreme DEHYDRATION, and very high blood glucose levels. Symptoms may include increased thirst, increased urination, nausea, lethargy, confusion, and seizures. Diabetic coma is usually seen in people who have not yet been diagnosed with diabetes or those who have neglected their diabetes. Older people and those with kidney insufficiency or congestive heart failure are particularly at risk for diabetic coma. Certain medications that impair glucose tolerance or increase fluid loss may also precipitate a diabetic coma, as may infection, stroke, or recent surgery.

Diabetic coma is generally the result of a combination of excess glucose and dehydration stemming from an inability to consume enough water. When dehydration occurs, the kidneys try to conserve fluid, which leads to an increase in glucose levels and even more dehydration. The blood becomes much more concentrated with sodium, glucose, and other molecules, which draw even more water into the bloodstream. The result is a vicious cycle of ever-increasing dehydration and ever-rising glucose levels. Preventive measures include good control of diabetes and recognition of early signs of dehydration. Once a person is in a diabetic coma, the goal of treatment is to correct dehydration through intravenous therapy while treating the high glucose levels with short-acting insulin. More than half the people who experience diabetic coma die as a result.

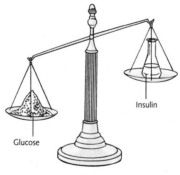 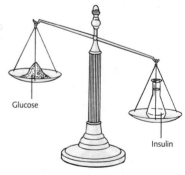

DIABETIC EMERGENCIES
In a person with diabetes, the balance of insulin and glucose in the blood is not maintained. Diabetic coma occurs when a person's blood glucose levels are high (hyperglycemia) and insulin levels are low. Another diabetic emergency—hypoglycemia, which can lead to insulin shock—occurs when blood glucose levels dip too low and insulin levels are too high.

Diabetic retinopathy

See RETINOPATHY, DIABETIC.

Diagnosis

The act or process of determining a disease process by history, physical examination, and often laboratory testing (such as blood studies, urinalysis, and imaging studies). For some diseases (such as breast cancer or colon cancer), early diagnosis can make the difference between cure and serious illness or death. High cholesterol levels and symptomless diseases, such as hypertension (high blood pressure), are also important to detect and treat at an early stage. Many tests are used as aids in diagnosis.

Diagnosis-related group

See DRG.

Diagnostic imaging

Techniques that allow internal areas of the body to be visualized through X rays, magnetic fields, and radio-frequency waves and sound waves to produce pictures of the structures and tissues of the body. Computer-enhanced images are often used to improve imaging techniques and aid in diagnosis.

Among the currently used diagnostic imaging techniques that produce images of the whole body or body structures are CT SCANNING (computed tomography scanning), which uses X rays to produce cross-sectional images; ULTRASOUND SCANNING, which uses high-frequency sound waves; and MRI (magnetic resonance imaging), in which powerful magnetic fields and radio-frequency waves are used.

Dialysis

A medical therapy for eliminating toxic waste products that accumulate in the bloodstream because of inadequately functioning kidneys. Dialysis uses a membrane that permits different substances to diffuse or pass through at different rates, filtering and purifying the blood. Dialysis is necessary in cases of KIDNEY FAILURE. It is also used to remove drugs from the body after a poison is ingested or after a drug overdose. Although dialysis helps eliminate waste products and maintain fluid balance, it does

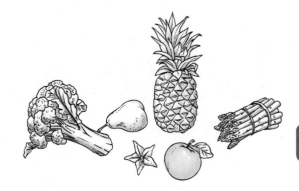

RECOMMENDED FRUITS AND VEGETABLES
A person undergoing dialysis needs the nutrients found in fruits and vegetables, but should choose carefully to limit intake of fluids (to reduce fluid accumulation) and potassium (which must be cleared by dialysis). Recommended fruits and vegetables (low in both fluid and potassium) include apples, pears, star anise, pineapple, broccoli, and asparagus.

not replace the endocrine function of the kidneys.

When the kidneys are healthy, they have a vital role in eliminating waste products created by organs and cells during the normal metabolic processes of the body. Kidney function is essential to maintaining fluid balance, regulating electrolyte balance and acid-base balance, and preventing waste products from building to toxic levels.

When the kidneys are unable to function at more than 10 to 15 percent of normal capacity, kidney dialysis or a KIDNEY TRANSPLANT is essential for survival. Dialysis is not a cure for kidney failure and does not eliminate toxins as expertly as natural, healthy kidneys, but it enables people with kidney failure to survive.

Several conditions and diseases may impair kidney function. High blood pressure, which damages the small blood vessels in the kidneys, can interfere with function or cause kidney failure. Diabetes mellitus can also affect the blood vessels and glomeruli (the filtering units of the kidneys), resulting in kidney failure.

There are two types of dialysis, HEMODIALYSIS and PERITONEAL DIALYSIS. In hemodialysis, blood is pumped from the body into a filter consisting of a membrane made up of many tiny plastic capillaries. Toxic waste products in the blood can diffuse across the capillary membranes, and the purified blood is then returned to the body. Hemodialysis is generally performed in a dialysis center three times a week; each session lasts about 4 hours. In peritoneal dialysis, fluid is drained out of and back into the abdomen via a technique that uses the peritoneum (the membrane that lines the abdominal cavity) to filter waste products. Peritoneal dialysis

can be performed at home but must be accurately and carefully done. The risks involved include PERITONITIS and damage to the peritoneum, which limit the diffusion of waste products across the peritoneum.

Dialysis machine

Also known as an artificial kidney, dialyzer, or hemodialyzer; a machine used for DIALYSIS that takes over the function of the kidneys when they are unable to filter toxic waste products from the blood. If the kidneys fail, toxic substances in the blood can accumulate and cause UREMIA, which, if untreated, leads to death. Dialysis can be a lifesaving procedure when the kidneys are incapacitated by disease.

A new kind of dialysis machine called a bioartificial kidney is being developed and uses living kidney cells to duplicate nearly all the functions of a healthy kidney.

Dialyzer

See DIALYSIS MACHINE.

Diaper rash

Skin irritation caused by prolonged dampness and the contact between a baby's skin and feces or urine. Factors that contribute to bright red skin on a baby's bottom include infrequently changed diapers and plastic pants that lock in moisture. Other causes of diaper rash include irritants such as laundry detergents and yeast infections.

Most diaper rashes respond well to simple home treatment. Doctors recommend keeping the baby's skin clean and dry, changing diapers frequently, applying ointment such as zinc oxide to prevent further irritation, and, when convenient, allowing the baby to go without a diaper. After changing, the diaper area should be gently rinsed (not scrubbed) and patted dry. Diaper rashes caused by yeast infections are treated with over-the-counter or prescription antifungal creams or ointments. Avoid products that contain alcohol or perfumes. When a diaper rash is persistent or severe or if fever, boils, blisters, or pus accompany it, contact a doctor.

Diaphoresis

Sweating, particularly profuse perspiration. Diaphoresis can occur with a fever and is a symptom of many diseases, such as hyperthyroidism.

Diaphragm muscle

The large sheet of muscle that divides the chest (thorax) from the abdomen and provides most of the power that moves air in and out of the lungs. The diaphragm is attached to the spine, ribs, and sternum, forming the floor of the chest cavity. In a resting position, the diaphragm curves up into the chest cavity. During inhalation, the diaphragm contracts, flattening and moving downward as much as 3 to 4 inches. This change in the shape of the chest lowers its internal pressure and draws air into the lungs. During exhalation, the diaphragm relaxes and rises into its former position, while pressure in the lungs increases, and air is forced out of the

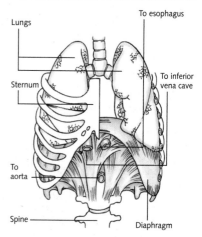

MUSCULAR SHEET
The diaphragm arches over the abdominal cavity, forming the powerful, muscular floor of the chest cavity. Three openings in the diaphragm provide passage for the esophagus, the aorta, the inferior vena cava (vein from the abdomen and lower limbs to the heart), and several nerves.

lungs. Contraction and relaxation of the muscles between the ribs add to the diaphragm's action.

Diaphragm, contraceptive

A birth control device that fits over a woman's cervix and keeps sperm from entering. See CONTRACEPTION, BARRIER METHODS.

Diarrhea

FOR SYMPTOM CHART
see Diarrhea, page 34

Abnormal increase in the frequency, fluidity, and volume of bowel movements. More than three soft, loose, or watery bowel movements in a day constitute diarrhea. In a healthy adult, most cases of diarrhea last from 24 to 48 hours and are not serious. Diarrhea can be more dangerous to infants and older people because of an increased risk of dehydration, upsetting body chemistry and depleting important body salts. Left untreated, it can lead to shock. Persistent or severe diarrhea requires medical attention. A sudden onset after years of regularity can suggest a serious digestive disorder, such as colon cancer. Diarrhea accompanied by symptoms such as weight loss, abdominal pain, or rectal bleeding requires a doctor's attention.

CAUSES
Under normal circumstances, the colon absorbs water from food residue, leading to semisolid feces. When the small intestine becomes inflamed, it fails to absorb food and instead secretes additional water and salts into the digestive tract. The colon cannot absorb the excess water, resulting in diarrhea. Most frequently, diarrhea is due to a viral infection or a change in diet. Sometimes, it can be traced to changes in the bacterial population of the digestive tract due to taking antibiotics or to foreign travel. Another cause can be increased frequency or intensity of contractions in the digestive tract, causing food to pass too quickly through the colon. Other common causes include food poisoning, GASTROENTERITIS, CELIAC DISEASE, LACTOSE INTOLERANCE, MALABSORPTION, DIVERTICULAR DISEASE, INFLAMMATORY BOWEL DISEASE, IRRITABLE BOWEL SYNDROME, anxiety, overconsumption of

alcohol, and reaction to medications. See also DIARRHEA, E. COLI; DIARRHEA, TRAVELER'S.

DIAGNOSIS AND TREATMENT
If symptoms last longer than 48 hours, it is important to seek medical attention. For moderate cases, the doctor may try to treat the symptoms and observe the person. In more severe cases, the doctor will conduct a physical examination and may order such tests as blood tests, stool analysis, a lower GASTROINTESTINAL (GI) SERIES (an X-ray procedure also called a barium enema), and SIGMOIDOSCOPY and COLONOSCOPY (examinations of the rectum and colon using flexible viewing tubes passed through the anus).

The symptoms of diarrhea provide clues to its cause. Diarrhea accompanied by nausea and vomiting is usually due to gastroenteritis. Bloody diarrhea that lasts for more than a few days is a sign of inflammatory bowel disease, while mucus is associated with irritable bowel syndrome, inflammatory bowel disease, and cancer. Loose, yellow, greasy, strong-smelling feces that are hard to flush are a symptom of malabsorption. Food poisoning, food allergy, drug toxicity, or anxiety can bring on watery diarrhea.

Doctors advise resting and drinking clear fluids until diarrhea subsides. Because watery diarrhea can rapidly cause a loss of body fluids and crucial body salts, oral rehydration fluid may be needed; available over-the-counter at pharmacies, this specially prepared solution contains water, salts, and glucose. Other over-the-counter medications may relieve symptoms. In severe cases, the doctor may prescribe drugs that slow intestinal activity and ease cramping. To prevent diarrhea, it is important to wash hands thoroughly after using the toilet and before preparing food. When diarrhea is due to underlying problems, it is important to seek treatment.

Diarrhea, E. coli

Escherichia coli (E. coli) diarrhea, frequent, liquid bowel movements caused by E. coli bacteria, which normally inhabit the digestive tract of humans without harm. However, a strain of E. coli (enterohemorrhagic) that is most commonly associated with contaminated hamburger meat causes bloody diarrhea and sometimes death. Another type of *E. coli* bacteria is responsible for many cases of traveler's diarrhea (see DIARRHEA, TRAVELER'S).

Contaminated hamburger meat is the most common source of *E. coli* infection. There have also been instances of apple cider contamination. In day care centers, human transmission of *E. coli* has taken place through contact with fecal matter. Three to four days after exposure to the enterohemorrhagic *E. coli* bacillus, watery diarrhea develops. In most people, this rapidly progresses to bloody diarrhea. Other symptoms include nausea, vomiting, and a low-grade fever. Symptoms generally last for a week, followed by spontaneous recovery. However, a life-threatening complication called HEMOLYTIC-UREMIC SYNDROME (HUS) occurs in approximately one in ten cases. This syndrome, which affects primarily very young children and older people, can lead to KIDNEY FAILURE.

DIAGNOSIS AND TREATMENT

The presence of bloody diarrhea suggests a diagnosis of *E. coli* infection. Stool analysis can confirm the diagnosis. However, if stool samples are taken after 48 hours of infection, culture results may be negative or inconclusive.

Dehydration due to *E. coli* diarrhea is treated with oral rehydration fluid, a solution that contains water, salts, and glucose that is available over-the-counter at pharmacies. In severe cases, intravenous fluids are required. Medications to reduce the contraction of the intestines should not be used in cases of bloody diarrhea. Treatment of HUS is with clotting factors, plasma exchange, and kidney DIALYSIS. Prevention of *E. coli* diarrhea is with careful hygiene and thorough cooking of all meat and poultry products.

Diarrhea, traveler's

Diarrhea caused by ingesting contaminated water or food while traveling in areas with poor sanitation. Abdominal cramps, fever, dehydration, nausea, and vomiting may also occur. In many cases, over-the-counter medications control diarrhea. DEHYDRATION can be treated by drinking adequate clear liquids. Because watery diarrhea can rapidly cause a loss of body fluids and crucial body salts, it is best to drink oral rehydration fluid (a solution of water, salts, and glucose that is available over-the-counter at pharmacies). A doctor may prescribe an antibiotic for more severe cases.

Persistent diarrhea may require testing to determine its cause. Tests may include analysis of a stool sample, blood tests, a lower GASTROINTESTINAL (GI) SERIES (an X-ray procedure also called a barium enema), and SIGMOIDOSCOPY or COLONOSCOPY, in which the colon and rectum are examined by using a slim, flexible, lighted tube inserted through the anus.

If a bacterial infection or parasite is the cause, the doctor will prescribe medication. (See also DYSENTERY; AMEBIC DYSENTERY.) To prevent diarrhea, doctors recommend that travelers use bottled water, avoid fresh fruits, and eat only thoroughly cooked foods. Thorough cooking destroys most infectious organisms.

Diastolic blood pressure

A measurement of the force exerted by the blood against the walls of the arteries when the heart relaxes between beats. The first measurement is called systolic blood pressure and is the top number or first number in a reading. Diastolic blood pressure is the second measurement (or bottom number) given in a blood pressure reading. See BLOOD PRESSURE.

Diathermy

Producing heat in a part of the body with a high-frequency electrical current, ultrasonic wave, or microwave radiation. Physical therapists use diathermy to relieve pain in joints and muscles. The heat that is generated can increase blood flow and help to reduce pain in people with arthritis, for example. Surgeons use a diathermy knife to coagulate bleeding vessels or to separate tissues without causing bleeding.

Diathesis

An inherited predisposition to certain diseases and conditions. For example, one type of hemorrhagic diathesis is an inherited predisposition to bleeding disorders such as HEMOPHILIA. Since males seem to be more susceptible than females, hemo-philia-related bleeding diathesis is most likely associated with the X chromosome.

Diazepam

See BENZODIAZEPINES.

Diclofenac sodium

See NONSTEROIDAL ANTI-INFLAMMATORY DRUGS.

Dicloxacillin

See PENICILLINS.

Didanosine (ddI)

An antiviral drug used in the treatment of HIV (human immunodeficiency virus) and AIDS (acquired immunodeficiency syndrome). Didanosine (Videx) stops the growth of the HIV. Didanosine is also called ddI. It is not a cure for AIDS, although in combination with other drugs, it can slow the disease process and prolong a person's life.

Diet, balanced

A diet that consists of adequate amounts of the seven essential substances: proteins, carbohydrates, fats, fiber, vitamins, minerals, and water in appropriate proportions. Proteins, carbohydrates, and fats contain calories and provide energy. A balanced daily diet for healthy individuals should derive 50 to 60 percent of calories from carbohydrates, no more than 30 percent (and preferably less) from fat, and 10 to 20 percent from protein. While fiber, vitamins, and minerals contain no calories, they are essential to good health. Two quarts (8 cups) of water should be drunk daily and can be in the form of beverages, soups, or other liquid foods. Beverages containing caffeine and alcohol promote water losses and should not count as sources of water.

A well-balanced diet is important for normal body function, growth and repair, and reproduction. It is required both for good health and the prevention of disease. Many common diseases, including heart disease, high blood pressure, atherosclerosis, diabetes, osteoporosis, and cancer, are affected by diet. Because no single

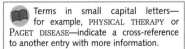

Terms in small capital letters— for example, PHYSICAL THERAPY or PAGET DISEASE—indicate a cross-reference to another entry with more information.

food supplies all the nutrients required for good health, doctors advise eating a balanced diet consisting of a wide variety of foods. At times, older people and those with chronic illnesses are unable to adhere to a balanced diet. In these cases, dietary supplements may be required. See also FOOD GUIDE PYRAMID.

Dietary assessment

The evaluation of an individual's diet to identify which nutrients are being supplied or neglected in the diet, related behaviors, and habits associated with disease. Dietary assessment is usually conducted by a registered dietician (RD). Once overall nutritional status is assessed, a personalized course of treatment is recommended.

Various instruments are used in dietary assessment. Dietary recalls are designed to assess food intake during the previous 24 hours. Food-frequency questionnaires ask about the specific consumption and portion size of foods and beverages over a defined period. A diet diary requires recording descriptions and serving sizes of what was consumed over periods from 3 to 7 days. Another effective tool is dietary risk assessment (DRA), which is used to assess behavior associated with coronary heart disease. This tool is simpler than the 7-day dietary recall and is often administered by people who are not trained in nutrition. The DRA contains 31 food frequency questions, 11 food preparation questions, and 7 attitude and misconception questions.

Dietary reference intakes

Current standards for the components of a healthy diet in the United States and Canada. The National Academies of Science released new dietary reference intakes (DRIs) in 1997 to update food allowances originally set in 1941. DRIs reflect the shift in health concerns that has taken place since then. In the 1940s, the emphasis was on the prevention of nutrient deficiencies. The current focus is on the benefits of healthful eating, such as decreasing the risk of chronic diseases including osteoporosis, heart disease, and hypertension.

DRI STANDARDS

DRIs, which can be used to plan or assess diets, apply to the healthy general population. The DRI standards include a number of measurements that have a bearing on health.

■ *Estimated Average Requirement (EAR)* The daily dietary intake that is sufficient to meet the nutrient requirements of 50 percent of the individuals in an age and sex group.

■ *Recommended Dietary Allowances (RDAs)* The daily dietary intake that is sufficient to meet the nutrient requirements of nearly all individuals in an age and sex group. An RDA can be set only if an EAR has already been accurately set.

■ *Adequate Intake (AI)* A substitute for the EAR, used when insufficient scientific evidence is available to correctly calculate an EAR.

■ *Tolerable Upper Intake Level (UL)* A new guideline that has been set in response to the growing popularity of dietary supplements and food fortification. UL is the highest level of daily nutrient intake that is likely to pose no risks of adverse health effects to most of the population.

Dietetics

The study of the kinds and quantities of foods needed to maintain health and manage diseases.

Diethylstilbestrol (DES)

A synthetic estrogen drug thought to prevent miscarriage that was commonly given to pregnant women from 1938 until 1971. DES has not been prescribed for that purpose since the early 1970s, when it was discovered the drug could cause cervical, vaginal, or uterine cancer and other birth defects in the daughters of women who took it. While it is still considered a dangerous drug to take during pregnancy, DES is prescribed for other conditions, such as inoperable, progressive breast cancer and prostate cancer.

Dietician, registered

A food and nutrition expert who has completed the academic and practice requirements established by the Commission on Dietetic Registration, the credentialing agency of the American Dietetic Association. A registered dietician (RD) specializes in evaluating diets, assessing nutrition status, and planning diets with appropriate variety and proportion of foods, based on an individual's or a population's needs. Diets are planned for people with specific diseases and conditions, as well as for weight gain or loss. RDs must demonstrate knowledge of food and nutrition by passing an examination. An RD must also engage in ongoing professional development. Many states regulate and certify dieticians. In addition to private practice, RDs work at hospitals, wellness programs, as teachers in medical schools, and in research at food and pharmaceutical companies.

Differentiation

The process of change during embryo development that leads to specialization among cells. During embryo development, cells differentiate, or change from a generalized form, or stem cell, into specialized forms intended for specific tissues, organs, or other body parts. For example, a stem cell may differentiate into a liver cell or a heart muscle cell. Differentiation is the normal process by which cells mature. Cancer cells are less differentiated than normal cells, and they are graded according to the extent of their differentiation. A poorly differentiated cancer is one in which the cells differ greatly from the normal cells found in an organ. Typically, the presence of cancer with poorly differentiated cells indicates a poorer prognosis than does cancer with well-differentiated cells.

Diffusion

The intermingling of substances, resulting in complete mixing. Diffusion involves the random movement of molecules or other small particles in a solution, tending toward uniform distribution throughout the available volume with no addition of energy. Diffusion plays a role in many physical phenomena, such as the transfer of oxygen from air in the lungs to the bloodstream. Typically, substances diffuse from an area of high concentration to an area of lower concentration.

Diflunisal

A nonsteroidal anti-inflammatory drug (NSAID). Diflunisal (Dolobid), an aspirin derivative, is used to treat mild to moderate pain, osteoarthritis, and rheumatoid arthritis.

Digestion

The process by which the body converts food into materials that can be absorbed in the intestines. The DIGESTIVE SYSTEM comprises about half the body's internal organs. In digestion, a wide variety of complex plant and animal food sources are broken down into their basic chemical units. The digestive tract, is a series of joined and coiled tubes that extends from the mouth to the esophagus, stomach, small and large intestines, rectum, and anus. Food is propelled through the digestive tract by a rhythmic series of muscular contractions called peristalsis.

Other organs involved in digestion are the liver, gallbladder, and pancreas. The liver and pancreas secrete substances such as enzymes and bile that enter the digestive tract through ducts that open into the first part of the small intestine. The gallbladder stores bile, which it releases as needed to aid in fat digestion.

Food travels from the mouth through the esophagus to the stomach. In the stomach, a hollow sac that is the widest part of the digestive tract, foods are processed by mechanical agitation. Limited protein and fat digestion by enzymes also takes place there, and hydrochloric acid begins the process of protein digestion. After food is digested into small enough pieces, it passes out of the stomach into the duodenum, the first part of the small intestine. Most of the digestive enzyme activity occurs in the first two thirds of the small intestine. Eventually food is broken into molecules small enough to be absorbed. After absorption, nutrients are distributed throughout the body and used for growth, reproduction, and the maintenance of health. Fiber and waste are eventually expelled through the anus as feces.

Digestive system

The organs that take food into the body, break it down into chemical components, extract nutrients to provide energy for the body's cells, and rid the body of the waste products. Also known as the gastrointestinal system, the digestive system can be considered to be a long tube stretching the full length of the body from the mouth to the anus; related organs such as the LIVER, GALLBLADDER, and PANCREAS, assist in the digestive process along the way.

The upper part of the digestive tract works in part to physically break down food that enters the body in various forms. The more complex part of the digestive process involves the chemical breakdown of the food so that usable chemical nutrients can be absorbed into the bloodstream.

DIGESTIVE ORGANS

The MOUTH is the opening into the digestive system. Inside the mouth, the teeth grind food into a pulpy consistency, with the tongue acting to stir the mass and mix it with saliva. Saliva is secreted by three pairs of glands in the cheeks and under the tongue; the saliva makes swallowing easier by providing lubrication, and it rinses off the teeth, but it also contains a digestive enzyme that starts to break down starches in foods. From the mouth, the food is pushed back into the throat, or pharynx, and then into the esophagus by means of muscular contractions that involve a combination of voluntary activity and involuntary reflexes regulated by impulses from the brain. The swallowed food passes down the length of the esophagus, which stretches from the throat to the stomach, squeezed along by a series of rhythmic muscular contractions called peristalsis. At the end of the esophagus, a valve regulates the passage of food into the stomach and prevents regurgitation.

The STOMACH is the widest portion of the digestive tract. It is a muscular organ that can expand to hold and store as much as 3 pints of food at a time. Layers of muscles in the walls of the stomach contract to further physically break down food by churning it into a semiliquid called chyme. The lining of the stomach secretes stomach acids and digestive enzymes (proteins that promote chemical action) that process the food chemically. A valve at the base of the stomach, the pyloric sphincter, opens to allow quantities of the liquefied, partially digested food into the small intestine.

In the small INTESTINE, the actual absorption of nutrients into the

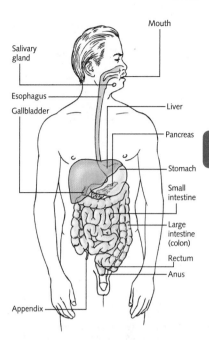

Mouth
Salivary gland
Esophagus
Gallbladder
Liver
Pancreas
Stomach
Small intestine
Large intestine (colon)
Rectum
Anus
Appendix

D

EATING, DIGESTING, ELIMINATING
Within the hollow organs of the digestive system, food is broken down and the nutrients are digested. Food passes through the system and is changed into smaller molecules of nutrients and waste through a combination of mechanical and chemical processes.

bloodstream takes place. The small intestine has three sections: the duodenum, the ileum, and the jejunum. In the first, shorter segment, the duodenum, the chemical breakdown of the food continues, aided by enzymes secreted into the duodenum from the liver, gallbladder, and pancreas (organs associated with the digestive process). The duodenum passes the food into the long, coiled part of the small intestine, where the final chemical breakdown occurs. The enzymes that act on the stomach contents are specialized to perform the chemical processes necessary to break down fats, carbohydrates, and proteins into forms that can be absorbed. The absorption into the bloodstream takes place through the thin intestinal walls.

At this point, the by-products that remain pass into the large intestine, which loops around the small intestine and then exits the body. The large intestine has three sections: the COLON; the cecum (a chamber in the colon); and the rectum. The colon has ascending, transverse, descending,

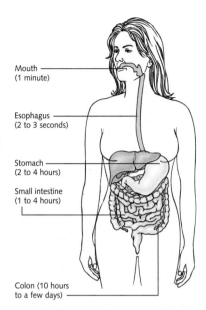

Mouth
(1 minute)

Esophagus
(2 to 3 seconds)

Stomach
(2 to 4 hours)

Small intestine
(1 to 4 hours)

Colon (10 hours
to a few days)

LENGTH OF THE DIGESTIVE PROCESS
The complex process of digestion takes as much as a day or more. The length of time required to complete the process differs with the type of food and the individual person. People in whom the digestive system works more slowly may be more prone to digestive disorders.

and sigmoid sections that loop around the small intestine. In the first part of the colon, the water content, vitamins, and minerals are absorbed from the digestive material. The solids that are left, called feces or stool, are waste that can be stored in the sigmoid colon before being expelled from the body via the rectum (the last part of the colon) and finally the anus (the opening to the outside of the body).

DIGESTIVE PROCESS
The chemical breakdown of food into absorbable forms of energy is accomplished by the digestive agents in the digestive tract. Carbohydrates, fats, and proteins are the major nutrients that must be processed for absorption. Carbohydrates are generally sugars and starches that are the body's main source of energy. Fats are a concentrated source of energy. Proteins (composed of building blocks called amino acids) are the main structural components of body cells and tissues. Vitamins and minerals are essential for various types of cell functioning, growth, and repair.

During digestion, carbohydrates are broken down into simple sugars (glucose, fructose, and galactose) to be used as energy. Fats are broken down into components called fatty acids that are absorbed and used for energy or stored. Proteins are dismantled into amino acids that can be absorbed and then rebuilt into proteins anywhere in the body. Vitamins and minerals can generally be absorbed without chemical breakdown.

Some of the mechanical aspects of the digestive process, such as parts of the swallowing mechanism and control of defecation, are under at least partially voluntary control. But much of the digestive process, including the mechanisms of appetite and hunger, are controlled by the autonomic nervous system, which regulates automatic, unconscious body functions.

Digital subtraction angiography

An X-ray procedure used to visualize blood vessels (both arteries and veins) through a series of computer images after they have been injected with a CONTRAST MEDIUM. Digital subtraction angiography (DSA) uses smaller amounts of injected contrast medium than traditional angiography but still produces high-quality images. This makes the technique especially appropriate for people in whom high-contrast examinations present risks. DSA subtracts the background of bone and soft tissue to provide an image of blood vessels after injection of a contrast medium.

Digoxin

A drug used to treat congestive heart failure and atrial cardiac arrhythmias. Digoxin (Lanoxin) is the most widely used cardiac glycoside (a chemical compound) derived from a plant, *Digitalis lanata* or *Digitalis purpurea*. It improves the force of ventricular contraction of the heart in a person with congestive heart failure. It is also used to treat atrial fibrillation and flutter (irregular heartbeat), as well as atrial tachycardia (rapid heartbeat).

Digoxin is available in a form that can be injected into a vein or occasionally into a muscle and as tablets, capsules, and liquid. The therapeutic dose is very close to the toxic dose, so digoxin should always be taken with care and monitored by a physician.

Dilation

Enlarging or expanding of something. Dilation takes place when a hollow organ or body cavity stretches or gets bigger. For example, dilation occurs when the pupils of the eyes widen in dimly lit surroundings.

Dilation and curettage

See D AND C.

Dilation and evacuation

See D AND E.

Dilator

An instrument used to enlarge an opening. A doctor may use a dilator to open the esophagus for people whose esophagus has been scarred so that food and fluids can pass through to the stomach.

Diltiazem

See CALCIUM CHANNEL BLOCKERS.

Dimenhydrinate

An antihistamine drug used to treat motion sickness. Dimenhydrinate (Dimetabs, Marmine) prevents nausea, vomiting, and vertigo (dizziness) associated with motion sickness. It is available without a prescription in capsules, tablets, and liquid form and by prescription as an injection.

Diphenhydramine

An antihistamine drug that has many properties. Diphenhydramine (Benadryl) is used to relieve symptoms of allergic reactions such as rash, hives, watery eyes, runny nose, itchy eyes, and sneezing. It is also used to treat motion sickness, anxiety, tension, and sleeplessness and to relieve certain side effects caused by some psychiatric drugs.

Diphtheria

An acute, contagious, bacterial illness that may affect the respiratory system or the skin. Symptoms of respiratory diphtheria include a fibrous membrane that forms on the tonsils, in the throat, and in the nose. The condition is spread by direct physical contact or by direct or indirect contact with respiratory secretions of an infected person. Respiratory diphtheria is potentially fatal and carries the risk of complications, including inflammation of the heart muscle, multiple nerve inflammation, and obstruction of the airway.

Symptoms of cutaneous diphtheria include open wounds on the skin that become infected with the diphtheria bacteria; it is spread by contact with an infected person's open sores. Serious complications and death occur much less frequently in the cutaneous form of diphtheria than with respiratory diphtheria. The infection is caused by toxin-producing strains of a specific bacterium, *Corynebacterium diphtheriae*, and is found in developing countries.

A vaccine has made respiratory diphtheria rare in the United States, although the illness may be carried without symptoms even in areas where most of the population has been immunized. Because immunity wanes over time, periodic booster vaccines are required to maintain sufficient levels of antibodies in the body to prevent infection.

Cutaneous diphtheria usually spreads most readily in areas where poor hygiene is prevalent. The infection tends to flourish in warm climates but is not limited to tropical areas, and there have been large outbreaks in temperate zones. Poverty and homelessness contribute to the spread of infection.

SYMPTOMS

The incubation period for diphtheria ranges from 1 to 4 days. Symptoms of respiratory diphtheria initially include a mild sore throat, difficulty swallowing, low-grade fever, fatigue, an increased heart rate, and an elevated white blood cell count. In children, symptoms may include nausea, vomiting, chills, headache, and high fever. Children may not have symptoms until the infection is well established.

The illness may remain mild or progress to include difficulty swallowing and breathing, extreme fatigue, and swollen lymph glands in the neck. In more severe cases, the neck tissue may become involved, causing the neck to enlarge. The airway may become completely obstructed, and there may be a bloody nasal discharge.

Symptoms of cutaneous diphtheria

include skin lesions, usually on the arms and legs, that become numbed or painful, swollen, red, and oozing. The nose, throat, ears, and genital tract may become infected, and rarely, the eyes may also become involved.

DIAGNOSIS AND TREATMENT

In cases of respiratory diphtheria, a characteristic membrane that forms on the respiratory system's structures can be clinically observed. A culture of the membrane or the tissue below it can be evaluated in a laboratory to isolate the organism and confirm a diagnosis. When cutaneous diphtheria is suspected, a culture may be taken from an infected skin lesion for laboratory evaluation.

People with symptoms of respiratory diphtheria are generally hospitalized in intensive care units (ICUs). Diphtheria antitoxin medication neutralizes the toxin produced by the bacteria, but only if it is not yet bound to cells. For this reason, this medication must be administered as soon as the illness is clinically diagnosed, without waiting for a laboratory confirmation. The medication can be effective when it is given within 48 hours. The dosage, which is based on several factors including severity of symptoms, may be given intravenously. Antimicrobial treatment, such as penicillin or erythromycin, must be given to destroy the disease-causing organism and prevent the disease from spreading.

Bed rest is essential to treatment, along with intensive nursing care emphasizing good nutrition, fluid intake, and possibly the person's need for oxygen. Potential respiratory and cardiac problems must be monitored. TRACHEOSTOMY may become necessary to allow breathing. Recovery is usually slow, and ongoing rest is generally advised. If inflammation of the heart muscle is involved, normal physical exertion may be dangerous until the person has completely recovered.

Treatment of cutaneous diphtheria is generally based on regular, thorough cleaning of skin lesions with soap and water and prescribed medication for a 10-day period.

Active immunization against the infection is offered by diphtheria-tetanus-pertussis (DTP) vaccines, which are routinely given to all chil-

dren, with boosters available to adults. Nevertheless, anyone who has had close contact with a person known to have diphtheria should be tested for the infection, regardless of previous immunization. People who have had contact with diphtheria should update their immunization status.

Diplopia

See DOUBLE VISION.

Disability

A physical or emotional condition that impairs the ability to function. Degrees of disability are highly variable. For example, with certain accommodations, a person with a minor disability (such as a learning disorder) can continue to lead a relatively normal life. Aids such as canes or wheelchairs can help people who have partial paralysis—for example, from a stroke or other condition that

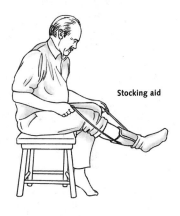

Stocking aid

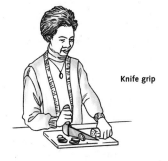

Knife grip

LIVING WITH ARTHRITIS
Many assistive devices are available to make life easier for a person with a disability such as arthritis. A "stocking aid" helps a person put on socks without bending over, and kitchen utensils with specially shaped handles make food preparation easier for someone with limited motion in the wrists and fingers.

limits mobility. However, someone who is disabled with a serious chronic illness (such as Alzheimer's disease) can require home health care or may need to enter a residential facility. In some cases, the government will help pay for the cost of caring for a person with a serious disability.

Discharge

Release from the hospital. Before departing, a person must have discharge orders from the doctor and a release form from the hospital business office. A discharge planner in the hospital can help plan for health care needs following release (such as entrance into another health care facility, arrangement for a visiting nurse, or the ordering of equipment such as a wheelchair).

Disclosing agents

Stains in tablet or liquid form that adhere to the plaque (SEE PLAQUE, DENTAL) on teeth. Plaque contains bacteria, mucus, and food particles that build up if the teeth are not brushed and flossed regularly. Dental plaque cannot be observed unless it is stained. When chewed, these tablets stain the plaque red so those areas of the teeth can be carefully cleaned with a toothbrush. Red disclosing agents may be purchased over-the-counter at pharmacies.

Disinfectants

Agents that destroy disease-carrying microorganisms. Disinfectants include heat, radiation, and chemicals, which may destroy, neutralize, or inhibit the growth of microorganisms. Disinfectants are used primarily on solid objects, such as food-preparation equipment and kitchen countertops.

Disk prolapse

See SLIPPED DISK.

Disk, intervertebral

The flat, circular structure firmly embedded between the vertebrae (bones of the spine) to serve as a shock absorber for the spine by separating the vertebrae and keeping the bony structures from rubbing together when a person moves and bends. Intervertebral disks are attached to the weight-bearing part of each vertebra by sheaths of muscle and by the ligaments that con-

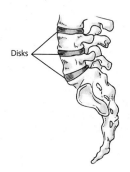

Disks

SHOCK ABSORBERS
The intervertebral disks act as cushions between the vertebrae. Each disk has a central core of gel, encased in a fibrous capsule. Ligaments running the length of the spine hold the disks in place.

nect the spinal bones. The characteristics of intervertebral disks change with advancing age. From childhood into early adulthood, the disks are soft, gel-filled sacs that begin to get firmer as a person gets older. In young adults, the blood supply to the disks has ended, the soft sacs are stiffening, and their structure is less elastic. By middle-age, intervertebral disks are tough, fibrous, and as inflexible as hard rubber. As a person ages, intervertebral disks can become more susceptible to damage from injury.

Diskography

An imaging technique used to locate the source of back pain caused by an injured disk. In diskography, a solution is injected into the specific disks believed to be causing pain, as well as into neighboring disks. A special X ray called a diskogram is taken, which is often used before back surgery to identify the exact area to be operated on. Diskography may be more painful than MYELOGRAPHY and requires experienced and expert technique for accurate results. Diskograms may be helpful for diagnosing sciatica, as they can reveal the extent of degeneration and damage of the offending disk.

Dislocation, joint

FOR FIRST AID
see Dislocations, page 1319

An irregularity in the close positioning of the two parts of a joint that prevents the joint from functioning normally. A dislocated joint may be

caused by trauma or may be present at birth. In some cases, a past injury to a jaw or shoulder joint weakens the joint so that it becomes dislocated spontaneously. The most common joint dislocation occurs in the shoulder and is usually caused by a person falling forward onto an outstretched hand or onto the shoulder itself. Torn ligaments, damage to the capsule that encases the joint, and injury to associated muscles, blood vessels, and nerves may be involved when the trauma to a joint is sufficiently severe to cause a dislocation. When shoulder or hip joints are dislocated, the nerves to the arm or leg extending from the joint can be damaged, and paralysis may occur. If spinal vertebrae are dislocated, the spinal cord can be damaged, resulting in paralysis below the point of dislocation. Symptoms of a joint dislocation include a misshapen appearance, pain, swelling, discoloration, and an inability to move the joint. A joint that is dislocated because of trauma is a serious injury and should be treated immediately. After giving the person a muscle relaxant, the doctor will gently rotate the dislocated joint back into place. In some cases, traction or surgery may be needed.

Disorientation

Loss of normal awareness of time, place, and identity. Disorientation can be caused by low blood pressure, fever, certain medications, delirium, dementia, and mental illness.

Displacement

The unconscious shift of an emotion from the original source of that emotion to an object, animal, or person perceived as less threatening. A person who releases the stress of the work day by yelling at a spouse or mistreating a pet is engaging in displacement. Displacement, one of the DEFENSE MECHANISMS, is an automatic, unconscious psychological process that protects an individual against stress and internal emotional conflict.

Dissociative disorders

A group of related abnormal emotional conditions in which an individual becomes detached from fundamental aspects of waking consciousness, such as personal identity, memory, or awareness of self and body. Dissociative disorders are thought to originate in overwhelming traumatic experiences, such as combat, physical or sexual assault, or severe accidents. Unable to integrate the trauma into his or her normal consciousness, the person detaches from the disturbing experience as a way of coping with it.

Dissociative disorders take a number of forms. In dissociative amnesia, the individual blocks out critical personal information, such as the memory of a trauma. The amnesia may be restricted to certain times or parts of an event, or it may affect life history as a whole or after a certain time. In dissociative fugue, which is very rare, the person suddenly and unexpectedly departs on a journey. Unaware of or confused about his or her identity, the person may adopt a new identity. Dissociative identity disorder used to be known as multiple personality disorder and is the best-known dissociative disorder. The individual with dissociative identity disorder has two or more distinct identities that surface regularly and control the person's actions, although the affected person knows little about the other identities. In dissociative personality disorder, the person feels apart from his or her body, moving through life like a robot or a character in a movie.

Since dissociative disorders usually arise from a traumatic experience, treatment typically consists of psychotherapy focused on that experience. People with dissociative disorders may also exhibit the symptoms of depression or anxiety and benefit from medications used to treat those conditions.

Distal

In anatomy, the portion of a body part located farther away from the point of origin or attachment. The elbow, for example, is distal to the shoulder, and the distal end of the thigh bone is part of the knee joint. The opposite of distal is PROXIMAL.

Disulfiram

An alcohol deterrent drug. Disulfiram (Antabuse) is used to help treat alcoholism. Disulfiram interacts with alcohol, even in small quantities, to produce unpleasant symptoms including facial flushing, dizziness, thirst, nausea, and vomiting. It is also used to treat nickel poisoning.

Diuretics

Drugs that cause the body to excrete water and salt. Diuretics have been used for centuries to treat edema, the accumulation of water in cells and tissues. They are still considered useful to treat HYPERTENSION (high blood pressure), especially among older people. Diuretics can significantly reduce the risk of stroke and, to a lesser degree, heart attacks caused by high blood pressure.

TYPES OF DIURETICS

There are three primary types of diuretics. The first, thiazides, are commonly used to treat high blood pressure (hypertension), whether taken alone to treat mild to moderate hypertension or used in combination with other drugs to treat more severe disease. There are many thiazides and thiazide-related drugs. Common examples include chlorthalidone (Hygroton), chlorothiazide (Diuril), and hydrochlorothiazide (Esidrix, HydroDIURIL).

Loop diuretics, so called because they work on the region of the kidneys called the loop of Henle, increase the excretion of water, sodium, potassium, calcium, and magnesium by decreasing the concentration and dilution of urine. They work very fast—within 20 minutes—and are the most potent diuretics available. Loop diuretics are particularly useful for medical conditions that have not responded to less potent diuretics. Examples include bumetanide (Bumex), furosemide (Lasix), and ethacrynic acid (Edecrin).

Potassium-sparing agents may be recommended to offset the effects of some diuretics, such as loop and thiazide, which tend to deplete the body's supply of potassium, which in turn can cause arrhythmias (disturbances in heart rhythm). Doctors may recommend potassium supplements to people taking diuretics, or they may prescribe a potassium-sparing agent, alone or in combination with a thiazide. Examples of potassium-sparing diuretics include amiloride (Midamor), spironolactone (Aldactone), and triamterene (Dyazide, Dyrenium).

Divalproex

See VALPROIC ACID.

Diverticular disease

The presence of small sacs (diverticula) in the walls of the lower end of the colon. Less frequently, diverticula develop in other parts of the digestive tract, such as the stomach, small intestine, and esophagus (see ESOPHAGEAL DIVERTICULUM). Diverticula are created by the bulging or protrusion of the inner lining of intestinal walls through the muscular layers of the wall. Occasionally, a blood vessel at the base of diverticula will erode, causing rectal bleeding. Diverticular disease includes both diverticulosis and diverticulitis. Diverticular disease is especially common in the United States, where the diet is typically low in fiber and constipation is a problem. Diverticula that develop in the colon mainly affect older people. Elsewhere in the digestive tract, diverticula are not related to age.

Diverticulosis refers to the presence of diverticula in the digestive tract. It is very common and about half of those older than age 60 experience it. Many people develop diverticula that produce no symptoms. Approximately one in five people with diverticulosis has abdominal pain, bloating, gas, constipation, or diarrhea. However, few people with diverticulosis ever develop diverticulitis. Left untreated, diverticulosis can lead to serious complications, such as an abscess.

Diverticulitis is the inflammation or infection of one or more diverticula. Inflammation leads to muscle spasm, severe abdominal pain, nausea, and fever. Cramps and tenderness may occur on the left side of the abdomen. The passing of gas or a bowel movement may relieve cramps temporarily. Stools usually become small, round, and hard. If diverticula bleed, red blood appears in the stools. Possible complications of diverticulitis include the development of a stricture, narrowing of the intestine (see INTESTINE, OBSTRUCTION OF); a fistula, an abnormal channel that forms between parts of the intestine; an abscess, a pus-filled sac around the diverticulum; and PERITONITIS, life-threatening inflammation of the membrane lining the abdominal cavity that occurs after an abscess bursts.

DIAGNOSIS AND TREATMENT

Diverticular disease is diagnosed by a complete physical examination and tests, such as blood tests, stool analysis, a lower GASTROINTESTINAL (GI) SERIES (an X-ray procedure also called a barium enema), and SIGMOIDOSCOPY or COLONOSCOPY (an examination of the rectum and colon using a flexible viewing tube passed through the anus). Because the symptoms of diverticular disease are similar to those of IRRITABLE BOWEL SYNDROME, it is important to differentiate between them in making the diagnosis.

In many cases, diverticulosis responds well to the adoption of a high-fiber diet. In diverticulitis, doctors often prescribe antibiotics, as well as antispasmodic drugs, to control abdominal pain. An attack of diverticulitis may require hospitalization. If the abdomen is distended and there is no passage of stool or gas, the contents of the stomach and intestine may need to be emptied by using suction. All fluids must be given intravenously for several days to allow inflammation to subside. In severe cases of diverticulitis, a COLEC-TOMY (the surgical removal of all or part of the colon) may be necessary. People with diverticular disease are advised not to eat poppy seeds, sesame seeds, or fruit with tiny seeds.

Diving medicine

A specialized form of medicine that treats DECOMPRESSION SICKNESS, based on hyperbaric oxygen therapy (HBO). During this therapy, scuba divers who have been affected by unreleased excess nitrogen in the bloodstream enter special hyperbaric chambers and are fitted with oxygen masks. This allows them to experience gradually decreasing pressure at a controlled rate that replicates the conditions of a safe ascent to the surface of the water. By combining increased air pressure with the inhalation of 100 percent oxygen, HBO allows the body to release the extra nitrogen at a healthful pace. When decompression sickness is treated promptly with HBO, the serious health risks associated with the extra nitrogen (confusion, paralysis, coma) can be prevented.

Dizziness

FOR SYMPTOM CHART
see Dizziness, page 36

A feeling of faintness or an inability to maintain normal balance while sitting or standing. Most causes of dizziness are minor, such as a bout of flu or a cold. Other common causes include infection or injury of the inner ear (which controls balance), low blood pressure, standing up too quickly from a sitting or lying position, alcohol intoxication, medications (particularly tranquilizers, narcotics, sedatives, and drugs used to treat high blood pressure), migraine, hyperventilation, severe pain, injury, fright, or strenuous coughing. Serious causes of dizziness include anemia, heart disease, cardiac arrhythmia, and central nervous system abnormalities. Medical attention is rquired only when dizziness is accompanied by a complete loss of consciousness, when other symptoms are present (such as tingling or chest pain), when the cause appears to be medication-induced, or when light-headedness persists for 3 weeks or longer. If medical examination reveals possible neurological problems, further testing probably will be done.

DNA

See DEOXYRIBONUCLEIC ACID.

DNA fingerprinting

A laboratory procedure in which individuals are identified by their DEOXYRIBONUCLEIC ACID (DNA). DNA fingerprinting is based on the fact that everyone has a unique set of genes and DNA. The technique, also called DNA typing or DNA profiling, is used by forensic scientists and police laboratories as evidence in criminal proceedings or to establish paternity. A related type of DNA testing is used to diagnose inherited disorders, such as cystic fibrosis, hemophilia, and sickle cell anemia. To construct a DNA fingerprint, a tiny sample is taken from body tissue or fluid, such as hair, blood, or saliva. The sample of DNA is further divided into smaller pieces by enzymes and sorted according to size, using a process called ELEC-TROPHORESIS. The segments are marked and exposed on X-ray film, where they form a characteristic pattern of black bars—the DNA fingerprint.

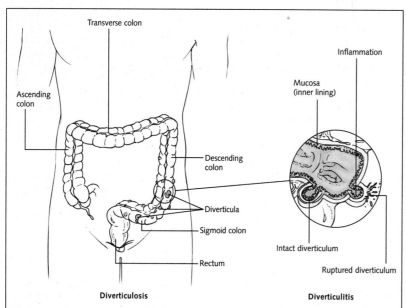

Transverse colon

Inflammation

Mucosa
(inner lining)

Ascending
colon

Descending
colon

Diverticula

Sigmoid colon

Rectum

Intact diverticulum

Ruptured diverticulum

Diverticulosis

Diverticulitis

TWO TYPES OF DIVERTICULAR DISEASE
Diverticula, which are little pouches or sacs, can develop when the inner lining (mucosa) of the intestine bulges through the outer wall. Diverticula are most likely to occur in a person who eats a low-fiber diet, which allows particles of fecal matter to lodge in the intestinal lining. The presence of diverticula is called diverticulosis, a condition that may not cause symptoms. But diverticulosis can develop into diverticulitis, a more serious condition involving inflammation. Diverticulitis can be very painful and can cause obstruction and rupture.

DNA forensic testing

The use of DNA FINGERPRINTING to identify suspects in criminal proceedings. Just as they collect fingerprints, criminal investigators routinely take biological tissue samples, such as bloodstains, semen, or saliva, from crime scenes. DNA evidence collected from a crime scene can link a suspect to evidence or eliminate a suspect.

DNR

A DO-NOT-RESUSCITATE ORDER (see also ADVANCE DIRECTIVES).

Do-not-resuscitate order

A type of advance directive, commonly known as a DNR, made by an individual or the person's physician, stating exactly under which circumstances the person should or should not be resuscitated (see ADVANCE DIRECTIVES).

Docetaxel

An anticancer drug. Docetaxel (Taxotere) is given intravenously to treat advanced breast cancer that has spread (metastasized). Docetaxel works by disrupting cell division.

Docusate sodium

A laxative. Docusate sodium (Colace, Senokot) softens stool to facilitate elimination for a person who should not strain, such as a person who has inflamed hemorrhoids. Docusate sodium is used to prevent and treat constipation and is available without prescription, but it is ineffective if used on a long-term basis.

Dofetilide

A drug used to treat atrial fibrillation or flutter; an antiarrhythmic agent. Dofetilide (Tikosyn) tries to normalize a person's heartbeat by changing some of the electrical currents that run through the heart. Dofetilide is recommended for use only when atrial fibrillation or flutter is very serious. It is often used in conjunction with an implantable defibrillator.

Donepezil

A drug used to ease Alzheimer's disease symptoms. Donepezil (Aricept) treats confusion and memory loss in people with Alzheimer's disease and slows disease progression.

Dong Quai root

An herbal medicine derived from the root of angelica, a kind of wild celery, used to treat menstrual and menopausal problems. Doctors in China use it to treat high blood pressure, poor circulation, and anemia because, they claim, it stimulates production of red blood cells; however, there is no clinical proof of its effectiveness.

Donor

A person who leaves instructions for his or her body or organs to be donated for medical use after death. To do this, a person fills out a Uniform Donor Card and has it signed by two witnesses. Some states also print legal donor cards on the backs of drivers' licenses. Because a surviving next of kin can elect to disallow even written instructions, doctors recommend that people openly discuss their wishes regarding organ donation with their families.

Dopamine

A NEUROTRANSMITTER in the brain that is involved in the control of movement. A depletion of dopamine produces symptoms of PARKINSON DISEASE, such as rigidity, tremors, and reduced movement. Dopamine is produced in an area of the brain called the substantia nigra. It is then transported to the basal ganglia (clusters of nerve cells deep within the brain) where it helps turn on neurons that affect muscle movement.

Doppler ultrasound

An ULTRASOUND SCANNING technique that produces images of structures inside the body and can provide information about blood flow rate at the same time. Doppler ultrasound creates an image of the area being scanned by processing the echoes produced by harmless, high-frequency sound waves as they strike moving material,

---

UNIFORM DONOR CARD

OF _____

(Print or type name of donor)

In the hope that I may help others, I hereby make this anatomical gift, if medically acceptable, to take effect upon my death. The words and marks below indicate my desires:

I give   (a) _____ any needed organs or tissues
        (b) _____ only the following organs or tissues

Specify the organ(s) or tissue(s)
for the purposes of transplantation, therapy, medical research or education:
        (c) _____ my body for anatomical study if needed
Limitations or special wishes, if any:

_____

Signed by the donor and the following two witnesses in the presence of each other:

_____   _____
Signature of Donor   Date of Birth of Donor

_____   _____
Date Signed   City and State

_____   _____
Witness   Witness
(Preferably next of kin)

This is a legal document under the Uniform Anatomical Gift Act or similar laws.

Courtesy of the Donor Network of Arizona

UNIFORM DONOR CARD
This card can be photocopied and filled in. When folded on the heavy line, and glued front to back, it can be carried in a wallet.

such as blood moving through the blood vessels. This information indicates flow through a blood vessel by interpreting the changes in the frequency of the sound.

Doppler ultrasound can provide important information about the blood vessels and the way blood is passing through them. It is commonly used to view the carotid arteries in the neck, which supply large amounts of blood to the brain. Doppler ultrasound can evaluate the flow and direction of blood surrounding the heart. In the abdomen, it can evaluate blood flow to the liver and other organs. Blood flow in the legs can be studied to identify blockage in the arteries or clots in the veins. During pregnancy, it is used to evaluate the development of the fetus.

HOW IT IS PERFORMED
A gel is applied to the skin of the area being examined, and an instrument called a transducer is moved over the skin surface. The transducer emits high-frequency sound waves. The sound waves bounce off the internal structures and produce echoes that are received by the transducer. The transducer converts the echoes into waveforms that can be recorded. The amplified waveforms are displayed on a monitor or on videotape. Color may be added to the images to offer more detailed information about the pattern and speed of blood flow. A doctor analyzes the waveforms.

At the same time, an audio receiver in the transducer amplifies the sound of flowing blood. The sound is transmitted by an audio speaker in the transducer. The level of this sound is interpreted to locate an obstruction of blood flow.

Dorsal

In anatomy, on or of the back of the body or an organ. Dorsal describes a position situated on or related to the back surface of the body or a body organ. The opposite of dorsal is VENTRAL.

Dorzolamide

A drug used as an eye drop to treat glaucoma. Dorzolamide (Trusopt) lowers eye pressure.

Dose

The quantity of a therapeutic agent to be taken at one time. Dose may refer to the quantity of a drug or amount of radiation.

Double vision

Seeing two images of a single object. Also known as diplopia, double vision is caused either by a defect in a single eye or by misalignment of both eyes.

TYPES AND CAUSES
In monocular (single-eye) double vision, the person continues to see two images through one eye even if the other eye is covered. Monocular double vision can have a number of possible causes: astigmatism (a lack of symmetry in the cornea of the eye); a thin, cone-shaped cornea (keratoconus); an abnormal thickening of the membrane (conjunctiva) that covers the inner surface of the eyelid until it extends over the cornea (pterygium); cataract (cloudiness and opacity in the normally clear lens of the eye); a dislocated lens, usually from trauma; a mass or swelling in the eyelid that exerts pressure on the eye; insufficient tear production (dry eye); and certain kinds of problems in the light-sensitive layer (retina) at the back of the eye.

In binocular double vision, covering one eye stops the diplopia. Binocular double vision arises from misalignment of the eyes and can be caused by any condition that affects the muscles that move the eyes. These diseases include crossed eyes (strabismus); damage to the nerves controlling the eye muscles because of tumor, infection, trauma, or stroke; blockage of the small blood vessels (microvascular infarction) that feed the nerves controlling the eye muscles; myasthenia gravis (a neuromuscular illness that causes muscles to weaken and tire easily); hyperactivity of the thyroid gland (Graves disease), which swells the tissue and muscles around the eyes; and trauma to the eye muscles, particularly fracture of the bones in the eye socket.

TREATMENT
Treatment of double vision depends on the cause. Astigmatism or keratoconus is usually remedied with corrective glasses or contact lenses. Abnormal growth of the conjunctiva is repaired surgically, as are dislocated lenses, cataracts, and some problems of the retina. Eyelid swelling may be treated with medicine or sur-

gery, depending on the underlying condition. Strabismus is usually repaired surgically during childhood. Conditions such as myasthenia gravis, Graves disease, and stroke are treated with medication. Microvascular infarctions, which are commonly seen in people with diabetes, often resolve on their own as the nerve regenerates, in which case double vision gradually clears up. Tumors of the brain are treated with surgery or anticancer medication. Trauma to the eye socket may heal without intervention, but severe fractures that entrap muscles or nerves require surgery.

Double-blind

A method that evaluates the effectiveness of a treatment or compares two treatments. In this type of trial, half the people receive the treatment of interest, while the other half receive a control treatment—often a PLACEBO. The goal is to discover in an unbiased way whether a treatment is effective. A double-blind study is the most rigorous type of clinical research, because neither the people in the study nor the researchers themselves know which treatment a person is receiving. In addition to reducing the risk of bias, the double-blind method can also eliminate the placebo effect, which is a positive or negative response to a treatment resulting from a person's expectations rather than from any real physical or chemical effect.

Douche

Cleansing the vagina by flushing it with water or chemicals. Douching is almost never recommended because the natural cleansing process of the vagina is adequate, and douching can facilitate the transport of infectious organisms into the uterus and irritate the vagina. Douching is not an effective method of birth control.

Down syndrome

A chromosomal abnormality that results in mental retardation and other complications. Down syndrome results from an extra copy of chromosome 21 and is also known as trisomy 21; children with Down syndrome have inherited 3 chromosomes 21, instead of the usual 2. Worldwide, an estimated 1 in every 600 to 1,000

COMPLICATIONS OF DOWN SYNDROME

All individuals with Down syndrome experience some degree of mental retardation. Early intervention can help them reach their full potential. Additional complications may include:

- Vision problems
- Hearing loss
- Frequent ear infections
- Increased susceptibility to infection
- Gastrointestinal obstructions
- Congenital heart defects
- Increased risk of developing leukemia

infants is born with Down syndrome; in the United States, about 5,000 babies are born with Down syndrome each year. The syndrome affects people of all races and economic levels. Women aged 35 or older have a significantly increased risk of having a baby with Down syndrome.

DIAGNOSIS AND TREATMENT

Children with Down syndrome have a characteristic appearance. Their heads may be smaller than usual and abnormally shaped. Facial features usually include a flattened nose and upwardly slanted eyes with a fold of skin at the inner corner. The hands are short and broad, with stubby fingers and a single crease across the palm. Growth and development are usually slower than normal, and most affected children do not grow to average adult height. The average mental age of people with Down syndrome is 8 years, although some individuals have almost normal intelligence.

Children with Down syndrome often have heart defects that may require surgical correction early in life. They are also more at risk for gastrointestinal abnormalities, such as blockage of the esophagus or the duodenum, that often require major surgery soon after birth. They have a much higher than average risk of developing childhood leukemia and are also at risk for developing epilepsy, hypothyroidism, and vision or hearing defects. The normal life span of people with Down syndrome is shortened by congenital heart disease and leukemia. Nevertheless, many people with Down syndrome survive

to age 60, and life expectancy continues to increase.

The diagnosis is usually suspected after a physical examination and confirmed with blood chromosome analysis. A chest X ray or echocardiogram can detect heart defects, and a gastrointestinal X ray can be used to find intestinal blockages. Down syndrome can be detected in a fetus in early pregnancy through AMNIOCENTESIS or CHORIONIC VILLUS SAMPLING.

There is no specific treatment for Down syndrome. Heart defects or intestinal blockages may require surgery. Special education and training and occupational and physical therapy are available in many communities for mentally retarded children.

Doxazosin

A drug that lowers high blood pressure. Doxazosin (Cardura) dilates arteries and veins and is used to treat high blood pressure and other conditions, such as a benign enlarged prostate. It also lowers cholesterol levels. Doxazosin belongs to a class of drugs called alpha-adrenergic blockers, or alpha blockers. It may cause low blood pressure and abnormal heart rhythms.

Doxepin

An antidepressant drug. Doxepin (Sinequan) is used to treat depression, anxiety, and sleep disorders. Doxepin has a sedative effect, although tolerance to the drug usually develops in a few weeks, and the drug becomes less effective.

Doxycycline

An antibiotic drug; a tetracycline. Doxycycline (Vibramycin, Doryx, Periostat) is used to treat chlamydial infections and traveler's diarrhea. It is also used to prevent infection in a woman who has been raped and possibly exposed to a sexually transmitted disease.

Drain, surgical

A device inserted during surgery to draw fluid from an internal body cavity to the surface. A surgical drain is used to prevent fluid from accumulating inside the body during an operation. A surgical drain can ensure that any fluid formed during the procedure will immediately pass to the surface and prevent infection

or a buildup in pressure. When necessary, suction can be applied to the drain to increase its effectiveness.

Surgical drains are used in several different types of surgery. One example of a surgical drain is a chest tube used to drain blood, fluid, or air from the lungs to permit the full expansion of the lungs. A colostomy is a surgical procedure that creates an opening in the abdomen for the drainage of feces from the colon after a surgical bowel resection. A surgical drain may be inserted into an infected ear canal so that fluid that has accumulated behind the eardrum can be suctioned out.

Dream analysis

The systematic study of the content of dreams as a way of understanding a person's unconscious mind. Dream analysis has been used in psychiatry and psychology since the time of Sigmund Freud, who called dreams the "royal road to the unconscious" and saw them as the acceptable expression of otherwise unacceptable and repressed emotions, particularly about sex. Contemporary psychoanalysts emphasize sexuality less, but still see dreams as symbolic representations of feelings and emotional conflicts in waking life. Dream analysis seeks to understand the symbols in dreams and make this understanding available to the individual as a way of improving his or her life.

Dreaming

A series of thoughts, emotions, or images experienced during sleep as real events. Most dreams are visual, but they can also involve the other senses, such as taste and hearing. Dreams occur during REM (rapid eye movement) sleep, a portion of the sleep cycle accompanied by fast, jerky eye movements and irregular heartbeat and breathing. REM periods last on average 10 to 20 minutes each and occur every 1.5 hours during the night. Dreaming is found in almost all mammals, but its function remains unclear. Depriving a person of dreams by waking when REM sleep begins causes irritability and restlessness and may lead to emotional problems. Dreams have been considered the bearers of special messages since ancient times, and many psychiatrists believe that dreams provide clues to a person's unconscious mind. Dreaming may also have a part in consolidation of information into long-term memory. See DREAM ANALYSIS.

Dressings

Materials used to cover and protect a wound; a dressing is also called a BANDAGE. Dressings vary in type and in the material used to make them. Some dressings are made of antiseptic gauze, for example, while others are made of dry gauze or absorbent cotton. A pressure dressing is one in which pressure is exerted on the area covered to prevent the buildup of fluids in underlying tissues or to stop bleeding; pressure dressings are used for burns and skin grafting. Depending on the location of the wound, dressings are held in place with tape, bandages, or binders.

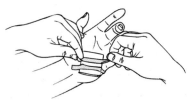

DRESSING A WOUND
For a wound that needs padding but does not require bandaging wrapped around the affected part, adhesive tape can hold the dressing in place. It is always important to thoroughly clean and dry a wound before dressing.

Dressler syndrome

A group of symptoms that often follow a heart attack or open-heart surgery. People who have had a heart attack or open-heart surgery frequently experience sharp, severe chest pain that may vary with breathing or changes in position. The symptoms occur because of pericarditis (inflammation of the membrane surrounding the heart), an increased white blood cell count, fever, pleurisy (inflammation of the membrane surrounding the lungs), and pneumonia. Dressler syndrome is also known as postmyocardial infarction syndrome. Symptoms usually improve with anti-inflammatory drugs.

DRG

Also known as a diagnosis-related group. DRGs are used in a payment system that determines how much MEDICARE or certain provider organi-

zations reimburse a hospital for a person's medical care. Under the DRG system, hospitals are reimbursed at a set rate according to factors such as a person's primary and secondary diagnosis, his or her age, the length of hospitalization, and what procedures are performed. The DRG system was established by amendments to the Social Security Act in 1983, with the goal of encouraging hospitals to manage patient care as efficiently as possible and to cut health care costs.

DRIs

See DIETARY REFERENCE INTAKES.

Dronabinol

A drug that controls nausea and vomiting and stimulates appetite. Dronabinol (Marinol) is used to treat or prevent nausea and vomiting caused by cancer drugs or when other drugs do not work. It is also used to increase the appetites of people with AIDS (acquired immunodeficiency syndrome). Dronabinol is a synthetic form of cannabis (marijuana).

Drooling

The flow of unswallowed saliva from the mouth, normal in children up to about age 1. In babies 3 to 4 months old, more saliva is produced than can be swallowed. Excessive drooling becomes even more common during teething. Most children no longer drool after the age of 4 years. Children who have neurological problems may drool because they have difficulty controlling the muscles and nerves involved in swallowing. Certain adult disorders such as Parkinson disease and facial paralysis can cause drooling. Poor-fitting dentures also can result in drooling.

Speech therapy can help a child learn how to control drooling. Medications are also sometimes helpful. In some cases, drooling is the sign of a more serious underlying problem. A sudden onset of drooling, especially if it is accompanied by difficulty swallowing, may indicate an infection of the tonsils, throat, or windpipe and requires medical care.

Drop attack

A type of SEIZURE that causes a sudden fall. This type of seizure may occur in a severe form of EPILEPSY called

Lennox-Gastaut syndrome. People who experience drop attack have a momentary loss of muscle tone that causes them to collapse to the ground.

Drowning

Suffocation or near-suffocation from submersion in water or other liquid. The immediate cause of drowning is a lack of oxygen. Many events can lead to drowning, including an inability to swim, boating accidents, panicked swimmers or those who have heart attacks while in the water, a blow to the head while in the water, drunkenness, and suicide. Symptoms of near-drowning include swollen abdomen; bluish skin on the lips and ears; cold, pale skin; confusion; cough with pink, frothy sputum; fever; lethargy; failure to breathe; shallow or gasping breathing; unconsciousness; vomiting; and chest pain. Although people who are drowning usually cannot shout for help, there are signs of drowning, such as a fully clothed swimmer, uneven swimming motions of a tired swimmer, and a swimmer whose head shows above the water though his or her body does not.

In a near-drowning emergency, quick action and first aid can prevent death. Whenever possible, a rescue should be attempted by boat or by using a throw rope attached to a life ring or life jacket that can be thrown to the drowning person, who will then be pulled in to shore. Only very strong swimmers who have had training in water rescue should attempt to swim out to retrieve a drowning person. Once rescued, ARTIFICIAL RESPIRATION (or rescue breathing) must be started immediately if the person is not breathing, even if this involves performing this maneuver in the water. It is wise to perform the HEIMLICH MANEUVER first to clear the airways of water. If the person cannot be aroused or is not breathing or moving, CARDIOPULMONARY RESUSCITATION (CPR) should be started. As soon as possible, the person must be checked by a doctor because lung complications are common. Although it is possible to revive a drowning person even if he or she has been in cold water for a long time, 8,000 people die by drowning in the United States each year.

Drowning, dry

A form of DROWNING in which no fluid enters the lungs. The primary cause of death by drowning is a lack of oxygen. In dry drowning, even though water does not enter the lungs, there is a fatal lack of oxygen. This may be due to a person's strong laryngeal reflex, which diverts water from the lungs to the stomach, but impairs breathing nevertheless.

Drowsiness

A decreased level of CONSCIOUSNESS characterized by sleepiness and trouble remaining alert. A simple case of drowsiness can be caused by a lack of sleep. However, drowsiness may be a medically significant symptom. Abnormal drowsiness may also be a sign of a head injury, high fever, HYPOGLYCEMIA (low blood sugar level), HYPERGLYCEMIA (high blood sugar level), MENINGITIS (inflammation of the membranes, or meninges, that surround the brain and spinal cord), or liver failure. Alcohol use or drugs—prescription, nonprescription, or an illegal narcotic—may also produce drowsiness. If a person who is drowsy fails to awaken after being shaken, pinched, or shouted at, the situation is a medical emergency and immediate professional help must be sought.

Drug

In medicine, a drug is a compound used to treat disease, injury, or pain. A drug may also be any substance intended for use as a component of a medication. A drug can cause addiction or a change in consciousness. Alcohol and tobacco are legal drugs that are widely abused.

Drug abuse

The use of illegal drugs or the use of a legal drug in excessive quantities or for purposes other than those for which it is normally intended. Commonly abused illegal drugs include cannabis (marijuana; hashish; THC, or delta-9-tetrahydrocannabinol), narcotics (heroin, morphine, methadone, codeine), cocaine, amphetamines ("speed"), hallucinogens (PCP, or "angel dust"; LSD, or lysergic acid diethylamide; psilocybin; mescaline), and inhalants (model glue, spray paint, gasoline, aerosol propellants). Legal prescription drugs, such as painkillers, tranquilizers, benzodiazepines, chloral hydrate, barbiturates, and preparations containing hydrocodone, can also be abused. Legal over-the-counter medications and products, including laxatives, nasal sprays, cough medicine, alcohol, and tobacco, can be abused as well.

Drug abuse may lead to drug dependence (see DRUG ADDICTION), which involves a compulsive craving for the drug, tolerance for its effects, and unpleasant or even dangerous symptoms if the drug is withdrawn. Depending on the drug, abuse can result in disease—such as hepatitis or AIDS (acquired immunodeficiency syndrome) from sharing contaminated needles—depression and other psychological problems, and fatal overdose. Risk factors predisposing a person to drug abuse include a lack of mental or emotional resources for dealing with stress, a low tolerance for frustration, and tension or distress. Treatment depends on the drug being used and the level of abuse.

Drug addiction

A disorder involving physical and psychological dependence on a drug or drugs and characterized by tolerance (the need to consume larger and larger amounts of the drug to feel its effects), physical symptoms if the drug is withdrawn, or both. Drug addiction poses serious health risks because of its long-term physical effects, disruption of family and work life, and the symptoms of drug withdrawal, which can range from highly unpleasant to fatal. In most cases, the disorder begins as drug abuse—the use of illegal drugs, or the use of a legal drug in excessive quantities or for purposes other than those for which it is intended—and progresses over time into addiction.

SYMPTOMS, AND EFFECTS

The signs of addiction and its physical and psychological effects depend on the particular drug involved. Some addictive drugs are legal substances used inappropriately, such as sedatives; others are illegal. Addiction to alcohol is known as ALCOHOL DEPENDENCE.

■ *Central nervous system depressants* Popularly known as "downers," these drugs include prescription medications such as SEDATIVES, BARBITURATES (such as phenobarbital or secobarbital), HYPNOTIC DRUGS (often used as sleeping aids), and antianxiety agents (such as the benzodiazepines, which include diazepam [Valium], chlordiazepoxide hydrochloride [Librium], and alprazolam [Xanax]). INHALANTS, such as model glue and aerosol propellants, also depress the central nervous system. The effects of these drugs are similar to those of alcohol intoxication: coma or drowsiness, slurred speech, lack of coordination, impaired memory, confusion, tremor or poor muscle tone, agitation, paranoia (extreme suspicion or feelings of being persecuted or pursued), and inappropriate emotions. All of these drugs pose the risk of death from overdose.

■ *Central nervous system stimulants* Stimulants accelerate body functions, producing agitation, rapid speech, irritability, difficulty concentrating, and often a pattern of heavy use for several days (called a "run") followed by a physical and emotional letdown (a "crash"). The most commonly used

---

MANAGING MEDICATIONS

Always follow a doctor's or a pharmacist's instructions for proper drug use. Taking the correct dosage at the proper time each day is important. Make sure the doctor is aware of other medications being taken. Also, remember to:

- Take all of the prescribed medication.
- Never take a prescription that was prescribed for another person.
- Keep lids and caps closed tightly to prevent children from accidental poisoning.
- Do not consume alcohol with medications; the mix can be dangerous.
- Keep drugs stored in a high, cool, and dry place. Bathroom medicine cabinets are subject to warm, moist conditions, which can reduce a drug's effectiveness.
- Throw away all damaged pills or capsules.
- Discard all medications past the expiration date, as well as any that are more than 1 year old.

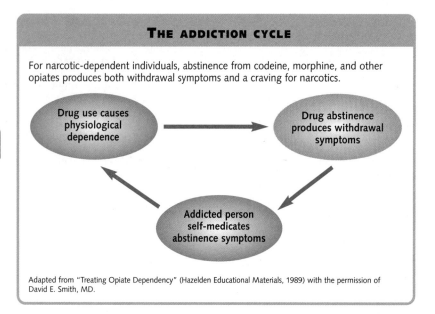

THE ADDICTION CYCLE

For narcotic-dependent individuals, abstinence from codeine, morphine, and other opiates produces both withdrawal symptoms and a craving for narcotics.

Drug use causes physiological dependence → Drug abstinence produces withdrawal symptoms → Addicted person self-medicates abstinence symptoms →

Adapted from "Treating Opiate Dependency" (Hazelden Educational Materials, 1989) with the permission of David E. Smith, MD.

addictive central nervous system stimulants are amphetamines ("speed") and cocaine ("coke").

Amphetamines, which can cause a euphoric state lasting for several hours, produce a very strong psychological dependence. Tolerance develops rapidly with repeated use, but the compulsion to use the drug remains. Since amphetamines produce less physical dependence than many other addictive substances, withdrawal causes fewer, milder symptoms.

Cocaine, which can be inhaled or injected as a powder or smoked in the form known as crack, releases hormones that raise body temperature, heart rate, and blood pressure, producing a euphoria in which the person feels powerful, in control of his or her surroundings, and sexually energized. Although often regarded as a safe recreational chemical, cocaine is highly addictive and dangerous, carrying a risk of death from seizures, respiratory failure, stroke, cerebral hemorrhage (bleeding in the brain), or heart failure even with a modest dose. Addiction disrupts sleeping and eating patterns and is psychologically disturbing, causing irritability and diminishing the ability to concentrate.

■ *Narcotics* Narcotics include drugs produced from the opium plant (the opiates, such as morphine and heroin) and synthetic compounds (opioids) such as codeine and methadone that mimic the effects of the opiates. Certain narcotics are used medically for pain control, anesthesia, and cough suppression. People who abuse narcotics are most likely to use heroin, which is an illegal drug usually injected into a vein but may be smoked or snorted. Narcotics cause central nervous system depression, often with agitation; anxiety; impulsiveness; fear of failure; low self-esteem, hopelessness, and aggression; reduced tolerance to frustration; inability to cope; and a need for immediate gratification. Narcotic users tend to associate with other people who abuse drugs. Inadequate sterilization of needles used to inject heroin can cause local or systemic infections, including tuberculosis, hepatitis, and HIV (human immunodeficiency virus) infection. Narcotics produce physical and psychological dependence. See WITHDRAWAL SYNDROME, OPIATES.

■ *Cannabis compounds* The leaves and flowers of the marijuana plant (*Cannabis sativa*) are smoked in cigarettes and pipes, or they are cooked into brownies or other foods. Concentrated marijuana resin is made into hashish, which is usually smoked. The active agent in marijuana, delta-9-tetrahydrocannabinol or THC, is used for certain medical purposes and sometimes sold illegally. Smoking marijuana (called a "joint") or hashish causes faster absorption than ingestion of the drug. Cannabis produces euphoria and relaxation, similar to moderate intoxication with alcohol. Thinking, perception, judgment, and coordination are all impaired. There can be severe psychological effects, including paranoia (feelings of suspicion or persecution) and delirium (extreme agitation and confusion), in individuals who are mentally or emotionally unstable. People who are addicted to cannabis lose interest in everyday events and have little or no ambition to achieve even simple goals, such as holding a job. They can suffer from increased heart rate, conjunctivitis (eyes reddened by inflammation), and decreased lung function from smoking. Withdrawal symptoms include sweating, tremors, nausea, vomiting, diarrhea, irritability, and difficulty sleeping (insomnia).

TREATMENT

Drug addiction can be treated with a variety of medical, behavioral, and supportive therapies. The goals of treatment are to keep the person off the drug, to improve his or her ability to function, and to address the medical and social complications of drug addiction. Most programs begin with detoxification, a 4- to 7-day medical process, usually in a hospital setting, in which a person addicted to drugs is withdrawn from the addictive substance under the care of a doctor. The goal of detoxification is to manage the symptoms of withdrawal and prevent serious medical problems. Following detoxification, the person can enter a treatment program. The type of treatment depends on the individual, the drug or drugs involved, and available resources. Short-term treatment programs last fewer than 6 months and include residential therapy (in which the individual lives in a special facility to receive treatment), medication therapy, and outpatient therapy. Outpatient therapy consists primarily of individual or group counseling.

Longer-term treatment programs last more than 6 months. The most common are methadone-maintenance treatments that involve giving a supportive dose of methadone to people addicted to heroin; the methadone blocks heroin's effects but produces no euphoria. Therapeutic communi-

DRUGS OF ABUSE

Addiction to drugs involves physical, psychological, and emotional dependence. Some people become addicted to so-called recreational drugs, the use of which may be legal or illegal. The great danger of drug addiction lies in the compulsion to continue taking the substance, regardless of the health or social consequences. A woman who abuses drugs during pregnancy not only hurts herself, but may seriously damage the fetus.

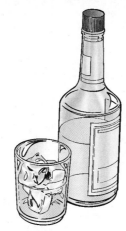

ALCOHOL
Because alcohol is widely available and socially acceptable, addiction may be difficult to identify. Genetic factors may have a large role in addiction to alcohol.

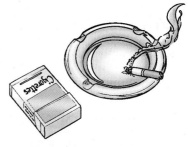

TOBACCO
Tobacco is the most widely abused legal drug in the United States. It is extremely addictive and damaging to a person's health.

SIGNS OF DRUG ABUSE OR ADDICTION IN ADOLESCENTS

Apart from actually seeing a teenager use drugs or come home "high," drug abuse or addiction may be hard to recognize. A number of changes may signal trouble, such as:

- A sudden dislike of school, excuses to stay home, an unprecedented drop in grades, or dropping a school sport without explanation.
- Declining health, particularly listlessness, apathy, or a severe lack of stamina.
- A change in appearance, particularly a lack of interest in clothing and current fashion.
- Unusual demands for privacy. An adolescent may refuse to say what he or she is doing away from home or may have long unexplained stays in the bedroom or bathroom.
- Peculiar behavior. The teen may demand money, be irritable, or have unexplained displays of anger.

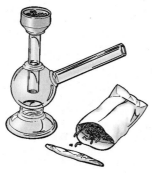

MARIJUANA
Smoking marijuana damages the lungs in a similar way to tobacco. Heavy use of marijuana tends to lead to loss of energy and drive.

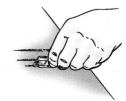

COCAINE
Cocaine and its derivative, crack, are potent drugs that act as stimulants and wear off quickly—leading to more use. Long-term use can cause anxiety and aggression.

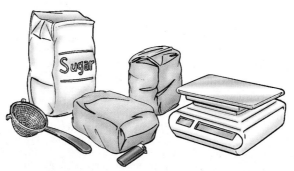

HEROIN
Heroin use can cause profound medical conditions such as coma, respiratory failure, and shock. Use of contaminated needles can spread infectious diseases such as AIDS (acquired immunodeficiency syndrome) and hepatitis.

ties offer highly structured, residential treatment programs over a 6- to 12-month period. These programs are particularly useful for people with long-term addictions.

Drug approval process

In the United States, a rigorous systematic procedure by which the Food and Drug Administration (FDA) determines whether a drug is safe and effective. The US system of approval is considered the most stringent in the world. Only five in 5,000 compounds get to the point of being tested in humans, and only one of those five is approved. On average, it takes 12 years for an experimental drug to reach US consumers.

The process of drug testing has many steps. The first step is preclinical testing in the laboratory to determine whether the compound has an effect on the targeted disease. After that, an Investigational New Drug Application is filed with the FDA to request permission to test in humans. Clinical trials, phases 1 through 3, test the new drug in humans to determine whether it is effective and safe for use. (See CLINICAL TRIAL.) Then a New Drug Application is filed with the FDA, with all the scientific information that has been obtained about the drug. Finally, the drug becomes approved by the FDA, which can require additional clinical trials (phase 4) to evaluate the long-term effects of the drug.

Drug dependence

See DRUG ADDICTION.

Drug eruption

A skin reaction that is caused by taking a medication. Drug eruptions are caused by a sensitivity or allergy (see ALLERGIES) to some medications. Symptoms range from a mild rash to life-threatening ANAPHYLAXIS. Penicillin and related drugs are the most common causes of allergic reactions. Other drugs that can cause reactions include sulfa drugs and antiseizure drugs. Many medications also cause PHOTOSENSITIVITY (heightened sensitivity to the sun).

It is sometimes difficult to distinguish a drug eruption from other skin problems. To make a diagnosis, the doctor will ask about any history of allergies and any recently introduced medications. It is essential to identify and avoid all medications that cause reactions. If a person has allergic tendencies, the introduction of a new medication must be closely monitored. Treatments to control rashes include corticosteroids and antihistamines.

COMMON DRUG RASHES

The red, itchy, round swellings of HIVES are a common drug reaction. Hives develop when natural chemicals including histamine are released in response to an allergic reaction. Any new medication that causes hives should be discontinued at once, and a doctor should be contacted. Hives are treated with over-the-counter antihistamines and sometimes stronger prescription medications. Hives with breathing problems or swelling in the throat are an emergency that requires immediate medical care.

SEVERE DRUG REACTIONS

The rash, called erythema multiforme, is a type of severe drug reaction. A central lesion is surrounded by rings of paleness and redness in a bull's-eye pattern. Rashes typically appear on the legs, arms, palms, hands, or feet. Lesions sometimes contain blisters and may itch. Erythema multiforme minor (a milder form of the disease) most commonly occurs in children and young adults. Approximately nine of ten cases are associated with herpes simplex or mycoplasma (a bacterium) infections.

In erythema multiforme major (the more severe form of erythema multiforme; also called Stevens-Johnson syndrome), extensive rashes of various sizes and shapes appear on the skin. Erythema multiforme major also involves the mucous membranes. There may be symptoms such as fever, joint aches, and a general feeling of illness, as well as involvement of the mucous membranes with mouth sores, eye burning, itching, and discharge. Medications that may cause erythema multiforme major include phenytoin and sulfonamides.

Treatment includes stopping the offending medication, relief of symptoms, and prevention of infection. Mild cases typically resolve within 2 to 6 weeks, although they may recur. Very severe cases of erythema multiforme major may evolve into toxic epidermal necrolysis (see NECROLYSIS, TOXIC EPIDERMAL). In toxic epidermal necrolysis, large blisters blend together, resulting in shedding of the skin and mucous membranes. Toxic epidermal necrolysis requires hospitalization in an intensive care or burn unit. Treatment of toxic epidermal necrolysis includes relief of symptoms, immunosuppressive medications to manage inflammation, antibiotics to control secondary infections, and skin grafts. Systemic infection and shock due to loss of body fluids may result in death.

Drug sensitivity

An individual's response to a drug, or an antibiotic's effectiveness against a microorganism. In cancer treatment, drug sensitivity can be tested in people to determine which of the available compounds is likely to be effective in a particular person. The tests are performed on live tumor cells.

An antibiotic agent can be tested for sensitivity by combining it with colonies of microorganisms to see whether the agent inhibits their growth. Such a test determines the appropriate drug therapy for an infection. The test can also identify the drug resistance of an organism.

Drug testing

See DRUG APPROVAL PROCESS.

Drug treatment programs

A process involving medical, psychological, behavioral, therapeutic, and other interventions designed to help a person abstain from alcohol or drugs and function normally in society. A variety of treatment programs are available. The choice among them depends on the individual, his or her history and emotional state, the drug or drugs used, and available resources.

COMPONENTS

Most treatment programs begin with an evaluation process. The key issue is determining whether a person is abusing drugs or alcohol—that is, using too much too often and engaging in dangerous behavior, or using illegal substances, such as cocaine or amphetamines—or is dependent on one or more substances, which is indicated by tolerance, withdrawal symptoms if the substance is stopped, or both.

In the case of dependence, evalua-

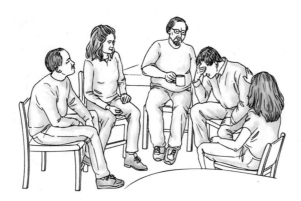

SUPPORT AND THERAPY After withdrawal from drugs, group therapy provides recovering addicts the opportunity to think through the underlying causes of their problems and to gain confidence and support from other people who are going through the same difficult process.

tion also involves determining the person's willingness to admit that he or she is dependent. Without acceptance of the dependence as a disease, recovery is unlikely. Depending on the substance or substances the person is using, he or she is evaluated for medical problems associated with the abuse or dependence, such as high blood pressure or liver damage.

If an individual is dependent, the next step is detoxification. This involves withdrawal from the substance in a supervised medical setting over a 4- to 7-day period. Often the person is treated with tranquilizers and sedatives to ease the physical symptoms of withdrawal, some of which, such as DELIRIUM TREMENS in alcohol withdrawal, can be dangerous and even fatal. Detoxification is not drug treatment, however, and by itself is unlikely to change long-term drug or alcohol use.

Following detoxification, the person enters a residential or day-treatment program that offers a variety of services and therapies designed to teach him or her how to live without alcohol or drugs, deal with the emotional issues underlying drug and alcohol use, and adopt a drug-free lifestyle. Services include medical assistance, counseling, vocational, educational, financial, child care, and housing combined in various ways to meet an individual's needs.

TYPES OF PROGRAMS

Outpatient or day-treatment centers allow the person to live at home and continue with work or school while undergoing a structured program of individual, group, and family therapy. The length of the program and the amount of time required per day vary from program to program.

Residential programs offer an intensive, live-in approach based on a modified 12-step approach (see TWELVE-STEP PROGRAM). The inpatient portion of the program, which takes place in a professionally staffed, secure facility, is followed by an outpatient phase involving therapy and participation in a self-help group such as ALCOHOLICS ANONYMOUS (AA), Narcotics Anonymous, or Cocaine Anonymous. Short-term residential programs last from 3 to 6 weeks, and long-term, up to 1 year.

Therapeutic communities (TCs) are full-time, residential, drug-free programs that use peer support, counseling, and work to help people learn how to live without substances. In many cases, people recovering from addiction serve as counselors. TCs usually require a commitment of 6 months to 1 year, and they are most useful for people who have been dependent over a long period and involved in crime because of their drug use.

Halfway houses are similar in that they rely on peer-group counseling within a residential setting while residents make the transition to individual living in the community, often following a residential treatment program. Residents usually stay in halfway houses for fewer than 90 days.

Medication maintenance programs serve people addicted to narcotics, such as heroin. One type of program, called agonist maintenance treatment, uses long-acting synthetic opiates, particularly methadone, which is administered orally at a dosage that prevents withdrawal symptoms, blocks the effects of illegal narcotic use, and decreases craving for the drug. People considered "stabilized" with methadone can function normally, take part in counseling, and avoid crime and violence. Another type of program, called antagonist treatment, uses naltrexone, an oral medication that blocks the effects of narcotics, particularly the euphoria they cause. As with methadone, people participating in antagonist treatment programs can function normally if they take part in counseling and avoid crime and violence.

EFFECTIVENESS

A number of factors influence the effectiveness of treatment programs. One is length of treatment. In most cases, 3 months is the necessary minimum. Medical treatment or maintenance alone, for example with methadone, is less effective than the same treatment combined with therapy and counseling, which help people build their skills for resisting the use of drugs, understand their own motivations toward drugs, and increase interpersonal skills. More than one round of treatment may be required. Treated individuals can have a relapse and return to treatment repeatedly before they are able to remain drug- or alcohol-free over the long term.

Drug trial

See CLINICAL TRIAL.

Drunk driving

Using a car or other motor vehicle while impaired by alcohol and not capable of handling the vehicle safely. Most states also apply drunk driving laws to operation of a motor vehicle under the influence of illegal or abused drugs, such as marijuana, narcotics, or tranquilizers, used alone or in combination with alcohol. In the United States, a driver with a blood alcohol concentration (BAC) of 0.08 percent or more is considered to have committed a drunk driving offense. At a BAC of more than 0.02 percent, critical driving skills are impaired and the driver poses a risk to his or her self and others. Drivers with high BAC are at increased risk for causing accidents, injuries, and death.

Approximately one in every five driving deaths involves a drunk driver. In most of these deaths, the alcohol level is considerably higher than the legal limit. The average BAC of fatally injured drivers is 0.17 percent, and almost half of fatally injured

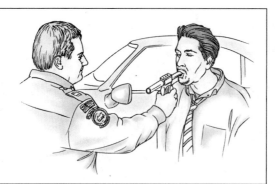

TESTING FOR BLOOD ALCOHOL LEVEL
The Breathalyzer is a roadside test to identify drunken drivers. By measuring the alcohol content in a person's breath, a law enforcement official can get an indication of the blood alcohol level. Even a small amount of alcohol can impair judgment, so it is best to avoid driving after drinking alcohol.

drunk drivers have a BAC of 0.20 or more. The legal consequences of drunk driving can be serious, particularly for repeated offenses: suspension or revocation of the driver's license for months or years, substantial fines and court costs, and jail time. Repeated drunk driving offenses are often a sign of ALCOHOL DEPENDENCE because they indicate the person's inability to stop or limit drinking despite adverse consequences. See ALCOHOL INTOXICATION.

Dry eye

Persistent failure of the tear glands to produce moisture of sufficient quantity or quality to wet and lubricate the eye normally. The principal symptoms of dry eye are a scratchy or sandy feeling in the eyes, stinging or burning, periods of excess tearing following sensations of dryness, a stringy discharge from the eye, and pain and redness. Contact lens wearers with dry eye usually find it more difficult to tolerate their lenses. The eyelids may seem heavy, and vision can become blurred, doubled, or decreased and highly sensitive to light. In extreme cases, dry eye can lead to ulcers of the cornea (the clear outer covering of the eye), which may result in perforation of the eyeball and loss of vision. Dry eye is more common in women (particularly after menopause) than men.

Dry eye can result from exposure to extremely dry climates. It may also be caused by certain medications, such as antihistamines (used for allergies), nasal decongestants, antidepressants, birth control pills, and tranquilizers. Dry eye becomes more common with age and to some degree is estimated to affect three of four people older than 65 years. Particularly when

accompanied by dry mouth, dry eye may be a symptom of systemic disease, such as RHEUMATOID ARTHRITIS, systemic lupus erythematosus, and SJÖGREN SYNDROME, all of which affect the body's lubricating glands.

Primary treatment consists of artificial tears, which usually contain methylcellulose and are available over-the-counter as eye drops. Sterile ointments may be used at night to prevent drying during sleep. Humidifiers, wraparound glasses for outdoor wear, and avoiding windy, dry conditions also help. In severe cases, the tear duct that carries tears away from the eye can be blocked with tiny plastic plugs to keep moisture in the eye.

Dry mouth

A symptom of certain diseases or a side effect of some medications usually caused by the failure of the salivary glands to function properly. The medical term is xerostomia. The purpose of the salivary glands is to secrete saliva and carry it through ducts into the mouth where it helps to keep delicate tissues and teeth moist and aids in chewing, swallowing, and digestion. While dry mouth is a symptom rather than a disease, it can present significant health problems. It may contribute to poor nutrition, tooth decay, and other infections of the mouth. It can also affect psychological well-being. In some cases, dry mouth is a perceived condition not related to problems with the function of the salivary glands. People who experience dry mouth should seek attention from a physician, a dentist, or both.

CAUSES

Dry mouth may be due to any number of medications, diseases, treatments,

or other causes. More than 400 different medications may cause dry mouth, including medication for high blood pressure, antidepressants, painkillers, tranquilizers, diuretics, and over-the-counter antihistamines. Cancer treatments may also play a part. RADIATION THERAPY can permanently damage salivary glands if radiation is applied in the area of these glands. Chemotherapy may alter saliva's composition, thus causing a person to experience dry mouth. Bone marrow transplants can also cause dry mouth. The symptoms of SJÖGREN SYNDROME, an autoimmune disorder, may include dry mouth. Nutritional deficiencies may be wholly or partially responsible for the sensation of dry mouth. Psychological symptoms and conditions, such as anxiety, mental stress, and depression, may be involved. Damage to the nerves that supply sensation to the mouth, usually caused by surgery in the head and neck area, can prevent them from signaling the salivary glands to secrete saliva, which results in dry mouth. The absence of normal sensation in the mouth, caused by stroke or Alzheimer's disease, can create a perception of dry mouth. Dry mouth is not considered a normal condition of aging. Older people who have dry mouth are usually experiencing symptoms of disease or side effects from medication.

TREATMENT

In addition to recommendations from a doctor or dentist who is treating a person for dry mouth, some self-help treatments may help relieve associated discomforts, protect the soft tissues in the mouth and throat, and prevent related health risks. Sipping water or sugarless beverages; pausing often during conversation to sip liquids; and avoiding dehydrating beverages such as coffee, tea, all alcoholic drinks, and caffeinated soft drinks may help. Smoking cigarettes or cigars and use of all other tobacco products should be avoided. Foods that may irritate the mouth—including spicy, salty, and very acidic dishes or beverages—should also be avoided. Keeping water at the bedside to sip during the night or first thing in the morning may prove helpful, and using a humidifier in the bedroom often helps. Drinking fluids frequently while eating can facilitate chewing and swallowing and enhance the flavors of foods. Because chewing helps stimulate saliva production, using sugarless gum can relieve dryness. Dissolving sugarless hard candies in the mouth, especially those with strong flavors such as cinnamon and mint, can help increase saliva flow.

To help maintain dental health, a person with dry mouth should brush his or her teeth at least twice a day and use dental floss and a fluoride-containing toothpaste daily. Avoiding foods that are sticky and sugary may help. People with dry mouth need to visit their dentist a minimum of three times a year for examinations, cleanings, and cavity treatment. The dentist may offer topical fluorides and remineralizing solutions to help keep teeth healthy or prescribe artificial salivas, which help lubricate the mouth.

DSA

See DIGITAL SUBTRACTION ANGIOGRAPHY.

DSM-IV

Abbreviation for *Diagnostic and Statistical Manual of Mental Disorders, Fourth Edition.* The DSM-IV is the standard classification of psychiatric disorders used by psychiatrists, psychologists, and other mental health professionals.

DTaP vaccination

A vaccine typically given at regular intervals during infancy and childhood that offers immunization against diphtheria, tetanus, and pertussis, which is also called whooping cough. Formerly called the DPT vaccine, a newer version called the DTaP was introduced in 1997 and is less likely to cause serious side effects such as fever, vomiting, and mild seizures. The "a" in the name DTaP stands for acellular, indicating that there are no whole bacteria in this vaccine, which contains only the parts of bacteria that can help children develop immunity. The older DPT contained the whole, inactivated pertussis bacteria, which may have been responsible for adverse side effects.

An infant is generally given an initial DTaP vaccination at the age of 2 months. The injections are repeated at the ages of 4 months and 6 months, in the period between 12 and 18 months, and again when the child is 4 years old. A booster vaccination is given at age 14 and every 10 years thereafter into adulthood.

Children who are moderately to severely ill should not be given the DTaP vaccine until they recover. The pediatrician should be advised about children who have had seizures or whose families have a history of seizures before the vaccine is given. A child who has previously had a severe reaction to DPT or DTaP vaccines should not be given the DTaP vaccine. It should not be given to children who have had swelling of the brain (a possible symptom of ENCEPHALOPATHY) within 7 days of any vaccination when it is known that the condition was not associated with another cause.

Potential adverse reactions have been primarily associated with the pertussis part of the vaccine, and the DTaP vaccination is much less likely to cause any side effects. There may be pain, swelling, and redness at the site of the injection, as well as a low-grade fever, drowsiness, vomiting, and fussiness in infants. The newer DTaP vaccine has dramatically reduced the rate of high fever and virtually eliminated the rate of seizures formerly associated with the DPT vaccine.

Dual diagnosis

The occurrence of both mental illness and alcohol or drug dependence in the same person. Some authorities estimate that as many as one of every two people with serious mental health problems is also dependent on drugs or alcohol and qualifies as having dual diagnosis. Alcohol is the most commonly used drug, followed by marijuana, cocaine, and prescription medications such as tranquilizers and sleeping aids. Dual diagnosis increases the risk of violence, particularly within the family, and of suicide.

The underlying cause of dual diagnosis is unclear. It may be that people with mental illness use alcohol and drugs in an attempt to alleviate their symptoms, or they may be genetically predisposed to both mental illness and drug dependence. Another theory is that because many people with mental illness have trouble supporting themselves, they live in marginal neighborhoods where drug use is common and, as a result, are exposed to that lifestyle. Dual diagnosis complicates treatment since it can be difficult to determine which symptoms are caused by mental illness and which by alcohol or drug dependence.

Dual-energy X-ray absorptiometry

The most complete and accurate imaging technique for measuring bone density. Dual-energy X-ray absorptiometry (DEXA) produces a measurement of bone density that can detect minute degrees (as little as 1 percent) of bone loss. DEXA is a painless procedure that uses very small amounts of radiation. The person undergoing the procedure, which takes from 3 to 15 minutes, lies on a table while a machine scans a hip or the spine.

DEXA is commonly used to confirm a case of OSTEOPOROSIS that is mild or asymptomatic or that has occurred after a bone fracture. Treating osteoporosis as soon as possible can prevent progressive bone deterioration. DEXA also offers physicians a baseline for treatment and is used during ongoing medical care to assess the response to treatment for osteoporosis. See Close-up on DEXA, page 484. See also BONE DENSITY TESTING.

Duct

In anatomy, a tube or other walled passage in an organ of the body. A duct is typically a narrow tubular passage through which fluid passes, such as those found in the gallbladder or glands.

Dumping syndrome

A condition in which sweating, faintness, and heart palpitations are caused by the rapid passage of food from the stomach to the upper intestine. Dumping syndrome affects primarily people who have had stomach operations.

Duodenal ulcer

A sore or wound in the mucous membrane lining the wall of the duodenum, the first part of the small intestine into which the stomach empties. Nine of ten duodenal ulcers develop on the duodenal bulb, the first part of the duodenum. Although variable in size, they are usually less than one-half inch wide. Men are more likely than women to develop duodenal ulcers.

SYMPTOMS AND CAUSES
Upper abdominal pain is the most

CLOSE-UP ON DEXA

This highly sensitive diagnostic technique measures changes in bone density and can detect small changes as early as 6 to 12 months following a previous measurement. Two X-ray beams are produced by the dual-energy X-ray absorptiometry (DEXA) scanner, one with a high level of energy and the other with a low level of energy. The amount of X-ray energy passing through bone varies with bone thickness. Bone density is determined by the amount of X-ray energy that is not absorbed as the two beams pass through a person's bones.

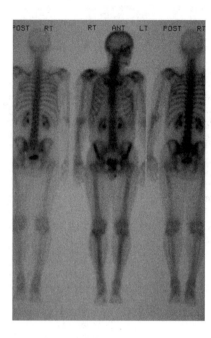

A TYPICAL RADIOGRAPH PRODUCED BY DEXA
In this full-body DEXA scan, the darker skeletal shadings indicate areas of greater bone density, while the lighter shadings indicate areas of reduced bone density.

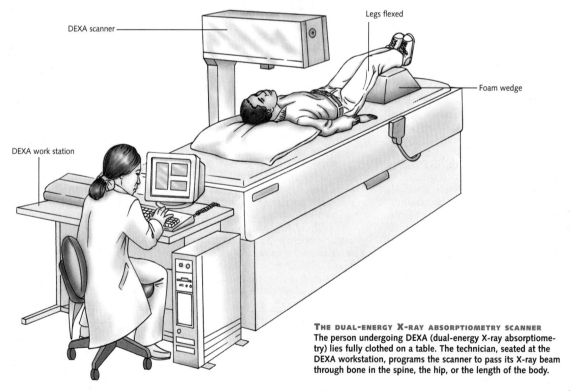

DEXA scanner

Legs flexed

Foam wedge

DEXA work station

THE DUAL-ENERGY X-RAY ABSORPTIOMETRY SCANNER
The person undergoing DEXA (dual-energy X-ray absorptiometry) lies fully clothed on a table. The technician, seated at the DEXA workstation, programs the scanner to pass its X-ray beam through bone in the spine, the hip, or the length of the body.

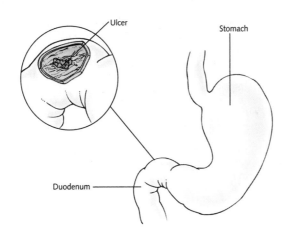

ULCER IN THE UPPER INTESTINE
The duodenum, which is the portion of the small intestine into which the stomach empties, is a common site of peptic (digestive tract) ulcers. The inner lining of the duodenum develops an ulcer (open sore) as the result of the corrosive action of stomach acids. Duodenal ulcers are probably caused by an infection with *Helicobacter pylori* (H. pylori) bacteria.

Ulcer

Stomach

Duodenum

common symptom of a duodenal ulcer. In some cases, a burning, gnawing pain is felt primarily in the back, between the shoulder blades. Pain typically occurs 2 to 3 hours after meals or in the early morning hours. Other symptoms may include nausea, vomiting, loss of appetite, and weight loss. However, these are generally more characteristic of gastric rather than duodenal ulcers.

Evidence strongly suggests that infection with the bacterium *Helicobacter pylori* (H. PYLORI) is responsible for the majority of ulcers. Other factors that may play a role are the long-term use of nonsteroidal anti-inflammatory drugs (NSAIDs), such as aspirin and ibuprofen, heavy use of alcohol, and smoking. Like *H. pylori*, any of these factors can damage the protective mucous lining of the duodenum, leaving it vulnerable to attack by acids and digestive enzymes secreted by stomach glands. A family history of peptic ulcer disease and experiencing stress may contribute to ulcer development.

DIAGNOSIS

Diagnosis is usually made after taking a medical history of symptoms and conducting a variety of tests. Because ulcer pain and nausea tend to follow a pattern, the doctor will want to know when symptoms occur and how they are relieved. Pain and nausea are typically eased by food, milk, antacids, or vomiting.

A duodenal ulcer may be diagnosed by tests, such as blood tests, breath tests, an upper GASTROINTESTINAL (GI) SERIES (an X-ray procedure also called a barium swallow), or GASTROSCOPY. Blood tests can detect the presence of

antibodies to *H. pylori*, while a urea breath test detects the presence of the actual bacteria. In a gastroscopy, the doctor uses a slim, flexible, lighted tube called a gastroscope to view, photograph, videotape, and possibly take a sample of tissue from the esophagus, stomach, and duodenum.

TREATMENT

Medications play a vital role in the treatment of duodenal ulcers. Over-the-counter or prescription antacids may provide temporary relief. However, because prolonged use of antacids can disrupt body chemistry, many doctors prefer to prescribe drugs that reduce acid secretion. These include histamine blockers, anticholinergic agents, and PROTON PUMP INHIBITORS. Some histamine blockers are available over-the-counter. There are also drugs that coat the lining of the duodenum and stomach with a protective layer that prevents acid from reaching the ulcer. No single medication has proven effective against *H. pylori*. However, a medical regimen called triple therapy (the use of three medications at once) can eradicate most cases of the bacteria; two medications are antibiotics and the third is usually a proton pump inhibitor. Lifestyle modifications, such as avoiding alcohol and smoking, are helpful. Because smoking decreases resistance to ulceration, smokers should quit. Eating a number of small meals a day rather than two or three large ones may sometimes be beneficial.

Possible complications of duodenal ulcers include bleeding, scarring, and PYLORIC STENOSIS. Pyloric stenosis is a condition in which the outlet from the stomach to the duodenum (the

pylorus) becomes partly or completely blocked. There is also a small risk that ulcers will penetrate or perforate the duodenal wall. Perforation is more common with duodenal than with gastric ulcers. However, duodenal ulcers are less apt than gastric ones to lead to cancer.

When a duodenal ulcer fails to respond to treatment or if complications develop, surgery may become necessary. The most frequently performed surgery for this type of ulcer is vagotomy, in which the vagus nerve is cut to reduce acid production. During the same procedure, the stomach outlet is often surgically widened (see VAGOTOMY). Less commonly, a surgeon performs a GASTRO-JEJUNOSTOMY to create a connection between the stomach and small intestine that bypasses the duodenum. In some cases, a GASTRECTOMY (surgical removal of part or all of the stomach) is required.

Duodenitis

Inflammation of the duodenum (the first part of the small intestine into which the stomach empties). Duodenitis frequently occurs in people who have duodenal ulcers. In some cases, duodenitis has no symptoms. Sometimes, there may be discomfort in the uppermost part of the abdomen, indigestion, nausea, or vomiting.

Duodenitis sometimes is accompanied by GASTRITIS (inflammation of the stomach lining). Infection with *Helicobacter pylori* (H. PYLORI), a bacterium, may play a role in duodenitis. Less commonly, inflammation of the duodenum is associated with Crohn disease, giardiasis, kidney failure, liver disease, pancreatic disease, or tuberculosis.

Duodenitis may be diagnosed by tests, such as blood tests, an upper GASTROINTESTINAL (GI) SERIES (an X-ray procedure also called a barium swallow), or gastroscopy, in which a slim, flexible, lighted tube called a gastroscope is used to view, photograph, videotape, and possibly take samples of tissue from the esophagus, stomach, and duodenum.

As with duodenal ulcers, antacids may offer relief of duodenitis. Although no single medication has been proved to be effective against *H. pylori*, a medical regimen called

D

triple therapy (the use of three medications at once) can eradicate most cases. Two medications are antibiotics and the third is usually one of the PROTON PUMP INHIBITORS. When an underlying problem is the cause, it must be treated appropriately.

Duodenum

The first part of the small INTESTINE; the duodenum extends below the stomach, curving around the pancreas before it empties into the jejunum (the second part of the small intestine). The duodenum receives secretions from the liver, gallbladder, and pancreas that aid in digesting the nutrients in food and preparing them for absorption into the bloodstream. See DIGESTIVE SYSTEM.

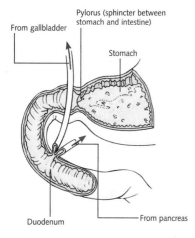

Pylorus (sphincter between stomach and intestine)

From gallbladder

Stomach

Duodenum

From pancreas

FIRST PART OF THE SMALL INTESTINE
Partially digested food from the stomach empties into the duodenum, the first of the three parts of the small intestine (followed by the jejunum and the ileum). The pancreas, gallbladder, and liver secrete digestive juices into the duodenum, beginning the process of nutrient absorption that occurs in the small intestine.

Dupuytren contracture

A disease that produces a rigid deformity of the hand, most commonly involving the inward bending of the ring finger and little finger, but sometimes progressing to involve all the fingers. Dupuytren contracture may involve one or both hands. The disease produces thickening and shortening of the tissues under the skin on the palm of the hand to the extent that the fingers' connecting tendons become increasingly immobile. As a result, the fingers bend toward the palm and cannot be straightened. Dupuytren contracture is painless and may progress slowly. The cause is unknown but the disease may be associated with alcoholism, liver disease, epilepsy, or diabetes mellitus. Dupuytren contracture generally occurs between the ages of 40 and 60 and is not associated with any work or occupational activities. The disease is more common and more severe in men and tends to affect those of Northern European origin more frequently. Treatment may include a surgical procedure.

Durable power of attorney

A legal document signed by a mentally competent adult, delegating decision-making responsibilities for his or her health care or property to another person or agent. It includes a statement specifying that the agent can continue to make decisions when the individual becomes incapacitated (see ADVANCE DIRECTIVES).

Dust diseases

Lung diseases caused by exposure to dust. Dust diseases are not caused by common kinds of household or outdoor dust, which consists of particles too large to settle in the lungs. The industrial and mining dusts that result in this group of diseases are made up of particles small enough to be inhaled into the lungs and become embedded in lung tissue. These dusts may have varying effects on the body that range from minor to severe injury and in some cases can cause death.

Some workers in manufacturing facilities or mines may be more affected than others by the associated dust in the workplace because of a variety of factors, including the general health status of the worker, his or her proximity to the source of dust, malfunctions of protective face masks, length of work hours, and length of time employed in the dust-producing environment. A worker may also be more susceptible if he or she performs more strenuous tasks and subsequently has a deeper and faster rate of breathing. When a person breathes through the nose, tiny hairs in the nostrils can filter out dust, whereas breathing deeply through the mouth is more likely to allow dust to get into the lungs.

CAUSES
Dust diseases are named for the type of dust that causes them. The most common of these is SILICOSIS, which is caused by the silica or quartz dust found in many kinds of mines, including coal and gold mines. Silicosis also results from working in foundries or doing work that involves sandblasting or making pottery. Silicosis may eventually damage and scar lung tissue. It may also lead to the development of emphysema and tuberculosis. Anthracosilicosis is another disease caused by breathing coal dust or silica.

ASBESTOSIS is caused by inflammation from inhaling asbestos fibers into the lungs. Berylliosis occurs when beryllium dust is inhaled. BAGASSOSIS results from breathing the dust given off by treated sugar cane. Breathing dust from moldy hay can produce a condition called FARMER'S LUNG. Iron oxide dust may cause siderosis, breathing dust from tin oxide can produce stannosis, and inhaling the dust from cotton processing may result in BYSSINOSIS.

SYMPTOMS AND TREATMENT
The course of a dust disease may be unpredictable. Some who are exposed to a disease-causing dust may not experience any effects, while others may become seriously ill from similar exposure. There may be no symptoms in the early stages of a dust disease, or symptoms may appear soon after onset. The first sign tends to be shortness of breath (see BREATH, SHORTNESS OF), which may occur years after the inception of the disease process. An affected person may then develop a cough. If the disease becomes severe, the lung damage it causes may prevent sufficient oxygen from getting into the bloodstream, causing blue discoloration of the lips and earlobes.

Dust diseases often weaken resistance to other diseases and make the affected person more susceptible to tuberculosis, lung cancer, pneumonia, chronic bronchitis, and emphysema.

The most effective treatment for dust disease is preventing further dust exposure. A doctor can determine what is required to eliminate or reduce an affected person's exposure to the dust responsible for the illness. In some cases, it may be essential for a person to seek alternative employment; in other cases, wearing a protective face mask while working may be sufficient.

Prevention of dust diseases can be undertaken by the industries with which this form of illness is most often associated. The exposure to dust in mining and manufacturing settings may be reduced by several means, including requiring all workers to wear protective face masks, having clean air piped into a closed hood over the workers' heads, removing dust (by suction) as it is produced, wetting down materials before beginning the work that produces dust, and using materials that do not involve harmful dust and cause disease.

Dust mites

Tiny insects that are related to spiders and ticks and can cause allergic reactions in sensitized people who inhale their microscopic body parts or fecal matter. Dust mites, which live on fabrics such as mattress bedding, upholstered furniture, stuffed animals, and carpeting that collect dust, may produce mild symptoms of allergic rhinitis or bring on bronchial ASTHMA attacks. The allergen produced by dust mites may be linked to skin disorders in infants, children, and adolescents. Dust mite allergies can be associated with persistent skin lesions.

The mites are so tiny that about 100 to 500 individual mites can exist in a single gram of dust. Female dust mites lay 25 to 30 eggs that produce new mites every 3 weeks. While it was once believed that people were allergic to dust, it is now known that it is the dust mites inhabiting the dust that cause the reaction.

Dust mites thrive in warm, humid conditions. They consume more food and develop more quickly when the humidity is above 70 percent, and they cannot flourish in very dry climates or at altitudes more than 3,000 feet above sea level. The mites live on a diet composed of microscopic skin scales from humans and pets that are continually shed naturally. People who have disorders such as ringworm and scabies, which produce large amounts of skin scales, may attract a greater number of dust mites. The insects do not bite or spread disease and are not harmful to people who are not sensitized to them. Their numbers have increased during the past two to three decades, during which time homes and other indoor structures have become more tightly constructed, providing less ventilation, and are kept warmer during cold weather. Dust mites thus proliferate during the winter months and are more keenly experienced as irritants by people who spend more time indoors. They also live in the nests of birds and small mammals.

CONTROL AND PREVENTION

The most effective approach to reducing allergic reactions to dust mites is to remove or limit the use of carpeting, especially wall-to-wall carpeting, and upholstered furniture. Wooden furniture with fewer upholstered surfaces is a good alternative, as are wood floors and area rugs that can be cleaned.

If it is not possible to replace wall-to-wall carpeting or upholstered furniture, vacuuming the house regularly with a water-filter attachment on the vacuum cleaner is sometimes beneficial. Treating carpets and furnishings with a spray containing tannic acid may also be helpful. The use of this spray has not been confirmed to be effective, but it is believed to be beneficial because it may chemically change house dust and neutralize the protein in the mites that produces allergic reactions. Benzyl benzoate, a powder that is applied and then vacuumed up, may be used in conjunction with tannic acid sprays to kill the dust mites.

A home dehumidifier or air conditioner in warm, damp climates may help reduce humid indoor conditions in which dust mites thrive. Dust mites grow poorly when the humidity is below 50 percent. If an air conditioner is used, the filter should be regularly cleaned.

Air cleaners and filters are not considered effective enough at ridding indoor air of dust to be worth the expense. The most effective of these have high-efficiency particle-arresting (HEPA) filters that are capable of trapping very small particles of dust. Those that generate ozone gas may exacerbate allergy symptoms because the ozone can irritate the respiratory system.

The bedroom is usually the area of the house where the highest concentration of dust mites is found. They can be controlled in this room by regularly washing all bedding in hot water every week to 10 days. Walls, ceilings, closets, and all furniture surfaces should be cleaned or dusted weekly. Mattresses can be covered in specially made, airtight sheaths made of a polyurethane coating that is permeable to water vapor but blocks mites and their feces. Covering the bed with a bedspread to collect dust during the day, then removing it at night before retiring may also be helpful. Fiberfill pillows and comforters are better than feather- or down-filled bedroom accessories for people sensitive to dust mites. Pillows should be enclosed with the same airtight coverings as mattresses. Stuffed animals should be removed from the bedroom, and bed canopies and blankets with a deep, nappy texture should not be used. The heat from an electric blanket on a mattress surface helps reduce dust mite populations.

DXA

See DUAL-ENERGY X-RAY ABSORPTIOMETRY.

Dying, care of the

See END-OF-LIFE CARE.

Dysarthria

Difficult to understand, poorly articulated speech. A person with dysarthria has trouble speaking or pronouncing words because of damage to the muscular systems required for normal speech. This problem is generally noticeable in day-to-day conversation. Common causes of dysarthria include stroke, degenerative neurological disorders, alcohol abuse, and poorly fitted dentures. Causes of dysarthria can be diagnosed through a physical examination and tests such as cerebral angiography, electroencephalogram (EEG), MRI (magnetic resonance imaging), CT (computed tomography) scanning, and X rays. Treatment may involve referral to a speech pathologist. People with dysarthia may need to use alternative communication systems (for example, word boards, writing, and synthesizers) if they cannot be understood. Dysarthria is sometimes confused with aphasia, which is a deficit in understanding or producing language.

Dysentery

An intestinal infection characterized by bloody diarrhea and abdominal cramps. There may also be fever, dehydration, and excess mucus secretions from the anus. Dysentery is caused by ingesting food or water contaminated with either bacteria or amebae. Diagnosis is made through analysis of a stool sample and blood tests. Other tests may include SIGMOI-DOSCOPY and COLONOSCOPY (examinations of parts of the large intestine using special lighted tubes).

Treatment of bacterial dysentery, usually caused by infection with the *Shigella* bacillus or the *Campylobacter* bacterium, is with antibiotics. Treatment of amebic dysentery is with antiamebic drugs, such as metronidazole. In most individuals, oral fluids can maintain hydration. However, if dehydration is severe, intravenous fluids will be given. After treatment, follow-up stool samples may be required for 2 to 3 months to monitor and resolve the infection.

Dysentery is most common in developing countries with poor sanitation. The infection can be prevented in such areas by drinking only bottled water, avoiding fresh produce, and eating only thoroughly cooked foods. Thorough cooking destroys infectious organisms.

Dysequilibrium

A type of dizziness. In dysequilibrium, a person experiences balance problems when walking or standing (and not when sitting or lying down). This condition most often affects older people and is usually associated with other medical problems, such as a prior STROKE, PARKINSON DISEASE, peripheral neuropathies, severe arthritis of the knee or hip, or visual changes (for example, those following cataract surgery). Diagnosis is usually made through medical history and physical examination. Treatment of dysequilibrium involves correction or care of any underlying medical problems. Physical therapy or canes or other walking aids are often helpful. See also OSTEROARTHRITIS.

Dyshidrotic eczema

Irritation of the skin on the palms of the hands and the soles of the feet. Dyshidrotic eczema is characterized by clear, deep blisters that itch and burn. See also DERMATITIS.

Dyskinesia

An abnormal, involuntary movement such as twitching, nodding, or jerking. Dyskinesias range from mild to severe and from slow to rapid. These movements may develop as a side effect of a drug, such as levodopa (which is often prescribed to treat PARKINSON DISEASE), or they may be caused by a brain disorder.

Dyslexia

One of the LEARNING DISABILITIES characterized by difficulty with written symbols. Dyslexia is not necessarily linked with low intelligence.

CAUSES

Although its exact cause remains unknown, dyslexia may have educational, psychological, and biological components. Children with dyslexia may have trouble with certain teaching styles, such as those that emphasize the recognition of whole words rather than phonetics. Children who have family problems or difficult relationships with teachers may also be more prone to this problem. Finally, there is some evidence that dyslexia tends to run in families.

SYMPTOMS

Dyslexic children often have trouble with the mastery of early reading skills. In fact, the one trait shared by all dyslexic children is that they read at levels significantly lower than what is typical for their age and intelligence. Other common symptoms of dyslexia include problems with identifying single words, trouble understanding sounds, delayed spoken language, spelling problems, a tendency to transpose letters in words, confusion with directions and distinctions (such as right and left), and problems with mathematics.

DIAGNOSIS AND TREATMENT

Early evaluation and treatment of dyslexia are best; otherwise, a child can quickly fall behind in school. Unfortunately, many children experience repeated failures in school before they finally receive the necessary evaluation. Children suspected of having dyslexia must be tested by trained educational experts. Treatment of children with dyslexia should be tailored to each child's individual needs.

There are three general categories of treatment: developmental, corrective, and remedial. The developmental approach continues to use regular teaching methods, but emphasizes the necessity for small-group or tutorial sessions. The corrective reading approach also uses small groups in tutorial sessions, but with an emphasis on the child's particular interests. The hope is that this will motivate the child to use his or her own special abilities to overcome any impairments. The remedial approach stresses the use of individualized, structured techniques to correct a child's particular skill deficits.

Dysmenorrhea

A condition in which a woman experiences painful menstruation. See MENSTRUATION, DISORDERS OF.

Dyspareunia

A condition in which a woman experiences painful sexual intercourse. See INTERCOURSE, PAINFUL.

Dyspepsia

The medical term for INDIGESTION, general discomfort in the upper abdomen.

Dysphagia

See SWALLOWING DIFFICULTY.

Dysphasia

Impairment of the ability to speak or sometimes to understand language. Dysphasia is the result of brain injury. Aphasia is the absence of the ability to speak or understand language but is often used interchangeably with dysphasia to describe individuals with any type of language impairment.

Dysphonia

See HOARSENESS.

Dysphoria

A state of feeling unwell or unhappy; the opposite of euphoria.

Dysplasia

Abnormal cells that may precede the development of cancer. Dysplasia most often occurs in cells that reproduce rapidly. Dysplasia is classified as mild, moderate, or severe, depending on how abnormal the affected tissue appears under a microscope. For example, dysplasia can be found in the lungs and bronchi (tubes through which air passes into the lungs) of smokers. Normal bronchi are lined with cells that are covered by fine hairs lubricated by mucus. Over time, smoking causes these cells to undergo dysplasia, in which they lose their fine hairs and become flattened and cube-shaped. If smoking continues, cellular changes may evolve and cancerous cells may develop. Dysplasia can also be found in the cervix, where a Pap smear can detect abnormal, precancerous cells.

Dyspnea

The sensation of difficult, labored, or uncomfortable breathing. Dyspnea can vary widely in severity. It may be experienced as the result of many conditions, ranging from overexertion to serious illnesses, such as CHRONIC OBSTRUCTIVE PULMONARY DISEASE (COPD) or asthma. Other conditions that produce dyspnea include anxiety, interstitial pulmonary fibrosis, anemia, neuromuscular disorders, pneumonia, lung cancer, and heart disease.

TREATMENT

Doctors can generally identify the underlying problem causing this symptom by taking a medical history and performing a physical examination. Dyspnea most commonly results from conditions involving the heart or lungs. Anxiety and poor physical condition are also common causes of dyspnea.

Treating the underlying disease is the most effective and primary treatment for dyspnea; however, two types of medication, opiates and anxiolytics, may improve symptoms. Opiates can relieve breathlessness and may improve exercise performance, while anxiolytic medications help reduce anxiety, relieve the ventilatory response related to the available amounts of oxygen in the blood, and lower the intensity of the emotional reaction to breathlessness.

People who have lung conditions and diseases may sometimes experience relief from dyspnea with the use of a fan that produces a movement of cool air. Breathlessness related to COPD is sometimes improved by a course in retraining breathing, which teaches a person techniques to achieve slower, deeper breathing. A procedure

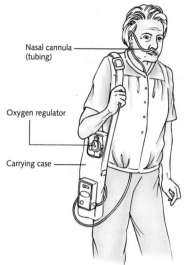

Nasal cannula (tubing)

Oxygen regulator

Carrying case

PORTABLE OXYGEN
Portability of an oxygen system is an important factor for an active person with dyspnea. Equipment that is meant to be carried weighs between 3 and 6 pounds. Larger systems can be pulled on a cart. Generally, a liquid oxygen system is the most portable but is more costly than compressed oxygen.

known as continuous positive airway pressure (CPAP) may relieve dyspnea during asthma attacks and during exercise for people with advanced COPD. Education about symptoms and techniques to promote relaxation and distraction from the discomfort of dyspnea is sometimes useful in coping with it.

Dysthymia

Chronic, persistent depressed mood; essentially a form of mild DEPRESSION. In adults, the depressed mood of dysthymia lasts for at least 2 years and is accompanied by two or more of the following symptoms: poor appetite or overeating, inability to sleep (insomnia) or too much sleep (hypersomnia), low energy or fatigue, low self-esteem, poor concentration, difficulty making decisions, and feelings of hopelessness. In the case of children, the mood may be expressed as irritability and needs to last only 1 year for a diagnosis of dysthymia to be made. People with dysthymia are able to function in day-to-day life, but usually only with difficulty and at reduced efficiency. Dysthymia may lead to and alternate with BIPOLAR DISORDER; if this occurs, the condition is

sometimes known as double depression. Dysthymia is more common among people whose immediate family members have major depressive disorder than among the general population and more common in women than men. Dysthymia usually begins in childhood, adolescence, or early adulthood and continues until it is treated. Treatment consists of psychotherapy, antidepressant medications, or both.

Dystonia

A neurological movement disorder that results in distorted or impaired voluntary movement. Dystonia often produces muscle spasms, irregular jerks, twisting and repetitive movements, or abnormal body positions. The disorder is often painful and may affect one part of the body, several parts, or the entire body. Focal dystonia, generally appearing during a person's 50s, is the term used to describe the disorder when a single part of the body is affected; an individual may have more than one focal dystonia. When the whole body is involved, the condition is termed generalized dystonia. This form of the disorder usually occurs during childhood. Dystonia may occur as the result of stroke, most commonly affecting an arm and leg on the same side of the body. Otherwise, the cause is unknown. Current research is exploring gene markers for some types of dystonia. Diagnosis depends on the parts of the body affected. There is no cure at present, although medication may help reduce spasm in selected cases.

Dystrophy

A progressive condition caused by defective nourishment of an organ or system. MUSCULAR DYSTROPHY is a group of disorders characterized by progressive skeletal muscle weakness. The most common muscular dystrophies seem to be linked to a genetic deficiency of the muscle protein known as dystrophin.

Dysuria

The medical term for painful or difficult urination. Dysuria is often a symptom of disorders such as cystitis, urethritis, or bladder stones or of a sexually transmitted disease, such as gonorrhea. See URINATION, PAINFUL.

E. coli

FOR FIRST AID
see Food poisoning, page 1322

A bacterium known as *Escherichia coli* that has hundreds of strains, some of which produce a powerful toxin that may cause severe illness. Most strains of *E. coli* are harmless and live in the intestines of healthy people and animals. *E. coli* is differentiated from other strains by specific markers found on its surface. It is also referred to as diarrheagenic *Escherichia coli* or non–Shiga toxin-producing *E. coli* and was first identified as a cause of food-borne illness in the United States in 1982. At that time, an outbreak of illness characterized by severe, bloody diarrhea was traced to hamburgers contaminated with this strain of *E. coli*. Since then, most infections have been associated with the ingestion of undercooked, contaminated ground beef.

CAUSES AND SYMPTOMS
The toxin-producing *E. coli* organism can live in the intestines of healthy cattle, and the meat from these cattle may become contaminated during slaughter. When the beef is ground, the organisms can be integrated into the ground beef. Contaminated meat has no unusual appearance or odor, and it is believed that only a very small number of organisms are required to produce illness. If contaminated beef has not been thoroughly cooked, *E. coli* can survive and cause infection when the beef is eaten. It is safest to use a meat thermometer and make sure the meat, such as a cooked hamburger, is well

ATTACHING TO HOST TISSUE
Under a microscope, *Escherichia coli (E. coli)* bacteria can be seen to have tiny hairlike structures called pili that attach to the surface of the host, such as the intestinal lining. Many strains of this bacterium live harmlessly in the intestines of people and animals, but some strains produce disease-producing toxins.

done and has reached an internal temperature of 155°F.

Because the *E. coli* bacteria may be present on a cow's udders or on dairy farming equipment, it may come into contact with raw milk. As a result, infection can also be caused by ingestion of unpasteurized milk or unpasteurized milk products.

Transmission of the illness may also occur via person-to-person contact in families and child-care facilities where there is exposure to the bacteria from loose stools of infected children. Living or working with toddlers who are not yet toilet-trained places people at higher risk of contracting the infection. Older children rarely carry the organism without symptoms, but small children may continue to shed the toxin-producing bacteria for several weeks after recovering from the infection.

The illness may also be contracted by drinking or swimming in water that is contaminated with human or animal fecal material. Drinking water that is inadequately chlorinated may cause infection. Becoming infected with *E. coli* has been known to occur as a result of ingesting certain foods that may have been improperly treated or washed, including fruit juice, unpasteurized apple cider, salami, sprouts, and lettuce.

Infection with *E. coli* causes intense bouts of diarrhea, which may be bloody, and abdominal cramps. There may or may not be mild fever and symptoms, which last 5 to 10 days. In a small number of cases, including people with weakened immune systems, children younger than 5 years, and older people, the infection can produce a complication in which the red blood cells are destroyed and the kidneys fail. This condition is called hemolytic-uremic syndrome; it is the principal cause of acute kidney fail-

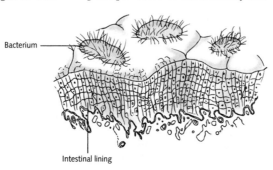
Bacterium / Intestinal lining

ure in children, and most cases are caused by *E. coli*.

DIAGNOSIS AND TREATMENT
The stool is cultured and tested for the causative strain of *E. coli* bacterium by SMAC agar, a test that detects the organism. Most people who become infected and who have diarrhea as their only symptom tend to recover without treatment within 5 to 10 days. Antibiotics have not been shown to diminish the infection or its symptoms, and antibiotic treatment may precipitate kidney complications. Antidiarrheal agents should be avoided as they may prolong the infection.

If the life-threatening complication hemolytic-uremic syndrome develops, the infected person is usually treated in an intensive care unit (ICU) and may require blood transfusions and kidney DIALYSIS. With treatment, most people survive this complication, but abnormal kidney function may persist for many years, sometimes requiring long-term dialysis. People who recover from hemolytic-uremic syndrome may have lifelong complications, including high blood pressure, seizures, blindness, and paralysis. If part of the colon, or large intestine, was removed, there may be lifelong effects from that surgery, such as chronic diarrhea.

E. coli diarrhea
See DIARRHEA, E. COLI.

Ear
The organ for hearing and balance. The structures of the ear are in three parts—the outer ear, the middle ear, and the inner ear. Most of these structures lie inside the skull. The outer ear receives sound waves from the environment and channels them to the middle ear, the middle ear transmits them to the inner ear, and the inner ear converts the sound waves into impulses that are sent to the brain.

OUTER EAR
The ear flap that is visible outside the head is only the first part of the outer ear. This external ear, called the pinna, consists of skin and cartilage that cups sound waves from the environment and funnels them into the ear canal just inside the head. The outer ear flap is really a continuation of the skin and cartilage that form the

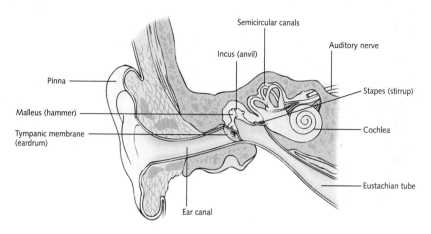

ANATOMY OF THE EAR

The structures of the ear gather sound waves and pass them through the hollow outer ear, through the vibrating ear drum and bones in the middle ear, and then into the fluid environment of the inner ear. There they are converted into nerve impulses that travel via the auditory nerve to the brain.

lining of the ear canal (also called the external auditory meatus). This skin produces ear wax (cerumen) and is covered with tiny hairs that trap dust and other foreign particles. The inner portion of the ear canal is lined with membrane and protected by bone. At the inner end of the ear canal is the eardrum, or tympanic membrane—a fibrous membrane stretched across the ear canal. When sound waves reach the eardrum, it vibrates to conduct the sound into the middle ear.

MIDDLE EAR

The middle ear is a cavity just behind the eardrum. Three tiny, separate bones reach across the cavity to the inner ear. Named for their shapes, they are commonly called the hammer, the anvil, and the stirrup (or the malleus, incus, and stapes). The hammer is attached to the ear drum on one end and is linked to the anvil on the other; the anvil links to the stirrup, and the stirrup lies against an opening to the inner ear called the oval window. The tiny, mobile bones of the middle ear carry the vibrations from the ear drum to the structures of the inner ear. The eustachian tube, which leads to the nasal cavities, opens into the cavity of the middle ear; although this passage to the outside is usually closed, it can be opened by swallowing or yawning to equalize pressure in the middle ear.

INNER EAR

The structures of the inner ear lie deep within the temporal bone of the skull. The oval window is covered by a delicate membrane called the inner ear membrane. Beyond this membrane are the two principal structures of the inner ear—the labyrinth and the cochlea. The labyrinth contains a series of passages that lead to the cochlea and a set of three looped tubes called the semicircular canals. The fluid-filled semicircular canals are concerned with balance. They are at right angles to each other, and the movement of the fluid within them monitors the movement and position of the head and sends this information to the brain through nerve fibers of the vestibular nerve.

The cochlea is a coiled, fluid-filled tube that curls around like a snail shell. Situated within the cochlea is the organ of Corti, which contains millions of tiny hair cells. Vibrations that reach the inner ear vibrate the oval window and move through the fluid in the cochlea, where they stimulate the hair cells. The bending of the hair cells converts pitch and volume information into nerve impulses that are transmitted to the auditory cortex of the brain through the eighth cranial nerve—the acoustic, or auditory, nerve. See HEARING.

Ear, discharge from

A symptom of infection in or damage to any of several parts of the ear. A discharge of blood or fluid from the ear following increasing pain and HEARING LOSS may indicate a ruptured or perforated eardrum (see EARDRUM, PERFORATED). A physician should be consulted immediately if these symptoms are present.

In some forms of acute OTITIS MEDIA (middle ear inflammation), pus fills the middle ear, putting pressure on the eardrum and causing it to rupture. The discharge is usually composed of blood and thick pus. Recurring ear infections of long duration can change the middle ear lining, causing a larger amount of a thicker fluid discharge. Ear discharge may also be caused by an infection of the ear canal, called SWIMMER'S EAR, or by an injury to the lining of the ear canal. Injury is often caused by attempts to clear wax from the ear by using an implement such as a hair pin. The discharge is usually yellow or yellow-green pus that has a foul odor and oozes from the ear. Sometimes the emission of pus helps relieve the pain of the infection. An ear discharge with similar characteristics may be produced by a fungus in the ear canal.

A physician should be consulted whenever there is a discharge from the ear. The discharge may be a symptom of a serious injury or infection that can result in permanent hearing loss. An OTOLARYNGOLOGIST (doctor specializing in medical conditions of the ear, nose, and throat) will be able to take a sample of the discharge to be cultured in a laboratory. Analysis of the culture can detect the kind of organism causing the infection. Depending on the type of infection producing the discharge, a doctor may prescribe antibiotics. In cases of swimmer's ear, a physician may remove the ear discharge and clean the ear with a suction device or cotton-tipped probe. Ear drops containing one of the CORTICOSTEROIDS and an antibiotic may be prescribed.

Ear, examination of

Observation, evaluation, and analysis of the ear by a physician, usually an OTOLARYNGOLOGIST (ear, nose, and throat specialist). A physical examination of the internal parts of the ear can be performed by using an OTOSCOPE (a lighted viewing instrument inserted into the outer ear). The doctor may pull the top of the ear up and back to straighten the canal and provide a clearer view of the entire ear canal. The otoscope allows the physician to view internal parts of the ear from the outer ear canal through the somewhat transparent eardrum. In more severe cases of ear infection, the ear examination may include taking a culture. Examining the ear with a binocular microscope is often helpful in difficult cases. When HEARING LOSS or symptoms including dizziness or ringing in the ears are present, AUDIOMETRY (hearing measurement tests) may also be recommended.

Ear, foreign body in

The presence of any object that is not part of the natural structure of the ear lodged inside the ear canal. Foreign bodies in the ears are usually small objects or pieces of objects, including earplugs, that are placed too deeply within the ear canal and cannot be readily removed. Other common foreign bodies include paper, toy parts, jewelry, cotton swabs, and eraser tips. Live insects may be particularly painful. Young children sometimes experiment with placing foreign bodies such as beads and beans in their ears where they can become firmly lodged or wedged in the small ear canal. Small button batteries are particularly dangerous because they can cause severe local injury to the ear; call a doctor immediately.

TREATMENT

Only a physician using the correct instrument—usually special tiny forceps or right-angle hooks—should attempt to remove foreign bodies from the ears. A doctor is often able to see the object by looking inside the ear canal or by using an OTOSCOPE (lighted viewing device used to examine the ear canal). Attempts to remove foreign objects from the ear at home are dangerous, especially if a household item is used as a tool. Such attempts can cause serious injury to the ear or push the object farther into the ear and complicate its removal. If a live insect gets stuck in the ear, it is safe to apply a few drops of mineral or baby oil into the ear canal to try to immobilize the insect until a doctor can remove it.

Terms in small capital letters—for example, PHYSICAL THERAPY or PAGET DISEASE—indicate a cross-reference to another entry with more information.

Earache

Pain in one or both ears, medically termed otalgia, which may be sharp and stabbing or dull and throbbing. When earaches are severe and persistent, an infection may be the cause. A physician should be consulted about a severe earache.

CAUSES

Any number of infections or conditions may cause an earache. Earaches are often symptoms of the common cold. If the pain of an earache becomes worse when the earlobe is pulled downward, an infection of the ear canal is probable. After airplane travel, pain in one or both ears accompanied by a blocked feeling in the ears may indicate damage to the middle ear caused by BAROTRAUMA. If, in addition to the earache, there is a sticky, yellow discharge from the affected ear or pain with movement of the outer ear, it may be the symptom of an inflammation of the ear canal (otitis externa, or SWIMMER'S EAR), or a more serious inflammation of the middle ear (OTITIS MEDIA). When the ear or ears ache and hearing is increasingly impaired over a period of several weeks or months, the cause could be blockage from a build-up of EARWAX. Ear pain can also be due to a sore throat or painful neck muscles. Pain in the teeth or jaw together with pain in the ear may mean that dental problems are causing the earache; a dentist should be consulted.

Eardrum, perforated

A hole, rupture, or tear in the tympanic membrane, commonly called the eardrum, which separates the ear canal and the middle ear. A decreased ability to hear and an occasional discharge often accompany a perforated eardrum. Any associated pain is usually not persistent.

CAUSES

Physical trauma, exposure to very loud noise, infection, or medical procedures are all possible causes of a perforated eardrum. The membrane may be ruptured as the result of a blow to the ear with a flat surface such as an open hand. Accidents while diving or water skiing, pressure changes from flying or scuba diving, or skull fractures can cause a ruptured eardrum. When harmful substances—such as acid or the hot slag

produced by welding—enter the ear canal, the eardrum may be perforated. Bobby pins, cotton swabs, or other objects pushed too far into the ear canal can perforate the eardrum. Being exposed to sudden explosions can cause the eardrum to rupture (see ACOUSTIC TRAUMA). Middle ear infections can cause a spontaneous tear in the eardrum. The perforation may be caused by a small hole remaining in the eardrum after a pressure-equalizing tube has been placed and subsequently either falls out or is removed by a physician.

The amount of HEARING LOSS is usually related to the size of the perforation and its location in the eardrum. In the case of a severe skull fracture, hearing loss may be severe if, in addition to the perforated eardrum, the sound-transmitting bones in the middle ear are disrupted or inner ear structures are injured. In cases of physical trauma or an explosion, the hearing may be significantly impaired, and ringing in the ears (see TINNITUS) can be severe, although hearing is usually partially restored and the ringing diminishes within a few days. If the perforation results in chronic infection, hearing impairment may be severe.

TREATMENT

A physician should be consulted if a perforated eardrum is suspected; he or she can diagnose the condition and recommend the appropriate treatment. A hearing test (see AUDIOMETRY) is generally performed before attempts are made to correct the perforation. When the perforation is very small, the physician often observes the condition over a period of time before beginning treatment. Most perforations of the eardrum will heal on their own, usually within a few weeks but possibly over several months. While the eardrum is healing, it must be protected from exposure to water and trauma. The doctor may also patch the eardrum during an office procedure performed with an instrument that resembles a microscope. The doctor places a chemical on the edges of the perforation and then puts a thin paper patch on the eardrum. Patching the eardrum in this way usually noticeably improves hearing. Some perforations may require three or four patchings before the rupture is completely closed. If the paper patch is not deemed a suitable course of treatment or if it proves ineffective, another surgical procedure will probably be recommended by the doctor.

Surgery to repair a perforated eardrum is called TYMPANOPLASTY. The procedure, done on an outpatient basis, involves placing tissue across the perforation to allow healing. This type of surgery is usually successful in closing the perforation and improving hearing.

Ears, pinning back of

See OTOPLASTY.

Earwax

Wax in the ear canal that is secreted by special glands in the skin lining the outer part of the canal. This wax, termed cerumen, traps dust and other particles to prevent them from going deeper into the ear where they might injure the eardrum and helps keep the ear canal dry by repelling water. It also has antibacterial properties. In most people, only small amounts of earwax are secreted. Usually, the wax migrates toward the outer ear canal, carrying dust and other particle debris with it to help clean the ear. When the wax reaches the outer part of the ear, it falls out or is washed or wiped off.

In some people, excessive wax builds up, sometimes as often as every few months. It becomes hardened and blocks the ear canal, causing discomfort. Wax blockage can impair hearing noticeably, create ringing in the ears, make the ears feel plugged, and sometimes even cause EARACHE or dizziness.

INVESTIGATION AND TREATMENT

It is dangerous to try to clean the ears using cotton-tipped applicators or metal implements, such as paper clips or hair pins. Doing so can injure the thin, fragile skin lining the ear canal, and it might injure or puncture the eardrum. It can also make the condition worse by pushing the wax deeper into the ears and packing it more tightly against the eardrum. Hearing can be impaired, and the wax might be more difficult to remove.

A physician may wash out the impacted wax. First, the accumulated wax is softened, then removed by

SYRINGING OF THE EARS with body-temperature water or saline. Usually, the ear is then treated with alcohol to absorb any leftover moisture, dry the ear canal, and destroy bacteria and fungi. Syringing of the ears should not be done on a person who has a perforated eardrum (see EARDRUM, PERFORATED) or has had mastoid surgery.

Other medical treatment options for people who have impacted earwax include vacuuming the wax with an electric suction device or removing it with a curet (a scoop-shaped instrument) or probe. Ear drops may be prescribed to soften the wax for 2 to 7 days before these removal techniques are attempted.

Over-the-counter ear drops to soften earwax are also available. They are not as strong as prescription softeners but can be effective. These drops should not be used if the eardrum is perforated. Softening agents sometimes make the ear seem more plugged, but only temporarily.

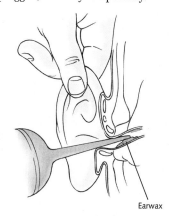

Earwax

CLEANING THE EARS
Accumulated earwax can be removed by applying a wax softener (baby or mineral oil or glycerin) with an eyedropper twice a day for 2 or more days, then washing the canal with body-temperature water or salt solution. With the head upright, pull the ear up and back, gently squirt the fluid into the ear, and turn the head to the side to drain the fluid from the ear into the sink.

Eating disorders

Abnormal and dangerous eating patterns that are caused by mental illness. There are two principal types of eating disorders. In ANOREXIA NERVOSA, the person is significantly underweight because of extreme dieting. In BULIMIA, the individual repeatedly indulges in out-of-control eating

binges, then rids the body of the food, usually by induced vomiting.

Eating disorders affect mainly adolescent and young-adult females who fear losing control, tend to be perfectionists, and base their self-esteem disproportionately on body shape and weight. Depression and anxiety often accompany eating disorders. Anorexia nervosa has serious physical consequences in young women, including disruption or stopping of menstrual periods, and can be fatal. Bulimia is less dangerous yet can lead to significant physical problems. Treatment consists of psychotherapy to address emotional conflicts and, in some cases, antidepressants or other medications.

Eaton-Lambert syndrome

A disorder in which ACETYLCHOLINE cannot be released from the nerve endings in the brain to cross the synapse and stimulate muscles to contract; also known as Lambert-Eaton syndrome, myasthenic-myopathic syndrome, and Eaton-Lambert myasthenic syndrome. This disorder differs from MYASTHENIA GRAVIS, in which acetylcholine is released but cannot bind with muscles to allow them to respond. Eaton-Lambert syndrome is most often associated with lung cancer, but can be caused by other forms of cancer or autoimmune diseases. People with Eaton-Lambert syndrome describe muscle weakness and severe fatigue (usually of muscles of the legs, arms, and trunk first). Unlike myasthenia gravis, facial weakness is rarely a symptom; dry mouth, loss of bowel or bladder control, muscle aches, and decreased reflexes may occur. The treatment of choice is to treat any present cancer. Immune suppressive therapy can sometimes be helpful.

Ebola virus

A family of viruses, which has four subtypes, three of which have been identified as a cause of disease in humans and one of which has caused disease in primates. The Ebola virus causes Ebola hemorrhagic fever (Ebola HF), a severe, often fatal illness, that was first recognized in 1976 and has appeared sporadically since then. The virus and the illness it causes are named after the Ebola River, where it was first recognized, in the Democratic Republic of the Congo (formerly Zaire) in Africa and southern Sudan. Much about the Ebola virus remains unknown, but it is believed to be carried by animal hosts or carriers that are native to the African continent.

Ebola HF diagnoses have been confirmed in several regions of Africa, but the illness has not been reported in humans in the United States. A subtype of the virus that affects only primates resulted in the deaths of monkeys imported from the Philippines for research in the United States and Italy. Although several research workers tested positive for the virus, they did not become ill.

HOW IT IS SPREAD

Humans do not carry the Ebola virus, and it is not known how they first contract the infection it causes. It is believed that the virus is spread via contact with an infected animal host. The virus may rarely be spread from one person to another via direct contact with the blood or body secretions of an infected person or by exposure to objects, such as needles, that have been contaminated with infected secretions.

Nosocomial transmission (spread of infection in health care settings) is known to occur in facilities in which patients are cared for by health care workers who do not take precautionary measures, including using masks, gowns, and gloves. The use of needles or syringes that are not disposed of following a single use and not sterilized can also spread the infection in hospitals and clinics.

The Ebola virus has been shown to spread via airborne particles in research settings, particularly among primates, but this transmission of the viral infection has not been known to occur among humans in day-to-day contact.

SYMPTOMS

The first symptoms of infection with the Ebola virus usually appear within a few days of infection, but may not appear until 10 days following infection. The most frequent symptoms include high fever, headache, muscle aches, stomach pain, nausea, fatigue, and diarrhea, with upper respiratory symptoms including cough and chest pain. Less frequent symptoms may include sore throat, hiccups, a rash on the trunk, eye inflammation (con-

junctivitis), jaundice, vomiting blood, and bloody diarrhea.

Within a week of symptoms, there may be blindness, internal bleeding, and bleeding around sores and mucous membranes. During the second week of infection, people infected with the virus either begin to recover or develop multiple organ failure. Severe chest pain, shock, and death may follow. Complete recovery takes a long time and may be complicated by several conditions, including HEPATITIS.

It is not understood why some people are able to recover from Ebola HF while others are not. Researchers have determined that, for unknown reasons, those who die of the infection have not developed an immune response to the virus.

DIAGNOSIS AND TREATMENT

Ebola HF can be diagnosed with blood tests within a few days of symptoms appearing. The tests used include electron microscopy, the antigen-capture enzyme-linked immunosorbent assay (also referred to as ELISA TEST), the polymerase chain reaction (PCR), or virus isolation tests. When Ebola HF is suspected in people who have died, the cause of death may be confirmed by immunohistochemical testing, virus isolation, or PCR.

There is no known cure or vaccine for Ebola HF, and no effective antiviral therapy exists. Treatment is generally based on supportive therapy, including the replacement of blood products and the maintenance of fluid and electrolyte balance, oxygen status, and blood pressure. An attempt is made to avoid invasive procedures that might further weaken the infected person. Complicating infections are treated as they occur.

PREVENTION AND OUTLOOK

Primary prevention measures present a challenge to medical authorities because how the Ebola virus originates before infecting humans and other primates is unknown. It is known that travel to sub-Saharan Africa or the Philippines or exposure to subhuman primates imported from these areas increases a person's risk of infection.

Because of the risk of an epidemic taking hold following a single infection, the medical goal is to stop or limit the spread of infection. This

requires timely, accurate diagnostic procedures and the immediate use of isolation precautions and barrier nursing techniques to prevent any person from coming in contact with the blood or secretions of an infected person. Protective clothing, including gowns, masks, gloves, and goggles, must be worn. Complete equipment sterilization and other infection-control measures must be followed. Infected individuals must be isolated and prevented from having contact with unprotected people. When Ebola HF causes death, direct contact with the body of the deceased must be avoided.

Researchers are investigating the development of diagnostic tools for early diagnosis of Ebola HF. Ecological investigations of the virus and monitoring of suspected at-risk areas are underway.

Ecchymosis

The oozing of blood from a blood vessel into the tissues, usually the result of a BRUISE. This causes a bluish discoloration of the skin.

ECG

Electrocardiogram; a recording of the electrical activity of the heart as a graph or series of waves on a strip of paper. The machine used to record the electrocardiogram is an electrocardiograph. The ECG is useful in determining whether heart rate and rhythm are normal and in detecting signs of a large number of conditions that affect the heart, such as current or past heart attack, angina, cardiomegaly (enlargement of the heart), tachycardia (heart rhythms that are abnormally fast), bradycardia (abnormally slow heart rhythms), insufficient oxygen supply as a result of coronary artery disease, myocarditis (inflammation of the heart muscle), pericarditis (inflammation of the membrane surrounding the heart), and congenital heart disease (heart defects present at birth).

An ECG is quick, painless, risk-free, and noninvasive; food and fluids are not restricted beforehand. The person removes clothing from the waist up, and electrodes (small, flat metallic devices that detect small electrical current) are attached to the skin. Depending on the purpose of the ECG, the number of elec-

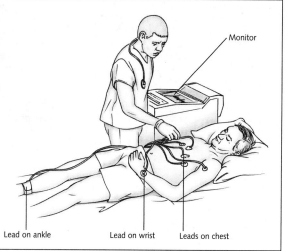

RECORDING HEART ACTIVITY
An electrocardiogram (ECG) is a recording of the electrical impulses that trigger heartbeat. For the procedure, electrodes, which are connected to the electrocardiograph by leads (insulated conductors), are attached to a person's chest, wrist, and leg. The ECG equipment painlessly records the electrical activity and can help diagnose heart problems and damage to heart muscle.

Monitor

Lead on ankle   Lead on wrist   Leads on chest

trodes varies between 3 to 5 and 12 to 15. Wires run from the electrodes to the electrocardiograph. The person lies still for about 60 seconds after the electrocardiograph is turned on, and the electrical activity of the heart is recorded.

A number of variations of the ECG are available if needed. An ECG may be given while exercising on a treadmill or a stationary bicycle to see how the heart behaves under stress (CARDIAC STRESS TESTING). The HOLTER MONITOR is a portable electrocardiograph used to record a continuous ECG over a 24-hour period. If an abnormality is suspected or detected on an ECG, other heart tests may be necessary.

Electrocardiogram is also abbreviated sometimes as EKG, after "elektrokardiogram," the spelling of the word used by Dutch electrocardiography pioneer Willem Einthoven. Electrocardiography refers to the study of the electrical activity of the heart using surface electrodes.

Echinacea

An herb used to stimulate the immune system. Echinacea grows wild in the Midwest and the Great Plains of the United States and was the favorite herb of Native Americans, who used it on the skin to treat snake bites, burns, boils, abscesses, and sores. It is claimed that echinacea, also known as purple coneflower, when taken orally, is able to mobilize white blood cells to swarm to areas of infection. There is no clinical proof of its effectiveness.

Echinacea should not be taken continuously for more than 8 weeks.

Echocardiogram

An image of the heart created by bouncing ultrasound waves off the heart and into a machine that translates the echoes into a computer-generated picture. Echocardiography is a method of visualizing the heart using ultrasound technology.

An echocardiogram allows doctors to see the heart while it is moving and to observe the main pumping chambers, the shape and thickness of the chamber walls, the valves, the outer covering, and the major vessels leading into and out of the heart. It is also possible to determine the volume and direction of blood flow through the heart. An echocardiogram is useful for determining the

size of the heart, its pumping strength, valve problems, damage to the heart muscle, abnormal blood flow patterns, structural abnormalities (such as enlargement of the heart, or cardiomegaly), and blood pressure in the pulmonary arteries (arteries leading to the lungs) (see HYPERTENSION, PULMONARY). A special technique, called Doppler echocardiography, can be used to measure the speed of blood flow through the heart. Another technique, called the TRANSESOPHAGEAL ECHOCARDIOGRAM, involves inserting a small transducer into the esophagus (the tube leading to the stomach). The transducer emits ultrasound waves that allow better images of the back of the heart.

An echocardiogram can be performed while a person lies still or after exercising (stress echocardiogram). If the person is resting, the transducer, which emits the ultrasound waves and captures the returning echoes, is held over the chest. For a stress echocardiogram, echocardiography is performed before and after exertion on a treadmill or a stationary bicycle.

A standard echocardiogram involves no special food or fluid restriction; the test is painless, noninvasive, and quick. It is commonly used in conjunction with other heart tests, such as an ECG (electrocardiogram), if a heart abnormality is suspected.

Echocardiography

A method of visualizing the heart by bouncing ultrasound waves off the heart and into a machine that translates the echoes into a computer-generated image. See ECHOCARDIOGRAM.

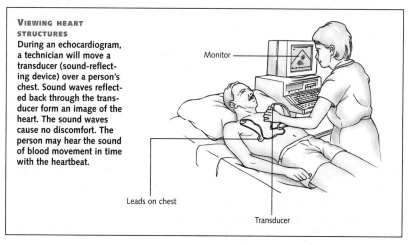

VIEWING HEART STRUCTURES
During an echocardiogram, a technician will move a transducer (sound-reflecting device) over a person's chest. Sound waves reflected back through the transducer form an image of the heart. The sound waves cause no discomfort. The person may hear the sound of blood movement in time with the heartbeat.

Monitor

Leads on chest

Transducer

E

Echolalia

Meaningless repetition of words, often in a mocking, mumbling, staccato, or parrotlike tone. In children, echolalia may arise as part of normal speech development that ceases as the child matures. It can also be a sign of autism, schizophrenia, Tourette syndrome, catatonia, or damage to the frontal lobe in the brain. In adults, echolalia is most often a symptom of schizophrenia. It sometimes occurs in certain forms of speech loss (aphasia) and dementia.

Eclampsia

A serious and rare condition of late pregnancy in which the mother develops seizures and can become unconscious, or comatose, and die. Eclampsia is almost always preceded by a condition called preeclampsia, in which the woman has swelling, high blood pressure, and protein in her urine. In about one pregnancy in 1,000, PREECLAMPSIA leads to eclampsia in late pregnancy, during labor or delivery, or after delivery. Eclampsia must be treated in the hospital to protect the lives of both the mother and the baby. The more severe the symptoms of preeclampsia, the more likely the condition will progress to eclampsia; eclampsia can often be prevented with early detection and treatment of preeclampsia.

ECT

Electroconvulsive therapy. Also known as shock or electric shock therapy, ECT consists of an electrical shock administered to the brain to induce a controlled seizure. ECT is used primarily as a psychiatric treatment for major depression that does not respond to antidepressant medication, particularly when there is a risk of suicide.

HOW THE PROCEDURE
IS PERFORMED

ECT is usually administered in a hospital or an ambulatory surgery setting. Since general anesthesia is used, the patient must refrain from eating or drinking after midnight the night before. After the patient's heart rate, body temperature, and blood pressure are checked, an intravenous tube is inserted into a vein, usually in the hand or lower arm, and a short-acting anesthetic is administered. Once the patient is asleep, a tube is inserted through the mouth and down the trachea (windpipe) to assist in breathing. Muscle-relaxant medications are given to prevent injury to the patient during the sudden, flailing movements that accompany the seizure.

Electrodes are attached to the head, on both the right and left side (bilateral ECT) or on only one side (unilateral ECT). A low-voltage electrical current is then sent into the brain for a half second or less. The result is a brain seizure, or convulsion, that lasts from less than 60 to 90 seconds. After the seizure ends, the anesthetic wears off and the patient awakens, typically within 5 to 10 minutes after the procedure began. In most cases, the person can return home following only a short recovery period.

Usually electroconvulsive therapy is given as a series of treatments. A typical program for depression consists of 6 to 12 treatments given over a 2- to 4-week period.

Complications of ECT include confusion or disorientation immediately following treatment, blood pressure abnormalities, headache, abnormally rapid heartbeat (tachycardia), or allergic reactions to anesthesia. Memory loss can also occur. Usually memory returns within 4 to 6 weeks of treatment; rarely the loss is permanent. The risk of memory loss is less with unilateral ECT, which, however, may be somewhat less effective than bilateral ECT.

EFFECTIVENESS AND CONTROVERSY

It remains unclear exactly why ECT works. Studies have shown that the seizures increase the activity of brain chemicals known as neurotransmitters, as do many antidepressant medications. ECT has other effects on the brain, however, and it may be that they also have a role in the therapy's effectiveness against depression.

A great deal of controversy has surrounded ECT, in part because the therapy was used indiscriminately after its introduction in the 1930s. Originally, the treatment was tried for many different types of mental disorders, and patients were not properly informed of the possible complications. As a result, many states today have laws stipulating the conditions under which ECT can be performed and require that patients be fully informed of the risks and benefits.

Several states also mandate reporting of ECT treatment. In addition, the treatment has been refined, and the procedure has been modified so that it is less physically demanding for the patient.

Antidepressant medications have made ECT less necessary than in the past. ECT remains an effective treatment for severe depression that does not respond to medication. In addition, ECT is effective in a few days, while medications usually take from 4 to 6 weeks to alleviate depression. Because severe untreated depression carries a high risk of suicide, ECT is an important treatment option. Antidepressant medications are often used preventatively after treatment since ECT does not prevent a reoccurrence of depression.

Ectoparasite

A parasite that lives on the exterior of its animal or human host. Ectoparasites may be organisms ranging in size from microscopic to those visible to the naked human eye. They can cause serious illness, such as Lyme disease (deer ticks and western black-legged ticks) and Rocky Mountain spotted fever (Lone Star ticks).

Ectopic

Occurring in an abnormal place or out of sequence. In an ECTOPIC PREGNANCY, the pregnancy develops outside the uterus. The most common site is within a fallopian tube. Symptoms include lower abdominal and back pain, nausea, vaginal bleeding, and breast tenderness. Rupture can lead to internal bleeding and shock. The usual treatment is surgical laparotomy (see LAPAROTOMY, EXPLORATORY) or LAPAROSCOPY.

Although the term "ectopic" is most commonly applied to ectopic pregnancies, other ectopic conditions can also develop. For example, an ectopic heartbeat is an arrhythmia (see ARRHYTHMIA, CARDIAC) involving small variations in a heartbeat. Ectopic CUSHING SYNDROME is caused by tumors.

Ectopic heartbeat

An abnormal heart rhythm, in which the heart contracts sooner than usual. It is the most common form of abnormal heart rhythm (see ARRHYTHMIA, CARDIAC) and the least serious. An ectopic heartbeat is also known as extrasystole. Ectopic heartbeats can give people the sensation that the heart skipped a beat. Occasional ectopic heartbeats are harmless and require no treatment other than to address the cause. Common causes include stress, lack of sleep, and using caffeine, alcohol, or tobacco. In some people, persistent ectopic heartbeat can produce spells of light-headedness, chest discomfort, or shortness of breath. If symptoms are troublesome or persistent, a medication that controls heart rhythm, such as a beta blocker, is typically prescribed.

Ectopic pregnancy

A condition in which a fertilized egg implants outside the uterus. Most ectopic pregnancies occur in the fallopian tubes, but can occur (less often) on the ovaries, cervix, and in the abdominal cavity. Many times, the cause of an ectopic pregnancy is unknown. However, some factors increase a woman's risk of having an ectopic pregnancy. For example, if a woman has had an inflammation of the fallopian tubes, known as SALPIN-GITIS, damage to tissues inside a tube, previous tubal surgery, or used an intrauterine device, her risk increases.

Symptoms of an ectopic pregnancy may include lower abdominal pain (usually concentrated on one side), vaginal bleeding, nausea, and vomiting. However, an ectopic pregnancy may cause no symptoms. Women with ectopic pregnancies often do not even know they are pregnant. Symptoms typically are experienced 6 weeks or more after a woman's last menstrual period. The greatest risk to the woman is when an ectopic pregnancy ruptures, and severe internal bleeding occurs. Abdominal pain will increase as blood builds inside a woman's abdominal cavity; she may experience shoulder pain, weakness, dizziness, or fainting.

DIAGNOSIS AND TREATMENT

When an ectopic pregnancy is suspected, a doctor performs a pelvic examination and usually orders blood tests and ULTRASOUND SCANNING. When it is suspected that an ectopic pregnancy has burst and internal bleeding is occurring, a culdocentesis may be performed. In this procedure, a needle is inserted through the vagi-

LOCATION OF ECTOPIC PREGNANCY
An ectopic pregnancy most often occurs in a fallopian tube (although it can locate in an ovary, the cervix, or even elsewhere in the abdominal cavity). Left untreated, an ectopic pregnancy will continue to grow and can rupture the fallopian tube, causing life-threatening bleeding.

Fallopian tube

Uterus

Fallopian tube

Ovary

Ovary

nal wall below the cervix and into the pelvic cavity to detect blood. A woman with a ruptured ectopic pregnancy needs immediate surgery to remove the embryo and repair or remove the damaged tissues of the fallopian tube. If an ectopic pregnancy has not ruptured or caused severe bleeding, and the fallopian tube has not ruptured, the embryo can usually be removed surgically by using a laparoscope, an instrument for viewing and treating internal organs. During LAPAROSCOPY, a doctor will remove the developing pregnancy by making a small incision in a woman's fallopian tube and scooping out the embryo. If, as a result of an ectopic pregnancy, a woman's fallopian tube has burst, it can sometimes be repaired. If damage to the tube is considerable and cannot be repaired, the tube will be removed in a procedure called SALPINGECTOMY.

In some instances, surgery may be avoided and medications given to halt the growth of an ectopic pregnancy. Medications are used only when the fallopian tube has not ruptured, there is no active bleeding, and the embryo is small. A woman who has had an ectopic pregnancy may have a future normal pregnancy, even if she has had a fallopian tube removed. If the remaining fallopian tube is healthy, a woman may be able to get pregnant. However, after having an ectopic pregnancy, a woman is at greater risk for having another.

Ectropion

Sagging and outward turning of the eyelid, usually the lower. The lining of the eyelid is exposed, and tears tend to flow out of the eye rather than across it. The eyelid is likely to crust over as mucus drains from the eye, causing irritation and pain. In severe cases, the clear outer covering of the eye (cornea) develops ulcers, leading to scarring and possible loss of vision. Ectropion usually develops with age, as muscles relax and weaken. It can also result from scarring of the eyelid caused by burns, injury, skin cancer, or eyelid surgery. The condition is also seen in children with Down syndrome because of malformation of a ligament in the eye socket. Artificial tears, which are available over-the-counter as eye

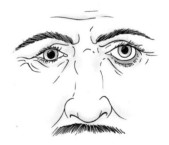

SAGGING LOWER LID
Ectropion becomes a problem because the lower lid cannot sweep across the cornea to help moisten it; resulting friction on the cornea can cause permanent damage. Surgery can correct the ectropion. After surgery, the person may wear a patch overnight and use antibiotic ointment for a week or so.

E

drops, can be used to alleviate dryness and prevent complications. Surgery to alleviate ectropion is effective and should be performed before permanent damage occurs. Usually done as an outpatient procedure under local anesthesia, the surgery tightens the ligament and tissues that hold the eyelid in place.

Eczema

See DERMATITIS.

Edema

Swelling in the body caused by a buildup of excess fluids. There is a constant exchange of fluid and nutrients between the small capillaries and the tissues they nourish. Edema can occur when increased pressure in the blood vessels disturbs the fluid exchange and forces more fluid out of the blood vessels and into the surrounding tissues. Edema can occur in different parts of the body and for various reasons, some of which are minor and others serious. Swelling in the feet and lower legs is common and can be caused by standing or sitting for a long time. People with varicose veins are particularly prone to develop leg swelling with standing. A serious cause of edema is congestive heart failure (see HEART FAILURE, CONGESTIVE), which can cause persistent swelling in the lower extremities and fluid buildup in the lungs (see PULMONARY EDEMA). Other serious causes of generalized edema include kidney failure, chronic liver disease (cirrhosis), and NEPHROTIC SYNDROME.

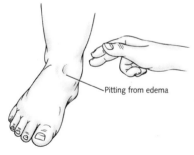

PRESSURE-SENSITIVE TISSUE
Edema usually develops first in the gravity-prone parts of the body, such as the foot and ankle, or the buttocks of a bedridden person. Because of poor blood flow, the tissue is oxygen-depleted. Even a small amount of pressure—the touch of a finger—may leave indentations (pitting) on the area.

EEG

See ELECTROENCEPHALOGRAM.

Efavirenz

A drug used to treat HIV (human immunodeficiency virus) infection. Efavirenz (Sustiva) is used with other drugs to treat HIV infection by suppressing RNA, the genetic material within the cell.

Efficacy, drug

The extent to which a drug produces a beneficial result under ideal circumstances. Much of the DRUG APPROVAL PROCESS involves testing to ensure that the drug under study has adequate effectiveness or efficacy.

Effusion

Fluid that accumulates in a body cavity. Effusion occurs when pus, serum, blood, lymph, or other fluid escapes into a body cavity as a result of inflammation or the presence of excess fluid in an organ or tissue. Types of effusion include hemorrhagic effusion, in which blood leaks into another body cavity; pericardial effusion, in which fluid accumulates in the sac surrounding the heart; and pleural effusion, in which fluid builds up between the layers of the pleural membranes surrounding the lungs.

Effusion, joint

The accumulation of fluid within a joint, such as the knee joint. Joint effusion may be caused by trauma, infection, gout, or arthritis. The resulting swelling may cause pain and restricted movement in the affected area. The escaped fluid is usually reabsorbed by the body within 1 to 2 weeks, after which the symptoms of joint effusion improve. Sometimes, withdrawing the fluid with a fine needle (aspiration) is necessary for analysis or to help relieve pressure. See also BURSITIS.

Egg

The female reproductive cell; the medical term is ovum. Produced in the OVARY, the egg is the largest cell in the human body, big enough to be seen with the naked eye. All of the eggs a woman will ever produce are present in her body at birth. But the ovaries only release one egg a month during a woman's reproductive years,

a process called OVULATION. The egg is released from a structure within the ovary called a follicle and then is swept into the fallopian tube to travel toward the uterus. If fertilized by a sperm cell from a male as a result of sexual intercourse, the cells of the fertilized egg can divide and multiply and develop into an embryo. Because of the unique way that both sperm and egg cells divide (MEIOSIS), a single egg contains only half as much genetic information as any other cell in the body. When a sperm and egg unite, the genetic material from each parent is mixed in the new cell that is formed. See CONCEPTION; REPRODUCTIVE SYSTEM, FEMALE.

Ego

The portion of the personality that exhibits reason and consciousness, processes thoughts and feelings, comprehends reality, and copes with life. In Latin, the word "ego" means "I," and the ego is central to a person's identity. In the writings of Sigmund Freud, whose work forms the basis of modern psychoanalysis (see FREUDIAN THEORY), the ego acts as a kind of a go-between to balance the demands of the instinctual self with those of morality and conscience.

Ehlers-Danlos syndrome

A group of hereditary connective tissue disorders characterized by defective collagen, the major structural protein of the body. Collagen is a tough, fibrous protein responsible for strengthening and holding cells together. In Ehlers-Danlos syndrome (EDS), defects of collagen cause abnormally loose and flexible joints that can become dislocated; unusually loose and stretchy skin; and fragile skin, blood vessels, membranes, and other tissues. Ehlers-Danlos syndrome is classified into six major subtypes, each of which is a distinct hereditary disorder. A parent with one subtype of EDS will not have children with a different subtype of the condition. The syndrome occurs among all ethnic groups in one of every 5,000 to 10,000 people, affecting males and females equally.

EDS is usually diagnosed from family history and clinical observation. Treatment depends on the subtype of the syndrome but is generally limited to managing symptoms. Skin wounds are common in several subtypes and must be repaired with care to avoid permanent disfigurement. Skin should be protected from sun exposure by use of sunscreen, and people with EDS must avoid activities that can cause joints to overextend or to lock. Bracing or surgical repair may help to stabilize loose joints.

The vascular type of EDS is the most serious subtype, because it can involve rupture of arteries or organs such as the intestines or the uterus. The skin is usually very thin and translucent in affected people, especially over the chest and abdomen, and minor trauma can lead to extensive bruising. Arterial rupture can cause sudden death.

Eisenmenger complex

A condition present at birth that combines pulmonary hypertension (high blood pressure in the arteries of the lungs) with a heart defect that mixes oxygen-rich and oxygen-poor blood, often giving the skin a bluish tint. Although people are born with Eisenmenger complex, symptoms usually first develop in the 20s and 30s. In addition to a bluish skin color, particularly under the fingernails and on the lips, early symptoms include fatigue, low tolerance for physical exertion, shortness of breath, and fainting. As the disease progresses and the heart muscle weakens, symptoms worsen. Irregular heart rhythm, chest pain, anemia, blood clots, kidney disease, heart failure, stroke, and sudden death can occur.

People with Eisenmenger complex are advised to adopt a heart-healthy lifestyle, by avoiding tobacco, high altitudes, dehydration, and situations that can lower blood pressure (such as saunas and steam rooms). Since the disease carries a high risk of death during pregnancy, women with Eisenmenger complex are counseled to avoid becoming pregnant. Antibiotics are prescribed for people with Eisenmenger complex before dental or surgical procedures to reduce the risk of endocarditis (inflammation of the lining of the heart, which usually involves the heart valves). Medications are generally used to help maintain a normal

heart rhythm and to strengthen the heart muscle.

Eisenmenger complex is the leading reason for performing combined heart-lung transplantation surgery. In this procedure, a person receives both lungs and the heart from a donor. Some persons in an advanced stage of the disease may also be treated with lung transplantation combined with surgical repair of the heart defect that mixes oxygen-rich and oxygen-poor blood.

Ejaculation

The discharge of semen from the opening in the end of the penis at the height of orgasm. Semen consists primarily of sperm, and its nutrients enhance the migration of the sperm to the female egg. Ejaculation is propelled by strong muscular contractions that squeeze the thick, white fluid out through the passageway in the penis that connects the sperm duct with the end of the penis (urethra).

EKG

See ECG.

Electra complex

A possessive, romantic attachment of daughter to father that, according to the theory developed by Sigmund Freud, is buried deep within the unconscious during childhood. The dilemma of attraction to the father is resolved by the girl's subsequent identification with her mother, from whom she learns moral values. This complex, an idea repressed into the subconscious, is named after a heroine from ancient Greek drama who lost her life because of her devotion to her father. The male equivalent to the Electra complex is the OEDIPUS COMPLEX.

Electric shock treatment

See ECT.

Electroacupuncture

See HOMEOPATHY.

Electrocardiogram

A recording of the electrical activity of the heart as a graph or series of waves on a strip of paper; commonly abbreviated ECG.

Electrocardiography

A testing method that records the electrical activity of the heart as a graph or series of waves on a strip of paper. See ECG.

Electrocautery

A surgical instrument that uses an electrical current to remove abnormal or diseased tissue or to control bleeding from small blood vessels. Also known as electrocoagulation, the device consists of a platinum wire that becomes white- or red-hot when an electrical current passes through it.

Electrocautery is commonly used to remove skin lesions. The area is anesthetized locally; then, the lesion is carefully cut away with a scalpel. Electrocauterization of the wound destroys any remaining abnormal tissue and seals blood vessels to stop bleeding. This type of procedure is usually done on an outpatient basis. Healing is normally complete within 2 or 3 weeks, with little or no scarring. Electrocautery is also used to help control bleeding in surgery; it is one of the techniques that make bloodless surgery possible.

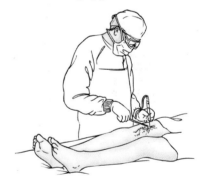

CAUTERIZING BLOOD VESSELS
Doctors use electrocautery to destroy tissue and seal off blood vessels to stop bleeding. For instance, it can be used to remove so-called spider veins (an overgrowth of tiny blood vessels). The electrical current, which closes the vessels with heat, can be applied through a needle or through a surgical knife (enabling a surgeon to make bloodless incisions).

Electroconvulsive therapy

See ECT.

Electrodiagnostic studies

Tests that are used to diagnose diseases of the nerves and muscles.

E

Electrodiagnostic studies record electrical activity in the body. They are used to evaluate symptoms such as numbness, tingling, pain, weakness, and muscle cramping. There are a number of possible electrodiagnostic tests. In an ELECTROMYOGRAM (EMG), a needle or needles are inserted into a muscle, which the person is then asked to contract. An EMG involves some discomfort when the needle is inserted, as well as muscle soreness later. EVOKED RESPONSES are painless tests that check nerve pathways. Nerve conduction studies show how the body's electrical signals travel through the body's nervous system. An ELECTROENCEPHALOGRAM (EEG) is also an electrodiagnostic test.

Electroencephalogram

Also known as an EEG, a neurological test in which the electrical activity of the brain is recorded and studied. The EEG is a useful tool in the diagnosis of medical problems, such as epilepsy, stroke, brain tumors, sleep disorders, and degenerative diseases. In this painless procedure, a person lies on a table and electrodes are attached to his or her scalp with a conductive paste. The brain's electrical activity is recorded on a long strip of paper or a computer screen. Abnormal activity is a sign of a possible problem. A regular EEG usually takes no longer than an hour. In a sleep EEG, a person is encouraged to sleep rather than merely relax. An ambulatory EEG is one in which an individual's brain activity is measured during normal activities.

Electrolysis

Removal of unwanted body hair through destruction of hair roots with an electric current. Men and women generally want to remove unwanted hair for cosmetic reasons. In electrolysis, a needle is inserted in the hair follicle, and an electric current is passed through it to destroy the hair at the root. Each hair is treated individually. The process is extremely time-consuming and can be painful. Because hair goes through dormant phases, many rounds of electrolysis must be performed to make even a small area of the body completely hair-free.

Electrolyte

A chemical substance capable of conducting electricity because it dissociates into electrically charged particles (ions) when dissolved or melted. Electrolytes are involved in metabolic activities and are essential to the normal function of all body cells, especially the heart's electrical system. The most important ions found in body fluids are those involving sodium, potassium, calcium, magnesium, chloride, bicarbonate, and phosphate. Electrolyte balance depends on adequate intake of water and electrolytes.

Electromyogram

Also known as an EMG, a test used to record the electrical activity of muscles. An EMG is most often performed when a person experiences numbness and weakness. In this test, a needle or needles are inserted into a muscle, which the person is then asked to contract. Abnormal findings may indicate diagnoses such as ALS (amyotrophic lateral sclerosis), muscular dystrophy, myasthenia gravis, or peripheral nerve damage. An EMG involves some discomfort when the needle is inserted, as well as muscle soreness later. An alternative to a regular EMG is a surface EMG (SEMG). This involves placing electrodes on the surface of the skin to detect electrical activity. Although this test may prove of some value in the future, at present it is considered less accurate. An EMG is often done in conjunction with nerve conduction velocity (NCV) tests, which show how well the nerve endings are working.

Electromyography

A diagnostic procedure, also referred to as EMG, that records and analyzes the electrical activity in muscles. The procedure involves the insertion of needle electrodes into a muscle. EMG allows a physician to examine individual parts of the muscle and explore changes that indicate disorders or pathology of the muscle tissue and its associated nerve. The procedure is used to diagnose neuromuscular disease.

Electrophoresis

A technique used in laboratories to separate electrically charged molecules, especially proteins. Electrophoresis is widely used to examine body chemicals, such as the different proteins found in blood serum, and is helpful for determining the cause of elevated serum protein levels. The method involves passing an electric current through a solution or other medium containing a variety of molecules. Each type of molecule will travel at a different rate, depending on its size and electrical charge, and separation is based on those differences. Similar molecules will group together on the medium, gradually separating into bands, which can be stained and visualized.

Elephantiasis

A disease spread by several different types of mosquitoes, including the one

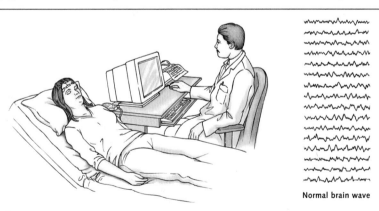

Normal brain wave

RECORDING BRAIN WAVES
An electroencephalogram (EEG) records the electrical activity of the brain to diagnose conditions such as epilepsy and sleep disorders. It cannot diagnose psychiatric disorders. The EEG recording shows normal brain waves of a sleeping person; abnormal activity is likely to be more sharply spiked and irregular.

that carries MALARIA. Elephantiasis occurs most commonly in central Africa and in southern and southeastern Asia. The disease is caused by a parasite that resides in the lymph nodes of humans, where the female worms produce an advanced stage of embryos, called microfilariae, that are released into the blood of affected humans. When mosquitoes feed on these people, the insects transform the ingested embryos into infective larvae.

The infection is transmitted to humans when the mosquito carrying these infective larvae feeds again on human beings. The larvae migrate to the lymph nodes, primarily those that drain the lower abdominal cavity and the legs. At this stage, the larvae reach sexual maturity. Repeated infections can produce blockage of the lymph nodes and ducts, causing an accumulation of lymph and swelling in the tissues of the scrotum and legs. This often results in enlarged disfigurations of the genitals and legs, creating a physical appearance that gives the disease its name, elephantiasis.

Elephantiasis is a parasitic infection that is also called bancroftian filariasis; it is diagnosed by the finding of the microfilariae, or by the advanced embryos in a blood smear.

ELISA test

A blood test that detects the presence of specific antibodies or antigens in the bloodstream. Enzyme-linked immunosorbent assay; (ELISA) testing is frequently used to diagnose Lyme disease and HIV (human immunodeficiency virus) infection.

Embolectomy

Surgical removal of a blood clot that has traveled through the bloodstream until it lodges in a blood vessel and blocks circulation. In some cases, the blocked section of blood vessel is removed and replaced, or it is bypassed by routing blood flow around the site of the blockage. See EMBOLISM for more information about the underlying disease process.

Embolism

Blockage of a blood vessel by a blood clot, fat deposit, or other material that has lodged in the vessel after traveling through the bloodstream. The medical

THE DANGER OF EMBOLISM
A pulmonary (lung) embolism often occurs when a blood clot in a deep vein breaks loose, travels through the bloodstream, and lodges in an artery supplying the lung. Blood flow to a portion of the lung is then cut off. Left untreated, the lung tissue may die from lack of blood supply, a condition called infarction. The clot may need to be removed surgically.

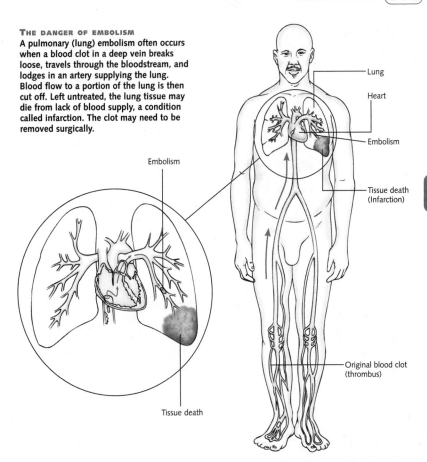

Embolism

Tissue death

Lung

Heart

Embolism

Tissue death (Infarction)

Original blood clot (thrombus)

E

importance of an embolism depends on the size of the blockage and the blood vessel it obstructs. Minor embolisms may produce no symptoms; major embolisms, such as those in the arteries of the heart or brain, can cause death by heart attack or stroke.

Most embolisms are caused by blood clots or detached fat deposits (plaques) that travel in the blood until they reach a medium- or large-sized artery, particularly in the neck, lungs, brain, intestine, legs, arms, or kidneys. Occasionally embolisms occur in the veins and capillaries. In addition to blood clots and plaques, globules of fat or bone marrow from a fractured bone, air or gas bubbles, clumps of bacteria, bits of tissue or tumor, and cholesterol crystals can cause embolisms.

A number of factors increase the risk of embolism. These include immobilization for long periods (such as transoceanic or transcontinental airplane flights), blood abnormalities present from birth or result-

ing from disease, some medications (such as birth control pills and hormone replacement therapy), surgery, trauma to the legs, fracture of the long bones of the legs or arms, advanced age (older than 70), and obesity.

Embolisms in the heart, brain, lungs, and kidneys can be life-threatening and require prompt emergency treatment. Those in the arteries of the limbs produce pain, numbness, tingling, splotches on the skin, muscular spasms, or paralysis. Left untreated, tissue death and gangrene can result. Embolisms in the veins may cause only local pain or swelling but can also result in sudden cardiac death.

Treatment depends on the location and size of the embolism and the condition of the person. Medications are used to break up blood clots in some cases and to prevent new ones from forming. Surgical removal of the embolism may be required or a doctor may insert a special thin tube into a blood vessel to break up or dislodge an embolism.

Embolization, therapeutic

Injection of a material such as gel foam or polyvinyl chloride into an artery to cut off the blood supply. The procedure may be used to stop internal bleeding or to cut off the blood supply to a tumor.

Embolus

A mass of clotted blood, fat, calcium crystals, air bubbles, or other material that moves through the bloodstream until it lodges in a narrower blood vessel and blocks circulation. See EMBOLISM for additional information.

Embryo

A fertilized egg from the time of CONCEPTION until the eighth week of PREGNANCY. Pregnancy begins with FERTILIZATION, the process in which the egg is united with a sperm. After fertilization, the egg (zygote) begins to divide into a cluster of cells, or blastocyst, which continues to divide as it moves down the fallopian tube toward the uterus. At conception,

---

DEVELOPMENT FROM ZYGOTE TO INFANT

The fertilized egg passes through several stages from zygote to infant:

- **Zygote:** A fertilized egg in the first 24 hours after fertilization
- **Blastocyst:** The mass of continually dividing cells up to 8 days after fertilization
- **Embryo:** The blastocyst after it attaches to the wall of the uterus from about 2 weeks after fertilization until the end of the seventh week after fertilization
- **Fetus:** 7 or 8 weeks after fertilization until birth
- **Infant:** After the birth

---

5 to 8 days after fertilization, the blastocyst implants itself in the wall of the uterus and becomes a developing embryo. After 8 weeks it is called a FETUS.

The outside layer of the blastocyst develops into the fetus's skin, hair, nails, tooth enamel, and parts of the nose, ears, and eyes. The middle

---

layer of cells becomes the fetus's heart, blood vessels, bone, muscle, cartilage, and connective tissue. The inside layer of cells eventually becomes the baby's bladder, tonsils, liver, pancreas, digestive tract, and respiratory tract.

By the end of the fifth week after conception, the arms and legs of the embryo have begun to form, and the eyes, nose, mouth, and umbilical cord begin to take shape. A 6-week-old embryo is about half an inch long, and its head, brain, spine, and nervous system are developing. Normally, the embryo's heart begins beating by the end of the sixth week.

Embryo transfer

The implantation of an embryo or embryos into a woman's uterus, typically 3 to 6 days after IN VITRO FERTILIZATION (fertilization outside the body). The procedure is performed with a small tube that is placed through the vagina into the uterus while the woman reclines on an examination table. Limited physical activity for 2 to 4 days is usually recommended. Pregnancy tests are given about 12 to 14 days after the procedure.

Embryology

The study of the origin, growth, development, and function of an organism from fertilization to birth.

Emergency

A medical crisis that threatens a person's life or limb(s) if appropriate care is not given within 2 hours. Medical emergencies are best identified according to these warning signs: fainting; shortness of breath or difficulty breathing; sudden dizziness, weakness, or change in vision; continuous bleeding; coughing up or vomiting blood; suicidal or homicidal urges; severe or persistent vomiting; high fever; pain or pressure in the chest or upper abdomen; confusion, lack of responsiveness, or unusual behavior; or sudden, severe pain anywhere in the body.

The definition of an emergency, according to the American College of Emergency Physicians is: "...medical conditions of recent onset and severity that would lead a prudent layperson, possessing an average knowledge of medicine and health, to

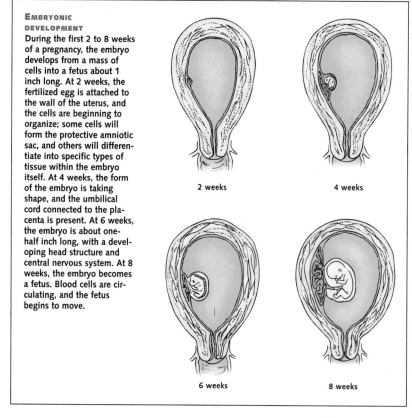

EMBRYONIC DEVELOPMENT
During the first 2 to 8 weeks of a pregnancy, the embryo develops from a mass of cells into a fetus about 1 inch long. At 2 weeks, the fertilized egg is attached to the wall of the uterus, and the cells are beginning to organize; some cells will form the protective amniotic sac, and others will differentiate into specific types of tissue within the embryo itself. At 4 weeks, the form of the embryo is taking shape, and the umbilical cord connected to the placenta is present. At 6 weeks, the embryo is about one-half inch long, with a developing head structure and central nervous system. At 8 weeks, the embryo becomes a fetus. Blood cells are circulating, and the fetus begins to move.

2 weeks

4 weeks

6 weeks

8 weeks

believe that urgent or unscheduled medical care is required."

Emergency childbirth

See CHILDBIRTH, EMERGENCY.

Emergency department

The department of a hospital that is continuously staffed 24 hours a day by specially trained personnel able to deal with any medical, traumatic, psychiatric, or environmental emergency. It is the center of activity for the region's ambulance system and regional disaster management. More than 100 million visits to emergency departments in the United States are made annually; about half of those visits are considered nonurgent.

Emergency medical technician (EMT)

A person trained to transport individuals to the hospital in an emergency; some emergency medical technicians, or EMTs, provide basic emergency first aid. EMTs have varying degrees of training depending on their individual jobs. Some are dispatchers, who answer calls for help and send ambulances and rescue vehicles to the site of an emergency, while others drive ambulances, assist with rescues, and perform basic emergency first aid. The highest level of EMT training is associated with a PARAMEDIC, who performs advanced medical procedures at the scene of an emergency or in the ambulance on the way to a hospital.

Emergency physician

A doctor with special training in the diagnosis and treatment of medical emergencies. Emergency physicians typically work in hospitals with people who have been injured in accidents or who have become sick very suddenly with such conditions as a heart attack or unexplained fever. Emergency physicians practice emergency medicine, a specialty developed out of the wartime experiences of physicians and paramedics on the battlefield who invented procedures and techniques that have been adapted for use in hospitals. The fundamental goal of emergency medicine is to save lives by beginning treatment

as soon as possible, preferably in the first minutes after a serious injury or illness.

Emesis

Forcible ejection of the contents of the stomach up through the esophagus and out of the mouth. See VOMITING.

Emetics

Agents that cause vomiting. Emetics are used to induce vomiting when poisonous or toxic substances have been consumed. They may act directly on the gastrointestinal tract by irritating portions of it, or they may work indirectly, by affecting areas of the brain that control vomiting.

Emetics that act directly on the stomach include IPECAC syrup, copper sulfate, and very large quantities of warm saltwater. The most commonly used of these direct emetics is ipecac syrup, which is available without prescription and generally induces vomiting within 20 minutes. Ipecac syrup also acts on the brain stem to induce vomiting. Indirect, or systemic, emetics include apomorphine, which acts through the blood on the part of the brain center that controls vomiting. Indirect emetics are no longer used in medicine.

Ipecac syrup may or may not be useful in cases of poisoning. For instance, emetics should never be used to treat poisoning by strong acids or petroleum distillates such as kerosene because vomiting in those cases would re-expose the gastrointestinal tract to the toxic substance. In most cases of poisoning, the use of activated charcoal (see CHARCOAL, ACTIVATED) is preferred to emetics. It is always advisable to call a poison center or a doctor before beginning treatment.

EMG

See ELECTROMYOGRAPHY.

Emotional deprivation

A lack of psychological nurturing and emotional stimulation, particularly during infancy and early childhood.

Emotional problems

Feelings such as anger, fear, sadness, excitement, love, or hate that are an abnormal response to a situation, cause the person significant distress,

and interfere with day-to-day functioning.

Empathy

Awareness and understanding of how another person thinks, feels, and behaves. People with autism, schizophrenia, and some other personality disorders often show a lack of empathy for others.

Emphysema

A chronic lung disease characterized by destruction of the walls of the alveoli, or air sacs, in the lungs, resulting in overinflation of the air sacs. Emphysema occurs gradually, usually as a result of years of exposure to cigarette smoke. The disease process occurs over time as the thin, fragile walls of the air sacs break down and the air sac tissue is destroyed. This irreversible damage interferes with the normal exchange between oxygen taken from the air breathed in and the carbon dioxide in the blood. Less oxygen is transferred from the lungs into the bloodstream, and overexpansion of the chest makes it difficult for a person to breathe and causes shortness of breath (see BREATH, SHORTNESS OF).

Early symptoms include feeling short of breath when active or during exercise. A characteristic cough is another sign of emphysema. Over time, even walking a short distance can produce significant difficulty breathing. As the lungs lose their elasticity, exhalation becomes particularly difficult, making emphysema one type of CHRONIC OBSTRUCTIVE PULMONARY DISEASE (COPD). Chronic bronchitis, also a type of COPD, may occur in combination with emphysema.

CAUSES AND TREATMENT

Most cases of emphysema are caused by smoking, which triggers the destruction of the elastic fibers of the lungs. An inherited deficiency of the protein alpha 1-antitrypsin (AAT) can lead to alpha 1-antitrypsin, a deficiency–related emphysema.

Because the disease is irreversible, medical care is centered on helping a person to live more comfortably with the symptoms and to prevent progression of the disease. Instructing a person with emphysema to quit smoking is the first and foremost element of treatment. When there is a tendency toward constriction or tightening of the airways, bronchodilators may be prescribed to relax and open air passages in the lungs. Secondary bacterial infections of the lungs, such as pneumococcal pneumonia, are treated with antibiotics.

Breathing exercises may be recommended as part of a program to rehabilitate the lungs and condition the rest of the body. These exercises involve the muscles used in breathing.

Surgery can be performed to reduce the volume of the lungs, a procedure in which the most severely diseased portions of the lung are removed to permit better functioning of the remaining lung and associated breathing muscles. Lung transplantation is a major procedure that can be beneficial in some cases.

Prevention of emphysema is best achieved by avoiding cigarette smoke entirely. Prompt SMOKING CESSATION is essential for those who have already acquired the habit. Once the disease is established, the goal becomes the

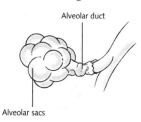

Centrilobular

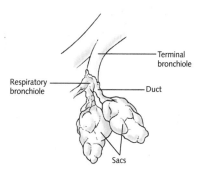

Alveolar duct

Alveolar sacs

Respiratory bronchiole — Terminal bronchiole

— Duct

Sacs

Panlobular

TWO TYPES OF EMPHYSEMA
In centrilobular emphysema, the ducts leading into the alveoli are damaged, but the alveoli are intact, so the person does not have symptoms. As the disease advances and the sacs of the alveoli are affected, the person develops symptoms. Finally, all the structures—bronchioles, ducts, and sacs—are damaged (panlobular emphysema).

prevention of secondary infections and further lung deterioration. A doctor generally recommends the maintenance of overall good health habits, including proper nutrition, adequate sleep, and regular exercise. Vaccinations against influenza and pneumococcal pneumonia are recommended. Colds and respiratory infections should be medically evaluated immediately.

Reduction or elimination of exposure to air pollution is also advised. When ozone levels are unhealthy, it is recommended that people with emphysema restrict outdoor activity to early morning or late in the day. When pollution reaches a dangerous level, outdoor activities should be avoided; weather forecasts usually include "ozone warnings" when needed.

Emphysema, subcutaneous

A rare condition produced by the presence of gas within the tissue beneath the skin. Subcutaneous emphysema is generally related to an unintentional introduction of air into tissues under the outer layers of skin. It also sometimes occurs as a result of gas production within a tissue, which occurs with gas gangrene. It often is associated with PNEUMOTHORAX.

Subcutaneous emphysema is diagnosed by a medical history and physical examination. It may be recognized by the appearance of a smooth, bulging protrusion on the skin. Upon pressure, this bulge produces a crackling sensation caused by gas being forced through the tissue. This symptom is generally preceded by more severe symptoms that are already being evaluated and treated. Most of the underlying conditions causing subcutaneous emphysema are serious and require hospitalization.

Empirical treatment

Medical care that is undertaken when a precise diagnosis is uncertain or cannot be determined. For example, for a person with a fever of unknown cause, a doctor may prescribe a course of antibiotics based on experience with comparable cases and clinical judgment as to what may be the most likely cause of the fever.

Employee assistance programs (EAPs)

A workplace-based, employer-funded treatment program for problems affecting a person's job performance, particularly a dependence on alcohol or drugs. EAPs, which began in the 1940s to help individuals whose alcohol use affected job performance, have grown to include a wider range of mental health issues. Since EAPs have been shown to be cost-effective in increasing productivity, they have been adopted by most Fortune 500 companies. By federal law, EAPs are confidential; an employee's participation in the program does not jeopardize employment. Most EAPs offer assessment of the issue by a trained counselor (either in person or over the phone), short-term counseling (no more than 10 sessions), and referrals to outside services for issues that need attention over a longer term. In addition, some EAPs offer consultation with attorneys for certain kinds of legal problems, financial consultation for personal money issues, and assistance with child and elder care.

SYMPTOMS OF ADDICTION AT WORK

Dependence on alcohol or drugs can cause a dramatic change in the person's ability to contribute to a company's mission. Managers or coworkers may notice a drop in productivity, loss in product quality, increased absenteeism, and depression or mood swings. The following signs may indicate a dependence problem:

- **Dramatic change in attendance or job performance**
- **Decline in personal appearance or hygiene**
- **Mood swings, including a change in attitude**
- **Pulling back from responsibility or social contact with fellow workers**
- **Unusual behavior**
- **Defensiveness and secretiveness about the abused substance, such as drinking at lunch and lying about it**
- **Increasing tardiness or use of "sick days"**

EMPLOYEE PROBLEMS

These are the most common workplace problems, according to a survey of employee assistance professionals.

- Family crisis
- Other problems
- Workplace/job conflict
- Substance abuse
- Alcoholism
- Stress
- Depression

Courtesy of International Employee Assistance Professionals Association, Inc.

Empyema

A collection of pus in a body cavity, particularly in the space called the pleural space, which is located between the lung and the membrane that surrounds it. This form of empyema is usually caused by an infection that spreads from the lung. The lung infection may be due to bacterial pneumonia, a lung abscess, trauma or injury to the chest, or surgical procedures performed on the chest. Prompt treatment of infections of the lungs can help prevent empyema.

A form of empyema called subdural empyema involves a collection of pus between the outer and middle membranes covering the brain. This may be caused by complications from sinusitis, ear infections, head trauma, surgery on the head, or BACTEREMIA. In children younger than 5 years of age,

subdural empyema is often due to bacterial meningitis. The symptoms include headache, lethargy, and seizures evolving over several days. Untreated, these symptoms can rapidly progress to coma and death. Subdural empyema is a medical emergency requiring immediate surgical draining of the pus surrounding the brain, as well as antibiotic therapy.

SYMPTOMS, DIAGNOSIS, AND TREATMENT

When empyema affects the area surrounding the lungs, the infected fluid in the pleural space may increase in volume to a pint or more. This accumulation of fluid can begin to put pressure on the lungs, which causes difficulty breathing, shortness of breath, and chest pain that worsens with deep inhalations. Other symptoms may include a dry cough, fever

and chills, excessive sweating (especially at night), malaise, and weight loss.

Empyema may be diagnosed by physical examination; the doctor will listen to the person's chest with a stethoscope. Other diagnostic tests include a chest X ray and a pleural fluid Gram stain and culture. Antibiotics are prescribed to treat the infection, and if necessary, a procedure called THORACENTESIS may be performed. Thoracentesis involves inserting a needle through the chest wall to drain the infected fluid. In some cases, the fluid may be too thick to be removed by this method, and surgery may be needed to drain the pus. During this procedure, a chest tube may be placed in the chest and remain there to continue to drain the fluid after surgery.

The inflammation produced by empyema may result in a complication that causes scarring and thickening of lung tissue, a condition called PULMONARY FIBROSIS, but empyema generally does not cause permanent lung damage.

Emulsion

A suspension of small globules of one liquid in a second liquid with which the first will not mix. Examples of emulsions include oil in vinegar and water in oil. In pharmaceutical preparations, mixtures of oil and water are sometimes united by a third substance.

Enabling

Behavior that helps or allows an individual who is dependent on alcohol or drugs to maintain that dependency. Enabling is also known as CODEPENDENCE.

Enalapril

A drug used to treat hypertension (high blood pressure) and congestive heart failure. Enalapril (Vasotec) is one of a class of drugs called angiotensin-converting enzyme, or ACE, inhibitors.

Enamel, dental

The hard, outer layer that covers and protects the teeth. Dental enamel is the hardest substance in the human body. Enamel protects the less durable, underlying parts of the teeth: the dentin, pulp chamber (see PULP,

DENTAL), root canals, and nerves. Eroded enamel allows decay-causing substances to penetrate the more vulnerable inner parts of the tooth; this leads to more severe decay and possible damage to the root canals and the nerves. The fluoride found in toothpaste helps to keep the enamel more resistant to decay.

Encephalitis

An inflammation of the brain that may be due to many different causes. Encephalitis may be caused by an injury to the head or brain, or it may be a complication of a viral, bacterial, or fungal infection. Two viral forms of encephalitis are herpes simplex, which when untreated can be fatal in an otherwise healthy person, and varicella-zoster, which can be fatal to people with weakened immune systems. In rare cases, MEASLES can cause a very serious form of encephalitis.

A virus that causes a form of encephalitis called arboviral encephalitis is chiefly transmitted to humans by mosquitoes, most frequently between the months of June and October. The common transmitters are infected birds including sparrows, blackbirds, pheasants, chickens, and pigeons. The birds usually carry the virus without developing illness. When mosquitoes feed on the infected birds, they become infected and spread the virus by biting horses and humans. Encephalitis cannot be spread person-to-person, nor can it be contracted by humans from horses.

There are several types of mosquitoborne encephalitis. Among the most recently identified is WEST NILE VIRUS, which usually affects older people and young children. Other common types in the United States are eastern equine encephalitis, which is the most serious and affects all age groups, particularly in New England; western equine encephalitis, which usually affects young adults and children younger than 1 year of age, particularly residents of the rural American West; St. Louis encephalitis, which primarily affects adults, especially older persons and people in low-income areas, especially near the Mississippi River; and La Crosse encephalitis, which primarily affects children younger than 16 years of age, especially those residing in rural

areas in the Great Lakes and mid-Atlantic regions of the United States. Venezuelan equine encephalitis is less common but has occurred in Texas.

SYMPTOMS, DIAGNOSIS, AND TREATMENT

The symptoms of encephalitis vary widely among people who have been bitten by infected mosquitoes. Most of these people do not contract the illness at all. Others have only flulike symptoms that resolve within a few days. These symptoms may include headache, drowsiness, and fever. When the infection is severe, a person may have an intense headache, stiff neck, high fever, nausea, vomiting, aching muscles, chills, sensitivity to light, and mental confusion. There may be behavioral and personality changes. Or, encephalitis may cause seizures, localized paralysis, partial or almost complete unconsciousness, and coma. These symptoms indicate a medical emergency, and the person should be treated in a hospital emergency department where appropriate measures can be taken.

Diagnosis is made after the person's blood samples are evaluated for antibodies to the agent causing the infection. CT (computed tomography) scans of the head are also used to diagnose encephalitis.

While there is no specific medical cure for mosquito-borne encephalitis, people can fully recover from the infection under a doctor's supervision with medical attention to symptoms and complete bed rest. Hospitalization may be necessary.

Encephalitis due to other viral infections, including herpes simplex and varicella-zoster, can be treated with antiviral therapy to shorten the course of the infection and prevent complications. Antibiotics and corticosteroid medications may be given to treat underlying infections.

The prognosis for people who have encephalitis varies according to a person's health status, age, immune status, and preexisting conditions, as well as the strength of the virus and the severity of the infection. Mental retardation and high mortality are associated with several forms of encephalitis, including eastern equine encephalitis and herpes simplex encephalitis. Persons older than

60 years who have St. Louis encephalitis are at higher risk of dying and may have long-term complications, including behavioral disorders, memory loss, and seizures. Western equine encephalitis and La Crosse encephalitis have low mortality rates, but the former may result in developmental delay, seizure disorder, and paralysis in children and parkinsonism in adults.

Encephalomyelitis

Inflammation of the brain and spinal cord that may occur as a complication of a viral infection. Encephalomyelitis is distinct from ENCEPHALITIS, which involves inflammation of the brain only. Both diseases can be serious and even life-threatening, especially in infants and older people. Many different viruses can cause encephalitis or encephalomyelitis, including herpes simplex, chickenpox, measles, mumps, Epstein-Barr, HIV (human immunodeficiency virus), polio, rabies, and mosquitoborne viruses. The bacterium that causes Lyme disease, *Borrelia burgdorferi*, also can cause encephalitis or encephalomyelitis. Symptoms include fever, headache, nausea, vomiting, lethargy, weakness, seizures, stiff neck, memory impairment, and confusion. Diagnosis and treatment require hospitalization. The doctor may order tests such as a lumbar puncture, CT (computed tomography) scanning, MRI (magnetic resonance imaging), or an electroencephalogram (EEG). Treatment includes drugs such as acyclovir and corticosteroids.

Encephalopathy

Any disorder of the brain that involves widespread dysfunction of brain activity. Encephalopathy is characterized by neurological symptoms, such as personality changes, behavior changes, and changes in consciousness. Signs include agitation, confusion, delirium, hallucinations, insomnia, nervousness, palpitations, unsteady gait, and abnormal eye movements. Symptoms may progress to unconsciousness and coma. Causes of encephalopathy include metabolic abnormalities, such as liver or kidney dysfunction, WERNICKE-KORSAKOFF SYNDROME (a brain disorder), lack of oxygen, toxins associated with metabolic abnormality, and diffuse brain damage. If the skin is jaundiced, liver disease may be responsible. Diagnosis usually requires tests such as blood analysis, CT (computed tomography) scanning, and an electroencephalogram (EEG). Hospitalization is usually required. Treatment of encephalopathy usually depends on the underlying cause.

Encopresis

Also known as soiling, a disorder in which children older than age 4 involuntarily pass feces into their clothing. Primary encopresis refers to the disorder in which the child has not yet achieved bowel control. Secondary encopresis occurs when a child who has previously established control loses it. Encopresis is most commonly caused by chronic constipation. Fecal soiling can also result from central nervous system disorders and defects in the nerves and muscles of the anus. Typically, hard stools build up in the bowel and become difficult to pass. Bowel movements are painful. The child may frequently pass watery, foul-smelling stools, which leak past the built-up hard stool. Constipation may be the result of stress, a reluctance to use the toilet, or an inability to sit still long enough to use it. Less commonly, it may be associated with an underlying medical condition such as an inadequate level of thyroid hormone or a weakness of the intestinal muscles. See also TOILET TRAINING.

To evaluate encopresis, a doctor will conduct a thorough physical examination, probing the abdomen to check for hard stool in the bowel. A rectal examination may also be performed to detect hard stools. Physicians sometimes recommend an enema, a rectal suppository, or a stool softener. With treatment, children outgrow encopresis. Because one in four children with this condition may have emotional problems, the pediatrician may also refer the child to a mental health professional. Children should attempt to move their bowels each day. Because eating can stimulate the colon, a child should be encouraged to have a bowel movement after meals. A high-fiber diet and plenty of liquids can soften the stool.

Endarterectomy

A surgical procedure to remove the buildup of fat and cholesterol in an artery and restore normal blood flow. Endarterectomy is most commonly performed on the carotid artery, which supplies blood to the brain, and is known as CAROTID ENDARTERECTOMY.

Endemic

A disease or condition persistently found in a given population or geographical area. An example of a typical endemic disease is the common cold, which affects a portion of the total population each year.

Endocarditis

Inflammation of the endocardium (lining that covers the inside of the heart) and usually the heart valves. The most common cause of endocarditis is infection by bacteria, particularly varieties that normally reside in the mouth, respiratory tract, and intestinal system. The disease can also be caused by fungi. Endocarditis is a serious disease that can cause major damage to the heart valves and is life-threatening.

Endocarditis affects people with underlying heart disease, particularly diseases or defects of the heart valves, heart disease present at birth (congenital), or a history of rheumatic fever. The disease also poses a risk for people who have had a heart valve replaced surgically. Blood tends to clot at damaged areas in the heart lining or around an artificial heart valve, and the clots trap infectious microorganisms, which multiply rapidly and infect the endocardium. Clots and clumps of microorganisms can break free, travel through the bloodstream, and block major blood vessels, most dangerously in the lungs (pulmonary embolism) or brain (stroke).

The symptoms of endocarditis may develop suddenly or slowly. They include fever, chills, weight loss, shortness of breath, fatigue, persistent cough, headache, and joint or chest pain.

Endocarditis is usually treated with antibiotics for at least 6 weeks. If damage to the heart valves is severe, surgery may also be required. Prevention is preferable to treatment. It consists of using antibiotics for those who have had endocarditis or are at

risk for developing it before any dental procedure (including teeth cleaning); before removal of the tonsils or adenoids; before examination of the respiratory tract with a rigid bronchoscope; or before surgery on the intestine, prostate, bladder, or female reproductive system. Maintaining good oral hygiene decreases the risk of developing endocarditis. Excessive alcohol use and intravenous drug use increase the risk of developing the disease.

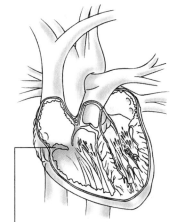

Tricuspid valve with vegetation, inflammation, infection

LIFE-THREATENING INFECTION
Endocarditis occurs when the endocardium (smooth lining of the heart) is damaged, and bacteria are present in the bloodstream. The endocardium becomes inflamed and infected, especially around the valves. Vegetation (a mixture of blood cells and bacteria) forms and interferes with heart function.

Endocrine glands

See ENDOCRINE SYSTEM.

Endocrine system

A group of glands and organs that secrete hormones (chemical messengers) directly into the bloodstream to help regulate many essential body processes, including metabolism, growth, and sexual functioning. (By contrast, exocrine glands secrete substances through ducts into or onto organs [see EXOCRINE GLAND].)

In the brain, the HYPOTHALAMUS secretes hormones that direct the production and release of hormones by another brain structure—the PITUITARY GLAND. The pituitary is sometimes called the master gland because it secretes hormones to stimulate other

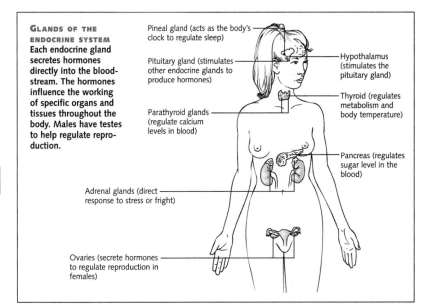

GLANDS OF THE ENDOCRINE SYSTEM
Each endocrine gland secretes hormones directly into the bloodstream. The hormones influence the working of specific organs and tissues throughout the body. Males have testes to help regulate reproduction.

Pineal gland (acts as the body's clock to regulate sleep)

Pituitary gland (stimulates other endocrine glands to produce hormones)

Parathyroid glands (regulate calcium levels in blood)

Hypothalamus (stimulates the pituitary gland)

Thyroid (regulates metabolism and body temperature)

Pancreas (regulates sugar level in the blood)

Adrenal glands (direct response to stress or fright)

Ovaries (secrete hormones to regulate reproduction in females)

glands throughout the body to produce specialized hormones—in effect orchestrating major body functions. The hypothalamus detects shortages or oversupplies of hormones in the blood and causes the pituitary gland to vary its gland-stimulating hormones accordingly.

The PARATHYROID GLANDS, located in the throat, make parathyroid hormone, which regulates the level of calcium, an essential nutrient, in the blood. The thyroid gland, which sits between the parathyroids, secretes thyroxine and triiodothyronine—hormones that regulate metabolism and body temperature—as well as calcitonin, which helps bones absorb calcium.

The adrenal glands, which are on top of the kidneys, produce corticosteroid hormones, which influence many body processes at a cellular level and are part of the body's response to stress; epinephrine, also called adrenaline, which helps the body respond immediately to stress and danger; and aldosterone, which controls the level of salt in the body.

The PANCREAS secretes insulin and glucagon, which control the levels of sugar, fats, and proteins in the blood. In women, the ovaries secrete estrogen and progesterone, the sex hormones that regulate reproductive function; similarly in men, the testicles produce testosterone, the sex hormone that directs sexual and reproductive functions.

Endocrinologist

A doctor trained in the diagnosis, treatment, and management of diseases and disorders of the endocrine glands, including the hypothalamus, pituitary gland, thyroid gland, parathyroid glands, thymus gland, adrenal glands, pancreas, ovaries in women, and testicles in men. Disorders that may be treated by an endocrinologist include growth hormone deficiency, thyroid disorders, adrenal disorders, menopausal difficulties, osteoporosis, cholesterol disorders, high blood pressure, and obesity.

Endocrinology

The field of medical science that concentrates on the endocrine glands, including the structure and function of these glands and the hormones they secrete. The endocrine system is composed of the hypothalamus, pituitary gland, thyroid gland, parathyroid glands, thymus gland, adrenal glands, pancreas, ovaries in women, and testicles in men. These glands regulate the flow of hormones throughout the body. Hormones have a role in almost every vital aspect of the function of the body, determining a person's rate of growth and maturation and directly influencing such important human characteristics as intelligence and physical agility. Hormones also have a role in a person's sexual drive.

Endodontics

The branch of dentistry concerned with the treatment of diseases or injuries that affect the nerves and pulp in teeth and the tissues in the gum. Endodontics primarily deals with the removal of dental pulp (ROOT CANAL TREATMENT). Root canal treatment is necessary when the dental pulp is injured because of deep decay or trauma. The pulp is removed; the canal is sterilized and then filled with a special medicated dressing. The tooth may then be restored like any other tooth.

Endodontist

A dentist who has received additional training to treat the nerves and pulp in teeth and gum tissue. Endodontists are trained and skilled in ROOT CANAL TREATMENT, as well as procedures that involve the root canals, nerves, blood supply inside the teeth, and the root tips of the teeth. A dentist in general practice may refer a patient to an endodontist when more extensive, specialized care is necessary.

End-of-life care

Care at the end of life that relieves symptoms but neither hastens nor postpones death. End-of-life care may include a medical decision to withdraw treatment or not to initiate a potentially ineffective treatment. End-of-life care may include stopping delivery of food and fluids by tube. In end-of-life care, it is acceptable to give high doses of pain medication even if it compromises respiration because the medical intention is clearly to relieve pain rather than to shorten life.

HOW HOSPICE CARE WORKS

In earlier times, most people died in their own homes surrounded by family and loved ones. Modern medical care of the 20th century resulted in many people spending their last days in a hospital. Renewed interest in home care for the dying spurred development in the field of HOSPICE care, which is a special course of treatment available to terminally ill individuals and includes their families as a part of the care team. Hospice care or palliative care allows people to spend their final days in their home or in a homelike setting with people who love them and

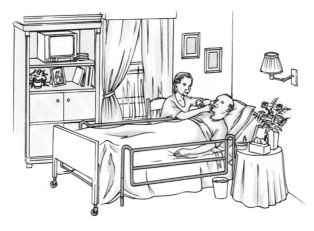

AT-HOME CARE
Hospice services may enable a terminally ill person to die at home. Hospice workers are available 24 hours a day to provide assistance and advice about relief of pain or other symptoms, to run errands, or to give family members a break from the demands of care.

where the focus is on relieving symptoms.

Most hospice care is provided at a person's home but may also be provided in a nursing home, assisted living residence, or residential hospice. Hospice care shifts the focus of attention from prolonging life to maximizing the quality of life remaining.

The purpose of hospice care is to help the person who is dying and the person's family handle the challenges of a terminal illness or condition during the final phase of life. The nature of these challenges may be physical, emotional, social, and spiritual. Hospices also offer bereavement services for grieving family members.

COSTS OF HOSPICE

Reduced medical expenses may be another factor in the choice of hospice care. The cost of end-of-life care is usually greatly reduced when a person moves from acute care to palliative care. Medicare and most private insurance plans, including managed care plans, cover hospice care. In some states, hospice care is covered by Medicaid. Some hospice programs provide care and services regardless of ability to pay. Hospices are usually run by nonprofit, independent organizations, and the programs may be affiliated with hospitals, nursing homes, or home health care agencies.

FAMILY AND VOLUNTEER INVOLVEMENT IN HOSPICE CARE

Hospice care is based on the concept of a cooperative effort among the dying person's family, friends, and a team of professional caregivers working together. A hospice team made up of professionals and trained volunteers is

led by the attending physician. A nurse usually organizes the daily care of the patient, while social workers and chaplains are generally available for counseling. Trained volunteers may perform a wide variety of roles that range from acting as companions to helping with light housekeeping, meal preparation, and errands.

The hospice team can offer instruction and support to family and friends who wish to care for a person at the end of his or her life. Hospice team members may have a more or less active role, depending on the needs and desires of the family.

Medical professionals suggest that adults in good health aged 18 years or older make decisions about their own end-of-life care. These decisions can be recorded as ADVANCE DIRECTIVES, which are legal documents that serve to communicate a person's wishes if he or she becomes unable to do so. Advance directives are fol-

lowed by health care personnel to the fullest extent possible and conform to a standard of reasonable medical practice.

Endogenous

Developing in or originating within the body. Endogenous cholesterol, for example, is cholesterol that is made inside the body rather than consumed in the diet.

Endometrial ablation

A surgical procedure used to treat abnormal bleeding from the uterus by eliminating tissue in the lining of the uterus. An alternative to HYSTERECTOMY, endometrial ablation is a relatively new approach to abnormal uterine bleeding, especially during menopause. An instrument called a hysteroscope is used to visualize the inside of the uterus and to cauterize (use heat to destroy cells and stop bleeding) its lining by one of several methods that may include laser or electronic heat probes. The advantages of endometrial ablation over a hysterectomy include shorter hospitalization and recovery time and fewer serious complications.

Surgery for uterine bleeding is always a treatment of last resort and, in most cases, is considered only when other treatments, such as HORMONE REPLACEMENT THERAPY, have failed. Some doctors are concerned about a possibility that endometrial ablation may promote cancer of the uterus by burying glandular tissue under scar tissue.

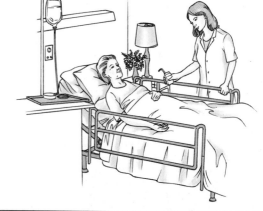

A NURSING HOME SETTING
End-of-life care in a nursing home or hospital setting is often provided by a separate organization whose employees work with the medical staff as well as the family. The focus of the care is on relieving the person's immediate discomforts (with medication, counseling, and other therapies) and supporting and counseling friends and family.

E

Endometrial biopsy

A procedure in which a tissue sample is taken from the lining (ENDOMETRI- UM) of a woman's uterus to examine it for signs of overgrowth or cancer. An endometrial biopsy may be recom- mended to evaluate abnormal bleed- ing, to screen for cancer of the uterine lining, or in an infertility evaluation, to help assess whether the uterine lining is normal.

To perform the procedure the doctor uses a speculum to open the woman's vagina and then stabilizes the cervix with a clamp. The woman may feel a pinching sensation when the clamp is applied. The doctor then inserts a long, thin, flexible tube into the uterus to remove a tiny piece of tis- sue. The tissue is sent to a pathologist for microscopic detection of any ab- normal or cancerous cells.

Endometrial cancer

A malignant growth of the uterus. Endometrial cancer, which usually develops after menopause, is the most common reproductive cancer in women. If detected and treated in an early stage, it is most often curable. Symptoms commonly include vagi- nal bleeding or spotting in a woman who has completed menopause or abnormal bleeding at any age, such as unusually heavy menstrual flow or bleeding between menstrual periods. Pain and discomfort are usually expe- rienced only in advanced stages of the disease. After menopause, any vaginal bleeding other than that asso- ciated with HORMONE REPLACEMENT THERAPY must be considered abnor- mal and should be reported to the doctor as soon as possible.

Endometrial cancer is most com- mon between the ages of 50 and 70 years and is rare in younger women. The risk factors for endometrial can- cer are related to increased exposure to the hormone estrogen. Obesity, for example, is a risk factor because fat cells convert certain hormones into excess estrogen. Starting menstrua- tion early or menopause late exposes women to estrogen over more years. Having irregular ovulation or men- struation subjects women to risk because the hormone progesterone does not adequately counterbalance the estrogen. The same is true for women who use long-term estrogen replacement therapy that is not com-

REMOVING TISSUE FOR BIOPSY
To do an endometrial biopsy, the doctor will widen the vagina with a speculum and then use a clamp called a tenacu- lum to hold the cervix steady. He or she will gently insert an instru- ment called a pipette, which is a small suction device, to remove a small piece of tissue from the lining of the uterus (the endo-metrium).

bined with progesterone. Women are also at risk if they have a history of infertility; POLYCYSTIC OVARIAN SYN- DROME; ENDOMETRIAL HYPERPLASIA; or cancer of the ovaries, breast, or colon.

Diagnosis can be made at an early, curable stage with the help of an endometrial biopsy. Sometimes vagi- nal ultrasound, performed for other reasons, inadvertently detects an abnormal thickening of the endo- metrium, a possible sign of endome- trial cancer. A biopsy can then be per- formed for diagnosis. A HYSTEROSCOPY can be used to examine the inside of the uterus for abnormalities. Treatment includes a HYSTERECTOMY to remove the cancer and find out whether it has spread to the lymph nodes or other organs. Some women with endometrial cancer require RADI- ATION THERAPY in addition to a hys- terectomy.

Endometrial hyperplasia

An overgrowth of the lining of the uterus. Endometrial hyperplasia is thought to result from a relative excess of estrogen and is sometimes considered a precancerous condition, especially in women who are begin- ning or have completed menopause. This condition is almost always non- cancerous in younger women, and it is easily treatable at all ages. Its most common symptom is abnormal vagi- nal bleeding. This can include any bleeding after menopause or unusual- ly long or heavy periods or bleeding between periods before menopause.

Diagnosis is usually made by

endometrial biopsy, which can help differentiate hyperplasia from endometrial cancer or polyps. A D AND C (dilation and curettage), in which endometrial tissue is scraped away, may be done to obtain cells for microscopic examination. A D and C can sometimes be used to eliminate the hyperplasia at the same time that the diagnosis is made. Sometimes, a doctor prescribes progesterone or birth control pills containing both estrogen and progesterone for young- er women with abnormal vaginal bleeding to attempt to regulate men- struation. The progesterone offsets the excessive estrogen supply. In a woman near or past menopause, progesterone may be used to treat hyperplasia. If bleeding continues, however, a hysterectomy may be required.

Endometrial polyp

A spongy growth attached to the inner lining of the uterus (ENDOMETRI- UM) by a stalk that protrudes into the uterine cavity. An endometrial polyp sometimes can extend through the cervix and may even reach into the vagina. While endometrial polyps can occur at any age, they occur most frequently during the 10 years before menopause or during menopause. Symptoms may include cramping, irregular menstruation, and bleeding after intercourse. If the polyp has become twisted or injured, it may become infected, producing a foul- smelling discharge. In some women, endometrial polyps cause no symp- toms at all.

A woman with symptoms of endometrial polyps will typically have a PAP SMEAR or a biopsy to rule out cancer, because similar symptoms occur for ENDOMETRIAL CANCER and cancer of the cervix (see CERVIX, CANCER OF). Once cancer has been ruled out, the doctor may recommend a D AND C (dilation and curettage) or HYSTEROSCOPY to examine the polyps and remove them. If more polyps develop or if abnormal vaginal bleeding continues, particularly in women who have gone through menopause, some doctors recommend HYSTEREC-TOMY (removal of the uterus). See also CERVICAL POLYPS.

Endometrioma

A cyst formed when endometrial tissue, which typically forms the lining of the uterus, becomes attached outside the uterus, usually to an ovary. Symptoms include severe pain in the lower abdomen, pain during sexual intercourse, irregular or delayed menstrual periods, or a dull ache or feeling of pressure in the lower abdomen. Endometriomas, sometimes called chocolate cysts because of their color, are a form of ENDOMETRIOSIS and are treated with the same methods.

Endometriosis

FOR SYMPTOM CHART
see Menstrual cramps or pain, page 16

A condition in which the type of tissue (endometrial) that normally lines the uterus is found outside the uterus, most often as a cyst on the ovaries, fallopian tubes, the ligaments attached to the uterus, or the exterior of the uterus. Less often, endometriosis occurs on the surfaces of the bladder, bowel, or vagina. The tissue grows and bleeds during MEN-STRUATION, just as it would if it were in the uterus. Endometriosis is common, especially among women in their 30s and 40s, although it can also occur in adolescent females. The condition affects about 10 percent of women who are of childbearing age.

Endometriosis frequently causes pain, especially just before or during the first few days of the menstrual period. It may also be associated with abnormal menstrual bleeding. The pain is usually mild but can be severe. Some women

who have endometriosis experience backaches or pain when they defecate or have sexual intercourse. The symptoms of endometriosis often worsen over time, although some women have no symptoms. Because endometriosis can cause infertility, women sometimes discover that they have it only when they visit a doctor to find out why they have not become pregnant.

The cause of endometriosis is unclear. It may be caused by menstrual blood backing up and carrying endometrial cells from inside the uterus into the fallopian tubes or elsewhere, where they attach and grow. Possibly, a flaw in the immune system allows endometrial tissue to grow outside the uterus more easily in some women than in others. Heredity probably plays a role, as a woman whose mother, sister, or daughter has endometriosis is more likely to develop it herself.

DIAGNOSIS AND TREATMENT

When endometriosis is suspected, based on symptoms and a pelvic examination, the doctor may perform a LAPAROSCOPY under general anesthesia to confirm the diagnosis. In this procedure, a small opening is made near the woman's navel, and a thin illuminated scope is inserted into the abdomen, enabling the doctor to see the pelvic organs. A tissue sample may be removed during a BIOPSY to check for cancer cells, although endometriosis is almost never cancerous. Abnormal endometrial tissue can be removed during a laparoscopy using additional tools that cut it out or burn it out with heat or a laser. Mild cases often require no treatment. For women with infertility problems or significant symptoms, endometriosis can be treated with hormone therapy, surgery, or a combination of both. Hormone therapy may include taking oral contraceptives (birth control pills); gonadotropin-releasing hormone (GnRH) agonists, hormones that stop the ovaries from making estrogen; danazol, a synthetic hormone that stops menstruation; or progestin, the hormone that regulates menstruation.

Extensive endometriosis may require a laparotomy, a procedure in which a bigger incision than for a laparoscopy is made, giving access

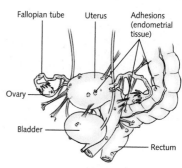

TISSUE OUTSIDE UTERUS
In endometriosis, bits of tissue from the lining of the uterus (endometrial tissue) escape from the uterus and attach on the ovaries, fallopian tubes, and other organs in the area. The tissue forms abnormal scars and scar tissues called adhesions. The tissue builds up and bleeds each month, just as it would in the uterus. Abnormal endometrial tissue usually can be removed with a laparoscope.

to a larger area for removal of endometrial tissue. If endometriosis returns after surgery and causes severe pain that is not controllable with medication, the doctor may recommend the surgical removal of the uterus (HYSTERECTOMY), the ovaries (OOPHORECTOMY), or both. Removing the uterus may dissipate the pain, while removing the ovaries eliminates the hormonal stimulus for endometriosis.

Endometritis

An inflammation of the endometrium, the lining of the uterus. Postpartum endometritis is a bacterial infection that typically develops in a woman several days after giving birth. It is the most common infection seen just after childbirth. Symptoms include fever, tenderness of the uterus, and tachycardia (an accelerated heart rate). Treatment includes bed rest, fluids given by mouth and by intravenous drip, and antibiotics.

The most common risk factor for endometritis is having had a CESARE-AN SECTION; endometritis is always much more severe for such patients. Poverty, poor nutrition, obesity, and having sexual intercourse near the end of a pregnancy all are risk factors for the infection. Endometritis may also be seen after other procedures in which the uterine cavity has been penetrated, such as a D AND E, a D AND C, or a HYSTEROSCOPY.

Endometrium

The tissue that lines the uterus. The endometrium is pink and velvety and consists of glandular tissue that undergoes cyclical monthly changes under the influence of hormones. After menstruation, it is thin, gradually becoming thicker until 1 week after ovulation. If conception does not occur, the endometrium sheds its surface during menstruation.

Endorphins

Hormones that are released by certain regions of the brain and function as chemical neurotransmitters to help control a person's response to pain and stress. Endorphins act as natural painkillers and can also help elevate a person's mood. Intense physical exercise can trigger the release of endorphins, producing a sense of well-being and suppressing sensations of pain. Feelings of euphoria sometimes experienced by athletes during intense levels of physical exertion are the result of endorphin release.

Endoscope

An instrument used to examine the interior of a body cavity. An endoscope may be inserted through a small incision or through one of the body's openings. Examples of endoscopes include the gastroscope, used to examine the inside of the stomach, and the auriscope or otoscope, used to examine the inside of the ear canal. An endoscope usually has a light at one end, and some have a miniature video camera that transmits an image to the doctor's eye. See ENDOSCOPY.

Endoscopic retrograde cholangiopancreatography

See ERCP.

Endoscopy

A procedure in which interior parts of the body are examined by using a slim, flexible, lighted tube called an endoscope. Endoscopy allows a doctor to view, photograph, and videotape the inside of the body without surgery. The procedure can detect abnormalities that do not appear on X rays. Causes of symptoms can be diagnosed, and tiny instruments may

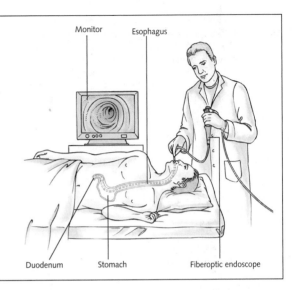

VIEWING THE UPPER DIGESTIVE TRACT To examine the upper digestive tract, the doctor inserts a flexible viewing instrument, called an endoscope, through the mouth and down into the esophagus, stomach, and duodenum. The endoscope images the digestive tract on a monitor, enabling the doctor to locate and diagnose disease. The doctor can also insert instruments through the tube to remove samples or to perform minor surgery.

Monitor   Esophagus

Duodenum   Stomach   Fiberoptic endoscope

be passed through the endoscope to perform minor surgery or remove samples of tissue for analysis (see BIOPSY).

Endoscopies are often performed to view the digestive tract, lungs, urinary system, and joints such as the knee. Commonly performed types of digestive tract endoscopy include gastroscopy and colonoscopy. Bronchoscopy is used to view the lining of the lungs, while cystoscopy is used to view the bladder. In some cases, instruments are inserted through natural openings in the body. For example, in gastroscopy, a gastroscope is passed through the mouth to examine the esophagus, stomach, and duodenum. In colonoscopy, a colonoscope is passed through the anus to view the inside of the digestive tract. Sometimes, such as for examination of the knee or arteries, a small incision is made and the endoscope is inserted through it.

During the procedure, the person wears a hospital gown and lies on an examination table. Depending on the type of endoscopy, a mild oral or intravenous sedative or local or general anesthesia may be given. Endoscopies generally last from 30 minutes to 2 hours.

Endothelium

The smooth layer of cells that forms the interior lining of the heart, the blood and lymphatic vessels, and the cavities of the body.

Endotoxin

A poisonous material shed by the outer membranes of certain types of disease-causing bacteria, particularly when they are disturbed or destroyed. Endotoxin is responsible for the symptoms arising from infection with these bacteria. Small amounts of endotoxin produce fever and lower resistance to infection. Large amounts can lead to internal bleeding, heart failure, low blood pressure, and severe diarrhea.

Endotracheal tube

A thin, flexible breathing tube inserted through the mouth or nose and into the windpipe (TRACHEA) past the vocal cords. An endotracheal tube is used to aid breathing during general anesthesia by attaching the exposed end of the tube to a ventilator, which pumps air into and out of the lungs of the person. It is also used after a traumatic injury to secure and protect the airway and help the person continue to breathe.

Most endotracheal tubes have a wraparound balloon at the end that is inflated below the vocal cords to seal the airway and prevent material regurgitated by the stomach from passing around the tube into the lungs, an event that can be life-threatening.

Inserting an endotracheal tube carries a slight risk of damage to the teeth or vocal cords. The most common complication is a mild sore

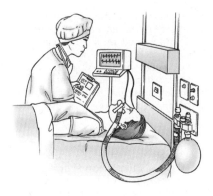

BREATHING WHILE ANESTHETIZED
To maintain breathing function for a person under general anesthetic, the doctor places an endotracheal tube through the mouth or nose and down the trachea (windpipe). The tube is attached to a ventilator that mechanically pumps air in and out of the lungs until the person has recovered and is able to breathe normally. The ventilator adjusts the air supply according to the person's requirements.

throat after the tube is withdrawn. This lasts for several days after surgery and usually has no permanent effect.

End-stage renal disease
See KIDNEY FAILURE.

Enema
A liquid instilled from a tube or syringe into the rectum. The liquid is retained for a predetermined time, until it is released by defecation or drained away following a procedure. Enemas are used for treatment of constipation or for medical diagnosis, such as a barium enema, a type of X-ray procedure of the lower gastrointestinal tract.

Energy
The calories provided by food used for the body's growth, tissue repair, and physical activity. In nutrition, calories represent the amount of energy contained in foods or the amount of energy expended by a person. To maintain a constant weight, the amount of energy or calories supplied by the diet should not exceed the amount of energy a person expends (see CALORIE REQUIREMENTS). Growth and recovery from injury, illness, or surgery increase an individual's energy requirements. Carbohydrates and fats

are the body's main sources of energy. Excess energy is stored in the body as fat.

When deprived of carbohydrates and fats, the body begins to break down proteins into glucose to produce energy. While protein contributes calories, it should not be the primary source of energy. To be used for energy, protein must be broken down, releasing nitrogen, which is then excreted in the urine. Excess protein increases the workload of the kidneys. However, sufficient protein should be consumed to provide a sufficient source of amino acids, an important building block of tissues and other vital compounds.

Energy medicine
Therapies intended to restore balance and harmony to the body by harnessing vital energy. Some energy therapies derive from ancient Asian medicine, such as CHINESE MEDICINE, based on the idea that a person can be physically, emotionally, and spiritually healthy only when his or her life force is in correct balance. The aim of all energy therapies is to restore and prevent imbalances in the life force.

LIFE FORCE
The life force is a concept with no real equivalent in Western cultures or in Western medicine. Chinese medicine calls it qi ("chee"); Japanese

practitioners of Shiatsu massage call it ki ("key"); and in ayurveda, which comes from India, it is called prana. Energy is thought to flow throughout the body, through a system of meridians, or channels, as a function of dual opposing forces, called yin and yang. Energy therapies seek to make the body's life force flow freely by bringing it into balance.

METHODS OF BALANCING THE LIFE FORCE
Some energy therapies seek to avoid ill health rather than to treat existing illness or symptoms. YOGA, T'AI CHI, and CHAKRA BALANCING, for example, all seek to achieve and maintain a state of peace and happiness so that ill health may be avoided. QIGONG is a form of energy medicine that literally means "working with energy"; it is an element of Chinese medicine that promotes health by strengthening the flow of qi, or energy, throughout the body.

Other remedies, such as ACUPUNCTURE, ACUPRESSURE, REFLEXOLOGY, REIKI, and THERAPEUTIC TOUCH, are intended to treat specific ailments or symptoms. These methods are used to adjust the flow of qi in particular body organs. Therapies are always individualized, and some can be taught to individuals so that they can practice them on their own. In all energy therapies, lifestyle and diet are important considerations.

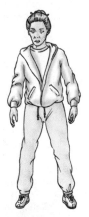

Opening posture: "Emptiness"

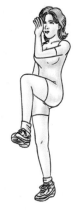

"Golden rooster stands on one leg"

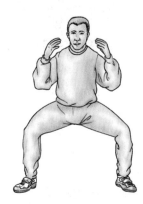

"The horse stance"

HEALING POSTURES
Qigong, an ancient Chinese practice, seeks to heal by harnessing the body's bioelectric energy through structured exercises or postures; relief of stress is a primary goal. A qigong master teaches the exercises to the person, who can then continue them at home. Qigong can be used to complement Western medicine.

E

Energy requirements

See CALORIE REQUIREMENTS.

Engagement

The first of eight stages of movement that a baby makes in childbirth. At the engagement stage, the baby's head typically settles against the top of the cervix. See DELIVERY, VAGINAL.

Enkephalins

Pain-relieving chemicals produced in the body. Enkephalins are located in the brain and spinal cord. Their function is to inhibit neurotransmitters in the passage of pain perception. This helps to reduce the emotional perception as well as the physical reality of pain.

Enlarged prostate

See PROSTATE, ENLARGED.

Enophthalmos

Backward displacement (inward sinking) of the eyeball into the socket.

Enoxaparin sodium

A drug that prevents blood clots during or after surgery. An anticoagulant, enoxaparin sodium (Lovenox) is used to prevent blood clots from traveling through the bloodstream to lodge in a small blood vessel. The drug is given as an injection.

ENT

Ear, nose, and throat physician or surgeon. See OTOLARYNGOLOGIST.

Entacapone

A drug used to treat Parkinson disease. Entacapone (Comtan) is used along with LEVODOPA AND CARBIDOPA to treat Parkinson disease because it increases levels of levodopa in the blood, which helps more of the drug get into the brain.

Enteric fever

See TYPHOID FEVER.

Enteritis

See CROHN DISEASE.

Enterocele

A condition in which a portion of the intestines bulges into the top of the vagina. An enterocele can cause lower back pain and pressure in the pelvic area. It is most common in women after menopause, particularly those who have given birth many times, are obese, or have conditions that cause chronic coughing, which puts pressure on abdominal muscles. Surgical repair is possible.

Enteroclysis

A fluoroscopic X-ray examination of the small intestine using a CONTRAST MEDIUM. In fluoroscopy, the gastrointestinal organs deep within the body can be seen as images projected onto a computerlike screen or monitor.

WHY IT IS PERFORMED

Enteroclysis is the most effective method of examining the inside of the small intestine to diagnose polyps, ulcers, tumors, adhesions, and partial bowel obstruction.

HOW IT IS PERFORMED

The person undergoing the test needs to follow a clear liquid diet and not smoke or take certain medications for at least 24 hours before the test.

To start the procedure, a tube is inserted into the nose or mouth. The tube is manipulated past the stomach and into the duodenum, which can cause discomfort. A pump infuses a contrast medium at a controlled rate through the tube. The flow rate of the contrast medium causes the small intestine to dilate at a site of obstruction. The movement of the contrast medium is visualized via images displayed on the monitor. X rays are made at intervals to establish a permanent film record.

Enterostomy

An operation in which a surgeon creates a connection between the small intestine and a stoma or opening in the abdominal wall, allowing for emptying of the feces into a bag attached to the skin. Less commonly, the stoma is created to accommodate a feeding tube. An enterostomy is sometimes referred to simply as an ostomy. An enterostomy is sometimes necessary in severe cases of intestinal disorders, such as CROHN DISEASE, COLITIS, and cancer.

An enterostomy is referred to as an ILEOSTOMY when the lower part of the small intestine (the ileum) opens through the stoma and a jejunostomy when the middle part of the small intestine (the jejunum) does so. Enterostomies can be temporary or permanent. If temporary, the stoma is surgically closed once the intestine has recovered from inflammation or surgery or when a feeding tube is no longer necessary. A permanent enterostomy requires keeping the stoma clean and regularly emptying of the bag of waste.

Enterotoxin

A bacterial toxin that causes an adverse reaction in the lining of the intestine. Enterotoxin is produced by certain types of bacteria, such as *Staphylococcus* (see STAPHYLOCOCCAL INFECTIONS). Reactions to enterotoxin infection include vomiting, diarrhea, cramps, and other symptoms of food poisoning. Only supportive care is required because the illness passes spontaneously.

Entropion

Inward turning of the eyelid. Entropion usually affects the lower eyelid and causes the skin of the eyelid and the eyelashes to rub against the surface of the eye. The rubbing can lead to excess tearing, crusting of the eyelid, mucus discharge, the feeling that something is in the eye, irritation of the clear outer covering of the eye (cornea), and impaired vision. Scarring of the cornea can result, which may lead to some vision loss. Entropion usually develops with age, as muscles relax and weaken. It can also result from scarring of the eyelid caused by burns, injury, skin cancer, or eyelid surgery. Artificial tears, which are available over-the-counter as eye drops, can be used to alleviate dryness and prevent complications. Surgery to alleviate entropion is effective and should be performed before

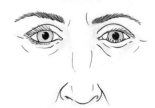

A ROLLED LOWER LID
Entropion, usually the result of aging, causes the lower eyelid to turn inward so that the lashes brush against the cornea. Surgery to tighten the lid can be done before the cornea is damaged. Recovery from the surgery takes about a week, and the eye will feel more comfortable.

permanent damage occurs. Usually done as an outpatient procedure under local anesthesia, the surgery tightens the ligament and tissues that hold the eyelid in place.

Enuresis

The medical term for involuntary BED-WETTING during sleep.

Environmental medicine

A branch of medicine concerned with illnesses that are caused by pollutants or toxins. These include problems such as food allergies (see FOOD ALLERGY) and HAY FEVER. In some cases, environmental practitioners use a variety of holistic and homeopathic treatments, as well as regular pharmaceutical therapies.

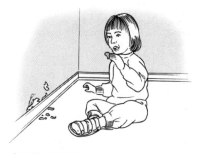

LEAD POISONING
The lead found in some paints is a widely publicized environmental toxin. Children may eat chips of peeling paint or inhale dangerous amounts of dust from lead-based paints. Treatment involves preventing further exposure and using chelating agents that bind to the lead in the body and carry it out in the urine.

Enzyme

A protein that promotes or accelerates a specific chemical reaction. Substances acted on by enzymes are called substrates. Most enzymes are manufactured in small quantities, and their function is to catalyze chemical reactions in cells. However, digestive enzymes are produced in large quantities by the salivary glands, stomach, pancreas, and small intestine. These enzymes act in the digestive tract to break down the fats, carbohydrates, and proteins in food into smaller chemical components that the body can absorb.

Enzyme therapy

The use of enzyme supplements to cure disease. Enzymes are catalysts for virtually all the chemical processes of the body, and digestive enzymes are essential for the breakdown of food into nutrients that can be absorbed and converted to energy. Enzyme therapy is based on the idea that since cooking and processing food destroys the enzymes in it, people should eat food raw or take supplements to restore the missing enzymes. Without enzyme supplements, believers in enzyme therapy contend that large amounts of undigested food accumulate in the body, where they rot, ferment, and contribute to many physical problems. This view is disputed by medical experts, who believe that the body's enzyme supply is adequate to digest the food consumed by most people and that enzyme supplements taken orally do not work.

Ependymoma

The third most common type of childhood brain tumor. An ependymoma develops from cells of the ependyma (the membrane lining the ventricles and the central canal of the spinal cord). Symptoms of this tumor include headache, vomiting, and an unsteady gait. Ependymomas are graded based on how abnormal their cells appear under the microscope. Tumors with cells that are more similar to normal cells are considered low-grade tumors, while very abnormal-appearing cells are considered high-grade tumors and represent more aggressive tumors with a poor prognosis. Treatment options include surgery, radiation, and chemotherapy.

Ephedrine

A popular nonprescription decongestant that acts by releasing epinephrine from nerve cells to relieve nasal congestion. Derived from *Ephedra*, the scientific name for an Asian plant, the decongestant acts as a stimulant and is often abused for that reason.

Epicondylitis

A painful condition caused by inflammation or minor tears of the tendons near the elbow, which are attached to muscles in the forearm. When the forearm muscles that flex the wrist are involved, the condition may be called GOLFER'S ELBOW. If the muscles that extend the wrist are involved, the condition is often termed TENNIS ELBOW. Elbow pain is caused by a movement that involves the combination of pressure on the wrist while it is being rotated. The combined movements involved with overuse of the forearm muscles may occur during sports activities, including golf, tennis, or rowing, or in the course of everyday activities, such as the use of a manual screwdriver. Forceful and repetitive gripping, particularly with the elbow extended, may cause this condition. The most effective preventive measure is for a person to hold the wrist in a stable and neutral position when the forearm muscles are engaged, when force is being used, or when pressure is applied to the wrist. Treatment includes rest, cold packs, ultrasound, splinting, nonsteroidal anti-inflammatory drugs (NSAIDs), corticosteroid injections, and elbow stretching exercises. Sometimes, a surgical procedure to release the affected tendons may be necessary.

Epidemic

An extensive outbreak of a disease, most commonly a contagious or infectious disease, that usually spreads rapidly within a community or region and affects a large number of people at the same time. Epidemics tend to occur suddenly and involve more cases of disease than could be anticipated. The cause of the rapid spread of a disease may be person-to-person contact (especially when overcrowding occurs) or contamination of the public drinking water or general food source.

Epidemiology

The study of the occurrence and distribution of diseases in large populations, including the conditions influencing the spread and severity of disease. Epidemiology is a medical science that investigates and traces the general causes of disease within a given population or among several populations, as well as the source of isolated outbreaks of a specific disease.

Epidemiology undertakes to discover the direct relationship between causative agents and the illnesses they produce, for example, the association of microorganisms, including viruses and bacteria, with infectious diseases. Epidemiological researchers also conduct investigations into the causes of chronic diseases such as heart disease and cancer. As a result of these investigations, it has been

E

discovered that elements of a person's eating habits and other behaviors are linked to certain chronic diseases.

Among the discoveries made in the field of epidemiology in recent decades are the causes of sudden outbreaks of previously unknown illnesses. For example, epidemiologists discovered a new microorganism that had not been previously identified and was found to be the cause of LEGIONNAIRES DISEASE. Epidemiology is the medical science responsible for the identification of the retrovirus now known as HIV (human immunodeficiency virus) as the main cause of AIDS (acquired immunodeficiency syndrome).

Epidermal cyst

A closed sac filled with oily or fatty fluid and debris; also known as a sebaceous cyst. Epidermal cysts commonly develop on the face, neck, upper chest, and back. They are usually benign (not cancerous) and do not require treatment. However, in some cases, epidermal cysts grow large and painful or become infected. Treatment is with antibiotics and, as necessary, surgical incision and drainage or surgical excision (cutting out the cyst).

Epidermis

The outer layer of the SKIN. The epidermis itself has four layers, from the outside in: horny, granular, spiny, and basal layers. Cells in the basal layer divide constantly to form new cells, which push up toward the surface. Typically it takes 4 weeks for cells to move from the basal layer to the granular and another 2 weeks to reach the top layer, where they flake off after another 4 weeks.

Epidermolysis bullosa

A rare inherited disorder characterized by blistering of the skin from very minor injuries. In all types of epidermolysis bullosa, the genetic defects prevent the various layers of the skin from adhering properly to each other, creating areas of structural weakness. The fragile skin that results is apt to become blistered from mild friction, even from everyday activities. Blisters can form outside of the body and on the inside of the mouth, the inside of the throat, and on the lining of the eyes and the anus. Epidermolysis bullosa appears in about one of 100,000 babies born in the United States.

Epidermolysis bullosa exists in three main types. Symptoms are of varying severity, even within types. Blisters on the skin may affect specific areas of the body, such as the feet and hands, but can appear all over the body. In milder forms of epidermolysis bullosa, blisters may heal normally without damaging the skin permanently, while in other forms, blisters may leave permanent scars that fuse fingers together or scar the hands and reduce movement. Epidermolysis bullosa can be life-threatening in early infancy. Blisters and scarring in the mouth and throat can lead to infection, anemia, and malnutrition. There is no cure for epidermolysis bullosa; the prognosis can range from mildly disabling to severely debilitating or fatal. People with milder forms may only have periods of temporary disability. The more severe forms can be devastating, and families often require counseling.

Epididymal cyst

See SPERMATOCELE.

Epididymis

A twisted duct, attached to the back side of each testicle within the scrotum. The epididymis, about 20 feet long, connects the vas efferens (tube emerging from the testicle) with the vas deferens (a tube or duct leading into the urethra). Sperm produced in the testicle move into and through the epididymis, where they mature over the next 10 to 20 days until they have the ability to move and fertilize an egg if released. See REPRODUCTIVE SYSTEM, MALE.

Epididymitis

Infection and inflammation of the epididymis, the tubular structure on the upper part of the testicle. If the testicle is also inflamed, the condition is known as epididymo-orchitis. Epididymitis is caused by bacteria from SEXUALLY TRANSMITTED DISEASES, such as gonorrhea, chlamydia, or infections of the urinary tract or prostate that infect the epididymis. It can also be a complication of surgical removal of the prostate (called a prostatectomy) or the use of a tube for urination (catheter). Symptoms can include pain, usually quite

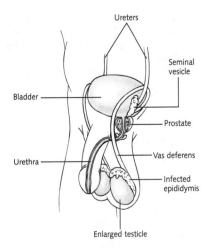

INFECTION OF THE EPIDIDYMIS
The epididymis, a structure on top of each testicle in which sperm mature, can become infected and inflamed. The infection can easily spread to a testicle, causing enlargement. The infection, called epididymitis, can occur as a result of a sexually transmitted disease, other infection, or surgery.

severe and aggravated by bowel movements, and may reach into the groin and lower abdomen. Other symptoms include rapid, painful swelling of the back of the scrotum and testicle to as much as twice the normal size in only 3 to 4 hours; a temperature of up to 104°F; discharge from the penis; and pain during urination or ejaculation. Tests are performed to determine the bacterial cause of the infection, which is treated with appropriate antibiotics.

A man with epididymitis should rest in bed for 3 to 4 days, with the affected testicle supported by a small pillow or rolled towel. Ice bags in the first 24 hours, followed 1 day later by warm compresses, can help to relieve pain. Pain medication can be prescribed to control discomfort and fever; if pain is severe, the doctor may prescribe a local anesthetic. Stool softeners can be given to lessen pain during bowel movements. Sexual activity should be avoided. Symptoms usually resolve within 2 weeks, but it may take 4 to 6 weeks for the epididymis to return to normal size. Complications are unusual; infertility can result if the epididymis on each of the testicles is involved. Prevention depends on the type of bacteria causing the infection. If the cause is sexually transmitted, safer sexual practices can lower risk. If the epididymitis results from infection of the urinary tract or prostate, antibiotics are prescribed.

Epidural abscess, spinal

An accumulation of pus, due to a bacterial infection, that collects in the space between the spinal bones and the outermost of the three membranes that cover the spinal cord. The organisms that commonly cause spinal epidural abscess also cause acute infection of the middle ear and sinusitis. Because these bacterial infections are generally treated with antibiotics, spinal epidural abscesses are very rare.

When a pus-filled abscess forms on the spine, it may exert pressure on nerve tissue as the volume of pus within it increases. This can cause muscle weakness in the legs and a lack of sensation in the lower body. General symptoms from the bacterial infection can include fever, confusion, and sometimes delirium or seizures.

The tests that may be used to diagnose a spinal epidural abscess include blood tests to identify the bacteria, CT (computed tomography) scan of the spine, MRI (magnetic resonance imaging) of the spine, and MYELOGRAPHY, an X ray of spinal tissues and structures after injection of a contrast dye.

Treatment includes surgical drainage of the abscess and antibiotics. Despite treatment, spinal cord injury may cause permanent weakness and loss of sensation.

Epidural steroid injection

An injection of a small amount of cortisone and an anesthetic into the bony spinal canal to reduce the inflammation of the nerves in the spine and ease the discomfort of lower back pain. Although cortisone is a strong anti-inflammatory medication, the procedure is not always successful, and that is especially true for people with long-standing back pain. Epidural steroid injections tend to be given, often in a timed series, if more conservative measures are not effective in relieving back pain. The injections are sometimes given to try to avoid back surgery.

Epiglottis

The lidlike structure that closes over the opening of the larynx (voice box) during swallowing to prevent food from entering the trachea (windpipe). The epiglottis, made of cartilage, tilts downward during swallowing, while the opening between the vocal cords shuts tightly. Together these actions prevent food from going down the trachea.

Epiglottitis

A rare but serious inflammation of the epiglottis that can cause a child to suffocate if not treated immediately. The valve at the top of the windpipe (trachea) becomes swollen due to infection and can obstruct breathing. The bacteria *Haemophilus influenzae* type b is the most common cause. Children between the ages of 2 and 6 are most susceptible. The first signs of infection are a sore throat and high fever, rapidly progressing to noisy, hoarse, and labored breathing called STRIDOR. Swallowing may become so difficult that a child drools.

Epiglottitis is a medical emergency that requires immediate attention at a hospital emergency department. After the condition is diagnosed, the child will be given antibiotics. To permit unobstructed breathing, it may be necessary to bypass the swelling by inserting a tube through the nose or the mouth into the trachea. Very severe cases may require a tracheostomy, in which a breathing

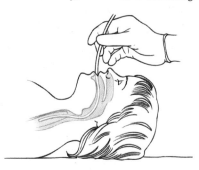

EPIGLOTTITIS: A RARE EMERGENCY
If the epiglottis (the valve at the top of the windpipe, or trachea) becomes infected, it can block the airway and restrict breathing. Immediate treatment in an emergency department is necessary. Antibiotics will be given to treat the infection, which is usually caused by flu bacteria (*Haemophilus influenzae* type b). To enable breathing, a tube may be passed through the nose, as shown, and down into the trachea.

tube is introduced into the trachea through a small incision in the neck.

Widespread immunization with the Hib vaccine (see VACCINATIONS, CHILDHOOD), which prevents infection due to *Haemophilus influenzae* type b, has made cases of epiglottitis very rare. The vaccine is given in a series of three or four shots, depending upon which of several types of Hib vaccine is used.

Epilepsy

FOR FIRST AID
see Seizures, page 1329

A neurological disorder characterized by two or more seizures, caused by abnormal electrical activity in the brain. A SEIZURE is a sudden and transient episode of uncontrolled electrical activity in the brain. Seizures may cause a series of involuntary muscle contractions or a temporary lapse in consciousness.

CAUSES

In epilepsy, clusters of nerve cells (neurons) sometimes signal or fire abnormally. When normal neuronal activity is disturbed, there may be unusual sensations, emotions, or behavior or there may be convulsions, muscle spasms, and loss of consciousness. The normal rate at which neurons signal is 80 times a second. In a seizure, they fire as many as 500 times a second. Not all seizures are epileptic seizures. For example, a child may have a single febrile seizure (see SEIZURE, FEBRILE) as a result of a high fever, and this does not mean that he or she has epilepsy. A person has to have two or more seizures before he or she is considered to have epilepsy.

About half of all cases of epilepsy have no known cause. In other cases, seizures are linked to infection, trauma, or other medical problems. Epilepsy may also run in families. In children, seizures are frequently associated with CEREBRAL PALSY and other neurological abnormalities. In people with epilepsy, seizures can be triggered by lack of sleep, alcohol consumption, stress, smoking, and

Terms in small capital letters—for example, PHYSICAL THERAPY or PAGET DISEASE—indicate a cross-reference to another entry with more information.

E

hormonal changes associated with the menstrual cycle.

TYPES OF SEIZURES

There are more than 30 different types of seizures. Seizures are divided into two main categories: partial seizures and generalized seizures.

■ *Partial seizures* More than half of people with epilepsy have partial seizures, in which the abnormal impulses arise in just one part of the brain. Frequently these seizures are identified by the part of the brain with which they are associated (for example, partial frontal lobe seizures). In a simple partial seizure, a person remains conscious but experiences unusual thoughts, movements, or feelings. These may include unexplainable sensations of joy or anger. Other simple partial seizures may be motor seizures that involve localized twitching of an arm or leg. In a complex partial seizure, a person experiences a change in or loss of consciousness. People who have this type of seizure may demonstrate unusual repetitive behaviors (such as blinks or twitches) called automatisms.

Partial seizures (especially complex partial seizures) are often preceded by auras. An aura is an unusual sensation that is a warning sign of an impending seizure. An aura may consist of dreamlike perceptions or visual disturbances, such as seeing stars or flashes. When it precedes a seizure, an aura is actually a simple partial seizure in which a person maintains consciousness.

■ *Generalized seizures* Unlike partial seizures, generalized seizures are caused by abnormal neuronal activity in multiple parts of the brain. These seizures may cause convulsions, massive muscle spasms, falls, and loss of consciousness. There are many different kinds of generalized seizures. In absence seizures (which were formerly called petit mal seizures), a person appears to be staring into space and may have only minimal twitching of muscles. Tonic seizures cause stiffening of the muscles, while clonic seizures cause repeated jerking movements. A person having an atonic seizure loses muscle tone and may fall down. Tonic-clonic seizures (which were formerly called grand mal seizures) cause stiffening, jerking, and a loss of consciousness.

DIFFERENT TYPES OF EPILEPSY

There are many different types of epilepsy. People with recurrent absence seizures have absence epilepsy or petit mal, a type of epilepsy that tends to run in families. Childhood absence epilepsy usually disappears at puberty. Frontal lobe epilepsy is characterized by clusters of short seizures that have a sudden onset and termination. Lennox-Gastaut is a severe form of epilepsy that can cause atonic seizures, which in turn cause sudden falls and are also called drop attacks.

Temporal lobe epilepsy (see EPILEPSY, TEMPORAL LOBE) is the most common type of epilepsy with partial seizures. This type of epilepsy usually begins during childhood. Temporal lobe seizures are frequently associated with auras. Over time, repeated temporal lobe seizures can cause a brain structure known as the hippocampus to shrink. The hippocampus, which is part of the brain's limbic system, is essential to normal memory and learning. Multiple seizures over the years may cause significant damage to the hippocampus, so to prevent these seizures, early diagnosis and treatment are vital.

DIAGNOSIS

Many different techniques are used to diagnose epilepsy. These include medical history; blood tests; electroencephalogram (EEG) monitoring; and neurological, developmental, and behavioral tests. An EEG, which measures the electrical activity of the brain, is among the most informative tests for evaluating possible epilepsy. Although many people with seizures have normal EEGs, the EEG can help confirm the diagnosis of epilepsy, classify the seizure type, and aid the doctor in selecting therapy. A number of imaging techniques are also used in diagnosis. The most commonly used brain scans are CT SCANNING (computed tomography scanning), MRI (magnetic resonance imaging), and PET SCANNING (positron emission tomography scanning). CT scanning and MRI reveal the structure of the brain. PET scanning and a special type of MRI known as a functional MRI are used to monitor the brain's activity and possible abnormalities in how it works. A relatively new brain scan called SPECT (single-photon emission computed tomography) may be used to locate problems such as seizure foci in the brain.

TREATMENT

Antiepileptic drugs are the first line of treatment. These include traditional alternatives such as carbamazepine, valproate, phenobarbital, and phenytoin, as well as newer drugs. Most adults with epilepsy are able to work and live normal lives. Certain occupations in which a loss of consciousness could be catastrophic (for example, airplane pilot or bus driver) are usually off limits to people with epilepsy. Most states deny driving privileges to people with poorly controlled epilepsy. However, people whose epilepsy is well controlled

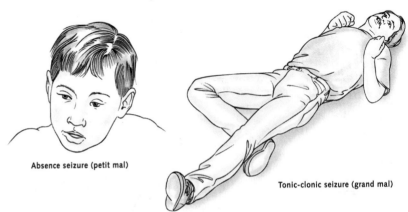

Absence seizure (petit mal)

Tonic-clonic seizure (grand mal)

TYPES OF SEIZURES
Different forms of epilepsy can be characterized by different types of seizures. A person having an absence (petit mal) seizure may stare into space and be unresponsive, but remain conscious. A person having a tonic-clonic (grand mal) seizure loses consciousness and twitches or stiffens. A typical seizure lasts 1 or 2 minutes.

with medications and who are seizure-free for a specified period (usually 2 years, depending on the state) may be permitted to drive.

Special drugs such as fosphenytoin are administered in hospital settings to treat STATUS EPILEPTICUS. This is the occurrence of repeated or prolonged epileptic seizures. Status epilepticus is a severe, life-threatening condition that must be treated as quickly as possible. The sooner medication is administered, the better the chance of recovery. A single medication can usually control the seizures of about 50 to 75 percent of people with epilepsy; for others, a combination of two or three drugs is needed to control seizures. When seizures cannot be adequately controlled with medications, doctors consider surgical alternatives such as temporal lobectomy (removal of the affected temporal lobe), hemispherectomy (removal of half the brain's cortex), or placement of a vagal nerve stimulator (an electric stimulator threaded under the skin, attached to the vagus nerve, which blocks seizures by providing a stimulation pulse to the brain).

Epilepsy, temporal lobe

Also known as TLE, the most common type of EPILEPSY with partial seizures. A SEIZURE is a sudden episode of uncontrolled electrical activity in the brain. TLE usually begins during childhood. Over time, repeated temporal lobe seizures can cause a brain structure known as the hippocampus to shrink. The hippocampus, which is part of the brain's limbic system, is essential to normal memory and learning. Multiple seizures over the years may cause significant damage to the hippocampus, so to prevent these seizures, early diagnosis and treatment are vital.

SYMPTOMS
TLE is classified as a partial seizure because the seizures begin in a focal area of the brain, the temporal lobe. Temporal lobe seizures are frequently associated with auras. An aura is an unusual sensation that is a warning sign of an impending seizure. It may consist of a strange feeling, abnormal perceptions, or visual disturbances, such as seeing stars or flashes. When

it precedes a generalized seizure, an aura followed by loss of consciousness represents the abnormal electrical impulses that start in a localized area of the brain.

DIAGNOSIS AND TREATMENT
Many different techniques are used to diagnose TLE. These include medical history; blood tests; electroencephalogram (EEG) monitoring; and neurological, developmental, and behavioral tests. An EEG, which measures the electrical activity of the brain, is very helpful for evaluating people with possible TLE. Although many people with seizures have normal EEGs, the EEG can help confirm the diagnoses of epilepsy, classify the seizure type, and aid the doctor in selecting therapy. A number of imaging techniques are also used in diagnosis. The most commonly used brain scans are CT SCANNING (computed tomography scanning), MRI (magnetic resonance imaging), and PET SCANNING (positron emission tomography scanning). CT scanning and MRI reveal the structure of the brain. PET scanning and a special type of MRI known as a functional MRI are used to monitor the brain's activity and possible abnormalities in how it works. A relatively new brain scan called SPECT (single-photon emission computed tomography) may be used to locate, for example, the focus of seizures in the brain.

Antiepileptic drugs are the first line of treatment. These include traditional alternatives such as carbamazepine, valproate, phenobarbital, and phenytoin, as well as newer drugs. In about 50 to 75 percent of people with TLE, seizures can be controlled with a single drug; in more severe cases, a combination of two or three drugs may be needed to control seizures. When seizures cannot be adequately controlled with medications, doctors consider surgical alternatives, including temporal lobectomy.

Epinephrine

A hormone secreted in the brain by the adrenal medulla; also known as adrenaline. Epinephrine is secreted in response to a low blood sugar level, exercise, and stress, causing increased cardiac output and other physiological changes known as the

"fight-or flight-response." Epinephrine can be produced synthetically for medical purposes.

Epinephrine is available both with and without prescription, by injection, and as an inhaler. Its chief use is to treat severe allergic reactions by opening the airways. People with known severe allergies to insect stings, certain foods, or specific drugs are encouraged to carry anaphylaxis (antiallergy) kits containing prefilled epinephrine syringes with them at all times (EpiPen, Ana-Kit). In an inhaler, epinephrine is used to treat bronchospasm associated with asthma. It is also used to treat cardiac arrest and forms of heart block. Epinephrine is also available in eye drops to treat glaucoma.

Epiphora

The excessive production of tears in one or both eyes. See TEARING.

Epiphysis, slipped capital femoral

The dislocation of the upper, wide end of the thighbone, a part of the bone that is still growing during early puberty. During the rapid growth phase in adolescence, the uppermost part of the thighbone, the ephysis, may be separated from the rest of the bone by cartilage. This causes the weakened bone to slip into an abnormal position. The symptoms include knee and hip pain, hip stiffness and restriction of movement, difficulty walking, limping, and an outward turning of the leg. Slipped capital femoral epiphysis is a rare disorder, most common among boys 11 to 16 years old. The disorder often occurs in overweight children and may be caused by trauma during contact

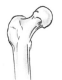

Healthy hip Slipped capital Distorted
femoral epiphysis femur head

MISALIGNMENT OF THE THIGHBONE
If the cartilaginous growth plate on the head (epiphysis) of the thighbone slips out of place and is left untreated, the dislocation distorts the head of the thighbone (femur) and causes a deformity of the hip.

sports or an injury due to a fall. The disorder is also known to be related to the effects of growth hormone on bone tissue during puberty. Diagnosis of the condition is made by a physical examination, which generally indicates decreased mobility of the hip. An X ray or CT (computed tomography) scan of the pelvis or hip can reveal the displacement. Surgery may be the only treatment to correct this disorder. In surgery, the displaced bone end can be moved into the proper position and fastened with metal pins. Complications include acute degeneration of the cartilage in the hip.

Episcleritis

Inflammation of one of the outer layers of the eyeball. The episclera lies between the sclera (the white, fibrous, covering of the eye) and the conjunctiva (the outer mucous membrane). Episcleritis can cause mild pain and tenderness and increases light sensitivity and tearing. The blood vessels in the episclera become prominent, making the eye look pink or bright red. Episcleritis is common, usually mild,

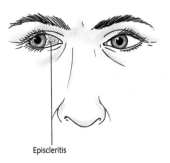

Episcleritis

EXTERNAL EYE INFLAMMATION
Episcleritis usually causes an area of redness in one or both eyes and some tenderness, especially when the eye is touched. There may be a raised lump. The cornea remains clear, and vision is not significantly affected.

and occurs most frequently in young adults. The cause is unknown, but the condition has been associated with a number of diseases, including rheumatoid arthritis, syphilis, Sjögren syndrome, herpes simplex virus, and tuberculosis. Rarely, episcleritis progresses to inflammation of the sclera (scleritis), which is more serious. Episcleritis usually runs its course without treatment in 2 weeks or longer, but the duration of the inflam-

mation can be shortened with artificial tears, topical antihistamine, or corticosteroid eye drops. Episcleritis tends to recur.

Episiotomy

A procedure during childbirth in which an incision is made in the mother's perineum (the skin between the vagina and the anus). The incision enlarges the vaginal opening and allows the baby to pass through it more easily without tearing the vaginal skin during delivery. The incision is stitched closed after the birth.

Episiotomies once were performed routinely during many deliveries because doctors believed that a clean cut would be easier to repair and quicker to heal than a jagged tear of the skin. Now, doctors typically perform an episiotomy only if it appears the baby is stretching the vaginal opening to the point that significant tearing of the skin is likely, or in a FOR-CEPS DELIVERY to prevent the forceps from tearing the skin. An episiotomy sometimes is done to avoid pressure on the baby's head if the baby is premature, or when a baby is in distress and must be delivered immediately. An episiotomy may be performed to ease the delivery when labor has been difficult and prolonged, and the woman is too exhausted to push the baby out. Episiotomies are more often performed during the delivery of a woman's first baby because her tissue has not been stretched previously.

To perform an episiotomy, a local anesthetic (painkiller) may be injected into the area where the incision will be made. The anesthetic does not affect the baby. If an epidural has been given for pain management, the woman may already have sufficient anesthetic for an episiotomy. Once the area is numb, the doctor inserts two fingers against the wall of the woman's vagina to protect the baby's head and prepares to make the incision. While the woman is having a contraction, the doctor uses surgical scissors to cut a small opening (an inch or two) either straight down between the vaginal opening and the anus or at an angle slightly to one side of the anus. After delivery, the opening is closed with stitches that dissolve over time. Additional painkillers may be needed while repairing the episiotomy. The area around the incision remains sore for a few days and should be cleaned with warm water after urinating or having bowel movements to help prevent infection.

Epispadias

A congenital defect in which the upper wall of the urethra is missing. This condition occurs more often in males than in females. The opening of the urethra may be anywhere on the top surface of the penis in males born with epispadias; usually it appears as a groove or cleft without a

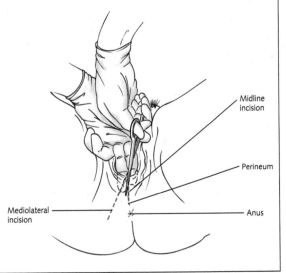

ENLARGING THE VAGINAL OPENING
To prevent tearing of the perineum (the area of skin between the vagina and anus) during childbirth, a doctor can cut the skin to create a larger opening. Protecting the baby's head with his or her fingers, the doctor cuts either straight down toward the anus or diagonally alongside the anus. The broken lines indicate both the so-called midline and mediolateral episiotomy incisions. The midline incision usually heals more easily.

Midline incision

Perineum

Anus

Mediolateral incision

covering. In females, the urethra may open into the clitoris or just above it. Epispadias may require surgery to repair the defect.

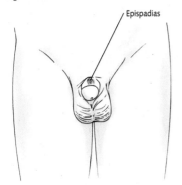

Epispadias

AN OPEN URETHRA
Epispadias can be surgically repaired so that the person will be continent and able to function sexually.

Epistaxis

See NOSEBLEED.

Epithelium

The layer of cells that covers the body and lines most of the structures within it. Epithelial cells thickly cover the skin; the layer may be only one cell deep in the delicate linings of body cavities, hollow organs, or structures such as blood vessels. Epithelial cells vary widely depending on the specialized function of the body part they cover.

Epstein-Barr virus

One of the most common human viruses and a member of the herpesvirus family. Epstein-Barr virus (EBV) was discovered in 1964. EBV affects people worldwide, infecting most people at some point in their lives. It is estimated that up to 95 percent of the US population between the ages of 35 and 40 years has been infected. Most infections with EBV cause no symptoms. Children sometimes acquire infection with EBV and have only mild, brief illnesses or are without symptoms altogether.

ASSOCIATED INFECTIONS

Epstein-Barr is the virus that most often causes infectious mononucleosis, particularly when infection occurs for the first time in adolescence or young adulthood. (See also MONONUCLEOSIS, INFECTIOUS.) When the symptoms of mononucleosis have subsided, the virus remains dormant or latent in throat and blood cells for the remainder of a person's life. It can reactivate without symptoms. People who have previously been infected with EBV are not at risk for contracting infectious mononucleosis when exposed to someone who has the illness.

Some cells of the body's immune system retain a lifelong dormant infection with EBV. Rarely, this dormant infection is believed to have a role in some cancers that are extremely uncommon in the United States: a cancer of the lymph glands in the jaw called BURKITT LYMPHOMA and a type of facial and oral cancer called nasopharyngeal carcinoma. EBV has been associated with Burkitt lymphoma in children in South Africa and with nasopharyngeal carcinoma in Asian populations.

Epstein-Barr virus may also cause hairy leukoplakia, a condition that produces a lesion that appears as a white patch, usually on the side of the tongue, and occurs most commonly in people with weakened immune systems. The condition responds to antiviral medication, but tends to return when this therapy is discontinued. There is no specific drug therapy for EBV.

Transmission of EBV requires direct contact with an infected person's saliva. The virus is not normally transmitted through the air or via blood contact. The virus is often found in the saliva of healthy people, who may carry and spread EBV intermittently over a lifetime.

ERCP

An acronym for endoscopic retrograde cholangiopancreatography. The procedure combines the use of X rays and ENDOSCOPY to view the stomach, duodenum, bile ducts, and pancreas. Endoscopy involves examination of the interior parts of the body using a slim, flexible, lighted tube that allows a doctor to view, photograph, videotape, and if necessary, take a sample of tissue (see BIOPSY). ERCP is used to investigate the cause of symptoms, such as jaundice (a yellowing of the skin and the whites of the eyes), upper abdominal pain, and unexplained weight loss. By using this procedure, doctors are able to diagnose problems in the liver, gallbladder, bile ducts, and pancreas.

Because the stomach and duodenum must be empty, there is no eating or drinking for 6 to 8 hours before ERCP. Shortly before the procedure, to reduce discomfort and gagging, the person's throat is sprayed with a local anesthetic. Additional pain medication or a sedative may help the person relax.

In ERCP, the endoscope is passed through the mouth, esophagus, stomach, and duodenum until it reaches the area where the bile ducts and pancreas open into the duodenum. The person is then asked to lie flat on his or her stomach, as a contrast dye is injected through the endoscope to make the bile ducts and surrounding organs show clearly on X rays. If the test reveals a gallstone or stricture (narrowing) of the ducts, additional instruments can be inserted to remove or work around the obstruction. Balloons can be inserted to dilate strictures. A sample of tissue or cells can also be taken at this time for later analysis.

ERCP takes from 30 minutes to 2 hours. There may be some discomfort when dye is injected into the ducts. Afterward, the only side effect in

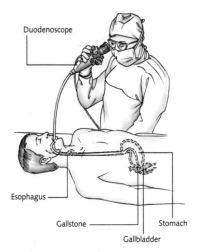

Duodenoscope

Esophagus

Gallstone

Stomach

Gallbladder

SOPHISTICATED IMAGING TECHNIQUE
Endoscopic retrograde cholangiopancreatography (ERCP) enables a doctor to examine the pancreas, bile ducts, liver, and gallbladder. The doctor inserts a flexible, lighted instrument called a duodenoscope down through the stomach into the duodenum (upper intestine). The duodenoscope provides a side-angled view into the opening where the bile and pancreatic ducts empty into the duodenum. ERCP can also be used to dislodge a gallstone from the bile duct and to perform other surgical procedures.

E

HEALING ERECTILE DYSFUNCTION

Erectile dysfunction is the frequent inability to attain, or sustain, an erection adequate for satisfactory sexual activity. It affects an estimated 20 million men in the United States. Typical causes of the disorder are medications for high blood pressure, an addiction to smoking or recreational drugs, partner conflicts, or depression. Physicians experienced in treating erectile dysfunction say that it can be treated successfully more than 95 percent of the time.

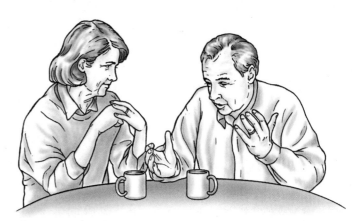

FRANK COMMUNICATION
Although erectile dysfunction is difficult to discuss, it is important to acknowledge its existence and not to allow embarrassment or guilt to delay treatment. A couple should discuss their feelings and reassure each other about their feelings of love. Couples who communicate and have a mutual commitment to improve their sexual relationship have the best chance of successful treatment.

MEDICAL RECOMMENDATIONS
The primary care physician will determine if a man has any medical conditions, such as certain heart problems, that might need attention before starting any treatment for erectile dysfunction. Once those possibilities are eliminated, the physician will probably refer the man to a specialist. An endocrinologist may be the appropriate choice if the condition is due to a hormonal problem. If the physician suspects another physical cause, a referral to a urologist may be in order. If psychological causes (such as depression, anxiety, or relationship problems) are more likely, he or she may suggest seeing a psychiatrist.

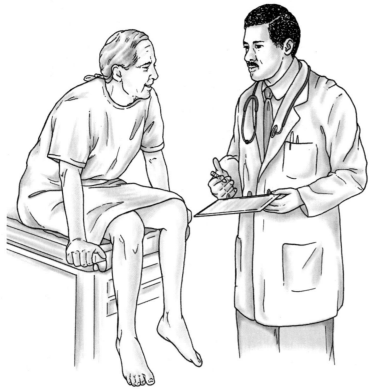

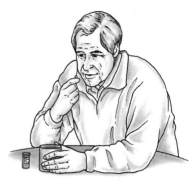

EFFECTIVE MEDICATION
Sildenafil (Viagra), the first pill to treat erectile dysfunction, was approved by the Food and Drug Administration in 1998. It is usually taken 1 hour before sexual activity, and it works by causing an increase in the blood flow to the penis.

most people is a mild sore throat. Rare complications may include PANCREATITIS (inflammation of the pancreas), bleeding, infection, and puncture of the duodenum. Following the procedure, it is usually necessary to rest an hour or two until medication wears off. If minor surgery, such as the removal of a gallstone, is performed through the endoscope, it may be necessary to stay in the hospital overnight.

Erectile dysfunction

Consistent inability to produce or maintain an erection of the penis sufficient to have sexual intercourse; also known as impotence. Erectile dysfunction is more common in older men, but it is not an inevitable consequence of aging. The cause can be either psychological or physical. Causes include relationship troubles, mental disorders (such as depression and anxiety), or severe guilt feelings. Physical causes include disease, such as diabetes mellitus, kidney disease, multiple sclerosis, coronary artery disease, alcoholism, medications (antidepressants, appetite suppressants), or injury to the genitals, pelvis, or spinal cord; smoking; and surgery, especially surgery of the prostate, bladder, colon, or spine.

To identify the cause of impotence, a doctor will conduct a thorough physical examination and talk to the man about his sexuality. The physician may also order laboratory tests to look for underlying disease. Treatment depends on the cause. Psychotherapy can help with psychological issues. Erectile dysfunction caused by medications can sometimes be resolved by changing to a different medication. Quitting smoking and abstaining from alcohol can also help. Prescription medications are available to help men produce and maintain erections. Some medications are taken by mouth a short time before sexual activity, for example, sildenafil; others are injected into the penis or are inserted into the opening at the end of the penis. Vacuum devices that produce an erection can also be used. In some cases, surgery is performed to place an inflatable implant in the penis (see PENILE IMPLANT). See also Healing erectile dysfunction, page 522.

Erection

The rising and hardening of the penis due to blood accumulating in its tissues. During sexual stimulation, blood fills the erectile bodies of the penis, which are closed by exit valves in the veins to keep the blood in rather than let it flow out. A similar process hardens and raises the clitoris. Erection is also used to describe the rising of other tissues, such as the nipple or fine hairs on the skin, that stand up from muscular contraction rather than from the accumulation of blood.

Ergocalciferol

See CALCIFEROL.

Ergometer

A device designed to measure the amount of energy used or amount of work done while a person is engaged in a specific task. An ergometer may be used to test the overall ability of the heart, lungs, blood vessels, and muscles to increase energy expenditure to meet the metabolic demands of physical work. Treadmills and stepping machines are examples of ergometers.

Erogenous zones

Areas of the body that respond with sexual arousal when touched, kissed, or otherwise stimulated. Although any part of the body may be sexually sensitive, some areas are typically more sensitive than others. Erogenous zones vary from person to person. They may include the lips, mouth, ears (especially earlobes), cheeks, neck, shoulders, breasts, nipples, waist, genitals, buttocks, anus, hands, fingers, insides of thighs, backs of knees, feet, and toes.

Eroticism

The sexual instinct or drive.

Erysipelas

An acute, red, raised, sharply demarcated rash caused by streptococcal bacteria (see STREPTOCOCCAL INFECTIONS). The rash can appear on the face and lower legs and occasionally on the arms. Streptococcus is the same bacteria that causes strep throat and some wound infections. Infection may occur in breaks in the skin caused by trauma, ulcers, or bites and occurs most often in older people and people with diabetes.

The onset of erysipelas is ordinarily abrupt. The rash is hot to the touch, has clearly defined margins, and spreads quickly. Affected areas are painful, shiny, and swollen and can contain fluid-filled bumps. There may also be swelling of the eyelids, fever, chills, fatigue, nausea, and vomiting. In severe cases, abscesses (pus-filled sacs) develop. Left untreated, bacteria begin circulating in the bloodstream and can cause BACTEREMIA (the presence of bacteria in the bloodstream), which in turn leads to SEPSIS, a potentially fatal condition. Diagnosis of erysipelas is made by identifying the characteristic rash. Treatment is with penicillin.

Erythema infectiosum

See FIFTH DISEASE.

Erythema multiforme

See DRUG ERUPTION.

Erythema nodosum

An inflammatory skin condition that is characterized by tender, red bumps or swellings under the skin, most often on the legs. Erythema nodosum occurs more frequently in women than in men. Although its exact cause remains unknown, half of all cases may be associated with infection with *Coccidioides, Mycoplasma, Streptococcus,* or *Yersinia*

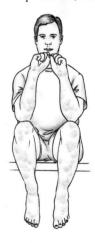

INFLAMMATION OF SOFT TISSUE
The swellings of erythema nodosum are very tender. The affected areas may be covered with scaly skin or may be more easily felt than seen. The lesions may change in appearance and color over a period of weeks, gradually fading to look like bruises.

E

organisms and diseases such as hepatitis B and tuberculosis. It may also occur as a reaction to drugs such as oral contraceptives or sulfonamides. Some cases have been linked with ulcerative colitis, leukemia, and sarcoidosis.

Erythema nodosum most commonly appears on the front of both legs (shins). The onset is characterized by hot, red, painful bumps that eventually fade to flat brown patches. Other symptoms may include fever, joint aches, and a general feeling of illness. Diagnosis is made according to the appearance of the skin and sometimes the results of a biopsy. It is essential to identify and treat any underlying infection or condition. Treatment includes bed rest. Doctors may prescribe nonsteroidal anti-inflammatory drugs to relieve pain and to control inflammation. Oral corticosteroids are prescribed in severe cases. Symptoms may last for up to 6 weeks.

Erythrocyte

A red blood cell. The erythrocyte is composed of hemoglobin, a protein that binds easily with oxygen and serves to transport it through the blood. Erythrocytes form in the bone marrow where they lose their nuclei before passing into the bloodstream, meaning that they cannot reproduce. Erythrocytes have a life span of about 120 days, after which they break down in the spleen and are destroyed. See BLOOD.

Erythrocyte sedimentation rate

See ESR.

Erythroderma

A skin condition characterized by redness and scaling over the entire body; also known as exfoliative dermatitis. Erythroderma usually occurs as a complication of another skin disease such as atopic dermatitis, psoriasis, or contact dermatitis. Less commonly, it is a symptom of a systemic disease such as leukemia or lymphoma.

Erythroderma commonly begins with isolated patches of scaly, red skin. These patches may enlarge until all of the skin is affected. The continuous peeling and flaking of skin results in a loss of body protein. In serious cases, the loss of normal skin can result in severe heat loss and a drop in body temperature. Secondary infections may occur; severe cases of erythroderma can become life-threatening. Treatment includes diagnosing and treating the underlying primary disease, preventing secondary infection, stabilizing body temperature, and maintaining fluid balance.

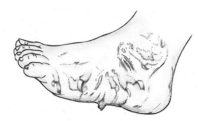

OVERALL SKIN CONDITION
Erythroderma, also called exfoliative dermatitis, causes dry flaking, scaling, and peeling of large portions of the skin all over the body. The skin underneath may be severely inflamed. The condition usually starts in small patches that enlarge and spread. The person may have chills because of the loss of the insulating effect of the outer layers of skin.

Erythromycin

An antibiotic used to treat a variety of bacterial infections. Erythromycin works by inhibiting the synthesis of some proteins in bacteria; it is active against many strains of bacteria as well as some bacterialike microorganisms, including *Chlamydia*. Based on its action against microorganisms, erythromycin is categorized as a macrolide antibiotic.

Erythromycin is used to treat pneumonias, whooping cough, legionnaires disease, middle ear infections, skin infections such as impetigo and acne, and other infections. Erythromycin is available as a skin cream for skin infections and as liquids and tablets for other infections. It is known by many brand names, including E.E.S., A/T/S, ERYC, and Erythrocin.

Erythropoietin

A protein secreted by the kidney that stimulates formation of red blood cells in the bone marrow. Epoetin, a manufactured version of human erythropoietin, is used to treat severe anemia in people whose kidneys are not working properly. Epoetin alfa (Epogen, Procrit) is given by injection.

Esalen massage

A form of massage therapy; sometimes called Swedish massage. Esalen massage focuses on relieving muscle tension, creating deep relaxation, achieving beneficial states of consciousness, and promoting general well-being.

Eschar

Discarded dead tissue. An eschar can be caused by a burn or cauterization. Acids, alkalis, solid carbon dioxide (dry ice), and metallic salts that damage the skin can cause an eschar.

Escherichia coli diarrhea

See DIARRHEA, E. COLI.

Escherichia coli

See E. COLI.

Esophageal atresia

A rare and severe birth defect in which an infant is born with part of the esophagus missing. The esophagus is a muscular tube that connects the throat to the stomach. In esophageal atresia, there is no passageway to the baby's stomach. Because the baby cannot swallow, food is regurgitated back into the mouth. If a segment of the esophagus is connected to the trachea (windpipe), food can enter the lungs. This results in coughing and severe breathing difficulties. Infants with this problem may turn blue from a lack of oxygen.

A baby with esophageal atresia cannot be fed by mouth. Nourishment is given intravenously until the condition is surgically corrected. Diagnosis is made through esophagoscopy (visual examination of the esophagus through a slim, flexible, lighted tube called a gastroesophagoscope). Surgery must be performed to join the separate sections of the esophagus. In some cases, more than one procedure is necessary to correct the problem. See GASTROSCOPY.

Esophageal dilation

Widening of the esophagus. The esophagus, part of the digestive tract, is a muscular tube that connects the throat to the stomach. Esophageal dilation may be performed to relieve blockage from noncancerous conditions, such as scar tissue or a cancerous tumor that blocks the esophagus but cannot be removed. Scarring and narrowing may occur due to prolonged use of nonsteroidal anti-inflammatory drugs (NSAIDs), the antibiotic tetra-cycline, or potassium supplements. A special type of dilation is required for ACHALASIA, a rare disorder of the esophagus that interferes with swal-lowing.

In some cases, doctors mechanically widen the esophagus using a special-ly designed flexible metal rod or tube called a bougie. Sometimes, the pas-sageway is enlarged with a water-filled rubber bag. A laser may also be used to relieve blockages and destroy cancerous tissue. See also ESOPHAGUS, CANCER OF THE; ESOPHAGEAL STRICTURE.

Esophageal diverticulum

An outward bulge in the esophageal wall. The esophagus, part of the digestive tract, is a muscular tube that connects the throat to the stomach. Bulges or diverticula in its walls are most commonly caused by weakness in the walls, scarring, or a failure of the esophageal muscles to relax dur-ing swallowing.

Diagnosis is usually made through an upper GASTROINTESTINAL (GI) SERIES (an X-ray procedure also called a bar-ium swallow) or esophagoscopy. There are three types of esophageal diverticula: the pharyngeal pouch, the midesophageal diverticulum, and the epiphrenic diverticulum. A pha-ryngeal (also called Zenker) diverticu-lum, is located in the back wall of the lower throat and must be surgi-cally removed. During the procedure, the surgeon also cuts the esophageal sphincter to weaken it and prevent the pouch from recurring. Mid-esophageal diverticula, which occur farther down in the esophagus, usual-ly cause no symptoms and require no treatment. Epiphrenic diverticula, found at the end of the esophagus, are often secondary problems associated with disturbances in the sphincter between the stomach and esophagus.

Esophageal reflux

A condition in which acid from the stomach flows up into the esophagus, a muscular tube that connects the throat to the stomach. Esophageal reflux, which affects almost a third of all Americans, is also known as acid reflux, reflux, and gastroesophageal reflux disease (GERD). HEARTBURN is the most common symptom of esophageal reflux. This burning sen-sation in the upper abdomen or chest often develops when an affected person eats, bends, or lies down. Heartburn is especially common at night when lying down after a heavy meal. Also known as acid indiges-tion, this problem is most common in older people and pregnant women. In some cases, heartburn is accompa-

PREGNANCY AND ESOPHAGEAL REFLUX

Reflux is common in the later months of pregnancy. Increased levels of the female hormone progesterone in a pregnant woman can cause the esophageal sphincter muscle to relax, allowing stomach acid to escape. The expanding uterus increases pressure in the abdomen and may also con-tribute to the condition.

Treatment is somewhat limited by safety concerns for the fetus. Lifestyle changes can help. Doctors recom-mend not eating before going to bed, avoiding alcohol and spicy foods or medications that may cause heart-burn, and raising the head of the bed by about a foot. Pregnant women should not smoke. Antacids that con-tain aluminum, calcium, or magne-sium are acceptable for use during pregnancy. However, sodium bicar-bonate is not.

For extreme cases that do not respond to lifestyle changes or antacids, doctors may prescribe hista-mine$_2$ (or H$_2$) antagonists, such as cimetidine, ranitidine, and famotidine. Proton pump inhibitors, commonly used when pregnancy is not involved, are used sparingly during pregnancy because their effects on the fetus are not yet fully known.

nied by a bitter or sour taste in the back of the throat. Belching may also occur.

Normally, the muscle at the junc-tion blocks the backflow of gastric acid from the stomach into the esoph-agus. If the lower esophageal sphinc-ter is weak or defective, acid can wash up into the esophagus. Greasy or fatty foods may contribute to weak-ening of the lower esophageal sphinc-ter muscle. Chocolate, spicy foods, and alcohol can cause local irritation. In some cases, a HIATAL HERNIA devel-ops, in which part of the upper stom-ach protrudes into the chest through the esophageal hiatus, the opening in the diaphragm between the esopha-gus and the stomach.

Persistent esophageal reflux can lead to inflammation, ulceration, and formation of scar tissue that lead to ESOPHAGEAL STRICTURE (narrowing). Other potential complications include dysphagia (difficulty in swallowing), and bleeding. Left untreated, esopha-

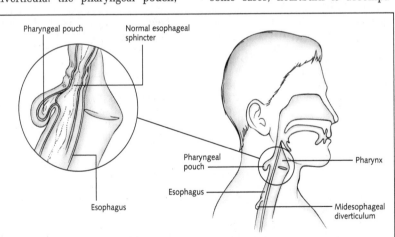

POUCHES IN THE ESOPHAGUS
Pouches, or diverticula, can form in several areas of the esophagus if the muscular wall of the esophagus bulges outward. A pharyngeal pouch forms at the back of the lower part of the throat (pharynx) if the action of the sphincter at the top of the esophagus becomes irregular. A midesophageal diverticulum is a similar pouch located farther down in the esophagus.

E

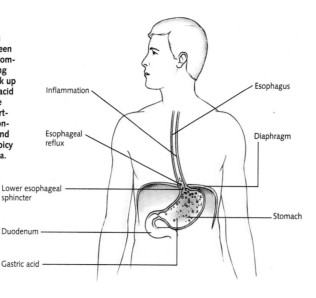

THE CAUSE OF HEARTBURN
Esophageal reflux occurs when the sphincter between the esophagus and the stomach malfunctions, allowing stomach acid to flow back up into the esophagus. The acid irritates the lining of the esophagus, causing heartburn. Fatty foods may contribute to the problem, and chocolate, alcohol, and spicy foods may irritate the area.

Inflammation

Esophageal reflux

Lower esophageal sphincter

Duodenum

Gastric acid

Esophagus

Diaphragm

Stomach

geal reflux increases the risk of esophageal cancer (see ESOPHAGUS, CANCER OF THE).

DIAGNOSIS AND TREATMENT
Diagnosis of esophageal reflux is usually made through an upper GASTROINTESTINAL (GI) SERIES (an X-ray procedure also called a barium swallow), GASTROSCOPY (visual examination of the esophagus, stomach, and duodenum with a slim, flexible, lighted tube), and esophageal manometry. In esophageal manometry, a small flexible tube is threaded through the nose into the esophagus and stomach to measure changes in pressure that occur during swallowing and the strength of the sphincter between the stomach and esophagus.

In many cases, simple modifications in lifestyle can control esophageal reflux. Avoiding spicy or greasy foods, chocolate, coffee, and alcohol sometimes can help. Smoking increases acidity in the stomach and inhibits the effectiveness of the lower esophageal sphincter. Reflux is more likely to occur when the stomach is full (as well as during pregnancy). Doctors recommend not smoking and losing weight for those who are overweight. It can be helpful to forgo eating 2 to 3 hours before bedtime and to eat several small meals a day rather than two or three large ones. Elevating the head of the bed 2 to 4 inches for sleeping can decrease heartburn at night.

When these measures prove insuffi-

cient, or if it is necessary to take antacids frequently, a doctor should be consulted. Persistent, uncontrolled esophageal reflux can lead to serious complications, such as esophageal stricture, bleeding, perforation, and a long-term increased risk for cancer. Prolonged use of antacids can disrupt body chemistry. To manage reflux, doctors can prescribe drugs that reduce acid secretion, such as histamine blockers, anticholinergic agents, and proton pump inhibitors. Medications are also available to speed the passage of food through the stomach. If symptoms persist or complications occur, surgery may be necessary.

Esophageal spasm

Irregular, uncoordinated spasms of the muscles in the wall of the esophagus (the tube that connects the throat and stomach) that cause intense chest pain and dysphagia (difficulty swallowing). Esophageal spasm is rare, and its cause is unknown, although it may be associated with stress. The condition is usually diagnosed through an upper GASTROINTESTINAL (GI) SERIES (an X-ray procedure also called a barium swallow) and esophageal manometry, which measures pressure within the esophagus. Attacks of esophageal spasm are intermittent, and the condition is difficult to control. In some cases, to treat the condition and relax the smooth muscle of the esophagus,

doctors prescribe calcium channel blocker drugs, medications that are also used to treat high blood pressure.

Esophageal stricture

A narrowing or obstruction of the esophagus (the tube that connects the throat and stomach) that may lead to dysphagia (see SWALLOWING DIFFICULTY). Esophageal stricture occurs as a result of the accumulation of scar tissue in the esophagus, as in CROHN DISEASE and persistent esophageal reflux (the backward flow of stomach acid up into the esophagus). Scarring and narrowing can also be due to prolonged use of nonsteroidal anti-inflammatory drugs (NSAIDs), the antibiotic tetracycline, or potassium supplements. Narrowing, blockage, and dysphagia less commonly are caused by tumors (see ESOPHAGUS, CANCER OF THE).

Esophageal stricture may be diagnosed by a physical examination, a medical history, and tests, such as an upper GASTROINTESTINAL (GI) SERIES (an X-ray procedure also called a barium swallow) or GASTROSCOPY (visual examination of the esophagus, stomach, and duodenum using a slim, flexible, lighted tube called a gastroscope). To treat esophageal strictures, doctors perform ESOPHAGEAL DILATION to widen the passageway and permit easier swallowing. The esophagus can be widened using a specially designed flexible metal rod called a bougie or a water-filled rubber bag. A laser may also be used to relieve blockages and destroy cancerous tissue. In some cases, more extensive surgery is required.

Esophageal varices

Large, swollen, varicose veins in the lower portion of the esophagus (the muscular tube that connects the throat to the stomach) that can erode and bleed into the esophagus and stomach. Esophageal varices are usually caused by portal hypertension (increased blood pressure in the portal vein, which carries blood from the intestines to the liver). Portal hypertension is usually due to liver disease. When a person has the severe liver disease CIRRHOSIS, blood flowing from the abdominal organs to the liver encounters increasing resistance and is diverted to the esophageal

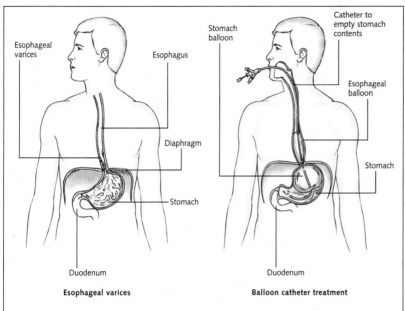

SWOLLEN VEINS IN THE ESOPHAGUS
Left untreated, esophageal varices can break and bleed into the stomach. Emergency treatment for ruptured esophageal varices involves threading a balloon catheter down the esophagus and into the stomach and then inflating the balloons to compress the bleeding veins. A tube drains blood from the stomach.

veins. Consequently, those veins swell and balloon into the esophagus.

DIAGNOSIS AND TREATMENT

Symptoms of esophageal varices include vomiting blood, black stools, and a dangerous drop in blood pressure. Varices may be diagnosed with a physical examination, taking a medical history, and tests, such as an upper GASTROINTESTINAL (GI) SERIES (an X-ray procedure also called a barium swallow) or GASTROSCOPY. In a gastroscopy, a slim, flexible, lighted tube called a gastroscope is passed through the mouth to view, photograph, and videotape the tissue. By using a tool that is threaded through the gastroscope, the doctor may take samples of tissue from the esophagus, stomach, and duodenum for analysis (see BIOPSY).

Esophageal varices are treated with the injection of a solution that shrinks and blocks off affected veins or by banding the veins. Because new varicose veins often form, repeated injections or banding may be necessary to control severe recurrent bleeding. If veins burst, immediate medical attention is necessary. Often, a blood transfusion is required, and the doctor may use a balloon catheter to compress the veins and control bleeding. If bleeding continues to be a problem, an ESOPHAGECTOMY (partial removal of the esophagus) may be necessary.

Esophagectomy

Partial or total removal of the esophagus (the tube that connects the throat and stomach). An esophagectomy is usually performed to treat esophageal cancer (see ESOPHAGUS, CANCER OF THE). In some cases, an esophagectomy is performed to control severe recurrent bleeding caused by ESOPHAGEAL VARICES (large, swollen, varicose veins in the esophagus).

An esophagectomy is a major operation. Generally, it involves removing a tumor along with the surrounding tissue and nearby lymph nodes. In most cases, the stomach can be joined to the remaining part of the esophagus. If necessary, the surgeon may use tissue from another part of the digestive tract (such as the colon) to form a new passageway from the throat to the stomach.

Some people may require intravenous feeding for several days before and after an esophagectomy. Antibiotics are usually necessary to prevent or treat infection. Following surgery, special coughing and breathing exercises must be practiced to keep the lungs clear. Doctors also prescribe medication to control pain and discomfort. In some cases, CHEMOTHERAPY or RADIATION THERAPY are recommended after cancer surgery.

Esophagitis

See ESOPHAGEAL REFLUX.

Esophagogastro-duodenoscopy

See GASTROSCOPY.

Esophagogastroscopy

See GASTROSCOPY.

Esophagogram

A series of X rays of the esophagus. An esophagogram is also known as a barium swallow or an upper GI series (see GASTROINTESTINAL [GI] SERIES).

Esophagoscopy

See GASTROSCOPY.

Esophagus

The muscular tube that passes from the throat (pharynx) to the stomach. When food is swallowed, the upper portion of the esophagus relaxes so that the food can move into it. Then the food is automatically passed down to the stomach by rhythmic waves of muscular contractions (peristalsis). Cells in the lining of the esophagus secrete mucus so that the food pieces slide down smoothly. At

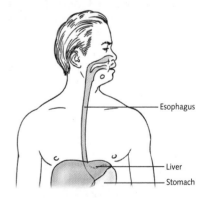

HOW FOOD IS SWALLOWED
Chewed food moves the length of the esophagus (from the throat to the stomach) through a combination of gravity, rhythmic muscular contractions called peristalsis, and lubrication from mucous glands in the esophageal wall. The process is carefully coordinated so that swallowing does not interfere with breathing.

the lower end of the esophagus, a sphincter relaxes as food approaches, allowing it to enter the stomach. This sphincter controls the amount of food that enters the stomach at one time. Gastroesophageal reflux disease (GERD; see ESOPHAGEAL REFLUX) is caused by a dysfunction of the sphincter valve; too much acid moves into the esophagus and causes heartburn. See also DIGESTIVE SYSTEM; SWALLOWING.

Esophagus, cancer of the

An uncommon cancer that can occur in any part of the esophagus (the tube that connects the throat and stomach). Small tumors in the esophagus do not usually cause symptoms. As a tumor grows, dysphagia (difficulty swallowing) is often the first symptom of cancer. At first, it may be difficult to swallow foods, such as raw vegetables or chunks of meat. As time goes on and the tumor grows, it becomes difficult to swallow even liquids. Difficulty in swallowing requires a physician's attention. Other symptoms of cancer of the esophagus include coughing, hoarseness, choking on food, indigestion, heartburn, vomiting, and weight loss.

Cancer of the esophagus most frequently appears in people age 55 or older. Men are affected twice as often as women. Heavy use of alcohol and tobacco increase the risk of developing this disease. A history of persistent, untreated ESOPHAGEAL REFLUX, in which stomach acid frequently backs up into the esophagus, also increases the risk of this cancer.

DIAGNOSIS AND TREATMENT

The diagnosis of cancer of the esophagus is based on a physical examination, medical history, and a number of tests. Initially, a series of X rays of the esophagus known as a barium swallow or upper GASTROINTESTINAL (GI) SERIES may be done. The doctor may also order blood tests, GASTROSCOPY (visual examination of the esophagus, stomach, and duodenum using a slim, flexible, lighted tube called a gastroscope), and other visual imaging tests of the esophagus, chest, and upper abdomen.

Treatment depends on the size and location of the tumor and how advanced it is. Early diagnosis improves the likelihood for a cure. An ESOPHAGECTOMY is usually performed to treat esophageal cancer. In this major operation, the tumor is removed along with tissues surrounding the esophagus and nearby lymph nodes. Usually the stomach can be joined to the remaining part of the esophagus, or tissue from another part of the digestive tract (such as the colon) may be used to form a new passageway from the throat to the stomach. CHEMOTHERAPY and RADIATION THERAPY may be recommended before or after surgery.

When a tumor blocking the esophagus cannot be surgically removed, ESOPHAGEAL DILATION may be used. In this procedure, doctors mechanically widen the esophagus using a specially designed flexible metal rod or tube called a bougie. Sometimes, the passageway is enlarged with a water-filled rubber bag. A laser may also be used to relieve blockages and destroy cancerous tissue.

Esotropia

A type of crossed eyes (strabismus), in which one or both eyes may turn inward toward the other. This can lead to diplopia (double vision) or AMBLYOPIA. See also STRABISMUS.

ESR

A medical test measuring the rate at which red blood cells settle through a column of liquid. The erythrocyte sedimentation rate (ESR) test is commonly performed to identify or monitor inflammatory diseases such as rheumatoid arthritis, rheumatic fever, or subacute bacterial endocarditis (heart valve inflammation). An elevated sedimentation rate usually indicates an acute inflammatory process occurring in the body as a result of infection or other disease.

Estradiol

A hormone used to treat a lack of estrogen. Estradiol is chiefly produced in the ovaries, but also is produced in the placenta, testis, and adrenal cortex. When estrogen is lacking in a woman after menopause or removal of the ovaries, estradiol may be prescribed for hormone replacement therapy. It is also used to treat prostate cancer, osteoporosis, and other conditions.

Estradiol is available in several forms: it can be taken orally, by injection, as a vaginal cream, or in skin patches. It is sold under many brand names, including Alora, Climara, Gynodiol, Estrace, and Vivelle. Estradiol is a component of the oral contraceptive desogestrel (Desogen, Mircette, and Ortho-Cept).

Estriol

An estrogen hormone usually obtained from the urine of pregnant women. Pregnant women may be tested for estriol levels based on the results of an AFP TEST (alpha-fetoprotein test). AFP is a protein produced by the growing fetus. If a pregnant woman has a lower-than-normal level of AFP, she will be given a PAN-AFP, or triple screen test, which detects estriol, AFP, and human chorionic gonadotropin, another hormone. The results of these tests can predict the risk of Down syndrome in a fetus.

Estrogen

The key female sex hormone produced primarily in the ovaries. Estrogen exists in several forms, including estradiol, estrone, and estriol. Estrogen is responsible for the development of women's sexual characteristics; it governs the monthly thickening of the endometrium that results in monthly periods; and it controls the quantity and quality of cervical and vaginal mucus necessary to transport sperm. Some types of adrenal hormones are converted to estrogen by fat cells. Small amounts of estrogen are produced in men in the testes and adrenal glands to balance testosterone. Estrogen helps to keep the brain cells of both men and women healthy.

Estrogen replacement therapy

See HORMONE REPLACEMENT THERAPY.

Estrogen, conjugated

Female sex hormones used to treat symptoms of menopause. Conjugated estrogens are also used to treat vaginitis, osteoporosis, and breast and prostate cancer. Conjugated estrogens are available under several brand names, including Premarin, Prempro, Premphase, and Cenestin. While they are useful for treating symptoms of menopause, such as hot flashes and dizziness, the long-term use of estrogen is not without risk. Heart disease, stroke, blood clots, high blood pressure, gallbladder disease, and endometrial cancer are all associated with the long-term use of conjugated estrogens.

Estrone

See ESTROGEN.

Etanercept

A drug used to treat the symptoms of rheumatoid arthritis. Etanercept (Enbrel) is used in cases of moderate to severe rheumatoid arthritis. Etanercept is designed to block the action of tumor necrosis factor (TNF), a protein that causes the joint inflammation associated with rheumatoid arthritis. Because it compromises the ability of the body to fight infection, etanercept should not be taken by people with chronic infections or weakened immune systems.

Ethics, medical

The moral principles in the fields of medical treatment and research. Medical ethics are a subset of the field of bioethics. Issues in medical ethics encompass a number of professional fields, including medicine, law, sociology, philosophy, and theology. Ethical issues affect physicians and patients as well as society.

Medical ethics have their roots in the HIPPOCRATIC OATH, which has the prime directive that physicians should "do no harm." The first formal professional code of medical ethics in the United States was established by the American Medical Association in 1847. Since the 1950s, innovations in medical technology have given rise to more complex ethical issues associated with medical research and practice.

ISSUES OF MEDICAL ETHICS

Medical ethics must be considered in both patient care and medical research when addressing issues such as the importance and practicality of obtaining informed consent from patients about to undergo surgery and from participants in medical research (see INFORMED CONSENT FOR SURGERY or TREATMENT; INFORMED CONSENT FOR RESEARCH). For research protocols, federal law requires that human subjects give consent and that federally funded health research projects be reviewed by appointed review boards. These institutional review boards place an emphasis on protecting any human subjects who may be part of a research study.

Ethical issues involving the definition of DEATH became a matter of public debate with the advance of life-support technologies in the 1960s, which gave physicians the ability to artificially maintain heart and lung function. In refining the definition of death to accommodate these medical innovations, medical ethicists sought to ensure that a gravely ill person was afforded the right to be kept alive through technology, while the body of a deceased person would not unnecessarily occupy much-needed life-support equipment indefinitely.

Developments in reproductive medicine raised other ethical dilemmas such as the rights of humans to control their bodies and to control the embryos that women may carry. Infertility also involves issues of medical ethics including how sperm or egg donors may be chosen by potential parents and what procedures should be implemented for recruiting donors. Ethical considerations concerning the moral status of embryos have been brought to light because of the use of fetal tissue by biomedical researchers. Advances in diagnosing prenatal conditions and abnormalities in the first months of pregnancy have led to ethical considerations about the use of medically ascertained knowledge to terminate pregnancies based on predictions of the newborn's sex, potential disabilities, and perceived quality of life.

Economic issues often are involved in considerations of medical ethics. Providing scarce and costly lifesaving equipment and treatment, including organ transplants, was once based on a person's ability to pay. This approach has been replaced with national systems governing the distribution of organs for transplantation that are based on criteria such as a person's place on a waiting list and the severity of the person's illness.

Medical ethics questions often arise in establishing a balance between the rights of individuals and the interests of society. For example, people with dangerous infectious diseases who have religious or personal reasons for refusing traditional medical care may endanger the community. Questions involving the legalization of EUTHANASIA raise ethical questions about the basic moral obligation of physicians to do no harm.

Innovations in genetic technology, especially the identification of a number of genes that may lead to specific diseases or conditions, are certain to give rise to questions of medical ethics. For example, the issue involves determining whether a potential employer should be made aware of an individual's genetic predispositions. Ethical considerations arise even in the study of gene therapies to genetically engineer viruses and the production of organisms genetically identical to a parent, or cloning.

Ethylene glycol

A clear, odorless liquid with a sweet taste that can cause poisoning. Ethylene glycol is found in antifreeze, hydraulic brake fluids, and industrial solvents. Many cases of ethylene glycol poisoning occur because children drink large amounts of the sweet-tasting liquid. Alcoholics may also drink ethylene glycol as a substitute for alcohol.

By itself, ethylene glycol is not particularly toxic, but digestion by the body breaks it down into metabolites that are extremely poisonous. Even small amounts of antifreeze (less than 8 ounces) can cause kidney damage, especially to children, and death may occur within 24 hours. Anyone who suspects ethylene glycol has been consumed should call a POISON CENTER immediately. It is one of the most common causes of poisoning in pets.

Etiology

The science or study of the causes or origins of a disease.

Etretinate

A drug used to treat severe psoriasis. Etretinate (Tegison) is an oral retinoid, a class of drugs derived from retinoic acid (vitamin A1). Etretinate is not recommended for use by a woman who is pregnant because it can cause birth defects in a fetus.

Euphoria

An extreme feeling of mental and physical well-being, particularly when such a mood is not justified by external events. Euphoria can be brought on by drugs, especially opiates (such as heroin, morphine, and opium), amphetamines, cocaine, and alcohol. It also occurs in the state of abnormal excitement and energy known as MANIA.

Eustachian tube

The narrow channel connecting the middle ear with an area of the upper throat at the back of the nose. The basic functions of this tube are to replenish the air that is constantly in the middle ear and to equalize any pressure changes that may occur with changes in altitude. The tube performs these functions by periodically opening for a fraction of a second, then quickly closing, usually in response to swallowing and yawning. The eustachian tube also acts as a drainage passage and helps maintain hearing.

If an infection of the upper respiratory tract causes the tube to become inflamed and partially blocked, negative pressure in the middle ear can cause the eardrum membrane to suck in. The symptoms of this blockage are usually mild hearing impairment, ringing in the ears, and a feeling of fullness or pressure in the ears. Children sometimes experience no symptoms. Over time, these obstructions can draw fluid from the mucous membrane of the middle ear, resulting in OTITIS MEDIA (inflammation in the middle ear). This condition frequently occurs in children who have infections of the upper respiratory tract and often results in some degree of temporary hearing impairment. Sometimes failure of the eustachian tube to properly equalize middle ear pressure develops during air travel (see BAROTRAUMA).

If the tube becomes entirely blocked, small capillaries of the middle ear may rupture and bleed, filling the ear with blood. This produces HEARING LOSS and a sensation of being underwater. A physician should be consulted when these symptoms are present.

Euthanasia

Also known as physician-assisted suicide; formerly known as mercy killing. The intentional act of causing the painless death of a person with an incurable disease or condition. Many people involved in the "right-to-die" movement define euthanasia as the right of an individual, especially an individual who faces a possibly painful and prolonged death, to die in a dignified and controlled manner at a time of his or her choosing.

LEVELS OF EUTHANASIA

Euthanasia may be categorized into two levels. The first level affects people who are hospitalized and in the painful final stages of terminal illnesses such as cancer. This form of euthanasia involves the intentional administration of medications to cause death. The second and most controversial level of euthanasia involves individuals who may be in relatively good health and who want to end their lives before a debilitating or terminal illness, such as Alzheimer's disease or cancer, drastically impairs their quality of life.

The medical profession does not consider the removal of artificial life support (even nutrition or hydration) to be euthanasia.

THE DEBATE ON EUTHANASIA

Those in favor of euthanasia argue that people should be granted the right to die with dignity, with their senses intact and free of debilitating pain. They contend that the cost of ineffective care, such as medical treatment of people who are in a coma, is wasteful, and that it is inhumane to prolong suffering. If physician-assisted suicide were legalized, doctors would be allowed to offer relief to comatose and suffering people.

The arguments against euthanasia are centered on the "slippery slope" that doctors and policy makers will face in determining when euthanasia is acceptable. This position holds that physicians should not be placed in situations where it is acceptable for them to cause the ultimate harm of death, that no one policy could encompass the scope of the right to die, and that, because most of the people with a terminal illness are unable to express their true wishes effectively, it is too difficult to determine what those wishes are. Those against euthanasia advocate providing more supportive care to the dying. When people with chronic illnesses such as amyotrophic lateral sclerosis seek euthanasia, those against it advise counseling for depression.

Euthyroid

Characterized by normal thyroid gland function. Euthyroid refers to the normal performance of the thyroid gland as compared with hypothyroid (underfunctioning of the thyroid gland) or hyperthyroid (overfunctioning of the thyroid gland).

Eversion

An outwardly turned position of the sole of the foot. Eversion is caused by a deformity or a muscular weakness on the outer side of the lower leg. Eversion can also refer to the turning outward of an eyelid, for example.

Evoked responses

Tests that assess the ability of information to travel to the brain. There are three commonly used evoked response tests: visual evoked response (VER), brain stem auditory evoked response (BAER), and somatosensory evoked potential (SSEP). VER tests assess how well information travels from the eyes to the occipital lobes (visual cortex). Electrodes are placed on the scalp, and the person is asked to stare at a screen with an alternating checkerboard pattern. BAER tests are performed to assess neurological function and diagnose nervous system abnormalities. This test may also be administered to detect hearing loss, especially in infants and children. During the test, electrodes are placed on the scalp, and clicking noises or tones are sent through earphones. Electrodes detect and record the brain's response on a graph. Abnor-mal findings can indicate diagnoses such as hearing loss, multiple sclerosis, or a stroke or brain damage. SSEP tests assess how information travels from the hands or feet through the spinal cord and to the brain.

Ewing sarcoma

A type of malignant tumor that originates in bone. Ewing sarcoma chiefly occurs in children and adolescents, very rarely in adults. This type of sarcoma generally affects the marrow of the long bones, especially the leg and the upper arm. However, it can sometimes occur in bones of the face, the rib, or the pelvis. It is more common among boys than girls and rarely appears in black or Asian individuals. Symptoms include painful, tender swelling in the affected area, fever, and anemia.

Diagnosing Ewing sarcoma may require blood and urine tests, X rays of affected bones, CT (computed tomography) scans, and tissue biopsy. Treatment depends on the stage of the disease and may include surgery, radiation therapy, and chemotherapy. About 150 cases of Ewing sarcoma are diagnosed in the United States each year; two thirds of people with Ewing sarcoma survive more than 5 years after diagnosis.

Examination, physical

A thorough study of a person's state of health. The physical examination typically follows history-taking, in which a doctor listens to a person's concerns and asks questions. Examination usually includes inspection, palpation (direct feeling with the hand), percussion (striking parts of the body with short, sharp taps and feeling and listening to subsequent vibrations), and auscultation (listening with a stethoscope). If a person reports symptoms, the doctor will attempt to determine their cause. Tests may also be ordered to aid in diagnosis. One main objective of regular physical examinations, conducted at frequent intervals even when a person is feeling well, is the early detection of disease. In some cases, early diagnosis and treatment make the difference between cure and serious illness or death. See Focus: Physical examination, page 532.

Excision

Surgical removal of an organ or tissue by cutting out diseased tissue. An excision is used to remove tissue that is abnormal or diseased, such as a breast lump.

Excoriation

Peeling, chafing, or rawness of the skin. Excoriation may be the result of injury caused by trauma due to scratching or an abrasion or burn.

Exemestane

A drug used to treat breast cancer. Exemestane (Aromasin) works by inactivating aromatase, the principal enzyme that converts androgen to estrogen, the female hormone that is often responsible for producing the growth of breast cancer cells. Exemestane interferes in that process.

Exercise

Increased energy expenditure due to muscular activity, usually resulting in movement of the body or its parts. Exercise involves one or more organs and structures of the body and is important for overall health. Regular exercise gives improved balance and coordination, improved sleep, and a longer life expectancy. The specific benefits of an ongoing exercise program throughout a lifetime include the prevention or delay of serious diseases and conditions including coronary artery disease, stroke, the most common form of diabetes, some types of cancer, age-related bone loss, and osteoporosis. Exercising regularly aids in weight management because exercise helps regulate the appetite and reduce body fat.

Exercise should be geared to the physical condition and health of a person. Exercise specialists found in most community exercise facilities and private health clubs can help in the evaluation of the appropriate exercise for an individual, including the kind of exercise, the length and frequency of exercise sessions, and the level of intensity with which the exercises should be performed. Moderately intense exercises, such as walking, are a safe activity for nearly all individuals. Persons with known chronic disease or concerns about the safety of exercise for them should check with their doctor before starting an exercise program. Older persons and persons with risk factors for heart disease should check with their physician before starting a vigorous exercise program.

It is considered more beneficial in general to exercise consistently rather than to achieve a high level of intensity when exercising. As little as 30 minutes a day of exercise at a moderate intensity will gradually increase the fitness level of an individual and establish the known health benefits derived from regular exercise. The 30 minutes can be divided into three separate sessions throughout the day, each lasting 10 minutes, without diminishing the benefits. In addition to 30 minutes of moderately intensive aerobic activity on most days, it also is important to engage in 30 to 40 minutes of strengthening or resistance exercises (see EXERCISE, STRENGTHENING; EXERCISE, RESISTANCE) at least twice a week.

Exercise and aging

Exercise offers many benefits to people as they age because it prevents or delays many age-related physical diseases and disorders and helps maintain function. Regular physical activity is known to help prevent coronary artery disease, high blood pressure, stroke, diabetes, depression, and some cancers. Physical conditioning can also improve the quality of life as a person grows older by helping an individual retain the self-reliance and independence that are drastically altered by the effects of diseases such as osteoporosis and arthritis.

Healthy people who are older can

BENEFITS OF DIFFERENT KINDS OF EXERCISE

Exercise protects against disease, improves endurance, helps the body more efficiently process food, improves the quality of sleep, and helps reduce anxiety, stress, and depression. Here are the benefits of various types of exercise on the body:

- **Aerobic exercise** improves the health of the heart, lungs, and circulatory system. Stamina, metabolic rate, and endurance are increased in response to the demands of physical work. Examples: walking, running, bicycling.
- **Weight-bearing exercise** helps strengthen bones and prevents bone loss and osteoporosis. Example: walking.
- **Stretching exercise** increases the range of motion and suppleness of the joints, muscles, tendons, and ligaments, developing flexibility to keep joints healthy and functional. Example: yoga.
- **Anaerobic exercise** increases speed and muscle power; it is important for performance in some sports. Example: weight lifting.
- **Resistance or strengthening exercise** increases muscle mass, strength, and endurance; it adds support to joint structures and improves the ratio of muscle to fat in the body. Examples: isometrics, weight lifting.

FOCUS: PHYSICAL EXAMINATION

Doctors assess a variety of factors during a physical examination, each of which can provide vital clues about a person's health. The doctor's first step is to take the person's medical history—that is, to hear the person's complaints, if any, and to ask questions about the person's general medical condition, lifestyle, and family history of disease. The doctor also may offer recommendations about how to prevent development of medical problems.

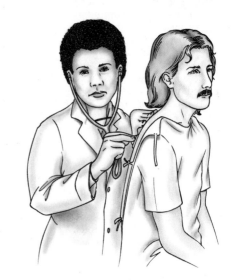

AUSCULTATION
Doctors usually use a stethoscope to listen to heart and lung sounds, a procedure called auscultation. Auscultation may be performed without a stethoscope as well.

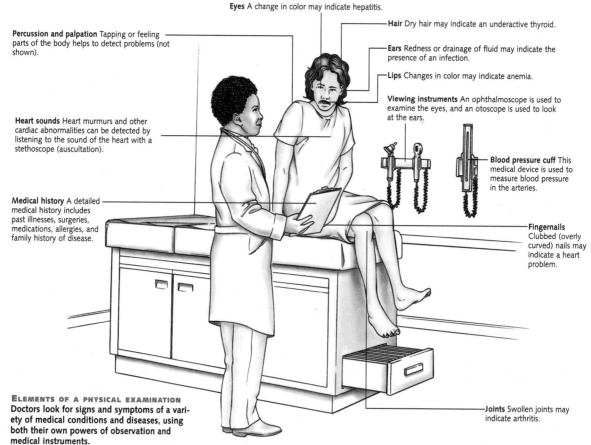

Eyes A change in color may indicate hepatitis.

Percussion and palpation Tapping or feeling parts of the body helps to detect problems (not shown).

Hair Dry hair may indicate an underactive thyroid.

Ears Redness or drainage of fluid may indicate the presence of an infection.

Lips Changes in color may indicate anemia.

Viewing instruments An ophthalmoscope is used to examine the eyes, and an otoscope is used to look at the ears.

Heart sounds Heart murmurs and other cardiac abnormalities can be detected by listening to the sound of the heart with a stethoscope (auscultation).

Blood pressure cuff This medical device is used to measure blood pressure in the arteries.

Medical history A detailed medical history includes past illnesses, surgeries, medications, allergies, and family history of disease.

Fingernails Clubbed (overly curved) nails may indicate a heart problem.

ELEMENTS OF A PHYSICAL EXAMINATION
Doctors look for signs and symptoms of a variety of medical conditions and diseases, using both their own powers of observation and medical instruments.

Joints Swollen joints may indicate arthritis.

derive many health benefits from moderate, regular exercise. Brisk walking on most days of the week offers these benefits and is an ideal exercise for an older person. Getting exercise from daily chores and recreational activities, including going up and down stairs, gardening, shopping, vacuuming, mowing the lawn, and social dancing, can be an important part of an overall physical activity program. The overall goal is to get about 30 minutes each day of some form of moderately intense activity. Strengthening exercises, including weight training, should be included at least twice weekly.

The benefits of exercising for people who have arthritis outweigh the risks, unless one or more joints are acutely inflamed. Guidelines for exercising with arthritis include starting the session gradually after massaging or applying heat to muscles and joints, taking a warm shower, or walking in place for a few minutes to warm up the body. The person should stop any specific exercise that causes pain, experiment to find the time of day when the least pain and stiffness are experienced, and take aspirin or another nonsteroidal anti-inflammatory drug (NSAID) 1 hour before exercising to minimize swelling and reduce pain. A person with arthritis should also avoid high-impact and stop-and-start exercises and stretch slowly without bouncing at the end of every exercise session, including walking.

Bone loss in women and muscle loss in men, once considered normal effects of aging, can be reduced by regular exercise, which can slow bone loss and reverse the loss of muscle by increasing muscle mass and strength. Because regular exercise increases the ability of the heart, lungs, and blood vessels to deliver adequate oxygen to muscles during physical activity, it slows the loss of aerobic capacity that normally occurs with the aging process.

The appropriate fitness level for an older person is one that provides the amount of energy required to perform everyday activities. The best level of fitness will promote enthusiastic participation in social and recreational activities and help a person avoid the debilitating consequences of aging. The goal of a personal exercise pro-

gram is to maximize individual potential in the four basic components of fitness: aerobic capacity, strength, flexibility, and weight control.

Exercise stress testing

See CARDIAC STRESS TESTING.

Exercise, aerobic

A form of physical EXERCISE that increases the heart rate and blood flow to deliver more oxygen to the working muscles. Aerobic exercise is physical exertion and repetitive motion of the large muscles, such as the leg muscles, that sustain increased heart, lung, and circulatory rates. These body systems supply the working muscles in the body with the amount of oxygen they require to continue functioning and to remove by-products and wastes of the metabolic process. A person's maximum aerobic capacity is a measure of the body's ability to accomplish this. Repetitive, sustained physical activities, such as brisk walking, jogging, running, swimming, rowing, hiking, bicycling, rope jumping, aerobic dancing and step aerobic classes, and cross-country skiing, are considered aerobic exercise and can increase a person's aerobic capacity.

Aerobic exercises are also called endurance or "cardio" exercises. It is recommended that people aim for an exercise schedule that includes 30 minutes of aerobic exercise every day; starting with a program of three aerobic sessions weekly and building up to daily activity may be advisable. Each vigorous aerobic session should be preceded by a 5-minute warm-up and followed by 5 to 10 minutes of cooling down and stretching. Warm-ups help the body adapt to higher levels of exercise, while cooling down and stretching may help avoid sore muscles and stiffness.

The health benefits of regular aerobic exercise are numerous. Aerobic activity enhances the efficient functioning of the heart and lungs, helping to increase the health of these organs, and helps prevent heart disease and stroke. It also improves flexibility in the muscles and joints and may help deflect the effects of arthritis. Combined with a healthy diet, aerobic exercise aids in controlling weight. Regular aerobic exercise low-

ers blood pressure and raises the "good" HDL (high-density lipoprotein) cholesterol levels. Regular aerobic activity also improves feelings of well-being and is known to help combat some forms of depression.

Exercise, anaerobic

Short-term EXERCISE that relies on anaerobic (meaning not requiring oxygen) metabolic processes for energy required to perform the activity. Examples of anaerobic exercise include short sprints, jumps, weight-resistance exercises (see EXERCISE, RESISTANCE), and doing lunges, squats, sit-ups, push-ups, and other activities that require shorts bursts of explosive movements. A good anaerobic exercise routine should include exercises that involve all the major muscle groups including the abdominals, legs, chest, back, shoulders, and arms. Anaerobic exercise can increase muscular strength and power; an example is weight lifting.

Exercise, resistance

Strength-building EXERCISE that requires the muscles to push against or resist the weight of an object or a force, such as gravity. Resistance exercise may also be called strength training, body building, body sculpting, and strengthening exercise. Lifting free weights or using weight machines involves the resistance of the muscles against the weight of what is being lifted or pushed. Calisthenics, including sit-ups, push-ups, and leg lifts, use the body's muscles to resist gravity. The weight machines at fitness centers, used

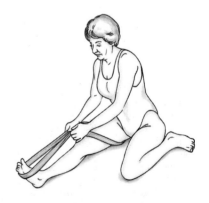

MAKING MUSCLES WORK
Resistance builds both strength and endurance and can be done at home or in a fitness center.

with the guidance of an instructor or trainer, offer one of the safest and most efficient forms of resistance exercise, which can also increase a person's endurance.

Exercise, strengthening

Physical activity that builds strength in the muscles. Strengthening exercises may also improve posture and balance, Exercises that strengthen muscles help support the joints, which can help reduce the symptoms of arthritis. Improved strength may help decrease the risk of injuries and improve a person's ability to perform many activities of daily life.

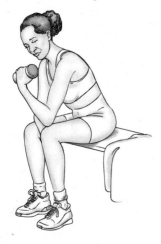

STRENGTHENING MUSCLES
Strengthening exercise increases metabolism and contributes to weight loss. A good strengthening workout, which often involves resistance exercise, involves all the major muscle groups.

Weight lifting, using either free weights or weight machines, sometimes called resistance training, is the most common and efficient exercise for building strength and increasing muscle mass. Lifting weights may also increase bone density and help prevent the amount of bone lost with aging. Other strengthening exercises include those that use the muscles to move the body's weight and resist gravity, such as push-ups, leg lifts, and other calisthenics or floor exercises.

A routine of strengthening exercises should incorporate the use of all the major muscle groups: the arms, shoulders, back, chest, legs, and abdominals. The routine should also

be balanced and work the muscles on opposite sides of the same joint equally. For example, the triceps (muscles on the underside of the upper arm) in addition to the biceps (muscles on top of the upper arm) should be exercised with the same amount of weight for the same number of repetitions. See also EXERCISE, ANAEROBIC; EXERCISE; and WEIGHT TRAINING.

Exercise, weight-bearing

Any physical activity that requires the body to support its weight, including many aerobic exercises (see EXERCISE, AEROBIC) as well as strengthening and resistance exercises (see EXERCISE, STRENGTHENING; EXERCISE, RESISTANCE). Exercise that is done in a standing position qualifies as weight-bearing exercise; swimming, cycling, and other exercises performed in a seated or prone position are not considered weight-bearing exercises. The principal benefit of weight-bearing exercise is that it strengthens the bones. When bones take on the weight of the body, the bone tissue builds density and

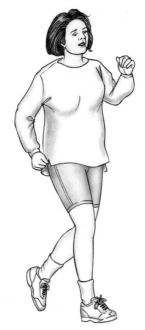

BUILDING STRONG BONES
Just as exercise builds muscle, weight-bearing exercise builds bone by making the bone tissue more dense, which is particularly important for women at risk of osteoporosis.

becomes stronger. Walking is a beneficial weight-bearing exercise because it places weight on the large bones of the legs and torso with little risk of injury. Weight-bearing exercise is especially recommended for women who are at risk for osteoporosis as it may help prevent this disease by increasing bone strength.

Exfoliation

Shedding skin cells or peeling off layers of skin. Exfoliation is a natural process. However, it can occur more acutely in cases of certain skin diseases or after a severe sunburn. Exfoliative skin preparations and roughly textured loofahs or sponges are sometimes used for cosmetic purposes to accelerate the shedding of skin cells.

Exfoliative dermatitis

See ERYTHRODERMA.

Exhibitionism

A mental illness characterized by highly arousing urges, fantasies, or actions involving the exposure of one's genitals to a stranger. Sometimes the person masturbates during exposure or a fantasy of exposure. Some people engaging in exhibitionism are aware of wanting to shock; others fantasize that the stranger will find the exposure sexually stimulating. Exhibitionism impairs the person's ability to function in a family, society, or work setting and usually causes significant distress. The disorder usually begins before age 18, almost always affects males, and appears to become less severe after age 40. It is difficult to treat unless the person is faced with arrest, divorce, or other negative consequences or unless the person is highly motivated to change.

Exocrine gland

A gland that releases substances through a duct or channel onto or into an organ or area of the body. For example, lacrimal ducts secrete tears onto the eye; the salivary glands secrete saliva into the mouth; sweat glands produce sweat on the skin; pancreatic tissue secretes digestive enzymes that are carried through ducts into the intestine. Exocrine secretions may be directed by hormones or by chemical neurotransmitters that function similarly to hormones. See ENDOCRINE SYSTEM.

Exophthalmos

Abnormal bulging of one or both eyes; also known as proptosis. Exophthalmic eyes blink infrequently and seem to stare. The most common cause is a hyperactive thyroid gland (hyperthyroidism), which swells tissues in the eye socket and pushes the eyeball forward (see GRAVES DISEASE). The condition can also result from bleeding behind the eye (usually from injury), inflammation or infection of the eye socket, tumors, or blood vessel abnormalities that cause blood to back up behind the eye. A bulging eye requires prompt professional evaluation.

Treatment depends on cause. Surgery is used to repair vessel abnormalities, remove tumors, or relieve pressure on the optic nerve. Control of hyperthyroidism with medication may improve exophthalmos from that cause. Sometimes radiation therapy is needed to control exophthalmos caused by Graves disease. Inflammation of the eye socket is treated with corticosteroid medications, which reduce swelling.

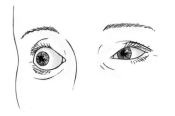

BULGING EYE
When the eyeball is pushed outward, usually as the result of swelling behind the eye, an unusual amount of the "white" of the eye is exposed. The eye will feel dry, and the person may have double vision or otherwise impaired sight. The eyelid may not close completely. Medical attention is important.

Exostosis

A growth on the surface of a bone. It typically occurs in the femur (thighbone) or tibia (shin). Usually, exostosis is noncancerous and involves bones that develop from cartilage, including those found in the ear. About 90 percent of all bone tumors are cases of exostosis, which affects twice as many men as women. Treatment is rarely necessary, except

when the bony growth is unsightly or pressing on a nerve.

Exotoxin

Poisonous proteins produced inside the cells of disease-causing bacteria and released into the bloodstream. Effects depend on the particular exotoxin, but exotoxins are among the most poisonous substances known. They can affect nerves and cause paralysis. They can also invade the intestinal tract, leading to diarrhea, fever, rash, and possibly TOXIC SHOCK SYNDROME. The most common cause for exotoxin production is FOOD POISONING.

Exotropia

A type of crossed eyes (strabismus), in which one or both eyes may turn outward. Exotropia may produce double vision or other types of vision impairment.

Expectorants

Drugs used to promote a productive cough. Coughs are productive (produce phlegm) or nonproductive (dry and hacking). Expectorants are the treatment of choice to help eject mucus and fluids from the lungs. The best natural expectorant is water. A person with mucus in the airway should greatly increase his or her consumption of fluids. Expectorants work by triggering the cough reflex to help get mucus up and out of the throat and chest.

Many expectorants are sold without prescription. Guaifenesin is the only expectorant classified as safe and effective by the Food and Drug Administration. Examples of guaifenesin include Robitussin, Hytuss, Naldecon Senior EX, and many others.

Expectoration

The act of discharging matter from the throat or lungs by coughing and spitting.

Expiration

The stage in respiration, or breathing, when air is expelled from the lungs. During this process, the diaphragm is pulled upward and the rib cage contracts, or moves downward.

Exploratory surgery

Any diagnostic procedure used to examine a portion of the body that is thought to be diseased. With sophisti-

cated X rays, such as CT (computed tomography) scans and MRI (magnetic resonance imaging) to aid in diagnosing a condition, exploratory surgery is performed less frequently. However, exploratory surgery is an option when a medical problem exists and the exact cause, extent of disease, or treatment cannot be determined without direct examination. An example is abdominal pain, which can come from multiple causes. In some cases, determining the cause of some otherwise unexplained abdominal pain may require opening the abdomen and physically examining the organ or bowel, which may be removed or repaired during the time of the exploratory surgery.

Explosive disorder

A mental illness characterized by repeated episodes of serious violence against people or property that occur with little or no provocation. The outbursts last from a few minutes to several hours and may be preceded by a change in mood, rapid heartbeat, confusion, or amnesia. Relief follows the violent episode, and the individual usually expresses upset, remorse, regret, or embarrassment. Since explosive disorder is very rare, little is known about the cause of the disorder. Similar outbursts can be caused by certain medications, illegal drugs, a serious head injury, epilepsy, Alzheimer's disease, or by a number of other disorders, such as attention deficit/hyperactivity disorder, mania, or psychosis.

Exstrophy of the bladder

An uncommon birth defect in which the bladder and urethra are turned inside out and are open to the outside of the body through a space in the lower abdominal wall. The bones of the pelvis are also separated. To reduce the risk of kidney infection and damage to the bladder lining, surgery to repair the defect is usually performed within 48 hours of birth. During surgery, the bladder is separated from the wall of the abdomen and closed. The urethra may be reconstructed at this time or closed in a second surgery. The pelvic bones may be repaired at the same time or in a later surgery. Follow-up operations are often needed, depending on

E

the severity of the defect and associated problems.

Extradural hemorrhage

See HEMORRHAGE, EPIDURAL.

Extrapyramidal system

The portion of the central nervous system that affects electrical impulses sent from the BRAIN to the skeletal muscles, influencing large muscle movements such as walking. The system connects nerves in the CEREBRUM with the basal ganglia (structures deep within the brain that coordinate voluntary muscle movement) and parts of the BRAIN STEM.

Extrovert

A personality type that is primarily concerned with and focused on external objects and actions and other people. Extroverts are generally at ease in social settings, unlikely to engage in solitary pursuits, and often avoid being alone. The opposite of extrovert is INTROVERT.

Exudate

Fluids such as pus that leak through vessel walls into adjoining tissues. Exudate is composed of white blood cells, proteins, and other substances. Fluids may leak from surgical incisions or sites of inflammation or infection.

Eye

The sensory organ of sight. The eyes focus light rays to perceive images and then convert these images into impulses that are transmitted to the brain.

The two spherical eyeballs lie within the skull, protruding through the eye sockets, but largely protected by bone. Inside the skull, the eyeballs are cushioned on all sides by fat. The EYELID protects the protruding portion of the eyes, trapping foreign particles in the eyelashes and TEARS and opening and closing reflexively to cover the eyeballs. The principal lacrimal glands, which produce and release tears, lie just inside the eye socket and drain onto an outer layer of the eye called the CONJUNCTIVA. The conjunctiva is a clear membrane that covers the entire front side of the eyeballs, extending somewhat back into the eye socket, and then folding back

out to form the inner lining of the eyelids. The eyeball can move freely within this seal. The conjunctiva contains glands that, along with the main lacrimal glands, secrete tears and mucus to continuously cleanse and lubricate the eyeballs.

Behind the conjunctiva is the SCLERA, the white of the eye, which forms a tough outer layer over the eyeball. In the center front of the sclera, the CORNEA is a transparent, protruding structure that is the main focusing lens for the eye. The cornea is cushioned by the aqueous humor, a thick transparent fluid that fills an area in the front part of the eye. The IRIS, which is the colored part of the eye, lies behind the aqueous humor. It is a ring of muscle fibers surrounding the PUPIL, which is an opening through which light rays can pass. The iris contracts or expands to control the size of the pupil, which determines the amount of light entering the eye. Behind the iris is the crystalline LENS, which adjusts the focus of the light rays. The shape of the crystalline lens is altered by a circle of muscle, the ciliary body, which surrounds the lens. Behind the crystalline lens, the hollow of the eyeball is filled with a clear, gelatinous substance called the vitreous humor.

The RETINA lines the back of the eyeball. The pattern of light or image focused by the cornea and the crystalline lens falls on the retina. This complex structure is composed of nerve tissue containing light-sensitive cells called rods and cones. The rods and cones translate the image on the retina into a pattern of nerve impulses that travel to the brain via the optic nerve, which extends from the back of the eye. The area of the brain that controls sight, the visual cortex in the cerebrum, interprets the impulses. To keep the retina supplied with oxygen and nutrients, a web of blood vessels surrounds the retina. See VISION.

Eye drops

Liquid medicine used to treat conditions of the eye. Eye drops are used for chronic conditions such as glaucoma and dry eye, and they are also used for the short-term treatment of allergies and infections. Doctors may use eye drops during an eye examination to enable them to dilate the pupil and view the interior of the eye.

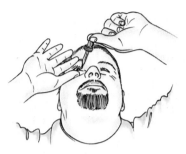

Technique for adult

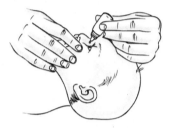

Technique for infant

ADMINISTERING EYE DROPS
The technique for applying eye drops effectively and comfortably is to pull down the lower lid to create a little pocket for the medication—not to drop the medication directly on the eye. For an infant or small child, an adult can give the eye drops the same way, resting the hand with the eye dropper on the child's forehead to help steady the child.

Eye drops must be given with care to prevent waste. One recommended method is for the person to lie down or sit with the head tilted back, then to pull the lower eyelid slightly away from the eye, thereby forming a little pouch into which one drop can be placed. The eyes should then be kept closed for 3 minutes to permit the medication to be absorbed. If more than one drop (or more than one medicine) is prescribed, it is advisable to wait at least 10 minutes before repeating the procedure. Eye drops are sterile, and the dropper should never touch the eye.

Eye injury

FOR FIRST AID
see Eye injuries, page 1320

Physical damage to the eye or its surrounding tissue as a result of accident or mishap. The structure of the face protects the eye from most injuries. The eyeball is set into a socket surrounded by a strong, bony ridge that

INSIDE THE EYE

Light waves from perceived objects pass through the cornea, anterior (front) chamber, pupil, and lens of the eye. These structures focus the light waves onto the retina, resulting in images that appear upside down. The retina then relays signals to the optic nerve. These signals travel through the optic nerve, through the middle of the brain, to the visual cortex where they are interpreted and experienced as sight.

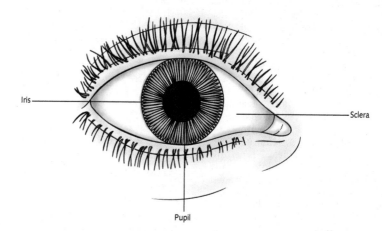

EXTERIOR OF THE EYE
The pupil of the eye is the round, black opening through which light passes to the retina. The iris is the circular, colored portion of the eye around the pupil. The sclera is the dense, curved membrane surrounding the iris and is commonly referred to as the "white of the eye."

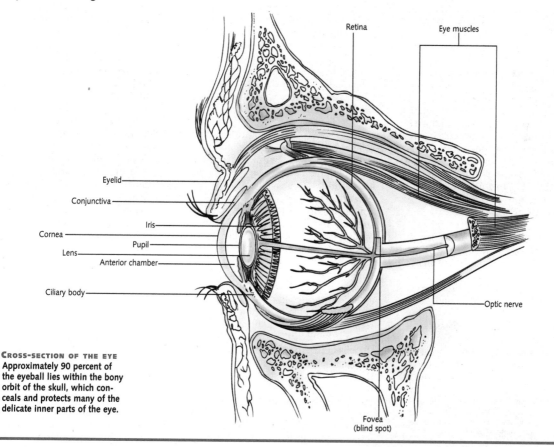

CROSS-SECTION OF THE EYE
Approximately 90 percent of the eyeball lies within the bony orbit of the skull, which conceals and protects many of the delicate inner parts of the eye.

can absorb considerable energy without serious damage. The eyelids close quickly as a barrier against foreign objects, and the eye itself tolerates light impact. Still, injuries to the eyes occur. The danger an injury poses to sight and the way it is treated medically depends on the type of injury.

FOREIGN OBJECTS

Foreign objects are the most common cause of eye injuries, and the foreign objects most likely to cause injury are contact lenses. Injury results if contact lenses are worn too long, cleaned improperly, or removed forcibly or ineptly. Another common source of such injuries is windblown sand and dirt, low-hanging tree branches, glass particles, metal shavings, and sawdust. Most foreign-object injuries are painful but minor. However, there is danger that a foreign body can damage the cornea (the clear outer covering of the eye), resulting in infection or scarring and vision loss. Symptoms of a foreign object include pain, a feeling of something in the eye, redness, bleeding from surface blood vessels, swelling of the eye and eyelid, and blurred vision. A foreign object in the eye needs to be removed, but this should be done only by a medical professional if the object is touching the cornea or is embedded in the eye or surrounding tissue. After removing a foreign body, treatment includes applying antibiotic ointment if the cornea has been scratched. With large abrasions, a patch is placed over the eye to allow healing, which is usually complete in 1 to 3 days.

BLUNT TRAUMA

A nonpenetrating force directed against the eyes—such as impact from a baseball or basketball, a fist, or a car dashboard—can force the eye back into the socket, possibly damaging the surface structures (eyelids, cornea, lens, sclera, and conjunctiva; see EYE for anatomical detail) and those at the back of the eye (retina and optic nerve). Bruising (black eye) and swelling result quickly from blunt trauma; broken blood vessels on the eye surface can give the eye a red appearance. A black eye usually

> Terms in small capital letters—for example, PHYSICAL THERAPY or PAGET DISEASE—indicate a cross-reference to another entry with more information.

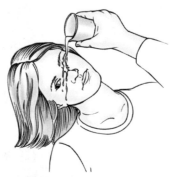

FLUSHING OUT THE EYE
A foreign object (such as an eyelash or a speck of dirt) that is floating on the surface of the eye is usually fairly easy to remove. If natural tearing does not wash the object out, tilt the person's head back and pour a gentle stream of water over the eyeball.

indicates superficial damage to the tissues surrounding the eye and usually heals on its own within 2 weeks. Damage to the interior of the eye is more dangerous; for example, bleeding in the interior of the eye, tearing of the iris, dislocation of the lens, or detachment of the retina can all cause loss of vision. Fracture of the bones of the eye socket causes vision problems if eye muscles or the optic nerve are involved. In very severe injuries, the eyeball can be ruptured.

Ice packs are used to reduce swelling and bruising from blunt trauma. Damage to the surface or interior of the eye may require surgical repair. Medication may be given to reduce swelling. Pain medications are often prescribed since eye injuries are painful.

PENETRATING INJURIES

An object that enters the eyeball or surrounding tissues is an emergency requiring the fastest possible treatment. Penetrating injuries include wounds from BBs, bullets, knives, nails, broken glass, and other sharp objects. First aid consists of placing a shield over the injured eye without touching the object, without trying to remove it, and without applying pressure to the object or the eye itself. If the object is large, a paper cone or cup is placed over it and taped in place. If it is small, both eyes are covered with a sterile cloth or dressing without applying any pressure to the eye.

BURNS

The eye can be burned by heat, by exposure to ultraviolet light, and by exposure to irritating chemicals, such as solvents, acids, garden chemicals, and cleaning products. Since the eyelids close very rapidly to protect the eyes, most heat burns affect the eyelids. Extreme heat can burn the eye itself. Treatment depends on the severity of the injury.

Chemical burns from alkaline substances (for example, lye) are generally more dangerous than acids. When the eye is burned with a chemical, the person tends to keep the eye closed because of the pain. This may trap the irritating substance against the surface of the eye, increasing the damage. The eye should be flushed with water immediately. Applying a cool compress can help relieve pain and swelling, but pressure should not be applied on the injured eye.

Eye tumors

Abnormal growth of tissue in the eyeball or its surrounding structures. Eye tumors can be benign, or noncancerous—that is, their growth is confined to a particular body structure and they do not metastasize or spread throughout the body. Some are malignant (cancerous)—that is, they can spread and threaten life.

RETINOBLASTOMA

This is a rare but dangerous cancer found in children, mostly those younger than 5 years. It affects the retina, the light-sensitive layer of nervous tissue at the back of the eye. Retinoblastoma may be inherited, or it can occur sporadically. Tumors found in young children are usually inherited, and the disease often affects both eyes. The sporadic form usually occurs from damage to a gene that suppresses tumor growth, affects one eye, and can occur in older children. Symptoms of retinoblastoma include whiteness in the pupil, a white glow in the eye, crossed eyes, redness and pain, poor vision, and a different-colored iris in each eye. Diagnosis requires a thorough examination of the eye when it is widely dilated. This is usually done under general anesthesia in a hospital setting. If a tumor is suspected, ultrasound scanning of the eye is generally performed, as well as a CT (computed tomography) scan of the head, eye sockets, and eyes to assess the size and extent of the tumor.

Treatment depends on the stage of

the cancer and whether one or both eyes are involved. If the tumor is small and confined to the eye, radiation therapy (use of X rays to kill cancer cells), cryotherapy (use of extreme cold to kill cancer cells), thermotherapy (use of extreme heat to kill cancer cells), laser surgery (to destroy blood vessels that nourish the tumor), or chemotherapy (cancer-killing medications) is used in order to preserve the eye. If the tumor is large and the eye cannot be saved, it is usually removed surgically. If both eyes are involved and the cancer has not spread beyond them, the eye with the larger tumor may be removed and nonsurgical therapy used on the remaining eye to preserve sight.

Survivors of the heritable form of retinoblastomas are at risk for developing other new tumors, especially osteosarcomas, after many years. Therefore, survivors need to be observed carefully throughout their lives. The siblings of a child with retinoblastoma need to be examined regularly since they are at risk for the disease. People who come from a family with retinoblastoma and who are planning to have children should consider GENETIC COUNSELING.

MELANOMA

Usually thought of as a cancer of the skin, melanoma can also occur in the eye. Melanoma is the most common malignant eye tumor in adults. Since this cancer arises in the choroid (the vascular layer under the retina), it is also known as choroidal melanoma. Melanoma is a particularly fast-growing and fast-spreading cancer, and it is often lethal. Melanoma in the eye can be a primary tumor, or it may have spread from another site in the body. Early symptoms are mild and often pass unnoticed. They include a small lesion in the iris or the conjunctiva (the membrane lining the eyelids and the exposed outer surface of the eye), change in iris color, poor vision in one eye, or a bulging eye. If the tumor is left untreated, it will eventually cause the retina to detach from the back of the eye, which results in distorted vision or blindness. Treatment depends on the size of the tumor and whether other sites in the body are involved. Small melanomas are treated with radiation therapy or laser surgery. Large tumors may require removal of the eye to

prevent spread of the cancer to the brain and other organs. Chemotherapy is usually advised if the cancer extends beyond the eye. Since skin and eyelid melanoma are related to sunlight exposure, wearing sunglasses and staying out of the sun are effective preventive measures for these types of cancer.

EYELID TUMORS

The most common tumor on the eyelids is the xanthelasma, which is a yellow-white, flat growth of fatty material. Xanthelasmas are benign and are usually removed only if they become cosmetically unappealing. Xanthelasmas may indicate elevated blood cholesterol levels, particularly in young people. Two kinds of skin cancer, BASAL CELL CARCINOMA and the less common SQUAMOUS CELL CARCINOMA, can develop on the eyelids. If a growth on the eyelid fails to disappear within several weeks, a biopsy may be indicated. If the growth is cancerous, it is removed surgically.

ORBITAL TUMOR

Tumors can arise in the bones, muscles, and fat surrounding the eye, or they may develop in surrounding structures, such as the sinuses or brain cavity, and invade the eye socket (orbit). Orbital tumors appear in both children and adults, and most of these growths are benign. The principal symptom of an orbital tumor is a bulging eyeball.

Most orbital tumors in children result from abnormal development, such as cysts on the lining of bone or blood vessel tumors. Orbital tumors in childhood are rare.

In adults, the most common benign tumor of the eye socket is a blood vessel abnormality, such as a hemangioma. Less commonly, tumors arise from the nerves, fat bodies, or sinuses. Some of these tumors can be cancerous; the most common cancerous tumor of the orbit in adults is LYMPHOMA. Rarely, cancerous eye tumors can also result from the spread of cancer elsewhere, such as the breast or prostate, or from invasion of the eye socket by skin cancers in surrounding tissues.

Eye, examination of

A series of tests performed to measure the eyes' ability to see clearly and to screen for common eye diseases. If one sees normally, an eye examination

every 3 to 5 years during adulthood until age 50 years is recommended. After that, the eyes should be examined more frequently, including checks for glaucoma, a disease that causes loss of vision as a result of damage to the optic nerve often as a result of high pressure in the eye. If one wears or needs glasses, examinations should be conducted at least every 2 years, or more often if recommended by an eye specialist. Contact lens wearers should be examined at least once a year. Young children's eyes are usually examined during well-child examinations, but unless a vision problem is suspected, a child's visual acuity is usually examined for the first time between ages 3 and 5 years.

HISTORY

In the first portion of the examination, the eye specialist (an ophthalmologist or an optometrist) is likely to begin with a series of questions about the person's family history and the person's own medical history. The eye specialist will inquire about diseases that affect the eyes, such as diabetes mellitus, types 1 and 2; glaucoma; and high blood pressure (hypertension), and about any medications taken. The eye specialist will also ask if there is any family history of eye diseases, such as glaucoma. Finally, the eye specialist will make sure there are no current visual problems, such as double vision, blurred vision, light sensitivity, or pain.

VISUAL ACUITY

This part of the examination assesses the sharpness of vision. The most common test for visual acuity is performed using a Snellen chart, which shows letters arranged in lines of increasingly smaller size. Each row is designated by a number corresponding to the distance in feet from which a person with normal vision can read all the letters of the row. For example, the letters in the "40" row are large enough for a person with normal vision to read from 40 feet. By convention, vision is measured at a distance of 20 feet. If a person can read the "20" row, he or she is said to have 20/20 vision. Acuity is scored as a set of two numbers, such as 20/20. The first number represents the distance from the chart in feet, and the second number represents the smallest row of letters that a person can read from the testing distance. For example, if a person whose vision is less sharp can only read from 20 feet that which a person with normal vision can read from 60 feet, visual acuity would be scored as 20/60. Special charts with numbers instead of letters are used for people who cannot read, and children are tested with charts that replace letters with shapes. If one wears glasses or contact lenses, visual acuity will probably be measured with one of these forms of correction.

As part of this phase of the examination, the eye specialist will test the movements of the eyes, typically by moving a light or object across one's field of vision and asking the person to follow it. Color blindness is assessed with Ishihara color plates, which determine color vision based on the ability to see patterns or numbers in a series of multicolored charts. People who are color blind cannot see the numbers, or they perceive different numbers from those seen by people with normal vision.

EXTERNAL EXAMINATION

The eye specialist can also examine the external parts of the eye with a slit lamp, a table-mounted microscope combined with a special light source. The person being examined is seated with his or her chin placed on a chin rest. Light is projected by a slit beam, which allows the eye specialist to examine the eye through the

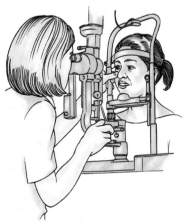

SLIT-LAMP EXAMINATION
The slit lamp is a fundamental tool for eye examinations. The device enables the doctor to direct a beam of light into a person's eye and view the features of the eye through a microscope. Within the lamp, the light passes through a slit that the doctor can vary in width to study the eye in different ways.

microscope. The combination of the slit beam of light and the magnification allows a detailed examination to be made of the eyelid, cornea, iris, and lens.

INTERNAL EXAMINATION

The eye specialist can look inside the eye with an instrument known as the ophthalmoscope. This is a handheld device that combines a magnifier with a strong, focused light source that shines through to the back (fundus) of the eye and allows the specialist to examine its structures, such as the optic disc, the retina (the thin light-sensitive layer of nervous tissue that relays visual information to the brain), and blood vessels. Dilating drops are usually placed in the eye to allow easier examination. The fundus can provide clues to the health of the eye and often of the whole body. Changes in blood vessels in the retina can indicate the severity of hypertension. Small particles in these same vessels signal the formation of plaques or clots containing cholesterol and indicate an increased risk for heart attack or stroke. Changes caused by diabetes mellitus and tears or holes in the retina are visible through the ophthalmoscope.

The eye specialist also examines the portion of the retina known as the optic disc (or optic nerve), which is the point where the optic nerve joins the retina. The shape and color of the optic disc can indicate eye disease, particularly glaucoma. Changes in the optic disc may also occur in people with extremely high blood pressure or brain tumors.

ADDITIONAL TESTING

The pressure inside the eye is routinely tested. This is technically known as tonometry. The most common tonometry device places a small plastic tip against the cornea (the clear outer covering of the eye). This displaces a small area of the cornea, and a reading of the pressure in the eye may then be obtained. Less common and less accurate is pneumotonometry, a test that directs a quick puff of air against the surface of the eye.

If the eye specialist suspects breaks in the cornea (the clear covering on the exposed portion of the eye), he or she may examine it with the aid of FLUORESCEIN strips. The fluorescein collects in any breaks in the cornea

and can be seen in cobalt-blue or fluorescent light.

Eye, foreign body in

See EYE INJURY.

Eye, prosthetic

An artificial, cosmetic replacement for an eye lost to trauma or surgery; also known popularly as a glass eye. Although glass was used in the past to fashion prosthetic eyes, it is rarely used now. Since the middle 1980s, the most widely used materials are hydroxyapatite, an inert porous substance, and porous polyethylene. The material is shaped into a sphere, then wrapped in sclera (the tough, white, fibrous outer covering of the eye) obtained from a cadaver. The wrapped sphere is inserted surgically into the eye socket, and the muscles that move the eye are connected to it. Once the area heals after surgery, blood vessels penetrate the sphere so that it becomes an integral part of the eye socket and moves normally with the remaining natural eye. Prosthetic eyes achieve good cosmetic results in most cases, with a relatively small number of complications, such as bulging or sinking of the prosthesis within the eye socket or poor coordination of movement with the other eye.

Eyelid

Two folds of skin that protect the surface of each EYE. Under the skin lie layers of dense fibrous tissue and muscle. The upper and lower eyelids close quickly as a reflex action to shield the eye against harsh light and foreign objects. They also secrete an oily component of tears. Their constant blinking action moves tears over the surface of the eyes to keep them moist and clean. The eyelashes along the edge of each eyelid are actually three to four rows of hairs that help sift out dust and other materials before they reach the eye. The eyelid itself is held in position by ligaments attached to the eye socket of the skull. The eyelids can also close tightly and push the eyeball back into the socket to prevent injury.

Eyelid surgery

A procedure that tightens bagging or drooping eyelids by removing excess tissue; also called blepharoplasty. Typically, eyelid surgery is performed for cosmetic reasons; baggy eyelids make an individual look older and more tired than he or she feels. Cosmetic eyelid surgery can be performed alone or along with another cosmetic surgery, such as a FACE-LIFT. In some cases, drooping eyelids interfere with vision, primarily to the sides. In such cases, eyelid surgery is medically indicated as a way of correcting the impairment.

THE PROCEDURE

Eyelid surgery is most commonly performed with a patient under local anesthesia, coupled with CONSCIOUS SEDATION, in the office of a physician or at a surgery center. No hospital stay is required. The patient is awake, but relaxed and insensitive to pain during the procedure. Some surgeons prefer to use general anesthesia so that the person sleeps through the procedure. Even with general anesthesia, the procedure is performed as ambulatory surgery, so that the patient goes home the same day.

After the patient is under anesthesia, the surgeon makes an incision that follows the natural contour of the eyelid—in the crease of the upper eyelid, and just beneath the lashes in the lower eyelid. The incision may stop at the edge of the eyelid or extend beyond the outer corners of the eye. Through the incision, the surgeon divides the skin from the underlying fatty tissue, cuts away excess fat, and trims extra skin and muscle as needed. The incisions are sutured with very delicate stitches.

In some people with bagging lower eyelids from which no skin needs to be removed, the surgeon can use a technique called transconjunctival blepharoplasty. The incision is made on the inside surface of the eyelid, the conjunctiva. No visible scar remains after healing.

Eyelid surgery can take from 1 to 3 hours, depending on the difficulty of the procedure or whether one or both eyelids are being repaired.

BEFORE AND AFTER SURGERY

Blood and urine laboratory studies may be required before or after surgery, and the person is usually screened for undetected conditions that may affect safety and outcome, such as high blood pressure or diabetes. As with any surgery that involves anesthesia, the person must have nothing to eat or drink after midnight on the night before. The surgeon may also provide instructions about medications or nutritional supplements that should be avoided or added in preparation for surgery.

After the procedure is completed, the surgeon lubricates the eyes with ointment and may apply bandages to the sutured incisions. As the anesthesia wears off, the eyes feel tight and sore, a discomfort that can be controlled with prescribed oral pain medication.

To reduce swelling and bruising, the patient is advised to keep his or her head elevated for several days and to apply cold compresses to the eyes. Bruising varies with the individual—peaking within the first 48 hours and lasting from 2 weeks to a month.

During the first few weeks of healing, eye drops may be required to clean and lubricate the eyes. The eyes may tear, and vision may change because of a heightened sensitivity to light, blurring, or double vision. These effects are temporary and typically cease within a few weeks. Usually people who have had eyelid surgery can read or watch television within 2 or 3 days, but contact lenses cannot be worn for about 2 weeks. After that time, they may be worn, but they may be uncomfortable until healing is complete.

Stitches are removed from 2 days to a week after surgery; if dissolvable sutures have been used, they will disappear in the same period. The scars remain slightly pink for up to 6 months. The scars fade into white lines that are nearly invisible. Since nicotine inhibits blood flow to the skin, scarring tends to be more pronounced in smokers.

Physical activity should be minimized for 3 to 5 days after surgery, and most people can return to work in a week to 10 days. Strenuous exercise like running, bending, and lifting must be avoided for 3 weeks because it can raise blood pressure and cause the eyelids to swell. Abstinence from alcohol is also advised, since alcohol promotes fluid retention in the body, leading to swelling.

POSSIBLE COMPLICATIONS

Eyelid surgery is usually free of complications. In some cases, however, blood can gather under the skin and form a swelling known as a HEMATOMA. Typically the blood is absorbed within a few days, and no permanent damage is done. In very rare cases, severe bleeding or hemorrhaging leads to the loss of vision.

Another severe and rare complication is called ECTROPION. If too much skin is removed from the lower eyelid or if the eyelid has become weak, the eyelid turns out and down following surgery. When this happens, tears fall from the eyelid but fail to travel over the eyeball and lubricate it. This situation may resolve by itself. In severe cases, surgery is required to correct the ectropion.

Eyelid, drooping

Also known as ptosis or BLEPHAROPTO-SIS, drooping of one or both upper eyelids can be an acquired or congenital condition. There are many different causes of drooping eyelids. It sometimes can be associated with eye movement abnormalities or pupillary problems. These include injuries, tumors, inflammation, and disease (such as diabetes mellitus, type 1 or type 2; myasthenia gravis; or HORNER SYNDROME). In some cases, aging is the cause. The upper eyelid is normally lifted by the levator muscle; over the years, the attachment of the levator muscle to the lid may weaken. It is important to diagnose and treat the underlying cause of a drooping eyelid. Outpatient surgery under a local anesthetic is usually recommended to correct the problem.

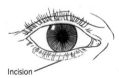 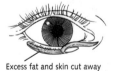 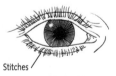

Incision | Excess fat and skin cut away | Stitches

REPAIRING SAGGING EYELIDS
Blepharoplasty of the lower lids is usually done to make the eyes look younger. The incision is made close to the lower eyelash line; excess fat is separated from underlying muscle and removed along with excess skin; and the incision is closed with a row of stitches.

Fabry disease

A very rare genetic disorder characterized by widespread damage to blood vessels. Its symptoms include edema (swelling), high blood pressure, enlargement of the heart, and stroke. It is an X-linked recessive trait, which means that only men get the full disease, while women are carriers. Carriers usually do not have symptoms themselves but can pass the disease on to their children.

Face-lift

A surgical procedure to remove fat and skin and tighten muscles and underlying tissues in the face. Because a face-lift is intended to give a more youthful look, it is a type of cosmetic surgery. Results from a face-lift are best in people who are of normal weight and have a well-defined facial bone structure. Most people who undergo the procedure are in their 40s to 60s, but the procedure has also been successful in people in their 80s.

THE PROCEDURE

Face-lifts are most commonly performed with local anesthesia, coupled with CONSCIOUS SEDATION, in the office of a physician or in a surgery center with no hospital stay. The patient is awake, but drowsy and insensitive to pain during the procedure. Some surgeons prefer to use general anesthesia, allowing the patient to sleep through the operation. Even with general anesthesia, the procedure is typically performed as AMBULATORY SURGERY so that the patient goes home later on that same day. The exception is for people with diseases such as high blood pressure or diabetes that may require monitoring of the patient after surgery, necessitating a short hospital stay.

The surgeon begins by making an incision that starts above the hairline, in the scalp above the temple. The incision is extended along the contour of the face in front of the ear and behind the earlobe into the scalp. If the skin in the neck area is to be tightened as part of the procedure, another incision is made under the chin.

Small blood vessels, severed by the incisions, are carefully clamped and tied to prevent blood from gathering under the skin, a condition that promotes the growth of scar tissue during healing.

Working through the incisions, the surgeon separates the skin from the fat and muscle tissues that underlie it. The muscle and the membrane that enclose it are tightened. The skin is then pulled back, and the excess is cut away. Fat may be trimmed during the procedure or suctioned, particularly as a way of reshaping the chin or neck.

Tissue layers are secured in place, and the incisions are closed with sutures. Scalp incisions may be closed with small metal clips. In some cases, a small tube is placed under the skin of the lower portion of the scalp to drain blood or fluid. Bandages may be wrapped loosely around the face to reduce bruising and swelling.

BEFORE AND AFTER SURGERY

Blood and urine laboratory tests may be required before surgery, and the person is screened for undetected conditions that may affect safety and outcome, such as high blood pressure or diabetes. As with any surgery that involves anesthesia, the person must have nothing to eat or drink after midnight the night before the operation. The surgeon may also provide instructions about medications or nutritional supplements that should be added or avoided in preparation for surgery. Smoking should be avoided because nicotine restricts blood flow to the skin, slows healing, and increases scarring.

Discomfort following face-lift surgery is generally not severe and can be controlled by oral prescription pain medications. Depending on the rate of healing, bandages are removed 1 to 5 days after surgery, drain tubes in 1 to 2 days, and stitches or metal clips in 5 to 10 days. If dissolvable sutures have been used, they will disappear or fall away in the same period. The scalp heals more slowly than the face. Stitches or clips in that area may be left in place longer.

Usually 1 or 2 days must pass before a person who has had a face-lift can move around easily; rest is advised for the first week. The person should sleep with his or her head elevated to prevent fluid from gathering in the face and scalp, which would cause increased swelling.

Most people are able to return to work in 10 days to 2 weeks. Camouflaging makeup can be worn to cover bruises or swelling. Restrictions include avoiding strenuous activity for the first 2 weeks and abstaining from alcohol, steam baths, and saunas for several months.

During the initial period of healing, swelling or puffiness, bruising, and sensations of numbness, tingling, and stiffness in the skin are common. Bruising disappears by the end of the third week; numbness and tingling can last up to several months. Since face-lift scars are hidden in the scalp and the creases of the face, they are largely invisible and disappear into thin white lines within several months to a year. Following a face-lift, the hair around the temples, surrounding the scalp incisions, may be thin for several months.

Complications of face-lift surgery include HEMATOMA (a small pocket of blood collected under the skin), which must be removed by a surgeon. The facial muscles may be weakened; this effect may be temporary or, rarely, permanent. Poor healing is most likely in people who smoke. Infections can occur but are rare in healthy individuals.

Because aging continues after surgery, a face-lift does not permanently reshape the face. It reverses the process but does not stop it. As a result, some people decide to have the procedure repeated 7 to 15 years later.

Facial palsy

An abnormal neurological condition characterized by weakness or paralysis of the facial muscles. One common form of facial palsy is BELL PALSY, a condition caused by damage to or dysfunction of the facial nerve. Although the cause of the nerve inflammation of Bell palsy is usually not identified, it is sometimes caused by a virus, such as the one that causes cold sores and fever blisters. Other possible causes of facial palsy include strokes, tumors, and infections (such as shingles). Any case of facial weakness, paralysis, or palsy calls for prompt and careful evaluation by a physician. Treatment of facial palsy depends on its underlying cause.

THE STEPS IN A FACE-LIFT

A face-lift can tighten loose skin and sagging muscles on the face, jaw, and neck. A face-lift cannot stop the aging process, but it can create a more youthful appearance. Some people decide to have the procedure done again in 7 to 15 years in an effort to maintain the desired effect.

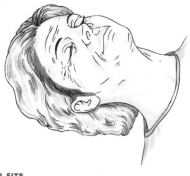

INCISION SITE
An incision is made along the hairline in the scalp area and in front of the ear and behind the earlobe.

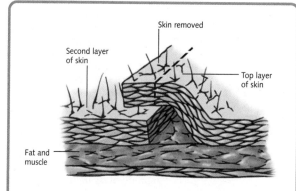

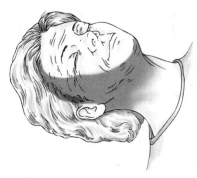

SKIN TO BE TIGHTENED
The surgeon separates the skin in the shaded area from underlying fat and muscle. Next, excess fat may be suctioned away. Then the surgeon pulls the skin tight on the face, trims excess skin, and stitches the skin in place.

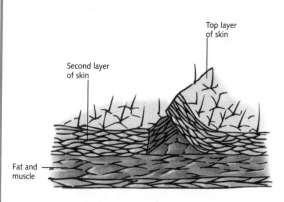

SEPARATING THE SKIN
During a face-lift, the top layers of skin are separated from underlying fat and muscle in a technique called undermining. Excess skin is then removed, and the top layer of excess skin is carefully stitched to the second layer of skin, to give a smoother appearance.

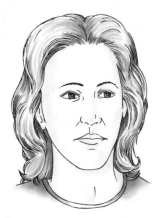

AFTER THE SURGERY
The skin is smoother after the face-lift. Very tiny stitches are used that are intended to fade with time and not leave noticeable scarring.

F

F

Facial spasm

An involuntary, repetitive, spasmodic movement of the facial muscles. The most common facial spasms are eye blinking or squinting, twitching around the mouth, and wrinkling of the nose. While their cause remains unknown, facial spasms usually increase in severity during stressful periods. Facial spasms most often occur in childhood, but some persist in adulthood. Facial spasms, although annoying, are rarely caused by severe problems. Although a facial spasm is commonly called a TIC, tics can also refer more generally to involuntary, repetitive movements anywhere in the body. Treatments of facial spasms include muscle relaxants, anticholinergic agents, and dopamine agonists, but the most effective treatment is injection of botulinum toxin type A (Botox).

Facies

A medical term used to describe facial appearance, which is sometimes affected by a disease or disorder.

Factitious disorder

The intentional feigning or production of physical or psychological symptoms out of a deep-seated need to assume the sick role. A person with factitious disorder may make up the complaint and support it with lies and fabrications or inflict injuries on his or her own body, such as injecting saliva under the skin to produce abscesses. In some cases, psychological complaints are the main concern; in others, physical complaints predominate; in yet others, both physical and psychological symptoms appear. The motivation of a factitious disorder is not to gain some advantage, such as avoiding jury duty or military service. Rather, the individual has an unconscious need to be cared for as a sick person. The disorder may cause the person to seek unneeded medical tests and exploratory surgeries. Factitious disorder is thought to be rare and to occur more commonly in males than females.

Factor IX deficiency

Hemophilia B, or Christmas disease, a genetically inherited bleeding disorder characterized by inadequate amounts of clotting factor IX in blood plasma. Factor IX, also known as plasma thromboplastin component (PTC), is involved only in blood coagulation (clotting). Hemophilia B occurs in only about 70,000 men worldwide at any given time and occurs a fifth as frequently as does hemophilia A (factor VIII deficiency). Factor IX deficiency affects males only; females who inherit the condition are carriers. Carriers are usually, but not always, symptom-free. People with factor IX deficiency may need supplementary factor IX or fresh frozen plasma if they have a bleeding injury or are undergoing surgery.

Factor VII deficiency

A bleeding disorder characterized by inadequate amounts of the plasma protein factor VII, an important clotting protein; also known as extrinsic factor deficiency. Factor VII deficiency may be either acquired via a vitamin K deficiency or inherited. Symptoms include bleeding into joints and muscles, excessive menstrual bleeding and bruising, and bleeding of the mucous membranes. Treatment with normal plasma, concentrates containing factor VII, or recombinant factor VII is generally effective.

Factor VIII deficiency

A genetically inherited bleeding disorder characterized by inadequate amounts of clotting factor VIII in blood plasma. Factor VIII deficiency is the cause of the bleeding disorder known as hemophilia A (see HEMOPHILIA). Factor VIII, also known as antihemophilic factor (AHF), is a substance involved exclusively in blood coagulation (clotting). Factor VIII deficiency is inherited as a sex-linked recessive trait; only males can inherit the disorder. Females may carry the disorder and pass it on to their sons; their daughters can also be carriers. All daughters of affected males are carriers, but men cannot pass the disease on to their sons. Hemophilia A occurs in one in 10,000 males in the world, or approximately 350,000 men at any given time. People with factor VIII deficiency may need treatment with factor VIII if they are actively bleeding or undergoing a surgical procedure. The condition has no cure and often requires counseling to address physical, emotional, and psychological challenges.

Fad diets

Weight-loss plans that may not be based on scientific findings. In the past, examples have included a high-protein low-carbohydrate regimen and an all-grapefruit diet. Fad diets often are unhealthy because they lack many vitamins, minerals, and other nutrients. A balanced diet is required to provide the necessary nutrients for growth, tissue repair, and physical activity. See also DIET, BALANCED; WEIGHT LOSS.

Fahrenheit scale

A scale used to measure temperature. In the Fahrenheit scale, the point at which water freezes is 32°, while the point at which it boils is 212°. The Fahrenheit scale is named after its inventor, a German physicist, and is used mainly in the United States.

Failure to thrive

A lag in growth and development behind the expected rate for a child's age and sex. It most often affects children younger than age 5, especially those 2 and younger. Failure to thrive, also called FTT, refers to a cluster of symptoms rather than a specific disease. Among those symptoms are the failure to gain weight

COMPARING CELSIUS AND FAHRENHEIT		
EVENT	DEGREES CELSIUS	DEGREES FAHRENHEIT
Absolute zero	−273.15	−459.67
Freezing point of water	0	32
Normal body temperature	37	98.6
Boiling point of water	100	212

and length. A steady weight gain is essential in infants and toddlers, indicating that they are obtaining the proper care and nutrition for normal growth and development (see GROWTH, CHILDHOOD). Except for a small loss of weight in the first few days of life, babies normally do not stop growing or lose weight. Affected children are usually underweight for their age and sex. They may be shorter than normal and have smaller heads. Physical characteristics are often accompanied by developmental delays. For example, a failure to thrive may cause children to sit up, crawl, or walk later than their peers (see WALKING, DELAYED).

A physical examination can reveal clues to an underlying disease. For example, a heart murmur may suggest a heart disorder. Other causes can be detected by their symptoms, such as foul-smelling stools, which may indicate that an infant is not absorbing nutrients. Emotionally neglected children may bang their heads on the sides of cribs or rock back and forth, attempting to stimulate themselves (see ABUSE, CHILD; HEAD BANGING). Some cling inappropriately to caregivers. In severe cases, children who fail to thrive are limp. Their skin is pale and dry. When failure to thrive is due to a chronic disease, children also exhibit the symptoms of that disease.

CAUSES
Frequently, failure to thrive is due to inadequate nutrition. Commonly, difficulty with feeding prevents the infant from getting adequate nutrition. For example, new parents may be nervous during feeding, or an infant with colic may be fussy and unable to eat all that he or she needs. Some breast-fed infants may not be getting enough milk. Other times, lack of money may influence the amount of nourishment that a child receives.

Physical problems can interfere with a baby's ability to take in or digest food. A mother's poor prenatal habits (such as smoking or using alcohol) can contribute to problems with digestion and normal growth. PREMATURE BIRTH, a cleft lip and palate, and chronic disorders—such as DOWN SYNDROME; DIABETES MELLITUS, TYPE 1; or CYSTIC FIBROSIS—may all bear on a baby's ability to thrive. Almost all

serious pediatric diseases can slow growth and development. Most of them have clear symptoms or can be detected during a physical examination.

Insufficient emotional stimulation can cause failure to thrive. A lack of nurturing can lead to depression and loss of appetite in a child. Poverty, ignorance, inexperience, stress, and drug or alcohol dependence can all affect parents' ability to provide adequate emotional stimulation and nutrition for their children. Failure to thrive has been observed in infants adopted from countries in political or economic upheaval.

DIAGNOSIS
When a baby's growth does not reflect normal gains in weight, length, and development on standardized growth charts, a physical examination can help determine whether an underlying illness is responsible. The child's eating patterns and medical history will be checked for nutritional needs and for illnesses that may be contributing to the problem. Blood, urine, and stool tests may be ordered, and sometimes a short period of hospitalization may be necessary. When there is no detectable physical reason, the pediatrician will search for emotional or social disturbances in the family.

TREATMENT
Underlying diseases or disorders must be treated appropriately. Breast-feeding mothers may need to improve their diets to increase the quantity and quality of their milk. Enriched formulas or high-calorie diets may be prescribed. When physiological causes can be excluded, the doctor may refer parents to a social worker or mental health professional. Good PRENATAL CARE and counseling new parents about their child's needs can help prevent failure to thrive. When diagnosed and treated early, most children catch up to their peers in physical and emotional growth.

Fainting

FOR FIRST AID
see Fainting, page 1321

Temporary loss of consciousness. Fainting occurs when there is an insufficient supply of blood to the brain for a short period, which happens when blood vessels in the body

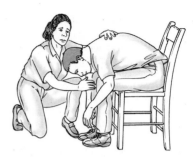

FEELING FAINT
A person who feels as if he or she might faint may be able to prevent it by sitting down and placing the head between the knees. A person with a heart problem or breathing difficulties should lie down with the legs elevated.

widen, causing blood to drain away from the brain. Fainting is characterized by a sudden pallor, or pale skin; nausea; sweating; loss of consciousness; and twitching or brief convulsive movements. By itself, fainting is not harmful, and, as a general rule, the person who has fainted will recover quickly with no lasting effects. Sometimes, however, a fainting spell is a signal of a serious condition, such as an injury from a fall.

Fainting can have many causes, among them standing at attention, rising quickly after lying down, wearing a too-tight collar, low blood pressure, abnormal heart rate or rhythm, severe pain or fright, alcohol or drug use, strenuous coughing, or hyperventilation (fast, shallow breathing).

Immediate first aid for fainting includes having the person lie down with legs elevated 6 to 12 inches. Assisting the person to a cooler environment may also be beneficial. Medical assistance should be sought at once if the person is having difficulty breathing, has chest pain, does not arouse promptly, or was injured by falling during the fainting spell.

Faith healing

The restoration of physical, emotional, or spiritual health by invoking the intervention of divine power through the laying on of hands or other means. Faith healing is a feature of some religions. Some faith healers believe that all disease has its source in the disorder of the mind or spirit, such as the CHRISTIAN SCIENCE belief that disease is the result of "ignorance of true reality." Other faith

F

healers believe that disease is caused by demons, and they practice healing techniques in which the divine Spirit is believed to triumph over evil ones. In less extreme forms of faith healing, prayer is used by people who are sick, either as a supplement to traditional medical treatment or as a last resort when conventional medicine has failed.

Two states of faith healing have been identified. In one, the healer enters an altered state of prayerful consciousness in which he or she joins with the person to speed up ordinary healing; no touching is involved, and the faith of the healer is considered the channel of cure. In the other type, the healer touches the person, transmitting a flow of energy through his or her hands to the diseased area of the person's body; this "laying on of hands" is an ancient practice and was known among the ancient Greeks and Romans.

Fallen arches

See FLAT FEET.

Fallopian tube

Either of two passages that extend from each OVARY to the uterus; medically called the oviducts. Each tube fans out at the end closest to the ovary, and the open end has hairlike projections reaching toward the ovary. In a mature woman, the ovary releases an egg once a month (a process called OVULATION), and the egg is waved into the fallopian tube by these projections. The egg travels along the tube toward the uterus, aided by muscular contractions. If sperm are present in the tube as a result of sexual intercourse, the egg

can be fertilized, and the fertilized egg will continue to the uterus. See REPRODUCTIVE SYSTEM, FEMALE.

Fallout

The descent to Earth of radioactive particles following a nuclear explosion. Radioactive fallout, which can cause cancer, may travel thousands of miles and spread across a wide geographic area.

Falls, in older people

The most common type of injury in older people. Falls are both more common and more serious for older people than for others and frequently result in fractures. Each year, one fourth of adults older than age 65 who live at home fall. Older adults in hospitals and nursing homes fall even more frequently. Falls or the complications resulting from them account for more than half of the accidental deaths among older people. Especially vulnerable are people who are alone; they may fall and not be discovered at once. Such serious complications as hypothermia, pneumonia, or muscle damage can develop. As a precaution, an older person who lives alone can carry a cellular phone, an attention-getting device such as a whistle, or a monitor that can be activated to alert a friend or family member of an injury.

Physiological changes associated with aging contribute to falls in older people. Typical examples include impaired vision or hearing, poor balance, slowing reflexes, loss of muscle strength and flexibility, DEMENTIA, chronic diseases such as OSTEOARTHRITIS or diabetes mellitus (see DIABETES MELLITUS, TYPE 2), infection, and low

blood pressure. Tranquilizers and high blood pressure medications can cause side effects such as dizziness, blurred vision, sleepiness, and problems with balance that can lead to falls. Because many prescription drugs interact with alcohol, an older person who both drinks and takes medications is at increased risk for falling.

A broken bone that results from a fall can be a critical injury for an older person. In hip fractures, hospitalization and surgery usually are required. Older people who normally live at home may require institutional care for more than a year after a hip fracture. The mortality rate for people in the year following a hip fracture is more than 20 percent greater than for people the same age and sex without a hip fracture. Fractures occur more commonly in older individuals because their bones are more likely to have been weakened by OSTEOPOROSIS, a disease in which bone density declines and bones become increasingly fragile and brittle. Women are more likely than men are to develop osteoporosis. Broken hips, which are actually thighbones (femurs) broken near the top, are especially common in older people. If a fracture is suspected, an older person should be taken at once to an emergency room for X rays.

TREATMENT

A thorough physical examination by a doctor, including a complete understanding of why a person fell, is necessary after a fall. Even minor falls can lead to extensive injury in older people. If the head has been hit, dangerous bleeding can occur within the skull. To assess the damage, a doctor conducts a careful examination and may order imaging studies of the injured area. These may include X rays of bones, CT (computed tomography) scanning, or MRI (magnetic resonance imaging) to rule out a head injury.

To further reveal underlying conditions that have a role in falls, a physician may recommend various tests. They may include hearing and vision tests; basic analyses of blood and urine; an electrocardiogram (ECG or EKG); a mental status examination; and neuropsychological tests of memory, problem solving, and language. A common clinical test is to observe a patient "get up and go." The physician watches the individual sit, stand up, walk, and turn

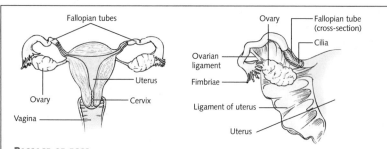

Fallopian tubes · Ovary · Fallopian tube (cross-section) · Cilia · Ovarian ligament · Uterus · Fimbriae · Ovary · Cervix · Ligament of uterus · Vagina · Uterus

PASSAGE OF EGGS
The fallopian tubes, about 4 or 5 inches long, extend from the ovaries into the cavity of the uterus. In a mature woman, an egg produced in an ovary is drawn into a fallopian tube by fiberlike projections at the end of the tube called fimbriae. Tiny hairs (cilia) lining the tube fan the egg along toward the uterus.

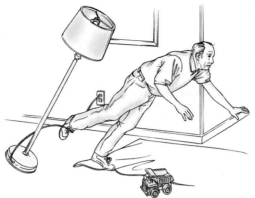

REMOVING HAZARDS
Most household falls can be prevented. Electrical cords should run under carpeting or be affixed to walls or mopboards. Throw rugs should be removed or tacked down. Members of a household that includes an older person should be particularly alert to tripping hazards, such as toys, shoes, or other obstacles left on the floor.

around. This inspection can help detect whether dizziness, poor balance, poor vision, neuropathy, arthritis, or muscle weakness contributed to the fall. The doctor may prescribe a hearing aid (see HEARING AIDS), new glasses, or a walker. Adjustments to types or dosages of medications may be made. An occupational therapist or nurse can help detect unsafe factors in the home and suggest preventive remedies such as removing loose carpets or installing safety bars in the bathroom. Physical therapy may be prescribed to improve a person's gait, muscle strength, and balance.

Inpatient and/or outpatient rehabilitation is usually necessary after a fracture. Rehabilitation involves regaining physical strength and range of motion, overcoming the fear of falling, and taking action to prevent future falls. Inactivity during the healing period can result in a loss of muscle strength and flexibility. Staying as active as possible helps maintain strength. Even a short time in bed can lead to weakness, stiffness, and a loss of balance.

After a fall, the support of family and friends is important. If hospitalized, an older person should be returned home as soon as is practical. Home health aides or physical therapists can regularly provide rehabilitation help at the patient's home. Social support and familiar surroundings can help prevent a downward spiral of decreased activity, fear of falling, diminished self-esteem, and reclusiveness that affects some older people after a serious fall. See also HOME HEALTH CARE FOR OLDER PEOPLE.

PREVENTION
Regular exercise has been found to help older people maintain strength,

and it reduces the number of falls. The use of walkers or canes, when necessary, also diminishes the risk of falling. Shoes should fit well and have firm soles and low heels. Long shoelaces, which can easily become untied, should be avoided. Learning to rise slowly from chairs and beds can prevent falls. Getting up too swiftly can cause a momentary drop in blood pressure and dizziness. If a new medication is prescribed, an older person should carefully monitor its effects and discuss any concerns with the physician. Physical therapy may be helpful for improving balance and gait. Eyeglass and hearing aid prescriptions should be kept up-to-date.

Adjustments can be made in and around the home to ensure safety. Low, soft chairs are examples of environmental impediments that should be replaced if possible. Changes may include replacing low, soft chairs with higher, firmer ones; repairing uneven sidewalks; improving light-

ing; installing night lights and banisters; marking top and bottom steps with white tape; tacking down carpets; minimizing clutter; attaching loose wires to walls or moldings; and removing raised doorway thresholds. Frequently used items, such as dishes, pots, and food, should be within easy reach. Safety bars or handrails can be installed near the bathtub and toilet. Also helpful are nonslip mats inside and outside the bathtub and raising the toilet seat's height. A chair may be useful in the shower stall.

False memory

A memory that distorts an actual experience or that is a fictional creation of the imagination. In some cases, false memory involves errors in remembering details of events. Dreams can be confused with reality and later recalled as if they were actual events. False memories may also arise from prodding or leading impressionable individuals, particularly children.

In recent years a considerable debate has arisen over false memory in relation to childhood sexual abuse. In a number of high-profile legal cases, individuals who remembered long-repressed instances of sexual abuse brought charges as adults against the people who allegedly perpetrated the abuse. Some authorities argued that the long delay in recovering the memory was the result of selective amnesia surrounding the trauma (see DISSOCIATIVE DISORDERS). Others maintained that recovered memories were inherently false and that they often came from overeager prodding by therapists convinced that sexual abuse had

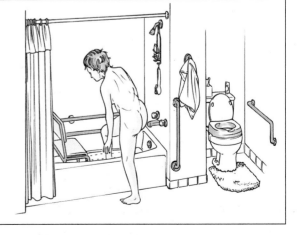

HELP IN THE BATH
A wide variety of equipment is available to prevent falls in or near the bathtub or shower. Treads on the bottom of the tub reduce slipping. Handrails for the side of the tub or the wall are inexpensive and easy to install. A waterproof chair makes a shower easier for someone who cannot stand for long periods of time.

F

indeed occurred. The issue remains a matter of controversy among specialists in the field.

False teeth

Artificial teeth used to replace natural, permanent teeth that are missing or have been removed by a dentist during a tooth extraction. See BRIDGE, DENTAL; DENTURES; and IMPLANTS, DENTAL.

Famciclovir

An antiviral drug used to treat herpes zoster (shingles). Famciclovir (Famvir) is sometimes used to treat genital herpes. Famciclovir works by interfering with the reproduction of DNA in the herpesvirus, but it has less effect on DNA in uninfected body cells.

Familial

Occurring more frequently among members of a family than would be expected by chance. The term is often used incorrectly to mean "genetic."

Familial hyper- cholesterolemia

An inherited tendency to have dangerously high blood CHOLESTEROL levels. Since high cholesterol levels increase the risk of ATHEROSCLEROSIS (artery disease), people with this condition have a greater than normal incidence of heart attack. Familial hypercholesterolemia may be indicated by a history of early heart attack in close blood relatives, particularly parents or siblings. If blood tests show elevated cholesterol levels, a program of appropriate diet (including restricted intake of fats and cholesterol), exercise, and cholesterol-lowering drugs (statins) will decrease the risk of heart attack.

Familial Mediterranean fever

A rare inherited intestinal disorder characterized by recurrent fever and inflammation. Familial Mediterranean fever (FMF), also called periodic peritonitis, chiefly affects people of Mediterranean ancestry, including Sephardic Jews, Arabs, Armenians, and Turks. It may be inherited as an autosomal recessive trait, involving a gene on chromosome 16. FMF usually first appears between ages 5 and 15. Symptoms usually include fever, inflammation of the lining of the abdominal and chest cavities, pain and swelling in the joints, and sometimes skin rashes. Attacks usually last 24 to 48 hours and, although varying in frequency, occur every 2 to 4 weeks.

FMF is usually diagnosed through a process of elimination. Its symptoms are similar to those associated with appendicitis, pancreatitis, and intestinal obstruction. Laboratory tests and X rays may be used to eliminate other diagnoses. FMF is incurable; treatment is aimed at relieving symptoms and reducing frequency of attacks. Colchicine is a medication that may decrease frequency of attacks.

Family medicine

Also known as family practice, the medical specialty that provides continuing and comprehensive care for a person or family. Family medicine combines the biological, clinical, and behavioral sciences. Its broad scope of care encompasses all organ systems and diseases and wellness and prevention of illness for people of any age and either sex.

Family physician

A doctor who is educated and trained in family medicine or practice. Family physicians provide continuing and comprehensive care for a person or family. They treat all organ systems and diseases and extend care to people of any age and either sex.

Family therapy

A form of psychological counseling that focuses on the entire family rather than an individual and is based on the belief that a person's emotional problems can best be understood and treated in the context of family behavior and communications. For example, depression in an adolescent child may be viewed as a response to family issues, such as marital stress between the parents, rather than as a mental illness affecting only one person. A variety of therapeutic techniques can be used, including behavioral, cognitive, and interpersonal. Family therapy is used by psychiatrists, psychologists, social workers, and other mental health workers in the treatment of a wide variety of emotional problems and mental illnesses.

Famotidine

A drug used to treat ulcers, gastroesophageal reflux disease (GERD), heartburn, acid indigestion, and stomach conditions that cause acid to build up. It is also used to stop the production of stomach acid during surgery. Famotidine is a histamine$_2$ (H$_2$)-receptor antagonist that works by inhibiting the production of stomach acid and other secretions.

Famotidine (Pepcid, Pepcid AC) is effective for treating the symptoms of ulcer and preventing complications. It is the most powerful of the four available H$_2$-receptor antagonists. Famotidine is available with and without prescription, although the nonprescription form is recommended only for indigestion and heartburn.

Fanconi anemia

See ANEMIA, FANCONI.

Fanconi syndrome

A rare metabolic disorder that is associated with the loss of a number of minerals or nutrients in the urine, including amino acids, glucose, and phosphate. It can lead to rickets and failure to grow in children. Fanconi syndrome may be inherited or acquired later in life. When Fanconi syndrome is acquired later in life, the kidney damage may be caused by exposure to agents such as cadmium, lead, mercury, and outdated tetracycline medications.

Fantasy

A daydream of an imagined situation or series of events. Fantasy can serve as a way of rehearsing or planning for the future, or it can provide an escape from reality. In extreme cases, people live in a world of fantasy to escape the emotional conflicts or problems posed by the real world.

Farmer's lung

A dust disease caused by inhalation of dust from moldy hay. Farmer's lung results from a reaction to exposure to a fungus known as *Thermoactinomyces vulgaris (T. vulgaris)* and occurs primarily in people who are sensitive to it. The symptoms may be acute, producing a flulike illness with a cough that resolves within a few days after exposure. Symptoms generally appear within 4 to 12 hours following exposure but may also occur chronically and include breathlessness caused by exertion, a productive cough, and weight loss.

Farmer's lung can be diagnosed by abnormalities that appear on a chest X ray. Blood test results may reveal antibodies to *T. vulgaris*, and pulmonary function test results show restriction in lung function in the early phase of the disease and restriction combined with obstruction in disease that has progressed over time. Treatment consists of terminating a person's exposure as soon as possible to the moldy hay dust that causes the disease. In the early stages, significant improvement or complete recovery is expected. Farmer's lung can progress to more serious conditions, including PULMONARY FIBROSIS, if exposure continues.

Farsightedness

A focusing (refractive) error of the eyes that makes it difficult to see close objects clearly; also known as hyperopia. In most cases of farsightedness, the eyeball is shorter from front to back. As a result, the distance between the lens and the retina (the thin layer of light-sensitive tissue at the back of the eye that relays visual information to the brain) is too short to focus incoming light rays. Farsightedness can also result from weakness of the lens and cornea (the clear covering on the exposed surface of the eye) in focusing (see PRESBYOPIA). In both types of farsightedness, close objects are blurry. Eyestrain and headache may result, particularly after close work such as reading.

Farsightedness is generally present at birth. Children often overcome mild farsightedness through the natural accommodation of the eye (changes in shape of the lens to see close objects). This ability diminishes with age, so that glasses or contact lenses are commonly needed by farsighted adults. Such corrective lenses bend incoming light so that it focuses correctly on the retina.

Farsighted people often have a narrower than normal angle between the iris and the interior surface of the cornea, which increases the risk for closed-angle GLAUCOMA, a potentially sight-threatening disease. Regular testing for glaucoma is advised. See Correcting farsightedness, page 550.

Fascia

Any fibrous connective tissues that lie under the skin, cover muscles or muscle groups, or enclose internal organs. Fascia surrounds many structures in the body to provide support and protection.

Fasciculation

The twitching of an isolated muscle, which may or may not be related to a neuromuscular disorder.

Fasciitis

A painful inflammation of the fibrous connective tissue, called fascia, that encloses the muscles. The condition often affects the tissues in the lower legs as a result of overuse or intense sports activities. A common form of fasciitis, called plantar fasciitis, involves the long band of connective tissue on the bottom of the foot, producing a sharp pain in the heel. This form of fasciitis can be caused by overuse during athletic activity. Treatment usually involves rest, applying ice for pain relief, the use of special inserts into the heel portion of shoes, exercises to increase strength and flexibility of the foot, and corticosteroid injections. In severe cases, surgery may be necessary. See FASCIOTOMY.

Fasciotomy

Surgery involving an incision made into the fascia, or fibrous connective tissue, that encloses the muscles. The goal of the procedure is to relieve the pressure on the muscles that are causing pain. The surgery may be used to treat muscle swelling, often in the lower legs, from intense athletic activity. Endoscopic plantar fasciotomy is an outpatient surgical procedure involving two small incisions on the foot. With the use of specialized small instruments, the surgeon can see the structures inside the foot on a video screen. The procedure is generally not considered until it has been demonstrated that the symptoms of fasciitis will not respond to more conservative treatments, including orthotics (shoe inserts), cortisone injections, and physical therapy.

Fasting

Not eating or eating fewer calories than the body needs at rest. During fasting, the body compensates by slowing the metabolic rate (a measurement of the body's need for calories to sustain basic functions while at rest).

Prolonged or severe fasting can slow the metabolic rate and reduce maintenance requirements to as low as 500 calories a day. When the metabolism slows this much, the body is not burning sufficient calories to warm itself (even in summer). Fatigue, depression, constipation, and dry skin and hair are consequences of a severely reduced metabolic rate. Doctors caution that fasting should never be used to lose weight. A drop in the metabolic rate eventually produces a frustrating plateau in weight loss, since energy requirements become lower. When a normal diet is resumed, the reduced metabolism results in a more rapid weight gain than before fasting. Very-low-calorie diets are associated with health hazards including an increased risk for sudden death. People who need to fast for religious reasons and have diabetes mellitus or a history of heart problems should talk to their doctors about fasting.

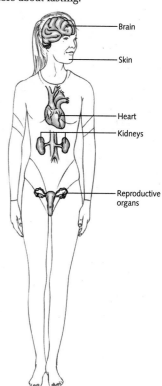

EFFECTS OF FASTING
Prolonged fasting has harmful effects on many organs and systems in the body. For example, heart irregularities and a halt in the production of sex hormones can result from the drastically lower metabolic rate caused by fasting.

F

CORRECTING FARSIGHTEDNESS

When the eye is too short from front to back or the cornea is too flat, light rays focus behind the retina, causing difficulty seeing near objects. The symptoms usually do not appear in childhood because the eye accommodates for the condition by changing the shape of the lens. As a person ages, accommodation becomes less effective, and corrective lenses to change the point of focus become necessary.

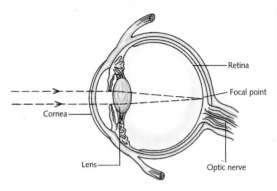

NORMAL EYE
In normal vision, light passes through the cornea and lens to its proper focal point on the retina.

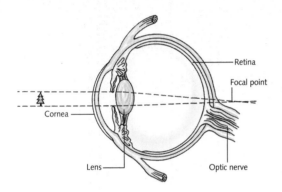

FARSIGHTED (HYPEROPIC) EYE
Farsightedness results when the focal point of light rays falls beyond the retina.

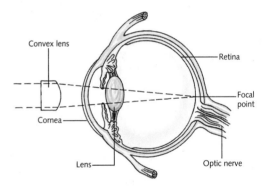

CONVEX LENS CORRECTING FARSIGHTEDNESS
Eyeglasses or contact lenses refocus light rays so that the focal point falls on the retina.

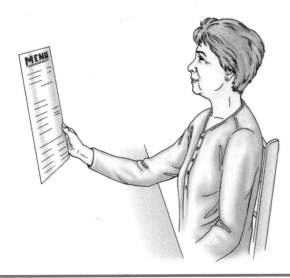

CORRECTING FOR PRESBYOPIA WITHOUT CORRECTIVE LENSES
People with presbyopia, a condition similar to farsightedness that shifts the focal point of images beyond the retina as a result of a loss of elasticity of the lens, can sometimes correct for blurred close vision by holding objects at arm's length.

Fat, body

Body tissue consisting largely of masses of fat cells; adipose tissue. Body fat is formed as a thick layer under the skin and normally occurs around the kidneys and in the buttocks, thighs, and abdomen, where it serves as an insulating layer and to store energy. When a person regularly eats more than he or she needs, it is converted into fats and is stored in adipose tissue.

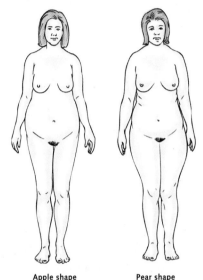

Apple shape   Pear shape

APPLE OR PEAR BODY SHAPE
Distribution of body fat seems to be a risk factor for heart disease, type 2 diabetes mellitus, high blood pressure, and some cancers. A person who tends to accumulate fat around the waist and abdomen (an apple shape) is at increased risk compared with a person whose fat tends to collect in the hips and thighs (pear shape).

Fatigue

Tiredness, lethargy, exhaustion, or lack of energy. Fatigue is usually a normal response to rigorous physical activity, stress, or a lack of sleep. However, it may also be a symptom of a physical or psychological disorder. People who experience unexplained fatigue are advised to see their doctors for a physical examination.

Fats and oils

Fats are nutrients found in animal products and plant foods such as nuts, whole-grain cereals, seeds, avocados, and olives. Fats should constitute no more than 30 percent of an individual's total intake of calories each day. In addition, no more than 10 percent of daily calories should come from saturated fat. To lower the risk of heart disease and other health problems, doctors recommend that individuals reduce their total fat intake and replace some saturated fats with unsaturated fats. For individuals with atherosclerosis (arterial blockage from fat deposits), a diet even lower in fat content may be recommended.

No diet should be entirely fat-free. Fat is a source of stored energy for the body, and small quantities are needed for growth and repair. Fats or lipids also promote absorption of the fat-soluble vitamins A, D, E, and K in the intestines. However, fat contains more calories per unit than any other food, and every gram of fat has more than double the number of calories than in a gram of protein or carbohydrate. Most Americans consume too many fatty foods. Excess fat is stored in the body as fatty tissue, and fat contributes to serious health problems such as high blood pressure, elevated blood CHOLESTEROL levels, heart disease, diabetes, and an increased risk of cancer.

TYPES OF FATS AND OILS

All fats and oils are mixtures of fatty acids: monounsaturated, polyunsaturated, and saturated. However, not all fats affect the body the same way. Certain fats are more healthful than others; fish oils and pure vegetable oils are healthier choices than animal fat, dairy fat, and hydrogenated oils. Some fats have specific benefits. For example, some monounsaturated fats, such as olive oil and avocados, may lower the risk of cardiovascular disease. For optimum health, in addition to keeping overall fat consumption low, doctors advise reducing intake of saturated fats and trans-fatty acids and primarily using unsaturated fats. Unsaturated fats, found in plants and fish rather than animal sources, are divided into two groups—monounsaturated and polyunsaturated.

■ ***Saturated fats*** Fats that are solid at room temperature consist primarily of saturated fat. The saturated fat in foods such as butter, cream, and well-marbled meat contributes to the formation of artery-clogging plaque. The amount of saturated fat in the diet can be more damaging to blood cholesterol levels than cholesterol in foods such as egg yolks. Common dietary sources of saturated fats include animal products such as meats, poultry, and dairy products, as well as coconut and palm oils. These fats (along with trans-fatty acids) are most responsible for high blood cholesterol levels and an increased risk of heart disease. For many people, the best way to lower harmful blood cholesterol levels is to reduce saturated fat in the diet.

■ ***Trans-fatty acids*** These fats are made in the hydrogenation process that solidifies liquid oils for use in preparation of many types of food products. Hydrogenated vegetable oils give certain processed foods a longer shelf life. Also known as trans fats, trans-fatty acids are similar to saturated fats. They contribute to increased levels of harmful low-density lipoprotein (LDL) cholesterol, promote clogged arteries, and

F

THE LOW-FAT DIET

A low-fat diet is beneficial for good overall health. To cut back on dietary fat, a person should:

- Choose low-fat or fat-free cheeses, sour cream, salad dressing, and mayonnaise.
- Serve more whole grains and fresh vegetables with main courses.
- Drink low-fat or skim milk.
- Choose lean instead of fatty cuts of meat.
- Limit meat serving size to that of a deck of cards.
- Remove the skin from poultry and fish.
- Trim the fat from beef and pork before cooking.
- Bake, broil, or boil foods instead of frying them.
- Use a nonstick pan.
- Use cooking oil spray in place of cooking oil.
- Cook with olive or canola oil rather than palm oil, lard, shortening, or butter.
- Season dishes with fresh herbs instead of bacon or butter.
- Drain the fats from meats, after cooking.
- Cool soups and gravies and skim fat off the top before serving.
- Serve sorbet and fresh fruit instead of high-fat desserts.

increase the risk of heart disease. Varying amounts of trans-fatty acids can be found in stick margarine, crackers, cookies, doughnuts, and deep-fried foods. Because of the health risks associated with them, the Food and Drug Administration has proposed that, like saturated fat content, trans-fatty acid content be included on the Nutrition Facts panel of food labels.

■ *Monounsaturated fats* Mono-unsaturated fatty acids lower levels of harmful LDL cholesterol and have no negative effect on the helpful HDL (high-density lipoprotein) variety. Fat calories in the MEDITERRANEAN DIET, which has long been associated with good health and low rates of heart disease, come principally from olive oil, a good monounsaturated fat source, rather than from meat and dairy products, which contain large amounts of saturated fat. Canola and avocado oils are also good sources of monounsaturated fats, as are a variety of nuts: almonds, hazelnuts, maca-damias, pecans, and pista-chios.

■ *Polyunsaturated fats* Found in corn, safflower, soybean, and sunflower oils, polyunsaturated fats lower total blood cholesterol even more than monounsaturated fats. However, they do so by lowering helpful, heart-protective HDL as well as harmful LDL cholesterol. Omega-3 fatty acids, another type of polyunsaturated fat, are found in deep-water fish such as salmon and tuna. Omega-3 fatty acids are believed to

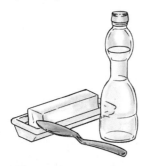

CHECK NUTRITION LABELS CAREFULLY
Saturated fats are generally solid at room temperature; a good example is butter. Oils may contain saturated fats (coconut and palm oils), monounsaturated fats (olive and canola oils), or polyunsaturated fats (corn and safflower oils). Monounsaturated and polyunsaturated fats in the diet help lower cholesterol and prevent heart disease.

prevent blood cells from adhering to the inside of blood vessels and the buildup of plaque. Several studies have linked eating fish rich in omega-3 fatty acids several times a week with a reduced risk of dying of heart disease. These fatty acids are also vital for brain and eye development.

Fatty acids

Acids containing carbon, hydrogen, and oxygen that are found in fat. Some fatty acids cannot be manufactured by the body and must be consumed in food. These include linoleic, linolenic, and arachidonic acids, which are known as the essential fatty acids. Monounsaturated, poly-unsaturated, and saturated fatty acids make up all FATS AND OILS, but one type usually dominates in a particular fat or oil. For example, monounsaturated fatty acids dominate in olive oil, polyunsaturated fatty acids in corn oil, and saturated fatty acids in lard, or pork fat.

FDA

See FOOD AND DRUG ADMINISTRATION.

Febrile seizure

See SEIZURE, FEBRILE.

Fecal impaction

An accumulated hard mass of feces in the rectum. Fecal impaction results from CONSTIPATION (infrequent bowel movements in which the feces are hard and dry). An ENEMA may be needed to help a person have a bowel movement. If this proves unsuccessful, a physician may remove it manually. Fecal impaction can be a symptom of a more serious disorder, especially when additional symptoms, such as weight loss, abdominal pain, or rectal bleeding, are present. People with limited mobility, such as bedridden individuals, are more likely to develop fecal impaction.

The cause of fecal impaction and constipation is identified through a complete physical examination and tests. Testing may include blood tests, a lower GASTROINTESTINAL (GI) SERIES (an X-ray procedure also known as a barium enema), and SIGMOIDOSCOPY and COLONOSCOPY (examinations of the rectum and colon using flexible viewing tubes passed through the anus). In many cases, only simple

treatment is required. Physicians advise adding fiber-rich vegetables, fruits, and bran to the diet, drinking plenty of fluids, and responding promptly to the urge to defecate. Because regular use of LAXATIVES can make the colon inactive, they should be taken sparingly, if at all. Constipation that is due to an underlying problem, such as hemorrhoids or irritable bowel syndrome, requires appropriate treatment.

Fecalith

A hard, stonelike mass of feces. A fecalith can be responsible for blocking the appendix and causing acute appendicitis.

Fecal-occult blood test

A screening test to detect the presence of nonvisible (occult) blood in the feces. In a fecal-occult blood test, chemically sensitive paper is used to detect blood in a stool sample. In the laboratory, a stool sample is placed on a white chemical strip. When a chemical substance is dropped on the strip, the strip turns blue if blood is present. Blood in the feces can be a sign of serious disorders of the digestive system, including COLITIS, CROHN DISEASE, and colorectal cancer (see COLON, CANCER OF THE; RECTUM, CANCER OF THE). Doctors recommend annual fecal-occult blood testing for individuals older than age 50. This test is also done regularly for people with iron-deficiency anemia.

Feces

Excrement or stool discharged from the anus in a bowel movement. Feces are the solid waste that remains after food is broken down in the digestive tract (see DIGESTIVE SYSTEM). Feces are composed of a mixture of undigested and indigestible materials that include vegetable fibers (roughage), bile pigments, mucus, bacteria, and dead cells from the lining of the intestine. Feces that are an unusual color, contain blood, or are foul-smelling can be a symptom of a digestive disorder (see FECES, ABNORMAL; FECES, BLOOD IN THE).

Most people form and pass feces once a day. However, as many as three bowel movements a day or as few as three a week are considered normal. In general, the more frequent the bowel movements, the softer and looser the feces. A change in the pattern of bowel movements can be the sign of a problem. See also BOWEL MOVEMENTS, ABNORMAL.

Feces, abnormal

A sign of a disorder in the digestive system. There are many types of abnormal feces. Infrequent bowel movements that are hard and dry are the symptoms of CONSTIPATION. Three or more loose bowel movements a day are considered DIARRHEA. Chalk-colored feces may be a symptom of hepatitis (inflammation of the liver). Loose, greasy, strong-smelling feces that float may be due to MALABSORPTION (impaired absorption of nutrients through the small intestine). Malabsorption can be a sign of such problems as CELIAC DISEASE (an inflammation of the small intestine due to a protein found in grains), CROHN DISEASE, or PANCREATITIS (inflammation of the pancreas). Floating feces that are hard to flush are due to gas within the feces.

Even when abnormal feces are not apparent, doctors recommend that people older than age 50 have a regular rectal examination and fecal-occult blood test (a test for traces of hidden blood in the feces). People who experience blood in the feces should seek immediate medical attention (see FECES, BLOOD IN THE). Possible tests to detect the cause of abnormal feces include a GASTROINTESTINAL (GI) SERIES, GASTROSCOPY, PROCTOSCOPY, SIGMOIDOSCOPY, and COLONOSCOPY.

Feces, blood in the

A sign of a possible gastrointestinal disorder. In many instances, blood in the feces is due to a minor problem, such as HEMORRHOIDS. Sometimes, it is caused by a more serious disorder, such as COLITIS, CROHN DISEASE, or colorectal cancer (see COLON, CANCER OF THE; RECTUM, CANCER OF THE). Doctors recommend that anyone who experiences blood in the feces seek immediate medical attention.

Blood in the feces may be visible, or it may be mixed in with the feces and not be apparent. Therefore, doctors advise individuals older than age 50 to have a regular FECAL-OCCULT BLOOD TEST to test for hidden traces of blood. A rectal examination is also recom-

mended. Blood in the feces varies in color and consistency. Bright red blood is likely to have originated close to the anus. Sticky, partly digested blood that ranges from dark mahogany to jet black is called MELENA. Melena, a sign of dangerous internal bleeding higher in the digestive tract, is considered a medical emergency. Possible tests to determine the cause of blood in the feces include a GASTROINTESTINAL (GI) SERIES, GASTROSCOPY, PROCTOSCOPY, SIGMOIDOSCOPY, and COLONOSCOPY.

Feeding, infant

In a baby's first 4 to 6 months, either breast milk or formula can provide full nutrition. While breast milk provides a baby with the most complete nutrition possible, nutritious commercial formulas are also available. Cow's milk should not be given to babies younger than 1 year of age. Babies should be fed on demand. The younger and smaller an infant, the more frequently he or she needs to eat. Newborns do not take a great deal of formula or breast milk. A baby's first feeding may only be a half ounce. By the third day, an infant drinks about 2 ounces of formula every 3 to 4 hours. At first, breast-fed babies' feedings may be less than 2 hours apart. By 1 month of age, breast-fed infants usually take 3 to 4 ounces of breast milk every 2 to 3 hours. Gradually, babies take larger amounts of breast milk or formula and go longer between feedings.

To feed the baby, the parent or caretaker can gently stroke the baby's cheek to stimulate the rooting reflex that causes the baby to search for and suckle on the bottle or breast. Breast-feeding babies need to nurse for 20 minutes at a time, alternating sides with each feeding. Bottle feedings usually take from 10 to 20 minutes. See Burping a baby, page 554.

Although babies lose some weight after birth, most regain their birth weight by 2 weeks of age. In most cases, the baby correctly determines how much food he or she needs. A baby's weight gain is the best guide to whether food intake has been adequate. A rule of thumb is that infants double their birth weight at about 6 months, triple it at 12 months, and quadruple it by 2 years.

SOLID FOODS

At around 4 to 6 months of age, solid foods are introduced. Most pediatricians recommend a single-grain, iron-fortified cereal, such as rice cereal, as the first solid food. New foods—pureed table food or jarred baby foods—are slowly added, one at a time. Meanwhile, the baby continues getting most nutrients from formula or breast milk. To detect possible allergic reactions, several days are allowed to elapse between the introduction of each new food. At 9 or 10 months, the baby can eat certain foods with his or her fingers. Finger foods must either dissolve in the baby's mouth, like crackers, or be easy to swallow, like cheese. Because they can cause choking, hot dogs cut into round pieces, whole grapes, raisins, raw carrots, popcorn, nuts, or large chunks of meat are not appropriate finger foods. Babies are more interested in playing than eating at this time, and messy mealtimes are normal. Parents should praise babies for their efforts.

Feldenkrais method

A form of "body education" that teaches efficient and coordinated use of the body. See BODYWORK. The goal of the Feldenkrais method is to reduce stress on joints, increase flexibility, and expand the range of motion. The method was invented by an Israeli nuclear physicist following his own knee injury when he developed a way to restore function without pain. The Feldenkrais method teaches students to attend to messages communicated by their bodies and to substitute free-flowing movements that relax tense muscles. The method is popular with dancers, actors, and other performers. People with conditions such as back pain, chronic fatigue, fibromyalgia, stroke, and neurological and musculoskeletal disorders, are most likely to benefit from this method of movement.

Fellatio

Oral stimulation of a man's penis with a partner's mouth and tongue. See ORAL SEX.

Felodipine

A drug used to treat hypertension (high blood pressure). Felodipine (Plendil) is in the class of drugs called calcium channel blockers.

BURPING A BABY

Burping a baby to expel excess gas during and after feeding helps relieve discomfort and reduces spitting up. Several different positions may help the baby burp. Always use a towel under the baby's mouth, and pat the child's back gently. Sometimes, it takes several minutes before the baby burps.

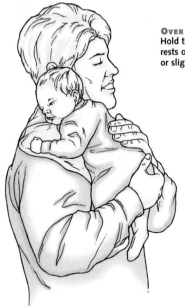

OVER THE SHOULDER
Hold the child so that his or her head rests on your shoulder, facing backward or slightly to the side.

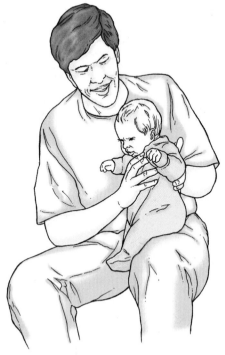

SITTING UP
Sit the baby on one leg, leaning him or her forward slightly and supporting his or her chest and chin from the front with one hand, while patting with the other hand.

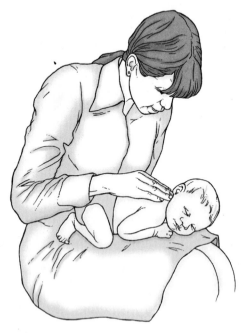

STOMACH DOWN
Lay the infant facedown across your lap, with his or her stomach on one leg and head on the other. Position your leg so that the baby's head is slightly raised. Turn the baby's head to the side, and pat his or her back gently.

F

Felodipine lowers blood pressure by relaxing the heart's vascular smooth muscle in order to reduce vascular resistance.

Female genital mutilation

The ritual cutting of parts of a girl's genitalia. A traditional practice in parts of Africa and Asia, female genital mutilation (FGM) marks a girl's achievement of womanhood. Sometimes known as female circumcision, the practice generally destroys a woman's capacity to feel sexual pleasure. Three main types of FGM are practiced: type 1, CLITORIDECTOMY, involves removal of the clitoris; type 2 includes clitoridectomy plus removal of the inner LABIA; and in type 3, the outer labia are stitched to form a hood of skin covering the URETHRA and part of the vaginal opening. All three methods have been associated with immediate and long-term health consequences, including excessive bleeding and shock at the time of circumcision, and the formation of abscesses, keloids (see KELOID), cysts, and scar tissue. Women who have undergone FGM often experience psychological trauma, recurrent urinary tract infections, DYSMENORRHEA (painful periods), chronic pelvic inflammatory disease, and painful sexual intercourse. The American Medical Association and the World Health Organization have condemned FGM as a form of child abuse and called on physicians not to perform the ritual.

Female sex hormones

See ESTROGEN; PROGESTIN.

Fentanyl

A narcotic pain reliever. Fentanyl (Duragesic, Sublimaze) is used as a short-acting pain reliever and as an adjunct to general anesthesia for surgical procedures. It works by altering the person's perception of painful stimuli, relieving pain that is moderate to severe. Like morphine, fentanyl is a central nervous system and respiratory depressant and should not be used by people with respiratory diseases or head injuries.

Fentanyl is also available as a skin patch for the management of chronic pain when other pain relievers have not worked.

Ferrous sulfate

A dietary supplement used to treat iron deficiencies and iron deficiency anemia. Ferrous sulfate (Feosol, Fero-Folic, ViTelle, Irospan, Vi-Daylin) contains the iron needed for the formation and function of red blood cells that carry oxygen through the bloodstream. Ferrous sulfate is available without a prescription, but it should not be used for long periods without the approval of a doctor because the body rids itself of iron very slowly. Excessive amounts of iron can be dangerous.

Fertility

The biological capacity to reproduce. Human fertility varies with age. A woman's fertility begins with the onset of menstruation, peaks when she reaches her 20s, then declines gradually as she approaches menopause, the phase when a woman stops menstruating and ovulating. There are many conditions that may diminish a person's fertility. These include diseases of the reproductive system, failure of ovulation, severe medical conditions, medications, heredity, exposure to toxins, and harmful lifestyle habits.

Fertility drugs

See GNRH.

Fertilization

The union of an egg with a sperm. Fertilization produces the first cell of a zygote, with half of the genes from the mother and half from the father. The zygote becomes an embryo, which then develops into a fetus.

FESS

Functional endoscopic sinus surgery; a surgical treatment that uses endoscopes (lighted viewing devices of varying sizes for operating inside a cavity of the body) and is performed to promote sinus drainage. Reoccurring or untreated infections of the sinuses may produce scarring that narrows or closes the openings of one or more sinuses. When the openings are partially or fully blocked, the sinuses cannot drain properly. A surgeon performs FESS to clear the tiny nasal passage that has become blocked and allow the sinuses to drain. This procedure is not performed unless medical treatment has failed, usually including multiple courses of antibiotics, decongestants, nasal corticosteroid sprays, and possibly allergy shots and vaccinations.

HOW IT IS PERFORMED

A surgeon specializing in otolaryngology (division of surgery dealing with ear, nose, and throat problems) inserts an endoscope and delicate cutting tools into the nostrils and blocked sinuses. While looking through the endoscope or observing an image projected on a monitor by the endoscope, the surgeon removes whatever is blocking the sinus opening—including infected sinus membranes, polyps, and small bone fragments—and enlarges the opening. He or she may then insert a small vacuum to drain accumulated fluids from the sinus. There is usually only mild to moderate postoperative pain or swelling, and natural drainage and sinus function are restored. Complications are rare but can be

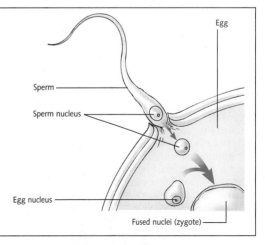

JOINING OF EGG AND SPERM
Fertilization takes place when a sperm penetrates the wall of an egg and the nuclei of the two sex cells join to create a single new cell. The egg and sperm cell each contain 23 chromosomes—half the number of any other cell in the body. Upon fertilization, the newly created cell contains the full complement of 46 chromosomes, with half the genetic material from each parent.

Egg

Sperm

Sperm nucleus

Egg nucleus

Fused nuclei (zygote)

F

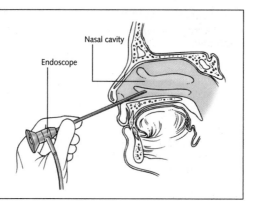

REMOVING SINUS BLOCKAGE
Functional endoscopic sinus surgery (FESS) is a technique to clear tiny passages in the sinuses to permit drainage. After a local anesthetic has been given, the doctor uses an endoscope (a lighted, hollow viewing instrument) to insert tools through the nostrils and into the sinus cavities. The surgeon clears out infection, polyps, or bone fragments that plug the passages and vacuums out fluids.

Nasal cavity

Endoscope

serious. Finding a surgeon who is experienced in FESS is strongly recommended.

WHAT TO EXPECT
An evaluation precedes the decision to perform FESS. During this evaluation, the physician uses an endoscope to examine the interior of the nose, after applying a decongestant and local anesthetic. A CT (computed tomography) scan is also requested to confirm the diagnosis and so that the surgeon can refer to it during the procedure.

FESS is generally performed in a hospital, although a hospital stay following the operation is not always required. Some people are able to return to their normal activities the day after surgery. In preparation for the procedure, the patient will usually be sedated and given a local anesthetic. The operation takes 30 to 90 minutes. Postoperative antibiotics and painkillers will be prescribed. Some nasal crusting, discomfort, and nosebleeds may persist for a few weeks, requiring visits to the physician to have dried blood and other secretions removed. In some cases, sinus blockage recurs, and the procedure must be repeated.

Fetal alcohol syndrome
A group of birth defects that occur as a result of excessive alcohol consumed by a mother during pregnancy. Birth defects associated with fetal alcohol syndrome include growth and mental retardation, DEVELOPMENTAL DELAY, and abnormalities of the heart, head, face, skeleton, and nerves. Babies with fetal alcohol syndrome are also likely to be premature, of low birth weight, and unusually

fussy. The syndrome is associated with higher than normal infant mortality. Fetal alcohol syndrome is the most common identifiable cause of mental retardation in the United States and the third most common cause of birth defects, after Down syndrome and spina bifida.

The more a mother drinks during pregnancy, the more likely her baby is to develop fetal alcohol syndrome. Drinking heavily during the first trimester leads to the most severe problems. Babies have a 10 percent risk of developing the syndrome if their mothers drink more than an ounce of alcohol, or two drinks, a day; the risk doubles at two ounces of alcohol per day. Because of the concern that even small amounts of alcohol can cause neurological abnormalities, standard medical practice is to advise pregnant women to abstain altogether from alcohol throughout pregnancy.

SYMPTOMS
The symptoms of fetal alcohol syndrome may appear different in different babies, depending on how much alcohol their mothers consumed in pregnancy. In mild cases, symptoms include irritability, difficulty in focusing attention, mild developmental delay, and sometimes hyperactivity. More severely affected babies may show developmental delay, hyperactivity, attention-deficit disorder, seizures, and severe mental retardation. Physical abnormalities associated with the syndrome include a small head, short upturned nose, narrowly spaced eyes, thin upper lip, clubfoot, characteristically creased palms, and cardiac defects.

DIAGNOSIS AND TREATMENT
Although it may be emotionally difficult for her, a mother who has consumed more than two drinks a day during pregnancy needs to tell the doctor. The diagnosis of fetal alcohol syndrome is based on growth rate, central nervous system involvement, and the presence of characteristic features. Newborns exposed to alcohol just before birth may show signs of withdrawal after delivery, including jitteriness, tremors, seizures, abnormal reflexes, disturbed sleep, decreased sucking, and low Apgar scores (a system for assessing the condition of newborns). In many cases, the signs of fetal alcohol syndrome are subtle and may not emerge until the child is of school age, when learning problems or learning disabilities emerge.

Fetal alcohol syndrome is not only a disorder of childhood. A progression of the developmental and cognitive handicaps associated with the disorder persists into adulthood. Major psychological problems and lifelong adjustment problems, including poor judgment, distractibility, and inadequate social skills, are characteristic of adults who had fetal alcohol syndrome. Although the condition can be prevented, it has no cure. Treatment consists of providing good nutrition and treating complications. Children with learning disabilities may need to attend special schools.

Fetal distress
Signs during labor that the well-being of a fetus may be compromised. An early sign of fetal distress can be a deceleration of the fetal heartbeat as a contraction ends. Other signs include contractions of the uterus in abnormal patterns and a variety of fetal heartbeat abnormalities. The presence of meconium (a waste product from the baby) in the amniotic fluid is also an indication that the fetus is in distress.

Doctors and midwives often use FETAL MONITORING during labor to permit early detection of abnormalities that may endanger the fetus. The presence of more than one sign of fetal distress on the fetal monitoring tracing generally calls for taking a sample of the baby's blood from its scalp to test for pH level, a measure of acidity and alkalinity. A low pH level (less than 7.0) calls for immediate intervention, including CESAREAN SECTION. Intermediate levels require close monitoring and intervention as needed.

Fetal monitoring

Methods used by doctors to check a baby's heart rate and assess the baby's health before birth. Fetal monitoring is routinely used during labor to establish how the fetus is reacting to the stresses of labor. It is used throughout pregnancy to assess the health of the fetus if the woman has previously had a stillbirth, has symptoms of PREECLAMPSIA, or when the growth of the fetus has been slower than expected. There are two types of fetal monitoring: internal and external. No known risks are associated with external fetal monitoring. A minor risk of infection exists with internal fetal monitoring.

In external monitoring, a doctor presses a stethoscope or a handheld ultrasound device to a pregnant woman's abdomen to listen to a baby's heartbeat. To provide precise and continuous electronic monitoring, belts that measure the baby's heart rate and the length and frequency of contractions are placed around a woman's abdomen. The belts are connected to a machine that records and prints the information. For many situations, such as checking on the well-being of a fetus or evaluating the frequency of contractions, external monitoring is sufficient. However, in other situations a more accurate assessment may be necessary, and a doctor may recommend internal fetal monitoring.

Internal fetal monitoring gives a much more precise picture of a baby's heart rate and the strength of the mother's contractions. Internal monitoring devices are attached to equipment that records and prints the data. To internally monitor a fetus, an electrode is inserted through the mother's vagina and cervix. The electrode is attached to the baby's scalp to monitor the baby's heart rate. If a fetus has an abnormal heart rate, a blood sample may be taken from its scalp to check the oxygen supply. Internal fetal monitoring requires the rupturing of the amniotic sac, so it is usually done only when a woman is in labor. A pressure catheter (a long thin tube) may be inserted into the uterus to measure the length, intensity, and frequency of contractions.

SPECIAL TESTS

Women who have a high risk for problems during pregnancy, for example, or women with high blood pressure, diabetes, too much or too little amniotic fluid, kidney or heart disease, multiple fetuses, or a post-

TYPES OF FETAL MONITORING

During labor, instruments may be used to monitor the fetus's movements and heart rate and record the length, frequency, and sometimes the intensity of the mother's uterine contractions. The goal is to make sure the fetus is getting enough oxygen. Information obtained through either external or internal monitoring is transmitted to an electronic monitor and printer.

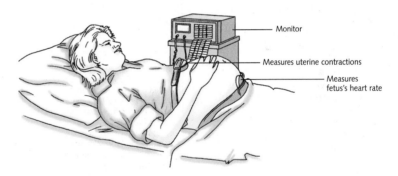

Monitor

Measures uterine contractions

Measures fetus's heart rate

EXTERNAL FETAL MONITORING
Two recording devices are belted around the pregnant woman's abdomen while she lies in bed.

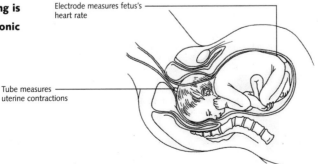

Electrode measures fetus's heart rate

Tube measures uterine contractions

INTERNAL FETAL MONITORING
An electrode that measures the fetus's heart rate is attached to the fetus's scalp through the woman's vagina and cervix. Periodically, a thin tube is inserted through the vagina into the uterus to measure the mother's contractions. Internal monitoring is invasive, but it gives more accurate readings of the fetus's heartbeat.

term pregnancy, all may require special fetal monitoring. In these cases, a doctor may order various tests beyond what is typically done to ensure the health of the fetus.

■ *Ultrasound examination* An ultrasound is a test in which the echoes of sound waves directed at the fetus are used to create a picture. Doppler ultrasound tests use sound waves to create signals of the fetal heartbeat. An ultrasound is done by moving a handheld transducer over a woman's abdomen or by placing a probe inside a woman's vagina. Ultrasound examinations help doctors to gain information about a fetus's growth, health, and anatomical structure. Most pregnant women in the United States have an ultrasound at least once during their pregnancy. It is the first step in screening for possible complications.

■ *Nonstress test* This test measures the heart rate of a fetus in response to its own movements. For this test, which takes from 20 to 40 minutes, a belt is placed around the abdomen of the woman. She presses a button every time she feels the fetus move. This information is recorded and helps provide an indication of fetal health.

■ *Biophysical profile* A combination of a nonstress test and an ultrasound, a biophysical profile involves five factors: heart rate, breathing, muscle tone, body movement, and amount of amniotic fluid. Each item is given a score. The total score may indicate whether a woman will need special care or whether an early delivery should be planned.

■ *Contraction stress test* This test measures the response of the fetal heart to contractions of the uterus. A normal response means the fetus is receiving enough oxygen. To perform a CONTRACTION STRESS TEST, mild contractions may be induced either by using the hormone oxytocin or by having the woman massage one of her nipples (which causes the uterus to contract). This test can take from 1 to 2 hours.

Fetal tissue research

Also known as fetal nerve cell transplantation. Researchers have studied the implantation of fetal cells and stem cells into the brains of individuals with a degenerative brain disorder

to treat diseases such as Parkinson disease. The controversy regarding this approach to treatment centers on the source of the fetal tissue and the ongoing ethical debate about abortion. See also ETHICS, MEDICAL.

Fetishism

A psychiatric disorder involving intense, repeated sexual urges or fantasies focused on nonhuman objects, most often articles of clothing (such as shoes, undergarments, or boots). A person with fetishism often masturbates while holding or smelling the desired object or asks a sexual partner to wear it. In many cases the person can function sexually only if the object is present. Fetishism usually begins in adolescence and is likely to continue throughout life.

Fetus

The product of CONCEPTION, from the eighth week of pregnancy until birth. Before the eighth week, the fertilized egg is considered an EMBRYO. A fetus in the eighth week is about 1 inch long, with all major internal organs formed and clearly visible arms, legs, and joints. Blood cells have developed, and blood is circulating in primitive blood vessels. Fingers and toes are distinct but are still joined by webs of skin. The eyes, nose, and mouth are recognizable, the ears have begun to develop, and movement by the fetus can be detected. The fetus will grow rapidly and be ready to be born at about 40 weeks after conception.

Fever

FOR FIRST AID
see Fever, page 1321

Body temperature above the normal range, which is an orally taken body temperature of 98.6°F to 100°F in adults aged 18 to 40. Fever in children is measured at higher values because children have a slightly higher normal body temperature. A child is diagnosed with a fever when he or she has a temperature above 100.4°F when measured rectally, 100°F when measured orally or in the ear, or 99°F when measured under the arm.

Body temperature tends to be lowest in the morning and highest in the late afternoon. Accordingly, an adult may have a fever with a body temperature above 98.9°F at 6:00 AM and above 100°F at 4:00 PM. Some people, particularly those who smoke cigarettes, have a normal oral temperature of up to 100.3°F.

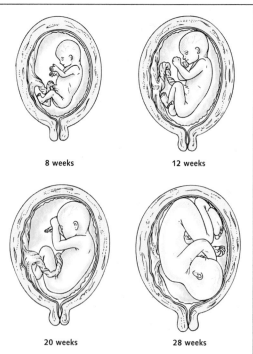

FETAL DEVELOPMENT
At 8 weeks, the embryo is called a fetus. It is about 1 inch long and weighs about seven hundredths of an ounce. Facial features are becoming recognizable, and blood is circulating. At 12 weeks, the fetus is perhaps 3 inches long and weighs about half an ounce. Its head is disproportionately large; it can move its limbs and make sucking actions, and genitals have formed. At 20 weeks, the fetus is 10 inches long and about 11 ounces. The limbs have lengthened, and teeth and hair are beginning to form. The fetus now sleeps and wakes and hears sounds. At 28 weeks, the fetus is 14 to 15 inches long and has grown rapidly to a weight of about 2 or more pounds.

8 weeks

12 weeks

20 weeks

28 weeks

CAUSES OF FEVER

The hypothalamus gland in the brain sets the body's temperature within a normal range when a person is healthy. When the body is invaded by infectious viruses, bacteria, or fungi or by toxins or abnormal chemicals produced by tumors, the body's immune response is triggered by small molecules called pyrogens, which cause the hypothalamus to raise the body's temperature.

Fever may last 24 hours or several weeks, depending on the cause. An elevated body temperature may be caused by any number of conditions or illnesses. These include common infectious diseases such as colds, flu, and gastroenteritis; less common infectious diseases such as those contracted in areas of poor sanitation; chronic inflammatory conditions such as rheumatoid arthritis; and severe illness such as pneumonia. Other causes of high fever include severe trauma such as the fever that may be caused by invasive surgery; the excessive loss of body fluids that causes dehydration; inflammation of blood vessels caused by a blood clot; a malignant tumor; adverse reactions to certain medications and immunizations; and the ingestion or inhalation of toxins.

HYPERTHERMIA is a condition that occurs when the body overheats, usually due to overexertion or exposure to hot environmental conditions. Symptoms may include confusion, lethargy, loss of consciousness, and inability to sweat despite an extremely elevated body temperature. This condition is treated differently from other causes of fever; a person experiencing hyperthermia must be cooled immediately; he or she should be taken to a cool place and fanned, the person's clothing should be removed, and a wet sponge should be used to keep the person's skin damp and cool. Emergency medical care should be sought.

Symptoms that accompany fever can sometimes lead to a diagnosis. For example, when vomiting and diarrhea occur with fever, the symptoms may indicate gastroenteritis. Symptoms including coughing, discolored phlegm, and wheezing with fever may signal bronchitis or pneumonia.

In some instances, fever persists for several weeks and no cause for a fever can be determined by medical testing. This is referred to as a fever of unknown origin, and may occur when an infection is present but the harmful organism causing the fever cannot be identified. A fever of unknown origin may also result from tumors or from autoimmune or genetic disorders.

SYMPTOMS

The symptoms experienced when a person has fever include sweating, chills, shivering, headaches, aching muscles, loss of appetite, general weakness, fatigue, and possibly restlessness, dehydration, and rash. When fevers reach a very high level, symptoms may include confusion and other signs of mental dysfunction, extreme sleepiness, irritability, and seizures. When triggered by fever, seizures are called febrile seizures and affect a small percentage of young children who have a rapid rise in their temperature. Febrile seizures are characterized by rigid muscles and other signs of seizure generally lasting less than 10 minutes and followed by a lengthy episode of sleep. A pediatrician should be informed immediately when a child has a febrile seizure.

Most fevers are caused by bacterial or viral infections such as influenza, measles, or tonsillitis, but fever can also occur along with noninfectious conditions such as dehydration, heart attack, and tumors in the lymphatic system.

DIAGNOSIS

The cause of fever is diagnosed by medical history, physical examination, and evaluation of symptoms. A medical history may include the time the fever began, immunization status, recent travel, exposure to people who are ill, medications taken, illegal drug use, dietary history, exposure to animals, sexual history, allergies, recent surgeries, and underlying illnesses or medical conditions.

A physical examination may include observing the skin for signs of rash or infection and examining the person's lymph nodes for signs of swelling. The eyes may be examined for discoloration, and the heart and chest are listened to with a stethoscope. Signs of infection are looked for in the throat and mouth. The abdomen may be checked for abnormalities in the gallbladder, intestines, or appendix. The limbs may be evaluated for problems with the joints, such as arthritis. The genitals may be examined for signs of sexually transmitted diseases.

Diagnostic tests may be performed to rule out problems with the nervous system, including encephalitis and meningitis. Laboratory examinations of blood, urine, stool, or spinal fluid may be undertaken. X rays, scans, liver tests, and biopsies may be necessary to determine why a person has a fever.

TREATMENT

When a fever is mild (below 102°F), it is generally treated by increased intake of fluids, which act as internal coolants and replenish vital salts; by restricting the person's diet to easily digestible foods; by bed rest and sleep to slow body functions and reduce the body's core temperature; and by taking medications that reduce fever. Adults may take nonsteroidal anti-inflammatory drugs (NSAIDs), such as aspirin or ibuprofen, which stop the hypothalamus from raising body temperature.

Children may take acetaminophen or ibuprofen, which should lower the body temperature by about 2 degrees within 1 hour. Aspirin should not be taken by children younger than 18 years, as this medication is linked to Reye syndrome, a life-threatening neurologic disorder. Children with fever may be made more comfortable with tepid water sponge baths. Rubbing alcohol sponge baths should not be used.

There is some controversy over taking medication to reduce body temperature, as fever is believed to help the body fight infection. Some health practitioners recommend using fever-reducing medication only when fever is severe. A sustained body temperature of 106°F or above may result in brain damage.

Most fevers are due to common infections and tend to improve either on their own or when the underlying cause of infection is treated. Antibiotics may be prescribed to treat bacterial infections, and antifungal medication may be given if the infection is caused by a fungus. Medication and other treatment may be given for nausea and diarrhea. Fever warrants medical attention

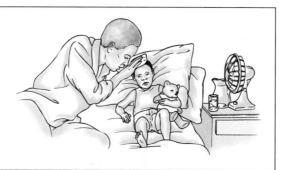

LOWERING A FEVER
To lower a fever in a child, let him or her rest and give plenty of fluids. To reduce fever and chills, give acetaminophen or ibuprofen. Never give aspirin to a child younger than 18. Sponging or bathing the child with tepid (99°F) water will help cool the skin and reduce the fever. Keep the room cool but not uncomfortable.

when it exceeds 103°F in an adult or 101°F in an infant. A physician should be notified if milder fever persists for more than 24 hours or if associated symptoms become worse. A fever of 105°F or higher or a fever accompanied by seizures, unconsciousness, a stiff neck, difficulty breathing, severe pain, swelling, blood in the stool, repeated vomiting, a discolored or foul-smelling discharge from the vagina or penis, or urinary tract symptoms requires immediate medical attention. A mild fever in people with serious medical conditions, including cancer, diabetes mellitus, and HIV (human immunodeficiency virus) infection, indicates a need for timely medical attention. A woman who has a fever and is pregnant should also seek medical attention.

In combination with other symptoms, a fever may indicate the need for emergency medical care. When a fever is accompanied by severe headache and a stiff neck, meningitis may be the cause and emergency attention is essential. When either chest pain or difficulty breathing is associated with fever, emergency care is required. It is considered a medical emergency when fever is present with blood in the stool, urine, or mucus. A person should be taken to an emergency medical facility if fever is accompanied by agitation or confusion with no apparent cause.

Fever blister

A localized viral infection caused by the herpes simplex virus type 1. Fever blisters, also called cold sores, usually involve small areas of skin on the border of the lip. They may also occur inside the mouth, on the gums or tongue, or on the inner surface of the cheeks. The virus that causes

them is passed from person to person by direct contact with an infected person's skin or saliva.

A primary infection, which may not cause symptoms, occurs when the virus first invades the skin, usually in childhood. In some people, especially children, the primary infection produces symptoms including fever, sores in the mouth, and sore throat. Most people eventually contract the infection, with or without symptoms, by adulthood. Following the primary infection, the virus persists in the nerves near the affected skin in a dormant stage that is intermittently reactivated. Reactivation of the virus produces a fever blister and may be caused by any of several different factors including fever, emotional stress, poor nutrition, dental procedures, and sun exposure.

The first symptom of a fever blister is a sensation of tingling and itching in the affected skin. Swelling and redness in the area then occur, followed by the eruption of one or more tiny blisters. The blisters open up, produce fluid, and become painful sores, which usually crust over within 4 days, then form scabs, and in most cases, heal completely within 8 to 10 days.

Fever blisters are diagnosed by examination and a medical history that explores factors that may have triggered the reactivation of the virus. When it is medically significant to confirm a diagnosis, cells scraped from the infected area may be tested.

Fever blisters can be treated with antiviral medications, including acyclovir, but the use of antiviral medications does not significantly reduce how long symptoms last and is generally only recommended to suppress recurrences in people with weakened immune systems. Keeping the area

clean, avoiding contact with the hands, and using a soothing lip balm is usually the recommended course of treatment. If a fever blister limits the ability to speak, obstructs swallowing, or is accompanied by fever or headache, a doctor should be consulted.

Several different vaccines are now being developed against the herpes virus that causes fever blisters. However, the vaccine will only be useful for preventing infection in people who have never been infected. People in whom the virus is dormant have a lifelong risk of developing fever blisters.

Feverfew

An herbal remedy used for migraine, fever, and inflammation. Feverfew is a member of the chrysanthemum or sunflower family and has been used for centuries to reduce fever. Feverfew is thought to act in a way that is similar to aspirin, which inhibits chemical compounds that promote inflammation. It also may have a favorable effect on blood platelets, and it may be effective in the prevention and treatment of migraine headaches. Feverfew is also used to treat arthritis.

Fexofenadine

A drug used to treat seasonal allergies. Fexofenadine (Allegra) is a nonsedating antihistamine used to treat symptoms of hay fever, including sneezing, runny nose, watery eyes, and itchy throat. It is also used to treat certain cases of hives or itching skin. Unlike other antihistamines, fexofenadine is not likely to cause drowsiness.

Fiber, dietary

Nondigestible substances found in plant foods such as fruits, vegetables, and grains. Dietary fiber, a valuable component of a healthy diet, consists of the parts of plants that cannot be broken down by enzymes in the digestive system. A diet high in fiber helps maintain proper bowel function and prevents intestinal disorders ranging from constipation to irritable bowel syndrome. It may also reduce the risk for cardiovascular disease, cancer, and diabetes. In the intestines, fiber absorbs water. This adds bulk to stools and makes them softer, larger, and easier to expel. High-fiber foods include fruits and vegetables (especially with edible skins on), nuts, dried beans, and whole-grain breads and cereals. Although fiber itself provides no nutrients, the foods that contain it are rich in valuable vitamins and minerals.

TYPES OF FIBER

Based on its capacity to dissolve in water, dietary fiber is considered either soluble or insoluble. Both types of fiber are found in fiber-rich foods. Insoluble fiber is more abundant in the food supply than soluble fiber.

Soluble fiber is found in the greatest amounts in oatmeal, oat bran, barley, dried beans, and psyllium. Fiber extracted from psyllium, a type of grass, is a component of many over-the-counter stool softeners and laxatives. However, a diet naturally rich in fiber is a better choice to maintain regularity. The health benefits of soluble fiber are related to its viscosity as a gel and its breakdown into certain fatty acids by bacteria in the large intestine. In combination with a diet low in saturated fat and cholesterol, soluble fiber can also help lower total cholesterol levels and thus reduce the risk of heart disease. It also slows carbohydrate absorption, which helps regulate the blood sugar level.

Insoluble fiber does not mix with liquid and passes through the digestive tract largely intact. Examples of insoluble fiber include the stringy filaments in celery or cabbage. Whole-grain breads, wheat bran, and fruit and vegetable skins are all good sources of insoluble fiber. Eating these foods can promote regularity and protect against a range of bowel disorders.

ADDING FIBER TO THE DIET

Doctors recommend that people consume 20 to 35 grams of fiber each day. About one fourth of the total fiber consumed should be soluble fiber. However, many American adults consume much less than this. High-fiber foods are those that contain at least 2 grams of fiber per serving. Medical experts advise increasing fiber intake by eating high-fiber cereals, fruits with the skins on, popcorn, whole wheat bread, and vegetables. Food choices should include 1 to 2 daily servings of good sources of soluble fiber.

It is best to add fiber gradually to the diet. A sudden increase in fiber intake can lead to FLATULENCE (gas) and bloating. Drinking plenty of water can help to alleviate side effects, especially if fiber sources are whole-grain breads and cereals, which have a low water content. Fruits and vegetables have a higher water content, but lower concentrations of fiber than whole grains. Without adequate water, fiber, which increases the water-holding capacity of stool, can be constipating. Because fruits, vegetables, and grains provide a variety of health benefits in addition to fiber, doctors recommend that people get fiber from these natural sources rather than from dietary supplements.

Fiberoptics

Transmission of an image through bundles of thin, flexible glass or plastic threads that convey light by total internal reflection. In medicine, fiberoptics has led to the development of ENDOSCOPY (a procedure in which interior parts of the body are examined using a slim, flexible, lighted tube called an ENDOSCOPE). Doctors use endoscopes to view, photograph, videotape, and treat the inside of the body without surgery. One bundle of fibers sends light to the far end of the tube, while another bundle carries back images to the physician performing the procedure. The flexibility of the fibers permits an endoscope to be passed through the esophagus, stomach, duodenum, and lower digestive tract.

Fibrillation

An extremely fast, chaotic heartbeat. Fibrillation reduces or eliminates the ability of the heart chamber to pump blood effectively, depending on what portion of the heart is affected. Fibrillation in the atrium (upper chamber) of the heart is known as ATRIAL FIBRILLATION. Fibrillation in the ventricle (lower chamber) is known as VENTRICULAR FIBRILLATION.

Fibrinolysis

The process by which enzymes break down a blood clot. Fibrinolysis means "fibrin dissolving"; fibrin is a principal component of blood clots. Fibrinolysis occurs continuously in nature, but it is increased by such fac-

tors as intense exercise, certain medications, bacterial infection, and a low blood sugar level.

Fibroadenoma

A benign fibrous growth in the breast. Fibroadenomas are firm, solid lumps that contain no fluid and are usually freely movable when touched. They are common, appearing most frequently in young women, usually within 20 years of puberty. Typically, fibroadenomas are first detected by a woman herself. Discovery of any breast lump requires a doctor's examination to rule out the possibility of breast cancer. Ranging from the size of a pea to that of a lemon, fibroadenomas cause no nipple discharge or pain. Most women who get a fibroadenoma do not get another, although some women have several. Their cause is unknown.

Fibroadenomas are not related to breast cancer. Although they require no treatment, fibroadenomas frequently are removed when a doctor is unable to distinguish a fibroadenoma from a more serious cause of a breast lump, such as cancer, without microscopic examination. The surgery is usually performed with the use of a local anesthetic and does not require a hospital stay.

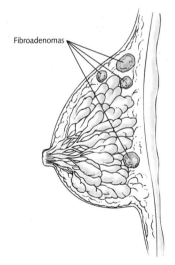

Fibroadenomas

NONCANCEROUS GROWTH
A fibroadenoma is a common breast lump of unknown cause that is not related to cancer in any way. Many fibroadenomas require no treatment at all. But some growths are removed surgically if they are difficult to distinguish from other, harmful growths.

Fibrocystic breasts

FOR SYMPTOM CHART
see Breast pain or lumps, page 22

Multiple painful, benign lumps and cysts in the breasts. Fibrocystic breasts are most common among women between the ages of 30 and 50 years and are rare in women after menopause. The condition is very common and most likely is linked to estrogen. A fibrocystic breast contains small, nodular lumps and cysts that can be detected through self-examination. Pain and lumpiness in the breasts occurs and increases toward the end of the menstrual cycle, when the cysts tend to enlarge. The size of the lumpy areas commonly fluctuates, and lumps may appear and disappear rapidly. Symptoms usually subside after menopause.

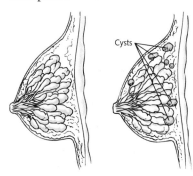

Normal breast   Fibrocystic breast

NONCANCEROUS, PAINFUL LUMPS
A fibrocystic breast contains small, benign cysts that give the breast a lumpy texture. The cysts tend to enlarge and become painful toward the end of the woman's menstrual cycle and can appear or disappear quickly. The lumps are not a sign of any underlying disease, but are probably linked in some way to estrogen. The condition tends to subside after menopause.

A woman whose breasts contain fibrocystic lumps can be treated with needle aspiration, in which the lumps are drained. While fibrocystic breasts are not cancerous, there is a risk of breast cancer in women who have atypical cells lining the cysts. Women with fibrocystic breasts should examine their breasts carefully each month just after menstruation and inform their doctors of any new lumps. To rule out cancer, the doctor may order a biopsy, in which tissue from the lump is examined microscopically. Mammography is also used to assess lumps, but is not always accurate in detecting cancer.

To avoid the pain associated with fibrocystic breasts, doctors recommend wearing bras with good support and avoiding consumption of caffeine, thought by some to have a role in the condition. When symptoms are severe, doctors sometimes prescribe DIURETICS, DANAZOL, or PROGESTERONE.

Fibroid, uterine

Benign growths in or on the uterus. Uterine fibroids, also known as myomas or leiomyomas, are the most common type of abnormal growth in a woman's pelvis. They occur in about 25 percent of women and are most common between the ages of 30 and 40 years. Among black women, fibroids are more common, occur at younger ages, and grow more rapidly. Most fibroids, even large ones, produce no symptoms, although some women experience pain in the abdomen and lower back, abdominal pressure, and more frequent urination. Changes in the amount, frequency, and duration of menstruation also may occur. Because fibroids sometimes block the entrance to a fallopian tube or distort the inner surface of the uterus, they can cause miscarriages and infertility.

The reason fibroids develop is unknown, although estrogen appears to promote their growth and development. When estrogen is plentiful, such as during pregnancy, fibroids often grow larger, shrinking when estrogen production drops. Fibroids vary in size from that of a pea to that of a grapefruit, sometimes growing so large they are mistaken for a pregnancy. They may become part of the inner or outer walls of the uterus, or they may hang from stems inside or outside it. They can also grow within the uterine wall. Fibroids rarely become cancerous, and then usually only after menopause.

Diagnosis is based on clinical examination of the fibroids and, at times, on techniques such as ULTRASOUND SCANNING, LAPAROSCOPY, HYSTEROSCOPY, or HYSTEROSALPINGOGRAM. Treatment is not always necessary unless the fibroids cause excessive pain or bleeding, or if the doctor cannot distinguish the fibroid from a cancerous tumor. When required, fibroids are removed surgically, through myomectomy (removal of only the fibroids) or hysterectomy (removal of the uterus).

Fibroma

A benign or nonmalignant tumor composed largely of fibrous connective tissue. These smooth, usually painless, growths under the skin or in

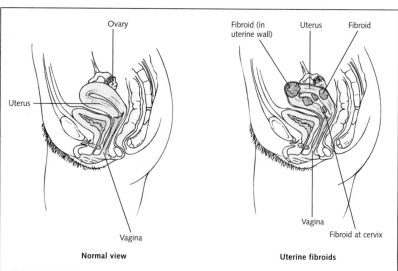

Normal view   Uterine fibroids

UTERINE FIBROIDS
The smooth outline of the uterus in the normal view contrasts with the changes that occur when fibroids grow in the uterus, uterine wall, or cervix.

the bone are often caused by injury or infection. Doctors recommend medical evaluation for any unexplained lump or swelling.

Fibromyalgia

A common condition that produces stiffness and pain in the fibrous tissues deep in the muscles. Aching and fatigue along with a slight swelling of the muscles may also be symptoms. Some people may have tension headaches, numbness or tingling of the extremities, and symptoms usually associated with irritable bowel syndrome. Sometimes called fibrositis, fibromyalgia produces multiple tender areas in specific muscles, including those of the neck, shoulders, upper back, lower back, and hips. The cause is unknown, but it does not affect joints. Sleep disturbance, clinical depression, and emotional stress may be associated with the condition. Many people who have fibromyalgia have disruptive sleep patterns.

Other contributing factors include immune or endocrine abnormalities, altered serotonin levels, or other biochemical abnormalities in the central nervous system. People with rheumatoid arthritis, spinal arthritis, or Lyme disease may also develop fibromyalgia.

DIAGNOSIS AND TREATMENT

Fibromyalgia is diagnosed on the basis of symptoms, especially persistent, widespread muscular pain, and the physician's discovery of tenderness in specific areas of muscle. Laboratory tests and X rays may be ordered to exclude conditions such as hypothyroidism, lupus erythematosus, rheumatoid arthritis, and infections, all of which may mimic fibromyalgia. While there is no cure for the condition, it often improves on its own and does not damage the muscle tissue. Pain can sometimes be managed with aspirin or other nonsteroidal anti-inflammatory drugs (NSAIDs) and by taking hot baths. If pain is severe, an injection of the anesthetic lidocaine or a corticosteroid may also prove helpful, but these treatments may not be effective. Massage, stretching, and range-of-motion exercises may help relieve symptoms. A physician may treat fibromyalgia with medications that promote sleep and relax muscles or with antidepressant medications. Physical therapy may be prescribed. When factors such as stress or depression are involved, psychological counseling may be appropriate.

Fibrosarcoma

A rare cancer involving connective tissue around a muscle, tendon, or bone. Fibrosarcoma of soft tissue generally originates in the fibrous tissue of the arms, legs, or trunk, often deep within the thigh. Soft-tissue fibrosarcomas most often appear in men in their 40s or 50s. Fibrosarcoma of the bone generally affects the pelvis, leg, arm, or hip. It can occur at any age but is rare in childhood and adolescence. Most fibrosarcomas of the bone occur in adults aged 30 to 40 and appear most commonly in the long bones, particularly of the leg.

Fibrosis

An abnormal increase in the amount of fibrous connective tissue in an organ, body part, or tissue. Fibrosis occurs normally in the formation of scar tissue or as a reaction to foreign bodies in the tissue. CYSTIC FIBROSIS is a life-threatening inherited disorder that causes severe lung damage and nutritional deficiencies.

Fifth disease

FOR SYMPTOM CHART
see Rashes in infants and children, page 50

The most common infection caused by parvovirus B19; also called erythema infectiosum. Fifth disease is an illness that produces a mild fever and a redness of the skin formed by tiny red eruptions that may vary in intensity. This gives the person with the infection a "slapped cheek" appearance that may progress from a pale rosy hue to a bright red. Eventually, a lacy, netlike pattern of color develops on the skin of the face, arms, and trunk. Fifth disease gets its name from being one of the five common childhood infections that cause fever and a rash. The others are MEASLES, MUMPS, CHICKENPOX, and RUBELLA (German measles). Fifth disease is the least serious of the five and most commonly occurs in the winter and spring. This rash is less common in adults, who are more likely to experience joint pain and swelling with the infection. The joints of the hands, wrists, and knees on both sides of the body are most commonly affected, and these symptoms may improve within a week or persist for several months.

HOW IT IS SPREAD

Parvovirus B19 infects only humans. The virus is present in an infected person's respiratory secretions, including saliva, sputum, and nasal

---

DIAGNOSING FIBROMYALGIA

To be diagnosed with fibromyalgia, a person must have a history of widespread pain on both sides of the body, above and below the waist, for at least 3 months. The person will also have at least 11 to 18 "tender point" sites on areas of the body that are painful when pressed.

But how does a doctor diagnose fibromyalgia, a form of arthritis that mimics conditions such as chronic fatigue syndrome, hypothyroidism and hyperthyroidism, lupus erythematosus, and even depression?

Unfortunately, there is not a diagnostic marker in the blood of people with fibromyalgia, and no evidence of the condition appears on X rays. Diagnosis is typically made on the identification of several symptoms and on the exclusion of other possible conditions.

Because fibromyalgia has been recognized only since the early 1980s, studies show that it generally takes an average of 5 years from the time people start experiencing symptoms until the time the disease is diagnosed. Some of those symptoms include muscle pain, insomnia, fatigue and sleep disturbance, depression and anxiety, headaches, morning stiffness, numbness and tingling in the hands and feet, circulatory problems, irritable bowel syndrome, and cold intolerance.

Researchers know little about what causes fibromyalgia but are interested in similarities between the condition and chronic fatigue syndrome, another disease of unknown origin. Scientists are also looking into what effect, if any, hormones might have in people who have the condition.

F

mucus before a rash develops. During this early part of the illness before the rash appears, an infected person may have symptoms of a common cold and can spread the illness to others who are susceptible and come in contact with the infected secretions. Frequent hand washing is recommended to prevent spreading the infection. There is no vaccine to prevent infection with the parvovirus.

The incubation period of the virus is usually 4 to 14 days after exposure, but it may be as long as 20 days. By the time the rash has appeared, there is generally no risk of the infection being contagious.

Some adults and children who become infected with the parvovirus do not become ill, and some acquire a nonspecific illness that is not characteristic of fifth disease. People who have been infected with parvovirus B19 develop immunity to the disease and cannot contract fifth disease.

DIAGNOSIS AND TREATMENT
Fifth disease is often diagnosed by observation of the characteristic rash during physical examination by a doctor. A blood test confirms the diagnosis.

The illness is usually mild, and symptoms generally improve on their own in healthy children and adults within 10 days. During the course of the illness, fever, pain, or itching can be treated. Adults with joint symptoms may need to rest, restrict activities, and use aspirin or ibuprofen.

People who have certain medical conditions may develop acute, severe anemia from parvovirus B19 infection; symptoms include paleness, weakness, and fatigue. This group may include persons with sickle cell disease or other types of chronic anemia and people who have weakened immune systems from illnesses such as cancer, leukemia, or HIV (human immunodeficiency virus) infection or because they are recipients of organ transplants. A woman who is pregnant may occasionally develop serious complications from the infection. In these cases, medical treatment is necessary.

If the infection causes severe ane-

mia, hospitalization and blood transfusions may become necessary. In people with deficient immune systems, immune globulin treatment can help eliminate the infection.

Fight-or-flight response

Response of the sympathetic nervous system to a life-threatening event. The fight-or-flight response prepares the body to fight an enemy or flee from a dangerous situation by secreting the hormone adrenaline, which increases the heart rate and the flow of blood to the brain and muscles, raises the blood sugar level, and dilates the pupils. The fight-or-flight response is designed to help people and animals summon extra strength and energy needed to cope in a life-threatening situation.

When people react to situations that are not truly life-threatening by triggering the fight-or-flight response, the response represents a false alarm. Too many such false alarms take a toll on the body and can lead to stress-related physical disorders, such as migraine headache, panic disorder, insomnia, heart disease, high blood pressure, and sexual dysfunction.

Filariasis

A parasitic disease caused by microscopic, threadlike worms that live in the human lymph system. Filariasis, also known as lymphatic filariasis, is found in the tropics and subtropics, particularly central and western Africa. It is spread from an infected person via mosquito bites. The microscopic worms circulating in the infected person's blood enter and infect the mosquito when the insect feeds on the person's blood. When the infected mosquito bites another person, the microscopic worms pass through the skin and travel to the lymph vessels, where they grow into adults, subsequently mate, and release millions of microscopic worms into the blood.

Lymphatic filariasis is not contracted from the bite of a single mosquito, but rather from many mosquito bites occurring over a period of several months. While long-term residents of affected areas may be at greatest risk for the infection, short-term visitors are not considered to be at risk.

SYMPTOMS
Symptoms are not usually experi-

enced until the adult worms have died. The disease is not life-threatening but may permanently damage the lymph system and the kidneys. Impairment to the lymph system causes lymphedema, which is produced by fluid accumulation and swelling in the arms, breasts, legs, and male genitalia. Swollen areas may expand to several times their normal size. Decreased function of the lymph system impairs the body's ability to fight germs and infections. An increase in bacterial infections in the lymph system and skin can cause the skin to become hardened and thickened. Combined with swelling of the lower extremities, this condition is called ELEPHANTIASIS.

Filariasis is diagnosed by evaluation of blood test results. There is no cure for the disease. Medication can kill all the microscopic worms circulating in the blood and some, but not all, of the adult worms. Yearly doses of this medication may help prevent infection and can also prevent infected persons from transmitting the disease via mosquito bites, but the medicine will not diminish symptoms in those who are already infected.

Filgrastim

A drug used to prevent infection in people with cancer. After chemotherapy, which often depresses the production of anti-infective white blood cells (WBCs), filgrastim may be prescribed to stimulate the production and activity of WBCs, returning the WBC count to pretreatment levels. It is also used to treat people with AIDS (acquired immunodeficiency syndrome) or aplastic anemia.

Filling, dental

The restorative material used to fill a dental cavity caused by TOOTH DECAY or to replace part of a chipped or BROKEN TOOTH. Dental fillings are placed in partially decayed or broken teeth after the decay has been removed, and the teeth have been cleaned and prepared by a dentist. The fillings may be composed of silver amalgam (see AMALGAM, DENTAL) or of tooth-colored materials, made of dental composite (see BONDING, DENTAL) or ceramic. The filling material is determined by the dentist based on a number of factors. Amalgam fillings are considered the most durable and may be the

Terms in small capital letters— for example, PHYSICAL THERAPY or PAGET DISEASE—indicate a cross-reference to another entry with more information.

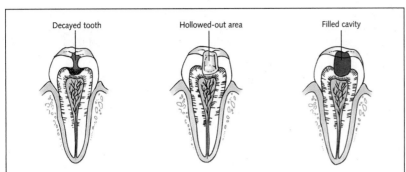

REPAIRING A DECAYED TOOTH
A dental cavity is usually caused by bacteria that have eaten through the protective enamel on a tooth. Left untreated, the decay will progress into the nerve-laden pulp of the tooth, causing pain and perhaps loss of the tooth. Cleaning out the decay and filling the cavity with an inert material halts the spread of the decay. First, the dentist removes decayed tissue and then drills a hole that will securely hold a filling. Then the dentist fills the hole with one of a variety of filling materials.

preferred choice for the biting surfaces of the back teeth. Composite fillings can be matched to the natural tooth color and offer a more acceptable appearance than amalgam fillings on the front teeth. Initially, composite fillings may be sensitive to extremes in temperature, and they may discolor more readily with tobacco or staining beverages such as coffee, tea, and red wine. Ceramic fillings are generally used in larger areas where teeth need to be restored. They are typically fabricated as dental inlays or onlays in a dental laboratory and require more complex procedures than amalgam or composite fillings. They offer the natural appearance of composite, but are more durable and less likely to become discolored. Ceramics are the most expensive option in filling material.

Film badge
A small pack of sensitive photographic film worn as a badge. A film badge indicates how much radiation the person wearing the badge has been exposed to over time. Technicians and radiologists wear film badges to make sure they are not overexposed to radiation.

Finasteride
A drug used to reduce the size of an enlarged prostate gland in men and to improve urine flow. Finasteride (Proscar) works by decreasing the level of an androgen (male sex hormone) that stimulates development of the prostate gland. Finasteride (Propecia) is also used to treat male pattern baldness. This drug is intended for use only by men. Women who might be pregnant are warned never to come in contact with it, even in the amount that may be in semen from the male sexual partner, because of the risk of causing an abnormality in the fetus.

Finger
Any of the five digits on the hand. The thumb contains two bones, and each of the other fingers contains three bones (phalanges.) Hinge joints between these bones, controlled by tendons, allow the fingers to bend or straighten. The fingers are finely tuned grasping devices, and the range of motion of the thumb is much wider than in any other primate. An artery, a vein, and a nerve run down each side of the finger. The nail, actually a specialized type of skin cell at the end of the finger, protects the highly sensitive fingertip. The skin on each fingertip is loaded with sensory nerve cells that make the area extremely sensitive to touch. The skin on the surface of the fingertip is grooved to help the fingers achieve a good grip.

Finger joint replacement
See JOINT REPLACEMENT, FINGER.

Fingerprint
A unique pattern of lines and swirls in the skin found at the end of each finger. When the fingertips are used to touch certain surfaces, they leave an impression of the characteristic pattern of lines. Because they are unique, these impressions can be used to identify the person to whom they belong. Individual fingerprints are recorded by making an ink impression for the purpose of identification.

Fistula
Abnormal passageway between two hollow organs or leading from a hollow organ to the outside of the body. A fistula is often caused by infection or injury, as when an abscess in the rectum bursts, thereby creating an opening between the anal canal and the surface of the skin. A fistula may also develop as a complication of surgery or may be congenital (present at birth).

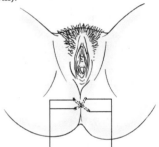

Fistulas (broken lines indicate internal paths)
Exterior view

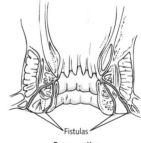

Fistulas
Cross-section

ANAL FISTULA
Generally, an anal fistula creates a primary opening inside the anal canal and a secondary opening on the outside of the body. The internal course of a fistula can be predicted from the location of the external opening. A cross-section shows the paths of typical fistulas.

Fitness
The capacity to perform physical activity. There are several types of fitness, and these include aerobic capacity, muscular strength, muscular endurance, and flexibility. Fitness

is partly determined by inheritance but is mainly developed as the result of physical activity. Aerobic capacity is developed by activities that increase the heart rate, such as walking, jogging, swimming, cycling, and sports that involve running or constant movement, such as basketball, soccer, tennis, and squash. Muscular strength and endurance are developed by resistance exercise, which can involve free weights or weight machines. Flexibility is developed by exercises that stretch the muscles and connective tissues around the joints.

The amount of fitness developed is dependent on the total amount of EXERCISE in which a person participates. The total amount of exercise is determined by the frequency, intensity, and duration of exercise sessions. Therefore, the same total amount of exercise can be obtained over a week by exercising 3 days for 1 hour per day or by exercising 6 days for 30 minutes per day, if the intensity is similar in both examples.

A minimum of 3 days per week is recommended for aerobic exercise, and a minimum of 2 days a week is recommended for resistance exercise training. It is not clear how many days per week are required for flexibility exercise, but 3 to 5 days is a reasonable target.

The maintenance of a healthy body weight appropriate to a person's age, height, and skeletal structure is another element of overall fitness. Weight control is a natural result of regular exercise when combined with a healthy diet. See also Total fitness, page 567.

Fitness testing

Assessments to determine a person's level of FITNESS. Fitness testing may begin with recording basic information such as age, height, weight, blood pressure, and medical history. A body composition test may be performed to determine the body's ratio of fat to lean tissue. The person being tested may be requested to perform a number of activities or exercises that measure his or her aerobic capacity, muscular strength and endurance, and flexibility.

Fixation

A failure to develop past a particular stage in normal psychological growth (see CHILD DEVELOPMENT) or an abnormally close and suffocating attachment to another person, usually a figure from childhood.

Flail chest

A chest wound involving three or more ribs broken in two or more places, thus destabilizing a segment of the chest wall. Flail chest, which usually occurs after a severe crushing chest injury, is characterized by motion that is the reverse of normal—the loose chest segment moves inward when the person breathes in, outward when he or she breathes out; thus, the chest is not moving air effectively. Other symptoms include shortness of breath, extreme pain, and bluish skin. Flail chest is a medical emergency requiring immediate attention.

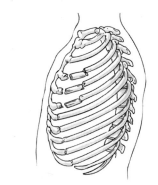

Flail chest (side view)

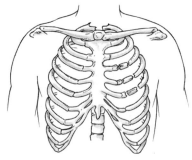

Flail chest (front view)

UNSTABLE CHEST WALL
When ribs are broken in several places on the same side of the chest, a portion of the muscular chest wall will move independently of the rest of the wall. The motion interferes with the mechanics of breathing and is a severe medical emergency.

Flat feet

A structural disorder of the feet in which the curve of the long arch flattens. The term fallen arches may sometimes be used to describe flat feet. Flat feet are considered normal in young children since everyone has flat feet at birth, and the arch of the foot develops slowly over the first 6 years of life. In adults, the condition may cause pain in the feet and can be associated with pain in the ankle, knee, or lower back.

Because flat feet prevent an even distribution of body weight on the bottom surface of the foot during walking, running, and other activities, the condition can contribute to the severe heel pain of plantar FASCIITIS. Custom-made orthotic devices inserted in the shoes may help distribute weight more evenly and relieve the discomfort of plantar fasciitis. Flat feet may also contribute to HALLUX VALGUS or bunions.

The most common cause of flat feet is aging. With time, the ligaments that hold the foot's arches up become loose or stretched. Without proper support, the arches collapse and the feet flatten. Excess body weight and lack of exercise contribute to flat feet. There may be several other causes of the condition. Standing for long periods of time without sufficient support of the feet is a contributing factor. A first line of treatment for flat feet is the use of properly fitting footwear to support the arch. Over-the-counter shoe inserts designed for arch support or custom-molded orthotic devices fitted by a podiatrist, orthopedist, or orthotist may be helpful. If all other attempts at treatment fail and the condition is impeding daily activities, surgery can reconstruct the bone and soft tissue in the feet to correct the abnormality.

Flatulence

The expulsion of air from the digestive tract through the anus. Flatulence is also known as flatus. Lower intestinal gas is the result of bacterial fermentation of food residue in the colon. Approximately a half quart of gas is produced by the body each day. Gas consists primarily of nitrogen and carbon dioxide, along with smaller amounts of methane and hydrogen. While these gases have no

TOTAL FITNESS

Regular, varied physical activity improves overall health and reduces the risk of many health problems. There are three kinds of physical exercise—aerobic, strength, and flexibility—each providing different benefits. Combining exercise with a balanced diet is the best way to achieve and maintain a healthy body weight. Regular exercise also enhances emotional well-being by improving sleep and reducing stress, depression, and anxiety.

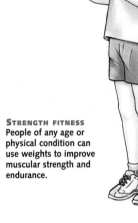

STRENGTH FITNESS
People of any age or physical condition can use weights to improve muscular strength and endurance.

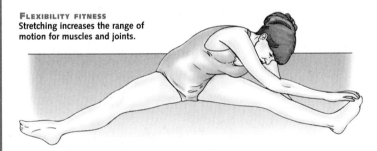

AEROBIC FITNESS
Swimming is an excellent aerobic exercise that conditions the heart and lungs. Another good choice is walking.

FLEXIBILITY FITNESS
Stretching increases the range of motion for muscles and joints.

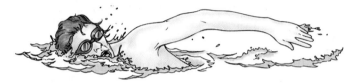

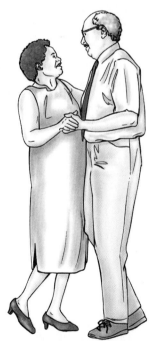

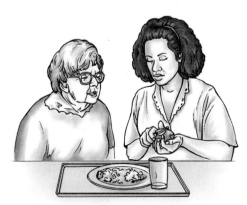

FITNESS AND NUTRITION
Combining exercise with a balanced diet is the best way to achieve and maintain a healthy body weight.

FITNESS AND WELL-BEING
Enjoying an activity such as dancing helps people feel better physically and emotionally.

F

odor, flatus may also contain the odorous gas hydrogen sulfide.

The more fiber that is eaten, the more gas is produced. Fiber-rich foods, such as bran, beans, cabbage, and broccoli, contain complex sugars that cannot be completely digested in the small intestine. Instead, undigested food is fermented by bacteria in the large intestine, or colon. In some cases, flatulence is a sign of LACTOSE INTOLERANCE. In this condition, the body lacks the enzyme lactase and is unable to digest the sugar found in milk and other dairy products. When undigested sugar passes into the colon, bacteria ferment it, causing excessive gas and diarrhea.

Management of flatulence depends on its cause. It is often helpful to eat fewer gas-producing foods or to exercise more to encourage passage of gas through the digestive tract. In some cases, medications are recommended or prescribed to relieve gas. For lactose intolerance, doctors suggest decreasing the intake of milk and dairy products or taking a supplement containing lactase, the enzyme that digests milk sugar. Flatulence is rarely a symptom of a serious disease. However, if gas is excessive or accompanied by other symptoms, such as bloating, abdominal pain, or changes in bowel movements, doctors may recommend a variety of tests to discover the underlying cause. See also BOWEL MOVEMENTS, ABNORMAL; FECES, ABNORMAL.

Flatus
See FLATULENCE.

Flatworm
A group of flat-bodied, unsegmented worms, most of which are parasitic. Some flatworms live in fresh water, in wetlands, and in salt water; they are rare in the United States. Humans are affected by them through contact with contaminated water. Other types of flatworms spend part of their lives living in animals and the other part living in humans. They enter humans when infested animal meat is ingested. Tapeworms and flukes (see TAPEWORM INFESTATION; FLUKE) are members of the flatworm group.

Flexibility training
Physical activity based on stretching movements, which are designed to increase the range in which a person can bend and stretch his or her joints, muscles, and ligaments. Exercises that stretch the muscles may also help relieve certain kinds of pain: lower back pain may be alleviated or prevented by stretching the hamstring muscles (at the back of the thigh) and the lower back muscles; calf cramping may be prevented by regularly stretching the calf muscles. With age, the muscles weaken and the joints become less flexible. Flexibility training can help overcome these aspects of aging.

Stretching exercises are most effective when performed following aerobic exercise (see EXERCISE, AEROBIC) or strengthening exercises when the muscles are warmed up and more supple. The muscles used during exercise are the ones to emphasize when stretching because these muscles tend to shorten and tighten during exercise. The back and chest muscles should always be stretched because these muscles keep the torso flexible and support the spine. To increase flexibility, stretching sessions following exercise should last at least 5 to 10 minutes, and each stretch should be held for at least 30 seconds.

While everyone can improve the flexibility of the spine, torso, and limbs by regularly doing stretching exercises, some people tend to be more flexible than others, and this may vary in different areas of the body. Flexibility training may be frustrating for those whose muscles and joints are inherently less supple, but injuries can result if a person extends stretching movements beyond a normal level of comfort. Stretching should offer a pleasant sensation and should not cause pain. A certified exercise trainer or physical therapist can demonstrate appropriate flexibility exercises.

Floaters
Small specks, threads, circles, cobwebs, clouds, or other shapes moving in a person's field of vision. Floaters are most easily seen against a plain background, like a blank wall or the sky. They are actually small clumps of material that form inside the clear jellylike fluid (vitreous) filling the cavity of the eye and cast shadows on the retina (the thin layer of light-sen-

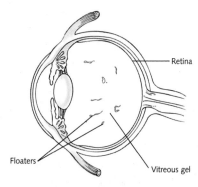

FLOATING PARTICLES IN THE EYE
Floaters (cellular debris adrift in the eye) may take months to disappear from a person's line of vision. The loose debris is never reabsorbed by the eye; it just settles into the bottom of the fluid-filled eye cavity. A person may see floaters suddenly when he or she bends over or does somersaults for exercise.

sitive tissue at the back of the eye). Floaters usually appear during middle age, when the vitreous liquefies and pulls away from the retina. This condition is known as posterior vitreous detachment, and the strands in the vitreous and attachments to the retina float freely and result in floaters. Floaters may be annoying, but they require no treatment. If a new floater appears suddenly, if the number of floaters increases, or if quick flashes of light also appear, these symptoms can signal damage to the retina (see RETINAL DETACHMENT), which requires prompt medical attention to prevent vision problems.

Floppy infant
A group of symptoms giving a child a floppy, loose-limbed appearance. All newborns are somewhat floppy because their muscles are still developing. However, infants who are especially limp should be examined by a physician promptly, since floppiness can be a sign of serious illness in infants.

Floppiness can be a result of PREMATURE BIRTH or oxygen deprivation at birth. Babies who were oxygen-deprived at birth may also experience additional problems such as seizures and irregular heartbeat. An affected baby may require care in a neonatal intensive care unit. If the infant's condition returns to normal within a week, the likelihood of normal development is excellent. In babies older than 4 months, a floppy appearance can be a sign of a neuromuscular problem. Both situations require a pediatrician's care.

Floss, dental

A soft, nylon string that is inserted between the teeth, and particularly at the base of the teeth below the gum line, then manipulated to slide up and down against the tooth surface to remove food particles and plaque (see PLAQUE, DENTAL) and to stimulate the gum. Dental floss may be waxed or unwaxed. The wax helps the floss slide more easily through the spaces between the teeth but adds bulk to the string. Unwaxed floss may be preferable when the teeth are very close together. The daily use of floss is essential to ORAL HYGIENE because floss removes plaque from places on the teeth that a toothbrush cannot reach. The regular removal of plaque deposits helps to prevent TOOTH DECAY and gum disease. A dentist, dental hygienist, or dental assistant can provide instructions on proper flossing techniques, based on the teeth and the presence of bridges, dentures, or other dental restorations. Gums may be sore with slight bleeding during the first week of flossing.

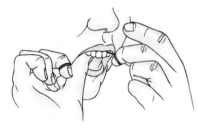

DAILY FLOSSING
Good flossing technique involves inserting a lengthy piece of clean dental floss between adjacent teeth and moving the floss up and down against the surfaces of each tooth with a sawing motion to remove debris and stimulate the gums. Daily flossing removes food particles and other substances that a toothbrush cannot reach.

Flow cytometry

A method for measuring components or structural elements of cells, primarily by optical means. In flow cytometry, a cytometer, a device for counting cells, projects a beam of laser light through a liquid stream containing cells or other particles. When the intensely focused light strikes the stream, cellular elements give out sig-

nals that are picked up by detectors. The signals are converted for computer storage and data analysis, which eventually yield information about various cellular properties. The biophysical properties of the cells in the stream can be measured at rates exceeding 1,000 cells per second. Because cytometry allows many cells to be studied quickly, irregular cells can easily be identified.

In flow cytometry, selected cells can be removed from the stream for study. Flow cytometers are found in all major biological research institutions and most medical centers, where they are used for diagnosis and research. Flow cytometry is currently the preferred method of monitoring CD4 lymphocyte levels in the blood of people with AIDS (acquired immunodeficiency syndrome).

Flu

A contagious disease caused by a virus. See INFLUENZA.

Fluconazole

An antifungal drug used to treat yeast infections. Fluconazole (Diflucan, Triflucan) is used to treat oral candidiasis (thrush) and cryptococcal meningitis, opportunistic infections often seen in people with AIDS (acquired immunodeficiency syndrome). Other infections against which fluconazole is effective include esophageal candidiasis, systemic candidiasis, and vaginal candidiasis. It is also used to prevent infection in people undergoing bone marrow transplantation.

Fluctuant

Wavelike motion felt during physical examination when a bodily structure containing fluid is palpated, or examined with the hands and fingers. When physical examination shows that an abnormal body structure is fluctuant, this means that it is filled with fluid rather than a solid mass.

Fluke

A member of the flatworm group; also called *Trematoda*. Flukes are parasitic and maintain complicated life cycles residing in animal tissues of two or more hosts. A subgroup of flukes, called the liver fluke, is found most commonly in China. This flat-

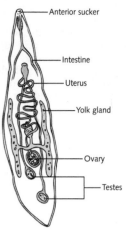

HARMFUL FLATWORM
One type of fluke, the Chinese liver fluke, attaches to the walls of the ducts in the liver. Although these flatworms are primitive animals, they have complicated life cycles and are very harmful to their host organisms—which can be sheep or people.

worm infests sheep and can be transmitted to humans who ingest plants that have been contaminated by the larvae of the fluke. The ingested worm larvae settle inside the bile ducts of the liver and cause jaundice, or yellowing of the skin and the whites of the eyes. Schistosomiasis is a fluke infestation that is spread via contact with contaminated water in tropical regions.

Fluocinolone

A corticosteroid used to treat skin disorders and inflammatory eye, ear, and nose disorders. Fluocinolone (Fluonid, Flurosyn, Synalar, Synemol, Derma-Smoothe/FS) is available as a cream, gel, lotion, ointment, and shampoo.

Fluorescein

An orange dye used in eye examinations to detect foreign bodies or injury to the cornea (the clear outer covering of the exposed surface of the eye). Fluorescein is placed in the eye with a dropper or a strip of blotting paper, and one must blink to spread the dye. The surface of the eye is then illuminated with a cobalt-blue light, which causes the fluorescein to glow green. Since the dye accumulates in regions where the corneal surface is disturbed by injury or infection, it allows the eye specialist to detect defects in the cornea. Fluorescein is also used in tonometry, the most common test for checking eye pressure (see EYE, EXAMINATION OF). Fluorescein may be used after contact lenses are prescribed to determine whether tear flow under the lens is adequate. Application of fluorescein to the eye is painless. The dye is also used to study blood vessels in the eye. See FLUORESCEIN ANGIOGRAM.

Fluorescein angiogram

A diagnostic test that uses a dye to analyze circulation in the eye. Eye drops that dilate the pupil are administered to the person being tested, who then places his or her chin on a support that holds the head steady during the test. Pictures of the interior of the eye are taken with a special camera. Next, fluorescein dye is injected into a vein in the arm or hand. More photographs are taken right after the injection; additional pictures may be taken 20 minutes and 1 hour later as well. The dye, which glows green under special light, outlines the blood vessels of the eye and allows the eye specialist to visualize them and to detect areas of leakage. The fluorescein angiogram is useful for diagnosing a number of eye diseases that affect the back (fundus) of the eye, including diabetic retinopathy (see RETINOPATHY, DIABETIC), damage from high blood pressure (hypertension), MACULAR DEGENERATION, OPTIC DISC EDEMA, and RETINITIS PIGMENTOSA, and for determining the effectiveness of treatment.

A fluorescein angiogram may cause a slight sting at the site of the injection and mild nausea when the dye is injected. These sensations usually pass quickly. People who are highly sensitive to the dye may experience vomiting, dry mouth or increased salivation, metallic taste, dizziness, fainting, hives, sneezing, or an accelerated heartbeat, but these side effects rarely occur. Such reactions are more likely to occur in people who are sensitive to iodine. Vision may be blurred for 12 hours after the test because of the eye drops used to dilate the pupils.

Fluoridation

The addition of FLUORIDE to the public water supply as a way to decrease the incidence of TOOTH DECAY. Fluoridation has been endorsed by the American Dental Association since the first community fluoridation program began in 1945. Adding fluoride to public water effectively reduces tooth decay in children, adolescents, and adults. The fluoride works its way into the developing enamel and makes a tooth more resistant to decay. The range in the concentration levels of fluoridation in public water in the United States depends on such factors as climate and the amount of fluoride naturally present in the water supply.

Fluoride

A naturally occurring mineral known to help prevent TOOTH DECAY. Fluoride strengthens the enamel on the surface of the tooth and makes the teeth more resistant to decay. Fluoride is added to many public water supplies in the United States; this process is known as FLUORIDATION. Fluoride is also an ingredient in toothpaste and mouthwash. Topical fluoride in a solution or gel may be applied to the teeth at home or in a professional office setting by a dentist, dental hygienist, or dental assistant. In addition to being available in fluoridated water, fluoride may be obtained in over-the-counter tablets, drops, lozenges, and some beverages.

Fluoroquinolones

Antibiotics used to treat bacterial infections in many different parts of the body. Fluoroquinolones work by killing bacteria or preventing their growth. They are powerful fluorinated antibacterials with broad-spectrum activity able to treat infections of bones and joints and infections in the respiratory, genital, and gastrointestinal tracts.

The first five fluoroquinolones were introduced in the United States in the mid-1980s. Ciprofloxacin (Cipro) and ofloxacin (Floxin) were most widely used because they were known to be effective against the widest range of infections. Within the last few years, five new fluoroquinolones have been introduced to the United States, including and gatifloxacin (Tequin), grepafloxacin (Raxar), levofloxacin (Levaquin), sparfloxacin (Zagam), and trovafloxacin mesylate (Trovan). The newer drugs need be taken only once a day.

Fluoroquinolones are widely used to treat bacterial infections in livestock as well as in humans. There is some concern that their use in livestock may contribute to increased resistance in food-borne bacteria, such as *Salmonella*.

Fluorosis

A condition that changes the color and texture of the tooth enamel (see

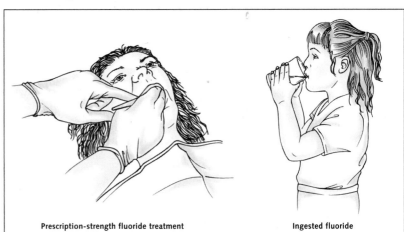

Prescription-strength fluoride treatment Ingested fluoride

EFFECTS OF FLUORIDE
Fluoride chemically "remineralizes" tooth enamel, which loses minerals to bacteria and sugar in the mouth. In a child younger than 6, ingested fluoride (as from drinking water) is actually incorporated into the teeth and decreases mineral loss. In an adult, fluoride—in water, toothpaste, or applied in a dentist's office—disrupts bacterial mineral loss and speeds the process of remineralization.

ENAMEL, DENTAL) as a result of excessive exposure to FLUORIDE. Most cases of fluorosis are caused by higher than necessary concentrations of naturally occurring fluoride in drinking water. Fluorosis may cause the tooth enamel to become darkened, pitted, mottled, or spotted with opaque white patches. Although all the teeth are involved in fluorosis, changes in coloration and structure of the enamel may affect only a few teeth and may range from white surface spots to yellow or brown pitting. When these changes are not cosmetically acceptable, or in severe cases of fluorosis that cause the tooth enamel to crack or chip off, dental bleaching, composite bonding, or dental crowns (see BLEACHING, DENTAL; BONDING, DENTAL; and CROWN, DENTAL) may become necessary.

Fluoxetine

A drug used to treat depression, bulimia, and obsessive-compulsive disorder. Fluoxetine (Prozac) is the best-known member of the class of drugs known as selective serotonin reuptake inhibitors (SSRIs), which work by increasing the amount of serotonin, a substance known to enhance a person's mood, at the nerve endings in the brain.

Fluoxetine is approved by the Food and Drug Administration for the treatment of major depression, bulimia (an eating disorder), obsessive-compulsive disorder, and premenstrual dysphoric disorder. Because people who take fluoxetine sometimes lose weight, doctors occasionally prescribe it for that purpose.

Flurbiprofen

See NONSTEROIDAL ANTI-INFLAMMATORY DRUGS.

Flush

Also known as BLUSHING; a sudden reddening of the face, neck, and sometimes upper chest. Flushing is usually a normal response to embarrassment, anger, or other strong emotion. However, it may also be associated with a high fever, MENOPAUSE, ROSACEA, a drug reaction, or food allergies.

Flutamide

A drug used to treat prostate cancer. Flutamide (Eulexin) is an antiandro-gen drug that works by inhibiting the uptake of the male hormone androgen. Because prostate cancers are sensitive to androgens, flutamide interferes in the growth of these tumors.

Fluticasone

A corticosteroid (see CORTICOSTEROIDS) used to treat asthma attacks and certain skin disorders. Fluticasone is available as an inhalant for the treatment of asthma (Flovent); as a nasal spray to treat symptoms of rhinitis, such as runny nose and postnasal drip (Flonase); and as a skin cream or ointment to treat skin disorders (Cutivate).

Fluvastatin sodium

A drug used to lower cholesterol and other fats in the blood. Fluvastatin sodium (Lescol) helps to prevent heart attacks and strokes by lowering blood cholesterol levels.

Fluvoxamine maleate

A drug used to treat obsessive-compulsive disorder. Fluvoxamine maleate (Luvox) is a selective serotonin reuptake inhibitor (SSRI) that is thought to improve behavior associated with obsessive-compulsive disorder in children, adolescents, and adults.

Folic acid

A water-soluble B vitamin essential to growth and cell repair. (See also VITAMIN B.) Adequate folic acid is required for a healthy pregnancy, DNA and RNA synthesis, and building red blood cells. A combination of folic acid and vitamins B6 and B12 can reduce the blood level of HOMOCYSTEINE, an amino acid that is associated with an increased risk of diseases related to the heart and blood vessels. Adults require at least 400 micrograms (0.4 milligrams) of folic acid daily. These minimal requirements double during pregnancy. In the United States, the most common dietary sources of folic acid are fortified commercial cereals, enriched breads, fruits, orange juice, and dried beans. Most folic acid in foods occurs as folate. Good dietary sources of folate include leafy green vegetables, liver, mushrooms, oatmeal, peanut butter, soybeans, and wheat germ.

PREGNANCY AND FOLIC ACID

A lack of folic acid is one of the most common vitamin deficiencies and can result in serious problems such as BIRTH DEFECTS, anemia, and elevated homocysteine levels. During pregnancy, folic acid is required for the proper development of a baby. Folic acid deficiency is associated with severe birth defects of the brain and spine known as neural tube defects. Because adequate folic acid is critically important in the first weeks of pregnancy, doctors advise women to get adequate amounts of folic acid when they are planning to become pregnant. To reduce the risk of neural tube defects, in January 1998 the Food and Drug Administration ordered the fortification of all flour and grain products with folate.

FOLIC ACID AND HOMOCYSTEINE

Homocysteine is a natural by-product of the breakdown of protein in the body that is harmless in small amounts. Recent studies have related elevated homocysteine blood levels to an increased risk for a range of ailments, including heart attack, stroke, venous thrombosis (blood clots in the legs), early miscarriage, neural tube defects including spina bifida and anencephaly, premature delivery, low birth weight, preeclampsia (high blood pressure during pregnancy), and dementia from Alzheimer's disease.

Dangerously high levels of homocysteine are believed to be due to two dietary factors: a high intake of animal protein and low intake of B vitamins. Following consumption of animal protein, homocysteine builds up in the blood if the amino acid methionine cannot be converted to cysteine because of an insufficient amount of enzymes. Folic acid, B6, and B12 are crucial to ensuring adequate amounts of these enzymes. Cutting back on animal protein and consuming adequate folic acid and vitamins B6 and B12 can control homocysteine levels.

Folic acid deficiency

A lack of folic acid is one of the most common vitamin deficiencies and can result in serious problems such as anemia, elevated homocysteine levels, and, in pregnant women, fetal birth defects. Adults require at least 400 micrograms of folic acid daily, which usually is found in foods as folate. See FOLIC ACID.

Follicle

A pouchlike depression or pore, such as the openings in the skin through which hair grows.

Follicle-stimulating hormone

See FSH.

Folliculitis

An inflammation and infection of the hair follicles that is usually caused by bacteria. Folliculitis may be a mild and superficial condition, or it may be more severe and involve deeper infection of the skin, particularly in bearded areas where the hair follicles are numerous and deep in the skin.

Folliculitis may appear following or in association with a skin infection. A skin blister containing pus initially surrounds the hair follicle. The hair may be easily removed, but new blisters will develop. Oral antibiotic medication is used to treat folliculitis and may be used with topical antibiotics and antiseptics.

A condition known as "whirlpool folliculitis" can be acquired from sitting in hot tubs, Jacuzzis, warm swimming pools, and baths. The infection is caused by bacteria called *Pseudomonas,* which produce an extensive, itchy rash that is usually in areas covered by a bathing suit. Associated symptoms may include headaches, dizziness, sore throat, and abdominal cramps.

Fomite

A physical object or surface that transmits an infectious agent from one person to another. A fomite may be a vehicle for larger, visible organisms, such as a comb carrying head lice. It may also be a tiny dust particle that is contaminated by droplets of infected saliva coughed into the air by a person who has an infectious cold virus. When a susceptible person comes in contact with a fomite, he or she can contract the infection present on the infected object or surface.

Fontanelle

One of two soft areas on an infant's head where the skull bones have not yet joined. The fontanelle that is located at the top of an infant's head usually closes by 14 months. In most children, the fontanelle at the back of the head is closed at birth. In others, it

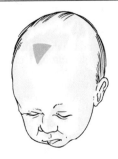

Site of anterior fontanelle

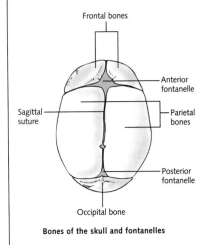

Bones of the skull and fontanelles

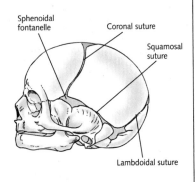

A side view of fontanelles

closes by 3 or 4 months of age. Normal handling and washing of an infant does not harm the fontanelles. A baby's soft spot normally bulges when he or she is crying. However, a fontanelle that is firm and bulging when a baby is not crying can indicate that the brain is under pressure from HYDROCEPHALUS, an accumulation of fluid; an infection; or a tumor. A sunken fontanelle may indicate DEHYDRATION. It is important to consult a pediatrician in these cases.

Food additives

Chemicals added to food as preservatives, sweeteners, colorants, flavorings, or antioxidants. Food additives are used in the processing of many foods, including baked goods, dressings, hot dogs, bologna, salami, canned vegetables, dried fruit, fruit juices, jams and jellies, relishes, teas, and processed seafood products. Thousands of food additives exist, and most are safe. Some, however, cause adverse reactions in susceptible individuals. Signs of a problem include headaches, hives, abdominal cramps, diarrhea, chest tightness,

FOOD ADDITIVES AND ADVERSE REACTIONS

Individuals with sensitivities to food additives can check food labels for additives under their specific names.

- **Aspartame (sweetener)**
- **Benzoates (preservative)**
- **BHA and BHT (antioxidants)**
- **FD&C dyes (colorants)**
- **MSG (flavoring)**
- **Nitrates and nitrites (preservatives)**
- **Parabens (preservatives)**
- **Sulfites (preservatives)**

light-headedness, lowered blood pressure, and weakness. An allergist can help individuals identify food additives to which they are sensitive.

Food allergy

A specific response of the immune system to a specific food or food component to which a person is sensitized. Food allergies result when the immune system produces a large number of antibodies to attack the food that a person has ingested. This response releases HISTAMINE, which causes the symptoms of food allergies. Food allergens are generally proteins within the food that are not completely broken down by the digestive process. They may then be released from the gastrointestinal lining, enter the bloodstream, and cause allergic reactions throughout the body. This is the reason a reaction to a food allergen that is ingested may be experienced in the skin or the respiratory system.

An allergic reaction to a food may begin at the first bite with an itching sensation in the mouth. ANAPHYLAXIS can occur when sensitized people eat peanuts, fish, eggs, or grains. The most common symptoms of food allergies include abdominal pain, diarrhea, nausea, and vomiting. Hives and swelling beneath the skin, or eczema (see DERMATITIS) may also result from food allergies. There may be swelling of the lips, eyes, face, tongue, and throat. Nasal congestion and asthma may be symptoms of the allergy, and sometimes the affected person faints. If these symptoms are severe, or if anaphylaxis results, immediate emergency medical attention is essential and may be lifesaving.

DIAGNOSIS AND TREATMENT

Diagnosing a food allergy is generally aimed at pinpointing the specific food or food components that produce the allergic reaction and distinguishing a food allergy from FOOD INTOLERANCE. This requires a comprehensive review of a person's medical history, including a family history of allergies, and a physical examination. A person who seems to have a nonsevere food allergy may be requested by the physician to eliminate suspected foods entirely for 1 or 2 weeks, then add them back gradually one food at a time. This is called food elimination and may prove beneficial in identifying the culprit.

Another approach that may be used when it is not clear which foods are responsible involves keeping a detailed food diary for several weeks that itemizes a history of symptoms, when they occur, which foods seem to cause problems, and the amount of food eaten when an allergic reaction is experienced.

A skin scratch test involves introducing a small amount of food extract into the surface of the skin. If this activates the immune system to produce a skin reaction, it may be that the food is causing the allergy. Because food that causes a mild skin reaction may not prompt the symptoms of a food allergy when ingested, the results of a skin scratch test are not always reliable.

In some cases, a double-blind challenge test may offer more accurate results. This involves giving doses of suspected foods in disguised forms so that neither the person being tested nor the person administering the test knows what food is being eaten. The test is time-consuming and difficult to administer, but may offer more conclusive results.

Blood tests called immunoassays that check for antibodies specific to certain foods can be useful for excluding possible food allergens.

Treatment of food allergies is based on learning which foods cause them so they can be avoided. In some cases, it is a simple matter of eliminating these foods from the diet. Avoiding foods or food components that cause allergies is more difficult when the food allergen is a common food that is not easily avoided in everyday life or in social situations. Avoidance can be complicated if the culprit is an ingredient in many common foods, and it is not always easily identified in prepared foods.

Not everyone remains allergic to particular foods over a lifetime. Children often outgrow food allergies by the age of 6 years. Adults can also become less sensitive to foods they were allergic to as children. Milk, eggs, and soy products are foods that people of all ages often lose their allergic reactions to, whereas peanuts, walnuts, fish, and shellfish tend to cause more persistent food allergies.

Food and Drug Administration

Also known as the FDA, a regulatory government agency that is part of the US Department of Health and Human Services. The mission of the FDA is to promote and protect the public health by helping safe and effective products reach the market in a timely manner and by monitoring products for continued safety once they are in use. The FDA regulates products ranging from complex medical devices and lifesaving drugs to food ingredients and cosmetics. It is charged with protecting American consumers by enforcing the Federal Food, Drug, and Cosmetic Act and related public health laws.

Food Guide Pyramid

A chart developed by the US Department of Agriculture to illustrate the relative amounts of the different foods that should be consumed daily to achieve a balanced diet. The Food Guide Pyramid promotes balanced meals, moderation, and variety in food choices, with special emphasis given to grain products, fruits, and vegetables. The pyramid image is used to represent relative amounts that individuals should consume from each food group, with the base (bread, cereal, rice, pasta) being the group with the most daily servings, and the top (refined sugars and fats and oils) being the least needed. The pyramid divides foods into six groups and indicates how many servings from each group should be eaten daily. Because women are generally smaller and require fewer calories than men, the lower number is usually more appropriate for them. See more on the Food guide pyramid on page 574.

DIETARY GUIDELINES FOR GOOD HEALTH

In addition to the Food Guide Pyramid, the US Department of Agriculture provides federal dietary guidelines. The current guidelines are as follows:

1. Let the pyramid guide your food choices.
2. Keep food safe to eat.
3. Aim for a healthy weight.
4. Be physically active each day.
5. Choose a variety of grains daily, especially whole grains.
6. Choose a variety of fruits and vegetables daily.
7. Choose foods that are low in saturated fat and cholesterol and a diet moderate in total fat.
8. Choose beverages and foods that limit your intake of sugars.
9. Choose and prepare foods with less salt.
10. If you drink alcoholic beverages, do so in moderation.

F

F

THE FOOD GUIDE PYRAMID

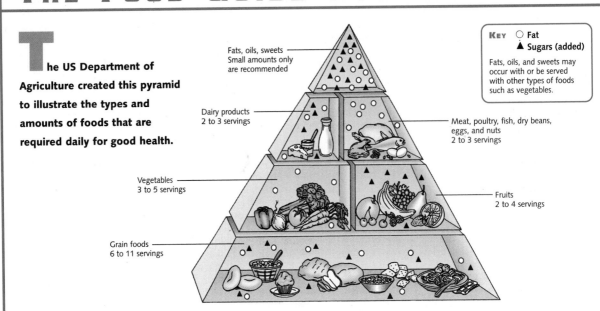

The US Department of Agriculture created this pyramid to illustrate the types and amounts of foods that are required daily for good health.

Fats, oils, sweets
Small amounts only
are recommended

KEY ○ Fat
▲ Sugars (added)

Fats, oils, and sweets may occur with or be served with other types of foods such as vegetables.

Dairy products
2 to 3 servings

Meat, poultry, fish, dry beans, eggs, and nuts
2 to 3 servings

Vegetables
3 to 5 servings

Fruits
2 to 4 servings

Grain foods
6 to 11 servings

SERVING SIZE

The following amounts count as a single serving:

Fats, oils, sweets: as little as possible

Dairy: 1 cup of milk or yogurt; or 1½ ounces of natural cheese; or 2 ounces of processed cheese

Meat and other protein sources: 2 to 3 ounces cooked lean meat, poultry, or fish (½ cup of cooked dry beans, 1 egg, or 2 tablespoons of peanut butter = 1 ounce of lean meat)

Vegetable: 1 cup of raw leafy greens; or ½ cup of other vegetables, cooked or raw; or ¾ cup of vegetable juice

Fruit: 1 medium apple, banana, or orange; or ½ cup chopped, cooked, or canned fruit; or ¾ cup of fruit juice

Grains: 1 slice of bread; or 1 ounce of ready-to-eat cereal; or ½ cup of cooked cereal, rice, or pasta

SERVING SIZES

The Food Guide Pyramid is designed to help consumers understand food portions and make more healthful choices. A serving of lean meat, poultry, or fish consists of 2 to 3 ounces. However, most restaurants and fast-food outlets offer servings 2 to 4 times this size. Eating the recommended 6 to 11 servings of grains, 3 to 5 servings of vegetables, and 2 to 4 servings of fruit every day may seem excessive. However, serving sizes are small. For instance, a single large baked potato counts as 2 to 3 servings of a vegetable, and a half cup of cooked vegetables constitutes 1 serving.

■ *Bread, cereal, rice, and pasta* Foods from this group, the base of the pyramid, consist of the grain products that provide carbohydrates, vita-

mins, minerals, and fiber and should be the basis for most meals. At 6 to 11 servings, this is the largest recommended food group. A slice of bread, an ounce of ready-to-eat cereal, or ½ cup of pasta or rice each constitutes a single serving.

■ *Vegetables* Three to 5 servings of vegetables are recommended each day. This group is low in fat and high in vitamins, minerals, and fiber. Single serving amounts include a cup of raw leafy vegetables such as lettuce, ½ cup of other vegetables, either raw or cooked, or ¾ cup of vegetable juice.

■ *Fruits* The Food Guide Pyramid suggests 2 to 4 servings of fruit every day. As well as being low in fat, fruits provide vitamins, minerals, and fiber. Single serving amounts consist of one medium-sized piece of fresh fruit; ½

cup of cooked, chopped, or canned fruit; or ¾ cup of 100 percent fruit juice.

■ *Meat, poultry, fish, dried beans, eggs, and nuts* Foods from this group provide protein. Two to 3 servings each day should add up to a total of 5 to 7 ounces. These are very small servings compared with past ideas about protein requirements and the amounts typically served in restaurants. Servings may be 2 to 3 ounces of meat, fish, or poultry; ½ cup of cooked dry beans; 1 egg; or 2 tablespoons of peanut butter.

■ *Milk, yogurt, and cheese* Foods from this group provide calcium, protein, vitamins, and minerals. Low-fat or nonfat dairy products are best. The pyramid recommends 2 to 3 servings from this group each day, which may include a cup of milk, a cup of yogurt, 1½ ounces of natural cheese, or 2 ounces of processed cheese.

■ *Fats, oils, and sweets* The smallest proportion of energy should be derived from fats, oils, and refined sugars. A large amount of these items in the diet provides the body with unnecessary energy and few nutrients. However, they can be enjoyed in moderation.

Food intolerance

A response to food that may produce symptoms similar to those of a FOOD ALLERGY but does not involve the immune system or the production of antibodies in the body. Food intolerance is usually caused instead by a missing digestive enzyme, irritable bowel syndrome, emotional anxiety, or contamination of the food eaten. The symptoms generally experienced occur primarily in the gastrointestinal system and may include nausea, vomiting, abdominal pain, and diarrhea. Physical and emotional stresses can affect digestion and prompt adverse reactions.

Food intolerance may be difficult to diagnose in part because a person may be sensitive to a substance or ingredient used in the preparation of the food rather than the food itself. Lactose-containing foods, wheat, certain vegetables, wine, monosodium glutamate, sulfites, and salicylates fall into this category. Lactose is a sugar found in milk that the body may not be able to digest properly. People who are lactose intolerant may find that hard cheeses, yogurt, and sour cream, which are dairy foods in which the lactose is already digested, can be tolerated. Some people are intolerant of broccoli and peas, which produce intestinal gas. Food intolerance to mushrooms and wines can result in indigestion and diarrhea.

Ingredients in foods that are less easily recognized include monosodium glutamate (MSG), a flavor enhancer often used in Chinese cooking and in some prepared foods and seasoning mixtures. MSG can cause flushing, headache, and a numb sensation in the mouth. Sulfites are used to help sanitize and preserve certain foods, including wine, salads, fresh and dehydrated fruits, seafood, potatoes, dehydrated soups, maraschino cherries, and some soft drinks. People who have asthma are more

likely to have a food intolerance to sulfites. Intolerance to salicylate is uncommon, but this ingredient is found in many foods, including fruits, vinegar, cider, wine, tartar sauce, ketchup, corned beef, and pickles. Salicylate is also found in avocado, corn, cucumbers, peppers, white potatoes, and olives. Tea, root beer, some fermented and distilled alcoholic beverages, and wintergreen- and mint-flavored foods may also contain salicylate.

Food poisoning

An illness with vomiting, diarrhea, and abdominal pain that is caused by ingesting contaminated food or liquid. The contaminants can be bacterial or viral and can cause outcomes ranging from upset stomach to death. Food poisoning may occur in isolated cases or as an epidemic when a number of people consume the same contaminated food. Food poisoning can be caused by contamination during the slaughter of an animal or later during its preparation. Bacteria from an infected sore on a cook's finger may contaminate food. When food is left at room temperature, bacteria can multiply. Undercooked meats, inadequate refrigeration, raw eggs, and poor hygiene all can lead to food poisoning. See also GASTROENTERITIS.

The signs of food poisoning vary according to their cause. In addition to vomiting, diarrhea, and pain, symptoms may include severe cramping, fever, and chills. Types of bacterial food poisoning include botulism, *Escherichia coli* (E. COLI), CAMPYLOBACTER, LISTERIOSIS, and SALMONELLA. Toxins produced by STAPHYLOCOCCAL INFECTIONS can also cause food poisoning. In healthy adults, mild attacks often clear up spontaneously. However, food poisoning poses a special danger to very young children, older people, pregnant women and their fetuses, and anyone with a compromised immune system.

DIAGNOSIS AND TREATMENT
In many cases, food poisoning that resolves on its own goes undiagnosed. However, diarrhea that persists for longer than 48 hours or is accompanied by other symptoms (such as fever, chills, or vomiting) requires medical attention. The doctor will diagnose its cause according

SIGNS OF FOOD POISONING

Different kinds of toxins produce different symptoms; medical attention is required for all cases of food poisoning.

- **Botulism: Dizziness, headache, blurred or double vision, muscle weakness, and difficulties swallowing, talking, and breathing. Symptoms follow within 12 to 36 hours after eating (usually) home-canned food. Botulism is very serious and is often fatal.**
- **Mushroom poisoning: Dizziness, difficulty breathing, abdominal pain, diarrhea, bloody diarrhea, vomiting, sweating, salivation, and tears. Symptoms arise minutes to 24 hours after eating mushrooms.**
- ***Salmonella* poisoning: Abdominal cramps, diarrhea, fever, chills, headache, vomiting, and weakness. Symptoms arise 6 to 24 hours after eating contaminated food.**
- ***Staphylococcus* poisoning: Abdominal cramps, nausea, vomiting, diarrhea. Symptoms arise 2 to 6 hours after eating contaminated food that, typically, was not properly refrigerated.**

to symptoms, a physical examination, and tests, such as stool analysis.

Treatment varies according to the cause of the problem. Generally, doctors advise rest and drinking clear fluids until symptoms subside. Because diarrhea can quickly deplete body fluids and crucial body salts, oral rehydration fluid (see REHYDRATION FLUID, ORAL) may be required. Specially prepared commercial solutions containing water, salts, and glucose are available over-the-counter at pharmacies. In serious cases of DEHYDRATION, intravenous fluids are required.

Over-the-counter medications may relieve symptoms of diarrhea. In severe cases, the doctor may prescribe narcoticlike or antispasmodic drugs to slow intestinal activity and ease cramping. However, medications to reduce the contraction of the intestines should not be used in cases of bloody diarrhea.

RISK FACTORS AND PREVENTION
To prevent food poisoning, all meats must be thoroughly cooked to destroy

F

F

PREVENTING FOOD POISONING

About 6 million cases of food poisoning are diagnosed in the United States every year. Millions more go unreported because the symptoms of abdominal pain, cramps, and diarrhea are confused with those of "stomach flu." The food supply is not sterile, but normally our bodies are able to fight off tiny amounts of bacteria in our food. However, if bacteria are allowed to multiply through poor food handling, then the immune system is susceptible.

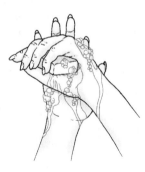

HAND WASHING
Hands should be washed well in hot, soapy water for 30 seconds before preparing food and after touching raw meats. This includes washing the backs of the hands, wrists, between the fingers, and under the fingernails.

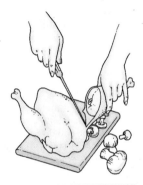

PREVENTING CROSS-CONTAMINATION
The juices from raw meats must not come in contact with raw fruits and vegetables; about half of supermarket chickens are infected with *Salmonella* or *Campylobacter*. Clean utensils and surfaces thoroughly before using them to prepare other foods. Use separate boards and knives for poultry or meats and for other raw foods.

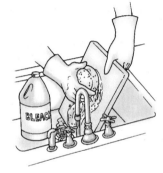

WASHING THE CUTTING BOARD
The cutting board should be cleaned well with a solution of hot water and bleach, especially after handling any raw meats. Experts are evenly divided on the merits of wooden versus plastic cutting boards. The important point is to keep the boards clean.

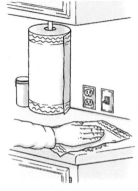

CLEANING THE KITCHEN COUNTER
Paper towels are good for avoiding cross-contamination in the kitchen because they are not reused. Kitchen sponges and dish cloths provide a perfect environment for bacterial growth. If you prefer sponges, clean them often in the dishwasher, or heat them for 60 seconds at the high setting in the microwave.

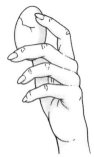

CHECKING AN EGG FOR CRACKS
After examining eggs for cracks, the safe cook discards any that are not intact. *Salmonella* bacteria can infect eggs through tiny imperfections.

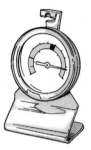

MAKING SURE FOOD IS KEPT COLD
To keep food safe, a constant temperature of 40°F or below should be maintained in the refrigerator section and −10°F or below in the freezer compartment.

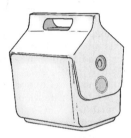

TRANSPORTING FOOD ON HOT DAYS
In hot weather, it is advisable to take a cooler to the supermarket to keep refrigerated and frozen foods cold during the ride home. Visiting the frozen food aisles last will help keep frozen items at the right temperature.

infectious organisms. Precooked and partially cooked foods also need to be completely reheated. To make certain that it heats through, frozen food such as poultry must be fully thawed before cooking. To avoid cross-contamination, vegetables and fruits must not be prepared on the same kitchen surfaces as raw meats. Cutting boards and knives used in the preparation of raw meat, poultry, and fish need to be scrubbed with very hot water and soap. Individuals, especially food handlers in restaurants, must wash their hands scrupulously after using the toilet and before preparing food.

Food poisoning, E. coli

Poisoning caused by eating foods contaminated with E. COLI (*Escherichia coli*), a bacteria strain that produces a powerful toxin that causes an estimated 25,000 cases of food poisoning in the United States each year. A person can also have traveler's diarrhea from a less serious form of *E. coli.* The bacteria live in the intestines of healthy cows, and contamination of meat sometimes occurs during slaughter when intestinal fecal matter is mixed with meat ground into hamburger. Bacteria on a cow's udders or milking machines can sometimes contaminate raw milk. Other examples of food poisoning with *E. coli* have been identified, including an outbreak caused by unpasteurized apple juice and cider made from fallen apples contaminated with feces, and another caused by alfalfa sprouts and lettuce grown in sewage-contaminated water.

The symptoms of *E. coli* food poisoning occur 12 hours to 7 days after a contaminated food is eaten. Severe abdominal cramps and profuse watery diarrhea that can progress to bloody diarrhea are typical symptoms. Little or no fever is seen, and in most cases, the best treatment will be to let the food poisoning run its course, taking care to replace lost fluids by drinking small but frequent sips of water or an electrolyte replacement solution. In about 2 to 7 percent of people with *E. coli* food poisoning, HEMOLYTIC-UREMIC SYNDROME will occur, in which red blood

cells are destroyed and kidney failure develops. This disorder, which is particularly dangerous in children younger than 5 and older people, is treated with blood transfusions and kidney dialysis.

FOOD POISONING WARNING

E. coli food poisoning is often caused by meat that is inadequately cooked or eaten too rare. Food poisoning involving *E. coli* can also occur when a person drinks contaminated water or eats produce grown in or washed with contaminated water.

Preventive measures include:

- Washing the hands before, during, and after food preparation
- Washing all utensils, cutting boards, and other tools used to prepare food
- Cooking meats and poultry thoroughly
- Never leaving cooked food at room temperature for more than 2 hours
- Avoiding eating rare meats
- Avoiding unpasteurized milk products and fruit juices
- Rinsing fruits and vegetables thoroughly with fresh tap water

A MEAT THERMOMETER
Using a meat thermometer helps ensure that meat is adequately cooked and bacteria have been killed.

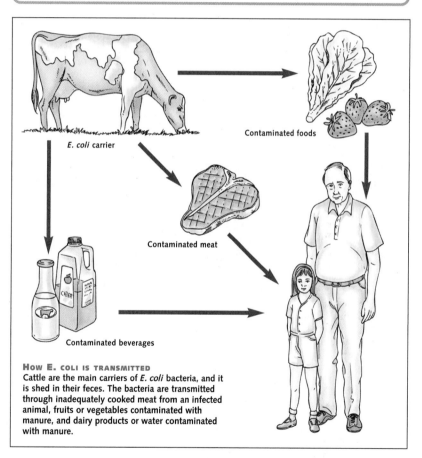

HOW E. COLI IS TRANSMITTED
Cattle are the main carriers of *E. coli* bacteria, and it is shed in their feces. The bacteria are transmitted through inadequately cooked meat from an infected animal, fruits or vegetables contaminated with manure, and dairy products or water contaminated with manure.

E. coli carrier

Contaminated foods

Contaminated meat

Contaminated beverages

Food poisoning, seafood

Poisoning caused by eating fish or shellfish that have been inadequately preserved. Several types of seafood poisoning have been identified.

F

SOME RISKY SEAFOOD

Food poisoning can be caused by eating inadequately preserved seafood. Because parasites may be present, consumption of raw fish in the form of sushi or ceviche is riskier than eating cooked fish. To minimize the risk, a person should not eat raw or marinated seafood that has not been adequately frozen to destroy parasites. Commercially frozen fish are essentially free of parasites.

Ciguatera, for instance, is a type of food poisoning found in tropical waters in which large fish over 6 pounds eaten by vacationers and other recreational fishermen have fed on small fish that in turn have fed on toxic microplankton. The symptoms of ciguatera begin within 6 hours of eating the toxic fish and include nausea, cramping, and vomiting, followed by headache and tingling or numbness of the lips, tongue, and mouth.

Another type of seafood poisoning is scombroid poisoning, which occurs when scombroid fish such as tuna, bluefish, mackerels, and mahimahi (dolphins) are not kept frozen after capture. In this type of poisoning, bacteria on the surface of the fish convert an amino acid to histamine, which can cause an allergic reaction when the fish is eaten by humans. The symptoms appear within 2 hours after the fish is eaten and include burning of the mouth and throat, dizziness, flushing, nausea, and headache, which may be followed by hives, facial rash, diarrhea, and abdominal cramps, usually lasting about 4 to 6 hours and rarely exceeding 24 hours. The condition is usually treated with an antihistamine.

Food-borne infection

A sickness that is a result of eating food contaminated by pathogens. Symptoms may include nausea, vomiting, cramps, bloody diarrhea, fever, chills, weakness, and headache. Pathogens can occur in a broad cross-section of food. For instance, bacteria such as E. COLI do not appear just in meat; the bacteria have also been found in apple juice, lettuce, alfalfa sprouts, and potato salad. Food-borne infection is often caused by the mishandling of food, such as chopping vegetables on the same board on which raw meat was cut without first thoroughly washing the board. However, it can also be due to problems during commercial food processing.

Food-drug interaction

An event in which foods and drugs consumed at about the same time alter the ability of the body to use one another; a side effect caused by the interplay of foods and drugs. Certain foods are known to interact with specific drugs in undesirable ways. For example, grapefruit juice and some drugs used to treat high blood pressure do not mix well. The juice has an ingredient that can increase the blood concentration of calcium channel blockers, thereby leading to headaches and light-headedness. Because of their high acidity, orange juice and orange soda interact with the proper absorption by the body of antibiotics such as penicillin and erythromycin, thereby making the drugs less effective.

Food-drug interactions vary according to dosage and the person's age, sex, and general health. It is advisable to carefully follow any instructions from a doctor or pharmacist about consuming particular foods while taking medication.

Foot

The mobile structure, beginning at the ankle, that supports and stabilizes the weight of the body and helps propel the body forward in walking or running. At the ankle, the two bones of the lower leg (the tibia and fibula) join with the seven bones of the ankle. The ankle bones are called the tarsals. The ankle allows the foot to move up and down and to rotate from side to side. Below the ankle another 19 bones, the metatarsals and the phalanges, are held together by strong ligaments to form the rest of the foot and the toes. The toes lack the wide range of motion found in the fingers, providing instead the smooth, rolling support needed for balance and walking. The big toe, like the thumb, has only

---

MONITORING FOOD CHOICES WHEN TAKING MEDICATIONS

Foods that are known to interact adversely with specific drugs include the following:

- Foods high in vitamin K (spinach, cauliflower, brussels sprouts, potatoes, vegetable oil, and egg yolks) should be consumed in moderation while taking anticoagulants (warfarin).
- The high acidity of citrus juices and soft drinks may interfere with the absorption of certain antibiotics (penicillin and erythromycin) and reduce the effectiveness of methenamine, a drug used to treat urinary tract infections.
- The consumption of foods containing tyramine can result in potentially life-threatening elevations in blood pressure when taken in conjunction with monoamine oxidase inhibitors; tyramine is a chemical commonly found in alcoholic beverages, specifically wine, and in aged cheeses, chocolate, beef and chicken livers, pickled herring, brewer's yeast, avocados, sauerkraut, sour cream, and fava beans.
- High-fiber foods (oatmeal, bran muffins) have been found to interfere with the absorption of the heart drug digoxin and tricyclic antidepressants.
- Licorice or licorice cough drops may exaggerate the effects of diuretics or digoxin.
- Foods rich in calcium (milk, cheeses, ice cream) can decrease the effectiveness of tetracyclines and ciprofloxacin.
- High-sodium foods (bacon, cold cuts, canned fish, salted breads, buttermilk) should be eaten in moderation while taking antihypertensive medications; excess sodium intake can result in elevated blood pressure and increased water retention. Foods with excessive sodium can also cause severe potassium deficiencies and electrolyte disturbances while taking diuretics (potassium-wasting furosemide and hydrochlorothiazide).
- Potassium-rich foods (bananas, figs, wheat germ, dried fruits, salt substitutes) should be limited while taking amiloride, triamterene, or spironolactone; cardiac problems can result from retaining excess potassium.

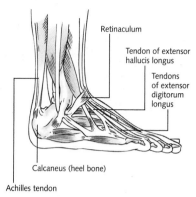

STRUCTURE OF THE FOOT
The bones and muscles of the foot work together to achieve the strength and flexibility required to support and balance the weight of the body and to provide the leverage for walking. Bands of tendons wrap around the ankle, connecting the muscles that work the foot and the toes.

two bones, while the other toes, like the rest of the fingers, have three. While the foot functions to hold up the weight of the standing body, the arch of the foot—formed by the bones and their binding of ligaments—provides a cushion and keeps a person's weight from pushing the foot flat against the ground. During walking, the arch helps roll the weight onto the big toe, which moves the body forward.

Footdrop

An abnormal neuromuscular condition often caused by damage to the nerve that extends into the foot. The nerve can be directly damaged in the leg or at the level of the lower back, or it can be indirectly damaged by injury to the central nervous system that blocks messages to the nerves in the leg. In footdrop, there is an inability to flex the foot. Consequently, it catches on the ground when walking. Most cases of footdrop are caused by external pressure or trauma to the peroneal nerve. Footdrop can also be caused by neuritis (inflammation of a nerve), multiple sclerosis, neuropathy (loss of sensation), or spinal cord problems (for example, a protruding disk pressing on a nerve). Treatment depends on the underlying cause. A footdrop splint can be used to keep the foot in a fixed position while walking.

Foramen

An opening, such as a hole in a bone through which a nerve passes. There are a number of different foramens in the body. For example, the foramen magnum is a large opening at the base of the skull through which the spinal cord passes.

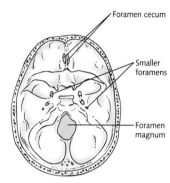

PASSAGES THROUGH THE SKULL
Foramens (or foramina openings) in the base of the skull allow for the passage of nerves and blood vessels. The largest opening, the foramen magnum, allows the spinal cord to pass from the spinal column into the brain.

Forceps

A medical instrument designed to grasp an object so it can be held firmly or pulled. Forceps come in many varieties and are used by doctors and dentists to perform such tasks as extracting teeth or gently pulling a newborn out of a woman's vagina. A small forceps is called a tweezers, which is frequently used at home to remove splinters or to shape the eyebrows by removing individual hairs.

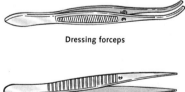

Dressing forceps

Utility forceps

GRASPING INSTRUMENTS
Various types of forceps enable doctors to perform difficult grasping tasks. Dressing forceps, with curved tips, are used for applying sterile dressings or holding body tissue during surgical procedures. Utility forceps, with pointed ends, are also used for holding tissues for suturing or dissection.

Forceps delivery

A birth in which forceps (tonglike instruments) are used in the delivery of a baby. The forceps blades are placed on both sides of the baby's head; gently, the baby is pulled from the womb. Forceps are used during a prolonged labor or when a baby, far along in the birth canal, needs to be delivered quickly because of fetal distress. Forceps typically are used in a breech birth or when the baby's heart rate indicates that delivery should be accomplished quickly; when the contractions fail to push the baby down the birth canal; or when the mother is too exhausted to push or has a medical problem that keeps her from bearing down.

A forceps delivery can be performed safely only under certain conditions: the cervix is fully dilated; the amniotic sac membranes are ruptured; the widest part of a baby's head is engaged (has started to descend through the pelvic canal) and is in or near the lower pelvis; the doctor is certain of the baby's head position; the pelvis is wide enough for a baby's head to pass through; and the woman's bladder is empty. Before the forceps are used, the woman is given an anesthetic for pain control, and an episiotomy is usually performed.

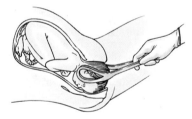

ASSISTING A BIRTH WITH FORCEPS
To accomplish a delivery using forceps, the doctor inserts the forceps into the vagina on either side of the baby's head. Then the doctor pulls gently on the baby's head, in concert with the mother's efforts to push during contractions. When the baby's head is outside the mother's body, the forceps are removed and the baby is guided out by hand.

Forensic medicine

The branch of medicine that applies medical knowledge to legal areas, chiefly to criminal cases. Forensic medicine is usually used to study injuries related to accidental trauma, chemicals, and violence, in order to establish the cause of a sudden or

F

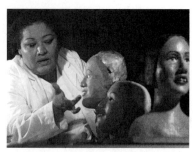

FIGHTING CRIME WITH MEDICINE
A forensic specialist creates a model of a murder victim's face and head, using teeth recovered from the body. The model will help with the identification of the victim.

unexpected death. In cases in which the paternity of a child is disputed, forensic experts may evaluate DNA and establish blood type. Forensic medicine is also involved in establishing the time of a death, rape, or injury or other data needed in court cases.

Forensic experts may be physicians, usually pathologists, or other professionals with special training in various forensic sciences, such as psychiatry, toxicology, firearms examination (wound ballistics), trace evidence, forensic serology, and DNA technology. A forensic PATHOLOGIST may look into the identity of the deceased (particularly when the remains are reduced to a skeleton or severely decomposed), the time of death, and the manner of death (disease, accident, suicide, or homicide), in addition to the cause of death. Specimens, such as hair, blood, semen, and saliva, may be collected for use as evidence, including DNA evidence. If the death was a result of injury, the forensic pathologist will try to find out how the injury was inflicted (by gun, knife, or chemical, for example).

A clinical forensic pathologist may examine living patients who are victims of rape or other injury and also may evaluate whether a victim's injuries are consistent with police reports. In forensic medicine, a forensic pathologist usually acts as a case coordinator for the medical and scientific assessment of a death. The forensic pathologist explores the medical history of the deceased, correlates all the information, reports the findings to law enforcement officials,

and may be subpoenaed to testify in criminal cases.

Foreplay

Sexual activities such as fondling, body massage, kissing, and oral sex that precede SEXUAL INTERCOURSE. Extended foreplay can help many men and women achieve orgasm.

Foreskin

The loose fold of skin that covers the tip (or glans) of the penis; also known as the prepuce. During the first months or years of a boy's life, the foreskin naturally separates from the tip of the penis. If the penis becomes erect, the foreskin moves back to expose the tip. The foreskin may be surgically removed in a procedure called circumcision. See CIRCUMCISION, MALE.

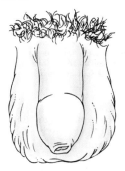

RETRACTABLE SHEATH
An intact foreskin loosely covers the head of the penis. It naturally separates from the tip during the first months or year's of a boy's life. Until the skin is fully retractable, washing externally is adequate to keep the penis clean. After that, washing under the foreskin during a bath is a good hygienic habit.

Formaldehyde

A gaseous compound that is a strong disinfectant. Formaldehyde is used in solution as a disinfectant and as a preservative and fixative for laboratory specimens. As a gas, formaldehyde is both toxic and carcinogenic (cancer-causing) if inhaled or absorbed through the skin. Inhaling formaldehyde can exacerbate asthma. Before its poisonous qualities were known, formaldehyde was used to disinfect and sterilize hospital rooms and mattresses.

Formula, chemical

A symbolic representation of the composition of a chemical com-

pound. A chemical formula uses numbers and other symbols to represent the elements that make up a particular compound, including those used as medication. A common example of a chemical formula is H_2O, which represents water (2 atoms of hydrogen plus 1 atom of oxygen equals 1 molecule of water). In clinical medicine, a chemical formula is often used as an abbreviation in a patient's medical chart.

Formulary

A list of approved pharmaceutical products; a collection of formulas for medicinal preparations. In hospital or managed care settings, the formulary is a list of drugs, procedures, and guidelines that is continually revised to maintain a database of approved drugs, their properties, and other information associated with them—all reflecting the current clinical judgment of the medical staff.

Fosinopril

A drug used to treat HYPERTENSION and heart failure. Fosinopril (Monopril) is an angiotensin-converting enzyme (ACE) inhibitor. It lowers blood pressure by preventing certain enzymes from narrowing blood vessels.

Fracture

FOR FIRST AID
see Fractures (broken bones), page 1323

The medical name for a broken bone, referring to a break or crack in a bone or in cartilage. There are two basic types of fracture: a compound, or open, fracture and a simple, or closed, fracture. A compound or open fracture involves a broken bone that ruptures the skin, exposing the bone. This is a more serious fracture, which requires emergency medical attention, because it allows germs to reach the bone and cause infection. A simple or closed fracture is a broken bone that does not break through the skin and is not visible on the surface. The term single fracture indicates that one break has occurred in a bone; multiple fractures means more than one break in the same bone. A fracture is called complete if the bone is broken straight through, and incomplete, or greenstick, if the break does not extend through the complete width of

TYPES OF BONE FRACTURE

An oblique bone fracture is an angled break across the bone, usually the result of a direct blow. A spiral fracture, caused by violent twisting, is a break that goes around and down the length of the bone. In a comminuted or crush fracture, the bone is broken into pieces by a blow. In a compound fracture, the force of the break knocks apart the broken ends of the bone and layers of skin are penetrated.

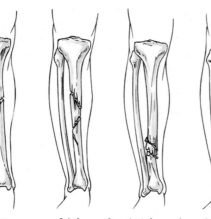

Oblique   Spiral   Comminuted or crush   Compound

the bone shaft, sometimes involving bending or crushing of the bone. Greenstick fractures most commonly occur in young children whose bones are more pliable. A fracture near a joint but outside the joint itself is called an extra-articular fracture; when the break involves the bones of the joint, it is called an intra-articular fracture.

CAUSES AND SYMPTOMS

The cause of most fractures is excessive force or pressure on the bone produced by the trauma of a fall, by the physical contact of certain sports, or by the impact of a heavy, fast-moving object. Simple and seemingly safe activities, like ball-throwing, may sometimes involve sufficient force to fracture a bone. The usual symptoms of a bone fracture include intense localized pain, tenderness, swelling, and possibly a deformed appearance.

TREATMENT

When the skin has been ruptured in open or compound fractures, antibiotics may be administered to ward off potential infection. In many cases, the break in the bone leaves two bone segments that are separated by the fracture but remain in the proper anatomical relationship to each other. When the fractured bone or bones are not properly aligned, which is called a displaced fracture, treatment includes realignment of the sections of broken bone in a procedure medically termed reduction. This may be achieved by stretching, traction, or external manipulation. In some cases, surgery may be necessary to realign and attach the bone segments, a procedure called open

reduction in which screws, wires, or metal plates are used to join the sections of bone. The aligned bones' position is held in place by a plaster cast or a splint worn externally to hold the bones immobile. This encourages healing by allowing new tissue created by the body to reattach the broken bone segments. The newly created tissue contains minerals that harden into new bone. See also ARM, FRACTURED; LEG, FRACTURED; JAW, FRACTURED; HIP, FRACTURED; and RIB, FRACTURED.

Fracture, dental

A break or crack in the crown or root of a tooth. Usually caused by an accident or fall, a dental fracture may involve only the enamel on the surface of the tooth, or it may affect the inner structures, such as the dentin and pulp. Premolars and repaired molars are vulnerable to vertical fractures, which extend through the crown to the root. Teeth that have received root canal treatment and crowns supported by posts may also be more prone to vertical fractures. These fractures can be caused by trauma caused by excessive pressure when biting. Fractures in the teeth may be clearly visible, or they may not be detectable, even with X rays. The only symptom may be pain when chewing. These fractures may be treated with composite bonding or veneers. When part or all of a tooth or teeth is fractured, the teeth may need fillings, crowns, or implants. If the fracture is very severe or if the tooth splits, tooth extraction may be necessary.

Fragile X syndrome

An inherited genetic condition that is a leading cause of mental retardation. Fragile X syndrome results from an altered gene on the long arm of the X chromosome. Fragile X syndrome is transmitted from mother to son, never from father to son. Mothers are carriers of the condition, and their sons are at risk of being affected with the disorder, while their daughters are at risk for being carriers and are usually only mildly affected intellectually. A male with fragile X syndrome inherited it from his mother, who had a 50 percent chance of passing it on to her baby, since she has two X chromosomes. Some males who are unaffected by the disorder are carriers of the fragile X gene and will pass the chromosome to all of their daughters but none of their sons. Fragile X affects boys more often than girls and occurs in approximately one of every 1,250 males.

Physical features associated with fragile X syndrome include a long, narrow face and prominent ears, jaw, and forehead. Enlarged testicles and loose finger joints are also seen in some cases. The physical features are more noticeable after puberty and are often less prominent in females. Half the girls who are affected intellectually have prominent ears and loose finger joints.

DIAGNOSIS

Developmental delay is a common sign of fragile X syndrome in early childhood. Delayed speech and language skills and behavioral difficulties such as hyperactivity and short attention span occur frequently. Some children with fragile X syndrome may also demonstrate autistic-like behavior, such as unusual hand gestures, repetitive speech, and refusal to interact with others.

DNA testing is used to diagnose fragile X syndrome. Laboratory analysis of blood cells will identify those with fragile X chromosomes. Testing can identify males who have the syndrome and females who are carriers. Fragile X syndrome is inherited from a parent who is a carrier. Since the pattern of inheritance in fragile X is complicated, it is important for people in affected families to receive GENETIC COUNSELING, in which they can learn their risk of carrying the gene and passing it on to their children.

F

About 80 percent of boys with fragile X syndrome are mentally retarded. Although IQ seems to diminish throughout childhood, mental impairment can range from severe retardation to low-normal intelligence. Men and boys with fragile X syndrome are usually friendly and sociable, although they tend to interact in unusual ways, such as avoiding eye contact, having temper tantrums, and flapping or biting their hands during conversation with others. Girls are much less likely to have cognitive defects: about 30 percent with the genetic condition also have some degree of mental retardation.

TREATMENT

Fragile X syndrome does not have a cure. Medical care is recommended for related conditions. Medication is often given to treat attention deficits, hyperactivity, aggressive behavior, and other problems. Special education in speech therapy, physical therapy, and vocational preparation may be necessary. Education has been found to help individuals function at a higher level.

Normal XY chromosome   Fragile XX chromosome

ALTERED X CHROMOSOME
Fragile X syndrome is so named because an abnormal gene on the X (female) chromosome has a fragile connection to the rest of the body of the chromosome. The syndrome has a more profound impact on males because they have only one X chromosome, while a female has two.

Freckle

A small, flat, brown or tan, benign (not cancerous) spot occurring on sun-exposed skin. Freckles are most common in fair-skinned people, especially those with red hair, and most commonly occur on the face, arms, and upper trunk. They are a sign of sun damage. Freckles increase in number and darken with sun exposure. They require no treatment. However, people who develop freckles are advised to use protective sunscreen because they are more susceptible to developing skin cancer.

Free-floating anxiety

A severe, overall, and general sense of unease and apprehension unrelated to any event, situation, or thought. Symptoms include increased heart rate and breathing, sweating, trembling, fatigue, and weakness accompanied by feelings of impending danger and fear.

Freudian theory

A conceptual approach to understanding psychological development and treating mental illness based on the clinical work and writings of Sigmund Freud. Freud was the founder of psychoanalysis, which is a widely used and highly influential technique for revealing the deep self and resolving psychological issues. Freudian theory is based on a number of Freud's central ideas about the structure and function of the human mind.

THE UNCONSCIOUS

According to Freudian theory, the unconscious mind works in ways different from those that characterize conscious, waking experience. The unconscious mind can take thoughts and feelings that belong together and shift them out of context, dramatize thoughts in the form of images rather than abstract ideas, and represent one person or object with the image of another person or object. Recognizing how the unconscious mind works makes it possible to understand seemingly incomprehensible psychological events, such as dreaming. In Freud's view, dreams prevent unacceptable and disturbing thoughts, usually related to conflicts arising in early life, from becoming conscious, and thereby dreams protect sleep. By understanding how the unconscious mind transforms these disturbing thoughts, a psychoanalyst can help a person interpret dreams as a way of uncovering unconscious psychological material.

INSTINCTUAL DRIVES

Freudian theory assumes that unconscious conflicts such as those incorporated into dreams involve drives, or instinctual impulses, that begin in childhood. Many of these drives center on sexuality. Freud saw adult sexuality as the result of a complex process of development that begins in childhood, involves a variety of body areas (oral, genital, and anal), and corresponds to different stages in the child's relationship to his or her parents. Centrally important is the Oedipal conflict, which occurs at approximately 4 to 6 years of age. The child forms a strong emotional attachment and sexual desire to the parent of the opposite sex and enters into conflict with the parent of the same sex as a rival for the desired parent's affections. How the child resolves this conflict and how parents and other adults respond to and deal with the child at this time have a significant role in determining the individual's psychological maturity and his or her ability to form love relationships in later life.

ID, EGO, AND SUPEREGO

In Freudian theory, the psychic system has three component parts. The first, the id (Latin for "it") includes the sexual and aggressive drives that arise from the body rather than the mind. These drives want immediate satisfaction, which is perceived as pleasure. Thus the id is dominated by the pleasure principle and moves toward immediate gratification.

The second part, the ego (Latin for "I"), determines how that need for pleasure is satisfied. The ego contains the conscious mental processes, such as thinking, perception, and muscular control, that assess what is happening in the surroundings and direct responses to it. Since, for reasons of survival, the ego must often stand in the way of the id's drive toward immediate satisfaction, the ego develops DEFENSE MECHANISMS against internal emotional conflicts, such as repression (excluding unacceptable desires from consciousness), projection (ascribing unacceptable desires to someone else), and reaction formation (behaving consciously in a way directly opposite to the unacceptable desire).

Often an id impulse is unacceptable because of the prohibitions or demands laid upon the individual by others, particularly parents and parentlike figures such as teachers and members of the clergy. The sum total of these exterior rules and expectations forms the third part of the psyche, the superego (Latin for "above I"). The individual typically experiences his or her failure to meet the demands

SIGMUND FREUD (1856–1939)

Born in what is now the Czech Republic, Freud spent most of his career in Vienna, where he trained as a physician and practiced as a neurologist after becoming fascinated by neurological research as a medical student. Later, Freud studied in Paris with Jean Charcot, who was using hypnosis with mentally ill patients. Troubled by his inability to develop physical explanations for psychological symptoms, Freud delved more and more into the workings of the psyche. His research and clinical work led to the publication of a number of important books, such as *The Interpretation of Dreams* (1900), *Three Contributions to the Sexual Theory* (1905), and *Ego and Id* (1923), in which he explained his developing theory of psychoanalysis.

Although widely reviled by most doctors at the time, Freud's thinking strongly influenced the work of other leading psychiatrists, such as Carl Jung, Otto Rank, and Alfred Adler. In 1910 the International Psychoanalytic Association was founded as a worldwide professional organization for psychiatrists following Freud's ideas. After World War I, Freud did little clinical work and devoted his writing increasingly to the application of his ideas to religion, mythology, art, and literature. Following the Nazi occupation of Austria in 1938, Freud fled with his family to London, where he died the following year.

of the superego as shame or guilt. Since the superego begins to form during the Oedipal conflict, it has a power much like that of the id, is in part unconscious, and can cause feelings of guilt not justified by any objective transgression or wrongdoing.

Psychological symptoms, such as depression or hysteria, form because of conflicts among the three parts of the psyche. If the ego cannot handle the sometimes contradictory demands of the superego, the id, and the outside world, the ego expresses the tensions of this unresolved conflict as psychological symptoms.

ANXIETY

Anxiety rouses the individual to protect himself or herself against danger by means of defense mechanisms. According to Freud, these dangers are fear of abandonment by a loved one, the risk of losing the loved one's love, retaliation or punishment, and reproach by the superego. Anxiety felt in response to these psychological dangers has a role in the development of psychological symptoms.

Friedreich ataxia

Also known as spinocerebellar degeneration, an inherited disease characterized by progressive dysfunction of the cerebellum, spinal cord, and peripheral nerves. Friedreich ataxia is the most common form of inherited ATAXIA; hereditary ataxias are a group of diseases affecting the nervous system and consequent problems with balance, gait, movement, and speech.

SYMPTOMS

In Friedreich ataxia, damage to structures in the cerebellum and spinal cord results in a gradual loss of coordination and balance. Symptoms generally begin in childhood or in the early teen years. One of the earliest symptoms is an unsteady gait that makes walking difficult. The ataxia gradually worsens and spreads to the arms and trunk. Later symptoms include muscle weakness, eye tremor, speech problems, clubfoot, hammer toes, flexion (involuntary bending) of the toes, foot inversion (turning in), and scoliosis (curving of the spine to one side). Severe scoliosis can affect breathing, and there may also be chest pain and heart palpitations. Most people with this disease eventually are confined to a wheelchair.

DIAGNOSIS AND TREATMENT

Diagnosis is made through careful physical examination, medical history, and tests such as electromyography and genetic testing. There is no cure. Physical therapy, braces, and surgery may be helpful in coping with orthopedic difficulties.

Related problems, such as heart disease and diabetes mellitus, type 2, are treated with medications. How-ever, heart disease may progress into life-threatening heart failure. Medication can help with some of the symptoms of Friedreich ataxia but does not cure the disease.

Frontal lobe syndrome

A mental illness characterized by a change in personality and behavior and often caused by tumor, injury, stroke, or disease in the frontal lobe region of the brain or in a nerve pathway leading to or from it. Typical symptoms, which can be variable and subtle, include apathy, poor attention, emotional outbursts, lack of impulse control, impaired ability to anticipate events or consequences, self-neglect, depression, changes in gait, and lack of bladder or bowel control (incontinence). Treatment depends on the cause.

Frostbite

FOR FIRST AID
see Frostbite, page 1324

A condition occurring when areas of skin and underlying tissue freeze in cold weather. Frostbite is classified into four degrees of severity:

- First-degree frostbite, or frostnip, is a superficial injury in which the skin turns white and is temporarily numb. No blistering is likely.
- Second-degree frostbite is deeper and more serious; outer skin layers are frozen and hard, while underlying tissue is still intact. Blistering is likely to occur.
- Third- and fourth-degree frostbite freeze all layers of the skin and the underlying tissues. The skin becomes solid and hard and appears blue and white and blotchy. Skin may blister. If blood vessels freeze, gangrene (dead tissue) may appear and amputation may be necessary.

Frostbite usually occurs without pain in its later stages.

Frostbite should not be treated until it is certain that the area will not refreeze. Any wet or old clothing should be removed. First aid measures include immersing affected areas for 20 to 30 minutes in water that is warm rather than hot or applying warm cloths to frostbitten areas such as the ears, nose, and cheeks. Affected areas should not be rubbed. Warming is complete when the skin is soft and sensation is restored. Warm fluids should be consumed.

Prevention of frostbite includes avoiding going outdoors in extreme cold and high winds, not wearing wet

INJURIES FROM THE COLD

Depending on the degree of frostbite or frostnip, the body shows certain symptoms and responds predictably to rewarming.

CONDITION	SKIN SURFACE	TISSUE UNDER SKIN	SWELLING	BLISTERS	SYMPTOMS AFTER REWARMING	COMPLICATIONS (LONG-TERM)
Frostnip (early frostbite)	Soft, mild redness	Normal	None	None	Resolution of symptoms	None
First-degree frostbite (superficial frostbite)	Soft, redness, numbness	Normal	Mild, transient	May be present on back of ear, usually absent on fingers and toes	Itching, burning, deep pain, resolution of numbness, increased blood flow	None
Second-degree frostbite	Firm, white, or waxy numbness	Firm	Present	Present, with clear or milky fluid	Itching, burning, deep pain, resolution of numbness, increased blood flow	Numbness, cold sensitivity, sweating
Third-degree frostbite	Hard, pale, blue in appearance, numbness	Hard and woody texture	Moderate	Present, deeper blisters with purple (bloody) fluid	Bluish color to skin persists	Skin ulcers, severe cold sensitivity, arthritis, sweating
Fourth-degree frostbite	Hard, numbness	Hard, skin shrivels, damage to muscle and bone can occur within 3 to 6 weeks	Moderate, gangrene can develop once swelling subsides	Usually not present	Painless after rewarming, symptoms progress	Amputation, bone injury (in children), depigmentation of darker skin

Compiled by Jerrold B. Leikin, MD

clothes outdoors, and not wearing tight clothing and boots that can restrict circulation. People with diseases that affect the blood vessels, such as diabetes mellitus, type 1 (insulin dependent) and diabetes mellitus, type 2 (non–insulin dependent), are at particular risk for developing frostbite, as are people who smoke or drink alcoholic beverages before going out into the cold. Wearing many layers of dry polyester, goose down, polypropylene, or wool clothing, as well as suitable clothes for cold weather, including mittens, hats that cover the ears, and scarves, can help protect the skin from frost-bite. Cotton is the least effective material for preventing cold injuries.

Frottage

A mental illness characterized by a person touching a nonconsenting person sexually and rubbing against his or her genitals. In most cases, this behavior occurs in crowded places such as busy sidewalks, movie theaters, or packed subway trains, where the person is more likely to escape arrest. Typically, the person rubs his or her genitals against the thighs or buttocks of the victim while fantasizing an exclusive, loving relationship with the nonconsenting person. The person then tries to escape the victim's detec-tion after the episode occurs. This disorder is most likely found in men between the ages of 15 and 25 and declines as the person ages. Frottage is also known as frotteurism.

Frozen section

A laboratory technique used to freeze a fresh sample of tissue removed during surgery. The tissue sample from a biopsy is frozen; then, it is sliced thin and examined under a microscope. Frozen section is used primarily for preliminary diagnosis of disease and during cancer surgery to determine whether enough tissue has been removed to treat the tumor.

F

Frozen shoulder

A painful condition, medically termed adhesive capsulitis, resulting in greatly restricted mobility of the shoulder joint. The immobility tends to occur at a level or point in the range of motion at which the shoulder cannot be moved, either by the person experiencing frozen shoulder or by another person manipulating the arm in the shoulder joint. At this blocked level of movement, there may be increased pain. The pain may be intensified at night.

Frozen shoulder may be the result of an injury to the shoulder or injury to another body part that prevents normal movement of the shoulder. Frozen shoulder is sometimes caused by the arm being kept in a sling for a few weeks, with prolonged restriction of shoulder movement. Frozen shoulder has also been known to follow recovery from a heart attack and to occur following surgery for conditions not involving the shoulder. In many cases, the cause is unknown. One theory suggests the involvement of an autoimmune reaction, in which the body's defense system erroneously perceives a threat from its own tissues and begins to attack them. The tissues of the shoulder's joint capsule respond to the attack with a severe inflammatory reaction. Normally the tissue that encloses this joint capsule is loose and allows the shoulder a wide range of relatively unrestricted movements. When this tissue becomes inflamed, it sticks together and limits or prevents movement of the shoulder.

DIAGNOSIS AND TREATMENT

Frozen shoulder is diagnosed from symptoms, history, and physical examination. In general, routine X rays will not reveal the problem, but an ARTHROGRAM can reveal scarring and contraction of the shoulder joint capsule. Frozen shoulder may be distinguished from a torn rotator cuff by the greater range of motion possible in the latter condition when another person moves the joint. MRI (magnetic resonance imaging), which can determine an underlying condition in the soft tissues of the shoulder, may be ordered to confirm a suspected diagnosis.

Recovery from a frozen shoulder may take months. Anti-inflammatory medication is often prescribed to decrease the inflammation. Physical therapy, emphasizing stretching exercises, may be prescribed to regain movement in the shoulder. Specific exercises, performed four times daily, may be required. Injected cortisone with a long-acting anesthetic can help to control pain and inflammation to assist the person in stretching. Manipulation of the shoulder allows a doctor to stretch the joint capsule and break up scar tissue in the capsule, which increases the possibility of movement in the shoulder. This procedure is done under general anesthesia and may have to be repeated, but generally improves the shoulder's mobility. There is also an operation that involves surgical release of contracted soft tissues.

Fructose

A simple SUGAR or monosaccharide. Pure fructose naturally occurs in fruits, where it combines with glucose to form sucrose. It can be refined and added to foods and beverages as high-fructose corn syrup or in its crystalline form. Fructose is approximately one and a half times sweeter than sucrose (table sugar), so less can be used to achieve the same desired sweetness.

Like other sugars, fructose is a carbohydrate that provides calories but few other nutrients. The Food Guide Pyramid advises consumers to have the smallest proportion of their diet derived from fats, oils, and refined sugars. When consumed from its natural sources, such as fruits, fructose does not need to be restricted since natural sources also provide fiber, vitamins, and minerals.

Frustration

The emotional tension that arises when impulses, actions, or desires are blocked or thwarted.

FSH

Follicle-stimulating hormone. FSH is a hormone released by both women and men from the pituitary gland at the base of the brain.

In women between puberty and menopause, the monthly menstrual cycle begins when FSH is released and transported by the blood to one of the ovaries. FSH stimulates the ovary to release a mature egg in the process called ovulation. FSH also signals the ovary to begin forming a follicle, which is a tiny cavity that holds and supports each egg. The female hormones estrogen and progesterone and a small amount of male hormones, called androgen hormones, are produced and secreted in response to stimulation of FSH. These hormones have a vital role in the reproductive cycle.

In men, FSH stimulates the testicles to produce sperm.

Fugue

Sudden, unexpected travel away from home or work accompanied by an inability to remember some or all of one's past and either confusion about identity or the assumption of a new identity. The travel may last only hours or days and cover short distances, or it may extend to weeks or months and thousands of miles. Individuals in a fugue state do not appear to be abnormal and do not attract attention. When the individual recovers and returns to normal consciousness, he or she may have no memory of events during the fugue. Fugue is thought to represent a response to the overwhelming emotional trauma of an insurmountable crisis and can also be associated with epilepsy or head injury. Fugue is one of a group of mental illnesses known as DISSOCIATIVE DISORDERS.

Functional endoscopic sinus surgery

See FESS.

Functional improvement

The progress toward normalized activity in the musculoskeletal, neuromuscular, cardiovascular, or respiratory system of an individual who has been debilitated by disease or injured. Functional improvement of the joints, muscles, and other body structures and organs may be attained through PHYSICAL THERAPY and instructions in how to do appropriate strength, flexibility, and endurance exercises.

Fundoplication

Surgery that creates a new junction or valve between the ESOPHAGUS and the STOMACH by wrapping the uppermost portion of the stomach (the fundus)

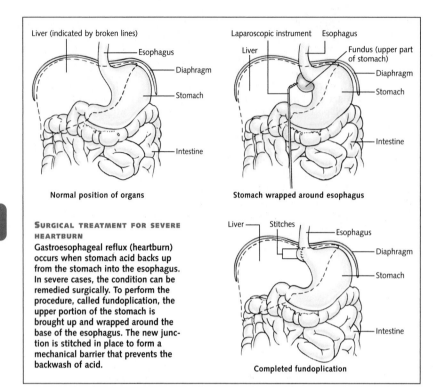

Liver (indicated by broken lines)

Esophagus

Diaphragm

Stomach

Intestine

Normal position of organs

Laparoscopic instrument   Esophagus

Liver

Fundus (upper part of stomach)

Diaphragm

Stomach

Intestine

Stomach wrapped around esophagus

Liver — Stitches

Esophagus

Diaphragm

Stomach

Intestine

Completed fundoplication

SURGICAL TREATMENT FOR SEVERE HEARTBURN

Gastroesophageal reflux (heartburn) occurs when stomach acid backs up from the stomach into the esophagus. In severe cases, the condition can be remedied surgically. To perform the procedure, called fundoplication, the upper portion of the stomach is brought up and wrapped around the base of the esophagus. The new junction is stitched in place to form a mechanical barrier that prevents the backwash of acid.

around the lower end of the esophagus. Fundoplication is performed to treat gastroesophageal reflux disease (GERD), a common cause of severe heartburn. See ANTIREFLUX SURGERY.

Fundoplication can be performed through either a foot-long abdominal incision or with the aid of a laparoscope, a tiny telescopic camera that gives the surgeon an inside view of the abdomen. The LAPAROSCOPIC SURGERY requires four or five incisions, each about one-half inch long, to allow the insertion of the laparoscope and surgical instruments.

The actual procedure in both open and laparoscopic surgeries is the same. The surgeon detaches the bottom of the esophagus from the tissue that holds it in place. The upper portion of the stomach is then wrapped around the base of the esophagus and stitched into place. This forms a new "valve" between the esophagus and the stomach and helps to prevent acidic stomach juices from washing back into the esophagus.

The open incision requires a hospital stay of 5 to 7 days and a recovery period of 4 to 6 weeks before normal activities can be resumed. Fundoplication performed with the use of laparoscopy reduces the hospital stay to 1 or 2 days; full recovery is 1 or 2 weeks. With either type of surgery, the patient will likely be on a diet of clear liquids on the day after surgery, with solid food being introduced back into the diet on about the third day after surgery. Within a week, the person should be eating normally.

Fungal infections

See MYCOSIS.

Fungi

A diverse group of organisms that obtain food by absorbing nutrients directly. Fungi are found wherever other forms of life are found. With BACTERIA, they are responsible for the decay and decomposition of organic matter. Fungi may also cause mold-related illnesses in people who spend substantial amounts of time in water-damaged buildings. Some fungi are parasites on living organisms, including humans, and can cause serious infections and diseases. Fungi also have beneficial medical uses. An alkaloid in one fungus may be used to stimulate uterine contractions in childbirth. Antibiotics such as penicillin, which are now produced by nonfungal microorganisms, were originally derived from a fungus. The antifungal antibiotic griseofulvin is made from fungi, and the immunosuppressant medications cyclosporine and tacrolimus, which are used in organ transplantation, are both derived from fungi. See also MYCOLOGY.

Furosemide

A drug used to treat fluid retention associated with heart failure. Furosemide (Lasix) is a diuretic ("water pill") given by tablet, liquid, or injection to decrease the amount of water retained in the body by increasing urination. By eliminating water from the body, blood pressure can also be reduced. A person taking furosemide needs to be monitored by a doctor since the drug can lower potassium to dangerously low levels.

Furuncle

See BOIL.

G

G6PD deficiency

Glucose-6-phosphate dehydrogenase enzyme deficiency. A common inherited disorder that can cause anemia. Deficiency of G6PD leads to an abnormal rupture of red blood cells, or hemolytic anemia, which can result in a low red blood cell count. The abnormal gene responsible for this condition is located on the X chromosome. G6PD deficiency is found more often among males than females, since males have only one X chromosome. G6PD deficiency is more common among blacks, Italians, Greeks, Asians, and people of Mediterranean ancestry. Approximately 10 to 14 percent of black American males are affected.

Individuals with G6PD deficiency may not become anemic or have symptoms unless the red blood cells are exposed to certain chemical compounds such as antimalarial drugs, sulfa drugs (antibiotics), anti-itching drugs, and others that have oxidant properties, meaning they can damage the red blood cells. Fava beans and mothballs also contain oxidants and can trigger the breaking up of red blood cells. Symptoms may include fatigue, pale skin color, shortness of breath, rapid heart rate, jaundice (yellow skin color), dark urine, and enlarged spleen. Treatment involves discontinuing the offending drug or compound, and recovery is usually complete. Blood transfusions are sometimes needed when the anemia is severe.

GABA

The acronym for gamma-aminobutyric acid, an inhibitory NEUROTRANSMITTER that has a role in EPILEPSY (a disease in which neurons in the brain signal abnormally, leading to seizures). GABA inhibits or decreases neuronal activity in the brain. When there is an insufficient level of GABA, abnormally high levels of neuronal activity can lead to a seizure.

Gabapentin

An anticonvulsant drug used to treat seizures associated with epilepsy.

Gabapentin (Neurontin) is usually taken with other drugs to control seizure disorders.

Gait

The manner in which a person walks. Problems with gait can be a sign of an orthopedic problem or of neurological disease. A gait that is unsteady or uncoordinated may be caused by muscle spasms and nerve damage that were caused by problems such as a cerebral palsy, stroke, ALS (amyotrophic lateral sclerosis), multiple sclerosis, Parkinson disease, head trauma, brain abscess, or brain tumor. A person who staggers may be intoxicated with alcohol or drugs, or he or she may have a cerebellar disease. It is important to diagnose and treat the underlying causes of gait problems.

Gait training

A type of physical therapy used to help a person walk again after any orthopedic or neurological illness or when he or she has a chronic instability of gait.

Galactorrhea

Breast milk production at any time other than just before and after childbirth. The milk is usually whitish or gray-green and leaks out of both breasts. Galactorrhea, which can occur in men, though rarely, may be caused by excessive amounts of estrogen, a pituitary tumor called a prolactinoma, hypothyroidism, or as a side effect of medication, including oral contraceptives. It is sometimes associated with absence of menstrual periods (see AMENORRHEA).

Diagnosis is based on a physical examination and review of medical history to rule out pregnancy or medication as the cause. Blood tests for hypothyroidism and prolactin level may be done. A CT (computed tomography) scan of the hypothalamus and pituitary gland may be done. Galactorrhea is serious only if it is caused by a pituitary tumor, which can be treated with medication, surgery, and radiation.

Galactosemia

A rare genetic disorder of carbohydrate metabolism. Galactosemia can be caused by any of three defects in galactose metabolism. (Galactose is a sugar derived from the milk sugar, lactose.) The most common version (classic galactosemia) is caused by a deficiency in a certain enzyme and is associated with liver disease, cataract formation, and mental retardation. Treatment consists of removing galactose-containing foods from the diet, especially milk. Eliminating dietary galactose usually leads to improvement in all features except mental retardation.

Gallbladder

A pear-shaped organ of the DIGESTIVE SYSTEM, located just below the LIVER. The gallbladder stores and concentrates bile produced in the liver, then

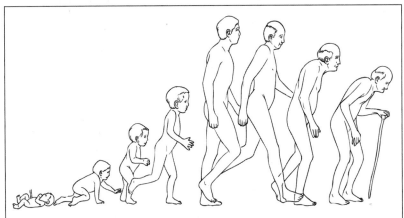

GAIT AND POSTURE
As a growing child develops the skills to walk, he or she assumes a characteristic posture and gait. As the individual ages, the gait and posture change as a result of both neurological and orthopedic factors. Stride shortens, the foot flattens, and the forward arm swing decreases.

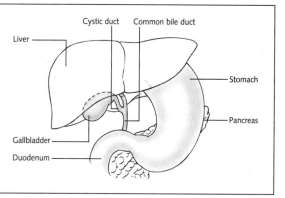

STORAGE OF BILE
The muscular gallbladder, located just under the liver, holds and concentrates bile produced in the liver. When a person eats, the gallbladder contracts to squeeze the bile into the small intestine, where it aids in the digestion of fats. The bile flow is channeled through a series of ducts called the biliary system.

releases it into the duodenum, the first part of the small intestine. The gallbladder is a thin-walled, flexible sac of fibrous tissue enclosed by smooth muscle and lined with mucous membrane. It connects with the liver via the common hepatic duct. When bile (a substance necessary for digestion) reaches the gallbladder, it is mostly water. In the gallbladder, this bile solution is concentrated down to pigment, cholesterol, and bile salts that aid in the digestion of fats and proteins. Concentrated bile flows from the gallbladder to the cystic duct, then into the common bile duct, and from there into the duodenum. If the person consumes food that contains a high proportion of fat, the small intestine secretes a hormone that contracts smooth muscle in the gallbladder's walls and causes the release of the additional bile needed for digestion. Although the gallbladder has a useful role in digestion, it is not absolutely necessary because the liver can secrete bile directly into the duodenum. As a result, the gallbladder can be removed without harm when, for example, GALLSTONES form.

Gallbladder cancer

A rare cancer that originates in the gallbladder. Gallbladder cancer affects women more often than men, and blacks and Native Americans more than whites; it mostly occurs in people age 65 or older. A high percentage of people with gallbladder cancer have a history of gallstones. Symptoms are much like those for other gallbladder diseases, typically, intense abdominal pain and indigestion. An individual who experiences abdominal pain, unintentional weight loss, diminished appetite, fever, nausea, or jaundice (yellowing of the skin and the whites of the eyes) should contact a doctor.

Diagnosing the disease is difficult because the organ is hidden behind other organs. Sometimes, cancer is diagnosed only after the gallbladder has been removed for other reasons. X rays and other tests can be used to investigate, although surgery is the only method likely to identify the cancer clearly. The only known cure is surgical removal of the gallbladder, if the cancer has not yet spread to other organs. Because gallbladder cancer is so uncommon, and because its symptoms resemble those of more common diseases, it is often not found until it has spread to nearby tissues, such as the liver, stomach, or lymph nodes. Treatment involves pain relief and the restoration of normal bile flow from the liver into the intestines by insertion of a stent (tube). Radiation therapy or chemotherapy may be used, but in general, the prognosis for patients with advanced gallbladder cancer is poor.

Gallium scan

A NUCLEAR MEDICINE scanning procedure involving the injection of radioactive gallium. Gallium is a rare bluish white metallic element that accumulates in areas of inflammation and certain tumors. A gallium scan is generally used to help diagnose Hodgkin disease and to locate abscesses, inflamed areas, and some types of tumors. The entire body is scanned at intervals of 6, 24, 48, and 72 hours after gallium has been injected. Areas that show a high concentration of gallium indicate abnormalities that require further evaluation.

Gallstones

Hard masses made primarily of cholesterol that commonly develop in the GALLBLADDER where BILE is stored. Less commonly, gallstones form in the bile ducts leading from the liver to the small intestine. They occur more frequently in women than men, especially women who are overweight.

Gallstones usually result from an imbalance in the chemical composition of bile. They range in size from that of a grain of sand to that of a golf ball. The gallbladder may contain one stone or hundreds of them. Most are composed of cholesterol, a fatlike substance that is excreted by the liver. Excess dietary cholesterol may be a factor in stone formation. At times, bilirubin and calcium salts also make up gallstones.

SYMPTOMS AND CAUSES

More than half of the individuals who have gallstones do not have symptoms. However, at times, gallstones leave the gallbladder and become lodged in the bile duct. This condition, which is known as BILE DUCT OBSTRUCTION, leads to BILIARY COLIC, or severe pain in the upper middle or right part of the abdomen. CHOLECYSTITIS, or inflammation of the gallbladder, may develop as the result of a gallstone lodging in the cystic duct and blocking the flow of bile from the gallbladder to the intestine.

Biliary colic occurs when the gallbladder and bile duct muscles contract in an attempt to propel a lodged stone from the duct into the intestine. The resulting pain may radiate to the back and is often accompanied by nausea and vomiting. Attacks of biliary colic typically last from 2 to 5 hours.

Pain from a gallstone may disappear if the stone falls back into the gallbladder or is forced through the duct into the intestines. If the obstruction of the bile ducts persists and prevents bile from entering the intestines, increased pressure in the liver can result in jaundice (a yellowing of the skin and the whites of the eyes). Cholangitis (inflammation and infection of the bile ducts) may also develop. Less frequently, pancreatitis (inflammation of the pancreas) occurs as a result of gallstones.

DIAGNOSIS AND TREATMENT

Gallstones may be diagnosed through

ULTRASOUND SCANNING or ERCP (endoscopic retrograde cholangiopancreatography), a procedure in which a viewing tube called an endoscope is passed from the mouth through the stomach into the intestines. Contrast material (dye) is injected into the bile duct to make it visible on X rays. If the test reveals a gallstone lodged in a duct, tiny instruments can be threaded down the endoscope to remove it. Less commonly, CHOLECYSTOGRAPHY (an X ray of the gallbladder and common bile duct after they have been filled with a contrast dye) and CHOLESCINTIGRAPHY (visual examination of the gallbladder and bile ducts by scanning with a radioactive substance) are performed to diagnose gallbladder problems.

In a laparoscopic CHOLECYSTECTOMY, the gallbladder is removed using a fiberoptic viewing instrument called a laparoscope and several small incisions. This is the preferred surgical treatment of symptomatic gallstones. Because the laparoscopic treatment results in less postoperative pain and disability, a shorter hospital stay, and a more rapid recovery, it has largely replaced open cholecystectomy, which requires a long abdominal incision. In about 10 percent of cases that begin as laparoscopic procedures, it becomes necessary to complete the operation as a traditional open surgery because of technical difficulties or complications.

Various other treatments are recommended for gallstones. In rare cases, drugs are prescribed to dissolve stones. Sometimes, stones are pulverized by LITHOTRIPSY, or shock waves that are passed through the skin. Often, these techniques are used together. However, gallstones recur in about half of the people who have nonsurgical treatment.

Complications of gallstones can require additional treatment. For example, cholangitis requires immediate removal of the stone and intravenous antibiotics to combat the infection. When tests reveal gallstones that do not cause symptoms, it is up to the individual physician to determine whether treatment is necessary.

Gambling, addictive

A pathological inability to restrain the impulse to gamble that results in severe personal, domestic, and vocational consequences, sometimes ending in financial ruin or divorce. Addictive gambling is also known as compulsive gambling or pathological gambling. Addictive gambling, which typically begins in adolescence, is considered an addiction because the attraction to the gambling behavior has the same characteristics as addiction to alcohol or a drug: loss of control, preoccupation, narrowing of interests, dishonesty, guilt, and repeated relapse.

SYMPTOMS

A person who is an addictive gambler becomes preoccupied with gambling and spends most of his or her time gambling, planning the next round of gambling, or figuring out ways to raise money to gamble. Many people with the disorder say they gamble because they love the "action," but they may need to place larger and larger bets to achieve the same feeling of euphoria. Some people who are addictive gamblers seek to escape depression or problems at home. Others may try to cut back or control their gambling, but continue to gamble anyway. They often "chase" their losses — that is, put down bigger and bigger bets or take higher and higher risks to pay off a loss. Lying to cover up the extent of gambling is common, as is illegal activity to obtain money, such as embezzlement, forgery, or writing bad checks. Typically a person who is an addictive gambler asks family and friends for bail-out money to pay off debts, then uses the funds to continue gambling. The gambling continues despite its effects on family relationships, career, or educational opportunity.

Two of three people with this disorder are males. Women who gamble addictively are more likely to do so to escape depression or home problems, while men are usually interested in the euphoric mood that comes from gambling. Individuals with the disorder are often highly competitive, energetic, restless, and easily bored. Excessive concern with approval by others and extravagant generosity are common. It is estimated that one of five people who are addictive gamblers have attempted suicide.

COURSE OF THE DISEASE

Some medical experts describe addictive gambling as a four-phase process. In the first, or winning stage, the individual first gambles occasionally, then increases the amount of gambling, often because of a big win. He or she feels omnipotent and unreasonably optimistic and brags about winning while minimizing losses. This stage can last for months or years. The second, or losing, stage often begins with a losing streak that prompts the individual to keep placing bets, often with borrowed money to recover the loss. The person is likely to lie and cover up, ignore family and work obligations, and become irritable, restless, and withdrawn. While the spouse may be aware of the loss, usually he or she does not realize how large the loss is. In the third, or desperation stage, the person may gamble away a bailout intended to pay off the debt, engage in illegal activities to raise gambling funds, suffer a loss in reputation, and

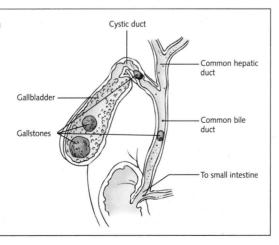

WHERE GALLSTONES LODGE
Gallstones travel out of the gallbladder and either pass out of the body unnoticed or lodge somewhere between the gallbladder and the small intestine. If the stone blocks the cystic duct, pressure will build up in the gallbladder, causing pain and infection. If the stone blocks the common bile duct, it will inhibit drainage of bile from the liver to the intestine, causing jaundice and fever.

Cystic duct

Common hepatic duct

Gallbladder

Common bile duct

Gallstones

To small intestine

G

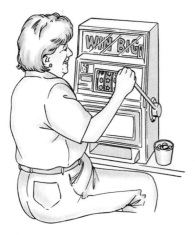

COMPULSIVE BEHAVIOR
Addiction to gambling resembles other addictions in terms of both symptoms and treatment. Compulsive gambling behavior leads gradually to loss of control over other areas of the addicted person's life. Overcoming a gambling addiction requires giving up the behavior and getting therapy for underlying problems.

become alienated from family and friends. Suicide may be attempted in the fourth, or helplessness, stage. Alcohol or drug abuse is more likely at this point, as are divorce and emotional breakdown.

TREATMENT
Addictive gambling is often associated with denial that the gambling is in fact addictive and pathological. Many people with this disorder enter treatment at the insistence of others, but effective treatment can begin only when the individual recognizes the problem. Options include individual and group psychotherapy, as well as self-help support groups such as Gamblers Anonymous, which is a TWELVE-STEP PROGRAM similar to Alcoholics Anonymous.

Gamete intrafallopian transfer
See GIFT.

Gamma globulin
A protein found in the blood that helps fight infection; also, a substance prepared from a mixture of proteins in the fluid portion of blood.

Terms in small capital letters—for example, PHYSICAL THERAPY or PAGET DISEASE—indicate a cross-reference to another entry with more information.

Gamma globulin contains antibodies, which are proteins formed in the liver, spleen, bone marrow, and lymph glands. The antibodies in gamma globulin target proteins (called antigens) found on the surface of invading organisms, such as viruses and bacteria, that cause infections. For each antigen, there is a specific antibody circulating in the blood for a period of time after a person has recovered from an infection. Gamma globulin can be used to quickly boost short-term immunity and improve the immune systems of people who have serious infectious illnesses, including hepatitis A and measles.

Gamma globulin medication is usually given by injection in a doctor's office. People being treated with gamma globulin should advise their physicians about past reactions to it, as well as problems with their immune system or heart.

Gamma knife radiosurgery
A technique developed in the 1990s that delivers a high dose of radiation to a precise target in the skull without cutting into the area. Gamma knife radiosurgery is used in neurological procedures, along with a local anesthetic, for treatment of malignant brain tumors, benign brain tumors, vascular abnormalities in the brain, and trigeminal neuralgia (a painful nerve disorder of the face).

Ganciclovir
A drug used to treat or prevent infections caused by cytomegalovirus (CMV). Ganciclovir (Cytovene, Vitrasert) is used to treat CMV infections associated with HIV (human immunodeficiency virus) infection and to prevent CMV infections in people who have had organ transplants. It works by interfering in DNA replication by the virus and is given by injection.

Ganglion
A cyst that most commonly appears under the skin on the side of the wrist, hand, or the top part of the foot. Ganglia vary in size. They occur when a gel-like substance that leaks from a joint capsule accumulates and balloons out to form an external swelling or cyst. The cyst has a rubbery texture and may be firm to the touch. Ganglia are generally harmless and painless or only mildly painful, and they rarely impede movement of the wrist or foot. If one is located on the upper surface of the foot, it may interfere with wearing shoes. Any swelling on the skin's surface requires medical attention, and a ganglion is no exception. A doctor may determine that no treatment is necessary, or the decision may be made to aspirate or draw fluid from the cyst and sometimes to inject a corticosteroid drug. If these treatments are not successful and if the ganglion is painful or obstructive, surgery to remove it may be considered. When surgical removal is contemplated for cosmetic reasons, it should be noted that a small scar will replace the removed cyst.

Gangrene
A condition in which a tissue of the body dies because of blockage of arterial blood supply. Gangrene develops, most commonly in the extremities, when the blood supply to the affected body part is cut off due to infection, a blood clot in an artery, vascular disease such as arteriosclerosis, trauma due to accident or surgery, severe frostbite, or the vascular collapse that may accompany diabetes mellitus. Gangrene is most dangerous when it affects the intestines or stomach.

Symptoms may include blackened skin with underlying dead tissue of the muscle and bone, crinkling of the skin, swelling, pain or numbness in the affected area, fever, and possibly a discharge from open sores.

The two forms of gangrene, dry gangrene and wet gangrene, each have different causes and symptoms. Dry gangrene is a chronic condition that occurs when arteries become blocked and the tissues are deprived of blood. This form of gangrene may be caused by arteriosclerosis, frostbite, injury, or it may be a complication of diabetes.

Wet gangrene is an acute form of the condition in which the dead tissue becomes infected with bacteria as a result of the contamination of an open sore or wound with infected material. This form produces a foul-smelling, gaseous discharge and is also referred to as gas gangrene. Associated symptoms include high fever, severe pain, acute anemia, and prostration. This form requires urgent surgery and antibiotic therapy.

TREATMENT

Gangrene is generally curable in the early stages. It is treated in a hospital setting with efforts to improve circulation to the impaired area and surgery to remove the dead tissue, sometimes by amputation when necessary. Antibiotics are given intravenously in the early stages of gangrene to fight infection. Pain relievers and anticoagulants to prevent blood clotting are also given. Bed rest is required until healing begins.

Wet gangrene can be fatal and, in severe cases, may necessitate amputation. Other possible complications of gangrene include blood poisoning, shock, and a blood-clotting disorder called disseminated intravascular coagulation.

Risk factors for gangrene include poor blood circulation, diabetes mellitus, advanced age, smoking (which impairs circulation), and alcohol abuse (which interferes with blood-vessel function).

Ganser syndrome

A psychiatric syndrome in which a person gives approximate or near-miss answers to questions he or she appears to understand. As an example, the question "When does Santa come?" brings the answer "Halloween." This behavior is known technically as "Vorbeireden," which is German for "talking around the point." Ganser syndrome is associated with emotional disorders that involve the disturbance of fundamental aspects of waking consciousness, such as personal identity, memory, or awareness of self and body (see DISSOCIATIVE DISORDERS).

Garlic

A plant used as a spice and as a medicinal herb to lower cholesterol levels and blood pressure. Garlic contains a compound called allicin that is known to lower cholesterol and blood pressure. Allicin may also stimulate the immune system and have antibiotic properties. Garlic has been used as a medicinal herb for thousands of years and is commonly used in Chinese medicine.

Gastrectomy

Surgical removal of the stomach. A partial gastrectomy is the removal of part of the stomach, and a total gastrectomy is the removal of the entire stomach. A partial removal is most commonly performed to treat noncancerous stomach or duodenal ulcers, as well as stomach cancer that is low in the stomach near the duodenum. A total gastrectomy is required in some cases of stomach cancer and when ulcers that fail to respond to nonsurgical treatment bleed uncontrollably or perforate the stomach wall. The advent of new medical treatments for ulcer disease has made surgical remedies less common.

Before the procedure, the stomach is emptied through a nasogastric tube (a thin, flexible, plastic tube that is threaded through the nose into the stomach). The tube remains in place during and for a period after the operation. Gastrectomy is done in a hospital under general anesthesia. After making an incision in the upper abdomen, the surgeon removes all or part of the stomach. In a partial gastrectomy, the healthy remaining edges are joined together, maintaining a passageway for food. Surgery takes 2 to 4 hours.

After surgery, the patient receives nutrients intravenously as the gastrectomy heals. Often, digestive secretions will be drained using a nasogastric tube. In a few days, the digestive tract recovers sufficiently to allow slow resumption of eating and drinking. Doctors may prescribe drugs to control side effects, such as nausea, vomiting, and diarrhea. In cases of cancer, CHEMOTHERAPY and RADIATION THERAPY are recommended. Maintaining normal nutrition is more difficult after a total than after a partial gastrectomy and may require more modifications in diet.

Gastric

Pertaining to, relating to, or originating in the stomach.

Gastric erosion

A superficial raw area in the mucous membrane that lines the stomach. Gastric erosion is a relatively common problem. The main symptom is bleeding of the affected area, although symptoms may not always be present. In rare severe cases, bloody vomiting may occur. Unlike a GASTRIC ULCER, there is no danger of gastric erosion penetrating or perforating the stomach lining. However, if internal bleeding persists, anemia will eventually result.

Gastric erosion is sometimes caused by the use of nonsteroidal anti-inflammatory drugs (NSAIDs), such

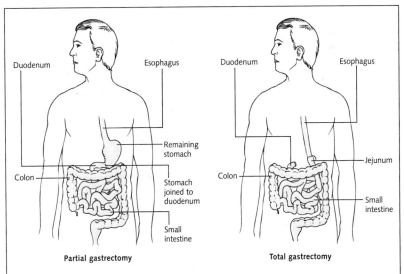

Duodenum   Esophagus   Duodenum   Esophagus

Remaining stomach

Colon   Colon   Jejunum

Stomach joined to duodenum   Small intestine

Small intestine

Partial gastrectomy   **Total gastrectomy**

PARTIAL OR TOTAL REMOVAL OF THE STOMACH
Gastrectomy is a surgical procedure to remove part or all of the stomach to treat stomach cancer or severe ulcers. In a partial procedure, the lower portion of the stomach is removed and the remaining portion is stitched to the duodenum (the upper part of the small intestine). In a much more rare total gastrectomy, the entire stomach is removed and the esophagus is stitched to the jejunum (the midsection of the small intestine).

as aspirin and ibuprofen, which irritate the stomach lining. These drugs are often used to alleviate musculoskeletal problems, such as arthritis. Use of corticosteroid drugs prescribed for problems such as asthma or colitis can also lead to gastric erosion. The bacterium *Helicobacter pylori* (H. PYLORI), which has been implicated as the likely cause of peptic and gastric ulcers, may also contribute to the problem. *Helicobacter pylori* may damage the protective mucous lining of the stomach, leaving it more vulnerable to attack by harsh acids and enzymes. Gastric erosion also develops in people recovering from severe injuries or burns and in those under prolonged stress.

Gastric erosions are diagnosed by a GASTROSCOPY (visual examination of the esophagus, stomach, and duodenum through insertion of a slim, flexible, lighted tube) or an upper GASTROINTESTINAL (GI) SERIES (an X-ray procedure also known as a barium swallow). Treatment depends on the underlying cause. For example, a physician may prescribe alternative drugs that are less irritating to the stomach lining or recommend taking drugs with an antacid or acid-suppressing medication. Although no single medication has proven effectiveness against *H. pylori*, a medical regimen called triple therapy (the use of three medications; two are ANTIBIOTICS and the third is usually one of the PROTON PUMP INHIBITORS) can eradicate most cases of the bacteria.

Gastric lavage

See STOMACH PUMPING.

Gastric ulcer

A sore or wound in the mucous membrane lining the stomach. Gastric or stomach ulcers are a form of PEPTIC ULCER DISEASE. Gastric ulcers can develop anywhere in the stomach, but are most often located on the stomach's lesser curve or in the lower half of the stomach. They vary in size from one fifth of an inch to 3 inches long. Men and women are equally susceptible to gastric ulcers. Upper abdominal pain is the most common symptom of a gastric ulcer. The pain tends to be intermittent, burning, and gnawing and occurs a half hour to 2 hours after meals. Occasionally, it spreads to the lower part of the chest.

Weeks of periodic discomfort may be followed by pain-free periods. Other symptoms include nausea, vomiting, and loss of appetite and weight.

CAUSE AND DIAGNOSIS

Although the exact cause of gastric ulcers remains unknown, evidence strongly suggests that in most cases infection with the bacterium *Helicobacter pylori* (H. PYLORI) is responsible. Other factors that have a role are long-term use of nonsteroidal anti-inflammatory drugs (NSAIDs), such as aspirin and ibuprofen, heavy use of alcohol, and smoking. Like *H. pylori*, these damage the protective mucous lining of the duodenum, leaving it more vulnerable to attack by harsh stomach acids and enzymes. A family history of peptic ulcer disease and frequently experiencing stress can make individuals more susceptible to ulcers.

Diagnosis is based on a variety of investigations, including blood tests, breath tests, an upper GASTROINTESTINAL (GI) SERIES (an X-ray procedure also called a barium swallow), or GASTROSCOPY (a visual method that can also take samples of tissue from the esophagus, stomach, and duodenum). The tissue can be tested for cancer and *H. pylori*. Blood tests can detect the presence of antibodies to *H. pylori*, while a urea breath test detects the presence of the actual bacteria. Knowing when the symptoms occur and how they are successfully relieved is important in diagnosing a gastric ulcer because ulcer pain and nausea tend to follow a pattern. They are typically eased by food, milk, antacids, or vomiting.

TREATMENT

Medications have a vital role in treating gastric ulcers. For many years, over-the-counter or prescription antacids have been used to neutralize stomach acid and relieve symptoms. However, because prolonged use of antacids can disrupt body chemistry, today many doctors prescribe other medications. These include drugs that reduce acid secretion, such as histamine blockers, anticholinergic agents, and proton pump inhibitors. Some histamine blockers are now also available over-the-counter. There are also drugs that coat the lining of the duodenum and stomach with a protective layer that prevents acid from reaching the ulcer. A medical regimen called

triple therapy (the use of three medications at once) can eradicate most cases due to *H. pylori* bacteria; the three medications are two ANTIBIOTICS and usually one of the PROTON PUMP INHIBITORS. Lifestyle modifications are also useful. Doctors recommend avoiding excessive alcohol and tobacco use. Because smoking increases acidity in the stomach, smokers should quit. Eating a number of small meals each day rather than two or three large ones may also be beneficial.

Possible complications of gastric ulcers include bleeding, scarring, and PYLORIC STENOSIS, a condition in which the outlet from the stomach to the duodenum [the pylorus] becomes partly or completely blocked. There is a greater risk with gastric ulcers than with duodenal ones that cancer will develop. However, there is less risk that gastric ulcers will penetrate or perforate the wall of the stomach. When a gastric ulcer fails to respond to treatment or if complications develop, surgery may become necessary. The most frequently performed surgery for gastric ulcers is a partial GASTRECTOMY, in which the lower part of the stomach is removed.

Gastritis

Inflammation of the mucous membrane lining the stomach. Gastritis may be sudden and acute, or chronic (persistent over a long period). In most cases, it exhibits no symptoms, but can cause indigestion, nausea, and vomiting. Gastritis is occasionally accompanied by GASTRIC EROSION, a superficial raw area in the mucous membrane that lines the stomach. Contributing factors can include bacteria, viruses, and substances that damage the protective mucous lining of the stomach, leaving it more vulnerable to attack by harsh acids and enzymes. As with PEPTIC ULCER DISEASE, the bacterium *Helicobacter pylori* (H. PYLORI) is believed to have a role in gastritis. Inflammation may also be linked to the use of nonsteroidal anti-inflammatory drugs (NSAIDs), such as aspirin, which irritate the stomach lining. These drugs are often used to alleviate musculoskeletal problems, such as arthritis. Gastritis may also occur as a result of alcohol use, heavy smoking, or as a side effect of other drugs, including certain anticancer medications.

DIAGNOSIS AND TREATMENT

Gastritis is diagnosed by physical examination, medical history, gastroscopy (visual examination of the esophagus, stomach, and esophagus through a lighted tube), or an upper GASTROINTESTINAL (GI) SERIES (an X-ray procedure also called a barium swallow).

Treatment of gastritis depends on its underlying cause. For example, a physician may prescribe antiarthritis medications called COX-2 inhibitors that are less likely to cause gastrointestinal side effects than are ordinary NSAIDs. Or the physician may recommend taking the medication with an antacid or acid-suppressing medication. Although no single medication has proven effectiveness against *H. pylori*, a medical regimen called triple therapy (the use of three medications at once) can eradicate most cases; the medications include two ANTIBIOTICS and usually one of the PROTON PUMP INHIBITORS. Alcohol and smoking should be avoided.

Gastroenteritis

Inflammation of the stomach and intestines as a result of infection. Gastroenteritis is very common, especially in children. While not usually serious, very young children and older people are at greater risk for complications, such as dehydration or electrolyte imbalance. The symptoms of gastroenteritis range from mild to severe and include nausea, vomiting, and diarrhea; profuse diarrhea can be accompanied by severe cramping, vomiting, weakness, and fever. Persistent diarrhea may also lead to DEHYDRATION, upsetting body chemistry and depleting important body salts. Left untreated, dehydration can lead to shock. Diarrhea remains a frequent cause of death in many parts of the world.

Most frequently, gastroenteritis is due to a viral infection. A virus can spread by droplets when an infected person coughs or sneezes or by contact with contaminated items. Viruses, such as the adenovirus, coxsackievirus, and rotavirus, are common causes of gastroenteritis. They enter the digestive tract and multiply, causing inflammation and other symptoms. Sometimes, gastroenteritis is due to eating or drinking contaminated food or water. Food poi-

soning may occur in a lone individual or as an epidemic when a number of people consume the same contaminated food. It results from ingesting either a toxin formed by bacteria or an infectious organism that is in the food. In some cases, gastroenteritis can be attributed to changes in the bacterial population of the digestive tract due to taking antibiotics or traveling to a foreign country. See also DIARRHEA, E. COLI; DIARRHEA, TRAVELER'S.

DIAGNOSIS AND TREATMENT

Within 48 hours, most cases of gastroenteritis clear up without medical intervention. If symptoms persist, medical attention is necessary. The doctor can diagnose the cause of gastroenteritis by asking questions, such as what was eaten, where it was eaten, and whether others also are ill. Tests, such as stool analysis, are sometimes performed to make sure there is not another more serious cause of symptoms.

To treat gastroenteritis, physicians advise resting and drinking oral rehydration fluid, a commercial product that contains water, salts, and glucose. Homemade rehydration solutions also work well. Over-the-counter medications may relieve diarrhea. If gastroenteritis is caused by bacteria, antibiotics may be prescribed. No specific treatment exists for viral gastroenteritis. However, in severe cases, the doctor can prescribe drugs that slow intestinal activity and ease cramping, or antiemetic drugs to control violent vomiting.

To prevent gastroenteritis, doctors recommend eating only foods that have been prepared under hygienic conditions. Hands must always be washed with soap and very warm water after using the toilet and before preparing food. When traveling in areas where conditions may be unsanitary, it is best to drink only bottled water, avoid fresh fruits, and eat only thoroughly cooked foods because high temperatures destroy infectious organisms.

Gastroenterologist

A physician who specializes in the diseases, disorders, and conditions of the gastrointestinal tract from the mouth to the anus, including diseases of the liver, gallbladder, and pancreas. Most gastroenterologists are

board-certified in both internal medicine and gastroenterology. Gastroenterologists often use various visualizing tools to examine the lining of the gastrointestinal tract and to take samples for laboratory analysis. They also advise on diet and lifestyle as they relate to the health of the digestive tract.

Gastroenterology

The study of diseases, disorders, and conditions of the gastrointestinal tract, including the esophagus, stomach, small intestine, colon, liver, gallbladder, pancreas, and bile ducts.

Gastroesophageal reflux disease (GERD)

See ESOPHAGEAL REFLUX.

Gastrointestinal (GI) series

A series of X rays using the contrast medium barium. An upper GI series uses X rays to diagnose problems in the esophagus, stomach, and duodenum (the first part of the small intestine into which the stomach empties). This series is also known as a barium swallow. A lower GI series uses X rays to examine problems in the large intestine, which includes the rectum and colon. This series is often called a barium enema.

An upper GI series can detect problems, such as a blockage, abnormal growth, ulcer, hernia, or accumulation of scar tissue. To prepare for the test, an individual drinks a chalky barium solution that coats and outlines the walls of the esophagus, stomach, and duodenum. Barium makes the linings of these organs show up more clearly on X rays. In some cases, the doctor also uses an X-ray machine known as a fluoroscope to follow the path of barium to the stomach as a person swallows. An upper GI series takes 1 to 2 hours. There is little discomfort, although barium may cause constipation and white stools for a few days following the procedure.

A lower GI series can reveal problems such as abnormal growths, ulcers, polyps, diverticula, and inflammation. Because it requires an empty colon, a restricted diet is required for a few days before the procedure. An enema or laxative may also be given. In the test, a thick liquid containing barium is inserted anally and passes into the colon and rectum. Air may be pumped into the colon to help provide better contrast, and then, X rays are taken. The barium causes a sense of pressure and fullness in the abdomen, sometimes causing discomfort. Although rare, there may be an urge to have a bowel movement. After X rays are taken, the patient defecates. Additional X rays may then be taken of the empty colon. A lower GI series takes 1 to 2 hours. Constipation and white or gray color in the stool may persist for a few days after the procedure.

Gastrointestinal system

See DIGESTIVE SYSTEM.

Gastrointestinal tract

See ALIMENTARY TRACT; DIGESTIVE SYSTEM.

Gastrojejunostomy

A surgically created connection between the stomach and small intestine that is specifically designed to bypass the duodenum (the first part of the small intestine into which the stomach empties). A surgeon performs a gastrojejunostomy to prevent gastric acid from causing further irritation to a DUODENAL ULCER.

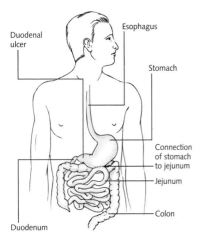

Esophagus

Duodenal ulcer

Stomach

Connection of stomach to jejunum

Jejunum

Colon

Duodenum

BYPASSING A DUODENAL ULCER
In a person with a duodenal ulcer, a surgical procedure called a gastrojejunostomy can be done to connect the stomach directly to the jejunum, the midsection of the small intestine, so that gastric acid will not pass through the duodenum and irritate the ulcer.

Gastroscopy

A procedure in which the linings of the esophagus, stomach, and duodenum are examined by using a slim, flexible, lighted tube called a gastroscope. Gastroscopy is a type of ENDOSCOPY that enables the physician to view, photograph, and videotape the inside of the body without surgery. The procedure is also known as upper endoscopy, esophagogastroduodenoscopy, esophagogastroscopy, and esophagoscopy, depending on what is being examined. A gastroscopy may be performed to help determine the cause of dysphagia (difficulty swallowing), nausea, vomiting, INDIGESTION, ESOPHAGEAL REFLUX (the backward flow of stomach acid into the esophagus), bleeding, abdominal pain, or chest pain. Gastroscopy may also be used in the emergency diagnosis and management of bleeding. By using this procedure, the physician can detect abnormalities that may not appear on X rays.

HOW IT IS DONE

Food and liquids should not be consumed for 6 to 8 hours preceding gastroscopy in order to empty the stomach and duodenum. To reduce discomfort and gagging, the throat is sometimes sprayed with a local anesthetic shortly before the procedure. Additional pain medication or an intravenous sedative is used during the examination. In the procedure, the gastroscope is passed through the mouth and the throat to the esophagus, stomach, and duodenum. The scope inflates the stomach to increase visibility. If an abnormality is present, the doctor can take a small tissue sample through the instru-ment for further analysis.

A gastroscopy takes about 20 minutes. After the procedure, it is usually necessary to rest an hour or two until medication wears off. The only side effect of a gastroscopy is a mild sore throat. However, rare complications may include bleeding and puncture of the stomach lining.

Gastrostomy

A surgical procedure in which an external opening, or STOMA, is created in the stomach. The stoma provides a passageway through the abdominal wall for a temporary or permanent tube. The tube may be used for either feeding or drainage.

Gatekeeper

A primary care provider, usually a family physician, internist, or pediatrician, who provides primary health care services to people enrolled in health insurance plans. A gatekeeper is generally responsible for coordinating a person's overall health care. In health plans that use a gatekeeper, the doctor, except in time of an emergency, is consulted before using services such as laboratory testing or being referred to a specialist. Gatekeepers are sometimes called care coordinators. There are some who prefer the term "gate openers" so as not to associate the process with denial of treatment, but rather with providing appropriate and timely health care services.

Gaucher disease

An inherited illness caused by a gene mutation. In Gaucher disease, an enzyme defect results in the body's inability to break down a key fatty substance. Gaucher disease is inherited as an autosomal recessive trait, meaning the parents carry it but do not have it. It is common among Ashkenazi Jews of central or eastern European descent, occurring in one of 500 babies. The disease can appear at any age, and the later in life the first symptoms appear, the less severe the disease usually will be.

People with Gaucher disease lack the enzyme needed to break down the fatty substance called glucocerebroside into glucose and a fat called ceramide. Glucocerebroside accumulates and is consumed by macrophages, specialized scavenger cells. These enlarged macrophages, called Gaucher cells, tend to gather in the spleen, liver, and bone marrow. When an organ containing Gaucher cells becomes enlarged and impaired, symptoms develop.

The nature and severity of the symptoms vary widely, depending on the organ involved. When Gaucher cells accumulate in the spleen, for example, it becomes enlarged and overactive. An enlarged spleen may make a person look overweight or pregnant. An overactive spleen breaks down red blood cells faster than they can be produced, leading to a deficiency, or anemia. People with anemia often feel weak and lack energy. The spleen may also break down platelets too rapidly, leading to easy bruising. When

Gaucher cells accumulate in the liver, it can become enlarged and function abnormally. Some people will develop cirrhosis, or scarring, of the liver. Gaucher cells that accumulate in the bone marrow can result in the bones becoming prone to infection, thinner or weaker than normal, or so brittle that they break easily. People with Gaucher disease often complain of general bone and joint pain.

Symptoms appear in varying degrees and may include a lack of energy and stamina, enlarged spleen or liver, pain, compression of the lungs, growth retardation in children, pain and degeneration of joints, loss of bone density, disruption of kidney function, jaundice (yellow skin color), purplish red spots around the eyes, frequent nosebleeds and bruises, abnormal blood counts, loss of appetite, and intestinal complaints.

Until recently, treatment was limited to symptom management, including bed rest, pain medication, oxygen therapy, and sometimes surgery to remove damaged organs or reduce pressure on bones. It is now possible to supplement or replace the enzyme needed to break down glucocerebroside in people with some types of Gaucher disease. Enzyme replacement therapy is given intravenously every 2 weeks and can stop or reverse symptoms completely. This treatment is relatively new and very expensive, but has been found to be safe and effective.

Gauze

A thin, loosely woven surgical dressing usually made of cotton. Gauze has been used for wound care for centuries because it is absorbent yet permits moisture to escape. Gauze dressings are available in many forms and sizes and are used as a bandage and in dressings and surgical sponges. When used during surgery, gauze is sterilized with antiseptics.

Named for Gaza, the city where it was first manufactured, gauze is available as sponges, pads, ropes, ribbons, strips, and on rolls. Gauzes vary in the tightness of their weave, ranging from heavyweight to lightweight gauze. Woven gauzes are made of cotton and woven like fabric, while nonwoven gauzes are usually made of synthetic fibers pressed together to resemble woven fabric.

Gay

A slang term for homosexual. See HOMOSEXUALITY.

G-CSF

Granulocyte colony-stimulating factor; a chemical that fosters the development of the white blood cells known as granulocytes. This growth factor is used to treat people with leukopenia (a very low white blood cell count), particularly after bone marrow transplant or intensive chemotherapy for cancer.

Gem therapy

See CRYSTAL THERAPY.

Gemfibrozil

A drug used to lower both cholesterol and triglyceride levels. Gemfibrozil (Lopid) is an antilipemic drug to reduce the risk of heart disease by treating hyperlipidemia (high blood triglyceride level) and hypercholesterolemia (high blood cholesterol levels) when diet and other drugs have not been effective.

Gender-identity disorder

Acting and presenting oneself as a member of the opposite sex, combined with strong feelings of discomfort in one's physical gender, for a period of at least 2 years. This rare disorder appears in both children and adults. Children with the disorder want to be the opposite sex, express revulsion at their own genitals, dress in the clothes of the opposite sex, play games and pursue pastimes typical of the opposite sex, and strongly prefer friendships with the opposite sex. Adults typically want to be rid of their genitals, desire to live as a member of the opposite sex, believe their emotions and feelings are more like those of the opposite sex than their own, and may be erotically oriented to either same-sex or opposite-sex relationships. They also seek to rid themselves of the obvious characteristics of their sex by taking hormones, having facial hair removed, or seeking sex-change surgery. Both children and adults tend to be socially isolated by peer pressure and rejection and to experience depression and anxiety as a result.

The course of the disorder depends on when it begins. In boys, the disorder usually begins between 2 and 4 years of age and is typically resolved by adolescence. However, in a minority of cases, the disorder continues into adulthood. These individuals usually seek sex-reassignment surgery as adults. If the disorder begins in late adolescence or adulthood, the degree of cross-gender identification is more changeable, and the individual is less likely to seek surgery as a solution.

The cause of gender-identity disorder is not fully understood. Theories linking the disorder to inherited abnormalities, imbalances in hormones, and defective bonding in early childhood have been proposed. Treatment often consists of family and individual psychotherapy. Sex-change surgery is an option for some individuals, but emotional problems may continue.

Gene

The fundamental unit of genetic inheritance within a chromosome; a segment of DEOXYRIBONUCLEIC ACID (DNA) containing a sequence of biochemical information that determines a particular genetic trait. The sequence is called the genetic code. Each DNA molecule contains many genes and is located within the cell nucleus. Each gene contains the instructions to synthesize a specific protein that has a specific function. RIBONUCLEIC ACID (RNA) works as a messenger that carries the genetic instructions to a site in the outer cell where protein is manufactured. Every human cell holds within its nucleus more than 80,000 genes. Genes con-

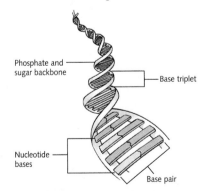

Phosphate and sugar backbone

Base triplet

Nucleotide bases

Base pair

BASIC UNIT OF HEREDITY
Genes direct the function of all body organs and processes by regulating the production of many types of essential proteins.

tain all of the information needed to direct the body to function properly.

Gene mapping

The construction of detailed guides that plot the type and location of genes on chromosomes. One goal of the HUMAN GENOME PROJECT, a long-term international research program, is to create accurate genetic maps of the human genome, or the complete set of chromosomes inherited by humans from their parents. The human genome is estimated to contain 50,000 to 100,000 genes, making up the complete set of instructions for the development and functioning of a human being.

Two types of mapping have been developed by the Human Genome Project: gene mapping and physical mapping. Gene mapping identifies the relative order of genes along a chromosome, while physical mapping involves more precise methods, making it possible to place genes at specific distances from one another on a chromosome. Both types of mapping use genetic markers, particular physical or molecular characteristics that differ among individuals and are passed from one generation to the next.

Gene therapy

Changing the function of some genes in order to treat, cure, or prevent disease. Gene therapy is a largely experimental approach to the treatment of disease that involves replacing or counteracting a person's faulty gene. Potentially, it may be an alternative way to aid the production of proteins such as insulin and growth hormones. Gene therapy is intended to correct certain diseases at their most fundamental level and has been compared to the transplantation of a tiny organ. Now that one of the genes associated with diabetes mellitus type 2 has been identified, for example, it may be possible to treat diabetes with a new or treated gene transplanted into the appropriate chromosome. The transplanted gene may permanently restore an individual's ability to produce insulin.

Research into gene therapy has been limited to the targeting of specific cells known as somatic (body) cells. The recipient's genetic makeup is altered by the treatment, but the change is not passed along to subse-

quent generations. Methods of gene therapy that would pass altered genes to future generations (germline gene therapy) have not been developed.

A significant challenge is the safe and efficient delivery of genetic material to the appropriate cells of the person. One strategy currently in use involves chemical delivery vehicles called vectors, which enclose therapeutic genes and deliver them to specific cells where they can become a new part of the host cell's DNA. Many of the vectors use modified viruses, life forms that can efficiently enter target cells and deliver genetic material. Gene therapy involves splicing the therapeutic genetic material into the virus's DNA, taking advantage of the virus's delivery system.

Early experiments in gene therapy were designed to treat two genetic disorders: an inherited form of immune deficiency in children and a disorder resulting in extremely high levels of serum cholesterol in both children and adults. Experiments have also been designed to treat cystic fibrosis, in which therapeutic genes are delivered to the person's lung tissue by viruses known to cause respiratory disease, during which there may be some risk of viral infection. Gene therapy is also being investigated for heart disease, cancer, and infectious diseases such as AIDS (acquired immunodeficiency syndrome). In studies, gene therapy has been used to treat single-cell defects such as hemophilia, muscular dystrophy, and sickle cell anemia, but the therapies remain largely experimental.

General anesthesia
See ANESTHESIA, GENERAL.

Generalized anxiety disorder
See ANXIETY DISORDERS.

Generic drug

A drug that is not protected by a trademark; the scientific name for a drug as opposed to its proprietary or brand name. Generic drugs contain identical active ingredients and amounts as the brand-name equivalents, but they are usually less expensive.

Genetic code

The biochemical language by which all known organisms transfer genetic

information. DNA (DEOXYRIBONUCLEIC ACID) uses the genetic code to communicate the information or instructions that allow specific genes to function. A genetic code is present in all animals, plants, fungi, bacteria, and viruses.

The code is read and communicated in a series of chemical reactions involving DNA and a genetic messenger called RNA (RIBONUCLEIC ACID). DNA is a two-stranded molecule. Each strand is made up of four chemical substances called nucleosides, or bases: A (adenosine), T (thymidine), C (cytidine), and G (guanosine). These chemicals occur in specific sequences that run in opposite order on the two strands. One strand of DNA has distinct sections that contain the information needed to replicate genes, while the other strand contains information to be decoded by RNA. The strands connect via bonds between the A, T, C, and G chemicals called base pairs. To make a protein, the strands separate; the DNA translates the genetic code through the base pairs to a new strand of messenger RNA, which then moves outside the cell nucleus to the cytoplasm where RNA directs the production of protein according to the genetic code.

Genetic counseling

A process in which individuals or families at risk for genetic disorders can learn about the disorders and the options for dealing with them. Genetic counseling is intended to help individuals or families understand the role a genetic disorder may have in their family, help them make informed choices in deciding how to cope with the risk and the disorder, and help them find appropriate medical care and other services.

Because many birth defects are the result of inherited genetic disorders, couples with family histories of birth defects or genetic disorders such as Down syndrome, Tay-Sachs disease, sickle cell anemia, mental retardation, or spina bifida should consult genetic counselors before starting families. Women who become pregnant after age 35 and those who are married to relatives of women who have had multiple miscarriages should also receive counseling. Genetic counseling can help couples assess their risks of having children with genetic disorders.

GENETIC COUNSELORS

Genetic counselors are health professionals with experience in counseling in addition to specialized training in the field of medical genetics. Most genetic counselors have master's degrees in genetic counseling. Trained genetic counselors provide information and support to persons and families who have relatives with birth defects or inherited disorders. They also provide assistance in helping families locate appropriate services, such as special education or financial aid.

Genetic disorders

Medical conditions caused by errors in genetic material. Some genetic disorders cause medical problems that are apparent at birth, while others do not show up until later in life. Some genetic disorders, such as CYSTIC FIBROSIS, can be so severe that they ultimately cause death, while others, like color blindness, produce mild symptoms. Genetic disorders can be rare or common. They can be caused by an error in the DNA of a single gene; by abnormalities of entire chromosomes; by combinations of genes and environmental factors, such as diet or chemical exposure; or by mutations in MITOCHONDRIA (self-reproducing parts of cells).

Genetic engineering

Alteration of an organism's hereditary material to eliminate undesirable characteristics or to create desirable new ones. Examples of genetic engineering include selective breeding of plants and animals and the creation of hybrids by combining elements of different strains or species to create new ones. Genetic engineering is used to increase food production, to produce vaccines and other drugs, and to help eliminate industrial waste.

The first technique used to engineer genetic material was selective breeding of plants and animals to increase crop yield and improve nutrition. Corn, for example, has been bred selectively for thousands of years to make its kernels bigger and to expand its nutritional content. Animals have been bred selectively for food or for other purposes, such as the develop-

ment of champion racehorses or show dogs. Hybridization, or cross-breeding, has been performed for at least 3,000 years. Hybrids featuring the most desirable qualities can be created from members of the same species with different characteristics or from members of different species. Mules, for example, are created by breeding female horses with male donkeys.

The newest method by which genetic engineering is implemented is RECOMBINANT DNA, or gene splicing. In this method, one or more genes of an organism are introduced into a second organism. If the DNA is incorporated into the second organism, recombined DNA is said to exist. This technique is involved in the development of GENE THERAPY.

Genetic probe

Fluorescence in situ hybridization (FISH) testing. A test of DNA (deoxyribonucleic acid) designed to identify the presence of genetic defects in a person or, usually, a fetus. In a genetic probe, a particular fragment of DNA is examined for genetic markers, specific base sequences (chemical configurations) that have been associated with a genetic defect. Genetic probes can be used to detect the presence of DOWN SYNDROME, CYSTIC FIBROSIS, TRISOMY 21 SYNDROME, TRISOMY 13 SYNDROME, and TRISOMY 18 SYNDROME and such chromosomal abnormalities as KLINEFELTER SYNDROME and TURNER SYNDROME.

Various techniques are used in genetic probes. In one, enzymes are used to break down the chromosome (taken from a cell of the fetus or individual being tested). The resulting fragments are then placed in a filter with a radioactively labeled sequence of DNA (from another source) that is coded to bind to the genetic marker for the suspected defect. Special techniques detect whether the chromosome fragment binds to the marker. If it does, most likely the person or fetus has the defect. GENETIC COUNSELING is generally the next step.

Genetic screening

Medically testing members of a population for individuals who have genes associated with a disease; a form of preventive medicine. Because many diseases are passed from generation

to generation, genetic screening is used to detect disease by identifying persons who are at risk.

Various types of genetic screening are used. Prenatal screening, such as AMNIOCENTESIS, is used to determine whether a fetus is at risk for various genetic diseases or traits. In newborn screening, blood tests are performed on babies shortly after birth to detect certain congenital disorders, including PKU (phenylketonuria), HEMOGLOBINOPATHY, and CONGENITAL HYPOTHYROIDISM, which can be treated before symptoms appear. Sometimes blood or tissue samples are taken from a healthy person who may be a carrier of an inheritable genetic trait, such as SICKLE CELL ANEMIA or TAY-SACHS DISEASE, and may pass it along to offspring. Susceptibility screening tests individuals for their genetic susceptibility to environmental hazards or other toxic substances to which they may have been exposed. Screening is also done to detect the presence of genes for a specific inherited illness, such as Huntington disease, or for genes associated with a risk for developing cancer, such as breast cancer or colon cancer.

Genetics

The branch of biology that is concerned with genes and heredity. Genetics involves the study of the origin of an individual's characteristics and the manner in which they are passed along to offspring. Characteristics are determined by the way an individual's genes, inherited from the parents, interact with the environment throughout development. For the most part, genes are inherited without mishap, but sometimes changes, or genetic defects, occur unexpectedly. Medical genetics is the study of the relationship between heredity and disease.

Genetics, behavioral

A specialized area of psychological research that studies the role of inherited traits in shaping individual personality. Many behavioral genetics studies focus on twins. Identical twins who are raised together share the same genetic makeup and the same home environment, while fraternal twins raised together share the same home environment but not the same genetic makeup. Certain studies have also focused on identical twins who grew up in different homes. These research projects allow geneticists to determine how much of individual personality arises from inheritance (sometimes called "nature") and how much comes from environmental influences in upbringing (sometimes referred to as "nurture.") Studies comparing behavioral traits in identical and fraternal twins have found that about 40 to 50 percent of differences in personality are due to genetics and that environment accounts for about 30 percent. One of the most surprising findings of behavioral genetics is that parental behavior, apart from extremes of abuse and neglect, has relatively little effect on personality. Environmental influences, such as school and friends, may have more of an impact. However, these effects may also be subtly genetic, since people tend to seek out or create environments to which they are predisposed by their inherited personality characteristics.

Behavioral genetics has also been important in determining the patterns of inheritance governing psychiatric disorders and mental illness. The major mental illnesses, such as schizophrenia and bipolar disorder, appear to be largely inherited.

Genital herpes

See HERPES, GENITAL; SEXUALLY TRANSMITTED DISEASES.

Genital ulceration

A lesion or sore on the external genitals, including the vulva, labia, penis, and anus. Genital ulcerations are caused by one of several infectious organisms, most of which are spread by sexual contact. They require medical attention to prevent the development of later complications and should not be self-treated.

The more common infections that can cause a genital ulceration include SEXUALLY TRANSMITTED DISEASES, LYMPHOGRANULOMA VENEREUM (LGV), CHANCROID, and SYPHILIS. See also CHANCRE.

Genital warts

Warts that develop in the genital area, including the urethra and the rectum,

that are caused by HUMAN PAPILLOMAVIRUS (HPV). Genital warts are one of the most common of the SEXUALLY TRANSMITTED DISEASES. See also CONDYLOMA ACUMINATUM.

Genitalia

The male and female reproductive organs, both external and internal. The male genitalia include the penis, testicles, prostate gland, seminal vesicles, and system of ducts. The female genitalia include the ovaries, fallopian tubes, uterus, vagina, mons pubis, clitoris, and labia. See REPRODUCTIVE SYSTEM, FEMALE; REPRODUCTIVE SYSTEM, MALE.

Genotype

The entire genetic makeup of an individual. See also PHENOTYPE.

Gentamicin

An antibiotic used to treat a wide variety of bacterial infections. Gentamicin (Garamycin and others) works by inhibiting bacterial protein synthesis. It is available as an ointment to treat eye infections, as a skin cream or ointment to treat skin infections, and as an injection to treat serious infections.

Gentian violet

A green to purple dye that is an effective medication against infections of certain kinds of bacteria, fungi, and parasitic worms. Gentian violet is applied directly to infected surface tissues, such as skin and mucous membranes, and given orally for infestations of pinworms in the intestine and liver infections. The dye is also used to stain bacteria for viewing under a microscope (see GRAM STAIN).

Geographic tongue

A condition producing a maplike appearance on the TONGUE due to the breakdown of PAPILLA (tiny surface cell projection that coats the tongue) producing smooth, dark or bright red patches with sharp, raised margins on some areas on the tongue's surface. There may also be deep crevices on the tongue. These patches may change from day to day or remain the same. They may intermittently disappear and then recur. Causes of the condition are unclear. A person who has geographic tongue usually does not have any symptoms but may find

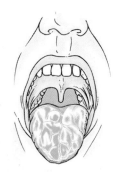

GEOGRAPHIC TONGUE
A geographic tongue is so named because the surface has smooth areas and crevices that make the tongue look something like a map. The appearance is caused by the breakdown of the tiny bumps (papillae) that form the surface of a normal tongue. The smooth areas may change from day to day. The condition is harmless and painless, and the cause is not known.

contact with certain foods or substances mildly painful. Even toothpaste can cause soreness. Although uncomfortable, the condition is considered harmless. No specific treatment is available, but avoiding spicy foods, hot foods and beverages, alcohol, and tobacco can help prevent discomfort.

Geriatric care manager

A private case or care manager who helps caregivers locate and coordinate health and social services. Usually a nurse or social worker with special training in geriatrics, a geriatric care manager will evaluate an older person's situation, make recommendations for care, and arrange services. Areas covered may include the person's health care needs, housekeeping, and diet. For a monthly fee, the care manager will continue to monitor services and report to the family. Sometimes, care managers are employed by HMOs (health maintenance organizations) to supervise care of clients. See also CAREGIVING FOR OLDER PEOPLE.

Geriatric medicine

A medical specialty concerning the treatment of older people. While older adults experience many of the same illnesses and conditions as younger people, their response to diseases often differs. Changes due to aging in many of the body's organs create unique circumstances. As a consequence, some infections or injuries that are not life threatening to a younger person can be fatal to an older one if not treated aggressively. Also, because the body changes with age, medications are used in different dosages in geriatric medicine.

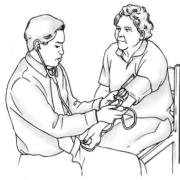

GERIATRICS
The treatment of older people is now a medical specialty. Aging causes the body to respond differently to disease and to medication, so diagnosis and treatment may differ from those for a younger person. A doctor who specializes in geriatrics has specifically studied aging and its effects on the body.

Geriatrician

A physician specializing in GERIATRIC MEDICINE, the medical specialty concerned with the treatment of older adults and the conditions associated with AGING.

Germ

Any tiny, living, disease-causing agent; the term often describes disease-producing microorganisms, such as bacteria and viruses. The germ theory of disease was proposed in the later half of the 19th century when Louis Pasteur's research suggested that human diseases were caused by specific microorganisms called germs.

Germ cell tumor

A tumor that develops typically in the reproductive tissues that become egg cells or sperm cells. Germ cell tumors are a type of ovarian or testicular cancer. About 95 percent of all testicular cancers are germ cell tumors. A small group of cancers known as extragonadal germ cell tumors, which do not involve reproductive tissue, have been identified in recent years. These tumors develop in the central nervous system and

account for about 2 percent of all brain tumors in the United States. Usually they occur in adolescence and young adulthood.

Germ cell tumors sometimes can be identified through two blood tests—the alpha-fetoprotein (AFP) and the human chorionic gonadotropin (HCG) tests. They are usually treated with chemotherapy. They constitute one of the few groups of solid tumors that can be cured with chemotherapy even after the disease has metastasized (spread) to other organs. Certain combinations of drugs will cure up to 70 percent of patients with metastatic germ cell tumors.

German measles

See RUBELLA.

Gerontologist

A specialist in the scientific study of all aspects of the aging process, from clinical, biological, historical, mental, and sociological perspectives.

Gerontology

The scientific study of all aspects of the aging process, from clinical, biological, historical, mental, and sociological perspectives.

Gerson therapy

Dietary therapy in which the body's self-healing abilities are thought to be boosted by the consumption of large doses of enzymes and other nutrients. Gerson therapy was developed in the 1920s by Max Gerson, a medical doctor who believed that degenerative diseases such as cancer, tuberculosis, severe headaches, arthritis, and diabetes mellitus are caused by toxic, degraded food, water, and air. He believed that the increased cancer rate was due to agricultural fertilizers and food processing.

Gerson therapy seeks to restore health by the daily consumption of about 20 pounds of fresh, organically grown fruits and vegetables, chiefly used to make fresh raw juice consumed 13 times per day. Solid food is eaten raw or cooked, and animal fats, sodium, and excess protein are avoided.

Gerson therapy also uses intensive DETOXIFICATION to eliminate wastes from the body, on the principle that degenerative disease makes the body progressively unable to do so. Gerson

advocated using COFFEE ENEMAS, self-administered several times a day, though the safety of such enemas has not been proven. The dietary regimen is intended to flood the cells of the body with easily assimilated, wholesome nutrients that strengthen the immune system, while the detoxification program allegedly eliminates toxins that interfere with healing.

Gestalt theory

An approach to understanding human psychology that holds that experience affects the entire body and mind and can be understood only in terms of the total effects throughout the person's being in the present time. Gestalt therapists focus on the here and now, deal with the past only insofar as it affects the present, and make their patients aware of physical events such as muscle tension and breathing patterns, as well as thoughts and ideas. (This is in contrast with FREUDIAN THEORY, which concentrates on childhood experiences and memories.) Gestalt in German means "complete form" or "entire shape."

Gestation

Pregnancy; the period of time during which a fetus develops in the uterus, from conception to childbirth. The average time span for gestation is 266 days, or 38 weeks, from the date of fertilization. Since that date is rarely known, doctors traditionally measure gestation from the beginning of the mother's last menstrual period, calculating the baby's due date as 280 days, or 40 weeks, from that point. A pregnancy that results in a birth within 2 weeks of the predicted due date is called a term pregnancy.

Gestational diabetes

A form of diabetes that has its onset or is first diagnosed during pregnancy. In this condition, the pancreas is unable to produce enough insulin to counteract the hormones produced during pregnancy that increase the sugar level in the blood. Women who are older than 30 years, obese, have a family history of diabetes, or have had problems with a pregnancy before, such as a stillbirth or an unusually large baby, are considered to be at risk for gestational diabetes.

About 5 percent of pregnant women develop this condition, usually between the 24th and 28th weeks of pregnancy.

DIAGNOSIS AND TREATMENT

Gestational diabetes is diagnosed with a GLUCOSE TOLERANCE TEST. In this test, the woman drinks a sugar solution, and an hour later, her blood sugar level is measured. If the level is high, a more extensive test, the 3-hour glucose tolerance test, may be used to confirm the diagnosis. For the 3-hour test, the woman consumes a diet high in carbohydrates for 3 days in order to stimulate the pancreas to produce as much insulin as it can. After that, she fasts overnight; her blood sugar level is tested the next morning. Then, she drinks another sugar solution, and her blood sugar level is measured 1, 2, and 3 hours later. If two of the four blood sugar levels are abnormal, the diagnosis is confirmed. Women considered to be at risk for gestational diabetes are likely to be given the 1-hour glucose tolerance test during the first trimester of pregnancy and again between the 24th and 28th weeks.

TREATMENT

Gestational diabetes is initially treated with diet and exercise. A diet low in fat and high in dietary fiber, with a total daily intake of 1,800 to 2,400 calories, is essential to controlling diabetes. Participating in daily exercise, such as swimming, walking, or stationary bike riding, is also important. Women with gestational diabetes may need to check their blood sugar levels four times a day throughout pregnancy. For women whose blood sugar level remains high after 1 to 2 weeks of diet and exercise, insulin may be required. After delivery, women with gestational diabetes are at risk for developing diabetes in the future and should be monitored. Risk factors that can be modified, such as obesity and a sedentary lifestyle, should be addressed.

Gestational trophoblastic disease

A group of pregnancy-related conditions in which abnormal growths develop inside the uterus from abnormal fetal tissue. The conditions include a hydatidiform mole, a type

of tumor, and the cancer CHORIOCARCINOMA, both of which involve trophoblasts, cells that make up one of the layers of the placenta. Symptoms include vaginal bleeding and excessive morning sickness early in pregnancy. The doctor may find that the uterus is larger than expected for the stage of the pregnancy, and there may be no detectable fetal heartbeat. Urine tests and blood tests usually show higher than normal levels of human chorionic gonadotropin, a hormone secreted by cells in the placenta.

Gestational trophoblastic disease is usually treated by removing the contents of the uterus during a D AND C. If a woman has completed her childbearing years, a hysterectomy may be performed. After both procedures, the woman's blood is tested for human chorionic gonadotropin every 1 to 2 weeks until levels are normal, and thereafter at 3-month intervals for 6 to 12 months to make sure the tumor has been completely removed from the uterus. Choriocarcinoma is also treated with CHEMOTHERAPY, almost always successfully. Women who have had a trophoblastic disease should wait at least a year after treatment before becoming pregnant again.

GI series

See GASTROINTESTINAL (GI) SERIES.

Giant cell arteritis

See ARTERITIS, GIANT CELL.

Giardiasis

A disease caused by the microscopic parasite called *Giardia lamblia* (*G. lamblia*) that lives in the small intestines of humans and animals. The cysts of the parasite in its infectious stage are passed out of the body in bowel movements. These cysts are environmentally resistant and can live outside a person or animal for long periods. *Giardia lamblia* exists throughout the world and is found in soil, food, water, and on contaminated surfaces. *Giardia lamblia* is one of the most common causes of waterborne illness in humans living in the United States. It is spread when a person accidentally ingests the parasite.

HOW IT IS SPREAD

Infection may occur by one of several different ways. Transmission sometimes occurs by direct person-to-person contact, particularly in mental

institutions and day care centers and among sexual partners, especially promiscuous male homosexuals. Infection rates are high in people who have had stomach surgery, who have chronic pancreatitis, and who have hypogammaglobulinemia.

A person may acquire giardiasis by swallowing water containing cysts of the parasite while swimming in lakes, rivers, springs, ponds, or streams contaminated by sewage or fecal material from animals or humans. The infection may be acquired from swimming pools, as the cysts are resistant to routine levels of chlorination.

The illness may also be contracted by eating uncooked, unwashed food that is contaminated with *G. lamblia*. The parasite can be acquired from contact with surfaces contaminated by fecal matter from an infected child or adult. These surfaces may include bathroom fixtures, diaper-changing tables, diaper pails, and young children's toys. A person's hands may become contaminated if good hygiene and hand washing are not practiced, particularly after using the toilet or changing an infant's diapers.

In countries where public sanitation standards are poor, open sewers in city streets and contamination of drinking water may be sources of infection. Giardiasis frequently occurs in countries in which public drinking water is chlorinated but poorly filtered and in communities where the use of human feces for crop fertilization is common. Visitors to these regions may acquire "traveler's diarrhea," which is often giardiasis. In more developed countries, drinking water may be contaminated when septic systems are located near wells. In rural areas, well water can become contaminated if animal waste seepage contaminates a well, particularly if the well is poorly constructed, if the casings are cracked, or if the well is too shallow.

It is believed that giardiasis infects beavers in the wild and that campers who drink water from streams may be infected in this way. Streams may also be contaminated from human feces, and stream water should always be treated before drinking. Boiling water kills the infectious cysts of the parasite, and commercially available filters remove the cysts from drinking water. Iodine disinfec-

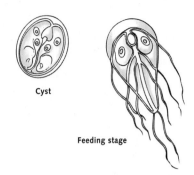

Cyst

Feeding stage

A HARDY, COMMON PARASITE
The one-celled parasite that causes giardiasis is protected by an outer shell that enables it to live outside a host for long time. When it passes into a host organism, it breaks out of this cyst and goes into its active, mobile feeding stage.

tion requires 8 hours to destroy the cysts.

SYMPTOMS, DIAGNOSIS, AND TREATMENT
Not every person who becomes infected with giardiasis has symptoms, and a person with a mild infection may not have any symptoms at all, or mild symptoms may include intermittent flatulence and watery diarrhea, mild abdominal cramps, and bloating. The illness may have a chronic phase in which these symptoms are experienced periodically. In more serious, acute infections, the symptoms can include severe and chronic diarrhea, abdominal cramps, and nausea. Associated symptoms may include fever, chills, malaise, and headaches. Symptoms of giardiasis usually appear within 1 to 3 weeks after ingestion of the parasite and may last 4 to 6 weeks or longer, at which point dehydration and malabsorption of sugars and fat lead to weight loss.

Diagnosis is generally made by laboratory evaluation of a stool sample that reveals the presence of the parasite's cysts or trophozoites, which are another infectious stage of the parasite's life cycle. When the illness is chronic, it can be difficult to diagnose and may require a person who is suspected of having an infection to submit several stool samples over a period of several days. In some cases, samples of the contents of the upper small intestines may be obtained by drawing fluid (aspiration) using an ENDOSCOPE. Blood tests may be used to detect the parasites.

The illness is treated with one of several prescription medications available. Oral METRONIDAZOLE is considered effective, as is oral furazolidone, which is available in liquid form for young children. It is recommended that people who have acquired the infection without symptoms be treated to help prevent spreading it to others.

GIFT
Gamete intrafallopian transfer. GIFT is an ASSISTED REPRODUCTIVE TECHNOLOGY (ART) in which sperm and unfertilized eggs (gametes) are placed in a fallopian tube for normal fertilization. The advantages of this procedure over IN VITRO FERTILIZATION are that embryos develop in their natural environment and reach the uterus at the right time. This is the only ART officially approved by the Roman Catholic Church because fertilization occurs within the body (in vivo).

Gilbert disease
An inherited disorder in which bilirubin is not properly processed in the liver for excretion in the feces. Bilirubin is a by-product of the breakdown of the hemoglobin in red blood cells. The condition is usually diagnosed in the teens or early adulthood. Symptoms are rare, but mild JAUNDICE may appear, particularly if the individual is under stress or is not eating. Jaundice may fluctuate and appear from time to time throughout the person's life, but it will rarely cause health problems. Gilbert disease is more common in males and affects between 2 and 7 percent of the adult population in the United States; it is most commonly recognized when elevated levels of serum bilirubin show up in blood tests in the absence of other illnesses. Gilbert disease is a benign liver disorder that requires no treatment.

Gingiva
The medical term for the gums. The tops of the teeth, or natural crowns, develop within the gingiva, grow outward from it, and are attached by the CEMENTUM, or tissue covering their roots. The gingiva has a rich supply of blood vessels that become red and inflamed if not properly cleansed and stimulated by flossing and using a rubber pick.

Gingivectomy
A minor surgical procedure to remove deep pockets of infected gum tissue or to surgically trim excess gum tissue that has grown over part of the natural crown in a tooth. During the procedure for periodontal pockets, the pocket is cleaned and its soft tissue wall is removed to decrease the depth of the pocket. The purpose of a gingivectomy is to remove extra tissue so that the gum can reattach to the tooth or teeth more securely. The depth of the gum pocket must be reduced so that the patient can brush properly. A gingivectomy may be needed to treat gum inflammation caused by plaque (see PLAQUE, DENTAL). Other causes may include poor ORAL HYGIENE, certain medications, hormonal changes, and irritation from crowns, bridges, or orthodontic braces (see CROWN, DENTAL; BRIDGE, DENTAL; and BRACES, DENTAL). A gingivectomy is performed as an in-office procedure with local anesthesia to prevent pain. After surgery, the gums are sutured and packed with a puttylike material to allow healing. The periodontal packing is generally left in place for 1 or 2 weeks, and this packing does not usually interfere with speaking and eating. If laser surgery is used in a gingivectomy, postoperative pain may be reduced, but the healing time may be extended.

Gingivitis
See PERIODONTAL DISEASE.

Ginkgo biloba
Extracts from the leaves of the ginkgo tree used as an herbal medicine. The ginkgo tree is known to have existed for 300 million years, surviving the Ice Age in China, where it is revered. The ginkgo tree was brought to the United States in 1784. Ginkgo biloba is the most popular herbal medicine in several European countries. The active components of ginkgo leaves are molecules called flavonoid glycosides attached to sugars unique to ginkgo.

Ginkgo biloba is used to treat many conditions. Its chief attributes include the claim—as yet clinically unproven—that it stabilizes tissue membranes, particularly in the brain, and enhances the use of oxygen and glucose. Ginkgo biloba is associated with the ability to prevent metabolic disturbances resulting from insufficient blood supply to the brain. It may also stimulate the system that regulates blood vessel tone, clearing toxic substances accumulated as a result of insufficient oxygen. Its primary clinical use has been in the treatment of vascular problems, such as insufficient artery function in the brain caused by atherosclerosis (hardening of the arteries). By increasing cerebral blood flow, ginkgo biloba may reduce symptoms associated with aging, including short-term memory loss and depression.

Ginseng

A root used as an herbal remedy for various conditions. Ginseng contains steroidlike substances called ginsenosides and panaxosides that are said to stimulate the immune system and to possess antistress properties. Ginseng is cultivated in Korea, Russia, Siberia, China, Japan, and the United States. It is used to treat fatigue, stress, and diabetes and to speed recovery from illness. Ginseng has few toxic side effects and has been used for thousands of years, although some of the claims made for it have never been clinically proven.

Gland

An organ or collection of cells forming a structure that produces and releases chemical substances, principally hormones and enzymes. The substances are released into the system of the body by the glands for a variety of purposes.

As a group, the endocrine glands make up the endocrine system, including the hypothalamus, pituitary gland, thyroid gland, parathyroid glands, thymus gland, adrenal glands, pancreas, ovaries in women, and testicles in men. This system is the chemical control center of the entire body. The ductless glands in this system secrete hormones directly into the bloodstream. The hormones regulate the function of specific tissues or organs and have a role in many vital activities of the body. The pituitary gland is the principal regulator in the system, sending out hormones that control the functions of many of the other glands, including the thyroid, adrenals, ovaries, and testicles. See also EXOCRINE GLAND.

Glands, swollen

Enlarged lymph nodes, also called lymph glands. Swollen glands that enlarge suddenly and feel painful are usually caused by a localized or systemic infection or by an injury. Enlarged glands may also be a sign of a dental abscess. The swelling may also be caused by a reaction to certain medications or vaccines, or it may be caused by sores in the mouth or impacted teeth. When the swelling is gradual and painless, it may result from a tumor.

The lymph glands usually become swollen when the body attempts to fight off the invasion of infectious organisms. The glands are part of the lymphatic system, which produces various blood cells and is important to protecting and maintaining the body's fluids. The glands also have an essential role in defending the body from infection. Some invading organisms that cause illness and infection spread through the lymphatic system and reach the lymph nodes, where they are attacked by a type of white blood cells called lymphocytes. This defensive response is what causes the nodes, or glands, to swell.

Sore, swollen glands usually begin to improve within a few days. Lymph glands generally swell rapidly during the early stages of fighting infection and tend to take longer to return to their normal size. Medical attention is recommended if the glands do not decrease in size over a period of several weeks, if swollen glands are red and tender, if they are located behind the ears in association with a scalp infection, or if they continue to swell for 2 to 3 weeks. If it appears that the swollen glands are the result of a bacterial infection, treatment usually consists of a course of antibiotics.

Glass eye

See EYE, PROSTHETIC.

Glasses

Lenses worn in front of the eyes to compensate for refraction errors. The name comes from the fact that glass was originally used for corrective lenses. Today most glasses have plastic or polycarbonate lenses because these types of lenses are lighter in weight and shatter-resistant. Some lenses use materials that are denser than the usual optical plastics and allow lenses with very strong corrections to be thinner, lighter in weight, and more cosmetically appealing. Coatings added to lenses provide ultraviolet light protection, provide scratch resistance, and reduce reflection and glare.

The shape and thickness of the lens depends on the type and degree of vision error. Lenses for people who are nearsighted subtract focusing power from the eye to allow incoming light to focus on the retina (the thin layer of light-sensitive tissue at the back of the eye) rather than in front of it. Lenses for people who are farsighted add focusing power to bring the focal point forward to the retina. Lens power is measured in diopters, which are negative for nearsightedness and positive for farsightedness. Cylindrical lenses, which curve more in one direction than the other, are used to correct astigmatism, a defect in vision caused by uneven curvature of the eye's clear outer surface (cornea). Prism lenses help the two eyes converge on the same point, usually to prevent double vision.

Multifocal lenses include corrections for vision at different distances. The most common multifocal lens is the bifocal, which has an upper portion for distance vision and a lower for close-up viewing. Trifocals place a lens for intermediate viewing (between 18 and 24 inches) between the distance and close-up lenses. Progressive lenses have no sharp line separating the different viewing areas of the lens. The distance lens melds gradually into the close-up lens and provides an intermediate viewing distance.

Glaucoma

An eye disease characterized by damage to the optic nerve and loss of vision. Often glaucoma is a result of high pressure in the eye. This type of glaucoma results from an abnormality in the space in the front of the eye known as the anterior chamber. The anterior chamber is filled with a fluid (aqueous humor) that bathes and nourishes nearby tissues and is produced continuously. In the normal eye, aqueous humor flows into and out of the anterior chamber in equal amounts, maintaining a constant pressure. In high-pressure glaucoma, the fluid drains more slowly than it flows in, causing a buildup of pressure. Over time, this pressure damages the nerve and impairs the ability to see. Damage caused by glaucoma is irreversible, and untreated glaucoma can eventually lead to blindness. Glaucoma may also affect eyes with normal pressures. Glaucoma affects approximately one in every 100 Americans and is most likely to occur in people older than 50 years.

TYPES

■ *Chronic (open-angle) glaucoma* This is the most common form of the disease. It takes its name from the fact that the angle between the iris and cornea (the clear covering on the exposed portion of the eye) remains open and looks normal. For some still-unknown reason, the drainage system in the front of the eye (the trabecular meshwork) is blocked or fails to function properly. Pressure rises slowly in the eye, gradually affecting the optic nerve. The early stages of the disease are painless and produce no symptoms. Visual loss becomes apparent only as nerve damage progresses and blind spots appear in the field of vision. Peripheral vision (vision to the sides) is affected first, followed by central vision. In most cases, chronic glaucoma affects both eyes.

■ *Acute (angle-closure) glaucoma* This form of the disease comes on very suddenly, causing significant pain and visual effects. The name comes from the fact that the angle between the iris and the cornea closes and prevents normal drainage of aqueous humor. Acute glaucoma usually affects only one eye. An attack of acute glaucoma occurs most commonly during conditions in which the pupil is dilated, such as in a darkened movie theater or as a result of stress. The eye turns red, looks swollen or cloudy, and becomes so painful that nausea and vomiting often result. Vision blurs, and halos may appear around lights. An acute glaucoma attack is an emergency that requires immediate attention. Untreated, the eye can be permanently damaged in as little as 1 or 2 days. Laser surgery is used to clear the blockage and restore normal flow of aqueous humor.

■ *Secondary glaucoma* This form of the disease develops as a complication of other diseases or medical conditions. Secondary glaucoma is associated with advanced cataracts (cloudiness in the lens of the eye); eye surgery;

inflammation of the eye (uveitis); certain eye tumors; traumatic eye injuries; diabetes mellitus, type 1 and type 2; and corticosteroid medications. In one form of the disease, pigmentary glaucoma, pigment flakes off the iris and blocks the trabecular meshwork.

■ *Congenital glaucoma* This form of the disease is present in newborns at birth. It results from abnormal development of the eyes that results in a drainage defect. Children with congenital glaucoma usually have obvious symptoms, such as cloudy eyes, sensitivity to light, buphthalmos ("ox eye"), and excessive tearing. Surgery to repair the faulty drainage may be effective. Cases of glaucoma at birth have a poor prognosis.

RISK FACTORS AND SCREENING

Acute glaucoma is most common in older people and in people who are farsighted. Chronic glaucoma is most common among people older than 50 years with a family history of the disease; those who are of African or Asian descent; those with nearsightedness, previous eye injury, or diabetes mellitus; and those who have used corticosteroid medications for a long period. There are no effective measures for preventing glaucoma. Rather, the key is detecting the disease in its early stages and beginning treatment before severe damage occurs.

Chronic glaucoma can be detected in a standard eye examination. There are four parts to the screening. The first test is an inspection of the eye with an instrument known as an ophthalmoscope, which has a magnifier and a light source to allow the eye specialist to look into the eye and examine its interior. Glaucoma changes the shape and color of the optic nerve in characteristic ways that can often be seen through the ophthalmoscope. This test is important since in some cases optic nerve damage develops even when the pressure inside the eye is normal. The second test (TONOMETRY) measures the pressure inside the eyeball. In air tonometry, a puff of air is directed onto the cornea to measure pressure. This test causes a short-lived sensation on the surface of the eye, but it is painless. Applanation tonometry, which is more accurate, measures pressure by displacing a certain area of the cornea. The third test, the visual field test, checks how

well the eyes can see throughout the full range of peripheral vision. In the computerized version of this test, the person being tested places his or her chin on a stand in front of a computerized screen. Every time the person being tested sees a light, he or she presses a button. The printout reveals the visual field, which is useful for detecting the mild impairment of vision to the sides that characterizes early glaucoma. The fourth test (GONIOSCOPY) evaluates the angle of the eye to determine if it is open, narrow, or closed. This is done by placing a special lens (gonioprism) against the eye.

The frequency of glaucoma testing depends on risk factors. People who have no risk factors and are younger than 45 years should be tested every 4 years. Testing every 1 to 2 years is recommended for people in the same age group who have risk factors. For people 45 years or older, testing every 2 years for those with no risk factors is advised; for those with risk factors, testing at least every year is best.

TREATMENT

With acute (angle-closure) glaucoma, treatment usually consists of surgery (iridotomy) to open the closed angle as soon as possible. In most cases this is done with a laser, which eliminates the need to make an incision in the eye. Surgery is also the usual treatment for congenital glaucoma.

For chronic (open-angle) glaucoma, medicated eye drops are usually the first form of treatment. Various forms of medication are used. Some slow

---

ACUTE GLAUCOMA ATTACK

When acute glaucoma occurs, normal drainage of the fluid inside the eye suddenly stops, causing a sharp rise in pressure within the eye and rapid destruction of the optic nerve. Emergency medical attention is needed because permanent blindness can result in as little as 1 or 2 days. Here are the warning signs:

- **Sudden, severe pain in the eye and face**
- **Loss of vision**
- **Cloudy, blurry vision with halos around lights**
- **Red eye**
- **Dilated pupil**
- **Nausea and vomiting**

Close-up on Glaucoma

The most common form of glaucoma, chronic (open-angle) glaucoma, is painless and without symptoms in its early stages. Persons with glaucoma are often unaware they have the disease until they experience vision loss; by the time this occurs, however, damage to the optic nerve is usually quite advanced and irreversible. Regular glaucoma screening, including examination of the optic nerves, intraocular pressure measurement, and a visual acuity test, is the only way to prevent the disease from reaching its advanced stages.

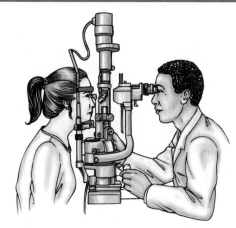

GOLDMANN APPLANATION TONOMETER
An eye specialist measures intraocular pressure using an instrument called the Goldmann applanation tonometer.

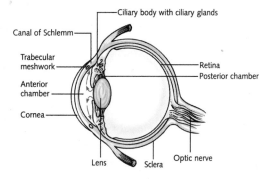

FLOW OF AQUEOUS HUMOR
In a normal eye, the ciliary body produces aqueous humor in the posterior chamber. The aqueous humor flows through the pupil to the anterior chamber, passes through a network of fibers called the trabecular meshwork, and drains out through the canal of Schlemm (the circular canal between the iris and cornea).

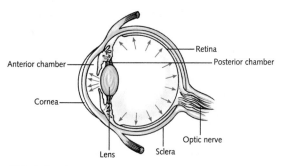

HIGH-PRESSURE GLAUCOMA
The obstructed flow of aqueous humor causes a buildup of pressure within the eye. Over time, this can damage the weakest point of the eye, the site in the sclera (the white membrane that forms the outer layer of the eyeball) at which the optic nerve joins to the eye.

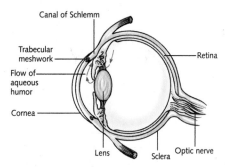

OPEN-ANGLE GLAUCOMA
While the exact cause of open-angle glaucoma is unknown, the flow of aqueous humor is obstructed somewhere at the level of the trabecular meshwork just before the canal of Schlemm.

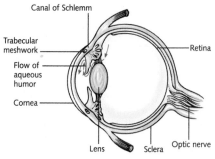

ANGLE-CLOSURE GLAUCOMA
The iris blocks the trabecular meshwork, obstructing the flow of aqueous humor. This is a medical emergency.

the production of aqueous humor, while others increase the flow of aqueous fluid out of the eye. In both cases, the net result is decreased pressure within the eye. If the medication fails to work or the side effects are intolerable, laser surgery is an option. This procedure, called trabeculoplasty, focuses a laser beam on the trabecular meshwork and increases the fluid flow out of the anterior chamber. Trabeculoplasty takes from 10 to 15 minutes, can be performed in a doctor's office, and is essentially painless. Complications are rare. Eye drops still need to be used after a trabeculoplasty.

The third alternative is traditional surgery or trabeculectomy. After administering a local anesthetic, the eye surgeon removes a small portion of the trabecular meshwork and creates a new channel for draining aqueous humor. The procedure is safe and often results in a reduction or discontinuation of the need for previous glaucoma drops. It can increase the risk of cataracts, and in some cases a second surgery is needed later to reopen the drain if scar tissue closes it.

Glioblastoma multiforme

The fastest-growing and most malignant type of BRAIN TUMOR; a type of GLIOMA. Glioblastoma multiforme is a malignant tumor of nervous tissue, usually found in the cerebrum. The tumor grows very rapidly, spreading throughout the brain. Symptoms can include seizures and signs of brain disturbance. Glioblastoma multiforme accounts for about 30 percent of all primary brain cancers and affects mostly adults of middle age or older. The tumors are treated with surgery or surgery with radiation therapy.

Glioma

A brain tumor arising from the glial cells, which form the supporting tissues of the central nervous system. Gliomas are known by the names of the several cell types from which they develop. The most common gliomas are astrocytic tumors, arising from star-shaped cells called astrocytes. Like other brain tumors, gliomas can lead quickly to an increase in pressure inside the skull. Symptoms resulting from the pressure and the tumor can vary greatly, depending on the location and size of the growth. They may include headache, vomiting, double vision, partial paralysis, loss of sensation, seizures, and personality changes.

Brain tumors are diagnosed using imaging procedures, such as CT (computed tomography) scanning and MRI (magnetic resonance imaging). Treatment is usually surgical removal of the tumor, often followed by radiation therapy. Success of the treatment depends on the location and accessibility of the tumor and the degree to which it has infiltrated various parts of the brain. Gliomas can vary greatly in their rate of growth and degree of malignancy. Some gliomas are rapid growing and tend to be fatal, while others have a survival rate of 50 percent after 5 years.

Glipizide
See SULFONYLUREA.

Global warming

An average increase in the Earth's temperature, which in turn causes changes in climate. A warmer Earth may lead to changes in rainfall patterns and a rise in sea level and may have a wide range of effects on humans, wildlife, and plants.

Like the glass in a greenhouse, certain gases that occur naturally in the atmosphere tend to trap the sun's heat. This natural GREENHOUSE EFFECT helps keep the Earth's average temperature at a comfortable 59°F. Without the greenhouse gases, the Earth would be at or below zero and extremely cold.

The problem the environment and people on Earth now face is that human activities are causing some greenhouse gases, such as carbon dioxide, to build up in the atmosphere. The burning of fossil fuels such as gasoline, oil, coal, and natural gas emits more carbon dioxide into the atmosphere, which, over many years, can change the global average temperature and bring about a major climate change.

Rising global temperatures, scientists say, will raise sea level and change precipitation and other climate conditions to ultimately alter forests, crop yields, and water supplies. Global warming could threaten human health through increases in heat-related mortality and illness resulting from expected increases in heat waves. Deaths, injuries, psychological disorders, and exposure to chemical pollutants in water supplies could increase if extreme weather events, such as storms and floods, become more frequent, according to the US Environmental Protection Agency (EPA).

The EPA is asking cities and states across the United States to pursue programs and policies that will result in a reduction of greenhouse gas emissions.

Globulin

One of a group of simple proteins that are soluble in salt solutions. Globulin is present in the blood as the serum globulins, which include the alpha, beta, and gamma globulins. Some globulins function as antibodies, while others transport lipids, iron, and copper in the blood.

Globus hystericus

The medical name for the lump-in-the-throat feeling that commonly accompanies crying, depression, anxiety, grief, and emotional conflict. There is no actual lump in the throat, but the sensation can make swallowing difficult or unpleasant. Medical attention is needed only if the condition persists. Treatment depends on the underlying psychiatric disorder.

Glomangioma
See GLOMUS TUMOR.

Glomepiride
See SULFONYLUREA.

Glomerulonephritis

The group of kidney diseases characterized by inflammation of the glomeruli (the filtering units of the kidneys). Glomerulonephritis can result in the gradual and progressive destruction of the glomeruli. The damaged structures within the kidney may result in excessive leakage of protein into the urine and may affect the capacity of the kidneys to filter toxic waste products, water, and salt.

The damaged glomeruli associated with glomerulonephritis may also permit red blood cells and other substances to leak into the urine, making the urine a reddish or darker color. When large amounts of protein are lost in the urine, fluid retention and high blood cholesterol levels may result.

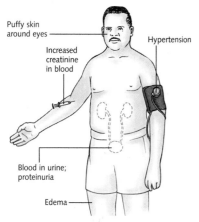

SYMPTOMS OF GLOMERULONEPHRITIS
Although a person with mild glomerulonephritis may have not symptoms, a more advanced case may produce such symptoms as puffiness around the eyes; high blood pressure (hypertension); blood in the urine; excessive protein in the urine (proteinuria); excessive creatinine (a substance usually eliminated by the kidneys) in the blood; and swelling (edema) in the abdomen or legs.

SYMPTOMS, DIAGNOSIS, AND TREATMENT
In mild cases, there may be no symptoms of glomerulonephritis. Symptoms that can develop include high blood pressure, swelling around the eyes, aching in the lower part of the back, reduced urination, and dark or reddish urine. If large amounts of protein are lost in the urine, generalized swelling may result, especially in the face, abdomen, lower legs, ankles, or feet.

To make a diagnosis, the doctor will look for signs of water retention such as weight gain and swelling and perform a physical examination including a blood pressure evaluation. Urinalysis, urine sediment evaluation, blood and urine tests to measure kidney function, and a KIDNEY BIOPSY may be part of a diagnostic evaluation.

Treatment generally includes diuretics (medications that aid in the excretion of salt and water) if there is swelling, high blood pressure medication, and dietary changes. It may be necessary for the person to take immunosuppressive medications to decrease the activity of the immune system. If glomerulonephritis results in a loss of the filtering function of the kidneys, resulting in KIDNEY FAILURE, medical treatment may include DIALYSIS or a KIDNEY TRANSPLANT.

CAUSES
Glomerulonephritis can have a number of causes, including STREP THROAT, particularly in young children. Rarely, it may result from other bacterial or viral infections, especially mumps, measles, mononucleosis, and HIV (human immunodeficiency virus). Immune system abnormalities, autoimmune diseases such as lupus erythematosus, and inflammation of small blood vessels are other possible causes. Sometimes there is no identifiable cause.

See also NEPHRITIS and GOODPASTURE SYNDROME.

Glomerulosclerosis

Scarring of the tissue that makes up the glomeruli (the filtering units of the kidneys). Diabetic glomerulosclerosis is generally the result of diabetes mellitus. Focal segmental glomerulosclerosis involves damage to kidney tissue caused by deposits in parts of the glomeruli. Interference with the filtering function of the kidneys results in blood and protein in the urine and can progress to KIDNEY FAILURE. Glomerulosclerosis is sometimes associated with severe GLOMERULONEPHRITIS. Although some types of glomerular disease respond to corticosteroid therapy, glomerulosclerosis usually does not.

Glomus tumor

A skin-colored or dusky blue, firm, ball-like swelling of the skin; also known as a glomangioma. Glomus tumors are usually extremely tender and tend to occur under the fingernails. They contain many blood vessels and glomus cells (smooth muscle cells). Treatment is through surgical removal.

Glossectomy

Partial or complete surgical removal of the tongue to treat cancer of the tongue. After the surgery, the remaining tongue usually becomes stronger and larger, and rehabilitation programs can help regain some speech and chewing ability, depending on the amount of tongue tissue removed.

Glossopharyngeal nerve

The ninth cranial nerve (see CRANIAL NERVES) that connects the BRAIN STEM to the back of the tongue, larynx (voice box), and salivary glands. The glossopharyngeal nerve performs both sensory and motor functions and is responsible for taste on the back third of the tongue, feeling and sensation in the pharynx (throat), swallowing, and the secretion of saliva. It also directs movement of the throat muscles and serves as the nerve supply to the middle ear and eustachian tube, which passes from the nose to the middle ear.

Glottis

The opening between the vocal cords, inside the larynx (voice box). The opening and closing of the glottis by the vocal cords is part of the production of speech sounds. The glottis also closes reflexively during SWALLOWING to keep food and other foreign matter out of the lungs. See SPEECH MECHANISM.

Glucagon

Substance used to treat severe hypoglycemia (low blood sugar level). Glucagon is a hormone that stimulates release of glucose from the liver. It is given by injection to reverse severe insulin-induced hypoglycemia. Glucagon may also be used before X rays of the gastrointestinal tract as a diagnostic aid, and it formerly was used to reverse a coma induced as part of insulin coma therapy, a treatment for schizophrenia that is no longer used in the United States.

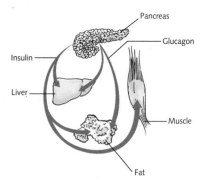

HOW INSULIN AND GLUCAGON BALANCE EACH OTHER
The pancreas secretes both glucagon (which stimulates the release of glucose from the liver) and insulin (which promotes the storage of glucose in the liver as glycogen, or in fat tissues to be available as energy for muscle). When blood glucose is low, the pancreas secretes glucagon to raise the level; when blood glucose is high, the pancreas secretes insulin to bring it down.

Glucocorticoids

See CORTICOSTEROIDS.

Glucosamine-chondroitin

A popular nutritional supplement used to treat osteoarthritis. Both glucosamine and chondroitin are found naturally in the joints, where they are assumed to be involved in joint repair: glucosamine is thought to stimulate the formation of cartilage, and chondroitin is believed to stimulate cartilage repair and inhibit enzymes involved in the breakdown of cartilage.

Both glucosamine and chondroitin are sold as nutritional supplements rather than as drugs because neither has been evaluated or approved by the US Food and Drug Administration. Some research has been performed on the ability of glucosamine to relieve the pain of osteoarthritis and to expand the range of motion of affected limbs. The results of these studies suggest that the supplements may lessen pain in 30 to 50 percent of people with osteoarthritis. People taking glucosamine and chondroitin are encouraged to buy high-quality products from a reliable source because the quality and effectiveness of unregulated supplements can vary significantly.

Glucose

A simple sugar or monosaccharide that is the body's chief source of energy. Most carbohydrates are broken down by digestive enzymes into glucose. After digestion, glucose passes into the bloodstream where it is used by cells for energy and growth. In order for glucose to enter most cells, insulin (a hormone produced by the pancreas) must be present. However, in a person with type 1 diabetes (see DIABETES, MELLITUS, TYPE 1), the pancreas produces insufficient insulin. Consequently, glucose accumulates in the blood, flows into the urine, and passes out of the body. People with type 1 diabetes require daily insulin injections.

Many foods (especially fruits) are naturally high in glucose. In nature, glucose combines with fructose to form sucrose and with galactose to form lactose. Pharmaceutical preparations of glucose are widely used in hospitals to provide nutrition via intravenous infusions. Glucose is also added as sucrose to processed foods to make them sweeter.

Glucose metabolism

The chemical processes through which the body makes use of glucose. Glucose, a simple sugar or monosaccharide, is the body's chief source of energy. Many foods, especially fruits, are naturally high in glucose. In nature, glucose combines with fructose to form sucrose and with galactose to form lactose. When consumed, CARBOHYDRATES are broken down by digestive juices into glucose. After being eaten, almost all carbohydrates absorbed from food as glucose pass through the liver, where some is stored as glycogen while the rest enters the blood as glucose where it can be used by cells for energy and growth. When the glucose level in the body drops, the pancreas releases glucagon, a hormone that stimulates the liver to break down stored glycogen into glucose and release it into the bloodstream to raise blood sugar levels. Carbohydrates that are not used for energy or stored in the body as glycogen are converted into fat.

CARBOHYDRATES AND INSULIN

Complex carbohydrates (starches) provide more lasting sources of energy than simple carbohydrates (sugars) because they are absorbed and released into the blood more slowly. Simple sugar carbohydrates such as sucrose and lactose are rapidly broken down by the body and take only minutes to reach the bloodstream as glucose or galactose. Simple sugars from fruit reach the bloodstream more slowly because the fiber in fruit slows absorption. Complex carbohydrates generally take more time to be converted into glucose because digestion is more complex for these larger molecules.

Following digestion, glucose passes into the bloodstream to be used by the brain, muscles, red blood cells, and fat tissue. However, in order for glucose to enter cells, the pancreas must release the hormone known as insulin. Specific insulin receptors on cells bind insulin, which signals the cell to increase the uptake of glucose into the cell and metabolize glucose. Glucose metabolism provides energy to muscle cells for movement, while in fat cells, excess energy is converted into body fat.

FAULTY GLUCOSE METABOLISM AND DIABETES

Diabetes mellitus is a disorder of glucose metabolism. In diabetes, the body either produces too little insulin (type 1) or is resistant to insulin (type 2), causing elevated levels of glucose in the blood. Excess glucose can also pass into the urine. Monitoring blood sugar levels is the most common way to detect diabetes. In individuals with type 1 diabetes, the body cannot make use of the glucose and loses its primary source of fuel.

Diet, exercise, and regular blood glucose testing are the basis for manage-

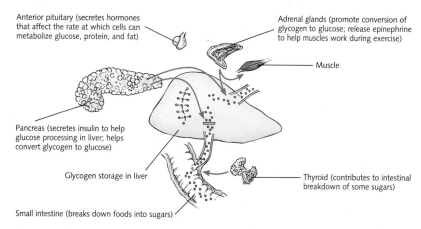

Anterior pituitary (secretes hormones that affect the rate at which cells can metabolize glucose, protein, and fat)

Adrenal glands (promote conversion of glycogen to glucose; release epinephrine to help muscles work during exercise)

Muscle

Pancreas (secretes insulin to help glucose processing in liver; helps convert glycogen to glucose)

Glycogen storage in liver

Thyroid (contributes to intestinal breakdown of some sugars)

Small intestine (breaks down foods into sugars)

HOW THE BODY PROCESSES GLUCOSE
With the help of other organs, the liver controls glucose levels in the blood by either storing excess glucose as glycogen to bring the level down or by converting glycogen back into glucose and releasing it to bring the level up.

ment of diabetes. Some experts believe that a diet following the GLYCEMIC INDEX—a ranking of foods based on their immediate effect on blood sugar level—can help control the disease. If diet and exercise cannot control the blood sugar level, medications or insulin injections may be necessary. Despite the availability of these pharmacological agents, diabetes remains a leading cause of death and disability in the United States. Complications include diabetic retinopathy (an eye disorder), peripheral neuropathy (a nerve disease), chronic kidney failure, and KETOSIS (an abnormal accumulation of ketones in the body caused by a deficiency or inefficient use of carbohydrates). Attempts to keep the blood sugar level near normal lessen the risk of these complications. See DIABETES, MELLITUS, TYPE 1; DIABETES, MELLITUS, TYPE 2; and DIABETES, GESTATIONAL.

Glucose meter

A device that enables people to monitor their blood glucose levels on a regular basis. Glucose meters are generally used by people with type 1 diabetes and sometimes by people with type 2 diabetes who require insulin (see DIABETES MELLITUS, TYPE 1; DIABETES MELLITUS, TYPE 2). The person using the meter extracts a drop of blood, usually by pricking a fingertip, and places it on a specially coated strip. The strip is inserted into the glucose meter, which offers a digital reading of the blood sugar level in about 60 seconds.

Glucose meters, when used properly, are considered the most accurate form of self-monitoring of the blood sugar level. The meters come in a variety of sizes and weights; many are conveniently small and lightweight, and some offer the advantage of storing readings for up to several weeks. A health care professional or diabetes educator can help a person decide which meter is most appropriate for his or her daily needs and can also instruct a person in the use and maintenance of the meter. Care must be taken to keep the meter calibrated by regularly testing it for accuracy according to the manufacturer's instructions. The meters can be purchased over-the-counter or at diabetes supply stores.

Glucose tolerance test

A test of the body's ability to process glucose, a form of sugar that is the chief source of energy. The test involves ingesting a measured amount of glucose and monitoring subsequent levels of glucose in the blood and urine. See GLUCOSE METABOLISM.

Glue sniffing

Inhaling the vapors of model glue and similar chemicals for their mind-altering effects. Technically, glue is a solvent, and inhaling the vapors of other solvents, such as paint thinner and dry-cleaning fluid, produces similar effects. Glues contain a chemical that can cause cardiac, kidney, and brain abnormalities. See INHALANTS.

Gluten

A protein found in grains such as wheat, rye, and barley. Gluten gives bread dough its tough, elastic character. In CELIAC DISEASE, the lining of the small intestine is damaged by an allergic reaction to gluten.

Gluten intolerance

See CELIAC DISEASE.

Gluten-sensitive enteropathy

See CELIAC DISEASE.

Glyburide

An antidiabetic drug. Glyburide (DiaBeta, Glynase PresTab, Micronase) is a member of a class of drugs called sulfonylureas. The drug is used in addition to diet to lower blood glucose levels in people with diabetes mellitus who are not dependent on insulin injections to maintain their blood sugar level. Glyburide works by stimulating the release of insulin from functioning beta cells in the pancreas.

People who take glyburide must follow prescribed diet and exercise regimens. They will also have to monitor their blood glucose and urine glucose levels. Glyburide is not effective for treating type 1 (juvenile-onset, or insulin-dependent) diabetes.

Glycemic index

A ranking of food sources of carbohydrates based on their immediate effect on blood sugar levels. A high glycemic index indicates rapid absorption of glucose from that food,

while a low glycemic index indicates a slow absorption of glucose. See GLUCOSE METABOLISM.

Glycerol

A clear, viscous liquid produced as a by-product in the making of soap; a component of fats. Also known as glycerin, glycerol is used by pharmaceutical companies as an emollient in many skin preparations, as a laxative, and as a sweetening agent.

Glycogen

A carbohydrate made up of glucose. Glycogen is the principal form in which carbohydrate is stored in the body, the same way that starch is stored in plants. Glycogen is stored in the liver and the muscles and is readily broken down into glucose.

Glycosuria

A metabolic disorder that produces the excretion of abnormally large amounts of GLUCOSE in the urine; also known as renal glycosuria. In pathologic glycosuria, large amounts of glucose appear in the urine for considerable periods. Pathologic glycosuria usually results from diabetes mellitus and occurs when the pancreas fails to produce sufficient INSULIN. This causes an abnormally high blood sugar level, leading to frequent or continuous elimination of glucose in the urine. When the blood sugar level is normal, glycosuria may be caused by the failure of certain cells in the kidneys to reabsorb glucose as urine is produced.

Temporary or alimentary glycosuria may occur when large amounts of carbohydrates are ingested and the body cannot convert the excess amount to glycogen or fat. The glomeruli (the filtering units of the kidneys) become overloaded and unable to filter the extra carbohydrates, which are excreted as glucose in the urine. Emotional stress may also be associated with temporary glycosuria because stress causes abnormal secretion of stress hormones (such as epinephrine,) which can stimulate the breakdown of glycogen and release glucose from the liver.

GM-CSF

Granulocyte-macrophage colony-stimulating factor; a chemical that fosters the development of the white blood cells known as granulocytes and of macrophages, cells found throughout the body that attack invading microorganisms and other foreign matter. This growth factor is used to treat people with leukopenia (a very low white blood cell count), particularly after bone marrow transplant or intensive chemotherapy for cancer.

GnRH

Gonadotropin-releasing hormone. GnRH is secreted by the hypothalamus. Release of GnRH signals the pituitary gland to secrete gonadotropic hormones, including FSH (follicle-stimulating hormone) and LH (luteinizing hormone) into the bloodstream. Gonadotropic hormones are essential for male and female fertility. They stimulate cell activity in a woman's ovaries and a man's testicles.

Women who are unable to conceive may be given synthetic GnRHs that mimic the action of natural GnRH. Synthetic GnRHs such as leuprolide acetate are used as fertility drugs that can help regulate a woman's menstrual cycle and promote ovulation at the right time for fertilization. Synthetic GnRHs may be prescribed to women as an adjunct to other assisted reproductive technology methods.

Synthetic GnRHs may also be used to treat endometriosis, a condition in which the tissue lining the uterus is implanted elsewhere in the body. They are generally not prescribed for longer than 6 to 9 months because they lower estrogen levels, which can reduce bone density in women with a history of low bone density. Medications called GnRH agonists mimic menopause by blocking the production of estrogen and may be prescribed for the treatment of fibroids (noncancerous growths in or on the uterus). These medications are taken by injection or nasal spray for 3 to 6 months.

Goiter

A painless enlargement of the thyroid gland that causes a visible swelling in the neck. Most goiters are not associated with excess production of thyroid hormone and are only rarely malignant (cancerous). A goiter can be barely noticeable or as large as a grapefruit.

CAUSES

Disorders associated with an enlarged thyroid gland include HYPERTHY-

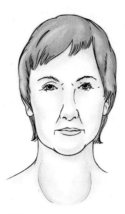

ENLARGED THYROID GLAND
A goiter, the result of an enlarged thyroid gland, looks like a swelling in the neck. Treatment may involve thyroid hormone medication to shrink the swelling. A large goiter can press on the esophagus or trachea, causing difficulty swallowing or breathing. In such cases, surgery may be recommended.

ROIDISM (overactivity of the thyroid gland), HYPOTHYROIDISM (underactivity of the thyroid gland), a thyroid nodule, and certain forms of THYROIDITIS. The enlargement may also occur as a side effect of mood-stabilizing medications such as lithium and of a diet deficient in IODINE.

DIAGNOSIS AND TREATMENT

Goiter is diagnosed by physical examination, a blood test to evaluate thyroid hormone levels, radionuclide scanning to assess the activity of the thyroid gland, and occasionally ultrasound.

A small goiter that does not affect thyroid function usually requires no treatment. Goiters of this type may shrink on their own or disappear completely with time. When this does not occur naturally or if the gland continues to enlarge, synthetic thyroid hormone medication may be prescribed to signal the pituitary to make less TSH (thyroid-stimulating hormone). Suppressing TSH levels has the effect of stabilizing the size of the thyroid gland and preventing further enlargement. If TSH therapy is ineffective and the goiter continues to grow, surgery may be considered.

Otherwise, treatment is generally directed at the specific cause of the goiter. If hyperthyroidism is involved, radioactive iodine may be administered to help shrink the goiter. Surgery is necessary if a large goiter compress-

es or displaces the trachea and esophagus, causing difficulty breathing and swallowing. In this case, the goiter may cause coughing, voice alteration, or choking during sleep. If a goiter compresses blood vessels in the neck, surgery is necessary. When a goiter becomes large enough to be disfiguring, it usually also compresses vital structures in the neck. In such instances, surgery may be considered. However, in some unusual cases, a goiter becomes large enough to be a cosmetic problem without causing associated medical difficulties.

Although goiters are rarely associated with cancer, if cancer is suspected, surgical removal is the standard medical treatment.

Gold compounds

Drugs used in the treatment of rheumatoid arthritis and other conditions. Gold compounds, such as gold sodium thiomalate (Myochrysine) and aurothioglucose (Solganal) are given by injection to treat rheumatoid arthritis not adequately treated by other anti-inflammatory drugs. Gold sodium thiomalate is also used to treat psoriatic arthritis and Felty syndrome, a form of rheumatoid arthritis that includes splenomegaly (enlarged spleen) and leukopenia (reduced white blood cell count).

Gold compounds are thought to work by altering the immune system to reduce inflammation. Gold compounds are associated with serious side effects and must be taken only under close medical supervision. People taking gold compounds must stay out of direct sunlight if possible, in addition to wearing protective clothing and using a sunblock product with a sun protection factor (SPF) of at least 15.

Golfer's elbow

An overuse injury, most commonly caused by the repetitive force placed on the tendon that attaches to the inside part of the elbow joint during a golf swing. The part of the elbow joint involved in golfer's elbow is called the medial epicondyle, and the medical term for golfer's elbow is medial epicondylitis.

Muscles of the forearm that allow the wrist to bend are called wrist flexors. These flexor muscles join together and form the common ten-

G

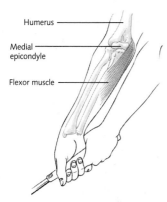

STRAIN ON THE INNER ELBOW
The flexor muscles in the forearm attach to the inner knob (medial epicondyle) of the bone of the upper arm (humerus) at the elbow. Golfer's elbow is an inflammation or small tear in the tendon that attaches these muscles to the bone.

don, called the medial flexor, at the elbow. When the wrist flexes or the hand grips firmly, the wrist flexors contract and pull against the elbow's medial flexor tendon. The repetitive use of hand tools such as a chain saw or an ax to chop wood may also engage this tendon and result in the same overuse injury.

Symptoms of golfer's elbow may include tenderness and pain on the inside of the elbow, which tends to become worse when the wrist is bent. The pain may spread into the forearm. Any activity that involves flexing the wrist or gripping with the hand will engage the flexor muscles and increase the elbow pain. The condition is usually diagnosed by physical examination. Because the symptoms rarely mimic a pinched nerve in the elbow, tests may be required to examine the nerve and rule out that cause of pain.

Self-help treatments for golfer's elbow include icing the sore area to decrease inflammation and relieve pain. An elbow strap or brace may help decrease symptoms. Exercises that help maintain muscle strength without overstressing the tendon may be helpful as the area heals and the pain lessens. Nonsteroidal anti-inflammatory drugs (NSAIDs) such as aspirin or ibuprofen may be recommended to reduce inflammation. In some cases, cortisone may be injected into the inflamed area to decrease inflammation and pain. If other treat-

ments fail and golfer's elbow persists, an outpatient surgical procedure may be performed under general or local anesthesia. The goal of the surgery is to release the tendons involved and to remove any bone spurs that may have formed on the medial epicondyle of the elbow. Complete healing following surgery takes up to 3 months.

Gonadotropin hormones

The hormones regulating the levels of estrogen and progesterone in the body. The hypothalamus produces GnRH (gonadotropin-releasing hormone) in response to declining levels of estrogen at the end of the menstrual cycle. When estrogen levels are low, production of GnRH increases markedly.

Gonadotropin-releasing hormone works through the two gonadotropins: follicle-stimulating hormone, or FSH, and luteinizing hormone, or LH. These hormones are produced by the pituitary gland in both men and women. They regulate the menstrual cycle by stimulating the ovaries to produce and release eggs during ovulation. In men, they regulate the production of sperm and testosterone in the testicles.

Gonadotropin-releasing hormone
See GNRH.

Gonads
The sex glands—the ovary in the female and the testicle in the male—that produce reproductive cells and sex hormones. In a woman, the ovaries produce eggs and the female hormones estrogen and progesterone; in the male, the testicles produce sperm and the male hormone testosterone. See REPRODUCTIVE SYSTEM, FEMALE; REPRODUCTIVE SYSTEM, MALE.

Gonioscopy
Ocular examination of the front portion (anterior chamber) of the eye. Gonioscopy is used primarily for viewing the angle between the iris (the colored part of the eye) and the cornea (the clear outer covering on the exposed part of the eye). This examination is important in diagnosing and managing GLAUCOMA, a disease in which the pressure inside the

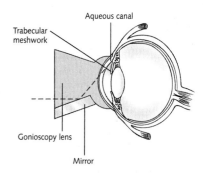

THREE-MIRRORED LENS
When fluid leaves the eye, it normally moves through the trabecular meshwork, or drainage angle. If the trabecular meshwork is obstructed, fluid cannot easily leave and internal eye pressure rises, causing glaucoma. To examine the trabecular meshwork, which is hidden from plain view, gonioscopy is performed. A gonioscope, a handheld lens with tilted mirrors, is used to examine the angle at which aqueous (fluid) drains out of the trabecular meshwork. Without the use of a gonioscope, an eye specialist cannot accurately diagnose the type of glaucoma (open-angle versus angle-closure).

front chamber of the eye often rises and damages the optic nerve. Since the angle cannot be observed directly, the gonioscope uses a modified contact lens with mirrors and a special lamp to allow the eye specialist to look inside the anterior chamber, examine its structures, and measure the angle. Before the procedure, the eye is numbed with anesthetic drops, and a cushioning agent (in drop form) is added to position the lens correctly over the cornea and maintain com-

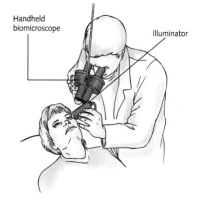

DIRECT GONIOSCOPY
During direct gonioscopy, anesthetic drops are applied to the eyes and a gonioscopy lens mounted on a handheld biomicroscope is placed directly on the cornea. This enables the doctor to see the trabecular meshwork.

fort. After the procedure, the eye is rinsed and the cornea inspected. Gonioscopy is performed as part of the initial diagnosis of glaucoma and at regular intervals afterward to gauge the progression of the disease and assess the effectiveness of treatment.

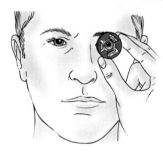

INDIRECT GONIOSCOPY
In indirect gonioscopy, a gonioscope is positioned before the eye to provide the eye care specialist with views of the trabecular meshwork.

Gonorrhea

One of the SEXUALLY TRANSMITTED DISEASES; caused by the bacterium *Neisseria gonorrhoeae*, which thrives in moist body areas including the vagina, penis, throat, eye, and rectum. Gonorrhea is one of the most common infectious diseases in the United States. It can affect anyone of any age, but is most common among sexually active adults between the ages of 20 and 30.

The predominant means of transmission is sexual intercourse. Gonorrhea can be contracted via penile-vaginal, oral-penile, oral-vaginal, or penile-anal sexual contact. Self-infection can occur if infected genitals are touched and contact is made with the eye or mouth. Rarely, gonorrhea is transmitted through kissing if there is an open cut or sore on the lips or inside the mouth. A newborn can be infected during childbirth if the mother has gonorrhea.

SYMPTOMS

Many people carry the bacteria that cause gonorrhea without any symptoms; about 20 percent of infected men have no symptoms. When there are symptoms, they include inflammation of the urethra. In men, this may cause a discharge from the tip of the penis, ranging from a clear or milky fluid to a yellowish green, puslike discharge. The head of the penis may turn red. There may be frequent

urination, blood in the urine, and a stinging sensation during urination. The man may also have swollen glands (see GLANDS, SWOLLEN) in the groin.

Gonorrhea usually causes inflammation of the cervix in women, but most women do not experience symptoms and are unaware of the infection until complications occur. If symptoms are experienced, they generally include a vaginal discharge, low-grade fever, irritation of the external vaginal area, a burning sensation when urinating, and abnormal menstrual bleeding.

When the infection occurs in the throat, it may cause a sore throat. Anal infections may not produce pain, or the person can have pain, itching, redness, and a discharge of pus or blood in the affected area.

Symptoms may be experienced at any time between 1 day and a few weeks after a person has become infected. Gonorrhea persists until it is treated; without treatment a person can have serious complications. In women, the infection can spread to the fallopian tubes and ovaries. If the infection spreads to the uterus or other internal sexual organs, it can cause PELVIC INFLAMMATORY DISEASE (PID), which is a major cause of infertility.

In men, the infection may spread up the urethra and into the prostate gland, seminal vesicles, and epididymis (the tube in which sperm mature), producing pain, chills, and fever. If the epididymis is scarred,

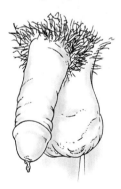

GENITAL DISCHARGE
In men, gonorrhea causes inflammation of the urethra, sometimes causing a dripping, puslike discharge from the end of the penis. In women, the disease may inflame the cervix, leading to a discharge from the vagina. In many cases, gonorrhea does not have any symptoms.

infertility can result. In rare cases, untreated gonorrhea in men leads to septic arthritis. If the eyes become infected and are untreated, gonorrhea can cause blindness. The skin and joints can become infected if the bacteria spread into the blood, a condition called disseminated gonorrhea.

DIAGNOSIS, TREATMENT, AND PREVENTION

The infection is detectable within 2 to 6 days after the bacteria invade the urethra. A sample is taken from the area of possible infection and evaluated for bacteria in a laboratory. Once diagnosed, the infection is considered treatable, but gonorrhea is becoming more resistant to antibiotics such as penicillin and tetracycline, which have been commonly used in treatment. The choice of treatment generally depends on the sex and age of the infected person, as well as the body area affected. Gonorrhea and CHLAMYDIA tend to occur simultaneously and may be treated together.

To prevent reinfection and potential transmission to others, all sexual activity should be stopped until treatment is completed. To avoid contracting gonorrhea, sexual relationships should be approached responsibly. Condoms should be used during all sexual activity, and the number of different sex partners should be limited.

Good Samaritan laws

State laws that offer immunity from legal liability to health care professionals who volunteer to offer emergency care in a good-faith effort to help a person who is injured or otherwise debilitated by a medical condition. Under these laws, the health care professional must use reasonable and sensible judgment in providing care that uses the resources available at the time.

Good Samaritan laws do not provide complete protection from malpractice claims; the care provided must meet reasonable standards and take into consideration the setting and situation. States have different guidelines for health care professionals, but it is generally accepted that a health care professional should not leave an injured person until care can be transferred to an equally competent professional.

G

The law in some states stipulates that it is a punishable offense not to offer aid, even for people who are not health care professionals. For example, in Minnesota it is a misdemeanor not to offer help to a person in an emergency, providing the aid does not endanger the person offering it. But the state of Michigan does not require anyone, even health care professionals, to offer help to strangers.

Goodpasture syndrome

A rare autoimmune disease characterized by inflammation of the glomeruli (the filtering units of the kidneys) and bleeding from the lungs. Goodpasture syndrome is a form of rapidly progressive GLOMERULONEPHRITIS that results in a continuous decrease in kidney function. It is more common in males and tends to affect men in their 20s. There is a genetic predisposition, and the risks for developing the disorder are increased by smoking.

CAUSES

Goodpasture syndrome results from the abnormal reaction of the immune system against normal body tissues. Antibodies deposit in the membranes of the filtering tissue of the kidneys and in the alveoli of the lungs, which are tiny sacs that exchange oxygen and carbon dioxide between the lungs and the bloodstream. The exact cause of this autoimmune activity is unknown. It may sometimes be triggered by a viral infection or by inhaling gasoline or hydrocarbon solvents.

SYMPTOMS, DIAGNOSIS, AND TREATMENT

The first sign of Goodpasture syndrome is often coughing up blood caused by bleeding within the lung tissues. The resulting hemorrhage can be mild but it may be life-threatening. Excretion of protein and blood in the urine results from inflammation of the kidneys. The syndrome can rapidly progress to KIDNEY FAILURE, resulting in associated anemia.

Conclusive diagnosis is made by biopsy of the lungs or kidneys. A physician may prescribe corticosteroids or cyclophosphamide to control symptoms. An additional treatment option is the removal from the blood of antibodies that may have a role in the cause of the disorder.

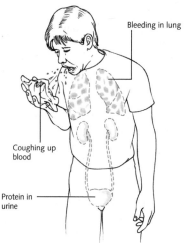

Bleeding in lung

Coughing up blood

Protein in urine

SYMPTOMS OF GOODPASTURE SYNDROME
The first symptoms of Goodpasture syndrome may be vague: fatigue, nausea, difficulty breathing. But other more specific symptoms include coughing up blood; damaged lung tissue, apparent in X rays; and excessive protein in the urine (proteinuria), caused by kidney damage.

Goserelin

A drug used in the treatment of advanced cancer of the prostate and the breast and advanced endometriosis (tissue from the lining of the uterus growing outside of the uterus). Goserelin (Zoladex) is given by injection under the skin to reduce symptoms of these advanced conditions. Goserelin is a luteinizing hormone-releasing hormone (LHRH) that acts on the pituitary to decrease the release of follicle-stimulating hormone (FSH) and luteinizing hormone. In men, the result is dramatically lowered levels of testosterone in the blood. Goserelin injections are usually given every 28 days for about 6 months.

Gout

A form of arthritis that produces sudden and severe attacks of pain, swelling, and tenderness in joints. Gout most commonly affects the large joint of the big toe but also occurs in the knees, ankles, hands, and wrists. The attacks, which often resolve within 5 to 10 days, are usually interspersed with periods when there are no symptoms. The discomfort of gout is associated with excess amounts of uric acid in the blood, a condition called HYPERURICEMIA.

Uric acid is normally formed when the body breaks down waste products. Under healthy conditions, the uric acid is dissolved in the blood and excreted by the kidneys into the urine. Excess uric acid in the blood is the result of increased production of uric acid or the inability of the kidneys to excrete uric acid efficiently.

When extra uric acid circulates in the bloodstream, sharp, needlelike crystals may form in a joint and its surrounding tissues. These crystals cause the area to become painful and swollen. In cases of chronic gout, the joint may become deformed and eventually be destroyed by the crystals.

DIAGNOSIS AND TREATMENT

Gout is diagnosed by physical examination and medical history. Blood tests may be done to measure the uric acid levels in the blood, but the results of these tests may not be conclusive. The most accurate procedure for diagnosing gout involves the removal of fluid from an affected joint to examine it for uric acid crystals.

Gout cannot be cured, but several treatments are available; medication and dietary guidelines are the primary approaches. Medications may include NONSTEROIDAL ANTI-INFLAMMATORY DRUGS (NSAIDs) to help relieve pain and swelling. COLCHICINE may be used to relieve discomfort and help prevent future attacks. Uricosuric medications, which promote the excretion of uric acid in the urine, may be used to lower the uric acid level in the blood by increasing the amount of uric acid passed in the urine. ALLOPURINOL can reduce the amount of uric acid in the blood and urine by slowing the rate of uric acid production.

Dietary guidelines are a useful adjunct to medication for controlling gout. Recommendations include reducing intake of foods containing purines. When foods containing purines are metabolized, uric acid is produced. Purines are substances that occur naturally in the body as well as in certain foods. Foods high in purines include liver, brains, kidneys, sweetbreads, anchovies, herring, mackerel, seafood, beans, oatmeal, spinach, and cauliflower. All meats, fish, and poultry contain some purines. Abstaining from drinking alcohol is recommended for people who have gout because excessive alcohol use can inhibit the excretion of uric acid, possibly leading to a buildup of uric acid and an attack of gout. Drinking plenty of water is also recommended to help dilute the uric acid.

Losing weight gradually is recommended to reduce the burden of weight on the affected joints. Rapid weight loss and fasting are to be avoided because they can cause an increase in uric acid level.

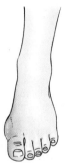

SWOLLEN, PAINFUL JOINTS
Although gout is a form of arthritis that can attack other joints, it almost always affects the joint at the base of the big toe. The joint becomes swollen and tender; the pain can be so sudden and extreme that even the weight of a bed sheet on the toe is painful. An attack may last 3 to 10 days.

Gout therapies

Treatments used for GOUT. Gout is a painful arthritic disease in which increased levels of uric acid in the blood are deposited within joints and tissues. The primary therapy for gout is drug therapy, first for acute attacks and second, to prevent their recurrence.

Acute attacks of gout are usually treated with anti-inflammatory drugs such as COLCHICINE or indomethacin. Long-term drug treatment to reduce the risk of future attacks of gout will most often include colchicine and some NONSTEROIDAL ANTI-INFLAMMATORY DRUGS (NSAIDs). In chronic cases of gouty arthritis, ALLOPURINOL and one of the SULFA DRUGS, probenecid, may also be prescribed.

Grafting

Transplanting a portion of skin, bone, or other tissue from one part of the body to another. Grafting is used to replace diseased or injured tissue with healthy tissue from the same body. For example, skin grafts are used to replace skin that has been burned or removed surgically.

Graft-versus-host disease

A rejection response that follows certain BONE MARROW transplants (see TRANSPLANT SURGERY). In graft-versus-host disease, the donor's immune cells in the transplanted marrow make antibodies against the tissues of the person receiving the transplant. Bone marrow transplants are performed in cases of LEUKEMIA and other types of bone marrow malignancy. They are also used to treat metastatic breast cancer and aplastic anemia. The infected bone marrow is destroyed by drugs or radiation and is replaced with compatible marrow from a donor. Every effort is made to match the tissues of the donor and recipient. However, only identical twins have identical tissue types, so some degree of graft-versus-host disease is seen as an expected complication of bone marrow transplantation. Treatment involves a careful balance of drugs that suppress the immune response but do not damage the new marrow.

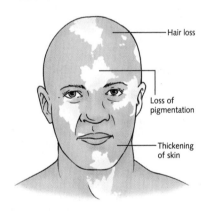

IMMUNE REACTION
Graft-versus-host disease occurs when tissue is grafted or transplanted or when blood is transfused and the body attacks the new cells. After a bone marrow transplant, the disease causes hair loss, loss of skin pigmentation, and thickening of skin (scleroderma). The disease is treated with corticosteroids, immunosuppressants, cyclosporine, or other medications.

Gram stain

A widely used method for adding a color stain to normally colorless bacteria so they can be viewed and identified under a microscope. The bacteria are treated first with a dye called GENTIAN VIOLET and then with a solution of iodine, potassium, and water. Next, the bacteria are rinsed in alcohol, and a red dye is applied. The bacteria are then viewed under a microscope to see which color they have absorbed. If they are purple from the gentian violet, the bacteria are gram-positive. If they have absorbed the red dye, they are gram-negative. Gram-positive bacteria can usually be controlled with penicillin and similar antibiotics, while gram-negative bacteria resist these medications. The difference in dye absorption reflects differences in the structure of the outer wall of the bacteria and also indicates their susceptibility to medication.

Grand mal seizure

An older term for a tonic-clonic SEIZURE. See EPILEPSY.

Granulation tissue

Rough, pink tissue that forms around the edges of a wound as a normal part of healing. Granulation tissue contains new connective tissue in the form of small, grainy particles, as well as a great many tiny blood vessels, or capillaries.

Granulocyte

A type of white blood cell named for its grainy appearance. The grains are granules of powerful chemicals the granulocytes use to attack invading microorganisms and foreign matter. Granulocytes have key roles in the inflammatory reactions to disease and infection. There are three types of granulocytes: neutrophils, eosinophils, and basophils, all named for the way they react to the laboratory stains used to make them visible under a microscope. Neutrophils attack invading microorganisms by engulfing or swallowing them, then releasing the chemicals in their granules. Eosinophils and basophils rely on releasing the chemicals in their granules.

Granuloma

A diseased growth characterized by a mass of GRANULATION TISSUE (tissue that develops in a wound during the healing process). Types of granuloma include GRANULOMA ANNULARE, GRANULOMA INGUINALE, and PYOGENIC GRANULOMA. In granuloma annulare, round (annular) skin lesions resembling ringworm most commonly appear on the hands and feet. Treatment is typically with prescription corticosteroid creams or ointments. In severe cases, the doctor will prescribe oral medications. Granuloma inguinale, one of the SEXUALLY TRANSMITTED DISEASES (STDs), causes the erosion and destruction of genital tissue. This disease, commonly found in tropical areas, is rare in the United States. In pyogenic granuloma, small, elevated, vascular lesions appear on the skin following an injury. Although harmless, they bleed easily. Many disappear without treatment, while others must be removed using a method such as cauterization, freezing, or lasers.

Granuloma annulare

A benign (not cancerous) rash characterized by papules (small superficial bumps on the skin) that occur in a ring shape. The papules are frequently located on the backs of the hands and feet, or the arms and legs, of children and young adults. The rash can appear in only one spot or occur all over the body; there are usually no other symptoms. The cause of granuloma annulare is unknown.

Granuloma inguinale

One of the SEXUALLY TRANSMITTED DISEASES; caused by a bacterial infection of the genital skin. Granuloma inguinale occurs most frequently in tropical and subtropical regions and is almost never seen in the United States. Incubation of the disease varies from 1 week to 3 months. The primary symptom is a painless, red, nodulelike lesion that appears on the penis, scrotum, groin, or thighs of men and on the vulva, vagina, or perineum in women. If the infection has been spread via anal sex, the lesion may appear on the anus and buttocks. The lesion slowly enlarges to become bright red, moist, raised, soft-surfaced, ulcerated plaques that produce a foul odor; eventually, the lesions may spread over the entire genital area. If the infection spreads into the blood, it may reach the bones, joints, or liver. Left untreated over time, the infection can cause ANEMIA, declining health with severe weight loss, and even death.

Diagnosis is made by physical examination and observation of the characteristic lesions. The diagnosis of granuloma inguinale is confirmed by microscopic examination of smears taken from scrapings of the lesions that are treated with a special stain.

Antibiotics, including tetracyclines, macrolides, and trimethoprim-sulfamethoxazole, have been used successfully to treat granuloma inguinale. Other medication options include aminoglycosides, quinolones, or chloramphenicol. The course of therapy may last as long as 4 weeks, but symptoms should improve within 7 days. People who have HIV (human immunodeficiency virus) infection may require longer treatment.

Extensive granuloma inguinale is slow to heal, and symptoms may recur, prolonging the need for antibiotic therapy. The disease can cause scarring. An infected person should be medically monitored for a period of 6 months following apparently successful treatment, and sexual contacts of an infected person should be examined for lesions.

Graves disease

An autoimmune disease that affects the thyroid gland, skin, and eyes. Graves disease may also be referred to as diffuse toxic GOITER. It is rarely life-threatening and can affect men or women of any age, but is most common in women between 20 and 60 years of age.

SYMPTOMS

Graves disease is characterized by specific symptoms that may or may not occur in everyone with the disorder. The symptoms include an enlarged thyroid gland; bulging eyes; sudden weight loss; and warm, moist skin. It also causes red, thick, swollen skin on the shins and sometimes on the top of the feet.

In a condition called Graves ophthalmopathy, tissues behind the eyes retain fluid, causing the tissues and eye muscles to swell. This pushes the eyeball forward in the orbit, making the eyes bulge outward. The eyelids may widen, and the eyes may appear red and swollen. The exposed surface of the eyeball can become dry, causing increased tearing. A person with Graves disease may experience discomfort in one or both eyes, light sensitivity, blurred or double vision, inflammation, and decreased eye movement. In severe cases, vision may be impaired.

Other symptoms include nervousness, irritability, sensitivity to heat, increased perspiration, thin skin, brittle hair, shakiness, weight loss despite increased appetite, increased heart rate, palpitations, irregular heart rhythm, elevated blood pressure, insomnia, confusion, an increase in bowel movements, weakened muscles in the upper arms and thighs, and light or irregular menstrual periods in women.

CAUSES

Graves disease occurs as a result of the immune system's abnormal attack on the thyroid gland, the tissue behind the eyes, and the skin of the lower legs. An antibody that is mistakenly produced by the immune system overstimulates the thyroid gland, which becomes enlarged and produces more thyroid hormones than the body needs. These conditions cause hyperthyroidism. The normal influences of the thyroid hormones on the rate of metabolism, temperature, muscle tone and strength, and overall mood are disrupted.

What produces this autoimmune response is not known. Medical researchers believe that the likelihood of developing Graves disease may be determined by a combination of factors, including a person's heredity, immune system function, sex, and age.

DIAGNOSIS AND TREATMENT

Graves disease is diagnosed by a complete medical history, physical examination, and a few simple tests. Blood samples are taken for laboratory analysis to measure the amount of thyroid hormone in the bloodstream. THYROID SCANNING using a radioactive substance is used to produce an image of the thyroid gland and to observe its functioning.

Treatment for Graves disease varies depending on several factors including a person's overall health, age, medical history, and individual symptoms, as well as the degree of hyperthyroidism. Other considerations include the physician's judgment regarding the course of the disease and the person's tolerance for certain medications, procedures, and therapies.

Antithyroid medications may be

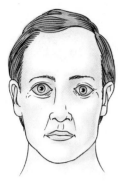

BULGING EYES

A typical symptom of Graves disease is bulging eyes. The bulging is caused by inflammation and fluid retention in the tissues behind the eyes that push the eyeball forward. The eyes may tear excessively, and double vision may be a problem. But vision is rarely impaired permanently.

prescribed that inhibit the synthesis of thyroid hormone by the thyroid gland, thereby helping to lower the level of thyroid hormones in the blood. The BETA BLOCKERS, which block some of the actions of excess thyroid hormones on the body, may be used to control symptoms such as palpitations or a rapid heart rate, tremor, and excessive perspiration. Radioactive iodine, administered either by pill or in liquid form, decreases thyroid gland activity by damaging cells in the thyroid gland and destroying some of the gland's tissue. Surgery to remove part of the thyroid gland may also be useful to treat Graves disease effectively. For patients undergoing surgery or radioactive iodine treatment, careful monitoring of the thyroid hormone level is important, and hormone therapy may be needed to maintain the proper balance of thyroid hormones in the body.

People with Graves disease may also need treatment for the many symptoms and discomforts related to the disease. A doctor may prescribe creams or ointments to reduce the redness and swelling of the skin. If Graves ophthalmopathy occurs, cool compresses, sunglasses, and lubricating eyedrops may be recommended. Elevating the head of the bed helps reduce pressure and swelling. Prisms for eyeglasses can sometimes help correct problems with double vision that can occur with Graves disease.

Medical treatments for eye disorders associated with Graves ophthalmopathy include corticosteroid medications or orbital radiation therapy to shrink the engorged tissues surrounding the eyes. For severe cases, orbital decompression surgery can improve vision and increase the space behind the eyeball, allowing it to move back into a protected position in the orbit. Surgery on the eye muscles may be needed to correct double vision. Surgery to reposition the eyelid when the front surface of the eyeball is too exposed may also be performed.

Graves disease, eye

Swelling and bulging of the eyes caused by excessive production of thyroid hormones; also known as Graves ophthalmopathy. The thyroid gland, located to the front and sides of the windpipe (trachea) just above the breastbone (sternum), produces thyroid hormones that control important body processes, such as the rate of metabolism, body temperature, and muscle tone and vigor. In Graves disease, the thyroid gland becomes overly active (hyperthyroidism) and produces excessive levels of hormones. In addition to changes in the eye, symptoms of hyperthyroidism include weight loss, irritability, shifts in menstrual patterns, less tolerance of heat, moist skin, and irregular or accelerated heartbeat. Research indicates that Graves disease results from a disorder of the immune system. It may develop in either sex and at any age, but is most common in women between the ages of 20 and 60 years. Treatment consists of medication to block the effects of thyroid hormones, destruction of a portion of the thyroid with radiation, or surgical removal of part of the thyroid. Some eye symptoms may be present during periods of normal levels of thyroid hormones.

SYMPTOMS

Graves disease can cause the tissues behind the eyes to retain water, causing the tissues and muscles attached to the eyeball to swell and push the eye forward in the socket. The eyes look red and swollen, and they bulge prominently. The space between the lids may widen, drying the front portion of the eye. The eyes may tear excessively; become inflamed, uncomfortable, and sensitive to light; move only with difficulty; and cause blurred or double vision.

TREATMENT

Until the hyperthyroidism of Graves disease is controlled, treatment consists of cool compresses to soothe and moisten the eyes, sunglasses to dim light, and eye drops for added moisture. In some cases, anti-inflammatory medications are prescribed to reduce swelling. Radiation therapy can also help control swelling. Control of Graves disease usually resolves eye symptoms; if it does not and the eyes remain swollen and bulging, a number of options are available. In cases of double vision, prisms can be added to glasses to align the eyes and help them converge on a single point. Double vision can also be treated with surgery that moves and reattaches the muscles controlling the eyeballs and brings them into better alignment. If the opening between the eyelids remains too wide and causes irritation, the eyelids can be repositioned surgically. Both eye muscle and eyelid surgery are usually performed on an outpatient basis under local anesthesia, and the person undergoing these procedures can go home the same day.

In rare cases, a procedure called orbital decompression surgery is performed to remove the bone between the eye socket and the sinuses. This enlarges the socket, providing room for the eye to move back inside it. A short hospital stay is required for orbital decompression surgery. Complications can include double vision, persistent numbness in the lip, leaking of the cerebrospinal fluid that surrounds the brain, and infection.

Gravida

In medicine, a pregnant woman. The term derives from gravid, meaning pregnant, while gravidity is the total number of normal and abnormal pregnancies a woman has had. A woman having her first pregnancy is

> Terms in small capital letters—for example, PHYSICAL THERAPY or PAGET DISEASE—indicate a cross-reference to another entry with more information.

G

a primigravida, while one who has had many pregnancies is a multigravida. Sometimes a Roman numeral follows the word to indicate a woman's number of pregnancies. For example, gravida I refers to a woman in her first pregnancy.

Gray matter

Gray nervous tissue in the brain and spinal cord composed primarily of neuron cell bodies and unmyelinated axons. Gray matter is located in the cortex of the cerebrum, cerebellum, and core of the spinal cord. Nuclei in the gray matter of the spinal cord act as centers for all spinal reflexes.

Greenhouse effect

The rise in temperature that the Earth experiences after gases in the atmosphere, such as water vapor, carbon dioxide, nitrous oxide, and methane, trap energy from the sun. Without these gases, heat would escape back into space and the Earth's average temperature would be about 60°F colder. These greenhouse gases, much like a greenhouse that traps heat from the sun to keep plants warm enough to live in the winter, cause the world to heat up so that the Earth is warm enough for humans to live comfortably. But if the greenhouse effect intensifies, it could make the Earth warmer than needed and cause serious problems for humans, plants, and animals. See GLOBAL WARMING.

Grieving

The normal emotional response to the loss of a valued relationship through death or dissolution, such as separation or divorce. Grief reactions vary markedly from person to person and may last anywhere from a few weeks to years, depending on the closeness and length of the relationship and the personality style of the grieving person.

Symptoms and signs include tightness or pain in the chest or throat; disturbed sleep patterns; weight loss or gain; poor concentration; difficulty completing tasks; disorientation to space and time; headaches, digestive upset, and other physical complaints; withdrawal from social activity; lack of interest in normal routines; sighing; periods of teariness or crying; anger, resentment, and bitterness;

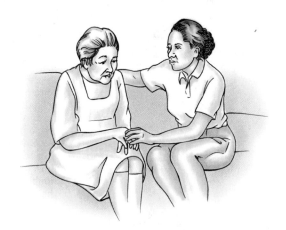

COMFORTING A GRIEVING PERSON
Every person grieves individually and at his or her own pace. A friend, counselor, or member of the clergy cannot entirely relieve the grief but can provide a listening ear and a reassuring presence. Another person can also help ensure that the grieving person is eating regularly and getting adequate rest.

sexual disturbances or lack of erotic interest; and mood swings.

STAGES

Typically, the grieving person passes through a series of stages as the loss has its full emotional impact and as the individual comes to terms with the loss. There is no set time for how long a person spends in any given stage. Also, the grieving individual may move back and forth between two or more stages or not follow the traditional order of grieving.

In the first stage, called denial and protest, the grieving person may have trouble believing that the death or loss has occurred. He or she feels confused, has great difficulty concentrating, and misses much of what is said in conversation. This stage usually occupies the first days or weeks after the death or loss.

Despair is the second stage. As the full pain of the loss is felt, the grieving person has recurring dreams about the dead or lost person and may even hear his or her voice. Anger is common, and it may be expressed toward inappropriate people, such as the dead person's physician or other family members.

The third phase, depression, lasts the longest, typically for months. The grieving person may have difficulty sleeping through the night or may want to do nothing but sleep. Social withdrawal is commonplace. Usually there is little motivation to perform ordinary tasks inside the home and even less interest in activities outside it.

In the final phase, resolution and acceptance, the unpleasant symptoms of grief resolve. He or she can

talk about the departed person without crying or feeling guilty and has the capacity to take pleasure in life again. While difficult emotions may be roused from time to time, the individual is able to continue with his or her life despite the death or loss.

ABSENT GRIEF

Grief that is not expressed openly comes out in other ways, often only over time. The grieving person may seem oddly euphoric or begin to experience physical symptoms similar to those of the person who died. Sometimes behavior becomes erratic and unpredictable on the anniversary of the person's death or birthday. The grief may also be shifted onto another, minor loss.

TREATMENT

Since grief is a necessary emotional process following the death or loss of someone close, it needs to be experienced rather than prevented. Treatment is recommended only if the depressive symptoms escalate into a major depressive episode or in cases of absent grief, in which the emotional response is thwarted. Support groups, counseling from members of the clergy or mental health workers, and support from family and friends can help ease the symptoms of grief and allow the individual the full, necessary expression of emotions.

Grip

Grasping or seizing; functional position of the hand. Grips can vary, depending on the work the hand is doing. Grasping involves the entire hand, while pinching involves the thumb and a finger. Three types of grip have been identified: the hook grip, in which the fingers are curled toward the palm in order to grasp something; the power grip, in which the fingers are curled around an item with counter pressure coming from the thumb; and the precision grip, in which an object is grasped with the tips of one or more fingers and the thumb.

A person's grip can be affected by disease. Grip strength is lost by some people with muscular dystrophy, because their muscles easily become fatigued. A weak grip is a common symptom among people who have CARPAL TUNNEL SYNDROME; in this case, the weakened grip is caused by difficulty in bringing the thumb across the palm of the hand to meet the other fingers.

Griseofulvin

An antifungal drug used to treat infections such as fungal infections of nails and hair follicles. Griseofulvin (Fulvicin P/G and Fulvicin U/F, Grifulvin V, Grisactin, Gris-PEG) works by interfering with the fungal cell division and may inhibit DNA replication. Griseofulvin is available as tablets, capsules, and liquid.

Groin

The region of the body where the lower abdomen joins the top of the thigh.

Groin strain

A pulled muscle that occurs suddenly during vigorous activity in a fall, twisting injury, or during a fast run. A groin strain causes pain in the area just below the crease between the lower abdomen and the thigh. What distinguishes a groin strain, or groin pull, is that the pain comes on suddenly. Pain in the groin area that develops gradually over several weeks, without a preceding single event, may be a symptom of a stress fracture in the hip and requires immediate attention from a physician with expertise in sports medicine. A groin strain may be treated for the first 48 hours with ice, nonsteroidal anti-inflammatory drugs (NSAIDs), and gentle stretching exercises when symptoms allow. The upper leg may be wrapped with an elastic bandage

to support the area during healing. In an older person, a groin strain may be more severe and take longer to heal. If pain persists, a doctor should be consulted.

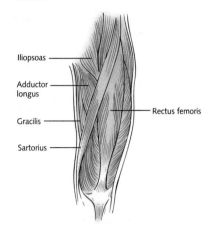

A PULLED GROIN MUSCLE
There are five muscles in the thigh. A strain or tear in any of these muscles—most frequently the adductor longus—causes groin pain.

Groin, lump in the

A raised swelling of variable size that may be tender. A lump in the groin may be due to any number of causes, including an infection, an abscess, a mole, a localized response to irritation, and trauma to the area. If the lump is sore, the cause is probably a hernia infection, which can be cured with antibiotic medication. Any lump in the area of the groin should be medically evaluated and diagnosed by a physician to determine the specific cause and the appropriate treatment.

Group A streptococcus infection

Disease resulting from a pathogenic bacterium. Group A streptococcal bacteria (group A strep) are also known as *Streptococcus pyogenes* and are frequently found in the mouth. Infections caused by this bacteria often involve the throat as in STREP THROAT, which is the most common bacterial throat infection and tends to affect children between the ages of 5 and 15 years. Consequences of strep throat include SCARLET FEVER, the kidney condition poststreptococcal GLOMERULONEPHRITIS, and acute

RHEUMATIC FEVER, which affects the heart after a strep throat infection. A group A streptococcal infection may also cause skin conditions such as IMPETIGO. In rare instances, group A strep may spread below the skin and cause serious soft tissue infections of the muscle. This severe invasion by the strep bacteria, sometimes called "flesh-eating disease," can cause a person to lose a limb or to develop liver and kidney abnormalities, and it may be even fatal. It is uncertain how or why these deep-tissue infections occur.

Streptococcal infections are contagious, and the bacteria are commonly passed from person to person via fluid droplets in coughs and sneezes. Group A strep may be easily spread among children via kissing or the sharing of eating utensils and drinking cups. Streptococcal bacteria can also contaminate food, water, and milk.

The infections are usually diagnosed by bacterial culture of a swab taken from the throat or skin lesions and are treated with antibiotics.

Group therapy

A technique for dealing with emotional issues in which a professionally trained therapist meets with a group of people with similar problems. Group therapy is widely used and has been a standard treatment for at least 50 years. Studies show that group therapy is as effective as, and sometimes more effective than, individual therapy. Depending on the problem, group therapy can be used alone or in combination with individual therapy.

A typical therapy group consists of a therapist and six to eight people with similar emotional issues. Issues around which groups are formed include addiction to alcohol or drugs, problems of aging, chronic medical illness such as cancer, grief and bereavement, and sexual orientation. The therapist guides the discussion and provides professional knowledge and expertise as needed.

Many people find group therapy helpful because they discover they are not alone in their problems. In addition, group therapy provides increased feedback and may help individuals see how others deal with similar situations and problems.

G

G

Growing pains

Arthritislike pains that occur, usually in the arms and legs of children 6 to 10 years old. The pains appear to be unrelated to growth but may be the result of fatigue, emotional difficulties, poor posture, or other problems. Children always outgrow growing pains. If a child experiences severe growing pains, or if pains are accompanied by swelling, a physician should be consulted to rule out other causes. Relaxation exercises and stretching are sometimes used to relieve the pain.

Growth

The process of developing to full size or to maturity. All living things gradually grow in size as they mature and develop. Growth is a term also used to characterize an abnormal development, such as a cancerous growth or tumor.

Growth hormone

A substance produced by the pituitary gland that is necessary for human growth; also known as human growth hormone, somatotropin, or somatotropic hormone.

Growth hormone acts on the hard and soft tissues of the body to stimulate their growth and maintain appropriate size once growth is achieved. By increasing the rate at which amino acids enter cells and are built up into proteins, growth hormone causes the cells to grow and multiply. Human growth hormone also influences the metabolism of fats, causing cells to switch from using carbohydrates for fuel to burning fats for energy. It also accelerates the rate at which glycogen stored in the liver is converted into glucose and released into the blood to stimulate the liver's secretion of a hormone that enables bone formation.

The release of growth hormone by the pituitary gland is increased by physical exercise and stress, as well as by insulin, estrogen, and a decreased intake of sugar. Release of growth hormone is decreased by somatostatin, a peptide produced by the hypothalamus.

Disturbances in the synthesis of growth hormone can produce conditions affecting a person's physical size. Unusually TALL STATURE is caused by an excess of growth hormone during childhood. ACROMEGALY results from an overproduction of growth hormone during adulthood. Unusually SHORT STATURE occurs when insufficient growth hormone is produced during the childhood years.

When overproduction of growth hormone causes unusually tall stature or acromegaly, the syndrome can be treated by administering the growth hormone–inhibiting protein, somatostatin. Genetic engineering can now produce human growth hormone medications to treat children with deficiencies in growth hormone. Recently, growth hormone was approved for treatment of short stature associated with Turner syndrome (a genetic disorder affecting girls and women with only one X chromosome) and for treatment of chronic kidney disease.

Growth hormone is sometimes used by athletes in an effort to improve performance by increasing lean body mass and reducing body fat. Clinicians are studying the effects of growth hormone in people who are frail or older. Risks of growth hormone therapy include generalized swelling, carpal tunnel syndrome, enlarged breasts in older men, and diabetes. Growth hormone may also be potentially useful for treating other conditions associated with a wasted state such as cancer or AIDS (acquired immunodeficiency syndrome).

Growth, childhood

An important measure of a child's health; physical growth follows a similar pattern in most children. With some variation in the first year of life, girls and boys grow at the same rate. Boys are usually slightly larger, except briefly at PUBERTY. The rate of growth is fastest during embryonic and fetal development and remains fast during infancy until it slows at about age 2 or 3. The onset of puberty triggers another dramatic growth period that lasts until full adult height is reached in the late teens. Factors that influence growth usually can be categorized as either environmental or hereditary. Environmental factors may include nutrition and emotional welfare. Genetic traits, ethnicity, and hormones are considered hereditary influences. General health also influences growth.

STAGES OF GROWTH

Healthy infants and toddlers steadily gain weight, except for a small loss of weight in the first few days of life. By 2 weeks of age, healthy babies return to their birth weight. In the first year, babies triple their birth weight and grow up to 12 inches longer. Between their first and second birthdays, children grow approximately 5 inches and gain 5 to 6 pounds. It is not normal for a baby to stop growing or to lose weight. An infant who does not gain weight as expected may not be receiving adequate nutrition. (See also FAILURE TO THRIVE.) After age 2, most children grow at a rate of about 2 inches and about 5 pounds a year until the adolescent growth spurt. Different parts of the body grow at different rates. A newborn's head is nearly one fourth of his or her length. After the first year, other parts of the body grow more rapidly in proportion, and by adolescence the head represents only one eighth of body size.

A growth spurt occurs at puberty, prompted by the body's increased output of sex and growth hormones. This adolescent growth spurt occurs in girls between ages 11 and 14, and in boys, 13 and 16. Children reach most of their adult height during this time. In the first 2 years of the growth spurt, girls grow 3 inches a year. After they begin menstruating, growth slows to an inch or two a year. Girls usually reach their maximum adult height by about age 15. Boys grow approximately 4 inches a year for 2 years, usually reaching their adult height by age 19. Girls gain 15 to 20 pounds in the initial stage of their growth spurt, and boys gain about 30 pounds. Because girls begin their growth spurt earlier than boys do, they are briefly larger than boys.

MONITORING GROWTH

Doctors use growth charts to monitor children's growth rates. At each visit, the pediatrician will measure a child's height and weight and plot these measurements on a growth chart. Measurements will be compared with those of past visits to make sure a child is growing properly.

A CHILD'S CHANGING BODY

Height is an important indicator of a child's growth and health. Doctors usually use growth charts to determine whether a child's growth is within the normal range. It is important to remember that children vary a great deal in their pattern of growth. As long as a child is growing steadily, his or her height relative to other children is not especially significant.

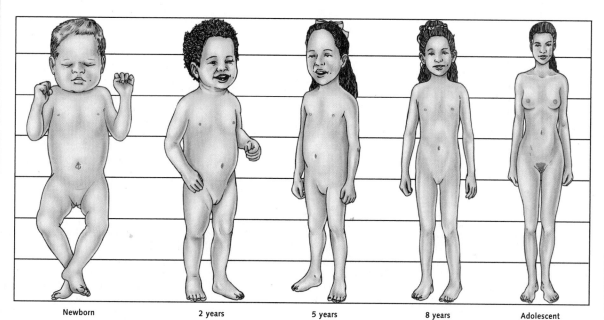

Newborn   2 years   5 years   8 years   Adolescent

THE GROWING BODY
As a child grows, his or her overall height increases at a fairly steady rate. But different parts of the body grow at different rates, so body proportions change significantly. A newborn's head, for instance, comprises nearly one fourth of his or her height. By adolescence, the head is only about one eighth of the child's height. A newborn's legs are only about three eighths of his or her total height, while a teenager's legs are nearly half.

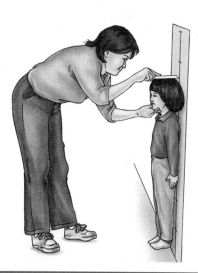

MEASURING HEIGHT
A doctor measures a child's height as part of a routine well-child visit. Parents can also measure their child's height at home to keep track of the rate at which the child grows.

If a child's growth rate suddenly changes or lies significantly above or below the norm, the doctor will order tests such as X rays to determine the cause. Unusually rapid growth may indicate a pituitary gland disorder. Slowed growth may indicate a number of illnesses or poor nutrition. Height is usually a function of heredity; that is, short parents have short children. Less commonly, a short stature or weight problem is due to factors such as growth hormone deficiency, a problem with thyroid hormones, or celiac disease, a digestive disorder in which the body does not absorb essential nutrients.

Guaifenesin

An expectorant drug (cough syrup) used to loosen mucus in the lungs. Guaifenesin is found in many products sold without prescription to help loosen mucus so that it can be coughed up. Products containing guaifenesin must be taken with a full glass of water, which helps break up mucus and clear congestion.

Guillain-Barré syndrome

Also known as GBS, a rare, potentially life-threatening, inflammatory disorder of the peripheral nerves. The onset of GBS is typically sudden and unexpected.

CAUSES

Guillain-Barré syndrome is characterized by progressive muscle weakness and paralysis. In fact, it is the most common cause of acute paralysis in young adults. The weakness and paralysis of GBS are caused by the loss of myelin, the sheath that normally coats nerve cells. Guillain-Barré syndrome is thought to be an autoimmune disorder (in which a person's own immune system reacts against his or her own tissues). Two out of three cases occur after a viral infection such as an upper respiratory infection. Other occurrences take place following a bacterial infection or medical procedure. Some vaccinations have also been associated with the onset of GBS.

SYMPTOMS

Guillain-Barré syndrome can affect people of any age. Symptoms may develop over a few hours or a few weeks. The earliest signs are often

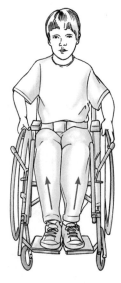

PROGRESSIVE PARALYSIS
The symptoms of Guillain-Barré syndrome—numbness, tingling, and muscle weakness leading to paralysis—begin in the leg nerves and spread quickly up to other parts of the body. Most people recover completely, and an exercise program can help them recover muscle strength.

weakness or tingling in the legs. Over time, weakness and tingling spread to the arms and upper body. There may be an overall feeling of weakness, such as when a person has a virus. In a mild case of GBS, the symptoms progress no further than this. In moderate cases, the ability to walk is impaired. This requires medical attention.

A severe case of GBS is characterized by problems with breathing, blood pressure, and heart rate. A person may become totally paralyzed. This is a medical emergency, and immediate hospitalization is required. In the hospital, the person will be placed in the intensive care unit and may require the use of a ventilator to assist with breathing.

DIAGNOSIS AND TREATMENT

Diagnosis of GBS is based on symptoms and physical examination. Individuals will have evidence of weakness without sensory loss, and reflexes will be absent. The doctor may also conduct tests, such as electromyography (see ELECTROMYOGRAM) or analysis of cerebrospinal fluid, to confirm the diagnosis and rule out other causes of symptoms.

There is no cure for GBS, and those who are diagnosed with it generally recover with or without treatment. However, early treatment can help prevent progression to complete paralysis and the need for a ventilator to assist with breathing. There are two primary treatments: plasmapheresis and intravenous immunoglobulins. Plasmapheresis is a blood-cleansing technique. Immunoglobulin, a substance naturally manufactured by the body's immune system, contains antibodies from blood donors; these appear to block the person's own antibodies. Other supportive therapies include rehabilitation therapy to help people with GBS recover neurological function.

Guilt

A painful, inwardly directed emotion resulting from the perception that an individual has violated his or her conscience or principles. Guilt leaves the person feeling worthless, low, and in need of punishment.

Gulf War syndrome

A nonscientific term referring to unexplained illnesses of veterans who served in Operation Desert Shield and Desert Storm during the Persian Gulf War. Symptoms generally include fatigue, joint pain, skin rash, memory loss, and diarrhea. These problems may have been caused by exposure to environmental hazards, such as chemical warfare agents. The exact cause of the syndrome is unknown.

Gum

The pink, soft tissue in the mouth that surrounds the teeth. The gum, which is medically called the gingiva, lies close to the teeth to help prevent infection. The gum is secured to the jaw bone by ligaments. Fibrous tissue in the gum serves as part of the support structure that holds the teeth in place. Healthy gums are firm and pale pink and do not bleed easily. If bacteria build up under the gums, a substance called plaque forms that can ultimately pull the gum away from the teeth. Careful, regular brushing and flossing are needed to avoid inflammation of the gums (gingivitis) or a more advanced stage of gum disease called periodontitis (see PERIODONTAL DISEASE).

Gumma

A firm, tumorlike growth of the tissues, which is called a granuloma, and is usually caused by SYPHILIS. A gumma tends to appear during the late stage of the illness, referred to as tertiary syphilis, most frequently occurring in the liver. Gumma often appears as a skin lesion on the scalp, face, chest, and legs. It may also occur in the brain, testes, heart, skin, or bone. The growth usually contains a painless mass of dead, fiberlike tissue that may be swollen. Treatment is with antibiotics; usually a single dose of penicillin. For people allergic to penicillin, other antibiotics are available to treat gumma. Penicillin or other antibiotic treatment will kill the syphilis bacterium and prevent further damage from the gumma.

Gynecologist

A doctor who specializes in gynecology, the care of the female reproductive system, and diagnosis and treatment for the diseases and disorders that affect it. Gynecologists treat conditions related to breast and reproductive organ health, fertility, menstruation, sexual function, hormones, and menopause, and they provide contraception and may perform elective abortion and treat women during other types of abortion. Gynecologists are usually also trained as obstetricians, specialists who handle issues related to PREGNANCY and CHILDBIRTH. Physicians who are trained in both OBSTETRICS and gynecology are called obstetrician-gynecologists, or ob-gyns for short.

Gynecology

The medical specialty focused on women's reproductive health, including diagnosis and treatment for the diseases and disorders that affect it. Special areas of concern are fertility, methods of birth control, hormonal function, menopause, the reproductive organs, and breast health.

Gynecomastia

Male breast enlargement. In gynecomastia, breast tissue responds to both androgen hormones (male hormones, including testosterone) and estrogens (female hormones). It results from an increase in the ratio of estrogen to testosterone, which may be due to an increase in estrogen or a decrease in androgen hormone levels. As men age and testosterone levels fall, gynecomastia may be a relatively normal finding.

Certain medications—such as estrogens for prostate cancer, spironolactone for high blood pressure, and digitalis for heart conditions—may increase the size of a man's breasts. Medications account for 10 to 20 percent of cases of gynecomastia.

Marijuana use can cause breast enlargement in men as a result of marijuana's effects on hormone receptors.

Illnesses such as chronic liver disease that disturb the normal balance between male and female SEX HORMONES in men result in a man's breasts growing larger. Rarely, tumors of the endocrine glands that produce female hormones may cause gynecomastia. Breast cancer in men is uncommon but does occur. Symptoms of breast cancer in men include breast enlargement on only one side, hardened breast tissue, a deformed nipple, and bleeding from the nipple.

Newborn boys may have temporary breast enlargement as a result of exposure to the mother's estrogens during development in the uterus. Gynecomastia occurs temporarily in many boys during puberty and may last for months or years without persisting into adulthood. Obese adolescent boys may appear to have gynecomastia if excess fatty tissue enlarges the breasts. If the nipple area is firm and sensitive, gynecomastia is usually the cause.

Treatment depends on the underlying cause. If a drug is responsible, an alternative medication may be tried. If there is no disease, swelling usually subsides without treatment in about 3 months. If the swelling is bothersome, cosmetic surgery is an option but is rarely needed.

G

H. pylori

Helicobacter pylori; a bacterium believed to cause duodenal ulcers, gastric ulcers, and gastritis. Ulcers are sores or open wounds in the linings of the small intestine (duodenum) and stomach. Gastritis is an inflammation of the lining of the stomach. *Helicobacter pylori* infection is implicated in these conditions because it burrows beneath the surface and damages the protective mucous linings, increasing vulnerability to harsh stomach acids and enzymes. Because the bacteria do not disappear spontaneously, treatment is necessary.

Infection with *H. pylori* sometimes has no symptoms. Other times symptoms are those of the diseases it causes. Duodenal and gastric ulcers typically cause upper abdominal pain. Pain from a duodenal ulcer usually occurs 2 to 3 hours after a meal or in the early morning. The pain of a gastric ulcer tends to occur a half hour to 2 hours after a meal and may spread to the lower part of the chest. Other symptoms of ulcer disease include nausea, vomiting, loss of appetite,

and weight loss. Gastritis may cause no symptoms, or at other times, indigestion, nausea, and vomiting.

Helicobacter pylori infection is usually acquired in childhood, although uncertainty exists concerning how it spreads. The United States has a lower incidence of *H. pylori* than that in many other countries, possibly due to higher standards of sanitation. Diagnosis is based on blood tests that can detect antibodies signifying the presence of *H. pylori*; a urea breath test, which detects the actual bacteria; an upper GASTROINTESTINAL (GI) SERIES (an X-ray procedure also known as a barium swallow); or GASTROSCOPY, in which a lighted tube is used to view, photograph, videotape, and sometimes take a sample of tissue from the esophagus, stomach, and duodenum.

Although no single medication has proven effective against *H. pylori*, a 2-week medical regimen called triple therapy (the use of three medications at once) usually succeeds at eradicating this infection. Triple therapy combines medications such as bismuth subsalicylate, tetracycline, and metronidazole. For people with disease that does not respond to metronidazole, clarithromycin can be substituted. New drug therapies and combinations continue to surface. For example, dual therapy with amoxi-

cillin and metronidazole has emerged as an alternative to triple therapy.

Habituation

A therapeutic technique used to eliminate or reduce the frequency of a problem behavior by purposely repeating the stimulus for that behavior again and again. Repeating the stimulus over and over gradually robs it of meaning, lessens the anxiety it causes, and makes it less likely to trigger the problem behavior. Habituation is commonly used in COGNITIVE-BEHAVIORAL THERAPY.

Haemophilus influenzae

A bacterium that is a common cause of bacterial PNEUMONIA. *Haemophilus influenzae* is so named because it was erroneously associated with an influenza outbreak during the 19th century. Strains of the bacteria commonly colonize the upper airways of adults and may colonize the lower respiratory tract of people with chronic BRONCHITIS. The bacteria are often implicated in exacerbated cases of chronic bronchitis.

Strains of the bacteria containing the type b polysaccharide capsule (Hib) tend to cause the most severe illness, including meningitis and epiglottitis, in children 3 to 5 years old. These diseases, along with bacterial pneumonia, are now extremely rare in the United States and other developed countries because of widespread use of the Hib vaccine.

Hair

Long, slender, threadlike filaments that grow from the skin. Made of a protein called keratin, hair on the head shields the scalp and head from temperature extremes and conserves heat. Hair also grows on the entire skin surface, where it helps prevent microbes or foreign matter from entering the skin. The only areas of the body where hair does not grow are the palms of the hands and the soles of the feet, the backs of the fingertips, the lips, and some parts of the genitals.

What is commonly called hair is actually only the hair shaft, which protrudes above the surface of the skin. The root of the hair lies below the skin surface, in the layer called the dermis, originating in a structure

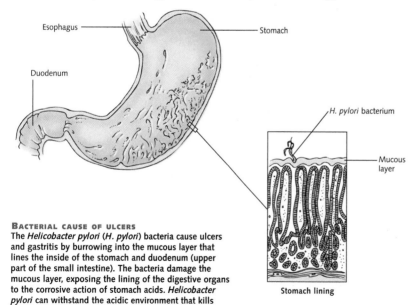

BACTERIAL CAUSE OF ULCERS
The *Helicobacter pylori* (*H. pylori*) bacteria cause ulcers and gastritis by burrowing into the mucous layer that lines the inside of the stomach and duodenum (upper part of the small intestine). The bacteria damage the mucous layer, exposing the lining of the digestive organs to the corrosive action of stomach acids. *Helicobacter pylori* can withstand the acidic environment that kills other bacteria because they secrete an enzyme that neutralizes the acids.

Esophagus — Stomach

Duodenum

H. pylori bacterium

Mucous layer

Stomach lining

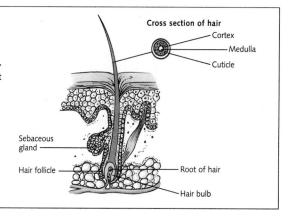

STRUCTURE OF HAIR
The visible hair shaft is composed of dead cells, pushed up through the skin by the living root of the hair deep in the dermis. The root is nourished by the bloodstream to produce new hair. The hair shaft has three layers: the inner medulla, present only in thick hairs; the strong, colored cortex; and the colorless, protective layer called the cuticle.

Cross section of hair
Cortex
Medulla
Cuticle
Sebaceous gland
Hair follicle
Root of hair
Hair bulb

called the hair follicle. The root of a new hair stimulates the development of a hair bulb, which brings keratin (a protein found in skin, hair, and nail cells) to the growing hair. The keratin and dead hair cells continually push toward the surface of the skin, forming the hair shaft. The shaft has three microscopic layers: the hollow inner core called the medulla, long fibrous cells called the cortex, and scaled cells on the outside called the cuticle.

Sweat (sebaceous) glands in the skin produce an oily secretion that gives hair its sheen and helps waterproof it. Small involuntary muscles attached to the hairs cause the hair to stand on end in response to certain emotions, such as fear. The tingling feeling associated with "goose bumps" is the sensation caused by these muscles as they stand the hairs on end. Body hair is fine, soft, and almost colorless until puberty. During puberty, hair on some parts of the body becomes darker, coarser, and longer.

An individual hair on the head grows for 2 to 5 years and then retreats into a rest stage during which the bulb shrinks back from the root and hair begins to travel toward the skin surface. When a hair falls out, a new hair grows behind it. Scalp hair grows at a rate of about one-half inch per month.

Hair texture and color depend on a person's heredity. Hair texture is determined by the shape of the follicle from which the hair grows. Hair color is caused by the amount and type of melanin, the same pigment that darkens skin, present in the hair shaft. The more melanin, the darker the hair. With age, the cells in the

hair follicles slow their production of melanin; without pigment, the hair becomes white. Gray hair is usually white hairs mixed with darker hairs; it is rare to have truly gray hair.

Hair removal

Excess hair (see HIRSUTISM) may be due to elevated androgen levels or an underlying endocrine disorder, which should be treated with appropriate medication. There are other causes. Hair can be removed for cosmetic reasons in a number of ways.

Shaving with a shaver or razor is the most common way to remove hair. It is relatively fast, efficient, and inexpensive. However, to prevent problems such as skin irritation or infected hair follicles (see SHAVE BUMPS), it is important to use the proper techniques. If an electric shaver is used, skin should be dry. If a blade is used, skin should be dampened and lubricated with shaving cream or gel. Doctors recommend shaving in the direction the hair grows. Both the area to be shaved

and the razor should be clean. Many people prefer to use disposable razors for sanitary reasons and convenience; these razors should be replaced frequently. Applying moisturizer directly after shaving can reduce irritation. Cosmetics or deodorants should not be applied to freshly shaven skin.

Depilatories (chemical hair removers in the form of a cream or paste) break down the hair so that hairs break and can be wiped off. Depilatories may cause irritation but are useful when skin problems such as warts prevent the skin area from being shaved.

Waxing and tweezing remove hair from beneath the surface of the skin. The effects of waxing last longer than those of shaving or depilatories. However, waxing can be painful and irritating to the skin and should be done only by a professional. Some people regularly pluck their eyebrows with tweezers to reshape them. Tweezers are also used to remove hair from the ears or nose. Plucking can be painful, and hairs usually grow back 2 to 12 weeks later.

ELECTROLYSIS and LASER SURGERY for hair removal last longer than other methods of hair removal. Electrolysis is a time-consuming, labor-intensive, painful, and expensive process. In this procedure, each hair follicle is charged with an electric current, which kills hair at its root. Repeated treatment is required to clear even a small area of skin to remove hairs that were dormant at the time of previous therapy.

Using lasers is the newest method of hair removal. In this type of surgery, lasers are used to damage hair follicles. The ideal candidate for laser hair removal has fair skin and dark

HAIR REMOVAL BY LASER
Laser surgery removes hair painlessly by damaging the "growth zone" of the hair follicle. The laser beam is directed through the skin, using melanin (a pigment in skin and hair) as the target. Melanin is always more dense in hair than in skin and is most dense in the bulb of the hair follicle. While electrolysis works on one hair at a time, laser surgery works on a larger area.

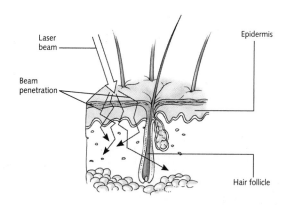

Laser beam
Epidermis
Beam penetration
Hair follicle

H

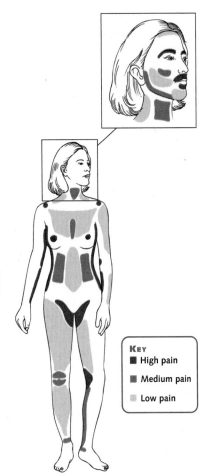

SKIN SENSITIVITY TO PAIN
Hair removal by electrolysis, waxing, or tweezing is painful, and the degree of pain a person perceives varies depending on the area of the body that is affected. Pain is a protective mechanism, and the skin contains many specialized pain receptors—especially around delicate structures such as the eyes.

brown or black hair, since lasers target dark-colored hair better than light-colored hair. Side effects of laser therapy may include redness and pigmentation changes. Treatment lasts about 3 months.

A cream that slows the rate of hair growth may be prescribed in conjunction with other hair-removal methods.

Hair transplant

A surgical procedure to remove small portions of hair-bearing scalp and relocate them to a bald area on the head of a person. Hair transplants are usually performed as COSMETIC SURGERY for the baldness that develops as a result of aging, hormonal changes, or from a family history of hair loss. Hair transplantation can also be used for baldness caused by traumatic injuries or burns. In almost all cases, hair transplantation requires a series of procedures rather than just one operation.

Hair transplants are more common in men than in women since men are more likely to be affected by a receding hairline and pattern baldness, the kind that leaves the top of the head completely or partly hairless. Women after menopause are more likely to experience thinning all over the scalp rather than pattern baldness.

Hair transplants are most successful in people with a dense growth of hair on the back of the head that serves as a donor site. Although transplanting hair can reduce thinning and add hair cover to bald areas, it will not restore the original thickness or fullness of the hair. In addition, a hair transplant should not be performed until the person is sure his or her baldness has stopped. If baldness continues to progress after transplantation, the result can be an unusual pattern on the scalp.

THE PROCEDURE

Hair transplants are performed in the office of a physician or at an outpatient surgical center. The patient returns home the same day as the procedure is completed. Local anesthesia with CONSCIOUS SEDATION is standard; the patient is awake, but relaxed and pain-free.

Before the surgery begins, the donor area on the scalp is trimmed to allow the surgeon easy access to the grafts. Once the anesthetic has been given, the surgeon removes the grafts. The size of the graft and the technique of removal vary with the type of graft. Punch grafts are taken with a tubelike instrument that removes hair, skin, and underlying tissue. Each punch graft contains 10 to 15 hairs. A scalpel is used for the other types of grafts: micrografts (one or two hairs each, with underlying tissue); minigrafts (two to four hairs); slit grafts (four to ten hairs); and strip grafts (long and thin, 30 to 40 hairs). As the grafts are removed, the surgeon may inject the donor site with small amounts of saline solution to maintain normal skin strength.

Next, the grafts are relocated to the bald area of the scalp. Punch and minigrafts are placed in small holes that are incised into the scalp; slit and strip grafts are placed into small slits made with a scalpel. The surgeon places the grafts in such a manner that the new hair will grow in a normal direction. The scalp is closed with fine sutures at both donor and recipient sites: one for a punch graft and several for a slit or strip graft.

After the transplant procedure is complete, the surgeon cleans the scalp and covers it with gauze. A pressure bandage that is to be worn for a day or two may also be added.

The number of grafts, transplanted in a single procedure, varies with the type of graft. With punch grafts, the average is 50. Since micrografts are much smaller, as many as 1,500 can be moved at one time. Because there

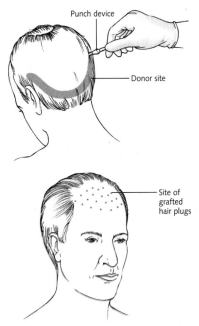

PUNCH GRAFT TECHNIQUE
To transplant hair using punch grafts, the surgeon first removes plugs of hair-bearing skin and underlying tissue from the "donor site" on the hairy part of the scalp. The skin from which the grafts are taken is stitched together to close the holes; the resulting scars are invisible under the hair. The plugs of hair, each containing about 15 strands, are inserted into new holes created in the area of the scalp to be covered. The grafts are positioned to duplicate the growth pattern of the original hair.

FLAP TECHNIQUE
To transplant a hair flap, a flap of bald scalp is removed and a flap of scalp with hair is lifted from an adjacent donor site. Without being entirely removed, the donor flap is shifted into the bald area and sutured in place. The flap of hair receives its blood supply from the portion of tissue that remains attached. The scalp from the donor site is stitched back together.

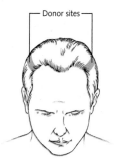

Donor sites

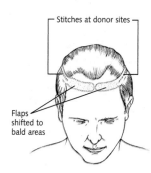

Stitches at donor sites

Flaps shifted to bald areas

is a limit as to the number of grafts that can be transplanted in any single procedure, the full hair transplantation process almost always takes more than one surgery. The surgery can be repeated at an interval of several months, with the total time taking up to 2 years. Follow-up surgery may also be needed to correct unevenness, replace failed grafts, or fill in the hairline.

It is normal for grafted hair to fall out about 6 weeks after surgery. Normal hair growth resumes approximately 5 or 6 weeks later and progresses at the usual rate of one-half inch per month.

SURGICAL ALTERNATIVES

An alternative technique to grafting involves relocating a section of scalp with hair to a bald spot. The surgeon first removes a section of bald scalp. A hair-bearing flap of a matching shape is cut from an adjacent portion of the scalp. This incision does not completely free the flap from the underlying tissue. Rather, one end is left in its original position as the flap is shifted into the originally bald area and stitched in place.

Flap surgery may be combined with scalp reduction techniques or tissue expansion. In the latter, a balloon-type device is inserted under the skin of a portion of hair-bearing scalp next to a bald area. Salt water is added to the device for several weeks to stretch the skin and cause it to grow. When the skin has been stretched enough, in about 2 months, flap surgery is performed to move the hair-bearing scalp into the bald area.

In scalp reduction, a section of bald scalp is cut out; then, the adjacent hair-bearing scalp is loosened, brought up and forward, and stitched

in place. The shape of the removed section of scalp varies with the pattern and degree of baldness. Scalp reduction can be used on the top or back of the head, but it is not useful for creating a frontal hairline.

The advantage of these more extensive surgical techniques is that they produce desired results faster than hair transplants. One flap can cover as much of an area as 350 plug grafts. The disadvantage is that the surgery is more extensive, usually demands deeper sedation during surgery with more discomfort during healing, and requires a longer recovery period.

BEFORE AND AFTER SURGERY

Blood and urine laboratory tests may be required before surgery, and the person is screened for undetected conditions that may affect safety and outcome, such as high blood pressure and diabetes. As with any surgery that involves anesthesia, the person must have nothing to eat or drink after midnight the night before surgery. The surgeon may provide instructions about medications or nutritional supplements that should be avoided. Smoking should be avoided before and after the procedure because nicotine restricts blood flow to the skin, slows healing, and increases scarring.

Discomfort after surgery typically consists of mild pain that can be controlled with oral pain medications prescribed by the surgeon. Temporary swelling and bruising are normal.

Bandages, if used, are removed the day after surgery, and stitches are taken out within a week to 10 days. If dissolvable sutures have been used, they will disappear in about a week. Gentle washing of the hair is allowed on the third day.

Strenuous activity increases blood flow into the scalp and should be avoided for the first 2 to 3 weeks to prevent bleeding. Some surgeons also recommend abstinence from sexual activity for the first 10 days since it increases blood pressure and can lead to bleeding. Most hair transplant recipients are able to go back to work and return to light physical activities within 5 to 7 days.

Possible complications involve infection of the surgical site and excessive bleeding. Scarring is rarely a problem since the surrounding hair is used to camouflage thin spots. Some transplant plugs or slices may not graft and have to be replaced in a later procedure.

Halitosis

See BAD BREATH.

Hallucination

False perceptions in any of the senses in a person who is awake, but the perceptions are not based on an external reality. Examples include hearing voices of the dead, feeling as if insects are crawling under the skin (formication), or seeing visions of people who are elsewhere. Hallucinations are sometimes but not always a sign of a severe mental disorder. Hallucinations may be due to an adverse effect of a medication, substance abuse, or drug withdrawal.

Hallucinogenic drugs

Chemical substances that can alter a person's perception of reality and cause hallucinations and other alterations of the senses. Hallucinogenic substances are found in nature, in plants, fungi, and animals; and they have been used throughout history in a wide variety of highly advanced and preliterate cultures.

Drugs classified today as hallucinogens include LSD (lysergic acid diethylamide); DOM (2,5-dimethoxy-4-methylampheamine); DMT (N,N-dimethyltriptamine); psilocybin; and mescaline, derived from peyote cactus. All hallucinogens are classified as controlled substances under schedule I (drugs with high abuse potential).

EFFECTS OF HALLUCINOGENIC DRUGS

The physical and psychological effects of hallucinogenic drugs are caused by an increase in the level of the neurochemical serotonin in the brain, combined with an inhibition of the rapid firing of neurons containing serotonin. As the serotonin level in the brain rises, the activity of affected neurons decreases. In this way, hallucinogens cause both physical and psychological effects on humans.

Physical effects of hallucinogenic drugs include dilated pupils, elevated body temperature, increased heart rate and blood pressure, loss of appetite, sleeplessness, tremors, headache, nausea, sweating, heart palpitations, blurring of vision, memory loss, trembling, and itching. The psychological effects include hyperawareness of sensation, altered thinking and self-awareness, hallucinations (seeing and hearing things that are not real), and illusions (erroneous sensory perception of objects or sounds).

Sensory alterations associated with hallucinogenic drugs include complicated phenomena described as "seeing sounds" and "hearing colors." Such experiences are of great interest to brain scientists, as is the fact that hallucinogenic drugs can cause temporary symptoms of psychosis, or loss of contact with reality. The study of hallucinogenic drugs has gone on for more than a century and is considered to represent the beginning of modern "biological psychiatry," which seeks to comprehend human behavior by understanding how the brain functions.

Negative reactions to a hallucinogenic drug may include psychological symptoms of panic, confusion, suspicion, anxiety, and loss of control, in addition to all the physical and psychologic symptoms listed. Long-term effects of the drugs can be serious as well: people may experience flashbacks, mood swings, impaired thinking, sudden outbursts of violence, and depression that may lead to suicide.

USE OF HALLUCINOGENS

According to the National Institute on Drug Abuse (NIDA), between 13 million and 17 million people in the United States have used a hallucinogenic drug at least once. The NIDA also reports that the use of the hallucinogenic drug LSD by high school seniors decreased from 9.4 percent in 1999 to 8.1 percent in 2000. The number of high school seniors using cocaine dropped from 6.2 percent to 5 percent in that same time period.

Hallux

The medical name for the big, or first, toe.

Hallux rigidus

A form of degenerative arthritis in the bottom joint of the big toe. Hallux rigidus causes a prominent outgrowth of bone at the back edge of the joint. It usually occurs in young adults; the joint may become fused or partially fused, and the toe loses some of its ability to bend at its juncture with the foot. With hallux rigidus, extending the toe is generally limited and painful, while the toe can flex more normally. Since extension of the big toe is necessary for walking properly, hallux rigidus may restrict a person's ability to walk normally. Typically, a person with this condition will favor the outer part of the foot when walking to avoid moving or pressing on the painful, affected joint. The mechanics of walking are then performed entirely by the other four toes, resulting in an unnatural and painful gait. A splint for the toe is available, and its use can restrict toe motion and provide some relief. Nonsteroidal anti-inflammatory drugs (NSAIDs) and wearing a hard-soled shoe may be of some help. In severe cases, surgery may be necessary.

Hallux valgus

A deformity of the foot caused by an osteoarthritic degenerative condition in the joint of the big toe. It is characterized by the big toe moving inward toward the second toe and sometimes overlapping it or becoming positioned under it. With time, the condition becomes increasingly painful. Hallux valgus is more common in women and tends to be inherited. It is aggravated by the wearing of high-heeled or ill-fitting shoes, particularly those with a narrow, pointed toe box. An inflamed and painful BUNION almost always develops at the site of the affected joint.

To diagnose hallux valgus, the doctor will perform a physical examination and order an X ray of the foot. Orthotic devices, corrective footwear, and physical therapy may be prescribed to treat the condition. Medication, including aspirin and other nonsteroidal anti-inflammatory drugs (NSAIDs), may be recommended to control inflammation and pain. Corticosteroids may be injected into the joint to reduce inflammation. When more conservative treatments fail and the condition is severe enough to restrict daily activities, surgery may be considered. Managing the discomforts associated with hallux valgus includes wearing soft leather, low-heeled shoes with a wide toe box; placing a protective, adhesive ring or cap around a bunion to reduce the pressure from shoes; and applying ice and resting the affected foot.

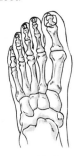 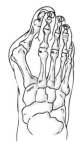

Healthy foot   Foot with hallux valgus

DEFORMITY OF THE BIG TOE JOINT
A person with hallux valgus has a big toe joint that has shifted outward, causing the toe itself to turn inward and perhaps overlap or lie under the second toe. The condition may result in bunions, which are tender, inflamed lumps on the ball of the distorted joint.

Haloperidol

An antipsychotic drug. Haloperidol (Haldol) is used to treat symptoms of mental and emotional disorders and Tourette syndrome (a neurological disorder characterized by tics); it is also used for people with severe agitation or behavior problems. Haloperidol is thought to have antipsychotic effects because it blocks dopamine receptors in the central nervous system.

Haloperidol is available in tablet or liquid form for the long-term treatment of psychotic illnesses and Tourette syndrome. The drug can be given by injection to help control severely agitated people. Long-term use of haloperidol is associated with a risk of developing a serious side effect called tardive dyskinesia (TD), characterized by uncontrollable muscle movements. People taking haloperidol should be in close contact with their doctors, who will be alert to any signs of the problem.

Halothane

See ANESTHESIA, INHALATION.

Hamartoma

A benign (not cancerous) tumorlike growth consisting of normal mature cells in abnormal numbers or distribution. For example, a lung hamartoma contains normal pulmonary tissue, such as smooth muscle and collagen, growing in a disorganized manner. Because hamartomas generally cause no harm and because of the risks involved, surgical removal is generally not done.

Hammer toe

A condition in which a toe becomes deformed in such a way that it bends downward or becomes clenched like a claw. It is painful and causes a reduction in the person's ability to move the toe, sometimes making it uncomfortable and difficult to walk and almost impossible to jog or participate in sports. It may be caused by poorly fitting shoes, which crowd the toes and push them into irregular positions. Bunions can create pressure on the toes next to the big toe, leading to the development of hammer toes. Muscle and nerve damage in the feet as a result of diabetes mellitus may also contribute to the condition. Switching to properly fitting

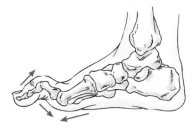

DEFORMITY OF THE TOE JOINT
A hammer toe bends upward at the middle joint, forcing the tip of the toe and the joint at the base of the toe down. Over time, the muscles that straighten the toe tighten and fail to stretch.

shoes or using a prescribed orthotic shoe insert can sometimes correct hammer toes. In some cases, corrective surgery is necessary.

Hamstring pull

An injury involving a strain in one or more of the three muscles located at the back of the thigh. The hamstring muscles run between the buttock and the knee, where they are connected to the bones of the lower leg. These muscles allow the knee to flex and the hips to extend. A hamstring pull often occurs following participation in strenuous sports or other activities involving the heavy use of leg muscles. The symptoms include a sharp pain in the back of the thigh, swelling and weakness in the upper leg, an inability to bend the leg, and discomfort and difficulty walking or sitting down. Hamstring pulls and their complications can be prevented by stopping to rest at the first sign of pain in the muscles behind the thigh. Warming up and stretching the hamstring muscles before participating in athletic activities can be helpful in preventing this injury. Treatment is centered on resting the leg as much as possible. In some cases, painkilling medication and physical therapy may be recommended.

Hand

The most flexible part of the skeleton, extending from the wrist to the tips of the fingers.

The framework of the hand is its bone structure. The hand begins where the two bones of the forearm (the radius and the ulna) join with four of the eight carpal bones that form the wrist. The other four carpal bones join the metacarpal bones that underlie the palm. They connect to the bones of the fingers and thumb (phalanges.) Ligaments join the bones of the hand together.

Muscles that move the hand and wrist are in the forearm and are connected to the bones of the hands by tendons. The tendons are encased in protective membranes called tendon sheaths. The sheaths contain a lubricant that gives the tendons the movement to extend, flex, and rotate the fingers. There are also shorter muscles within the hand itself. The tendons and muscles in the thumb allow

it to be brought close to the index finger and to move to a right angle to the palm—a range of motion found in no primate other than humans. As a result, the human hand has unique gripping and grasping capabilities.

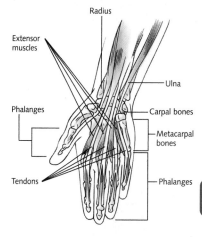

STRUCTURE OF THE HAND
The muscles and bones of the human hand—connected to the arm at the rotating wrist joint—provide tremendous flexibility, finely tuned dexterity, and precise grasping skills.

Hand-foot-and-mouth disease

An illness caused by a virus (COXSACKIEVIRUS) that primarily affects young children, particularly those in day care centers or nursery schools. Hand-foot-and-mouth disease may also affect adults and occurs most commonly in the summer and early fall. The virus may be spread by the fecal-oral route (as when a person fails to wash the hands properly after using the rest room), by respiratory secretions, by person-to-person contact, by saliva on the hands or children's toys, and by direct contact with the skin blisters caused by the virus. The incubation period is 3 to 5 days. The disease can be spread for several weeks after symptoms begin.

Symptoms often appear to be those of a common cold with an associated rash that lasts for 7 to 10 days. The rash may appear as ulcers inside the mouth, on the inner cheeks, gums, and sides of the tongue. It may also appear as blisters or bumps on the hands, feet, and other parts of the body.

There is no specific treatment for the virus that causes hand-foot-and-mouth disease. Recommended practices for preventing infection include washing hands well after using the rest room or handling soiled diapers; covering the mouth and nose when coughing or sneezing, and instructing children to do this; washing toys and other surfaces that have had contact with children's mouths and saliva; and making sure that children with fever or ulcers in the mouth are excluded from group settings.

Hangover

The unpleasant symptoms that result from drinking an excessive amount of alcohol. Symptoms usually include nausea, headache, dizziness, irritability, thirst, and fatigue. A hangover may also involve tremor, pale skin, unsteady walking, vomiting, heartburn, and loss of appetite. Hangover is caused by the body's metabolism of the alcohol and other chemicals, known technically as congeners, that occur in alcoholic beverages. Intense hangover symptoms usually begin approximately 14 or 15 hours after the first drink and can last up to 24 hours. There is no cure except time; the only treatment is over-the-counter pain medications, fluids to help offset dehydration, and rest. Frequent hangovers can be a sign of alcohol abuse or dependence; medical attention is recommended.

Hansen disease
See LEPROSY.

Hantavirus infection

An acute infection caused by the hantavirus, which is transmitted from rodents to humans. Hantaviruses have been found in wild rodents, including deer mice, rats, and moles throughout the world. Rodents transmit hantavirus via the respiratory route, and humans contract it through inhalation of infectious airborne droplets of saliva or urine or through dust from feces of infected wild rodents, especially deer mice. The virus is sometimes transmitted when broken skin comes into contact with contaminated material or when contaminated food or water are ingested. Person-to-person transmission is also possible, but has not occurred in North America.

PREVENTING INFECTIONS CARRIED BY RODENTS

Rodents carry viruses that can be dangerous to humans. Preventing rodent infestation in the home and work environment is the first step in preventing hantavirus infections. Key points include:

- Storing all food in sealed containers and screening or sealing possible points of entry into buildings can help avoid exposure to rodents, as can professional extermination.
- When working in areas where rodent excretions may exist, HEPA (high-efficiency particulate air) masks can be used to trap dust and prevent inhalation of dust particles that cause infection.
- Wearing latex, rubber, or vinyl waterproof gloves during contact with rodents or their excretions helps prevent direct contact with infectious material.
- Pouring bleach over a trapped rodent and its urine and droppings before removal can disinfect a possibly infected animal and its excretions.
- Dead rodents and all materials used in clean-up, including gloves, should be placed in a plastic bag, the opening should be tied or sealed, and the bag should be placed in another plastic bag to be tied or sealed; the bags should be disposed of in an outdoor garbage can or buried.
- Disinfectant should be used on the area where the rodent was found, and the hands should be washed thoroughly.

CLINICAL SYNDROMES
Hantavirus infection can cause either of two major clinical syndromes, both of which are rare: hemorrhagic fever with renal syndrome (HFRS) and hantavirus pulmonary syndrome (HPS). The virus produces a persistent infection and is shed in the urine, feces, and saliva.

Milder cases of HFRS generally come on suddenly with high fever, headache, backache, and abdominal pain. Small internal hemorrhages in the eyes, on the roof of the mouth, and as a rash on the trunk of the body occur by the fourth day of infection. In some cases, a toxic condition causes mental disability, and rarely, there are neurologic complications such as seizure and bladder paralysis.

Hemorrhagic fever with renal syndrome may follow a more severe course involving abrupt symptoms such as fever, chills, backache, abdominal pain, and muscle aches. A low heart rate associated with high fever occurs. There is often a diffuse reddening of the face that resembles sunburn. Small internal hemorrhages may develop on the palate, in the armpits, and in the membrane lining the eye. By the fifth day of infection, blood pressure may fall dramatically and shock can occur.

Hemorrhagic fever with renal syndrome is diagnosed by urinalysis and treated with intravenous ribavirin over a period of a week. Complete recovery may take several weeks to several months. The risk of death is low, and most people recover completely without lingering effects. Residual liver dysfunction sometimes occurs, and renal dialysis may become necessary.

There are mild cases of HPS, but more severe forms of the illness can be extremely serious and carry a 50 to 75 percent mortality rate. Symptoms begin as a flulike illness with fever, chills, muscle aches, headache, stomach pain, nausea, vomiting, coughing, and shortness of breath. The infection progresses rapidly, sometimes within a few days of the first symptoms, to an abnormal fall in blood pressure and an accumulation of fluid in the lungs resulting in fatal respiratory failure.

Early diagnosis may be made by chest X rays and blood tests. People who are diagnosed with HPS are hospitalized in intensive care units where they are treated for shock and given continuous oxygen. Intravenous ribavirin is sometimes used, but its effectiveness is undetermined. With treatment, the condition of some infected people improves rapidly within 5 to 7 days, and they are able to leave the hospital within 2 to 3 weeks and have no residual effects.

Hardening of the arteries
See ATHEROSCLEROSIS.

Hashimoto thyroiditis

A slowly developing and persistent autoimmune disease caused by the action of certain antibodies that attack the tissues of the thyroid gland; also known as chronic lymphocytic or autoimmune thyroiditis. The disease tends to occur more often to women in their 30s and 40s and especially in women older than 50 years. Hashimoto thyroiditis can eventually cause HYPOTHYROIDISM (underactivity of the thyroid gland). In Hashimoto thyroiditis, thyroid tissue is invaded by white blood cells called lymphocytes. The invasion produces inflammation, degeneration, and scarring of the tissue within the thyroid gland, gradually decreasing the gland's ability to produce and release hormones.

SYMPTOMS

The initial inflammation is generally mild and causes few symptoms. People with Hashimoto thyroiditis may not be aware that they have it for many years. Eventually, the inflammation within the thyroid gland may destroy a sufficient amount of thyroid tissue, producing hypothyroidism. At this point, Hashimoto thyroiditis produces symptoms associated with low levels of thyroid hormone, including fatigue, sensitivity to cold, forgetfulness, slow heartbeat, and psychological depression. Constipation, weight gain, and muscle cramps may be experienced. The skin may become dry and coarse and the hair dry and brittle.

Tissue inflammation may enlarge the thyroid gland, causing a feeling of fullness or tightness in the throat and a noticeable swelling at the front of the neck. There may be difficulty swallowing solid food and fluids.

DIAGNOSIS

Hashimoto thyroiditis may be detected early on by the presence of thyroid antibodies in blood, but it is usually discovered during a routine physical examination when a doctor notes an enlargement of the thyroid gland. The thyroid may also feel lumpy or nodular. A thyroid biopsy of one of the thyroid nodules may be ordered. However, thyroid enlargement or nodules do not occur in everyone with Hashimoto thyroiditis.

If there are other symptoms of the disease, blood tests may be performed to measure hormone levels. A low level of the thyroid hormone THYROXINE and an elevated level of TSH (thyroid-stimulating hormone), along with the presence of thyroid antibodies, can confirm the diagnosis.

TREATMENT

In people with normal thyroid hormone levels and a normal or modestly enlarged thyroid gland, treatment consists of regular physical examinations and blood tests to measure thyroid hormone levels.

There is no cure for Hashimoto thyroiditis. Treatment primarily consists of compensating for low thyroid function. If hypothyroidism is present, oral thyroid hormone medication is generally prescribed in incremental doses until the thyroid hormones reach a normal level in the bloodstream, at which time the symptoms of Hashimoto thyroiditis usually disappear. Doctors usually continue to monitor thyroid hormone and TSH levels in the blood to maintain the correct dosage of the medication. When there is insufficient thyroid hormone, the TSH blood levels become elevated, indicating the need for a higher dose of thyroid hormone. When the dose of thyroid hormone is excessive, the TSH blood levels become abnormally low, and the amount of thyroid hormone medication is decreased.

RISK FACTORS

Thyroid disturbances and autoimmune diseases tend to run in families. A person who has relatives with other forms of hypothyroidism or HYPERTHYROIDISM (overactivity of the thyroid gland), including GRAVES DISEASE, is at greater risk for Hashimoto thyroiditis. Other autoimmune conditions that may be associated with Hashimoto thyroiditis are type 1 diabetes mellitus, pernicious anemia, alopecia areata (patchy hair loss), vitiligo (white spots on the skin), and prematurely gray hair. When any of these diseases or disorders are noted by a doctor in a person's medical history, blood tests may be performed to check thyroid hormone levels. Screening techniques such as these tests to detect mild hypothyroidism early on can help a doctor diagnose and begin treating Hashimoto thyroiditis before it becomes more serious. Regular visits to a doctor for thyroid examinations, blood tests, and adjustments in thyroid hormone medication dosages can prevent the progression of more debilitating symptoms associated with hypothyroidism.

Hatching, assisted

A type of fertility technique that improves the ability of some embryos to implant during IN VITRO FERTILIZATION; also known as assisted zona hatching. In assisted hatching, a small opening is created in the thick, transparent outer membrane (zona pellucida) of the embryo, increasing the chance that the membrane will be shed and implantation of the embryo in the uterus will occur. In the procedure, an embryo is placed in a petri dish and the membrane is dissolved with a chemical. The embryo is then placed in an incubator and transferred to the woman's uterus a few hours later. The technique is generally used by couples whose previous attempts at ASSISTED REPRODUCTIVE TECHNOLOGY inexplicably failed or whose fertility is limited by advancing age.

Hatha yoga

A slow-paced, physical form of yoga. Hatha yoga is the most familiar form of yoga in the United States. In hatha yoga, ancient postures ("asana"), breathing exercises ("pranayama"), and purification practices ("kriyas") are performed to reduce stress and boost energy. Hatha yoga is also used to reduce mechanical stresses that cause physical pain. The traditional purpose of yoga is to attain enlightenment through meditation. Hatha yoga is sometimes called "meditation in action," a discipline that goes beyond physical exercise to realign the person with the flow of nature. See YOGA.

Hay fever

A set of symptoms caused by the immune system's response to inhalation of tiny airborne pollens of certain seasonal plants. Hay fever is caused by the body's antibodies reacting with the inhaled pollen, a reaction that causes HISTAMINE to be released. The histamine promotes an inflammatory response in the linings of the nose, sinuses, eyelids, and eyes. Inflammation in the sinuses causes congestion, and the nose begins to produce excess mucus. Inflamed mucous mem-

H

COPING WITH ALLERGIES

Avoidance of pollens is not always possible, but there are several things people with hay fever can do to minimize the effects of exposure. People with allergies should:

- Avoid outdoor activities between 5 AM and 10 AM when pollen counts tend to be highest. The pollen count drops in the mid- to late-afternoon hours. Wearing a dust mask during yard work may be helpful, even when the concentration of pollen in the air tends to be low, because raking and mowing stir up pollen on the ground.
- Use an air-conditioner indoors even when cool air is not desired. The fan setting on an air conditioner will help filter out pollen inside the house. Air conditioner filters should be cleaned monthly.
- Avoid drying laundry outdoors on a line where airborne pollen will cling to it. It is best to use an indoor line or a clothes dryer.
- Take a thorough shower after spending time outdoors during allergy season. Pollen can cling to the skin and hair, causing symptoms long after a person has come indoors.
- Avoid, as much as possible, exposure to other inhaled irritants, including dust, smoke, insect sprays, air pollutants, and tar fumes, all of which can intensify hay fever symptoms.

---

branes result in an itchy sensation that occurs in the eyes, nose, throat, and the roof of the mouth. The eyes may feel irritated and teary. The nose is stuffy or runny. Sneezing can become frequent and violent and may occur repetitively as often as 20 times in a row. The medical term for hay fever is allergic rhinitis.

What makes some people sensitized to airborne pollens is not entirely understood. In part, it is an inherited trait that involves the immune system's response. A person who has family members with allergies is at a higher risk for hay fever. Having other allergic conditions, including dermatitis and asthma, also predisposes a person to this allergy. Symptoms may be year-round or have a seasonal variation.

DIAGNOSIS AND TREATMENT

If the symptoms of hay fever interfere with daily activities, it may become necessary to consult an ALLERGIST. This physician will generally take a full medical history to determine the specific allergens that are causing the symptoms. The affected person may be requested to keep a detailed account of symptoms, including the time of year, time of day, severity, and duration of congestion, sneezing, tearing eyes, and runny nose. Skin scratch tests may be performed to identify the pollens to which a person is sensitive.

Hay fever is best controlled by avoidance of the pollens that produce symptoms. An allergist may prescribe antihistamines, decongestants, and a corticosteroid nasal spray. Eye drops may

also be prescribed. Using over-the-counter nasal sprays and drops is usually not recommended as these products relieve congestion only temporarily and can cause nasal symptoms to worsen over the long-term.

While there is no cure for hay fever, a series of injections or allergy shots to desensitize an affected person to the specific pollen or pollens may be beneficial. This process is called immunotherapy and involves the person receiving injections of increasing amounts of an extract of the pollen allergen over a period of time until the person becomes desensitized to it. This can take up to 2 years, is often expensive, and may not be effective for everyone. This option may be tried if avoidance measures are not effective and medications are causing adverse side affects.

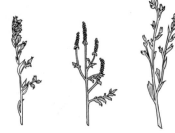

| Golden rod | Ragweed | Sage bush |

COMMON HAY FEVER TRIGGERS
Pollen-bearing grasses, including golden rod, ragweed, and sage bush, are common causes of hay fever. An allergic person inhales the pollen, and the body produces antibodies. The immune response leads to inflamed mucous membranes in the nose, eyelids, eyes, and bronchial tubes.

HCG
See HUMAN CHORIONIC GONADOTROPIN.

HDL
High-density lipoprotein. See CHOLESTEROL.

Head and neck cancer
A broad category of tumors that arise in the head and neck area, including tumors in the mouth, tongue, lips, gums, sinuses, salivary glands, throat, and larynx (voice box). Symptoms can include swelling or sores in the mouth that do not heal; pain, swelling, or obstruction of the nose; chronic sinus trouble that is unresponsive to antibiotics; paralysis of one side of the face; ear pain; pain when swallowing; bloody nasal discharges; persistent hoarseness; difficulty breathing; and double vision.

Head and neck cancers account for between 5 and 10 percent of all malignancies. They are three times more likely to develop in men than in women and are most common after age 50. Individuals who smoke or drink alcohol are at greatest risk of developing head and neck cancer. Cancer of the nasopharynx (the area above the soft palate) has been linked to Epstein-Barr virus (EBV) infections. Oral cancers are sometimes discovered by dentists during routine examinations. Specific diagnostic testing depends on the location of the cancer and can include X rays, MRI (magnetic resonance imaging) and CT (computed tomography) scanning, and biopsy. Surgery is often the first choice for treatment, although radiation therapy is sometimes as effective and may better preserve the appearance and function of the affected area of the head or neck. Chemotherapy, usually in combination with radiation, is sometimes used.

Head banging
Repetitive banging of the head against the side of the crib, most common in infants between ages 5 and 11 months. Some normal bruising may occur, but lacerations or skull injuries may indicate child abuse and need to be investigated. Boys are more likely than girls to be head-bangers. In some cases, the behavior may indicate discomfort due to an ear infection or teething.

Other times, it is a way of getting attention. Less commonly, head banging is a sign of a more serious problem such as a FAILURE TO THRIVE, AUTISM, or neglect (see ABUSE, CHILD).

Children who bang their heads rarely cause themselves serious harm, and the behavior usually passes within a few months. However, a rare but serious result of head banging can be the formation of cataracts, the loss of transparency in the eye's lens. Periodic eye examinations are necessary for chronic head-bangers. Doctors advise diverting a head-banging baby's attention with soothing music or by holding and comforting the baby. Padded crib sides can decrease both the risk of injury and the noise.

Head injuries

FOR FIRST AID
see Head injuries, page 1324

Any injury that results in damage to the brain or trauma to the head. Head injuries, also called traumatic brain injuries, are quite common. Each year, an estimated 2 million people in the United States have head injuries. Most of these are mild, with symptoms that disappear over time with treatment, but many—500,000 to 750,000—are severe enough to require hospitalization. Head injuries are most common among males aged 15 to 24, but persons of any age can be affected, with some head injuries causing permanent disability.

SYMPTOMS

The signs and symptoms of head injury may occur immediately or may develop slowly over several hours. Anyone who has received a bump on the head should be watched closely for a day because symptoms are sometimes delayed. The person may get better right away, only to get worse later. The many possible symptoms of head injuries include the following: loss of consciousness; bleeding; slowed breathing; confusion; seizures; skull fracture; fluid drainage from the nose, mouth, or ears that is either clear or bloody; headache that may be severe; increased drowsiness; slurred speech; stiff neck; and swelling at the site of the injury. Additional symptoms include scalp wounds, vomiting that may be severe and persistent, irritabil-ity, personality changes, change in pulse rate, and pupils of unequal size.

TYPES OF HEAD INJURIES

There are two basic types of head injuries: closed head injuries and penetrating head injuries.

■ *Closed head injuries* A closed head injury happens when a head that is moving is stopped suddenly. A person in a car whose head hits the windshield when the car makes a sudden stop may sustain a closed head injury. Another type is a concussion, a blow to the head that causes a temporary loss of consciousness. Another type occurs when a solid object hits the head with sufficient force to smash the bone of the skull into the brain. Closed head injuries can occur without direct trauma to the skull if the brain undergoes a rapid forward or backward motion— as in whiplash, which is caused when vehicles come to a sudden stop. Neck injuries may occur, too.

■ *Penetrating head injury* Penetrating head injuries happen when fast moving objects penetrate the skull. A bullet entering the brain is an example of a penetrating head injury.

TREATMENT

The first step in treating head injuries is to provide emergency medical attention when appropriate. Anyone who has had a head injury, even a very mild one, should refrain from vigorous activity for 24 hours.

PREVENTION

Head injuries can be prevented, particularly by wearing helmets when biking, in-line skating, snowboarding, or motorcycling and by wearing a seatbelt when in an automobile. It is wise to avoid riding a bicycle at night.

DANGEROUS HEAD INJURIES

Head injuries can be very serious if there is bleeding or swelling inside a person's brain, which is impossible for a layperson to detect. Emergency assistance is indicated for these pronounced symptoms:

- **There was loss of consciousness.**
- **The person is confused or has lost his or her memory.**
- **There is clear or bloody discharge coming from the ears, nose, or mouth without a visible external source such as a cut.**
- **There are seizures.**
- **The person reports changed vision or speaks differently.**
- **The person reports having a severe headache.**
- **The person vomits more than twice after the injury.**
- **Uncontrolled bleeding occurs.**

Here are other instances when a person with an injury needs immediate medical assistance to rule out head injury:

- **The fall was greater than the person's height.**
- **A person is found unconscious.**
- **An automobile accident caused severe force to the head or upper body.**
- **A gunshot wound penetrated the head.**
- **A car crashed, and the driver or passengers were not wearing seat belts.**
- **A person was thrown from a moving vehicle.**
- **A person was injured severely enough to damage his or her hard hat or helmet.**
- **A person was struck by lightning.**

H

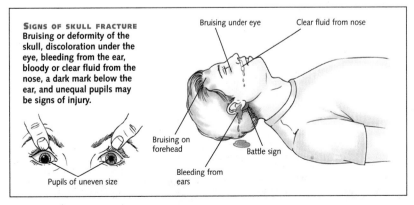

SIGNS OF SKULL FRACTURE
Bruising or deformity of the skull, discoloration under the eye, bleeding from the ear, bloody or clear fluid from the nose, a dark mark below the ear, and unequal pupils may be signs of injury.

Bruising under eye

Clear fluid from nose

Bruising on forehead

Battle sign

Bleeding from ears

Pupils of uneven size

Head lag

The backward flopping of the head when an infant is placed in a sitting position. Weak neck muscles make the baby unable to hold up his or her head until age 4 months. After that, head lag is a sign of possible DEVELOPMENTAL DELAY, a failure to develop physical and intellectual skills at the normal time for the child's age and sex. Head lag can be the sign of a serious problem such as CEREBRAL PALSY.

Headache

FOR SYMPTOM CHART
see Headache, page 38

Pain in the head. Approximately seven of ten people get headaches. A headache may be located in any part of the head and may even extend to the neck. The problem can be acute (short and isolated) or chronic (a common occurrence). Most headaches are painful and annoying but can be easily relieved with aspirin or acetaminophen. However, in some cases head pain becomes severe and debilitating, and occasionally a headache is a symptom of a serious underlying medical problem. The most common types are tension headaches and migraines. See also MIGRAINE.

CAUSES

Tension headaches are traditionally attributed to tensing of the facial, scalp, or neck muscles, while migraine pain is associated with alternate constriction and relaxation of blood vessels in the brain. While these factors indeed have a role in headache pain, in recent years researchers have also focused attention on alterations in nerve pathways and imbalances in brain chemistry. The trigeminal nerve system seems to be a major pain pathway for headaches; SEROTONIN, a neurotransmitter or nerve chemical, regulates pain messages passing through the trigeminal nerve system. A malfunction or chemical imbalance in this system is believed to be an underlying cause of headaches.

TYPES OF HEADACHES

It is important first to separate primary headaches from secondary headaches (those caused by another medical condition, such as a tumor). Primary headaches are common and tension headaches and migraines; other types include cluster headaches, sinus headaches, and rebound headaches.

Tension headaches are the most common primary headache. They are characterized by a feeling of dull pain that affects the entire head. The pain is typically described as a tightness or bandlike constriction, which is usually dull and does not throb. Tension headaches are commonly triggered by stress, fatigue, depression, or anxiety. Other causes include excessive alcohol or caffeine use, excessive smoking, eye strain, overexertion, colds or flu, and working for an extended period with the head held in one position (as at a computer).

Migraine headaches are characterized by throbbing pain that commonly begins on one side of the head. Some are preceded by fatigue, depression, or an AURA (an unusual sensation that may consist of tingling or numbness, strange tastes or odors, restlessness, confusion, or visual disturbances, such as seeing flashing lights). Migraine attacks occur on a sporadic basis and may last several hours to several days. Their pain may become disabling. In addition, there may be other symptoms, such as nausea, vomiting, dizziness, chills, loss of appetite, irritability, fatigue, and sensitivity to light and sound. These headaches may be triggered by factors such as hormonal fluctuations (including PREMENSTRUAL SYNDROME), allergic reactions, stress, foods that contain the amino acid tyramine (such as red wine, aged cheese, and smoked fish), chocolate, food additives, bright lights, and loud noises. Migraines run in families, and women are three times more likely to have them than are men.

Cluster headaches are rare and intensely painful. They are characterized by burning or boring pain that generally occurs at night, waking a person from sleep. Pain is usually located behind or around one eye. Cluster headaches tend to occur in groups or clusters for a period of time (which can be as short as days or as long as months) and then disappear. They may or may not return at a later time. This type of headache affects primarily men, especially heavy smokers.

A sinus headache may develop when the sinuses become infected or inflamed. (See SINUSITIS.) Pain typically comes on quickly in the nasal area

HEADACHE AS WARNING SIGN

In certain cases, a headache is a warning sign of a potentially serious underlying problem. Doctors recommend immediate medical evaluation in the following cases:

- **Any headache accompanied by a loss of consciousness**
- **A headache characterized by sudden, violent pain, which may be a symptom of a ruptured aneurysm**
- **A headache that worsens over time and is accompanied by nausea and vomiting**
- **A headache that is accompanied by nausea, vomiting, fever, and a stiff neck, which may be a symptom of meningitis**
- **A headache that is associated with abnormal neurological functions (such as changes in speech, vision, balance, movement, and sensation), which may indicate a stroke**
- **A headache after any head injury, even a minor one**
- **A change in headache patterns**

and worsens over time. A sinus headache usually follows a bad cold and is accompanied by a fever. While many people have head pain in the area of the sinuses, most do not have sinus headaches; these are usually migraine or tension headaches.

Rebound headaches may develop when a person takes medication for headaches more than two or three times a week. When analgesics are overused to treat headaches, the body adapts and grows dependent on them. Rebound headaches may vary in timing and intensity, but can occur as often as daily. There may be nearly constant low-grade pain, with occasional episodes of more intense pain.

DIAGNOSIS AND TREATMENT

Doctors advise people who have chronic or severe headaches to seek prompt medical evaluation and treatment. Diagnosis of headache type is based on the nature of the pain, its frequency and duration, location, severity, and accompanying symptoms. Tests such as CT SCANNING (computed tomography scanning) and MRI (magnetic resonance imaging) may be performed to rule out any serious underlying causes of symptoms, such as a ruptured ANEURYSM, BRAIN TUMOR,

TYPES OF HEADACHES

Headaches are traditionally classified by how severe the pain is and by patterns of pain. The frequency and duration of headaches provide doctors with information to help them distinguish benign or non-serious headaches from head pains that may be associated with more severe disorders.

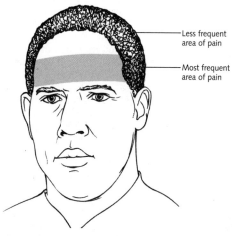

Less frequent area of pain

Most frequent area of pain

TENSION HEADACHE
Pain associated with tension headaches is most frequently described as a bandlike sensation around the head or as a feeling of weight pressing down on the entire top half of the head.

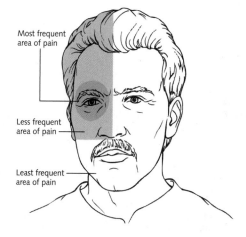

Most frequent area of pain

Less frequent area of pain

Least frequent area of pain

CLUSTER HEADACHE
Cluster headache pain is almost always one-sided; the most common sites of pain are around the eye, the temple, and the side of the head.

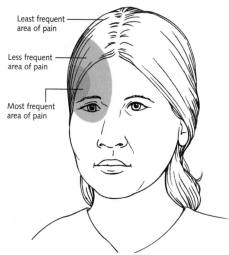

Least frequent area of pain

Less frequent area of pain

Most frequent area of pain

MIGRAINE HEADACHE
Migraine pain is throbbing, usually on one side of the head, and is frequently concentrated at the temple or the base of the skull.

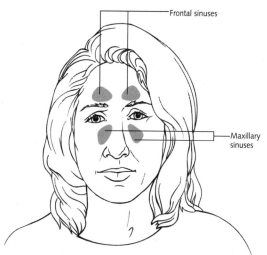

Frontal sinuses

Maxillary sinuses

SINUS HEADACHE
Sinus headaches can occur in any of the sinus cavities of the face or head.

H

H

or temporal arteritis (see ARTERITIS, GIANT CELL).

Home care for mild-to-moderate headaches includes rest, ice or heat packs, hot showers, massage, and over-the-counter pain relievers, such as aspirin, acetaminophen, or ibuprofen. To prevent rebound headaches, only the minimal necessary dose of medication should be taken. Doctors recommend strategies such as exercise, meditation, relaxation therapy, and biofeedback to control stress. People who have migraines benefit from napping in a dark, quiet room.

It is also important to identify and avoid the triggers of headaches (such as alcohol, caffeine, smoking, and certain foods). This is particularly important in the case of migraine headaches. To identify triggers, it is useful to maintain a headache diary (a calendar record of headaches, associated symptoms, and environmental factors, such as diet, menstrual cycles, and sleep patterns).

Doctors treat chronic or severe headaches with two categories of medications: abortive (to relieve pain and other symptoms) and prophylactic (to prevent headaches from developing). Abortive medications include triptans (such as sumatriptan and zolmitriptan), vasoconstrictors (such ergotamine tartrate), lidocaine nasal drops, muscle relaxants, narcotic analgesics, and aspirin and other nonsteroidal anti-inflammatory drugs (NSAIDs). Prophylactic medications include tricyclic antidepressants, serotonin antagonists, cardiovascular drugs (beta blockers and calcium channel blockers), antiseizure drugs (such as valproic acid), riboflavin (vitamin B2), and magnesium. Preventive medication is usually recommended only for people who have frequent attacks and for people in whom headaches are so severe that they prevent normal activity.

For sinus headaches, doctors recommend use of decongestants or antibiotics and in some cases draining the affected sinus. Because serious complications may develop, headaches resulting from temporal arteritis (a type of arterial inflammation) require careful medical evaluation and treatment with corticosteroid medications. A person who has rebound headaches must be weaned from reliance on analgesics.

This process is easier under a doctor's supervision, as he or she can recommend treatments to help with drug withdrawal. Any medical conditions that underlie headaches (for example, depression, anxiety, or other emotional problems) also require appropriate treatment.

Healing

The act or process through which a person regains the normal structural and functional characteristics of health and well-being after an illness or injury.

Healing touch

See ENERGY MEDICINE; THERAPEUTIC TOUCH.

Health

A state of physical, mental, and social WELL-BEING; the absence of disease. Many factors determine a person's state of health. These include both genetic components and lifestyle choices.

Health food

A general term often used to refer to foods that are unprocessed, whole, or organically grown or that are free of additives, hormones, antibiotics, pesticides, and waxes. Health foods have become increasingly available in most supermarkets as well as specialty stores. Because there is no standard, legal definition of health foods or natural foods, it is important to read the labels of foods touting health benefits. Doctors recommend close evaluation of the fat, calorie, sugar, and salt content of health food. For example, additive-free ice cream may still be high in fat, and granola is often heavily coated with sugar and high in fat.

Health law

The field of law that deals with the legal issues associated with health care, including the interrelationships among health care professionals, patients, and the parties who are financially responsible for health care services. Both government (through Medicare and Medicaid) and private organizations (such as the Joint Commission on Accreditation of Healthcare Organizations) heavily regulate the health care industry. Health law also covers health care

business associations, both profit and not-for-profit.

Health law is considered a rapidly changing area of legal practice. In 1976, the American Bar Association (ABA) developed a health law forum; in 1996, health law became a section of the ABA.

Health maintenance organization

See HMO.

Hearing

The ability to perceive and identify sound. All sources of sound send vibrations or sound waves through the air. These sound waves are funneled into the outer EAR opening and travel through the ear canal to the eardrum, causing this thin membrane to vibrate. These vibrations are passed through small bones in the middle ear to fluid in the inner ear. The vibrating movement of the fluid stimulates hairlike projections called hair cells to transform the sound wave vibrations into electrical nerve impulses and sends them to the hearing nerve in the inner ear. This nerve transmits the impulses to the brain. In the brain's hearing centers, the nerve impulses are identified and interpreted as individual sounds that are understandable to the person listening to them. Hearing is supplemented by vibrations conducted through the bones of the skull into the inner ear. A person hears his or her own voice via these vibrations within the skull.

The ability to hear ranges rather widely from person to person. Anything that interferes with the delicate hearing apparatus can contribute to HEARING LOSS. Various ear infections, physical trauma to the ear, and abnormal ear structures can all affect hearing. Acute or chronic inflammation of the middle ear, called OTITIS MEDIA, may cause inflammation and affect the eardrum's mobility so that hearing is impaired. Serous otitis media involves a buildup of fluid in the middle ear that can interfere with hearing. Deformed structures in the middle ear, such as those associated with OTOSCLEROSIS may also be responsible for loss of hearing. Inner ear diseases such as MENIERE DISEASE can cause hearing loss. Defects in the ear's structures, which may be present at birth, can cause impaired hearing. A perforated eardrum (see EARDRUM, PERFORATED), earwax, or foreign objects in the ear (see EAR, FOREIGN BODY IN) are also causes of decreased hearing ability.

Being in the water, especially during prolonged swimming, is one of the causes of acquired ear disease, which may impair hearing (see SWIMMER'S EAR). Rapid or extreme changes in air pressure, both at high altitudes during flying and at depths underwater when scuba diving, can affect the middle ear and impair hearing (see BAROTRAUMA). Sound itself can be the cause of hearing loss when it is sudden and excessively loud (see ACOUSTIC TRAUMA). When hearing is impaired, corrective implements and devices may be used to improve a person's ability to hear (see HEARING AIDS; ASSISTIVE LISTENING DEVICES; and COCHLEAR IMPLANT).

Hearing aids

Electronic devices, consisting of four miniature components—a microphone, amplifier, receiver, and battery—that bring amplified sound to the ear of a person whose hearing is impaired. On most hearing aids, sound level controls are adjustable. Some hearing aids have directional microphones. The amplifier is made up of electronic circuits, acting something like a computer chip. The miniature receiver and battery of the hearing aid are enclosed in either a small chassis or shell, worn behind or inside the ear. When HEARING LOSS is due to malformation of the ear canal or functional problems in the middle ear, an additional component, a small vibrator held behind the ear with a headband, may be necessary. This vibrator is clamped against the mastoid bone (back portion of the bone that contains the inner ear) and conducts sound through the bones of the head to the inner ear. For people with profound DEAFNESS whose auditory nerves are functional, a surgically implanted device may provide limited sound perception and serve as an aid to lip-reading or may even allow a person to understand while on the telephone (see COCHLEAR IMPLANT).

HOW THEY WORK

Hearing aids increase the volume of sound electrically through their vari-

ous components. The tiny microphone transforms sounds into electrical signals. The amplifier increases the strength of the signals, and a tiny speaker delivers the sound to the ear. Batteries lasting 1 or 2 weeks provide the electrical power.

WHAT TO EXPECT

Purchasing a hearing aid is best done after a doctor's evaluation and medical recommendation. People who experience hearing loss are usually referred by their physician to an AUDIOLOGIST (professional trained in evaluating the cause of hearing impairment and fitting hearing aids) to have their hearing tested (see AUDIOMETRY).

If it is determined that a hearing aid will be beneficial to a person with impaired hearing, the audiologist or a hearing aid dealer will evaluate and fit the person with the appropriate device.

Hearing aids are fitted to an individual's ears, and the person's hearing is then evaluated under various noise conditions. The person is generally given instructions on care and use, a suggested wearing schedule, and recommended communication strategies with hearing aids.

Hearing tests performed while a person is wearing a hearing aid are called real-ear measurements. This evaluation allows an audiologist to make necessary adjustments in the hearing aid and assure optimal amplification by fine-tuning the aid to individual need.

Hearing aids may be more helpful for certain types of hearing loss or impairment than for others. If hearing loss is consistent at all frequencies, a hearing aid offers the person enhanced sound perception and sound discrimination. People with MENIERE DISEASE, for example, often benefit.

In cases of age-related hearing loss (see HEARING LOSS, IN OLDER PEOPLE), when impaired hearing is most severe at higher frequencies of sound, special hearing aids that magnify only the high frequencies may or may not be of help. People who are overly sensitive to loud sounds may also find hearing aids of little benefit.

TYPES OF HEARING AIDS

There are several options in hearing aids, depending on the extent of hearing loss or impairment, as well as the size and shape of the ear canal. Some

hearing aids have special "telecoil," or "T" switches, to augment sound during telephone conversations; but with newer phones, this is less often possible. Two basic kinds of hearing aids are available.

Behind-the-ear (BTE) hearing aids consist of a microphone, amplifier, speaker, and battery, all contained in a small, lightweight plastic chassis, or case, worn behind the ear or attached to the earpiece of eyeglasses. This case is connected by a short tube to an earphone that fits into the outer part of the ear, sealing it so that all the amplified sound enters the ear.

In-the-ear (ITE) hearing aids are most often prescribed, probably because their small size makes them convenient and unobtrusive. ITE aids are contained in a shell, or case, small enough to be worn inside the ear. The case is molded to seal the ear canal so that no sound is lost. This kind of hearing aid is easy to insert in the ear and has easily adjustable volume controls. Even smaller versions of ITEs are called half-shell or in-the-canal (ITC) hearing aids. The least visible hearing aids are worn completely in-the-canal and are called CICs. See Types of hearing aids on page 636.

Hearing loss

Partial or total loss of the ability to perceive and identify sound. There are four general categories of hearing loss: conductive hearing loss, sensorineural hearing loss, mixed hearing loss, and central hearing loss (see DEAFNESS). Each hearing loss can be distinguished from the other by the evaluation of hearing test results (see AUDIOMETRY).

Conductive hearing loss includes impairments to hearing caused by any interference with the structures and mechanisms that conduct sound waves from the external environment to the fluid in the inner ear. Possible causes of conductive hearing loss range from simple disorders such as impacted EARWAX, to more serious problems such as fluid in the ear, perforated eardrum (see EARDRUM, PERFORATED), OTOSCLEROSIS (abnormal bone growth in the inner ear), or a benign cyst or tumor in the ear. These hearing losses can usually be corrected by medical treatments or procedures, including surgery.

TYPES OF HEARING AIDS

Some types of hearing loss can be corrected with a hearing aid, a device that amplifies sounds. If a doctor or audiologist recommends a hearing aid, tests will be done to determine the appropriate kind of hearing aid for an individual. A wax mold will be made of the ear, and a hearing aid will be custom-made for the individual's ear. Once fitted, a hearing aid should be tested and adjusted regularly to ensure that it is working properly.

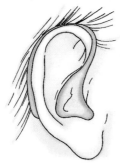

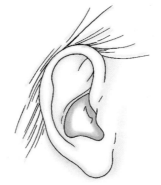

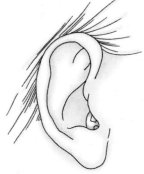

BEHIND THE EAR
In a behind-the-ear (BTE) hearing aid, all the components of the device are inside a plastic unit that fits behind the ear or attaches to a pair of glasses. A wire carries sound from the unit to an earphone that is molded to the inside of the ear. This type of device is somewhat more visible than other models, but it is stable and tends not to whistle as some models do.

IN THE EAR
An in-the-ear (ITE) device is the most common type of hearing aid. It is remarkably small and unobtrusive but is somewhat more expensive and difficult to fit.

COMPLETELY IN THE CANAL
A completely in-the-canal (CIC) hearing aid is made to fit all the way into the ear canal, so that it is almost invisible. Once in, it must be removed with a handle. These aids are considerably more expensive and difficult to fit, and it is less convenient to adjust them or change batteries. But their invisibility makes them very popular. They are appropriate for someone with a mild to moderate hearing loss.

HOW A HEARING AID WORKS
In a person wearing a hearing aid, sound waves from the environment enter a miniature microphone that amplifies them and sends them down the ear canal. The sound waves are transmitted through the structures of the middle ear to the fluid-filled cochlea in the inner ear. There the sound waves are converted to nerve impulses that are carried along the auditory nerve to the brain, where they are interpreted as sound.

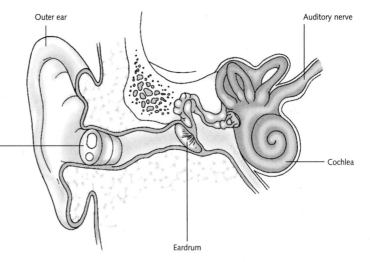

Outer ear

Auditory nerve

In-the-canal aid

Cochlea

Eardrum

Sensorineural hearing loss is also called perceptive hearing loss. The possible sources of this type of hearing loss include problems in the inner ear, problems with the nerve that transmits impulses from the inner ear to the brain, and problems with the brain's functioning. Although there may be wide variations in the degree of loss, aging is the most common cause of this kind of hearing loss (see HEARING LOSS, IN OLDER PEOPLE). Exposure to sudden, extremely loud noise such as explosions or gunshots can also produce this kind of hearing loss (see ACOUSTIC TRAUMA). "Rock and roll deafness," caused by exposure to overly amplified music at concerts or by listening to music at high volumes through earphones, is a form of sensorineural hearing loss experienced by young people. Unlike conductive hearing loss, sensorineural hearing loss is often permanent; it is difficult to treat medically and cannot be corrected surgically. In many cases, special devices can enhance sound for people who have sensorineural hearing loss (see HEARING AIDS; ASSISTIVE LISTENING DEVICES; and COCHLEAR IMPLANT).

Hearing loss, in older people

A common problem of aging. About one third of Americans between the ages of 65 and 75 and half of those older than 85 experience age-related hearing loss (presbycusis). It is more common among men than women and may run in families. It can affect both ears but not necessarily equally. With age, the inner and middle ear gradually degenerate. Tiny hair cells in the cochlea (in the inner ear) that are critical for normal hearing die and cannot grow back. Some older people become hearing impaired from earlier damage due to loud noise, injury, or disease. Others experience declines in hearing attributable to both degeneration and injury. Hearing loss in older people is important to diagnose and treat. Older people with unrecognized hearing loss can be mistaken for being confused or unresponsive. Left untreated, the condition may lead to depression and feelings of isolation. Even patients with dementia may show some improvement if a hearing loss is corrected.

DIAGNOSIS AND TREATMENT

Symptoms of age-related hearing loss include an initial decrease in the ability to hear high-pitched sounds, eventually followed by loss of the lower range; difficulty hearing speech, especially amid background noise; and loss of sound clarity. Older people who have difficulty hearing should see their doctor for a thorough physical examination and a hearing test. Often, the hearing test is performed by an audiologist, a health professional trained in testing hearing. Hearing tests, which are painless, measure a person's ability to hear sounds at different pitches and loudness. Older people are sometimes referred to an otolaryngologist, a medical doctor who specializes in the treatment of disorders of the ear, nose, and throat.

Because some causes are treatable, it is important to determine whether a hearing problem is due to factors other than aging. For example, hearing loss is sometimes due to a viral or bacterial infection or occurs as a side effect of medications. Wax also accumulates more quickly in the ears as people grow older and can cause hearing problems. Earwax softeners may control this condition, or a doctor can flush wax out of the ears. When hearing loss is permanent, hearing aids amplify sounds and can significantly improve hearing. An audiologist can advise the specific model and design that best fit a person's needs. It is important to get a hearing aid with controls that are easily managed by an older person. See also HEARING AIDS.

Hearing tests

See AUDIOMETRY.

Heart

The hollow, muscular organ that pumps blood throughout the body. Lying in the chest midway between the sternum (breastbone) and the spine, the heart sits slightly left of center. At each beat its tip strikes the inner surface of the chest wall, sometimes producing visible movement and allowing it to be felt by hand. In an adult, the heart is a little larger than a clenched fist, weighing about 1 pound.

STRUCTURE AND FUNCTION

The heart is a four-chambered organ composed of specialized muscle tissue called myocardium. The interior surfaces of the heart are lined with a smooth membrane called the endocardium; the entire heart is contained in a strong sac called the pericardium.

Each side of the heart is composed of an upper chamber called the atrium and a lower chamber called the ventricle. The right and left sides act as separate pumps. On the left side, blood rich in oxygen from the lungs is pumped from the atrium to the ventricle, then into the aorta to be transported throughout the body via arteries. On the right side, depleted blood that has traveled throughout the body discharging oxygen and other nutrients returns to the heart, via the vena cava, into the right atrium and then into the right ventricle. From there, it flows via the pulmonary artery into the lungs, where it is reoxygenated. This oxygen-rich blood is returned through the pulmonary veins into the left atrium. See CARDIOVASCULAR SYSTEM.

Each of the heart's four chambers has a one-way valve (see HEART VALVE) controlling blood flow in the right direction, to ensure the intricate sequence of the heartbeat. The heart cannot extract oxygen and nutrients from itself, and so the organ has its own circulatory system. The right and left coronary arteries— so named because the network of arteries around the heart form a crown—branch off the aorta very close to where it leaves the heart wall. These arteries divide into smaller and smaller vessels. After the blood has released its oxygen to the heart muscle, it travels back toward the right atrium through the cardiac veins.

HEARTBEAT

An individual heartbeat is timed by electrical impulses from the heart's pacemaker, which is called the sinoatrial node. A heartbeat occurs in three carefully synchronized phases: the diastole, the atrial systole, and the ventricular systole. In the diastole, or resting phase, the heart's two upper chambers or atria, fill with blood. Oxygen-rich blood flows into the left atrium, and at the same time, oxygen-poor blood fills the right atrium.

The sinoatrial node generates impulses that stimulate the atrial systole. In this second phase, the two

HOW THE HEART WORKS

The pulmonary veins deliver oxygen-rich blood from the lungs and deposit it into the left atrium of the heart. Then the atrium channels the oxygen-rich blood into the left ventricle, where it is pumped through the main artery of the body, the aorta. The aorta divides into smaller arteries that carry blood to every organ and tissue in the body. At the same time, the body's tissues deposit waste material into the blood. The oxygen-depleted blood is pumped back into the right atrium, where it is channeled to the right ventricle. The right ventricle pumps blood into the pulmonary artery and then to the lungs, where waste material leaves the blood as carbon dioxide and oxygen enter.

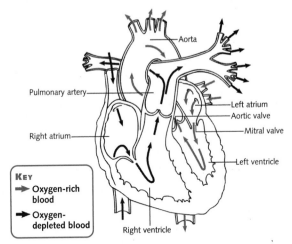

KEY
➡ Oxygen-rich blood
➡ Oxygen-depleted blood

HOW THE HEART PUMPS BLOOD
The heart delivers blood to every organ and tissue in the body. The right side of the heart pumps blood from the veins to the lungs, where the blood is oxygenated. The left side of the heart pumps oxygen-rich blood through the aorta and out to the rest of the body.

CROSS-SECTION VIEW OF THE HEART
The heart is a muscular organ that is approximately the shape and size of an average adult male fist. The parts of the heart and their functions are noted.

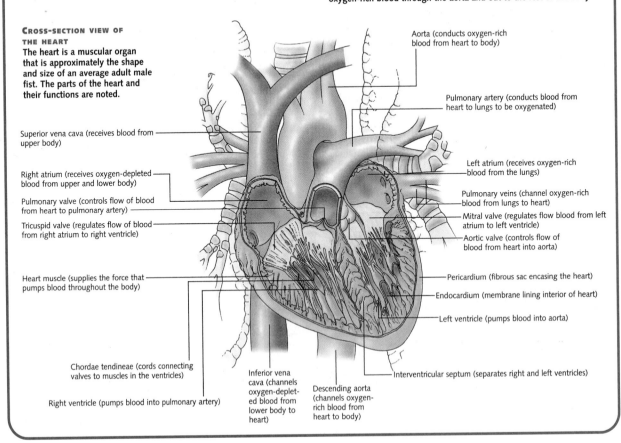

atria simultaneously squeeze blood into the two lower chambers of the heart, the ventricles. The electrical impulse moves to the atrioventricular node, signifying the final phase, the ventricular systole. In this phase, the heart empties as the left ventricle squeezes oxygen-rich blood into the aorta, while the right ventricle squeezes oxygen-depleted blood into the pulmonary artery.

HEART RATE AND CARDIAC OUTPUT

There are two important measures of the activity and efficiency of the function of the heart: heart rate and cardiac output. The heart rate is the number of times the heart beats per minute, and cardiac output is the volume of blood it pumps out with each contraction, multiplied by the number of beats per minute. At rest, the heart rate is 60 to 80 beats per minute, and the cardiac output is about 10 pints per minute. When greater demands are made on the heart, such as during strenuous exercise, the heart rate can increase to as much as 200 beats per minute, and the cardiac output can increase to about 100 pints per minute. This increased output meets the muscles' increased need for blood and the oxygen it brings.

Two factors accomplish changes in heart rate and output. First, a greater volume of blood flowing into the heart from the muscles causes the ventricles to expand and then more powerfully contract to push the blood out in the final phase of the heartbeat. Second, the autonomic nervous system, which directs automatic body functions, is involved with regulating heart function. The autonomic nervous system includes sympathetic and parasympathetic activity. Parasympathetic nerves control the heart at rest, slowing or inhibiting the heart rate. When demand on the heart is increased, the sympathetic nerves speed up the heart rate in two ways: the nerves act directly and immediately on the heart to allow it to speed up, and the nerves stimulate the secretion of the hormone epinephrine (or adrenaline) to cause a more sustained activity. The change from parasympathetic to sympathetic activity can be triggered by increased exercise, fear or anger, or a medical cause such as low blood pressure.

Heart attack

FOR SYMPTOM CHART
see Chest pain, page 24

FOR FIRST AID
see Heart attack, page 1325

A total or near-total blockage of one of the coronary arteries that supply the HEART with oxygen; known medically as myocardial infarction. In most cases, the blockage is caused by a blood clot that forms at a point in the artery narrowed by fatty deposits (plaque; see ATHEROSCLEROSIS). A spasm in an artery can also trigger a heart attack, although this is less common. Since the coronary arteries provide the heart muscle with its oxygen supply, tissue downstream from the blockage can die. The severity of the attack depends on the amount and location of affected heart tissue. Heart attack is one of the leading causes of sudden death and disability in the United States.

SYMPTOMS AND DIAGNOSIS

The pain accompanying a heart attack is often severe and sudden and classically described as comparable to someone "sitting on my chest." Typically, the pain begins in the chest, radiates through the upper body into the neck, arm, shoulder, or jaw, and does not go away with rest. While the pain accompanying a heart attack is often more focused and localized in men than in women, the symptoms can vary tremendously. For example, in older persons and in people with diabetes mellitus, a heart attack may occur with no pain, in which case it is called a silent heart attack.

With or without pain, a heart attack may also cause intermittent or constant pressure or squeezing in the chest, shortness of breath, palpitations (a fast or irregular heartbeat), an abnormally fast or weak pulse, fainting, fatigue, heavy sweating, nausea, or a gray color in the face.

If a heart attack is suspected, the doctor typically requests an electrocardiogram, which records the electrical activity of the heart and often shows evidence of the attack. Blood tests that screen for enzymes released in the blood during a heart attack are also used in diagnosis. Other tests, such as echocardiogram and radionuclide scanning, may be used to assess damage to the heart muscle, the blood

SIGNS OF A HEART ATTACK

There are three classic warning signs of a heart attack. Although different people experience different symptoms, one or more of the following is likely to occur if a heart attack is taking place:

- **Uncomfortable pressure, fullness, squeezing, or pain in the center of the chest that lasts more than a few minutes. The pain may also go away, then return.**
- **Pain that radiates from the chest to the shoulders, neck, or arm (usually the left). In women particularly, it may affect the jaw.**
- **Chest pain accompanied by light-headedness, fainting, nausea, or shortness of breath.**

A number of other symptoms occur less commonly but may also indicate heart attack:

- **Unusual pain in the chest, abdomen, or stomach**
- **Nausea or dizziness without chest pain**
- **Shortness of breath or difficulty breathing without chest pain**
- **Anxiety, fatigue, or weakness lacking apparent cause**
- **Cold sweating, palpitations, or pallor**

If one or more of these signs is present, emergency medical help should be sought immediately. The earlier a heart attack is treated, the higher the chance of survival.

flow through the heart, and the status of the heart valves.

TREATMENT

Since a heart attack is not an instantaneous event but develops over several hours, prompt emergency medical attention is critical for survival and limiting the damage. The initial treatment for a person who has had a heart attack can include medications that dissolve the blood clot, prevent new clots from forming and causing additional attacks, and reduce stress on the heart. These medications include beta blockers, angiotensin-converting enzyme (ACE) inhibitors, anticoagulants, nitrates, aspirin, and "clotbusters" (such as streptokinase, urokinase, and tissue plasminogen activator).

Other treatments may be used depending on the location and sever-

H

HEART ATTACK TIMELINE

The first hour immediately after a heart attack occurs is often called the "golden hour." It is the span of time during which it is essential to get medical attention. If the flow of blood is not restored within the first hour after a heart attack, starved heart muscle begins to die from the inside out, and permanent damage and death can result.

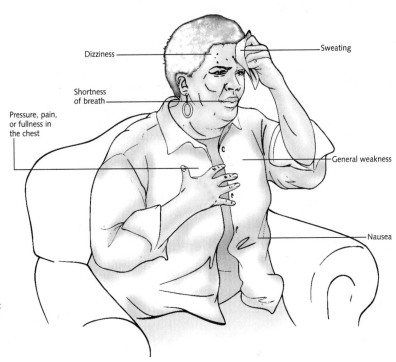

HEART ATTACK SYMPTOMS
Not all of the symptoms of heart attack are experienced during an actual attack, but these areas of the body may be affected.

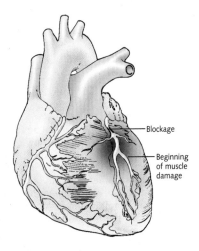

HEART DAMAGE 1 HOUR AFTER HEART ATTACK
Blockage of a coronary artery causes reduced blood flow to the heart, which in turn causes heart attack symptoms. Permanent heart damage can be minimized if the person gets immediate medical attention, ideally within the first hour.

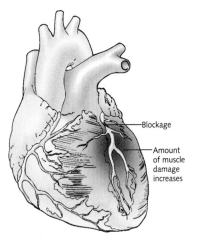

HEART DAMAGE 3 HOURS AFTER HEART ATTACK
Mild-to-moderate damage to heart muscle usually occurs if blood flow is not stabilized and restored within the golden hour.

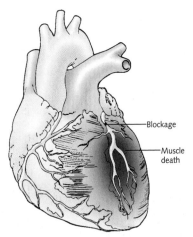

HEART DAMAGE 6 HOURS AFTER HEART ATTACK
Muscle death occurs throughout the area of ischemia (reduced blood flow) if adequate blood flow is not restored within 6 hours of the onset of a heart attack.

When a heart attack occurs, it is critical to react immediately. Even a short delay can be the difference between life and death. If a heart attack is suspected:

- Medical attention should be obtained as quickly as possible. The quickest way is to call 911 or your emergency number.
- An aspirin tablet should be taken. Aspirin helps dissolve blood clots and prevent new blood clots from forming.
- Cardiopulmonary resuscitation (CPR) should be used if the person having a heart attack becomes unconscious. CPR can help prevent brain death if the heart stops beating before emergency personnel arrive.

ity of the coronary artery blockage. One option is BALLOON ANGIOPLASTY. An inflatable device on the end of a catheter (long, thin tube) is threaded through a blood vessel into the heart and then inflated to press the plaque against the artery wall and widen the narrowed area. A stent (a thin cylinder of wire mesh) is often inserted to hold the artery open. In some cases the blockage may be remedied by open surgery on the heart (BYPASS SURGERY).

A heart attack typically requires a hospital stay of 3 to 7 days, depending on the severity of the attack and the invasiveness of the treatment. After release from the hospital, people who have had a heart attack usually undergo CARDIAC REHABILITATION, a medically supervised program designed to speed recovery and improve mental and physical functioning. In addition, beta blockers, ACE inhibitors, aspirin, and cholesterol-lowering agents are often prescribed to reduce the risk of future heart attacks.

COMPLICATIONS

For those who survive a heart attack, a number of complications can develop because of damage to the heart. The heart may lose some of its pumping efficiency, leading to congestive heart failure (see HEART FAILURE, CONGESTIVE). Cardiac arrhythmias (abnormal heart rhythms) may also result. The most severe of these, VENTRICULAR FIBRILLATION, can cause sudden death.

Part of the heart muscle may fail, leading to leakage between the two ventricles (lower chambers) of the heart, damage to the mitral valve between the upper and lower heart chambers, or rupture of the ventricle. Some people who have experienced a heart attack can develop pericarditis (inflammation of the membrane that surrounds the heart). Moreover, if blood flow through the heart is sluggish, clots can form, travel through the bloodstream, and lodge in other organs, such as the brain or kidneys, where they can cause severe or life-threatening damage.

PREVENTION

A number of risk factors increase the chance of having a heart attack. These include advancing age, male sex, smoking, high blood cholesterol levels, diabetes mellitus, uncontrolled hypertension (high blood pressure), lack of exercise, ANGINA, and obesity. Except for age and sex, most of these risk factors can be controlled by lifestyle or medication and their contribution to the risk of heart disease reduced. Prudent measures to avoid a heart attack include abstinence from tobacco use; eating a low-fat diet rich in fruits, vegetables, and whole grains; controlling diabetes and hypertension; exercising regularly; and maintaining a healthy body weight. Stress management and including sufficient B vitamins in the diet can also be preventive.

Heart block

A slowing of electrical impulses in their normal conduction pattern from the atria (upper chambers) of the heart to the ventricles (lower chambers). The delay in electrical communication between the top and bottom of the heart can slow the heartbeat to an abnormally low rate (bradycardia).

There are a number of possible causes for heart block. A lack of sufficient oxygen to the heart (cardiac ischemia) from coronary artery disease or past heart attack is one cause. Myocarditis (inflammation of the heart muscle), rheumatic fever, heart surgery, electrolyte imbalances in the blood, aging, and heart medications (such as beta blockers and calcium channel blockers) can also cause heart block. Heart block may also be congenital (present at birth).

Heart block is graded by the severi-

ty of the blockage. In first-degree heart block, electrical impulses are slowed, but they still travel from the atria to the ventricles. This condition usually produces no symptoms and requires no treatment. If medication is the cause of heart block, changing medication or its dosage may remedy the problem. In second-degree heart block, some electrical signals fail to travel from the atria to the ventricles, resulting in missed heartbeats. Symptoms may be unnoticeable, but dizziness, fatigue, or light-headedness occurs in pronounced cases. In third-degree heart block, no signals reach the ventricles from the atria, and the ventricles beat according to their own rhythm, which is insufficient to provide the body with enough blood. Dizziness, breathlessness, seizures, and loss of consciousness can result, possibly leading to cardiac arrest (complete stoppage of the heart). An artificial PACEMAKER, which regulates heartbeat, is used to treat severe second-degree and third-degree heart block.

Heart disease, congenital

An abnormality or malformation of the heart or the blood vessels connected to the heart that is present at birth. Congenital heart disease affects approximately 1 in every 100 newborns. Some types of congenital heart disease cause no symptoms during infancy and are not detected until later in life, while others can result in death soon after birth if left untreated. The causes of congenital heart disease are unknown. Current research suggests that contributing factors may include genetic abnormalities (such as DOWN SYNDROME), certain medications taken during pregnancy, alcohol or drug abuse during pregnancy, and viral infections of the mother, particularly German measles (rubella).

There are many types of congenital heart disease, some of which are rare.

VENTRICULAR SEPTAL DEFECT

Ventricular septal defect is the most common form of congenital heart disease. It consists of an opening in the wall, or septum, dividing the ventricles (lower chambers) of the heart. As a result of this defect, an increased amount of blood under high pressure flows into the lungs. Symptoms

H

depend on the size of the defect. If it is small, the only sign may be a murmur (an abnormal sound) that a doctor usually detects with a stethoscope. If the defect is large, pulmonary hypertension (abnormally high blood pressure in the pulmonary artery), difficulty with feeding, heavy sweating, slowed growth, repeated lung infections, and heart failure can develop in the infant. Since as many as half of all ventricular septal defects close on their own during the first year of life, medication is used initially to alleviate symptoms. If the defect does not close, surgery to close the opening is performed.

ATRIAL SEPTAL DEFECT

If an opening exists between the atria (upper chambers) of the heart, the disease is known as an atrial septal defect. This defect is more commonly occurs in newborns with Down syndrome. Often there are few or no symptoms early in life. The defect can be repaired surgically, usually when the child is between 1 and 6 years of age.

PATENT DUCTUS ARTERIOSUS

In a newborn, the blood vessel known as the ductus arteriosus connects the pulmonary artery (the artery to the lungs) with the aorta, which carries blood to the rest of the body. Normally, the ductus arteriosus closes immediately after birth, but in premature newborns and some full-term infants the vessel remains open. A small opening produces no symptoms, while a large one results in a heart murmur, retarded growth, and pulmonary hypertension. Sur-gery is performed to close the vessel when the baby is 1 or 2 years old. Patent ductus arteriosus is most common in the babies of women who had rubella during pregnancy and babies born at a high altitude. It occurs more often in girls than in boys.

COARCTATION OF THE AORTA

Coarctation of the aorta refers to severe narrowing of the main artery leading from the heart to the body, usually just past the point at which the artery that supplies the upper body branches off. This results in

> Terms in small capital letters—for example, PHYSICAL THERAPY or PAGET DISEASE—indicate a cross-reference to another entry with more information.

lower blood pressure in the lower body and higher blood pressure in the upper body, along with a number of other complications. Signs of the disease include cyanosis (a bluish tint to the skin) in the lower body, high blood pressure in only the upper body, and weak pulse in the groin along with strong pulse in the neck. Symptoms can include dizziness, headache, cramps in the legs with exercise, fainting, and nosebleeds. Surgery is the usual treatment. The procedure may be performed as soon as the condition is detected or delayed until childhood. In some cases, balloon angioplasty—which involves threading a catheter (long, thin tube) with an inflatable tip into the artery and expanding it—is used in place of surgery.

PULMONARY STENOSIS

Stenosis (narrowing) of the valve leading to the artery that connects the heart to the lungs results in pulmonary stenosis. Symptoms depend on the degree of obstruction. If it is mild to moderate, there may be no symptoms. Severe obstruction produces cyanosis and heart failure. In the worst cases, congestive heart failure (see HEART FAILURE, CONGESTIVE) develops within a month of birth. Children with mild to moderate stenosis can live normal lives but require regular medical examinations. Severe stenosis requires surgical widening of the valve.

AORTIC STENOSIS

In aortic stenosis, the narrowing occurs in the valve leading into the aorta, a defect occurring more often in boys than in girls. Unless the stenosis is severe, most children with aortic stenosis show no symptoms, and the problem is detected during a routine physical examination as a heart murmur. Children with mild to moderate stenosis require regular medical examinations to detect any worsening of the disease. Severe aortic stenosis can be repaired surgically.

TETRALOGY OF FALLOT

Not one defect but four in combination ("tetra-" means four in Greek) and named after the French physician who first described them, tetralogy of Fallot consists of a large ventricular septal defect, pulmonary stenosis, enlargement of the right ventricle, and a rightward shift in the position of the aorta. Blood flow to the lungs is

decreased, leading to an insufficient supply of oxygen to the body and cyanosis. Surgery is performed to correct the defects. Often more than one operation is needed because of the complexity of the disease.

TRANSPOSITION OF THE GREAT VESSELS

Another complex congenital heart disease, transposition of the great vessels refers to abnormal anatomy in which the aorta arises from the right ventricle and the pulmonary artery from the left—rather than the normal (opposite) arrangement. As a result, a portion of the blood circulates through the lungs without ever flowing to the rest of the body, while another portion of the blood circulates through the left side of the heart and into the body without passing through the lungs and picking up oxygen. This congenital heart disease produces bluish skin coloring and it usually causes death within the first year of life if not treated. Several surgical procedures are available to remedy the disease.

Heart disease, ischemic

Disease caused by blood flow to the heart muscle that is insufficient to meet its oxygen needs. The shortfall in blood flow and oxygen supply occurs because of obstruction in one of the coronary arteries, the blood vessels that provide oxygen to the heart muscle. The obstruction can be caused by a buildup of fatty material (plaque; see ATHEROSCLEROSIS), a blood clot, or a spasm in the artery. Minor episodes of ischemic heart disease usually cause little long-term damage to the heart, but more severe events can trigger a HEART ATTACK, result in an abnormal heart rhythm (see ARRHYTHMIA, CARDIAC), or cause a fainting spell or cardiac arrest.

The most common symptom of ischemic heart disease is pain or pressure (see ANGINA) that may radiate through the upper body into the neck, back, arms, shoulders, or jaw. In women, the pain tends to be less focused than in men and more difficult to recognize. In some cases there is no pain, in which case it is called silent ischemic heart disease.

Treatment for ischemic heart disease begins with medications that reduce the heart's need for oxygen by lowering the heart rate, reducing blood pressure, and relaxing the blood vessels. The three main classes of drugs used to achieve these effects are calcium channel blockers, beta blockers, and nitrates. Aspirin and other medications that help prevent the formation of blood clots are commonly used to reduce the risk of heart attack. Exercise and stress management may help. In more advanced cases, an invasive technique such as BALLOON ANGIOPLASTY or BYPASS SURGERY can improve the flow of blood to the heart muscle.

The risk of ischemic heart disease increases in people who use tobacco, have high cholesterol levels, have uncontrolled diabetes mellitus or hypertension (high blood pressure), avoid exercise, or are obese. Quitting smoking, controlling diabetes and hypertension through lifestyle changes and medication, exercising, and maintaining a healthy body weight are effective preventive measures.

Heart failure, congestive

A serious, potentially life-threatening condition in which the heart cannot pump enough blood to meet the body's demand for oxygen. The name comes from the fact that the pumping failure often results in pulmonary edema (a buildup of fluid, or congestion, in the lungs). As the heart begins to fail, it works harder and harder to compensate, a response that worsens the disease over time. Congestive heart failure can occur at any age, but it is most common in people older than 70, in whom it is a leading cause of death and disability. Usually the disease is chronic, or long-term. Acute congestive heart failure can result from a coronary event such as a heart attack or cardiac arrhythmia (abnormal heart rhythm) and constitutes a medical emergency. Once it is detected, the symptoms of congestive heart failure may be improved with lifestyle changes, medications, and, sometimes, surgery. However, the 5-year survival rates are still poor.

CAUSES
In most cases, heart failure begins slowly, with only minor symptoms that a person may fail to notice or choose to ignore. Since the heart pumps with decreasing efficiency, it works harder to compensate for the shortfall in function. Over time, this creates a vicious cycle that causes further impairment and progressive worsening of the heart failure.

Congestive heart failure can affect the left side of the heart, which pumps blood into the body; the right side of the heart, which pumps blood into the lungs; or both sides of the heart. Usually the disease affects the left side of the heart first, then progresses to involve the right side. Left-sided congestive heart failure results in shortness of breath, dizziness, fatigue, coughing, and sometimes lung congestion. Right-sided heart failure, also known as cor pulmonale (Latin for "lung-affected heart," because it is often associated with severe lung disease), typically causes fluid buildup in the veins and swelling in the feet and legs.

As congestive heart failure forces the heart to work harder, a number of changes occur in the body. The walls of the heart muscle may thicken and then enlarge as the heart dilates in an attempt to increase its pumping ability. The heartbeat may become abnormally fast (tachycardia), again as an attempt at increasing the pumping volume of the heart. The ventricles (lower chambers) may lose their ability to pump from continued overwork. In response to reduced output of the heart, the kidneys may retain water and salt, worsening the fluid buildup and potentially leading to kidney failure.

Congestive heart failure can result from a number of causes, including narrowing of the arteries that supply blood to the heart muscle (see CORONARY ARTERY DISEASE), HYPERTENSION (high blood pressure), cardiomyopathy (impaired heart muscle function), defects in the heart's valves, heart defects present at birth (see HEART DISEASE, CONGENITAL), diabetes mellitus, and severe lung disease, such as emphysema. Less common causes are rheumatoid arthritis, systemic lupus erythematosus, hyperthyroidism (an overactive thyroid gland), and abuse of alcohol or illegal recreational drugs, such as cocaine and amphetamines.

RISK FACTORS AND SYMPTOMS
The risk of developing congestive heart failure increases with a number of factors, including smoking, obesity, sedentary lifestyle, high salt

---

CONGESTIVE HEART FAILURE

Early treatment is the key to improving survival with congestive heart failure. The presence of any of the following symptoms is a signal to get medical attention as soon as possible:

- **Fatigue, weakness, and inability to exert or exercise**
- **Shortness of breath almost as soon as exercising begins**
- **Shortness of breath that wakes a person up at night**
- **Swelling in the legs, ankles, or feet**
- **Rapid weight gain, such as a pound a day for 3 days**
- **Swollen neck veins**

---

intake, uncontrolled hypertension, cardiac arrhythmia, severe lung disease, infection, emotional distress, certain medications, thyroid disease, and heart attack.

Shortness of breath is one of the earliest symptoms of heart failure, resulting in fatigue even from ordinary activities and little or no tolerance for exercise. Edema (swelling) in the legs is another common symptom. Neck veins may bulge, and fluid buildup in the abdomen can cause bloating, pain, or nausea. Some people with the disease experience confusion, and others may experience palpitations (a racing, uncomfortable heartbeat).

A doctor may detect other key signs, such as a heart murmur (a signal of valve problems), the sound of fluid in the lungs, fast or irregular heartbeat, swelling in the liver or abdomen, enlargement of the heart, and leg swelling. Several tests may be used in the diagnosis of congestive heart failure, including electrocardiogram (to measure the heart's electrical activity), echocardiography (to visualize the heart via ultrasound), chest X ray, and radionuclide imaging tests.

TREATMENT
The sooner congestive heart failure is detected, the less damage is done to the pumping function of the heart. Although the disease cannot be cured, it can be managed successfully, particularly with early detection.

Lifestyle changes are an important part of treating congestive heart failure. Measures such as quitting smoking, abstaining from alcohol con-

H

sumption, reducing salt intake, reducing body weight to a healthy range, eating a low-fat diet, avoiding excess fluids, resting regularly during the day, and exercising at an appropriate level determined by a doctor can help.

Medications are commonly used to relieve symptoms and to compensate for the effects of the disease. Diuretics help the body eliminate excess salt and fluid, which reduces swelling and congestion. Digoxin helps the heart muscle contract more strongly, increasing its pumping efficiency. Angiotensin-converting enzyme (ACE) inhibitors dilate (widen) the blood vessels, which reduces the resistance to blood flow and eases the pumping load on the heart. Beta blockers slow or prevent progression of the disease by lowering the heart rate, reducing the workload of the heart, and decreasing the risk of irregular heartbeat. Cardiotonic drugs, which are administered intravenously in a hospital, increase the force of the heart's contractions, allowing the heart to beat more effectively.

If coronary artery disease is the underlying cause of the congestive heart failure, BALLOON ANGIOPLASTY can be used to widen a narrowed artery. The point of narrowing may be kept open with the placement of a stent (a small cylinder of wire mesh). In more serious cases, direct surgery may be used to repair the causative problem. This can include coronary artery BYPASS SURGERY, repair or replacement of defective heart valves, and implantation of a pacemaker to correct an abnormally slow heartbeat. In the most extreme cases, heart transplant may offer an option.

Heart murmur

An abnormal blowing, whooshing, or rasping sound in the heart that is detectable with a stethoscope. A heart murmur results from vibrations caused by abnormal blood flow patterns.

A heart murmur may or may not indicate heart disease. Children, in particular, have so-called innocent heart murmurs that are common and harmless. Innocent heart murmurs usually disappear as the child ages; occasionally they persist into adulthood. In other cases, a heart murmur can signal a heart problem, such as a structural irregularity in a heart chamber or a narrowing of one of the heart's valves. Tests such as an echocardiogram are often performed after a heart murmur is detected to determine the cause and assess the need for treatment.

Heart rate

The number of heartbeats per minute; also known as pulse.

Heart transplant

A surgical procedure to remove an irreparably diseased heart and replace it with a healthy heart from a recently deceased person. Performed since 1967, heart transplants are now the third most common form of transplantation surgery, following only kidney and cornea transplants. Heart transplant surgery extends the lives of people who would otherwise die within a short time due to advanced heart disease.

RECIPIENTS AND DONORS

People most likely to benefit from a heart transplant are those younger than 65 who have an irreversible, untreatable heart condition that is likely to result in death within 2 or 3 years. In addition, the transplant candidate must be free of other conditions that can shorten life or interfere with the medications required after transplantation, such as addiction to drugs or alcohol, liver or kidney failure, obesity, infection, certain kinds of cancer, or an unwillingness to adhere to a strict medical regimen. The most common causes for heart transplant are advanced blockage of the arteries supplying oxygen to the heart (CORONARY ARTERY DISEASE), CARDIOMYOPATHY (impaired heart muscle function), heart disease present at birth (see HEART DISEASE, CONGENITAL), defective heart valves, and inability of the heart to meet the body's need for oxygen (heart failure).

In some cases, the heart is transplanted along with the lungs. This procedure is used primarily with persons who have abnormally high blood pressure in the lungs (HYPERTENSION, PULMONARY) or EISENMENGER COMPLEX, a congenital condition that combines pulmonary hypertension with a heart defect.

Donor hearts are taken from people who have consented to the use of their organs after death and who have died of an illness or accident that has left the heart intact and undamaged. After death, the donor's heart and blood are checked for blood type and evidence of infection, such as HIV (human immunodeficiency virus) and hepatitis. The blood type of the donor and the recipient need to be the same to give the best chance of success. In addition, the size of the heart matters. An exact match is not required, but the size of the donor heart needs to be proportional to the recipient's body frame.

THE SURGICAL PROCESS

Adding a person to the list of those waiting for a heart transplant requires a thorough medical evaluation to determine suitability. Once an eligible recipient is added, he or she has to wait until a suitable donor is found. Often the wait is long, since there are 10 to 20 times more eligible recipients than willing donors in any given year.

During the waiting period, transplant candidates need to follow a series of steps to prepare for surgery. These include quitting smoking, avoiding the use of alcohol or drugs other than prescribed medications, exercising regularly to build strength and stamina, and controlling diabetes mellitus and hypertension.

Heart transplant surgery must be performed on short notice, since the donor heart can survive outside the body for only 4 to 6 hours. Recipient candidates keep a suitcase packed and carry a pager so that they can receive and act on the message to come to the hospital immediately at any time.

Once the transplant recipient is prepared for surgery and given a general anesthetic, the chest is opened by cutting through the sternum (breastbone) and separating the ribs to expose the heart. The recipient is then connected to a heart-lung machine, which takes over the functions of providing oxygen to the blood and pumping that blood through the body. Next, the surgical team removes the diseased heart by separating it from the major vessels. The donor heart is positioned, and the major blood vessels are attached to it. Finally, the chest incision is closed, and the new heart is started. Often the warmth of blood passing through the transplanted heart prompts it to start beating. If it does not respond, an electrical shock is used to initiate a heartbeat.

RECOVERY AND MAINTENANCE

The condition of a person who has received a heart transplant is carefully and continuously monitored following surgery. Usually the heart transplant recipient can get out of bed within 3 or 4 days and will typically stay in the hospital for 10 to 14 days, with up to 21 days required in some cases.

Heart transplant surgery entails two principal risks. The first is rejection of the donated heart. To the recipient's immune system, the donor heart looks like an invading microorganism, and it tries to attack with antibodies. Left unchecked, the antibody attack will damage the heart and eventually cause it to fail. To prevent rejection, the heart transplant recipient is prescribed medications that suppress the immune reaction. In addition, the recipient is checked at regular intervals (blood tests and microscopic samples of heart tissue are taken) to see if rejection is occurring.

Immunosuppressive drugs lead to the second risk: an increased susceptibility to infection. Heart transplant recipients need to take extra precautions against infection, such as avoiding public places during flu season and immediately reporting any sign of infection, such as redness, swelling, or fever.

Heart transplant recipients continue taking immunosuppressive medications for as long as they live. These drugs cause side effects, such as trembling of the hands, elevated blood cholesterol levels, and hypertension (high blood pressure), which may in turn be treated with other drugs.

OUTCOMES AND COMPLICATIONS

Most recipients of a donated heart live significantly longer than they would have without the transplant. Many return to most of their routine activities, including moderate exercise, and some go back to work.

Apart from the ongoing risks of rejection and infection, certain problems tend to develop over the long-term. Heart transplant recipients commonly develop widespread narrowing of the coronary arteries as a result of fat deposits (coronary artery disease). However, since the nerves from the heart are severed during the surgery, they do not experience the

ANGINA that is a common symptom of coronary artery disease. As a result, heart transplant recipients have to be monitored regularly for the condition by means of cardiac catheterization (see CATHETERIZATION, CARDIAC). Immunosuppressive drugs also increase the risk of developing cancer, particularly cancer of the skin and the lymphatic system.

Heart valve

The structure at the exit of each of the four chambers of the HEART that allows blood to flow out, but prevents backflow. The mitral valve separates the left atrium of the heart from the left ventricle. The tricuspid valve divides the right atrium from the right ventricle. The pulmonary valve controls blood flow from the right ventricle into the pulmonary artery, which leads into the lungs. The aortic valve performs the same function between the left ventricle and the aorta, the artery that leads to the rest of the body.

Heart valves open and close in synchrony at each stage in the heartbeat. When the atria contract, the mitral and tricuspid valves open, allowing blood to enter the ventricles. The aortic and pulmonary valves close, keeping the received blood in the ventricles. As the ventricles contract, the mitral and tricuspid valves close, preventing backflow into the atria. The aortic and pulmonary valves open to allow blood to enter the arteries.

DISORDERS

The valves of the heart can be defective at birth (see HEART DISEASE, CONGENITAL), or they can become narrowed, a condition called stenosis (see STENOSIS, VALVULAR), or become unable to prevent backflow, called insufficiency or incompetence. The mitral valve and the aortic valve are the most common sites of disease, probably because they are under the greatest strain from the left ventricle. MITRAL VALVE PROLAPSE (MVP) is the most common valve disorder, usually an inherited structural defect in which the walls of the valve are thickened and elongated and cannot prevent backflow. The condition is rarely serious and usually found in slender young women. AORTIC STENOSIS is an abnormal narrowing of the aortic valve, usually caused by deposits of calcium as a result of aging.

Heart valve surgery

An operation to repair or replace one of the four valves in the heart. In the normally functioning heart, the flaps of each of the four valves—pulmonary, mitral, aortic, and tricuspid—allow blood to flow in only one direction as it travels to and from the lungs and to and from the body. Stenosis (narrowing) of a valve limits normal blood flow, while regurgitation (leaking) lets blood flow in the wrong direction. Left untreated, severe valve problems can lead to life-threatening disease, such as heart failure.

Heart valve surgery is an open-heart procedure. That is, the chest is opened and the heart exposed, while a heart-lung machine takes over the function of oxygenating the blood and pumping it to the body. The procedure is performed under general anesthetic through an incision in the sternum (breastbone). The ribs are spread to expose the heart.

In some cases, the surgeon can repair a damaged valve. Widening the valve opening with a scalpel repairs stenosis, and a ring may be inserted to support the valve and help it function properly.

Other cases require surgical removal and replacement of the valve. Two types of replacement valves are used. Bioprostheses are made from animal or human tissue, while mechanical valves are constructed of plastic or metal. Mechanical valves are extremely durable, but blood tends to clot around a mechanical valve, either clogging the valve or raising the risk of embolus (a clot) that travels through the bloodstream and lodges in the brain or another organ—for example, the lung. As a result, the person receiving a mechanical valve must take anticoagulant medications to prevent clots. Bioprostheses rarely require anticoagulation, but they are less durable. The choice between a bioprosthesis and a mechanical valve depends on the age, sex, and general health of the person requiring heart valve surgery. In general, bioprostheses are preferred in people older than 70 and women who plan to become pregnant (anticoagulation must be avoided during pregnancy). Mechanical valves are a practical option for younger people who do not need to avoid anticoagulation.

In recent years, a catheter-based procedure called VALVULOPLASTY has

REPLACING HEART VALVES

If a damaged heart valve cannot be repaired, it can be replaced with a mechanical device, an animal valve (most often from a pig or cow), or a human valve from a deceased donor. Heart valve surgery is generally very successful. After surgery, the person will stay in a critical care unit for several days and will remain in the hospital for 1 to 2 weeks. He or she will be fully recovered in several weeks to several months.

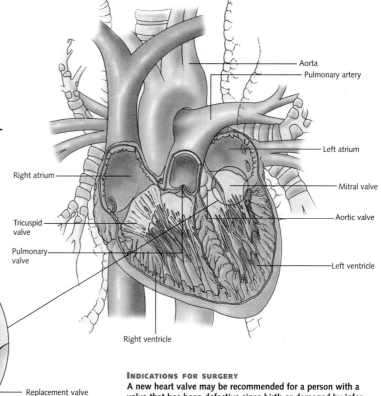

Aorta
Pulmonary artery
Left atrium
Right atrium
Mitral valve
Aortic valve
Tricuspid valve
Left ventricle
Pulmonary valve
Right ventricle

Replacement valve

INDICATIONS FOR SURGERY

A new heart valve may be recommended for a person with a valve that has been defective since birth or damaged by infection, calcification (usually from aging), or some medications.

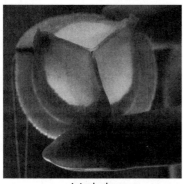

Animal valve

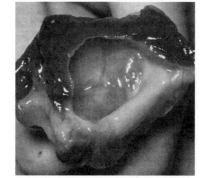

Human valve

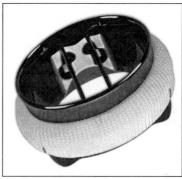

Mechanical valve

TYPES OF REPLACEMENT VALVES

An animal heart valve (mounted on a frame) is readily available, requires short-term medication to prevent clotting, and is relatively durable for natural tissue. A human heart valve is durable and does not necessitate medication, but availability may be a problem. On average, both animal and human heart valves last about 10 years. Mechanical heart valves are readily available and tend to be more durable, lasting on average 15 years or longer; however, the person also must take drugs for a lifetime to prevent blood clotting.

replaced many heart valve surgical repairs. In addition, new minimally invasive techniques allow replacement of defective heart valves through a much smaller incision in the chest and heart. Minimally invasive techniques cause less pain and shorten recovery, but the procedure is more complicated and takes longer to perform.

Heart, artificial

A mechanical device that substitutes for, or augments, the normal blood-pumping function of the heart. Still experimental, artificial hearts are generally seen as a temporary solution to prolong the life of a person with advanced heart disease who is waiting for a heart transplant and might otherwise die.

Heartburn

A burning sensation in the upper abdomen and chest. Also known as acid indigestion, heartburn is most common in older people and pregnant women. Burning chest pain is sometimes accompanied by a bitter or sour taste in the back of the throat. Heartburn is the most common symptom of ESOPHAGEAL REFLUX (the backward flow of acid from the stomach up into the esophagus). Simple modifications in lifestyle can control most cases of heartburn. Doctors recommend avoiding foods and beverages that contribute to the problem (such as spicy or greasy foods, chocolate, coffee, and alcohol); not smoking; losing a few pounds if overweight; and not eating 2 to 3 hours before going to bed. Over-the-counter antacids may also provide relief. If these measures prove insufficient, or if it is necessary to take antacids very frequently (more than 3 or 4 times a day), it is important to see the physician. Esophageal reflux may require further treatment with prescription medication or, rarely, in severe cases with surgery.

Heart-lung machine

A device that takes over the functions of the heart and lungs during open-heart surgery. The heart-lung machine consists of a pump, which circulates the blood and substitutes for the heart, and an oxygenator, which, taking over for the lungs, removes carbon dioxide from the blood and adds oxygen. Because the heart-lung machine is keeping the person under-

going open heart surgery alive, the surgeon can stop the heart to work on it without causing bleeding. When surgery is complete, the heart is restarted, either from the stimulus of blood flowing through it or by electrical shock, and the person undergoing surgery is disconnected from the heart-lung machine.

Heart-lung machines can result in complications, particularly small blood clots that may lodge in the heart, brain, or kidney and cause a heart attack, stroke, or kidney failure. Powerful anticoagulants are used to lower the chance of clotting, but a small risk remains. To minimize this danger, surgeons are developing minimally invasive heart surgery techniques, which allow the surgeon to work on the beating heart, making the heart-lung machine unnecessary.

Heart-lung transplant

A surgical procedure to remove a diseased heart and lungs and replace them with a healthy heart and lungs from a recently deceased donor. Heart-lung transplant is performed only on those who have both severely diseased lungs and advanced heart disease, are likely to die soon without the procedure, and have no other life-threatening diseases, such as diabetes mellitus. See HEART TRANSPLANT.

Heat cramps

A condition caused by prolonged activity in high temperatures that produces the sudden development of cramps in the skeletal muscles. Loss of water and salt (sodium chloride) through profuse perspiration obstructs the ability of the body to release heat, causing the muscles to cramp. A person who has heat cramps should stop exercising and move to a cool place. Tight clothing should be loosened, and the feet should be raised. Water, and electrolyte solution, if available, should be given to the person. Cooling off and drinking water are important to help prevent heat stroke.

Heat disorders

A group of physical disorders brought on by prolonged exposure to hot temperatures, insufficient fluid intake, and failure of the body to successfully regulate its internal temperature. Heat disorders, which usually

result in HYPERTHERMIA, include HEAT CRAMPS, HEAT EXHAUSTION, and HEAT STROKE. These conditions can be serious and even life-threatening if prompt action is not taken to manage them. Heat disorders are especially serious in older people.

HEAT CRAMPS

The least severe of the three heat disorders, heat cramps are the first sign that the body is having trouble coping with increased temperatures. These painful, involuntary muscle spasms usually occur when a person is exercising heavily in a very hot environment. Excessive perspiration (electrolyte loss) and insufficient fluid intake also contribute to the problem. The muscles most commonly affected include those in the calves, abdomen, and arms.

Treatment of heat cramps consists of moving out of the sun or the hot environment and resting, drinking water or sports drinks, and gentle stretching and massage.

HEAT EXHAUSTION

This is a more serious and complex condition. Like heat cramps, heat exhaustion is linked to heavy exercise, high temperatures, excessive perspiration, and inadequate fluid intake. However, symptoms come on suddenly and resemble those of shock. They include nausea, faintness, a rapid heartbeat, low blood pressure, a low-grade fever or a subnormal body temperature, ashen appearance, and cool, moist, pale skin. Heat exhaustion requires prompt attention; otherwise, it can develop into the still more serious heat stroke. People who have symptoms of heat exhaustion must be moved from the sun into the shade (or from the hot environment to a cooler area) and carefully laid down with their legs slightly elevated. Every effort must be made to lower the person's body temperature. This includes having the person drink cool (not cold) fluids such as water or sports drinks; loosening clothing; and fanning the person and spraying him or her with cool water. If the fever rises above 104°F, or if symptoms such as fainting, confusion, or seizures develop, immediate emergency medical assistance should be sought.

HEAT STROKE

Also known as sunstroke or heat hyperpyrexia, heat stroke is a severe

H

and potentially fatal condition. Sunstroke is a type of heat stroke. As with other heat disorders, it can occur when a person exercises or works too strenuously in hot weather or a hot environment without replenishing body fluids. Particularly susceptible to heat stroke are older people and individuals who have an impaired ability to sweat. Other risk factors include obesity, alcohol use, DEHYDRATION, and cardiovascular disease.

The primary symptom of heat stroke is a spike in temperature to greater than 104°F. When a person experiences heat stroke, he or she loses the normal mechanisms for coping with heat stress, such as temperature control and sweating. Fainting is often the first symptom in older people. Other signs include hot, dry skin; rapid heartbeat; rapid and shallow breathing; low blood pressure; irritability; and cessation of sweating. Changes in mental status range from personality changes to confusion to, rarely, coma. Immediate emergency medical assistance is required. In the meantime, individuals should be cooled down as much as possible.

Heat exhaustion

FOR FIRST AID
see Heat exhaustion, page 1326

A condition in which the body produces heat faster than it can sweat it off; overexposure to heat. Heat exhaustion is characterized by cool, moist, pale skin; headache; nausea and vomiting; weakness; and dizziness or fainting.

Risk factors for heat exhaustion include cardiovascular disease, high temperatures or humidity, sweat gland dysfunction, alcohol use, excessive exercise, and wearing too much clothing in hot weather. People are at particular risk of heat exhaustion if they are older, obese, or take drugs that impair heat regulation, such as amphetamines, phenothiazines, or ANTICHOLINERGIC AGENTS, such as an antihistamine.

Heat exhaustion should be taken seriously. Once the signs of heat exhaustion appear, the person's condition can worsen rapidly. The person should be moved to the shade or a cooler area. A person with heat exhaustion should take a tepid (medi-

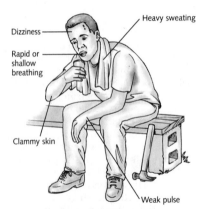

SIGNS OF HEAT EXHAUSTION
A person with these signs of heat exhaustion should move to a cool place; remain quiet; loosen clothing; apply cool, wet cloths to the forehead and body; and drink water or half-strength sports drinks. If the person does not recover within an hour, medical attention is necessary.

um cool) bath or cool, wet cloths should be placed on the person's forehead and body. The person should also drink a lot of cool water or an electrolyte replacement solution, slowly. If the person shows any signs of confusion or loses consciousness, medical attention must be sought.

Measures can be taken to prevent heat exhaustion. In very hot weather people should sip water or sports-related beverages frequently, whether thirsty or not. Light-colored, loose-fitting clothing and wide-brimmed hats should be worn. Sunscreen and umbrellas should be used to avoid the heating effects of the sun. Exercise should be light and gradual,

with increased fluid intake. Frequent rest is recommended.

Heat stroke

FOR FIRST AID
see Heat stroke, page 1326

A condition caused by overexposure to heat in which the body stops sweating. Heat stroke is a life-threatening illness that can cause shock, brain damage, and death. The signs of heat stroke include extremely high body temperature, often as high as 106°F; red, hot, dry skin; progressive loss of consciousness; rapid pulse; confusion; and rapid, shallow breathing. Symptoms include weakness and fatigue, headache, dizziness, blurred vision, and vomiting.

All cases of heat stroke require emergency medical attention. First-aid measures include removing any tight or heavy clothing and applying cool sponges or cool packs made with towels soaked in cool water to the person's skin. Rubbing alcohol (isopropyl alcohol) should not be applied, and the person should not be given anything to eat or drink.

Heat treatment

The use of an electric heating pad, hot-water bottle, hot compresses, a heat lamp, a hot tub, hot baths, or hot showers to promote healing. Heat treatments increase blood flow to an area, which can help augment natural healing. Heat treatments are sometimes used to treat back pain. Care should be taken not to use heat treatment too soon after an injury (such as in the first

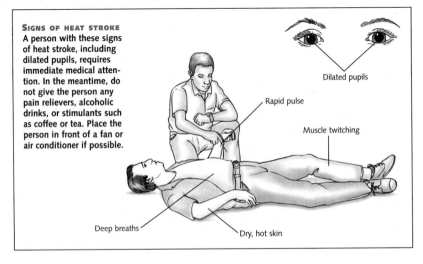

SIGNS OF HEAT STROKE
A person with these signs of heat stroke, including dilated pupils, requires immediate medical attention. In the meantime, do not give the person any pain relievers, alcoholic drinks, or stimulants such as coffee or tea. Place the person in front of a fan or air conditioner if possible.

24 hours), since it can increase swelling and pain from increased blood flow. Heat treatment must be used cautiously to prevent burns.

Heimlich maneuver

FOR FIRST AID
see Choking (Heimlich maneuver), page 1318

An emergency technique for dislodging an object stuck in the windpipe. The Heimlich maneuver is used to

---

STEPS IN A HEIMLICH MANEUVER

To perform the Heimlich maneuver, a person should:

- Stand behind the person choking and wrap his or her arms around the person's waist, bending the person slightly forward
- Make a fist with one hand and place it slightly above the person's navel
- Grasp the fist with the other hand and press hard into the abdomen with a quick, upward thrust
- Repeat until the object is expelled from the airway

An adult who is choking can perform the Heimlich maneuver on himself or herself if help is not available. The person should:

- Position his or her fist slightly above the navel
- Grasp the fist with the free hand and thrust upward into the abdomen until the object is expelled
- Alternative: a person who is choking can lean over the back of a chair or table edge and press his or her upper abdomen against the edge with a quick thrust
- Repeat until the object is expelled from the airway

---

prevent suffocation when a person is CHOKING and unable to breathe, cough, or speak. The universal sign for choking is a hand clutched to the throat, with thumb and fingers extended. It is advisable to learn how to perform the Heimlich maneuver in a first-aid course.

Helicobacter pylori
See H. PYLORI.

Hellerwork
See ROLFING.

Helmets, sports

Protective covering worn during vigorous athletic activities to prevent head injuries. Helmets are the single most important piece of protective gear used in sports. Research has established that the wearing of helmets saves lives by reducing the risk of head injuries. Sports helmets should be worn while riding bicycles or motorcycles, when using in-line skates, and when playing football or other contact sports.

Sports helmets are scientifically developed to provide several layers of protection, including a rigid outer shell, an inner layer intended to absorb impact, comfort padding, and a chin strap retention system to keep the helmet in place during an accident. Helmets are designed to absorb the shock of a crash, to withstand a blow from a sharp object, and to stay fastened without breaking or stretching. Sports helmets are the safety equivalent of motor vehicle seat belts and should always be used.

Hemangioblastoma

A rare brain tumor composed of blood vessel cells. Hemangioblastomas are usually slow growing and benign. They most commonly occur in the cerebellum, retina of the eye, and spinal cord. Treatment requires removing the entire tumor surgically.

Hemangioma

A common tumor that develops at or soon after birth consisting of a proliferation of blood vessels. There are two primary types: capillary hemangiomas and cavernous hemangiomas. Capillary hemangiomas are slightly raised and bright red and are caused by blood vessels near the surface of the skin. Cavernous hemangiomas are blue and are caused by blood vessels that are located deeper in the skin. The incidence of hemangiomas is slightly higher in females and premature infants.

Hemangiomas can occur anywhere on the face or body. Usually a child has only one, but it is possible to have two or three hemangiomas. Rarely, multiple lesions may develop, and some may occur internally. Unlike other types of birthmarks,

hemangiomas may grow rapidly; some can be 3 inches in diameter or larger. They usually stop growing after the first year of life and then slowly begin to shrink and turn white. By age 5 years, half of all hemangiomas are flat. Nine of ten hemangiomas are completely flat by the time a child is 9 years old. Although a faint mark may remain, hemangiomas usually disappear on their own without treatment. It is impossible to know how large a hemangioma will grow or if it will disappear completely.

It is essential for a child's doctor to monitor the growth of a hemangioma. This is particularly important when hemangiomas are located over the genitals or rectum or near the eyes, nose, or mouth. Medical attention is also necessary when rapidly growing or shrinking hemangiomas cause bleeding, bruising, or open sores. Medical options include systemic corticosteroids and LASER SURGERY that destroys the blood vessels. However, both involve serious side effects that must be discussed with a physician.

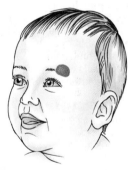

HARMLESS BIRTHMARK
The appearance of a hemangioma on an infant may be alarming, but the growth is usually harmless. Most hemangiomas grow rapidly, stabilize, and then gradually disappear, leaving only very faint traces. Laser surgery is used only if the growth is obstructing a vital structure such as the eye.

Hemarthrosis

The presence of blood within a joint, usually the result of a moderately severe injury that causes bleeding into the joint. In hemarthrosis, the blood accumulates in the joint within a few hours of the injury, and the joint becomes swollen, stiff, and painful. Hemarthrosis may also occur spontaneously in people who have a blood clotting disorder, such as hemophilia, or people who are taking blood-thinning medication. The knee joint may be affected by hemarthrosis when a ligament in the area (usually the anterior cruciate ligament, or ACL) is ruptured or torn, when the joint capsule of the knee is torn, when the kneecap is dislocated, when a tendon in the thigh is ruptured, or if there is a fracture within the joint. Cells in the joint capsule will slowly absorb any remaining blood. A large hemarthrosis may require aspiration, in which a fine needle is used to draw the fluid out of the joint.

Hematemesis

See VOMITING BLOOD.

Hematocrit

The proportion or percentage of the blood's volume taken up by red blood cells; abbreviated Hct. Hematocrit is usually included as part of standard blood testing (see BLOOD TESTS), and it is useful for detecting and diagnosing a variety of diseases that affect or involve the blood. The test is made by filling a specially marked tube with a sample of blood, then placing the tube in a centrifuge to separate the red blood cells from the plasma (liquid portion of the blood). The level of red blood cells read against the marks on the tube indicates the hematocrit.

Hematologist

A doctor who specializes in studying blood and blood-forming tissues and in diagnosing and treating the diseases that affect them.

Hematology

The branch of medical science that studies blood and blood-forming tissues, such as the bone marrow, and the diseases that affect them.

Hematoma

A collection of blood, usually clotted, in a body part as a result of ruptured or injured blood vessels. The medical importance of a hematoma depends on its location and size. A small hematoma under a fingernail resulting from an injury will heal on its own within a few weeks. A hematoma on the outer surface of the brain, called an epidural hematoma, may lead to death if not treated.

Hematopoietic progenitor cells

Cells that have the capacity to develop into red blood cells, white blood cells, and platelets and have a key role in hematopoiesis (producing blood cells). Hematopoietic progenitor cells are located principally in the red bone marrow, which in adults is restricted to the pelvis, ribs, spine, skull, sternum (breastbone), humerus (upper arm bone), and femur (thigh bone).

Hematospermia

Blood in the semen. Hematospermia is occasionally associated with other symptoms, including pain with urination, ejaculation, or bowel movement; swelling or tenderness in the groin or scrotum; back pain; and fever. The condition may be a sign of infection, obstruction, or injury in the male reproductive tract or of prostate cancer. Treatment depends on the underlying cause, but hematospermia is most often a benign, self-limiting condition.

Hematuria

Blood in the urine. Small amounts of blood make urine look smoky or cloudy; large amounts turn it dark red or a tea-colored brown. Hematuria is abnormal and can be a sign of serious disease; it requires prompt attention from a physician. Depending on the cause, hematuria may be accompanied by other symptoms, such as pain on urination, aching in the abdomen or back, fever, frequent and urgent need to urinate, increased or decreased thirst, decreased appetite, nausea, vomiting, or diarrhea. Hematuria combined with pain in the side below the ribs may indicate a stone in the ureter (the tube connecting the kidney and bladder) or a kidney tumor. Infection, tumor, kidney stone, or blood vessels broken by the strain of urinating with an enlarged prostate are other possible causes. Certain kidney diseases, sickle cell anemia, injury to the urinary tract, a number of medications, an abnormally high concentration of calcium in the urine, and strenuous exercise can also cause the condition.

A person seeking medical attention for hematuria will need a physical examination and a medical history. The history will include questions about the time pattern of the hematuria, including the color of the urine

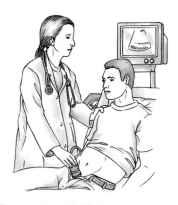

DIAGNOSTIC ULTRASOUND
The presence of blood in the urine (hematuria) requires immediate attention to determine the cause. Ultrasound of the lower abdomen, including the bladder, is a painless procedure that enables the doctor to see irregularities in the bladder. The technician moves a transducer over the person's abdomen and watches an image on a monitor.

and frequency of urination throughout the day, medications and foods taken, accompanying symptoms, allergies, recent injuries or surgeries, and any changes in sexual activity. Diagnostic laboratory tests may be performed, including blood tests, analysis of the urine, and an examination of the bladder, kidneys, and lower abdomen by X ray, visual instrument (cystoscope), ultrasound, or CT (computed tomography) scan. In some cases, a sample of tissue, or a biopsy specimen, may be taken.

Treatment of hematuria depends on the underlying cause. Exercise-induced hematuria clears up with rest; drinking adequate fluids during exercise often eliminates the problem. Infections can be treated with antibiotics. Stones may pass out of the system on their own, or they may require removal (see CALCULUS, URINARY TRACT). Tumors are managed with surgery or medication, depending on their type and extent.

A few conditions can mimic hematuria. Some people pass red urine after eating beets or rhubarb. Food colorings used in baked goods, soft drinks, and other items may produce red urine, particularly in children. In women, bleeding from the vagina is sometimes confused with hematuria.

Heme

A compound of iron that combines with a protein (globin) to form hemoglobin, the oxygen-carrying pigment that gives red blood cells their color.

Hemianopia

Blindness in half of the normal visual field. Hemianopia may affect one eye or both eyes. Whenever partial or complete blindness develops in one or both eyes, it is important to seek prompt medical attention. There are many possible reasons for the loss of sight. In the United States, the most common are injuries; diabetes mellitus, type 1 and type 2 (see RETINOPATHY, DIABETIC); and MACULAR DEGENERATION (a blood vessel disorder in which the central part of the retina in the eye deteriorates). Among the many other possible causes of vision loss are vitamin A (beta carotene) deficiency, retinitis pigmentosa, retinoblastoma, lead poisoning, glaucoma, trachoma, and progressive multifocal leukoencephalopathy (PML).

Hemiballismus

An involuntary movement disorder characterized by irregular and uncontrollable flinging and jerking motions on one side of the body. Hemiballismus is a symptom of a brain disorder, most commonly a STROKE.

Hemicolectomy

Surgical removal of part of the colon. A hemicolectomy (see also COLECTOMY) is usually performed to treat colon cancer, COLITIS, or DIVERTICULAR DISEASE or to remove colon tissue damaged by a blockage. In hemicolectomy, the diseased segments of the colon are removed and the remaining healthy parts are joined together.

Hemiparesis

Weakness on one side of the body. Hemiparesis and HEMIPLEGIA (paralysis on one side of the body) commonly occur as a result of a STROKE. Weakness or paralysis may affect only an arm, a leg, the face, or one entire side of the body and face. A person who has a stroke in the left hemisphere of the brain may exhibit right-sided paresis or paralysis; a person who has a stroke in the right hemisphere may have problems with the left side of the body.

Hemiplegia

PARALYSIS or weakness on one side of the body. Hemiplegia is one of the most common effects of a serious STROKE. Weakness without complete paralysis is called HEMIPARESIS.

Hemizygote

An individual who has only one instead of a pair of a particular gene. Males are hemizygotes for all the genes on the X chromosome because they have only a single X chromosome, unlike females, who have two.

Hemochromatosis

An inherited disorder in which the body absorbs too much iron from food. In healthy individuals, iron that the body does not need is excreted. In individuals with hemochromatosis, it accumulates throughout the body, primarily in the liver, pancreas, heart, and skin, and damages tissue in those organs. Symptoms include fatigue, abdominal pain, and JAUNDICE (a yellowing of the skin and the whites of the eyes). Skin color may change to gray or bronze. Left untreated, hemochromatosis can lead to serious health disorders, such as CIRRHOSIS (a severe liver disease), liver cancer, liver failure, diabetes, and heart problems. Hemochromatosis in which abnormal skin color is combined with diabetes is sometimes called bronze diabetes.

Diagnosis is based on blood tests that measure the level of iron in the body. In some cases, a LIVER BIOPSY is performed to measure the extent of liver damage. Treatment involves drawing blood to remove excess iron from the body. In the first 18 months of treatment, blood is drawn more frequently. Subsequently, blood is drawn every 2 to 6 months for the rest of an affected person's life.

Hemodialysis

A medical procedure that cleans and filters the blood by removing waste products and fluid from the blood through a dialysis machine.

The purpose of hemodialysis is to rid the body of harmful waste products, extra salt, and excess fluids. Hemodialysis becomes necessary when the kidneys are impaired by disease or injury and are unable to excrete nitrogen-containing waste products and regulate pH and electrolyte concentration. The procedure helps control blood pressure and helps the body maintain the proper balance

CREATING AN ACCESS SITE

Ongoing hemodialysis requires that large amounts of blood be removed, cleaned, and returned as often as three times a week, so a permanent site for accessing a vein and an artery is created surgically in the arm.

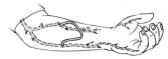

A SURGICAL SOLUTION
One approach to provide access for hemodialysis is to connect a vein and artery with a plastic tube.

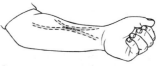

ARTERIOVENOUS FISTULA
Another approach is to surgically connect an artery to a vein, which forms a large blood vessel that bulges under the skin. One needle is inserted into the vessel to remove blood, and another is inserted into the vessel to return blood to the body.

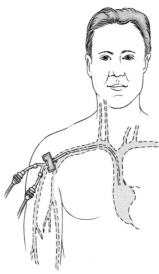

INTRAVENOUS CATHETER
A flexible tube called an intravenous catheter, commonly used when emergency hemodialysis is required, provides temporary vascular access until a permanent access site is created. An intravenous catheter has two chambers that permit a two-way flow of blood; for hemodialysis, it can be placed in the neck, chest, or leg near the groin.

EXPLAINING HEMODIALYSIS

During hemodialysis, blood is removed, filtered by a machine, and returned to the body as a treatment for kidney failure. This process requires a delivery system to circulate the blood, a site on the body to remove and return the blood, and a filtering mechanism (dialyzer) to clean the blood.

H

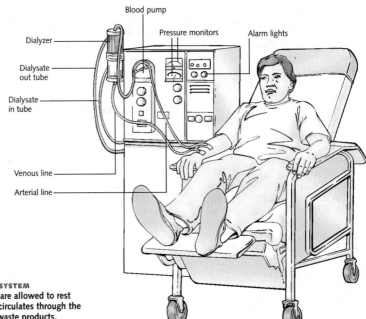

- Dialyzer
- Dialysate out tube
- Dialysate in tube
- Venous line
- Arterial line
- Blood pump
- Pressure monitors
- Alarm lights

THE HEMODIALYSIS DELIVERY SYSTEM
People undergoing hemodialysis are allowed to rest comfortably while arterial blood circulates through the dialyzer and returns cleansed of waste products.

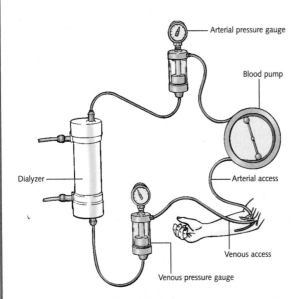

- Arterial pressure gauge
- Blood pump
- Arterial access
- Dialyzer
- Venous access
- Venous pressure gauge

FILTERING THE BLOOD
The dialyzer removes blood from the body, cleans wastes from it, and returns the cleansed blood to the body. An arterial pressure gauge and a venous pressure gauge are monitored to make sure the person's blood pressure does not rise or fall too drastically.

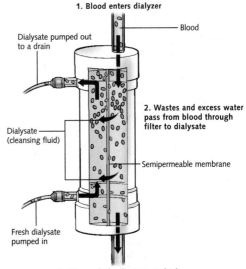

1. Blood enters dialyzer

- Blood
- Dialysate pumped out to a drain
- Dialysate (cleansing fluid)
- **2. Wastes and excess water pass from blood through filter to dialysate**
- Semipermeable membrane
- Fresh dialysate pumped in

3. Cleansed blood returns to body

HOW THE DIALYZER WORKS
Blood passes through a tube into the dialyzer, the part of the hemodialysis delivery system that is commonly known as the artificial kidney. Within the dialyzer is a semipermeable filter with tiny pores that permits wastes and excess water to pass from the blood into a cleansing fluid called dialysate, but prevents the blood and dialysate from mixing.

of potassium, sodium, and chloride. In hemodialysis, the blood is taken out of the body, passed through a dialysis machine, and returned to the body.

HOW IT WORKS

Hemodialysis uses a dialysis machine to clean the blood. A temporary catheter such as a large intravenous line may be inserted into a large blood vessel in the shoulder or neck. The procedure is performed by creating an opening to a blood vessel. The site and type of blood vessel opening varies, depending on the person's condition and the expected duration of dialysis. Two needles are inserted into this opening to transport the blood to the machine and return it to the body. The dialysis machine contains narrow hollow fibers that are only slightly thicker than a strand of hair; these fibers serve as a dialysis membrane. As the blood flows through the fibers, waste products pass through the walls of the fibers and into a surround-ing solution called dialysate. The dialysate bathes the fibers and allows the waste products to diffuse across the membrane into the dialysate. In addition to waste products, extra fluid can be removed through dialysis. The newly cleaned blood then flows through another set of tubes in the dialysis machine and back into the body.

HOW IT IS PERFORMED

Hemodialysis is generally performed three times a week in 2- to 4-hour sessions. The procedure is usually performed at an outpatient dialysis center. In rare cases, the procedure may be done at home with help. Both the person being treated and his or her helper must receive special training. The advantages of home hemodialysis include scheduling (according to a doctor's recommended schedule), convenience, and greater sense of control over the treatment. Disadvantages may include stress on family members, need for special training, space required to store equipment at home, and greater cost (less of the cost is covered by insurance).

The procedure is commonly done at a hospital or dialysis center by nurses or trained technicians. This setting provides the person being treated with access to skilled medical professionals throughout the procedure and the support of other people undergoing the same treatment.

It may take several months for an individual to become adjusted to hemodialysis. Although there is usually no pain or discomfort associated with the treatment, physical movement is restricted during the procedure because the person is connected to the dialysis machine. Generally, a comfortable chair is provided so the person being treated can sleep, read, write, talk, or watch television.

POSSIBLE COMPLICATIONS

Rapid changes in fluid and chemical balance may occur during treatment, producing muscle cramps and a sudden drop in blood pressure, which may result in weakness, dizziness, or nausea. Side effects such as these should be reported to a doctor immediately. They can often be avoided if a proper diet and medication schedule are followed.

Dietary recommendations for people being treated with hemodialysis include eating balanced amounts of foods high in protein and limiting fluid intake and foods containing the mineral phosphorus (such as milk, cheese, nuts, dried beans, and soft drinks). Intake of potassium-containing foods such as salt substitutes, certain fruits and vegetables, and chocolate should be regulated carefully because too much or too little potassium can be harmful to the person's heart. Salt and salt-containing foods should always be avoided in people undergoing hemodialysis. See also DIALYSIS.

Hemodialyzer

See DIALYSIS MACHINE.

Hemoglobin

The pigment in BLOOD that transports oxygen. Hemoglobin is formed in bone marrow and is found in all red blood cells. Hemoglobin is a large, complex molecule consisting of a protein component (globin) and an iron-bearing component (heme). It makes up about 33 percent of a red blood cell. The globin is composed of several hundred molecules of amino acids (the building blocks of proteins), arranged in chains. The chains of protein enclose a molecule of heme, which has an atom of iron at its center to which oxygen adheres. Oxygen-bound hemoglobin is called oxyhemoglobin, and it gives blood its red color.

The oxygen clings to the hemoglobin until the blood has penetrated into the capillaries, when hemoglobin displays its remarkable ability to release oxygen in exactly the amount needed by the body tissue it serves. When the tissue surrounding the thin-walled capillaries has less oxygen than the blood, the hemoglobin releases its oxygen molecules and they move into the tissues. Without oxygen, the hemoglobin immediately absorbs carbon dioxide, the waste product of body cell activity. This oxygen-poor blood returns to the lungs. In the lungs, where the concentration of oxygen is higher than in the blood, the iron in the hemoglobin acts as a magnet for oxygen, pulling in as much as the red blood cell can carry.

When hemoglobin is carrying oxygen, its concentration of oxyhemoglobin gives it its bright red hue, the color of blood in the arteries. When it releases oxygen, the pigment changes to a bluish purple—the color of blood in the veins.

Because iron is a key component of hemoglobin, it is important that the diet contain sufficient iron. Readily absorbable iron is found in red meat (especially liver), fish, chicken, turkey, eggs, peas, beans, potatoes, and rice. Iron is added as a supplement to many bakery products, but the form used is absorbed poorly, as is the iron in many vegetables.

Hemoglobinopathy

Inherited disorders involving abnormal hemoglobin molecules. Hemoglobin binds oxygen in red blood cells, facilitating its distribution throughout the body. Abnormal hemoglobin is generally less efficient than normal hemoglobin at carrying oxygen to the cells of the body. People with hemoglobinopathies may have mild to moderate anemia and occasional attacks of pain. The most common types of hemoglobinopathy are hemoglobin C disease, hemoglobin S-C disease, hemoglobin E disease, and SICKLE CELL ANEMIA; altogether, more than 400 variant forms of hemoglobinopathy have been identified.

Hemoglobin C involves the production of abnormal hemoglobin. Symptoms do not always occur but may include mild anemia, an enlarged spleen, and episodes of jaundice (yellowing of the skin). Gallstones may develop and require treatment. The disorder is most common among blacks, especially those from Ghana. About 2 percent of American blacks have hemoglobin C. Treatment is not usually required. Folic acid may aid the production of normal red blood cells and reduce symptoms of anemia. People with hemoglobin C can lead normal lives. Because hemoglobin C is an inherited disorder, a family history of the disorder is the chief risk factor. Couples with family histories of the disorder are encouraged to seek genetic counseling to determine their risk for passing it to their children.

In hemoglobin S-C, the affected person inherits the sickle cell trait, or hemoglobin S, from one parent and hemoglobin C from the other parent. People with hemoglobin S-C have mild to moderate anemia and may have occasional attacks of acute pain. They are also likely to have slightly shorter than normal life spans. Hemoglobin E occurs chiefly in people of Southeast Asian ancestry. It causes mild to moderate anemia.

SICKLE CELL ANEMIA

Sickle cell anemia is caused by an abnormal form of hemoglobin called hemoglobin S. Under certain conditions, hemoglobin S changes the shape of red blood cells from round to crescent or sickle shaped. These sickled cells can become trapped in the small blood vessels in different organs of the body, resulting in a lack of oxygen to the tissues. People who have inherited hemoglobin S from both parents develop sickle cell anemia, while those who have inherited hemoglobin S from only one parent carry the sickle cell trait, meaning they have no symptoms but are at risk for passing the disease on to their children.

The disease occurs primarily in people of African heritage. In the United States, one of 400 blacks is affected. Sickle cell anemia produces a chronic anemia that can become life-threatening when red blood cells break down (hemolytic crisis) or when bone marrow fails to produce blood cells (aplastic crisis). Repeated crises can damage internal organs. Sickle cell anemia is associated with periods of acute pain caused by the lack of oxygen. Genetic counseling is recommended for carriers of the trait to identify couples at risk for transmitting the disease to their children. Individuals may be screened to find out whether they are carriers. Prenatal diagnosis is now possible to identify children with sickle cell anemia. The disease has no cure and can shorten the life span.

Hemoglobinuria

The presence of hemoglobin in the urine without the simultaneous presence of red blood cells. Hemoglobin is the oxygen-carrying pigment that gives red blood cells their color. Under normal circumstances, red blood cells break down after a life span of approximately 120 days. The breakdown process occurs largely in the spleen. Breakdown in the blood vessels releases free hemoglobin, which is then bound by another protein for reprocessing into new blood cells. If, however, the breakdown process in the blood vessels occurs faster than the protein binding, free hemoglobin appears in the urine and can be detected with a laboratory test. Hemoglobinuria can signal a variety of diseases, primarily hemolytic anemia, glomerulonephritis, sickle cell anemia, thalassemia, and malaria.

In the rare disorder known as paroxysmal nocturnal hemoglobinuria, red blood cells break down abnormally and produce urine that is dark in the morning and lighter as the day progresses. Symptoms also include pain in the back and abdomen, headache, shortness of breath, and easy bruising. The exact cause of this disease is unknown.

Paroxysmal cold hemoglobinuria is a disorder in which antibodies form on exposure to cold temperatures and cause the breakdown of red blood cells, which discolor the urine. Other symptoms include chills, fever, leg pain, back pain, abdominal pain, headache, and malaise (a general feeling of illness or discomfort). This rare disease is associated with illnesses such as advanced syphilis and some viral infections. Treatment of the underlying infection often resolves the hemoglobinuria. Drugs that suppress the immune system can also be prescribed.

Hemolysis

The breaking up or destruction of red blood cells, characterized by liberation of hemoglobin into blood plasma. Hemolysis, which usually causes anemia, can result from defects in the red blood cells and from poisoning, infection, the action of antibodies (see ANTIBODY), and mismatched blood transfusions. The Rh factor in newborn babies can result in hemolysis if the mother's red blood cells are Rh negative while the baby's are Rh positive. Antibodies formed in the mother's blood in response to the baby's red blood cells will destroy the baby's red blood cells. If not prevented, hemolysis caused by the Rh factor will cause very severe anemia in the baby or even stillbirth.

Hemolytic disease of the newborn

A disease most commonly caused by RH INCOMPATIBILITY, a situation in which the mother's blood develops antibodies in reaction to the blood of the fetus. The antibodies enter the bloodstream of the fetus and combine with the red blood cells there, causing them to break down (hemolyze) more quickly than usual. The disease occurs when an Rh-negative mother is pregnant with an Rh-positive fetus; the fetus can develop anemia from the loss of red blood cells and JAUNDICE from its body's inability to process the destroyed cells, all of which may lead to a stillbirth. A less severe effect of hemolytic disease on the newborn is to cause swelling. Giving blocking antibodies to an Rh-negative mother prevents her from developing antibodies to the baby's blood in most cases. Blocking antibodies are usually given at the beginning of the third trimester and again within 72 hours of delivery.

AMNIOCENTESIS can detect Rh-factor problems in advance, and close monitoring of fetal development will enable the doctor to prepare for potential problems. Fetal blood sampling may be indicated as well. If the fetus shows signs of severe disease, a fetal blood transfusion may be given. This can be done by injecting blood into the umbilical cord of the fetus or into its abdominal cavity.

Hemolytic-uremic syndrome

A serious disease that involves the destruction of red blood cells, damage to the walls of the blood vessels, and failure of the kidneys. The disease is most likely to occur in children between the ages of 1 and 10 after a serious stomach and intestinal infection. The cause of the infection is often *Escherichia coli* (*E. coli*), a bacterium found in contaminated meat, dairy products, and fruit juice. Hemolytic-uremic syndrome occurs only rarely in adults.

The first stage of hemolytic-uremic syndrome is marked by severe digestive symptoms, such as abdominal pain, vomiting, and bloody diarrhea. Usually this stage ends after 2 to 3 days, but the child remains pale, tired, and irritable. Toxins produced by the bacteria in the intestinal system enter the bloodstream and destroy red blood cells, causing small, unusual bruises in the skin or hemorrhages in the mouth. The damaged red blood cells can clog the small passageways of the kidneys, forcing them to work harder and less effectively. Urine production falls. Fluid accumulating in the body raises the blood pressure and causes swelling, particularly of the hands and feet. The nervous system can be affected, leading to seizures, lethargy, and temporary blindness.

Once hemolytic-uremic syndrome begins, there is no cure. Treatment consists of supporting the child with fluids, salts, and blood transfusions as needed. In some cases, dialysis is required to augment the kidneys. Medication may be used to lower blood pressure and treat nervous system symptoms.

Of 20 children who contract hemolytic-uremic syndrome, 1 or 2 will die during the acute phase of the disease. Of those who survive, 2 to 6 will have some degree of progressive kidney impairment, which may lead to the need for regular dialysis or a kidney transplant.

Prevention is the most effective solution to hemolytic-uremic syndrome. Undercooked hamburger and unpasteurized fruit juices have been implicated in several recent outbreaks of the disease. Thorough cooking of all meats and consumption of pasteurized juices are prudent measures for preventing the *E. coli* infection that can cause hemolytic-uremic syndrome.

Hemophilia

An inherited disorder that causes the blood to clot ineffectively and can result in extensive bruising and bleeding. Because of the way in which it is inherited, hemophilia affects males almost exclusively. Individuals with hemophilia used to die at a young age, but with current treatments, the life span is nearly normal.

Hemophilia results from a deficiency in a protein required for clotting. The three different types of hemophilia result from deficiencies in three different proteins.

TYPES

■ *Hemophilia A* Also known as classical hemophilia, hemophilia A is the most common form, accounting for 80 to 90 percent of cases of hemophilia. It is caused by a deficiency of the coagulation protein known as factor VIII. The severity of the disease depends on the degree of deficiency. In the mildest cases, serious bleeding occurs only after an accident or surgery. In the most severe cases, bleeding can occur spontaneously deep in the body. People with moderate to severe forms of the disease have many large unexplained bruises, suffer pain and swelling in the joints from bleeding, bleed internally, and bleed uncontrollably after even minor injury or surgery. Repeated bleeding into the joints can cause severe pain and weakness; bleeding into the muscle is painful and may lead to wasting and numbness from nerve damage. Deformity and crippling can result. Serious episodes present a medical emergency when bleeding occurs in the head, neck, or digestive system. Prompt treatment with intravenous factor VIII is needed to prevent permanent injury and death.

■ *Hemophilia B* Also known as Christmas disease, hemophilia B arises from an inherited deficiency in coagulation factor IX. It is less common than hemophilia A and generally considered less serious. Like hemophilia A, hemophilia B ranges from mild to severe, reflecting the degree of factor IX deficiency.

■ *Hemophilia C* The most recently discovered and the rarest form of the disease, hemophilia C is also the least serious, causing only a mild bleeding disorder that responds well to treatment. Most do not discover they have the disease until they experience exaggerated bleeding after an accident or surgery. Sometimes hemophilia C causes nosebleeds and hemoglobinuria (hemoglobin in the urine). Unlike hemophilia A and B, hemophilia C can be inherited by women, in whom it may produce extremely heavy menstrual bleeding. Hemophilia C, also known as Rosenthal syndrome, results from an inherited deficiency in coagulation factor XI.

HEMOPHILIA AND HEREDITY

The genes that carry hemophilia A and B are sex-linked recessives transmitted on the X chromosome. Women have two X chromosomes. As a result, women with a hemophilia gene on one X chromosome are usually protected against the disease by the normal gene on the other. These women have no symptoms of hemophilia but are carriers of the disease, who can pass it on to their children. Men, however, have only one X chromosome, inherited from their mothers. If this X chromosome carries the hemophilia gene, the man is almost certain to have the disease, since there is no normal gene to counterbalance the hemophilia gene's effect. Among the children of a woman who is a carrier, each son has a 50 percent chance of having hemophilia, and each daugh-

H

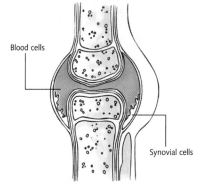

Blood cells

Synovial cells

BLEEDING IN THE JOINTS
In a person with hemophilia, bleeding into joints (hemarthrosis) can occur, either as a result of injury, or spontaneously. The accumulation of blood causes painful swelling and inflammation of the joint lining. The joint may stiffen, in part because the scar tissue caused by the inflammation affects the ability of the synovium (joint lining) to smooth the movement of the joint structures.

ter has a 50 percent chance of being a carrier. Typically hemophilia passes from grandfather to grandson through a woman who is a carrier.

The male children of a man with hemophilia cannot inherit hemophilia from him since he passes only his Y chromosome on to them, but his daughters inherit his X chromosome and become carriers. A woman can inherit hemophilia only if her father has the disease and her mother is a carrier. Since this happens very rarely, few women ever have hemophilia.

Not all cases of hemophilia are inherited. About 1 in 3 cases results from a spontaneous mutation in the gene in a person whose ancestors show no sign of the disease. The mutated gene is then passed on to subsequent generations.

DIAGNOSIS AND TREATMENT
The most severe cases of hemophilia are recognized early in childhood. If a male baby is circumcised, for example, the prolonged bleeding can indicate the disease. The milder forms may become apparent only when the child is hurt or undergoes surgery, such as a tooth extraction. The presence and type of hemophilia are determined by blood tests that identify the missing coagulation factor.

In mild cases of hemophilia A, slow injection of the drug desmopressin (DDAVP) can be used to stop bleeding episodes. The drug mobilizes the available factor VIII in the blood. In more severe cases of hemophilia A and in hemophilia B, treatment for bleeding episodes consists of transfusing the person with the missing coagulation factor in concentrated form. People with particularly severe disease may need regular preventive transfusions. Transfusions are also useful for preparing a person for dental work or surgery. Hemophilia C is managed with periodic transfusions of fresh frozen blood plasma.

People with hemophilia need to avoid situations such as contact sports and medications such as aspirin that make bleeding more likely. Immunization against HEPATITIS B is important because of regular exposure to blood products, which can transmit the infection. Since hemophilia is an inherited disease, anyone who comes from a family with hemophilia and is considering having children should seek GENETIC COUNSELING.

Hemorrhage

FOR FIRST AID
see Bleeding, page 1315

A loss of a large amount of blood in a short time. BLEEDING can be arterial (from an artery) or venous (from a vein). The BLOOD LOSS may be due to internal bleeding, as from the intestine or stomach; external bleeding from an injury; or loss of blood volume and body fluid associated with diarrhea, vomiting, dehydration, or burns. If the heart is unable to supply enough blood, hypovolemic shock can occur, with symptoms that may include a rapid or weak pulse, pale skin, cool or moist skin, rapid breathing, anxiety, overall weakness, and low blood pressure. Emergency medical attention must be sought. In the meantime, the person should be kept warm and covered and assisted to lie down with his or her feet slightly elevated (unless there is a severe head, back, or leg injury). If there is an external wound, sterile dressings and steady, firm, direct pressure should be applied.

Hemorrhage, cerebral

Also known as an intracerebral hemorrhage, a cause of STROKE in which blood vessels within the brain leak blood into the brain itself. A cerebral hemorrhage is a potentially life-threatening condition that requires immediate medical attention. Hemorrhage may be caused by trauma or by an abnormality such as an ANEURYSM (abnormal ballooning of a weakened

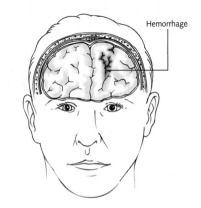
Hemorrhage

BLEEDING IN BRAIN TISSUE
A cerebral hemorrhage occurs when a blood vessel ruptures and bleeds within brain tissue. The hemorrhage can take place anywhere in the brain.

area in the wall of an artery). It can also be associated with HYPERTENSION (high blood pressure). Blood irritates brain tissue and causes swelling or edema; blood can also form into a mass or HEMATOMA. Either condition puts further pressure on brain tissue.

Internal bleeding can occur anywhere in the brain. The extent of BRAIN DAMAGE depends on the location and the extent of tissue affected. Symptoms commonly include severe headache; nausea and vomiting; changes in consciousness, such as sleepiness, apathy, stupor, or loss of consciousness; vision changes; numbness or tingling; difficulty speaking or understanding speech; problems with swallowing; abnormal taste; loss of motor skills, coordination, or balance; and seizures.

Immediate medical attention is required to diagnose and treat a cerebral hemorrhage. Diagnostic tests may include MRI (magnetic resonance imaging), CT (computed tomography) scanning, angiography, functional MRI, and magnetic resonance angiography. (See BRAIN IMAGING.) Blood tests are also important. Treatment varies but usually includes lifesaving interventions and supportive measures. Surgery may be required to remove a hematoma or repair damage. Possible medications include corticosteroids, diuretics, anticonvulsants, and analgesics. Rarely, blood products and intravenous fluids may be necessary to counteract loss of blood. Outcomes vary widely. Even with prompt treatment, death may occur. A person may recover completely or have permanent brain damage.

Hemorrhage, epidural

Also known as an extradural hemorrhage, bleeding that leads to a collection of blood outside the dura, which

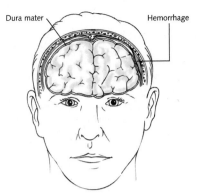

BLEEDING UNDER THE SKULL
Rarely, a skull fracture or other head injury can cause bleeding between the inner surface of the skull and the dura mater—the outermost of the three protective membranes covering the brain. The resulting pooling of blood can put pressure on the brain itself.

is the outside covering of the central nervous system. An extradural hemorrhage is often the result of head injury and is most commonly caused by tearing of the middle meningeal artery. Symptoms include headache, drowsiness, confusion, seizures, and weakness on one side of the body. These symptoms may occur from within minutes to several hours to a few days after the initial injury. Hospitalization and surgery to remove the clotted blood and relieve pressure in the brain are necessary. The surgery usually involves making a small hole in the skull called a burr hole. Early identification and treatment of an extradural hemorrhage usually results in a good long-term outcome.

Hemorrhage, intracerebral

See HEMORRHAGE, CEREBRAL.

Hemorrhage, intraventricular

Also known as IVH, bleeding from fragile blood vessels in the brain. Intraventricular hemorrhages are most common in premature infants born more than 8 weeks early. The vast majority occur during the first week of life. Symptoms of IVH include breathing problems, weak pulse, low blood pressure, paleness, seizures, and HYDROCEPHALUS (excessive accumulation of cerebrospinal fluid in the skull).

IVH is diagnosed and monitored in infants through ultrasound scanning.

The goals of treatment are to prevent bleeding and to keep the infant stable. Any related problems, such as infections or seizures, are dealt with appropriately. A blood transfusion may be necessary. Treatment for hydrocephalus includes spinal taps to remove fluid and relieve pressure on the brain. If this proves insufficient, it may be necessary to surgically place a temporary or permanent tube in the brain. Infants with severe IVH are more likely to experience developmental problems as they grow.

IVH can also occur in adults as an extension of an intracerebral hemorrhage. Blood extends into the ventricle and can cause a clot that obstructs flow of the cerebrospinal fluid, leading to hydrocephalus.

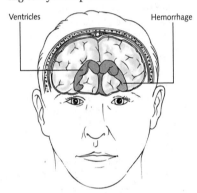

BLEEDING IN BRAIN VENTRICLES
Usually as a result of injury at birth or thereafter, bleeding can occur in the fluid-filled spaces (ventricles) in a newborn baby's brain. The blood vessels in the brain of a developing infant—particularly a premature infant—are especially fragile. More rarely, this type of bleeding can occur in an adult.

Hemorrhage, subarachnoid

Bleeding into the space between the brain and the arachnoid membrane (the middle membrane covering the brain). This is a life-threatening condition that can lead to STROKE, SEIZURE, BRAIN DAMAGE, or death. It may result in permanent brain damage caused by ischemia (loss of blood flow) or bleeding into the brain tissue. Most often, a subarachnoid hemorrhage is caused by a cerebral ANEURYSM that has ruptured or burst. However, it may also be a result of other blood vessel abnormalities (such as an ARTERIOVENOUS MALFORMATION) or trauma.

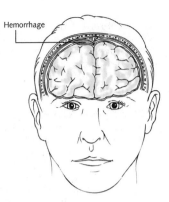

BLEEDING BETWEEN BRAIN MEMBRANES
Bleeding in the space between two of the brain's three protective membranes—the middle, weblike arachnoid layer and the inner pia mater, which adheres to the surface of the brain—is called subarachnoid hemorrhage. The collection of blood causes pressure on the brain.

H

SYMPTOMS

The primary symptom of a subarachnoid hemorrhage is the sudden onset of a severe headache. This may be accompanied by nausea, vomiting, fainting, a decreased level or loss of consciousness, breathing problems, difficulties with speech, trouble swallowing, confusion, irritability, vision problems, loss of movement or sensation, muscle aches, stiff neck, or a seizure.

DIAGNOSIS AND TREATMENT

Immediate medical attention is required to diagnose and treat a subarachnoid hemorrhage. Diagnostic tests may include neuromuscular examination, CT (computed tomography) scanning, MRI (magnetic resonance imaging), and angiography. (See BRAIN IMAGING.) A spinal tap will reveal the presence of blood in cerebrospinal fluid.

Treatment varies, but usually includes lifesaving interventions and supportive measures. Surgery is usually required to remove large hematomas or repair damage. Analgesics and antianxiety drugs are prescribed to relieve headache. Other possible medications include antihypertensives to control high blood pressure, anticonvulsants to control seizures, and calcium channel blockers to prevent cerebral VASOSPASM. In this common complication, the smooth muscles in the blood vessel contract, narrowing the blood vessel and impeding blood flow, creating a greater risk of further tissue damage. Outcomes of subarachnoid hemorrhage vary widely. Even with prompt treatment, death may occur. A person may recover completely or have permanent brain damage.

Hemorrhoidectomy

Surgical removal of HEMORRHOIDS, swollen or enlarged veins in the anal canal. Doctors use a number of different methods to remove painful or bleeding hemorrhoids. In a traditional hemorrhoidectomy, the veins are stretched and surgically cut at the base. This procedure is done in a hospital, and medication is given to cope with pain during the first bowel movements after the operation. It is more common, however, for hemorrhoids to be removed in outpatient procedures that may not even require anesthesia. In ligation, a flexible band is placed tightly around the base of each hemorrhoid. The lack of blood flow painlessly withers the hemor-

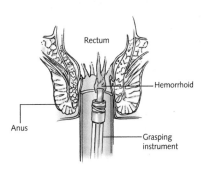

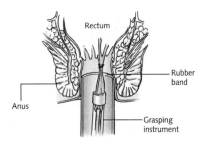

SURGERY FOR HEMORRHOIDS
Hemorrhoids are often removed in an outpatient procedure that involves closing off the hemorrhoid's blood supply with a rubber band. First the doctor uses a special instrument to enter the anus, grasp the hemorrhoid, and pull it downward. Then the doctor places a rubber band around the hemorrhoid that cuts off the blood supply. The hemorrhoid will shrivel in a few days and be eliminated in a bowel movement.

rhoid within a few days. Other options include destroying hemorrhoids with a laser; CRYOSURGERY (destroying by freezing); sclerotherapy (shrinking the hemorrhoids by injecting chemicals); or shrinking them with electric currents.

Hemorrhoids

Swollen or enlarged veins in the anal canal. Hemorrhoids are a common problem in both men and women after age 50. Also known as piles, hemorrhoids can be internal or external. Internal hemorrhoids arise near the beginning of the anal canal and cannot be seen with the naked eye. External hemorrhoids are visible as a bulge under the skin outside the anus.

Hemorrhoids often cause no problems. However, bleeding is a common symptom. Traces of bright red blood may appear on toilet paper or in the toilet. When they protrude from the anus, hemorrhoids tend to produce itching and a mucous discharge. In some people, hemorrhoids cause painful bowel movements. Hemorrhoids that contain a blood clot (thrombosed) are especially painful. Fear of pain can lead to postponing defecation, which worsens the situation, as the stool left in the rectum becomes drier and harder.

The primary cause of hemorrhoids is persistent straining to move the bowels, often related to a diet low in fiber and consequent constipation. Nonfibrous stools are dry and hard, and require straining to pass. Hemorrhoids are particularly apt to bulge when a constipated person strains to have a bowel movement. Obese people and people with advanced cirrhosis (a severe liver disease) are at special risk of developing hemorrhoids. Pregnant women are prone to hemorrhoids temporarily until several weeks after childbirth. Heredity and aging also have a role in hemorrhoid development.

DIAGNOSIS AND TREATMENT
Generally, hemorrhoids are not serious. However, in some cases, rectal bleeding may be due to cancer of the colon or rectum rather than hemorrhoids. Therefore, individuals who experience rectal bleeding should seek prompt medical attention even when they believe that bleeding is from hemorrhoids. Diagnosis is con-

> **HEMORRHOID CARE**
>
> These measures can be taken to reduce the pain and itching of hemorrhoids (if pain persists, a doctor should be contacted):
>
> - Using an over-the-counter hemorrhoid medication
> - Eating a high-fiber diet
> - Soaking in a hot bath for 20 minutes three times a day
> - Holding an ice pack against the anal area
> - Gently cleansing the anal area with moist toilet paper after defecating
> - Avoiding sitting or standing for long periods
> - Lying down as often as possible
> - Using a stool softener
> - Exercising regularly

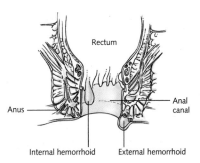

TWO TYPES OF HEMORRHOIDS
External hemorrhoids form on the rim of the anus, while internal hemorrhoids develop inside the anal canal and sometimes hang downward out of the anus as a result of bowel movements or childbirth. Either type can cause itching, pain, or bleeding.

firmed with a rectal examination and tests, such as SIGMOIDOSCOPY (a diagnostic procedure that allows the physician to see upward into the rectum and the sigmoid colon using a lighted tube).

Often, the only treatment required for hemorrhoids is adding more fiber and fluid to the diet. Doctors recommend eating fiber-rich fruits, vegetables, and whole grains and drinking six to eight glasses of water a day. This will soften stools, make them easier to pass, and decrease the pressure on hemorrhoidal veins. Responding promptly to the urge to defecate is also important, as is good hygiene. Doctors advise people with hemorrhoids to use moist, soft toilet paper and to pat rather than wipe after a bowel movement. Warm baths or sitz baths, cold packs, and over-the-counter medicated suppositories or creams can be beneficial home treatments.

When symptoms such as bleeding and pain persist, or when an internal hemorrhoid has prolapsed or fallen out of the anus, further treatment may be necessary. Options include destroying hemorrhoids with a laser, which seals blood vessels as it cuts the hemorrhoid; CRYOSURGERY (removal by freezing); sclerotherapy (injection of a chemical solution into hemorrhoids that causes them to shrink); shrinking swollen veins with electric currents; and HEMORRHOIDEC-TOMY (the surgical removal of hemorrhoids).

Hemosiderosis

An accumulation of iron in the tissues, a condition that causes no disease. Hemosiderosis can result from repeated transfusions needed in the treatment of certain diseases. If the accumulating iron causes tissue damage, the condition is known as HEMOCHROMATOSIS.

Hemostasis

The process of stopping BLEEDING after an injury, either by surgery or by the body's own BLOOD CLOTTING process. Bleeding can be arterial (from an artery) or venous (from a vein). There may also be minor bleeding from capillaries. Physicians recommend emergency medical attention for any case of severe bleeding. To prevent shock following an injury, the person must be kept warm and covered and lie down with his or her feet slightly elevated (unless there is a severe head, back, or leg injury). Sterile dressings and steady, firm, direct pressure should be applied to the wound.

Hemothorax

Blood that has collected in the space between the chest wall and the lung, an area called the pleural cavity. Hemothorax may be caused by cancer, a pulmonary embolism, chest surgery, tuberculosis, or tissue death in the lung, but it is most commonly caused by trauma or injury to the

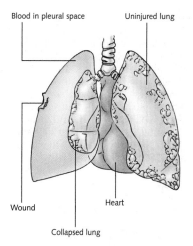

Blood in pleural space   Uninjured lung

Wound

Heart

Collapsed lung

BLEEDING INTO LUNG CAVITY
Hemothorax is mostly commonly caused by injury to the chest, as when a broken rib pierces lung tissue or an artery. In such a case, blood can pool in the pleural cavity and cause shock or even respiratory failure. Preventing injury, by wearing seat belts, for example, is one way to prevent hemothorax.

chest. The injury may cause a rib to pierce or tear lung tissue or a nearby artery, which causes blood to pool in the pleural cavity. A large hemothorax can produce shock in a person who has experienced trauma, and it may also be associated with a collapsed lung. Respiratory failure can result if a large amount of blood gathers in the pleural cavity.

Symptoms of hemothorax include chest pain, shortness of breath, rapid heart rate, anxiety, restlessness, and temporary cessation of breathing. It can be diagnosed by a physical examination using a stethoscope, which will reveal a decrease or lack of breathing sounds in the area where the hemothorax is present. Tests, including a chest X ray, thoracentesis (inserting a needle into the pleural cavity), and pleural fluid analysis, may be performed to confirm the diagnosis. Treatment is based on stabilizing the condition of the affected person, stopping the bleeding, and removing the blood present in the pleural cavity. A chest tube may be inserted through the chest wall to drain the blood. The tube is left in place temporarily to aid in the reexpansion of the lung. Surgery may be necessary to treat the injury that has caused the hemothorax. Complications include shock, fibrosis, or scarring of the membranes of the pleural cavity.

Henoch-Schönlein purpura

An allergic reaction most commonly observed in children that causes a skin rash and other visible marks; also known as anaphylactoid purpura. There is no way to predict who will develop Henoch-Schönlein purpura, and no way to prevent it. Boys are more frequently affected than are girls, and most cases occur between the ages of 2 and 7. Serious complications, including kidney failure, may occur as a result of Henoch-Schönlein purpura.

Purpura is a bleeding disorder that occurs when capillaries rupture, causing blood to accumulate in surrounding tissues. In Henoch-Schönlein purpura, lesions appear on the lower abdomen, buttocks, and legs. The rash first looks red and itchy like hives, but within a day or two develops into purplish or brownish bruises. Joint pain and swelling are also common, especially in the knees and ankles. Pain may be so severe that a child cannot walk. Other symptoms may include severe abdominal pain, fever, headache, loss of appetite, and blood in the urine or feces.

Although its cause is not fully understood, Henoch-Schönlein purpura most often appears several weeks following an upper respiratory virus infection (see COLD, COMMON; VIRUSES). The illness appears to be due to a reaction involving antibodies (special proteins of the immune system) manufactured to fight a cold.

DIAGNOSIS AND TREATMENT
Diagnosis is based on symptoms, medical history, and blood and urine test results. Imaging studies such as X rays or CT (computed tomography) scanning sometimes are used to detect possible complications in organs such as the kidneys or bowel. Hospitalization may be necessary because of the potential for serious complications. A RHEUMATOLOGIST (a specialist in the conditions of the joints and related structures) may be consulted. No specific medication has been found to cure Henoch-Schönlein purpura. Acetaminophen or ibuprofen (not aspirin) can relieve pain and inflammation in joints. For some children, the doctor may prescribe one of the CORTICOSTEROIDS such as prednisone. Follow-up may include periodic blood and urine tests to monitor the kidneys.

H

H

Most children recover completely from Henoch-Schönlein purpura. The illness may last for several months, with symptoms coming and going. A recurrence is likely in half of all cases. Although rare, complications such as kidney failure and hypertension may develop. Most pediatricians will monitor the blood pressure and perform urinalysis every month for 2 years in children who have had Henoch-Schönlein purpura.

Heparin

An anticoagulant drug used to prevent formation of blood clots in blood vessels. Heparin works by interfering with the blood clotting process specifically by accelerating the natural anticlotting process.

Heparin is given before and after open-heart surgery to prevent clot formation in blood vessels. It is also used to treat cardiovascular and pulmonary disorders such as deep vein thrombosis and pulmonary embolism, as well as for prevention of clots after hip surgery. Heparin (Heparin Lock Flush, Hep-Lock) is administered by injection.

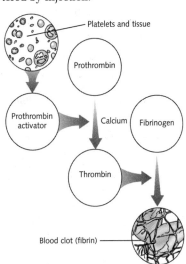

HEPARIN INHIBITS BLOOD CLOTTING
Blood clots when platelets and damaged tissue cells release a substance called prothrombin activator, which sets off a cascade of chemical interactions. Prothrombin produces thrombin, which acts on fibrinogen to form fibrin, which has a threadlike structure that traps red blood cells to form a clot. Heparin interferes with this process by inhibiting the formation of thrombin from prothrombin.

Hepatectomy, partial

The partial removal of the liver. A surgeon may perform this operation when cancer is contained within one lobe of the liver, in the absence of CIRRHOSIS (a severe liver disease), jaundice (a yellowing of the skin and the whites of the eyes), and ascites (an abnormal collection of fluid inside the abdominal cavity). In a partial hepatectomy, an entire lobe of the liver is removed (see LOBECTOMY, LIVER) or the area around the tumor is removed (a wedge resection). Complete removal of a tumor usually offers the best survival rate from liver cancer.

Hepatectomy, total

See LIVER TRANSPLANT.

Hepatic

Pertaining to, relating to, or originating in the liver.

Hepatitis

Inflammation of the liver that can lead to swelling, tenderness, and permanent damage. When hepatitis harms the liver, it can no longer perform key functions at peak efficiency. Severe cases of hepatitis can lead to life-threatening liver failure. Even without symptoms, hepatitis may be causing serious damage, such as scarring to the liver. Hepatitis is most commonly due to a virus, although certain drugs, poisons, or chemicals can also cause it.

TYPES OF HEPATITIS

Hepatitis may be sudden (acute) or long-lasting (chronic). In the initial infection, acute viral hepatitis can range from causing no symptoms to severe disease. If the virus persists in the blood for 6 months or more after the initial infection, it is considered chronic. Liver damage can occur as a result of either acute or chronic hepatitis. However, most acute cases of viral hepatitis are mild and self-limiting, and liver damage is more often associated with long-term, chronic hepatitis.

At least five different viruses are currently known to cause liver inflammation: A, B, C, D, and E. In the United States, infection with the A, B, and C viruses is most common. The hepatitis D virus coinfects with the hepatitis B virus or infects individuals already chronically infected with the hepatitis B virus. Hepatitis is

less commonly due to drug use, metabolic disorders, or autoimmune diseases. Excessive alcohol consumption is a very common nonviral cause of liver inflammation. While all strains of hepatitis cause liver inflammation, there are also significant differences.

■ *Hepatitis A* Also known simply as infectious hepatitis, HEPATITIS A typically produces mild, flulike symptoms, such as nausea, loss of appetite, muscle and joint pain, a low-grade fever, weakness, and headache. A frequent childhood illness, this virus is shed in the stool and passed from person to person via contaminated food or water.

■ *Hepatitis B* Infection with the HEPATITIS B virus (HBV) can be either acute or chronic. Approximately one in ten people with an acute viral infection eventually develops more serious, chronic hepatitis B. Symptoms can include nausea, loss of appetite, muscle and joint pain, fatigue, weakness, and a low-grade fever. HBV can lead to life-threatening chronic active hepatitis, cirrhosis, liver cancer, and liver failure. It is spread through contact with infected blood and other body fluids. Unprotected sex with an infected partner, sharing of contaminated intravenous (IV) needles, and passing from mother-to-newborn are common means of transmission.

■ *Hepatitis C* The HEPATITIS C virus (HCV) is viewed as the most serious hepatitis virus. Like HBV, HCV is spread through contact with contaminated blood and other body fluids. HCV is believed to be transmitted sexually and through contaminated needles. Hepatitis C provides the greatest risk for chronic liver disease and can lead to progressive, life-threatening chronic active hepatitis, cirrhosis, liver cancer, and liver failure.

■ *Hepatitis D* Also known as delta hepatitis; the HEPATITIS D virus (HDV) affects only people who already have hepatitis B. When HDV infection accompanies chronic hepatitis B, the results are more severe than for either chronic hepatitis B or C.

■ *Hepatitis E* Also known as epidemic non-A, non-B hepatitis, HEPATITIS E is transmitted through the intestinal tract. It spreads through drinking water in unsanitary areas, and outbreaks have not occurred in the United States.

■ *Alcoholic hepatitis* Excessive alcohol consumption can lead to this type of hepatitis. A mild case of liver inflammation may cause no symptoms. More serious cases may result in losses of appetite and weight, weakness, fatigue, nausea, vomiting, and pain above the liver. Severe alcoholic hepatitis, a life-threatening condition that requires hospitalization, is characterized by fever, bleeding in the gastrointestinal tract, ascites (accumulation of fluid in the abdomen), and eventual liver failure. The pain of alcoholic hepatitis can be difficult to distinguish from that of other conditions, such as gallstones. However, tests such as blood studies and X rays can identify the problem. Although recovery is common, scarring of the liver is a permanent result. See also LIVER DISEASE, ALCOHOLIC.

SYMPTOMS
Many people with various types of hepatitis experience no symptoms. However, doctors caution that even when symptoms are absent, progressive liver damage may occur. Signs of hepatitis vary according to its cause and whether the disease takes on an acute or chronic form. Symptoms commonly include severe fatigue, weakness, muscle and joint pain, a low-grade fever, headache, nausea, vomiting, diarrhea, abdominal discomfort, and loss of appetite. Some individuals develop jaundice (a yellowing of the skin and the whites of the eyes), which may be accompanied by pale stools, dark urine, and itching. Rashes and memory loss occur in a number of chronic cases.

Acute hepatitis refers to liver inflammation and symptoms that are short-term. A mild case of acute hepatitis may cause no symptoms at all or vague flulike symptoms that last from several days to several weeks. On the other hand, sometimes (as in an acute attack of chronic hepatitis B with hepatitis D) symptoms such as fatigue, nausea, and joint pain are severe and debilitating. Such cases can lead to permanent liver damage, liver failure, and the need for a liver transplant.

Chronic hepatitis also can exhibit a range of symptoms, although sometimes no symptoms are apparent. Chronic active hepatitis is a continu-

ing inflammation of the liver that damages liver cells. It can cause extreme weakness and disability and can lead to serious, potentially life-threatening complications. These include cirrhosis, liver cancer, and liver failure.

DIAGNOSIS AND TREATMENT
A diagnosis of hepatitis is made by physical examination, medical history, and blood tests. A medical history is especially important, because certain individuals (for example, IV drug users or people with multiple sexual partners) are at higher risk than others. When symptoms are not present, blood tests administered during the course of a routine physical examination may reveal elevated liver enzymes, which can be a sign of hepatitis. Over time, blood tests are repeated at regular intervals to monitor the progression of the disease. To determine the extent of liver damage, doctors often perform a LIVER BIOPSY.

Treatment of hepatitis depends on its cause and whether the disease is acute or chronic. In acute cases of hepatitis A, B, and C, doctors recommend bed rest, a balanced diet, and avoiding alcohol. Infants born to HBV-infected mothers should receive hepatitis B immune globulin within 12 hours of birth. Drugs such as interferon and lamivudine have met with some success in treating chronic hepatitis B. In cases of chronic hepatitis C, the combination of the drugs interferon and ribavarin is the only known effective treatment. The decision about whether or not to undertake this regimen must be made in consultation with one's physician because there are serious side effects. If hepatitis destroys a major portion of the liver and prevents it from functioning properly, a liver transplant may be considered.

RISK FACTORS AND PREVENTION
Certain groups are at special risk of hepatitis. These include people who have sex with an infected person or multiple partners, infants born to infected mothers, IV drug users, people with hemophilia, health care workers (who may accidentally stick themselves with a contaminated needle), and day care workers who handle soiled diapers. Today, however, methods exist to prevent most cases. For example, because blood banks in the United States now routinely screen for

hepatitis B and C, the risk of contracting these viruses from blood transfusions is considered minimal.

Good personal hygiene and proper handling of food can stop the spread of hepatitis A. People who are infected with hepatitis A must not prepare or handle food that is to be eaten by others. For those traveling to a country where this virus is common and for people otherwise at risk, doctors recommend vaccination against hepatitis A.

Immunization is also available for hepatitis B and is recommended for all children beginning at birth. Older children who have not been immunized should receive a series of three shots when they are 11 or 12 years old. Because unprotected sex is a major means of HBV transmission, doctors also recommend vaccination for adults who have multiple sexual partners. Immunization is also recommended for people with bleeding disorders such as hemophilia.

Currently there is no vaccine to prevent hepatitis C. To guard against this and other forms of hepatitis, doctors advise against getting tattoos and body piercings in unsanitary establishments. Intravenous drug users should not share needles. Health care workers who have contact with blood and blood products should be immunized against hepatitis B and take appropriate precautions to protect themselves from exposure to body fluids. Although the risk is slight, the personal items (such as razors and toothbrushes) of an infected person should not be shared.

Hepatitis A
Inflammation of the liver due to infection with the hepatitis A virus (HAV). The infection is sudden and acute and does not cause chronic or long-lasting disease. Initially shed in the stool, this virus is spread through food or water contaminated by feces. It is frequently a childhood illness and can occur in nurseries and day care centers where diapers are frequently changed.

The major symptoms of HAV infection include nausea, loss of appetite, muscle and joint pain, a low-grade fever, weakness, and headache. Jaundice (a yellowing of the skin and the whites of the eyes) develops in many infected adults, although rarely

H

in children. Some infected individuals may have very mild symptoms or none at all. Diagnosis is made by physical examination, medical history, and blood tests. Infection with HAV usually passes in 6 to 8 weeks with no treatment other than bed rest, a balanced diet, and avoiding alcohol. However, a lack of energy and prolonged fatigue may last for weeks or months. In rare cases, severe hepatitis A results in liver failure.

PREVENTION

Good personal hygiene, such as washing hands after using the bathroom, and proper handling of food can effectively prevent the spread of hepatitis A. People who are infected with HAV should not prepare or handle food that is to be eaten by others. Doctors recommend an HAV vaccine (introduced in 1995) for travelers to areas in which hepatitis A is endemic. To be effective, the vaccination must be given at least 1 month before possible exposure. Immunization is also advised for homosexual men who have sex with more than one partner, for intravenous (IV) drug users, for people with chronic liver disease or bleeding disorders such as hemophilia, for those who experience occupational exposure to HAV, and for children who live in high-risk communities. The vaccine can be used to control outbreaks of hepatitis A. When several cases of HAV infection are diagnosed in a community, immune globulin should be administered to everyone who may have been exposed to the virus.

Hepatitis B

Inflammation of the liver due to infection with the hepatitis B virus (HBV). The infection can be sudden and acute or chronic and long-lasting (the virus persists in the blood 6 months or more after the initial infection). In the United States, hepatitis B is most common in older adolescents and adults. In nine of ten affected people, the condition improves spontaneously; only a few develop chronic HBV infection. Of these, about half have active symptoms in addition to carrying the virus. Elsewhere in the world, HBV more frequently occurs in infants, in whom it is much more likely to become chronic.

SYMPTOMS AND CAUSES

Some people with hepatitis B virus experience no symptoms at all. Others have problems such as nausea, loss of appetite, muscle and joint pain, fatigue, weakness, and a low-grade fever. As time goes on, an enlarged liver and jaundice (a yellowing of the skin and the whites of the eyes) may develop. In some cases, severe, acute flare-ups of HBV are triggered by infection with hepatitis D virus (see HEPATITIS D). Hepatitis B is highly infectious during the 6- to 12-week incubation period (the time between initial exposure to the virus and the development of symptoms). Even after acute symptoms disappear, some individuals with HBV continue to be contagious and some people become lifelong HBV carriers.

When an acute case lasts longer than 6 months and enters the chronic stage, it can cause a progressive, life-threatening destruction of liver cells. Possible consequences include CIRRHOSIS (a severe liver disease in which healthy cells are destroyed and replaced by scar tissue), liver failure, and an increased risk for developing liver cancer. Contact with infected blood and other body fluids is the primary cause of hepatitis B. Risk groups include people who have multiple sexual partners (particularly homosexual men who do), intravenous (IV) drug users who share needles, health care workers, people who get tattoos or body piercings with improperly sterilized equipment, and those with bleeding disorders such as hemophilia. The virus can also be passed from an infected mother to her infant during childbirth.

DIAGNOSIS AND TREATMENT

Diagnosis of HBV is made by physical examination, medical history, and blood tests. Because the disorder commonly causes no symptoms, it is often detected through abnormal liver function results obtained during the course of routine blood tests. Treatment of acute cases consists primarily of bed rest, a balanced diet, and avoiding alcohol. Infants born to infected mothers should receive hepatitis B immune globulin within 12 hours of birth. Drugs such as interferon and lamivudine have had some success in treating chronic hepatitis B. However, interferon must be self-injected and has severe flulike side effects,

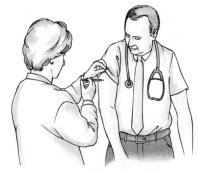

PREVENTING HEPATITIS B
Health care workers are at risk of contracting hepatitis B from infected patients and from accidentally sticking themselves with a contaminated needle. To avoid getting the disease and passing it to others, doctors and other health care professionals are vaccinated regularly.

such as fever, muscle aches, and chills. Lamivudine is now available in oral form. If HBV destroys a major portion of the liver and prevents it from functioning properly, a liver transplant may be considered.

PREVENTION

Because a vaccine for hepatitis B exists, HBV is preventable. In the United States, immunization with the hepatitis B vaccine (see VACCINATIONS, CHILDHOOD) begins at birth. Older children who have not yet been vaccinated should receive a series of three injections when they are 11 or 12 years old. Adults with multiple sexual partners or who live in a household with a carrier of chronic HBV and those with bleeding disorders (such as hemophilia) should be immunized. Pregnant women in the United States are now routinely tested for hepatitis B. This has helped to eliminate the passage of the virus from mother to infant. To guard against HBV, doctors advise people who use IV drugs not to share needles or to have unprotected sex with infected or multiple partners. Tattoos and body piercings should take place only in sanitary establishments. Although the risk is slight, personal items (such as razors and toothbrushes) should not be shared with an infected person.

Hepatitis C

Inflammation of the liver due to infection with the hepatitis C virus (HCV). Hepatitis C is more likely than any other type of hepatitis to lead to chronic hepatitis (meaning that the virus persists in the blood 6 months or more after the initial infection). Nearly nine of ten people who contract hepatitis C retain evidence of it indefinitely and are carriers of the virus. Until 1992, when a screening test was developed to identify blood donors with HCV, it was possible to contract this virus through a blood transfusion. This is no longer the case. Although many people never discover exactly how they contracted the virus, hepatitis C most frequently occurs in intravenous (IV) drug users who share needles; people who get tattoos or body piercings with poorly sterilized equipment; health care workers; and those with bleeding disorders such as hemophilia. It is not common for hepatitis C to spread through sexual activity with an infected person or from an infected mother to an infant.

SYMPTOMS AND DIAGNOSIS

Many people with hepatitis C experience no symptoms at all. They can have the disease for many years without being aware of it. However, about one in four affected people develops acute flulike symptoms within 6 months of exposure. Possible symptoms include nausea, loss of appetite, muscle and joint pain, fatigue, weakness, and a low-grade fever. As time goes on, an enlarged liver and jaundice (a yellowing of the skin and the whites of the eyes) can develop. Dark urine, pale stools, and itching may accompany jaundice. Rashes and memory loss also develop in some chronic cases. Possible complications of chronic HCV include CIRRHOSIS (a severe liver disease in which healthy cells are destroyed and replaced by scar tissue), liver failure, and an increased risk for liver cancer.

Diagnosis of hepatitis C is made by physical examination, medical history, and blood tests. Because the disorder commonly has no symptoms, it is often detected through abnormal levels of liver enzymes obtained during the course of routine blood tests. Typically, the elevated enzymes are alanine aminotransferase (ALT) and aspartate aminotransferase (AST), which leak out of injured liver cells into the blood.

TREATMENT AND PREVENTION

Bed rest, a balanced diet, and avoiding alcohol may relieve acute symptoms. However, treatment decisions regarding chronic hepatitis C are difficult, particularly for those who experience no symptoms. The course of the chronic disease varies from person to person. The majority of those chronically infected will not sustain any long-term liver damage. However, about two in ten persons develop the permanent scarring of the liver that is typical of life-threatening cirrhosis.

The only cure for chronic infection with HCV is a complicated and lengthy regimen of interferon injections and ribavarin capsules. These drugs must be taken for a year or more. Interferon is self-injected several times each week; in many people, it causes devastating, flulike side effects (including fever, chills, and body aches) and severe depression. Many find that they cannot tolerate the regimen. Treatment is not universally successful, and in many cases, the infection returns.

Eventually, if hepatitis C destroys a major portion of the liver and prevents it from functioning properly, a liver transplant may be required. Hepatitis C is currently the most common reason for liver transplants in the United States. Because there is no vaccine against hepatitis C, prevention is key. To guard against this virus, doctors advise people not to share IV needles and caution that tattoos and body piercings must take place only in sanitary establishments. Health care workers who have contact with blood and blood products should exercise appropriate precautions. In addition, although the risk is slight, personal items (such as razors and toothbrushes) should not be shared in the home of an infected person.

Hepatitis D

A liver infection that occurs only in people who are already infected with the hepatitis B virus (HBV). Like HEPATITIS B, this infection is spread primarily through contact with infected blood and through sexual activity. In the United States, hepatitis D (also known as delta hepatitis), which is caused by the hepatitis D virus (HDV), is responsible for about 2 percent of all cases of acute viral hepatitis. Elsewhere in the world, this disease is more common.

Infection with HDV affects the body in two ways. It may occur simultaneously with acute hepatitis B, in a condition called coinfection. The likelihood of recovery from coinfection is excellent. Only a small percentage of people eventually develop chronic infection, in which the virus persists in the blood 6 months or longer after the initial infection. However, HDV infection can also develop when HBV infection enters a chronic stage, in a condition known as superinfection. Superinfection with chronic HDV is a more serious disease than either chronic hepatitis B or C. It is more likely to lead to severe acute hepatitis, which can result in liver failure.

Symptoms include nausea, loss of appetite, muscle and joint pain, fatigue, weakness, and a low-grade fever. With time, there may be an enlarged liver and jaundice (a yellowing of the skin and the whites of the eyes). Urine may grow darker in color while stools are pale. Eventually, HDV infection can lead to CIRRHOSIS (a severe liver disease in which healthy cells are destroyed and replaced by scar tissue) and an increased risk of liver cancer. Even when symptoms are not present, a person with chronic HDV is a carrier of the virus.

Diagnosis of HDV is made by physical examination, a medical history, and blood tests. Treatment consists of bed rest, a balanced diet, and avoiding alcohol. Interferon, a drug that is useful in eradicating chronic hepatitis B and C, has not been found helpful in the treatment of hepatitis D. If HDV infection destroys a major portion of the liver and prevents it from functioning properly, a liver transplant may be considered. However, even when a transplant is successful, cirrhosis may recur.

Hepatitis E

Inflammation of the liver due to infection with the hepatitis E virus (HEV). This virus is also known as epidemic non-A, non-B hepatitis; it is transmitted through the intestinal tract. No outbreaks of HEV have occurred in the United States. The disease occurs mainly in areas with poor sanitation. Epidemics have been reported in Asia and South America, where the virus spreads through fecally contaminated drinking water.

Hepatitis E is an acute, short-lived disease. After an incubation period of 2 to 8 weeks, there are symptoms such as fever, nausea, loss of appetite, and discomfort in the upper right area of the abdomen. Jaundice (a yellowing of the skin and the whites of the eyes) may also develop. In most cases, hepatitis E is mild and disappears within a few weeks with no lasting effects. However, although it does not become a chronic disease, in some cases, hepatitis E destroys so many cells that it causes liver failure. Pregnant women are more at risk of this complication with HEV than with other types of hepatitis.

Hepatitis E is diagnosed by physical examination and blood tests. Treatment consists of bed rest, a balanced diet, and avoiding alcohol. There is no vaccine for HEV. When traveling, the best way to prevent infection with hepatitis E is to use only sterilized water and beverages.

Hepatitis, chronic active

A continuing inflammation of the liver that damages liver cells. In viral hepatitis, chronic means the virus persists in the blood for 6 months or more. Although severe cases of acute (short-lived) hepatitis can also be serious, chronic active hepatitis is far more likely to cause serious problems. It is more likely to lead to complications such as life-threatening cirrhosis (a severe liver disease in which healthy cells are destroyed and replaced by scar tissue), liver cancer, and liver failure. Eventually, if chronic active hepatitis destroys a major portion of the liver and prevents it from functioning properly, a liver transplant may be required.

Chronic active hepatitis may be caused by viral infection, drug ingestion, metabolic disorders, or autoimmune diseases. Very commonly, it is due to infection with the hepatitis B (HBV) and C (HCV) viruses. Hepatitis C is many times more likely than hepatitis B to lead to chronic infection. Hepatitis D, a liver infection that

> Terms in small capital letters—for example, PHYSICAL THERAPY or PAGET DISEASE—indicate a cross-reference to another entry with more information.

occurs only in people who are already infected with HBV, can also have a role in chronic active hepatitis. When hepatitis D occurs along with chronic HBV infection, the resulting superinfection is a more severe illness than either chronic hepatitis B or C alone. The risk of progressive, life-threatening chronic active hepatitis is also greater in people who are infected simultaneously with the B and C viruses.

Hepatitis, nonalcoholic steatohepatitis

See NONALCOHOLIC STEATOHEPATITIS.

Hepatitis, viral

Inflammation of the liver that is caused by viral infection. Viruses, the most common cause of HEPATITIS, can cause minimal symptoms or can damage liver cells so that they can no longer work properly. Severe cases of viral hepatitis can lead to life-threatening LIVER FAILURE. There are many viruses currently known to cause liver inflammation, including HEPATITIS A, HEPATITIS B, HEPATITIS C, HEPATITIS D, HEPATITIS E, hepatitis F, and hepatitis G. The Epstein-Barr virus (EBV) and cytomegalovirus can also cause hepatitis. Researchers continue to discover other viruses that cause hepatitis.

Hepatoma

A tumor originating from liver cells that is usually malignant. Athletes who use anabolic steroids are at increased risk for developing hepatomas. Hepatomas usually develop in livers that are damaged by hepatitis B or C or cirrhosis, a condition most commonly caused either by viral infection or excessive consumption of alcohol. Benign hepatomas can be removed surgically. Common symptoms of a malignant hepatoma (hepatocellular carcinoma) include bloating, abdominal pain, fever, weight loss, nausea, and decreased appetite. In advanced stages of the disease, symptoms can include ascites (swelling of the abdomen from fluid), jaundice (yellowing of the skin and the whites of the eyes), and swollen legs. Liver cancer is not common in the United States, although it may be the most common cancer worldwide. It is not generally diagnosed early and often reaches an advanced stage before symptoms

develop and a doctor is consulted. Diagnosis of liver cancer usually requires a biopsy. Frequently, the serum alpha-fetoprotein level is elevated. Early-stage hepatomas can be removed surgically, or destroyed by injecting alcohol, using cryotherapy (freezing), or by embolization, in which a substance is injected into the artery supplying blood to the tumor in order to block the blood flow. Current treatments of advanced liver cancer are not particularly effective; the primary goal is the relief of symptoms. Some patients can be treated with liver transplantation.

Hepatomegaly

Swelling or enlargement of the liver. Among the causes of hepatomegaly are liver congestion due to heart failure, obstruction of the veins that drain the liver, a cyst or tumor, or a fatty liver due to alcoholic liver disease (see LIVER DISEASE, ALCOHOLIC), or metastatic liver disease, in which cancer from another part of the body spreads to the liver. A physical examination, medical history, and various laboratory and imaging tests can detect the underlying cause of hepatomegaly. The treatment of an enlarged liver is determined directly by its cause. For example, heart congestion responds to diuretics, while a fatty liver requires complete abstinence from alcohol. Weight reduction helps those who are obese.

Herbal medicine

The use of leaves, flowers, fruits, stems, bark, and roots of plants to prevent, relieve, and treat illness. Herbal medicine, also called herbalism, herbology, or botanical medicine, is the oldest form of health care known to human civilization. Plants contain many biologically active ingredients and have been used throughout the world to treat disease. Scientists have isolated the medicinal properties of many botanicals, analyzing and extracting their components. Herbal medicine has a significant role in CHINESE MEDICINE and AYURVEDA.

HERBAL PREPARATIONS

Herbs and herbal compounds are available in many forms. Common preparations that are available in health food stores include the following:

■ Tinctures: concentrated extracts of herbs containing alcohol; very

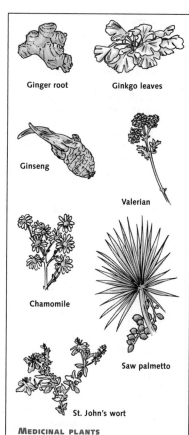

MEDICINAL PLANTS
Plants sometimes used as remedies include ginger root (nausea); ginkgo (circulation and memory); chamomile (gas); valerian (tension, insomnia); ginseng (fatigue, diabetes); saw palmetto (urinary and prostate problems); and St. John's wort (depression). Herbal remedies may interact with prescription or nonprescription drugs that a person is taking.

strongly flavored but cost-effective and easy to administer
- Extracts: similar to tinctures but may not contain alcohol; herb may be extracted with water
- Capsules and tablets: ground or powdered raw herb made into pills; less potent than extracts or tinctures
- Teas: loose herbs that can be steeped in hot water to produce medicinal beverages aimed at specific complaints
- Lozenges: herbal-based, naturally sweetened lozenges intended to suppress cough or fight colds
- Ointments, salves, and rubs: herbal-based skin creams that soothe minor burns, warm aching muscles, or treat infections or wounds

USING HERBAL REMEDIES SAFELY

Alternative therapies may have many advantages, but they also pose certain risks. Alternative medicines and therapies can interfere with standard medical treatments or mask a more serious problem, which is why it is important to tell your doctor if you are using alternative remedies.

People taking medication for long-term health problems, such as hypertension or diabetes mellitus, should be especially careful to check with a doctor to learn whether their medications interact with supplements or herbs they may be taking.

Alternative treatments may also delay treatment of a more serious condition or disease. For example, taking an herb for pain could delay addressing the real source of a person's pain, potentially permitting a condition or disease to become worse because it is unchecked or untreated.

In some cases, alternative supplements can directly harm a person. Ephedra (also called ma huang), an herbal diet pill, can cause a dangerous interaction and lead to heart trouble when mixed with decongestants, which also contain stimulants. Because alternative medications are classified as supplements, the US Food and Drug Administration does not regulate them. As a result, quality controls for the therapies are not uniform throughout the industry. These therapies may sometimes contain ingredients not shown on the label, or concentrations of the active ingredient can vary depending on the manufacturer. Just as with conventional medication, there is an optimal dose for alternative medications. Taking too much of an alternative remedy may cause a person harm.

Many common alternative therapies do not mix with over-the-counter and prescription medications. Here are some examples:

- Ginkgo biloba, used to protect the heart and circulatory system and to improve memory, adds to the anticoagulant effect of drugs, such as aspirin and warfarin, and may cause excessive internal bleeding.
- Ephedra, a stimulant used in over-the-counter herbal diet pills, may cause heart attack, seizure, or sedation when combined with common decongestants that contain pseudoephedrine (such as Sudafed, Actifed, and Sinutab) or when taken with caffeine.
- Ginger, often used to combat motion sickness and nausea, may lead to excessive thinning of the blood when used with warfarin, a blood thinner.

REGULATION OF HERBAL MEDICINE

In the United States, herbal remedies are not classified as drugs but as foods or dietary supplements. As a result, the Food and Drug Administration (FDA) does not regulate herbal remedies or oversee the research that would establish their effectiveness and safety. However, the FDA does restrict the claims that manufacturers of herbal remedies can make in labeling their products. Manufacturers cannot claim that an herbal remedy can diagnose, treat, cure, or prevent any disease. When it is known that a particular herbal substance has an effect on the body, such as the effect of calcium on the growth of bones, manufacturers may point that out.

As a result of the absence of FDA regulation, herbal remedies are available in unpredictable strengths, and varying quantities of active ingredients may be used in their preparation. Manufacturers often do not test ingredients to make sure they are free of

PLANTS AS PHARMACEUTICALS

At least a quarter of all conventional pharmaceuticals are derived from plant materials that have been purified to create commercial drug products. Many drugs considered to be conventional medications were originally derived from plants. These include the following:

- Aspirin, which as salicyclic acid, was originally derived from white willow bark and the meadowsweet plant
- Quinine, from cinchona bark, used for muscle cramps and malaria
- Morphine and codeine, from the opium poppy
- Vincristine, an anticancer drug, from rosey periwinkle
- Digitalis, used to regulate heart rhythm, from the purple foxglove

H

contaminants, and some ingredients may not be listed on the product label. Research into product effectiveness is minimal. The standards of quality have not kept pace with popular interest in herbal remedies, although use has been increasing. Many medical schools now teach students about herbal medicine.

Heredity

The genetic transmission of characteristics or traits from one generation to the next; the genetic makeup of an individual, derived from ancestors.

Heritability

The proportion of a certain characteristic or trait, such as intellect, that can be attributed to genetic factors rather than to environmental ones.

Hermaphroditism

A genetic abnormality in which a person is born with both male and female sex organs. The cause of this abnormality is not well understood. In one form of the disorder, during embryonic development, abnormalities in cell division occur that provide the baby with cells with 46 XY chromosomes as well as cells with 46 XX chromosomes. Typically, in an individual with hermaphroditism, the penis is small or incomplete and one or both testes may or may not appear, while a uterus, oviducts, and a vagina are present. Various patterns occur: a hermaphroditic baby can have an ovary on one side and a testis on the other; a testis on one side and an ovo-testis, containing both ovary and testis, on the other side; or an ovary on one side and an ovo-testis on the other.

When a baby is born with hermaphroditism, a pediatric endocrinologist, a specialist in the hormonal problems of infancy, should be consulted. The correct assignment of the baby's sex can be made only after thorough testing and evaluation. This process is critical because the baby's future life and emotional health are at stake. Hormones can be given to males to increase the size of the penis. Reconstructive surgery is also an option.

Hernia

Protrusion of an organ or tissue through a weak spot in a muscle or other tissue that normally contains it.

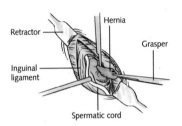
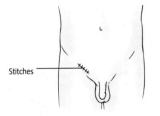

REPAIR OF AN INGUINAL HERNIA
An inguinal hernia, in which a portion of the intestine protrudes into the lower abdomen just above the thigh, is common in men because a loop of intestine can easily push into the inguinal canal through which the testicles descend. The problem can be repaired with surgery to push the distended intestine back into place. The incision in the groin is stitched shut at the end of the procedure.

The muscles and connective tissues are ordinarily firm enough to hold organs in place. However, when muscles grow slack due to disease or injury, tissue may bulge through the weak point. Although hernias can occur anywhere in the body, they are most common in the abdominal wall. Herniation may also occur internally where it cannot be detected by external examination.

A bulge or swelling is often the only sign of a hernia. Bulging usually develops slowly over a period of weeks. However, at times, it occurs suddenly, for example, when muscles are damaged by lifting a heavy object. Additional symptoms may include heaviness, tenderness, or aching at the location of the hernia. A person who has a hiatal hernia, in which the stomach protrudes through the diaphragm into the chest, can experience heartburn, especially at night or after a heavy meal.

Most abdominal hernias are diagnosed by a physical examination. A truss can be worn to keep a hernia in place. However, surgery is generally the best treatment. (See HERNIORRHAPHY.) Most hernias are reducible, meaning that the surgeon can push tissue back into its proper location. Loose muscles or other tissues are

then sewn together. If the tissue is very weak, the surgeon may use a synthetic mesh to reinforce it. Without surgery, hernias generally grow worse and develop complications. STRANGULATION, in which the protruding tissue becomes trapped, cutting off its blood supply, and obstruction may occur. If a herniated intestine becomes obstructed, intestinal contents become blocked (see INTESTINE, OBSTRUCTION OF.) Both conditions require immediate medical attention.

Herniated disk

See SLIPPED DISK.

Herniorrhaphy

An operation in which a HERNIA (a protrusion of soft tissue through other tissue, usually muscle, that normally contains it) is surgically corrected. It is the typical treatment for most hernias. In a herniorrhaphy, a small incision is made in the skin over the hernia. Through this opening, the surgeon pushes tissue back into its proper location and sews loose muscles together. In some cases, a plastic mesh or sheet is inserted to reinforce a weak muscle or one that has been replaced by scar tissue.

The location and severity of the hernia determine the extent of surgery. Surgery generally takes less than an hour. In many cases, the operation is performed in a hospital outpatient surgery unit under local anesthesia. More extensive surgery is done in a hospital under general anesthesia, and a short hospital stay is required. After the procedure, doctors prescribe medication to control pain. Many individuals go home on the same day of the operation and can resume most normal activities within a few days. However, heavy lifting must be avoided for up to 8 weeks after surgery.

Herpangina

An acute infectious disorder characterized by fever and ulcerated blisters on mucous membranes inside the mouth. Herpangina is most commonly caused by a COXSACKIEVIRUS, but may also be caused by other intestinal viruses. The disorder tends to occur in infants and children, spreading rapidly within a group.

Symptoms include a sudden onset of fever with sore throat, headache, and loss of appetite. Often pain is experienced in the areas of the neck, abdomen, and extremities. There may be vomiting and seizures in infants. Within a few days of initial symptoms, small grayish, blistering sores with red borders appear inside the mouth on the soft palate, uvula, or tongue and on the tonsils. These sores usually become shallow ulcers within 24 hours and heal in the following 1 to 5 days. In most cases, all symptoms have improved within 7 days. Complications are rare, and lasting immunity to the infectious agent is established.

Herpangina is diagnosed by a clinical history of symptoms and observation of the characteristic sores in the mouth. Blood tests may be used if it is necessary to diagnose the cause of infection. There are no medications to treat this viral disorder, so the infected child's symptoms are treated as recommended by a physician.

Herpes B virus

A member of the herpes group of viruses that is carried by rhesus and other Asiatic macaque monkeys. Herpes B virus is also referred to as Herpesvirus simiae and can cause serious disease, including ENCEPHALITIS. It is transmitted to humans from infected monkeys. Transmission via person-to-person contact has been documented in only one case.

Herpes B virus is believed to be transmitted to humans by exposure to the contaminated saliva of an infected primate that may occur when a person is bitten or scratched by a monkey. Symptoms generally occur within 1 month of exposure and may include blistered lesions on the skin and pain and numbness at the site of the bite or scratch. The infection may progress to encephalitis. The antiviral medication acyclovir has been successful in treating early stages of mild infections.

The risk of acquiring herpes B virus from monkeys is minimal even among people who work with primates. This may be due to several factors, including infrequent shedding of the virus by monkeys, immunity to the virus in many people who have had herpes simplex viral infections, and infections without symptoms.

Because of the risk of serious complications from the infection when it causes symptoms, preventive guidelines must be strictly followed by people who regularly handle macaque monkeys.

Herpes encephalitis

An acute inflammatory disease of the brain caused by direct viral invasion of the herpes simplex virus. Herpes encephalitis produces swelling of the brain tissues and small hemorrhages throughout the brain's hemispheres, the brain stem, cerebellum, and sometimes the spinal cord. When the brain is directly invaded by the herpes virus, nerve tissue is destroyed.

Symptoms may include fever, fatigue, vomiting, confusion, delirium, and a stiff neck and back. Repeated seizures occurring during the early stages of infection are characteristic of herpes encephalitis, as differentiated from bacterial and other viral forms of the disease. There may also be signs of brain dysfunction, including altered consciousness, personality changes, and partial paralysis.

Early MRI (magnetic resonance imaging) can exclude other possible causes of symptoms, such as a brain abscess or tumor, and detect inflammation of areas of the brain that suggest a diagnosis of herpes encephalitis. Evaluation of samples of spinal fluid from a LUMBAR PUNCTURE can also indicate the infection. These findings can prompt immediate antiviral therapy before the infected person lapses into coma. Early treatment can prevent deterioration of the nervous system and permanent damage to the brain. Intravenous acyclovir is generally given when herpes simplex encephalitis is suspected or cannot be excluded from diagnostic findings. Children and young adults respond better to treatment than older adults. Infants are more likely to have permanent brain damage.

Herpes gestationis

An itchy rash that develops in the second or third trimester of pregnancy and usually disappears by 3 months after childbirth. The rash consists of fluid-filled blisters that can occur anywhere on the skin. Herpes gestationis is linked with premature birth. It often recurs in subsequent pregnancies, with menstruation, or while taking oral contraceptives. The cause of herpes gestationis is not known. (It is not related to genital herpes.)

Herpes keratitis

Painful inflammation and ulceration of the outer surface (cornea) of the eye because of infection with the herpesvirus; also known as a dendritic (tree-shaped) ulcer because of its characteristic shape. Most herpes infections of the eye are caused by type 1 herpes simplex virus, the type of herpesvirus that causes fever blisters and cold sores. The infection is usually acquired during childhood and may lie dormant for years until it causes an outbreak. Herpes keratitis inflames the white of the eye and can scar the cornea, leading to vision loss and possible blindness. Prompt treatment with antiviral drugs (eye drops or pills) can prevent the infection from penetrating more deeply into the eye surface, where it is difficult to control and more likely to result in permanent damage. People who have had one outbreak of herpes keratitis are likely to have another, often as a result of fever, stress, exposure to sunlight, or eye injury. Herpes keratitis is the most common infectious cause of corneal blindness in the United States.

Herpes zoster

See SHINGLES.

Herpes, genital

One of the SEXUALLY TRANSMITTED DISEASES (STDs); typically caused by the herpes simplex virus type 2 (HSV-2). Genital herpes is a chronic, lifelong, viral infection that affects millions of people. Genital herpes is spread from person to person via sexual activities that include vaginal and anal intercourse. In addition to direct contact with the genitals of infected people, genital herpes may be transmitted via oral-genital contact with people who are infected with orolabial herpes (see HERPES, OROLABIAL), which is usually caused by herpes simplex virus type 1 (HSV-1).

An infected person can spread genital herpes when he or she has symptoms and also when there are no visible symptoms. The virus may be transmitted by people who are not

H

aware they are carrying the infection. During the 1980s and the 1990s, the incidence of genital herpes infections increased in the United States, with dramatic increases among young adults between the ages of 20 and 29 years and among white adolescents.

HSV-2 thrives in warm, moist areas and may be spread by contact with contaminated towels that are wet or damp, but this is rare. The virus is destroyed by high temperatures, so it cannot survive in hot tubs.

A woman who is pregnant and has an HSV-2 infection can spread the infection to her newborn during childbirth. This is the single greatest danger of genital herpes because the infant may contract an infection of the skin, mouth, lungs, or eyes. If the virus spreads through the infant's bloodstream, serious infections of the brain, such as HERPES ENCEPHALITIS, and other vital organs can occur. For this reason, a CESAREAN SECTION is generally performed if a woman has an outbreak of genital herpes when her baby is due.

SYMPTOMS

Most people who are infected with HSV-2 have no symptoms. When there are associated symptoms, they generally appear within 1 week of exposure, but may occur within 2 to 20 days following exposure. The symptoms are usually mild and may include itching and burning sensations in the genital area. Tiny, red, painful blisters emerge soon after the first symptoms are experienced. The blisters turn yellow and break open, causing ulcerations on the skin, which is particularly painful during urination. While the blisters are present, there may be swollen glands in the groin, and the infected person may experience headaches, fever, and general malaise. Some people with genital herpes acquire a FEVER BLISTER near the mouth.

For women, genital herpes may infect the larger genital area and cause more severe symptoms, including increased pain when urinating. Also, the infection may spread into the vagina and up to the cervix, which may increase the risk of cervical cancer. For this reason, women with the infection should have a PAP SMEAR every 1 to 2 years to screen for this cancer. Women who are pregnant and who experience symptoms of genital herpes should seek a medical evaluation immediately.

Men who have genital herpes usually get the characteristic blister or blisters on the head of the penis and may have a discharge from the penis. The virus may spread to the testicles, and irritation from clothing that comes in contact with blisters or ulcers can increase pain.

Symptoms tend to be most severe with the first infection of HSV-2; many infected people never have a repeated episode of the infection. The infection that causes genital herpes often persists over a lifetime, however, and some people may have as many as 4 to 5 recurrent infections each year. Patterns of recurrence vary from one individual to another, but the recurrent episodes of symptoms tend to follow sexual intercourse or sun exposure, or they occur during periods of emotional or physical stress.

The symptoms of newborns infected with HSV-2 usually occur within 9 to 11 days of birth. The symptoms may include skin blisters and reddened eyes with a discharge from the eyes. If the virus spreads through the infant's bloodstream to the brain, lethargy, irritability, and seizures can occur. If the lungs become infected, the baby may have difficulty breathing and require a ventilator to assist breathing.

DIAGNOSIS AND TREATMENT

Genital herpes is diagnosed by taking a sexual history and a clinical history of symptoms and by performing a physical examination during which the characteristic blisters or ulcers on the genitals can be observed. Symptoms can include swollen glands in the groin and fever blisters surrounding the mouth. Scrapings of the affected skin area or a small amount of fluid collected from the blisters may be cultured in a laboratory to confirm the diagnosis.

A blood test to determine which type of herpes a person may be infected with is available. Tests for other STDs may be performed because genital herpes predisposes a person to the risk of syphilis, gonorrhea, chlamydia, chancroid, and HIV (human immunodeficiency virus).

There is no cure for genital herpes, but when recurring episodes cause disturbing symptoms, the infection can be treated with oral or topical antiviral medications such as acyclovir, famciclovir, and valacyclovir, which may shorten the duration of symptoms. Taking oral antiviral medications every day can prevent frequent recurrences in addition to decreasing the severity of their symptoms. Daily oral medication is particularly helpful for decreasing the frequency of recurrences in people who experience 6 or more episodes of genital herpes per year. When HSV-2 infection spreads into the bloodstream causing widespread infection, intravenous antiviral medication may be necessary.

If antiviral therapy is not indicated, treatment may be directed at relieving discomfort and preventing a secondary bacterial infection. Keeping the genital area, as well as undergarments, bath towels, and bed linens, scrupulously clean is essential. Taking a hot bath to which salt has been added 2 to 3 times daily and applying a cold pack to the affected area after bathing may also decrease the symptoms and associated discomfort. Taking over-the-counter painkillers such as nonsteroidal anti-inflammatory drugs (NSAIDs) or acetaminophen can help relieve pain. Touching the open sores with the hands should be strictly avoided.

PREVENTION

As with all STDs, genital herpes can be prevented by approaching sexual relationships responsibly. This includes limiting the number of sex partners, using latex condoms during sexual activity, and avoiding sexual contact if an infection is even suspected. Men and women who believe they may have contracted genital herpes should inform their sex partner or partners and visit an STD clinic, hospital, or see a physician.

Herpes, orolabial

An acute viral infection caused by the herpes simplex virus type 1 and characterized by blisters in or around the mouth and lips. Orolabial herpes may or may not be related to genital herpes (see HERPES, GENITAL). Initially, the infection causes symptoms that include swelling, burning, or soreness in areas inside the mouth and on the outer skin surfaces of the mouth and lips. Clusters of tiny blisters with red bases then

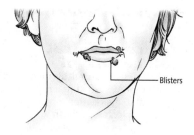

FEVER BLISTERS
The herpes virus causes fluid-filled blisters on the mouth and lips, often called fever blisters or cold sores. The fluid in the blisters is highly contagious, so a person with an outbreak should not kiss other people; share eating or drinking utensils; or share soap, washcloths, towels, or cosmetics.

erupt on the hard palate, gums, or border of the lip. The throat may also be involved. The blisters break and produce irregular, red ulcerations with swollen borders. The broken blisters eventually begin to crust over.

Orolabial herpes usually occurs for the first time as a primary infection in children and young adults. Symptoms are generally most severe with a primary infection, which may be preceded by high fever, sore throat, and headache and followed by red, swollen, bleeding gums. The infection tends to recur, often in association with emotional or physical stress, fever, menstruation, gastrointestinal disturbances, infection, the common cold, fatigue, or sun exposure. Symptoms usually last about 2 weeks, during which time the infection is contagious. Orolabial herpes may be contagious without symptoms as well.

DIAGNOSIS AND TREATMENT
Orolabial herpes may be diagnosed by a doctor after he or she physically examines the characteristic lesions inside the mouth and on the lips. The diagnosis may be confirmed by scraping the base of a blister, applying the smear to a slide and adding a certain stain, and examining it microscopically for the presence of the herpesvirus. The smear may also be stained with an antibody specific for herpes simplex virus type 1 and type 2. The swab may also be cultured for the virus.

Oral or topical antiviral medications such as acyclovir can help prevent spread of the infection and may be prescribed if the infected person or

a household contact has a weakened immune system or if outbreaks are unusually severe or frequent. However, these medications have not been shown to benefit persons who have typical orolabial herpes by decreasing the severity of symptoms or limiting their duration. Topical anesthetics may help relieve pain caused by lesions inside the mouth. Home remedies commonly used include oral doses or topical applications of lecithin, lysine, and vitamin E. In controlled studies, these remedies have shown some benefit. See also FEVER BLISTER.

Heterosexuality

Enduring erotic, emotional, romantic, or sexual attraction to members of the opposite sex. Most men and women are heterosexual. Heterosexuality, like the other sexual orientations, is an inborn predisposition. Heterosexuals are sometimes referred to as "straight."

Heterozygote

An organism that possesses two different forms of a GENE that controls a specific inherited TRAIT, in contrast to a HOMOZYGOTE.

HGE

See HUMAN GRANULOCYTIC EHRLICHIOSIS.

HHV-8

See HUMAN HERPESVIRUS 8.

Hiatal hernia

Protrusion of part of the stomach upward into the chest through an opening in the diaphragm. A hiatal hernia can develop when there is a defect or opening (hiatus) in the diaphragm at the junction of the esophagus and stomach. Hiatal hernias are most common in people who are overweight or who smoke.

Hiatal hernias are very common and are not fundamentally dangerous. In many cases, there are no symptoms at all. However, hiatal hernia is associated with ESOPHAGEAL REFLUX (the backward flow of acid from the stomach up into the esophagus). Persistent reflux can lead to complications such as inflammation and ulceration. Its most common symptom is heartburn, a painful, burning sensation in the upper abdomen or chest. Heartburn occurs

most frequently when an affected person eats, bends, or lies down and is especially troublesome at night and after heavy meals.

Diagnosis of a hiatal hernia is made by obtaining an accurate medical history and tests, such as an upper GASTROINTESTINAL (GI) SERIES (an X-ray procedure also called a barium swallow) and gastroscopy (visual examination of the esophagus, stomach, and duodenum with a lighted tube called a gastroscope). In many cases, simple lifestyle modifications control symptoms. Doctors recommend avoiding very large meals, spicy or greasy foods, chocolate, coffee, alcohol, and smoking. Elevating the head of the bed, avoiding lying down after eating, and not eating just before bed may reduce acid reflux. Obese people can manage symptoms by losing weight. Antacids

H

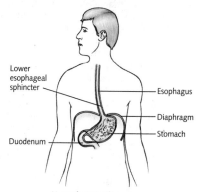

Normal stomach anatomy

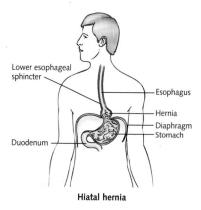

Hiatal hernia

A COMMON HIATAL HERNIA
In a person with a hiatal hernia, the upper part of the stomach bulges up into the chest through an opening (hiatus) in the diaphragm. Hiatal hernias are relatively common and may not cause any symptoms, but they often cause heartburn. Surgery to correct the hernia is necessary only if troublesome symptoms persist.

are often helpful, although prolonged heavy use can disrupt body chemistry. Stronger prescription medications, such as histamine$_2$ (H$_2$) blockers or proton pump inhibitors, are also available to reduce secretion of acids. However, if symptoms persist or complications occur, surgery may be necessary. See HERNIORRHAPHY.

Hib vaccine

The vaccine that induces antibodies that help prevent infection with *Haemophilus influenzae* type b, a bacterium that causes several types of dangerous infections in children (see VACCINATIONS, CHILDHOOD).

Hiccup

An involuntary contraction of the diaphragm, followed by the closing of the epiglottis over the vocal cords, producing a characteristic sound. Most hiccups last for only a few minutes. Although not normally a cause for concern, hiccups that persist can lead to exhaustion. Hiccups are caused by a temporary irritation to the diaphragm or the nerves that control it. Occasionally, they are due to a nervous disorder. In rare cases, hiccups are associated with serious diseases such as hepatitis (inflammation of the liver), inflammation of the esophagus due to causes such as persistent

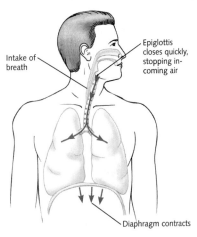

Intake of breath

Epiglottis closes quickly, stopping incoming air

Diaphragm contracts

WHAT IS A HICCUP?
A hiccup occurs when a person's diaphragm (the sheet of muscle between the chest and the abdomen) involuntarily contracts, causing the person to automatically take in breath. The epiglottis (a structure over the opening to the larynx) automatically shuts, stopping the column of incoming air and making the characteristic hiccup sound.

esophageal reflux (the backward flow of acid from the stomach up into the esophagus), or kidney failure.

HIDA scan

Hepatobiliary iminodiacetic acid scan. A HIDA scan assesses the excretory system of the liver after injection with the radionuclide iminodiacetic acid (IDA). A HIDA scan is a screening procedure used in NUCLEAR MEDICINE to examine the liver, gallbladder, and duodenum. After the acid is injected into the bloodstream, it is taken up by the liver, allowing the liver to be seen on a scan, and secreted into the bile so that the bile ducts and duodenum can be visualized.

Hidradenitis

Inflammation of the glands of the hair follicles (called sebaceous glands) and sweat glands in the skin. Doctors believe that hidradenitis is an inflammatory disease originating in hair follicles. This condition most commonly affects the armpits, where painful abscesses may form and secondary infections can develop. Treatment includes prescribed antibiotics and hot packs. In severe cases, surgery may be required.

High blood pressure

A popular name for the medical term HYPERTENSION.

Hip

FOR SYMPTOM CHART
see Hip pain, page 42

The joint that connects the bone of the upper leg to the pelvis and largely supports the weight of the upper body. The hip is a stable ball-and-socket joint. The round end of the upper thighbone (femur), fits into a rounded hollow in the pelvis called the acetabulum. The acetabulum is a deep cavity enclosing about two thirds of the head of the femur. Three strong ligaments attach the femur to the pelvis and contribute to the joint's stability. Because the hip is a ball-and-socket joint like the shoulder, it allows a limited range of movement. But because the head of the femur is held deeply within the pelvis, its range of movement is less than that of the shoulder. The hip is the most commonly replaced joint in the body. See JOINT REPLACEMENT, HIP.

Hip replacement

See JOINT REPLACEMENT, HIP.

Hip, congenital dislocation of

A birth defect caused by incomplete development of the hip joint. Congenital dislocation of the hip is usually detected at birth or shortly thereafter. Newborns with hip dislocation are usually fitted with a brace that positions the top of the femur (thighbone) in the hip socket. The brace is usually worn for 6 to 8 weeks. Failure to treat congenital hip dislocation can lead to permanent hip disability.

Hip, fractured

A serious injury involving a broken bone of the hip. Hip fractures are almost always surgically repaired. Traction may be used to repair a broken hip bone, but only when surgery is inadvisable. The lengthy confinement to bed involved in traction poses several serious risks, including pneumonia.

Most hip fractures occur in one of several specific bones of the hip. The upper part of the thighbone below the hip joint, called the femoral neck, is often the bone that breaks, especially in people in their late 70s. If the bone is still properly aligned after it has broken, a surgical procedure that involves inserting metal screws into the bone to hold it firmly together while it heals may be recommended. This approach to treating a fractured hip is called open reduction with internal fixation and is usually appropriate for younger people. When the two broken ends of the bone are not properly aligned or when they are damaged, the top part of the femur bone may be removed and replaced with a prosthetic segment of bone. The procedure, usually performed in older people, is called hemiarthroplasty. Another possible surgical treatment for a fractured hip is complete replacement of the upper part of the thighbone and the socket part of the ball-and-socket hip joint with an artificial hip or prosthesis. This procedure is generally performed when the joint has already been damaged by arthritis or a previous injury. The implantation of a prosthesis to repair a fractured hip is commonly recom-

REDUCING THE RISK OF HIP FRACTURES

Many hip fractures in people over 60 happen as a result of a fall, with most occurring at home. In one study, more than half of the participants said they had fallen because of common household hazards, such as steps and stairs, chairs and other furniture, and loose mats or flooring. Outside the home, the main causes of hip fractures included irregular pathways, steps, wet or slippery surfaces, and pets.

Although many of the hazards identified cannot be avoided, such as irregular walkways or a dog darting out underfoot, there are ways to reduce the risk of falling. Here are some ways to reduce the risk of hip fractures:

- Add handrails to staircases.
- Make sure there is adequate lighting on stairways.
- Relocate furniture that gets in the way of everyday tasks.
- Place nonskid mats under area carpets.
- Move loose electrical cords.
- Consider trying T'ai chi or weight training to improve balance.

A person who falls repeatedly for no apparent reason should see a doctor to rule out silent stroke, anemia, a heart rhythm disturbance, or a reaction to medications.

mended for people who are older or when the broken bones are not aligned.

Hip fractures may also occur in the wider part of the upper thighbone that protrudes outward to form the external shape of the hip. A fracture in this area is repaired with a metal screw called a compression hip screw that is inserted across the break in the bone. A metal shaft is attached to the screw and positioned along the length of the thighbone to stabilize the bone. The metal screw compresses the broken bone pieces as the bone tissue heals and allows the edges to grow together.

WHAT TO EXPECT

People who are recovering from surgery to repair a fractured hip are generally in the hospital for less than a week. Within 24 hours of surgery, most people are able to move, with assistance, to a sitting position in a chair. Assisted standing and walking are also sometimes possible a day after the procedure. People who walked well before the surgery are often walking again within a few days. Physical therapy may be prescribed to help recover total mobility. Moving around following surgery for a fractured hip is important to preventing further complications, including blood clots and infections. Walking aids, such as a cane, walker, or crutches, are usually necessary for a few months following surgery. Complete recovery may take as long as a year.

PREVENTION

Strengthening exercises, including

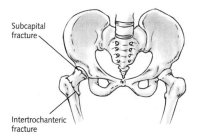

Subcapital fracture

Intertrochanteric fracture

COMMON SITES OF HIP FRACTURE
A subcapital fracture is located just under the head of the thighbone, 1 to 2 inches from the joint, and an intertrochanteric fracture is just above the angle of the femur, 3 to 4 inches from the joint.

T'ai chi and weight training, can help improve balance and prevent falls. For women, hormone replacement therapy may contribute to bone strength and prevent osteoporosis. Staying active and in good health is important to prevent hip fractures and for a complete recovery if a fracture should occur. People who fall repeatedly should consult with a doctor for a medical evaluation to rule out silent stroke, anemia, a reaction to medications, a disturbance of heart rhythms, or some other impairment.

Hip, snapping

A chronic and painful condition caused by the abnormal movement of a tendon involved in the hip joint. This tendon attaches the hip bones and is responsible for the movement of the hip joint, which allows the leg to flex forward. As a result of the irregular motion of the tendon when the hip joint moves, a snapping noise is heard and a sensation of snapping is experienced by the person who has this condition. Snapping hip may be associated with underlying tendinitis or bursitis in the hip area. Related conditions may be determined after an evaluation of MRI (magnetic resonance imaging) results. When the condition is disabling, a surgical procedure to release the involved tendon may correct it.

Hippocratic oath

An oath of professional conduct attributed to Hippocrates, an influential Greek physician of the fifth century BC. The oath outlines the nature of a doctor's role in society at the time. In general, when taking the oath, physicians swear to practice medicine to the best of their ability and for the benefit of patients and, above all, never to do anyone harm.

Hirschsprung disease

A genetic disorder in which a lack of nerve cells in a portion of the colon prevents normal bowel movements. Hirschsprung disease is caused by a failure of nerve cells to develop in a small segment of the end part of the colon, usually near the anus. The absence of nerve cells in the colon inhibits peristalsis, the rhythmic contractions that move stool through the colon. In the newborn, symptoms include the failure to pass meconium, the first stools of the newborn, within 24 hours of birth; a distended belly; dehydration; and weight loss. Hirschsprung disease is suspected in older children who have histories of constipation and bowel problems from birth. The disease occurs in one of every 5,000 live births and is 4 to 5 times more common in boys than girls.

Diagnosis can be made by physical examination, rectal biopsy, and other tests. The most effective treatment is a temporary colostomy, an operation in which the damaged part of the colon is removed and the undamaged portion is connected to a surgically made hole (stoma) in the abdomen. The infant can then have normal bowel movements by passing stool into a disposable pouch covering the stoma. When the baby is 12 to 18 months old, the colon is reconnected and the stoma is closed in a second operation, after which the baby will be able to move his or her bowels normally.

Hirsutism

Excess facial and body hair in women. Hirsutism typically means the growth of thick, dark hair in areas on a woman's face or body where it is not wanted. Hirsutism is not a disease, and the underlying cause is not usually a serious disorder. The principal problems associated with hirsutism are aesthetic.

Excess hair growth is usually an inherited condition that tends to occur in both male and female family members. Women of southern European or Middle-Eastern heritage may tend to develop darker hair and more hair on the face and body than women of northern European ancestry.

The fine, light hairs on the face and body may become noticeably darker and coarser, and most women will show increased facial hair growth with advancing age, especially after menopause. The decrease in female hormones at this time tends to affect hair growth.

Growth of body hair in females commonly begins at puberty, when the normal secretion of androgen hormones produces the beginning of hair growth in the pubic area and the armpits. Mild cases of hirsutism may develop at any age. Hirsutism is generally caused by increased production of a group of male hormones called androgen hormones or by an increased sensitivity of the hair follicles to androgen hormones.

Certain antiseizure medications such as PHENYTOIN SODIUM may result in excess hair growth on the body. Anorexia nervosa can be associated with an excess of fine body hair. In some cases, tumors of the adrenal glands or ovaries produce hirsutism. In many cases, there is no known cause for the condition.

MEDICAL EVALUATIONS AND TREATMENT

If a woman experiences a sudden increase in hair growth or if hirsutism cannot be controlled by standard cosmetic approaches, an evaluation by an ENDOCRINOLOGIST is recommended. It is rare for the condition to be related to serious underlying hormonal conditions. However, if hair growth is severe and accompanied by menstrual problems, male-pattern hair loss, or deepening of the voice, elevated androgen hormone levels may be suspected.

An endocrinologist will use screening techniques to rule out serious underlying abnormalities, explain treatment options, and offer treatment for hirsutism by prescribing medication that can reduce the effect of excess androgen hormones on the skin. Oral contraceptives that contain the hormones estrogen and progestin may prove effective for controlling hirsutism by suppressing androgen hormone levels. The diuretic spironolactone blocks the effects of androgen hormones on the hair follicle. Because these are powerful medications that have possible side effects and may take a long time to become effective, cosmetic approaches to treating hirsutism are often preferable or may be used in conjunction with medical therapy. If a woman with hirsutism is overweight, losing weight may lessen hair growth by decreasing androgen hormone production by fat tissue.

Histamine

A chemical that is released by mast cells in the immune system and can act as an irritating stimulant. Histamine is considered responsible for most of the swelling and itching symptoms of HAY FEVER and other allergies. The mast cells lining the skin and the respiratory and gastrointestinal tracts release histamine when an ALLERGEN enters the body. The function of histamine is to combat the allergen, which the body perceives as harmful.

Histamine may be released in the lungs, where it can cause excess mucus secretion and a swelling of the airways' lining that causes the passages to narrow. This produces symptoms such as wheezing, coughing, and shortness of breath. In the nose and sinuses, released histamine causes a runny nose, tearing eyes, and itching sensations in the nose, throat, and eyes and on the roof of the mouth. Histamine released into the skin results in hives and rashes. Within the digestive system, a person may have abdominal pain, cramps, and diarrhea, When the entire system becomes overwhelmed by an excessive release of histamine, the life-threatening medical emergency known as ANAPHYLAXIS occurs.

Antihistamine drugs, which are available over-the-counter or by a doctor's prescription, are a type of medication that combats the effects of histamine, thus preventing the symptoms that typically arise when a susceptible person is exposed to allergens.

Histamine$_2$ blockers

A class of drugs used to treat conditions in which the stomach produces too much hydrochloric acid; histamine$_2$ (H_2) receptor antagonists. H_2 blockers are used to treat stomach ulcers (gastric ulcers and duodenal ulcers), as well as other stomach disorders caused by excess stomach acid, such as heartburn caused by acid that moves back into the esophagus.

H_2 blockers are available by prescription to treat benign stomach ulcers. Some preparations are also available without prescription, but those products come in smaller doses and are intended to treat heartburn, sour stomach, and acid indigestion only.

H_2 blockers include the drugs cimetidine (Tagamet, Tagamet HB), famotidine (Pepcid, Pepcid AC), nizatidine (Axid, Axid AR,), and ranitidine (Zantac, Zantac 75).

Histocompatibility antigens

Substances that help the body identify tissue as its own or as foreign. Histocompatibility antigens also help determine whether tissue or organ transplants will be accepted or rejected. Histocompatibility means "tissue compatibility." If a tissue donor and recipient are histocompatible, as is the case with identical twins, a transplanted organ or tissue will be accepted easily. However, if donor and recipient are not histocompatible, transplants may be rejected by the recipient's immune system because they are identified as foreign and dangerous.

Histologist

A medical scientist who specializes in histology, the study of the microscopic structure, composition, and anatomy of body tissues.

Histology

The branch of medical science that studies the microscopic structure, composition, and anatomy of body tissues.

Histopathology

The branch of medical science that studies the microscopic structure, composition, and anatomy of diseased tissues.

Histoplasmosis

A disease primarily affecting the lungs that is caused by the fungus *Histoplasma capsulatum*. Histoplasmosis occurs when soil that is contaminated with bird or bat droppings, which contain histoplasmosis spores, is disturbed and the airborne spores are inhaled. The disease is most common in the eastern areas of the United States along the Ohio and Mississippi River valleys, as well as in Central and South America, Africa, India, and Southeast Asia. In these areas, construction or agricultural workers and people who explore caves, who are exposed to accumulations of bird or bat droppings, are at higher risk. Infants, young children, and older people are more susceptible to severe histoplasmosis, particularly if they have chronic lung disease.

SYMPTOMS AND TREATMENT

Most people who become infected have no immediate symptoms. If symptoms appear, they generally begin within 3 to 17 days after exposure, with an average incubation period of 10 days. Acute histoplasmosis causes a flulike syndrome and affects the lungs, causing malaise, fever, chest pains, respiratory symptoms, and a dry cough. A chest X ray may reveal a characteristic pattern of the disease. In its chronic form, histoplasmosis bears a clinical resemblance to tuberculosis; this form can become more severe over months or years.

Chronic histoplasmosis can result in permanent lung damage. A form of the disease in which organs in addition to the lungs are affected is called disseminated histoplasmosis. This form can be fatal if untreated. The mortality rate is higher for people who have cancer or HIV (human immunodeficiency virus) infection or are transplant recipients.

Mild disease tends to improve on its own without treatment. Severe cases of acute histoplasmosis and cases of chronic or disseminated histoplasmosis are treated with antifungal medications. Once a person has been infected, he or she has partial protection against ill effects if reinfected.

History-taking

The collection of information regarding a person's physical status and function. The medical history is a vital part of any patient evaluation. Physicians take a person's history in order to diagnose and treat disease, usually along with performing a physical examination (see EXAMINATION, PHYSICAL). Information includes facts about present symptoms as well as past illnesses, surgeries, allergies, hospitalizations, immunizations, family history of illness, transfusions, screening tests, and other conditions.

Histrionic personality disorder

A mental disorder marked by a constant pattern of excessive emotions and attention-seeking behavior that usually begins in early adulthood. People with this disorder often dramatize their everyday concerns, exaggerate their feelings or concerns in colorful speech, use clothing or hairstyles to draw attention to themselves, and consider relationships closer than they really are. They may also exhibit inappropriate sexual behavior or other provocative behavior. Often, people with the disorder act out a role for themselves (such as a "victim" or "princess"). While people with histrionic personality disorder may be at greater risk for attempting suicide, the risk of actual suicide is unknown. Treatment consists of behavioral therapy.

HIV

Human immunodeficiency virus; a virus that attacks the body's immune system and leads to associated infections and malignant tumors. HIV is the virus that leads to acquired immunodeficiency syndrome, which is known as AIDS. HIV was identified in 1984 as the cause of the widespread epidemic of severe immunosuppression called AIDS. Because HIV destroys the body's ability to fight off disease, common infections from which healthy people generally recover can prove fatal to people who have contracted the virus.

HIV infection is caused by one of two related retroviruses, HIV-1 and HIV-2, that produce a wide range of conditions varying from the presence of contagious infection with no apparent symptoms to disorders that are severely disabling and eventually fatal. HIV-1 has been identified as the predominant cause of AIDS throughout the world. HIV-2 seems to be less virulent and is largely limited to western Africa.

HOW IT IS SPREAD

HIV transmission requires contact with body fluids containing infected cells or infected plasma. These fluids include blood, semen, vaginal secretions, and breast milk. The most common means of transmission is by direct transfer or exchange of bodily fluids as a result of either sharing contaminated needles with an infected person or having sexual relations with an infected person.

The greatest risk of being infected with HIV is through genital intercourse, particularly penile-anal intercourse. The risk is increased by sexual practices that may cause damage to membranes of the vagina or anus before or during intercourse. Using latex condoms or vaginal barriers, such as a diaphragm, decreases but does not entirely eliminate the risk of being infected. Oil-based lubricants decrease the protective function of latex condoms, and natural membrane condoms may not provide protection.

Sexual practices that do not involve exposure to bodily fluids are considered safe and do not generally spread HIV infection. Oral-genital sexual activities are relatively safe but do not always protect a person completely from infection. The use of a DENTAL DAM may offer some protection during oral-genital or oral-anal activities.

HIV infection may be spread by contact with lesions caused by other SEXUALLY TRANSMITTED DISEASES (STDs) including chancroid, herpes simplex, syphilis, and trichomoniasis. People who have these STDs may be more susceptible to HIV infection.

HIV-infected cells in blood can be

transferred during a blood transfusion or by accidental injection. The use of enzyme-linked immunosorbent assay (ELISA) to screen blood donors has dramatically reduced the risk of acquiring HIV by transfusion. The risk of contracting HIV infection from a blood transfusion has been further reduced by current mandated screening for HIV antibody and p24 antigen in blood donors.

Transmission from HIV-infected health care personnel to their patients is rare because procedures to prevent the infection's spread have been identified and are in use. Transmission via saliva or airborne droplets produced by coughing or sneezing has not been known to occur. It is known that HIV is not transmitted via casual contact or by close, nonsexual contact such as may occur in work, school, or home settings.

SYMPTOMS

An infection with HIV may not produce symptoms, or symptoms may develop within a general range of 7 to 9 years. HIV does not cause most of the symptoms associated with AIDS, which are caused by an infection or other condition that is acquired because the body's weakened immune system cannot provide sufficient defense. These symptoms may include severe weight loss, fever, headache, drenching night sweats, fatigue, severe diarrhea, shortness of breath, and difficulty swallowing. Untreated, such symptoms may last for weeks or months at a time and may persist indefinitely.

DIAGNOSIS AND TREATMENT

An HIV diagnosis can be made by evaluating the results of a blood test that looks for the presence of antibodies to HIV. It can take anywhere from 6 weeks to 3 months following infection for the body to produce these antibodies to HIV. It is generally recommended that a person who suspects he or she has been exposed to HIV have the blood test within this time frame and again in 6 months. Early on, before HIV infection causes symptoms, a decline in the number and immunological abnormalities in the function of T helper cells occur and can be detected. Lymphocytes are white blood cells that have an important role in the body's immune system. It is believed that the CD4 lymphocytes are key to maintaining immunity against viral infections.

There is no cure for HIV infection. The first line of defense against the infection is for those who have a positive diagnosis of HIV to inform their sex partners and anyone with whom they have shared needles and syringes; all of these people should be tested for HIV. Health departments can offer help in contacting people who may have become infected.

A severely weakened immune system is indicated by the T-cell count of an infected person going below 200. At this point, anti-HIV therapy is generally initiated. Antiretroviral medications are the basis of treatment for the viral infection. This therapy uses three classes of medication: the nucleoside analogs (zidovudine [AZT], didanosine [ddI], zalcitabine [ddC], stavudine [d4T]), abacavir; nonnucleoside reverse transcriptase inhibitors; and protease inhibitors. When used in combination, these have been shown to prolong life and reduce the progression to AIDS. When given to pregnant women, AZT has been shown to make a significant reduction in the risk of passing HIV to an unborn baby. Combination therapy is thought to be even more effective.

Treatment for HIV infections is complex. The major emphasis of treatment is finding effective combinations of antiviral medication that the person can tolerate over an indefinite period of time. A major emphasis of the treatment is placed on the prevention of opportunistic infections that can prove fatal to a person whose immune system is compromised. *Pneumocystis carinii* pneumonia (PCP), tuberculosis, and systemic fungal infections pose serious risks for people with HIV infection. The infections can be effectively prevented with medication, which may be lifesaving for people with HIV.

RISKS AND PREVENTION OF HIV INFECTION

It is possible to become infected with HIV by performing oral sex, and the risk is increased if there are cuts or sores around the mouth or throat, if there is ejaculation into the mouth, and if the partner has another sexually transmitted disease in addition to carrying the HIV virus. Since blood, semen, preseminal fluid, and vaginal fluid are all possible carriers of the virus, the cells in the mucous lining of the mouth can transmit HIV to the lymph nodes or the bloodstream. A latex condom used on the penis of a male partner is known to decrease the risk of transmission during oral sex, but is not foolproof. Similarly, a latex barrier, such as a dental dam, or the use of plastic food wrap as a barrier can help prevent risk during oral sex with a female partner.

HIV can be transmitted to a woman during unprotected vaginal intercourse via tears in the lining of the vagina or direct absorption of the virus through the mucous membranes lining the vagina. The male may be infected during unprotected vaginal intercourse by HIV entering the body through the opening at the tip of the penis, called the urethra, or through open cuts or sores on the penis. The correct and consistent use of latex condoms can help prevent the infection, but condoms do not offer complete protection.

Unprotected anal sex is considered high-risk behavior for HIV infection because the lining of the rectum is thin and can allow the virus to enter the body via the partner's semen. Also, the partner may become infected through exposure to the virus via the urethra or open abrasions on the penis. Latex condoms are helpful in reducing the risk but are more likely to be ruptured during anal sex. Use of a water-based lubricant in addition to the condom may decrease the likelihood of breakage.

The practice of safer sex reduces possible exposure to the HIV virus that can cause AIDS. Safer sex is defined as abstinence from any behavior that may expose a person or his or her partner to bodily fluids.

Intravenous injections involve blood being introduced into the needles and syringes being used. When needles are shared, HIV can be transmitted from one person's blood to another's as infected blood may be injected directly into the bloodstream. Other paraphernalia involved in illegal drug use can spread HIV infection, as any reused materials—including syringes, water, bottle caps, or spoons used to dissolve drugs in water or heat drug solutions—may carry the blood-borne virus. Skin-popping and the injection of any

TRANSMITTING HIV

HIV (human immunodeficiency virus) can be spread by exchange of bodily fluids during sexual contact; by blood-to-blood contact (such as transfusions); or by blood-contaminated needles. A woman can pass the virus to her fetus during pregnancy or to her child during breast-feeding.

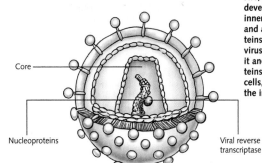

Core

Nucleoproteins

Viral reverse transcriptase

COMPONENTS OF HIV
HIV, the deadly virus responsible for developing AIDS, is composed of an inner core with genetic information and a protective outer shell of proteins (nucleoproteins). The AIDS virus weakens the immune system as it anchors itself to the receptor proteins on the surface of the helper T cells, the white blood cells that aid the immune system.

H

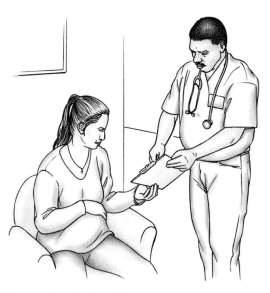

MOTHER-TO-CHILD TRANSMISSION
A woman who is pregnant and HIV-infected can transmit the virus to her fetus while she is pregnant or during delivery. To prevent transmitting the virus, the woman should be taking anti-AIDS (acquired immunodeficiency syndrome) medications while pregnant and through delivery.

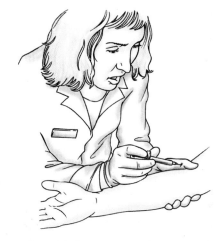

ACCIDENTAL NEEDLE STICK
Occasionally, health care workers will draw blood from an HIV-infected person and injure themselves with a needle containing that patient's infected blood.

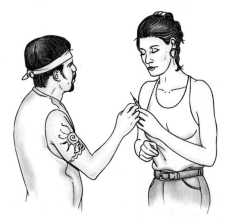

SHARING NEEDLES
The AIDS virus can be transmitted when an infected person shares a contaminated needle with another person.

medication also carry the risk of HIV infection when sterile syringes and needles are not used.

The risks of HIV infection associated with sexual contact are increased when a person has an STD. STDs may produce irritation of the skin including abrasions and sores that allow HIV to enter the body during sexual contact. Sexually transmitted diseases may also produce an immune response in the genital area that promotes HIV transmission. A person infected with HIV and an STD is up to five times more likely to transmit the virus via sexual contact than a person carrying only the HIV virus. Medical treatment of STDs can be an effective approach to reducing the risk of HIV infection.

Hives

Pink, itchy, round swellings that can occur anywhere on the body; also known as urticaria. Each individual hive disappears in 24 hours or less. Hives develop when natural chemicals including histamine are released in the skin. Most commonly, this occurs in response to an allergic reaction to a food, medication, pollen, or infections. Less frequently, hives are due to nonallergic causes such as autoimmune disease.

The best treatment for hives is to find the cause and eliminate it. Unfortunately, this is not always possible. Hives are usually treated

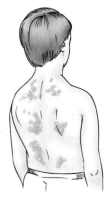

AN ALLERGIC RASH
Hives usually break out within an hour of each exposure to a specific substance, so many people can determine the allergy fairly easily and avoid the agent. However, some people have chronic hives (lasting 6 weeks or more) without an evident cause; antihistamines are the treatment. Most cases of hives disappear on their own within 6 months.

with over-the-counter antihistamines. For persistent or severe cases, it is important to consult a doctor. Prescription medications may be necessary to control the problem. Emergency medical care is required when hives are accompanied by breathing problems or swelling in the throat.

HLA types

Types of human leukocyte antigens (HLAs) on white blood cells. The HLA system is the main group of histocompatibility antigens, a group of proteins that is naturally present in tissues and has an important part in the body's immune system. The HLAs, which are inherited, may predispose a person to specific diseases or conditions, such as rheumatoid arthritis, inflammatory bowel disease, multiple sclerosis, or other autoimmune disorders. HLA types also have an important role in transplant surgery—laboratory studies of the HLA types are used to determine tissue compatibility between donors and recipients for transplants. Because only identical twins have identical tissue types, tissue typing can find close but not perfect matches between donors and recipients. However, the closer the matches, the less chance of complications.

HME

See HUMAN MONOCYTIC EHRLICHIOSIS.

HMG

See HUMAN MENOPAUSAL GONADOTROPIN.

HMO

The abbreviation for a health maintenance organization, or a MANAGED CARE plan that provides medical services to members on a prepaid basis. A person pays an HMO a set monthly premium regardless of the amount of services he or she requires. Medical care is usually coordinated by one primary care doctor, who makes referrals as necessary to specialists within the HMO. In most HMOs, people must receive care from the doctors and hospitals that participate in the plan's network. In others, point-of-service options allow members to see doctors or go to hospitals outside the network. However, this is usually at a significantly increased cost.

HNPCC

See COLON CANCER, HEREDITARY NON-POLYPOSIS.

Hoarseness

FOR SYMPTOM CHART
see Hoarseness or voice loss, page 31

An abnormal harshness or distortion in the voice. Hoarseness, medically termed dysphonia, can make the voice sound breathy, strained, or rasping. It can also result in changes in volume or in pitch, ranging from high to low. These changes in the sound of the voice are generally caused by disorders involving the vocal cords, or sound-producing parts of the larynx (voice box).

CAUSES
The most common causes of hoarseness are not serious. They include swelling due to inflammation (see LARYNGITIS) and irritation due to vocal abuse—for example, yelling at sporting events. These episodes of hoarseness usually do not last longer than a few days.

When hoarseness lasts longer than a few days, it is often caused by prolonged overuse or abuse of the voice. Excessive or improper use of the voice can result in VOCAL CORD NODULES (small, benign growths on the vocal cords) sometimes called singers' nodes, which cause hoarseness. Vocal abuse may also cause extensive swelling and the development of a POLYP (small, protruding growth).

Many people experience hoarseness with advancing age. Hoarseness in older people and in many younger adults may also be a symptom of gastroesophageal reflux (rising of stomach acid into the throat where it irritates the vocal cords), even in the absence of symptoms of heartburn. In this case, there may be discomfort in the throat, and the voice may tend to be more hoarse in the morning with gradual improvement over the course of the day.

Smokers experiencing hoarseness should consult an otolaryngologist (ear, nose, and throat specialist), since smoking is the leading cause of throat cancer. Other causes of hoarseness include allergies, thyroid problems, neurological disorders, and physical trauma to the voice box.

Phases in the cycle of menstruation may also contribute to hoarseness.

WHEN TO SEEK TREATMENT

When hoarseness persists for more than 2 weeks or when it does not seem to be caused by an infection such as the common cold or a respiratory tract infection, an otolaryngologist should be consulted. Other symptoms accompanying hoarseness that require medical attention include persistent throat pain, coughing up blood, difficulty swallowing, and a lump in the neck.

The physician will evaluate the symptom of hoarseness by taking a history of the symptom and the person's general health and by observing the vocal cords, possibly with a fiberoptic scope (small, flexible, lighted viewing instrument passed through the nose). Special tests to evaluate the voice may be recommended to help establish a diagnosis and determine treatment.

Treatment will depend on the cause of hoarseness. Resting the voice or modifying voice use are often recommended. Speech-language pathologists may help people who experience hoarseness by means of specialized behavior therapy, which can alter their method of speaking and, in most cases, resolve problems such as vocal cord nodules. Surgery may be necessary if hoarseness is caused by nodules or polyps and does not respond to speech therapy.

SELF-HELP AND PREVENTION

Several strategies can help prevent hoarseness and diminish its severity. These include not smoking and avoiding secondhand smoke, avoiding the dehydrating effects of alcohol and caffeine, increasing water intake, humidifying the home, avoiding spicy foods, not using the voice for too long or at too high a volume, seeking professional voice training, and resting the voice by not speaking or singing when hoarse.

Hodgkin disease

A type of LYMPHOMA; cancer of the lymphatic tissue. Hodgkin disease is an uncommon lymphoma, accounting for less than 1 percent of all cases of cancer in the United States. All other lymphomas are called non-Hodgkin lymphomas. Hodgkin disease is commonly characterized by painless enlarged lymph nodes (see LYMPH NODE) in the neck, underarm, or groin; weight loss; recurrent fevers; night sweats; and anemia. There are no benign forms of the disease. It can start in the lymph nodes, the bone marrow, or the spleen. Because Hodgkin disease develops in lymphatic tissue, which is present throughout the body, it spreads easily and progressively from one group of lymph nodes to the next. Eventually, it can spread to almost every part of the body. Diagnosis depends on a biopsy of part or all of a lymph node.

Treatment is based on the extent of the disease, taking into consideration the number and location of lymph nodes affected and whether the disease has spread. Early-stage Hodgkin disease can be cured with radiation therapy; even advanced disease can be cured with various chemotherapy regimens. Individuals whose disease recurs after treatment with chemotherapy may still be cured with a bone marrow transplant. The disease occurs most often during early adulthood (ages 25 to 30) and then again in later adulthood (older than age 55). About 10 to 15 percent of all cases are found in children younger than 16. Siblings of individuals with the disease have a higher than average chance of developing it. The infectious agent known as the Epstein-Barr virus is associated with an increased chance of developing Hodgkin disease.

Holistic medicine

Any approach to healing that addresses the whole person, including the mind, body, and spirit. Holistic medicine integrates both traditional and alternative therapies to prevent and treat disease, but its hallmark is its emphasis on promoting health and wellness. Health, to holistic medicine, is the free and unobstructed flow of life-force energy through mind, body, and spirit. One example of holistic medicine is ANTHROPOSOPHICAL MEDICINE.

THE WHOLE PERSON

In holistic medicine, diagnosis and treatment plans depend on a complete and thorough evaluation of the person. Such an approach requires analysis of the following considerations: physical status, nutritional needs, environmental factors, emotional concerns, social network, spiritual values, and lifestyle choices.

The holistic approach to health care seeks to help people achieve the best possible state of wellness by attending to all aspects of health.

HOLISTIC PHILOSOPHY

Holistic medicine emphasizes education and personal responsibility for making the effort to achieve balance and wellness. Holistic health is viewed as a daily concern: people are expected to make healthy choices every day, not just when they are sick. The person and the health care provider work together as partners to identify the root cause of the person's problems, using symptoms as a guide to the cause. Treatments are selected that support the body's natural healing processes whenever possible.

Holistic medicine encompasses all modalities of diagnosis and treatment, including drugs and surgery, when no safe alternative exists. Any health care professional can become a holistic practitioner after qualifying as a doctor of medicine or provider of CHIROPRACTIC, MASSAGE THERAPY, NATUROPATHY, or psychology. In addition to adherence to holistic philosophy, responsible holistic practitioners are fully licensed in conventional or alternative health care methods.

Holter monitor

A portable device for recording and analyzing the electrical activity of the heart over an extended period, usually 24 to 48 hours. Holter monitoring is also known as ambulatory ELECTROCARDIOGRAPHY, since it allows continuous recording of the electrical activity of the heart, even as the person being monitored goes about his or her daily tasks. The Holter monitor is particularly useful for detecting heart problems such as arrhythmia (irregular heartbeat) or angina (pain) that can come or go and may escape detection in the standard electrocardiogram. It is also used to assess the effectiveness of medications used to control heart rhythm. A person using a Holter monitor is usually asked to keep a diary of activities and physical symptoms, such as pain or rapid heartbeat, to allow the doctor to relate those events to the recorded electrical patterns of the heart.

H

The battery-powered Holter monitor varies in size and is usually worn as a wristwatch or on a belt around the waist. Small electrodes taped to the chest and connected by wires to the monitor convey data about the heart's activity, which are recorded on tape or a computer chip.

Holter monitoring is painless and carries no risk. A person wearing a Holter monitor can engage in all normal activities except bathing or showering, sleeping under an electric blanket, or entering areas in which high voltage, metal detectors, or large magnets are present.

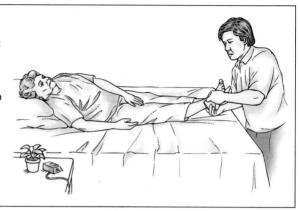

ASSISTANCE IN THE HOME
For someone who is not fully mobile, a home health professional can monitor his or her condition and provide necessary medical care such as dressing wounds or changing bandages.

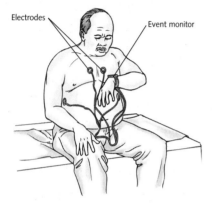

Electrodes

Event monitor

MONITORING THE HEART AT HOME
The Holter monitor, which records heart activity over a period of 24 hours or more, is lightweight and painless. While wearing the device, the person can follow a normal routine. He or she is asked to keep a diary of activities and is taught how to use an event monitor (wristwatch style) to record symptoms.

Homatropine hydrobromide

A drug used to relax pupil eye muscles during eye examinations. Homatropine (Isopto Homatropine) is given as eyedrops. Relaxed eye muscles allow the pupil to dilate, or widen, which allows the eye doctor to examine the interior of the eye. Homatropine is also used to treat eyes that are inflamed.

Home health care

Health care in the home that is ordered by a physician for the treatment of an illness or injury. Home health care services include physical, occupational, and speech therapy; skilled nursing care; the use of medical equipment such as oxygen and wheelchairs; and other services and supplies. Some home health care (such as skilled nursing after a recent hospitalization) is covered by Medicaid, Medicare, or private health insurance. However, services such as light housekeeping and help with grocery shopping are generally not covered.

Home health care for older people

Medical services provided to older people in their homes under the direction of a physician. Nurses, therapists, and other health care professionals perform various levels of skilled care. They can assess health; give injections and medications; administer physical, occupational, or speech therapy; and teach caregivers how to care for older family members. Home health care allows older people, even some who are seriously ill, to remain living at home. In some cases, this type of care is partially covered by Medicare.

Home health care often requires the use of assistive devices, including walkers, crutches, canes, a PROSTHESIS, or a WHEELCHAIR. (See also WALKING AIDS.) Other specialized equipment may include a hospital bed, an intravenous setup, oxygen (see OXYGEN, SUPPLEMENTAL), or monitoring devices. Medicare and Medicaid partially cover the cost of some devices if a physician prescribes them.

Home health care agencies, which can be private or government sponsored, can also arrange for less intensive forms of care in the home. For instance, home health aides provide assistance with personal care such as bathing, dressing, laundry, shopping, and cooking. Homemaker services are available in many communities to help out with minor repairs or housecleaning. Services such as Meals-on-Wheels deliver hot, nutritious meals

HOME HEALTH AIDES
A home health aide can help an older person remain in his or her home longer by providing such everyday services as grocery shopping, cooking, or laundry. Aides are often trained to help with bathing, dressing, and toilet needs. They may work through a home health care agency, which provides many levels of services, or they may be volunteers from religious or civic organizations.

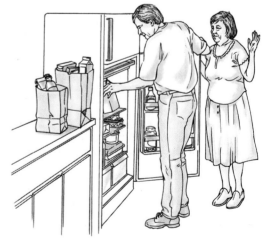

to those who can no longer shop for groceries and prepare meals. Medicare and Medicaid usually do not reimburse for these types of less skilled home health services. However, home-delivered meals are often subsidized and inexpensive, and many services are available for free or at a low cost from religious institutions, veterans' or social groups, or local civic organizations.

Home pregnancy tests

Kits that can be purchased without a prescription to help diagnose pregnancy. Home tests are similar to the pregnancy tests performed by doctors, but the results may not be as accurate. Several different types of home pregnancy testing kits are available; they all involve the detection of a hormone called HCG (HUMAN CHORIONIC GONADOTROPIN) in the woman's urine. HCG is produced in large quantities by the developing placenta during the first few weeks of pregnancy and is evident in the woman's urine. Home pregnancy tests can detect HCG as early as the first day of a missed menstrual period. Most tests involve dipping a chemically coated stick into a sample of the woman's urine and watching for a color change on the stick. It is important to follow the instruction to use a first-of-the-morning urine sample because the urine has a higher concentration of HCG then.

The result will be either positive or negative. If the test is done correctly, a positive result almost always means that the woman is pregnant. A woman with a positive result should see a physician to confirm the result. If the home pregnancy test registers negative, it may mean that the woman is not pregnant; but it also may mean that a pregnancy is in its early stages, and the HCG level is not yet high enough to show up in the urine. A woman who is pregnant may show a negative result if the test is performed incorrectly, or if the urine tested was not a first-of-the-morning sample. Such an error can result in a pregnant woman neglecting to take the proper dietary and lifestyle precautions indicated for pregnancy. A woman may choose to repeat the home test or to have her doctor confirm its result. See also PREGNANCY TESTS.

Homeopathy

A system of medicine developed in Germany based on the belief that disease is cured by a substance that creates symptoms similar to those experienced by the person being treated. The three principles that govern homeopathic medicine are the law of similars, the single medicine, and the minimum dose. According to the law of similars, "like cures like," which means that an illness can be treated by giving persons small doses of substances that produce effects similar to those of the illness itself.

The principle of the single medicine dictates that a single medicine should cover all the symptoms a person is experiencing, whether physical, emotional, or behavioral. Homeopathic remedies are made by crushing plant, animal, or mineral substances in tiny amounts and mixing them with solvents, such as grain alcohol. The extract that results from this process is then diluted with water many times. Once a remedy has been properly diluted, it can be administered in tablet, ointment, or liquid form.

Homeopathic medicine followers believe in using the smallest possible dose of any medicine and prescribing it only a few times. The homeopathic practitioner waits to see what effect the medicine has before proceeding further. Because homeopathic remedies combine varying substances, it has not been possible to verify their safety or effectiveness via clinical research or study.

Homeostasis

The maintenance of stable internal physiological or psychological conditions by the body. Organisms attempt to maintain relatively stable internal environments whenever possible. For example, a high level of carbon dioxide in body fluids will automatically trigger a person to breathe faster in an attempt to restore the carbon dioxide level to normal.

Homocysteine

An amino acid found in the blood. At high levels, homocysteine is associated with increased risk of heart attack and stroke. Homocysteine levels can be kept within normal limits through a diet that includes folic acid found in leafy green vegetables, oranges, and fortified cereals; vitamin B6 found in meats and fortified cereals; and vitamin B12, which is found in meats, potatoes, bananas, and fortified cereals. These nutrients seem to help convert homocysteine in the blood into other substances that do not cause heart disease.

Homocystinuria

A rare genetic disorder that expresses itself in infancy and is characterized by an excess of the amino acid homocystine in the urine. Homocystinuria is associated with developmental delay, failure to thrive, neurological abnormalities, and dislocation of the lenses of the eyes. Newborns with homocystinuria appear normal, with only vague symptoms, including failure to grow and to gain weight as expected. Increasing problems with vision may lead to the diagnosis, often around age 3. Intelligence may be normal, although some children with homocystinuria are mentally retarded. Children with this condition may have skeletal abnormalities, such as scoliosis (curvature of the spine); seizures; osteoporosis (loss of bone density); and a tendency to develop blood clots that can lead to life-threatening complications such as STROKE.

Homocystinuria is a metabolic disorder in which enzymes needed to convert an essential amino acid (methionine) to homocystine are inadequate. Essential amino acids are required for proper growth and development. Treatment may include high doses of vitamin B6 to lower blood methionine levels, although only about half of affected people benefit from this approach. A diet restricted in methionine and protein, supplemented with cystine, is often recommended for infants with the condition. Genetic counseling to discuss recurrence risks and testing options is recommended for parents with family histories of homocystinuria.

Homosexuality

Enduring erotic, emotional, romantic, or sexual attraction to members of the same sex. Homosexual men are commonly called gay and homosexual women, either gay or lesbian. Homosexuality appears in all cultures and societies, socioeconomic and educational levels, and religious

H

and ethnic groups. It is generally thought that about one of every ten persons is homosexual. Like hetero-sexuality (erotic orientation to mem-bers of the opposite sex), homosexu-ality appears to result from an inborn physiological predisposi-tion, not from sexual abuse, poor parenting, or contact with homosex-ual people. Therapeutic efforts to change homosexuals into heterosex-uals rarely if ever succeed. Although some religious groups condemn homosexuality as morally perverse, it is considered a normal sexual ori-entation, not a disorder or a sign of a disorder.

Homozygote

An individual who has two identical copies of the same gene, which may lead to a particular trait or disease.

Hookworm infestation

A condition that occurs when one or two species of nematodes, or round-worms, enter the human body. Hookworm infestation is a common cause of iron deficiency anemia among people who live in regions with a warm, humid climate, such as the tropics. The infestation generally occurs when a person's bare skin makes direct contact with hookworm larvae. This is most likely to happen when walking barefoot on soil or a beach contaminated with hookworms from dog or cat feces.

Adult hookworms are parasites that live in the small intestine of humans where they attach to the intestinal wall. Blood is lost at the site of this intestinal attachment, and this is the cause of anemia in people who have a hookworm infes-tation. The hookworms' eggs are passed in the stool, and given a favorable environment including moisture, shade, and warmth, they will hatch within 1 to 2 days, releas-ing larvae. The larvae grow in the feces or soil, becoming filariform lar-vae, which are infective, after 5 to 10 days. In this infectious stage, the lar-vae can survive 3 to 4 weeks under favorable conditions and will pene-trate the skin of a human host or car-rier when they come into contact with it. The larvae are then carried through the veins to the lungs. From the lungs, they go up the bronchial

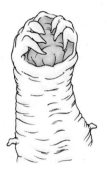

INTESTINAL PARASITE
The hookworm is so named because it attach-es to the intestinal wall by sinking microscopic "teeth" into the membrane. The blood loss from the attachment can cause anemia. The parasite is now extremely rare in the United States, but still is found in tropical areas of Europe, Africa, Asia, and South America.

tree to the throat, where they are swallowed and descend into the small intestine. In the intestine, they develop into adult worms where their life cycle begins again.

SYMPTOMS, DIAGNOSIS, AND TREATMENT

In addition to iron deficiency anemia, hookworm infestation may produce skin irritation with intense itching at the sites where the worm larvae pene-trate the skin and respiratory symp-toms during the larvae's migration into the lungs. There may be heart prob-lems if the larvae travel to the heart. The presence of hookworms in the intestine can cause gastrointestinal disturbances, in addition to nutritional deficiencies and metabolic disorders.

Hookworm infestation is diagnosed by evaluation of a stool specimen and the finding of hookworm eggs. Medications including mebendazole, pyrantel pamoate (also called pyran-tel embonate), and albendazole are generally used to treat a hookworm infestation.

Hormone replacement therapy

A treatment in which a woman's declining hormone levels are supple-mented with additional hormones. The treatment, also known as HRT and as estrogen replacement therapy, is used to address the short-term symptoms of menopause, such as hot flashes, night sweats, and sleep dis-turbance, and for its potential bene-fits such as reducing the risk of

OSTEOPOROSIS. From puberty until menopause, the ovaries produce estro-gen which causes the endometrium to thicken each month. If pregnancy does not occur, the endometrium is shed during the monthly period. As a woman ages, the ovaries gradually stop making enough estrogen to thicken the uterine lining, and even-tually, the monthly period stops. When this happens, a woman is said to have experienced menopause.

Hormone replacement therapy for a woman with an intact uterus consists of estrogen combined with progestin, a synthetic form of another import-ant female hormone, progesterone. Progestin lowers the risk of cancer of the endometrium, the lining of the uterus. Estrogen alone is usually pre-scribed for a woman who has had a hysterectomy.

BENEFITS OF HRT

Hormone replacement therapy can relieve the symptoms of low estrogen, such as hot flashes, vaginal dryness, and sweating. It also improves the thickness and elasticity of the skin. The principal benefit of the treatment is that it prevents osteoporosis.

■ *Heart disease* The leading cause of death for women over 65 is heart dis-ease. Once the ovaries stop making estrogen, a woman's risks for a heart attack and stroke increase over time until they equal those of a man. It was once thought that women who used HRT reduced their risk of fatal heart disease significantly because of the beneficial effect that HRT has on fats in the bloodstream. Estrogen low-ers levels of LDL (low-density lipopro-tein cholesterol, which is associated with atherosclerosis (hardening of the arteries), while it raises levels of HDL (high-density lipoprotein) cholesterol, which removes LDL cholesterol from the blood. But now doctors and researchers have evidence that sug-gests HRT may actually contribute to a woman's chances of having a heart attack or stroke or being diagnosed with breast cancer. The risks of taking HRT may outweigh the benefits in many cases and the decision to take HRT should be evaluated on an indi-vidual basis. Women in menopause at risk for heart disease should con-tinue to focus on proven treatments to reduce the risk of cardiovascular dis-ease, including medication to control high blood pressure, control of high blood cholesterol levels, and weight loss for obesity. Alternatives to HRT that may provide relief of menopausal symptoms include antidepressants, herbal remedies, and soy products.

■ *Osteoporosis* After menopause, women's bones slowly become more fragile and lose strength, sometimes resulting in osteoporosis. Hormone replacement therapy is the best way to slow bone loss after menopause. Estrogen preserves bone and works with other hormones to increase bone mass. It also helps bones to absorb calcium, which helps build strength. However, for those individuals who want to avoid the potential risks of taking HRT for the 5 to 10 years required to protect against the bone-crippling disease, doctors can prescribe other medications to reduce the risk of osteoporosis.

■ *Symptoms of menopause* Estrogen decreases the occurrence of hot flashes and is considered the most effective treatment for this uncomfortable symptom. Estrogen can also reduce vaginal dryness, which may help with the pain and discomfort some women in menopause experience during sexual intercourse. Estrogen also restores the elasticity of urinary tract tissues and reduces the incidence of urinary incontinence. It was thought that estrogen protects against ALZHEIMER'S DISEASE, which is more common in women than men; however, studies have shown that HRT causes dementia and memory loss.

SIDE EFFECTS

Like all medications, HRT has drawbacks. Estrogen may cause bloating, nausea, breast tenderness, and headaches. The use of estrogen alone can cause the lining of the uterus to overgrow and can increase the risk of endometrial cancer. Taking a preparation of HRT that includes progestin, a synthetic hormone that acts like progesterone, protects the uterine lining from excessive growth. However, progestin can cause resumption of menstruation. Women report various other side effects from taking progestin, including water retention, bloating, irritability, mood swings, and anxiety. Women who take HRT almost double their risk for developing gallstones.

When weighing the risks of heart disease and breast cancer against the benefits of HRT, each woman should review her health history and discuss the question with her doctor. A woman who takes hormones after menopause should have regular medical checkups, including a pelvic examination, Pap smear, blood pressure check, and mammogram. Erratic or unusual vaginal bleeding should be reported to the doctor.

FORMS OF TREATMENT

In addition to estrogen, a woman needs to take progestins to protect against cancer of the uterus, unless her uterus has been removed. The most common form of HRT is a hormone pill taken either every day or for 25 days each month. Progestins can be taken in combination with estrogen daily or for 10 to 14 days each month. In women taking the combined hormones, irregular bleeding is common during the first few months, but most women stop bleeding after 1 year. Adhesive transdermal patches (skin patches) containing time-release hormones can be placed on a woman's buttock and replaced every 3 to 4 days, at a slightly different site each time. Estrogen can be supplied in a cream to reduce vaginal dryness, but this form of therapy will not relieve any other menopausal symptoms.

To eliminate symptoms of menopause, such as hot flashes, entirely, HRT should last about 1 year. However, if treatment is stopped abruptly, the symptoms may return after a few months.

Hormone therapies, alternative

The use of natural alternatives to hormone replacement therapy for symptoms associated with menopause. Some plant compounds can produce estrogenlike and progestinlike effects in humans and are used to treat menopausal symptoms by women who do not wish to take hormone replacement therapy. Herbal remedies for symptoms of menopause have long been a part of traditional Asian medicine.

Herbal and nutritional remedies used in menopause include Native American black cohosh, a hormone stabilizer; chasteberry, used for severe symptoms; Siberian ginseng for energy; dong quai, to maximize effects of other herbs; and soy isoflavones to reduce symptoms and lower blood pressure. Natural progesterone cream may be applied to the skin to address severe symptoms. Alternative therapy for menopause emphasizes the importance of paying careful attention to diet, exercising regularly, and taking vitamins and minerals such as vitamins C and E, calcium, and magnesium. Sexual dysfunction associated with menopause may be treated with arginine, an amino acid, and the herb yohimbine, used to treat impotence in men.

Hormones

Chemicals produced by glands in the ENDOCRINE SYSTEM and released directly into the bloodstream to perform specific functions elsewhere throughout the body. Hormones balance each other in the bloodstream and control many vital functions of the body. Interference or disturbance in a person's hormonal equilibrium can affect normal growth and overall health and may sometimes endanger survival.

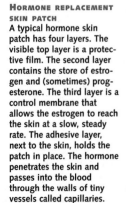

HORMONE REPLACEMENT SKIN PATCH
A typical hormone skin patch has four layers. The visible top layer is a protective film. The second layer contains the store of estrogen and (sometimes) progesterone. The third layer is a control membrane that allows the estrogen to reach the skin at a slow, steady rate. The adhesive layer, next to the skin, holds the patch in place. The hormone penetrates the skin and passes into the blood through the walls of tiny vessels called capillaries.

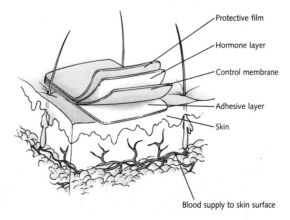

Protective film
Hormone layer
Control membrane
Adhesive layer
Skin
Blood supply to skin surface

The endocrine glands involved in the production and release of hormones include the hypothalamus, pituitary gland, thyroid gland, para-thyroid glands, adrenal glands, pancreas, ovaries in women, and testicles in men.

Hormones produced by the hypothalamus include CRH (corticotropin-releasing hormone), which stimulates the pituitary to release ACTH (adrenocorticotropic hormone); gonadotropin-releasing hormone GNRH, which signals the pituitary to secrete gonadotropic hormones into the bloodstream; and TRH (thyrotropin-releasing hormone), which stimulates the pituitary to produce and release TSH (thyroid-stimulating hormone). The hypothalamus controls hormonal secretions from the pituitary gland through direct nerve connections and through specialized nerve cells. The hypothalmus also produces two other hormones, ADH (antidiuretic hormone), which controls the volume of urine excreted by the body, and oxytocin, which stimulates contraction of the uterus in preparation for labor.

The hormones produced by the pituitary gland, which is considered the control center of the endocrine system of glands, include those that control skeletal growth (GROWTH HORMONE), regulate thyroid function (TSH), affect adrenal activity (ACTH), influence the reproductive system (FSH [follicle-stimulating hormone] and LH [luteinizing hormone]), and stimulate the formation of milk in a nursing mother (PROLACTIN). Pituitary hormones stimulate pigment cell function and influence blood pressure and urine production.

Hormones produced by the thyroid regulate all aspects of cell metabolism (THYROXINE and triiodothyronine) and regulate calcium levels in the blood (CALCITONIN). The secretion of thyroid hormone by the thyroid gland is primarily controlled by the pituitary. PARATHYROID HORMONE, released by the parathyroid glands, balances the concentration of calcium and phosphate in the bloodstream.

The hormones produced and released by the pancreas (INSULIN and GLUCAGON) influence the metabolism of carbohydrates in the body. Also, insulin is important in protein and fat metabolism.

The adrenal cortex (the outer layer of the adrenal glands) produces ALDOSTERONE, which helps balance the concentration of salts and water in body fluids and regulates blood pressure. The adrenal medulla (the inner layer of the adrenal glands) produces and releases EPINEPHRINE, which elevates the blood sugar level and stimulates the circulatory system and the sympathetic nervous system. Other adrenal hormones are NOREPINEPHRINE, which increases blood pressure, and CORTISOL, which helps maintain blood pressure and reduces inflammation. Little is known about how the adrenal hormone DHEA (dehydroepiandrosterone) works in the body.

The testicles produce ANDROGEN HORMONES, such as TESTOSTERONE, which influence the development of the secondary sexual characteristics in men. The ovaries produce ESTROGEN and PROGESTERONE, which interact with pituitary hormones to control ovulation and the menstrual cycle in women. The placenta also produces progesterone during pregnancy.

The mucous membrane of the small intestines secretes hormones during digestion to control the movement of various structures involved in digesting food. These hormones also stimulate digestive juices and liver bile, as well as certain secretions of the pancreas. Gastrin is a hormone secreted by the stomach that also has a role in digestion, including the stimulation of insulin secretion by the pancreas and signaling the stomach wall to contract.

Horn, cutaneous

A skin-colored projection made up of hardened keratin, the principal com-

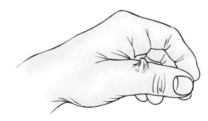

HARD, CONE-SHAPED GROWTH
Most cutaneous horns are benign, but a doctor will usually do a biopsy to rule out squamous cell carcinoma. These growths usually occur on sun-exposed skin, but may occur on protected areas. No treatment is required for a benign cutaneous horn, but it may be removed for cosmetic reasons.

ponent of skin, hair, and nails. Cutaneous horns most commonly appear on the head or face. Often they accompany ACTINIC KERATOSIS.

Horner syndrome

A set of physical changes that includes drooping eyelid (ptosis), sinking eyeball, narrowed pupil, and facial dryness. Horner syndrome occurs as a result of damage to the sympathetic division of the autonomic (involuntary) nervous system. It has many possible causes, including injury to the spinal cord, vascular disease, and tumors in the neck or chest that impinge on nerves. Diagnosis entails detailed and rigorous evaluation and may require tests such as imaging studies of the head, neck, and chest. Treatment depends on the underlying cause.

Hospice

A facility or a program that provides a combination of housing, medical care, and personal services for people with terminal diseases. A hospice facility offers a comforting, homelike environment as an alternative to spending the last weeks or months of life in a hospital. In hospice programs, the emphasis shifts from finding a cure to maximizing the quality of remaining life. Emotional, social, and spiritual support is emphasized, while medical care may consist primarily of the relief of pain and symptoms. Grief counseling is often provided for the family. Most hospices are operated by independent, nonprofit organizations. Some are affiliated with hospitals, nursing homes, or home care agencies.

Hospice programs also offer assistance to help keep a person with an illness in his or her home environment. In this instance, hospice workers help a person's caregiver manage the illness. Support may consist of skilled nursing assistance, training caregivers, providing support services (for example, physical therapy), and assisting with providing medical equipment, such as a hospital bed, if needed.

Hospitals, types of

Hospitals are classified in a number of different ways. For example, there are government hospitals run at the federal, state, county, and municipal levels; teaching hospitals, which usually have a close affiliation with universities and medical schools; and hospitals that are owned and operated by religious orders. Hospitals can also be considered for-profit or nonprofit, based on their corporate structure and tax status.

In recent years, for-profit hospitals such as investor-owned hospital corporations have acquired a number of nonprofit hospitals and converted them to for-profit status. This trend was brought about by a decline in the financial condition of many nonprofit community hospitals. Their financial deterioration was triggered by factors such as a decrease in the demand for traditional hospital services, since more tests and procedures are performed on an outpatient basis; increased competition from provider networks; and difficulties in dealing with CAPITATION.

In addition to ownership and tax status, hospitals can be classified according to the types of services provided and average length of stay. Today the majority of hospitals are short-term acute care facilities. Most long-term care now takes place at long-term care facilities (see LONG-TERM CARE FACILITY). Some hospitals are best known for their areas of specialization, such as burn centers, children's hospitals, or psychiatric facilities.

Host

A living human or other animal on which a PARASITE lives. A host may support a parasite externally, as on the skin, or internally, as in the intestines. Living plants are also sometimes hosts. The host may experience serious disease as a result of infestation with a parasite. In some cases, a parasite destroys its host and is itself killed in the process. In other instances, a parasite may move from one host to another, thereby transmitting disease among its hosts; parasites can also live in or on a host without having a significant effect on the host's health.

Hot flashes

A symptom of MENOPAUSE or PERI-MENOPAUSE in which a woman experiences fluctuations in body temperature. Three quarters of women in menopause get hot flashes, also

called night sweats, although they can happen at any time of day. During a hot flash, the skin, particularly on the head, neck, and upper chest, becomes uncomfortably warm and perspires. The heart may race or skip beats, and the woman may feel dizzy. Hot flashes can last from 1 to 5 minutes and may be followed by chills. Some women get chills before a hot flash.

While the cause of hot flashes is not completely understood, they appear to result from fluctuating levels of circulating estrogen, a common occurrence of menopause. Estrogen regulates the amount of blood flow to the skin, which, in turn, affects body temperature. Hot flashes can be treated with HORMONE REPLACEMENT THERAPY. If other factors prohibit a woman from having hormone replacement therapy, her doctor may prescribe clonidine, a medication for high blood pressure that can reduce hot flashes.

Avoiding caffeine (in coffee, tea, chocolate, cola soft drinks, and some over-the-counter pain relievers and cold remedies), alcohol, spicy foods, sugar, and hot soups or drinks may help reduce the intensity of hot flashes. Some women have more hot flashes when they are under stress and can reduce the incidence of hot flashes by practicing stress reduction techniques and getting regular exercise. Eating soy products and sweet potatoes, which are rich in phytoestrogens, is thought by some doctors to help alleviate the symptoms of menopause.

HPV

The virus that causes common warts. See HUMAN PAPILLOMAVIRUS.

HRT

See HORMONE REPLACEMENT THERAPY.

HSG

See HYSTEROSALPINGOGRAM.

Human chorionic gonadotropin

A hormone produced in the early weeks of pregnancy by the placenta. Human chorionic gonadotropin, or HCG, stimulates the ovaries to produce the hormones ESTROGEN and PROGESTERONE for the first 10 to 12 weeks of pregnancy. The hormones

are needed to maintain the endometrium (the uterine lining), in which the embryo grows and is nourished. After about 12 weeks, the PLACENTA becomes the major source of progesterone, a hormone essential to the maintenance of the pregnancy and prevention of miscarriage. Human chorionic gonadotropin also stimulates the male fetus's testicles to produce TESTOSTERONE, which stimulates the development of the fetus's sex organs. The tests used to confirm a pregnancy all involve detecting HCG in the woman's urine or blood.

Human Genome Project

An international collaboration in which the entire genetic blueprint of a human being has been mapped. Since its inception in 1990, the goals of the Human Genome Project have been to identify all the genes present in the nucleus of a human cell; to establish where those genes are located on the chromosomes in the nucleus, using GENE MAPPING; and to determine the genetic information encoded by the order of DNA's (see DEOXYRIBONUCLEIC ACID) chemical subunits. The goal of the project is to associate specific traits and inherited diseases with particular genes at certain locations on the chromosomes. Completion of the project is expected to launch research that will lead to an unprecedented understanding of the organization of human genes and chromosomes and, ultimately, to new approaches to the treatment and prevention of disease.

The human genome is made up of between 50,000 and 100,000 genes located on 23 pairs of chromosomes. Each human chromosome contains more than 250 million DNA base pairs, arranged in a particular sequence that provides the unique code for each gene. The human genome is made up of 3 billion pairs of bases. The DNA being analyzed in the Human Genome Project comes from small samples of blood or tissue obtained from many people. Even though each individual's genes are made of unique DNA sequences, the variation between any two individuals is small, which means that humans are more alike than they are different.

The Human Genome Project includes a bioethics component to

consider the ethical, legal, and social issues involved in unraveling the GENETIC CODE. Issues under study include fairness in use of genetic information, privacy and confidentiality, commercialization of products associated with genetic information, and reproductive issues. The Project announced that it had successfully completed mapping the entire human genome in 2000. See page 73 for more on the Human Genome Project.

Human granulocytic ehrlichiosis

An infection in humans that is transmitted by the black-legged tick (*Ixodes scapularis*) and the western black-legged tick (*Ixodes pacificus*) in the United States. Human granulocytic ehrlichiosis (HGE) is an illness that resembles ROCKY MOUNTAIN SPOTTED FEVER. Unlike Rocky Mountain spotted fever, which is caused by bacteria of the *Rickettsia* genus, HGE is caused by bacteria of the *Ehrlichia* genus.

Transmission of the bacteria that cause the illness begins 36 hours or more after an infected tick has begun to feed. It is believed that the number of deer ticks in the upper midwestern United States that carry the bacteria that cause HGE is comparable to the number that carry the bacteria that cause LYME DISEASE. Because the incidence of HGE infection from tick bites is much lower than that of Lyme disease in affected areas, and because of other characteristics of HGE, it is believed that the bacteria in HGE are less efficiently transmitted to humans than those of Lyme disease.

A person with the infection may have no symptoms, but most people have a sudden fever, chills, headache, muscle pain, and malaise that occur about 12 days after a person has been bitten by the infected tick. Other symptoms may include abdominal pain, vomiting, and diarrhea. Clots throughout the blood vessels and coma may result. Unlike Lyme disease, rashes, arthritis, and seizures rarely occur with HGE.

Specific blood tests and polymerase chain reaction analysis are used to establish a diagnosis of HGE early on. Diagnostic tests may also reveal blood abnormalities, including a deficiency of white blood cells and platelets, and abnormal liver function.

In many cases, when there is a suspicion of HGE, treatment will begin before diagnosis is confirmed by test results. Quick action may prevent serious complications of the infection, including a viral or a fungal SUPERINFECTION, and even death. Tetracycline, doxycycline, or chloramphenicol may be given orally or intravenously.

Human herpesvirus 8

A virus that has a key role in the development of KAPOSI SARCOMA, a type of cancer characterized by skin tumors that affects many people who have AIDS (acquired immunodeficiency syndrome). Human herpesvirus 8 (HHV-8), also called Kaposi sarcoma herpesvirus (KSHV), has been shown by blood studies to be tightly linked to the risk of Kaposi sarcoma. Infection with this virus precedes tumor development, and the tumors have cells that are infected with HHV-8.

Research suggests that HHV-8 is spread by sexual transmission. Latent infection with the virus is associated with several uncommon syndromes involving the proliferation of lymphocytes (white blood cells that are important to immunity) that occurs in people who have AIDS.

There is also evidence that HHV-8 infection may be linked to cases of Kaposi sarcoma that are not associated with AIDS or HIV (human immunodeficiency virus) infection. Human herpesvirus 8 has been found to exist in people who have Kaposi sarcoma, but who are HIV-negative. Infection with this virus may increase the risk for Kaposi sarcoma, independent of HIV or AIDS.

Human immunodeficiency virus

See HIV.

Human menopausal gonadotropin

The most potent fertility drug. Human menopausal gonadotropin is prescribed for women who are not ovulating and have not responded to treatment with clomiphene, a drug that stimulates ovulation. This drug, also known as HMG, may contain both FSH (follicle-stimulating hormone) and LH (luteinizing hormone), or FSH alone.

Human menopausal gonadotropin is extracted from the urine of menopausal women and supplements or replaces the gonadotropins of the woman taking it to stimulate development of follicles to produce eggs in the ovaries; HMG is given in daily injections, usually by an infertility specialist. Side effects include breast tenderness, bloating, mood swings, and abdominal pain. The most serious side effect is hyperstimulation syndrome, in which multiple follicle cysts develop in the ovaries, causing swelling and pain, which may be severe enough to require hospitalization. Multiple births, mostly twins, occur in 10 to 20 percent of women who take this drug.

Human monocytic ehrlichiosis

A disease caused by bacteria in the *Ehrlichia* genus that is carried and transmitted to humans by ticks, probably the dog tick or Lone Star tick. Human monocytic ehrlichiosis (HME) commonly occurs as an acute infection without long-term consequences. The bacterium that causes HME, *Ehrlichia chaffeensis*, is primarily transmitted by the Lone Star tick. This tick is found in the region of the United States that is south of a line that intersects with the southern border of New Jersey and the western border of Texas, as well as throughout the high plains.

For many people, exposure to the bacteria does not cause symptoms. Other people who are infected may have mild symptoms that appear within a week of a tick bite. Symptoms may include fever, severe headaches, malaise, muscle pains, chills, and a rash. Nausea, vomiting, confusion, and joint pain may also occur. Symptoms usually improve on their own without treatment.

In some instances, however, particularly among people who are older and those with weakened immune systems, symptoms are severe and the infection is life-threatening. Immediate antibiotic treatment at the first suspicion of HME infection is essential to prevent death.

DIAGNOSIS AND TREATMENT

The initial diagnosis is based on a person's symptoms and routine laboratory test results that may show a low white blood cell count, a low platelet count, and elevated liver enzyme levels. Diagnosis can be confirmed with a polymerase chain reaction (PCR) analysis performed within the first 10 days of infection or an immunofluorescent assay, done after 21 days of infection. In severe cases, blood smears may be examined for abnormal cells within the affected blood cells.

Treatment is based on antibiotic therapy such as oral tetracycline or doxycycline, usually for a period of 7 to 10 days. If there is suspicion that Lyme disease has also been transmitted, the course of antibiotic therapy may last as long as 28 days. The symptoms of HME infection usually subside within 1 or 2 days after treatment begins.

Human papillomavirus

The virus that causes warts. Human papillomavirus (HPV) infects only the topmost layer of the skin and is responsible for the appearance of skin growths called warts that may appear anywhere on the outer surface of the body, including the moist mucous membranes near the mouth, anus, and genitals.

There are 70 different types of HPV, each of which causes the eruption of warts in a distinct area of the body. One virus type produces the relatively small, painless warts with rough surfaces that occur on the fingers and face, while another is the cause of the painful, larger plantar warts that appear on the soles of the feet. Small, painless warts are more common on the hands of children, while plantar warts occur most frequently among teens and young adults.

There are 25 different types of human papillomavirus responsible for producing warts on the skin of the sex organs and anus; these are called GENITAL WARTS. At least five of the HPV types that cause genital warts have been linked to cervical cancer (see CERVIX, CANCER OF) and less commonly to SQUAMOUS CELL CARCINOMA of the penis, vagina, anus, and vulva. Infections with the human papillomaviruses that produce genital warts are considered SEXUALLY TRANSMITTED DISEASES, as they are transmitted via sexual contact.

All the virus types in the HPV group are spread by direct contact with infected sites on the skin where warts have appeared or by contact with a surface that has been contaminated by contact with warts. A person can spread warts from one part of his or her body to another by touching the warts or the infected area, then touching another area. A newborn can contract the infection when passing through the birth canal. Plantar warts are often spread from one person to another by contact with bathroom floors where people go barefoot, especially in gyms and dormitories. It may take as long as 3 to 4 months or even 2 years for a person who has had contact with HPV to develop warts.

SYMPTOMS

The singular symptom of HPV infection of the skin is the appearance of warts; however, it is possible to have the infection without any symptoms, especially when it occurs in the genital area. When warts occur, their appearance varies depending on the specific type of human papillomavirus that caused them and their location on the body.

The common skin warts that generally affect the hands, face, skin, or scalp, tend to occur most frequently at sites of previous trauma to the skin. These warts are painless. They are usually no larger than ¼ inch, rounded, and firm. They tend to be similar in color to the person's skin, ranging from pale white or pink to beige or brown. The surface may be smooth or roughly abraded. Flat, flesh-colored warts may sometimes itch. They tend to occur most commonly on the upper portions of the body, specifically the face, neck, chest, forearms, wrists, and hands.

Plantar warts are thick overgrowths of skin on the soles of the feet. What distinguishes them from callused skin is that they may have a small, dark center and can be quite painful.

Genital warts are painless and tend to occur as clusters of up to 10 small, pink growths with rough surfaces. In men, they tend to appear at the tip of the penis and in the opening of the urethra. Genital warts in women usually occur first on the skin surrounding the opening of the vagina and on the folds of skin around the vagina; they tend to spread up into the vagi-

na and may progress to the cervix, or the opening to the uterus. Genital warts may also be located in and around the entrance to the anus, particularly among people who have anal sex.

DIAGNOSIS AND TREATMENT

Warts are diagnosed by a doctor's physical examination of the affected skin. When genital warts are discovered on the exterior areas of a woman's genitals, a physician may use a lighted magnifying instrument called a colposcope to view the interior areas of the vagina and the cervix. A Pap smear is done to test for cervical cancer, and in some cases, a biopsy of overgrown cervical tissue may be performed. There are now DNA tests to detect an HPV infection in women without symptoms; these tests are done on cells scraped from the cervix.

About half of all common warts disappear without treatment within a period of 6 months to 1 year. Others may persist for 2 years or longer. There are over-the-counter topical treatments that may be recommended by a physician. These remedies are composed of strong chemicals that dissolve the wart's cells slowly and may take weeks or months to completely destroy the skin growths. They cannot be used by people who have diabetes mellitus (type 1 or type 2), poor circulation, or signs of infection on the skin where the warts are located.

Over-the-counter remedies should not be used for warts located on the face, genitals, or anus. These warts should be examined by a doctor who may prescribe a medication for a person to use at home.

Sometimes, the doctor may remove warts in the office; these medical treatments tend to be faster acting, more efficient, and more permanent than over-the-counter remedies. Surgical removal of warts involves cutting away the growth in a single office procedure. This offers the best immediate result. Warts can also be cauterized electrically in an outpatient procedure. Cryosurgery, which freezes the warts, or strong topical medications, such as acids or podophyllin, may also be used. Other medical treatments for warts include interferon injections or laser therapy. These treatments may require several office visits to remove the warts

H

completely and permanently. Warts can grow back after they have been successfully removed. This is because it is difficult to be certain that all the human papillomavirus has been removed from the infected skin. See also CONDYLOMA ACUMINATUM; PENILE WARTS.

Humidifier lung

A disease of the alveoli, or air sacs, of the lungs that is caused by inhaling mold spores contained in airborne water droplets from a humidifier. Humidifier lung occurs when the water reservoir of a humidifier becomes contaminated with a variety of mold spores. The mold can contaminate warm or cool air humidifiers used in the home or workplace.

Initial symptoms include fever, cough, and shortness of breath, which may be mistaken for pneumonia. If a humidifier is being used, it is important for the affected person to inform the doctor. Once this connection is made, blood tests can reveal antibodies against the molds.

Treatment is generally based on prevention of further exposure to the mold causing the disease. Corticosteroids are sometimes necessary for brief courses of treatment. Frequent cleaning of the humidifier's water reservoir and daily changing of the water can keep mold spores from contaminating the appliance.

Huntington chorea

Also known as Huntington disease, a progressive brain disease involving degeneration of nerve cells in the cerebrum. Huntington chorea is a genetic disorder caused by a faulty gene on chromosome 4. "Chorea" is from the Greek word for "dance" and refers to the involuntary, uncontrollable movements characteristic of the disease. These include facial grimacing and quick jerking and flinging movements of the body. The other primary characteristics of Huntington chorea are progressive mental deterioration, including the loss of cognitive functions, such as judgment and speech, and personality changes. These symptoms may begin with moodiness and progress to paranoia. The onset of Huntington chorea typically occurs between age 35 and 50 years. Diagnosis is made by genetic testing, MRI (magnetic resonance imaging) findings of wasting (atrophy) in a specific part of the brain, and clinical examination. Medication may lessen the symptoms of Huntington chorea, but there is no treatment for the mental deterioration. Most affected people eventually require institutional care.

Huntington disease

See HUNTINGTON CHOREA.

Hurler syndrome

An inherited metabolic defect in which the body is unable to make an enzyme called alpha-L-iduronidase. The enzyme helps the body break down sugar molecules called mucopolysaccharides, which are essential building blocks of connective tissue. In Hurler syndrome, the mucopolysaccharides accumulate in cells, where they cause progressive damage. As more and more cells are damaged, symptoms appear. Newborns with the disorder appear normal at birth, and symptoms emerge by the end of the first year of life. Symptoms include the development of coarse, thick features, prominent dark eyebrows, increased body hair, cloudy corneas, progressive stiffness of the joints, deafness, and mental retardation. Hurler syndrome occurs in an estimated one of 250,000 babies born.

Hurler syndrome damages many organs of the body, including the heart and heart valves. Most children with Hurler syndrome die before adolescence, usually of heart failure or respiratory infection, and there is no cure for the disorder.

Hurler syndrome is a recessive genetic disorder. An individual must inherit an abnormal copy of the Hurler syndrome gene from each parent to have the disease. Parent carriers of the disease have no symptoms. If a couple has a child with the disease, there is a one in four chance that each subsequent child will have the disorder. The condition can be diagnosed prenatally through amniocentesis. Genetic counseling is important for parents with family histories of the syndrome.

Hydatid disease

A rare, potentially fatal disease in humans caused by infection with the larval stage of a microscopic tapeworm found in foxes, coyotes, dogs (especially sheep dogs), and cats. Hydatid disease is also referred to as alveolar hydatid disease and hydatid cyst disease. In humans, the disease is caused by cystlike tapeworm larvae that are transmitted by animals. The larvae grow slowly in the body, producing parasitic tumors that usually form in the liver, but may also develop in the lungs, brain, and other organs. Left untreated, the infection can cause death.

The infection is caused by the tapeworm *Echinococcus multilocularis*, which is prevalent among wild foxes and coyotes and is found in the north central region of the United States from eastern Montana to central Ohio and in Alaska. Cases of human infection have been identified in Minnesota, Alaska, and the province of Manitoba in Canada.

Transmission of the tapeworm in humans is rare. Wild foxes, wolves, and coyotes, as well as some domestic cats and dogs, become infected without symptoms or ill effects when they ingest the tapeworm's larvae in infected rodents, field mice, or moles. Domestic dogs are more susceptible to infection than cats, but because they are less likely to eat rodents, they are infected less often. The tapeworm matures and lays eggs in the intestines of an infected fox, coyote, or cat. The eggs, which are passed in the stool of the infected animal, are too tiny to see and tend to adhere to anything they contact, including vegetation that humans consume.

People can become infected with hydatid disease by accidentally ingesting the eggs of the tapeworm in a hand-to-mouth transfer or contamination. This can occur in the course of eating vegetation gathered in the wild, including grasses, herbs, greens, or berries, that has been contaminated by the microscopic, adherent eggs in the feces of an infected fox or coyote. A person may also become infected by handling domestic dogs or cats whose fur becomes contaminated when they pass the eggs in their stool. Their fur can also become infected by "scent rolling" in the feces of wild animals.

SYMPTOMS, DIAGNOSIS, AND TREATMENT

There may not be any symptoms of hydatid disease in an infected person for many years. The tumorlike or cystlike tapeworm larvae that grow in the body develop slowly. Usually the liver is affected, but the infection may spread to other organs. As the cysts grow, an infected person may experience discomfort or pain in the upper abdomen, weakness, and weight loss. These and other symptoms can mimic those of liver cancer and CIRRHOSIS of the liver.

Hydatid disease is diagnosed by blood tests that reveal the presence of the parasite or antibodies to it. Surgery to remove the parasite cyst mass is the most common treatment for the disease, but it may not be completely effective and medication may be required to prevent regrowth of the cyst.

Hydatidiform mole

An abnormal pregnancy, also called a molar pregnancy, which probably results from the fertilization of a so-called empty egg, an egg without chromosomes. In this condition, the fertilized egg degenerates and the placenta grows into a mass of tissue resembling a cluster of grapes. Hydatidiform moles are rare, occurring only once in every 2,000 pregnancies, and are more common in older women. When a woman has a hydatidiform mole, the uterus expands much faster than it would during a normal pregnancy. Fetal movement and a heartbeat are absent. Some women may have vaginal bleeding or expel grapelike clusters of tissue from the vagina, or they may have severe nausea and vomiting, high blood pressure, and a fast heart rate.

A hydatidiform mole produces unusually large amounts of a hormone called HCG (HUMAN CHORIONIC GONADOTROPIN), which can be detected by testing a woman's blood or urine. ULTRASOUND SCANNING can be used to visually detect a hydatidiform mole, which appears as an abnormal placenta and no fetus. A doctor can remove a hydatidiform mole by suctioning out the contents of the uterus, in a procedure similar to a D AND C (dilation and curettage). After removal of a hydatidiform mole, follow-up examinations and blood tests are conducted to be sure that the growth does not come back or that a cancerous growth does not develop.

Hydralazine

A drug used to treat high blood pressure and congestive heart failure. Hydralazine (Hydra-Zide, Apresoline) is in a class of drugs called vasodilators that lower blood pressure by causing blood vessels to dilate, or widen. It is available in tablet form and by injection.

Hydramnios

An excessive amount of AMNIOTIC FLUID surrounding the fetus. This condition occurs in the middle or late stages of pregnancy and is usually harmless. In most cases, the uterus swells to a size only slightly larger than normal and the woman experiences either no symptoms or a gradual onset of breathlessness, indigestion, and tension in her abdominal muscles. In some cases, swelling is pronounced; symptoms, including nausea, may begin suddenly, and there is risk of premature labor.

Hydramnios occurs in women with diabetes mellitus (see DIABETES MELLITUS, TYPE 1; DIABETES MELLITUS, TYPE 2), in those carrying multiple fetuses, or when the fetus has a malformation of the spine, gastrointestinal system, or brain. Pregnancies in which RH INCOMPATIBILITY is a problem are also associated with hydramnios.

Diagnosis is based on a combination of a physical examination and ultrasound to rule out fetal malformations. Most cases require no treatment, but in severe cases, in which there is a risk of premature labor or other complications, the doctor may order bed rest and close monitoring. Sometimes, AMNIOCENTESIS will be used several times throughout the pregnancy to remove excess fluid.

Hydrocele

Accumulation of fluid in a male's scrotum, the protective pouch of skin that contains the testicles. Hydrocele at birth results from incomplete closure of the canal that links the scrotum with the abdomen during development of the fetus. This kind of hydrocele is sometimes accompanied by a loop of intestine protruding into the scrotum (HERNIA). Hydrocele can also occur in adults, but less frequently, and it may be caused by inflammation inside the scrotum or injury damaging the flow of blood or lymph in the testicle. Hydrocele

without hernia in newborns often repairs itself within the first year of life. In adults and newborns with a hernia, hydrocele can be repaired surgically. Sometimes a hydrocele found in an adult without symptoms, may require no treatment.

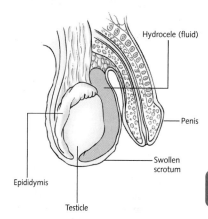

FLUID IN THE SCROTUM
The testicle is cushioned in a thin layer of fluid within the scrotum. Excess fluid can accumulate, causing swelling. The accumulation may resolve on its own, without symptoms, or the fluid can be drained surgically. Hydrocele in a newborn usually disappears within the first year.

Hydrocephalus

A disorder characterized by the presence of excessive fluid in the brain. Cerebrospinal fluid (CSF) is formed in the brain, where it circulates throughout the brain and the spinal canal, eventually being reabsorbed into the circulatory system. If the circulation or absorption of CSF is blocked or excessive fluid is produced, excess fluid accumulates and puts pressure on the brain ("water on the brain"). The pressure forces the brain against the bones of the skull, damaging or destroying brain tissue.

Symptoms vary, depending on the age at which hydrocephalus develops and the cause of the obstruction. In newborns, hydrocephalus is often a genetic birth defect. The head will be abnormally enlarged, and there may be bulging at the soft spots of the head (fontanelles). Other symptoms include spastic muscles, irritability, temper tantrums, delayed development, slow growth, lethargy, difficulty feeding, loss of bladder control, and decreased mental function. Older children may have headaches, vomiting, crossed eyes, loss of coordination, and confusion. Hydrocephalus can develop in adults, after either a head injury or an infection such as meningitis.

Treatment of hydrocephalus depends on the time of onset and its cause. Surgery to remove the obstruction is the primary treatment whenever possible. If removal of the obstruction is not possible, a tube placed within the brain may allow CSF to bypass the obstructed area. Untreated hydrocephalus has a poor prognosis, but depending on the cause, treatment can help most people live a fairly normal life. Hydrocephalus occurs in about one of every 1,000 children, and in adults is most common among the elderly. It can result from interactions between genetic and environmental factors. Same cases are inherited with significant risks of recurrence in a family. A genetic counselor can help assess those risks.

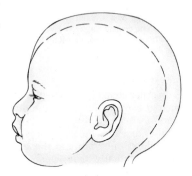

EXCESS FLUID IN THE BRAIN
In a child with hydrocephalus, the head will be abnormally enlarged by the pressure of excess cerebrospinal fluid (liquid that lubricates the brain). The dotted line indicates the normal shape of a child's skull.

Hydrochloric acid

A strong acid produced by the stomach that helps to break down food into chemical components usable by the body. Cells in the stomach glands are stimulated to secrete hydrochloric acid, or HCL, by the presence of a hormone called gastrin. Hydrochloric acid converts pepsinogen secreted by stomach cells into pepsin, an enzyme that helps the body digest protein. HCL also kills bacteria and other microorganisms that may accidentally be ingested with food.

Hydrochlorothiazide

A diuretic drug used to treat high blood pressure and excess fluid retention. Hydrochlorothiazide increases the production or amount of urine by promoting the passage of sodium and water through the kidneys, thereby decreasing blood volume and forcing excess liquid and sodium out of cells and tissues where they have accumulated. These activities of hydrochlorothiazide lower blood pressure and relieve edema associated with heart failure.

Hydrocodone

A narcotic painkiller. Hydrocodone is chemically similar to codeine, but more powerful and addicting. It is also used as a cough suppressant. Hydrocodone is available as a syrup, as pills, and as a liquid and in combination with acetaminophen. It is manufactured under many brand names, including Hycodan, Hydrocet, Lortab, Norco, Vicodin, and Triaminic.

Hydrocortisone

See CORTICOSTEROIDS.

Hydrogenated fats and oils

Substances made through the hydrogenation process that solidifies liquid oils for use in food products. See FATS AND OILS.

Hydronephrosis

Dilation or widening of the kidney caused by total or partial blockage of the urinary tract. As the urine backs up, pressure inside the kidney increases, distending the collecting system. Hydronephrosis is not a disease itself but the result of a disease blocking the urinary tract, such as a stone in the kidney, ureter (the urine tube connecting the kidney and bladder), or bladder; a urinary tract infection; or an enlarged prostate. Depending on where the obstruction is located, one or both kidneys can be affected. Hydronephrosis may produce no symptoms, but sometimes continuing or intermittent pain in the abdomen or side below the ribs can be symptoms of an obstruction. The condition is usually diagnosed by ultrasound scanning. Hydronephrosis can also occur before birth and is sometimes diagnosed while the fetus is still developing. In newborns whose hydronephrosis has been identified before birth, treatment can begin in the first few days of life.

Treatment is aimed at resolving the underlying cause. Medication can be used to combat the infection, and surgery may be needed to remove tumors or stones or to repair anatomical defects. Prompt treatment is necessary. If the condition persists, hydronephrosis can severely and permanently damage the kidney. Persistent hydronephrosis in both kidneys leads to kidney failure, which can be life-threatening.

Hydrops

An abnormal accumulation of fluid in fetal tissues. This condition can be detected by ultrasound and can include scalp edema (accumulation of fluid), ASCITES (abdominal edema), and fluid in the lungs. Fetal hydrops can be caused by viral infections, such as CYTOMEGALOVIRUS, and can lead to serious birth defects, including severely impaired intellectual or motor abilities. Termination of the pregnancy may be an option.

Hydroquinone

A medication used on the skin to lighten or bleach freckles and brown patches ("liver spots"). Hydroquinone (Eldopaque Forte, Eldoquin Forte, Lustra, Melanex, Solaquin Forte) is available as a cream, a lotion, a gel, and a solution for applying to the skin. The fading of darkened skin spots is a temporary effect.

Hydrotherapy

The use of water, such as in exercise pools, whirlpool baths, and showers,

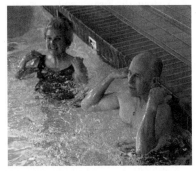

WATER THERAPY
Exercising in water provides a person with easy mobility and buoyancy. Hydrotherapy can soothe joint and muscle pain and promote relaxation.

to treat muscle and joint pain and other problems. Hydrotherapy can promote mobility of an injured area because water provides buoyancy and neutralizes gravity. Bathing an injury in alternating hot and cold water can stimulate blood flow to the area and aid in healing. Warm to hot water is known to promote muscle relaxation and may help relax the entire body, especially in combination with massage and stretching.

Hydroxychloroquine sulfate

An antimalarial, anti-inflammatory drug. Hydroxychloroquine sulfate (Plaquenil Sulfate) interferes with the DNA protein synthesis of the microorganisms associated with malaria to prevent attacks of the disease. Because of its anti-inflammatory effects, hydroxychloroquine sulfate is also used to treat rheumatoid arthritis and lupus.

Hydroxyzine

An antihistamine with many effects. Hydroxyzine hydrochloride (Atarax) and hydroxyzine pamoate (Vistaril) have antianxiety, sedative, fever-reducing, and antinausea properties. Hydroxyzine is used to treat anxiety, tension, nervousness, nausea, vomiting, allergies, skin rash, hives, and itching. It is available in tablets, capsules, liquid, and by injection.

Hygiene

The science and practice of promoting and preserving health. The term "hygiene" is often used synonymously with "cleanliness."

Hymen

A thin membrane stretching across the opening of the vagina, just inside the inner lips (labia minora). The hymen has a small hole in the center that allows menstrual blood and other discharges to flow out. The hymen is easily stretched or torn, often by the use of tampons or sexual activity. In rare instances, the hymen not does have an opening, a condition called imperforate hymen. A physician has to make an incision in the hymen to allow normal menstruation. Once torn, remains of the hymen form a ring of tissue around the vaginal opening. See REPRODUCTIVE SYSTEM, FEMALE.

Hyoid

Bone at the base of the tongue. The hyoid bone is a small, isolated, U-shaped bone that forms the center part of the hyoid arch supporting the tongue.

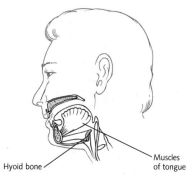

Hyoid bone

Muscles of tongue

SUPPORT FOR THE TONGUE
The hyoid bone actually "floats" at the back of the mouth, independent of other bones of the skull or jaw, to anchor and support the muscles of the tongue.

Hyperacidity

Excessive production of gastric acid by the stomach. Hyperacidity can often be a factor in a DUODENAL ULCER or a GASTRIC ULCER. Hyperacidity may also play a role in indigestion.

Hyperactivity

A state of excessive muscular activity characterized by constant fidgeting or moving, wandering, incessant talking, easy distractibility, or difficulty with quiet behavior such as reading. See ATTENTION DEFICIT/HYPERACTIVITY DISORDER.

Hyperacusis

A rare hearing disorder producing extreme sensitivity to noise, including normal environmental sounds, affecting people of all ages and usually accompanied by ringing in the ears. The disorder may affect one or both ears. People who have hyperacusis have difficulty tolerating sounds that do not seem loud to others—for example, the sounds made by running water from a faucet, by a car's engine when driving, by footsteps on leaves, or by handling paper. The condition is usually caused by sudden or prolonged exposure to loud noise (see ACOUSTIC TRAUMA) or by head injury. It may be related to a breakdown in the fibers of the hearing nerve that originates in

the brain and regulates or inhibits incoming sound. Hearing tests (see AUDIOMETRY) usually indicate normal hearing for people with hyperacusis, possibly because all of the hearing nerve fibers have not been damaged, leaving some hearing mechanisms intact and functional. People with symptoms of this disorder may be given a sound tolerance test before taking hearing tests because loud sounds on some tests may be painful and could aggravate their problem. Few treatments are available for hyperacusis. One promising treatment involves listening to a specific kind of white noise at barely audible levels for a period of time every day in order to retrain the damaged hearing nerves to tolerate normal levels of sound.

Hyperaldosteronism

See ALDOSTERONISM.

Hyperalimentation

See PARENTERAL NUTRITION.

Hyperbaric injuries

See DECOMPRESSION SICKNESS.

Hyperbaric oxygen treatment

A system of increasing the oxygen supply to the tissues by providing oxygen at a higher-than-normal atmospheric pressure. Hyperbaric oxygen treatment is used to treat people with gas GANGRENE, carbon monoxide poisoning (see POISONING, CARBON MONOXIDE), DECOMPRESSION SICKNESS, and smoke inhalation (see INHALATION, SMOKE). In a hyperbaric chamber, a person is exposed to up to three times the normal atmospheric pressure.

Hyperbilirubinemia

An excessively high concentration of the compound bilirubin in the blood. Bilirubin is produced during the breakdown of hemoglobin, the blood pigment that transports oxygen. When red blood cells are destroyed, the bilirubin that results from the breakdown of hemoglobin is transported to the liver and excreted as part of the bile into the gallbladder and small intestine. If an obstruction is blocking the bile ducts or gallbladder, the level of bilirubin in the blood increases. Abnormally high levels of bilirubin cause jaundice, a yellowish

H

discoloration of the skin and the sclera (white of the eyes), which can be a sign of liver or gallbladder disease.

Hypercalcemia

An excessively high concentration of calcium in the bloodstream. Symptoms include fatigue, muscle weakness, depression, lack of appetite, nausea, and constipation.

Hypercholesterol-emia

An abnormally high level of the waxy fat known as CHOLESTEROL in the blood. Hypercholesterolemia is a key factor in hardening of the arteries (see ATHEROSCLEROSIS); increases the risk of angina, heart attack, and stroke; and poses a significant threat to health.

Cholesterol in the blood is measured in terms of milligrams (mg) of cholesterol per deciliter (dL) of blood. Hypercholesterolemia is defined as a blood cholesterol level of 240 mg/dL or higher. Total cholesterol levels less than 200 mg/dL are considered desirable, and those between 200 mg/dL and 239 mg/dL are borderline high.

TYPES OF CHOLESTEROL

Cholesterol is a waxy fat that has a variety of essential roles in the structure and metabolism of animal cells, including those in the human body. Approximately 80 percent of the cholesterol in the body is synthesized in the liver. The remainder comes from eating animal products such as meat, eggs, seafood, milk, and cheese.

Since cholesterol does not dissolve in the blood, it is transported through the bloodstream in combination with specialized transport proteins. The protein-cholesterol complexes are known as lipoproteins. Two principal types of lipoproteins are high-density lipoproteins (HDLs) and low-density lipoproteins (LDLs).

In assessing hypercholesterolemia, a doctor measures not only the total cholesterol level, but also the levels of HDL and LDL. HDL is stable, moves easily through the blood, and helps to prevent artery disease by carrying excess cholesterol to the liver, where it is removed from the bloodstream. HDL is often called "good" cholesterol. LDL cholesterol contains more fat than protein and tends to stick to artery walls and build up the deposits (plaques) that can lead to heart attack

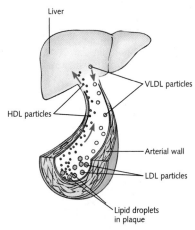

NORMAL CHOLESTEROL TRANSPORT
The liver sends out some cholesterol to be used or stored in the form of VLDL (very-low-density lipoprotein). Some VLDL is converted into LDL (low-density lipoprotein), which can be deposited on arterial walls as harmful plaque. But some of the cholesterol in plaque can be absorbed by HDL (high-density lipoprotein), returned to the liver, and excreted as bile.

or stroke. LDL is commonly known as "bad" cholesterol. In general, HDL levels should be higher than 40 mg/dL, and LDL levels should be 129 mg/dL or lower. An LDL level between 130 mg/dL and 159 mg/dL is considered borderline high, an LDL level between 160 and 189 mg/dL is considered high, and an LDL level of 190 mg/dL or greater is considered very high and places people at increased risk of developing atherosclerosis.

Some doctors also look at LDL and HDL as a proportion of total cholesterol. According to the American Heart Association, total cholesterol should not be more than five times the HDL level. This can also be stated as a ratio of total cholesterol to HDL of 5:1. Ratios of 4:1 or 3:1 are more desirable, while those of 6:1 or 7:1 place people at above-average risk for developing heart disease.

CAUSES

Diets high in fat are a leading cause of hypercholesterolemia. If a substantial proportion of daily calories comes from animal products or from saturated fats (see FATS AND OILS), the blood cholesterol level usually rises. This is especially true when a person is obese. Lack of exercise and smoking are also factors in elevating the LDL level relative to the HDL level.

Hypercholesterolemia can also result

from certain inherited conditions. The most widespread genetically based cholesterol disorder is familial hypercholesterolemia. Persons with this condition may have a blood cholesterol level over 500 mg/dL, develop visible waxy plaques (xanthomas) under the skin, and develop atherosclerosis before puberty. Men with this disorder can have heart attacks as early as their 20s; in women, heart attacks may occur about 10 years later.

DETECTION, TREATMENT, AND PREVENTION

Regular screening of blood cholesterol levels should begin in men and women older than 20. Screening at 5-year intervals is advised unless a person's cholesterol level is abnormally elevated, in which case more frequent screening is warranted. If a family history of early heart attack indicates possible familial hypercholesterolemia, screening can begin earlier and can be repeated more often.

If hypercholesterolemia is discovered, initial treatment consists of changes in diet to reduce the amount of cholesterol and saturated fat. Such a diet is rich in fruits, vegetables, and grains and low in meat, fats and oils, and dairy products. People with the disease should also quit smoking, increase their level of exercise, and lose weight if they are overweight or obese.

Should these measures fail to control the condition, medications are used to reduce the cholesterol level. The most widely prescribed drugs are the statins, which reduce both total cholesterol and LDL levels. Aspirin use may also be advised to reduce the risk of blood clots that can form in arteries clogged with plaque and cause a heart attack or stroke.

The risk of developing hypercholesterolemia decreases in people who eat a low-fat diet, exercise moderately and regularly, control their body weight, and abstain from tobacco use. In addition, research indicates that moderate consumption of alcohol may have a preventive effect.

Hyperemesis

Excessive vomiting that can result in severe dehydration and weight loss. Symptoms of hyperemesis may include a rapid pulse, a drop in blood pressure, dry mucous membranes in the mouth and elsewhere, a loss of skin elasticity, and confusion. Forceful vomiting can lead to RETINAL HEMORRHAGE, which impairs vision, or to rips in the digestive tract, which cause the vomiting of blood. HYPEREMESIS GRAVIDARUM is excessive vomiting during pregnancy.

Hyperemesis gravidarum

Persistent intractable vomiting, usually beginning in early pregnancy, leading to weight loss and dehydration. This condition is uncommon and is associated with obesity and carrying twins. As a general rule, persistent nausea and vomiting begin in the first trimester, ending at about the 28th week. Both the mother and fetus may experience serious nutritional consequences, and hospitalization may be necessary to restore normal metabolic balance and prevent serious liver damage. Administration of intravenous fluids to the mother may be required to correct dehydration. There is no clear cause of this disorder, and psychological factors can play a role, particularly when the pregnancy is unwanted.

Hyperglycemia

High blood sugar. Hyperglycemia may be caused by INSULIN RESISTANCE, by an insufficient supply of insulin from the pancreas, or by other factors involving the inability of the body to respond to insulin. Factors that contribute to hyperglycemia include overeating, inactivity, illness, stress, certain medications, and hormone disorders. Hyperglycemia may be mild or severe. The symptoms can vary and may include extreme thirst, frequent urination, fatigue, blurred vision, and unexplained weight loss.

CAUSES

Hyperglycemia occurs as a result of a disruption in the normal blood sugar level in the body. Hormones produced by the pancreas enable the body to utilize glucose, a simple sugar that supplies energy to all the cells. Normally, the pancreatic hormones regulate the use of glucose by the body by balancing the concentration of glucose in response to food intake, physical exertion, stress, infection, or other events and conditions.

Insulin is produced by the pancreas when the concentration of glucose in the blood increases, which occurs normally after eating. The insulin stimulates muscle, fat, and other cells to absorb the glucose they require to fuel everyday functions. If there is a surplus of glucose, it is stored in the form of a starch called glycogen in the liver. Another hormone produced by the pancreas, GLUCAGON, breaks down glycogen in the liver and releases it into the bloodstream when the cells need more fuel. This raises the concentration of sugar in the blood.

If the system of balancing the blood sugar level fails, the absorption of glucose by the cells and the liver is decreased. Glucose builds up in the blood when the cells cannot use it for fuel, and it is not stored in the liver. The resulting condition is excess glucose in the blood. When this is caused by problems with insulin activity, either due to an insufficient supply of insulin or a resistance to it, the condition produces diabetes mellitus (see DIABETES MELLITUS, TYPE 1 and DIABETES MELLITUS, TYPE 2).

Other disorders or conditions that may cause or be associated with hyperglycemia include ACROMEGALY, HEMOCHROMATOSIS, CUSHING SYNDROME, HYPERTHYROIDISM (overactivity of the thyroid gland), and surgical removal of the pancreas.

Hypergonadism

A rare condition marked by the overstimulation of cells in the testicles (see TESTICLE) in men and boys. It causes precocious sexual development and excessive growth. Hypergonadism causes early puberty in young boys. In men, symptoms may include male-pattern hair loss, excessive body hair growth, and acne. The resulting overgrowth of cells can produce enlarged muscles. When increased levels of excess testosterone are metabolized to estrogen, men with hypergonadism may develop enlarged breasts.

Hyperhidrosis

A disorder characterized by excessive perspiration. It may occur in one part of the body (such as the armpits) or all over the body. Hyperhidrosis can affect the hands, the armpits, or the feet. Perspiration is the way the body regulates temperature and is normally controlled by the sympathetic nervous system. Odor occurs because of the interaction between perspiration and bacteria that normally live on the skin. Excessive sweating and subsequent body odor can pose social problems that interfere with daily life. Although the exact cause of hyperhidrosis remains unknown, stress, emotion, or exercise can bring on the condition. Excessive sweating can also occur spontaneously.

A number of treatments are available for hyperhidrosis. A doctor can prescribe topical aluminum chloride preparations or anticholinergic medications. Iontophoresis (introducing ions [see ION] of soluble salts into body tissues through electrical stimulation) may also dramatically reduce sweating. Botulinum toxin injections decrease sweat secretion. When hyperhidrosis fails to respond to medical treatments, surgery may be performed to remove part of the main sympathetic nerve.

Hyperkeratosis

Thickening of the skin. Hyperkeratosis is the result of overgrowth of the keratin layer of the skin and can result in formation of a callus (see CALLUS, SKIN).

Hyperlipidemias

A group of diseases that involve abnormally elevated levels of lipids (fats) in the blood. Hyperlipidemias are key factors in hardening of the arteries (see ATHEROSCLEROSIS); they increase the risk of angina, heart attack, and stroke; and they are a significant threat to health. Some hyperlipidemias are inherited. Others are acquired as a result of disease, lifestyle, or medication.

TYPES AND LEVELS OF BLOOD LIPIDS

The lipids found in the blood include cholesterol, cholesterol compounds, phospholipids, and triglycerides. Since lipids do not dissolve in blood, they are transported through the bloodstream in combination with specialized transport protein molecules. The resulting compounds are known as lipoproteins. Most of the cholesterol in the blood takes the form of high-density lipoprotein (HDL) or low-density lipoprotein (LDL). Triglycerides are found in chylomicrons and in lipoproteins that also contain cholesterol.

A high level of cholesterol, elevated

triglyceride levels, or both in the blood are associated with an increased risk for the development of plaques (fatty deposits) in the arteries, which can lead to angina, heart attack, and stroke. The level of lipids in the blood is measured by drawing blood from a vein, usually in the arm, and determining the amount of fat it contains. The accurate determination of whether triglyceride levels are elevated requires that a person take a fasting blood test.

Cholesterol in the blood is measured in terms of milligrams of cholesterol per deciliter of blood. Too much cholesterol, known technically as HYPERCHOLESTEROLEMIA, is defined as a blood cholesterol level of 240 milligrams per deciliter (mg/dL) or higher. Total blood cholesterol levels below 200 mg/dL are considered desirable, and those between 200 and 239 are considered borderline high. In addition to the total cholesterol level, the levels of HDL and LDL are also measured. HDL helps to prevent artery disease by carrying excess cholesterol to the liver, where it is removed from the bloodstream. HDL is often called "good" cholesterol. LDL cholesterol contains more fat than protein and tends to stick to artery walls and build up the deposits (plaques) that can lead to heart attack or stroke. LDL is commonly known as "bad" cholesterol. In general, HDL levels should be higher than 40 mg/dL, and LDL levels should be lower than 130 mg/dL. An LDL level between 160 and 189 mg/dL is considered high, while an LDL level of 190 or more is considered very high. High or very high levels of LDL may indicate an increased risk of atherosclerosis even when the total cholesterol level is less than 240 mg/dL.

Triglycerides are also measured in milligrams per deciliter of blood. Less than 150 is normal; between 150 and 200 is borderline; over 200 is high; and over 500 is very high.

FAMILIAL AND ACQUIRED HYPERLIPIDEMIAS

If hyperlipidemia is caused by a genetic factor, it is said to be familial. An example is familial combined

hyperlipidemia, a disease that results in high cholesterol and triglyceride levels, which appear during adolescence and continue throughout life, raising the risk of early coronary artery disease or heart attack.

Hyperlipidemias caused by factors that are not inherited are said to be acquired. Acquired hyperlipidemia can arise from diabetes mellitus, certain kinds of kidney disease, and hypothyroidism (an underactive thyroid gland). Medications can be another cause. Birth control pills, certain hormones (corticosteroids and estrogen), some diuretics (which increase urine production), and beta blockers (drugs that lessen the workload of the heart and lower blood pressure) can raise blood lipid levels. Lifestyle, particularly diet, can also cause acquired hyperlipidemia. Diets that are high in saturated fats (see FATS AND OILS) and cholesterol (from meat and dairy products) increase the risk of developing acquired hyperlipidemia. Heavy habitual alcohol use and obesity are also risk factors. Smoking reduces the HDL level and may also contribute to developing acquired hyperlipidemia.

TREATMENT AND PREVENTION

Changing diet is the first step in treatment of both familial and acquired hyperlipidemia. Total calories, saturated fat, and cholesterol are reduced by following a diet that is rich in fruits, vegetables, and whole grains and low in meat, fats, oils, and dairy products. Reducing weight to a healthy level is important for obese individuals. Alcohol use should be restricted, usually to two drinks per day for men and one for women. If the level of triglycerides is elevated, sugar intake may also need to be reduced. Exercise can also be beneficial, both by reducing body weight and by increasing the level of HDL in the blood.

If dietary changes do not lower blood fat levels to the normal range, statin medications, such as simvastatin and atorvastatin, may be used to reduce both total cholesterol and LDL levels. Aspirin may also be prescribed to reduce the risk of blood clots, which can form in arteries clogged with plaque and thereby cause a heart attack or stroke. In addition, medications may be used to control any contributing conditions,

such as diabetes mellitus, kidney disease, or hypothyroidism. Since hyperlipidemia increases the risk of heart attack and stroke, detecting and controlling hypertension (which increases the risk of heart attack and stroke) is also important.

Hyperlipidemia can be prevented by following sensible lifestyle precautions, such as adhering to a low-fat, heart-healthy diet; participating in regular exercise; moderating alcohol use; maintaining a healthy body weight; controlling diabetes; and abstaining from tobacco use.

Hypernephroma
See RENAL CELL CARCINOMA.

Hyperopia
See FARSIGHTEDNESS.

Hyperparathyroidism
A disorder in which overactive parathyroid glands, located on the thyroid gland in the neck, produce excessive parathyroid hormone, which stimulates the release of calcium from the bones and produces an elevated calcium level in the bloodstream. Women tend to be affected more than men, and the risk increases with age, becoming most common in women aged 60 years or older. Hyperparathyroidism can lead to bone-weakening diseases such as OSTEOPOROSIS and OSTEOMALACIA. It is associated with kidney failure, which makes the body resistant to the activity of the parathyroid hormone. Excess calcium excreted into the urine by the kidneys may cause kidney stones.

The parathyroid glands secrete parathyroid hormone, which balances calcium and phosphorus in the body. Parathyroid hormone regulates the release of calcium from the skeletal bones and controls calcium absorption in the intestine and its excretion in the urine. When calcium levels in the blood are decreased, parathyroid hormone is normally secreted to restore the proper balance.

CAUSES

The condition is most frequently caused by an ADENOMA, a benign (not cancerous) tumor of the parathyroid glands. Enlargement of the parathyroid glands is the next most common cause. Only rarely does the disorder result from cancer of the parathyroid glands. The cause of the

Terms in small capital letters— for example, PHYSICAL THERAPY or PAGET DISEASE—indicate a cross-reference to another entry with more information.

tumor and gland enlargement are unknown.

The tumor or enlargement causes the glands to secrete excess parathyroid hormone. The excess hormone disrupts the balance of calcium and phosphorus levels in the blood, and the blood calcium level rises, resulting in a condition called HYPER-CALCEMIA.

The excess parathyroid hormone also stimulates the release of extra calcium from the bones into the bloodstream and enhances the amount of calcium absorbed by the intestine from food sources. Chronic hyperparathyroidism can lead to thinning of the bones. If there is increased calcium in the urine, kidney stones may result. The excess parathyroid hormone also reduces phosphorus levels in the blood by promoting the excretion of phosphorus.

SYMPTOMS

The symptoms of hyperparathyroidism may be minor or severe, or there may be no noticeable symptoms. Mild symptoms include body aches and pains, depression, and muscle weakness. When hyperparathyroidism is more severe, abdominal pain, nausea, vomiting, fatigue, increased thirst, frequent urination, confusion, and impaired memory may be experienced. Thinning of the bones may occur without apparent symptoms and can increase the risk of fractures. Kidney stones may develop as a result of increased calcium and phosphorus excretion in the urine. Excess parathyroid hormone also increases the risk of developing peptic ulcers, high blood pressure, and pancreatitis.

DIAGNOSIS AND TREATMENT

In a person who does not have symptoms, hyperparathyroidism is usually detected during a routine blood test that reveals elevated calcium in the bloodstream. If hyperparathyroidism is suspected to be the cause of hypercalcemia, the diagnosis can be confirmed with a blood test to measure the amount of parathyroid hormone in the bloodstream.

A diagnosis of hyperparathyroidism may be confirmed by a complete medical history, physical examination, DIAGNOSTIC IMAGING (including X rays of the bones), and blood tests in which the levels of calcium, phosphorus, and parathyroid hormone are measured.

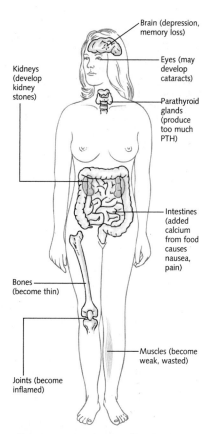

EFFECTS OF HYPERPARATHYROIDISM
Parathyroid hormone (PTH) normally regulates the release of calcium from bones, the absorption of calcium in the intestine, and the elimination of calcium via the kidneys. When the parathyroid glands produce too much PTH, excessive calcium is released from the bones and builds up in the blood and urine.

Once the diagnosis has been made, bone density tests may be ordered to assess any possible damage or weakening from calcium deficiency and to determine the risk of fractures. Specialized urine tests can reveal possible kidney damage. Abdominal X rays, CT (computed tomography) scans, or ultrasound may detect kidney stones.

Although surgery is the only cure for hyperparathyroidism, most doctors recommend surgery only for those with symptoms or signs of the disease. Other indications for surgery include a moderately high calcium level, deteriorating kidney function, younger age, and osteoporosis. In mild disease when calcium levels are only slightly high and the kidneys and bones are not affected, the dis-

ease can be managed without surgery. Clinical evaluations and measurements of calcium levels and kidney function should be performed at 6-month intervals, abdominal X rays to check for kidney stones once a year, and bone density tests once every 1 or 2 years.

If there are no signs that hyperparathyroidism is worsening with time, the person is advised to drink plenty of water, exercise regularly, and avoid taking diuretics such as thiazides. Because the calcium level may rise with gastrointestinal disorders, people with mild hyperparathyroidism are advised to seek medical attention if they experience vomiting or diarrhea.

In more advanced or severe cases, surgery is the only treatment available and is almost always effective. Complications of surgery are unusual but, in rare instances, there is damage to nerves controlling the vocal cords, and speech is affected. A chronically low calcium level occurs in a small percentage of people who undergo this surgery; they are given calcium and vitamin D therapy.

Hyperplasia

An abnormal increase in the number of normal cells in an organ that results in the organ becoming larger than normal. Hyperplasia is not necessarily a cancerous condition, although it may sometimes become cancerous.

Hyperplasia, endometrial

See ENDOMETRIAL HYPERPLASIA.

Hyperplasia, gingival

Swelling, inflammation, and irritation of the gums. Gingival hyperplasia may be caused by a buildup of plaque (see PLAQUE, DENTAL), which results in inflamed, swollen gums. Daily brushing and the use of dental floss will remove plaque and keep gums healthy. The condition may also be associated with vitamin deficiencies, certain antiseizure and antihypertensive medications, some glandular disorders, and blood diseases. People who have diabetes and pregnant women may be more susceptible to gingival hyperplasia because of hormonal changes. If the gums bleed

H

or the condition becomes more severe, PERIODONTAL DISEASE may be developing. A dentist should be consulted to discuss treatment options; he or she may offer a referral to a PERIODONTIST (gum specialist). Often, a gingivectomy has to be performed to eliminate deep periodontal pockets and the inflamed tissue.

Hyperpyrexia

An extremely elevated body temperature that sometimes occurs in acute infectious diseases (see FEVER). Hyperpyrexia most commonly affects infants and young children. To prevent seizures (see SEIZURE, FEBRILE), it is important to lower the child's temperature as rapidly as possible. This may be accomplished with tepid baths and giving the child acetaminophen. Aspirin must never be given to children because it is associated with a rare but life-threatening disorder known as REYE SYNDROME. In malignant hyperpyrexia (see HYPERTHERMIA, MALIGNANT), a person has a severe uncontrollable fever while undergoing general anesthesia or while taking muscle relaxants or major tranquilizers. This condition is a medical emergency.

Hypersensitivity

An excessive or abnormal reaction of the immune system to a specific stimulating or provoking agent or antigen. Hypersensitivity describes the process of interaction between a particular antigen and the body's antibodies or lymphocytes. The degree of hypersensitivity may be based on the amount of time required for the reaction to occur, the type of antigen introduced, or organ involvement in the reaction.

Hypersplenism

Increased activity by the spleen, a large organ in the upper left part of the abdomen that has an important part in filtering the blood and providing immunity. Hypersplenism usually results from another malady, such as liver disease (for example, cirrhosis), certain blood diseases (including leukemia and anemia), or infectious or parasitic diseases (such as tuberculosis or malaria). Symptoms include enlargement of the spleen, pain in the upper left side of the abdomen next to the stomach, and premature feelings

of fullness after meals because of the spleen's pressure on the stomach. In many cases of hypersplenism, the blood is deficient in one or more types of blood cells. Most people with hypersplenism require treatment for the underlying disorder. In some cases, the spleen is removed surgically, a procedure known as a splenectomy. Radiation of the spleen is also sometimes used to shrink the organ.

Hypertension

The medical term for high blood pressure. High blood pressure and hypertension are interchangeable terms used to describe blood traveling through the arteries at a pressure that is consistently too high to maintain good health. Although hypertension often causes no symptoms, it is dangerous. Left untreated, the disease leads to severe and possibly life-threatening damage to the heart, kidneys, and arteries.

Hypertension is the most common chronic disease affecting people in the United States. The incidence of the disease increases with age. In addition, hypertension is more common among blacks than whites. Among blacks, the disease is often more severe and tends to appear earlier in life than among whites. Hypertension is more common among men than women in young adulthood and early middle age. Later in life, it affects women more than men.

BLOOD PRESSURE

Blood pressure measures the force exerted by the blood against the walls of the arteries. It results from two forces. One is the force of the heart as it contracts; the other is the resistance of the arteries to blood flow, which is a function of their flexibility and size. In general, the more blood the heart pumps with each beat and the narrower and less flexible the blood vessels, the higher the blood pressure.

Blood pressure is measured in millimeters of mercury (mm Hg) and given as two numbers that are written like a fraction, such as 125/75 mm Hg. The first, larger number, representing the blood pressure when the heart is contracting, is called the systolic pressure. The second, smaller number, representing the pressure between beats when the heart is relaxed, is called the diastolic pressure.

Blood pressure lower than 120/80 mm Hg is considered normal for cardiovascular health. A person with readings of 120-139/80-89 mm Hg is considered to have PREHYPERTENSION. Blood pressure that is consistently over 140/90 mm Hg indicates stage 1 hypertension. Blood pressure above 160/100 mm Hg is stage 2 hypertension.

Blood pressure rises and falls during the day in response to a number of variables, such as emotions, fatigue, stress, and physical exertion. As a result, blood pressure readings should be taken in a relaxed setting while the person is at rest. Any abnormal reading should be confirmed with follow-up readings over subsequent days and weeks. (For more information about how to take a blood pressure reading, see BLOOD PRESSURE.)

TYPES OF HYPERTENSION

Blood pressure results from the complex interaction of several factors, including the function of the kidneys, various hormones, and the condition of the arteries; therefore, it is often impossible to determine the exact cause of hypertension in a given person. When a cause cannot be established, a person is considered to have essential hypertension. Essential hypertension occurs in approximately 19 of every 20 people with the disease. The remaining 1 of 20 has an identifiable cause of his or her hypertension, such as medications (for example, oral contraceptives and nasal decongestants), certain kidney diseases (such as glomerular nephritis), and diseases of the adrenal glands (for example, Cushing syndrome). Hypertension with an identifiable cause is called secondary hypertension, in which case remedying the underlying problem usually returns the person's blood pressure to normal.

Older people with hypertension often have a form of the disease known as isolated systolic hypertension in which systolic pressure is 140 mm Hg or above and diastolic pressure is under 90 mm Hg. Isolated systolic hypertension was once thought to be a normal part of aging that did not require treatment. Recent research has shown, however, that treatment with medication significantly reduces the risk of stroke for people with isolated systolic hypertension.

Malignant hypertension is a form of hypertension in which blood pressure suddenly rises to extremely high levels. Malignant hypertension is more likely to occur in people who already have hypertension, particularly as a result of kidney disease, and is most common among young black men and among women who experienced toxemia during pregnancy. Malignant hypertension is a life-threatening medical emergency that requires hospitalization and treatment to prevent or minimize damage to the heart, kidneys, brain, and blood vessels.

SYMPTOMS

The majority of people with prehypertension or early stage hypertension cannot tell they have the disease because they usually experience no symptoms. Symptoms occasionally appear in a minority of people with stage 1 or stage 2 disease, but they are more likely to occur in those with advanced hypertension. Symptoms include fatigue, confusion, nausea or upset stomach, vision changes, excessive sweating, pale or red skin, nosebleeds, anxiety or nervousness, palpitations (the sensation of an unusually fast or irregular heartbeat), ringing or buzzing in the ears, erectile dysfunction, impotence, headache, and dizziness. However, even people with advanced hypertension may not have symptoms, which is why regular blood pressure checks are so important to early detection and treatment.

RISK FACTORS

Increasing age is a principal risk factor for essential hypertension. The disease is more common among blacks than whites. Obesity, a sedentary lifestyle, a diet high in salt, excessive use of alcohol, diabetes mellitus, smoking, and gout all increase the chance of hypertension. The chance of developing hypertension is greater among those who have one or both parents with the disease. Emotional issues, particularly the way in which a person responds to stress, may also contribute to the development of hypertension.

COMPLICATIONS

Left untreated, hypertension causes damage to various parts of the body or target organs, which can lead to disability or death.

BLOOD PRESSURE LEVELS

The Seventh Report of the Joint National Committee on Prevention, Detection, Evaluation, and Treatment of High Blood Pressure provides the following classifications for blood pressure levels.

CLASSIFICATION	SYSTOLIC (MM HG)	DIASTOLIC (MM HG)
NORMAL	less than 120	less than 80
PREHYPERTENSION	120-139	80-89
STAGE 1 HYPERTENSION	140-159	90-99
STAGE 2 HYPERTENSION	more than 160	more than 100

■*Heart and artery disease* The leading cause of death in people with hypertension is complications associated with CORONARY ARTERY DISEASE. Hypertension accelerates the buildup of fatty plaques in the arteries (see ATHEROSCLEROSIS), which can narrow or block the arteries that supply oxygen to the heart muscle. Heart-related chest pain (ANGINA) or a heart attack can result.

In addition, hypertension forces the heart to work harder to maintain a flow of blood to the body. To compensate, the heart may enlarge, thicken, or stiffen, reducing its ability to pump effectively, a condition called CARDIOMYOPATHY. Cardiomyopathy carries an increased risk of sudden death and heart attack. Also, when the heart pumps inefficiently and cannot push out all of the fluid returning to it from the body, fluid may accumulate in the lungs, legs, and feet. The result is congestive heart failure (see HEART FAILURE, CONGESTIVE), which can lead to disability and even death.

Hypertension can also cause an artery to balloon outward, a malformation known as an aneurysm. Rupture of an aneurysm in a major blood vessel, such as the aorta, usually results in sudden death.

■*Stroke* Hypertension is the leading risk factor for stroke, which occurs when there is blockage or rupture of a blood vessel in the brain.

■*Kidney disease* The extensive beds of microscopic blood vessels in the kidney are highly vulnerable to damage from hypertension. The resulting disease makes it more difficult for the kidneys to control the balance of salt, acids, and water in the body and to filter out impurities. Ironically, this damage may further increase blood pressure, which accelerates damage to the kidneys, creating a vicious cycle that can result in complete kidney failure.

■*Vision loss* Like the kidney, the retina (light-sensitive layer at the back of the eye) is easily damaged by high blood pressure. Over time, the damage can degrade vision and even lead to blindness.

TREATMENT

When a doctor determines that a person has consistently high blood pressure, he or she next determines whether the disease is essential or secondary. This requires a review of a person's medical history and laboratory tests to look for kidney disease or other potential underlying causes. If hypertension is secondary, treatment is directed at the underlying cause. If it is essential, treatment consists of lifestyle changes and, if these fail to control the blood pressure, medications.

Lifestyle changes include quitting smoking, losing weight (particularly in the abdomen), limiting alcohol use to two drinks per day for men and one for women, exercising regularly, and changing diet. Research has shown that a diet rich in fruits, vegetables, whole grains, and low-fat or nonfat dairy products and low in meat, fats, oils, and salt significantly reduces blood pressure. Stress management techniques, such as meditation, are also helpful.

In some cases, lifestyle changes are sufficient to control hypertension. If they are not, medication can make a difference. A number of different drugs are available, depending on

H

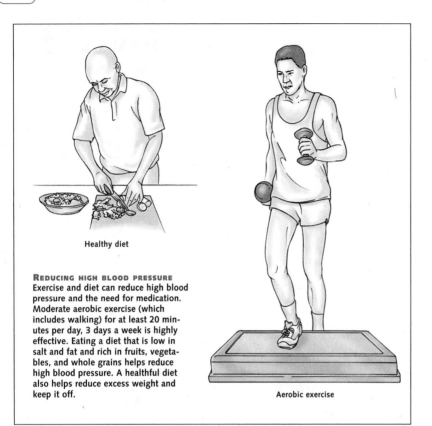

Healthy diet

REDUCING HIGH BLOOD PRESSURE
Exercise and diet can reduce high blood pressure and the need for medication. Moderate aerobic exercise (which includes walking) for at least 20 minutes per day, 3 days a week is highly effective. Eating a diet that is low in salt and fat and rich in fruits, vegetables, and whole grains helps reduce high blood pressure. A healthful diet also helps reduce excess weight and keep it off.

Aerobic exercise

medical history and the severity of the hypertension. Diuretics promote the production of urine in the kidneys, helping to rid the body of excess fluids and minerals, particularly sodium. They may cause abnormally low potassium levels and require the use of potassium supplements. Alpha blockers and beta blockers inhibit certain receptors in the nervous system, helping arteries relax and decreasing the force of the heartbeat, thereby reducing blood pressure. Beta blockers are particularly useful for people who already have heart disease. Angiotensin-converting enzyme (ACE) inhibitors reduce the activity of chemicals that cause blood vessels to constrict, allowing the blood vessels to relax and dilate (widen), easing the passage of blood through them. Angiotensin II receptor blockers (ARBs) are among the newest antihypertensive drugs. Calcium channel blockers, which relax the heart and blood vessels, are commonly used to lower blood pressure.

PREVENTION
The likelihood of developing hypertension can be reduced by following sensible lifestyle precautions, such as a low-fat, heart-healthy diet; salt intake restriction; regular exercise; moderation of alcohol use; maintaining healthy body weight; and abstinence from tobacco use.

Hypertension, pulmonary

A serious disease in which blood pressure in the arterial network supplying the lungs with blood (pulmonary arteries) is abnormally high. In people with pulmonary hypertension, pulmonary artery blood pressure is approximately two or more times higher than normal. The condition arises because the blood vessels in the lungs have narrowed, restricting blood flow. As a consequence, blood pressure in the pulmonary arteries rises, and the right ventricle (a lower chamber) of the heart has to work harder to pump blood into the lungs. The valves on the right side of

the heart may begin to leak (called regurgitation), and the right side of the heart may thicken, enlarge, and fail to pump properly, a condition known as COR PULMONALE.

There are two kinds of pulmonary hypertension. Primary pulmonary hypertension has no known cause and is very rare. Secondary pulmonary hypertension arises as a result of another condition or disease, such as a heart defect, chronic lung disease, pulmonary embolism (a blood clot in the lungs), or the use of certain drugs, particularly cocaine and some diet aids. Obesity, air pollution, living in high altitudes, and physical inactivity are known risk factors. Primary pulmonary hypertension is most common in women between 20 and 40 years old, but it can affect both sexes at any age, including children.

Symptoms include bluish skin, chest pain, coughing (sometimes with blood), swollen neck veins, dizziness, fainting, enlarged liver, shortness of breath, swollen ankles or feet, swollen abdomen, and fatigue. Pulmonary hypertension is often difficult to diagnose because symptoms may come on slowly and vary greatly among individuals.

There is no cure for pulmonary hypertension, but the disease can often be managed effectively. Lifestyle changes are important. These include avoiding strenuous physical activity, alternating short periods of regular exercise with rest, eating a healthy diet, and restricting salt intake. Supplemental oxygen may also be recommended. A number of medications are also available: anticoagulants to reduce the risk of blood clots, calcium channel blockers to lessen the workload on the heart, cardiotonics to strengthen the heartbeat, diuretics to eliminate extra fluid from the body, and vasodilators to relax blood vessels and improve blood flow. In extreme cases, in which disease is advanced and death likely, a heart-lung transplant may be considered.

Hypertensive hemorrhage

Bleeding caused by hypertension (high blood pressure). Hypertensive hemorrhage typically occurs in the blood vessels of the brain and is also known as cerebral hemorrhage. Chronically high blood pressure can weaken small blood vessels in the brain, leading them to swell, burst, and leak blood into the surrounding area. The blood irritates the brain tissues causing swelling, and the blood collects into a mass known as a hematoma. The swelling and the hematoma eventually destroy the affected brain tissue. The severity of the hemorrhage and the symptoms it causes depend on the location and extent of the bleeding. Symptoms can come on suddenly or gradually. They include rapid loss of function on one side of the body, changes in vision, numbness, tingling, difficulty speaking or swallowing, difficulty reading or writing, loss of coordination or balance, seizure, headache, nausea or vomiting, and change in consciousness, such as extreme apathy or sleepiness. Surgery to remove the hematoma is performed if the damage is likely to cause death or major disability. Medications are also used to control blood pressure, reduce swelling in the brain, stop seizures, and reduce pain.

Hyperthermia

An abnormally high body temperature; also used to describe deliberate elevation of the body temperature for therapeutic purposes. See also HEAT DISORDERS.

Hyperthermia, malignant

Also known as malignant HYPER-PYREXIA; an inherited condition that causes a severe uncontrollable fever when a person is under general anesthesia (see ANESTHESIA, GENERAL) or taking muscle relaxants. This condition is often associated with diseases such as MUSCULAR DYSTROPHY. In most cases, malignant hyperthermia is diagnosed the first time a person undergoes anesthesia. Symptoms include muscle rigidity and a high fever; muscle destruction and death due to acute renal failure can result if the person is not treated immediately with medications such as dantrolene. Malignant hyperthermia can be prevented by the person taking appropriate medications before anesthesia.

Hyperthyroidism

A condition produced by excess thyroid hormone in the bloodstream, which leads to overactivity of the metabolism of the body. The three most common causes of hyperthyroidism are GRAVES DISEASE; toxic multinodular GOITER, in which several nodules on a diffusely enlarged thyroid gland become overactive; and toxic ADENOMA, in which a benign nodular growth secretes excess hormone. THYROIDITIS can cause temporary hyperthyroidism, as does taking too much oral thyroid hormone medication. Rarely, hyperthyroidism is caused by excess thyroid hormone secreted from abnormal tissue growth in a woman's ovaries.

Graves disease, an autoimmune disorder, is the most common cause of hyperthyroidism. Antibodies against the thyroid gland interrupt the ability of the thyroid gland to regulate hormone secretion and cause it to produce excess hormone. It may be hereditary and is most common in young to middle-aged women, but the cause is unknown. A benign (not cancerous) thyroid tumor or nodule that secretes excess thyroid hormones in an uncontrolled manner is another principal cause of hyperthyroidism. It is not known why the thyroid nodules become overactive and result in hyperthyroidism. Thyroiditis associated with hyperthyroidism may be caused by an infection; however, the specific virus or bacteria has not yet been identified.

SYMPTOMS

The symptoms of hyperthyroidism can vary from person to person. They can include nervousness, irritability, increased perspiration, thinning of the skin, brittle hair, shakiness, increased heart rate, palpitations, elevated blood pressure, more frequent bowel movements, increased appetite, unexplained weight loss, insomnia, confusion, irregular menstrual periods, sensitivity to light, and weakness in the large muscle groups of the upper arms and thighs.

DIAGNOSIS AND TREATMENT

A complete medical history, physical examination, and DIAGNOSTIC IMAGING for hyperthyroidism are generally used to diagnose the disorder. The procedures include blood tests to measure the levels of thyroid hormone in the bloodstream and THYROID SCAN-NING using a radioactive substance to produce an image of the thyroid gland and assess its activity. This scan differentiates overactivity in the entire gland from overactivity in one or more nodules, as well as the inflammation of thyroiditis. A sensitive blood test for measuring TSH (thyroid-stimulating hormone) in the bloodstream can confirm the diagnosis.

The goal of treating hyperthyroidism is to restore thyroid hormone to normal levels. Treatment decisions depend on a person's general health and medical history, the type and severity of hyperthyroidism, a person's tolerance or preference among the various treatment options, and the doctor's expectations of how the disease will progress.

Treatment includes antithyroid medications to lower the level of thyroid hormones in the blood, radioactive iodine taken as a pill or liquid to destroy thyroid cells and slow production of thyroid hormones, and surgery to remove an overactive nodule or nodules or larger areas of thyroid tissue. It is common after surgery or radioactive iodine treatment for the remaining tissue to not make enough thyroid hormone and, over time, cause HYPOTHYROIDISM (underactivity of the thyroid gland). The individual will then need treatment with thyroid hormone supplements.

Drugs that block the activity of thyroid hormones in the body, which are known as BETA BLOCKERS, are generally used to control symptoms such as palpitations, increased heart rate, and excessive perspiration. Beta blockers do not lower high levels of thyroid hormones, but they are useful for reducing symptoms until treatment aimed at lowering thyroid hormones take effect.

Hypertonia

An abnormal increase in muscle tone. Hypertonia is a symptom of certain genetic disorders and may result in arm or leg deformities. When hypertonia is caused by damage to the central nervous system, it is usually called spasticity.

Hypertrophy

Enlargement or overgrowth of a body part or organ due to an increase in the size of its cells. Organs such as the

H

heart, liver, and muscles are prone to hypertrophy, a condition that can cause medical problems. Treatment is aimed at the underlying cause.

Hyperuricemia

A condition in which blood levels of uric acid become elevated. Uric acid is a waste product of normal metabolic processes. Hyperuricemia is the result of too little uric acid being excreted or too much being produced. Excessive amounts in the bloodstream can lead to GOUT. Diuretics such as hydrochlorothiazide and others in the thiazide class, which are taken for high blood pressure, may cause hyperuricemia in some people. ALLOPURINOL is one medication commonly used to treat hyperuricemia. It works by inhibiting the synthesis of uric acid.

Hyperventilation

Excessive, rapid, deep breathing that leads to reduced carbon dioxide in the blood. Hyperventilation usually occurs in people who are anxious or tense, but it may be a symptom of specific disorders, including asthma, croup, severe pain, chronic obstructive pulmonary disease (COPD), pneumonia, diphtheria, pleurisy, and other diseases. People who hyperventilate may complain of numbness or tingling in the lips, mouth, hands or feet; they may have muscle twitching; or they may faint. Hyperventilation usually occurs in young adults, more often in women than in men. If symptoms persist for more than 15 minutes despite breathing into a paper bag, or if the person complains of chest pain, medical help should be sought. If no medical problem is found, relaxation techniques are often the mainstay of therapy.

Hyphema

Bleeding within the front portion (anterior chamber) of the eye. A hyphema usually results from a blunt or penetrating injury to the eye. It can also be caused by certain medical conditions, including severe inflammation of the iris (the colored portion of the eye), an abnormal blood vessel, or cancer of the eye. If a person with a hyphema remains upright for a while, a blood level appears in front of the iris. A hyphema carries a risk of acute GLAUCOMA, which causes

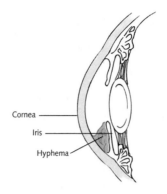

BLEEDING IN THE EYE
Hyphema, or bleeding between the cornea and the iris, usually as the result of injury, makes the eye appear filled with blood and causes pain and blurred vision. Immediate medical treatment is necessary.

pressure inside the eyeball to rise suddenly and damages the optic nerve. Hyphemas need prompt evaluation by an eye specialist to determine the causes of the bleeding and assess its severity. Emergency treatment is indicated if severe pain or nausea and vomiting are present.

In mild cases, a hyphema resolves on its own within a few days. With more pronounced bleeding, bed rest, patching of both eyes, limitation of movement, and sedatives are often prescribed. If pressure within the eye increases, an eye specialist may remove the blood surgically.

Hypnosis

A sleeplike mental state in which the individual is unusually open to suggestion and may behave, think, or perceive in uncharacteristic or seemingly impossible ways. Under hypnosis, consciousness is reoriented from the outside world to mental, sensory, and physiological experiences. Hypnosis is usually induced by a hypnotist who engages the attention of the individual with monotonous, repetitive commands. It can also be self-induced by focusing on breathing or silently repeating a monotonous phrase. Contrary to popular belief, hypnosis cannot be used to make someone perform actions against his or her will.

The depth of hypnosis depends largely on the person being hypnotized. Practically everyone can be hypnotized, but only a small number of people can be hypnotized deeply. In a typical light hypnotic state, the

individual is aware of his or her actions and can remember them on returning to ordinary consciousness. In a deep trance, the individual is unaware and loses memory of what happened (hypnotic amnesia).

Hypnosis has been used medically for pain control in cancer, childbirth, burns, and minor surgery. It can also be used to help frightened children tolerate potentially painful medical procedures, such as needle sticks for blood specimens, stitches, spinal taps, or injections. Hypnosis can also be used to treat anxiety, posttraumatic stress, conversion disorders, and morning sickness in pregnancy. It is also a useful therapeutic technique for helping people remember forgotten actions, stop smoking, control overeating, overcome abnormal fears (phobias), and resolve insomnia. But it is not used to replace anesthesia during surgical procedures.

Exactly what causes a person to become hypnotized remains unclear. Some researchers believe that hypnosis is a special and unusual state of consciousness that taps into aspects of the mind not normally accessible. Others maintain that hypnosis simply refocuses ordinary consciousness and does not represent a special state of mind.

Hypnotic drugs

Drugs used to decrease the time needed to fall sleep. Hypnotic drugs prescribed to treat insomnia, or sleeplessness, include BENZODIAZEPINES; novel nonbenzodiazepine hypnotic drugs, including ZOLPIDEM and ZALEPLON; ANTIDEPRESSANTS at low doses; the hormone MELATONIN; and chloral hydrate.

Nonprescription hypnotic agents are also available to induce sleep; most of them contain antihistamines. While some people find that these agents make them drowsy and help them fall asleep, they are associated with side effects and can cause next-day "hangover."

Benzodiazepines are more effective sleep inducers, but they are associated with the risks of overdose, addiction, and withdrawal. The relatively new nonbenzodiazepine hypnotic drugs have a very short duration of effect and are less likely to cause daytime sleepiness or hangover effects. Chloral hydrate is considered a weak hypnotic, but it is very addicting.

Hypoaldosteronism

A condition resulting from a deficiency of the hormone ALDOSTERONE, which is normally produced by the adrenal cortex (the outer layer of the adrenal glands). Hypoaldosteronism produces biochemical changes in the body that result in a low level of sodium in the blood combined with an increased level of potassium. The condition is often associated with kidney disease, especially in people with diabetes mellitus (see DIABETES MELLITUS, TYPE 1 and DIABETES MELLITUS, TYPE 2). In this instance, it is caused by low levels of RENIN and ANGIOTENSIN (enzymes involved in regulating blood pressure) combined with inadequate secretion of aldosterone. In other cases, hypoaldosteronism is the result of a hereditary defect in an enzyme involved in aldosterone production. Symptoms include general weakness and an increased risk of serious heart rhythm abnormalities, which can be fatal. Administering fludrocortisone, a synthetic MINERALOCORTICOID, is the most common treatment because oral aldosterone cannot be properly absorbed by the body.

Hypochondriasis

A persistent and abnormal preoccupation with physical health combined with the fear that one is suffering from a grave or major undetected illness, even though medical evidence to support that worry is lacking. An individual with this mental illness (commonly called a hypochondriac) misinterprets a sign or symptom as proof of disease, continues in the belief that disease is present despite medical reassurance, and suffers significant distress or impairment in social, occupational, or family settings because of the preoccupation with disease. Symptoms are often vague and ambiguous, and they may change over time. In many cases, people with this disorder go from doctor to doctor seeking a diagnosis and believe they are not getting proper care.

Hypochondriasis has no specific cause, but often appears in the relatives or friends of people who have actually suffered the feared disease. It occurs equally commonly in men and women. It can be associated with panic attacks.

Hypochondriasis can lead to serious complications in addition to the pain and discomfort the individual feels from the symptoms. Repeated diagnostic tests to determine the cause of the complaints can be risky and expensive. Because people with the disorder have a history of unsubstantiated complaints without physical evidence, physicians may miss the appearance of a real disease. Family and work life can be seriously disturbed by the preoccupation with sickness. In severe cases, a person with hypochondriasis may become an invalid. Other disorders, including anxiety and depression, are common.

Treatment consists of developing a relationship with one medical provider to prevent unnecessary testing, reassuring the patient that follow-up will control symptoms, encouraging discussion about causes of stress, and teaching new ways of dealing with worries. Family involvement in treatment is often helpful.

Hypogamma- globulinemia

An antibody deficiency that involves low levels of gamma globulin in the bloodstream and is characterized by both an immune system disorder and an autoimmune disorder. Gamma globulin is a class of immunoglobulin, IgG, that includes four kinds of antibodies. Normally, these antibodies enter tissue spaces and coat antigens, which makes the antigens readily absorbed by other cells involved in the immune system. In hypogammaglobulinemia (HGG), this function is disrupted. There is a depressed antibody response, and some of the antibodies that are produced attack the body's own tissues. Sometimes certain blood cells, including red blood cells, white blood cells, and platelets, are attacked and destroyed.

Hypogammaglobulinemia is also known as common variable immunodeficiency because the symptoms and results vary among people who have it. Evidence of the disorder usually appears in infancy or early childhood, but may not become apparent until adulthood, and is then referred to as late-onset or adult-onset immunodeficiency. This group of antibody deficiency disorders is usually inherited.

SIGNS, SYMPTOMS, AND DIAGNOSIS

Infections experienced by people with hypogammaglobulinemia frequently involve the respiratory tract (recurrent ear infections, chronic sinusitis, recurrent pneumonia, and bronchiectasis) and the gastrointestinal system (diarrhea caused by the poor absorption of protein, fat, and certain sugars). People with hypogammaglobulinemia may be particularly predisposed to infection caused by exposure to certain bacteria, such as *Campylobacter* or *Yersinia*, or parasites, such as *Giardia lamblia*. There is also an increased frequency of autoimmune disorders, such as rheumatoid arthritis, pernicious anemia, idiopathic thrombocytopenic purpura, and autoimmune neurological disorders, such as Guillain-Barré syndrome. Finally, people with hypogammaglobulinemia have an increased risk of developing malignant tumors in their 50s or 60s.

Hypogammaglobulinemia is sometimes suspected in children or adults who have a medical history of recurrent infections that involve the ears, sinuses, airways, and lungs. The diagnosis can be confirmed by blood tests that reveal a low level of immunoglobulins in the bloodstream. People who have been completely immunized against polio, measles, diphtheria, and tetanus have extremely low or absent antibodies to the microorganisms that cause these diseases. To determine what kind of antibodies a person can produce and in what quantities, vaccines may be used to measure the immune system's ability to produce antibodies. This may help a doctor determine whether a person might benefit from injections of GAMMA GLOBULIN.

TREATMENT

The goal of treatment is to prevent new infections and stop the development of chronic lung disease. An individual who has hypogammaglobulinemia can almost always benefit from injections of gamma globulin, providing there is no significant defect in a certain lymphocyte. Gamma globulin is extracted from human plasma and consists primarily of immunoglobulin G, or IgG, as well as all the necessary antibodies present in a normal human system. The immunoglobulins have been modi-

H

fied so that injections can be made directly into the veins.

In the presence of bacterial infections, including those associated with chronic sinusitis and chronic lung disease, long-term treatment with broad-spectrum antibiotics is generally required. If BRONCHIECTASIS occurs, physical therapy and POSTURAL DRAINAGE, involving physical therapy of the lungs, are generally necessary to remove pus from the airways and lungs. People with hypogammaglobulinemia must also be carefully observed for the possible development of malignant tumors, particularly of the gastrointestinal or lymphoid tissues.

Hypoglycemia

FOR FIRST AID
see Diabetic coma, page 1319
see Hypoglycemia, page 1326

Low blood sugar. Hypoglycemia occurs when the blood level of glucose becomes too low to supply the need for fuel in the body. In people who take insulin, hypoglycemia is sometimes referred to as an insulin reaction because it is a response to excessive insulin in the bloodstream. It is generally defined as a blood sugar level lower than 60 milligrams per deciliter (mg/dL). It most commonly occurs in people with type 1 diabetes (see DIABETES MELLITUS, TYPE 1), especially when meals are skipped or not eaten at properly scheduled times, when physical exercise is unusually long or strenuous, when alcohol is consumed on an empty stomach, or when the dosage of insulin or other diabetes medication is not properly adjusted. Sometimes hypoglycemia may occur in people with type 2 diabetes (see DIABETES MELLITUS, TYPE 2) if they take certain diabetes medications or insulin.

Symptoms of hypoglycemia include nervousness, shakiness, fatigue, increased perspiration, sensation of cold, hunger, confusion, irritability, and impatience. The most immediate treatment is to eat something that quickly raises the blood sugar level, such as glucose tablets, sugar-containing hard candy, fruit juice, or soda. If untreated, hypoglycemia can lead to seizures, unconsciousness, and even death.

Some people who experience hypoglycemia are not aware of the usual symptoms. They need to measure their blood glucose more frequently, especially when they exercise, drive, or operate dangerous machinery.

Medical help is essential if a person with hypoglycemia loses consciousness or is unable to swallow. GLUCAGON can be injected to quickly raise blood sugar.

In rare instances, some individuals experience a low level of glucose when fasting. Pancreatic disorders, such as an adenoma that secretes too much insulin, can cause a low blood sugar level. Hypoglycemia can also occur with inadequate pituitary gland function or severe liver disease.

Less common is a reactive hypoglycemia in which people experience symptoms of low blood sugar a few hours after eating. Another type of hypoglycemia occurs in people who have had all or part of their stomachs removed, leading to abnormally rapid movement of food into the intestines. Rapid absorption of carbohydrates can stimulate excessive insulin secretion, causing hypoglycemia. People with type 1 diabetes occasionally have a late but excessive release of insulin after a carbohydrate-rich meal. The glucose level may be elevated 2 hours after eating but drop below normal later as the delayed but increased insulin production begins to have an effect.

Hypogonadism

A condition produced by a decrease or total lack of the secretion of hormones from the testicles (see TESTICLE) in men and boys and the ovaries (see OVARY) in women and girls. Hypogonadism results from a deficiency of two hormones from the PITUITARY GLAND—FSH (follicle-stimulating hormone) and LH (luteinizing hormone) or the failure of the testes or ovaries to make hormones.

FSH and LH have an essential role in stimulating the testicles and the ovaries to secrete the SEX HORMONES that make possible a person's normal sexual development at puberty. Two gland disorders may result in the deficiency that produces hypogonadism. Damage to the pituitary gland can inhibit the stimulation of the sex hormones, resulting in delayed puberty and the development of secondary sexual characteristics. Failure of the HYPOTHALAMUS to produce LH-RH (luteinizing hormone–releasing hormone) can result in a failure to stimulate the sex hormones in the pituitary gland.

CAUSES
Failure of the testes or ovaries to produce the sex hormones or a lack of the hormones that stimulate them may be caused by CRANIOPHARYNGIOMA (a brain tumor that develops near the pituitary), a tumor in the area of the hypothalamus, Kallmann syndrome (a hereditary absence of the front part of the pituitary gland), rare chromosomal defects, and head injuries. Hypogonadism may also be associated with alcoholism and other chronic illnesses, including kidney disease and SICKLE CELL ANEMIA.

Diseases of one or both testicles, including MUMPS, may interfere with production of the male hormone TESTOSTERONE and lead to hypogonadism. Other elements that may temporarily or permanently impair the synthesis of testosterone and result in hypogonadism include physical trauma to the testicles and certain medications and therapies, including X-ray therapy and chemotherapy for the treatment of cancer.

SIGNS AND SYMPTOMS
The signs of hypogonadism depends on the stage of life in which the condition originates. In males, if the appropriate sex hormones are not released during early fetal development, the external genitals may be affected, leading to a condition in which the sex of the newborn is not obvious.

If a deficiency of the male hormone androgen occurs at puberty, the physical changes characteristic of this phase do not take place. The signs of hypogonadism in men may include decreased muscle mass and failure to develop secondary sexual characteristics such as pubic hair. A disturbance of skeletal development may cause unusually long arms and legs.

When hypogonadism occurs during adulthood, male sexual potency and fertility are decreased. A man's beard and pubic hair may grow sparsely, his skin may become thinner, his hips may widen, and he may experience enlarged breasts and OSTEOPOROSIS (loss of bone mass). A man may also experience weakness, a loss of interest in sexual activity, and an inability to achieve an erection or to ejaculate.

TREATMENT

The treatment of hypogonadism is generally based on its cause. A complete evaluation by an ENDOCRINOLOGIST (a specialist in the hormone-producing glands) can determine the source of the disturbance and the appropriate course of treatment. The male sex hormone testosterone may be administered, generally by intramuscular injection. GNRH (gonadotropin-releasing hormone) taken by nasal inhalation offers another treatment option. Females may be treated with estrogen and progesterone. Conventional endocrinological treatment is usually successful in eliminating all or most of the symptoms of hypogonadism when it is initiated at the onset of the disorder causing the abnormalities.

Hypohidrosis

An abnormal condition characterized by inadequate perspiration. Hypohidrosis leads to heat intolerance and extreme discomfort after physical exertion or after eating hot or spicy foods. It is often accompanied by other abnormalities in the growth of body structures or cells.

Hypomania

An abnormally expansive, elevated, highly energized, or irritable mood that comes on quickly, lasts for at least 4 days, and represents a distinct change from the person's normal, day-to-day mood. The change in mood is accompanied by inflated self-esteem or grandiosity, a decreased need for sleep, rapid and loud speech, far-fetched ideas, distractibility, increased involvement in goal-directed activities such as business or artistic ventures, and excessive involvement in pleasurable activities that can have painful consequences, such as sexual affairs, buying sprees, or reckless driving. Hypomania is usually not severe enough to cause difficulty in work, social, or school settings, and it does not cause hallucinations (such as

hearing the voices of the dead) or delusions, such as believing that one is someone else. Hypomanic episodes can last for several weeks or months and are often preceded or followed by a period of depression. In some cases, hypomania progresses to the more extreme mood change known as MANIA and may have a role in the development of BIPOLAR DISORDER.

Hypoparathyroidism

A condition caused by a deficiency of PARATHYROID HORMONE in the blood as the result of damaged or absent parathyroid glands, which are located on the thyroid gland in the neck. Hypoparathyroidism may be produced by the surgical removal of the parathyroid glands, damage to the glands caused by parathyroid disease, infection, hemorrhage, or structural and functional damage due to physical trauma. Symptoms of hypoparathyroidism include numbness, tingling, and muscle cramps and twitching; seizures can also occur. Insufficient levels of parathyroid hormone can cause hypocalcemia (low levels of calcium in the blood). Hypoparathyroidism may be treated with vitamin D and calcium supplements.

Hypophysectomy

The surgical removal of the hypophysis (pituitary gland). Hypophysectomy is usually performed to slow the

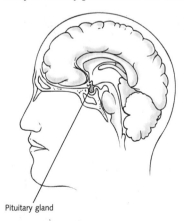

Pituitary gland

REMOVAL OF PITUITARY GLAND
The hypophysis, or the pituitary gland, can be surgically removed to treat cancer or serious hormonal disorders. After surgery, hormone replacement medication compensates for the loss of pituitary function.

growth of some cancers such as breast, ovarian, and prostate cancer. It is also used to eradicate pituitary tumors, which cause the majority of disorders of the pituitary gland.

Hypophysectomy is indicated when the hormonal activity or size of the pituitary tumor makes its removal necessary due to severe and possibly life-threatening hormonal disorders or to the pressure the tumor exerts on surrounding tissues. It is the usual treatment for disorders such as CUSHING SYNDROME and ACROMEGALY. Hypophysectomy is also sometimes performed to treat a PROLACTINOMA or a CRANIOPHARYNGIOMA.

The safest, most effective, and least disfiguring type of hypophysectomy is a transsphenoidal hypophysectomy. In this procedure, a surgeon removes the pituitary gland through an incision in the upper portion of the nasal passages. If this approach is not possible because of the size or position of the tumor, the surgeon must perform a craniotomy, which involves making an incision in the front portion of the skull.

Hypopituitarism

A disorder resulting from a deficiency in one or more of the pituitary hormones. The tendency for hypopituitarism may be inherited.

Hypopituitarism can be caused by a tumor on the pituitary gland or by inflammation of the gland. It may develop after a serious head injury that damages the pituitary gland. Sometimes the cause is unknown. If there is excessive overgrowth of the pituitary gland during a woman's pregnancy and the gland remains enlarged after childbirth, the woman may experience hypopituitarism.

The pituitary gland acts as a master control in the endocrine system, stimulating and regulating many important body functions. Because the production and activities of hormones released by other glands are stimulated by the hormones from the pituitary gland, their functions may be affected by an underproduction of the pituitary hormones. This may result in hypopituitarism producing symptoms of other disorders, including HYPOTHYROIDISM (underactivity of the thyroid gland) and ADDISON DISEASE.

H

The effects of hypopituitarism depend on which of the pituitary hormones are deficient. A life-threatening inability of the body to respond properly to physical stresses, including injury and illness, is caused by deficiency of the pituitary hormone that controls adrenal function. Impairment of the growth hormone results in problems with physical development, including unusually SHORT STATURE. Loss of sex hormones can cause absent menstrual periods in women and a loss of fertility and sex drive in men. Hormone replacement therapy can help to overcome these problems.

Hypopituitarism is diagnosed by blood and urine tests to measure hormone levels. When warranted, DIAGNOSTIC IMAGING, including MRI (magnetic resonance imaging), may be performed to detect tumors and other tissue overgrowth that may be causing or contributing to the disorder.

Hypoplasia

The failure of an organ to develop completely and reach its normal adult size; also refers to the lack of complete development of tissue in the body.

Hypoplasia, enamel

The incomplete development of tooth enamel (see ENAMEL, DENTAL) that produces abnormal tooth color and shape. Enamel hypoplasia may affect a single tooth with mild discoloration or white spotting, or the surface of many teeth may be deeply pitted. The enamel may be yellowish; the surface may flake and chip or show surface wrinkling. Enamel hypoplasia may be due to heredity or caused by environmental conditions, such as vitamin deficiencies, illness with high fever when the teeth are forming, certain venereal diseases, and FLUOROSIS. Trauma at birth and local infections of an abscessed primary tooth may also cause the condition. Dental treatments for enamel hypoplasia depend on the severity of the condition. Bonding, veneers, and crowns (see BONDING, DENTAL; VENEERS, DENTAL; and CROWN, DENTAL) may help to correct cosmetic problems. Partial or complete DENTURES or dental implants (see IMPLANTS, DENTAL) may be options in

more severe cases when tooth loss is involved.

Hypoplastic left heart syndrome

A serious congenital disease (present at birth) in which severe malformation of the chambers, valves, and blood vessels on the left side of the heart prevents blood from being pumped efficiently into the rest of the body. Before the 1990s, babies with hypoplastic left heart syndrome usually survived for only a few weeks. Now such infants can be treated by HEART TRANSPLANT or the Norwood procedure, a series of three open-heart surgeries performed from infancy through the toddler years. Chances for survival past childhood for those with hypoplastic left heart syndrome who have undergone either heart transplant or the Norwood procedure remain unknown.

Hypospadias

A developmental abnormality in males in which the urethra opens on the underside of the penis. Surgery to correct the birth defect is usually successful.

Hypotension

FOR SYMPTOM CHART
see Dizziness, page 36

FOR FIRST AID
see Fainting, page 1321

Low blood pressure. Physicians define hypotension as blood pressure below 90/60 millimeters of mercury (mm Hg) (see BLOOD PRESSURE for details on how blood pressure is measured). People whose blood pressure is consistently borderline low or slightly low usually exhibit no symptoms and do not require treatment. However, particularly in older persons, hypotension can indicate problems with the heart or nervous system, such as hypothyroidism (an underactive thyroid), diabetes mellitus, heart disease, hypoglycemia (low blood sugar), liver disease, or anemia. Hypotension can also result from the overdosing of medication to control blood pressure, high or low body temperature, substantial blood loss, allergic reaction (for example, to a bee sting), severe blood infection, or dehydration. Temporary hypotension

can result from heavy menstrual bleeding, unusually hot weather, overheating (for example, from too much time in a hot tub, a sauna, or the sun), or sudden emotional shock. Symptoms of hypotension include dizziness or light-headedness, fainting, blurry vision, lack of concentration, cold and clammy skin, nausea or stomach upset, muscle weakness, weak and rapid pulse, headache, and fast and shallow breathing. If blood pressure falls so low that the oxygen supply to the brain and other organs is insufficient, the person may lose consciousness or go into shock.

Postural hypotension refers to a situation in which blood pressure drops suddenly when a person stands up. Light-headedness or dizziness follow, and fainting may occur. Postural hypotension is most common in older people, and it is worsened when a person is hungry, thirsty, tired, or overheated. Postural hypotension increases the risk of a bad fall, a serious health risk in older people.

Treatment of hypotension depends on the underlying cause. If hypotension results from another disorder, treatment of that problem may resolve the hypotension. Hypotension can also be managed by raising blood pressure with increased fluid and salt intake and medication. People with postural hypotension are advised to get up slowly and in stages, to avoid going too long without food or drink, to wear support stockings, and to spend only short periods in the sun.

Hypothalamus

A structure located near the center of the base of the BRAIN. The hypothalamus directs the workings of the AUTONOMIC NERVOUS SYSTEM, which regulates vital, involuntary functions such as blood pressure, sleep, body temperature, appetite, and thirst. The hypothalamus also directs the hormonal activities of the PITUITARY GLAND.

The hypothalamus has nerve connections to most other regions of the nervous system. The hypothalamus controls the SYMPATHETIC NERVOUS SYSTEM, which prepares the body for a response to stress—the so-called fight-or-flight mechanism. When a person becomes alarmed or excited, the hypo-

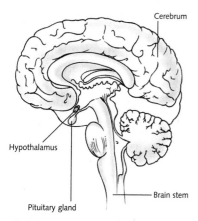

LOCATION OF HYPOTHALAMUS
The hypothalamus, about the size of a large grape, is located in the forebrain, just above the pituitary gland. Its nerve connections extend throughout the body, enabling the hypothalamus to direct the overall fight-or-flight response to stress.

thalamus triggers responses all over the body—the heart beats faster, breathing increases, the pupils of the eyes widen, saliva production in the mouth decreases, blood flow to the muscles increases, and the adrenal glands produce the hormones epinephrine and norepinephrine.

The hypothalamus also controls body temperature. When body temperature is low, it switches on mechanisms—such as narrowing blood vessels, increased burning of fat, and shivering—to produce heat. When the body temperature is high, these mechanisms slow down, and other processes, such as sweating, increase.

The hypothalamus also receives and transmits information from internal organs about the level of sugar (glucose) in the blood to regulate appetite and about the body's water content to regulate thirst. The hypothalamus is involved in regulating sleep, mood, emotions, and sexual drive.

The hypothalamus directs the activity of the powerful ENDOCRINE SYSTEM (hormonal system) by stimulating and inhibiting production of hormones by the pituitary gland. Specialized blood vessels carry hormones and nerve pathways carry nerve signals from the hypothalamus to the nearby pituitary gland. In response to each of these mechanisms, the pituitary gland produces hormones that stimulate other hor-

mone-producing glands throughout the body. Some of these hormones are involved in growth and development, the function of the reproductive organs, body metabolism, skin pigmentation, and pregnancy and breast-feeding in women.

Hypothermia

A condition in which the body temperature drops below 95°F. Hypothermia is usually caused by prolonged exposure to cold and occurs when more heat is lost than the body can generate. The onset of symptoms of hypothermia is usually slow and includes a gradual loss of mental and physical ability. The person with hypothermia may be entirely unaware of the condition. Other symptoms include apathy, lethargy, confusion, large pupils, drowsiness, loss of coordination, weakness, slow pulse, dizziness, slurred speech, and uncontrollable shivering. People who are very old, very young, very thin, hungry, tired, or under the influence of alcohol or drugs are most likely to experience hypothermia, as are those with heart or circulation disorders.

Hypothermia commonly happens when a person falls overboard from a boat, is outside in winter with an uncovered head, or wears wet clothes for long periods in windy, cold weather. Excessive physical exercise in cold weather, inadequate

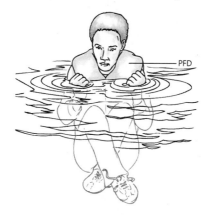

PFD

SURVIVAL IN COLD WATER
Use of a personal flotation device (PFD) greatly increases survival time in cold water; it supports even an unconscious person and enables the person to remain still to conserve heat. The heat escape lessening posture (HELP), bringing the limbs up against the body, also maximizes survival time.

fluid intake, or inadequate diet can also contribute to hypothermia.

Emergency treatment includes getting the person out of the cold and into warm, dry clothing. If it is not possible to get indoors, the person's head should be covered, and the person should be insulated from the cold ground. Warm drinks not containing alcohol may be given, unless the person is vomiting. The person's arms or legs should not be massaged. Emergency medical assistance should be sought.

Hypothyroidism

A condition resulting from a deficiency of the thyroid hormone THYROXINE. The thyroid, located in the front of the lower part of the neck, produces thyroxine to regulate the metabolism of the body. When this hormone is decreased to abnormally low levels, there is a slowing of the metabolism. The decrease in energy production disrupts many vital functions, including heart rate and ability to regulate temperature. Older people tend to be more susceptible to hypothyroidism.

CAUSES
Almost all cases of hypothyroidism are caused by underproduction of thyroxine as a result of a disorder within the thyroid gland that inhibits its ability to make enough thyroid hormone. This may be due to complications of thyroid surgery or treatments for HYPERTHYROIDISM (overactivity of the thyroid gland), including radioactive iodine therapy. Autoimmune disorders that make antibodies which attack the thyroid gland may also cause hypothyroidism. Rarely, a congenital defect in the gland may cause hypothyroidism in newborns. Transient episodes of hypothyroidism are generally caused by inflammation of the tissue or viral infections of the thyroid gland.

Less commonly, hypothyroidism may result when the hypothalamus or pituitary gland is not functioning properly. The hypothalamus stimulates the pituitary to release TSH (thyroid-stimulating hormone) in a chain reaction that activates the thyroid hormone. When there is a disruption in this chain reaction, the thyroid gland may be capable of functioning properly but is not receiving the

H

signal from the pituitary gland to produce thyroxine. This is called secondary hypothyroidism and is usually the result of impaired pituitary function caused by a tumor, an infection, SARCOIDOSIS, or spreading cancer. In rare instances, secondary hypothyroidism is caused by impairment of the hypothalamus.

SYMPTOMS

Symptoms of hypothyroidism differ among individuals, depending on the severity of thyroxine deficiency. The symptoms of a mild insufficiency may include sensitivity to cold temperatures, dry skin, constipation, and forgetfulness. Symptoms of more severe hypothyroidism include (in addition to the mild symptoms) chronic fatigue, muscle stiffness and cramping, poor appetite combined with weight gain, hair loss, hoarseness, decreased heart rate, and depression and other psychological problems. Untreated, advanced hypothyroidism may produce MYXEDEMA. Symptoms of myxedema include lack of facial expression; thinning hair; swelling around the eyes; enlarged tongue; shortness of breath; severe lethargy; cool, thickened skin; dementia; and even coma.

Newborns with hypothyroidism may have a hoarse cry and difficulty feeding; they are often constipated and less active. Untreated, this congenital form of hypothyroidism produces unusually SHORT STATURE, thin hair, bulging abdomen, delayed dental development, and impaired mental functioning. In an older child, hypothyroidism causes delayed puberty and symptoms similar to those of an adult.

DIAGNOSIS AND TREATMENT

When hypothyroidism is suspected, a doctor evaluates the person's medical history and conducts a physical examination. As part of the examination the doctor feels the thyroid gland, which may be enlarged. The skin, hair, abdomen, heart, neurological system, and musculoskeletal system are also examined carefully.

Blood samples are taken to measure the levels of thyroid hormones and TSH in the bloodstream. An elevated TSH level indicates an abnormally functioning thyroid gland. The blood may also be tested for cholesterol and for other abnormalities associated with hypothyroidism. Cardiac tests,

including an electrocardiogram, may be done if there are physical findings involving the heart.

Temporary hypothyroidism caused by inflammation or infection of the thyroid gland is generally not treated because hormone levels return to normal within months.

Chronic forms of hypothyroidism from other causes are lifelong disorders that are usually treated with synthetic forms of thyroxine such as LEVOTHYROXINE, liothyronine, and liotrix. Dosages must be adjusted carefully to prevent hyperthyroidism caused by excess amounts of thyroxine. If the hypothalamus or pituitary gland is involved, hydrocortisone (see CORTICOSTEROIDS) may need to be taken to prevent the risk of adrenal deficiency caused by replacing the depleted thyroxine.

Thyroid hormone replacement therapy usually relieves symptoms of hypothyroidism quickly. People of advanced age and people with heart problems may need to take the hormone replacement in small, progressive increments to prevent overstimulation of the heart, so they will experience improvement more gradually. Early signs of hypothyroidism in infants and children are immediately and consistently treated with thyroid hormone replacement therapy; serious symptoms such as problems with short stature, maturation, and mental development are all prevented by early treatment. In the United States, most states now recommend routine screening for hypothyroidism in the neonatal period.

Hypotonia

Decreased muscle tone. Hypotonia most commonly occurs in infants and causes an affected baby to seem exceptionally floppy—like a rag doll. The condition may be the result of a serious underlying problem such as cerebral palsy, Down syndrome, Tay-Sachs disease, or muscular dystrophy. When hypotonia involves one part of the body as a result of injury, the affected part is said to be flaccid or weak.

Hypotonia in infants

Decreased muscle tone in infants, usually indicating the presence of genetic, muscle, or central nervous

system disorders. Infants who are hypotonic feel floppy when held, and when at rest, they lie with their limbs loosely extended, unlike infants with normal muscle tone, who tend to flex their elbows and knees. Hypotonic infants often display poor or no control of their heads. Hypotonia can be a symptom of DOWN SYNDROME, MYASTHENIA GRAVIS, PRADER-WILLI SYNDROME, WERDNIG-HOFFMANN DISEASE, MARFAN SYNDROME, MUSCULAR DYSTROPHY, TAY-SACHS DISEASE, TRISOMY 13 SYNDROME, and CONGENITAL HYPOTHYROIDISM.

Hypovolemia

An abnormally low circulating blood volume. BLOOD LOSS in hypovolemia may be due to internal BLEEDING from the intestine or stomach; external bleeding from an injury; or loss of blood volume and body fluid associated with problems such as diarrhea, vomiting, dehydration, or burns. If the hypovolemia is severe, hypovolemic shock can occur, with symptoms that may include a rapid or weak pulse, feeling faint, pale skin, cool or moist skin, rapid breathing, anxiety, overall weakness, and low blood pressure. Emergency medical attention must be sought. The person should be kept warm and assisted to lie down with his or her feet slightly elevated (unless there is a severe head, back, or leg injury). If there is an external wound, sterile dressings and steady, firm, direct pressure should be applied.

Hypoxia

An inadequate supply of oxygen to the tissues. A lack of oxygen causes changes in breathing and neurologic symptoms that range from headaches and confusion to, rarely, a loss of consciousness. Hypoxia can be acute and severe, as when a person has an airway obstruction, acute hemorrhage, or cardiorespiratory failure. These conditions lead to a rapid depletion of oxygen to the tissues and a loss of consciousness. Chronic hypoxia, which may be due to the effects of emphysema or another lung disease, causes persistent fatigue and mental sluggishness and gradual damage to internal organs such as the heart. Cerebral hypoxia, in which circulatory failure deprives the brain of oxygen, causes irreversible brain damage after 4 to 6 minutes.

Hysterectomy

A surgical procedure in which a woman's uterus is removed. Hysterectomy is the second most common major surgical procedure performed on women in the United States, although the number of procedures performed has been declining. Hysterectomies are performed for a number of reasons. They may be done to treat fibroid tumors, excessive bleeding, endometriosis, or prolapse of the uterus or to remove a cancerous growth.

There are different types of hysterectomies. In a subtotal hysterectomy, only the body of the uterus is removed, leaving the cervix. In a total hysterectomy, the entire uterus and the cervix are removed. Radical hysterectomies involve removal of the uterus, cervix, surrounding tissue, lymph glands, part of the vagina, and sometimes the fallopian tubes and ovaries.

THE PROCEDURE

A woman may have an abdominal hysterectomy (in which an abdominal incision is made to remove the uterus) or a vaginal hysterectomy (in which the uterus is removed through the vagina). An abdominal hysterectomy will likely be done if a woman's uterus is enlarged or cancerous or if her ovaries also need to be removed. In an abdominal hysterectomy, an incision is made into the abdomen, either horizontally along the upper

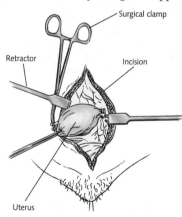

ABDOMINAL HYSTERECTOMY
For an abdominal hysterectomy, an incision is made in the abdomen and the uterus and cervix are cut away and removed. The vagina is sutured shut at its top end. If necessary, the ovaries and fallopian tubes are similarly cut away and removed. An abdominal hysterectomy is done if the uterus is enlarged or cancerous.

> ### WHEN IS A HYSTERECTOMY NECESSARY?
>
> A hysterectomy is major surgery and should be performed only after a clear diagnosis has been made. In the past, hysterectomies were done to treat symptoms such as bleeding or pain. But now the doctor will want to know what disease or abnormality is causing the symptoms before hysterectomy is considered. Women who have other serious medical problems have an increased risk of complications from a hysterectomy and should explore possible alternatives. The procedure is not an appropriate treatment for symptoms of menopause or premenstrual syndrome.
>
> Hysterectomy is indicated for early-stage cervical cancer, endometrial cancer, and most cases of ovarian cancer. However, not all cancers, fibroids, and other disorders require a hysterectomy. Alternative treatments and less invasive surgical procedures may be appropriate alternatives to hysterectomy. Women need to discuss alternatives, such as hormone therapy and laparoscopic surgery, with their doctors. Second opinions can be very helpful.

pubic hairline or vertically between the navel and pubic hair. The uterus is exposed and cut from the ligaments and other tissues that hold it in place. If necessary, the ovaries and fallopian tubes also may be removed. The cervix is then freed from the bladder, and the cervix and uterus are cut away from the vaginal wall and removed.

A woman's uterus may be removed through the vagina if it is not swollen by disease. Recovery from a vaginal hysterectomy is much faster, because there is no abdominal incision. In a vaginal hysterectomy, the labia and vulva are retracted to give access to the vagina. An incision is made in the front wall of the vagina, through which the bladder is moved aside to expose the uterus. The ligaments and tissues that hold the uterus in place are cut, and it is removed. A particular challenge of vaginal hysterectomy is avoiding damage to the urinary tract. A vaginal hysterectomy can also cause a shortening of the vagina, which later can lead to pain during intercourse.

Under some conditions, a laparoscopically assisted vaginal hysterectomy is performed. Combining laparoscopic surgery (surgery done using a viewing instrument) with a vaginal approach can allow a woman who might otherwise require a large abdominal incision to benefit from the shorter recovery period of a vaginal approach.

Following the procedure, a woman will be in the hospital for several days. At first, she may have a catheter inserted into her bladder, and she may receive fluids intravenously. After discharge from the hospital,

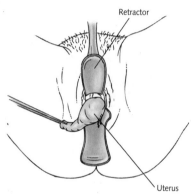

VAGINAL HYSTERECTOMY
For a vaginal hysterectomy, the vaginal opening is held opened with retractors, and an incision is made in the vaginal wall. The bladder is moved aside, and the uterus is cut away and removed through the vagina. A vaginal hysterectomy, which is easier to recover from because there is no abdominal incision, can be done if the uterus is not diseased.

painkillers are usually prescribed. A follow-up examination at the doctor's office is usually conducted 4 to 6 weeks after surgery. After that, she can usually resume sexual intercourse and other normal functions. If her ovaries have been removed, the woman's estrogen supply will be severely reduced, and menopause will begin.

Hysteria

An emotional disorder in which the person develops one or more dramatic physical symptoms, such as blindness, paralysis, altered consciousness, or abdominal pain; the symptoms are not due to organic or physical disease but can be traced to unconscious psychological reasons. The technical term "hysteria," which is distinct from the popular word meaning an emotional outburst, is used rarely in contemporary psychiatry. Rather, the various types of hysteria are recognized as separate disorders. They include CONVERSION DISORDER (in which physical symptoms mimic a major disease but lack physical basis), DISSOCIATIVE DISORDERS (in which consciousness is altered, as in amnesia), FACTITIOUS DISORDER (in which the person feigns the symptoms of disease out of a psychological need to be sick), and SOMATIZATION DISORDER (in which the individual is preoccupied with physical symptoms at times of stress).

Hysterosalpingogram

An X-ray procedure (also called an HSG) used to visualize the uterus and fallopian tubes. Via a thin tube, a special dye is injected through the cervix into the uterus. X rays are then taken to trace the dye as it moves through the uterus and fallopian tubes. A hysterosalpingogram may be done for either infertility or recurrent miscarriages, because blockages in the fallopian tubes or abnormalities of the uterus can result in infertility or miscarriage.

Hysteroscopy

A surgical procedure in which a hysteroscope (a thin, telescopelike instrument) is inserted through a woman's vagina and into the uterus to allow the doctor to view and treat a condition in the uterus. A hysteroscopy may be done in a doctor's office or in an operating room with local, regional, or general anesthesia. In some cases, little or no anesthesia may be needed. A diagnostic hys-

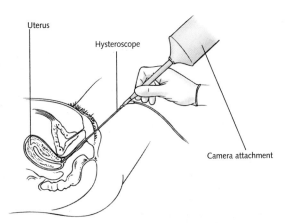

VIEWING THE UTERUS
A hysteroscopy allows the doctor to look inside the uterus to evaluate problems and treat some conditions. The hysteroscope is a lighted, tubular instrument that is inserted into the vagina. A liquid or gas is injected through the uterus to expand it for a better view. Instruments (such as a laser) can be passed through the hysteroscope to perform some procedures.

teroscopy is a safe procedure that poses little risk.

Hysteroscopy can help diagnose or treat a problem. It is useful for evaluating abnormalities in the uterus and can also be used to confirm the results of other tests. Sometimes a hysteroscopy is used in conjunction with another test or procedure. For example, it may be done before a D AND C (dilation and curettage) procedure or at the same time as a laparoscopy. Conditions for which a diagnostic hysteroscopy may be done include abnormal uterine bleeding, infertility, repeated miscarriages, a displaced IUD (intrauterine device), or for the detection of scar tissue or abnormal growths, such as polyps or fibroids. Sometimes treatment can be combined with a diagnostic procedure. For example, polyps and adhesions (scar tissue) in the uterus can be removed by using a hysteroscope.

SURGERY AND RECOVERY

Before the procedure, a woman may receive a sedative to help her relax. A local anesthetic may be injected around the cervix to numb it. Another drug may be used to block the nerves that receive sensation from the pelvic area. When local and regional anesthesia are used, a woman will remain awake during the procedure. If general anesthesia is used, she will be unconscious. The cervix may need to be dilated before insertion of the hysteroscope into the uterus. A gas is released through the hysteroscope to inflate the uterine cavity to allow a better view of the inside of the uterus.

When a local anesthetic has been used, a woman can usually return home after a short recovery period. After general anesthesia, the recovery period is longer. A woman may feel some discomfort until her body absorbs the gas released during the procedure. Some women feel sick and have vaginal bleeding or cramps for 1 or 2 days following the procedure. Fever, severe abdominal pain, or heavy vaginal bleeding or discharge should prompt an immediate visit to the doctor.

Iatrogenic

Any undesirable condition occurring as a result of a treatment or medicine. Iatrogenic disease is one caused inadvertently by a doctor, surgeon, diagnostic procedure, or medication, such as an infection acquired during the course of treatment or the side effect of a medication.

Ibuprofen

See NONSTEROIDAL ANTI-INFLAMMATORY DRUGS.

ICD

Implantable cardioverter defibrillator. See DEFIBRILLATOR.

Ichthyosis vulgaris

A condition characterized by dry, rectangular scales on the skin that is most pronounced on the legs. Ichthyosis vulgaris is the result of a hereditary skin defect that causes excessive accumulation of scales on the skin. Symptoms vary in severity. Mild cases cause primarily cosmetic problems. More serious ichthyosis leads to painful, bleeding cracks in the skin that can become infected if left untreated.

Dermatologists diagnose ichthyosis according to its characteristic appearance. The goal of treatment is to reduce scaling and add moisture to the skin. Topical keratolytics (such as lactic acid and alpha-hydroxy acids) reduce scaling. Effective moisturizers contain urea and petrolatum and should be applied immediately after bathing to help moisturizers penetrate the skin.

ICSI

Intracytoplasmic sperm injection. An IN VITRO FERTILIZATION procedure in which a single sperm is injected into an egg through the thick, transparent membrane surrounding it using a delicate microscopic technique.

Icterus

Another term for JAUNDICE, a yellowing of the skin and whites of the eyes.

Id

In FREUDIAN THEORY, the unconscious part of the self that is the seat of instinctual drives, particularly aggression and sex. These drives cause a person to seek immediate satisfaction, which is perceived as pleasure. The id is dominated by the pleasure principle and moves the person to strive toward immediate gratification.

Idiopathic

Of unknown cause. An idiopathic disease is one that develops for no apparent reason or cause. An example is essential HYPERTENSION, or high blood pressure for which no clear cause can be found. Even when the reason for a disease remains unknown, there may still be a recognizable pattern and progression of symptoms, and it may still be treated and cured.

Idiopathic thrombo-cytopenic purpura

See ITP.

Ileal pouch–anal anastomosis

A surgical procedure in which the colon and rectum are removed and part of the ileum (the lowest part of the small intestine) is used to construct an internal pouch in which waste collects. Ileal pouch–anal anastomosis is performed to treat large-bowel disease such as ulcerative COLITIS. This procedure ensures a high degree of continence and an acceptably low number of daily bowel movements.

A light or liquid diet is prescribed for several days before surgery. At this time, antibiotics and bowel-cleansing enemas are administered to rid the intestine of bacteria. The operation is done in a hospital under general anesthesia. The surgeon removes the diseased colon and fashions a pouch from the ileum. A temporary ILEOSTOMY allows the discharge of feces through a STOMA (an artificial opening created in the abdominal wall) into a device that adheres to the skin.

Following surgery, nutrients are given intravenously while fluid is drained from the abdomen and tissue heals. Once there is output through the ileostomy, a light diet is prescribed. Usually, the individual can

return home 5 to 8 days after surgery; the ileostomy is generally closed 3 months later, once the intestine has recovered from initial surgery. Continence improves substantially during the first year after surgery. The most common complication is inflammation of the pouch.

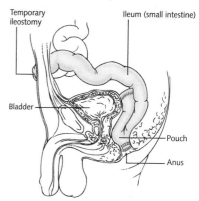

REMOVAL OF THE COLON
Ileal pouch–anal anastomosis is major surgery usually done in two operations. In the first procedure, the colon and rectum are removed. The surgeon constructs a pouch from part of the ileum, as shown here, and attaches the pouch directly to the anus. To allow the pouch to heal, the upper part of the ileum is temporarily brought through the abdominal wall (a procedure called an ileostomy) so that waste can be passed into a collection bag.

Ileitis

See CROHN DISEASE.

Ileostomy

A surgical procedure in which a stoma, an artificial opening, is created in the abdominal wall. After an ileostomy, the lower part of the ileum (the small intestine) opens through the stoma to allow the discharge of feces into a device attached to the skin. An ileostomy is different from a COLOSTOMY, in which the colon opens through a stoma.

An ileostomy is generally done in conjunction with another surgical procedure being done to treat a serious digestive disorder such as colon cancer (see COLON, CANCER OF THE), COLITIS, or DIVERTICULAR DISEASE. The operation is done in a hospital under general anesthesia. Ileostomies can be temporary or permanent. When temporary, the stoma is surgically closed once the intestine has recovered from inflammation or surgery. The stoma is usually placed on the lower right quarter of the abdomen in an ileostomy. See also COLECTOMY; ILEAL POUCH–ANAL ANASTOMOSIS.

Digested food passes through the stoma and is collected in an odor-free device called a pouch or appliance. The device is not bulky and cannot be detected through clothing. Instruction on keeping the stoma clean and how to empty the pouch is necessary. In a continent ileostomy, an internal pouch is created from a person's intestine. Instead of wearing an external appliance, the individual periodically drains the contents of the internal pouch through a tube. It may take several months to adjust to the new hygienic habits required after an ileostomy. Eventually, the routine takes no longer than did visits to the bathroom before the procedure.

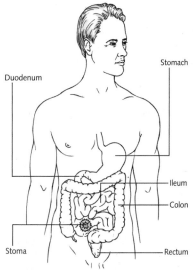

HOW AN ILEOSTOMY WORKS
An ileostomy is a procedure to bring the ileum (the part of the intestine just above the colon) through an opening in the abdominal wall so that waste can pass into a collection bag without passing through the lower digestive tract. To perform the procedure, the surgeon creates an opening (stoma) in the abdominal wall, brings the ileum through the opening, and stitches the rim of the ileum to the abdominal wall. The person wears a bag that covers the stoma, so that waste flows into the bag where it collects before being disposed of.

Ileum

The final and longest portion of the small INTESTINE; an important part of the DIGESTIVE SYSTEM. Together, the duodenum, the jejunum, and the ileum compose the small intestine. The ileum, about 12 feet in length, passes from the jejunum to the large intestine, or COLON.

The function of the ileum is to absorb nutrients from food that has been broken down in the stomach and first parts of the small intestine. The muscular layers of the ileum wall are very thin, and the inner layer (like all of the small intestine) contains millions of villi and microvilli (tiny projections with maximum surface area) that absorb the nutrient molecules into the minute vessels of the blood and lymphatic systems.

Ileus, paralytic

A serious condition in which the muscles of the small intestine become paralyzed and fail to function normally. Paralytic ileus may develop following abdominal surgery or in people who are otherwise severely ill. (See also PSEUDO-OBSTRUCTION.) It can be caused by inflammatory conditions such as a perforated ulcer, acute diverticulitis, or acute CHOLECYSTITIS.

In paralytic ileus, a person is unable to pass gas or propel intestinal contents and have a bowel movement. It can sometimes mimic an obstruction or other blockage of the intestines. Retained gas distends the abdomen and intestines; as the swollen abdomen presses against the chest, breathing can become difficult. Fever, vomiting, and persistent abdominal pain may occur. Even if pain lessens, treatment is required to prevent potentially life-threatening complications.

Paralytic ileus is treated by decompressing the intestine. A long tube is passed into the mouth and through the stomach into the intestine to suck out accumulated air and fluid. After abdominal surgery, some degree of ileus is anticipated and routinely treated. When severe conditions such as diverticulitis or perforation give rise to ileus, they may require emergency surgery.

Illness

Sickness, disease, or poor health. Many factors determine a person's susceptibility to illness. These include both genetic components and environmental influences. Although a person cannot control genetic pre-disposition, he or she can make intelligent decisions about diet, exercise, and habits such as smoking, drinking, and sexual activity. Proper lifestyle choices can help prevent many diseases. Doctors also recommend having regular checkups in order to diagnose illnesses as early as possible. For certain diseases, such as breast cancer or colon cancer, early detection can make a critical difference in outcome.

Illusion

A misperception of an external stimulus. For example, during alcohol withdrawal, some alcoholics will see shadows on a wall as insects or rodents. Illusions are often associated with LSD (lysergic acid diethylamide) use. An illusion differs from a HALLUCINATION in that the perception is false but the stimulus itself is real.

Imipramine

An antidepressant drug. Imipramine (Tofranil) is a tricyclic antidepressant that works by enhancing the action of the neurochemicals serotonin and norepinephrine in the central nervous system. Imipramine is also used to treat bed-wetting in children older than 6 years.

Immobility

The state of being unable to move independently as a result of disability or disease. Immobile persons must rely on caregivers to help them change position frequently in order to prevent problems such as pressure sores.

Immune globulins

Proteins obtained from human plasma; passive immunizing agents. Immune globulins are prepared as a sterile solution of globulins containing many antibodies that are normally present in adult human plasma. Immune globulins are used to boost immunities in people whose own immune systems are compromised, such as by HIV (human immunodeficiency virus) infection, leukemia, lymphoma, aplastic anemia, and other conditions involving bone marrow failure.

Immune globulins are used to protect immunocompromised people against hepatitis A and B, measles, pertussis (whooping cough), poliomyelitis, varicella (chickenpox), human rabies, and tetanus. They are also given to people who are not immunocompromised: for example, immune globulins are recommended for newborn babies exposed to chickenpox and for mothers who contract chickenpox shortly before or after delivery. The duration of the immunity provided by immune globulins is immediate, but it lasts for only a few months.

Immune response
The body's defense against a foreign substance, or antigen, that has entered or been introduced into the system. In an immune response, the immune system examines antigens and, under normal conditions, identifies them as "self" or "nonself." Nonself cells are attacked and destroyed by antibodies produced by certain LYMPHOCYTES in response to a specific antigen on the surface of the nonself cell. When a faulty or mistaken identification is made, the immune response may be activated against self cells, resulting in AUTOIMMUNE DISORDERS.

The immune system's response the first time an antigen is encountered is called the primary immune response. The response that occurs the second and subsequent times an antigen is encountered is called the secondary immune response. The secondary immune response is shorter, faster, and broader than the primary immune response.

Immune serum globulin
See IMMUNOGLOBULINS.

Immune system
The complex set of mechanisms by which the body prevents or fights infection by disease-causing microorganisms such as bacteria, viruses, and fungi. The immune system also fights abnormal cells such as cancer cells. The immune system must first identify organisms or cells as harmful or abnormal, and then fight them. Some of these defenses are innate, while others are acquired as the body encounters specific organisms and responds to them.
NATURAL IMMUNITY
The body has many natural, or innate, protections against infection.

These mechanisms are called the nonspecific immune system because they respond to any invading organism in the same way. Some of them are physical barriers or chemical defenses in body structures. Most microorganisms cannot penetrate the skin; they can enter the body only through the mucous membranes like those that line the mouth. The oil in the skin and sweat act to destroy some microbes, and in the mouth, saliva is similarly toxic. The respiratory tract, starting at the nose, traps many more would-be invaders. The hairs in the nose trap organisms, and the sneeze reflex expels them. In the mucous membranes that line the throat and other passages in the respiratory tract, mucus stops the microbes, and tiny hairs called cilia move them out; coughing also expels them. In the digestive system, stomach acids and helpful bacteria in the intestines ward off disease-causing organisms, and the urinary tract and vagina also contain disease-fighting bacteria.

In addition to these mechanisms, inflammation is a basic body response to infection. If an organism does get into the bloodstream, as when injury breaks the skin, some white blood cells release chemicals that cause the blood vessels to widen and increase blood flow. The area becomes red, swollen, and warm. White blood cells called phagocytes are drawn to the infected site, and the phagocytes surround the microbe and absorb it. The phagocyte then dies, and accumulated debris is called pus. A different type of phagocyte cleans up the debris. This mechanism is called the inflammatory response.

Another natural mechanism is a type of white blood cell called a killer cell, which chemically destroys disease organisms and cancer cells. Interferon, part of a natural immune response, is a type of specialized protein that the body produces to defend against viruses. The interferons prevent the virus from multiplying.
ADAPTIVE IMMUNE SYSTEM
If the nonspecific immune system fails to destroy disease organisms, the body can send in a different kind of cell that can recognize specific organisms and develop a specialized defense. The basic functional cell of

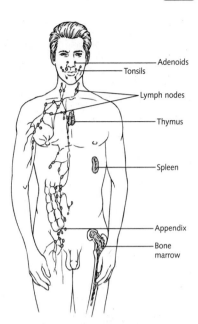

ORGANS OF THE IMMUNE SYSTEM
The lymphatic system, composed of clusters of lymph nodes connected by lymphatic vessels, carries disease-fighting white blood cells (lymphocytes) throughout the body. The thymus maintains lymphocytes while the spleen contains white blood cells. The tonsils and the appendix are made of lymphoid tissue. White blood cells are produced in the soft marrow of the bones.

the adaptive immune system is the lymphocyte, a type of white blood cell. There are two types of lymphocytes that are involved in two means of adaptive immune response: B cells, which perform in antibody defenses, and T cells, which perform in cellular defenses.

An ANTIBODY is a protein produced by B cells to fight a specific invading microbe. The antibody recognizes a protein, called an ANTIGEN, on the invading cell and binds to its specific shape. This binding process destroys the organism. After the infecting organism is destroyed, some of the B cells or lymphocytes develop a memory for the shape of the antigen. If that organism ever infects the body again, the B cells can immediately make antibodies to fight it. The body has developed IMMUNITY to that microorganism.

T cells are lymphocytes that have completed their development in the thymus, an organ of the lymphatic system located in the upper chest. In cellular defenses, one type of T cell called a helper T cell identifies antigens of a specific invading organism and summons killer T cells. The killer T cells multiply aggressively and chemically destroy the disease-causing microbes. Some of the T cells retain memory of the organism so that the body has built-in immunity in case of another infection. See ALLERGIES; IMMUNIZATION; and IMMUNE SYSTEM DISORDERS.

If the immune system mistakenly identifies the body's own cells or tissues as harmful and attacks them, the result is one of the AUTOIMMUNE DISORDERS.

Immune system disorders

Disorders caused by problems with the body's mechanisms for protecting itself against viruses, bacteria, and other foreign substances. Immune system disorders result in conditions in which some portion of the IMMUNE RESPONSE is weak or absent. They occur when there is a breakdown in the complex network of specialized cells and organs that normally defends the body against invasions by harmful agents. These agents, or antigens, include bacteria, viruses, fungi, and parasites. The immune system works as the body's mode of defense by seeking out and destroying the antigens as they enter or are introduced into the body.

In one form of immune system disorders, called AUTOIMMUNE DISORDERS, the immune system mistakenly identifies the body's own normal cells or tissues as foreign and attacks these cells and tissues as though they were antigens. Multiple interacting factors may contribute to the development of autoimmune diseases. These factors may include genetic predisposition, immunologic abnormalities, and even microbial infections. Furthermore, combinations of these factors may lead to a great variety of abnormalities in disease processes.

Many diseases and conditions are known or believed to be associated with immune deficiency disorders. They include the following: ADDISON DISEASE, ANKYLOSING SPONDYLITIS, HEPATITIS, celiac sprue, CREST SYNDROME, CROHN DISEASE, discoid lupus, FIBROMYALGIA, GRAVES DISEASE, GUILLAIN-BARRÉ SYNDROME, HASHIMOTO THYROIDITIS, hemolytic

anemia, idiopathic pulmonary fibrosis, insulin-dependent diabetes (see DIABETES MELLITUS, TYPE 1), JUVENILE RHEUMATOID ARTHRITIS, lupus (see LUPUS ERYTHEMATOSUS, SYSTEMIC), MULTIPLE SCLEROSIS, PSORIASIS, RAYNAUD PHENOMENON, REITER SYNDROME, RHEUMATIC FEVER, RHEUMATOID ARTHRITIS, SARCOIDOSIS, SCLERODERMA, SJÖGREN SYNDROME, ulcerative colitis (see COLITIS), VASCULITIS, and VITILIGO.

Immunity

The body's ability to defend itself against potentially harmful foreign substances and cells called antigens. Immunity invokes the IMMUNE RESPONSE, which includes both nonspecific and specific components. It initially activates nonspecific immune responses followed by highly specific responses that are exactly matched to the specific threats presented. Immunity is associated with the body's defense against disease-causing agents, problems with organ transplants and blood transfusions, and diseases resulting from an overreaction to antigens, such as occurs in AUTOIMMUNE DISORDERS, and underreaction, such as with AIDS (acquired immunodeficiency syndrome).

HOW IT WORKS

When microorganisms are able to penetrate the body's barriers, including the skin and mucous membranes of the respiratory, digestive, or urinary tracts, inflammation occurs. This inflammatory response often prevents the spread of infectious agents, including viruses, bacteria, and fungi. If it cannot prevent these agents from spreading, a system of proteins referred to as the "complement system" assists in the destruction of foreign cells to complement the immunity activity.

Immunity is based on the production of antibodies that are specifically matched to specific antigens. The antibodies bind to the antigens and inactivate or destroy them. One form of immunity is termed antibody-mediated immunity. It is regulated by B cells, which originate as lymphocytes in the bone marrow and produce antibodies that can defend cells in the body infected by viruses and bacteria. These antibodies can also protect against parasites, fungi, and protozoa and kill cancerous body

cells. T cells are lymphocytes that have migrated to the thymus and circulate in the blood to help the body's defenses. T cells may be referred to as helper cells or suppressor cells.

Immune responses are initiated by the recognition of a foreign antigen. This leads to the activation of lymphocytes that respond to elimination of that antigen. The mechanism of this specific immunity is divided into three phases. The cognitive phase consists of the binding of foreign antigens to specific antibody molecules or the surface of B lymphocytes. This is followed by the activation phase, in which B lymphocytes differentiate to antibody-secreting cells that eliminate the antigen. The third phase is the effector phase, which requires the participation of nonlymphoid cells. For example, antibodies bound to foreign antigens can be eliminated by phagocytes. There may be activation of plasma proteins, which may help to eliminate antigens.

CATEGORIES OF IMMUNITY

Immunity offers the body protection from infection by the response of the immune system. There are four categories of immunity designated by their origins. Active immunity is the immune response to an infectious substance of an immunologically healthy person. When the immune system of an immunologically healthy person responds to a VACCINATION, the term for this is acquired immunity. Innate immunity is the protection present from birth that is activated in a consistent manner when it is required. Passive immunity is the protection that results from the transfer of antibodies from one person to another, as when a mother passes her antibodies to an unborn fetus.

Immunization

The process of inducing the protection of antibodies to create IMMUNITY as a preventive measure against particular infectious diseases. Immunization is accomplished when a person has a VACCINATION that introduces antibodies into the body or prompts the body's immune system to create its own antibodies. The antibodies are generally administered as a VACCINE that consists of a suspension of whole or partial bacteria or viruses that have been treated to prevent them from causing disease in the person being immunized. The vaccine is given to elicit an immune response in the body and prevent a person from becoming infected with a particular disease. Not all immunizations are entirely safe for everyone, and some may not be completely effective, but they have provided widespread protection from disease in many parts of the world and continue to do so. While there are risks involved in immunization, the benefit of disease prevention has been found to clearly outweigh the risks.

Immunizations given routinely in the United States include vaccines against measles, mumps, and rubella; against tetanus, diphtheria, and pertussis, called the DTaP vaccine (see DTaP VACCINATION); against hepatitis B for those at risk of exposure; against influenza A, for those at high risk of serious consequences from flu infection, particularly those older than 65 years; against pneumococcal pneumonia, for those at risk; and varicella vaccine for those at risk. See also TRAVEL IMMUNIZATION.

Immunoassay

Any one of several techniques for identifying and measuring the number of chemical substances that use the specific binding between an antigen and its corresponding antibodies. Immunoassays are diagnostic tools that can quantify the body's response to infection. Antigens are foreign substances or organisms in the blood that can cause infection and disease. Antibodies, the body's natural defense against infection, are complex substances that are prompted to form in response to the presence of foreign substances or organisms—including antigens—and serve to neutralize or destroy them. Immunoassay is also the technique for evaluating urine drug screens. Examples of immunoassays are enzyme immunoassay, radioimmunoassay, and fluoroimmunoassay.

Immunoglobulins

Proteins produced in the blood by the immune system. Many immunoglobulins are antibodies. Antibody molecules can be divided into distinct classes and subclasses based on their size, charge, solubility, and behavioral characteristics. In humans, the classes of antibody molecules are IgG, IgM, IgA, IgE, and IgD. These immunoglobulins each have a different role in the immune system's strategy to defend the body from invasions of harmful antigens. IgG has four kinds of antibodies, all of which can enter tissue spaces and coat microorganisms with a substance called complement to increase the rate at which they are attacked by other cells in the immune system. IgM generally remains in the bloodstream where it is effective at destroying bacteria. There are two kinds of antibodies in the classification called IgA, and they are concentrated in body fluids, including tears, saliva, and secretions in the respiratory system and gastrointestinal tract; they are able to protect the body from antigens attempting to enter a system via these fluids and secretions. IgE normally occurs in only trace amounts. IgE possibly evolved as a defense against parasites, but it is the antibody that overreacts to nonharmful substances that can cause severe allergic reactions. IgD is located within the membranes of B cells and works to regulate the cell's activation.

Immunologist

A physician trained in the medical specialty of the immune system's normal functions and possible disorders. An immunologist diagnoses, manages, and treats conditions and diseases related to the immune system. This physician has completed training to become an internist or pediatrician and has then completed at least two additional years of study and training, called a fellowship, in the medical specialty known as IMMUNOLOGY. Immunologists can then take an examination from the American Board of Allergy and Immunology (ABAI) to become ABAI-certified. Many immunologists manage and treat allergic diseases and may be referred to as allergists.

Immunology

The branch of science concerned with the study of the immune system and the various aspects of IMMUNITY and immune responses. Immunology is an area of scientific and medical study that analyzes the immune system and how it functions and explores ways in which it can be stimulated to protect against disease. The science is concerned with the specific responses made by LYMPHOCYTES (one type of white blood cells) to foreign substances and the interactions between antigens and antibodies. The study of immunity involves investigating the responses of lymphocytes that are beneficial in preventing infections and the treatment of infections caused by microorganisms.

Immunotherapy, allergen

A process of exposing the body to small, injected amounts of a particular allergen in gradually increasing doses until the body builds up immunity to the allergen. See DESENSITIZATION, ALLERGY.

Impaction, dental

Teeth embedded in the gums or jawbone that have not erupted because of a physical obstruction or overcrowding. An impacted tooth fails to erupt or erupts only partially because it is blocked by bone or gum tissue, or because it is jammed against another tooth. Some teeth tend to be involved more frequently. The teeth usually include the third molars (also called wisdom teeth), the upper canines (eye teeth), and the second premolars (teeth between cuspids and molars). SUPERNUMERARY TEETH (extra teeth) may also be involved. The wisdom teeth often only partially erupt, and the surrounding gum is susceptible to infection. They may sometimes erupt normally if left untreated.

CAUSES

Impaction may be caused by an insufficient space for the tooth to erupt into the area that normally holds the teeth. Heredity might be a factor in a child who has a small, narrow jaw with inadequate room for permanent teeth. In some cases, the problem will correct itself as the upper and lower jaws mature and become large enough to provide space for the emerging tooth or teeth.

The misdirection of the evolving tooth bud before its full development may cause the impaction, or it may be caused by a lack of space in the dental arch. Another cause may be a permanent tooth that develops slightly out of place in the jaw and becomes

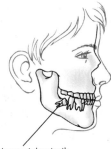

IMPACTED WISDOM TOOTH
Impacted lower wisdom tooth

The wisdom teeth commonly become impacted because of lack of room in the jaw. An impacted tooth fails to emerge through the gum because it is blocked by bone or gum tissue or by other teeth. The tooth can emerge at an angle instead of growing straight up, and some wisdom teeth emerge only part way through the gum, with some gum tissue remaining over the crown of the tooth.

impacted against another tooth as it attempts to emerge. The failure of teeth to erupt at the gum line can give rise to cysts and tumors around the follicle in the gum where the tooth should have erupted or around the tooth itself.

TREATMENT
X rays are used to diagnose dental impaction. Surgical removal of impacted teeth may be recommended if the teeth cannot be saved. The procedure is generally performed by an oral surgeon with the use of anesthesia. Impacted wisdom teeth are generally soft tissue impactions, which involve making a surgical incision in the gum tissue to allow the oral surgeon to grasp the tooth to be removed. If the teeth are deeply embedded in the jawbone or gum tissue, it may be necessary to remove surrounding bone and soft tissue to gain access to the tooth and remove it. If a tooth is completely embedded in bone and cannot emerge because of its misdirected position or being jammed against an adjacent tooth, removal can involve an incision through the gum, the elevation of a flap of gum tissue, and the removal of the covering bone. The exposed tooth may have to be removed in smaller pieces.

In most cases, impacted wisdom teeth that have been removed do not require replacement. When some impacted teeth are removed, howev-

er, they must be replaced to prevent adjoining teeth from tilting toward the vacant space and to prevent the corresponding tooth or teeth in the opposite jaw from emerging into the empty place. DENTURES, bridges, or dental implants (see BRIDGE, DENTAL; IMPLANTS, DENTAL) are commonly used to replace impacted teeth that are removed from other areas of the mouth.

Impairment

Damage, injury, or deterioration that affects the structure or function of normal physical or psychological abilities. Often the term is used to refer to sensory deficits, as in taste or hearing impairment. The degree of impairment is variable. For example, taste impairment ranges from an inability to perceive certain sensations (such as sweet or salty) to a complete loss of taste. Impairment also implies an increased risk for being involved in an accident because of a medical condition.

Imperforate anus

See ANUS, IMPERFORATE.

Imperforate hymen

A solid membrane covering the opening of the vagina. Normally, the hymen is perforated during early development in the womb, and it generally gets torn during vigorous childhood activities, but sometimes, a girl is born with no opening in her hymen. If this condition is noticed in infancy or childhood, a doctor can remedy this by cutting an opening in the central part of the membrane.

If the condition is not noticed before puberty, however, menstruation may have begun and menstrual blood may have accumulated in the vagina, blocked by the imperforate hymen. Early symptoms may include mild abdominal cramps and fatigue, but the girl may not realize she has begun to menstruate, since no blood has appeared. The vagina can hold a large volume of blood without stretching, and the girl may experience no other symptoms for some time. Eventually, however, the vagina becomes stretched and the accumulated menstrual blood can back up through the cervix and into the uterus. At that point, symptoms will

include lower abdominal and lower back pain, difficulty in urinating, and pain when defecating. Treatment involves surgical removal of a large central portion of the membrane.

Impetigo

A contagious, superficial skin infection. Impetigo is caused by *Staphylococcus* and *Streptococcus* bacteria, and most commonly occurs on unexposed areas of the arms, legs, and face. Impetigo can be found on normal, healthy skin, particularly on the legs of children, or it may sometimes follow a minor trauma that breaks the skin. It may also follow pediculosis, scabies, herpes simplex, herpes zoster (shingles), fungal infections, and insect bites.

The infection appears as groups of lesions that vary in size and form. The skin elevations may take the form of pea-sized, pus-filled, inflammatory pustules, or they may be larger and circular, resembling RINGWORM. The infection develops quickly into yellowish, circular lesions that become crusted over.

A clinical examination of the characteristic lesions is the basis for diagnosis. Impetigo is generally treated with the prescription ointment mupirocin, which is applied three times a day to affected areas. If there is no improvement after using this medication or there are more than a few lesions, an oral antibiotic such as cloxacillin or a cephalosporin may be prescribed. With treatment, recovery from impetigo is usually prompt.

Risks of untreated impetigo include cellulitis, lymphangitis, and furunculosis in adults. In children, prolonged persistence of lesions can occur and may cause changes in the skin's pigmentation with possible scarring. Children with untreated impetigo are also at risk for acute glomerulonephritis, which can follow an infection caused by a specific strain of the bacteria.

Implant

Any material placed inside the body to repair or replace damaged tissues or organs, deliver drugs or hormones, or improve appearance. Implants include artificial joints, screws, and pins to hold broken bones together; synthetic lenses used to replace lenses affected by cataracts (see cataract surgery); patches for strengthening hernia repairs; pacemakers (see pacemaker) to control heartbeat; and artificial heart valves. In a procedure called BRACHYTHERAPY, radioactive seeds are often implanted in the prostate gland to emit low-energy radiation for treatment of localized prostate cancer.

Implantable bone conduction hearing device

See COCHLEAR IMPLANT.

Implantation, egg

The process in which a fertilized egg attaches itself to the lining of a woman's uterus. Once the egg has been implanted, it is referred to as an EMBRYO. See CONCEPTION; PREGNANCY.

Implants, dental

An artificial tooth root that is surgically anchored into the jaw, or placed over it, to replace a permanent tooth, a dental bridge (see BRIDGE, DENTAL), or full DENTURES. There are two kinds of dental implants: the most common implant can be embedded directly into the jawbone to function as the natural roots of a tooth. The other kind of implant consists of a custommade, thin metal framework that fits over the existing bone and is placed under the membrane that covers the bone; this form of dental implant is used when there is insufficient jaw structure to hold the implant. Implant material is composed of metallic and bonelike ceramic materials that are compatible with human body tissue and unlikely to be reject-

ed by the gum and bone tissue. These materials bond with bone.

Dental implants are permanent and stable, and they do not require adjoining teeth to support them. Dental implants are a good solution to lost or removed teeth because they look and feel like natural teeth. People who are in good health and have the proper bone structure and healthy gums may be good candidates for dental implants. Implants may be an attractive option for people who cannot wear dentures. Bruxism (involuntary teeth clenching) or diseases, such as diabetes, may make a person a less viable candidate for dental implants. People who use tobacco or drink alcohol may not be good candidates for this procedure.

WHAT TO EXPECT

The procedure is generally performed in a dental office using local anesthesia. A dentist with special training in implant therapy, who may be a specialist in ORAL SURGERY or PROSTHODONTICS, performs surgery on the gum and bone in order to anchor the artificial root into the jawbone or on top of it. Painkilling medications may be prescribed to reduce the soreness following the surgery. Once the screws and posts have been surgically placed, the healing process may take as long as 6 months for the bone to bond with the implant. The fitting of the replacement teeth on top of the implant may take as long as 2 months.

If the implant will be positioned over the bone instead of being inserted into it, the complete procedure usually involves two surgical operations. The first uncovers the underlying bone so that an accurate impression (see IMPRESSION, DENTAL) of the

bone may be taken. After the implant has been made from a dental impression in a dental laboratory, a second operation is performed to position the implant over the bone.

Risks of the surgery include sinus perforation, infection, and paresthesia (pins and needles sensation). The success rate for implants depends on the purpose and location of the tooth. Teeth that are implanted in the front area of the lower jaw are the most successful, followed by those implanted on the sides and in the back of the upper jaw.

There may be long-term dietary restrictions following dental implants. Good oral hygiene is essential to maintaining successful dental implants. Using dental floss around the implanted teeth, rinsing with an antiseptic mouthwash, and brushing at least twice a day are important. A dentist may recommend special athome cleaning techniques, and professional cleanings may be increased to as many as four times a year. The goal is to maintain healthy gums and bone so that they can hold onto the implants.

Impotence

The inability to produce or maintain an erection of the penis. See ERECTILE DYSFUNCTION.

Impression, dental

An imprint of the teeth, the gums, and sometimes the palate. A dental impression creates a mold of a hard plaster or another substance. The reproduction created from a dental impression is generally used to construct crowns, bridges, inlays (see CROWN, DENTAL; BRIDGE, DENTAL; and INLAY, DENTAL), or full or partial DENTURES that closely resemble the form and size of the natural teeth.

Dental impressions are taken with small mouth trays that are filled with a puttylike substance. The trays are placed in a person's mouth and pressed against the upper teeth and the lower teeth, alternately, and held in place a short time until the soft material in the tray has begun to harden. When removed, the rubbery substance in the tray has taken the form of the teeth or gums in the area to be fitted with dental restorations (see RESTORATION, DENTAL).

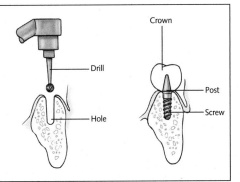

A PERMANENT ARTIFICIAL TOOTH
The dentist drills a hole in the jawbone where the root of the natural tooth was and inserts a screw topped with a temporary cap that remains in place during the healing process. The gum is stitched over the cap and allowed to heal for several months, while the bone grows around the screw, stabilizing it. After complete healing, the dentist makes an incision in the gum, removes the cap, and screws in a metal post that holds the custom-made tooth in place.

Crown

Drill

Hole

Post

Screw

In situ

The earliest stage of cancer, in which the disease has not spread beyond its original site or layer of cells. In situ cancer also is known as stage 0 cancer. Surgical removal of cancer in situ is usually the cure. Cancers known to have an in situ stage are those affecting the anus, bladder, breast, cervix, colon, endometrium (lining of the uterus), esophagus, lung, rectum, stomach, and skin (melanoma).

In vitro fertilization

A method of ASSISTED REPRODUCTIVE TECHNOLOGY for treating infertility. In vitro fertilization (IVF) involves several steps leading to the fertilization of one or more of a woman's eggs outside her body. An egg or eggs are removed, fertilized in the laboratory, and reinserted into the woman's uterus or fallopian tube. IVF was widely used in animal research long before it was first successfully applied to human reproduction in 1978.

The potential for a continuing pregnancy as a result of IVF depends on many variables, including the age and reproductive health of both the woman considering this procedure and her male partner. Success depends on the cause of the infertility and the age of the woman. Thorough medical evaluations are necessary to predict the probability of pregnancy for any given woman.

HOW IVF IS PERFORMED

A 2-week program of intensive preparation generally precedes IVF. Daily injections of hormone medications are usually given to a woman to stimulate the development of multiple eggs. If hormones are not used, usually only a single developed egg may be retrieved. The optimal time to retrieve the eggs is just before ovulation when the eggs are mature enough to be fertilized. This ideal phase for fertilization is identified by the physician through blood tests and through ultrasound scans of the follicles in the ovaries where the eggs are developing.

There are two methods for recovering eggs from a woman's body. The most commonly used technique is ultrasound-guided needle aspiration egg recovery, which is performed on an outpatient basis using local anesthesia in a procedure called trans-

CANCER IN SITU
Cancer (carcinoma) in situ describes cancer cells that have not spread beyond their original site into neighboring tissues. Early-stage breast cancer can occur in either the milk ducts or (less commonly) in breast lobules, but surrounding tissues and structures are healthy. At this early stage, the cancer cells can be surgically removed.

Healthy lobule

Lobular carcinoma

Lobules

Milk ducts in the breast

Ductal carcinoma

Healthy duct

vaginal oocyte retrieval. This procedure uses ultrasound images to allow the doctor to visualize the eggs and to guide a needle through the vaginal wall to retrieve the eggs from the ovary. During this procedure, the woman typically experiences mild discomfort similar to what may be felt during a Pap smear. A less commonly used technique is called laparoscopic egg recovery and involves surgery requiring a small abdominal incision through which the eggs may be retrieved.

After removal, the eggs are placed in a fluid medium in a laboratory. An embryologist examines the fluid from the follicles under a microscope to determine their readiness for fertilization. Semen from a woman's male partner is washed and incubated and, when the woman's eggs are ready, the sperm is placed with the eggs for about 18 hours. After this, the eggs are removed and placed into a special growth medium, a nutrient mixture that imitates the environment of the fallopian tubes. At this time, the eggs divide two or three times as they develop into preimplantation embryos, or pre-embryos. After approximately 40 hours, the pre-embryos are examined by an embryologist to see whether their fertilization and development are normal and whether they are ready to be implanted in the uterus. If multiple pre-embryos are viable, the woman may elect to have extra embryos

frozen for a future EMBRYO TRANSFER procedure.

The pre-embryos are transferred to the uterus of the woman from whom the eggs were retrieved or to the uterus of another recipient if an egg donor was used or a surrogate mother is the carrier. A special catheter is used to transfer the pre-embryos through the vagina into the uterus. There is minimal or no discomfort; the woman receiving the transfer is required to lie quietly following the procedure. Often, several fertilized eggs are transferred to enhance the possibility of a viable pregnancy. Daily progesterone supplementation may be given to the woman who has received the embryos. See also Steps in IVF, facing page.

In vivo

Occurring in the living body.

Incest

Sexual contact between family members so closely related that marriage between them is legally or culturally barred. Legally defined, incest refers to the prohibition of marriage between close relatives, such as between siblings, cousins, parents, and children; child protection laws prohibit sexual contact between adult and child family members. Incest takes place in families of all races, income levels, and religious and educational backgrounds. It most often occurs between older male relatives and minor-aged

Steps in IVF

n vitro fertilization is the process of fertilizing a woman's egg outside her body. The process may be used if a woman has difficulty conceiving because of a blockage in a fallopian tube, endometriosis, a cervical mucus problem, or a male fertility problem such as low sperm count.

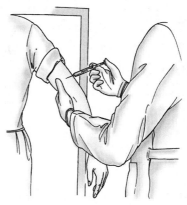

STEP 1: STIMULATING OVULATION
The first step in the in vitro process is the injection of a medication that induces ovulation. The dosage of medication is intended to produce multiple eggs.

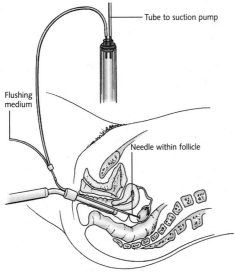

Tube to suction pump

Flushing medium

Needle within follicle

STEP 2: REMOVAL OF EGGS
After several eggs have been produced, the eggs are harvested from the ovary with an aspiration needle. This is done just before ovulation.

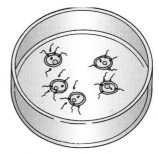

STEP 3: FERTILIZATION BY SPERM
The eggs are fertilized by depositing them with healthy sperm into a petri dish.

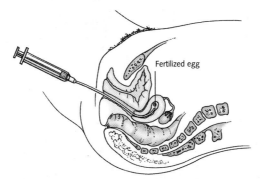

Fertilized egg

STEP 4: REINTRODUCTION OF FERTILIZED EGG
After the eggs are fertilized, they are evaluated and one to four of the healthiest fertilized eggs are introduced into the woman's uterus. This step in the process may be delayed by freezing and storing the eggs for future use.

girls, and in most cultures is considered a form of child abuse. Federal child abuse laws mandate reporting any sexual contact between an adult and child to child protection agencies. Sexual contact can include fondling of the genitals, using sexually suggestive language, prolonged kissing, and oral or anal sex, or intercourse.

Often adults who were incestuously abused as children conceal it for many years. They later report having felt guilty or considered themselves at fault. While some women who were subject to incest as children do not experience long-term injury, others have long-lasting psychological problems, including depression, substance abuse, eating disorders, and difficulties having intimate relationships as adults. Psychological counseling, support groups, or psychotherapy may help victims of incest overcome its lasting effects.

Incidence

A rate that measures the frequency with which a condition or disease occurs in a group of people during a specified period of time. To calculate incidence, the number of new cases of the disease (for example, 100 in a year) is divided by the total population (for example, an average of 10,000 through the year) to find the rate (0.01).

Incision

A precise cut made into body tissue with a sterile surgical knife. The incision is made to expose tissue inside the body so that the surgeon can repair or remove a diseased organ. The type, size, and depth of the incision depends on the surgical procedure being performed.

Incompetent cervix

Abnormal weakness in a woman's cervix that can result in recurrent miscarriages. If the cervix is weak, after the 12th or 14th week of pregnancy the weight of the developing fetus and the amniotic fluid around it can force the cervix open, allowing the fetus and placenta to drop down prematurely and cause a MISCARRIAGE. To help hold the baby in, a stitch may be placed at the opening of the cervix to hold it together firmly (see CERCLAGE, CERVICAL). The stitch is removed at the start of labor or

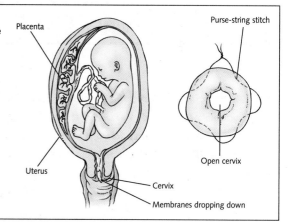

A WEAKENED CERVIX
If the cervix (the neck of the uterus) is unusually weak, the weight of a growing fetus will gradually cause the cervix to widen during pregnancy. The membranes surrounding the fetus can drop down through the cervix and rupture, causing a miscarriage. To prevent the miscarriage, a doctor can make a drawstring-like stitch (called a purse-string stitch) around the cervix to keep it closed until late in the pregnancy.

Placenta

Purse-string stitch

Uterus

Open cervix

Cervix

Membranes dropping down

around the 37th or 38th week of pregnancy, so the woman can deliver the baby.

Incontinence, fecal

The inability to retain feces in the rectum and control defecation. Fecal incontinence is less common than urinary incontinence. Temporary fecal incontinence can occur at any age during bouts of severe diarrhea. Chronic inability to control the bowel occurs more frequently in older people because the efficiency of muscle sphincters declines with age.

In young children, fecal incontinence may represent resistance to toilet training. In older children, it can signal stress or a psychological disorder. With adults, the condition is found among older individuals or people with nervous system disease or damage, such as stroke, multiple sclerosis, or diabetes. It can also occur in people with dementia, who may lack the cognitive ability to control the urge to defecate until an appropriate time. Fecal incontinence also can occur if the anal sphincter muscles are damaged by childbirth, trauma, cancer of the rectum, or surgery or if the nerves controlling the sphincter muscles fail to function properly. Fecal impaction (accumulation of hard feces in the rectum) can cause incontinence when fluid and new feces pass around the impacted mass.

Treatment of fecal incontinence varies according to its cause. Diagnosis of the cause is made by a complete physical examination and tests that may include a lower GASTROINTESTINAL (GI) SERIES (an X-ray

procedure also called a barium enema); a SIGMOIDOSCOPY or COLONOSCOPY, in which a lighted viewing tube is used to examine the gastrointestinal tract; and manometry, in which sphincter tone is measured. If impaction is the cause, an ENEMA or manual removal of the mass is necessary. When an underlying condition, such as a gastrointestinal disease or too little fiber in the diet, is the cause, the doctor will recommend appropriate treatment. For chronic fecal incontinence, waterproof undergarments with absorbent pads can be worn to prevent soiling. Anyone who experiences fecal incontinence or other changes in bowel habits after years of regularity should seek prompt medical attention, especially when additional symptoms, such as weight loss, abdominal pain, or rectal bleeding, are present.

Incontinence, urinary

Inability to control the bladder. Incontinence is not used to describe the normal lack of control in newborns and toddlers; the term applies only to individuals who are old enough to have voluntary control.

Lack of bladder control affects 10 to 20 percent of people older than 65, and it is twice as common in women as in men. The amount of urine lost involuntarily can range from a few drops to complete emptying of the bladder. Temporary urinary incontinence can result from urinary tract infections, infection in the vagina, severe constipation, or the side effects of medications. The incontinence disappears when the underlying condition resolves or the medication is changed. Persistent urinary incontinence continues and often worsens over time.

TYPES OF URINARY INCONTINENCE

In stress incontinence, the most common variety, sudden physical pressure on the abdomen, such as laughing, coughing, sneezing, lifting, or running, causes urine to leak. Stress incontinence is caused by the stretching of pelvic muscles during childbirth, weight gain, and certain surgeries. The muscle that holds urine in the bladder (urinary sphincter) is too weak to retain urine during physical stress. Stress incontinence is more common in women and often worsens after menopause.

In urge incontinence, the interval between the desire to urinate and the loss of urine is so short that the person may not be able to get to the bathroom in time. Large volumes of urine may be expelled every few hours. Urge incontinence is usually caused by infection of the bladder, nerve damage or disease (such as stroke or Parkinson disease), alcohol, and certain medications (such as antidepressants, beta blockers, antihistamines, cold medications, and diuretics).

In overflow incontinence, the bladder feels constantly full; yet, the person cannot urinate or produces only a small amount of urine despite considerable strain and effort. Overflow incontinence is rare in women. Diabetes, an enlarged prostate gland, or blockage because of tumors or stones are possible causes. Overflow incontinence requires prompt treatment because the backup of urine can produce permanent kidney damage, called HYDRONEPHROSIS.

DIAGNOSIS AND TREATMENT

Determining the cause of urinary incontinence requires a physical examination and a medical history. Laboratory tests may also be ordered, including urinalysis, a urine culture (to check for infection), cystoscopy (visual inspection of the inside of the bladder), X rays with contrast dyes, and studies of urine flow, retention, and loss.

For temporary incontinence, treatment consists of identifying the cause, commonly an infection, and resolving it, usually with antibiotics. For persistent incontinence, a number of therapies are available, depending on the cause of the condition and the severity of symptoms. KEGEL EXERCISES can strengthen pelvic muscles and help to restore control. The doctor may suggest restricting fluids and a frequent voiding schedule to be followed. BIOFEEDBACK, a learned method of positive reinforcement, can be used at the same time to retrain the bladder for better control. Medications that increase the strength of the urinary sphincter may be prescribed; these include estrogen, alpha-adrenergic blockers, and beta-adrenergic blockers. Surgery is usually recommended only if there is an abnormality of the muscles surrounding the bladder. The simplest procedure, used to treat stress incontinence, consists of injecting a natural protein material (collagen) into the urethra to enlarge it and allow it to stay closed under stress. This procedure is performed on an outpatient basis. Complications include infection, urine retention, and temporary erectile dysfunction in men. More complex procedures require hospital stays. These include surgeries to compress the urethra (used almost entirely in women), implanting an artificial urinary sphincter, or a procedure to raise the bladder. Possible complications include damage to the urinary tract and infection.

PREVENTION

Maintaining overall muscle tone and performing Kegel exercises can help to prevent symptoms from developing. Such pelvic-strengthening exercises during and after pregnancy are important preventive measures for women.

Incubation period

The period of time that begins when a person is first exposed to an infection and ends with that person's first signs or symptoms of infection. The incubation period is the process of disease development. It covers the phase between the initial invasion of an infectious agent into the body and the point in time when the disease has physical manifestations or symptoms. The length of an incubation period for a given disease can vary from one individual to another depending on a number of factors, some of which are unknown.

When a person comes into direct or indirect contact with an infected person or an object or surface contaminated with an infectious agent, the disease process begins. It may take time for the infectious substances or organisms to attach to the cells in the body that they can invade. In the case of a virus, there will be several generations during which the virus will have to replicate itself before it is present in sufficient numbers to cause illness.

Indigestion

Also called dyspepsia. General discomfort in the upper abdomen. Nausea, heartburn, upper abdominal pain, gas, belching, a sour taste of acid, or an uncomfortable feeling of fullness or bloating after a meal may all occur with indigestion. Often, indigestion worsens during times of stress. Many people have minor indigestion when they eat too fast or eat

MUSCULAR CONTROL OF THE BLADDER
The most common type of incontinence, stress incontinence, is generally caused by weakening of the pelvic muscles surrounding the urethral sphincter, which relaxes or contracts to control flow of urine from the bladder. When the muscles weaken, the pressure of displaced organs on the urethral sphincter makes urinary control more difficult. Additional pressure from sneezing, coughing, or jumping may cause leakage.

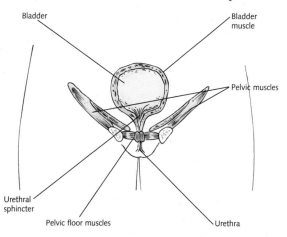

Bladder

Bladder muscle

Pelvic muscles

Urethral sphincter

Pelvic floor muscles

Urethra

foods that cause gas. To control the problem, doctors recommend eating more slowly and relaxing for a half hour after a meal; avoiding foods and drinks that have caused indigestion in the past; practicing stress management techniques; using acetaminophen instead of aspirin, which can irritate the stomach lining; stopping smoking; drinking alcohol only in moderation; and using over-the-counter antacids to relieve occasional heartburn.

Indigestion that becomes more frequent, persistent, or intense or occurs for no apparent reason requires medical attention. Indigestion may be the sign of a more serious underlying disorder, such as PEPTIC ULCER DISEASE, in which sores develop in the mucous membranes lining the duodenum, stomach, lower esophagus, or small intestine. Inflammation of the gallbladder or its lining, inflammation of the esophagus, liver disorders, or, rarely, stomach cancer can also cause indigestion. Occasionally, heart problems can cause symptoms that mimic indigestion. To find out the cause, doctors may order tests, such as blood tests, stool sample analysis, ultrasound scanning, an upper gastrointestinal (GI) series (also known as a barium swallow), or gastroscopy (visual examination of the digestive tract through insertion of a slim, flexible, lighted tube). Treatment varies according to the underlying cause of indigestion.

Indinavir

A protease inhibitor drug used to treat HIV (human immunodeficiency virus) infection. Indinavir (Crixivan) is an antiviral agent that prevents HIV from multiplying, thereby reducing the amount of active virus in the body. Indinavir is not a cure for HIV or AIDS (acquired immunodeficiency syndrome) but is part of a "cocktail" of drugs that work together to reduce the amount of the virus in the blood to undetectable levels, making HIV a manageable chronic illness rather than a fatal disease.

Indomethacin

See NONSTEROIDAL ANTI-INFLAMMATORY DRUGS.

Induction agents

A medication used to bring on (induce) the loss of pain and con-

sciousness in general anesthesia (see ANESTHESIA, GENERAL). In some cases, the induction agent is given through a small tube in the vein of the arm or hand of a person. Sometimes, the patient inhales the medication as a gas (see ANESTHESIA, INHALATION).

Induction of labor

The use of artificial methods to start labor intentionally. In general, induction is indicated when continuation of the pregnancy represents a significant risk to the mother, fetus, or both. This is especially true if the pregnancy has gone beyond term; the mother has developed an illness due to the pregnancy, such as PREECLAMPSIA (high blood pressure brought on by pregnancy); the fetus is endangered or has died; or the mother has a pre-existing health condition that makes induction safer than continuing the pregnancy.

Labor can be induced in different ways. The woman may be given OXYTOCIN, a hormone that signals the uterus to contract. Oxytocin is usually given slowly, with the dose increased over time, if necessary. The woman's contractions and the response of the baby will be carefully monitored while the oxytocin is given. If oxytocin does not induce labor, or if the baby must be delivered immediately, a CESAREAN SECTION may be performed.

If a woman's cervix has undergone the changes that normally occur before delivery (a thinning, softening, and widening process referred to as ripening), the doctor may rupture the membranes surrounding the fetus to help begin labor. The fluid that is released contains prostaglandins that may stimulate the uterus to contract.

There are some risks associated with inducing labor. The baby can be endangered if too much oxytocin is given and contractions are too strong. The placenta can separate from the wall of the uterus, depriving the baby of oxygen, once the amniotic sac is ruptured and the amount of amniotic fluid suddenly drops (a rare occurrence). The mother and baby are at increased risk for infection after the amniotic sac is ruptured, although the risk is not significant for the first 12 to 24 hours following the rupture. Prolonged oxytocin administration can result

in fatigue of the uterus, which could increase the chance of bleeding after delivery.

Infant mortality

A rate determined by dividing the number of deaths among children younger than 1 year of age within a given period by the number of live births within that same period. Infant mortality is usually stated as the number of deaths per 1,000 infants per year. In the United States, for example, the infant mortality rate in 2000 was 6.6. This means that for every 1,000 infants born during 1998, 6.6 died. Infant mortality is an important measure of a nation's overall health and the effectiveness of its health care system. Many poorer countries have infant mortality rates higher than 100. This means that 1 or more infants of every 10 die before they reach their first birthday. In countries with effective health care systems, infant mortality is 15 or less per 1,000.

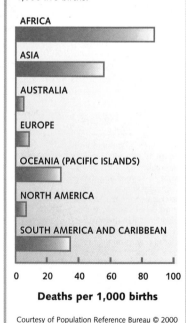

INFANT MORTALITY AROUND THE WORLD

Mortality in the first year of life varies from continent to continent. The rate is the number of infant deaths per 1,000 live births.

AFRICA
ASIA
AUSTRALIA
EUROPE
OCEANIA (PACIFIC ISLANDS)
NORTH AMERICA
SOUTH AMERICA AND CARIBBEAN

0   20   40   60   80   100

Deaths per 1,000 births

Courtesy of Population Reference Bureau © 2000

Infantile spasms

Seizures in which a baby suddenly and briefly shakes or tenses his or her body several times a day. A spasm may also include difficulty breathing or a loss of consciousness. This type of SEIZURE can occur until approximately 18 months of age. In some babies, no reason is ever found for the seizures and they disappear. Other times, infantile spasms are due to serious underlying problems such as brain damage or CEREBRAL PALSY. In such cases, other types of seizures follow as children grow older and are usually accompanied by some type of DEVELOPMENTAL DELAY.

DIAGNOSIS AND TREATMENT

After a seizure, tests are performed to determine the cause. The tests may include a complete physical and neurological examination; blood tests; an electroencephalogram, a recording of electrical impulses in the brain; imaging studies of the brain such as CT (computed tomography) scanning and MRI (magnetic resonance imaging); and on occasion, a SPINAL TAP. Additional tests may be performed to detect conditions related to seizures, such as meningitis, encephalitis, or a brain tumor.

During seizures, a child is at risk of being injured by nearby objects, which should be removed. The child should not be restrained during a seizure. Although infantile spasms can be alarming to parents, in many cases they spontaneously disappear over time. In other children, underlying causes such as infections or tumors can be diagnosed and treated. In the absence of treatable underlying causes, seizures can usually be controlled with anticonvulsant drugs.

Infarction

An area of tissue that dies because of blockage of the artery supplying it with blood. The usual cause of an infarction is a blood clot, which can form at the site of the blockage (a thrombus) or develop elsewhere in the body, then travel through the bloodstream until it lodges in a blood vessel (an embolus). Infarction in the heart (technically, myocardial infarction) is known as a HEART ATTACK.

Infection

The invasion and multiplication of infectious microorganisms in body tissues. An infection may not cause symptoms, or it may produce signs and symptoms caused by the microorganisms' injury to the body's cells or by the body's response to the invasion, which is the production of antibodies and inflammatory cells that are prompted by the specific cause of the infection. A common symptom of infection is FEVER.

When the body's defense system is effective, the infection may remain localized and temporary, producing only mild, treatable symptoms. If the infection persists and spreads, it can progress to an acute or chronic disease. Local infections can also become body-wide, affecting many organs, if the microorganisms spread to the bloodstream or the LYMPHATIC SYSTEM.

Infections are commonly caused by BACTERIA or one of the VIRUSES and can be diagnosed by laboratory evaluation of blood samples. The tests can reveal the presence of a strain of one of these microorganisms or their corresponding antibodies and identify them. Once diagnosed, most infections can be treated with medication, often ANTIBIOTICS. See also COLD, COMMON; INFECTIOUS DISEASE; INFLUENZA; PNEUMONIA; SEXUALLY TRANSMITTED DISEASES; VACCINATION; VACCINATIONS, CHILDHOOD. See also Preventing infection, page 720.

Infection, congenital

Infection that affects an unborn fetus at any time during a pregnancy up through and including the time of delivery. Congenital infections exist at birth and are generally caused by viruses such as cytomegalovirus (CMV), herpesviruses, German measles, parvovirus, chickenpox, and enteroviruses.

A virus that infects a pregnant woman may be passed to the fetus either directly through the placenta or during childbirth as the newborn passes through the birth canal. An infected woman who is pregnant may have mild, flulike symptoms caused by the virus, or she may not have any symptoms. Even if a pregnant woman with a viral infection feels sick, her immune system may prevent the virus from affecting the fetus.

SIGNS AND COMPLICATIONS

Congenital infections in a fetus or newborn usually occur without symptoms initially, but eventually cause serious medical and developmental problems that appear months or years later. There are some congenital infections that result in severe birth defects and may cause death.

Diagnosis can be difficult. An obstetrician may be able to diagnose an infection in a pregnant woman based on her symptoms and blood tests or based on physical findings in the fetus as evaluated by ULTRASOUND SCANNING. A pediatrician may diagnose a congenital infection in a newborn based on signs, physical findings, and blood tests. In some cases, even sophisticated medical diagnostic tests do not reveal congenital infections.

Medical complications of congenital infections are related to the type of virus involved. Cytomegalovirus infections can cause brain damage associated with calcifications in the brain, a disorder in which the brain does not grow properly and the head is smaller than normal, a condition called MICROCEPHALY. CMV infections may also be associated with groin hernias and a condition called hydrocephalus in which extra fluid accumulates in the cavities of the brain. Medical complications that may be caused by rubella, or German measles, include diabetes mellitus and heart problems. Herpes is associated with chronic, recurring eye and skin infections in newborns.

A broad range of developmental disabilities are also associated with congenital infections. These are generally due to the infection's effect on the developing brain and the sensory organs of the fetus. Hearing loss is the most common among the developmental complications due to congenital infections and is associated with CMV and rubella infections in particular. Loss of hearing may be present at birth and during infancy when it is difficult to detect, or it may develop later in childhood and become progressively more severe. Visual impairments associated with herpesviruses and German measles are due to the development of cataracts in the eyes or eye tissue destruction. If brain damage has occurred, there may be varying degrees of mental retardation, including learning and behavioral disorders, or autism.

PREVENTING INFECTION

Disease-causing organisms, such as bacteria, viruses, and fungi, can be inhaled from the air, ingested in food or water, picked up from direct contact with an infected person, or contracted from an insect or animal carrier. Many common infectious diseases can be avoided if the means of transmission are understood and good hygiene is practiced.

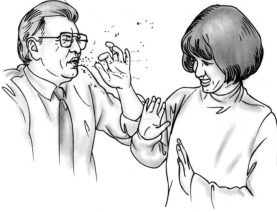

COUGHING OR SNEEZING

A person who has an infection, such as the common cold or a virus, should make sure to cover his or her mouth when coughing or sneezing to minimize the chance that people close by will become directly infected and get sick.

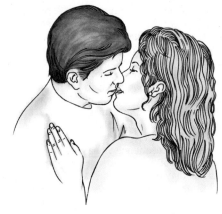

SKIN-TO-SKIN CONTACT

Kissing a person who has a cold or the flu virus is another direct transmission route for an infection. Intimate contact with people who have respiratory infections should be avoided.

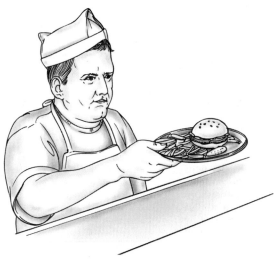

HANDLING FOOD

Professional food handlers should not touch food that others will be eating to avoid indirectly transmitting infection. At home, a person with an infectious illness should avoid handling food or using dishes or utensils that others will be using.

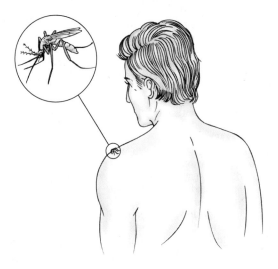

INSECT BITES

Biting insects can be carriers of diseases that are dangerous to people. For example, the West Nile virus, which can be deadly, is transmitted by mosquitoes.

TREATMENT

It is important that complications associated with congenital infections be identified as early as possible to allow interventional therapy to begin immediately. Surgery and other medical procedures can sometimes treat complications, including brain disorders. Early screening for vision and hearing problems is especially important. Serious developmental disabilities are often exhibited early in life, but newborns without symptoms or "silent" congenital infections may not show signs of disability until months or years later.

Infectious disease

An illness caused by an organism, such as bacteria, that enters the body, then grows and multiplies in the cells, tissues, or cavities of the body. An infectious disease may also be referred to as a contagious disease or a communicable disease. Infectious disease may be spread by direct or indirect contact with an infected person or by a common vehicle such as food or water. It may also be airborne or vector-borne, which usually means transmitted by insects.

The organisms that cause infectious disease are called pathogens. Depending on the interaction between the pathogen and its human host, infection can be silent or without symptoms, or it can be overt, which means signs and symptoms of infectious disease occur in the infected person. Silent infectious diseases without symptoms can often be spread to others, as HIV (human immunodeficiency virus) infection is spread during its early phase.

Infectious disease can be acute, a disease of short duration that may or not have symptoms, and is contagious only for a short time. INFLUENZA is an example of an acute infectious disease. Infection may also be chronic, which refers to a longer duration caused by the continual reproduction of pathogens. Chronic infectious disease is contagious for as long as the infection lasts. Hepatitis B and C can be chronic infectious diseases; *Haemophilus influenzae* type b (Hib) is an acute or chronic disease that can cause ear infections, meningitis, and arthritis.

Despite the perception that infectious diseases have been conquered by modern medical techniques, including the introduction of antibiotics to fight bacterial infections and vaccinations that offer protection from many serious childhood infections, infectious diseases continue to cause many deaths. New infectious diseases and new strains of known diseases are constantly emerging. Infectious disease is the leading cause of death worldwide; the infectious diseases AIDS (acquired immunodeficiency syndrome), PNEUMONIA, and influenza are among the leading causes of death in the United States.

Infectious mononucleosis

See MONONUCLEOSIS, INFECTIOUS.

Inferiority complex

The feeling that one is so much less able and competent than others that it spawns helplessness rather than a willingness to strive. In the theory of psychologist Alfred Adler, all humans begin life with feelings of inferiority, and the desire to overcome these feelings by proving oneself superior to life's obstacles is a central motivation. If the feelings of inferiority win out over the urge toward superiority, an inferiority complex results.

Infertility

The inability of a man and woman of reproductive age to produce offspring after unprotected sexual intercourse. A couple should seek help for infertility if the woman is younger than 35 years and has not become pregnant after having unprotected intercourse when ovulating for 1 year. If the woman is older, but still of childbearing age, most experts recommend that help be sought after no more than 6 months of unprotected sexual intercourse. There are many possible factors that may contribute to or cause infertility.

Primary infertility is the medical term for women who have never conceived a child. Secondary infertility is the term for women who have delivered one or more children and then have been unable to become pregnant. Infertility in women increases as they get older and is considered a part of the natural aging process. The decline in female fertility begins in the mid-20s and accelerates dramatically after about age 35.

A man is considered infertile when he has no sperm or his sperm are not capable of fertilizing an egg. This inability to fertilize an egg can be caused by conditions resulting in an insufficient amount of viable sperm, abnormal sperm structure, or insufficient ability of the sperm to move.

Female factors and male factors each account for approximately 40 percent of identifiable infertility causes. The cause of infertility is unknown in 10 to 15 percent of all couples.

CAUSES OF INFERTILITY

Four general conditions interfere with a couple's ability to conceive a child: the inability of a man to produce healthy sperm or a woman to produce healthy eggs; the inability of gametes (sperm and eggs) to get close enough to allow fertilization to occur; the inability of a fertilized egg to become successfully attached to the lining of a woman's uterus; and the inability to carry a pregnancy to its full term.

The root of female infertility is often the failure of a woman's fertility hormones to transmit chemical signals at exactly the right time for conception to take place. This can produce a lack of ovulation or an irregular pattern of ovulation, which results in irregular menstrual periods. Problems involving female hormone disorders are commonly, and often successfully treated with fertility drugs.

Another major cause of female infertility is ENDOMETRIOSIS, a condition that results when tissue from the lining (the endometrium) of the uterus grows outside the normal location in the uterus. The tissue fragments may cause scarring at the ends of the fallopian tubes or on the ovaries. When bands of scar tissue form, the sperm may be blocked from entering the fallopian tubes where they can fertilize an egg. In most cases, endometriosis may be treated with medication or surgery.

Commonly identified causes of male infertility are VARICOCELE and PROSTATITIS. Varicoceles are varicose veins near one or both of a man's testicles. They cause an increased temperature in the testicles that may damage sperm.

Varicoceles can be surgically corrected. Prostatitis is a bacterial infection of the prostate gland that may not produce noticeable symptoms but can be treated with antibiotics.

SEXUALLY TRANSMITTED DISEASES (STDs) are a leading cause of infertility in both men and women. In the United States, CHLAMYDIA and GONORRHEA are the two major infections that most often lead to infertility. In women, pelvic infections that are STDs may not cause noticeable symptoms. Consequently, these infections may not be recognized and treated. This can produce scarring of the upper reproductive tract, specifically of the fallopian tubes. In men, STDs can cause scarring of and damage to reproductive structures, including the delicate tubes (vas deferens) of the ejaculatory tract.

STDs can cause PELVIC INFLAMMATORY DISEASE (PID) in women, and a single episode of the disease, which may become chronic, can often cause infertility. PID produces an inflammation that may involve the fallopian tubes, uterus, and ovaries. PID may also occur after abortion, childbirth, D AND C (dilation and curettage), or the use of an INTRAUTERINE DEVICE.

The inability of a woman's ovaries to produce mature eggs (anovulation) causes female infertility. Certain severe illnesses can contribute to anovulation. A disorder involving hormonal imbalances and anovulation called POLYCYSTIC OVARIAN SYNDROME is involved in 5 to 10 percent of women with ovulation problems. In the United States and other developed countries, anovulation is occasionally the result of excessive weight loss and extreme physical exercise regimens. Obesity can also be a factor. Abnormal body weight (either underweight or overweight) can be a factor in infertility. The restoration of normal weight and the use of fertility medications can often re-establish fertility in affected women. In some cases, the cause of the failure to ovulate cannot be identified.

A pregnancy that develops outside the uterus, called an ectopic pregnancy, usually occurs in a fallopian tube. The surgical treatment of this complication may permanently damage the affected tube, blocking the egg and sperm from meeting, resulting in infertility. Rarely, disorders of a woman's uterus result in infertility. These disorders may include scar tissue that obstructs the uterine cavity and enlarged fibroids that distort the shape of the uterus to the extent that an embryo cannot be implanted.

The fertility of men and women whose mothers took the medication diethylstilbestrol (DES) may be affected as a result of their exposure to DES in the uterus. Some daughters of women who took DES have abnormal fallopian tubes or misshapen uteruses or vaginas, as well as other reproductive abnormalities, and may have higher risks of ectopic pregnancy, premature delivery, and miscarriage. Men born to mothers who took DES during pregnancy can have missing reproductive system ducts.

Genetic factors can have a role in male infertility, in some cases involving defects of a man's Y chromosome that produce abnormalities in the development of the sperm-producing system. Other factors linked to male infertility include undescended testicles, disorders of the HYPOTHALAMUS or PITUITARY GLAND, testicular damage from diseases such as mumps, chemotherapy or radiation treatments for testicular cancer, and severe trauma to the testicles.

A couple's ability to reproduce may be diminished or prevented by reasons that include exposure to environmental or other toxins, medications, and lifestyle. A reproductive specialist may recommend changes in behavior if smoking, drinking alcohol, or other lifestyle factors are thought to be contributing to infertility. See INFERTILITY TREATMENTS.

FERTILITY TESTING

Comprehensive testing may be required to explore the reason or reasons why a couple is unable to conceive. A fertility specialist uses fertility testing to look for the possible cause of a couple's infertility and to diagnose disorders that may be medically treated.

If a complete medical history and physical examination do not reveal the reason for infertility, a specialist may begin testing. Usually the first step is obtaining a semen specimen from the male partner and testing it for sperm viability. Sperm is generally evaluated for motility (ability to move), shape, speed, and ability to travel in straight lines—characteristics that affect the sperm's ability to fertilize an egg. Semen can also be cultured for infections. Semen analysis is usually ordered first to rule out sperm abnormalities before beginning the more extensive testing of the woman partner.

Both partners may have thyroid gland function tests and blood screening tests to check blood type, measure cell count and cholesterol levels, and determine whether viral infections are present. The woman's blood may be tested for levels of progesterone, a hormone that increases in the bloodstream after ovulation, to determine that ovulation has occurred. A man's blood may be tested for chromosome irregularities and the levels of hormones that stimulate the function of the testicles. High levels of gonadotropic hormones are an indication that the testicles are no longer producing sperm, an untreatable condition. If excess numbers of certain antibodies against sperm are detected in a man's blood, treatment may be possible.

X rays of a woman's uterus and fallopian tubes may reveal anatomical irregularities that prevent conception. A woman's cervical mucus may be cultured to rule out the presence of fertility-diminishing infections, including gonorrhea and chlamydia.

An investigation of the structure and function of the fallopian tubes may involve the use of a HYSTEROSALPINGOGRAM, an image produced by a diagnostic procedure in which dye is introduced through the vagina into the uterus and fallopian tubes. This procedure is generally performed to detect anatomical abnormalities that may interfere with conception and to verify that the fallopian tubes are open. Another diagnostic technique that may be used is LAPAROSCOPY, the insertion of a special viewing telescope into the abdomen so that the internal pelvic organs can be inspected. Dye can be injected, and the tubes can be observed directly. This test allows the physician to see whether the fallopian tubes are open, to observe any adhesions, and to note uterine abnormalities.

Terms in small capital letters— for example, PHYSICAL THERAPY or PAGET DISEASE—indicate a cross-reference to another entry with more information.

An endometrial biopsy may be performed. In this test, a tiny fragment of the uterine lining is removed and examined under a microscope for indications of ovulation and to assess the ability of the uterine lining to support pregnancy.

Tests and examinations timed to evaluate the function and condition of the reproductive system may be performed. A woman's cervical mucus may be tested during her most fertile day, usually at the midpoint in her menstrual cycle. A postcoital test of the cervical mucus may reveal the vitality and motility of a man's sperm in his partner's cervical environment. In rare instances, a woman's cervical mucus produces antibodies to her partner's sperm, repelling the sperm and impairing fertility.

The ovaries and uterine lining may be evaluated by ultrasound examination during the middle of the menstrual cycle to monitor the follicle development and to confirm that an egg has been released from the follicle. At this time the ovaries may be checked for ovarian cysts and the uterus checked for fibroid tumors. Blood screens for normal production of fertility hormones at the right times in a woman's cycle may be performed. Levels of the female hormone estradiol may be evaluated to indicate the number and condition of a woman's eggs. Testing levels of FSH (follicle-stimulating hormone) can reveal whether a woman's ovaries are functioning properly; an elevated FSH level may signal menopause. Hormone screening may be performed on men to test whether male hormone levels are normal.

Infertility treatments

Nonmedical or medical therapy for individuals who are unable or have a diminished capacity to conceive. When a specific disease or disorder that causes infertility is diagnosed, a physician may treat the underlying disorder. Some conditions are treatable only with ASSISTED REPRODUCTIVE TECHNOLOGY (ART).

When the cause of infertility is not a disease or functional problem, the solution may lie in coordinating sexual activity with the woman's most fertile period. Monitoring the basal body temperature is one approach. A woman's basal, or resting, body temperature is taken and recorded early in the morning while she is still in bed. A rise in temperature usually indicates that ovulation has occurred. This information may allow a couple to time sexual intercourse to coincide with the woman's production of eggs. A more accurate procedure is performed with an LH (luteinizing hormone) detection kit, which enables a couple to predict impending egg release 24 hours before ovulation occurs.

When a woman's cervical mucus produces antibodies to her partner's sperm, infertility treatments that bypass the cervix, such as IN VITRO FERTILIZATION (IVF), may be tried. When a couple's infertility involves a man's low sperm count, a specialized form of IVF involving a procedure called ICSI (intracytoplasmic sperm injection) may be implemented. In this procedure, a physician uses a glass needle to place individual sperm into each of several eggs that have been removed from a woman's ovaries. If fertilization takes place, the resulting embryo can later be introduced into the woman's uterus.

Other treatments for male infertility may include medications to correct hormone deficiencies or infections. Surgical treatment of a VARICOCELE is performed less frequently now that IVF is more successful. When the cause is unexplained or related to premature or delayed ejaculation, low sperm count, or poor quality sperm, sperm may be inseminated into a woman's cervix or uterus. In some cases, a previous VASECTOMY may be reversed surgically.

Fertility drugs are used to treat women who are having difficulty conceiving because of irregular or absent ovulation. These drugs do not improve the fertility of women who ovulate normally but may allow more controlled timing for artificial insemination. The appropriate hormonal medication and the correct dosage are determined on the basis of several evaluations, primarily blood tests. Medications that induce ovulation may be prescribed for women using other ART methods. For example, with ARTIFICIAL INSEMINATION, medication may be used to produce more than one egg during a woman's cycle to increase the possibility of fertilization. However, artificial insemination also increases the possibility of multiple births. A woman is usually instructed to keep a record of menstrual periods, ovulation, and episodes of intercourse. The physician will periodically review this record, treat any health problems, and monitor the effects of any prescribed medication.

There are several different fertility drugs. CLOMIPHENE CITRATE stimulates ovulation in women who have long intervals between menstrual periods and who menstruate infrequently. There may be a slight increase in a woman's risk of ovarian cancer if this medication is taken for longer than 1 year. Human menopausal gonadotropin is the most potent of the fertility drugs and is taken by women who are not ovulating and have not had a successful response to clomiphene citrate. It may contain

FSH (follicle-stimulating hormone) alone or a combination of FSH and LH. This medication must be monitored carefully with frequent ultrasound examinations and estradiol blood tests to avoid multiple births. Bromocriptine may be prescribed for women whose irregular ovulation is related to disorders of the pituitary gland.

Surgical procedures are sometimes necessary to treat female infertility. If endometriosis is thought to be the cause of female infertility, a surgical technique called LAPAROSCOPY is often performed. During laparoscopy, as much displaced endometrial tissue as possible is removed from elsewhere in the body; postoperatively, medications may be given to shrink the remaining tissue and suppress the growth of new tissue.

Large or numerous fibroids (noncancerous tumors) in a woman's uterus may prevent pregnancy. Myomectomy, a surgical procedure to remove the fibroids, may be done, leaving the uterus intact, which can enhance the possibility of pregnancy for the affected woman.

Fallopian tubes that are blocked by scar tissue, often caused by pelvic inflammatory disease, may be surgically opened. The degree of scarring and the age of the affected woman are important factors in determining the likelihood that the surgery will improve fertility. The type of surgery performed depends on the location and extent of the scar tissue causing blockage. If a tube is blocked near its opening into the uterus, a procedure called TUBAL CANNULATION may be performed. This involves inserting a thin, flexible tube, called a cannula, into the blocked tube. Tubal reanastomosis involves surgical removal of the area of the fallopian tube where scar tissue is blocking the tube and rejoining of the two severed ends of the tube. This scar tissue is most often the result of a previous tubal ligation.

Surgery to reshape an abnormally shaped uterus that cannot support a pregnancy to term is sometimes performed, usually when all other possible causes of infertility have been rejected.

Infestation

The presence of an organism, such as a parasite, living in or on a host body. An

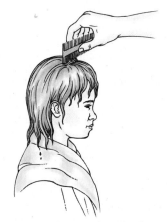

NIT COMB
Infestation with head lice is relatively common among school-aged children. After treatment with a specially formulated shampoo, a fine-toothed comb may be helpful to remove the dead lice and eggs from the hair shafts and scalp. Combs and towels must be thoroughly washed after use.

infestation with lice is an example of a parasite that lives on the outside of the body, while tapeworms are parasitic organisms that live inside the body in the intestines. Superficial infestations usually do not cause serious symptoms unless they transmit infections; some ticks can transmit LYME DISEASE and other infections, and certain mosquitoes carry the organisms that cause MALARIA. Infestations that occur inside the body may cause mild symptoms that are not detected unless the organisms infest vital organs or multiply, in which case they can cause serious complications

Most of the dangerous or life-threatening forms of infestation are rare in the United States. Getting rid of parasitic infestations generally requires medical treatment, as humans do not normally have sufficient natural defenses against these infestations. Parasite-killing medications are considered highly effective; most medications are available by prescription.

Infiltrate

Any substance that enters a cell, tissue, or organ under abnormal circumstances (noun) or to penetrate (verb). Examples of infiltrates are blood cells, cancer cells, fat, starch, and calcium and magnesium salts. Intravenous fluid that leaks out of a vein is said to infiltrate, or penetrate, tissue surrounding the injection site.

Inflammation

Redness, swelling, heat, and pain in a tissue that comes from the body's protective response to chemicals, or physical injury, or to infection. When body tissues are damaged, specialized mast cells (see MAST CELL) release chemical substances such as HISTAMINE. Histamine increases blood flow to the damaged tissue, which causes redness and heat. It also makes the capillaries leaky, so fluid oozes out of them and into the tissues, causing localized swelling. A person feels pain from the stimulation of nerve endings by the inflammatory chemicals. Inflammation is accompanied by a flood of white blood cells into the affected area, as part of the body's effort to expel invasive microorganisms and repair damaged tissue. Although inflammation is an essential element in the body's response to injury and infection, sometimes it brings an unwanted reaction. For example, in allergies, the body mistakenly identifies normal substances as intruders and in an inflammatory response attempts to expel them. This results in uncomfortable symptoms that may include nasal congestion or skin rashes. Treatment is with medications such as antihistamines and corticosteroids.

Inflammatory bowel disease

A general term used to refer jointly to chronic ulcerative COLITIS and CROHN DISEASE. The two diseases share many similarities. Both cause recurrent bouts of intestinal inflammation, and their onset is typically between ages 15 and 30 but may begin at any time. Symptoms include diarrhea, fever, and abdominal pain. Both diseases damage the digestive tract, can cause complications in other parts of the body, and can increase the risk of colon cancer. Treatment usually involves the use of medications that reduce inflammation.

There are also differences between ulcerative colitis and Crohn disease. Crohn disease can occur anywhere in the digestive tract, from the mouth to the anus. It most frequently affects the junction between the large and small intestines. Inflammation caused by ulcerative colitis affects the colon only. Crohn disease occurs as "skip lesions," in which some segments of the intestine are inflamed, while other parts remain healthy. Inflammation caused by ulcerative colitis is pervasive and affects the entire colon.

The exact causes of ulcerative colitis and Crohn disease remain unknown. However, heredity appears to play a role in both conditions. Contributing factors are thought to include exposure to an infectious agent and an abnormal immune reaction in the body. Ulcerative colitis is slightly more common than Crohn disease in the United States.

Infliximab

A drug used to treat Crohn disease, a chronic inflammation of the small intestine and bowel, and rheumatoid arthritis. Infliximab (Remicade) works by neutralizing tumor necrosis factor, a substance involved in the inflammatory process. It is only given by injection and is prescribed in people whose condition has not been helped by other medications.

Influenza

FOR SYMPTOM CHART
see Coughing, page 28

An acute, contagious infection caused by a virus that primarily affects the respiratory tract, but may also affect the musculoskeletal, gastrointestinal, and nervous systems. Influenza, which is also called flu, occurs in outbreaks with variable severity in the United States, usually during the winter months between October and May, generally peaking in intensity from late December through early March.

There are three types of influenza viruses (A, B, and C), that cause influenza. A and B influenza occur almost every winter in the United States and are sometimes associated with hospitalization and death. Type C influenza produces a mild infection that may or may not cause symptoms and does not occur in widespread outbreaks.

Infection with an influenza virus does not give a person lasting immunity, so people are susceptible to episodes of influenza throughout their lives. This is because the viruses that cause influenza constantly alter themselves via changes in their viral genetic material, a process called mutation.

These mutations create subtle differences in the virus that are significant enough to allow them to evade the defenses of the body's immune system that were developed during previous infections with the influenza virus. Large numbers of people can have insufficient immune protection from influenza, particularly when it is caused by a significantly altered virus. These viruses can be responsible for epidemics of influenza that may cause many deaths. In the late 1950s the "Asian flu" caused 70,000 deaths in the United States; in the late 1960s the "Hong Kong flu" caused 34,000 deaths in the United States.

SYMPTOMS AND DIAGNOSIS

Severity of symptoms varies with the type of virus that causes influenza as well as with the age and health of the person infected. There may be no symptoms, they may be mild to severe, or the flu may cause serious illness and death. A person with influenza may experience some or all of the following symptoms: moderate to high fever (temperature between 101°F and 103°F); chills; sore throat; cough; runny nose; general aching in the muscles; headache; loss of appetite; fatigue and weakness; diarrhea; burning of the eyes; and dizziness. If there is fever, it generally subsides within 2 or 3 days. Symptoms may last only 24 hours or as long as 2 weeks, but the worst symptoms are generally gone within 2 to 6 days, with feelings of fatigue for several days after. Influenza is contagious as long as the person has symptoms.

The symptoms of influenza may be very similar to those of the common cold (see COLD, COMMON), but there are characteristic differences. The onset of a cold is gradual, and the primary symptoms are sneezing and nasal congestion. Symptoms of influenza tend to develop suddenly, are more severe, and typically include fever, coughing, and muscle aches.

Influenza is diagnosed by an evaluation of symptoms, the taking of a medical history, and a thorough physical examination. Further testing may distinguish the flu from a cold, from severe STREP THROAT, or from the early stages of bacterial pneumonia, which is the most common serious complication of influenza. Blood tests and chest X rays may be performed. A sample of coughed-up

mucus, called a sputum culture, may be ordered to check for bacterial growth. Laboratory testing to identify the specific type of flu virus may be done if there is risk of a serious influenza epidemic.

TREATMENT AND PROGNOSIS

Treatment of influenza is usually based on easing the symptoms and preventing complications. The body can become so weakened by the flu that it cannot summon defenses against secondary bacterial infections. Physicians generally recommend reduced activity for the duration of severe symptoms and for at least 2 days after the fever has subsided. Other recommendations may include drinking at least 6 cups a day of clear fluids and, when necessary, taking over-the-counter painkillers and nasal decongestants. Prescription antiviral medications are effective only when taken during the first 48 hours of infection. Rimantadine and amantadine can prevent influenza virus A from multiplying in the body, which may help lessen the severity of symptoms and the duration of the illness. The newer antiviral medications, such as oseltamivir phosphate and zanamivir, are effective, work against influenza A and B, and seem to be better tolerated than other antiviral medications.

Most people fully recover from influenza. Others may develop serious, even life-threatening complications, such as pneumonia, requiring hospitalization. Medical attention is extremely important if certain flu symptoms, such as fever and coughing, get worse, or if blood or thick and foul-smelling mucus are coughed up. Other dangerous symptoms associated with influenza that require immediate help include chest pain and shortness of breath.

PREVENTION

Since the influenza viruses are often spread through direct contact, including shaking hands and touching contaminated surfaces, frequent hand washing during a known outbreak or flu season may be helpful in avoiding infection.

The influenza vaccine is a powerful medical preventative and is considered highly effective for preventing the flu or diminishing its severity. A new vaccine is made yearly to offer protection against the influenza viruses that are anticipated to cause illness in a given year. Correct timing of the flu vaccine increases its effectiveness because the body needs time to build up antibodies in response to the vaccine. The level of antibodies is usually greatest 1 or 2 months after vaccination. For this reason, it is recommended that people be vaccinated at the onset of flu season, between October and November. The protective effects of the vaccine may not last throughout the flu season for people who are vaccinated earlier than this.

People at high risk for flu infection should receive the influenza vaccine yearly. This group includes people aged 50 years or older; people who have chronic diseases, particularly diseases of the heart, lungs, or kidneys; people who have diabetes mellitus or anemia; people with immune-suppressing illnesses; people who take medication that suppresses the immune system; residents of assisted-living centers and nursing homes; health care workers; people who are in close contact with those at high risk for influenza; and healthy children 6 to 23 months old when possible. Infants are at risk for hospitalization from flu.

Informed consent for research

An essential ethical and legal element in clinical research stipulating that a person who participates in a clinical research project must be given all available, relevant information about the research before he or she makes the decision to participate. Informed consent is common practice in all clinical trials and has been required by law since the 1970s for any research project that receives federal funding.

Specifically, informed consent for research indicates that participants receive certain information before they agree to be part of a research project. This information must include the purpose of the study, whether the research is expected to benefit participants, what the alternatives are, and what risks might be encountered. The information given to prospective participants must also include details about procedures, treatments, and tests that may be involved.

THE ELEMENTS OF INFORMED CONSENT FOR RESEARCH

An informed consent form to be signed by a participant must include the following:

- An explanation of the purpose of the research and of the procedures the participant will undergo
- A full description of anticipated possible risks or discomforts
- A description of potential or expected benefits, if any, to the participant or to others
- A disclosure of alternative treatments the participant might seek instead
- A statement assuring the confidentiality of records
- An explanation of compensation for injury if the research poses more than a minimal risk
- A list of names of people who can be contacted to obtain more information about the project and the rights of the participants
- A statement stipulating that participation is voluntary and that the participant may choose to withdraw at any time

---

Key information must be listed on an informed consent form (see box, The Elements of Informed Consent for Research) to be signed by participants. A participant in a medical research project need not remain in the study, and is free to withdraw at any time.

Informed consent for surgery or treatment

A consent form a person signs before undergoing a surgical procedure and some diagnostic treatments or tests. Health care professionals are required to provide a careful explanation to the person of what to expect, potential benefits and risks, and any alternative options to the

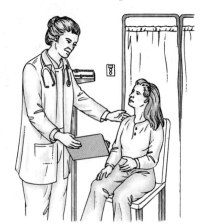

SIGNING A CONSENT FORM
Signing a consent form is the last step in the informed consent process—the process by which doctors and other medical staff explain treatment options and answer a patient's questions so that he or she can make an informed decision. Patients are always entitled to ask questions so that they feel educated and reassured when they sign the form.

surgery or treatment. The person is asked to sign a form that states that he or she understands the procedure or test and the risks involved.

Infrared

A form of radiation that emits energy as electromagnetic waves just beyond the limit of the red portion of the spectrum's visible rays. Infrared wavelengths are shorter than radio wavelengths and longer than those for light, and they may be detected as heat. Special infrared heat lamps used in PHYSICAL THERAPY emit natural, safe, short-wave infrared heat for the temporary relief of pain associated with many conditions, including muscular pain, sore muscles, arthritis, bursitis, backache, tennis elbow, aching joints, and related pains.

Ingrown toenail

A toenail that grows into the surrounding skin or tissue of the toe. The big toe is most commonly affected by ingrown toenails, which may be caused by improper trimming of the nails, wearing shoes that are too tight, or trauma. Symptoms include pain, swelling, redness, and the discharge of pus. Home care includes soaking the affected foot in warm water and placing a small piece of clean cotton under the corner of the nail. A doctor may prescribe antibiotics to control any infection. If the problem worsens, minor surgery may be necessary to remove part of the toenail. Prevention consists of trimming toenails straight across, leaving toenails at a moderate length, wearing shoes that fit properly, and keeping the feet clean and dry. Doctors advise those who have diabetes mellitus or other circulatory ailments to seek prompt treatment for ingrown toenails or other foot sores because they are much more prone to infections, which are difficult to treat, because of a reduced blood supply.

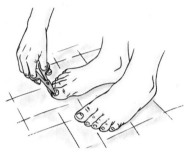

PREVENTING INGROWN TOENAILS
Cutting the toenails straight across, with no rounded corners, reduces the likelihood of ingrowing. The nail should extend past the skin, level with the top of the toe. Because chipping can contribute to the risk of ingrowing, it is important to use sharp scissors and to avoid picking at or tearing nails.

Inguinal

Having to do with the groin. An example of an inguinal structure is the inguinal ligament located in the groin. The inguinal canal is a passage in the lower abdominal wall that contains the spermatic cord in men and the round ligament in women. Because this passage creates a weakness in the abdominal wall, it is the most common site for HERNIA, the protrusion of an organ or tissue out of the body cavity in which it normally lies. An inguinal hernia, or rupture,

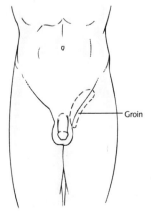

— Groin

GROIN AREA
The inguinal, or groin area is located between the lower abdomen and the thigh.

occurs in the lower abdomen when the intestine or its covering, the omentum, protrudes through the inguinal canal. An inguinal hernia can be caused by continual straining.

Inhalants

Breathable chemicals that produce psychoactive, or mind-altering, effects. Using these drugs is also known as glue sniffing and solvent abuse. Inhalants are not usually thought of as drugs since they are produced for very different purposes.

There are three principal categories of inhalants: solvents, such as paint thinners, degreasers, dry-cleaning fluids, gasoline, model glue, correction fluid, felt-tip pen ink, and electronic cleaners; gases, such as aerosols and propellants (for example, in whipped cream dispensers), spray paints, deodorants, and medical anesthetic gases (such as nitrous oxide, ether, and chloroform); and nitrites, including cyclohexyl nitrite (generally available), amyl nitrite (available only by prescription), and butyl nitrite (now illegal).

Inhalants may be sniffed from an open container or from a rag ("huffed" in street parlance) that is soaked in the material and held to the face. Sometimes the inhalant is placed in a bag to increase the concentration of vapors. When inhaled, the chemicals enter the bloodstream through the capillary surface of the lungs and reach the brain rapidly. Inhalants are often used together with alcohol.

Inhalants have effects like anesthetics and slow the body down. At low doses they may make the user feel stimulated. At higher doses they lead to a loss of inhibition. A high enough dose will cause a loss of consciousness. Many users experience distorted perceptions of space and time, headache, nausea and vomiting, slurred speech, loss of coordination, and wheezing. Many inhalants produce tolerance, forcing the user to use more to achieve the desired effect.

Even one-time use of inhalants carries a risk of sudden death from heart failure. Death can also result from suffocation when inhalant vapors are highly concentrated and too little oxygen reaches the lungs or when the individual vomits while unconscious and inhales vomit into the lungs.

Prolonged use can cause damage to the brain, nervous system, lungs, and kidneys; chronic headache; partial or complete loss of smell or hearing; nausea; nosebleeds; irregular heartbeat; violent behavior; chemical imbalances in the body; and incontinence (loss of control over bladder and bowel).

Most inhalant users are between 7 and 17 years of age. Besides intoxication, signs of use include a characteristic rash around the nose and mouth and the smell of paint or solvents on skin, clothes, or hair.

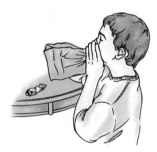

Inhaling fumes to get high

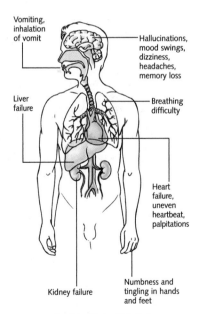

Vomiting, inhalation of vomit

Liver failure

Kidney failure

Hallucinations, mood swings, dizziness, headaches, memory loss

Breathing difficulty

Heart failure, uneven heartbeat, palpitations

Numbness and tingling in hands and feet

Possible effects of inhalants

ABUSE OF INHALANTS
Because inhalants are generally legal, nonmedical products, children have access to them and may try to misuse them to get "high." The abuser may be unaware of the extreme danger of sudden death; the chemicals in concentrated form can stop the heart or cause organ damage throughout the body.

Inhalation

The act of breathing in air. Inhalation therapy is the breathing in of substances such as oxygen or drugs in order to improve poor respiration or clogged airways.

Inhalation, smoke

Excessive breathing of smoke during a fire. The inhalation of smoke can cause serious lung damage. Many people who die from fire accidents have both smoke inhalation and burns; injury from smoke inhalation is responsible for as many as 75 percent of fire-related deaths in the United States. Closed-space fires, or fires in an enclosed area, increase the risk of smoke inhalation. Smoke inhalation injury happens because smoke contains toxic fuel by-products and sometimes contains fine solid particles, all of which can injure the lungs. Smoke inhalation symptoms include irritated eyes, gasping for breath, and coughing up black sputum.

Emergency treatment for smoke inhalation includes moving the person to a smoke-free area a safe distance from the fire and keeping as low to the ground as possible. The air at floor level is less toxic. If the person has not inhaled too much smoke, long, deep breaths of fresh air may help stop the coughing and clear the lungs. If the smoke is particularly dense, any rescue effort must be made by someone wearing proper breathing equipment. If the person is breathing, he or she should be made comfortable. ARTIFICIAL RESPIRATION

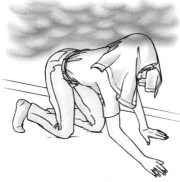

SURVIVING A FIRE
A person caught in a fire should crawl beneath the smoke, where the air is cleaner and cooler, to the nearest exit. To avoid smoke inhalation, he or she should drape a damp towel over the head if possible.

should be started if the person is not breathing. Emergency medical assistance must be obtained by dialing 911 or the emergency number for your area.

Inhalation, toxic gas

Excessive breathing of poisonous fumes. Toxic gas inhalation can result from breathing a number of different fumes, including cyanide or carbon monoxide, which is produced by gasoline-burning engines, defective cooking equipment, charcoal grills, and fires. If inhaled in large amounts, carbon monoxide will replace the oxygen in the bloodstream and reduce the supply of oxygen to the cells in the body. Symptoms of toxic gas inhalation include pale or bluish skin, headache, nausea, vomiting, and confusion. People who have inhaled poison gas need fresh air as soon as they can safely be moved. Emergency medical assistance must be sought.

Inhaler

Device used to deliver medication in an aerosol form that can be inhaled by people with asthma or other respiratory diseases. Inhalers are small, portable, and practical. They are used to deliver measured doses of drugs that improve breathing by dilating the airways. The types of antiasthma medication that are delivered by inhalers include BRON-CHODILATORS, CORTICOSTEROIDS, and CROMOLYN SODIUM.

Inheritance

The acquisition of characteristics or qualities by genetic transmission from parent to child; that which has been transmitted from parent to child.

Inhibin

A hormone produced by the testicles. Inhibin works with the hormone TESTOSTERONE to regulate the rate of sperm development.

Inhibition

Blocking of a physiological process. Also, an unconscious psychological process that restrains or suppresses a person's actions, emotions, or thoughts. Diseases such as dementia and alcoholism can cause reduced inhibition.

Injectable contraceptives

See CONTRACEPTION, HORMONAL METH-ODS.

Injection

The act of forcing a drug or other substance physically into the body by syringe or by catheter. Drugs may be injected under or through the skin or into a body cavity, a vein, or the tissues. Injection involves drawing up or loading the correct dose of a drug into a syringe, and injecting the drug into the body via a thin needle.

People with diabetes are often required to inject themselves with insulin one or more times each day. Insulin is usually injected subcutaneously (under the skin). A suitable site for the injection is usually an area with some fatty tissue, such as the abdomen, buttocks, thighs, or upper arms. See Types of injections on page 729.

Inkblot test

See RORSCHACH TEST.

Inlay, dental

A custom-made dental filling used to restore a badly decayed tooth. Dental inlays may be made of gold, porcelain, or composite. Inlays are generally used to support the biting surfaces of the back teeth that are being treated for tooth decay. Inlays may be made of gold because it is the hardest of the filling materials. For cosmetic reasons, however, porcelain or composite inlays may be more appropriate.

Gold inlays are generally used when a significant area of the tooth has been lost through decay. After the decay has been drilled away and the remaining hole shaped by a dentist, an impression (see IMPRESSION, DENTAL) is taken of the tooth structure. A temporary filling is placed in the tooth, and the impression is made to fit the cavity exactly. This usually takes about a week. The dentist applies a thin layer of cement over the base of the cavity and on the underside of the inlay to seal the tooth and permanently attach the inlay. Gold inlays are considered among the most durable options in dental restorations (see RESTORATION, DENTAL) for large cavities.

TYPES OF INJECTIONS

A thin needle and syringe are used to inject anesthetics, therapeutic drugs, nutrients, blood, blood plasma, and allergy-test substances. There are several different types of injections.

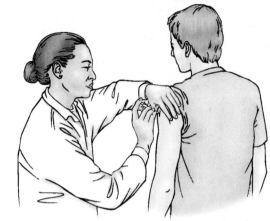

INTRAMUSCULAR
An intramuscular injection may be given when the drug has to be absorbed quickly. It is used for pain medications and for immunizations.

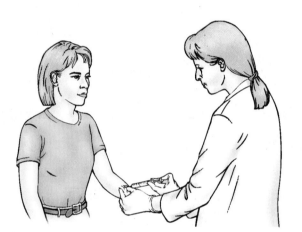

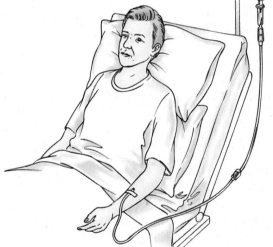

INTRADERMAL
An intradermal injection is directed into the tissues under the skin. It is used for tuberculosis testing.

INTRAVENOUS
An intravenous injection might be given to a person experiencing an allergic reaction.

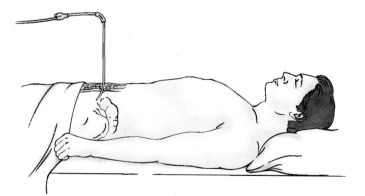

INTRAPERITONEAL
An intraperitoneal injection is given directly into the abdominal cavity. It is used to give antibiotics to treat infections and serious wounds.

Inoculation

The introduction into the body of microorganisms, such as bacteria or viruses, that have been modified or killed, for the purpose of stimulating resistance to specific diseases. Inoculation is usually accomplished by injection and may also be referred to as immunization or vaccination. The treated microorganisms trigger the body's immune system to form antibodies so the body can respond immediately if there is contact with the disease-causing agent.

Over a period of years, inoculations have significantly decreased the number of deaths caused by serious illnesses, including smallpox, diphtheria, poliomyelitis, tetanus, and certain types of meningitis.

There are two types of immunizations achieved by inoculation: active immunization and passive immunization. The active type injects all or part of a disease-causing microorganism, called an ANTIGEN, or a modified version of the antigen into the body to prompt a defensive response from the immune system that develops over several weeks. The immune system recognizes the antigens as foreign and forms antibodies or white blood cells called lymphocytes to attack the antigens. This type of inoculation can provide complete protection for many years or partial protection that allows the immunized person to contract the illness, but in a less severe form. In some cases, repeated inoculations, or booster shots, are required at certain intervals to maintain immunity.

A method of active immunization that protects against viral diseases involves injecting a person with live organisms that have been altered so they do not cause disease. This type of inoculation is used in vaccines against serious diseases, including poliomyelitis (in rare special cases), yellow fever, measles, and smallpox. The active type of inoculation that protects against bacterial diseases, including typhoid fever, whooping cough, and diphtheria, uses dead organisms that can no longer cause disease but still contain antigens. Another form of active immunization involves giving a person an injection of the chemicals that the bacteria produce rather than the bacterial organism itself. The toxins are treated with chemicals that render them no longer toxic, but leave their antigens intact. This method of inoculation is used to protect against toxic diseases, including tetanus and botulism.

Passive immunization involves the injection of antibodies obtained from the blood of an actively immunized human being or animal instead of injecting an antigen. This form of inoculation provides immediate, but temporary immunity that usually only lasts for several weeks to months. This form of inoculation can save the life of a person who has been infected with a potentially fatal organism, such as the virus that causes rabies.

Inoperable

A condition or disease state that most probably will not be improved or cured by using a surgical procedure. The term is often used to describe very advanced cancer or cancer situated in tissue that is not surgically accessible. People with inoperable tumors can be treated with other therapies, such as radiation, chemotherapy, or hormones.

Inorganic

In chemistry, a compound that does not contain carbon. The term "inorganic" is used to refer to matter that is not animal or vegetable.

Inpatient treatment

Medical care that takes place in the hospital and requires at least one overnight stay.

Insanity

A legal term describing a mental illness or impairment that leaves a person unaware of his or her actions. Insanity has no psychiatric or medical meaning. The legal definition of insanity varies depending on state law. In an insanity defense, a person charged with a criminal act argues that he or she is not guilty of the crime because of not comprehending the wrongfulness of the act at the time it was committed.

Insects and disease

Many insects are carriers of serious infections that can cause illness in humans. Viruses transmitted from insects to humans are called arboviruses. There are at least 80 different arboviruses that cause disease in humans. They are transmitted most commonly by mosquitoes and ticks. Mosquitoes often contract the virus by feeding on birds, then transmit it to domestic animals, such as horses, and to humans. Arboviruses most commonly cause infections without symptoms. They may also cause minor, nonspecific illnesses with fever. There are three separate syndromes caused by arboviruses: arthralgia-arthritis, hemorrhagic disease, and aseptic meningitis-encephalitis, which includes WEST NILE VIRUS, a potentially fatal, mosquito-borne illness that has caused brain infections and deaths in several areas in the United States and in central Europe.

The most common approach to controlling the spread of these viruses is to control the mosquito population by eliminating stagnant water in populated areas, by using larvacides to kill the insects' eggs, and by spraying particular pesticides to kill the mosquitoes. See also ENCEPHALITIS, YELLOW FEVER, DENGUE, LYME DISEASE, ROCKY MOUNTAIN SPOTTED FEVER, and MALARIA.

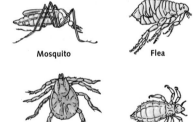

Mosquito   Flea

Tick   Louse

DISEASE-CARRYING INSECTS
Different insects carry specific diseases or cause specific medical problems. Some mosquitoes carry West Nile virus, yellow fever, malaria, and encephalitis. Fleas cause dermatitis and other skin irritations. Ticks carry Rocky Mountain spotted fever, Lyme disease, and Colorado tick fever.

Insecurity

An emotional feeling that makes a person feel unprotected or uncertain about what to do in a given situation. Insecurity is normal among children, adolescents, and adults in a new situation or at times of crisis or high stress, such as natural disaster, a death in the family, divorce, job loss, or serious disease.

Insemination, artificial

A procedure in which sperm (from the woman's partner or from a donor) is inserted with a syringe into a woman's vagina, cervix, or uterus during ovulation to try to impregnate her. Artificial insemination is sometimes used when for unknown reasons a woman has been unable to become pregnant, when abnormalities of the cervix have prevented sperm from entering the uterus, when sexual intercourse is impossible, or when a low sperm count or immunologic problems make special processing of the semen desirable. Donor insemination may be used when a husband or male partner is unable to produce viable sperm or at the request of a single woman or lesbian couple.

In the procedure, the man's semen is introduced with a syringe into the woman's cervix or, less often, into her vagina or uterus, as close to the time of ovulation as possible. The woman remains lying on her back for 20 minutes after the procedure to allow the sperm time to move toward the upper part of the fallopian tubes, where fertilization occurs. Usually the sperm are treated to enhance the chances that they will successfully fertilize the egg. For example, the semen of a man with a low sperm count may be

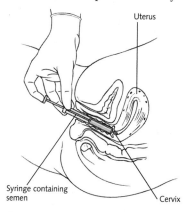

INJECTING SPERM DIRECTLY INTO UTERUS
For artificial insemination, a man's semen is injected into a woman's cervix (or sometimes into her vagina or uterus) around the expected time of ovulation. To increase the chances of fertilization, the semen usually has been treated to enhance viability of the sperm. After the injection, the woman remains lying on her back for about 20 minutes to give the sperm a chance to move toward the fallopian tubes, where fertilization usually occurs.

treated to increase the concentration of sperm. Sometimes the woman is given fertility drugs that cause more than one egg to mature at the time of artificial insemination to help increase the chances of fertilization.

About one in five women who are artificially inseminated become pregnant on the first try. The chance of becoming pregnant increases with subsequent attempts. By the sixth try, artificial insemination results in pregnancy in eight out of ten women who have no infertility risk factors, such as having problems ovulating.

Insight

The awareness and comprehension of the origin and importance of one's own feelings, attitudes, actions, and emotional symptoms. Psychotherapy often seeks to support and deepen insight, thereby allowing the person to see his or her issues more clearly and take steps to resolve them. In problem solving, insight refers to a sudden perception that results in a correct solution.

Insoluble fiber

See FIBER, DIETARY.

Insomnia

Difficulty getting to sleep or remaining asleep. Insomnia is a very common problem that can be short and self-limiting or may persist for years. Its causes range from stress and depression to physical pain (such as the chronic discomfort of arthritis) and SLEEP DISORDERS, such as RESTLESS LEG SYNDROME. Symptoms include difficulty falling asleep, waking frequently during the night, waking abnormally early in the morning and being unable to return to sleep, feeling tired during the day, and feeling restless and anxious as bedtime approaches. It is important to diagnose and treat the underlying cause of insomnia. In some cases, sleeping pills are helpful. However, they should be used on a temporary basis only. Regular use can make a person dependent on sleeping pills.

Good sleep hygiene is the best way to cope with insomnia. This means getting up at a regular time every morning, even on weekends; trying not to nap during the day; avoiding caffeine, alcoholic beverages, nicotine, and strenuous exercise for 4 to 6

hours before bedtime; consuming a light snack (but avoiding heavy meals) before retiring; and minimizing noise, light, and extreme temperatures in the bedroom. If a person is unable to sleep, it is best to leave the bedroom and engage in a quiet activity elsewhere. If sleeplessness persists, professional help should be sought.

Inspiration

The inhalation of air into the lungs. Inspiration involves contraction of the diaphragm and enlargement of the chest area as the walls of the lungs' air sacs expand with the intake of air.

Instinct

An inborn tendency to behave in a certain way. Hunger and thirst are examples of natural instincts.

Institutionalization

The placement of a person in a psychiatric hospital, prison, or other large institution. Today physicians and health care insurers consider it more beneficial to care for people with long-term illnesses in community settings rather than in large institutions. Institutionalization is most commonly used in response to severe psychiatric problems or medical conditions that require care beyond that which can be provided in the community, including severe mental retardation and marked autism.

Insulin

A hormone found in animals and humans; also an antidiabetic drug. Defective secretion of insulin by the pancreas is the cause of diabetes mellitus (see DIABETES MELLITUS, TYPE 1; DIABETES MELLITUS, TYPE 2). Many people with diabetes must control their blood glucose level with insulin injections.

WHAT INSULIN DOES

Insulin is a hormone secreted by the pancreas in response to high levels of blood sugar. It helps the body convert food to energy and to store energy for later use. Insulin works by processing sugar or glucose into body cells to make fat, sugar, and protein. Insulin has a role in the process by which stored fat, sugar, and protein are used for energy between meals. Without insulin, glucose cannot get into body cells, and the cells cannot work properly.

TYPES OF INSULIN

Various types of insulin are available for people who are required to use it because diet, exercise, or oral medication does not adequately control their blood sugar levels or because they had bad reactions to oral medications.

Commercially available human insulin is identical to natural human insulin, although it is manufactured through genetic engineering, using RECOMBINANT DNA methods. Another form of human insulin is produced by chemically converting pork insulin into human insulin; this is known as semisynthetic insulin. Other forms of commercially available insulin come from the pancreas of pigs and cows.

All forms of insulin must be administered by injection. Because insulin is destroyed by stomach acid, it can-not be taken orally. An inhalant form of insulin is being developed.

POSSIBLE SIDE EFFECTS

The most common side effect experienced by people who inject insulin is a low blood sugar level when too much insulin is injected; other side effects include having a depression in the skin at the site of the injection and an accumulation of fat under the skin from repeatedly using the same injection site.

Insulin antibodies

Proteins produced by the immune system that react against INSULIN. Insulin antibodies sometimes develop in people who take insulin made from pork or beef. The antibodies attack this insulin because it is different from human insulin or because it contains impurities. Insulin antibodies prevent the insulin from functioning properly and may produce an allergic reaction to the insulin.

The allergic reaction may cause red, itchy skin in the area where the insulin was injected, white or red patches of skin all over the body, or changes in heartbeat or respiration. The allergy is generally treated by desensitization therapy or by replacing the insulin that causes the reaction with purified insulin.

Insulin pump

An appliance for delivering insulin to people with type 1 diabetes (see DIA-BETES MELLITUS, TYPE 1). An insulin pump is a small device that is worn outside the body. It fits into a pocket or can be attached to a belt. The pump steadily injects insulin into the body, usually in the abdomen, via a tube attached to a needle that is inserted under the skin. An insulin pump supplies insulin to the person with diabetes in a pattern that is similar to the way the pancreas normally releases insulin into the bloodstream of a person who does not have diabetes. Implantable insulin pumps are currently under development.

Insulin resistance

A condition in which the body does not respond properly to the activity of INSULIN even though the pancreas produces sufficient amounts. To maintain a normal blood level of glucose (sugar), the pancreas needs to release abnormally large amounts of insulin into the bloodstream to compensate for insulin resistance. The elevated levels of insulin may damage the blood vessels and increase the risk of heart disease even if the blood sugar level remains normal.

Insulin resistance is common in people with type 2 diabetes (see DIA-BETES MELLITUS, TYPE 2). In type 2 diabetes, the insulin-producing cells in the pancreas initially compensate for the insulin resistance. At some point, the pancreas begins to fail and, even though it may still make more than an average amount of insulin, it can no longer overcome insulin resistance in the body. Consequently, the blood sugar level rises. As the disease progresses, the insulin level may continue to drop and fall below normal.

Being overweight is associated with insulin resistance because fat cells do not respond well to insulin. Insulin resistance is associated with high blood pressure and high levels of fat in the blood. Aging is another factor that contributes to insulin resistance.

Lifestyle factors that help a person control insulin resistance include eating less fat and fewer total calories, drinking little or no alcohol, not smoking, and reducing stress. Recent research has demonstrated that in many cases exercising regularly to build muscle and reduce fat can help control insulin resistance even if the activity does not result in weight loss.

Insulinlike growth factor

A peptide hormone made by most tissues of the body and believed to be secreted by the liver and released into the bloodstream. Insulinlike growth factor I (IGF-I) is involved in various biological activities in the cells. These activities include MITOSIS (normal cell division) and may be similar to the action of INSULIN. IGF-I is important to human survival because it regulates normal growth. It is mainly active in adults; the main growth factor in fetuses is insulinlike growth factor II.

Insulinlike growth factor is known to inhibit the self-destruction of cells in certain muscle cells of the heart, making it important to the survival of these cells. The hormone may be administered as a treatment for a person who has MULTIPLE SCLE-ROSIS or other nervous system disor-

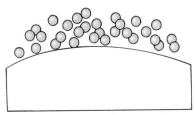

Type 1 diabetes

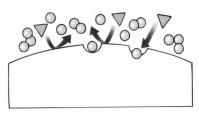

Type 2 diabetes

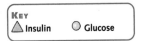

KEY
△ Insulin   ○ Glucose

ROLE OF INSULIN IN DIABETES
Insulin is a hormone that enables body cells to take in glucose (blood sugar) to use for energy. A person with type 1 diabetes produces too little insulin to allow glucose to enter a cell. In a person with type 2 diabetes, the cell resists the action of the insulin with the effect that glucose cannot enter the cell. In both types, the glucose gradually builds up in the bloodstream.

ders associated with injury to the spinal cord.

IGF-I may also be involved in tumor growth. Recent research has demonstrated that there is an association between higher concentrations of IGF-I in the blood and an increased risk of breast cancer in premenopausal women.

Insulinoma

A tumor of the beta cells that is found in the islets of Langerhans of the PANCREAS; also known as an insuloma or islet cell adenoma. An insulinoma is usually benign (not cancerous) but may be malignant (cancerous). In some cases, there is more than one tumor.

The specialized cells in the islet area of the pancreas produce INSULIN to regulate the metabolism of glucose in the body. Insulinomas produce an excess of insulin, causing an elevated level of insulin in the blood. This can lead to HYPOGLYCEMIA (low blood sugar).

SYMPTOMS, DIAGNOSIS, AND TREATMENT

Symptoms that may indicate an insulinoma include increased perspiration, rapid heartbeat, hunger, dizziness, headache, clouded vision, confusion, shakiness, seizures, and loss of consciousness. Severe hypoglycemia as a result of an insulinoma can cause coma.

If an insulinoma is suspected, MRI (magnetic resonance imaging) may be performed to determine the location of the tumor or tumors in the pancreas. Blood tests may be evaluated for levels of insulin in the bloodstream. Insulin C peptide in the blood may be measured after a person has fasted; a low blood sugar level after fasting can indicate an insulinoma.

Surgery is the most common treatment. Hypoglycemia may need to be treated and the blood sugar level stabilized before surgery. Usually only part of the pancreas is removed so that enough tissue is left to provide sufficient enzymes to avoid MALABSORPTION.

If the tumor cannot be found during surgery, the medication diazoxide, which inhibits the release of insulin, may be prescribed as an alternative treatment. Diazoxide must be taken along with a diuretic to prevent excess salt retention.

Integrative medicine

A blend of conventional medical practice with selected proven alternative therapies. Integrative medicine incorporates HOLISTIC MEDICINE, with its emphasis on person-centered care, and high-tech conventional medicine, with its focus on the cure of disease. With an eye to reducing health care costs, the National Institutes of Health (NIH) and other federal agencies have sponsored research to evaluate various components of integrative medicine. Alternative therapies under consideration include ACUPUNCTURE for chronic pain management; botanical medicine; YOGA; and MASSAGE THERAPY to boost the immune response; as well as several herbal remedies for chronic conditions.

Intelligence

The ability to comprehend, understand, and assimilate information. Because intelligence is an abstract general concept, it is difficult to define precisely. Most definitions of intelligence include abstract thinking, learning from experience, solving problems with insight, adjusting to new situations, and the ability to focus in order to achieve a goal.

THEORIES OF INTELLIGENCE

During the 20th century, scientists studying intelligence approached the issue in four basic ways.

■ **Psychometric approaches** The measurement of psychological traits or attributes is called psychometrics. Scientists studying intelligence psychometrically assume that intelligence is marked by differences among individuals. That is, one person may be more or less intelligent than another, and this difference is measurable. INTELLIGENCE TESTS are used to measure these differences, and the intelligence quotient, or IQ, is the best known intelligence measurement.

Various explanations have been developed to determine what intelligence tests actually measure. One school of thought maintains that a general ability underlies all specific intellectual abilities. Yet another school of thought argues that the various aspects of intelligence, such as verbal ability and spatial reasoning, are indeed separate. There is evidence to support both points of view, and the issue remains undecided.

■ **Neurological-biological approaches** Intelligence is obviously an aspect of the brain's structure and function. Researchers taking a neurological-biological approach to the study of intelligence look for aspects of the brain that are linked to intelligence. This approach holds that certain aspects of intelligence are independent of culture and, thus, the same in all humans. These shared aspects of intelligence are largely nonverbal, and they involve problem-solving capacities not measured by the intelligence tests used by psychometric researchers. So far, no specific neurological structures associated with intelligence have been found. This may change as brain anatomy and function are studied more closely.

■ **Developmental theory** The most famous proponent of this point of view is Jean Piaget, who saw intelligence as a special way for individuals to adapt to their environment. As individuals, particularly children, grow and develop, they constantly reorganize their psychological processes to come to terms with their surroundings. Adaptation becomes increasingly symbolic as age advances. This progression can be seen in Piaget's stages for the development of intelligence through childhood. In the sensorimotor period (birth to approximately 2 years), the child begins with simple reflexes and develops basic mental schemes to deal with the world. The preoperational period lasts from ages 2 to 7 years, as the child develops language and symbols (such as the alphabet and numbers), begins to think internally, can search for hidden objects, and understands past, present, and future. In the concrete operational period (approximately 7 to 11 years), the child can add, subtract, classify, and put objects in order, and he or she is more socially oriented than self-centered. With the formal operations period, beginning at approximately age 11 or 12 years, the child can think abstractly, reason deductively, develop and test hypotheses, and decide whether answers solve problems.

■ **Information-processing approaches** These theories look at the computer as a metaphor of the mind. In the same way that a computer has to manipulate individual bits and bytes of data, the human brain has to assemble a stream of information into a meaningful whole. To continue the metaphor, artificial intelligence programs provide insight into the actual workings of the brain. While these ideas are intriguing and promising, they have yet to generate a new understanding of intelligence.

FACTORS AFFECTING INTELLIGENCE
Research has shown that certain physical and cultural variables are associated with intelligence as measured by IQ. At least some aspect of intelligence is inherited; generally, higher-IQ parents, particularly mothers, have higher-IQ offspring. There is little or no connection between IQ and complications at birth, weight at birth, or childhood diseases, but malnutrition may lower IQ. Of environmental factors, the most important are family background and IQ. Income, education, occupational status, and home atmosphere affect IQ significantly. There is no clear connection between preschool enrichment programs or primary or secondary school quality and IQ. Girls generally have greater verbal intelligence than boys, who typically excel at visual-spatial thinking and mathematics during adolescence.

Intelligence tests

Question-and-answer devices used to measure the general intelligence of individuals. The most commonly used measurement of intelligence is the intelligence quotient, or IQ, which compares a person's intelligence with the average for his or her age. In most intelligence tests, an average score for a given age group is 100; an individual score between 90 and 109 is statistically average. Superior intelligence falls in the 120 to 140 range, with genius beginning at 140. Individuals with IQ scores from 80 to 89 are considered slow learners, and below 80 they are deficient in ways that usually cause school problems. Individuals with IQ scores below 70 are considered mentally retarded.

The most commonly used intelligence tests are the Wechsler Preschool and Primary Intelligence Scales (WPPS-R), Wechsler Intelligence Scale for Children-Revised (WISCR-R), the Wechsler Adult Intelligence Scale-Revised (WAIS-R), and the Stanford-Binet Intelligence Scale. Because IQ is measured against the average for the age, different tests are used for children and adults.

Controversy has arisen over the accuracy of intelligence testing, particularly the proven influence of education and social and cultural background on test scores. As a result, intelligence tests are often supplemented with other types of aptitude tests and measurements to provide a more accurate assessment.

Intensive care

See CRITICAL CARE.

Intensive care unit

The area of a hospital in which critical care is provided for people with life-threatening conditions. Types of intensive care units (ICUs) include medical, surgical, neurological, pediatric, neonatal (newborn), coronary care unit (CCU), and special burn units. ICUs are equipped to monitor blood pressure and heart rate, to provide oxygen and mechanical ventilation for the lungs, and to provide physical support for critical conditions. Neonatal ICUs are equipped to monitor infants' temperatures and the amount of oxygen in their blood. All intensive care units are staffed by nurses and physicians who have specialized training in critical care.

Intercostal

A term meaning between the ribs, such as the intercostal muscles that work with the diaphragm to help expand and contract the chest during breathing.

Intercourse, painful

Pain felt by a woman during arousal or during or after sexual intercourse. The pain may occur at the vaginal opening, in the vagina, or deeper in the pelvic cavity. Pain can arise from such problems as insufficient lubrication during sex; vaginismus (tightening of the muscles of the pelvic floor); infections of the organs and tissues of the reproductive system; endometriosis (a condition where the lining of the uterus grows outside the uterus); or scar tissue from infections, childbirth, or surgery. Pain can also be caused by infections in the bladder or urethra.

When a woman reports feeling pain during intercourse, a doctor will take a thorough history and perform a pelvic examination to help diagnose the cause of her pain. For undiagnosed persistent pain, a laparoscopy may be done to determine the cause of the pain. By inserting a laparoscope (a thin, light-emitting viewing tube) through the navel, a doctor can visually examine a woman's uterus, fallopian tubes, and ovaries. If no physical cause is found, a woman may need counseling to address issues that may make intimacy difficult and painful for her.

The condition can be made worse by emotional factors, such as having a history of sexual abuse or assault, domestic violence, or other personal problems. Women who experience painful intercourse suffer a major disruption in their lives and often benefit from treatments for its cause, the chronic pain itself, and from counseling for the emotional components of the condition.

Interferons

Substances produced by cells in the body to help fight infections and tumors. Interferons have been made synthetically since the late 1980s to treat certain cancers and other diseases using RECOMBINANT DNA technology. Naturally produced interferons are proteins secreted by cells in response to many triggers, or inducers, including viruses, parasites, and the proliferation of cells, both normal and malignant. Three major classes of interferons have been identified—alpha, beta, and gamma—all of them useful in the fight against infectious disease.

MANUFACTURED INTERFERONS
Several interferons made with recombinant DNA technology are available in the United States for treating infections. They also are currently used in the treatment of melanoma, certain leukemias, cancer of the skin and the cervix, Kaposi sarcoma, multiple sclerosis, and chronic viral hepatitis (hepatitis B and C), among others.

The Food and Drug Administration has approved these products for use in the United States. Interferon alfa-con-1 (Infergen) is used to treat chronic hepatitis B; interferon alfa-2a (Roferon-A) is used to treat chronic hepatitis C, hairy cell leukemia, and AIDS (acquired immunodeficiency syndrome)–related Kaposi sarcoma; and interferon alfa-2b (Intron A) is used to treat chronic hepatitis C and genital warts caused by the human papillomavirus. In addition, interferon alfa-n3 (Alferon N) is used to treat recurrent genital warts; interferon beta-1a (Avonex) is used to treat the relapsing form of multiple sclerosis; interferon beta-1b (Betaseron) is used to treat the relapsing form of multiple sclerosis; and interferon gamma-1b (Actimmune) is used to treat serious infections associated with chronic granulomatous disease, an inherited blood disorder.

Interleukins

A large group of hormonelike substances produced by white blood cells. Interleukins are part of the immune system and stimulate the body to fight infection and disease. They have become important in fighting some cancers.

Interleukin 1 (IL-1) is produced by a number of cells, including the white blood cells called T cells and B cells. IL-1 can set off a series of processes, including fever, that are involved in inflammation, a localized immune reaction. IL-1 also stimulates bone marrow growth.

Interleukin 2 (IL-2), also called T-cell growth factor, plays a central role in the regulation of the immune system by stimulating the growth and activities of a wide range of cells, some of which can kill cancer cells. Produced by T cells, IL-2 is used in immunotherapy, a developing area of cancer therapy. IL-2 is used in the treatment of kidney cancer and melanoma and is being investigated for possible use with other forms of cancer. Side effects can include fever, fluid accumulation in tissues due to leaking capillaries, and kidney function abnormalities. Interleukin 3 (IL-3) and other interleukins also are key to the immune system and are being researched as possible therapies for cancer.

Intermediate care facility (ICF)

Also known as an ICF, a type of NURSING FACILITY that provides food, lodging, and custodial care for people who are too ill or frail to care for themselves independently. Older people or those with serious illnesses or disabilities may enter intermediate care facilities, which provide regular (but not around-the-clock) nursing care. Some facilities also offer recreational programs. ICFs provide more services than assisted living facilities, which are geared toward more able and independent people; they provide fewer services than skilled nursing facilities, which are overseen by doctors, provide around-the-clock nursing care, and are meant for those who require more in-tensive medical and rehabilitative care.

Intermittent explosive disorder

See EXPLOSIVE DISORDER.

Intern

A RESIDENT in the first year of hospital training after medical school. An intern learns general medical practice and is only able to practice medicine under the supervision of an ATTENDING PHYSICIAN. Today interns are more frequently referred to as first-year residents.

Internal medicine

The branch of medicine concerned with the physiologic and pathologic characteristics of the internal organs of the body. Practitioners of internal medicine are known as internists; they specialize in the diagnosis and treatment of disorders of the internal organs.

Internist

A doctor who specializes in internal medicine, or the branch of medicine concerned with the physiologic and pathologic characteristics of the internal organs of the body. Internists diagnose and treat disorders of the internal organs and often provide a person's primary care.

Interstitial fibrosis of the lung

A disease in which the lung tissue becomes damaged by a known or unknown cause that produces inflammation of the lungs' air sac walls, which ultimately scars the interstitium (the tissue between the air sacs of the lungs). Interstitial fibrosis of the lung causes the tissue of the lung or lungs themselves to thicken and become stiff, which makes breathing difficult. Interstitial fibrosis of the lung is sometimes referred to as interstitial lung disease or simply PULMONARY FIBROSIS; all three terms describe the same condition.

Interstitial fluid

A clear liquid that bathes all the cells of the body. Interstitial fluid circulates outside the blood and lymphatic vessels; it is filtered from the blood in the

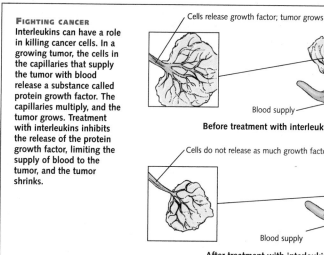
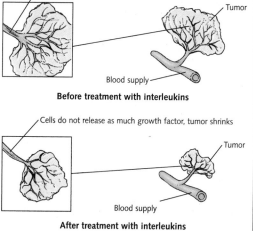

FIGHTING CANCER
Interleukins can have a role in killing cancer cells. In a growing tumor, the cells in the capillaries that supply the tumor with blood release a substance called protein growth factor. The capillaries multiply, and the tumor grows. Treatment with interleukins inhibits the release of the protein growth factor, limiting the supply of blood to the tumor, and the tumor shrinks.

Cells release growth factor; tumor grows

Tumor

Blood supply

Before treatment with interleukins

Cells do not release as much growth factor, tumor shrinks

Tumor

Blood supply

After treatment with interleukins

capillaries and returns to the blood-stream through the LYMPHATIC SYSTEM.

Interstitial nephritis

See NEPHRITIS.

Interstitial radiation therapy

See BRACHYTHERAPY.

Intertrigo

Inflammation and irritation of the skin caused by friction, moisture, bacteria, and yeast in skin folds. Intertrigo is most common in obese people and usually develops on the inner thighs, armpits, and underside of the breasts. This condition can be prevented by good hygiene, keeping the area dry, and losing weight. If a fungal infection develops, treatment is with a topical antifungal medication.

Intervention

A technique to encourage someone addicted to alcohol or drugs to enter treatment by telling that person to either recognize the disease or face its consequences, such as divorce or job loss. In most cases, individuals who are dependent on alcohol or drugs deny that a problem exists and are reluctant to face it. An intervention, in which the person is confronted with the abuse by loved ones, can help break down denial, which is the first step toward effective treatment.

Intervention studies

Research studies designed to determine the effectiveness of treatment in individuals with a particular disease or condition. The group being studied is known as the target population. The target population is divided into subgroups, one or more of which receives the treatment under study, while the others receive no treatment or the standard treatment. At the end of the study, differences in outcomes between the subgroups can provide a measure of the treatment's effectiveness. Intervention studies are commonly used to determine the effectiveness of new drugs and surgical procedures by comparing the outcomes achieved by the experimental procedure or medication with those achieved by standard treatment or no treatment at all.

Intestinal lipodystrophy

Also called Whipple disease, a rare disorder of the digestive system. Intestinal lipodystrophy is due to a bacterial infection. Its symptoms usually include abdominal pain, diarrhea, weight loss, joint pain, swollen lymph nodes, abnormal pigmentation, anemia, fever, and malabsorption of nutrients. Intestinal lipodystrophy most commonly affects middle-aged men. Treatment requires the long-term administration of antibiotics.

Intestine

The portion of the DIGESTIVE SYSTEM between the stomach and the anus, where absorption of nutrients into the bloodstream takes place. The intestine is in fact a long section of coiled tubing that has two parts—the small intestine and the large intestine—with different functions.

SMALL INTESTINE

The small intestine lies between the pyloric sphincter at the exit from the stomach and the first part of the large intestine (the cecum). The small intestine itself has three sections: the duodenum, the jejunum, and the ileum. Within the length of the small intestine, the chemical breakdown of food is completed and the usable components are absorbed into the bloodstream.

The walls of the small intestine are structured to perform its digestive functions efficiently. The intestinal wall has four layers: an outer protective layer (serosa); a muscular layer (muscularis); an inner layer containing blood vessels, lymphatic vessels, and nerves (submucosa); and a fourth layer that lines the inner walls and promotes absorption (mucosa). The surface of the mucosa is folded, and it has millions of tiny structures called villi that project into the intestine, much like the fibers of a carpet. The folds and villi together greatly increase the surface area of the lining of the intestine, so that maximum absorption can take place. The cells of the mucosa also secrete mucus to help pass food material along and digestive enzymes that continue the chemical breakdown of food. White blood cells in the mucosa prevent intestinal infection.

In the duodenum, which receives partially liquefied food material directly from the stomach, there are ducts that allow inflow of digestive enzymes from the LIVER and PANCREAS. The liver secretes bile, a substance that helps break down fats. Bile is stored in the GALLBLADDER (located just under the liver), which then releases it directly into the duodenum. Bile has pigments that give digestive waste products their brown color. From the pancreas, the duodenum receives enzymes that help break down fats, carbohydrates, and proteins and neutralize stomach

---

INTERVENING IN ADDICTION

Having an intervention is never easy, but it can be an effective way of putting an end to the destruction caused by dependence on drugs or alcohol. An intervention is an intensive process used for people with severe denial; it is often done when more routine attempts do not work and it is clear that the person with the addiction is in dire need of treatment. An intervention may work better when it is led by a professional who is accustomed to working with people who are addicted to drugs or alcohol. Here are some guidelines for people trying to help:

- It may be best to wait until the person with the addiction is sober before the issue is raised.
- The professional or designated individual hosting the intervention needs to explain that the dependent person has to get help or face the consequences, which may include the breakup of his or her marriage or family, loss of friendship, job termination, or chronic disease.
- Most important, the members of the intervention group must refuse to make excuses for the dependent person or to offer a second chance—moves that will be interpreted as tacit consent for the person to keep on drinking or using drugs.
- The addicted person should not be blamed. Blame is counterproductive and it misses the point. Dependence is a disease, not a moral weakness.

acids. The thicker muscular layer of the duodenum helps mix the food material and push it along into the jejunum. The jejunum, the second section of the small intestine, secretes enzymes that continue the chemical breakdown of food substances.

In the last section of the small intestine, the ileum, the actual absorption of nutrients occurs. The muscular layer is thinnest in the wall of the ileum. Each of the villi (the fiberlike projections) on the inner surface of the intestine contain a microscopic network of capillaries and lymphatic vessels that absorb the chemical components of foods and then transport them into the rest of the body.

LARGE INTESTINE

When digestive materials finally reach the first part of the large intestine called the cecum (a large pouch from which the appendix extends), nutrient absorption is complete. The undigested material that remains is composed of water, fibrous waste, and sloughed-off cells and mucus from the rest of the digestive tract. The function of the large intestine is to convert these waste materials into a form that can leave the body. In the COLON (the first and longest segment of the large intestine), water is absorbed. The amount of water absorbed depends on the length of time the wastes remain in the colon. The colon contains normal, helpful bacteria that extract the last vitamin and mineral content.

When the materials pass out of the colon, they are in a solid form called feces. The feces pass into the RECTUM, the final holding area, before moving out of the body through the anus. The rectum is a muscular structure that can expand to hold quantities of feces and keep them there until the reflex action of defecation starts. The rectum then provides the force required to push the feces toward the anus. The anus contains circular muscles that control the movement of feces. The muscles form two sphincters, one of which responds to involuntary reflex, and one of which is under voluntary control.

Intestine, obstruction of

A partial or complete blockage of the intestines that prevents the passage of the contents of the intestines. Obstruction of the intestine can be due to a number of different causes. Symptoms vary according to where the blockage occurs and may include severe abdominal pain, cramping, and distension. Abdominal distension due to obstruction is a medical emergency. Profuse vomiting and cessation of passing gas and feces are also signs. High-pitched BORBORYGMI (loud, rumbling, gurgling noises produced by the intestines) may indicate obstruction early on, as the bowel attempts to propel its contents around the obstruction.

The location of the obstruction can often be detected by the symptoms. When obstruction occurs high in the small intestine, vomiting is an early sign. Distension (an enlargement) of the abdomen becomes prominent with blockage of the large intestine because trapped feces, fluid, and gas cannot pass through the rectum; vomiting usually is minimal. Blockages can be partial or complete. With a partial obstruction in the small intestine, vomiting provides temporary relief of cramping. In partial obstruction of the large intestine, temporary pain relief comes with the occasional passage of gas and loose stools. Complete blockages anywhere in the digestive tract result in distension of the intestine above the affected site. The swelling develops

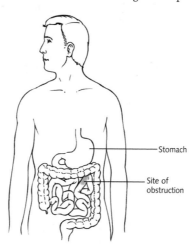

OBSTRUCTION IN SMALL INTESTINE
An obstruction high in the small intestine may cause vomiting; if there is any abnormal enlargement, it will be in the stomach or the small intestine leading out of the stomach.

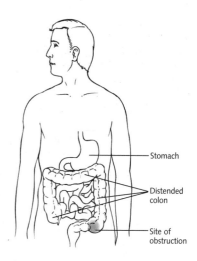

OBSTRUCTION IN LARGE INTESTINE
An obstruction in the large intestine causes stool and gas to back up, leading to considerable distension of the colon above the site of the obstruction

as gas builds up and is unable to escape.

CAUSES

The most common cause of obstruction of the small intestine is ADHESIONS. These bands of fibrous scar tissue bridge different bowel segments or attach the intestines to the abdominal wall following abdominal surgery or inflammation of the outer intestines and the abdominal wall. Although adhesions rarely cause serious problems, a loop of the small intestine can slip under an adhesion and become trapped. This leads to an obstruction inside the intestine. GANGRENE (death of tissue) can develop if the blood supply to the trapped part of the intestine is interrupted. Intestinal obstruction can result from VOLVULUS, in which a loop of the intestine becomes knotted or twisted and retains gas and feces. Distension, severe pain, and vomiting result. Gangrene may develop. In a strangulated HERNIA, protruding intestinal tissue can become trapped, cutting off its blood supply and obstructing intestinal contents. This condition requires immediate medical attention (see HERNIORRHAPHY). Obstruction of the large intestine may be due to colon cancer and may be the first sign of cancer. See COLON, CANCER OF THE.

DIAGNOSIS AND TREATMENT

Intestinal obstruction is diagnosed by

physical examination, X rays, and imaging studies, such as a lower GAS-TROINTESTINAL (GI) SERIES (an X-ray procedure that uses a contrast medium and is also called a barium enema). If the doctor suspects obstruction, hospitalization is necessary to find its cause and location. Intravenous fluids are given to prevent dehydration and shock. A long tube is passed through the mouth to decompress the intestines by removing fluid and air.

Often, surgery is needed to provide a diagnosis and to remove the obstruction. In cases of adhesions, the abdomen is opened and the adhesions are cut away to release the trapped intestine. If part of the intestine develops gangrene, that part is removed and the healthy remaining parts of the intestine are rejoined. Although more adhesions develop following surgery, most do not cause problems. Surgery is also the best treatment when colon cancer (see COLECTOMY) or volvulus (a twisted intestine) causes the obstruction.

Intestine, tumors of

Abnormal growths in the small or large intestine that may be benign (noncancerous) or malignant (cancerous).

TUMORS OF THE SMALL INTESTINE

Tumors of the small intestine grow slowly and are extremely rare. Although most are benign and without symptoms, 10 percent are malignant. Symptoms of a malignant tumor include fatigue, paleness, weight loss, abdominal pain, diarrhea, and blood in the feces. A history of CROHN DISEASE or CELIAC DISEASE increases the risk of malignancy. The tumors are generally diagnosed when a gastrointestinal (GI) series (a type of X-ray procedure) or colonoscopy is performed to determine the cause of the symptoms. If a tumor grows large enough, intestinal blockage can occur (see INTESTINE, OBSTRUCTION OF). Surgery is usually required to remove a malignant tumor or prevent obstruction. If tumors are too numerous or widespread for surgical removal, doctors may recommend CHEMOTHERAPY or RADIATION THERAPY. One or more of these treatments may also be ordered following surgery.

TUMORS OF THE LARGE INTESTINE

Benign tumors are more common than malignant growths in the large intestine. Most of these are polyps or abnormal tissue growths that arise from the intestinal wall and protrude into it. However, because polyps may become cancerous over time, doctors recommend their removal. See also COLON, CANCER OF THE; POLYPECTOMY; and RECTUM, CANCER OF THE.

Polyps may develop as a result of inflammatory diseases of the bowel, such as chronic ulcerative COLITIS and Crohn disease, or they may be hereditary. They are most common in countries where people consume a low-fiber, highly refined diet. Polyps usually cause no symptoms. Often, they are discovered during the course of a routine screening test such as a SIGMOIDOSCOPY (a procedure in which the rectum and sigmoid colon are examined using a slim, flexible, lighted tube inserted through the anus). Warning signs of cancerous tumors in the large intestine include blood in the stool and a sudden change in bowel habits.

Polyps are usually removed in a procedure called a colonoscopy (the viewing of the entire colon with a lighted tube). A colonoscopy can also be used to identify larger growths and to obtain a tissue sample to observe for cancer. For large growths, a more extensive operation called a laparotomy is necessary to identify and remove tumors. Tissues from abnormal growths are removed and examined under a microscope to find out whether they are cancerous. (See also BIOPSY.) Surgery may be necessary to remove a malignant tumor (see COLECTOMY). Doctors recommend regular screening colonoscopies for those who have had polyps because they are likely to recur. Colonoscopy may also be recommended for others at high risk for cancer of the colon.

Intoeing

Also called pigeon toes, an abnormality in which the leg or foot is slightly rotated, forcing the toes and foot to point inward. Many babies are born with feet that turn in. Intoeing is often the result of the child's position in the uterus and is usually not a serious problem, often correcting itself by about age 7. Severe cases may require surgery.

Intolerance

A physical reaction that may produce symptoms but does not involve the immune system. Intolerance may be due to emotional or physical stresses that trigger adverse reactions. These reactions are usually to food or other ingested substances and occur primarily in the digestive system. The symptoms of intolerance may be confused with those of ALLERGIES. Various diagnostic tests can distinguish between the two. See also FOOD INTOLERANCE.

Intracavitary therapy

Treatment directed into a body cavity. In intracavitary radiation, for example, radioactive substances are put directly into body cavities, such as the mouth, chest, vagina, or anus. The advantage to this method is that very high doses of radiation can be delivered directly to a tumor site while sparing surrounding tissue.

Intracerebral hemorrhage

See HEMORRHAGE, CEREBRAL.

Intracorneal ring

A small semicircle of plastic surgically implanted within the clear, surface layer (cornea) of the eye to treat nearsightedness. The ring spreads the cornea's layers apart, flattening its overall curve and reducing its focusing power. In most cases, this reduction decreases or eliminates nearsightedness by refocusing light onto the retina (the light-sensitive nerve layer at the back of the eye) rather than in front of it.

Intracorneal rings are inserted with the person awake. The eye is numbed with anesthetic drops and held open during the surgery to prevent blinking. Two small, tunnel-like incisions are made near the upper edge of the cornea, and the intracorneal rings are inserted. The incisions are closed with two small sutures, which are removed 2 to 4 weeks after the procedure.

The advantage to intracorneal ring surgery is that, unlike LASIK or PHOTOREFRACTIVE KERATECTOMY, the central cornea is not touched, reducing the risk of central scarring. In addition, the rings can be removed if necessary. The surgery can vastly improve vision in some cases of nearsightedness. The disadvantages of intracorneal ring surgery are greater discomfort during recovery, the risk of insufficient correction, and possible changes in vision, including glare and halos around light sources.

Intractable

Unstoppable. An intractable condition is one that cannot be cured or relieved, such as intractable diarrhea or intractable pain.

Intracytoplasmic sperm injection

See ICSI.

Intraductal papilloma

A small benign tumor growing in the cells lining a breast duct. Symptoms include a discharge from the nipple; the discharge may be clear and sticky, greenish yellow, or bloody. A discharge is normal in women who have recently been pregnant, but other women experiencing a nipple discharge should see their doctors right away. Because the symptoms of intraductal papilloma can resemble those of breast cancer, diagnosis will include a biopsy of the papilloma, a mammogram, and laboratory testing of the discharge, to rule out a diagnosis of cancer.

Intraocular lens implant

See CATARACT SURGERY.

Intraocular pressure

The force exerted by the fluid inside the eye pressing out against the eyeball. Normal intraocular pressure is between 10 and 21 millimeters of mercury. If intraocular pressure is abnormally high, it can result in a higher risk for developing GLAUCOMA, a disease that damages the optic nerve and can eventually lead to blindness.

Intrauterine device

A contraceptive device, usually made of plastic, that is placed inside the uterus for long periods. It interferes with the fertilization of eggs and the ability of fertilized eggs to attach to the wall of the uterus. See IUD; CONTRACEPTION, OTHER METHODS.

Intrauterine growth retardation

Stunting of fetal development. Newborns weighing less than 5 pounds and measuring less than 18 inches in length are considered to have intrauterine growth retardation (IUGR). This condition is usually caused by problems limiting the ability of the placenta to deliver nutrients to the fetus, such as when blood flow to some areas of the placenta is diminished. Intrauterine growth retardation is associated with severe PREECLAMPSIA, high blood pressure, hemorrhage, and PLACENTA PREVIA. Mothers with heart disease or diabetes mellitus and those who smoke, drink alcohol, take drugs, or are malnourished during pregnancy may deliver babies whose growth has been stunted.

Babies born with IUGR are less resistant to cold and are susceptible to HYPOGLYCEMIA. They have many more medical and developmental problems and have three times the risk of dying in infancy as babies born at normal weights. The risk for IUGR can be decreased with regular prenatal care. The uterus of the pregnant woman can regularly be measured by ultrasound, which can also be used with fetal heartbeat tests to monitor the fetus's health. If the fetus is not growing well because the placenta does not function properly, the doctor may induce labor early or deliver by cesarean section and let the baby develop in an intensive care nursery.

Intravenous anesthesia

See ANESTHESIA, INTRAVENOUS.

Intravenous pyelography

An X ray of the structures of the urinary system after the injection of an intravenous CONTRAST MEDIUM containing iodine into a vein. The contrast medium allows the kidneys, ureters, and bladder, which are normally not observable on X rays, to be visible for testing.

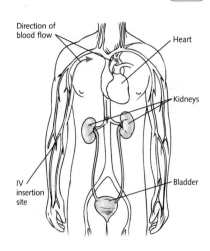

Direction of blood flow
Heart
Kidneys
IV insertion site
Bladder

IMAGING THE KIDNEYS AND URINARY TRACT
For intravenous (IV) pyelography, the person lies on an examining table and a dye is injected into the arm. The dye travels through the bloodstream, into the kidneys, and the bladder. The person is then asked to urinate, and the dye passes out of the body via the urinary tract. X rays are taken at 5- to 10-minute intervals to track the dye and obtain images of the structures.

WHY IT IS PERFORMED
Intravenous pyelography (IVP) is performed to locate tumors and other anatomical abnormalities of the kidneys, ureters, and bladder. It is also used to detect kidney and ureteral stones and to diagnose obstructions in the urinary tract.

HOW IT IS PERFORMED
The person undergoing the procedure may be asked to fast completely (no food or drink) for 8 to 12 hours before the procedure. Laxatives or enemas may be prescribed beforehand.

A baseline X ray is taken at the start of the procedure. A contrast medium is injected into an arm vein. People who have had an allergic reaction to the iodine contrast medium in the past should mention that fact to the physician or X-ray technician. X rays are taken periodically to track the contrast medium traveling through the kidneys and urinary tract. The person will be asked to urinate, and a final X ray will be taken to see if there is contrast medium remaining in the bladder.

Intraventricular hemorrhage

See HEMORRHAGE, INTRAVENTRICULAR.

Introvert

A personality type that is primarily concerned with and focused on internal events. Introverts tend to be withdrawn, shy, ill at ease socially, and interested in solitary pursuits. The opposite of an introvert is an EXTROVERT.

Intubation

An emergency medical procedure that involves inserting a tube through a person's mouth or nose into the trachea to allow the lungs to be manually or mechanically inflated. It also can be used to allow air to flow past a partial blockage of the throat, voice box, or windpipe. Intubation through the mouth or nose may be called tracheal intubation. It is performed if breathing has stopped or when a foreign object has been inhaled. STRIDOR, a crowing noise made during inhalation, is a sign of partial blockage of airflow in the upper respiratory system and may indicate the need for intubation. Intubation is also used when a person requires mechanical ventilation. This is common during general anesthesia. Intubation is also used as emergency treatment for people experiencing acute respiratory failure who need mechanical ventilation to assist their breathing.

Intussusception

A rare disorder in which part of an intestine retracts within itself, much as a telescope retracts. Intussusception most often occurs in the small intestine of babies 4 to 6 months old. Babies scream in pain when muscu-

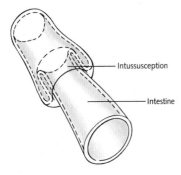

lar contractions occur in the telescoped portion of the intestine. Afterward, they become limp and pale, vomit, and pass bloody, mucous-filled stools. Babies who experience these symptoms require prompt medical attention. Diagnosis is made through a lower gastrointestinal (GI) series (an X-ray procedure also called a barium enema). The enema may force the telescoped portion back into place. If not, corrective surgery is recommended.

PAINFUL TELESCOPING OF INTESTINE
Intussusception affects babies only a few months old, comes on suddenly, and causes extreme pain. The child may become lethargic and vomit as the contents of the intestine back up. Immediate medical attention is required.

Investigational drug

A drug being studied that has not been approved for use by the Food and Drug Administration. Under certain circumstances, the use of investigational drugs is permitted for the treatment of serious or life-threatening conditions for which no alternative treatment exists. Four requirements must be met before an investigational drug can be used to treat patients: the drug must be intended to treat a serious or life-threatening disease, there cannot be a satisfactory alternative therapy available, the drug must already be under investigation or clinical trials must be completed, and the trial sponsor must be seeking approval to market the drug.

Involuntary movements

Uncontrolled, purposeless motions. TREMOR (involuntary, rhythmic muscle movement caused by alternate contraction and relaxation of the muscles) is the most common involuntary movement disorder. Others include CHOREA (involuntary, purposeless, rapid, jerking movements), ATHETOSIS (slow, writhing, continuous movements of the extremities), BALLISMUS (involuntary, irregular, and uncontrollable flinging and jerking movements), and tics (involuntary, repetitive muscle movements, such as blinking or twitching) (see TIC). In many cases, involuntary movements are a symptom of an underlying medical problem, such as PARKINSON DISEASE, MULTIPLE SCLEROSIS, head injury, or emotional disorders.

Iodine

A chemical element that is an important mineral in the human body. It is concentrated in the thyroid gland and is essential to the formation of the thyroid hormones, especially the hormone THYROXINE. Thyroid hormones maintain normal metabolism in the cells.

The principal dietary source of iodine is seafood. In areas where seafood is not available, iodized salt (table salt with added potassium iodide or other iodizing chemicals) can supply dietary iodine.

Radioactive iodine may be used as a medical treatment for HYPERTHYROIDISM (overactivity of the thyroid gland) or for thyroid tremors. It is given in the form of a clear, salty drink. Because iodine is essential to the thyroid hormones, the thyroid gland takes it in readily. The radioactive iodine becomes concentrated in the thyroid where it acts on the glandular tissue. Since the radioactive iodine concentrates in the thyroid, the overactivity of the cells can be controlled without exposing other areas of the body to radiation.

If too much radioactive iodine is taken, the hormone-producing cells of the thyroid gland are damaged and may become underactive. This results in HYPOTHYROIDISM (underactivity of the thyroid gland), which is treated with synthetic thyroid hormone medication.

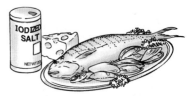

FOODS RICH IN IODINE
Good sources of iodine in the diet include seafood and dairy products. Today, iodine deficiency is rare because of the development of iodized salt, which is widely used in food processing and to season food at the table.

Ion

An atom that has lost or gained one or more electrons. Ions are electrically charged and therefore more active chemically. Ions are formed by electrolytes (see ELECTROLYTE).

Ipecac

A substance that when ingested induces vomiting; it is used to remove harmful or poisonous substances from the stomach and is commonly known as syrup of ipecac. When swallowed, ipecac irritates the stomach and acts on the brain stem to cause vomiting. Ipecac is available without prescription from any pharmacy.

Ipecac can be used by adults and given to children older than 6 months. The syrup should be stored at room temperature and will last several years. It should be taken with water.

Although ipecac is the safest way to induce vomiting, it should not be used by people who are unconscious or drowsy, by people with heart conditions, or by women during the third trimester of pregnancy.

Ipecac cannot be used in every poisoning emergency. Before using ipecac, it is wise to consult with a doctor or a specialist at a poison center.

Ipratropium

A bronchodilator delivered by INHALER for the relief of lung disease symptoms. Ipratropium (Atrovent) is used to open up narrow breathing passages and to control symptoms of asthma, emphysema, and chronic bronchitis. By increasing the flow of air into the lungs, ipratropium helps reduce coughing, wheezing, and shortness of breath.

IQ

Intelligence quotient, one measure of intelligence. See INTELLIGENCE TESTS.

Irbesartan

A drug used to control high blood pressure. Irbesartan (Avapro) is classified as an angiotensin II antagonist and has similar benefits to angiotensin-converting enzyme (ACE) inhibitors without producing a common side effect, a dry cough. Irbesartan causes blood vessels to dilate, or widen, thereby lowering blood pressure.

Iridectomy

A surgical operation to remove a portion of the colored portion of the eye (iris). Iridectomy is usually performed to alleviate the buildup of fluid in the eye in cases of angle-closure GLAUCOMA. It is also occasionally done to create an artificial pupil (opening in the iris).

Iridology

The analysis of patterns and structures in the iris of the eye to assess a person's general health and to detect certain forms of disease. The belief is that the iris is divided into six regions by which an iridologist can study the shape and color of the iris and correlate it to disease processes. Iridology is considered by those who practice it to be a safe, noninvasive, inexpensive diagnostic tool, one that can ascertain whether a person has a good constitution, whether he or she has nutritional imbalances, and whether toxic substances are present in the body. Iridology does not identify specific diseases but provides general information about body tissues. However, scientific investigations have failed to show any clinical effectiveness for iridology.

Iridotomy

A laser procedure in which a tiny hole is placed in the colored portion of the eye (iris). This is most often performed for angle-closure glaucoma.

Iris

The pigmented circular muscle that surrounds the PUPIL of the EYE and controls the amount of light entering it. The iris is made of thin layers of muscle that open or close the dark hole (the pupil) at its center in response to the intensity of surrounding light. In bright light and for near vision, the iris constricts the pupil. In dim light and for more distant vision, it widens (dilates) the pupil. Emotions can also affect the size of the pupil. For instance, the iris widens the pupil in response to fear or danger. The color of the iris, determined by heredity, depends on the amount of pigment cells it contains; blue eyes have less pigment than darker eyes.

Iron

An element essential to life. Iron is present in the adult body chiefly in the form of hemoglobin in the red blood cells, but also in muscles and other iron stores. Iron is essential to the transfer of oxygen from the lungs to the body tissues. If body cells do not receive adequate iron, the result is iron-deficiency anemia, which causes a person to feel weak and tired. People at highest risk for developing anemia include growing children between the ages of 6 months and 4 years; adolescents, especially girls; pregnant women; and women with very heavy menstrual periods.

The best dietary sources of iron are liver, lean red meat, poultry, fish, shellfish, and kidney. Iron can also be found in dried beans, fruits, and vegetables, although the absorption of that form of iron is blocked by other components of the diet, including all dairy products, tea, and whole grains. Iron is often added to enriched breads, cereals, wine, molasses, and dried fruits. Oral iron supplements are available without a prescription but should only be taken when recommended by a doctor.

Iron-deficiency anemia

See ANEMIA, IRON-DEFICIENCY.

Irradiation

Exposure to radiation. Medical irradiation is used for diagnostic or therapeutic purposes and may involve X rays or radioactive isotopes. See also NUCLEAR MEDICINE; RADIATION; and RADIATION THERAPY.

Irrigation, wound

To flush a cut area of the skin with a stream of liquid for the purpose of cleansing or medicating the area. Wound irrigation may be accomplished with clean, warm water or with a disinfectant such as hydrogen peroxide. To prevent infection, skin wounds should not be touched with the hands, particularly if the wounds are bleeding. Irrigating a wound allows the open skin surface to be cleaned or medicated without coming into physical contact with the possible contaminants carried on another person's hands. See also PUNCTURE WOUNDS.

Irritable bladder

FOR SYMPTOM CHARTS
see Urination in men, painful or frequent, page 56
see Urination in women, painful or frequent, page 57

Another name for urge incontinence, which refers to the involuntary loss of urine immediately after the need to urinate is felt. See INCONTINENCE, URINARY for details.

Irritable bowel syndrome

FOR SYMPTOM CHARTS
see Constipation, page 26
see Diarrhea, page 34

A condition characterized by any combination of symptoms, including abdominal pain, indigestion, bloating, diarrhea, and constipation, with no clear cause. Irritable bowel syndrome (IBS) can cause alternating bouts of diarrhea and constipation. In addition to pain, indigestion, and bloating, there may be excessive gas, nausea, abdominal distension, rumbling and gurgling, temporary relief of pain after passing gas or feces, mucus in the feces, and a feeling that the bowel is not emptying completely. Symptoms can be aggravated by anxiety. IBS, the most common disorder of the digestive tract, is not a chemical disease or due to a structural defect. It is a functional disorder that affects the muscles of the intestine and can be brought on or aggravated by emotional stress. Evidence suggests that increased responsiveness of the nervous system to normal stimuli is part of the cause. Food intolerance is another contributing factor. IBS is twice as common in women as in men and usually begins in early adulthood.

DIAGNOSIS
The symptoms of IBS are similar to those of many other gastrointestinal disorders. A sudden change in bowel habits after years of regularity can be a symptom of IBS or of a serious digestive disorder, such as colon cancer (see COLON, CANCER OF THE). As a result, the diagnosis of IBS is made by eliminating other possible causes of symptoms. The doctor typically orders a number of tests to rule out other underlying problems. Tests may include imaging procedures, such as ultrasound or CT (computed tomography) scanning, SIGMOIDOSCOPY (a procedure in which the rectum and sigmoid colon are examined using a slim, flexible, lighted tube inserted through the anus), barium X rays of the gastrointestinal tract, and stool analysis. When chronic symptoms include abdominal discomfort, problems with passing stools, and emotional stress, and tests do not reveal the presence of any other

disease, the diagnosis is most likely IBS.

TREATMENT
Although IBS has no cure, symptoms can be managed. Practicing relaxation techniques may reduce stress. A high-fiber diet that includes eight to ten glasses of liquid a day is recommended for constipation, and glycerin suppositories or enemas can be used in severe cases. For diarrhea, doctors advise resting and drinking clear fluids until symptoms subside. Watery diarrhea can cause dehydration and loss of crucial body salts, which may be restored with oral rehydration fluid (see REHYDRATION FLUID, ORAL). Gas-producing foods such as beans, cabbage, and onions should be avoided. Limiting dairy products may be helpful because LACTOSE INTOLERANCE can contribute to IBS. Smoking intensifies symptoms and should be eliminated.

Medications, such as antispasmodic drugs, mild sedatives, and tranquilizers, are recommended in some cases of IBS. Many individuals benefit from antidepressant drugs. Laxatives other than fiber should be used only cautiously and infrequently because they can worsen symptoms, and their long-term use may damage the colon.

Irritable colon

See IRRITABLE BOWEL SYNDROME.

Ischemia

A temporary shortage of oxygen in a part of the body caused by impaired blood flow. Ischemia is named by the location at which it occurs. Cardiac ischemia occurs in the heart, where it may cause ANGINA or a HEART ATTACK. Cerebral ischemia afflicts the brain, where it can lead to a TRANSIENT ISCHEMIC ATTACK or a STROKE. Ischemia in the kidney is renal ischemia; in the liver, hepatic ischemia. Ischemia in the legs results in CLAUDICATION, which causes pain and cramping with activity and can lead, in severe cases, to gangrene and amputation. The usual cause of ischemia is a buildup on the artery walls of fatty material known as plaque; the plaque narrows the artery and slows blood flow. If a blood clot forms at the site of the narrowing, the oxygen supply

may be completely interrupted, leading to the death of the affected tissue.

Ischemia can be treated with medication, such as beta blockers to decrease the workload on a heart affected by cardiac ischemia and aspirin to prevent blood clots. Surgery may also be used. See CAROTID ENDARTERECTOMY; BALLOON ANGIOPLASTY.

Risk factors associated with ischemia include a diet high in fats and oils, uncontrolled diabetes mellitus, uncontrolled high blood pressure, smoking, lack of exercise, and obesity. Minimizing these factors lowers the risk of ischemia.

Isoflurane

A gas that acts as a highly effective anesthetic agent when inhaled. Because isoflurane works rapidly, it can be used to begin, or induce, anesthesia, as well as maintain general anesthesia during surgery. Isoflurane is easily eliminated by the body and poses little risk to the liver and kidneys, which flush medications from the body.

Isolation

A method of preventing the transmission of infection in hospitals. Isolation procedures are generally used for the care of patients in acute-care hospital settings when serious symptoms come on suddenly.

One goal of isolation may be to prevent the spread of disease organisms from hospitalized patients to the hospital staff, visitors, and other patients. This kind of isolation is used with hospitalized patients who have highly contagious or dangerous infections. The procedures taken to contain or isolate the patients' infections and prevent their spread to uninfected persons may vary according to the specific infection. With certain severe respiratory infections, all visitors and staff wear face masks that cover the nose and mouth. This can be essential in certain cases, such as one in which a person has pneumonia caused by antibiotic-resistant bacteria. Gowns worn over street clothing and gloves may need to be worn by anyone in contact with patients who have infected wounds or serious and highly contagious gastrointestinal infections.

Protective isolation, on the other hand, seeks to protect hospitalized patients with weakened immune systems from exposure to contamination or infectious agents. Anyone who has contact with these patients must wear a gown to cover street clothing, a mask to cover the nose and mouth, and gloves to cover the hands to prevent unknown infectious agents from reaching the patient. In rare cases when a person's immune system is severely suppressed, the air the person breathes may need to be specially filtered to prevent infection. A person with such an immune disorder may have to be isolated in a specially constructed sterile room, or "bubble." See also NOSOCOMIAL INFECTIONS.

Isoniazid

An antibiotic used to treat tuberculosis (TB). Isoniazid (Laniazid, Nydrazid) is used to prevent TB in people who have been exposed to it but have no symptoms and in combination with other drugs to treat active disease. It is an antibiotic that works by interfering in the metabolism of the microorganism that causes TB.

Isoniazid is given as a tablet, a syrup, or by injection. It is administered together with vitamin B6 to prevent a number of side effects, including numbness, tingling, or unusual sensation such as prickling of the skin and stomach upset. Isoniazid may have to be taken for as long as 2 years to ensure that active disease has been adequately treated.

Isopropyl alcohol

A transparent, volatile, colorless liquid with disinfectant properties (see DISINFECTANTS); also called rubbing alcohol. Isopropyl alcohol is used as a solvent and disinfectant and as an antiseptic (see ANTISEPTICS) when applied to the skin. Rubbing alcohol, available over-the-counter, is a combination of 68 to 72 percent isopropyl alcohol and water.

Isopropyl alcohol is poisonous if a person ingests it. It should not be used as a bathing solution to cool children with a high fever. Symptoms of an overdose include labored breathing, lack of coordination, nausea and vom-

iting, low blood pressure, dizziness, and unconsciousness. If a person is suspected of drinking isopropyl alcohol, a POISON CENTER or hospital emergency department should be contacted immediately.

Isosorbide dinitrate

A drug used to relieve or prevent ANGINA (chest pain). Isosorbide dinitrate (Isordil, Sorbitrate, Dilatrate, and others) relieves angina pectoris by dilating or widening blood vessels and by relaxing the muscles in their walls, thereby improving oxygen flow and reducing chest pain.

Isotretinoin

A drug used to treat severe acne. Isotretinoin (Accutane) is prescribed only after milder medications, including antibiotics, have failed to clear up the acne. Isotretinoin works by shrinking oil glands within the skin, thereby diminishing the amount of oil they produce.

Isotretinoin is taken orally in capsule form. People who take it are warned that their acne may not improve immediately and that their skin may get worse before it gets better. Isotretinoin is known to cause severe birth defects, so women must not take it if they are pregnant, and they should not become pregnant while taking the drug.

Itching

See PRURITUS.

ITP

Idiopathic thrombocytopenic purpura; a condition of unknown cause in which the blood has an insufficient number of platelets and the person bruises excessively. ITP involves an abnormally low count of platelets in the blood, but numbers and quality of the person's other blood cells are normal. Platelets are tiny cells that help the blood form clots. When these blood cells are deficient, a person bruises easily and bleeds for a long time after being injured. Tiny red dots on the skin may appear, and when the condition is severe, the affected person may have uncontrollable nosebleeds and internal bleeding in the intestines.

While the cause of ITP is not known, it is known that people who

have the condition form antibodies that destroy the platelets in their blood as the result of an autoimmune disorder. One form of the condition affects children, typically between the ages of 2 and 4. This form results in sudden bleeding, in nosebleeds and bleeding gums, and in bruising and tiny red spots on the skin. These symptoms usually follow a viral infection by 2 weeks and typically improve on their own within about 3 weeks.

In contrast, the adult form is usually a chronic disease. It occurs primarily among young adults, with a peak incidence between ages 20 and 50. It occurs twice as often in women younger than 40 than in men. Increased bleeding and bruising are the characteristic signs, and in women, increased menstrual blood flow is another major symptom. Adults usually have a mild form of the condition that is not recognized until blood tests for other reasons reveal a low blood platelet count, which may persist for months. The spleen usually is not enlarged.

DIAGNOSIS AND TREATMENT

ITP is generally diagnosed by evaluating a medical history that indicates the typical signs, by a physical examination that may reveal a bleeding tendency, and by a blood test. Antibodies against platelets may help establish the diagnosis.

Treatment of children with ITP is aimed at managing the symptoms. Most children recover completely with no treatment because the disease usually resolves on its own.

In adults, ITP treatment is directed at increasing the platelet count by taking oral prednisone, a corticosteroid, for a month or longer. Approximately 80 percent of people will respond to treatment, and the platelet count will usually return to normal. If there is no response to prednisone therapy, surgical removal of the spleen may be necessary since the spleen manu-fac-tures most of the antibodies that destroy the blood platelets. Alternative therapies include high-dose intravenous

Terms in small capital letters— for example, PHYSICAL THERAPY or PAGET DISEASE—indicate a cross-reference to another entry with more information.

immunoglobulin and danazol. Immunosuppressive drugs may be helpful when all other treatments are ineffective.

Itraconazole

An antifungal drug used to treat serious fungal infections, particularly of the lungs. Itraconazole (Sporanox) is used to prevent and treat the fungal infections histoplasmosis and blastomycosis; both are diseases of the lung. A liquid form of the drug is used to treat candidiasis (thrush) in the mouth or throat. It has also been used to treat fungal infections of the nails. Itraconazole is also available in capsule form to treat oral candidiasis and fungal infections of the nails.

IUD

Intrauterine device. IUDs are small, usually plastic, devices containing copper or hormones that are placed in the uterus to interfere with ovulation and conception and to prevent pregnancy. The copper IUD releases a small amount of copper that changes the lining of the uterus to prevent fertilized eggs from implanting. The hormonal IUD releases small amounts of the hormone progesterone into the uterus. The hormone thickens cervical mucus, creating a barrier to sperm entering the uterus. It also affects the uterine lining in ways that prevent implantation of a fertilized egg. A hormonal IUD must be replaced every year; the copper

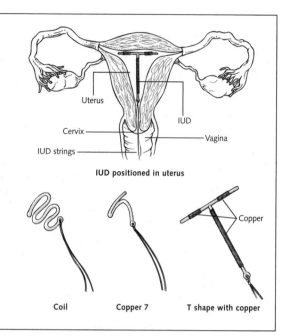

TYPES OF IUDS
An intrauterine device, inserted into the uterus by a doctor, changes the environment of the uterus so that sperm are unable to reach the fallopian tubes or so that fertilized eggs cannot implant in the uterus. Strings attached to the bottom of the device extend through the cervix down into the vagina; the woman wearing the device can locate the strings with her finger. Two basic types of IUDs—one containing copper and the other containing the female hormone progesterone—come in several typical shapes: the coil, the copper 7, and the T shape with copper.

Uterus

IUD

Cervix

Vagina

IUD strings

IUD positioned in uterus

Copper

Coil

Copper 7

T shape with copper

version can be kept in place for up to 12 years. The IUD is a highly effective method of contraception and is one of the safest. However, it is not recommended for women who have had a pelvic infection, an ectopic pregnancy, severe pain during menstruation, abnormal vaginal bleeding, or those who have multiple sexual partners (because of the risk of sexually transmitted diseases). IUDs tend to make pelvic infections worse and can render a woman infertile and increase the risk for an ectopic (tubal) pregnancy. See also CONTRACEPTION, OTHER METHODS.

IUGR

See INTRAUTERINE GROWTH RETARDATION.

IVF

See IN VITRO FERTILIZATION.

IVP

See INTRAVENOUS PYELOGRAPHY.

J

Jaundice

A yellowing of the skin and the whites of the eyes. Jaundice may also be associated with dark-colored urine, and it is a symptom of many liver disorders, including CIRRHOSIS, HEPATITIS, and LIVER CANCER. Also known as icterus, jaundice is usually a sign of a blockage of the bile ducts from the liver or disease within the liver. It is due to an excess of bilirubin (a normal by-product of the breakdown of hemoglobin from aging red blood cells) in the bloodstream. Normally, bilirubin is carried from the liver to the bile ducts to the small intestine, where it is broken down. Eventually, it is excreted in the stool. If this process is interrupted, excess bilirubin accumulates and causes jaundice.

Jaw

Usually refers to the lower jaw, called the mandible, the only movable bone in the face. The bone of the upper jaw, called the maxilla, extends all the way up to the eye sockets. Both the upper and lower jaw bones hold the teeth in position. The joint between the lower jaw bone and the skull is called the temporomandibular joint. Movement of the jaw is involved in chewing and biting and in speech production.

Jaw, dislocated

The displacement of the bones of the jaw's temporomandibular joint, which causes soft-tissue damage to the joint capsule and to the ligaments. Muscles connected to the joint may be strained, resulting in painful muscle spasms in the area of the jaw. When the jaw is dislocated, it is often impossible to close the mouth. A dislocated jaw may occur when the mouth is opened too wide during yawning, from a direct blow to the jaw, or from whiplash or other trauma to the neck and head area. The condition may be treated by manipulating the joint back into proper position, sometimes with the use of an anesthetic. Once the jaw has been properly realigned, a bandage may be used to hold it in place. Care must be taken not to open the mouth too wide for at least 6 weeks. A person whose jaw has been dislocated repeatedly should consult with a maxillofacial surgeon for possible treatment.

Jaw, fractured

A completely or partially broken lower jaw bone, or mandible. An inability to close the mouth or align the teeth properly, as well as a lower jaw that hangs without support, may all indicate a broken jaw. Other symptoms include severe pain in the area; swelling of associated muscles, tendons, and ligaments; or an apparent deformity of the jaw in complete breaks, which may cause the bone segments to separate. Other symptoms include tenderness with light contact and possibly a movable upper jaw, bleeding at the base of the teeth near the site of the fracture, and numbness at the site.

If a broken jaw is suspected, the person should seek immediate medical attention. Using a bandage to immobilize the jaw is the first line of emergency first aid for treating a fractured jaw. The most common cause of this injury is trauma from a direct blow to the jaw, as in contact sports such as boxing. Indirect stress on the jaw bone may be produced by intense muscle contractions, which can be sufficiently forceful to break the bone. A history of bone or joint disease and poor nutrition, specifically a deficiency of calcium in the diet, are risk factors for a fractured jaw. Diagnosis is made on the basis of a physical examination, special X rays, and possibly a CT (computed tomography) scan of the area. Surgery is often necessary to realign the segments of jaw bone and allow healing. In many cases, the jaw must be wired to the opposing jaw or otherwise immobilized for a period of up to 8 weeks. During this recovery period, only soft foods and liquids are permitted, and talking is often difficult.

Jealousy, morbid

An abnormally strong emotional reaction to the perceived, threatened, or actual loss of a loved person or object to someone else. Morbid jealousy most often arises in relationships between spouses or lovers when one partner senses that a competitor is winning the loved one's affections. Morbid jealousy can result in violence. It is estimated that one of every three to five murders involves jealousy.

Jejunal biopsy

A rarely performed diagnostic procedure in which a tissue sample from the jejunum (the part of the small intestine between the duodenum and ileum) is removed for analysis through a tube that enters the body orally. A jejunal biopsy is performed when an individual experiences symptom such as malabsorption (impaired absorption of nutrients through the small intestine), diarrhea, and weight loss. Eating and drinking are stopped for at least 8 hours before the procedure. To reduce discomfort, the throat is sprayed with a local anesthetic immediately before the procedure. A tube is inserted in the mouth and through the stomach into the small intestine.

A jejunal biopsy generally lasts 20 to 30 minutes. Afterward, it is necessary to rest an hour or two until medication wears off. In most people, the only side effect is a mild sore throat. However, rare complications include bleeding, bacterial infection causing fever and pain, and perforation of the bowel. Generally, duodenal biopsies are used instead of jejeunal biopsies because duodenal biopsies are simpler and usually provide similar types of information.

Jejunum

The midsection of the small INTESTINE. Together, the duodenum, the jejunum, and the ileum make up the small intestine. Cells in the lining of the jejunum secrete enzymes that combine with the secretions from the duodenum to break down nutrients at a cellular level. Absorption of fats into the bloodstream occurs primarily in the jejunum, as does the absorption of some carbohydrates, proteins, and vitamins.

Jet lag

A groggy, dragging, "out-of-sync" feeling that is caused by lost sleep when a person crosses time zones during air travel. Jet lag is most frequent when a person flies eastward, thus subtracting hours from his or her day. To minimize jet lag, doctors recommend resetting the body's clock to the sleep-wake pattern of one's destination several days in advance of departure; drinking plenty of fluids, avoiding the dehydrating effects of alcohol, and eating lightly; and exercising regularly, but not late in the evening.

Jock itch

A fungal infection of the groin; also known as TINEA cruris. Fungi thrive in the warm moist areas of the groin. Friction, poor hygiene, and prolonged moist skin increase susceptibility to the infection. Jock itch is a common skin disorder in men, especially in those who frequently wear protective athletic gear.

Jock itch is characterized by itching of the groin and a scaly red skin rash with sharply defined borders. Usually the genitals are not involved, but there may be itching and discomfort around the anus. Often the rash spreads in a circle, leaving normal-appearing skin in the center. The diagnosis is made through appearance of the skin. If necessary, a skin scraping or fungal culture can confirm the diagnosis.

Most cases of jock itch respond well to treatment with over-the-counter antifungal creams or powders such as clotrimazole or miconazole. It is also essential to keep the skin clean and dry. Severe infections require prescription topical or oral medications. Possible complications of jock itch include secondary bacterial infections and permanent skin discoloration.

Jogger's nipple

A painful irritation of the sensitive skin on a nipple that is usually caused by chafing from a sports bra during high-impact exercise, especially jogging or running. Women can help prevent jogger's nipple by wearing sports bras that are less likely to cause irritation. Synthetic fabrics do not stay as wet as cotton and are less likely to cause chafing from sweat. Sports bras with flat or covered seams are less abrasive against the nipples. Petroleum jelly or talcum powder may be applied to the area to help protect it. Specialty running stores often carry nonstaining lubricating products that are made for treating

jogger's nipple. The donut-shaped cushions made to treat corns on the feet offer good nipple protection for joggers and peel off easily after running or other high-impact activities.

Joint

The juncture of two bones. Some joints are fixed and immovable, but most have varying ranges of movement.

The individual bones of the skull join at fixed joints called sutures. The ragged edges of the bones tightly interlock to provide the greatest possible protection for the brain. Some other joints are capable of only slight movement; for example, the joints between the vertebrae move enough to allow the spine to be flexible, but are rigid enough to protect the delicate structure of the spinal cord.

Most of the joints in the body are movable, and the degree of mobility is determined by the function of the body part. The simplest type of movable joint is a hinge, in which one curved bone surface fits into another, allowing bending and straightening only. The finger and toe joints are hinges. Another type of joint, the pivot, allows rotational movement by means of a bone projecting into a circular bone; an example is the joint between the first and second vertebrae that allows the neck to turn partially. An ellipsoidal joint (in which an oval surface fits into an oval socket), such as the joint between the forearm and wrist, allows a wide range of movement, but only limited rotation. A ball-and-socket joint, in which a round head fits into a deep round cavity, allows the greatest range of movement. The hips and shoulders have such joints.

All movable joints have ligaments holding the bones together (external ligaments). Ligaments are made of tough connective tissue with very little elasticity. Some complex joints have internal ligaments that run between bones inside the joint. The entire joint is enclosed in a fibrous capsule that prevents the ends of the bones from dislocating. The capsule is strengthened with an inner layer of ligaments referred to as capsular ligaments. The lining of the joint capsule, called the synovial membrane, is lubricated by a secretion called

synovial fluid. The synovial fluid enables the ends of the bone to slide smoothly in the joint. The ends of the bones themselves are covered with a layer of smooth, hard connective tissue called the articular cartilage, which provides a good sliding surface. Some joints have additional disks of cartilage (menisci) that are attached just loosely enough to act as shock absorbers. Another form of protection within some joints is a cushioning sac of synovial fluid called a bursa. A bursa can be located anywhere in the joint where stress may occur.

Joint aspiration

A procedure that involves the withdrawal of synovial fluid, the fluid that lubricates the surfaces of the bones and provides nutrients to the cartilage inside a joint. Joint aspiration is also called arthrocentesis or a joint tap. It may be used as a diagnostic tool because an analysis of synovial fluid in a laboratory can establish the cause of swelling in a joint, distinguish between different forms of arthritis, and detect the presence of blood in the joint, indicating trauma or fracture. The procedure can also help diagnose septic arthritis and joint diseases associated with the presence of crystals in the joint, and it can be used to monitor the effects of antibiotics on septic arthritis. Joint aspiration may also be performed as part of a JOINT INJECTION evaluation or as a treatment to drain an excess accumulation of fluid from a joint.

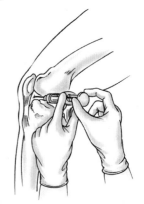

DRAINING FLUID FROM A KNEE JOINT
To perform joint aspiration, the doctor inserts a hollow needle into the joint space and withdraws fluid.

SEVEN TYPES OF JOINTS

Known as the place where two bones meet, joints are classified by their structure or the way they move. Movable joints slide over each other with little friction, while less mobile joints are more solidly linked by fibrous tissue or cartilage to provide stability or permit growth.

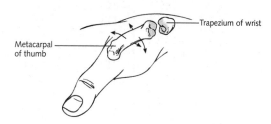

Metacarpal of thumb — Trapezium of wrist

SADDLE JOINT
The only saddle joints in the body are at the base of the thumbs. The bones can move back and forth and from side to side, but they have a limited ability to rotate.

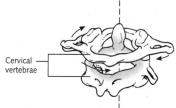

Cervical vertebrae

PIVOT JOINT
In a pivot joint, motion is limited to rotation, such as in the neck when a person rotates his or her head from side to side.

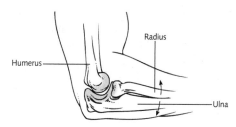

Pelvis

Femur

BALL-AND-SOCKET JOINT
A ball-and-socket joint, as in the hip, gives a person the greatest range of movement of all joint structures.

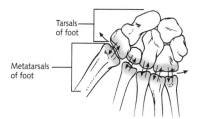

Tarsals of foot

Metatarsals of foot

GLIDING JOINT
Joints in the foot and wrist are examples of gliding joints. The surfaces of bones that meet in a gliding joint are almost flat, sliding over one another but with limited movement.

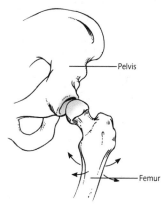

Radius

Humerus

Ulna

HINGE JOINT
One of the simplest joints, the hinge joint lets a person bend and straighten his or her arm. The knees and elbows and joints of the fingers are all hinge joints.

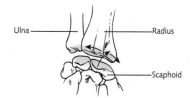

Ulna

Radius

Scaphoid

ELLIPSOIDAL JOINT
The radius bone of the forearm and the scaphoid bone of the hand meet in an ellipsoidal joint, which can be flexed or extended and moved from side to side.

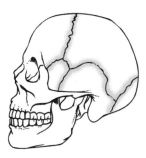

FIXED JOINT
The joints between the bones in the skull are examples of a fixed joint, which is firmly secured by fibrous tissue.

J

Joint aspiration is performed by a doctor in his or her office or at a hospital. The procedure takes from 3 to 5 minutes. The skin is first cleaned with an antiseptic, and a local anesthetic is applied on the skin or injected into the area. The needle is inserted and guided into the joint space, which may cause minor discomfort. Ice packs may relieve pain and swelling following the procedure.

Joint injection

A procedure to inject medication into an affected joint for the relief of inflammation, pain, and swelling. The corticosteroids called glucocorticoids, which include cortisone, are used for joint injections. The injections may be used to treat the joint pain caused by osteoarthritis and rheumatoid arthritis; bursitis of the shoulder, hip, or knee; frozen shoulder; tennis elbow; golfer's elbow; plantar fasciitis; carpal tunnel syndrome; and some forms of backache. Joint injections may decrease the time it takes to recover from an injury and are a source of pain relief during episodes of severe pain.

Joint injections are generally performed by a physician in his or her office. The procedure usually involves a local anesthetic, may involve JOINT ASPIRATION (in which fluid is removed from the joint with a fine, hollow needle), and takes about 15 minutes. The anesthetic may bring

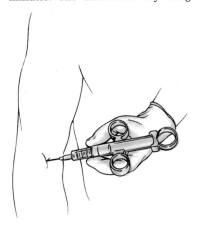

PAIN RELIEF FOR A JOINT
Corticosteroid drugs (identical to or related to hormones produced by the adrenal glands) can be injected into a joint to inhibit the white blood cells that cause swelling and inflammation and block substances called prostaglandins that trigger pain.

immediate pain relief that wears off before the corticosteroid medication takes effect. A significant improvement may be experienced within a few days and tends to last for a month or more.

Joint injections have an advantage over oral anti-inflammatory and pain-relieving medications because they place the corticosteroid medication directly into the painful area where it can reduce the inflammation causing the pain. No more than three or four injections are generally given within a year in one area of the body to avoid the risk of side effects, which may include permanent damage to a joint and the risk of rupturing a tendon. Other possible side effects associated with overuse of corticosteroids in joint injections include weight gain, thinning of the bones, high blood pressure, cataracts, diabetes, stomach ulcers, and psychiatric problems.

Joint replacement

A prosthetic device made of metal or a combination of metal with plastic or porcelain, which is used to replace an arthritic or damaged joint that has been removed. A joint is generally removed and replaced with a prosthesis because it is no longer functional, because of extreme pain, immobility, or both. Hip joint replacements, finger joint replacements, and knee joint replacements (see JOINT REPLACEMENT, HIP; JOINT REPLACEMENT, FINGER; and JOINT REPLACEMENT, KNEE) are the most common, but surgeons also perform joint replacements for ankles, elbows, and shoulders. In shoulder joint replacement surgery, the ball part of the ball-and-socket joint is replaced with a metal ball on a stem, which is inserted and sometimes cemented into the bone of the upper arm. The socket may be replaced with a plastic prosthesis, fixed in place with cement. This joint replacement is effective for pain relief but results for improved range of motion and function may vary.

Joint replacements are now common in younger people at earlier stages of joint disease. Substantial improvements in the replacements themselves, as well as techniques for securing them, have improved long-term results. However, the surgical procedure for replacing joints is considered only after more conservative

treatments have failed and after a careful evaluation of individual health risks.

Joint replacement, finger

A surgical procedure to remove diseased parts of the finger joint, usually the knuckle, and replace it with a prosthesis. The purpose of the procedure is to replace a finger joint that has been removed due to severe pain, deformity, and loss of function, generally as a result of arthritis. Polymer finger joint replacements offer relief from pain and an improved range of motion for most people, as well as improved appearance in the finger.

Joint replacement, hip

FOR SYMPTOM CHART
see Hip pain, page 42

A surgical procedure performed to replace the ball-and-socket joint of the hip with a specially designed prosthesis. A prosthetic hip joint replacement is implanted after removal of the diseased bone tissue and cartilage from the natural hip joint. Damage to the bone and cartilage, usually the result of degenerative osteoarthritis, can cause severe pain and prevent a person from using the joint. Other conditions that may lead to the need for this procedure include rheumatoid arthritis, injury, bone tumors, and avascular necrosis of the femoral head (insufficient blood supply leading to death of bone tissue). The extent of damage to a joint is diagnosed and evaluated by a physical examination, by X rays, and possibly by certain laboratory tests. If more conservative approaches cannot successfully treat the pain and lack of function in a hip joint, total hip joint replacement is considered.

HOW IT IS DONE
The structure of a hip joint replacement includes a metal ball attached to a metal stem that is fitted into the thighbone, and held there, usually with plastic bone cement. The metals used include stainless steel, alloys of cobalt and chrome, and titanium. A polyethylene socket is implanted into the pelvis to replace the damaged socket and to receive the prosthetic, ball-shaped head of the thighbone, forming a complete ball-and-socket

REPLACING A HIP JOINT

A hip joint replacement is a four-stage process that requires fitting a new head onto a damaged thighbone (femur) and preparing a new socket in the pelvic bone. The artificial joint then helps the person walk more easily and usually without pain.

STAGE 1
The surgeon exposes the hip joint and removes the arthritic head of the femur at the neck.

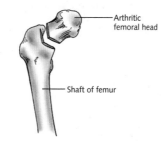

Arthritic femoral head

Shaft of femur

STAGE 2
The surgeon hollows out a channel in the femur with a filing instrument called a rasp and inserts the new metal head of the femur, which is on a long stem.

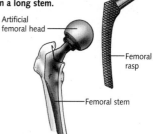

Artificial femoral head

Femoral rasp

Femoral stem

STAGE 3
The hip socket into which the femoral head will fit is smoothed out with a circular reaming tool, and a new cuplike socket component is inserted.

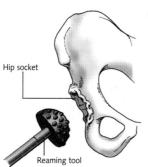

Hip socket

Reaming tool

STAGE 4
The person's bone grows around the new joint components so that they fit securely, and the new joint functions smoothly.

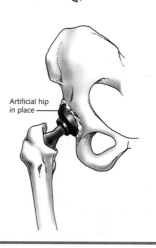

Artificial hip in place

J

joint. The goal of reconstruction of a hip joint using a prosthetic replacement is to restore normal and painless joint movement. The success of the procedure is largely based on a person's overall health and general activity level.

RECOVERY
People who receive total hip joint replacements are usually encouraged to stand and walk using a walking aid the day after surgery. There may be temporary pain in the joint due to healing tissues and muscles weakened from inactivity. The typical hospital stay following hip replacement surgery is a week or less. Full recovery usually takes from 3 to 6 months. Exercise and sometimes physical therapy are important elements of total recovery.

Joint replacement, knee

A surgical procedure to replace the knee joint with a specially designed prosthetic joint. The surface of the knee joint may be worn away by osteoarthritis, fractures, rheumatoid arthritis, or gout, making walking and normal daily activities difficult and painful. The first line of medical treatment for such symptoms includes recommendations for weight loss, anti-inflammatory medication, the use of support braces or orthotics (special shoe inserts), physical therapy, or injections with corticosteroids or one of the newer supplements. If full function without pain cannot be restored, if daily life is restricted, if pain is progressive and there is a constant need for pain medication, total joint replacement is usually considered.

HOW IT IS DONE
What is called a knee joint replacement is actually a resurfacing of the knee joint. There are several techniques for performing the procedure. The thighbone (femur) is covered with a metal sheath, and plastic is placed on the shin bone (tibia), using acrylic cement. Usually, the undersurface of the kneecap is also replaced with a plastic surface so that it fits smoothly with the metal-covered thighbone. The smooth, nonsticking surfaces replace the irregular arthritic surfaces so that the knee's movement and function are restored.

RECOVERY
Hospitalization following the surgery is usually between 4 and 6 days. Weight-bearing activity generally begins on the first postoperative day

with the use of a walking aid. Typically, a person who has had knee replacement surgery progresses from a walker to crutches to a cane within 3 to 8 weeks, at which time walking aids are no longer necessary. The success rate of the surgery is high. Many people who have received knee replacements enjoy walking, bicycling, golfing, and swimming. The replacement, however, is not designed to function for rigorous activities such as skiing, basketball, and racket sports.

Joule

The standard unit of work or energy; it is used in medicine to determine the extent of a person's electrical injuries. A joule is equal to the work done when the point of application of a force of 1 newton is displaced through a distance of 1 meter in the direction of the force. In electrical measurement, a joule is the work done per second when a current of 1 ampere flows through a resistance of 1 ohm. The symbol used for joule is J.

Jugular vein

The large vein that returns oxygen-poor blood from much of the head and neck toward the heart. The name "jugular" comes from the Latin word for throat. Below the base of the neck,

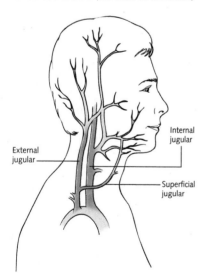

STRUCTURE OF THE JUGULAR VEIN
The largest of the three parts of the jugular vein is the internal jugular vein, which passes from the base of the skull down the side of the neck on either side. The external jugular veins and the superficial jugular veins share the job of carrying blood from the head back to the heart.

the jugular joins with the subclavian vein, which drains blood from the arm and shoulder, to form the brachiocephalic vein. The brachiocephalic vein connects with the superior vena cava, which enters the heart in the right atrium.

Jumper's knee

An irritation, sprain, or overuse of the large tendon that lies just below the kneecap. This tendon, called the patellar tendon, allows the knee joint to straighten and extend. Jumper's knee, medically termed patellar tendinitis, is caused by repeated pressure on the knee's tendon during activities that require frequent jumping, such as basketball, net ball, volleyball, long jumping, high jumping, and triple jumping. When a person lands on the ground during jumping movements, the pressure of the full body weight is exerted on the patellar tendon while it is in the extended position. Doing deep squats when weight lifting, running uphill, or rowing may also cause excessive pressure on the patellar tendon and produce jumper's knee. The resulting irritation of these activities causes symptoms of pain, swelling, and inflammation of the tendon. There may be tenderness at the bottom of the kneecap.

Self-care for the condition includes resting the overused tendon, icing to decrease swelling, and later, when swelling and pain are decreased, applications of heat to promote healing. A physician can diagnose jumper's knee by physical examination, which primarily shows extreme localized tenderness when touching the knee area. A doctor may recommend nonsteroidal anti-inflammatory drugs (NSAIDs) to control the inflammation. The use of knee braces or special straps to give support and compression to the knee as an aid to healing may also be recommended. Physical therapists can teach exercises to balance the muscles surrounding the knee joint, which can help maintain alignment of the kneecap. A physical therapist may also prescribe ice massage, electric stimulation therapy, or ultrasound treatments. Activities to avoid during the healing process include jumping, squatting, step-aerobics, and using stair-climber exercise machines.

When conservative rehabilitation of the condition is ineffective after a period of 8 to 12 weeks, cortisone injections into the tendon sheaths may be recommended. A surgical procedure to remove the scar tissue surrounding the patellar tendon may become an option if all other treatments have failed or if ultrasound testing reveals extensive degeneration of the tendon.

Jungian theory

An approach to understanding human psychology founded by Carl Jung, a Swiss psychiatrist who was an early pupil of Sigmund Freud (see FREUDIAN THEORY) but later broke with him. Jung called his theory analytical psychology.

Like Freud, Jung saw libido as central to human motivation, but he widened the concept to include not only sexuality but also all creative instincts and impulses. The libido, he believed, drives the individual toward psychological fulfillment, or what Jung called individuation.

In Jung's thinking, the unconscious mind is composed of two parts. The personal unconscious contains the results of a person's life history. The collective unconscious includes primordial images, or archetypes, common to all individuals in a particular culture or historical time. Archetypes function when the conscious mind is not engaged, as in sleep. Dreaming allows access to the archetypes in the form of the symbols and images that make up dreams, poetry, and art.

Jung divided individual personalities into two basic types. When the libido and general interest are focused outward, the person is an extrovert. When they are focused inward, the person is considered an introvert. In addition, each individual presents to the world a specific aspect of personality called the persona, which consists of the external role the person chooses to play in life rather than who he or she actually is.

Juvenile rheumatoid arthritis

A disease that can cause chronic inflammation of a child's joints and internal organs. Also known as JRA, juvenile rheumatoid arthritis most commonly begins between ages 2 and 5 or 9 and 12. It is unusual for symptoms to appear before age 1 or after age 16. The disease is more common in girls than in boys.

There are three types of juvenile rheumatoid arthritis. The most common form is pauciarticular JRA, in which joint inflammation occurs in four or fewer joints (usually the knees, ankles, or elbows). Only rarely do children with pauciarticular JRA have permanent joint disability. The second most common form is polyarticular, which affects five or more joints, including small joints in the fingers and hands. Least common is systemic JRA, the most serious type, which affects the internal organs as well as the joints. Between one third and one half of those with polyarticular or systemic JRA will develop a residual joint deformity and functional limitations. Although juvenile rheumatoid arthritis is a potentially disabling disease, most children who have had appropriate treatment recover from it completely, particularly those with pauciarticular JRA. In some cases JRA causes permanent damage.

The exact cause of juvenile rheumatoid arthritis remains unknown. Researchers believe that JRA is an autoimmune disorder triggered by viral infections in susceptible children. In autoimmune disorders, a defect causes the body's immune system (which defends the body against infection) to instead turn on itself. In children who are not susceptible to JRA, the same virus (see VIRUSES) would probably cause only a minor illness.

SYMPTOMS

An early warning sign of juvenile rheumatoid arthritis is joint stiffness in the morning. Other symptoms include a fever with no apparent cause, persistent joint stiffness, swelling, and pain. The skin over swollen joints may appear red and feel hot. A child's appetite may also be affected, leading to weight loss or gain.

Symptoms vary according to the type of JRA. Pauciarticular JRA is associated with eye inflammation

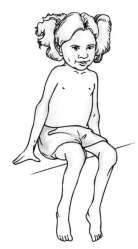

ARTHRITIS IN A CHILD
A child with juvenile rheumatoid arthritis usually has swollen joints in the knees, ankles, hands, and wrists. The muscles of the legs and arms may not be well developed because of decreased mobility.

that may lead to glaucoma or cataracts. Early diagnosis requires referral to an ophthalmologist, who will look for signs of telltale inflammation. In polyarticular JRA, children can develop lumps on affected joints due to pressure from objects such as shoes and chairs. In systemic JRA (sometimes called Still disease), children may have a high fever, chills, and swollen glands and feel ill overall. A rash of red spots may occur early in the disease. This very serious disease can also cause damage to the internal organs, including the heart, lungs, liver, and brain.

Juvenile rheumatoid arthritis is not uniformly painful. Children may experience periods of remission, in which symptoms recede and they feel much better. At other times there will be flare-ups when pain, stiffness, and inflammation are at their worst.

DIAGNOSIS AND TREATMENT

Juvenile rheumatoid arthritis can be difficult to diagnose. Sometimes there are no visible symptoms, and a child may not complain of pain. An

accurate diagnosis is more likely when a doctor is visited while typical symptoms are present. A doctor should be consulted if a child develops a limp or consistently favors one hand, arm, or leg over another. To make a diagnosis, the doctor will examine the child and take a medical history and may order X rays and blood tests. If the arthritis is severe, the child will likely be referred to a pediatric RHEUMATOLOGIST (a specialist in treating children's joints and related tissues).

Treatment varies according to the type of JRA but is generally directed toward reducing inflammation. Generally nonsteroidal anti-inflammatory drugs (NSAIDs), including aspirin, ibuprofen, naproxen, and several other medications, are recommended to relieve pain and swelling. This is one of the very few occasions in which aspirin is considered appropriate for use in children. Aspirin increases the risk of developing REYE SYNDROME (a rare childhood disorder that is potentially fatal to children younger than 18). To control symptoms, doctors may also prescribe one of the CORTICOSTEROIDS, gold therapy, or methotrexate.

When swollen or acutely painful, the joint needs to be rested. However, when symptoms are in remission, regular exercise is recommended. Neglecting to move the joint can cause the muscles around it to tighten and shorten, potentially leading to deformity and disability. A physician may refer a child to a physical therapist. Sometimes splints are necessary. In severe cases, the doctor may recommend surgery.

All children with JRA should see an ophthalmologist at least annually for a slit-lamp examination. A slit lamp is an instrument that helps an eye doctor detect early stages of inflammation. Children with pauciarticular JRA may need to be screened more frequently, since they are at greater risk for eye problems.

J

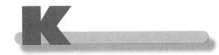

Kala-azar

See LEISHMANIASIS.

Kaposi sarcoma

A cancerous tumor primarily of the skin that may also involve intestines, lymph glands, and other tissues. In the United States, Kaposi sarcoma occurs almost exclusively in people with AIDS (acquired immunodeficiency syndrome), although it also occurs in older Haitian and Jewish men, younger patients in Africa, and individuals who have had kidney or heart transplants. The tumors chiefly arise in the skin, where they appear as irregular, slightly raised spots, ranging in color from purple to brown. Kaposi sarcoma can also appear in mucous membranes, the gastrointestinal tract, lungs, heart, lymph nodes, spleen, and adrenal glands.

Kaposi sarcoma was an extremely rare form of cancer until it was discovered in people with AIDS; today, it is found in approximately 15 percent of people with AIDS. A viral cofactor called Kaposi sarcoma–associated herpesvirus (KSHV) triggers Kaposi sarcoma. The number of cases seen in people with AIDS has begun to decline since the advent of highly active antiretrovirus therapy (HAART) with protease inhibitors. Treatment can also include chemotherapy or radiation therapy to individual skin lesions.

Kartagener syndrome

An inherited lung disease characterized by recurrent bronchial infections, male infertility, and a condition called situs inversus, in which the heart is found on the right side of the chest rather than the left. Other organs may also be reversed. In Kartagener syndrome, mucus transport in the lungs is ineffective. Mucus is normally carried through the lungs by microscopic hairlike projections called CILIA, which move in a coordinated way to force mucus from smaller to larger airways, where it can be expelled by coughing. In Kartagener syndrome, the cilia do not work prop-

erly, and as a result, mucus becomes stuck in the respiratory passages, where it becomes a breeding ground for bacteria.

Symptoms of Kartagener syndrome resemble the respiratory symptoms of CYSTIC FIBROSIS. They include respiratory distress in the newborn; recurrent episodes of OTITIS MEDIA (middle ear infections) that can result in deafness; clubbing of the fingers and toes; nasal polyps; and BRONCHIECTASIS, or chronic dilation of the bronchi caused by inflammation. Adults will also have sinusitis. The diagnosis is made by documenting the lack of mucus transport by cilia in the lungs, which is usually correlated with situs inversus. Electron microscopic examination of the cilia in the cells of the skin lining the nose confirms the diagnosis by demonstrating the defective structure of the cilia. Kartagener syndrome is uncommon, occurring in 1 of 20,000 to 40,000 births.

Karyotyping

Chromosome analysis. Medical diagnostic tests used to identify CHROMOSOMAL ABNORMALITIES as the cause of malformation or disease. Karyotyping can be conducted on samples of blood, bone marrow, amniotic fluid, or placental tissue. Cells are stained, viewed under a microscope, and then photographed to provide a karyotype showing the arrangement of the chromosomes, which sometimes can indicate the presence of abnormalities.

Chromosome analysis is usually used to evaluate suspected genetic abnormalities, detect chromosome abnormalities before birth, evaluate a couple with a history of miscarriages, or identify the chromosome present in a type of leukemia. Abnormal results may indicate DOWN SYNDROME, TRISOMY 18 SYNDROME, TURNER SYNDROME, KLINEFELTER SYNDROME, leukemia, and other disorders.

DIAGNOSTIC PRENATAL TESTING

Before diagnostic prenatal testing, screening tests are usually given to a pregnant woman to assess the risk for abnormalities in the fetus. Screening tests are noninvasive and most commonly involve ultrasound scanning or alpha-fetoprotein testing (see AFP TEST), in which a mother's blood is tested for substances that have passed from the fetal blood. Abnormal results may indicate an increased risk

of certain genetic defects, indicating a need for further prenatal testing for a definitive diagnosis.

Diagnostic prenatal testing is reserved for women who are at high risk for having a fetus with a genetic abnormality. Such women include those who are older than 35, who have a chromosomal abnormality, who have or whose mates have family histories of an abnormality, or who have had an abnormal screening test result.

Diagnostic testing is considered invasive; the two diagnostic testing procedures, AMNIOCENTESIS and CHORIONIC VILLUS SAMPLING, involve a risk of miscarriage. In amniocentesis, amniotic fluid, the liquid surrounding a fetus in the uterus, is extracted with a hypodermic needle. The fluid contains many fetal skin cells that can be cultured to produce a karyotype. Amniocentesis can detect Down syndrome and neural tube defects, including SPINA BIFIDA. In chorionic villus sampling, a small sample of the chorion, the tissue that later develops into the placenta, is taken from the embryo. These cells contain the same genetic information as the fetus. This test can detect Down syndrome and other abnormal chromosome conditions. Genetic counseling is recommended for pregnant women who are considering prenatal testing.

Kava

An herbal remedy used to reduce stress and anxiety; also known as kava kava. The kava plant is a member of the pepper family and is found in the South Pacific. Kava may relax the body and induce sleep, although the precise way in which it works is not entirely understood or proven. Kava is popular in Germany and other European countries. Kava may impair a person's ability to drive and can also cause hepatitis.

Kawasaki disease

A rare but serious childhood disease of unknown origin that causes inflammation of blood vessels. Also called mucocutaneous lymph node syndrome, it is accompanied by fever, swollen lymph glands, and a skin rash. Although inflammation weakens the blood vessel walls, in most cases, they return to normal on their own within a few months. However,

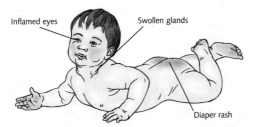

SYMPTOMS OF KAWASAKI DISEASE
Kawasaki disease, a rare but serious disorder, causes blood vessel inflammation. Symptoms include fever, redness, swelling, and dryness in the palms of the hands and soles of the feet; inflamed eyes and swollen, cracked lips; swollen glands in the neck; and a diaper rash.

Inflamed eyes — Swollen glands — Diaper rash

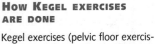

HOW KEGEL EXERCISES ARE DONE

Kegel exercises (pelvic floor exercises) can be done while standing, sitting or lying down. They can even be done in public because the contractions cannot be seen.

- First, the muscles are identified while urinating. Flow is started and stopped to get the feel of controlling the muscles.
- Then the same muscles used for urinating are tightened and held for 2 to 3 seconds at first, working up to 8 to 10 seconds. This process is repeated 10 times.
- The set of 10 contractions is repeated 5 times a day.
- Concentration should be on holding, rather than pulsing, the muscles.

at times blood vessel walls remain weakened and balloon out into an aneurysm. An aneurysm in the coronary arteries that becomes blocked or bursts can be fatal.

Kawasaki disease is most common in boys between ages 6 months and 5 years. Children of Japanese or Korean ancestry are more frequently affected. Researchers believe that a virus (see VIRUSES) or bacteria may cause Kawasaki disease, although its exact cause remains unknown. The disease, which is not contagious, occurs most frequently in winter and early spring. Symptoms include a high fever that persists for 5 days or longer and does not respond to antibiotics. Other signs include a measleslike rash that may be particularly severe in the diaper area of infants; reddened and swollen hands and soles of the feet; red, cracked lips; reddened eyes; swollen lymph glands in the neck (see GLANDS, SWOLLEN); and irritability, apathy, or crankiness. An affected child may complain of stomach pain, headache, or joint pain. Without treatment, a child may appear to improve after 2 weeks. However, internally, at that time, the disease begins to affect the heart. Coronary arteries may grow inflamed, and the child can develop a fast, irregular heartbeat (see ARRHYTHMIA, CARDIAC). A life-threatening aneurysm can occur at this time.

DIAGNOSIS AND TREATMENT
Early diagnosis and treatment are necessary to decrease the risk of aneurysm. No single test exists to diagnose Kawasaki disease. The diagnosis is made when typical symptoms are present and tests rule out other possible causes of disease. The doctor may order blood and urine tests, an echocardiogram to detect a possible aneurysm, an electrocardiogram to look for arrhythmias, and a chest X ray to examine the heart.

A child with Kawasaki disease

needs to be admitted to a hospital. Treatment consists of large doses of intravenous gamma globulin, a blood product containing human antibodies. The child will also be given aspirin for 8 weeks, in high doses for the first 2 weeks. Aspirin inhibits the tendency for blood to clot in damaged blood vessels. The outlook for complete recovery is good when Kawasaki disease is diagnosed and treated early. However, about 2 percent of children with this disease die from heart complications.

Kegel exercises
Exercises done by women to strengthen the pelvic floor muscles that control urine flow and support the bladder, uterus, vagina, and rectum. Kegel exercises (also called pelvic floor exercises) involve repeated tensing, holding, and releasing of the muscles. If done correctly and regularly, Kegel exercises may help a woman have a more comfortable childbirth, overcome urinary incontinence (lack of bladder control; see INCONTINENCE, URINARY), and increase sexual satisfaction.

STRENGTHENING PELVIC MUSCLES
Kegel exercises strengthen the muscles that control urination and help provide support for the pelvic organs. Specifically, the exercises isolate and work the muscles of the bladder wall and the sphincter that controls the flow of urine from the bladder into the urethra. During urination, the detrusor muscle of the bladder wall contracts to squeeze urine into the urethra, and the urethral sphincter muscle relaxes to allow passage. After urination, the sphincter tightens to contain urine, and the detrusor muscle relaxes to relieve pressure on the bladder.

Kegel exercises can be done anywhere. The muscles that need strengthening can be identified by starting and stopping the flow while urinating. The same contracting and releasing action can then be repeated throughout the day—no matter what else the woman is doing—in lying down, sitting, standing, or bending positions.

If a woman has trouble learning to do Kegel exercises, a nurse, physical therapist, or midwife may be able to assist her. Special BIOFEEDBACK equipment is sometimes used to help women learn to do Kegel exercises correctly.

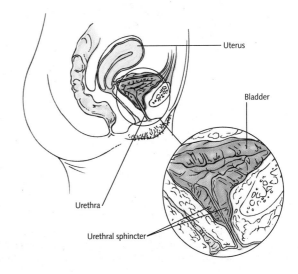

Uterus — Bladder — Urethra — Urethral sphincter

Keloid

A raised scar that extends beyond the original site of injury or that occurs around the incision line after surgery. Keloids are the result of an abnormal healing response and are caused by an excess buildup of collagen. Most keloids occur on the chest or on the earlobe after ear piercing. They may occur after an injury, surgical incision, or burn. Blacks are more frequently affected than whites. Although harmless, keloids can be unsightly, and some are itchy or tender.

Keloids can be treated with corticosteroid injections directly into the keloid and CRYOSURGERY (freezing with liquid nitrogen). Surgical removal can present a problem because a new surgical incision may create a new scar that in turn can lead to another keloid. Injecting corticosteroids or treating the site with radiation after surgery can help prevent the development of new scars.

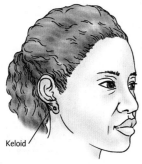

OVERGROWN SCAR TISSUE
A keloid is generally shiny, hard, and raised above surrounding skin. Sometimes, it is itchy or tender. These unsightly scar formations often form at the site of a body piercing. People with darker skin or a history of keloids can best prevent them by avoiding cosmetic piercing and elective surgery.

Keratin

A fibrous protein that is the major component of the epidermis (the outermost layer of skin) and of the nails and hair. Keratin acts as a protective barrier against harmful environmental influences.

Keratitis

Inflammation of the clear outer covering of the exposed portion of the eye (cornea). Inflammation can cause the cornea to scar and may lead to vision loss. The most common cause of keratitis is infection, usually from viruses.

Keratoacanthoma

A papule (small superficial bump on the skin) or nodule (solid mass of tissue) with a central crater that appears on sun-damaged skin. The papules or nodules may disappear on their own. Keratoacanthomas should be treated by a dermatologist because, although they are benign (not cancerous), they closely resemble tumors of SQUAMOUS CELL CARCINOMA.

Keratoconjunctivitis

Inflammation of the clear outer covering of the eye (cornea) and of the membrane lining the eyelids and covering the eye surface (conjunctiva). It can lead to visual impairment from scarring of the cornea. Keratoconjunctivitis can be caused by infection of the eyes with a virus that also causes headache and swelling of the lymph nodes. It can also be caused by autoimmune disease or allergies. Vernal keratoconjunctivitis involves the development of large bumps on the lining of the upper eyelid, itching, burning, foreign body sensation, excessive tearing and mucus production, and blurred vision. The disease primarily affects young men in warm climates and is particularly common in the Middle East during the spring.

Depending on severity, the disease is treated with topical corticosteroids to control inflammation and prevent scarring of the cornea. Atopic keratoconjunctivitis largely affects people with atopic dermatitis (eczema), an allergic skin disease. Symptoms include itching, burning, foreign body sensation, excessive tearing and mucus production, and blurred vision. The disease is treated with antihistamine and other allergy medications. In severe cases, suppression of the immune system with drugs is required to prevent scarring of the cornea and vision loss.

Keratoconjunctivitis sicca

See DRY EYE.

Keratoconus

A disease that involves a progressive, gradual thinning of the clear outer covering of the eye (cornea) and changes its shape from a dome to a cone; also known as conical cornea. The change in the cornea's shape causes nearsightedness (blurring of distant

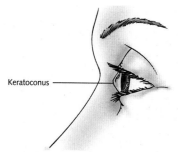

Keratoconus

MISSHAPEN CORNEA
In a person with keratoconus, the cornea bulges outward and becomes conical instead of rounded. As a result, the central portion of the corneal tissue thins out and eventually scars over, causing vision problems. The disorder affects women more often than men.

objects) and astigmatism (tilting and distortion of the field of view), which can range from mild to severe. Most cases of keratoconus begin in adolescence or early adulthood and progress over a 10- to 20-year period. Research indicates that keratoconus has a number of possible causes, including an inherited abnormality of the cornea, certain eye diseases (for example, retinitis pigmentosa and vernal keratoconjunctivitis), and some systemic diseases, such as Down syndrome. Some researchers believe that keratoconus is associated with excessive eye rubbing or the long-term wearing of hard contact lenses.

Treatment depends on the severity of the disease. Eyeglasses can correct nearsightedness and astigmatism in the early stages. In more severe cases, rigid contact lenses are used to flatten the surface of the cornea and provide improved vision. If vision remains badly impaired even with contact lenses, the person may need to undergo a corneal transplant. See KERATOPLASTY, PENETRATING.

Keratopathy

A noninflammatory disease of the clear outer covering of the eye (cornea). Keratopathy can occur as a result of aging, glaucoma, eye surgery, or exposure to extreme temperatures or light. See KERATOPATHY, ULTRAVIOLET.

Keratopathy, ultraviolet

Damage to the clear outer covering of the eye (cornea) from short-term exposure to intense light, such as strong sunlight or an arc welder's flame. Ultraviolet keratopathy is commonly known as snow blindness. Symptoms include reddening of the eye, severe pain, feelings of grit on the eye, tearing, sensitivity to light, and involuntary twitching of the eyelids. Treatment consists of antibiotic ointment, drops to relieve spasms in the ciliary muscles of the eye, covering the eyes, and administering medication to control pain. The condition usually resolves on its own within 1 to 3 days. The risk of ultraviolet keratopathy can be lowered by wearing a hat in bright sun and protecting the eyes with glasses that block out ultraviolet light.

Keratoplasty, conductive

A medical procedure that uses radiofrequency energy to heat and reshape the cornea, the clear front surface of the eye, and thereby correct hyperopia (FARSIGHTEDNESS). Approved by the Food and Drug Administration in 2002, conductive keratoplasty (CK) is considered innovative because it is less invasive than the other procedures used to correct vision by reshaping the cornea with lasers, such as PHOTOREFRACTIVE KERATECTOMY, laser in situ keratomileusis (LASIK), and laser thermal keratoplasty.

Before a person undergoes CK, an eye specialist places anesthetic drops into the eye. The eyelid is held open with a special instrument. The eye not having the procedure is taped shut. Then a microscope is placed over the eye, and the eye is marked with a rinse-away ink that guides the application of radiofrequency energy. During CK, the heat from a radiofrequency energy device is used to shrink the cornea at specific treatment spots, creating a band of tightening. This band of tightening steepens the cornea and allows light to focus precisely on the retina. The entire procedure takes about 5 minutes.

CK has been shown to be effective in reducing farsightedness between 0.75 and 3.00 diopters (a unit of measurement used to determine the extent of farsightedness, nearsightedness, or astigmatism of the eye) in people 40 years or older. People who undergo the procedure may no longer need to wear glasses or contact lenses to see clearly. CK is not recommended, how-ever, for women who are pregnant or nursing, nor is it recommended for people with a tendency to form scars or with severe dry eye, thin corneas, or KERATOCONUS. In addition, CK is not recommended for people with any disease that affects the body's ability to heal, such as AIDS (acquired immunodeficiency syndrome), RHEUMATOID ARTHRITIS, systemic lupus erythematosus (see LUPUS ERYTHEMATOSUS, SYSTEMIC), or MULTIPLE SCLEROSIS.

As with other medical procedures to correct vision, CK is not risk-free. A person who has undergone the procedure may be less dependent on eyeglasses or contact lenses but may still need them for reading. There is also a small risk that a person may lose some vision after the CK procedure. Since it is a relatively new procedure and the long-term effects are not yet known, it is important to discuss the risks and benefits with an eye care specialist before undergoing CK.

Keratoplasty, penetrating

Surgery to replace the clear outer covering of the eye (cornea). The donor cornea is taken from a recently deceased person who has agreed to donate his or her eyes after death. All donors are tested for HIV (human immunodeficiency virus) and hepatitis A, B, and C. Penetrating keratoplasty is performed in people who have had diseases or injuries that scar their own corneas and leave them with little or no vision. Penetrating keratoplasty is highly successful in restoring or improving sight.

Penetrating keratoplasty is usually performed with the person awake. Conscious sedation keeps the person relaxed, and the eye is numbed with a local anesthetic. The surgeon removes the central part of the diseased cornea with a circular cutting tool (trephine). The donor cornea is then set in the surgical opening and stitched in place with very small sutures. Following the procedure, eye drops are administered to promote healing. The sutures remain in the eye for months or even years and are removed in the eye surgeon's office. Complications from penetrating keratoplasty include rejection of the transplanted cornea (graft) and glaucoma.

Penetrating keratoplasty has the highest success rate of any transplant surgery. Rejection of the donor cornea can usually be stopped if medication is begun at the first warning sign. The warning signs consist of redness in the eye, pain, and increased sensitivity to light.

Keratosis

A skin growth caused by the overproduction of KERATIN, a protein found in skin, hair, and nails. Normally, keratin acts as a protective barrier against harmful environmental influences. An example of a benign (not cancerous) keratosis is SEBORRHEIC KERATOSIS, a skin tumor that commonly occurs after middle age. An ACTINIC KERATOSIS is a precancerous growth that occurs in sun-exposed areas of the body. Such growths appear as a result of long-term sun exposure and, if left untreated, can progress to SKIN CANCER.

Keratosis pilaris

A common benign (not cancerous) skin condition characterized by rough papules (small superficial bumps on the skin) that generally appear on the upper arms, thighs, and face. Keratosis pilaris is the result of dead skin cells or keratin accumulating around hair follicles. It usually improves or disappears with age. If keratosis pilaris is cosmetically disturbing, over-the-counter moisturizers or medicated creams may improve the appearance of skin.

Kerion

A tender, swollen mass of dandruff-like scales, broken stubbles of hair, and pustules (small pus-filled blisters) caused by a fungal infection of the scalp. Fever and enlarged lymph nodes in the neck and scalp may occur. It is often the result of a TINEA infection of the hair follicles and is treated with oral antifungal medication.

Kernicterus

A rare, potentially fatal neurological disorder in newborn infants caused by a toxic accumulation of BILIRUBIN in central nervous system tissues. Bilirubin is a normal by-product of the breakdown of red blood cells.

K

When the immature liver and kidneys of a newborn cannot process a large amount of this substance, the resulting condition is called hyperbilirubinemia. It is especially common in premature infants. Severe prolonged hyperbilirubinemia results in kernicterus. Hyperbilirubinemia is common in newborns; kernicterus is extremely rare. Jaundice—a yellowing of the skin and whites of the eyes—is an early warning sign of hyperbilirubinemia. Untreated bilirubin levels that remain high for a long period can cause mental retardation, CEREBRAL PALSY, delayed or abnormal motor development, DEAFNESS, perceptual problems (see PERCEPTION), and behavioral disorders. Severe cases of kernicterus can be fatal.

TREATMENT AND PREVENTION

Early identification and treatment of infants at high risk for kernicterus is essential, because appropriate treatments of hyperbilirubinemia can prevent kernicterus. Phototherapy, or exposure to ultraviolet light, is the treatment most often used to bring high bilirubin levels under control. Rarely some infants may need an exchange transfusion, in which the baby's blood is exchanged for donated blood.

Premature infants have the greatest risk of developing kernicterus. Although prematurity is sometimes unavoidable, pregnant women can help to ensure the health of a developing fetus by following a healthy diet and not smoking, drinking alcohol, or using narcotics (see PRENATAL CARE). Rh incompatibility between mother and fetus is another risk factor for kernicterus. However, the use of preventive measures in Rh-negative pregnant women has made kernicterus in full-term infants rare.

Ketoacidosis

FOR SYMPTOM CHARTS

see Urination in men, frequent or painful, page 56

see Urination in women, frequent or painful, page 57

An emergency medical condition usually occurring in people with type 1 diabetes (see DIABETES MELLITUS, TYPE 1) but that can also occur in people with type 2 diabetes (see DIABETES MELLITUS, TYPE 2). Ketoacidosis is an acute complication of diabetes. It begins slowly and starts when the blood sugar level becomes too elevated, a condition called HYPERGLYCEMIA (high blood sugar). As hyperglycemia progresses, glucose accumulates in the blood, and the cells become less able to utilize it. These cells begin to use stored fat for energy, causing the production and release of acids called ketone bodies. Glucose and ketones accumulate in the blood, making it more acidic.

Ketoacidosis occurs when diabetes is undiagnosed, untreated, or inadequately controlled. It may also occur in people whose diabetes worsens as a result of stress from an injury or illness. Bouts of diarrhea or vomiting that cause dehydration can lead to ketoacidosis. When these conditions affect a person with diabetes, it is important to monitor the glucose level in the blood and the ketone concentration in the urine to prevent the occurrence of ketoacidosis. Failure to receive scheduled insulin or getting an insufficient amount of physical exercise may also be associated with ketoacidosis.

Over the course of a few hours, a person with ketoacidosis typically experiences an unquenchable thirst and frequent urination. This may be followed by weakness and sleepiness. Subsequent signs may include nausea and vomiting, which may cause dehydration, as well as stomach pain. Other signs may include flushing of the face, dry skin and mouth, a weak but rapid pulse, and low blood pressure. The mouth may also have a sweet odor because of the waste product acetone being expelled through the lungs. In more advanced ketoacidosis, deep and rapid breathing occurs. If a person with diabetes shows these signs and does not receive insulin and fluids immediately, ketoacidosis can result in the loss of consciousness and ultimately death.

The first line of emergency treatment for ketoacidosis is to restore hydration by replacing fluid and electrolyte losses. This is generally accomplished by giving liquids containing isotonic saline and potassium intravenously. Insulin therapy is administered. Complete recovery from ketoacidosis is usually rapid when immediate medical treatment is given. People with diabetes should alert family and friends to the signs of ketoacidosis; they should also stress that professional medical care should be obtained for the person with diabetes immediately.

Ketoconazole

An antifungal drug available as a tablet, a shampoo, and a cream. Ketoconazole (Nizoral), taken as a tablet, prevents the growth of fungus or yeast in the body. The cream preparation of ketoconazole is used to treat athlete's foot, ringworm, "jock itch," "sun fungus," and yeast infection of the skin. The shampoo is used to treat dandruff.

Ketorolac

A nonnarcotic painkiller. Ketorolac (Toradol) is a nonsteroidal anti-inflammatory drug (NSAID) used to relieve moderate to severe pain, usually following a surgical procedure or an injury. It is not habit-forming, although it is often prescribed together with a narcotic to provide the best possible relief from pain. It may be injected or taken orally. Ketorolac has serious side effects and should not be taken for more than 5 days. Ketorolac is also available as an eye drop (Acular), to treat conjunctivitis and inflammation of the eye following cataract surgery.

Ketosis

An abnormal accumulation of ketones in the body caused by a deficiency or the inefficient use of carbohydrates. Ketones are a by-product of the metabolism of fatty acids. Ketosis occurs when glucose is unavailable for use as a source of energy, and the body instead uses fats, resulting in fatty acids being released into the blood where they are converted to ketones. See GLUCOSE METABOLISM.

Kidney

The major organ of the urinary tract, in which blood is filtered and waste products and excess fluid are excreted as urine. The two kidneys are located in the back of the abdominal cavity on either side of the spine, at about waist level. The right kidney is positioned under the liver; the left kidney, which sits slightly higher, is near the spleen.

How the Kidneys Work

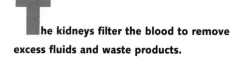

The kidneys filter the blood to remove excess fluids and waste products.

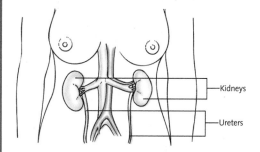

LOCATION OF THE KIDNEYS
The kidneys are located at the back of the abdominal cavity, above the waist. The right kidney lies below the liver, while the left kidney is located just below the spleen. The ureters carry the urine from the kidneys to the bladder.

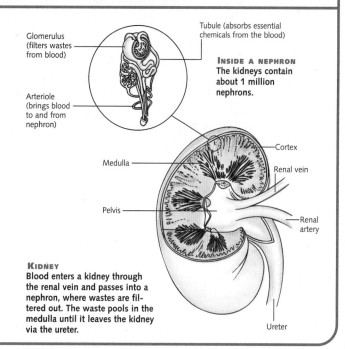

Glomerulus (filters wastes from blood)

Tubule (absorbs essential chemicals from the blood)

INSIDE A NEPHRON
The kidneys contain about 1 million nephrons.

Arteriole (brings blood to and from nephron)

Cortex

Medulla

Renal vein

Pelvis

Renal artery

Ureter

KIDNEY
Blood enters a kidney through the renal vein and passes into a nephron, where wastes are filtered out. The waste pools in the medulla until it leaves the kidney via the ureter.

K

STRUCTURE

The kidneys are wrapped in two layers of fat and held in place by strong straps of flexible connective tissue. This structure allows them to move with the diaphragm and abdomen as a person breathes yet protects them against impact. A tough layer of tissue called the renal capsule encloses the kidney for added protection.

Blood enters the kidneys through the renal arteries, which branch from the aorta (the main artery leading from the heart to the rest of the body). Inside the kidneys, the arteries subdivide until they are a network of tiny vessels called arterioles. An individual arteriole carries blood into the smallest functioning unit of the kidney called a nephron. A nephron consists of a structure called a glomerulus and an elongated structure called a tubule. Within the glomerulus, the blood is filtered and then released into a tubule. The tubule, which is surrounded by capillaries, reabsorbs some essential chemical components and allows others to flow back into the center of the kidney, called the medulla. In the medulla, which is a holding area, fluid containing wastes pools before passing out of the kidney into a ureter (the tube leading from the kidneys to the BLADDER).

FUNCTION

The blood that leaves the heart and passes into the kidneys via the renal arteries is rich in oxygen but contains the chemical waste products of body metabolism. Blood channeled into a nephron flows into the glomerulus, which conserves blood cells and proteins, but lets amino acids (the chemical components of proteins), glucose (blood sugar), mineral salts, fluids, and other by-products flow into the tubule. The tubule reabsorbs most of these essential substances, including amino acids, glucose, calcium, and phosphorus, in precisely the amounts the blood needs. These substances are returned to the blood supply via the capillaries that surround the tubule. (The filtered blood leaves the kidneys via the renal vein.)

The excess by-products, along with excess fluid, are carried, via the tubule, back into the medulla of the kidney and then are excreted in the waste liquid called urine. The filtering process in the kidneys is precisely calibrated to the requirements of the blood supply at the time and is remarkably flexible and efficient. Even though diet, fluid intake, and exercise vary significantly, the kidneys maintain constant levels of needed nutrients and fluid levels in the blood.

From the medulla, the pooled urine passes into the ureter and then into the bladder. The bladder holds the urine until it passes from the body via the urethra.

Kidney biopsy

The taking of a tiny sample of kidney tissue to help determine the cause of protein or blood in the urine or to monitor the effectiveness of treatments for kidney disorders. A kidney biopsy is done by inserting a sterile, narrow, hollow needle into a kidney to extract tissue, which is then examined by a pathologist under a microscope. A kidney biopsy is considered the most accurate assessment of abnormalities in kidney tissue.

A kidney biopsy is performed in a

hospital radiology unit by a nephrologist and a radiologist or radiology technician. The entire procedure may last 1 to 2 hours, or possibly longer, depending on the size and location of the kidney.

The person on whom the biopsy is being performed lies facedown, and an imaging technique such as X rays, ULTRASOUND SCANNING, or CT SCANNING (computed tomography scanning) is used to allow the nephrologist to visualize the kidney. The area is anesthetized, and the biopsy needle is passed through the skin to the kid-

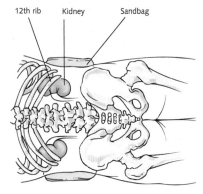

12th rib   Kidney   Sandbag

Preparation (view from above)

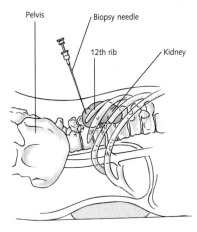

Pelvis   Biopsy needle

12th rib   Kidney

Biopsy (view from the side)

BIOPSY OF THE KIDNEY
For a kidney biopsy, the person lies on a table with a sandbag under the abdomen; X rays are taken, and a local anesthetic is given. The doctor makes a small incision under the 12th rib and inserts a biopsy needle. The person is asked to hold his or her breath, and the needle is passed into the kidney. A small piece of tissue is removed by an instrument passed through the needle.

ney, a procedure that may take about 15 minutes. The person who is undergoing the procedure must hold his or her breath as the needle is inserted and moved to make sure the kidney does not move.

A small piece of the kidney is taken up in the needle, a procedure that may need to be repeated until an adequate sample is obtained. There may be some pain during the procedure.

After the biopsy, the person must remain in a prone position for several hours to prevent excessive internal bleeding. It is common for the urine to be blood-tinged for the next 24 hours; this is not a sign of excessive bleeding. If the blood cell count and blood pressure are stable within 12 to 24 hours after the biopsy, the person may be discharged from the hospital.

A person who has had a kidney biopsy may experience a dull backache or mild discomfort in the area of the biopsy for several days after the procedure. These symptoms are typical and are caused by irritation of the back muscles and inflammation of the biopsy site. Abdominal pain or pain in the groin should be reported to a physician.

To avoid dislodging the small blood clot that forms over the biopsy site, the person should abstain from any physical activity that involves a bouncing motion for several weeks after the procedure. Preliminary results may be available within 2 to 3 days; final results are generally provided within a week. If a treatable problem is revealed, therapy is generally provided in the form of specific medication. Treatment may also be prescribed for risk factors that impact the kidneys, including high blood pressure or elevated blood cholesterol levels.

In a small number of cases, internal bleeding is sufficiently severe to require further treatment, and possibly a blood transfusion. There is a small risk of infection and of moderate to severe kidney damage.

Kidney cancer

A cancer that originates in the kidney. Kidney cancer accounts for between 2 and 3 percent of all cancers diagnosed in the United States.

Symptoms may include pain on one side of the back, blood in the urine, a mass in the abdomen or side, high blood pressure, and fever. Some people with kidney cancer also experience loss of appetite, nausea and vomiting, constipation, weakness, and fatigue.

Diagnosis of kidney cancer may include blood tests, ultrasound, urinalysis, CT (computed tomography) scanning and MRI (magnetic resonance imaging), and an IVP (intravenous pyelogram, or X rays of the kidney). Many tumors found in the kidney are benign (noncancerous); surgical biopsy is the only way to distinguish benign from malignant tumors. Kidney cancer is usually treated with surgery, radiation therapy, biological therapy, chemotherapy, or hormone therapy.

Kidney cancer occurs twice as often in men as women and is slightly more common in white men than black men. It develops most often in adults between the ages of 50 and 70 and is more common in urban, industrial areas. Smoking doubles the risk of getting the disease. Other risk factors associated with kidney cancer include exposure to asbestos and cadmium, a family history of the disease, long-term dialysis, obesity, and a diet high in fat.

Kidney cyst

A common, usually benign (noncancerous) lesion on the kidney. Kidney cysts are hollow, round growths that contain a watery fluid. About half of the people over age 50 in the United States have at least one kidney cyst.

Kidney cysts usually cause no symptoms but may sometimes cause blood in the urine, back pain, or abdominal pain if the cyst is unusually large. Kidney cysts are most commonly discovered in the course of ULTRASOUND SCANNING or CT SCANNING (computed tomography scanning) performed in connection with other conditions.

Treatment is not usually required. If a cyst becomes infected, antibiotics will be prescribed. Kidney function may be impaired if the cyst is abnormally large, but this is rare. A physician may choose to collapse or decompress a large kidney cyst by inserting a needle, guided by ultrasound or X rays, through the skin and into the cyst. See also POLYCYSTIC KIDNEY DISEASE.

Kidney failure

The inability of the kidneys to perform their normal function of filtering waste products from the blood. Kidney failure may be caused by infection, injury, exposure to toxins, kidney disease, and other diseases such as diabetes, systemic lupus erythematosus, or sickle cell anemia. Structural disorders obstructing the flow of urine from the kidneys may be associated with kidney failure. These disorders can include a stricture (narrowing), cancerous growth, or chronic obstruction of the urethra (the tube by which urine is excreted from the bladder) by an enlarged prostate gland.

Kidney failure may be acute or chronic. The acute form results in a sudden loss of kidney function. One cause of acute kidney failure is a prolonged severe drop in blood pressure that may occur in association with trauma or surgery. Severe infection or illness may also cause acute kidney failure. Acute kidney failure is potentially life-threatening and may require hospitalization and constant monitoring. In some cases of acute kidney failure, the kidneys are capable of resuming normal function within a period of several weeks to a few months. In these situations, transient DIALYSIS may be needed to remove toxic waste products until normal kidney function returns.

Chronic kidney failure involves the slow, progressive destruction of kidney function as a result of kidney disease. End-stage renal disease is chronic, irreversible kidney failure. It requires either dialysis or a KIDNEY TRANSPLANT for survival.

Kidney function tests

Diagnostic evaluations performed to determine the level of a person's kidney function. Kidney function tests involve taking blood and urine for analysis in a laboratory to check for substances that indicate the ability of the kidneys to filter the blood properly.

BLOOD UREA NITROGEN

Blood urea nitrogen (BUN) is used as an indicator of kidney function. In day-to-day cellular function, a nitrogen-containing waste product called urea is produced and found in the blood. Normally, the kidneys filter the urea from the blood into the urine. When the kidneys are not functioning properly, the blood level of the urea rises, indicating that the kidneys are not functioning properly.

CREATININE

Creatinine is a waste product of the normal breakdown of muscle during activity. It is removed from the blood by the kidneys and excreted in the urine. Elevated levels of creatinine in the blood indicate impaired kidney function.

CREATININE CLEARANCE

Creatinine clearance is a test that measures the ability of the kidneys to remove creatinine from the blood and excrete it in the urine; it is used to determine how well the kidneys are working. Creatinine is formed as a by-product of metabolism. If creatinine is not being adequately cleared from the blood, the creatinine blood level becomes elevated, indicating that the kidneys are not filtering properly. Urine samples are collected over a 24-hour period according to special instructions for timing the collection. A blood sample is also taken to determine the creatinine level in the blood. A calculation based on the amount of creatinine in the urine and in the blood can determine the rate of creatinine removal by the kidneys.

PROTEIN IN THE URINE

Normally, protein found in blood is not filtered or is filtered only in minimal amounts by the kidneys. In certain diseases, the kidneys allow more protein to leak into the urine (see PROTEINURIA). A doctor can use a urine dipstick test to test a small sample of urine for the presence of protein. In a dipstick test, a strip of cellulose is dipped into a sample of urine. The strip will change color to indicate the presence of protein in the urine. More accurate evaluation of protein in the urine requires collecting the urine for 24 hours and then testing the urine for protein.

Kidney imaging

Diagnostic scanning performed to detect anatomic abnormalities in the

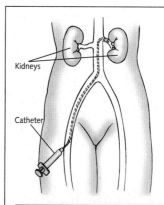

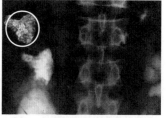

Kidney stone highlighted by arteriogram

SCANNING THE KIDNEY
For renal angiography, a catheter is inserted into an artery in the thigh and threaded up through the blood vessels into the kidney. A contrast medium (dye) is injected through the catheter to show blood flow through the kidneys and highlights any abnormality that obstructs it. The circle highlights a kidney stone.

kidneys. Kidney imaging may be done to detect a tumor, mass, cyst, or kidney stone or to locate a kidney during a kidney biopsy. It may also be performed to examine the blood vessels that supply blood to the kidneys. Specific types of kidney imaging include ULTRASOUND SCANNING, ANGIOGRAPHY, CT SCANNING (computed tomography scanning), and INTRAVENOUS PYELOGRAPHY.

Ultrasound scanning of the kidneys, also known as renal ultrasound, images kidney tissue as well as the size and shape of the kidneys. It is used to detect urinary tract obstructions, to locate a kidney for a biopsy, and to observe circulation in the arteries and veins of the kidneys by incorporating a special monitor that provides DOPPLER ULTRASOUND. Renal ultrasound works by passing a transducer over a kidney so that emitted sound waves are reflected off the kidney to transmit an image that can be viewed on a video screen. The images are studied by a radiologist who can provide a diagnosis by interpreting those images. Renal ultrasound takes 45 minutes or less and is painless.

In angiography of the kidneys, also known as renal angiography, a CON-TRAST MEDIUM is injected through a catheter that is threaded into the blood vessels of the kidneys. The contrast medium makes the blood vessels visible on a fluoroscope, a device that is equipped with a fluorescent screen. The images permit the detection of abnormalities that may affect the blood supply to the kidneys. Renal angiography is also used to determine whether a mass in a kidney is a tumor, cyst, or excess vascular tissue. The procedure lasts 3 to 4 hours and may be mildly uncomfortable.

CT scanning of the kidneys provides more accurate imaging of the kidneys than is provided by conventional X rays. A renal CT scan provides an image that allows a physician to evaluate the structure, size, and shape of the kidneys and to detect abnormalities. Renal tomography takes about an hour. If a contrast medium is injected, there may be minor discomfort and side effects.

Intravenous pyelography provides images of the kidneys and lower urinary tract. It is generally the first imaging test performed when an abnormality of the bladder or lower urinary tract is suspected. The person undergoing the procedure may be asked to fast for 8 to 12 hours before the procedure and may be given a laxative to empty the colon. A contrast medium is injected into the arm, and a series of X rays are taken periodically while the contrast medium travels through the kidneys into the ureters and the bladder. Abnormal readings are generally followed up with ultrasound or CT scans to more accurately diagnose initial findings. Intravenous pyelography takes about an hour and may involve minor discomfort and side effects such as flushing and nausea from injection of the contrast medium.

Kidney stones

FOR SYMPTOM CHART
see Urine discoloration, page 58

Also known as renal calculi; stones composed of abnormal chemical

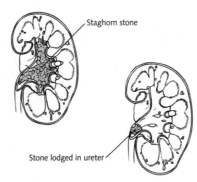

TYPES OF KIDNEY STONES
A so-called staghorn kidney stone fills the cavities of the kidney. More typically, stones are smaller and may pass out of the urinary tract without causing any symptoms. But a stone may pass into the ureter and lodge there, obstructing the flow of urine and causing pain.

deposits that form inside the urinary tract. Kidney stones are hard and may be the size of a grain of sand or larger than a marble. When they are very small, they pass out of the kidneys through the ureters (two narrow tubes, each connecting a kidney and the bladder) in the urine. If they are large, they may remain in the kidneys or travel into a ureter where they become trapped, causing a variety of symptoms that include extreme pain, blocked urine flow, and bleeding.

TYPES OF KIDNEY STONES
Kidney stones are common. The reason they form and their chemical composition vary from one person to another. Medically, they are grouped as calcium, struvite, uric acid, or cystine stones.

Calcium stones are composed of calcium oxalate or calcium phosphate. They are the most common kidney stones and occur more frequently in men and adults. They are often associated with elevated calcium levels in the urine, which may be caused by inherited factors. An abnormally low level of citrate in the urine can also cause calcium stones, as can HYPERPARATHYROIDISM, chemical imbalances after bowel surgery, or RENAL TUBULAR ACIDOSIS, which is a problem with the ability of the kidneys to maintain a normal acid-base balance.

Struvite stones are composed of magnesium and the waste product ammonia. They are associated with

bacterial urinary tract infections and are more common in women. This type of kidney stone often develops in people who must have a catheter in the bladder for long periods.

Uric acid stones result from an excessive concentration of uric acid in the urine and are often associated with GOUT. They are more common in men.

Cystine stones are made up of the amino acid cysteine, a building block of protein. They are rare and are generally caused by a genetic defect.

SYMPTOMS
Small kidney stones usually do not cause symptoms. When kidney stones enlarge and become trapped in a ureter, they can cause severe back pain or pain in the side. There may be nausea and vomiting, as well as blood in the urine. Pain closer to the groin indicates that the stone has traveled closer to the bladder, producing an increased urge to urinate and a burning sensation during urination.

DIAGNOSIS AND TREATMENT
Anyone with kidney stones, even very small ones that do not cause symptoms, should be examined by a doctor. A physician will take a general medical history and ask about changes in urine color and if there is a family tendency for kidney stones or gout.

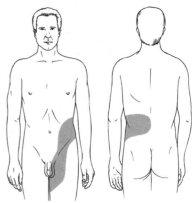

Site of pain—front   Site of pain—back

PAIN FROM KIDNEY STONES
Pain from kidney stones can be intense. It is felt in the area of the urinary tract and kidney on the side of the affected kidney. If the stone is lodged in the lower part of the ureter, the pain may extend all the way down along the inner thigh. The pain tends to come in waves and may be accompanied by nausea and vomiting.

If a kidney stone is not too large, pain medication may be prescribed until the stone is passed. This may be a matter of hours, days, or weeks. Smaller stones are usually flushed out through urination and should be saved and brought to a doctor for chemical analysis. The person will also undergo blood and urine tests to identify the possible cause of the kidney stones. Larger stones tend to remain trapped in a ureter where they obstruct the flow of urine and cause infection. When extreme pain is experienced, KIDNEY IMAGING such as INTRAVENOUS PYELOGRAPHY and ULTRASOUND SCANNING may be used to detect and locate a trapped kidney stone. If the stone is large and causing intolerable pain, infection, or heavy bleeding, it may be necessary to break up the stone in a procedure called LITHOTRIPSY. The stone will be chemically analyzed, and the person will have blood and urine tests to determine its cause.

Drinking 2 to 4.25 quarts of water daily reduces the risk of recurrence. Medication and changes in the diet may also be recommended to help prevent recurrence. Thiazide diuretic medications are prescribed to help prevent calcium stones. Uric acid stones may be treated with ALLOPURINOL and a diet low in foods (such as red meats, fish, and poultry) that contain purines.

Kidney transplant

A surgical procedure in which a healthy kidney is taken from one person (see NEPHRECTOMY) and placed in another person with end-stage renal disease (see KIDNEY FAILURE). A kidney transplant restores sufficient kidney function so that the person does not need dialysis.

HOW IT IS PERFORMED

Healthy kidneys may be taken from dead organ donors (within 48 hours of the donor's death) or from living donors, usually a blood relative. A donated kidney can be transported across the country in a refrigerated container.

Analyzing a variety of factors, including blood type and the nature of the antibodies in both donor and recipient, increases the likelihood of a successful transplant. Improvements in medications that suppress

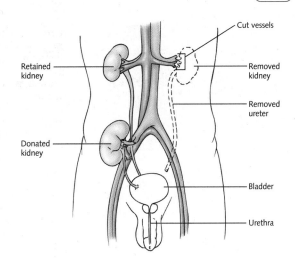

the immune system may make perfect matching less important.

The most current technique for removing a healthy kidney from a living donor is LAPAROSCOPY. Several dime-sized incisions are made in the abdomen and hollow tubes are inserted into the incisions. A fiberoptic camera placed in an incision transmits an image onto monitors that allow the surgeons to view the kidney. Surgical instruments for retrieving the kidney are placed in the other tubes. The kidney from the donor is encased in plastic and removed with a tool inserted into another incision about 2 inches wide. Recovery usually requires a 2-day hospital stay for the donor.

The healthy kidney is transplanted into the recipient through a surgical incision in the lower abdomen. The blood supply to the new kidney is established by attaching the veins and arteries of the recipient to the organ. The nearest ureter is also attached. Taking the healthy kidney from the donor and transplanting it into the recipient takes an average of about 3½ hours.

After the transplant, it is essential to assure that the body does not reject the donor organ. Medications and a special diet are to necessary to prevent rejection.

ELIGIBILITY

Not everyone who needs a kidney transplant to survive is a suitable candidate to receive one. Conditions that may cause a kidney transplantation to fail include infection, acute GLOMERULONEPHRITIS, and unstable coronary artery disease. In most areas of the United States, there is a shortage of donor kidneys and a long list of potential recipients waiting for them.

Kidney, polycystic

A genetic disorder characterized by the growth of multiple fluid-filled cysts in the kidneys. The cysts can slowly replace much of the kidney tissue, reducing kidney function and ultimately leading to kidney failure. Kidney failure, sometimes called end-stage renal disease or ESRD, must be treated with DIALYSIS or transplantation. Polycystic kidney disease (PKD) occurs in both children and adults. Infantile PKD, a severe childhood disorder, is an autosomal recessive disorder (neither parent has the disease, but both are carriers). Onset of adult PKD, an autosomal dominant disorder, usually does not occur until affected

K

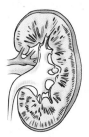 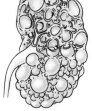

Healthy kidney   Polycystic kidney

FLUID-FILLED CYSTS
Healthy kidney tissue consists of tiny tubules and filtering units, supplied by capillaries, that enable the kidney to filter blood. In the kidneys of a person with polycystic kidney disease, clusters of fluid-filled cysts form and expand to gradually destroy the kidney tissue.

POLYCYSTIC KIDNEY DISEASE

Signs of adult polycystic kidney disease may include:

- **Pain in back or midabdomen**
- **Blood in the urine**
- **Excessive urination at night**
- **Kidney stones**
- **Hypertension (high blood pressure)**

individuals are in their teens or 20s. About 500,000 adults in the United States have adult PKD, which is usually inherited from a parent who has the disease.

SYMPTOMS AND DIAGNOSIS

Many symptoms are associated with infantile polycystic kidney disease. Infantile PKD is usually diagnosed shortly after birth. Symptoms include enlarged kidneys that produce abdominal distension, anemia, high blood pressure, kidney failure, and liver disease. The disease is very serious in childhood and can cause death in infancy or childhood.

Adult PKD is associated with high blood pressure and progressive loss of kidney function. Sometimes bleeding into a cyst occurs, which can cause pain in the back or midabdominal pain. Kidney stones occur more often in people with PKD than they do in people who do not have the disease. Most adults with the disease reach end-stage renal disease by their 40s or 50s, although some will experience only mild to moderate loss of kidney function throughout their lives. Adults with PKD frequently have cysts in the liver as well as the kidney, which can become infected and cause fever.

DIAGNOSIS AND TREATMENT

Diagnosis of polycystic kidney disease is made by ultrasound examination of the kidneys. CT (computed tomography) scanning and MRI (magnetic resonance imaging) may also be used to look for cysts. DNA blood tests are available to detect mutations in the gene for PKD. No treatment currently exists to prevent the cysts from forming or growing.

Treatment generally focuses on related symptoms. For instance, high blood pressure will be controlled with medication and diet to preserve kidney function, and urinary tract infections must always be treated promptly

to prevent kidney damage. Sometimes it is necessary to drain cysts when they cause pain, bleeding, infection, or obstruction. At other times, cysts grow large enough to affect neighboring organs, such as the liver, the pancreas, and the intestines, and it is necessary to drain the cysts. End-stage renal disease must be treated with dialysis or transplantation. Genetic counseling is recommended to individuals with a family history of PKD.

Kilocalorie

A measurement of energy used in nutrition. A kilocalorie (kcal) represents the amount of energy necessary to raise the temperature of 1 kilogram of water by 1 degree Celsius (centigrade). In popular, nonscientific usage, a kilocalorie is usually called a calorie.

Kilojoule

One thousand joules; a JOULE is a standard unit of work or energy.

Kleptomania

A rare mental illness characterized by a compulsive, uncontrollable desire to steal. Objects are not stolen because of monetary value and may in fact be worth little, indicating that a person with kleptomania does not intend to be criminal. A person with kleptomania feels a buildup of tension that is released when he or she steals, but the person often feels remorseful after the theft. The stealing is usually not planned in advance. A person with kleptomania may steal in obvious ways, with little concern about apprehension or legal consequences. The person is often caught in the act, possibly signaling a desire to be noticed and treated. The disorder usually begins in childhood or adolescence, may continue throughout life, and is often accompanied by depression, anxiety, and bulimia.

Klinefelter syndrome

A chromosome abnormality affecting only men due to the presence of an extra X chromosome. Klinefelter syndrome causes HYPOGONADISM (inadequate function of the sex glands that results in decreased production of sex hormones) and infertility. An

infant with Klinefelter syndrome appears normal at birth, but during puberty the secondary sexual characteristics fail to develop, at which point the problem becomes apparent. Testicular abnormalities result in infertility in most cases. Symptoms and associated conditions may include a small penis and small firm testicles; diminished pubic, facial, and body hair; sexual dysfunction; enlarged breast tissue (GYNECOMASTIA), tall stature, long legs and short trunk; learning disabilities; and emotional disorders. In some mild cases there may be few signs, except for infertility.

Diagnosis may involve tests to identify a low sperm count or abnormal levels of sex hormones. The diagnosis is established conclusively by blood chromosome analysis, which reveals the presence of the extra X chromosome (two Xs and one Y instead of one X and one Y).

Treatment may include testosterone therapy to improve the development of secondary sex characteristics and promote normal sexual function. Gynecomastia can be treated with plastic surgery if it is disfiguring. Counseling may be required to reinforce male identity and to adjust to the disorder. There is no treatment for the infertility associated with the syndrome.

Klumpke paralysis

Paralysis of the forearm resulting from injury to the lower brachial plexus. Klumpke paralysis is present from birth, most often with breech deliveries. It is often associated with other problems, such as HORNER SYNDROME.

Knee

The hinge joint between the thighbone (femur) and the shin (tibia). This powerful joint joins the two longest bones in the body and helps bear much of the weight of the upper body.

The knee joint, like many other joints, is encased in a tough capsule to help prevent dislocation. The outer layer of the capsule is composed of interwoven collagen fibers that provide both strength and flexibility. An inner layer of ligaments called capsular ligaments binds the bones togeth-

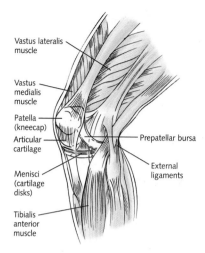

ANATOMY OF THE KNEE
The knee is one of the most complex joints in the body. It is a hinge joint that also rotates slightly. The thigh and calf muscles connect to the long bones of the leg, with the bony patella riding on the front of the knee joint. Ligaments stabilize the joint, cartilage smoothes its motion, and the bursae cushion it.

er and strengthens the joint capsule. The joint capsule is lined with the synovial membrane, which also encloses all ligaments and cushions of cartilage within the joint. The synovial membrane secretes a liquid called synovial fluid, which lubricates the entire joint.

Within the joint capsule, the two bones that connect at the joint are covered with a layer of articular cartilage. This cartilage is lubricated by synovial fluid, allowing the two surfaces of the bone to slide over each other with little friction. The bones are firmly connected by the internal ligaments. The knee joint is further padded and protected by pieces of cartilage called menisci that are more loosely attached to the inside of the joint capsule.

The kneecap (patella) is a disk of bone that lies in front of the knee joint. It is attached to the muscles of the upper and lower leg by tendons (tough but elastic fibrous cords that connect bone to muscle). The kneecap is cushioned above and below by an upper and a lower bursa (sac of synovial fluid) that prevent wear between the femur and the tendon attached to the kneecap, and the kneecap and the skin on top of it.

Another set of external ligaments connects the two long bones of the knee joint outside the joint capsule. These ligaments restrict the range of movement of the joint to prevent dislocation.

The muscles of the knee joint are the quadriceps muscles on the top of the knee, which straighten the knee joint, and the hamstring muscles at the back of the thigh, which bend it. The quadriceps muscle must remain slightly contracted whenever the body is standing upright. The design of the knees is such that the knee joints lock to help reduce the tension in the quadriceps.

Knee replacement
See JOINT REPLACEMENT, KNEE.

Knock-knees
Knees that touch due to an inward curving of the legs. Knock-knees help children maintain balance as they learn to walk and are normal between the ages of 2 and 6. Overweight children are more apt to develop them than are children of average weight. Knock-knees that persist into adolescence are usually an inherited prob-

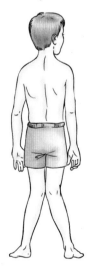

CHILDHOOD KNOCK-KNEES
In a child younger than 10 years, knock-knees are not a cause for concern; they are part of a normal stage of development as the child learns balance. Properly fitting shoes and plenty of exercise will help a child grow out of the knock-knees. If the condition is pronounced after the age of 10 or so, a pediatric orthopedist can be consulted for treatment to ensure that the knock-knees do not cause joint strain.

lem. In rare cases, they are the result of a more serious underlying condition, such as RICKETS (a vitamin D deficiency that causes bones to soften), a fracture, infection, tumor, or JUVENILE RHEUMATOID ARTHRITIS.

In most cases, knock-knees correct themselves over time and require no treatment. Providing children with shoes that fit correctly and ample opportunity to exercise are essential. If knock-knees persist after age 10, children are usually referred to a pediatric orthopedist for consultation and possible treatment. Braces (see BRACE, ORTHOPEDIC) or corrective shoes may be required to remedy the problem. Corrective surgery may also be necessary. In younger children, these measures are not recommended and may even cause physical or emotional damage.

Koilonychia
A condition in which thinning of the nail creates a flattened, concave, spoonlike shape. Koilonychia can be caused by a long-standing iron deficiency or an injury to the nail bed, but it is sometimes also inherited. The cause may be unknown.

Koplik spots
Tiny red spots with a white center most commonly found on the mucous surface inside the cheek and opposite the molar teeth. Koplik spots, which are the size of grains of sand, may appear less commonly on the inner surface of the lower lip and on the palate. The spots appear directly before the characteristic skin rash of rubeola, which is MEASLES, and are often the basis for an initial diagnosis of measles. They disappear once the rash, typical of the illness, begins.

Korsakoff psychosis
A mental illness marked by extreme confusion, mental impairment, memory loss, and symptoms of nerve damage. Also known as alcohol-induced persisting amnesic disorder, Korsakoff psychosis usually is caused from alcoholism but may also be a result of a brain tumor, a head injury, starvation, or a minor stroke. The person cannot remember recent events and invents plausible fictions to account for the gaps in memory, an

K

activity called confabulation. In its early stages, Korsakoff psychosis caused by alcoholism can be slowed by abstinence from alcohol and administration of vitamin B1 (thiamin). The loss of memory and intellect cannot usually be reversed.

Kyphoscoliosis

An abnormal and excessive backward and lateral curvature of the spine. Kyphoscoliosis is a combination of two spinal conditions: KYPHOSIS and SCOLIOSIS.

Kyphosis

An abnormal and excessive outward curvature of the vertebrae in the upper spine. It is usually painless unless severe, but can result in chronic fatigue in the back muscles. Kyphosis produces humpback, hunchback, or rounding of the shoulders and can occur in several different age groups. The back pain is usually worse when standing for a long time. Osteoarthritis, rheumatoid arthritis, rickets, and compression fracture may be associated with kyphosis. It is usually hereditary when present in young children. Women who are older and postmenopausal may develop a form of kyphosis called senile kyphosis or "dowager's hump," which is caused by osteoporosis. In adolescents, who are usually taller and heavier than their peers, it is called juvenile kyphosis and may be related to Scheuermann disease (an inflammation of the bone and cartilage of the vertebrae), tuberculosis, or tumors.

Kyphosis is diagnosed by physical examination, X rays, and in some cases, laboratory tests. Treatment generally emphasizes the use of orthotic braces or other devices for juvenile kyphosis, a back corset for older adults, and exercise routines to strengthen the muscles and ligaments associated with the spine and upper back. Medication may be prescribed to treat related conditions such as osteoporosis, ankylosing spondylitis, or tuberculosis. When kyphosis is severe, it may be treated by a surgical procedure involving spinal fusion, with or without the use of metal rods.

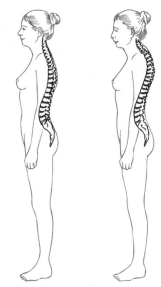

Healthy spine curvature   Spine with kyphosis

OUTWARD CURVATURE OF THE SPINE
Kyphosis in an adult may be caused by long-time poor posture (postural kyphosis) or by diseases such as arthritis or osteoporosis. Treatment may involve medication for underlying conditions, strengthening exercises for the spinal and abdominal muscles, or a brace or corset.

K

La Leche League

A volunteer organization that provides information and encouragement to women who breast-feed. The league was formed in the United States in 1956 by a small group of nursing mothers and has become an internationally recognized authority on breast-feeding. The league sponsors informal discussion groups, lectures, and conferences for parents and health care professionals, and it publishes books, pamphlets, and magazines to help nursing mothers.

Labetalol

An antihypertensive drug. Labetalol (Normodyne, Trandate) is used to treat high blood pressure. It works by preventing nerve impulses from exerting an excessive effect on the heart and blood vessels. The outcome is a slightly decreased heart rate and lower blood pressure.

Labia

Lips; usually refers to the lips of the vaginal opening that protect the female's external genitalia. The outer, thicker folds, which have hair and sweat glands, are called the labia majora. The thinner, inner folds, called the labia minora, form the hood over the clitoris. See REPRODUCTIVE SYSTEM, FEMALE.

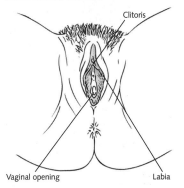

VAGINAL LIPS
The outer labia majora, the most visible parts of a woman's genitals, are folds of skin covering the muscle on either side of the entrance to the vagina. The labia minora lie just under the labia majora and meet just above the clitoris.

Labile

Unstable. In psychiatry and psychology, moods or behaviors that are changeable and unstable are called labile. Someone who is emotionally labile is capable of switching from anger to sadness to cheeriness rapidly. In medicine, the term "labile" is sometimes used to describe rapidly changeable blood glucose levels in people with diabetes and fluctuating blood pressure readings in those with labile hypertension.

Labor

FOR FIRST AID
see Childbirth, page 1317

A series of physiological changes in a woman that allow for the delivery of a fetus through her birth canal. Labor is divided into three stages: dilation and effacement (opening and thinning of the cervix), delivery of the baby, and delivery of the placenta. Changes in hormone levels appear to cause the start of labor, although the exact cause is unclear. The duration of labor varies for each woman and each birth. A first pregnancy typically results in the longest labor. Subsequent births usually will have shorter labors.

A definitive sign of the beginning of labor is experiencing contractions that progressively become stronger and more regular. Timing the contractions will indicate whether labor is progressing. Many doctors ask women to call when contractions are 4 to 5 minutes apart and have continued for an hour or more. When a woman is having regular contractions, a doctor will want to examine her to determine if her cervix has dilated. If it has not, she may be sent home to wait for her cervix to dilate.

In the ninth month of pregnancy, a woman may experience mild, irregular contractions known as Braxton Hicks contractions, which are not the beginning of labor, but a sign that the body is preparing for true labor. Another sign of labor is the passing of the mucus plug that has sealed off the cervix during pregnancy. A woman may notice mucus tinged with blood (called bloody show) when the plug passes from her body. Birth, however, may still be hours or even days away. A woman should notify her doctor if a significant amount of bleeding occurs, since bleeding can occasionally be a sign of a serious problem with the baby or the placenta. Rupture of the amniotic sac (the membranes that surround the fetus) usually occurs during labor, but can occur before. When a woman's water breaks, a clear fluid flows from her vagina as either a trickle or a gush of liquid. A doctor should be notified. If labor has not yet begun, the doctor may recommend inducing labor. Sometimes, contractions begin as a woman's water breaks.

STAGES OF LABOR
Labor has been established when a woman's contractions are strong enough to prevent normal activities and are no more than 5 minutes apart for an hour. The uterus contracts in a pattern, with mild and infrequent contractions at the start of labor that become more frequent and stronger as labor progresses over time. Labor proceeds in specific steps with distinct physiological characteristics.

■ *Stage one* Usually the longest for most women, this stage begins when a woman's cervix starts to dilate (open) and efface (thin), to permit the baby to pass through the cervix and into the birth canal. Dilation is expressed in centimeters, and effacement is expressed as a percentage. For example, during labor, a woman's doctor may say that she is 4 centimeters dilated and 80 percent effaced. The pain associated with labor varies from woman to woman. Generally, however, contractions at the beginning of labor are experienced as less painful than later contractions.

There are three phases of stage 1 labor: early, active, and transition. During the early phase, a woman's cervix dilates to 4 centimeters, and contractions occur at varying intervals. In the active phase, contractions are stronger and more frequent (coming every 5 minutes or less), as the cervix dilates from 4 to 8 centimeters. The transition phase brings the most intense contractions of labor (at intervals of every 2 to 3 minutes), as the cervix fully dilates to 10 centimeters. The baby descends into the vagina and the mother may feel the urge to push.

■ *Stage two* Birth occurs in this stage. A woman will be asked to bear down

STAGES OF LABOR

Labor has three main stages: dilation and effacement (the thinning and opening of the cervix), delivery of the baby, and delivery of the placenta.

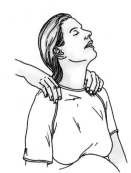

FIRST STAGE
In the first stage, which is usually the longest, the cervix becomes thinner and opens so that the baby can pass through. Contractions are usually mild at the beginning and gradually get stronger and more frequent. The woman's labor partner can help provide pain relief through a shoulder rub or back rub.

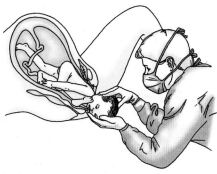

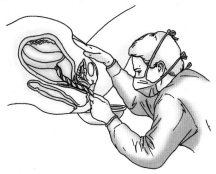

SECOND STAGE
The second stage is the delivery of the baby. Once the cervix is fully dilated, the woman can push with the contractions. It may take several minutes or a few hours until the baby is born. The doctor guides the baby's head and shoulders.

THIRD STAGE
The third stage of labor, in which the placenta (afterbirth) separates from the wall of the uterus and is expelled from the woman's body through contractions, is generally short but can last up to 30 minutes.

L

and push during contractions to assist in the delivery of her baby. Before pushing, a doctor will first confirm that the cervix has fully dilated. The length of this phase will depend on the frequency and intensity of a woman's contractions and her ability to bear down. Stage 2 labor may last 2 hours or longer for a first delivery and 1 or 2 hours if a woman has previously delivered a child. This stage ends when the baby is delivered.

■ *Stage three* In this stage, the afterbirth (the placenta and membranes surrounding the fetus) are delivered. The contractions in stage 3 labor are not as intense or painful as those of the first two stages of labor. During this stage, the placenta detaches from the uterine wall and is expelled from the woman's body with the aid of contractions. Sometimes, the woman may be asked to push gently to assist

in the delivery of the afterbirth. Stage 3 may last a few minutes to a half hour.

Labyrinthitis

An inflammation of the inner ear's system of fluid-filled tubes and sacs called the labyrinth. The symptoms of labyrinthitis depend on the severity and extent of the inflammation. HEARING LOSS or ringing in the ears may result if the inflammation affects the COCHLEA (hearing organ of the inner ear). Difficulty with balance, dizziness, and nausea may be experienced if the inflammation reaches the vestibular system (group of organs in the inner ear responsible for balance control and eye movements). Because the inner ear is so small (about the size of a dime), inflammation of the labyrinth often affects both the cochlea and the vestibular system at the same time and produces symp-

toms associated with both hearing and balance. These symptoms may be temporary (peaking during the first few days with gradual recovery) or long lasting, mild or intense, depending on the severity of any inflammation present. In the worst cases, there is an intense spinning sensation accompanied by nausea, vomiting, and an inability to walk, as well as profound one-sided hearing loss. It is important to seek medical attention promptly if these symptoms are experienced, because they can also be symptoms of a more serious condition such as stroke.

CAUSES

Labyrinthitis is caused either by bacterial or viral infections, often when an ear infection is left untreated. Bacterial infection of the labyrinth may also be caused by bacterial meningitis (inflammation of the protective sheath covering the brain).

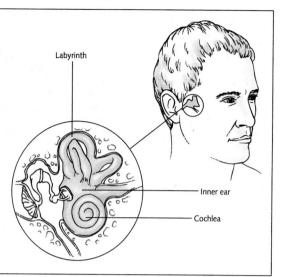

SITE OF LABYRINTHITIS
The labyrinth is a region of convoluted passages in the inner ear including the cochlea (the principal organ of hearing) and the vestibular system (a group of organs concerned with balance). Labyrinthitis is an inflammation of any of these organs. If the cochlea is inflamed, hearing loss or ringing in the ears may occur; inflamed semicircular canals may cause dizziness or loss of balance. The region of the labyrinth is very small (about the size of a dime), so infection can spread easily throughout the system.

Labyrinth

Inner ear

Cochlea

Rupturing of the membranes between the middle ear and the inner ear may also cause bacteria to infect the labyrinth. Among the common viruses associated with labyrinthitis are influenza, measles, mumps, German measles, herpes, hepatitis, polio, and Epstein-Barr.

Bacterial labyrinthitis is treated with antibiotics. The only treatment for the viral form, which is by far the most common, is bed rest, mild tranquilizers, and medication to relieve dizziness. Remaining as still as possible in dim lighting may help ease dizziness and nausea. Intravenous fluids may be necessary to treat dehydration due to vomiting.

Laceration

Wound in which the skin is opened or cut. Lacerations are commonly caused by sharp objects such as knives, scissors, or broken glass, although they can also be caused by a blunt object that splits the skin. Lacerations usually bleed heavily, and deep cuts can bleed severely. Deep lacerations can damage nerves and large blood vessels and may not be painful if nerves have been injured. Cuts that are less than ¼ inch deep and ½ inch long, with smooth edges not over any joint, can usually be treated at home without stitches by cleaning the wound thoroughly, applying antibiotic ointment, closing the wound with butterfly bandages, and applying a sterile dressing.

Lacrimal apparatus

A body system associated with the production and drainage of tears. The lacrimal apparatus is a protective device that keeps the eye moist and free of dust and other irritants. The tear-forming system includes the lacrimal glands, the eyelid margins, the conjunctival sac, and the tear drainage system.

The lacrimal gland secretes tears from its position at the upper and outer corner of the eye; the tears flow through ducts directed toward the eyeball. A stream of tears constantly washes over the front surface of the eyeball and is drained off through tiny openings in the inner corner of the eye, eventually reaching the nasal cavity.

Lacrimal gland

Any one of four tear-producing glands that lubricate and drain the EYE. Two glands lie in the upper, outer corner of the eye socket and drain onto the conjunctiva (the clear membrane covering the eyeball) when the eye is irritated or when the person is crying. Two accessory glands lie in the conjunctiva itself, supplying tears directly onto the membrane to maintain a constant film.

Tears keep the delicate structures of the eye moist and help rid the eye of microorganisms and foreign materials. Blinking action is lubricated by tears; excess fluid from blinking is drained off through a system of ducts into the nose. Tears drain out of the eye through the tear ducts located on the inner end of each eyelid. Tearing also has a part in the expression of emotion.

Lactase deficiency

A shortage of the enzyme lactase, which breaks down lactose (the predominant sugar in milk and other dairy products) so that it can be absorbed by the body. See also LACTOSE INTOLERANCE.

Lactation

The production and secretion of milk from the breasts after childbirth. The first 2 weeks following birth are crucial for establishing the milk supply, and therefore nursing must be initiated at that time. The breasts produce and secrete COLOSTRUM for several days before lactation begins. Colostrum provides the baby with essential nutrients and infection-fighting substances until the milk begins to flow. Milk production is a constant and efficient process; 2 hours after breast-feeding, 75 percent of the breast's milk will have been replenished. Lactation automatically adjusts to the baby's demand for milk, and the longer and more frequently a baby breast-feeds, the more milk will be produced. The baby's sucking stimulates milk production.

Lactic acid

A compound that forms in body cells as an end product of the metabolism of glucose. Lactic acid levels are normally raised during exercise, and lactic acid can accumulate in the muscles and cause cramps following strenuous exercise. People with severe infections or poisoning sometimes experience severe elevations of lactic acid, which is known as lactic acidosis.

During the fermentation of milk, LACTOSE (a sugar) is converted to lactic acid by bacteria such as *Lactobacillus*. Lactic acid is responsible for the preservation and flavor of cheese, yogurt, and other milk products and is an important food preservative.

Lactobacillus

Bacteria used as a food supplement to help control diarrhea. Lactobacillus (Lactinex) is a harmless bacterium that occurs naturally in unpasteur-

L

ized whole milk and yogurt. Lactobacilli produce lactic acid from the breakdown of carbohydrates responsible for making milk go sour. The bacteria are used commercially to prepare cheese and yogurt.

Doctors have used lactobacilli for years to help control certain kinds of diarrhea, especially that caused when oral antibiotics destroy the bacteria normally found in the intestine. There is little scientific information available to support its use in other illnesses, although claims have been made for lactobacillus as an immune system booster.

Lactose

The principal sugar in both human and cow's milk. Lactose is converted to lactic acid by bacteria such as *Lactobacillus*, resulting in the production of cheese and yogurt. In digestion, lactose is broken down into constituent sugars by lactase, an enzyme that is secreted in the small intestine. Some people, especially those of middle Eastern and African descent, have low or nonexistent levels of this enzyme and are therefore unable to absorb lactose; they are considered lactose-intolerant.

Lactose intolerance

The inability to digest lactose, the predominant sugar found in milk and other dairy products. Lactose intolerance is due to a shortage of the enzyme lactase, which breaks down lactose so that it can be absorbed by the body. Although virtually all infants are born with this enzyme, more than half of adults worldwide lack it. As many as 75 percent of African American, Native American, Mexican American, and Jewish adults are lactose-intolerant. Nine of ten Asian American adults are also likely to have the condition.

The symptoms of lactose intolerance develop 30 minutes to 2 hours after consuming products such as milk, ice cream, sour cream, or cheese. They include nausea, bloating, gas, and diarrhea. The severity of symptoms and the amount of lactose that can be consumed before develop-

> Terms in small capital letters—for example, PHYSICAL THERAPY or PAGET DISEASE—indicate a cross-reference to another entry with more information.

ing symptoms differs among individuals. A diagnosis of lactose intolerance is suggested by the appearance of characteristic symptoms after ingesting lactose and the resolution of symptoms by a lactose-free diet. Tests such as the lactose intolerance test and the hydrogen breath test or measuring stool acidity can be used to confirm a diagnosis. In the lactose intolerance test, the individual drinks a liquid that contains lactose, and samples of blood are taken over a period of time to see whether the body can absorb lactose. In the hydrogen breath test, undigested lactose leads to the formation of hydrogen, which is detectable on the breath. The stool acidity test measures the amount of acid created by undigested lactose.

Lactose intolerance is easily treated. By eliminating dairy foods from the diet one by one, the person can discover which foods cause discomfort and which ones can be tolerated. Many people can continue to enjoy dairy products if they consume them in small amounts or along with other foods. Others can take advantage of products such as lactose-reduced milk or tablets that help digest lactose. Because milk and dairy products are a rich source of calcium, doctors recommend that people who are lactose-intolerant consume other foods that are high in calcium but low in lactose. This is especially true for children, pregnant women, breast-feeding mothers, and postmenopausal women. Leafy green vegetables, dried beans, soybean (such as tofu), and fish (especially sardines) are good nondairy sources of calcium. When necessary, doctors can also prescribe calcium supplements.

Lactulose

A type of sugar used to treat constipation. Lactulose (Duphalac and others) is a sugar that is not metabolized and not absorbed by the body. The bacteria in the colon break it down into acids that pull water into the colon and soften the stool. Because lactulose also lowers ammonia in the blood, it is sometimes used to treat associated mental changes that can occur in people with cirrhosis of the liver.

Lagophthalmos

Inability to shut the eyes completely.

Laminectomy

The surgical removal of one or more pieces of bone from a vertebra. The purpose of a laminectomy is to relieve the pain caused by pressure on a nerve being compressed by bones in the spine from arthritis, trauma, or a cancerous tumor.

Lamivudine

An antiviral drug used to treat HIV (human immunodeficiency virus) and hepatitis B virus infections. Lamivudine (Epivir) is also known as 3TC and is one of a class of drugs called nucleoside analogue reverse transcriptase inhibitors. It is prescribed in combination with other antiretroviral drugs to suppress HIV; it works by preventing the virus from replicating itself and infecting new cells.

Lance

To pierce or cut an abscess or boil in order to release accumulated pus. Abscesses and boils (called furuncles) should never be lanced by a person at home; this can result in the spread of infection, which is usually caused by bacteria. Doctors lance lesions in sterile surroundings, inserting a drain if the infection is large or deep.

Lancet

A small, pointed, two-edged surgical knife. A lancet is used to open abscesses, for example.

Lanolin

A fatlike substance derived from the wool of sheep. Lanolin is used as the base for an ointment and as a skin moisturizer.

Lansoprazole

See PROTON PUMP INHIBITORS.

Laparoscopic surgery

An operation performed with the use of a fiberoptic device called a laparoscope (a viewing tube), which projects images onto a television monitor while the surgeon manipulates surgical instruments within the body. When patient safety allows it, laparoscopic surgery is preferred

LAPAROSCOPIC SURGICAL TOOLS

Depending on the procedure, the surgeon will attach one of five surgical tools used in laparoscopic surgery: a biopsy forceps, a scissors, a forceps, a cytology brush, or a wire loop. By manipulating one of the small instruments through a small incision, the surgeon is able to perform the necessary operation and offer the patient reduced postoperative pain and a quicker recovery.

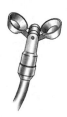 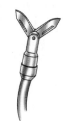 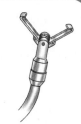

Biopsy forceps are used to remove a tiny tissue sample for testing; the tube is only ¼ inch wide.

Scissors are used to cut tissue as needed.

Forceps help the surgeon grasp or reposition tissue.

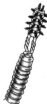 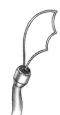

A cytology brush is used to remove cells from a suspected area for testing.

A wire loop is a cautery device that uses heat to cut tissue without causing bleeding in the patient.

INSTRUMENT HEADS
Laparoscopic procedures are performed with tiny instruments inserted into the body through tubes. These are just some of the small instruments the doctor might use in laparoscopic surgery.

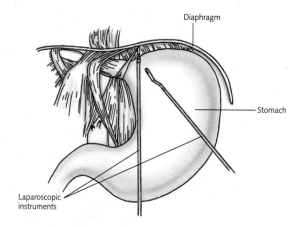

REPAIRING A HIATAL HERNIA: STEP ONE
The laparoscope and a tube are inserted into the abdomen. A wire loop is used to gently pull the stomach away from the opening in the diaphragm.

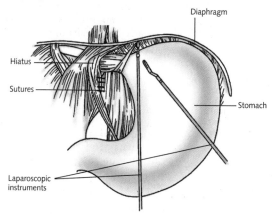

STEP TWO
The hiatus or opening in the diaphragm is closed with stitches.

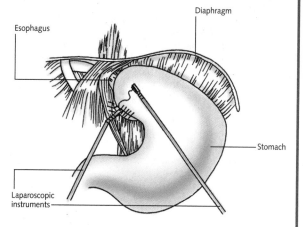

STEP THREE
The upper portion of the stomach is wrapped around the esophagus and stitched in place.

L

over more invasive open procedures because of the smaller incision, reduced postoperative pain, and quicker recovery.

Surgeons use the laparoscope for diagnosing infertility in women; removing a gallbladder; repairing hernias; removing a lung nodule; colon surgery; removing tumors or masses within the pelvis; ANTIREFLUX SURGERY; and voluntary sterilization in women (TUBAL LIGATION).

HOW IT IS DONE
Abdominal laparoscopic procedures are usually done with a patient under general anesthesia (see ANESTHESIA, GENERAL). A small incision is made in or just below the navel, and a needle is inserted into the abdomen. Carbon dioxide, pumped through the needle, inflates the abdomen and lifts the abdominal wall up and away from the internal organs.

Next, the surgeon makes a few small incisions into the abdomen, and hollow tubes called cannulas are inserted into the abdominal cavity to allow the laparoscope and other surgical instruments to be inserted into the inflated abdomen. Using the magnified television monitor image from the laparoscope to see the procedure, the surgeon completes the surgery and removes the cannulas and instruments. The carbon dioxide is released from the abdomen, which returns to its normal size. The incision is then sutured shut and bandaged.

WHAT TO EXPECT
Laparoscopic surgery requires that the patient fast from food and drinks after midnight on the day before surgery. Many laparoscopic procedures are performed as AMBULATORY SURGERY; the person enters the hospital or surgery center on the morning of the procedure and goes home later the same day. If a longer hospital stay is required, it is usually limited to 1 or 2 days.

Some discomfort and tenderness at the incision points can be expected during the first few days after surgery. The shoulders and chest may feel achy from the carbon dioxide pumped into the abdomen, but this pain goes away soon on its own. Patients can resume normal activity as soon as they are comfortable, with full recovery typically expected within 5 to 7 days.

Laparoscopy

A diagnostic and surgical procedure in which the abdomen is examined and sometimes treated, using a laparoscope, a fiberoptic viewing tube that transmits images to the surgeon on a screen. The laparoscope also enables a surgeon to perform various surgical functions. Laparoscopic surgery, which is done through a tiny incision, has replaced many operations that formerly were performed through abdominal incisions several inches long.

Laparoscopy is performed in a hospital or surgery center under general anesthesia. Imaging studies, such as CT (computed tomography) or ultrasound scans, direct the surgeon where to make the incision. The laparoscope is inserted through the incision into the abdomen, from which it sends clear images to a video monitor in the operating room. Tiny instruments are then passed down through the laparoscope to perform the necessary surgery.

Laparoscopic appendectomies and cholecystectomies (gallbladder removals) are more common than open versions of these operations. Laparoscopy generates less postoperative pain and disability, a shorter hospital stay, and a more rapid recovery.

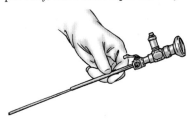

THE LAPAROSCOPE
In laparoscopy, a small incision is made in the abdomen, and the abdomen is filled with gas to expand the area. The laparoscope is inserted through the incision, and the doctor examines the internal organs by watching images on a monitor. For further surgical procedures, other instruments are inserted through other small incisions and the images from the laparoscope guide the operation.

Laparotomy, exploratory

An open diagnostic operation within the abdomen. An exploratory laparotomy is performed when noninvasive tests fail to reveal the cause of symptoms, such as inflamation, abdominal distension, pain, vomiting, and fever. In this operation, the surgeon makes an incision in the abdominal wall to examine the inside of the abdomen. Intestinal obstructions, ruptured ulcers, cancer, ovarian cysts, and ectopic pregnancies are commonly diagnosed by laparotomy. When operable tumors, obstructions, or other problems are discovered during a laparotomy, the surgeon removes or otherwise treats them during the procedure.

Larva migrans

An infestation with the larvae of roundworms that move through the tissues of the human body; the larvae are the immature forms of the worm. When the larvae migrate into the lungs, liver, brain, and muscles, the condition is called visceral larva migrans syndrome. When the eyes are affected, it is referred to as ocular larva migrans syndrome.

Roundworm parasites live in the small intestines of both dogs and cats and are transmitted to humans most commonly by dogs, their natural host. The infestation is carried in the feces of cats and dogs, especially puppies. Heavily infected dogs can pass millions of eggs in their feces every day. The infection is generally contracted by accidental oral contact with embryonated eggs, or larvae. Preschool children are most often affected, especially those with a history of ingesting dirt.

The larvae of the worms hatch in the small intestines of a person who has contracted the infestation. They do not mature into adults in humans, but persist in the body's tissues. Some larvae may remain trapped in the liver; other larvae migrate to the lungs and circulate to all the body's organs. The larvae can cause severe inflammation and scarring as they migrate through the body, and the immune system responds to their presence. The symptoms of visceral larva migrans can include loss of appetite, rash, wheezing, cough, abdominal pain, and neurologic problems. Severe infection with seizures, encephalitis, and heart failure can also occur. The syndrome is rarely fatal, but death is possible. Ocular larva migrans may cause the loss of vision in the affected eye.

Larva migrans can be prevented by

taking care to avoid direct physical contact with the fecal matter of household pets. Disposable gloves should be worn when changing kitty litter or cleaning up a pet's excretions. Dogs and cats should be dewormed by a veterinarian, and owners should not allow pets to defecate in public places, especially in areas where children play, such as playgrounds.

Larva migrans is usually diagnosed by blood tests and possibly chest X rays and other scanning techniques. Treatment is based on medications that kill parasitic worms, as well as treatment of associated conditions and symptoms. See also ROUNDWORMS and TOXOCARIASIS.

Laryngeal papilloma

A tumor on the larynx (voice box) that is usually benign and resembles a wart. Laryngeal papillomas are believed to be caused by a virus (see VIRUSES). They usually develop in groups and may cause difficulty breathing, in addition to hoarseness. They are common in children, especially boys, and often diminish spontaneously at puberty. Rarely, papillomas will grow large very quickly. In these instances, they may obstruct breathing and should be treated as soon as possible to prevent total blockage of the air supply. Because they grow in clusters, papillomas are difficult to remove completely in children without injuring the larynx. In recent years, laser treatment has yielded more satisfactory results than traditional surgical procedures for removing laryngeal papillomas. They often recur and require repeated treatment. Sometimes a TRACHEOSTOMY becomes necessary.

Laryngectomy

Surgical removal of all or part of the larynx (voice box) to treat cancer of the larynx. The procedure may involve complete or partial removal of the larynx and surrounding structures, depending on the location, size, and stage of the tumor, as well as the person's age and health. Radiation therapy may be given in combination with the surgery. Generally, laryngectomy is the only possible treatment for cancer of the larynx if the tumor is large or if previous radiation therapy has failed.

HOW IT IS PERFORMED
The surgery involves an incision in the front of the neck to open the trachea (windpipe) in a procedure called TRACHEOSTOMY. The incision is kept open, and a new airway is created to allow breathing by inserting a tube. The surgeon then may remove part of the larynx and, after the patient has recovered from surgery, take out the tube. Or, he or she may remove the entire larynx, leaving an opening in the neck, called a stoma, for breathing.

WHAT TO EXPECT
The first night after surgery is usually spent in the intensive care unit. The hospital stay after laryngectomy is about 5 to 7 days. While the lower part of the throat heals, the person cannot swallow food or liquid, so a small plastic feeding tube is placed into the stomach through the nose or the throat. Sometimes a tracheostomy tube is placed into the stoma on a temporary basis until the stoma can stay open without it.

If only part of the larynx (voice box) is removed, the person's ability to speak is preserved, but the voice may be weak and hoarse. Patients recovering from a partial laryngectomy can usually speak within a few weeks after surgery. After a total laryngectomy, normal speech is not possible,

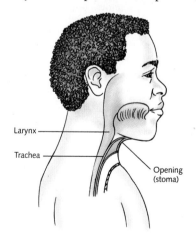

OPENING THE TRACHEA
Laryngectomy, performed to treat cancer of the throat, may require removal of the entire larynx. To enable the person to breathe and speak, the surgeon creates an opening (stoma) in the front of the throat. The top of the trachea is sewn to the rim of the opening to create a new airway through which the person will inhale and exhale.

Larynx
Trachea
Opening (stoma)

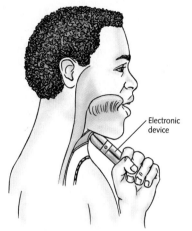

ELECTRONIC LARYNX
An electronic larynx enables a person without a larynx to speak. The electronic device emits a buzzing sound; the person holds it against his or her throat so that the buzz vibrates the air in the throat cavity. By moving the teeth and lips, the person shapes the buzz into speech sounds.

Electronic device

but various new ways of communicating can be learned, usually from a speech pathologist.

In most cases, people who have had a laryngectomy can eventually resume normal activities. Because it is dangerous for water to enter the windpipe and lungs through the stoma, special precautions must be taken when showering or shaving, and special equipment is required for swimming.

Risks for developing new cancers in the throat, mouth, or other areas of the head and neck are higher than average for people who have been treated for cancer of the larynx, so regular follow-up examinations are important. Support groups may help a person adjust during the recovery period.

Laryngitis

An inflammation of the mucous membrane of the larynx (voice box). Symptoms of laryngitis include hoarseness, gradual loss of voice, and throat discomfort. The cause of the inflammation is usually a viral infection but may also be due to bacterial infections. ALLERGIES can produce inflammation of the larynx, as can exposure to harsh chemicals. Overuse or abuse of the voice is another possible cause (see HOARSENESS).

If a virus (see VIRUSES) is the cause, the laryngitis will go away within a few days without treatment. If it lasts

L

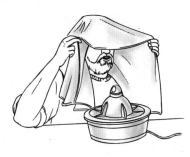

TREATING LARYNGITIS
If the membranes of the larynx are inflamed, it helps to keep them moist by inhaling steam. A steam-emitting appliance such as a vaporizer provides the moist air. The person can direct the steam toward his or her face by draping a towel over the head and holding it over the vaporizer like a canopy.

longer than a day or two, a physician should be consulted. Children whose laryngitis becomes a sharp, barking cough should be taken to a doctor immediately; their airways may be restricted, or they might have CROUP.

For laryngitis caused by bacteria, antibiotics may be prescribed. If allergies are the cause, antihistamines may be prescribed. If there is a serious allergic reaction and, in addition to laryngitis, there is difficulty breathing, one of the CORTICOSTEROIDS may be prescribed. Decongestants may inappropriately dry up the vocal cords and should be avoided.

PREVENTION AND SELF-HELP
When it is necessary to overuse or strain the voice—as may be occasionally required of teachers and lawyers, for example—it is beneficial to rest the voice afterward by not speaking at all or speaking at low volume only when necessary. (Whispering should be avoided as it strains the larynx.) Avoiding tobacco use and exposure to harsh, caustic chemicals may also help prevent laryngitis. Drinking at least six glasses of water daily, inhaling steam, and applying warm compresses to the throat may also help relieve the inflammation that produces laryngitis. If hoarseness continues for more than 2 weeks, a doctor should be consulted.

Laryngocele

An abnormal air sac attached to the larynx (voice box); an inherited condition. A laryngocele may become enlarged when there is pressure inside the larynx, such as when a per-

son coughs. When enlarged, a laryngocele may protrude on the outside of the neck, resembling a tumor. The condition may recur. The only treatment is a surgical procedure to remove the growth.

Laryngomalacia

The most common problem of the larynx (voice box) in infancy. As a result of soft or deformed cartilage or muscular weakness, portions of the upper part of the larynx collapse into the airway. The baby will make a wheezing or hoarse breathing sound known as stridor and will have some degree of difficulty breathing. The disease appears in the first few weeks of life and typically goes away in the first few months. Only rarely is treatment needed to protect the child's airway.

Laryngoscopy

An examination of the larynx (voice box) that includes the use of a slender, flexible medical instrument called a laryngoscope, which is threaded through the nose and down the back of the throat to the larynx. It is equipped with a light source and lenses for examination of the larynx. The laryngoscope is used to look for ulceration or inflammation of the vocal cords, to collect tissue samples, to locate and remove polyps or other growths, to photograph the vocal cords, or to evaluate the severity of a malignant tumor that has already been diagnosed.

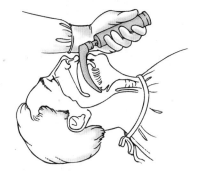

DIRECT LARYNGOSCOPY
Direct laryngoscopy enables the doctor to look for damage to the vocal cords, take images, or obtain tissue samples. A flexible laryngoscope can be used similarly. A doctor can view the larynx through a mirror held at the back of the person's mouth in a procedure called indirect laryngoscopy.

Laryngoscopy is performed in a hospital or outpatient surgery clinic by a surgeon. In preparation for the procedure, the nasal passages are usually cleared, decongested, and, with the throat, lightly anesthetized. The person undergoing the procedure may also be lightly sedated. Laryngoscopy generally takes about 45 minutes but may take longer depending on what the surgeon is doing. After a person has had a laryngoscopy, he or she may be kept in the hospital or clinic for 24-hour observation. Most people are able to return to normal activities within a few days of the procedure, although they may experience a lingering sore throat and cough up blood for a day or so. If there is fever, a large amount of blood, or other symptoms of infection, the doctor should be notified immediately.

Laryngospasm

A strong, rapid, involuntary contraction of the muscles in the larynx (voice box). In addition to producing speech, the larynx serves as a protective "gateway" between the upper airway (the mouth, nose, and throat) and the sterile lower airway (the trachea and lungs). As such, it prevents foreign material from entering the trachea and lungs. When an abnormal stimulus reaches the larynx, the muscles contract to prevent material from being inhaled into the lungs. In adults, gastroesophageal reflux disease (GERD; see ESOPHAGEAL REFLUX), a condition in which acidic contents of the stomach rise into the ESOPHAGUS, can be the cause of laryngospasm. In children, it may be caused by epiglottitis (inflammation of the flap of elastic cartilage overhanging the entrance to the larynx). The changes in chest pressure produced by laryngospasm can compromise the heart and lungs. A person experiencing laryngospasm should try to remain calm because anxiety can exacerbate the spasm. If the person loses consciousness, which almost never happens, emergency medical treatment is required. Usually the muscles relax before the person loses consciousness, and the condition is relieved.

Larynx

The organ in the throat responsible for voice production; commonly called the voice box. The larynx is a

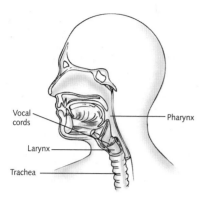

THE VOICE BOX
The larynx is the organ of the respiratory system that generates sound for speech. The larynx, located at the top of the trachea, is constructed of linking pieces of cartilage. The vocal cords, ribbons of tissue stretched between the pieces of cartilage, vibrate in the airstream coming from the lungs to produce sound waves.

structure of the RESPIRATORY SYSTEM, lying between the pharynx (throat) and the trachea (windpipe).

The larynx is constructed of cartilage lined with mucous membrane. The most prominent piece of cartilage is the thyroid cartilage (Adam's apple), which lies at the upper, outer part of the throat. It is connected to the trachea by the cricoid cartilage, which encircles the throat. Resting on the back side of the cricoid cartilage are two pieces called the arytenoid cartilages. Stretched between the arytenoid cartilage and the inside of the thyroid cartilage are two fibrous folds called the vocal cords, or vocal folds. When a person starts to speak, air is pushed out of the lungs and rushes up the trachea to the larynx. The airstream vibrates the vocal folds, producing sound waves that continue up into the mouth to be modeled into speech sounds.

The larynx also functions to prevent choking. Every time a person swallows food, the brain stem initiates reflexive action to keep food from entering the trachea. First, breathing stops temporarily. The epiglottis (a flap of cartilage at the back of the throat) drops down at the same time that the larynx moves up, sealing off the entrance to the trachea. The vocal folds also close, providing further protection. See SPEECH MECHANISM; SWALLOWING.

Larynx, cancer of

A cancer that develops in and around the larynx (the voice box). This cancer can be detected at an early stage if changes in the voice occur. Symptoms usually include hoarseness, pain, and difficulty swallowing. If untreated, as the cancer grows within the larynx, it may eventually cause discomfort in the ears or spitting up blood.

Diagnosis of cancer of the larynx usually includes an examination of the area using a laryngoscope, a thin, flexible, viewing instrument. A biopsy may be performed during the examination. Treatment of cancer of the larynx typically involves radiation therapy, especially in the early stages of the disease, because radiation offers the best chance of cure with preservation of the voice. Chemotherapy is also used to treat cancer of the larynx. If the cancer recurs after radiation, treatment may include surgical removal of the tumor using lasers or partial or complete removal of the larynx. When the entire larynx, including the vocal cords, is surgically removed, speech can be restored in a variety of ways that usually require retraining and practice.

Men are more likely to develop cancer of the larynx than women, and blacks more often than whites. Most cases of cancer of the larynx occur in adults, between the ages of 60 and 75. The two principal risk factors for cancer of the larynx are smoking and alcohol abuse. Smokers have five to 35 times the risk of developing the disease than nonsmokers; and heavy drinkers have two to five times the risk of nondrinkers. Other risk factors include inhaling wood dust, paint fumes, asbestos, and chemicals. Professional cooks have high rates of cancer of the larynx, probably

SIGNS OF CANCER OF THE LARYNX

The presence of any of these symptoms requires a doctor's attention:

- **Hoarseness that lasts longer than 2 weeks**
- **Lasting cough, sore throat, or earache**
- **Painful or obstructed swallowing**
- **Trouble breathing**
- **Lump on the neck**
- **Unexplained weight loss**

because they inhale large amounts of carcinogenic compounds formed during the cooking of meat.

Laser

A medical instrument that produces a very thin, powerful beam of light. Lasers are used by a surgeon to operate on small diseased areas without damaging delicate surrounding tissues. For instance, lasers are used to unblock coronary arteries and to remove certain kinds of birthmarks, warts, and tattoos. Lasers are also used in eye surgery to operate on the cornea and the retina; and they can be used to seal nerve endings to reduce postoperative pain.

The term "laser" stands for light amplification by stimulated emission of radiation. There are several types of lasers, each of which has a specific use. The color of the laser used is directly related to the surgery being performed and to the tissue being treated.

Laser in situ keratomileusis

See LASIK.

Laser resurfacing

A technique for removing fine wrinkles, scars, damaged skin, and uneven pigmentation from the face with a laser light source. Laser resurfacing, or laser peel, can be performed on the entire face or a specific portion, such as around the mouth or eyes. See LASER SURGERY.

Laser resurfacing accomplishes the same goals as a CHEMICAL PEEL or DERMABRASION. Damaged skin is removed layer by layer so that new skin can grow to replace it. In some cases, laser resurfacing reduces postoperative discomfort, bruising, swelling, and bleeding compared with other methods.

Like all skin-resurfacing techniques, laser resurfacing works best on patients with fair skin. People with olive, brown, and black skin have a greater risk for changes in skin pigmentation, no matter what type of resurfacing is used. Individuals who have taken ISOTRETINOIN (Accutane, used to treat severe acne) within 18 months, who are prone to abnormal or keloid scarring, or who have active skin infections in the area to be treated should not undergo laser resurfacing.

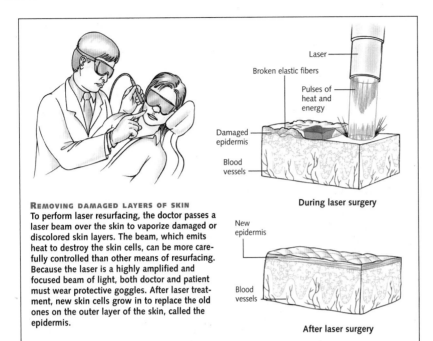

REMOVING DAMAGED LAYERS OF SKIN
To perform laser resurfacing, the doctor passes a laser beam over the skin to vaporize damaged or discolored skin layers. The beam, which emits heat to destroy the skin cells, can be more carefully controlled than other means of resurfacing. Because the laser is a highly amplified and focused beam of light, both doctor and patient must wear protective goggles. After laser treatment, new skin cells grow in to replace the old ones on the outer layer of the skin, called the epidermis.

Laser resurfacing can be performed alone or in conjunction with another cosmetic procedure, such as EYELID SURGERY.

The word "laser" is an acronym that stands for light amplification by stimulated emission of radiation. The laser device transforms ordinary light, which covers a wide range of frequencies, into a single-frequency, highly intense beam that focuses extreme heat and energy at close range. Depending on the materials used as amplifiers, a laser can destroy all tissue that it touches, or it can target tissue of a specific color or pigment.

THE PROCEDURE
Laser resurfacing is most often performed in a physician's office or outpatient surgery center. If the procedure is to be extensive, it may be preferable to have the procedure performed in a hospital. Pain control usually consists of local anesthesia combined with CONSCIOUS SEDATION, in which the patient is awake but drowsy, relaxed, and pain-free. General anesthesia, which puts the patient to sleep, may be used for extensive laser resurfacing.

During the surgery, the surgeon passes the laser carefully over the skin to vaporize layer after layer. This process is continued until the level that makes the wrinkle or scar less

apparent has been reached. In the case of deeper flaws, a second procedure can be performed at a later date. When the surgery is complete, the surgeon may treat the resurfaced skin with protective cream or ointment and apply a bandage. Laser resurfacing takes from a few minutes for a small area to 1 to 2 hours for a full-face procedure.

BEFORE AND AFTER SURGERY
As with any surgery that involves anesthesia, the person must have nothing to eat or drink after midnight the night before the procedure. The surgeon may also provide instructions about medications or nutritional supplements to be avoided in preparation for surgery. Smoking should be avoided before and after the procedure because nicotine restricts blood flow to the skin, slows healing, and increases scarring.

Mild swelling, soreness, itchiness, and oozing in the treated area are normal reactions during the first 48 to 72 hours after the procedure. They can be controlled with ice packs and oral pain medications prescribed by the surgeon. Any bandage applied after surgery should be replaced after 1 or 2 days. This bandage is then taken off in a week or slightly longer; often, a thin layer of ointment is applied to the skin at the same time.

Laser-resurfaced skin crusts as it heals. These crusts should not be removed until they fall off by themselves, typically within 10 days, or scarring can result.

The new skin that appears after the crusts detach is bright red to pink. After about 2 weeks, makeup can be applied to the new skin to conceal its color. In addition, the surgeon may prescribe medications that make the color subside more rapidly. In most cases, the redness is gone within 6 weeks, and the pinkness in 6 months.

For the 6 months following laser resurfacing, the new skin must be carefully protected from the sun with a hat and sunblock with a SUN PROTECTION FACTOR (SPF) of 30 or higher. Good-quality sunglasses that filter out all ultraviolet A and B rays are advised for resurfaced skin around the eyes.

Possible complications from laser resurfacing include burns caused by the heat from the laser, scarring, new skin that is either lighter or darker than the surrounding areas, and outbreaks of herpes simplex virus infections (see COLD SORE). If healing or pigmentation is abnormal, additional treatment may be needed. In some cases, resurfaced skin is very sensitive to makeup; usually this reaction disappears over time.

The full benefit of laser resurfacing appears about 6 months after the procedure when the skin looks smoother and younger. The results of the procedure are long lasting, but not permanent since the skin continues to age. Laser resurfacing can be repeated.

Laser surgery
The use of a concentrated, pulsating beam of light to perform surgical procedures such as shrinking or destroying tumors or lesions; cutting, burning, sculpting, or vaporizing tissue; and sealing blood vessels. The word "laser" is an acronym for: light amplification by stimulated emission of radiation. At high intensity, the concentrated beam of light released by a laser can destroy cells on which it is focused and cut through tissues without causing bleeding.

ADVANTAGES OF LASER SURGERY
When used as surgical tools, lasers cut through tissue without causing excessive bleeding. In fact, lasers can

even coagulate tissue to limit or stop bleeding. The precision of a laser and the intensity of the light enable surgeons to focus on small areas and hard-to-reach body parts, affording them a clear view of the area they are treating. By adjusting intensity, lasers can penetrate tissue as deeply as needed.

Laser surgery is often quicker than conventional surgery, and often the recovery period is shorter. Many times, laser surgery is performed using a local rather than a general anesthetic. Laser surgery, like any surgery, carries a risk of complications such as pain, infection, and scarring. In some cases, conventional surgery is preferable. For example, lasers can successfully remove spider veins, but conventional surgery is better for removing hemorrhoids and varicose veins.

SPECIAL APPLICATIONS OF LASER SURGERY

Because laser wavelengths can be adjusted to focus selectively, lasers are uniquely suitable to many forms of dermatologic or plastic surgery. For example, treatments for tattoo removal have traditionally been limited because of the likelihood of scarring. Now careful selection of specific wavelengths makes it possible to target and destroy the tattoo without harming nearby tissue. This same selective technique makes laser surgery particularly helpful for lighten-

ing or removing a BIRTHMARK (such as a port-wine stain) or other pigmented lesions, removing warts and hair, and LASER RESURFACING. Laser resurfacing is a highly controlled procedure in which a laser is used to vaporize superficial layers of facial skin. It successfully eliminates precancerous and benign (not cancerous) superficial growths and signs of sun damage or aging such as brown spots, lines, and wrinkles. Younger-looking skin then grows back on the fresh surface. The risk of scarring and other complications is significantly diminished. Laser surgery of the skin causes little pain or bleeding and may pose less risk of infection than other surgical methods.

Laser surgery is used to relieve the pressure of glaucoma and to treat diseases and disorders of the eyes such as retinal detachment, macular degeneration, and the blurred vision that occurs after cataract surgery. It is also used by ophthalmologists to correct common eye problems such as nearsightedness, farsightedness, and astigmatism through REFRACTIVE SURGERY. In the procedure called laser in situ keratomileusis (LASIK), a thin, circular, hinged cut is made in the surface of the eye after a local anesthetic has been applied. The surgeon lifts the flap and uses a special laser that emits no heat (heat would damage the eye) to shape the cornea under the flap. The reshaping improves vision by

allowing the cornea to focus more normally. LASIK procedures take about 20 to 30 minutes per eye and are performed on an outpatient basis.

Laser surgery is used to treat many different conditions, such as removing tumors and diseased organ tissues and shrinking or destroying abnormal tissue in various locations throughout the body. Surgeons use lasers to remove tumors from the brain, spinal cord, colon, esophagus, and vocal cords. Lasers can break up kidney stones and pulverize gallstones. They can also fuse herniated disks. Lasers can be inserted down an endoscope (a viewing tube) into the stomach to seal bleeding blood vessels. In gynecology, they are used to vaporize fibroid tumors, destroy precancerous lesions, and remove the excess tissue of endometriosis. Dentists use lasers to treat hard-to-reach cavities. In addition, new uses for lasers are constantly emerging. For example, in photodynamic therapy, laser therapy is combined with photosensitizing drugs to destroy tumors.

LASIK

Laser in situ keratomileusis; a surgical procedure that uses a laser to reshape the clear outer layer of the eye (cornea) in order to permanently correct vision problems. LASIK is used for people who are highly motivated to stop wearing glasses or contact lenses and who have nearsightedness (difficulty seeing distant objects), farsightedness (difficulty seeing close objects), or astigmatism (tilted and distorted vision caused by an abnormally shaped cornea). The procedure is not used to correct the difficulty in reading (presbyopia) common in people older than 45 years, since it results from age-related changes in the lens of the eye, not the cornea. LASIK has been approved for use in the United States since 1998.

PROCEDURE

The LASIK procedure is performed with the person awake. The eye is numbed with anesthetic eye drops, and an oral sedative may be given during the surgery. Working through a microscope, the surgeon uses a surgical instrument called a microkeratome to cut a tiny hinged flap in the surface of the cornea. The laser is then aimed at the area of the cornea under the flap to reshape it as needed

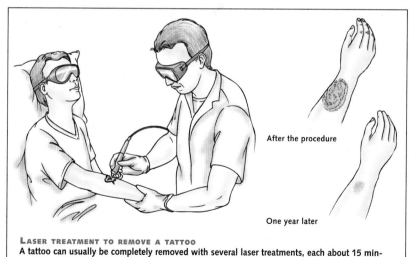

LASER TREATMENT TO REMOVE A TATTOO
A tattoo can usually be completely removed with several laser treatments, each about 15 minutes long. A local anesthetic is usually injected into the area first, and both the doctor and patient wear protective eye goggles. After the procedure, the skin will be raw and red; a year later, the hair will have grown back, and the tattoo will be nearly invisible.

After the procedure

One year later

THE MONOVISION OPTION

Almost everyone older than 40 years is subject to some degree of difficulty in reading, a problem that worsens with age. Progressive hardening of the lens of the eye (known technically as presbyopia) is not remedied by LASIK or other forms of refractive eye surgery, such as photorefractive keratectomy. As a result, a middle-aged person who undergoes LASIK will most likely still need reading glasses after the surgery.

An alternative is to have each eye corrected differently—one for distance vision, one for near—a correction called monovision. The brain learns over time which image from which eye to attend to, depending on the distance between the eye and the object being viewed. Not everyone finds monovision acceptable, however, and it should be discussed thoroughly with the eye specialist before surgery. People older than 60 years tend to adapt better to monovision.

---

to correct the person's vision. The flap is then put back in place, and it quickly reattaches to the rest of the cornea without stitches. A plastic or metal shield is placed over the eye to protect it during the immediate recovery period.

LASIK takes 10 to 15 minutes per eye. Usually, both eyes are operated on at the same time. Some surgeons prefer to operate on one eye and allow it to heal before correcting the other eye a few weeks later.

Following LASIK, the eye may sting or burn for a few hours, and vision is usually blurry for the first day. In most cases vision clears by the second day. Most people can return to work and normal activities, except for heavy lifting and contact sports, within 1 or 2 days. Swimming, hot tubs, and whirlpool baths must be avoided for 2 weeks to diminish the risk of infection.

OUTCOME, COMPLICATIONS, AND SUITABILITY

LASIK has generally good results, with most people able to see well enough after surgery to stop wearing contacts or glasses. In people with particularly severe nearsightedness or farsightedness, vision is usually improved, but glasses or contacts

may still be needed. The improvement appears within the first few days of surgery, but often vision continues to improve for up to 6 months.

Possible complications after LASIK include overcorrection or undercorrection of vision requiring repeated surgery (or enhancement), scarring or misshaping of the cornea, infection in the cornea, loss of sharpness in vision, difficulty with night vision because of the appearance of halos or starbursts around bright lights, sensitivity to light, dry eye, and problems with the flap. Most complications resolve soon after surgery, but they can be permanent.

LASIK cannot be performed until the person is at least 18 years old, since the eye continues to change before that age. In cases of severe nearsightedness, delaying surgery until the middle or late 20s is generally recommended because of continuing changes in vision. LASIK cannot be performed in women who are pregnant or breast-feeding; people who take certain prescription drugs, such as prednisone; or people who have certain diseases, such as rheumatoid arthritis and herpes infections of the eye. Caution should be used in persons with diabetes mellitus, type 1 and type 2, or glaucoma. In people with cataracts (cloudiness in the lens of the eye), surgical removal of the cataract with implantation of an intraocular lens can correct the refractive error, thus eliminating the need for LASIK.

Lassa fever

A serious systemic (body-wide) infection caused by a virus. Lassa fever involves most of the principal internal organs but not the central nervous system. A small rat found in Africa carries the virus that causes the illness; Lassa fever was first identified in Lassa, Nigeria, in 1969. Transmission to humans is believed to occur most commonly from contamination of food with rodent urine. Person-to-person transmission is known to occur via contact with urine, feces, saliva, vomit, or blood. Outbreaks in Nigeria and Liberia were hospital-associated and transmitted from one infected patient to hospital staff and other patients.

Symptoms occur within 24 days of exposure and initially include sore

throat, fever, chills, headache, muscle aches, and general fatigue. These symptoms can progress to loss of appetite, vomiting, and pains in the chest and upper abdomen. In some cases, there may be swelling of the face and neck, bleeding from the gums, rashes, cough, and dizziness. In some people, the infection progresses to a severe stage involving mental confusion, shock, agitation, fluids in the lungs, and seizures. There is a high risk of death.

Lassa fever is diagnosed by blood tests that show an elevation in antibodies, a urinalysis revealing protein in the urine, and chest X rays that show inflammation and fluid in the lungs. Treatment includes increasing fluids, usually with oral or intravenous rehydration (see REHYDRATION FLUID, ORAL). Ribavirin increase survival significantly if the medication is begun within 6 days after symptoms begin. Anti–Lassa-fever plasma is sometimes used in very ill patients.

Latanoprost

An antiglaucoma agent. Latanoprost (Xalatan) is used to decrease the pressure within the eyeball, which if left unchecked can damage the optic nerve and lead to loss of vision. It is given as an eye drop and works by increasing the flow of fluid out of the eyeball, which reduces pressure in the eye.

Lateral

The side of the body; the outer side of the body, the outer side of a body part, or a position or structure that lies away from the midline of the body. The lateral or outside part of a knee, for example, is that side farther from the other knee. The opposite of lateral is MEDIAL.

Lavage, gastric

See STOMACH PUMPING.

Laxatives

Foods or drugs that stimulate a person's bowels for the relief of constipation. Laxatives may be taken orally to help produce bowel movements, or they may be used rectally as enemas or suppositories to generate bowel movements in a short time. Laxatives should be used only to provide short-term relief, unless directed otherwise

L

by a doctor. A proper diet that includes whole grains, fruits, and vegetables, as well as 6 to 8 glasses of water or other liquids per day, is the most effective way to promote healthy bowel function. Exercise is also important. There are many different types of laxatives and dozens of laxative products on the market. Most laxatives are available without prescription.

BULK FORMERS

Bulk-forming oral laxatives work by absorbing liquid in the intestines, swelling into a soft, bulky stool. The bowel is stimulated normally by the presence of the bulky stool. Examples include psyllium and malt soup extract. These type of laxatives usually take 12 to 72 hours to have an effect.

HYPEROSMOTICS

Hyperosmotic laxatives work by drawing water into the bowel from surrounding tissues to produce a soft stool and increased bowel action. Hyperosmotic laxatives are available as oral and rectal products and are not intended to be used regularly on a long-term basis. Examples include "salts" (sodium phosphates), glycerin, and sorbitol. These types of laxatives take 1 to 2 hours to have an effect.

LUBRICANTS

Lubricant laxatives, such as mineral oil, are used to coat the bowel and the stool with a waterproof film that keeps moisture in the stool. This keeps the stool soft and makes its passage through the colon easier. Lubricants may be given orally or rectally. This laxative takes 6 to 8 hours to have an effect and is not recommended for children younger than 6 years.

STIMULANTS

Stimulant laxatives, also called contact laxatives, act on the intestinal wall to stimulate muscle contractions that move the stool mass through the intestines. Examples of stimulant laxatives include bisacodyl, dehydrocholic acid, senna, and castor oil. These laxatives may be given orally and can take from 1 to 10 hours to work.

STOOL SOFTENERS

Stool softeners, or emollients, encourage bowel movements by drawing water into the stool to prevent dry, hard stool. This type of laxative makes it easier to have a bowel movement but does not cause one directly. Stool softeners are given orally. An example of this type of laxative is docusate, which can take up to 72 hours to work.

Lazy eye

See AMBLYOPIA.

LDL

Low-density lipoprotein. See CHOLESTEROL.

Lead poisoning

Poisoning from an overdose of lead. Exposure to excessive amounts of lead can be very serious, causing brain damage. It is most common in young children. Symptoms of lead poisoning include poor appetite, vomiting, fatigue, weakness, abdominal pain, irritability, and seizures. People are exposed to lead from many sources, particularly through cracked paint chips and dust. Other sources of lead include drinking water, food, and soil that have been contaminated. Airborne lead enters the body through inhaling or swallowing lead dust or particles; lead can leach into drinking water from pipes; and it can be deposited on floors and other surfaces.

Treatment for lead poisoning should always begin with the advice of a poison center professional or a doctor. It is advisable to remove the person from the source of lead or vice versa. In cases of lead poisoning, CHELATION THERAPY may be used to help remove lead from the body.

Learning

Acquiring knowledge or developing the ability to perform new behaviors. The scientific study of learning focuses on behavior, specifically on how behavior changes as a result of experience.

SIMPLE LEARNING

The most basic forms of learning involve a single stimulus—that is, anything that can be perceived by the senses, such as sights, sounds, tastes, smells, and touches. In habituation, an individual becomes familiar with a repeated or prolonged stimulus and learns to ignore it. For example, a person who rents an apartment next to a railroad line may get little sleep the first night because of the noise from passing trains, but soon learns how to ignore the sound and sleep normally. Habituation allows an individual to focus only on the important stimuli that require attention and avoid continuous distraction by the ordinary or trivial. Sensitization, another form of simple learning, entails a heightened response after exposure to a particularly irritating or intense stimulus. For example, someone attending a rock concert may experience heightened sensitivity to all sounds for some time thereafter.

CLASSICAL CONDITIONING

Classical conditioning is a type of learning in which an unconscious or automatic response is connected with an external event not associated physiologically with that response. Classical conditioning is also known as Pavlovian conditioning because it was first described by the Russian physiologist Ivan Pavlov. Studying digestion in dogs, Pavlov noticed that when feeding time came each day, the dogs salivated at the sight of the laboratory assistants responsible for feeding, even before food was offered. Pavlov designed an experiment in which a bell was rung when the dogs were fed. After several repetitions, simply ringing the bell at any time of the day or night with no food present caused the dogs to salivate. Through classical conditioning, the dogs had associated the bell with food, and responded by salivating. Classical conditioning creates a new connection between the stimulus (bell) and the response (salivation). It occurs independent of rewards and punishments and of the action of the individual.

Once learned, a conditioned response will disappear over time if the stimulus is withdrawn. If the bell is rung repeatedly but no food is presented, the dog will stop salivating at the bell. This is known as extinction. The response, however, remains in the animal's memory and can be reactivated. If the bell is rung and food is again presented, the dog will begin to salivate again at the sound of the bell.

Classical conditioning is subject to what is called generalization and discrimination. If a child has been frightened by a large snake, the child may generalize the response and feel fear at the sight of any snake, no matter how small or harmless, or of an animal that has snakelike qualities, such

L

as a night crawler or lizard. By the same token, the child may realize that snakes in cages at the zoo or on the television pose no threat and experience no fear when he or she sees them. This ability to distinguish one stimulus from a similar stimulus is called discrimination.

Conditioning can have powerful effects on human behavior and feelings. For example, a person who has been through a traumatic experience, such as a severe car accident, may experience a powerful emotional response to the smell of gasoline. The gasoline serves as a stimulus that elicits an emotional response because of the conditioning that occurred at the time of the accident. Classical conditioning is thought to underlie many phobias (see PHOBIA), abnormal fears of people, objects, or situations.

OPERANT CONDITIONING

In operant conditioning, a behavior increases in frequency when it is followed by a reward (reinforcement) and decreases when it is followed by a punishment. The word "operant" refers to the fact that the person has to perform a behavior, or operate, before receiving the reinforcement or punishment.

Reinforcements can be positive or negative. Positive reinforcements increase a behavior because they result in something pleasant—food, drink, sex, praise, attention, power, or feelings of love. Negative reinforcements increase a behavior by taking away an unpleasant stimulus. If a painkiller removes the disagreeable sensation of a headache, an individual will probably use that same painkiller again the next time a headache begins. Similarly, driving under the speed limit is a way of avoiding the unpleasant stimulus, or negative reinforcement, of a traffic ticket.

Punishment, by contrast, weakens a behavior and decreases its frequency. Positive punishment delivers an unpleasant stimulus whenever the behavior occurs. A parent scolding a child for misbehavior is using positive punishment. Negative punishment involves removing a pleasant stimulus as a consequence of engaging in the unwanted behavior. Parents use negative punishment when they ground a high school–aged child for getting poor grades.

Severe punishment is usually counter productive, because the punished individual becomes angry, resentful, and aggressive. Often, severe punishment extinguishes more behaviors than the intended one. For example, a child who is punished for rough conduct in a basketball game may give up basketball altogether, rather than improve his or her play, to lower the risk of further punishment.

Shaping uses operant conditioning to help individuals learn behaviors they have never before exhibited. For example, shaping is used to teach severely retarded children how to speak. The children are rewarded for making any sound at all, then gradually rewarded only for sounds that more closely imitate the teacher's. Over time, the children can learn to form and pronounce words.

Like classically conditioned responses, those created by operant conditioning are subject to extinction if the reinforcement is withdrawn. Operant conditioning is also subject to generalization and discrimination. Techniques based on operant conditioning are used successfully in the treatment of emotional disorders and mental illnesses in what is known as BEHAVIOR THERAPY.

OBSERVATIONAL LEARNING

Much of what people learn comes from watching others and then imitating their actions. A number of factors come into play in learning by imitation or observation. The individual has to pay attention to specific details of what the other person (model) is doing. He or she must remember what the model did and have the physical and intellectual skills to reproduce the behavior. Finally, the person needs to be motivated to learn the behavior.

OTHER TYPES OF LEARNING

Language learning is extremely complex, involving shaping, reinforcement, observational learning, generalization, and discrimination. Some researchers maintain that children have an inborn capacity to determine word meanings, sentence structure, and grammar rules from the complex stream of spoken sounds. This indeed appears to be the case. If the areas of the brain responsible for speech are damaged, the person can no longer speak or understand language.

Reading is another important avenue of learning. Concept formation allows us to group various objects or ideas into a single category, a key ability in learning how to recognize stimuli never encountered before. Finally, motor skill learning applies to the acquisition of complex sets of coordinated physical movements, such as driving a car, typing on a computer keyboard, playing a musical instrument, dancing, or hitting a fastball. In many cases, once a motor skill is learned well, performance becomes automatic.

INFLUENCES ON LEARNING

Age has a role in learning. Both adults and children can learn a new language, but children usually become fluent faster and more easily. Otherwise, learning ability does not decline with age, except in the presence of age-related illnesses such as Alzheimer's disease. Motivation is also important. People who want to learn and are attentive learn faster. Experience with similar forms of learning also contributes to behavior. Someone who already plays two musical instruments will find it easier to learn a third instrument than will a person trying to learn to play his or her first instrument. INTELLIGENCE has a role, as does the presence of any LEARNING DISABILITIES or disorders.

Learning disabilities

A group of lifelong disorders that affect the ability to master basic skills such as reading, writing, doing mathematics, following instructions, and paying attention. Learning disabilities are among the leading reasons for failure in school. Although learning disabilities become more obvious when children of the same age are compared, they should not be confused with normal, different rates of development. Learning disabilities appear to be caused by a malfunction in the way a child's brain receives, processes, and communicates information. This difficulty with brain function interferes with the normal learning process. Most disabilities occur in children of average or above-average intelligence. Typically, achievement in a certain area lags behind what is expected based on the child's full intelligence. Global mental retarda-

THE QWIC dROWN 70X juMBed OV7r THE Lasy WHiTe POOBle

DYSGRAPHIA AND DYSLEXIA
A child with dysgraphia may have difficulty spelling or forming written letters and words. Letters may be inconsistently formed, written backward or in a combination of lower and upper case, or left incomplete. Dysgraphia is one part of dyslexia, which may interfere with reading and writing. The disability involves the way the mind interprets the written image, although intelligence may be normal or above normal.

tion is distinguished by a more uniform delay in all areas, as opposed to the scattered strengths and weaknesses in the learning-disabled child. In some cases, learning disabilities may also be related to hearing or vision problems, poor motivation, emotional difficulties, or mental retardation.

Certain factors make a child more likely to develop learning disabilities. These may include a history of premature birth, low birth weight, severe head injuries, poor prenatal habits in the mother (such as smoking, alcohol dependence, or drug abuse during pregnancy), stress before or after birth, infections of the central nervous system (such as meningitis), or treatment for cancer or leukemia. Learning disabilities appear to be more common in boys than in girls.

TYPES OF LEARNING DISABILITIES
Children who have learning disabilities may try very hard to concentrate on reading, writing, or math, but problems with brain function prevent them from succeeding. Common learning disabilities diagnosed in children include the following types:

■ *Dyslexia* A reading disability involving spatial impairment. In reading, a person may see words, letters, and numbers reversed. For example, a student may confuse "b" with "d" and "95" with "59." Consequently, he or she may have difficulty reading letters, sentences, paragraphs, or numbers. The problem is not with vision but in how the brain processes information.

■ *Dysgraphia* A writing disability whose major symptom is messy homework. Teachers may complain that they cannot read a child's handwriting. Children with dysgraphia have trouble forming letters and writing within a designated space.

■ *Language problems* A disability in which children have problems speaking or comprehending words or sentences. They easily get mixed up telling a story, frequently ask their teachers to repeat instructions, and often scramble the word order in their sentences.

■ *Dyscalculia* Inability to grasp basic mathematical concepts or perform calculations appropriate to one's age. Such children may be strong in other academic areas.

■ *Problems with time and place* Not understanding the concept of time; confusing yesterday with tomorrow or today. The concept of direction is also confusing. Children with this problem may easily get lost.

■ *Memory problems* Difficulty remembering even very recent events. Recalling classroom assignments or multiplication tables is a major challenge. Some children have problems remembering their own address and telephone number.

■ *Sensory integration dysfunction* Having difficulty interpreting sensory input such as the meaning of symbols or the rules of a game.

■ *Attention deficit/hyperactivity disorder* Inability to maintain attention and avoid being distracted. Children with this disorder often find it difficult to understand or follow instructions. They may make careless mistakes and fail to complete tasks. Some children also experience hyperactivity, a syndrome in which the child may be continuously overactive, fidgety, often impulsive, and likely to sleep less than their peers do (see ATTENTION DEFICIT/HYPERACTIVITY DISORDER).

DIAGNOSIS AND TREATMENT
Federal law requires that all schools test and provide help for children who have learning disabilities at no direct cost to parents. Diagnostic and remedial services are available to all children with learning disabilities from birth to age 21. Although children develop at their own pace, the lack of certain skills long before school age may indicate a learning disability. At 2½, a child should be able to speak in phrases, and by 3, form simple sentences. The speech of a 3½-year-old should be intelligible to people outside the family. By that age, a child should be able to sit still while being read a story. A child entering kindergarten is expected to tie shoes, button, hop, and cut with scissors. After age 5, the signs become subtle. More complex language skills are expected. Constant misuse of pronouns or poor syntax suggests a disability. School failure and lack of fine motor skills are common signs of a problem. A child suspected of having learning disabilities should be evaluated comprehensively by an expert. A child psychiatrist may work with school professionals and the family to coordinate the evaluation and educational testing. Eye and ear examinations are recommended to rule out physical causes of learning problems.

If a learning disability is diagnosed, recommendations will be made concerning appropriate school placement. A child may require assistance such as special education services or speech therapy. Sometimes individual or family psychotherapy is recommended, and medication may be prescribed for hyperactivity. Early diagnosis and treatment of learning disabilities are crucial and can help avoid later psychological trauma. Children with undiagnosed learning problems may feel bad about themselves and suffer from low self-esteem. They may fear going to school. Even though these children may be highly intelligent, their inability to succeed in school makes them feel stupid. Consequent anger and frustration may lead to emotional problems. Managing learning disabilities at home includes creating an atmosphere of understanding, love, and support. Knowing that parents care helps children feel better about themselves and increases their self-confidence.

L

Leech

A flat, ringed, carnivorous or blood-sucking worm. Leeches were once widely used for bloodletting (drawing blood from the body, particularly via the fingers or toes), and they are still used for medicinal purposes today. Leeches are used to relieve blood congestion in certain kinds of delicate surgery, such as microsurgery to replace a severed finger or other body part, because their use is less likely to cause infection than other techniques.

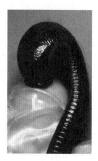

HELPFUL WORMS
Leeches can be useful during repair of severed arteries and veins. Fragile veins, are difficult to repair, and blood can clot at the injury site. Leeches can draw excess blood away from wounds while surgeons work, helping prevent further injury.

LEEP

Loop electrosurgical excision procedure. A procedure for diagnosing and treating abnormalities of the CERVIX. Using a colposcope (a small viewing tube), the doctor removes any apparent abnormal tissue from the cervix with a thin wire loop that sends out low-voltage, high-frequency radio waves. The tissue is then examined for cancerous cells under a microscope. LEEP, which is also known as LLETZ, or large loop excision of transformation zone, can be performed on an outpatient basis, using a local anesthetic.

LEEP is preferable to both LASER SURGERY and CAUTERIZATION because it can simultaneously diagnose and treat cervical abnormalities, such as precancerous conditions and early stage cancer of the cervix. The choice of procedure depends on how much abnormal tissue has to be removed and where on the cervix it is located.

Leflunomide

A drug used in the treatment of rheumatoid arthritis, an autoimmune disease. Leflunomide (Arava) can relieve some symptoms of rheumatoid arthritis, such as inflammation, swelling, stiffness, and joint pain. Leflunomide works by preventing the body from producing too many of the immune cells that cause the swelling and inflammation.

Leg ulcer

A slow-healing, open sore on the leg, often accompanied by swelling. Leg ulcers are typically caused by insufficient arterial blood supply or by inadequate drainage through the veins. This often painful and disabling condition is a common problem for older people. Frequently associated with varicose veins and other circulation problems, they can also be caused by trauma or bacterial infection. Poor circulation combined with long-term immobility can produce the leg ulcers often called bedsores or pressure ulcers. People with DIABETES MEL-LITUS, TYPE 2 have an increased susceptibility to the ulcers.

Leg ulcers, especially the nonvenous kinds, tend to resist treatment. Usually, treatment includes elevation of the leg two or three times daily. Elastic support and compression hosiery are also helpful. However, even when ulcers heal, they frequently recur. Consequently, in many cases, hospitalization and removal of diseased tissue are needed. For people with poor arterial circulation, surgery may be needed to improve the blood supply.

Leg, fractured

FOR FIRST AID
see Fractures (broken bones), page 1323

A break or crack in one of the bones of the leg. This occurs when a bone cannot withstand the physical force exerted on it. The shin (tibia) is one of the most frequently fractured bones. If the bones are healthy, a fractured or broken leg is usually the result of a powerful impact on the leg, such as from a motor vehicle collision. Older people are more likely to break a bone in the leg than younger people because a decreased calcium level leaves the leg bones weak and brittle, and age-related difficulty with balance and coordination can make falls more common. Pathologic fractures of the leg are principally caused by an underlying disease that has weakened the bones, such as bone cancer or osteoporosis. In this case, a bone of the leg may fracture as a result of minor impact or stress, or it may fracture spontaneously without any force exerted. In young children, whose leg bones are more flexible, an incomplete fracture of the leg, called a greenstick fracture, is more common.

DIAGNOSIS
A fractured leg is diagnosed by means of physical examination and the evaluation of X rays. The lower bone of the leg (tibia) may be broken straight across, which is called a transverse fracture, or on an angle, which is called an oblique fracture. A crush or comminuted fracture is one in which a section of the leg bone shatters into many pieces.

TREATMENT
As is true for fractured bones in other areas of the body, treatment emphasizes properly aligning the broken bone segments, followed by applying

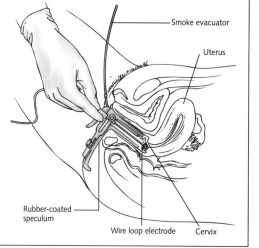

REMOVING A LESION ON THE CERVIX
During a LEEP procedure, the woman lies on an examining table and a speculum is inserted to open her vagina. A tube is connected to the speculum to remove the small amount of smoke and smoke odor that will be emitted during the procedure. A special sticky pad is placed on the woman's thigh to provide a safe return path for the electrosurgical current. The cervix is injected with anesthetic. Then an instrument tipped with a wire loop electrode is passed through the speculum and into the surface of the cervix. The current that passes through the loop generates heat to remove all the diseased tissue.

Smoke evacuator

Uterus

Rubber-coated speculum

Wire loop electrode   Cervix

a cast or splint to immobilize the bone and allow it to heal. The thighbone is one that is difficult to immobilize in this way because of the large muscles surrounding it. These muscles tend to pull the ends of the broken bone fragments over each other. To prevent this from happening when a bone of the thigh is broken, a system of weights, called traction, may be necessary to maintain the broken bone segments in alignment so they can heal properly. Tibial fractures usually require a long leg cast for 4 to 6 weeks. See also FRACTURE.

Leg, shortening of

A discrepancy in leg length, generally caused by a disease or fracture that interferes with normal bone growth during childhood. Possible causes include poliomyelitis (see POLIO) or a fracture that crossed the long bone's growing end in the thighbone or shinbone of one leg during childhood. If the shinbone (tibia) is affected, the shortening of the leg is called a tibial length discrepancy; if the thighbone (femur) is affected, it is called a femoral length discrepancy. A true leg-length discrepancy can be determined by an orthopedist's measurement of the legs. When both legs are of equal length but one leg appears shorter, called an apparent leg-length discrepancy, the condition may be caused by irregularities in the hip muscles (pelvic tilt).

Legg-Calvé-Perthes disease

See OSTEOCHONDROSIS.

Legionnaires disease

An infection caused by the bacterium *Legionella pneumophila* that may cause pneumonia. Legionnaires disease is also referred to as legionellosis. Although the infection and the bacteria that cause it had been in existence since 1947, they were identified and so-named in 1976 when 200 people attending an American Legion convention in Philadelphia became ill with pneumonia; 34 people died of the illness. It was discovered that the bacteria that caused these cases of illness had been spread by the inhalation of small droplets of water dispersed in the atmosphere from air-conditioning cooling towers.

The *Legionella* bacterium, which is common in the environment, is found predominantly in warm, stagnant water. The organisms can be found in some plumbing systems and hot water tanks, in the cooling towers and condensers of large air-conditioning systems, as well as in humidifiers, showers, and whirlpool spas. In nature, it is found in creeks and ponds. It is also found in soil at excavation sites. The disease is believed to be spread through the air from a water or soil source. There are no instances of infection stemming from air conditioners in automobiles or household window units, and the disease is not transmitted from one person to another.

The illness tends to occur sporadically and in outbreaks, most commonly during the summer months. When outbreaks erupt, local health departments conduct investigations to discover possible environmental sources of the infection. When discovered, appropriate prevention and control measures are recommended, including decontamination of water sources. Prevention is based on improving the design and maintenance of cooling towers and plumbing systems to limit the growth and spread of *Legionella* organisms.

SYMPTOMS

Symptoms generally occur 2 to 10 days following exposure to the bacteria, which sometimes cause a mild respiratory illness. People with mild infections usually recover within 2 to 5 days without treatment. In some cases, people infected with the bacteria do not develop any illness at all.

Infected persons have symptoms that can include muscle aches, diarrhea, fatigue, loss of appetite, headache, and abdominal pain. More serious illness tends to occur more frequently in men older than 50 years, particularly among those who smoke cigarettes and abuse alcohol. People with diabetes mellitus, chronic lung disease, or kidney infections, as well as people with cancer or immunodeficiency disorders, such as AIDS (acquired immunodeficiency syndrome), are also more susceptible. In the more severe form of legionnaires disease, the person may develop a cough that is either dry or produces sputum, followed by a high fever with a temperature of 102°F to

105°F, shaking, chills, disorientation, and extreme lethargy. These symptoms may progress to pneumonia. Severe cases may lead to death.

DIAGNOSIS AND TREATMENT

Pneumonia associated with legionnaires disease may be diagnosed by evaluation of chest X rays. There may be considerable lung damage and accumulation of fluid in the lungs. Laboratory tests that reveal improper kidney function may be included among diagnostic tools. Legionnaires disease may be difficult to differentiate from other illnesses such as influenza and other types of pneumonia, which often makes it necessary to perform other tests to confirm the diagnosis. These tests may include sputum cultures to test for the specific bacteria, urine samples to detect the presence of *Legionella* antigens, and blood tests, with blood samples generally taken 3 to 6 weeks apart, to compare antibody levels to the bacteria. Antibiotics are effective in treating the disease.

Leiomyoma

A noncancerous tumor of the smooth muscles that control the movements of the internal organs. Leiomyomas can occur in the bladder, breast, esophagus, and inside the uterus, as fibroid tumors. Cancerous tumors of the smooth muscle (leiomyosarcomas) are very rare, developing most often in the uterus, the rear area of the abdominal cavity, or the walls of the blood vessels.

Leishmaniasis

A parasitic infection spread by the bite of certain types of phlebotomine sand flies. Leishmaniasis, also called kala-azar, occurs most commonly in rural areas of tropical and subtropical countries ranging from Central America to western Asia; the infection is rare in the United States, but residents in rural southern Texas have developed a form of the infection. Certain sand flies become infected by feeding on an infected animal, usually a dog or a rodent, or on an infected person. They then transmit the parasitic protozoa *Leishmania donovani* to uninfected humans by biting them. The parasite attacks the body's phagocytes, the "hunter-killer" cells in the immune system.

L

L

SKIN INFECTION
Cutaneous leishmaniasis causes one or more skin lesions with a raised rim. The sores can be treated with medication. The infection is transmitted by a bite from a sand fly, but the sores may not appear until months after the bite. The infection is rare in the United States, occurring only in areas of south Texas.

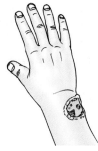

Typical wound

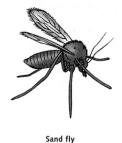

Sand fly

One bite from an infected sand fly is sufficient to cause the infection. The sand flies are tiny, about one third the size of a typical mosquito. They are most active from dusk to dawn. In unusual cases, the infection can be spread by a pregnant woman to her fetus. Blood transfusions and contaminated needles also carry the infection.

TYPES OF INFECTION
There are two types of leishmaniasis: cutaneous and visceral. Cutaneous leishmaniasis, the more common form of the infection, causes one or more skin sores that may change in size and appearance over time and may or may not be painful. The skin sores generally develop within a few weeks of a person being bitten, but may not appear until several months following a bite. They generally progress to a stage in which each sore has a raised edge with a central crater. The sores may form scabs. Some people experience swollen glands (see GLANDS, SWOLLEN) near the areas of the sores, under the arm if the sores are on the hand or arm, and in the groin if the sores appear on the legs or trunk. The skin sores usually heal over time without treatment; healing time may take months or even years, and the sores may leave scars.

Diagnosis may be made by examining cells from the skin sores under a microscope to detect the parasite. Untreated, cutaneous leishmaniasis may cause sores in the nose or mouth, resulting in mucosal leishmaniasis. This progression may not be noticed until several years after the skin sores have healed. Treatment is based on antiprotozoal medications.

Visceral leishmaniasis affects some of the body's internal organs, especially the spleen and liver, which may be enlarged by the infection. The bone marrow may also be affected.

The infection can produce swollen glands and is detected by abnormal results on blood tests. Red blood cells, white blood cells, and platelets may have low counts. Blood tests to look for antibodies to the parasite and for the parasite itself can also be helpful in diagnosing visceral leishmaniasis. The symptoms and signs of infection generally become apparent within several months of a bite, but in rare instances they may not appear for as long as several years. A person who becomes ill with visceral leishmaniasis may require hospitalization and intensive supportive care, in addition to treatment with antiprotozoal medication. Untreated, the infection can cause death.

Lens

The transparent structure within the pupil of the EYE that helps focus incoming light; also called the crystalline lens. Light entering the eye is bent (focused) first by the cornea, which directs the light through the pupil (the opening in the black center of the eye). The light then passes through the crystalline lens, which bends it into final focus. Held in place by fibers called the ciliary body, the crystalline lens thins to focus on objects in the distance and thickens for close vision.

Lens dislocation

Any condition in which the lens is out of its normal place behind the iris (the colored portion of the eye). Lens dislocation can be present at birth; it may develop as the result of diseases such as syphilis or Marfan syndrome that weaken the fibers holding the lens in place; or it can result from injury to the eye. The condition may affect either the natural lens or a synthetic one (intraocular lens implant)

placed in the eye during surgery to correct a cataract (clouding or opacity in the natural lens).

Treatment depends on the position of the dislocated lens and its effect on vision. If vision is not affected, the lens may simply be monitored from time to time. If vision is affected, the lens can be removed surgically. A synthetic lens is implanted in the normal lens position and takes over its function.

Lens implant
See CATARACT SURGERY.

Lentigo
See AGE SPOTS.

Leprosy
A chronic infectious disease caused by the parasitic bacterium called *Mycobacterium leprae*, which affects the peripheral nerves, skin, and mucous membranes. Leprosy is also known as Hansen disease and affects about 10 million people worldwide, most commonly in Asia and Africa, but also in Mexico, South and Central America, and the Pacific islands. There are a relatively small number of cases in the United States, almost all of them involving immigrants from developing countries who have settled in Texas, California, or Hawaii. Severe cases are more common in men than in women, and the peak ages of onset are in a person's 20s or 30s.

People with untreated leprosy retain a large quantity of the parasitic bacteria in the mucous membranes of the nose. The infection is believed to be transmitted by contact with respiratory or nasal droplets from an infected person. About half of all people who have leprosy have a history of intimate contact with an infected person. The bacteria are found in soil and insects, including bedbugs and mosquitoes, and these sources may have a role in transmission. A milder tuberculoid form of leprosy is believed to be noncontagious.

The incubation period generally averages from 5 to 7 years and can be as long as 40 years. The bacteria grow slowly, and, before signs and symptoms become apparent, an infected person may harbor many more of the infectious organisms than are present in any other bacterial infection.

CLINICAL TYPES
The majority of people exposed to

the parasitic bacterium that causes leprosy do not become ill, but tend to develop antibodies to the parasite in their blood as well as immune responses to it in the cells. In those who contract the disease, symptoms may vary. There are several types of leprosy.

Tuberculoid leprosy produces a rash and inflammation of peripheral nerves. Lepromatous leprosy causes symptoms including many severe ulcerations of the skin all over the body, inflammation of the eyes, and loss of body hair such as eyelashes and eyebrows. This type of leprosy may progress to include fever, anemia, glaucoma, loss of interior and exterior tissue of the nose, impotence and sterility, arthritis in the large joints, and severe inflammatory disorders of the nerves, kidneys, and lymph system. Borderline leprosy may evolve into one or the other of the two types.

DIAGNOSIS AND TREATMENT

Leprosy is diagnosed by physical examination of characteristic skin lesions and nerve damage. Examination of biopsy specimens of the lesions can confirm the diagnosis. Skin testing is not considered conclusive. Blood tests for antibodies to the bacteria are useful in monitoring the effects of treatment.

Minor skin inflammation associated with mild forms of leprosy is generally not treated or is treated with aspirin and short courses of PREDNISONE. For more severe cases, antimicrobial medications such as dapsone and antibiotic medications such as rifampin have been shown to be an effective cure. Other effective medications include clofazimine, ethionamide, minocycline, clarithromycin, and ofloxacin. Corticosteroids are generally included in the medical treatment of leprosy; prednisone therapy is helpful in treating nerve and skin inflammation. A combination of therapies is often recommended. THALIDOMIDE may be given for recurring cases, but not to women who may become pregnant. Surgical procedures may be used to correct functional disabilities associated with leprosy.

Leptin

A hormone important in the regulation of body weight. Leptin is produced by fat cells and is believed to have a role in appetite control and weight gain and loss. Research indicates that administering injections of leptin to obese people may help them lose body fat. Study results have been promising but inconclusive. In some people, leptin does not work at all.

Leptospirosis

Infections due to an organism in the *Leptospira* group that is carried in animals and shed in their urine. Leptospirosis is spread to humans by direct contact with contaminated urine or body tissue from an infected animal, most commonly a dog or rat. It is also transmitted indirectly by contact with contaminated water or soil. The organism gains entry into the human body via exposure to contamination by open skin abrasions or mucous membranes of the eyes, nose, or mouth. The infections are more common in men and may occur as an occupational hazard among farmers and sewer workers, but tend to be caused by incidental exposure during recreational activities, including swimming in contaminated water. Reported, diagnosed leptospirosis infections are rare in the United States and generally occur in the late summer and early fall.

Incubation is usually 7 to 13 days, but may range from 2 to 20 days. There may be abrupt symptoms including headache, conjunctivitis, severe muscle aches, chills, and a spiking fever. Excessive watering of the eyes is characteristic of the infection. After apparent recovery, symptoms may recur in 4 to 7 days, and signs of MENINGITIS may develop. Among the specific syndromes of leptospirosis, Weil syndrome, which may be potentially fatal in people who are older, has symptoms including jaundice, hemorrhage, anemia, disturbed consciousness, persistent fever, and kidney abnormalities. Aseptic meningitis and canicola fever are two other syndromes associated with the infection. Leptospirosis infections can cause abortion in a woman who is pregnant.

Leptospirosis is diagnosed by finding the suspect organisms in blood and urine samples. The infection is treated with antibiotic therapy, such as doxycycline. Higher doses of penicillin and ampicillin are given in more severe cases, along with fluid and electrolyte therapy.

Lesbianism

Sexual attraction and relations between women. See HOMOSEXUALITY.

No accurate estimates are available as to how many women are homosexual or bisexual (having sexual relationships with men and women). Sometimes people change sexual orientation during adulthood.

Negative social attitudes toward lesbianism—often on the part of family or employers—may pose challenges. Many lesbians develop a network of friends in the lesbian community that helps provide support.

Lesion

A wound, injury, or other pathologic alteration of an organ or tissue. Skin lesions include sores, rashes, and boils. Lesions can be benign or malignant (cancerous).

Lethargy

A feeling of dullness, sluggishness, weariness, and FATIGUE.

Leukemia

A malignant, or cancerous, disease that affects the blood-forming cells found in the bone marrow and the lymphatic system. Leukemia results in an abnormally high number of abnormal white blood cells (blasts). The blasts are cells that would develop into white blood cells but stop short in their development. High concentrations of blasts in the bone marrow, lymph nodes, and bloodstream can also impair the function of these tissues. Some types of leukemia may also affect the liver, spleen, or brain. In addition, overproduction of the blasts can crowd out normal cells in the bone marrow and decrease the number of red blood cells, platelets, and normal white blood cells formed by the bone marrow. This can lead to fatigue, weakness, increased bleeding and bruising from slow blood clotting, and a decreased ability to fight infection. Leukemia worsens over time and may result in death if left untreated.

In the United States, most types of leukemia are more common in men than in women and are found in more whites than in blacks. The risk of leukemia increases with age; more than five of ten cases occur in people older than 60. Although leukemia strikes ten times as many adults as

L

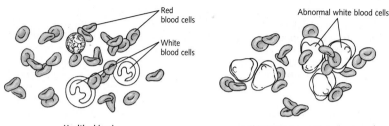

LEUKEMIA CELLS
Normal white blood cells (lymphocytes) are large and round. In a person with leukemia, the white blood cells are far more numerous and long-lived than normal, but they are underdeveloped. The person is less able to fight off infection, production of red blood cells is hindered, and blood clotting is affected.

children, it is the leading type of cancer among children. Leukemia causes more deaths in children younger than 15 than any other disease.

TYPES

Leukemia is classified according to two key characteristics. The first is the speed with which symptoms develop. In acute leukemia, symptoms begin very rapidly. Blast cells, which are immature and undeveloped, increase in number rapidly. People with acute leukemia almost always seek medical attention because they feel ill and become sicker over time. Almost all childhood leukemias are acute. In chronic leukemia, the number of blasts (immature cells) is lower and increases slowly. As a result, symptoms develop gradually. In the early stages, many people with chronic leukemia may not realize they are ill. Often the disease is discovered by a physician during a routine physical examination or blood test. Chronic leukemia usually has a slowly progressive course and is largely an adult disease.

The second way of classifying leukemia pertains to the type of blast. The abnormality can arise in either of the two main types of white blood cells: lymphoid or myeloid. If the leukemia affects the lymphoid cells, it is known as lymphocytic or lymphoblastic. If it affects the myeloid cells, it is known as myeloid or myelogenous.

There are four principal types of leukemia. Acute lymphoblastic leukemia is the most common type of leukemia in children, but can also affect adults, especially those older than 65. Acute myelogenous leukemia is found in both children and

adults, although it occurs most commonly in people who are middle-aged. Chronic lymphocytic leukemia is primarily a disease of people older than 65, occurring much less commonly in younger adults and almost never in children. Chronic myeloid leukemia is also primarily an adult disease that rarely afflicts children. Other less common leukemias include hairy cell leukemia (see LEUKEMIA, HAIRY CELL).

SYMPTOMS

Leukemia's symptoms vary somewhat between the different forms of the disease. Common symptoms include fever and chills; fatigue and weakness; frequent infections and poor wound healing; unusual bruising or bleeding; loss of appetite or weight; swelling or tenderness in the spleen (upper left abdomen), liver (upper right abdomen), or lymph nodes (such as in the neck, armpits, or groin); tiny red spots under the skin (called petechiae and caused by pinpoint hemorrhages); swollen or bleeding gums; sweating, especially at night; and pain in the bones or joints. Leukemia cells may invade the nervous system, producing headache, vomiting, lack of coordination or muscle control, blurred vision, and seizures. Leukemia cells can also gather in the testicles and cause painful swelling. In some cases, the lungs, digestive tract, and other organs are affected by the spread of the cancerous cells.

CAUSES

In most cases, the cause of leukemia is not known. As a result, little can currently be done to prevent the disease. One exception is smoking, which seems to have a causative role

in one of five cases of acute myelogenous leukemia in adults.

Exposure to large amounts of radiation is involved in a small number of cases of acute leukemia. There is no evidence that the small doses of X rays used in medical or dental care raise the risk of leukemia. Chemicals can also have a role. Exposure to benzene in particular has been shown to increase the risk of leukemia. The treatment for other types of cancer with radiation or chemotherapy increases the risk of leukemia later in life.

Genetics may also be a factor, since some families have more than the expected number of cases of the disease. Children with an inherited gene mutation known as Li-Fraumeni syndrome are at increased risk for leukemia.

DIAGNOSIS AND TREATMENT

Since the symptoms of leukemia can arise as the result of other diseases as well, a number of tests are needed to make the diagnosis. A blood test called a complete blood cell count is performed to determine the number of the different types blood cells. A blood smear can be examined under a microscope and may identify abnormal cells. If these tests point toward leukemia, a small sample (biopsy) of bone marrow and bone is taken and examined for leukemic cells. In some cases, a sample of the cerebrospinal fluid (the fluid that surrounds the spine and flows through the brain) is obtained with a needle to see whether the cerebrospinal fluid contains leukemic cells. Imaging studies, such as X rays, ultrasound scans, CT SCANNING (computed tomography scanning), and MRI (magnetic resonance imaging), may be used to see whether the leukemia is affecting the lymph nodes and internal organs.

Once the extent and type of the disease have been determined, treatment can begin. Treatment varies with the type of leukemia. In general, most leukemias are treated with chemotherapy, which involves the use of cancer-killing drugs. In some types of leukemia, particularly for leukemias that have not responded well to chemotherapy, bone marrow transplant is also used. For specific details on treatment and outcome, see the four principal types of leukemia: acute lymphoblastic leukemia (LEUKEMIA, ACUTE

LYMPHOBLASTIC), acute myelogenous leukemia (LEUKEMIA, ACUTE MYELOGENOUS), chronic lymphocytic leukemia (LEUKEMIA, CHRONIC LYMPHOCYTIC), and chronic myeloid leukemia (LEUKEMIA, CHRONIC MYELOID).

Leukemia, acute lymphoblastic

A rapidly developing cancer of the blood-forming tissues, particularly the bone marrow, that causes overproduction of immature white blood cells known as lymphoblasts. The disease is also known as acute lymphocytic leukemia because it affects the development in the bone marrow of the normal white blood cells known as lymphocytes. The lymphoblasts multiply rapidly and replace the lymphocytes. The abnormal cells also populate the bone marrow, causing the bone marrow to fail and the number of normal blood cells to decrease. Untreated, acute lymphoblastic leukemia leads to death within months, usually from infection (caused by poor immunity because of the low number of normal white blood cells) or bleeding (caused by the abnormally low number of platelets, which have a key role in blood clotting).

Acute lymphoblastic leukemia accounts for eight of ten cases of childhood leukemia. Most children affected by the disease are between the ages of 3 and 7. Acute lymphoblastic leukemia also occurs in adults, accounting for approximately one in five adult leukemias.

SYMPTOMS

Acute lymphoblastic leukemia is called acute because symptoms develop quickly and progress rapidly. Malaise (overall weakness), pallid skin, and fatigue are key signs of the disease. Infection can lead to chills and fever. Easy bruising, small spots of blood under the skin (known as petechiae and caused by pinpoint hemorrhages), and nosebleeds result from the low number of platelets. Weight loss and bone and joint pain may also occur. In children, the lymphoblasts often accumulate inside the brain and spinal cord and lead to seizures, blurred vision, and other nervous system symptoms.

CAUSES AND RISK FACTORS

Most cases have no apparent cause. Research studies indicate that, in at least a small percentage of cases, exposure to radiation, chemicals such as benzene, and certain drugs used to kill cancer cells (chemotherapy agents) may contribute to the disease. Genetic factors also seem to have a role, since people with Down syndrome have a higher than normal risk of developing the disease.

DIAGNOSIS, TREATMENT, AND OUTCOME

A type of blood test called the complete blood cell count is performed to count the different types of blood cells. A blood smear can be examined under a microscope to detect abnormal cells. If these tests point toward leukemia, a small sample (biopsy) of bone marrow and bone is taken and examined for abnormalities. If symptoms indicate that the brain and spinal cord are involved, a sample of the fluid that surrounds the spine and flows through the brain (cerebrospinal fluid) is obtained by performing a LUMBAR PUNCTURE (spinal tap), and is examined under a microscope for leukemic cells. Imaging studies, such as X rays, ultrasound scans, CT (computed tomography) scans, and MRI (magnetic resonance imaging), may be used to see whether the leukemia is affecting the lymph nodes and internal organs.

The goal of treatment in acute lymphocytic leukemia is remission, which means that the blood and bone marrow return to normal. The primary treatment is chemotherapy, or the use of drugs to kill cancer cells. The chemotherapy is divided into several phases. Initially, the person is hospitalized for 3 to 6 weeks for initial chemotherapy, or the induction phase, which uses a combination of three to eight drugs administered by mouth or into a vein. Since children are likely to have leukemia that affects the brain and spinal cord, chemotherapy agents are injected into the spinal fluid, and the brain is treated with radiation. This treatment is usually not needed in adults. If the individual is anemic (has too few red blood cells), he or she may need transfusions of red blood cells. If the platelet count is low and there is a risk of unusual bleeding, platelets are transfused. Antibiotics are often prescribed to prevent infection, and the person undergoing treatment may be isolated to reduce exposure to viruses, bacteria, and fungi that cause infections.

After the induction phase is complete, chemotherapy continues, usually on an outpatient basis. The purpose of this phase is to kill any cancer cells that have survived the induction phase and could cause a relapse. The person is then given maintenance therapy, which consists of low doses of cancer-killing drugs at regular intervals for 2 or 3 years.

If a relapse occurs (the leukemia returns), a second round of induction chemotherapy may be used. An alternative treatment is a bone marrow transplant (see BONE MARROW TRANSPLANT, ALLOGENEIC; BONE MARROW TRANSPLANT, AUTOLOGOUS), a rigorous and difficult therapy that makes it possible to use extremely large doses of chemotherapy drugs combined with radiation to eliminate the cancer.

Thirty or 40 years ago, acute lymphocytic leukemia was universally fatal within a few months. Now a substantial number of people remain in remission 5 years after diagnosis, which is considered a cure. Among children, eight of ten cases result in a cure. Among adults, however, only two or three of ten survive 5 years or longer.

Leukemia, acute myelogenous

A rapidly progressing cancer of the blood-forming tissues, particularly the bone marrow, that causes overproduction of immature white blood cells known as blasts. If the leukemia were not present, the blasts would go on to develop into the white blood cells known as granulocytes. The blasts multiply rapidly and replace the granulocytes, crowding out normal cells and causing the bone marrow to fail and the number of normal blood cells to decrease. Untreated, acute myelogenous leukemia leads to death within 3 to 4 months, sometimes in a matter of weeks, usually from infection (caused by poor immunity because of the low number of normal white blood cells) or bleeding (caused by the abnormally low number of platelets, which have a key role in blood clotting).

Acute myelogenous leukemia can occur at any age, but it primarily affects children younger than 1 year and middle-aged adults. It is the most

L

common type of acute leukemia in adults.

The name "myelogenous" means "produced in the bone marrow." This form of acute leukemia is also sometimes referred to as nonlymphocytic, monocytic, myelocytic, or granulocytic leukemia.

SYMPTOMS

Acute myelogenous leukemia is called acute because symptoms develop quickly and progress rapidly. Malaise (overall weakness), pallid skin, and fatigue are key signs of the disease. Infection can lead to chills and fever. Easy bruising, small spots of blood under the skin (known as petechiae and caused by pinpoint hemorrhages), and nosebleeds result from the low number of platelets. Swelling and bleeding of the gums is characteristic of this type of leukemia. Weight loss and bone and joint pain may also occur. Lymph nodes in the groin, armpit, and neck may become enlarged. The blasts often accumulate inside the brain and spinal cord and lead to seizures, blurred vision, and other symptoms.

CAUSES AND RISK FACTORS

Most cases have no apparent cause. Research studies indicate that, in at least a small percentage of cases, exposure to radiation, chemicals such as benzene, and certain drugs used to kill cancer cells (chemotherapy agents) may contribute to the disease. Genetic abnormalities may also have a role. Drugs used after organ transplantation to suppress the immune system and prevent rejection increase the risk of developing acute myelogenous leukemia, as do the blood diseases polycythemia vera, idiopathic THROMBOCYTOPENIA, and refractory anemia (see MYELOPROLIFER-ATIVE DISORDERS).

DIAGNOSIS, TREATMENT, AND OUTCOME

A type of blood test called the complete blood cell count is performed to count the different types of blood cells. A blood smear examined under a microscope can detect leukemic cells. The doctor also looks for certain chromosome abnormalities that may indicate leukemia or predict how a person will react to treatment. If these test results point toward the disease, a small sample (biopsy) of bone marrow and bone is taken and examined for abnormalities. When

symptoms indicate that the brain and spinal cord are involved, a sample of the cerebrospinal fluid (the liquid that surrounds the spine and flows through the brain) is obtained with a needle to be examined under a microscope for leukemic cells. Imaging studies, such as X rays, ultrasound scans, CT (computed tomography) scans, and MRI (magnetic resonance imaging), may be used to see whether the leukemia is affecting the lymph nodes and internal organs.

The goal of treatment in acute myelogenous leukemia is remission, which means that the blood and bone marrow return to normal. The primary type of treatment is chemotherapy, or the use of drugs to kill cancer cells. Typically several drugs are used in combination and administered by mouth or into a vein. If the person is anemic (has too few red blood cells), he or she is treated with transfusions of red blood cells. If the platelet count is low and there is a risk of unusual bleeding, platelets are transfused. Antibiotics are often prescribed to prevent infection, and the person undergoing treatment may be isolated to reduce exposure to infectious viruses, bacteria, and fungi. Chemotherapy results in remission of the leukemia in 70 to 80 percent of cases, with survival over the long-term achieved by 20 to 30 percent.

If a relapse occurs (the leukemia returns), another round of chemotherapy treatment may be used.

An alternative treatment is a bone marrow transplant (see BONE MARROW TRANSPLANT, ALLOGENEIC; BONE MARROW TRANSPLANT, AUTOLOGOUS), a rigorous and difficult therapy that allows the administration of extremely large doses of chemotherapy drugs combined with radiation to eliminate the cancer.

Leukemia, chronic lymphocytic

A cancer that involves proliferation of the white blood cells known as lymphocytes. Unlike normal lymphocytes, which are involved in maintaining the body's immunity against invading microorganisms and other foreign invaders, the cancerous cells have little immune function and tend to accumulate in the bone marrow, bloodstream, spleen, and lymph nodes.

Chronic lymphocytic leukemia is the most common leukemia in the Western hemisphere. It is primarily a disease that occurs among older individuals; 90 percent of cases occur in people older than 50. The disease affects twice as many men as women, a distinction not found in other types of leukemia.

SYMPTOMS

Chronic lymphocytic leukemia is called chronic because the disease tends to develop slowly and insidiously. Most cases are discovered through routine blood testing before any symptoms appear. As the disease progresses, symptoms begin, usually with fatigue and a decreasing ability to sustain exercise without tiring. Unusual bruising, pallid skin, jaundice (yellowish color of the skin and whites of the eyes), infection, bone tenderness and pain, weight loss, and swollen lymph nodes may occur. The spleen and sometimes the liver also enlarge. In advanced disease, cancerous lymphocytes may invade the testicles or ovaries, digestive system, skin, and kidneys.

CAUSES

Environmental factors such as radiation and exposure to toxic chemicals, which cause a small proportion of cases of other forms of leukemia, are not thought to be involved in this form of leukemia. Viruses may be responsible for the disease in some instances; research into this possibility is ongoing. Inherited defects in the immune system seem to predispose some people to chromic lymphocytic leukemia, but not everyone who inherits these defects develops the disease.

DIAGNOSIS, TREATMENT, AND OUTCOME

A type of blood test called the complete blood cell count is performed to count the different types of blood cells. A blood smear examined under a microscope can detect leukemia cells. If these test results point toward the disease, a small sample (biopsy) of bone marrow and bone is taken and examined for abnormalities. Imaging studies, such as X rays, ultrasound scans, CT (computed tomography) scans, and MRI (magnetic resonance imaging), may be used to see whether the leukemia is affecting the lymph nodes and internal organs.

Treatment of chronic lymphocytic

leukemia depends on the course of the disease, which varies markedly from person to person. Some live for years after the diagnosis with few symptoms and little or no treatment. In others, the disease worsens more quickly, and aggressive therapy is required.

The basic treatment for chronic lymphocytic leukemia is chemotherapy, or the use of cancer-killing drugs. Corticosteroid drugs such as prednisone are often combined with the chemotherapy to suppress the formation of abnormal lymphocytes. The complications of chemotherapy may leave the person undergoing treatment with too few red blood cells (anemia), which causes fatigue and weakness, and too few platelets (thrombocytopenia), which results in abnormal bleeding. Transfusions of red blood cells and platelets may be given to increase the number of normal blood cells. Radiation serves to shrink swollen lymph nodes and an enlarged spleen. If the spleen does not respond, it may be removed surgically, a procedure called splenectomy. In some cases, the abnormally high number of leukocytes turns the blood sticky and thick, which is an indication that treatment is needed.

Chronic leukemia is only rarely cured. Rather, treatment aims to control symptoms and allow the person to live as normally as possible.

Leukemia, chronic myeloid

A cancer characterized by an abnormal increase in white blood cells arising from rapid, malignant growth of blood-forming cells in the bone marrow. This cancer is also known as chronic myelocytic leukemia, chronic myelogenous leukemia, and chronic granulocytic leukemia. It is a progressive disease that can occur at any age but is most common among persons who are middle-aged. Once it is detected, chronic myeloid leukemia tends to remain in a long-lasting (chronic) phase that may last for several years, followed by a sudden acute attack known as a blast crisis, when the number of immature white blood cells (blasts) increases rapidly. The blast crisis is very difficult to treat and can result in death.

SYMPTOMS
The earliest signs of chronic myeloid leukemia are fatigue, shortness of breath following mild exercise, and fullness in the upper abdomen caused by an enlarged spleen. Because the enlarged spleen crowds the stomach, people with the disease may feel full after eating small amounts. Abnormal bleeding and bruising, swollen lymph nodes, tenderness in the sternum (breastbone), pallid skin, low fever, and enlargement of the liver are other possible symptoms.

CAUSES
Chronic myeloid leukemia has been associated with exposure to large doses of radiation and to benzene, both of which increase the risk of some other types of leukemia. Chronic myeloid leukemia is also associated with an inherited abnormality known as the Philadelphia chromosome, which is found in about 90 percent of people with the disease.

DIAGNOSIS, TREATMENT, AND OUTCOME
In approximately one of three cases, chronic myeloid leukemia is discovered before symptoms appear, usually though blood tests performed during routine physical examinations. A type of blood test called the complete blood cell count determines the number of the different types of blood cells. A blood smear examined under a microscope can detect leukemic cells. If test results indicate disease, a small sample (biopsy) of bone marrow and bone is taken and examined for abnormalities. Imaging studies, such as X rays, ultrasound scans, CT (computed tomography) scans, and MRI (magnetic resonance imaging), may be used to see whether the leukemia is affecting the spleen, lymph nodes, and liver.

Treatment of chronic myeloid leukemia aims to suppress the bone marrow with chemotherapy, or the use of cancer-killing drugs. A drug known as interferon is often combined with chemotherapy. This course of treatment reduces the number of abnormal white blood cells and controls symptoms, but it does not cure the disease. The drugs are usually given on an outpatient basis. The spleen may be removed to relieve symptoms, but this surgery does not extend survival. Recently, a new drug (STI571, the code name for imatinib mesylate) was approved for treatment of chronic myeloid leukemia. This drug interferes with certain types of cancer cells on a molecular level, preventing growth and proliferation. In some people with chronic myeloid leukemia, a return to normal blood counts is possible.

Bone marrow transplant (see BONE MARROW TRANSPLANT, ALLOGENEIC) from a donor is used for some people with the disease, particularly those who have not yet entered the blast crisis and are younger than 40. This treatment cures chronic myeloid leukemia in approximately half of the people who receive it.

Leukemia, hairy cell

A rare cancer of the blood-forming tissues, particularly the bone marrow. The number of all types of blood cells falls, while abnormal cells (known as hairy cells because of their unusual appearance under the microscope) proliferate in the blood and bone marrow. Hairy cell leukemia affects five times as many men as women, usually during middle age. Symptoms include fatigue, weakness, easy bleeding and bruising, recurrent infections, excessive sweating, swollen lymph nodes, and an enlarged spleen. The disease progresses slowly and is treated with chemotherapy (cancer-killing drugs) plus antibiotics to stop infections and transfusions of platelets to stop bleeding episodes. In many cases, the spleen is removed to resolve symptoms. Although the disease is not curable, most people with hairy cell leukemia live 10 years or longer after diagnosis.

Leukocyte

A blood cell that helps fight infection; also called a white blood cell. Any blood cell that contains a nucleus is a leukocyte. Leukocytes are capable of moving independently, as when they travel through blood vessel walls to a wound site to protect the body against foreign substances. Leukocytes are able to engulf foreign particles, such as bacteria, and this process causes an increase in the number of leukocytes in the blood during infection. Laboratory testing to determine whether infectious disease is present is based on the number of leukocytes in the blood.

In the healthy body, there are five

types of leukocytes: neutrophils, lymphocytes, basophils, eosinophils, and monocytes. Monocytes defend against infection by engulfing foreign substances of all sorts, while lymphocytes react to specific infectious agents. The neutrophils, basophils, and eosinophils are also involved in the immune response. Lymphocytes are either B cells, which produce antibodies, or T cells, which attack virus-infected or foreign cells. In disease, a variety of immature forms of red or white blood cells may also appear in the blood, as happens in leukemia.

Leukoencephalopathy, progressive multifocal

Also known as PML, an aggressive infection of brain cells caused by the JC virus (JCV). In PML, JCV infects and destroys the cells that produce myelin, the substance that forms the sheath that normally surrounds and protects nerve cells. This disease develops most frequently in people who have compromised immune systems as a result of HIV (human immunodeficiency virus) infection or long-term chemotherapy for cancer. Otherwise healthy people who are exposed to JCV rarely develop PML. The occurrence of PML in the presence of HIV constitutes a diagnosis of AIDS (acquired immunodeficiency syndrome), according to the Centers for Disease Control and Prevention (CDC).

The symptoms of PML include extreme weakness; HEMIANOPIA, or blindness in half of the normal visual field; mental impairment; lack of coordination; paralysis on one side of the body; and language difficulties. Diagnosis is usually made by a neurologist with the aid of tests such as MRI (magnetic resonance imaging) and CT (computed tomography) scanning. An examination of cerebrospinal fluid can help distinguish PML from other diseases with similar symptoms, such as multiple sclerosis. There is no known cure for PML, and the period between the onset of symptoms and death can be a matter of months. However, in some cases anti-HIV drugs, such as zidovudine (also known as AZT), have proven helpful.

Leukopenia

An abnormally low number of white blood cells circulating in the blood; commonly known as a low white blood cell count. Leukopenia is diagnosed by taking a sample of blood and counting the number of white blood cells per microliter (a millionth [1/1,000,000] of a liter). The normal white blood cell count is 4,000 to 10,000 per microliter of blood. The normal neutrophil (white cells that fight infection) count in whites is 1,500 per microliter of blood; in blacks, 1,200 per microliter. Mild neutropenia is 1,000 to 1,200 or 1,500 per microliter of blood depending on race; moderate, 500 to 1,000 per microliter; and severe, less than 500 per microliter.

Leukopenia usually occurs when white blood cells are used up at a rapid rate and production of new cells falls behind. This happens most commonly in response to medications, particularly those used to kill cancer cells. Leukopenia can also result from cancers affecting the bone marrow, where white blood cells are produced; because of enlargement of the spleen, which filters and retains white blood cells; or because of infection, including short-term viral illnesses, septicemia (bacterial infection of the blood), or HIV (human immunodeficiency virus) infection. Autoimmune diseases and nutritional deficiencies, such as a vitamin B12 or folate deficiency, can result in low white blood cell counts.

Since white blood cells have central roles in providing immunity against disease-causing microorganisms, leukopenia is a key problem in bacterial or fungal infection. Infection may appear as sores and inflammation in the mouth, severe sore throat, pneumonia, liver abscess, or gum infection, all accompanied by a temperature of 101°F or higher. In people with poorly functioning immune systems, such as those with cancer or HIV infection, these infections can be life-threatening. Treatment consists of antibiotics to combat the infection. If the leukopenia is severe, the growth factors G-CSF (granulocyte colony-stimulating factor) and GM-CSF (granulocyte-macrophage colony-stimulating factor), which stimulate white blood cell production, are given as medications.

Leukoplakia

Raised white patches on the inside of the cheek, tongue, or lips. In the mouth, leukoplakia may be due to irritation from poorly fitted dentures, chronic cheek biting, or tobacco. In its early stages, leukoplakia usually causes no symptoms and is diagnosed during the course of a routine physical or dental examination. Because it is a potentially cancerous condition, leukoplakia must be closely monitored by a physician; a biopsy may be necessary. Treatment consists of eliminating all tobacco products and other irritants.

Leukorrhea

A vaginal discharge consisting of mucus and pus cells. The discharge may be white or yellowish. Leukorrhea sometimes occurs at or just before each menstrual period.

Leuprolide acetate

A drug used in the treatment of prostate cancer. Leuprolide acetate (Lupron, Viadur) is used for people with advanced prostate cancer to decrease the production of testosterone, thereby reducing prostate cancer growth and relieving symptoms such as pain and difficulty in urinating. Leuprolide acetate is implanted in the upper arm once a year by a doctor to provide continuous treatment for 1 year. At the end of the year, the old implant is removed and replaced with a new one.

Levamisole

An anticancer drug. Levamisole (Ergamisol) tablets are used to treat cancer of the colon. It is usually given in combination with fluorouracil, another anticancer drug.

Levodopa and carbidopa

An anti-Parkinson drug combination. Levodopa and carbidopa are usually given in combination (Sinemet, Atamet) to treat Parkinson disease. Levodopa is the active ingredient that is converted into dopamine, which is a neurotransmitter in the brain. Increased amounts of dopamine in the brain relieve the symptoms of Parkinson disease. Levodopa is used to treat the stiffness, tremors, spasms, and poor muscle control associated with Parkinson disease.

Carbidopa makes levodopa more effective by preventing its conversion to dopamine before it crosses into the brain. Besides enhancing the effects of levodopa, carbidopa also makes it possible for lower doses of levodopa to be prescribed, thereby reducing side effects. Levodopa is associated with many side effects, including dizziness, stomach upset, irregular heartbeat, and mood changes.

Levofloxacin

An antibiotic used to treat pneumonia, bronchitis, urinary tract infections, and minor skin infections. Levofloxacin (Levaquin) is an antibiotic that works by interfering with bacterial DNA, preventing the bacteria from reproducing. Levofloxacin is active against bacteria, including *Streptococcus pneumoniae*, which is resistant to penicillin.

Levonorgestrel

An oral contraceptive; birth control pill. Together with ethinyl estradiol, levonorgestrel combines natural or synthetic estrogens and progestins that are similar to the natural sex hormones produced in a woman's body. Ethinyl estradiol is an estrogen, while levonorgestrel is a progestin. Together, these products can prevent ovulation and pregnancy, regulate menstrual flow, and treat acne or other hormone-related problems. The type and amount of each hormone varies among brands of oral contraceptives.

Levothyroxine

A thyroid hormone. Levothyroxine (Levothroid, Levoxyl, and others), a naturally occurring hormone produced by the thyroid gland, is associated with metabolism and energy. Levothyroxine is used to replace a thyroid hormone deficiency and to treat goiter, or enlarged thyroid gland, which can be caused by hormone imbalance, radiation, cancer, or thyroid surgery.

Lewy body dementia

A form of DEMENTIA in older people characterized by the presence of distinctive formations within brain cells called Lewy bodies. Dementia is a disorder in the brain that causes a progressive decline in memory and other intellectual functions. There are also behavioral changes and physical consequences. Symptoms of Lewy body dementia often resemble those of ALZHEIMER'S DISEASE. However, people with Lewy body dementia commonly tend to have muscular stiffness and poor balance due to problems in the central nervous system more than do those who have Alzheimer's disease. Gradually they become unable to perform the usual activities of daily life and eventually are incapacitated. Lewy bodies are sometimes found in the brains of people who have Alzheimer's disease or PARKINSON DISEASE.

LH

Luteinizing hormone; also known as luteotropin in females and interstitial cell–stimulating hormone in males. LH is produced by the pituitary gland. Together with one of the female SEX HORMONES called ESTROGEN, LH in women stimulates the follicles in the ovaries to release a developed egg. Another pituitary hormone, FSH (follicle-stimulating hormone), has previously prepared the follicles for the eggs in a chain of events called ovulation. LH also prepares the uterus to support a fertilized egg. Also in women, LH promotes the formation of the tissue in the ovary that secretes another female sex hormone, PROGESTERONE, and prepares the mammary glands for milk secretion.

In men, LH stimulates the interstitial cells in the testicles to produce and release large amounts of TESTOSTERONE, the major male sex hormone. Testosterone influences a man's body shape, voice, body hair, sex drive, and ability to achieve an erection.

LH-RH

Luteinizing hormone–releasing hormone. LH-RH is released in response to estrogen, progesterone, and testosterone; regulates the hormone levels; and triggers sexual and reproductive functions. LH-RH stimulates the release of LH (luteinizing hormone), the pituitary hormone that triggers a woman's ovaries to produce ESTROGEN, which stimulates female sex characteristics and the growth of the uterine lining in preparation for pregnancy. PROGESTERONE maintains pregnancy, in part by inhibiting FSH (follicle-stimulating hormone) and LH release. TESTOSTERONE in males stimulates male sex characteristics and promotes sperm production in the testicles.

Libido

The psychological, physical, and emotional energy that comes from instinctual drives, particularly sexual. The level of libido can vary with mood (such as anxiety and sadness), physical health, hormonal changes (such as during pregnancy and menstruation), and emotional states (such as anticipation, pursuit, or fantasy).

Lice, head

Small parasites that feed on blood from the scalp. Head lice are tiny gray insects (about the size of sesame seeds) that cause an intensely itchy scalp. Head lice are extremely contagious and affect primarily schoolchildren. However, lice on a child can quickly spread to family members of all ages.

Head lice are treated by applying over-the-counter or prescription shampoos or lotions to the scalp and hair. Directions on the label must be carefully followed for the product to be effective and safe. It is also important to remove nits. Nits are the scarcely visible, whitish eggs of lice. Nits can be seen firmly attached to hair shafts. Hair rinsed with a solution of 50 percent vinegar and 50 percent water may help loosen nits, which must then be removed with a fine-tooth comb or with the fingernails. Treatment should be repeated 1 week later. Sometimes lice will cause an allergic reaction in the form of a rash.

To prevent lice from reattaching to the hair of the scalp, clothes and

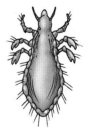

TINY BLOODSUCKERS
Head lice are tiny but visible on the scalp of an infested person. The nits, or lice eggs, are also visible as white flecks along hair strands. The first symptoms of the presence of lice are itching and the appearance of small, red bumps on the scalp, neck, and shoulders.

bedding must be washed in very hot water. Items that cannot be easily washed (such as stuffed animals) should be sealed in plastic bags for 3 weeks. Upholstered furniture and carpets should be vacuumed. To prevent lice from spreading, combs, brushes, and hats should not be shared with others.

Licensure, medical

The granting of a license allowing a person to practice medicine. Licensure is granted by a state agency, frequently a state board of medicine in the state where a person wishes to practice medicine. Generally, state boards meet at least once a year to examine applicants. To obtain a medical license, a person must have a diploma from an accredited medical college, pass an examination that reflects knowledge of his or her branch of medicine, and be of good moral character.

Lichen planus

A benign (not cancerous) skin condition consisting of shiny flat papules (small superficial bumps on the skin) that vary from pink to red to violet. The itchy bumps of lichen planus usually develop on the arms and legs but may occur anywhere on the body. On the scalp, lichen planus can cause hair loss. When it affects the mouth, whitish patches form inside of the cheeks. Lichen planus of the nail leads to brittle or split nails.

This condition is most common between the ages of 30 and 60 years. Although in most cases the cause remains unknown, lichen planus can occur as a reaction to a medication; there may be a link to hepatitis C. Diagnosis is made through physical examination, medical history, and sometimes a skin biopsy. Treatment of the rash is with topical and, in severe cases, oral corticosteroids. Retinoids (forms of vitamin A) and PHOTOTHERAPY (treatment with light) have also been used to treat this disorder. Antihistamines help control itching. Lichen planus may persist for weeks or months and can recur.

Lichen sclerosus

A skin disorder of the VULVA, or external female genitalia. The cause of lichen sclerosus is unknown. It can appear at any age but most often affects white women older than age

65. The skin surface of the vulva becomes thin, wrinkled, and papery and red or purple in appearance. The affected area can spread to include the skin at the top of the thighs and the inner buttocks, sometimes surrounding the anus. The skin under the arms, beneath the breasts, on the neck, on the back, and on the arms can be affected. The chief symptom is intense itching. Lichen sclerosus may develop into cancer, and a BIOPSY of affected skin is recommended for precise diagnosis. Treatment focuses on management of the itching, usually with creams containing CORTICO-STEROIDS. Ointments containing testosterone are also used.

Lichen simplex

A localized area of skin thickening caused by rubbing and scratching. The patches are thick, dry, and leathery and may be darker or redder than the surrounding skin. Lichen simplex is a localized form of DERMATITIS or NEURODERMATITIS. The areas most commonly affected are easily reached, such as the nape of the neck and the outer part of the lower legs.

Diagnosis of lichen simplex is based on the appearance of the skin and a medical history. Doctors may perform a skin biopsy to confirm the diagnosis. Sometimes lichen simplex is the result of chronic irritation. It may start with an insect bite or rough clothing that irritates the skin, which leads to an urge to rub or scratch the area. Or symptoms are brought on or aggravated by stress. Lichen simplex is sometimes associated with anxiety or depression, so it may be necessary to control underlying psychological problems with counseling and medication. Antihistamines to reduce itching and sedatives to reduce stress are sometimes prescribed. Depending on the severity, other treatments may include soothing lotions and topical corticosteroids. In severe cases, corticosteroids are injected directly into lesions to control inflammation and itching.

Lichenification

Thickening of the skin resulting in thick, dry, leathery skin. The markings of the skin may become prominent. Lichenification is the result of constant scratching and rubbing and is most often associated with DERMATITIS.

Licorice root

An herbal medicine. Licorice root is used to treat viral infections, including colds, AIDS (acquired immunodeficiency syndrome), and hepatitis; inflammation; menstrual and menopausal disorders; peptic ulcers; canker sores; herpes; eczema; and psoriasis. Licorice root has many possible medicinal actions, including antiallergic, antiviral, anti-inflammatory, and hormonal actions. Its major active component is glycyrrhizin. It should not be used at high doses or for a prolonged time because it can be toxic.

Life expectancy

The number of years a newborn can expect to live under current health conditions. Life expectancy is an indicator of general health conditions, such as access to health care, infant mortality, nutrition, and air and water quality. The longer the life expectancy, the better the health conditions. In preindustrial times, life expectancy averaged between 25 and 35 years; similar numbers are found

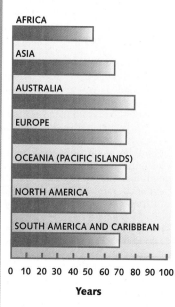

LIFE EXPECTANCY AROUND THE WORLD

The number of years a newborn boy or girl can expect to live varies from continent to continent.

AFRICA
ASIA
AUSTRALIA
EUROPE
OCEANIA (PACIFIC ISLANDS)
NORTH AMERICA
SOUTH AMERICA AND CARIBBEAN

0 10 20 30 40 50 60 70 80 90 100
Years

Courtesy of Population Reference Bureau © 2000

today in certain very poor countries, particularly those at war. In the industrialized nations, life expectancy generally exceeds 70 years during peacetime conditions.

Life support

A system involving equipment and procedures that provides all or some of the bodily functions necessary to maintain life. Life support may involve providing oxygen, nutrients, and water and eliminating carbon dioxide and other body wastes. The most commonly used form of life support is a ventilator, which is designed to breathe for a person with respiratory failure. Other forms of life support include nutrition and hydration provided through a tube surgically implanted in a person's stomach or inserted into a vein.

USE OF VENTILATORS

A ventilator helps maintain adequate tissue oxygenation and removes carbon dioxide from the lungs when the heart and lungs are unable to perform these functions. Brain stem cells can survive 15 to 20 minutes without oxygen, while cells in the cerebral hemispheres are destroyed within 4 to 6 minutes of oxygen deprivation. Respiratory distress and failure may be caused by long-term illness, traumatic injury, heart failure, respiratory disease, severe infection, and brain disorders.

When a person stops breathing, a mask connected to a bag containing air and extra oxygen is placed over the face; the air is forced into the lungs by pressure. If a person cannot breathe without assistance, intubation is implemented. In intubation, a tube is inserted into the mouth, guided into the trachea (windpipe), and attached to a ventilator, which supplies air and removes carbon dioxide from the lungs.

ETHICAL CONSIDERATIONS

A person's life may be artificially sustained by life support. Considerations about the withdrawal of life support are based on the feelings of a person's family and on the expressed wishes of the person requiring life support.

Mechanical ventilation is the form of life support most frequently withdrawn. It is usually withdrawn gradually, and sedatives and analgesics are often given to the person undergoing withdrawal. Without an

advance directive (see ADVANCE DIRECTIVES), physicians are generally reluctant to withdraw forms of life support. In medicine, it is considered ethically acceptable to withdraw life support when further care is futile and when withdrawal is consistent with the patient's express desires. See also EUTHANASIA.

Ligament

A strap of tissue that connects bones at joints. A type of connective tissue, ligaments are made up of interlocking fibers to form strong cords. Some ligaments are inside joints to stabilize the bones, and others connect the bones outside the joints to provide protection. Ligaments may allow some movement, as in the joints between the vertebrae, or may fix the joint so firmly that the bone will break before the ligament will detach. See JOINT.

Ligament injuries, knee

Stretching or tearing injuries, sometimes referred to as sprains, involving one of the knees' ligaments. The two cruciate ligaments are bands of soft tissue that attach the top of the shinbone to the bone that forms the kneecap in a crisscross pattern. The ligament that crosses in front, called the anterior cruciate ligament, is generally injured by sudden twisting motions that turn the knees in a different direction from the one in which the feet are planted, as may happen while skiing. The ligament that crosses in back, the posterior cruciate ligament, is apt to be stretched or torn by a powerful impact, as may happen during a motor vehicle collision or contact sports. The medial collateral ligament, on the inside of the knee, is generally injured by a violent twisting or stretching of the knee during sport activities, such as football or hockey.

SYMPTOMS

An injury to the cruciate ligament often produces a "popping" sound with swelling, but may not be painful. The leg may buckle or "give out" when weight is put on it. Diagnosis is made by physical examination and several tests exploring the knee's capacity to maintain its proper position when pressure is applied. MRI (magnetic resonance imaging) can detect a complete

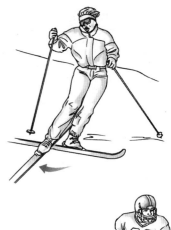

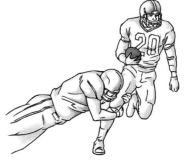

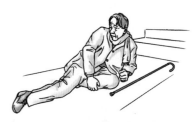

CAUSES OF KNEE LIGAMENT INJURY
In younger adults, sports injuries commonly damage ligaments in the knee. A skier may twist ligaments when the foot is planted firmly and the leg turns. A football player may violently twist the ligaments or take a direct blow that stretches or tears ligaments. In older people, falls often cause twisting of knee ligaments.

tear in the ligament; a partial tear can be detected by arthroscopy. See ARTHROSCOPIC SURGERY.

TREATMENT

Exercises to strengthen surrounding muscles and a protective knee brace may be prescribed for a partial tear of a cruciate ligament, but jumping is discouraged. Surgery is sometimes recommended when the ligament is completely torn, especially in the case of an active athlete or exerciser. Reconstruction is generally accomplished using a combination of open surgery and arthroscopic surgery. The surgeon may reattach the two ends of the torn ligament or graft on a healthy tendon to reconstruct the torn area. In the latter operation, a small incision is made in the leg and small tunnels are drilled in the bone to provide access for grafting the new ligament tissue. As the knee heals, the tunnels fill in and secure the tendon in place. Successful recovery following surgery involves a regular exercise and rehabilitation program for 4 to 6 months. Physical therapy may include the use of specialized equipment. Often, a normal life can be resumed.

With injuries to the medial collateral ligament, a pop may be heard and the knee may buckle to the side. There is often pain and swelling with this injury. Diagnosis involves a physical examination in which pressure is applied to the side of the knee to gauge the looseness of the joint and the amount of pain. Ice may be recommended to ease pain and swelling. Exercise may be prescribed to strengthen supporting muscles, and a sleeve-type brace may be worn to protect and stabilize the knee for 2 to 4 weeks while the injury heals; non–weight-bearing crutches are used during this time. If both ligaments are torn, surgical repair is usually necessary, with a return to full activity within about 9 weeks.

Ligation

Tying up or binding of a blood vessel to prevent bleeding of another structure. In surgery, ligation is used to close severed blood vessels and prevent bleeding. The surgeon uses a thread, usually made from silk or other material, to tie off a vessel or duct, such as in a TUBAL LIGATION, when fallopian tubes are tied off to prevent pregnancy.

Ligature

The material used in LIGATION, the tying off of a blood vessel or duct. The ligature is typically a length of threadlike material; it can be made of cotton, wire, silk, or any other suitable material. A soft, thin wire or elastic ligature is often used in orthodontic procedures.

Terms in small capital letters—for example, PHYSICAL THERAPY or PAGET DISEASE—indicate a cross-reference to another entry with more information.

Light therapy

The use of natural or artificial light to treat various ailments such as depression or sleep disorders by affecting chemicals in the brain and hypothalamus. Light therapy is used to treat people with seasonal affective disorder (SAD), which is thought to be a form of depression that occurs in winter and in the absence of adequate daylight. Light therapy is also used to treat workers who have shift-related sleep disorders. The most common form of light therapy is called bright-light therapy and involves sitting for about 15 to 20 minutes near a special light box fitted with high-intensity light bulbs that provide full-spectrum or white light. The light produced by the special box is about 15 times brighter than that found in a home or office.

Colored-light therapy is also used to bathe the skin in different shades of color, a practice thought to affect the neurochemicals produced in the brain. This form of COLOR THERAPY has been tested as a treatment for migraine headaches, among other disorders. The best way to get light therapy is to go outside for at least 30 minutes each day. Even if the sun is behind the clouds, it will provide the light the body needs. Sunlight is also important for proper metabolism of certain nutrients; however, it is vital to use sunscreen to protect the skin from cancers.

Light treatment

See PHOTOTHERAPY.

Lightning injuries

Injuries caused by lightning from thunderstorms. Lightning strikes about 1,800 people per year in the United States. It is the cause of more deaths—anywhere from 100 to 450 each year—than any other weather hazard. Types of lightning injuries include "flashes" and "jolts." Flashes are lightning strikes that surround a person very briefly, often blowing off the person's clothes but rarely leaving burns or other external signs of injury. Jolts of lightning can hurl a person through the air or cause the heart to stop beating. Other injuries can include severe burns, nervous system damage, broken bones, and loss of hearing or eyesight. Lightning can carry up to 50 million volts of electricity, which—if it could be harnessed—would be enough to serve 13,000 homes.

People at greatest risk of being struck by lightning are those who are outside during a storm and engaged in recreational activities. Joggers, hikers, campers, and golfers are at risk, as are boaters and swimmers. People holding onto metal objects, such as golf clubs or baseball bats, are at highest risk. Lightning injuries can be prevented by simple, common sense measures. If a storm is approaching, people should immediately seek shelter, because lightning can travel 10 to 12 miles ahead of the storm. If no shelter is available, a person should remove metal objects, crouch down in a ball position, and stay at least 15 feet away from other people. A person should not seek a tall tree to stand under during a lightning storm. The use of telephones and electrical equipment during a thunderstorm is not recommended, as lightning may strike outside electrical and phone lines, causing shocks to a person through the equipment.

Limb, artificial

A manufactured prosthetic replacement for an arm or leg, worn when all or part of the limb has been lost due to injury, accident, disease, or birth defect. A person requiring an artificial limb can discuss his or her needs and preferences with both the physician and the technician who will custom design the prosthesis.

An artificial limb is designed and constructed by first taking a plaster mold of the person's natural limb. Scanning lasers may sometimes be used to measure and reproduce the shape of the limb. The resulting measurements are used to shape the socket for the prosthesis, a critical element in the use of the limb. Areas of the socket that will contact or support the artificial limb and any forces exerted during movement are modified to provide greater comfort for the person wearing it. In the final fitting stages, the artificial limb is aligned properly and cosmetically shaped to duplicate the appearance of the natural arm or leg.

The traditionally designed artificial limb uses simple hinge joints, possibly with counterweight pendulums, while the newer "bionic" arms and

PREVENTING LIGHTNING INJURIES

Being struck by lightning is life-threatening because the electricity generated by the lightning disrupts the electrical activity in the brain that controls a person's breathing and heartbeat. The heat from the lightning can cause severe burns and internal injuries. The person may be thrown into the air by the force of the lightning strike, causing further harm.

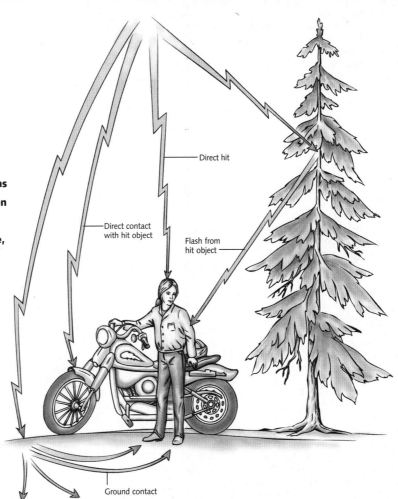

Direct hit

Direct contact with hit object

Flash from hit object

Ground contact

FOUR TYPES OF EXPOSURE
A person can be injured four ways in a lightning strike: a direct hit, contact with a hit object, a flash from a hit object, or contact with current in the ground. A person should not stand under a tree or hold onto a metal object, such as handlebars on a motorcycle or bike, during a lightning storm.

L

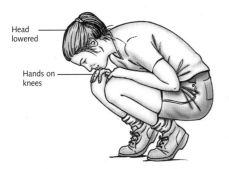

Head lowered

Hands on knees

PREFERRED POSTURE DURING LIGHTNING STORM
Crouching low with the head down decreases the chance of a lightning strike.

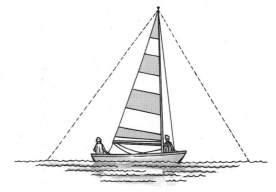

CONE OF PROTECTION AROUND SAILBOAT
A special grounded lightning mast may divert a lightning strike that would otherwise fall in a cone-shaped space surrounding the boat.

legs can be operated by electrical motors or other devices that are stimulated by nerve impulses from the person's remaining limb. A physical therapist can be helpful in teaching a person how to use a prosthesis. In the case of an artificial leg, physical therapy is important to learn how to walk with a new limb. With the currently available flexible materials and highly functional components of artificial limbs, most users can return to normal daily activities.

Limbic system

A group of structures within the brain that are associated with emotions and feelings such as pleasure, sexual arousal, sadness, anger, and fear. The limbic system has a role in the AUTONOMIC NERVOUS SYSTEM (the part of the nervous system that controls involuntary activities of body functioning) and in the sense of smell. Its components include the amygdala, cingulate gyrus, hippocampal gyrus, isthmus, and uncus. When the limbic system is damaged or diseased, there may be abnormal emotional responses, such as easily provoked rage; inappropriate crying or laughter; unwarranted fear, anxiety, or depression; or excessive sexual interest.

Limp

A characteristic, unsteady gait that favors one leg over the other because of pain or problems with the muscles or bones of the hips, legs, or feet. In adults, limping may also be related to pain or problems in the lower back. In children, limping can indicate a simple injury or bruise, a strain or fracture, ill-fitting shoes, a PLANTAR WART on the sole of the foot, a splinter in the foot, or an inflamed joint. But a child's limp may also be a sign of a more serious ailment requiring immediate medical attention. Swelling, redness, and warmth around the knee, ankle, and hip joints could be symptoms of RHEUMATIC FEVER or JUVENILE RHEUMATOID ARTHRITIS (JRA). Pain and tenderness over a bone in the leg or foot accompanied by fever could indicate a bone infection or OSTEOMYELITIS.

Lip

One of two soft folds that line the opening to the mouth. The lips move by the action of a muscle that circles the mouth. The lips are covered with thin skin and are lined with mucous membranes. The principal functions are to keep food in the mouth and to help produce speech sounds. Muscles at the outermost corners of the lips are responsible for facial expression.

Lip cancer

Cancer that usually occurs on the lower lip. Lip cancer is most common in white men older than 40 years and is most often caused by long-term sun exposure. Using tobacco and alcohol also contributes to lip cancer, as well as to other forms of ORAL CANCER. Often lip cancer is first detected by a dentist or physician during a routine examination. A biopsy is required to make the diagnosis.

Squamous cell carcinoma of the lip begins as actinic CHEILITIS (a sun-induced inflammation) or LEUKOPLAKIA (raised white patches). The most common symptom is an enlarging growth that at first is not painful. Over time, it becomes an infected open sore. There may also be numbness of the lower lip. Lip cancer may grow rapidly and invade other tissues. Treatment is with surgical EXCISION (cutting).

To prevent lip cancer, a person should use a sunblock or a lip balm with sunscreen and wear a wide-brimmed hat when outdoors. It is also important not to smoke and to avoid drinking alcoholic beverages.

Lipid-lipoprotein metabolism

The chemical processes through which the body uses, stores, and circulates lipids and lipoproteins. Lipids are a broad category of substances that includes fats and fatlike compounds such as sterols (including CHOLESTEROL). Phospholipids are a group of lipids that constitute an important component of the membranes that surround body cells. Lipoproteins are complex substances made of varying amounts of cholesterol, TRIGLYCERIDES, phospholipids, and protein. Apolipoproteins are the protein components of lipoprotein complexes. Because they are not soluble in water, lipids such as fats and cholesterol are carried in the blood in the form of lipoproteins. Fats are used for energy or stored in fat cells. Cholesterol is not used for energy, but as a building block for a wide range of compounds such as bile, estrogen, testosterone, and vitamin D.

Although not all lipids are fats, the two terms are often used interchangeably. A certain amount of fat and cholesterol is required by the body. However, eating too much fat, especially saturated fat, can raise blood cholesterol levels. (See also FATS AND OILS.) High cholesterol levels are associated with an increased risk of ATHEROSCLEROSIS, a condition in which blood vessels are narrowed by plaque accumulation and less and less blood reaches vital organs. Eventually, plaque accumulation can block arteries. Since blood carries oxygen and vital nutrients, this can cause problems such as angina or a heart attack.

ABSORPTION OF LIPIDS

Although most lipid digestion takes place in the small intestine, lipid digestion begins in the stomach, where the enzyme lipase begins to break down lipids, allowing them to mix with water-based digestive enzymes. In the small intestine, bile carries the lipids and water permitting the enzymes to further break down lipids into fatty acids to be absorbed. Salts in bile convert large droplets of fat into smaller droplets. This activity increases the surface area of droplets, allowing fat to mix with water, and lipids are then able to be digested by more lipase that is excreted by the pancreas. Lipase breaks down fats into glycerol (a sugar alcohol) and fatty acids.

Absorption of fats consumed in foods is usually complete. This is why little fat normally appears in the feces. Lipid absorption occurs mainly in the jejunum, part of the small intestine. Tiny fat globules pass first into the center of villi and then into large lymphatic channels, which allow circulation of lipids throughout the body.

Most lipids are then transported to the liver for further processing. In the liver, cells called hepatocytes convert the fats eaten in foods into lipids that can be stored by the body or used as fuel. Hepatocytes also have a key role in regulating cholesterol levels. All the cholesterol needed by the body is manufactured in the liver. However, the more dietary cholesterol from animal foods and saturated fat a person consumes, the more excess cholesterol the liver produces to make bile, since bile is needed for lipid digestion and absorption.

Lipids, including excess cholesterol, are transported through the bloodstream by special carriers called lipoproteins. The two most important carriers of cholesterol are low-density lipoprotein (LDL) and high-density lipoprotein (HDL). The relative levels of LDL and HDL have opposite effects on the heart. HDL is typically called "good" cholesterol because high levels of it have no apparent health risk. High levels of LDL, commonly referred to as the "bad" cholesterol, are associated with a buildup of plaque in the arteries, leading to atherosclerosis and heart disease. Fats produced in the liver are transported by VLDL (very-low-density lipoprotein).

Lipid-lowering agents

See CHOLESTEROL-LOWERING DRUGS.

Lipids

A broad category of substances in the body that includes fats and fatlike compounds such as sterols (including CHOLESTEROL). Although not all lipids are fats, the two terms are often used interchangeably. See also LIPID-LIPOPROTEIN METABOLISM.

Lipodystrophy, insulin

A small, harmless dent or lump on the skin's surface that forms when a person with diabetes repeatedly injects insulin at the same site. Lipodystrophy can be prevented by rotation of injection sites and, in some cases, by using purified insulin.

The areas of the body where insulin is most easily injected include the outer area of the upper arms, the region slightly above and below the waist (avoiding the 2-inch radius surrounding the navel), the upper part of the buttock behind the hip bone, and the front part of the thigh (about 4 inches below the top of the thigh to about 4 inches above the knee).

Changing the injection site in a regular pattern helps avoid lipodystrophy. It is recommended, however, that the injection always be given in the same body area at the same regularly scheduled time of day. For example, if the stomach is the site used for the morning injection, this area should always be the morning injection site. This helps synchronize the timing and action of insulin in the body.

Lipoma

A benign tumor that develops from fatty tissue. Most lipomas occur on the thigh, trunk, or shoulder, although they can develop in any fatty tissues. Lipomas are the most common benign soft-tissue tumors. They commonly appear as slow-growing soft swellings and usually require no treatment. See also LIPOSARCOMA.

Lipoprotein

A substance that is made of varying amounts of CHOLESTEROL, TRIGLYCERIDES, lipids, and protein. Since fats are not soluble in water, lipoproteins carry fats through the blood. See LIPID-LIPOPROTEIN METABOLISM.

Liposarcoma

A cancerous tumor that develops from fatty tissue. Liposarcomas are usually found in the thigh or the back of the abdominal cavity, chiefly in middle-aged men. Liposarcomas tend to be large and to recur. Some liposarcoma cells may travel to the lungs or to the interior surface of the abdomen. Treatment of liposarcoma varies among patients. Some tumors can be easily removed surgically, while others require more extensive surgery and aggressive chemotherapy, with or without radiation therapy. See also LIPOMA.

Liposuction

A surgery that uses a suction device to permanently remove unwanted deposits of fat tissue and reshape specific body parts. Also known as lipoplasty and suction lipectomy, liposuction can be performed on the abdomen and waist, hips, buttocks, back, chest, neck, chin, and cheeks. The procedure works best on healthy individuals with normal body weight, firm skin, and pockets of excess fat. There is no age limitation, although the less elastic skin of older people may not achieve the same results as the more elastic skin of younger adults.

THE PROCEDURE

If a small or moderate amount of fat tissue is to be removed from only a few sites, liposuction is usually done as AMBULATORY SURGERY in the office of a physician or an outpatient surgery center. That is, the patient returns home on the same day that the surgery is performed. If a large volume of fat is to be removed, such as greater than 4 liters of fat, a blood transfusion is usually necessary. In that case, an overnight stay in a hospital may be required.

Anesthesia varies with the extent of liposuction. In less extensive surgeries, with a smaller amount of fat to be removed from a few sites, local anesthesia (see ANESTHESIA, LOCAL), often with CONSCIOUS SEDATION, is used. The patient is awake, but relaxed and pain-free. Regional anesthesia, which blocks pain in a portion of the body, is suitable for more extensive procedures. If a large volume of fat is to be removed, general anesthesia, in which the person is put to sleep in a temporary unconscious state, is preferred by many surgeons and patients.

HOW IT IS DONE

The surgeon makes small (one-fourth inch) incisions in the skin area to be suctioned. The incision is placed so that when it heals, any scar will be difficult to detect. A narrow hollow tube, called a cannula, is inserted through the incision to dislodge fat cells, which are sucked through the instrument and into a container. Since fluid is removed from the body along with the fat, it is important that the patient be monitored carefully

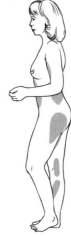

AREAS OFTEN TREATED BY LIPOSUCTION
Liposuction is most effective for small areas that are particularly resistant to fat reduction.

L

and receive intravenous fluids during and after surgery. Excessive fluid loss can lead to shock (see SHOCK, PHYSIOLOGICAL).

Once all the fat has been suctioned, small drain tubes may be inserted into the incisions, which are then closed with small stitches or sutures. In most cases, the liposuction procedure takes from 1 to 3 hours, depending on the number of sites and the volume of fat removed.

VARIATIONS

Many surgeons now favor combining the basic liposuction technique with fluid injection. A solution that contains salt, the local anesthetic lidocaine, and epinephrine (a medication that constricts blood vessels) is injected into the surgical site before the fat is removed. In addition to enhancing anesthesia, the solution reduces bleeding during surgery, makes suctioning easier, and decreases postsurgical bleeding.

In the tumescent technique, a very large amount of fluid is injected into the fat layer, as much as three times the volume of the fat to be removed. The fluid makes the surgical site look firm and swollen, or tumescent, which gives the technique its name. The tumescent technique often requires no additional anesthesia because of the solution's lidocaine content, but it may take slightly longer.

Another variation, called the superwet technique, utilizes less solution than the tumescent technique, typically a volume equal to the amount of fat to be suctioned. Conscious sedation or general anesthesia is usually necessary.

Ultrasound-assisted liposuction makes use of a special cannula that produces ultrasound waves, which liquefy the fat after dispersing the walls of fat cells. The fat is then suctioned. This technique is used in all parts of the body but is particularly useful in areas with large amounts of fibrous tissue, such as the upper back and the male breast. Because ultrasound-assisted liposuction is precise, it is also used in follow-up procedures to correct lumpiness or other problems that remain after an initial liposuction operation.

BEFORE AND AFTER SURGERY

Blood and urine laboratory tests may be required before surgery, and the

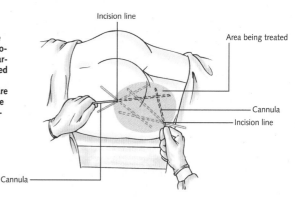

Incision line

Area being treated

Cannula

Incision line

Cannula

patient is typically screened for undetected conditions that may affect safety and outcome, such as high blood pressure or diabetes. As with any surgery that involves anesthesia, the person must have nothing to eat or drink after midnight the night before the operation. The surgeon may also provide instructions about medications or nutritional supplements that should be added or avoided in preparation for surgery.

After surgery, fluid drainage from the incisions is likely. If drain tubes have been inserted, they are left in place for about 48 hours and then removed. Pain, burning, tingling, swelling, soreness, and temporary numbness at the surgery sites are also to be expected. The pain can be controlled with prescription medications. To reduce swelling and facilitate a more even healing to minimize waviness in the skin, a snug elastic garment may be fitted over the surgical area and worn for a few weeks after surgery. Most bruising and swelling disappear within 3 weeks, but some swelling can remain for 6 months or longer. Stitches are removed after about a week or 10 days. If the sutures are dissolvable, they disappear in the same period.

Most people can return to driving and to work in a few days, and they begin to feel less tired (and less sore) within 2 weeks.

The improved body contour is usually apparent in 2 to 6 weeks, after most of the swelling has subsided. Once all swelling has disappeared, the final shape can be seen.

POSSIBLE COMPLICATIONS

Surgical risks for liposuction increase with the number of areas treated and with the volume of fat removed. Complications include infection, slow healing, damage to the skin or nerves, and waviness in the skin. Rarely, blood clots, perforation of organs with the cannula, or even death can occur. In the case of ultrasound-assisted liposuction, heat from the device can damage the skin or underlying tissues. In the case of the tumescent and superwet techniques, reaction to lidocaine and the collection of fluid in the lungs are potential risks.

Although liposuction scars are small and hidden from view in body folds and creases, the skin may heal in ways that leave it looking irregular or asymmetric. Numbness can also result, and skin pigmentation may rarely change. Additional surgery may be needed to repair unfavorable results.

Lipreading

Understanding speech by watching the movements of the lips rather than by listening to the sound. Lipreading is one of the processes by which an observer comprehends someone's spoken language when the observer is unable to hear what is being said. Also known as speechreading, it is commonly used by people with hearing loss to understand spoken language.

Lisinopril

An antihypertensive drug. Lisinopril (Prinivil, Zestril) is an angiotensin-converting enzyme (ACE) inhibitor used to treat high blood pressure, either alone or in combination with other high blood pressure medications. Lisinopril works by reducing the production of a substance that increases salt and water retention in the body and causes constriction of arteries, thereby driving up the blood pressure. Lisinopril may also be used to treat heart failure. If given within 24 hours of a heart attack, lisinopril may improve the person's chance of survival.

Lisp

The defective pronunciation of the sibilant letters s and z. See SPEECH DISORDERS.

Listeriosis

A serious bacterial infection that is common in livestock and infects humans when food contaminated with the bacterium *Listeria monocytogenes* is ingested. The bacterium that causes listeriosis is found in the intestines of several different animals, including nonhuman mammals, birds, arachnids, and crustaceans, as well as in soil and water.

Listeriosis bacteria are transmitted to humans by the ingestion of contaminated meat, dairy products, and raw vegetables. Raw and undercooked foods of animal origin and processed soft cheeses and cold cuts may be particularly vulnerable to contamination. Raw milk and products made from raw milk may be contaminated. The bacteria contaminate vegetables via the soil they grow in, especially when manure is used as fertilizer. Pasteurization and the usual heating methods for preparation of processed meats are generally sufficient to kill any bacteria present on these foods. However, contamination may occur after processing, and the bacteria can survive and grow under refrigeration. The peak period of infection occurs from July through August.

People in good health may ingest contaminated foods without becoming ill, but people in high-risk groups can acquire listeriosis after exposure to very few of the bacteria. People with weakened immune systems are highly susceptible to infection. Other persons most at risk include women who are pregnant, people who take glucocorticosteroid medications, older people, and people who have cancer, diabetes mellitus, or kidney disease. Butchers and slaughterhouse workers are at risk because of greater exposure to possibly infected animals.

SYMPTOMS AND DIAGNOSIS

An infected person has fever, muscle aches, and sometimes nausea and diarrhea. The infection can spread to the nervous system, possibly producing headache, stiff neck, confusion, loss of balance, and seizures. When infections occur in women who are pregnant, symptoms may be mild and flulike. Consequences during pregnancy can be serious, leading to premature delivery, infection of the newborn, or even spontaneous abortion and stillbirth.

Severe forms of the infection are rare but may produce bacteremia with high fever, meningitis, inflammation of the eyes, lymph node enlargement, and skin inflammation caused by direct contact with infected animal tissues.

A physical examination and clinical history of symptoms may be included in the initial diagnosis of listeriosis infections. Blood tests revealing the presence of antibodies to the bacteria within 2 to 4 weeks after symptoms begin are considered diagnostically conclusive.

The infection is treated with antibiotics such as penicillin, tobramycin, and erythromycin. When antibiotics are given promptly to a woman who is pregnant, infection of the fetus or newborn can be prevented. Babies who have been infected can also be successfully treated with antibiotics.

For some people who are at high risk, including older people and those with serious medical conditions, the infection can cause death, even with prompt treatment.

Lithium

An antimanic drug used to treat bipolar disorder, a psychiatric illness. Lithium (Eskalith, Lithobid) is an element found in nature that is similar to sodium and potassium. Although the mechanism by which it controls manic episodes is unclear, lithium is known to alter sodium transport and to regulate circuits in the brain, possibly by affecting the body's circadian rhythm (biological cycle over a 24-hour period). Lithium also enhances the amount of the neurotransmitters, norepinephrine and serotonin, in the brain.

Lithium is used to treat acute manic episodes in people with bipolar affective disorders. Maintenance therapy with lithium has been effective in preventing or diminishing the frequency of relapses in people with bipolar disorder who have a history of manic episodes. The drug must be taken under close medical supervision, because to be effective, plasma levels of lithium must be relatively close to toxic concentrations. To ensure that an adequate but nontoxic concentration has been reached, people who take lithium must have their blood tested regularly.

Lithotomy position

The position in which women lie on their backs with their legs or feet raised in stirrups, commonly used for gynecological examinations. The lithotomy position is also the traditional position for childbirth, because it allows a doctor or midwife easily to see the delivery and perform an EPISIOTOMY, if necessary. Some obstetricians think the lithotomy position may not be best for the baby and mother, because it slows the mother's return blood flow, lowers the supply of oxygen to the baby, makes pushing harder, and diminishes the effectiveness of uterine contractions (see CONTRACTIONS, UTERINE).

Lithotripsy

A procedure in which kidney stones are broken up into smaller pieces so they can be removed or flushed out in the urine. There are several ways of performing lithotripsy.

Extracorporeal shock wave lithotripsy (ESWL) is the most common approach to treating kidney stones. X rays or ULTRASOUND SCANNING helps the surgeon locate the stone. Most of the time, an anesthetic is required. The person being treated reclines in a container filled with water or on a soft cushion. Shock waves, generated outside the body, are used to break up the stones. The shock waves travel through the skin and other tissues to break the kidney stones into tiny sand-like particles that are then excreted in urine.

Percutaneous nephrolithotripsy is used to remove kidney stones when the stone is large or when ESWL cannot be effectively used because of the location of the stone. It is performed by passing a narrow tubelike instrument through a small incision in the back into a kidney. An instrument called a nephroscope allows the surgeon to locate and remove the stone. If the stone is very large, a small

L

PERCUTANEOUS LITHOTRIPSY
For percutaneous lithotripsy, to remove a large or awkwardly located stone, a small incision is made in the person's back and an instrument called a nephroscope is used to locate and remove the stone. If necessary, the stone will be broken up by ultrasound so that it can be removed easily.

ultrasonic or electrohydraulic energy probe may be used to fragment the stone; the small pieces are then removed. Percutaneous nephrolithotripsy generally requires a hospital stay of several days and may necessitate the placement of a nephrostomy tube, which is a small tube left in the kidney during the healing period.

Laser lithotripsy uses a laser to break up stones that have traveled to a ureter. The small fragments can then be flushed out in the urine.

Ureteroscopy uses a tiny fiberoptic telescope passed up a ureter from the bladder to view the kidney stone. The stone can then be either fragmented with a special instrument that produces a form of shock waves or removed intact with a small basketlike device. After the procedure, a small tube called a stent is left in the ureter for several days to aid in the healing of the ureter.

Live cell therapy

The use of live, healthy cells from embryos, thought to stimulate the growth and function of aging tissues. Live cell therapy involves the injection of live cells into the muscles of a person to "wake up" the person's own corresponding cells, creating new connective tissue in the process. Live cells are taken from shark, cow, and sheep embryos and are used to treat chronic skin disorders, muscular dystrophy, cancer, congenital defects, sexual dysfunctions, AIDS (acquired immunodeficiency syndrome), and many other diseases. Live cell therapy is one of the ANTIAGING THERAPIES not approved in the United States by the Food and Drug Administration.

Livedo reticularis

A skin reaction in which blotches develop in a netlike pattern on arms and legs. Livedo reticularis becomes more intense in response to cold temperatures. It is more obvious in pale skin and is more common in women than men. Blotches frequently occur in infants and children and are especially apparent at bath time. Livedo reticularis is due to changes in blood flow that lead to excess blood in the superficial veins. Blood is blue because of low oxygen content and stands in contrast to surrounding areas of normally pale skin. Livedo reticularis may be a benign (not cancerous) condition, but it is a blood vessel response to a disorder. It can be a sign of a more serious underlying illness, such as an infection, vascular problem, or connective tissue disorder.

Liver

An organ that performs complex functions relating to the processing, filtering, and regulating of chemicals in the blood. The liver also has a role in the digestive process. The liver—the largest organ in the body—lies in the upper right side of the abdomen, just under the diaphragm, over the intestine on the right side and the stomach on the left.

STRUCTURE

The liver has two lobes, right and left; the right lobe is the larger, and the left lobe tapers over the stomach. Three large blood vessels transport blood to and from the liver—two from the bottom of the organ and one from the top. The hepatic artery enters the underside of the liver from the heart, carrying oxygen-rich blood that travels to liver cells. The portal vein, also

entering from the underside, carries nutrient-rich blood from the digestive tract into the liver for processing. From the top side of the liver, the hepatic vein carries blood from the liver and into the vena cava, the major vein that drains into the heart. The hepatic duct, which leaves the liver from the underside, carries a liver secretion called bile to the GALLBLADDER for storage.

Liver tissue is composed of microscopic units called lobules. Each lobule contains liver cells called hepatocytes that do the liver's work; a branch of the hepatic artery, portal vein, and hepatic vein; and a bile duct. (Hepatic is a medical term that means related to the liver.)

FUNCTION

The numerous and complex chemical processing functions of the liver include manufacture, regulation, storage, filtering, and removal of waste products.

The liver manufactures chemical proteins to enrich the blood, such as albumin and globin. Albumin helps bind essential nutrients to blood cells; globin is a component of HEMOGLOBIN, which carries oxygen to red blood cells. Another protein made in the liver contributes to the body's defenses against infection. Clotting factors, also called coagulation factors, are produced in the liver to help prevent blood loss in case of injury.

The liver regulates the level of amino acids in the blood. (Amino acids are components of proteins, and proteins are the main structural elements of body cells.) If amino acid levels get too high, the liver filters them out and either stores them in some form or sends them to the kidneys to be excreted. Liver cells also regulate the levels of cholesterol (a fatlike substance) in the body. The liver manufactures blood cholesterol based in part on how much dietary cholesterol the person consumes in foods.

If levels of blood sugar (glucose) get too high, the liver cells remove it from the blood, convert it to another form called glycogen, and then store it. When blood glucose levels get too low and the body needs energy, the liver converts glycogen back into glucose and returns it to the blood supply. The glucose that is not stored in the liver is converted into fats that are sent out to be stored in body fat.

The liver also metabolizes toxic substances, including alcohol and other drugs, from the blood. After chemically detoxifying them, the liver cells secrete them into bile, which is then sent to the digestive system to be removed from the body.

Bile is a secretion of the liver composed of water, bile salts that help break down fats in the digestive system, pigments, and cholesterol, which helps carry fats throughout the body. Bile also contains the waste products of liver function. Bile is secreted into the network of bile ducts that penetrate the liver tissue and then exits the liver into the common hepatic duct that leads to the gallbladder. The gallbladder holds the bile until it is released into the small intestine. In the intestine, bile helps

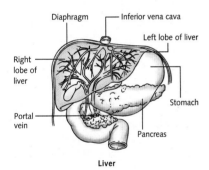

Liver

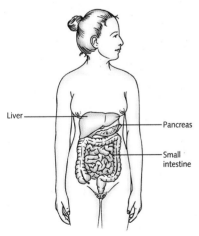

ANATOMY OF THE LIVER
The liver is a large, spongy organ of the digestive system lying over the stomach on the upper right side. It has right and left lobes. The portal vein carries blood from the digestive tract to the liver. The liver filters the nutrients in the blood and helps filter wastes, too.

break down fats and neutralize stomach acids. See BILIARY SYSTEM; BLOOD.

Liver abscess

A pus-filled sac in the liver that may be caused by an amebic infection, a bacterial infection, or trauma. Symptoms include night sweats, fever, chills, nausea, vomiting, loss of appetite, weight loss, and abdominal pain. Diagnosis is made through blood tests, X rays, and ultrasound scanning. Amebic dysentery should be suspected if a person has recently traveled to a developing country with poor sanitation. Depending on the underlying cause of an abscess, antiamebic drugs such as metronidazole or antibiotics are prescribed. For a liver abscess with a perforation (a hole in tissue), treatment is with needle aspiration (removal of fluid by suction), catheter drainage, or open surgical drainage.

Liver biopsy

A diagnostic procedure in which a needle is used to remove a small piece of the liver for testing. A liver biopsy is also known as a percutaneous liver biopsy (because a sample of tissue is obtained through the skin) or an aspiration biopsy (because the sample is suctioned through a needle). The tissue can also be obtained during a laparotomy (see LAPAROTOMY, EXPLORATORY), or through a laparoscopic procedure. The tissue is examined under a microscope for abnormalities or to assess the damage to the liver. This procedure may be performed in cases of HEPATITIS (inflammation of the liver), CIRRHOSIS (a severe liver disease), JAUNDICE (a yellowing of the skin and the whites of the eyes), HEPATOMEGALY (swelling or enlargement of the liver), repeated abnormal results of LIVER FUNCTION TESTS, abscesses, LIVER CANCER, or HEMOCHROMATOSIS (a disorder in which the body absorbs too much iron from food).

A liver biopsy can be done in a hospital on an outpatient basis. Food and drink must be avoided 4 to 8 hours before the test, and neither aspirin nor ibuprofen (which inhibit clotting function) should be taken for at least a week beforehand. In preparation, the doctor may perform platelet count and blood-clotting (prothrombin time) tests. A liver biopsy is not appropriate

for people who have clotting disorders, significant ascites (an abnormal collection of fluid inside the abdominal cavity), or tumors that are enlarged or are likely to bleed heavily.

An hour or so before the liver biopsy takes place, a person may be given a sedative to relax. During the procedure, it is necessary to lie completely still on the back with the right hand under the head. A radiologist may use CT (computed tomography) or ultrasound scanning to choose the location where the needle will be inserted, but often the site is determined by the technician tapping on the abdomen. A local anesthetic is given, and the patient is asked to breathe in, out, and then hold his or her breath as the needle is rapidly inserted and withdrawn from the chest wall. When the needle passes the phrenic nerve, there is a sensation resembling a punch to the right shoulder. After the test, pressure is applied to the site to stop any bleeding, and a bandage is placed over it.

Minor discomfort may be experienced during a liver biopsy. Acetaminophen (not aspirin or ibuprofen) can be taken to relieve soreness. The individual remains in the hospital for 4 to 8 hours while vital signs, such as pulse, temperature, and breathing rate, are monitored. The risks of a liver biopsy are slight, but include internal bleeding, the introduction of air into the chest cavity, and accidental puncture of an organ. If severe pain, difficulty breathing, or persistent bleeding is experienced after the test, the doctor should be contacted.

Liver cancer

Liver cancer is categorized as either primary or secondary. Primary liver cancer, which originates in the liver, is relatively rare in the United States. It is usually associated with a history of HEPATITIS B, HEPATITIS C, or some other chronic liver disease. Secondary liver cancer, the more common type, is metastatic, meaning that it has spread to the liver from other parts of the body (most commonly from cancer of the breast, lung, or intestinal tract). The symptoms of liver cancer include appetite loss, weight loss, fatigue, weakness, and abdominal discomfort. In the later stages, there may be jaundice (a yellowing of the skin

L

and the whites of the eyes) and ascites (an abnormal collection of fluid inside the abdominal cavity).

Diagnosis of liver cancer is made by physical examination and tests, such as a complete blood cell (CBC) count, liver function tests, imaging studies, and a LIVER BIOPSY. Because cancer is usually advanced once it has spread to the liver, the outlook is often poor, and LIVER FAILURE often results. However, if the cancer is localized in a small area, a surgeon may perform a partial removal of the liver (see HEPATECTOMY, PARTIAL). In some cases, RADIATION THERAPY and CHEMOTHERAPY are helpful.

Liver disease, alcoholic

Progressive liver damage due to excessive alcohol consumption. Alcohol abuse is a primary cause of liver disease in developed countries. Alcoholic liver disease progresses through three stages of rising severity: a fatty liver (in which fat accumulates inside liver cells), alcoholic HEPATITIS (inflammation of the liver due to excessive alcohol use), and finally CIRRHOSIS (a severe liver disease in which healthy cells are destroyed and replaced by scar tissue). Eventually, LIVER CANCER and LIVER FAILURE may result. Nonalcoholic steatohepatitis (NASH) has symptoms similar to those of alcoholic liver disease, but is not due to alcohol.

FATTY LIVER
Heavy use of alcohol causes an accumulation of fat in the liver. The body has no natural storage capacity for alcohol. Therefore, after alcohol is consumed, it is either excreted unchanged in the urine or breath or converted by liver cells into acetaldehyde, a toxic substance that can damage and eventually kill cells in the liver. People who have a fatty liver often experience no symptoms. However, the liver may be tender and enlarged, and results of LIVER FUNCTION TESTS are often abnormal. If alcohol use ceases, the problem is reversible. Fat disappears and the liver heals. If an individual continues to drink, however, irreversible scarring can develop.

ALCOHOLIC HEPATITIS
If, despite increasing signs of damage, a person continues to consume alcohol, alcoholic hepatitis can develop. As with a fatty liver, there may be no symptoms other than elevated liver function test results. However, inflammation causes individual liver cells to die, and eventually liver damage gradually worsens. Later symptoms may include losses of appetite and weight, weakness, fatigue, nausea, vomiting, and pain around the liver. Severe alcoholic hepatitis is a life-threatening condition characterized by fever, bleeding in the gastrointestinal tract, ascites (accumulation of fluid in the abdomen), and eventually liver failure.

Alcoholic hepatitis is sometimes difficult to distinguish from other gastrointestinal problems such as gallstones and viral hepatitis. X rays, blood analysis, and other tests are necessary for diagnosis. With hospitalization, most people recover from alcoholic hepatitis. Any further alcohol consumption is life-threatening, because the liver becomes permanently scarred. About a third of people with alcoholic hepatitis also have viral hepatitis C.

ALCOHOLIC CIRRHOSIS
The scarring or fibrosis of cirrhosis is the final stage of alcoholic liver disease. The seventh leading cause of death in the United States, cirrhosis obstructs blood flow through the liver. This prevents the liver from performing crucial tasks, such as the elimination of toxins, absorption of fats, manufacture of proteins, and storing and releasing of energy. Cirrhosis is a permanent and irreversible form of liver disease.

Symptoms of cirrhosis include JAUNDICE (a yellowing of the skin and the whites of the eyes), loss of appetite, gastrointestinal bleeding, and ascites (excess fluid in the abdomen). Possible complications are diabetes, kidney problems, ulcers, and bacterial infections. Although alcohol abuse is the most common cause of cirrhosis, genetic disorders or viral infections, such as hepatitis, can also cause it. Cirrhosis often leads to liver failure.

DIAGNOSIS AND TREATMENT
Alcoholic liver disease is diagnosed after repeated abnormal liver function test results, blood tests, CT (computed tomography) or ultrasound scanning, and often a liver biopsy, in which liver tissue is examined for unhealthy cells. Individuals with this disease must completely abstain from alcohol consumption. In some cases, although scarring is permanent and the liver afterward remains vulnerable to alcohol and infection, abstinence is sufficient to allow the liver to recover from damage. Sometimes, alcoholic liver disease progresses to life-threatening kidney failure, intestinal bleeding, or infection. If chronic liver failure develops, the only remaining option is liver transplantation. Success with a liver transplant depends on strict adherence to a treatment program. A transplant is considered only for those who have abstained from alcohol use for a minimum of 6 months.

RISK FACTORS AND PREVENTION
The amount of alcohol that causes liver damage varies. Significant permanent damage is most common in people who drink to excess for at least 5 or more consecutive years. Risk increases the more and the longer that one drinks. However, any amount of alcohol can potentially damage the liver, and even intermittent alcohol use can prove dangerous. Women are more sensitive than men to the effects of alcohol and typically develop liver problems, such as cirrhosis, more rapidly.

Liver failure

A condition in which a damaged liver can no longer meet the many demands placed upon it. Important functions of the liver include eliminating toxins, promoting absorption of fats, manufacturing proteins, and storing and releasing of energy. Liver failure, the final life-threatening stage of liver disease, means that the liver can no longer perform these vital tasks. Disorders that can result in liver failure include CIRRHOSIS (a liver disease in which healthy cells are destroyed and replaced by scar tissue), HEPATITIS (inflammation of the liver), severe alcoholic liver disease (see LIVER DISEASE, ALCOHOLIC), and LIVER CANCER.

The symptoms of liver failure include JAUNDICE (a yellowing of the skin and the whites of the eyes), HEPATOMEGALY (swelling or enlargement of the liver), loss of appetite, fatigue, weakness, malnutrition, confusion, and ascites (accumulation of fluid in the abdomen). Liver problems are diagnosed through blood tests, imaging studies such as ultrasound or CT (computed tomography) scanning, and a LIVER BIOPSY. In this type of biopsy, a needle is used to remove a small piece of the liver for diagnostic testing. The tissue is examined under a microscope to check for abnormalities and measure the amount of liver damage. (This is not an appropriate procedure for people who have clotting disorders, excess abdominal fluid, or tumors that are enlarged or contain many blood vessels that may bleed heavily.)

Early stages of certain types of liver disease (such as a fatty liver, the earliest level of alcoholic liver disease) are reversible. As with all liver ailments, complete abstinence from alcohol is an essential element of recovery. At other times, liver disease progresses to the permanent and irreversible scarring of cirrhosis. When a major portion of the liver is destroyed and the liver fails to function properly, the final treatment option is a liver transplant. Hepatitis C is currently the leading reason for liver transplants in the United States. Transplants are more successful when performed in cases of chronic liver failure that develops over time. When liver failure is sudden and acute and the transplant must be performed on an emergency basis, the outcome is less certain. A transplant is considered only for those who have abstained from alcohol use for a minimum of 6 months.

Liver fluke

A small flatworm that can invade the bile ducts of the liver. In the United States, the risk of infestation is confined to parts of the West and South and involves a specific type of fluke called *Fasciola hepatica*. This fluke is found in sheep feces and aquatic vegetation, especially watercress. An infestation can result in inflammation and obstruction of the bile ducts, enlargement of the liver, and jaundice (a yellowing of the skin and the whites of the eyes). Treatment is with medication. A different species of liver fluke that is associated with freshwater fish is common in far eastern Asia.

Liver function tests

Blood tests that assess the general health of the liver or biliary system. Abnormal results denote the possibility of liver damage or inflammation. Liver function tests, in combination with a physical examination and a medical history, are used to diagnose and plan treatment for a variety of liver diseases, including HEPATITIS (inflammation of the liver), CIRRHOSIS (a severe liver disease), and alcoholic liver disease.

Liver function tests include measurements of various enzymes, BILIRUBIN (a normal by-product of the breakdown of hemoglobin from aging red blood cells), and ammonia in the blood. The most common indicators of liver damage are the enzymes alanine aminotransferase (ALT) and aspartate aminotransferase (AST). Levels of these enzymes are elevated when they leak from injured liver cells into the blood. Because AST is also found in other organs, ALT is considered the more specific indicator of liver inflammation. The level of ALT is significantly increased in cases of acute viral hepatitis; however, it can remain in the normal range in a chronic liver disease such as cirrhosis. These enzymes formerly were commonly called SGOT and SGPT.

A test measuring levels of another enzyme, alkaline phosphatase (ALP), is used to detect obstruction in the biliary system. Comparing levels of gamma-glutamyl transferase (GGT) and ALP can help distinguish between liver and skeletal disease because ALP is elevated in the latter. The presence of excess bilirubin in the blood causes JAUNDICE (a yellowing of the skin and the whites of the eyes that is a symptom of many liver disorders). Liver disease may also cause high levels of ammonia, a protein by-product that is usually converted into urea and eliminated from the body.

Liver scan

A noninvasive technique used to record and display an image of the liver. Liver scans are useful in the diagnosis of problems such as abscesses and tumors. Before the test, a person receives an intravenous injection of a radioactive compound that is absorbed by the liver. A radiation detector records radiation emitted by the compound. The liver is photographed using a scintillation camera or X rays.

Liver transplant

Surgery in which a damaged liver is replaced with a healthy liver from a donor. Liver transplant surgery was first performed successfully in 1967. Technical modifications and the introduction of powerful immuno-suppressant drugs have made this complicated operation increasingly common and successful. Today, eight of ten people who undergo a liver transplant can resume their previous level of activity. The procedure is performed in cases of LIVER FAILURE, a condition in which the liver can no longer perform important functions, such as eliminating toxins, promoting absorption of fats, manufacturing proteins, and storing and releasing energy. Planned transplants for chronic liver failure are more successful than those performed on an emergency basis for acute liver failure.

Likely candidates for a liver transplant include those with disorders such as BILIARY CIRRHOSIS (a chronic liver disease that causes gradual, progressive destruction of bile ducts in the liver) and chronic active HEPATITIS (a continuing inflammation of the liver that damages liver cells; see also HEPATITIS, CHRONIC ACTIVE). HEPATITIS C cases currently account for the greatest number of liver transplants in the United States. In liver failure due to alcoholic cirrhosis (see LIVER DISEASE, ALCOHOLIC), a transplant is considered only for those who have abstained from alcohol use for a minimum of 6 months.

Liver donors are previously healthy people who, typically, have been pronounced brain-dead due to an accident. The liver is removed immediately after death and stored in a solution to preserve liver cells. Organ size and tissue type are significant factors in donor-recipient matching. Donors must be cancer-free, infection-free, and no older than age 55. Living donors may supply a lobe.

The transplant operation takes place in a hospital under general anesthesia. An incision is made in the upper abdomen. After cutting the hepatic artery, portal vein, and bile duct, the surgeon removes the diseased liver. The new liver is connected to the vena cava, the main vessel returning blood to the heart. The hepatic artery and portal vein are reconnected, and the donor bile ducts are joined to those in the body. The incision is closed, and large drainage

L

tubes are put in place. After a liver transplant, powerful immunosuppressive drugs are administered. Even though donated organs are matched as closely as possible, perfect matches are impossible. Drugs that suppress the immune system help to prevent rejection of the new organ by the patient's immune system. Although early immunosuppressive medications had many dangerous side effects, newer ones such as tacrolimus and cyclosporine, are much safer. People who receive cyclosporine need to be monitored closely because it can cause kidney problems. LIVER FUNCTION TESTS are performed regularly to monitor the new liver. Liver rejection and failure are uncommon after the first year.

Liver, cirrhosis of the
See CIRRHOSIS.

Living will
A document in which a person, while still mentally competent, directs his or her physician to withhold or withdraw life-sustaining treatment that would prolong life without the chance for meaningful recovery. A living will, a type of advance directive, normally becomes effective when a person is no longer capable of expressing his or her wishes and has become incapacitated or irreversibly unconscious or is in a persistent vegetative state (see ADVANCE DIRECTIVES).

LLETZ
See LEEP.

Lobe
One part of a clearly divisible organ; examples include the brain, lungs, and liver. A lobe may also be an extension of a structure, such as the earlobe.

Lobectomy
An operation to remove the lobe of an organ, such as the lung, liver, thyroid gland, or brain. A lobe is a clearly defined part into which such organs are divided. See LOBECTOMY, LIVER; LOBECTOMY, LUNG.

Lobectomy, liver
Surgical removal of one lobe or part of the liver. The liver is divided into

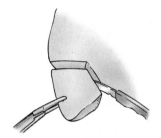

REMOVING A PART OF THE LIVER
A liver lobectomy is a procedure to remove one of the two lobes of the liver. It is done to remove a cancerous tumor, liver tissue damaged by injury, or a portion of a liver to be donated for a liver transplant.

two lobes by the gallbladder, with the left lobe being smaller than the right. In a lobectomy, one of the diseased lobes is removed and the other is left in place. The liver is the one internal organ that can regenerate; it grows back to its normal size within 6 to 8 weeks after surgery.

The most common reason for performing a liver lobectomy is to remove a cancerous tumor. This treatment is usually effective. If cancer has invaded the entire liver, a lobectomy is not a treatment option. Sometimes, the procedure is performed on patients with cancers that have spread beyond the liver as a way of alleviating symptoms caused by the tumor, even though a cure is not possible.

Benign, or noncancerous, tumors of the liver can also be treated with a lobectomy. A liver lobectomy may also be performed after an accident that damages a portion of the liver so severely that it cannot be saved. The procedure is also used to remove a portion of the liver from a donor who has agreed to donate his or her organ to another person. See LIVER TRANSPLANT.

THE PROCEDURE
A person being considered for a liver lobectomy as a treatment of liver cancer will be evaluated to ensure that the disease is confined to the liver. Typically, this screening consists of a CT (computed tomography) scan (a special type of X ray) of the abdomen, pelvis, and chest. A colonoscopy (an examination of the inside of the colon with a viewing tube) may also be performed since some liver cancers are caused by the spread of colon cancer.

A liver lobectomy is performed with the patient asleep and pain-free under general anesthesia. The proce-

dure typically takes 3 to 5 hours. It can usually be done without blood transfusions (see BLOODLESS SURGICAL TECHNIQUES). The patient spends about 5 days in the hospital after surgery and fully recovers in 6 to 8 weeks.

OUTLOOK
The only major side effect after surgery is postoperative pain, which can be relieved with oral pain medication. The person usually receives intravenous fluids for a few days, without eating or drinking, until full bowel function returns.

Lobectomy, lung
Surgical removal of one lobe of a lung. The right lung is divided into three distinct sections, or lobes; the smaller left lung has two lobes. A lung lobectomy involves the removal of one of these lobes, leaving the person with more lung tissue intact after surgery than would be the case with complete removal of the lung.

A lung lobectomy is usually performed to treat a malignant tumor. People with squamous cell carcinoma, large cell carcinoma, or adenocarcinoma (see LUNG CANCER) are candidates for surgery. Those with small cell carcinoma are seldom treated surgically because the disease moves too quickly and invasively to be totally removed. A lobectomy may also be used to treat a lung abscess, a severe, localized infection of the lung that can develop from inhaling contaminated material. If the abscess does not respond to antibiotics and drainage, a lobectomy may be needed.

A lobectomy is performed with the patient asleep and pain-free under general anesthesia. An incision is made in the chest; sometimes, a rib is removed for better access. The blood supply to the lobe to be removed is tied off with ligatures (see LIGATURE); then, the lobe is removed, along with any associated lymph nodes (see LYMPH NODE). Before the incision is sewn up, a tube is inserted into the surgical cavity to drain surgical air and fluids during healing. In certain cases, a lobectomy can be done by using a less invasive technique called video-assisted thoracic surgery, or VATS.

A lung lobectomy requires a hospital stay of 5 to 7 days, with a full recovery in about 4 weeks. Driving and vigorous exercise should be avoided until recovery is complete. Patients whose lungs were in good condition before the surgery usually have no impairment after a lung lobectomy. Those with tuberculosis, emphysema, or chronic bronchitis sometimes experience long-term shortness of breath. In patients with lung cancer, surgery may be followed by radiation therapy.

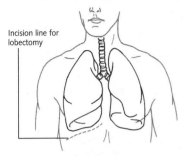

Incision line for lobectomy

Lungs before the procedure

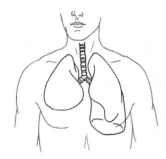

After lobectomy

REMOVAL OF A LOBE OF THE LUNG
For a lobectomy, an incision is made in the chest, and, if necessary, a rib may be removed to give the surgeon better access to the lung. Removal of only one of the lobes of the lung leaves some intact lung tissue on both sides, and an otherwise healthy person can recover with no impairment of lung function.

Lobotomy, prefrontal

A procedure, now considered obsolete, to cut the nerves connecting the frontal lobe to the rest of the brain. The procedure gained popularity in the mid-1930s and was hailed as a major step forward in treating patients with severe mental disease, such as SCHIZOPHRENIA and OBSESSIVE-COMPULSIVE DISORDER. The surgery had severe side effects, leaving patients with harmful personality changes. The development of effective medication for mental illness has made pre-

frontal lobotomy a treatment of last resort, used only with extremely severe disease that has failed to respond to any other treatment. The operation is now very rare, subject to review by state-appointed boards, and actually illegal in some parts of the United States.

Local anesthesia

See ANESTHESIA, LOCAL.

Lochia

The vaginal discharge that normally occurs after delivery of a baby. The lochia consists of mucus, blood, and tissue from the lining of the uterus. Usually, the lochia is bright red and as heavy or heavier at first than a menstrual period. The discharge then changes to pink, and then brown or yellow, tapers off and stops within 3 to 6 weeks after delivery. A sudden increase in the flow of lochia or the return of the bright red color can be signs that a woman is overexerting herself. A foul-smelling discharge or chills and fever may be signs of infection. A woman should contact her doctor immediately about any of these symptoms.

Lockjaw

See TETANUS.

Locomotor

Having to do with movement from one place to another; of or pertaining to locomotion. Locomotion in humans and other animals is possible because the locomotive system (consisting of bones, joints, and muscles) enables the body to move from place to place.

Loiasis

An infection caused by the larvae of a parasitic worm called *Loa loa*, which is transmitted to humans by the *Chrysops* fly. Flies become continually reinfected and spread the infection by biting infected humans, then transmitting the infection by biting uninfected humans. Loiasis is found principally in the rain forest and swamp forest regions of western Africa and is especially common in Cameroon and in the area of the Ogowe River. The infective parasitic larvae develop slowly into adult worms and then reproduce themselves inside the human body, residing and migrating through the upper

layers of skin. During their growth and development, they periodically travel through the deeper connective tissues below the skin and back to the skin's surface again.

Symptoms of loiasis are usually observed when the migrating adult worms appear near the surface of the skin, particularly around the eyes and the back of the hand and forearm. They can be removed at this time before damaging the membrane that covers the exposed surface of the eye. Swellings in the arms and legs may occur when the body's immune system responds to the internal migrations of the worms. The swelling may recur and cause connective tissue around the sheaths of the tendons to enlarge. These cystlike swellings can cause severe pain with movement. As the worms die off, they may cause chronic abscesses that form masses of scar tissue and overgrowths of fibrous tissue.

Loiasis can be treated with medications such as diethylcarbamazine, albendazole, or ivermectin. These medications kill or paralyze the worms or make them vulnerable to attack by the immune system.

Long QT syndrome

A rare, inherited, sometimes fatal disorder of the heart's electrical system. Heartbeat is controlled by electrical impulses that begin in a group of cells called the sinus node, which is located in the right atrium (upper right chamber) of the heart (see HEART for anatomical detail). The electrical signal moves across the atria (the two upper chambers of the heart), then to another group of cells called the atrioventricular (AV) node. The AV node connects to specialized fibers in the ventricles (lower chambers) of the heart that conduct the electrical signal and cause the ventricles to contract. The path of the electrical impulse through the heart muscle can be followed with an ECG (electrocardiogram) as a series of five waves identified as P, Q, R, S, and T. In long QT syndrome, the interval between the Q and T waves, which represents the time it takes for the ventricles to contract and rest before contracting again, is longer than normal. Under great emotional or physical stress, this abnormality may weaken the ability of the heart to maintain a nor-

L

mal rhythm and pump effectively. The result can be reduced blood flow to the brain, which may cause sudden fainting. People with this disorder may also develop a very fast heartbeat, which can accelerate to 350 beats per minute (ventricular fibrillation). This quickly tires the heart and, if untreated, causes it to stop pumping and death results.

Individuals with long QT syndrome must take care not to overexert or to engage in hard, strenuous exercise. Some prescription and over-the-counter medications that prolong the QT interval, such as certain antihistamines, antibiotics, and heart medications, have to be avoided. Beta blockers, a family of medications that slow heartbeat and decrease the number of nerve impulses affecting the heart, help protect against ventricular fibrillation under stress. If medication alone is insufficient, a PACEMAKER or an implantable DEFIBRILLATOR—devices that monitor the heartbeat and correct it if it becomes abnormal—can be put in place surgically. Emergency equipment should be kept on hand to prevent oxygen deprivation in the event of fainting or ventricular fibrillation.

Since long QT syndrome is inherited, there is no way to prevent it, and persons of both sexes are equally at risk. Early diagnosis and treatment offer the best protection against sudden death. Children of parents with the disease and those whose family members have had unexplained fainting spells should be tested for long QT syndrome.

Long-term care facility

A number of types of facilities designed for people who require custodial care for a longer period than is possible in a hospital. Long-term care is generally provided to people who have a chronic, progressive illness or disability. Many long-term care residents are older adults. The term nursing home is commonly used to describe these facilities but may be misleading. Some residents do not need nursing care, or their nursing care needs are minimal, while others may need extensive care. The expression long-term care encompasses all levels of care.

TYPES OF CARE FACILITIES

Long-term care options extend far beyond traditional nursing homes. Medicare and Medicaid programs use at least two designations to categorize long-term care facilities: skilled nursing facility and intermediate care facility. Some facilities may use different terms, and there are a number of types of facilities in addition to the government's designations. State authorities license most types of facilities. To qualify for Medicare or Medicaid reimbursement, those programs must approve the facilities.

■ *Nursing home* Also known as a nursing facility. A broad term for a facility that offers care for older people for a longer period than is possible in a hospital. Generally, the term applies to various levels of assisted living.

■ *Intermediate care facility* A government term for a residential facility for people who may need some health services; minimal nursing care; and limited help with eating, dressing, or getting around.

■ *Assisted living* Nonmedical housing with private apartment-style living and 24-hour services provided to individuals as required. Frequently used by older adults, this alternative is intended for those who cannot maintain their own households without assistance but do not require constant medical attention. In an assisted living arrangement, a staff oversees and monitors the needs of residents. Help is available for daily activities such as taking medications, bathing, grooming, dressing, and bathroom use. Services vary according to the facility but often include dining rooms, exercise classes, physical therapy, social programs, and recreational opportunities.

■ *Board-and-care homes* Group homes that provide rooms, meals, and limited assistance with daily activities such as bathing, grooming, dressing, and bathroom use. Board-and-care homes are an alternative for older people whose physical or mental ailments no longer permit them to live independently but who do not require constant medical attention. Although these are not medical facilities, staff provides protective supervision to residents, ensuring their safety and welfare. In some states, board-and-care homes are not licensed.

■ *Continuing care retirement communities* Often called CCRCs, these organizations provide a range of services and housing options on one campus. These include independent living, assisted living, and skilled nursing care. Older people may move from one component of a CCRC to another. For example, they may initially opt for independent living. As time goes on and more aid is required with daily activities such as bathing and dressing, an individual may move to assisted living. If skilled medical care is required, he or she may move to a nursing home on the same campus. Sometimes members of a married couple may reside in different areas, depending on the care each individual requires.

■ *Skilled care (or nursing) facility* An institution that provides physician coverage; 24-hour nursing services; and complete assistance with daily living, including feeding and hygiene. Long-term skilled care may also be administered in rehabilitation hospitals, psychiatric hospitals, hospitals for people with chronic diseases, and hospitals for those who are mentally disabled.

■ *Hospice* A facility or service that provides care for terminally ill people. The focus is on relieving pain, making an individual as comfortable as possible, and allowing people to spend meaningful time with family and close friends in a suitable environment. Care is available 24 hours a day. Hospice services may also be provided in a nursing home, hospital, or the individual's home.

CHOOSING A LONG-TERM CARE FACILITY

Those in need of a facility and their families should consult with a doctor or social worker to evaluate which type of long-term care facility is appropriate. Cost and location are major considerations. A facility that is convenient for family members to visit is desirable. Health professionals advise looking into facilities before the need arises; many of them have waiting lists, and choosing among them will be more difficult later in an emergency situation. Licenses and annual fire safety reports should be available for public inspection. State inspection reports, which assess how well the facility meets the state standards, should also be available to the public.

Adapting to a new environment can be challenging at any age. Older people need the support and reassurance of family and close friends at this time. Although it is normal for older people to be anxious about leaving their homes, many adjust very well to new living circumstances. The adjustment may be helped by a facility that allows residents to bring some of their possessions with them.

PAYING FOR LONG-TERM CARE FACILITIES

Long-term care for older people is costly. Except for specific LONG-TERM CARE INSURANCE, private insurance rarely covers long-term care. Public coverage of long-term care varies from state to state. Medicare helps pay some bills for eligible persons over 65. Most Medicare assistance is limited to 100 days. Medicaid may pick up some further charges for older people who have low incomes. Supplemental Security Income may cover part of the cost of board-and-care homes for low-income individuals in some states. In some cases, Medicaid may cover skilled care in a nursing home or other facility. However, to be eligible for Medicaid, an older person must deplete nearly all of his or her own income and assets. Coverage often depends on a recent hospitalization. The costs of continuing care retirement communities are considerable and usually must be paid by individuals.

Long-term care insurance

Private coverage for long-term custodial care in an assisted living center. Public programs offer minimal support for the significant expenses of a LONG-TERM CARE FACILITY. For example, Medicare will not pay for long-term custodial nursing home care. Although Medicaid does so, older people must deplete their assets to be eligible. Older people can buy long-term care insurance policies from private insurance companies. Eligibility, restrictions, costs, benefits, and the range of services covered vary among insurers. The coverage chosen determines the cost. In choosing a policy, important considerations are what conditions must be met to collect benefits, whether home care and hospice care are covered, and whether benefit amounts will increase over time to keep pace with inflation.

Loop electrosurgical excision procedure

See LEEP.

Loose bodies

A joint injury in which pieces of bone or cartilage break off into unattached fragments. Loose bodies usually cause pain, restricted range of motion, and increased damage to the joint. In the elbow, loose bodies can produce sensations of popping and catching in the joint. The fragments must be removed, usually by ARTHROSCOPIC SURGERY, to restore the joint's normal function and movement.

Loperamide

An antidiarrhea drug. Loperamide (Imodium, Kaopectate, and others) helps stop diarrhea by slowing the movements of the intestines, reducing the amount of fluid in the stool, and increasing the density of the stool. Loperamide is used to relieve the symptoms of acute and chronic diarrhea.

Loperamide in capsule form is available only by prescription, while liquid and tablet forms may be bought over-the-counter. Loperamide is usually used along with other measures to treat diarrhea. People with diarrhea must be careful to replace the lost fluid by drinking plenty of caffeine-free clear liquids. They must also avoid foods that may aggravate diarrhea, such as fruits, vegetables, fried or spicy foods, bran, candy, caffeine, and alcohol. Loperamide should be used with caution by people with liver or colon disease.

Loracarbef

See CEPHALOSPORINS.

Loratadine

An antihistamine. Loratadine (Claritin) is used to treat seasonal allergic rhinitis, or hay fever. Loratadine is a nonsedating, long-acting antihistamine that is also fast-acting: effects may be felt within 1 to 3 hours of taking a dose, and they may last more than 24 hours. Loratadine is used to relieve symptoms such as sneezing, runny nose, itching, watery eyes, and other allergy symptoms. It may also be used to treat hives (chronic urticaria).

Loratadine may cause dizziness or drowsiness, so people who take it are urged to use caution when driving or operating machinery. Alcohol can increase drowsiness and dizziness in people who are taking loratadine. Prolonged exposure to sunlight is also to be avoided because loratadine may increase the skin's sensitivity to sunlight.

Lorazepam

See BENZODIAZEPINES.

Lordosis

The abnormal curvature of the lumbar spine, or lower back. The curve of lordosis sometimes becomes more exaggerated when the abdomen is enlarged. This is an overcorrection in posture that helps maintain balance and may occur during pregnancy, with obesity, or when there are large tumors in the abdominal area. If the exaggeration of the curve is temporary, as in most of these cases, structural changes of the spine do not occur, and back problems do not result.

Hyperlordosis is a medical term for swayback, a common condition in young children, particularly girls, that improves by puberty. This condition may be caused by the rapid growth of the skeleton and insufficient stretching of surrounding soft tissues. Hyperlordosis is rarely a permanent condition caused by degenerative bone diseases, such as osteoporosis that affects the vertebrae or intervertebral disks. Treatments may include wearing a brace or lumbar

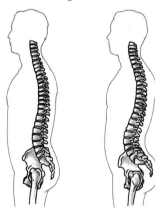

Healthy
spinal curvature

Spine with lordosis

INWARD CURVATURE OF THE SPINE
The spine naturally curves inward at the base of the neck and the base of the spine. Lordosis is an abnormal inward curvature that alters the relationship between the spinal column and the pelvis.

belt, and in severe cases, a surgical procedure may be recommended.

Losartan

An antihypertensive drug. Losartan (Cozaar) is a drug used to treat high blood pressure. It works by blocking the action of angiotensin, a hormone found in the body that causes blood vessels to tighten and salt and water to be retained. By blocking these actions, losartan lowers blood pressure. Losartan is also used together with diuretics to lower blood pressure.

Lou Gehrig disease

Amyotrophic lateral sclerosis, or ALS, the most common form of MOTOR NEU-RON DISEASE. Lou Gehrig disease is characterized by progressive loss of muscle function.

Lovastatin

A cholesterol-lowering drug. Lova-statin (Mevacor, Mevinolin) is used together with diet to treat people with primary hypercholesterolemia, or too much cholesterol. Lovastatin is also used to slow hardening of the arteries in people with coronary heart disease.

Keeping cholesterol levels normal is important to lower the risk of heart disease, particularly in people who are at risk. Lovastatin is usually pre-scribed only when a low-fat, low-cho-lesterol diet has failed to lower cho-lesterol levels enough. People who take lovastatin are still expected to maintain appropriate diet and exer-cise regimens to keep their choles-terol levels normal. The drug should be taken with meals and not be taken by a woman who is pregnant.

Ludwig angina

An acute bacterial infection that involves inflammation and swelling of the tissues of the neck, jaw, and the area below the tongue. Ludwig angi-na is a type of CELLULITIS that is the most common infection of the neck and surrounding tissues in adults; it is rare in children. It tends to occur following trauma or infectious condi-tions of the mouth, including infec-tion of the roots of the teeth that may be caused by a dental abscess. The associated swelling is rapid and can obstruct the airway.

The symptoms include neck pain and swelling, fever, weakness, ex-treme fatigue, and mental confusion.

Earache and drooling are sometimes associated with Ludwig angina. Breathing difficulty signals a medical emergency. Diagnosis is initially based on a physical examination revealing redness and swelling of the upper neck under the chin, possibly extending to the floor of the mouth. If the inflammation has spread to the tongue, it may be swollen or displaced in an upward position toward the rear of the mouth. A CT (computed tomog-raphy) scan can determine the extent of inflammation in the neck. Fluid from affected tissues may reveal *Streptococcus* or *Staphylococcus* bac-teria.

If the airway is blocked, emergency treatment may involve placing a breathing tube through the mouth or nose and into the trachea, or wind-pipe (a procedure called intubation) to allow the intake of air, or a surgical procedure called TRACHEOSTOMY, in which the airway is opened by inser-tion of a tube into the trachea through the lower front potion of the neck.

The infection can cause a general-ized infection or septic shock and may even be life-threatening if not treated promptly with antibiotics. Penicillin is usually given intra-venously until symptoms improve. Treatment of underlying causes of Ludwig angina, such as dental treat-ment of tooth infections, may be required.

Lumbar

Having to do with the lower back. The lumbar region of the human body is situated between the thorax, or chest, and the pelvis. This area includes the lower back and the loins, or the back and side of the body between the lowest rib and the pelvis. The word "lumbar" comes from the Latin word for loin.

The five lumbar vertebrae in the spinal column are those located between the thoracic or chest verte-brae and the sacral vertebrae (end-point of the vertebral column) and are sometimes referred to as L1 through L5. A lumbar puncture is a procedure in which spinal fluid is removed from the spinal column for diagnostic purposes. In this procedure, a hollow needle is inserted between the third and fourth lumbar vertebrae (L3 and L4), and a small quantity of spinal fluid is removed. Lumbar arteries are

those that arise from the aorta and supply the muscles of the loins, the skin of the sides of the abdomen, and the spinal cord.

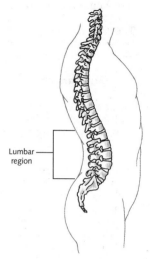

Lumbar region

LOWER BACK
The term lumbar is often used to describe the lower portion of the spine, between the ribs and the pelvis, composed of five vertebrae and the structures surrounding them. The term also describes other structures (nerves, muscles, blood vessels) or procedures performed in this general area.

Lumbar puncture

Also known as a spinal tap, a proce-dure that involves inserting a needle into the spinal canal to remove a sam-ple of CEREBROSPINAL FLUID (CSF). A lumbar puncture is most commonly performed to diagnose problems such as a subarachnoid hemorrhage (see HEMORRHAGE, SUBARACHNOID), ENCEPHALI-TIS, MENINGITIS, MULTIPLE SCLEROSIS, GUILLAIN-BARRÉ SYNDROME, REYE SYN-DROME, POLIO, and tumors or inflamma-tion of the brain or spinal cord. Less commonly, it is done to administer drugs, such as antibiotics or anesthet-ics, or to remove spinal fluid in order to decrease spinal fluid pressure.

A lumbar puncture can be performed in a doctor's office or in a hospital. It usually takes less than 20 minutes. In this procedure, a person typically lies on one side with the knees bent and pulled up and the chin touching the chest. Local anesthesia is injected into the lower back at the lumbar level. A needle is then inserted through the skin between the vertebrae into the spinal canal, and spinal fluid is removed for analysis. Following the

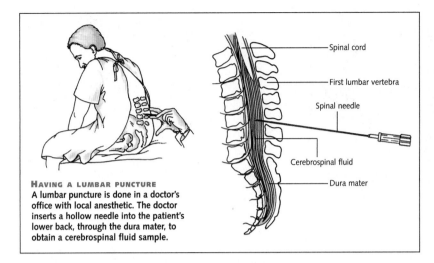

HAVING A LUMBAR PUNCTURE
A lumbar puncture is done in a doctor's office with local anesthetic. The doctor inserts a hollow needle into the patient's lower back, through the dura mater, to obtain a cerebrospinal fluid sample.

procedure, it is necessary to lie flat for 1 to 3 hours. The most common complication of a lumbar puncture is a headache.

Lumbosacral spasm

A tightening of the muscles that surround the lower part of the spine. Lumbosacral spasm can be prolonged or intermittent and is a common cause of BACK PAIN. It may result in temporary scoliosis, an S-shaped curvature of the spine. Treatment for back pain due to lumbosacral spasm depends on the cause, duration, and severity of discomfort.

Lumen

The space inside any tube or tubular body organ. A lumen may refer to a cavity or a channel within a body part. Examples of lumens include the spaces within intestines, blood vessels, and the airways used in breathing.

Lumpectomy

The removal of a lump in a woman's breast and some of the tissue around it to evaluate for or treat BREAST CANCER. In cases of breast cancer, a lumpectomy is usually followed by radiation therapy to the remaining part of the breast to reduce the chance of the cancer coming back. Most doctors also remove some of the lymph nodes under the arm. Many doctors now perform a lumpectomy for small tumors instead of a MASTECTOMY in women with breast cancer; a lumpectomy is less deforming than and as effective as a mastectomy in treating early breast cancer.

Lung

The major organ of the RESPIRATORY SYSTEM, in which oxygen from the air enters the bloodstream and is exchanged for the waste product carbon dioxide. The two lungs lie in the chest cavity, protected by the ribs. The upper end of each lung lies just above the collarbone, and the bottom ends rest on the diaphragm (the sheet of muscle that separates the chest cavity from the abdomen).

BREATHING, the mechanical drawing in and expelling of air, takes place by means of the rhythmic expansion and contraction of the spongy tissue of the lungs within the chest cavity. As air is drawn into the lungs during inhalation, the lungs begin to expand. The muscles between the ribs (intercostals) stretch to expand the rib cage, and the diaphragm also contracts up into the chest cavity. Each lung lies in two layers of membranous sac called the pleural membranes. One layer lies against the lungs, and the other layer lies against the inside of the rib cage. Between the two membranes is pleural fluid, which lubricates the surfaces of the membranes so that the lungs can expand and contract inside the chest cavity without friction. As air is exhaled from the lungs, the lungs deflate and the process is reversed: the intercostal muscles and the diaphragm relax, and the volume of the chest cavity decreases; air is expelled.

Air enters and leaves the lungs through the TRACHEA (windpipe). The trachea branches into two large bronchial tubes that lead directly into the lungs. Within each lung, the bronchial tube divides into three airways called main stem branches; each branch leads into one of three lobes (upper, lower, and middle) of the lung. The lobes subdivide into smaller areas called segments, with each segment supplied by an airway called a segmental bronchus. The bronchi continue to branch into successively smaller airways that penetrate the spongy lung tissue.

The smallest airways are the bronchioles, which end in tiny elastic air sacs called alveoli. An alveolus, the smallest functional unit in lung tissue, is covered by a net of capillaries. Through the walls of the alveoli and capillaries, oxygen passes from the air drawn into the alveoli into the blood, and carbon dioxide passes from the blood into the lungs to be expelled.

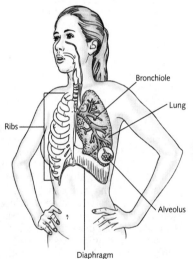

ANATOMY OF THE LUNG
The lungs lie in the chest, protected by the rib cage. The fundamental process of respiration occurs in the bronchioles, the smallest airways in lung tissue. A single bronchiole ends in a cluster of air sacs (alveoli). Through the walls of the alveoli, oxygen exchange with the bloodstream takes place at a cellular level.

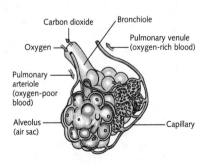

L

In medical terms, the mechanical process of breathing—inhaling oxygen and exhaling carbon dioxide—is called VENTILATION. RESPIRATION refers to the total process of bringing oxygen into the body, transporting it to the bloodstream in the lung tissue and exchanging it for the waste products of metabolism, absorbing oxygen into blood cells, and expelling the waste product carbon dioxide. The lungs are the principal organs involved in these processes. See also CARDIOVASCULAR SYSTEM.

Lung cancer

Cancer that originates in the lung. Lung cancer accounts for only about 15 percent of all new cancers in the United States, but is responsible for 25 percent of all cancer deaths, because it is frequently incurable. Early detection is difficult because symptoms often do not appear until the disease is advanced. Warning signs may include a persistent cough, coughing up blood, shortness of breath, hoarseness, persistent pain in the chest or upper back, and a persistent chest infection, such as pneumonia or bronchitis.

Lung cancer can take many years to develop. It commonly originates in the lining of the bronchi (the tubes that bring air from the windpipe to the lungs), but it can also start in other areas, such as the trachea, bronchioles, or alveoli. Once lung cancer develops, it can spread to other areas of the body and can be life-threatening. It often is not discovered until it has spread.

Tests used in the diagnosis of lung cancer include the following types of imaging tests: chest X ray; BRONCHOSCOPY, in which a narrow fiberoptic viewing instrument is used to examine the airways; CT (computed tomography) scanning and MRI (magnetic resonance imaging); and MEDIASTINOSCOPY, a procedure done under anesthesia in which a thin telescope is inserted through an incision in the neck. A needle biopsy of a lung lesion, in which a very thin needle is inserted through the chest wall, may also be used.

CAUSES

Most lung cancers are caused by smoking. Cancer-producing substances (see CARCINOGEN) in tobacco damage cells in the lung, and over time, the damaged cells may become

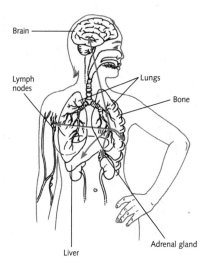

WHERE LUNG CANCER SPREADS
Lung cancer can spread to the bones, lymph nodes, liver, adrenal glands, and even the brain. Symptoms and treatment vary depending on where the cancer spreads. Some types of early stage cancer in the lung can be removed surgically, and radiation or chemotherapy can be used to treat cancer in the lungs or other areas of the body.

cancerous. People who smoke cigarettes, pipes, or cigars all have a considerably higher risk of developing lung cancer than nonsmokers; the longer they smoke, the more likely they are to develop the disease. Even people who do not smoke are at risk of developing lung cancer if they are exposed to secondhand or environmental tobacco smoke (the smoke left in the air by smokers).

Exposure to radon, an invisible, odorless, and tasteless gas, occurring naturally in soil and rocks, may cause lung cancer. People who work in mines are exposed to radon, and it is found in homes in some areas of the United States. Asbestos, a mineral formerly used in buildings as fireproof insulation, is a carcinogen. People who are exposed to asbestos are three to four times more likely to develop lung cancer than unexposed individuals.

TYPES OF LUNG CANCER

The two main types of lung cancer have different characteristics, requiring different treatment approaches. Most lung cancers—about 80 percent—are grouped as the non–small cell lung cancers, while most of the remaining lung cancers are considered SMALL CELL CARCINOMA, also called oat cell lung carcinomas.

■ *Small cell lung cancer* This disease is named for the relatively small size of its cancer cells. These cancer cells multiply quickly to the form large tumors, which spread to the lymph nodes and other organs, such as the bone marrow, brain, liver, and adrenal glands. Small cell lung cancer can spread to other organs at an early stage. Small cell lung cancer is usually caused by smoking; rarely does someone who has never smoked develop it. This type of cancer usually responds to chemotherapy and radiation therapy, although the response may last for only a limited amount of time. When small cell lung cancer is limited to the chest, it can be cured with radiation therapy and chemotherapy.

■ *Non–small cell lung cancer* The three main types of non–small cell lung cancer are named for the types of cells in which they develop: squamous cell carcinoma; adenocarcinoma; and large cell carcinoma. Surgery, chemotherapy, and radiation therapy are all used to treat all types of non–small cell lung cancers. Early-stage non–small cell lung cancers can be cured with surgery alone.

TREATMENT

Treatment of lung cancer depends on several factors, including the type of lung cancer, the stage of the disease, and the general health of the person. Different treatments, alone or in combination, are used.

■ *Surgery* Non–small cell lung cancers that have not spread can be surgically eliminated. Part of a lung along with the tumor (lobectomy) or the entire lung (pneumonectomy) may be removed. Because of their size or location, some tumors cannot be removed surgically. For some individuals in poor medical condition or with chronic lung conditions, surgery may not be an option. Small cell lung cancer is not usually treated with surgery.

■ *Chemotherapy* In this type of treatment, anticancer drugs are used to kill cancer cells throughout the body and may be used to control the growth of cancer or to relieve symptoms. Even after surgery has been used to remove a tumor, lung cancer cells may remain in the body, and chemotherapy may be used to control them. Chemotherapy does not cure non–small cell lung cancer that has spread to other organs.

■ *Radiation therapy* High-energy X rays can be used to kill cancer cells. Radiation therapy may be used before surgery to shrink a tumor or after surgery to destroy remaining cancer cells. Radiation can be administered externally, using a machine that focuses the radiation on the tumor area, or internally through a small container of radioactive material that is implanted directly into or near the tumor.

OUTLOOK

Lung cancer is more likely to be cured when the disease is diagnosed and treated before it has spread. Overall, 13 percent of people with lung cancer survive more than 5 years after diagnosis. However, those whose lung cancer was detected before it spread have a 5-year survival rate of between 33 and 80 percent. New treatments may eventually improve survival rates.

The best way to lower the risk of developing lung cancer is to stop smoking. There are no screening procedures, such as routine chest X ray, that have been of proven value in diagnosing lung cancer early. However, another imaging technique, CT (computed tomography) scanning, shows considerable promise.

Lung disease, chronic obstructive

See CHRONIC OBSTRUCTIVE PULMONARY DISEASE.

Lung imaging

Diagnostic techniques for viewing the lung tissue. Several procedures allow a doctor to examine the lungs. Chest X rays of the lungs may be taken from back to front and are sometimes supplemented with side views. X rays can help diagnose many serious diseases of the lungs and adjacent spaces, including pneumonia, lung tumors, collapsed lung, emphysema, and fluid in the pleural space. While X rays of the lungs may not reveal the exact cause of a condition or disease, they offer sufficient information to help determine the need for further testing to make a diagnosis.

CT SCANNING (computed tomography scanning) of the chest is a type of X ray that provides additional detail by creating several cross-sectional X-ray images of the lungs. A dye is sometimes administered orally or by injection to provide contrast for clarification of lung abnormalities. MRI (magnetic resonance imaging) produces images in great detail and is particularly useful for detecting blood vessel abnormalities. Ultrasound scanning is useful for detecting the presence of fluid in the pleural space, the space between the two layers covering the lungs. ULTRASOUND SCANNING may also be used to guide a needle into the space where the fluid is located to aspirate the fluid, or draw it out.

Nuclear scanning of the lung involves the use of short-lived radioactive materials to reveal air and blood flow through the lungs. It is helpful for detecting blood clots in an artery in the lungs, a condition called PULMONARY EMBOLISM, and may be used in preoperative assessments of lung cancer. A type of CT scanning called a spiral or helical CT is also useful for diagnosing a pulmonary embolism. ANGIOGRAPHY reveals the blood supply to the lungs and may be used to diagnose pulmonary embolism. However, since angiography is a more invasive procedure requiring the threading of a catheter into the pulmonary artery, it is reserved for cases in which the diagnosis remains uncertain after performing less invasive tests.

Lung surfactant

See SURFACTANT.

Lung transplantation

A complicated, high-risk surgical procedure in which a healthy lung or lungs replace damaged or diseased lungs. Lung transplantation is performed only as a lifesaving measure on people who have not responded to other treatment options, will not survive without the transplant, and have a high probability of a positive outcome from the transplant. Most people who successfully receive a transplanted lung or lungs can recover to live relatively normal lives, but long-term outcomes are not yet known. Single lung transplantation is more common than bilateral lung transplantation.

There are many limitations to lung transplantation. Finding appropriate donor lungs is difficult because the organs must match exactly the recipi-

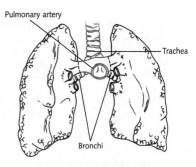

Pulmonary artery

Trachea

Bronchi

DOUBLE LUNG TRANSPLANT
The removal of both lungs, but not the heart, from a donor requires severing both atrial (heart) tissue and pulmonary (lung) arteries and veins—then reattaching or reconstructing both blood vessels and airways in the recipient. This elaborate surgery is becoming increasingly successful.

ent's body size, blood type, and tissue. The average waiting period for donor lungs is about 15 months. Immunosuppressant drugs used to prevent the body's immune system from rejecting the "foreign" tissue that is implanted are not uniformly effective. The costs associated with the entire procedure and subsequent care are extremely high.

The disease that most commonly results in the need for lung transplantation is chronic obstructive pulmonary disease (COPD). Other diseases that may ultimately be treated with the procedure include cystic fibrosis, pulmonary hypertension, pulmonary fibrosis, and emphysema.

Lung tumors

See LUNG CANCER.

Lung, collapsed

A physical event that occurs when air or gas collects in the chest cavity, exerting pressure on the lung and causing it to collapse. Collapsed lung is also referred to as PNEUMOTHORAX.

Lupus erythematosus, discoid

A form of lupus that most commonly causes red, round plaques (patches of thick raised skin) on the face, scalp, or ears. Lupus is an inflammatory autoimmune disease. It occurs when an unknown trigger causes the immune system to attack parts of the body as if they were foreign substances. Discoid lupus erythematosus

L

(DLE) is a less common and less severe form of lupus than systemic lupus erythematosus (SLE; see LUPUS ERYTHEMATOSUS, SYSTEMIC). While SLE can affect many organs in the body, DLE affects only the skin. DLE is suspected by its appearance and diagnosed through a biopsy of the rash. In DLE, the results of the blood test for antibodies typically used to detect SLE may be negative, or the antibodies may be present at a low level. Treatment of the skin rash is with corticosteroid creams or oral medications. Because sun sensitivity can be a problem, sunscreen, sunglasses, and protective clothing should be worn. In one of ten people, DLE progresses to SLE.

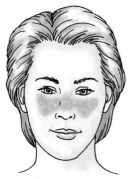

BUTTERFLY RASH
The most characteristic manifestation of discoid lupus erythematosus is a rash that covers the nose and flares out over the cheeks. The rash can also occur on the ears and scalp and, less commonly, on other parts of the body. The bumps are inflamed, scaly, and sometimes warty. Sunlight may aggravate the rash.

Lupus erythematosus, systemic

An autoimmune disorder that produces an uncommon form of arthritis that affects several tissues and internal organs. Systemic lupus erythematosus, which is commonly called SLE or lupus, causes the body's antibodies to damage cells and tissues in the body, which may include the joints, skin, kidneys, heart, lungs, pancreas, blood vessels, and brain.

Lupus occurs nine times more often in women than in men and occurs more frequently in African American than in white women. The causes of SLE may involve genetic, environmental, and hormonal factors. The disease usually begins when a person is between 20 and 40 years of age, but the onset may be difficult to pinpoint because symptoms vary widely. SLE can run in families, but the risk of developing the disease is low for children or siblings of an affected person.

SYMPTOMS AND DIAGNOSIS
Affected individuals may have a wide variety of symptoms that range from mild to severe. The most commonly experienced of these are extreme fatigue, painful or swollen joints due to arthritis, unexplained fevers, anorexia, anemia, skin rashes, and kidney problems. Skin rashes are common among those with SLE, and most have sun sensitivity. Characteristic features of these rashes may include a butterfly facial rash on the cheeks; a deeper, scarring rash on the exposed skin and scalp; and a blistering rash, which is rare. Like other rheumatic diseases, lupus can cause aches, pain, and stiffness in the joints, muscles, and bones. It is also characterized by intermittent episodes of symptoms, called flares, and periods of wellness, called remission.

Diagnosis is difficult because of the nature of the symptoms and is generally based on a medical history, a physical examination, and laboratory test results. The antinuclear antibody (ANA) blood test and other autoantibody blood tests may be useful in the diagnosis. Other tests may include an erythrocyte sedimentation rate (ESR) evaluation to indicate inflammation in the body, a urinalysis, skin or kidney biopsies, and a syphilis test, which may have a falsely positive result in some people with lupus who do not have syphilis.

TREATMENT
Treatment is aimed at preventing flares, treatment of flares when they occur, and minimizing the risk of complications. Nonsteroidal anti-inflammatory drugs (NSAIDs) such as aspirin or ibuprofen may be recommended to treat joint pain, fever, and swelling. Antimalarial medications may be beneficial because they may suppress parts of a person's immune response and prevent flares. Corticosteroid medications, such as prednisone, may be given orally, as skin creams, or by injection. Mainstays of treatment for lupus, these medications function by

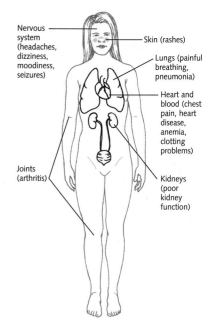

CHRONIC INFLAMMATION OF TISSUES
In a person with lupus, a combination of heredity, environmental factors, and hormones causes inflammation of tissues in different organs and parts of the body. The symptoms vary with the body part affected and can fluctuate within one person.

rapidly suppressing inflammation. Immunosuppressive medications may be prescribed to restrain the overactive immune system by inactivating or blocking the production of immune cells. These drugs may spare persons with SLE from the harmful effects of long-term corticosteroid treatment. When many body systems are affected, intravenous gamma globulin may be given to control severe bleeding, increase immunity, and help fight infection.

There is presently no known cure for lupus, but symptoms can be managed with medication. Most people who have lupus are able to live healthy, active lives.

Lupus pernio
A skin eruption characterized by small purple patches of thick raised skin on the head and neck. Lupus pernio is caused by SARCOIDOSIS (an inflammatory disease associated with an abnormal immune response).

Luteinizing hormone
See LH.

Luteinizing hormone–releasing hormone

See LH-RH.

Luxated tooth

A dislocated tooth that is usually caused by a direct blow to the mouth. When a permanent tooth has been dislocated, a dentist should be contacted immediately. The tooth may be reimplanted if it has been properly preserved. Storing the tooth in milk or saline, placing it under the tongue, or in the mouth between the gums and the inner side of the cheek, may help to keep it sound enough to be implanted back into the socket. The tooth should not be scrubbed clean so as not to disturb any tissue that is still on it. If a child has lost a permanent tooth and is unconscious, the tooth may be stored in a parent's mouth until the dentist can be seen. See also AVULSED TOOTH.

Lyme disease

FOR FIRST AID

see Bites and stings: tick bites, page 1315

A bacterial infection that is transmitted to humans by the bite of infected deer ticks and infected western black-legged ticks. Lyme disease is an inflammatory disorder that causes a rash, which may be followed by symptoms that appear weeks or months after the initial infection. The infection can affect the skin, joints, heart, and nervous system, with symptoms that persist for months or even years without treatment.

Lyme disease was named after the town of Lyme, Connecticut, where itwas first identified in 1976. Illness occurs most commonly in the spring and summer, particularly June, July, and August. Tick infestations can cause more than one person to acquire Lyme disease at the same time. However, the infection is not contagious among people in close contact.

The ticks that cause Lyme disease carry the bacterial spirochete called *Borrelia burgdorferi*. Also called Lyme borreliosis, Lyme disease is the most frequently diagnosed tick-borne disease in the United States. It is found most commonly in the northeastern, mid-Atlantic, and upper north-central regions of the United

---

PREVENTING LYME DISEASE

Lyme disease, an inflammatory disorder that usually starts with a rash, may quickly develop into other more serious symptoms that can cause damage to a person if not promptly treated. A person who thinks he or she might be in an area where Lyme disease is a concern should consider taking precautions.

- A vaccine that seems to be safe and effective is available and may be recommended to those who live in areas where contracting Lyme disease is a concern.
- Household pets should be kept free of fleas and ticks.
- Protective measures should be taken when time is spent outdoors in affected areas. These include wearing light-colored clothing so ticks can be seen before they bite, wearing long-sleeved shirts and long pants with pant legs tucked into tall boots or socks, and careful use of insect repellent.
- After possible exposure, the entire body should be carefully inspected to locate possible ticks.
- Attached ticks should be promptly removed, using tweezers to grasp the head of the tick at the skin's surface. (If no tweezers are available, the fingers should be covered with tissue for protection when removing a tick as contact with the tick's body fluids can transmit infection.) The tick should be pulled straight out from the site of attachment with a steady pull. The skin should be cleaned and disinfected with water, soap, and isopropyl alcohol, and a sterile bandage should be placed on the bite site.

States, where it is transmitted by the deer tick, and in Texas and several northwestern counties in California, where it is transmitted by western black-legged ticks. Both kinds of ticks are in the *Ixodes* group and are much smaller than common dog or cattle ticks. They are infectious in their larval and nymphal stages when they are the size of a pinhead and in the mature, adult stage when they are only slightly larger. The white-footed mouse is the primary animal reservoir for the bacterium that causes Lyme disease; deer ticks in their early stages feed on the mice. As adults, the ticks' preferred host is the white-tailed deer in the United States. Dogs may be incidental hosts and can develop Lyme disease if bitten by deer ticks.

The ticks feed on blood by inserting their mouthparts into the skin of an animal or person. They feed slowly and may remain attached to a person's skin for several days. Because of their small size, the *Ixodes* ticks may not be felt or noticed, even when they become engorged with blood. Transmission of the bacterium that causes Lyme disease does not occur until the infected tick has been feeding for 36 to 48 hours. The bacteria enter the skin at the site of the tick bite and spread in the lymph or through the blood to organs, structures, and other skin sites. The immune system's response to the infection then produces symptoms.

SYMPTOMS

There are three different stages of illness, with possible overlapping and apparent recovery between each stage.

The first stage occurs in as few as 3 days or as many as 28 days after exposure and may last for months. It begins with general flulike symptoms that may include fatigue, lethargy, headache, fever, chills, a stiff neck, aching muscles, possible muscle cramps, joint pain, backache, sore throat, swollen glands, abdominal pain, nausea, vomiting, dizziness, and a dry cough. Associated fever is usually mild but may be high, especially in children. Any or all symptoms may come and go, with fatigue and lethargy usually persisting.

During this first stage, most infected people develop an expanding, circular skin lesion surrounding the reddened site of the tick bite. This is usually less than 1 inch in diameter, but it can grow to 14 inches. It usually has the appearance of a red outer ring with a paler center and can be confused with RINGWORM. It may also have a dark red, hard center and form blisters that burst and develop a thick, dark scab, similar in appearance to a spider bite. The lesion at the site of the bite can sometimes remain small, repeatedly draining and scabbing over for several weeks. Periodic rashes may also appear, at different

OVERVIEW OF LYME DISEASE

Lyme disease is transmitted by the bite of certain ticks. This bite often leaves a rash and may lead to a broad range of symptoms.

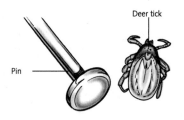

Pin

Deer tick

A HARD-SHELLED TICK
The deer tick is tan and about the size of a pinhead in the larval stage when it is most infectious.

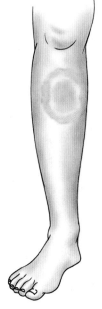

TYPICAL BULL'S-EYE RASH
A rash can develop and appear anywhere from a few hours to several weeks after a person is bitten by a tick. The red rash most often takes the shape of a "bull's-eye" surrounding the site of the bite.

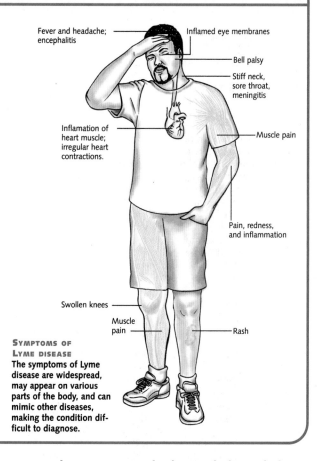

Fever and headache; encephalitis

Inflamed eye membranes

Bell palsy

Stiff neck, sore throat, meningitis

Inflamation of heart muscle; irregular heart contractions.

Muscle pain

Swollen knees

Muscle pain

Pain, redness, and inflammation

Rash

SYMPTOMS OF LYME DISEASE
The symptoms of Lyme disease are widespread, may appear on various parts of the body, and can mimic other diseases, making the condition difficult to diagnose.

---

times resembling hives, poison ivy, chicken pox, or insect bites. These rashes can be defined as circular or irregularly shaped areas of redness.

During stage two of Lyme disease, the nervous system and heart can become affected. Extremely severe headaches and neck pain with stiffness may be experienced for hours at a time. Some infected people develop sleep disturbances, poor concentration and memory, emotional instability, irritability, double vision, numbness and weakness in the extremities or the face, eye pain, and ear pain. Within several weeks of infection, a small percentage of infected people develop an unusually strong, rapid, or irregular heart beat; this symptom is generally temporary, lasting from 1 to 6 weeks, and seldom recurs.

Stage three of Lyme disease involves arthritic complications, experienced as joint pain that comes and goes, usually in the larger joints, such as the knees and hips. The symptoms may last for a few weeks to several months after the initial infection. In rare instances, ARTHRITIS may not appear for up to 2 years later. Attacks of associated joint pain may last for a few days and recur a few weeks later. Sometimes, the arthritis becomes chronic. Other ongoing symptoms may include chronic fatigue, psychological problems, or an illness resembling MULTIPLE SCLEROSIS.

DIAGNOSIS AND TREATMENT

Initial diagnosis may be made by a doctor's examination of the characteristic skin lesion and a clinical history that includes a reported tick bite or fleabite or residence in or travel to a suspected area. Blood tests for the bacteria that cause Lyme disease may be negative early in the course of the illness, but later antibodies to the bacteria may be found in the blood and can contribute to a diagnosis. When the joints have become involved, tests may be performed on the synovial fluid and membrane, and X rays may be evaluated. Other tests are sometimes done to differentiate Lyme disease from other disorders, especially JUVENILE RHEUMATOID ARTHRITIS in children and REITER SYNDROME and atypical RHEUMATOID ARTHRITIS in adults.

The success of treatment is improved by treating Lyme disease with antibiotics such as amoxicillin, doxycycline, or erythromycin as promptly as possible. A woman who is pregnant may be given amoxicillin. Most of the features and symptoms of the infection respond to antibiotic therapy, but recovery may be prolonged and extend beyond the period of treatment. If cardiac, joint, or neurological disease has developed, treatment with intravenous ceftriaxone or penicillin may be needed.

To relieve inflammatory and painful symptoms, nonsteroidal anti-inflammatory drugs (NSAIDs), including aspirin, may be recommended to infected persons older than 18 years. A temporary pacemaker may be required if there are significant cardiac symptoms. Swollen knee joints may be aspirated to remove excess fluid, and persistent arthritis of the knee may be treated with a surgical procedure called arthroscopic SYNOVECTOMY.

Lymph node

A small, hollow structure in a lymph vessel, generally occurring in clusters in some parts of the body. Lymph nodes contain concentrations of LYM-PHOCYTES, white blood cells that attack invading organisms such as bacteria and viruses. Lymphocytes travel in and out of the lymph nodes via lymph vessels to circulate freely throughout the bloodstream, searching for harmful organisms and repairing damaged cells. Inside the lymph nodes, the white blood cells trap and kill microorganisms. The lymph nodes are clustered at sites throughout the body where infection may enter, including the neck, armpits, abdomen, and groin. See LYMPHATIC SYSTEM; IMMUNE SYSTEM.

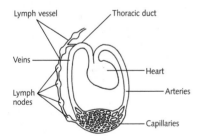

LYMPHATIC FLUID EXCHANGE
A lymph node is the smallest functional unit of the lymphatic system, which both drains fluids from body cells to be returned into the bloodstream and circulates lymphocytes (disease-fighting white blood cells) around the body. Fluid absorbed into the lymphatic system is filtered through at least one lymph node.

Lymphadenitis

An inflammation of one or more lymph nodes that may be caused by infection with bacteria, viruses, fungi, or other microorganisms that produce disease. Lymphadenitis occurs when these microorganisms are trapped in the lymph nodes, and white blood cells congregate to attack them. Pus, abscesses, and inflammation can occur as a result. The infection produces swollen, red areas of skin that are sometimes painful to the touch. Tuberculosis is a common cause of lymphadenitis, especially in the neck.

Lymphadenitis may be diagnosed by blood tests and a culture or biopsy of the person's lymph nodes. The treatment varies according to the microorganism that has caused the infection. Bacteria are a common cause and can be controlled within a few days with antibiotic therapy. Hot, moist compresses or a heating pad applied to the swollen, painful area, can help relieve discomfort. Aspirin or other nonsteroidal anti-inflammatory drugs (NSAIDs) may be recommended to treat associated pain. If there are abscesses, they may need to be surgically drained.

Lymphadenopathy

Abnormal enlargement of the lymph nodes. Lymphadenopathy most commonly occurs in the lymph nodes located in one area of the body, but it may also occur simultaneously in several unconnected areas. The disease is usually a result of a generalized infection in the body. The cause may be immediately obvious to a physician when diagnostic tests confirm a specific infection in the body. A common example of this is when a doctor palpates or feels the lymph nodes in the neck, finding them to be swollen and tender, and the result of a strep test is positive. In other cases, the cause of lymphadenopathy may be less clear, particularly when the swollen nodes are the only symptom or are one of several nonspecific symptoms. This may indicate that the lymphadenopathy is associated with serious illness, such as lymphoma, other malignant tumors, AIDS (acquired immunodeficiency syndrome), or major infection.

A complete medical history and a thorough physical examination are the initial basis for diagnosing the cause of lymphadenopathy. Usually this will produce a readily identifiable source of the problem such as an upper respiratory tract infection, pharyngitis, periodontal disease, conjunctivitis, lymphadenitis, tinea,

infected insect bites, a recent immunization, or some form of dermatitis. When no cause can be found, a surgical biopsy or fine-needle aspiration of the affected node or nodes may be recommended for diagnosis. Treatment of lymphadenopathy depends on the cause of the condition.

Lymphangioma

A benign (not cancerous) tumor in the skin composed of dilated lymph vessels. Lymphangiomas primarily occur on the arms and chest. They are usually removed by EXCISION (cutting away the tumor) for cosmetic reasons.

Lymphangitis

An inflammation of the channels of the lymph system that are located below the skin. Lymphangitis is commonly caused by *Streptococcus* bacteria that have entered the lymphatic channels through openings in the skin, such as abrasions, wounds, or infections on the extremities. CELLULITIS, an inflammation due to a bacterial infection of the skin and the tissues beneath the skin, is often involved.

Symptoms of lymphangitis include red, irregular, warm, and tender streaks that appear on the affected arm or leg near a skin lesion. The streaks appear to travel from the lesion toward the lymph nodes closest to the extremity involved, generally those in the armpits or the groin. The lymph nodes become enlarged and tender (see GLANDS, SWOLLEN).

Symptoms may include fever, chills with tremor, rapid heartbeat, and headache. In some instances, these symptoms can precede signs of local infection. They may be severe and may not be immediately perceived to be associated with what appears to be a minor skin wound or infection.

Diagnosis of lymphangitis is based on symptoms and signs. It may be possible to determine the infectious organism if cells can be cultured for laboratory evaluation. This can only be accomplished if there is pus, an open wound, or BACTEREMIA. It is important to treat lymphangitis promptly as there is a risk of bacteria spreading quickly through the lymph system. Also, cellulitis can progress to blood poisoning and tissue damage. In most cases, the infection and inflammation respond rapidly to antibiotic treatment.

Lymphatic system

A drainage system of vessels, glands, and ducts that channels a body fluid called lymph from tissues all over the body back into the bloodstream. The lymphatic system is a major part of the body's IMMUNE SYSTEM, which fights infection and cancer.

The lymphatic system is composed of a network of vessels running throughout the body, interspersed with small organs or glands called lymph nodes (see LYMPH NODE). In the course of normal body function, fluid passes through the walls of the capillaries in the circulatory system to provide body cells with oxygen and essential nutrients. Most of this fluid flows back through the capillary walls into the bloodstream laden with carbon dioxide and other waste products, but a quantity collects in body tissues and passes directly into the lymphatic vessels. These vessels carry the fluid back to the heart, just as the circulatory system does, but the fluid

in the lymphatic system is first filtered through the lymph nodes. In the lymph nodes, specialized white blood cells called lymphocytes destroy bacteria, viruses, and other harmful microorganisms and remove damaged cells. Lymphocytes can enter or leave the bloodstream through the lymph nodes to circulate throughout the bloodstream as well as the lymphatic system. Each lymph node includes its own artery and vein connecting it to the circulatory system.

Lymph nodes tend to be clustered throughout the body—for example, in the armpits and groin. When a particular part of the body is infected, the lymph vessels carry white blood cells and the harmful microorganisms to the lymph nodes closest to the site of the infection to be destroyed. The lymph nodes may become inflamed themselves as they fight off the invading organisms.

Lymphatic vessels also help absorb fats in the intestine. Within the walls

of the small intestine, a lymph vessel called a lacteal extends into the villi (tiny projections into the intestine through which nutrients are absorbed), where it absorbs fat globules. These fats are channeled into the lymphatic system to be emptied into the bloodstream for circulation throughout the body. See DIGESTIVE SYSTEM; INTESTINE.

Lymphocytes

A type of white blood cell that is the basic functional unit of the body's IMMUNE SYSTEM, which fights disease-causing microorganisms that invade the body.

There are about 1 trillion lymphocytes in the human body, all of which look identical under the microscope. They are differentiated by the distinctive molecules or markers they carry on their cell surface. These markers determine whether a lymphocyte is a B cell or a T cell, and within the two classes of cells, the markers determine specific behaviors of the cells.

Two types of lymphocyte work in different ways to destroy microorganisms: B cells manufacture antibodies, and T cells release toxic chemicals. These lymphocytes are "smart cells"—they recognize a specific invader and develop a specialized attack. This sophisticated response is part of the so-called adaptive immune system.

Most lymphocytes circulating in the body are T cells—white blood cells that have passed through the thymus gland during their development. In the thymus gland (an organ of the immune system located in the upper chest), the lymphocyte is specifically altered to perform the functions of the T cell. Two types of T cells work together. The helper T cell is critical to the immune response because it identifies the particular characteristics (antigens) of a disease organism or of body cells that have been damaged by infectious agents or cancer cells, and then it orchestrates the response from the second type of cell called a killer T cell. The killer cells travel to the site of infection, where they multiply rapidly. These new cells release a toxic substance called lymphokine that destroys the damaged cell and the invader.

B cells mount a so-called antibody defense against infection. Like helper T cells, B cells recognize antigens—

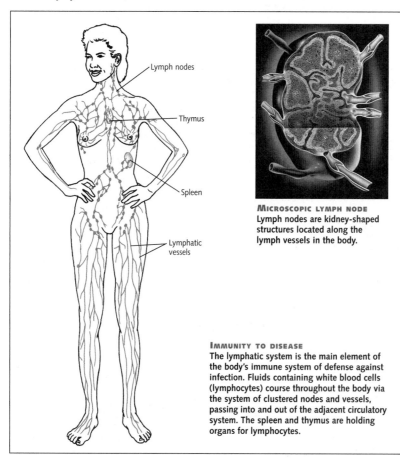

Lymph nodes

Thymus

Spleen

Lymphatic vessels

MICROSCOPIC LYMPH NODE
Lymph nodes are kidney-shaped structures located along the lymph vessels in the body.

IMMUNITY TO DISEASE
The lymphatic system is the main element of the body's immune system of defense against infection. Fluids containing white blood cells (lymphocytes) course throughout the body via the system of clustered nodes and vessels, passing into and out of the adjacent circulatory system. The spleen and thymus are holding organs for lymphocytes.

specific characteristics on the surface of a disease organism. In response, B cells multiply and transform themselves into plasma cells. The plasma cells manufacture antibodies (also called immunoglobulins) that are uniquely designed to attach to the specific antigen and destroy it.

After an infection has been successfully fought off, both T cells and B cells have the capacity to reserve some of their number to remain in the body as memory cells. These memory cells can quickly recognize the same invading organism if it enters the body again and multiply immediately to destroy it. This built-in protection against disease is called IMMUNITY. IMMUNIZATION works by infecting a person with a small amount of a prevalent disease organism so that the body fights it off and develops immunity. However, disease-causing organisms can develop new antigens (new strains of the organism) that the immune system cannot recognize. See LYMPHATIC SYSTEM.

Lymphogranuloma venereum

One of the SEXUALLY TRANSMITTED DISEASES (STDs); caused by specific types of the bacterium *Chlamydia trachomatis*. Lymphogranuloma venereum (LGV) occurs when these strains of bacteria invade and reproduce in the lymph nodes. This STD occurs mostly in tropical and subtropical areas; it is rare in the United States.

The incubation period of LGV is between 3 and 21 days. The first sign of infection is a small blister that forms in the genital area, possibly on the cervix or upper part of the vagina in women. The blister breaks open, then heals rapidly and may not be noticed. It is followed by enlarged, tender lymph nodes, or swollen glands (see GLANDS, SWOLLEN), on one side of the groin. This swelling develops into a large, tender mass within the tissues below the skin that produces inflammation of the skin's surface. A number of sores may develop on the skin's surface and produce a discharge containing pus or blood. Scars may form as the sores heal.

Other symptoms may include fever, malaise, headaches, joint pains, loss of appetite, and vomiting. Backaches may be experienced by women, and the infection's spread to the rectal wall in women or in persons who engage in anal sex may result in abscesses in the rectum, a narrowing of the rectal channel, and a rectal discharge that contains pus or blood. If the inflammation persists, it may obstruct the channels of the lymph system and can eventually produce genital ELEPHANTIASIS.

Diagnosis is made by a clinical history of symptoms and blood tests revealing elevated levels of antibodies. Antibiotic medications, including doxycycline, erythromycin, and tetracycline, taken for about 3 weeks can rapidly treat the early stages of LGV. Surgery may be required to treat abscesses, and plastic surgery can correct genital elephantiasis. A person who has received successful treatment will need further evaluation within 6 months. All sexual contacts of an infected person need to be informed of the disease and medically examined.

Lymphoma

A group of more than 24 types of cancers that develop in the LYMPHATIC SYSTEM, primarily in the lymph nodes and spleen. Different types of lymphoma behave differently. Some grow slowly, while others grow very quickly and can cause serious illness in a short time if they go untreated. Still others grow at moderate rates and are only moderately destructive. Lymphomas are classified by their appearance when examined under a microscope, and they are generally divided into two categories. If characteristic Reed-Sternberg cells are present, the lymphoma is HODGKIN DISEASE; all other lymphomas are considered non-Hodgkin lymphoma (see LYMPHOMA, NON-HODGKIN).

Lymphomas normally produce two types of symptoms: those related to the enlarged lymph nodes and generalized symptoms that affect the entire body. The first sign of lymphoma is usually an enlarged lymph node in the neck, the armpit, or the groin. The enlarged lymph nodes are usually at least an inch across, but are not typically tender or painful. Occasionally, they are mildly uncomfortable, particularly if they interfere with movement, as in the armpit or the neck.

Generalized symptoms include feeling unwell, sweating heavily during

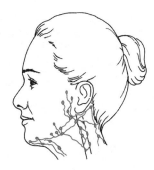

Normal lymph node cluster

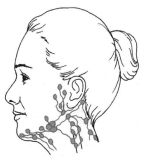

Swollen lymph nodes (lymphoma)

CANCER OF THE LYMPH SYSTEM
Lymph nodes are clustered in the neck, armpits, abdomen, and groin and contain white blood cells (lymphocytes) that fight disease-causing microorganisms such as bacteria and viruses. A cancer that strikes the lymph system (lymphoma) often first causes enlargement of the lymph nodes in, for example, the neck. This swelling is not necessarily painful. Lymphoma may also cause generalized symptoms (sweating, weight loss, and fatigue) that are felt throughout the body.

the night, and unintentionally losing weight and having lapses in energy and appetite. The causes of lymphoma are uncertain, although some forms are related to infection with the Epstein-Barr virus. Lymphomas are more common than usual in individuals who have weakened immune systems, such as people with AIDS (acquired immunodeficiency syndrome).

DIAGNOSIS AND TREATMENT
Diagnosis begins with a biopsy of an affected lymph node. The lymph node is removed and sent for microscopic examination, which may include analysis of the genes and chromosomes of the lymphoma cells in order to classify the type of lymphoma. If a lymphoma exists, further tests can detect whether it has spread beyond the lymph nodes. The tests

L

may include a chest X ray, an ultrasound scan of the liver, a bone marrow biopsy, a CT (computed tomography) scan or MRI (magnetic resonance imaging). Depending on the type of lymphoma and the extent of the disease, it may be treated with radiation, chemotherapy, immunotherapy, or bone marrow transplantation.

Lymphoma, non-Hodgkin

The cancers that develop in lymphatic tissue that are not HODGKIN DISEASE. Non-Hodgkin lymphoma accounts for about 5 percent of all cases of cancer in the United States. Symptoms usually include painless swelling of the lymph nodes in the neck, groin, or underarm. Other symptoms may include unexplained fever, night sweats, constant fatigue, unexplained weight loss, itchy skin, and reddened patches on the skin. Diagnosis requires several tests, including a biopsy of an affected lymph node. Blood tests, X rays, CT (computed tomography) scanning, and MRI (magnetic resonance imaging) are all used to find out the stage or extent of the disease.

TREATMENT

Treatment depends on the type of lymphoma and the extent of the disease. Staging, assessing the extent to which the lymphoma has developed, is an important part of planning the treatment. Staging non-Hodgkin lymphoma involves finding out the number and location of affected lymph nodes; whether they are above, below, or on the sides of the diaphragm (the tissue that separates the lungs and heart from the abdomen); and whether the disease has spread to the bone marrow, spleen, or to organs outside the lymphatic system, such as the liver. Non-Hodgkin lymphomas are categorized as low-, intermediate-, or high-grade, and their treatment varies accordingly.

■ *Low-grade lymphoma* Also known as indolent lymphoma, this type of lymphoma is slow-growing, and the affected lymph nodes sometimes fluctuate in size. Most low-grade lym-

phomas are widespread, and they are already generalized throughout the body by the time they are diagnosed. Although they grow slowly, they are almost always incurable. The disease can progress steadily throughout many years, while symptoms fluctuate and may even disappear from time to time. Treatment of low-grade lymphomas usually involves chemotherapy or radiation therapy when the person is experiencing symptoms. Once the symptoms have been controlled, treatment is stopped, until the symptoms reappear. In many cases, this intermittent treatment can continue for several years. Bone marrow transplantation (see BONE MARROW TRANSPLANT, ALLO-GENEIC; BONE MARROW TRANSPLANT, AUTOLOGOUS) is sometimes performed. A new therapy (immunotherapy) using antibodies that attack the cancerous cells has been shown to shrink lymphomas. Stage I (localized) low-grade lymphoma sometimes can be cured with radiation therapy alone.

■ *Intermediate- and high-grade lymphomas* Also known as aggressive lymphomas, these lymphomas progress more rapidly than low-grade lymphomas. Intermediate- and high-grade lymphomas can be cured with chemotherapy in about half of all cases. Intensive courses of several drugs are often necessary, requiring injections on different cycles for several weeks or months. This kind of treatment can be difficult for the person, who may experience many side effects and feel exhausted much of the time. Radiation therapy may be used to treat localized types of intermediate- and high-grade lymphomas, particularly if one large area of the body is affected.

RISK FACTORS

Doctors have identified several risk factors associated with non-Hodgkin lymphoma. Men are slightly more likely to get it than women; white people are more likely to get it than black people; and the likelihood of being diagnosed increases with age. The average age at diagnosis is 42. People with weakened immune systems have an increased risk for the disease. This group includes people with inherited immune deficiencies, people with HIV or AIDS (human immunodeficiency virus or acquired

immunodeficiency syndrome), and people taking immunosuppressive drugs after organ transplants. Viruses, including the Epstein-Barr virus, increase a person's chance of developing non-Hodgkin lymphoma. People who work with or are exposed to certain chemicals found in pesticides, solvents, and fertilizers may have a greater risk of developing non-Hodgkin lymphoma. The outlook for survival after diagnosis varies according to the type of non-Hodgkin lymphoma involved. About half those with the disease survive for at least 5 years after being diagnosed.

Lynch syndrome

See COLON CANCER, HEREDITARY NON-POLYPOSIS.

Lysis

A medical term for the destruction or dissolution of a cell or molecule by damage to its outer membrane. Lysis may be caused by chemical action, such as that of an enzyme, or physical action, such as heat or cold. Types of lysis include hemolysis, which is the breakdown of red blood cells with the release of hemoglobin into the surrounding liquid. The term "lysis" is also sometimes used to refer to sudden recovery from a fever.

Lysis of adhesions

A procedure to cut away scar tissue formed after earlier surgery. Those adhesions are most common in the abdomen. Because fibrous scar tissue is inelastic, adhesions in the abdomen can cause pain when they are stretched. In addition, adhesions involving the intestine can block or obstruct the digestive system, a condition that can be fatal if left untreated.

Lysis of adhesions is major surgery that requires general anesthesia. After the person is asleep and pain-free, either a large incision is made to open the abdomen and cut the adhesions free or the surgery is done less invasively through several small incisions with a laparoscope (a viewing tube). The choice of the open versus laparoscopic surgery depends upon the position and number of adhesions and other possible complications. Recovery after a laparoscopic procedure takes about 3 days versus an average of 7 days for open surgery.

L

Terms in small capital letters— for example, PHYSICAL THERAPY or PAGET DISEASE—indicate a cross-reference to another entry with more information.

Ma huang

An herbal supplement used as an energy booster. Ma huang is the Chinese name for *Ephedra*, the plant from which a drug (ephedrine) is derived that acts on the central nervous system much as amphetamines do—increasing blood pressure, speeding up the heart rate, and relaxing bronchial muscle. But the effects of ephedrine last about 10 times longer than those of amphetamines. Ma huang is marketed under many names as an aid to weight loss. It has been banned in several states and has been implicated in several deaths.

Macrobiotics

An extremely restricted diet plan based on organically grown whole grains, fresh vegetables, beans, and sea vegetables. No meat, animal fat, eggs, poultry, dairy products, refined sugar, strong alcoholic beverages, food additives, canned or frozen foods, or hot spices are consumed. Fish and seasonal fruits are for occasional use only. Macrobiotics also emphasizes chewing more (50 times per mouthful) and cooking on gas or wood stoves.

Because macrobiotics is a philosophical approach and not merely a diet, it also addresses lifestyle issues, stressing regular exercise, fresh air, positive outlook, cotton clothing, and using natural, nontoxic cosmetics and cleaning products. The macrobiotic approach views sickness as the body's attempt to return to a harmonious state with the natural environment. See more on page 911.

Macrocephaly

A congenital condition in which the head and brain are abnormally large in comparison with the rest of the body. Macrocephaly is associated with enlarged ventricles (HYDRO-CEPHALUS) or increased fluid and failure to develop parts of the brain (hydranencephaly).

Macroglossia

A congenital disorder in which the tongue is larger than usual. Macroglossia is seen in hereditary disorders such as Beckwith-Wiedemann syndrome (a genetic disorder related to glucose metabolism) and congenital HYPOTHYROIDISM. The symptoms of macroglossia include inarticulate speech and airway obstruction requiring surgery.

Macrolides

A class of antibiotics produced naturally by *Streptomyces*, a type of aerobic bacteria. The macrolides have a wide spectrum of activity and are used to treat infections in people who are allergic to penicillin. Among the infections treated with macrolides are *Streptococcus* infections, legionnaires disease, and chlamydial infections. Macrolides are also used to improve digestive activity in people with diabetes and to control severe cases of acne.

The macrolides currently available include azithromycin (Zithromax), clarithromycin (Biaxin), erythromycin, and many others.

Macular degeneration

A progressive disease of the eyes that affects the central portion of the retina (the light-sensitive layer at the back of the eye) and causes a gradual loss of vision. The central portion of the retina (macula) contains the greatest concentration of cones, the cells responsible for color vision and sharp, clear sight. The macula is the part of the eye that comes into play when one focuses or fixes on an object to see it clearly. In macular degeneration, the insulating layer between the retina and the underlying network of blood vessels (choroid) breaks down. Abnormal blood vessels may develop, which can rupture or leak blood and cause scar tissue to form; this, in turn, causes the macula to degenerate. Central vision fades as a result of this process, but vision to the sides (peripheral vision) remains unaffected. The disease may affect one or both eyes.

People with the disease are visually impaired but do not become totally blind, and they still have peripheral vision. However, as the disease progresses, they may lose the ability to drive and to read.

TYPES, SYMPTOMS, AND RISK FACTORS

There are two basic types of macular degeneration. In the dry (or atrophic) type, the degeneration usually proceeds slowly and vision loss is gradual. In the wet type, new blood vessels develop from the choroid, which can leak fluid under the retina, creating a large blind spot and rapid loss of central vision. Nine of ten cases of macular degeneration are the dry type.

The signs of macular degeneration are blurry or fuzzy vision, a dark or empty area in the center of the visual field, and the wavy appearance of straight lines (for example, sentences on a printed page, telephone poles along a road, or the sides of buildings). A diagnostic device called an Amsler grid, which consists of dark lines forming a square grid around a dot in the center, is used to diagnose and monitor the disease. Blurring of the grid or distortion of its lines into wavy, fuzzy, or missing areas can indicate macular degeneration. The eye specialist also inspects the back of the eye and may perform other tests, such as FLUORESCEIN ANGIOGRAM.

Most cases of macular degeneration are related to aging and are known as age-related macular degeneration. The disease affects one in six Americans between ages 55 and 64 years and one in four between ages 64 and 74 years. Certain rare hereditary forms of the disease occur at a younger age, even in childhood and adolescence.

Macular degeneration is more common in women and whites than in men, blacks, and Asians. People with light-colored skin and eyes are at greater risk. A hereditary factor is suspected even in age-related macular degeneration, since the disease tends to run in families. Other risk factors suggested by research and still under investigation include deficiencies of certain vitamins and antioxidants in the diet, uncontrolled high blood pressure, high blood cholesterol levels, exposure to ultraviolet light (primarily in the form of sunlight), smoking, and exposure to secondhand smoke.

TREATMENT AND PREVENTION

There is no proven treatment for dry macular degeneration. Rather, the person is taught how to adapt to the

FOCUS: MACULAR DEGENERATION

Macular degeneration is caused by a breakdown of the insulating layer between the retina (the light-sensitive layer at the back of the eye) and the choroid (the layer of blood vessels behind the retina). When fluid leaks into the choroid and forms scar tissue, destruction of the retinal nerve occurs. Central vision is subsequently affected while peripheral fields of vision are maintained.

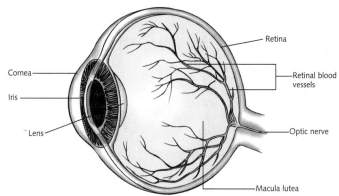

Cornea

Iris

Lens

Retina

Retinal blood vessels

Optic nerve

Macula lutea

MACULA LUTEA OF A NORMAL EYE
This yellowish depression on the retina just below the optic disc is the site of absorption of short wavelengths of light; it is believed that variations in coloring, size, and shape of the macula lutea may affect color vision.

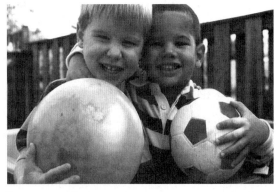

NORMAL VISION
This is an example of a scene as perceived by a person with normal vision.

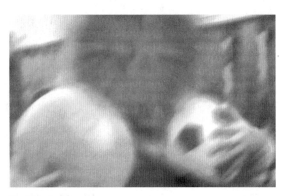

DISTORTED VISION
The same scene might look like this to a person with macular degeneration.

It was the best of times.
It was the worst of times.

No one would have believed in the last years of the nineteenth century that this world was being watched keenly and closely by intelligences greater than mans and yet as mortal as his own; that as men busied themselves about their various concerns they were scrutinized and studied, perhaps almost as narrowly as a man with a microscope might scrutinize the transient creatures that swarm and multiply in a drop of water.

DISTORTED TEXT
A block of text might appear like this to a person with macular degeneration.

M

loss of central vision with low-vision aids, such as magnifiers and reading lamps. Some research suggests that zinc diet supplements may slow progress of the disease. Studies of this possibility are continuing.

Some cases of wet macular degeneration can be treated with laser surgery. The eye surgeon focuses the laser beam on leaks in the choroid and seals them shut by coagulating the blood (photocoagulation). In many cases, this treatment cannot be used if leaks occur in the very center of the macula (the fovea, where the concentration of cone cells is highest), since more sight would be lost than gained from laser treatment. It also cannot be used if the choroid leaks cannot be visualized with diagnostic testing.

As a result, laser surgery is helpful for only one of two people with wet macular degeneration. Photodynamic therapy is a new procedure that may offer some benefit to those who cannot have laser surgery.

Certain possible risk factors for macular degeneration can be limited by lifestyle changes. Eating a diet low in cholesterol and rich in leafy dark-green vegetables, wearing sunglasses with ultraviolet protection, and avoiding tobacco may help delay or prevent the disease. See Focus: macular degeneration, page 818.

Macule

A flat skin spot about the size and shape of a freckle. A macule may be brown, blue, or red or a different color than surrounding skin.

Mad cow disease

Also known as bovine spongiform encephalopathy (BSE); a chronic, degenerative disorder that affects the central nervous system of cattle. Since 1996, concerns have arisen that there is a link between a disease in humans called new variant Creutzfeldt-Jakob disease and mad cow disease. Both are fatal brain diseases with unusually long incubation periods, and both are caused by unconventional transmissible agents. Mad cow disease has been a major public health problem in the United Kingdom. According to the Centers for Disease Control and Prevention, BSE is extremely unlikely to be a food-borne hazard in the United States.

Magnesium

A mineral essential in nutrition. Magnesium is important for healthy muscles, heart, and kidneys, and it is part of what makes up teeth and bones. Magnesium also activates many enzymes and is essential for healthy body functions. Adequate consumption of magnesium can reduce stress, insomnia, and feelings of depression.

Magnesium is available in many foods, and the best sources include blackstrap molasses, tofu, nuts, pumpkin seeds, green leafy vegetables, dried beans (legumes), whole grains, and soy flour. Other good sources include many cereals, whole wheat or oat flour, and bananas. Magnesium is also present in many herbs and spices, including coriander, dill weed, basil, cocoa powder, poppy seed, and tarragon.

Despite its ready availability in foods, some people in the United States do not get enough magnesium in their diets, and supplements are available. Magnesium is present in the laxative milk of magnesia, overuse of which can cause people to consume too much of the mineral, which can lead to serious health problems.

Magnet therapy

The use of magnetic devices placed on or near the body, thought by some to relieve pain and speed healing. Some people believe that fields produced by magnets can affect the func-

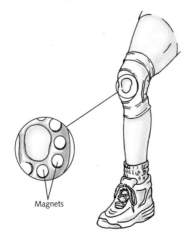

CLOSE-WRAPPED MAGNETS
In alternative medicine, magnet therapy is sometimes used for pain relief. Wraps are used to hold magnets close to joints or other areas of the body to direct the electromagnetic field.

tioning of cells to improve the working of the nervous system and internal organs. Magnetic devices come in many forms, including jewelry, shoe inserts, pillows, and mattresses. Magnet therapy is used to treat arthritis (especially osteoarthritis), insomnia, carpal tunnel syndrome, and headaches and is popular among professional athletes. It is controversial, in part because studies of the effects of magnet therapy on pain have produced contradictory results.

Magnetic resonance angiography
See MRI.

Magnetic resonance cholangiopancre-atography
See MRI.

Magnetic resonance imaging
See MRI.

Magnetic resonance spectroscopy
See MRI.

Malabsorption

Impaired absorption of nutrients through the small intestine. Malabsorption can be caused by enzyme deficiencies, pancreatic disorders, and intestinal diseases. See MALABSORPTION SYNDROME.

Malabsorption syndrome

Impaired absorption of nutrients in the small intestine. A number of diseases and conditions can damage the structure of the small intestine or diminish the presence of the enzymes that aid digestion. As a result, important vitamins, nutrients, and minerals fail to be absorbed by the body. Left untreated, serious long-term effects of malabsorption can include weight loss, fatigue, weakness, breathlessness, MALNUTRITION, iron-deficiency anemia (see ANEMIA, IRON-DEFICIENCY), vitamin B12–deficiency anemia, vitamin D deficiency, and death due to starvation.

SYMPTOMS AND CAUSES
Pale, greasy, foul-smelling stools are a common symptom of malabsorption. When fat passes through the intestine unabsorbed, stools tend to be greasy

M

and to float because of gas trapped within the stools. Additional symptoms include abdominal bloating, flatulence, and diarrhea. Signs of vitamin and mineral deficiencies due to malabsorption are a sore tongue, numbness and tingling sensations in the arms and legs, muscle cramps, and bone pain.

Conditions that commonly cause malabsorption include CELIAC DISEASE, CROHN DISEASE, LACTOSE INTOLERANCE, and LACTASE DEFICIENCY. Damage to the pancreas, which produces several enzymes essential for digestion, can also lead to malabsorption. Damage from celiac disease is due to the body's reaction to gluten, a protein found in grains such as wheat, rye, and barley. In Crohn disease, patches of the lining of the small intestine that normally absorb nutrients are destroyed by scarring. An insufficient amount of the enzyme lactase results in the inability to digest lactose, a sugar found in milk and milk products. Other possible causes of malabsorption are diabetes, pancreatitis (inflammation of the pancreas), and CYSTIC FIBROSIS (a genetic lung disorder). Malabsorption can also develop after digestive surgery (see BLIND LOOP SYNDROME).

DIAGNOSIS AND TREATMENT

Malabsorption is diagnosed by a complete physical examination and tests, such as stool analysis, blood tests, a GASTROINTESTINAL (GI) SERIES, and gastroscopy, in which the linings of the esophagus, stomach, and duodenum are examined by using a lighted viewing tube. If an abnormality is seen, a small tissue sample is taken for further analysis (see BIOPSY). In addition, a biopsy is performed on the duodenum. Once malabsorption has been diagnosed, treatment depends on its underlying cause. For example, the only effective treatment for celiac disease is avoiding all foods that contain gluten. Crohn disease is treated with anti-inflammatory drugs. People who are lactose intolerant should either avoid all dairy products or take tablets that contain lactase, the enzyme that makes digestion of milk possible. People with pancreatic insufficiency can take oral supplements of pancreatic enzymes that aid in digestion. To relieve symptoms, the doctor may also prescribe a low-fat diet that is high in protein and calories, along with vitamin and mineral supplements.

Maladjustment

In psychology, a person's failure to adapt his or her inner needs to the current life situation.

Malalignment

The abnormal positioning of the teeth in the jaw, producing an improper BITE. Malalignment, also called misalignment of the teeth, requires orthodontic treatment (see ORTHODONTICS) to correct the bite. If the condition is left untreated, the movement of the jaw may produce loosening or shifts in position of the opposing teeth or the adjacent teeth. The condition may also lead to headaches. See also MAL-OCCLUSION.

Malar flush

Sudden reddening of the skin around the cheekbones.

Malaria

A protozoal disease caused by a microscopic, single-celled parasite that is transmitted from person to person by a female *Anopheles* mosquito. Malaria is caused by infection with one of four different types of parasitic protozoa called plasmodia. Female *Anopheles* mosquitoes carry an infectious form of this parasite in their saliva. The parasite is transmitted to a person who has been bitten by an infected mosquito, and the parasite enters the person's bloodstream. Malaria begins when the parasites migrate through the bloodstream to the liver.

The parasites reproduce in the cells of the liver. After a week or two, parasites called merozoites are released from the infected liver cells. In some types of malaria, some infected liver cells may remain dormant for months. The released parasites invade immature red blood cells, where they mature and reproduce inside the cells. As they multiply within the red blood cells, the cells rupture and release more merozoites into the bloodstream. Once released, these parasites invade more red blood cells, causing them to rupture. When this episodic release occurs, this form of malaria results in repeated attacks of illness, possibly as often as every other day.

Some of the merozoites develop into another form of the parasite called gametocytes, which infect mosquitoes when they feed on a person who is infected with malaria. Inside the mosquitoes' bodies, the gametocytes evolve into an infectious form that transmits malaria to other people when they are bitten.

Another form of malaria occurs in a single episode of extremely severe illness that produces prolonged, irregular fever, chills, and trembling. This form of the disease, called falciparum malaria, results from infection by a certain species of plasmodia and is caused by the release of all of the parasites from the liver at the same time. The kidneys and brain may be affected, causing seizures, low blood pressure, and a low blood sugar level. Falciparum malaria must be treated immediately as it can cause death within a few hours.

When the plasmodia parasites destroy red blood cells, ANEMIA may develop, or the destroyed cells can develop into small masses that obstruct blood vessels and cause damage to the brain or kidney. Falciparum malaria carries the greater risk of obstruction of the blood vessels, which can be widespread and cause death.

The *Anopheles* mosquito that causes malaria exists most commonly in tropical and subtropical regions. There are an estimated 300 million cases of malaria worldwide each year. In the United States, malaria is very rare and generally occurs only when brought into the country from other regions, sometimes on airplanes and ships carrying infected mosquitoes. The *Anopheles* mosquito has been previously found in southeastern and western areas of the country, but has been mostly abolished from the United States by mosquito abatement programs. As more people travel to affected areas, the risk of person-to-person malaria transmission increases in countries where the disease is not commonly found. There have recently been as many as 1,100 cases of malaria each year in the United States and 1,000 cases a year in Canada.

SYMPTOMS

Symptoms of malaria tend to occur from 1 week to 1 month after a person has been bitten by a mosquito. In the less severe forms of malaria, symp-

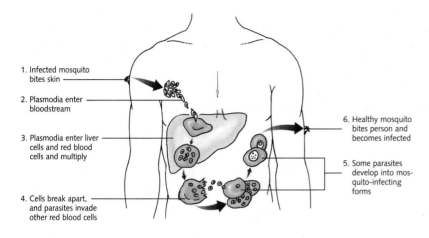

1. Infected mosquito bites skin

2. Plasmodia enter bloodstream

3. Plasmodia enter liver cells and red blood cells and multiply

4. Cells break apart, and parasites invade other red blood cells

6. Healthy mosquito bites person and becomes infected

5. Some parasites develop into mosquito-infecting forms

LIFE CYCLE OF A PARASITE
Mosquitoes carry the parasites (called plasmodia) that cause malaria in their saliva. When a mosquito bites a person, the infectious form of the parasite can be passed either way between them—from mosquito to the person, or from the person to the mosquito.

toms may include headache, fatigue, nausea, vomiting, and diarrhea lasting for 24 hours, followed by high fever, trembling, and chills lasting for 12 to 24 hours. Sudden chills may alternate with episodes of fever, marked by rapid breathing and an absence of perspiration. When the fever breaks, there is profuse perspiration. This syndrome is repeated each time the parasite is released again from the liver into the bloodstream, usually every 2 or 3 days. Untreated, symptoms associated with malaria may recur over a period of years. The immune system eventually establishes a defense against the parasite, and the number of recurrent bouts of disease diminishes.

Children who contract malaria tend to have a sustained high fever without chills. The elevated and prolonged fever may affect the brain, producing unconsciousness or seizures.

Falciparum malaria produces a single, extremely intense episode of alternating fever and chills that may last for 2 to 3 days and may be sufficiently severe to cause death.

DIAGNOSIS AND TREATMENT
Malaria is diagnosed by blood tests that can detect the plasmodia parasite. Several blood tests taken at given intervals may be required because the parasite is released intermittently into the bloodstream.

In the presence of severe symptoms, malaria may be treated immediately without waiting for blood test results.

There are several antiprotozoal medications that are effective against the illness. Chloroquine is a standard treatment for malaria, but the parasites in many areas are resistant to that drug. Quinine, mefloquine, pyrimethamine, sulfadoxine, and tetracycline are all effective when chloroquine is ineffective. Treatment is carefully monitored, as side effects, particularly nausea, occur with all protozoa-fighting medications.

There are antimalarial medications available, but a malaria vaccine does not yet exist.

Male sex hormones
See ANDROGEN HORMONES.

Malformation
Congenital defect resulting from abnormal prenatal development. Malformation can occur in a single organ or a larger area of the body and usually refers to a structural defect, such as a cleft lip. Malformation stems from abnormal differentiation of cells and tissues during early embryo development.

Malformation, congenital
A structural abnormality that is present at birth. Also known as BIRTH DEFECTS, congenital malformations include SPINA BIFIDA, CLEFT LIP AND PALATE, and structural defects of the heart.

Malignant
In medicine, the term used to describe a condition that becomes progressively worse over time and may result in death. In reference to a tumor, malignant signifies a cancerous growth or one that is likely to penetrate the tissues in the organ in which it originates. Malignant tumors tend to sink roots into the tissues around them, as well as to grow and spread. Malignant tumors invade surrounding tissues; nonmalignant cancers seldom spread to other parts of the body. Pathologists, doctors specializing in the study of diseased tissue, examine cancerous tissue microscopically to determine whether the tumor is fast-growing or slow-growing, grading the tumor according to its degree of malignancy. Some malignant tumors spread widely while the primary cancer remains small, escaping any notice. Other tumors grow locally quickly and are apparent right away. See METASTASIS.

Malignant melanoma
See MELANOMA, MALIGNANT.

Mallet finger
See BASEBALL FINGER.

Mallet toe
A deformity at the end of the toe that affects the movement of the toe, which may not be able to fully extend. Mallet toe can make walking uncomfortable and difficult. The toe can be tender to the touch, making closed shoes uncomfortable. The characteristic bony lump on top of the toe gives the toe a malletlike appearance. Mallet toe is frequently caused by wearing shoes that are too small. The second toe is most commonly affected. The first line of treatment emphasizes wearing well-fitted shoes. An orthotic appliance to be worn inside the shoes may be prescribed to properly position the toe, relieve the pressure on it, and ease the pain caused by walking. In some cases, corrective surgery is necessary.

Mallory-Weiss syndrome
A condition in which the lower end of the esophagus is torn by violent vomiting. This causes bleeding and

M

vomiting of blood. The esophagus usually heals on its own. The syndrome most frequently occurs in people with alcoholism, but may also be due to severe asthma, violent coughing, or epileptic seizures.

Malnutrition

A nutritional disorder that results from an imbalanced, inadequate, or excessive diet. Malnutrition may also be due to an underlying medical condition that interferes with the ability to obtain nutrients from foods, such as MALABSORPTION SYNDROME, in which the body becomes unable to absorb nutrients properly. In developing countries, the leading cause of death in children is malnutrition due to an inadequate intake of proteins, vitamins, and minerals. In the United States, malnutrition is more frequently associated with dietary imbalances.

Symptoms of malnutrition include unintentional weight loss, pale skin that bruises easily, thinness, bloating, rashes, changes in skin pigmentation, thin hair that falls out easily, bleeding gums, cracked lips, night blindness, abnormal sensitivity to light, anemia, diarrhea, disorientation, goiter, loss of reflexes, and muscle twitches. Diagnosis is often made through dietary assessment by a registered dietician, who can then recommend a diet to reestablish proper nutrition. In some cases, tube feeding or intravenous feeding is required (see PARENTERAL NUTRITION). Malnutrition can develop in people who consume too few or too many calories.

Undernutrition results from taking in too few nutrients or the body excreting them too rapidly. As a result, the body is not able to maintain healthy tissues and organ function. Factors such as chronic disease, infections, severe injury, substance abuse, diarrhea, and dieting can all have an impact on nutrient intake. For example, people with diseases such as cancer or AIDS (acquired immunodeficiency syndrome) may no longer be able to absorb or use vital nutrients. Certain groups require additional nutrients: infants, children, and pregnant women. In addition, many older people who do not take in adequate nutrients because of poor appetites, along with

people who lack the funds for a healthful diet, can become malnourished.

Overnutrition is more common than undernutrition in the United States. This condition is a result of factors such as overeating, consuming too many unhealthy foods, a lack of exercise, and taking too many dietary supplements. People who are obese or whose diets are high in fat and salt are particularly susceptible to this form of malnutrition. Despite an abundance of calories, these individuals can have vitamin or mineral deficiencies because of an unbalanced diet.

Malocclusion

An irregular alignment of the upper and lower teeth. Malocclusion is caused by any condition of the teeth or jaws that contributes to abnormal closure or meeting of the teeth and jaws during biting and chewing. When an abnormal BITE interferes with routine functioning of the teeth and constitutes a risk to the stability or health of adjacent or opposing teeth, orthodontic treatment (see ORTHODONTICS) is required to correct the condition. Malocclusion may also present a cosmetic problem that requires treatment.

CAUSES

Malocclusion usually begins in childhood with the normal development of the teeth and jaws. The causes of these problems may include nutritional deficiencies, hormonal imbalances, trauma, thumb-sucking, or heredity. Other causes may include the absence of some teeth, the presence of extra teeth, late eruption of permanent teeth or early loss of primary teeth, or ill-fitting dental restorations (see RESTORATION, DENTAL).

There are several types of malocclusion. A closed bite, also called a deep bite, involves the upper teeth covering the lower teeth when biting down. A CROSSBITE means some of the upper teeth are positioned inside the lower teeth when the jaws are closed. An open bite indicates that the front teeth are not coming together when biting down. An OVERBITE is when the upper teeth overlap the lower teeth when the jaw closes. Teeth that are crooked, overcrowded (see OVERCROWDING, DENTAL), or turned may also be called malocclusion.

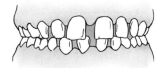

POOR CLOSURE OF THE TEETH
Misalignment of the upper and lower teeth can take many forms, and the resulting abnormal bite (meeting of the teeth) can be cosmetically unappealing or cause dental problems.

TREATMENT

Malocclusion may be a cosmetic problem that detracts from the appearance of a child or adult, or it may be diagnosed by a dentist who will offer a referral to an ORTHODONTIST (a specialist in treating malocclusion). An orthodontist can help to correct the positioning of the teeth by applying special fixed devices and appliances, called braces, to move the teeth into the proper alignment. The removal of some teeth and other surgical procedures may also be necessary, even with the use of braces. Common components of braces include brackets, the metal or ceramic pieces that are glued onto a tooth. The brackets serve to fasten the metal wire, called the arch wire, which moves the teeth. Plastic chains that stretch and attach the arch wires to the brackets to help move the teeth are called orthodontic chains. They may be available in several colors for children to choose from. Small, doughnut-shaped plastic pieces called ligating modules may also be used to hold the arch wires and the brackets on the teeth.

Braces require regular visits to the orthodontist. The length of time that a person may need to wear braces to correct malocclusion is determined by the orthodontist. The pressure applied to the teeth to move them into the correct position must be gradual, continual, and relatively gentle to prevent loosening of the teeth. For this reason, orthodontic appliances are generally worn for at least 2 years, and often longer. After they are removed, a removable dental retainer (see RETAINER, DENTAL) may be worn on the upper teeth to hold them in the correct position while the teeth become strongly attached to the jaw. The removable retainer is usually worn at night during sleep, but a person may also be instructed to wear the retainer during waking hours. A fixed retainer is often cemented on the lower teeth to keep them in place. This retainer often is worn indefinitely. It usually consists of two metal bands around the lower cuspids that are attached by a wire running behind the front teeth.

Malpractice

In medicine, a single act or ongoing conduct of a medical professional that does not meet established standards of care and that results in verifiable harm or damage to the person receiving treatment. Medical malpractice may involve an error or omission as a result of negligence, intentional wrongdoing, or ignorance.

LEGAL CONSIDERATIONS

As viewed by the legal system, medical malpractice involves the negligent conduct of a health care professional that directly results in death or injury to the person being treated. Cases in which professional judgment has detrimental results to the person under the professional's care may not necessarily be determined to be malpractice. To prove malpractice in such instances, there must be expert testimony about the acceptable standard of care as applied to the actions of the health care professional accused of malpractice, and testimony must demonstrate that there was a deviation from an acceptable level of care. This testimony can be countered by other experts.

Procedures for filing malpractice suits may vary from one state to another. In some states, an action for malpractice cannot be filed against a medical caregiver unless a written notice is offered to the physician or provider prior to filing the suit to provide an opportunity for settlement. Some states also require lawyers to certify that the malpractice case has been reviewed by a qualified physician who has determined that the malpractice action is justified.

Malpresentation

A position of the fetus immediately before childbirth that is not ideal and may cause problems during delivery. The part of the baby that is situated at the opening of the mother's pelvic cavity is called the presenting part and is normally the head, facing the mother's back. In some cases, a doctor

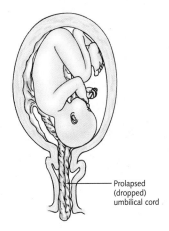

CORD PROLAPSE
Sometimes malpresentation in childbirth allows the umbilical cord to drop down into the cervix or vagina. In such a case, the baby's head may press on the cord, blocking his or her oxygen supply. To correct the problem, the doctor will reach into the vagina and manually move the baby's head off the cord. A cesarean section will be necessary to ensure a safe delivery.

Prolapsed (dropped) umbilical cord

can maneuver the fetus into the normal presentation position during the last few weeks of pregnancy, but in other cases, delivery may have to be by CESAREAN SECTION, forceps delivery, or vacuum extraction.

The most common malpresentations are BREECH PRESENTATION and occipital posterior presentation. In occipital posterior presentation, the baby's head is down but facing toward the mother's front, which is a difficult position in which to travel through the birth canal. Usually, the fetus rotates naturally to the correct position during delivery. If it does not, the doctor or midwife may deliver the baby vaginally, using forceps. In cases where a vaginal delivery is not considered safe, a cesarean section may be performed. Malpresentation can usually be diagnosed well in advance by pelvic examination, ultrasound, or X ray. Once a doctor has confirmed malpresentation, the mother will be monitored closely to see if the fetus spontaneously turns to the normal presentation. If it does not, careful management during labor is essential.

MALToma

Lymphomas that arise particularly in the gastrointestinal tract, but also in other organs. MALToma is a type of

LYMPHOMA that has only recently been recognized. (MALT stands for mucosa-associated lymphoid tissue.) It is associated with a particular bacterium and sometimes responds to treatment with antibiotics. MALTomas can also affect lymph nodes, where they tend to be localized and easily removed.

Malunion

A union of the fragments of a fractured bone in a crooked or faulty position. Tibial malunion can cause alignment problems in the ankles and knees. The condition may be treated by surgically refracturing and properly resetting the bone. Surgery may involve properly positioning the bone parts or bone grafting.

Mammary gland

See BREAST.

Mammogram

An X ray of a woman's breasts. Mammography is a safe, simple procedure requiring low doses of radiation. The resulting breast X rays, or mammograms, can help a doctor to diagnose breast cancer. Doctors recommend a mammogram for women younger than age 40 years for specific reasons (helping to evaluate an abnormality) or if there is a strong family history of breast cancer. Women ages 40 to 50 years should

M

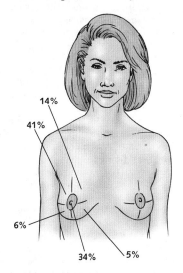

14%
41%
6%
34%
5%

WHERE BREAST TUMORS OCCUR
The percentages marked on the breast show where tumors are most likely to be found. Most tumors occur in the upper and outer quadrant or behind the nipple of each breast.

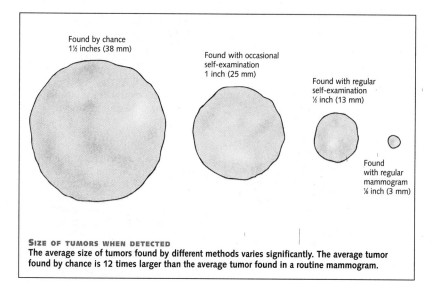

SIZE OF TUMORS WHEN DETECTED
The average size of tumors found by different methods varies significantly. The average tumor found by chance is 12 times larger than the average tumor found in a routine mammogram.

have a mammogram done every 1 to 2 years. Women older than 50 years should have a mammogram annually. Mammography exposes a woman's breasts to radiation; however, the dose is lower than the amount received naturally from the environment over a year's time.

An X-ray technician usually performs the mammography procedure, and a radiologist, a doctor specially trained in the use of X rays and other imaging techniques, interprets the results. Before having a mammography procedure, a woman should not wear powders, lotions, or deodorants because they can show up on the X ray. For each X-ray procedure, one of a woman's breasts is compressed between two flat, transparent plates. X rays may also be taken without the plates to obtain other X-ray views. The pressure of the plates may cause brief discomfort. Doctors recommend scheduling mammography at a time in the menstrual cycle when breasts are the least tender.

Some women rely on mammography alone to detect breast abnormalities. This tendency is dangerous because mammograms can sometimes miss breast cancers, even some cancers that can be felt. To decrease the risk of not detecting the disease, a woman should rely on a combination of methods to detect breast cancer, including regular self-examination, visits to the doctor, ultrasound scans, and mammography.

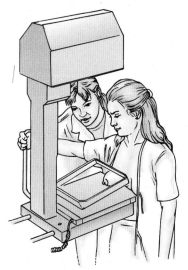

HOW A MAMMOGRAM IS TAKEN
For a mammography procedure, a trained technician positions a woman's breast between two transparent plates, and the breast is momentarily flattened so that an X-ray image can be taken. The procedure may be slightly uncomfortable, so it is best to schedule it at a time of the month when the breasts are least likely to be tender.

Mammography
See MAMMOGRAM.

Managed care
A health care system in which there is administrative control over primary health care services in a group practice. Medical care is usually coordinated by one primary care provider, who makes referrals as needed to specialists within the group. The goal of managed care is to streamline costs by emphasizing prevention and education and eliminating unnecessary services. Managed care has largely replaced the direct payment of a fee for services by a person to his or her physician. Instead, most people pay a set monthly premium to a health insurance organization regardless of the amount of services they do or do not require; the organization pays doctors and hospitals from premiums paid by subscribers. See also HMO and PPO.

Mandible
The bone of the lower jaw.

Mandibular orthopedic repositioning appliance
A type of splint worn on the lower jaw to correct a misalignment. This appliance, which may be referred to as MORA, is used to treat displacement of the lower jaw and to relieve temporomandibular joint disorder (TMJ; see CLICKING JAW). It may also be worn in combination with a MOUTH GUARD to help support the muscles and teeth of the lower jaw and to protect the lower teeth from physical injury during sports.

Mandibulofacial dysostosis
A birth defect (see BIRTH DEFECTS) characterized by a group of deformities affecting the size and shape of the ears, eyelids, cheekbones, and jaw. The condition is also called Treacher Collins syndrome. The extent of deformity varies from one individual to another. The syndrome is caused by a genetic abnormality. If neither parent of an infant born with mandibulofacial dysostosis shows signs of the syndrome, the abnormality is the result of a change in the genetic material at the time of conception; the exact cause of this change is unknown.

Physical features of mandibulofacial dysostosis may include downslanting eyes; notches in the lower eyelids; a prominent nose; a broad mouth; a small chin with a steeply angled lower jaw; underdeveloped, malformed, or prominent ears; and growth of hair extending in front of

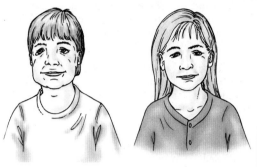

the ears. HEARING LOSS often accompanies the syndrome, and the person may also have problems breathing and eating. Less frequently, physical features include cleft lip or cleft palate, heart defects, and crossed eyes.

TREATMENT
Early diagnosis and treatment of hearing loss can prevent possible developmental and educational disabilities. The use of HEARING AIDS usually helps to correct hearing loss. Speech and language therapy may be required. Reconstructive facial surgery can improve the abnormal appearance of the face and close a cleft palate, which might interfere with the development of normal speech. GENETIC COUNSELING may be helpful to people with mandibulofacial dysostosis and their families. It is recommended that a craniofacial center (medical facility devoted to disorders of the skull and face) be consulted for help in coordinating evaluation and treatment, including referrals to support groups.

Mania
A mood state characterized by a persistently euphoric mood, decreased need for sleep, high physical energy, overspending, speeding while driving, increased sexual activity, rapid speech, loss of self-control and judgment, unrealistic beliefs in one's powers and abilities, racing thoughts, and disturbed appetite lasting for at least 1 week. Drug abuse, particularly of alcohol, cocaine, or sleeping medications, is common. Mania is a sign of BIPOLAR DISORDER. An underlying serious medical condition should be considered if mania occurs in an older person.

Manic-depressive illness
A mental disease characterized by extreme mood swings from high to low. See BIPOLAR DISORDER.

Manipulation
A technique used in the practice of CHIROPRACTIC, osteopathic medicine, and PHYSICAL THERAPY, which involves manual movements applied to the vertebrae of the spine and the body's joints and muscles. The basic premise of this technique is that this manipulation enhances the flow of nerve impulses to the brain and augments the body's natural ability to heal itself. Similar techniques of massage may be used in physical therapy to help improve or restore physical functioning to areas of the body debilitated by disease or injury.

Manometry
A technique for measuring changes in the pressure of gases or liquids as a result of biological or chemical actions. For example, in esophageal manometry, a tube is passed through the mouth or nose down into the stomach. To evaluate swallowing difficulties, pressure measurements are taken at intervals along the tube as a person swallows.

Mantoux test
See TUBERCULIN SKIN TEST.

Manual lymph drainage
The use of massage to reverse swelling by encouraging the drainage of lymph from tissues into the bloodstream. Lymphatic drainage is thought to encourage the transport of disease-causing substances to the lymph nodes, where they are inactivated. This process is thought to strengthen resistance to disease. Manual lymph drainage involves very light, rhythmic massage and is used in DETOXIFICATION or cases in which lymph circulation has been impaired by cancer, radiation therapy, or surgery.

MAOIs
See MONOAMINE OXIDASE INHIBITORS.

Marasmus
An especially severe form of malnutrition that develops from prolonged deficiency of caloric intake. Marasmus develops primarily in countries with famine conditions. It is always associated with protein deficiency, even when protein is being consumed regularly, because the body cannot metabolize protein without adequate caloric intake.

March fracture
A break or fracture of a bone that occurs as a result of prolonged or repeated marching, running, or other stress. March fractures can occur in any bone but most commonly appear in the metatarsal bones of the feet or in the lower leg. This kind of break is sometimes called a stress or fatigue fracture. It produces pain in the ball of the foot or in the leg and is made worse by activity. A person who spends a lot of time on his or her feet or has just begun a new program of running, jogging, or other exercise is a candidate for this type of fracture. X rays may not reveal a clear break in the bone, but rather a perceptible change in the tough membrane that covers the bone surface. A doctor may diagnose a march fracture on the basis of the X ray, bone scan, and clinical history. There are several approaches to the treatment of stress fractures. Bandages, braces, and crutches are the most common treatments. For stress fractures that are not as serious, a short-leg walking cast for 3 to 6 weeks may be recommended.

Marfan syndrome
An inherited disorder of the connective tissue primarily affecting the eyes and the skeletal, cardiovascular, and central nervous systems. Marfan syndrome is usually inherited from

M

a parent who has the condition, although in one third of cases, it occurs in a previously unaffected family as a spontaneous mutation. Marfan syndrome occurs in one of about 40,000 people. It is caused by a defective gene located on chromosome 15.

SYMPTOMS

People with Marfan syndrome usually have tall, lanky frames with long arms and slender, tapering spidery fingers (arachnodactyly). They tend to be nearsighted and have lenses of the eye that are slightly off-center. Curvature of the spine (scoliosis); flat feet; vision problems; thin, narrow face; small lower jaw; and sunken chest are also associated with the syndrome.

Serious problems associated with the syndrome are cardiovascular abnormalities, such as weakened walls of major arteries, including the aorta. The weakened walls of the aorta are at risk for tearing and leaking blood (aortic dissection). An ANEURYSM may also develop. People with Marfan syndrome are also at risk for problems involving the valves of the heart, usually the mitral and aortic valves. Blood can leak backward through a valve, which can place a burden on the heart and cause it to enlarge over time. The mitral valve is often oversized and subject to MITRAL VALVE PROLAPSE (MVP), in which the valve billows back into the left atrium of the heart.

TREATMENT

Marfan syndrome cannot be cured. Visual defects can often be corrected. Children with Marfan syndrome should be watched carefully throughout adolescence for signs of developing scoliosis. To prevent infection of the heart wall or valve, individuals should receive preventive antibiotics before dental procedures. Pregnancy, which puts extra strain on the heart and aorta, must be monitored very closely, particularly during labor and delivery. To avoid possible rupture of an aortic aneurysm, children with Marfan syndrome should avoid strenuous sports, especially contact sports like football or ice hockey, in which they might receive blows to the chest.

During medical examinations, chest X rays and echocardiograms are usually performed. Most people may need to take medication to lower the heart rate, blood pressure, or both, which reduces the risk of serious problems with the aorta. In cases involving major problems with the aorta or aortic valve, surgery may be required.

Marital counseling

Counseling or psychotherapy for a couple that focuses on the interactions between marriage partners. See COUPLES THERAPY.

Marsupialization

A procedure in which a cyst is cut open to drain its contents, and the edges of the incision are sewn to nearby skin to form a pouch. This procedure is used to drain a chronic or recurring Bartholin cyst (see BARTHOLIN'S GLANDS, DISEASES OF) and it preserves the affected gland's ability to continue to secrete mucus.

Masculinization

The normal process by which a male acquires sex-specific attributes during sexual maturation as a result of the response of the body to the male hormones called ANDROGEN HORMONES. Androgen hormones, including TESTOSTERONE, are produced in the testicles in response to stimulation by the pituitary hormone LH (luteinizing hormone).

Masculinization takes place as a male develops, beginning in the fetal stage when the testicles develop, due to the effects of androgen hormones. The elements of masculinization begin to occur in puberty as the secondary sex characteristics evolve. These characteristics include deepening of the voice, growth of facial hair, and large skeletal muscles. Male hormones ultimately determine a mature man's body shape, patterns of body hair, sex drive, and ability to achieve an erection.

Disorders of the adrenal glands, including tumors of the adrenal cortex (the outer layer of the adrenal glands), can cause disturbances in masculinization. Adrenal disorders may also cause masculinization in a woman, leading to the acquisition of male characteristics, including deepening of the voice, growth of body hair, and male-pattern hair loss. ALDOSTERONISM and CUSHING SYNDROME can also produce some masculinization factors in women, including hirsutism (excess facial and body hair).

Massage

A technique that may be used in PHYSICAL THERAPY or by a massage therapist involving a kneading with the hands of certain soft tissues of the body, especially the muscles, ligaments, and tendons. The purpose of massage is to promote relaxation of the body part being massaged and to relieve overall physical tension in the person receiving the massage. Muscles are relaxed by kneading the muscle tissue through the skin, most commonly in the areas of the neck, shoulders, and back, but also in other parts of the body. When muscles are compressed against underlying bone during massage, muscular tightness and spasm may be relieved. Massage also brings increased blood flow to the muscles involved, which warms and relaxes them.

Massage therapy

Holistic medical therapy that uses hands-on massage to promote healing. Massage therapy is used to improve blood circulation; to relax tense muscles and help stimulate weak ones; to stimulate secretions, such as lymph; to stimulate the nervous system; and to help release toxic metabolic by-products from body tissues. Massage therapy is thought to help restore healthy structure and function to the body, thereby promoting greater ease and wider range of

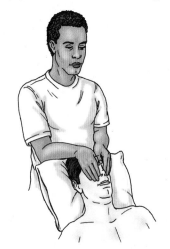

REIKI
Reiki, just one example of massage therapy, involves channeling the body's spirit and energy through gentle touch and massage. It is a form of meditation and philosophy with a healing component.

movement, more flexibility, and the release of chronic patterns of tension. All body systems are thought to benefit from the overall effects of massage therapy, as are the mind and spirit.

TYPES OF MASSAGE

There are several types and categories of massage used by massage therapists.

■ *Traditional European massage* This category includes Swedish massage, the most commonly used method in the United States, which includes stimulating blood circulation through the soft tissues.

■ *Contemporary Western massage* This category includes Esalen massage, the focus of which is on creating deep relaxation, beneficial states of consciousness, and general well-being.

■ *Deep tissue massage* This approach is used to release chronic patterns of tension by applying massage with greater pressure and at deeper layers than traditional massage.

■ *Trigger point massage* This form of deep massage applies concentrated finger pressure directly to individual muscles, to release "trigger points," which are intense knots of muscle tension that trigger pain in other areas of the body.

Massage is particularly effective for soft tissue damage, including sports injuries. See also BODYWORK.

Mast cell

A tissue cell that is part of the immune system and originates as a STEM CELL. Mast cells have an important role in the body's IMMUNE RESPONSE that occurs when foreign substances are perceived by the immune system to be harmful. The mast cells contain chemicals that are responsible for the symptoms of ALLERGIES. When allergens enter the body, they attach to antibodies located on the surface of mast cells. This attachment releases a signal that causes the mast cells to release certain chemicals, including HISTAMINE, that cause the symptoms of an allergy.

Mastectomy

Surgical removal of all or part of the breast, usually as a treatment for BREAST CANCER. The principal goal of surgery for breast cancer is to remove the primary tumor from the breast. Depending on the size and location of the primary tumor, any of four basic types of surgery will be selected: lumpectomy, partial mastectomy, subcutaneous mastectomy, and modified radical mastectomy. The selection of the procedure depends on the person's condition and preference.

In a lumpectomy, only the tumor and a small amount of surrounding tissue are removed. A small incision is made over the lump. A second incision is generally made in the armpit to remove some of the lymph glands on the affected side. A lumpectomy generally does not disturb the nipple unless the cancer is very close to it. The procedure leaves a barely noticeable scar and a small depression in the breast. The surgery usually is followed by radiation therapy and often by chemotherapy, to reduce the risk of recurrence. In patients with small tumors that have not spread, lumpectomy and radiation therapy offer the same chance for cure as a mastectomy.

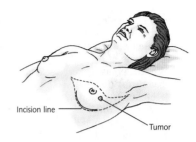
Incision line — Tumor
Before surgery

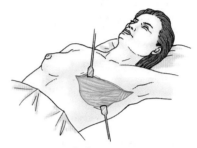
During surgery

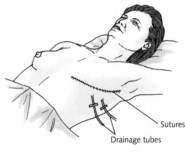
Sutures
Drainage tubes
After surgery

MODIFIED RADICAL MASTECTOMY
For a modified radical mastectomy, the incision is in the shape of an elongated oval. Some women choose to have breast reconstruction done at the time of surgery, while others wait until after recovery to decide. After the surgery, the incision is stitched shut; the scar is usually positioned so it is not visible under most necklines.

In a new technique called sentinel node biopsy, only a single lymph node, the first of the nodes that drain the breast tissue, is removed. The "sentinel node" is identified by injecting a dye.

In a partial mastectomy, a segment of breast tissue containing the primary tumor is removed, including the overlying skin, a portion of the tissue surrounding the tumor, and some of the underlying tissue. Some lymph glands in the armpit will also be removed, as in lumpectomy, and radiation therapy will usually follow

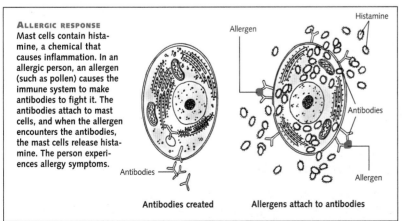
ALLERGIC RESPONSE
Mast cells contain histamine, a chemical that causes inflammation. In an allergic person, an allergen (such as pollen) causes the immune system to make antibodies to fight it. The antibodies attach to mast cells, and when the allergen encounters the antibodies, the mast cells release histamine. The person experiences allergy symptoms.

Allergen
Histamine
Antibodies
Antibodies
Allergen

Antibodies created   **Allergens attach to antibodies**

M

to reduce recurrence. Healing leaves a visible scar, and the breast is usually smaller after the surgery.

Subcutaneous mastectomy is used to prevent breast cancer in women at high risk for developing the disease. All the inner tissue of the breast is removed, leaving the nipple and as much skin as possible intact. The lymph glands in the armpit are examined and may be removed for biopsy. A silicone implant is inserted, to re-create the appearance of the original breast. Healing leaves a scar, usually under the breast. In a variant of this operation, sometimes called a simple mastectomy, the nipple and skin of the breast are removed as well, and the breast is reconstructed later.

In a modified radical mastectomy, the entire breast and all lymph glands under the arm are removed in a single block of tissue, if possible. The chest muscles are almost always left in place. Healing leaves a long scar across the chest, but the breast can usually be reconstructed later. BREAST RECONSTRUCTION uses some of the skin and underlying fat from a nearby site to cover a silicone implant. The nipple is reconstructed and stitched in place.

Radical mastectomy, in which the breast, lymph nodes in the armpit, and chest muscles are all removed, is almost never performed, because it is no more effective than a modified radical mastectomy.

Mastitis

An inflammation of the breast due to a bacterial infection; usually, but not always, found in breast-feeding mothers. Mastitis is caused by bacteria gaining access to the breast tissue through a crack or sore in the nipple. The infection is diagnosed by a physical examination—it is different from a plugged or blocked duct in the breast. Characteristic physical signs of mastitis include a swollen, hard, red area of the breast that is intensely painful, accompanied by fever. A low-grade fever may persist for 2 to 3 days, followed by an abrupt elevation in temperature, which indicates the presence of infection.

While other conditions, including a blocked duct, should not be treated with antibiotics, mastitis responds successfully to antibiotic therapy. In new nursing mothers, help with improved breast-feeding techniques may be necessary because poor draining of the breast often causes mastitis.

Mastocytosis

A disorder caused by the presence of too many mast cells (cells in the skin and elsewhere that produce histamine). Mastocytosis can be cutaneous (affecting the skin only) or systemic (affecting organs throughout the body). In young children, the most common skin form of mastocytosis is called urticaria pigmentosa, which usually resolves on its own. Chemicals released by mast cells in the skin cause allergic reactions such as hives and itching. Adults are more likely to develop systemic forms of the disease. When the disease is systemic or body wide, the gastrointestinal tract and the skeletal system are most commonly involved. Symptoms of this form of mastocytosis include nausea, vomiting, diarrhea, ulcers, bone pain, low blood pressure, faintness, and shock. Treatment is with antihistamines to prevent mast cells from releasing histamine, anticholinergics to reduce cramping, and topical corticosteroids to relieve the skin rash. Drugs (such as alcohol and codeine) that cause mast cells to release histamine should be avoided. In rare cases when mastocytosis is associated with cancer or a blood disorder, additional treatment may include corticosteroids or chemotherapy.

Mastoidectomy

Surgical removal of all or part of a honeycombed portion of the bone, called the mastoid process, that is located behind the outer ear. The mastoid process is connected to the middle ear, and an inflammation of the middle ear (OTITIS MEDIA)—generally a sign of infection—may spread to the mastoid (see MASTOIDITIS). If antibiotic treatment does not cure the infection, a physician may recommend complete mastoidectomy to remove the disease from the bone or partial mastoidectomy to remove part of the bone and drain the mastoid. Complications are rare but may include persistent ear drainage, hearing loss, paralysis of the face on the side of the surgery, and reinfection of the mastoid. Dizziness may be experienced for a short period following surgery. Loss of the sense of taste on the affected side may occur, usually lasting only a few weeks but in some cases, becoming permanent.

Mastoiditis

An inflammation of the honeycombed section of bone, called the mastoid process, located behind the outer ear. It is most commonly caused by the spread of bacterial infection of OTITIS MEDIA (middle ear inflammation) to the mastoid and generally affects children more than adults. When middle ear infections are untreated or inadequately treated, the infection can spread to the mucous membrane covering the mastoid process and the walls of the bone itself, where the infection deteriorates the bony honeycomb. Symptoms of mastoiditis, which last for at least 2 weeks, include earache, headache, and discharge of pus from the ear. High fever may occur with intermittent, sudden high increases. There may also be swelling, tenderness, and redness behind the ear.

Mastoiditis can be cured with antibiotics, but it is difficult to treat because the medication may not reach deeply enough into the mastoid, and infection tends to recur. Injected antibiotics may be given in addition to oral medication; repeated or long-term medication is often required. Surgical removal of part or all of the mastoid (MASTOIDECTOMY) may become necessary if antibiotic treatment proves unsuccessful. This condition has become extremely rare since the introduction of antibiotics to treat middle ear infections. Prompt and complete medical treatment of ear infections is the best way to prevent mastoiditis.

Mastopexy

See BREAST LIFT.

Masturbation

Touching the genitals and other sexually responsive areas of one's own body for pleasure, stimulation, and release of sexual tension.

Maternal mortality

A statistic determined by dividing the number of women who die during pregnancy or childbirth by the number of pregnancies during a given time period. Maternal mortality is an important indicator of a nation's overall level of health care and economic development. Particularly in developing countries, maternal mortality is underreported because of the lack of accurate hospital records and because of misdiagnosis of pregnancy-related deaths, particularly those related to abortion.

McArdle disease

An inherited metabolic disease characterized by abnormal storage of glycogen in the muscle tissue because of genetic enzyme deficiencies. The chief symptom of McArdle disease is muscle pain and stiffness following exercise and sometimes muscle cramps or weakness during exercise. People with McArdle disease lack the enzyme to metabolize glycogen, which is the main source of fuel for a brief, high-energy activity such as sprinting. McArdle disease is inherited as an autosomal recessive trait (see AUTOSOMAL RECESSIVE TRAITS).

McArdle disease is associated with several problems involving the muscles, including muscle fatigue, cramping, swelling, pain, tenderness, weakness, wasting, stiffness, and decreased stamina. Treatment includes the avoidance of strenuous exercise, which can lead to kidney damage as well as muscle pain and fatigue. People with the disease must always drink adequate water during periods of exercise.

Measles

FOR SYMPTOM CHART

see Rashes in infants and children, page 50
see Rashes in adults, page 52

A highly contagious, viral, respiratory infection that produces a characteristic rash. Measles, which is also called rubeola, usually spreads from person to person through contact with airborne respiratory droplets that occur when an infected person coughs or sneezes or via physical contact with items and surfaces that have been contaminated by the virus. This contact could include handling tissues used by an infected person, sharing eating and drinking items with a person who has measles, or touching the hands of an infected person who has touched his or her mouth or nose. Once contact has been made with the virus that causes measles, it enters the bloodstream and attacks the white blood cells. The infection is spread via the white blood cells to the respiratory tract, the skin, and other organs of the body.

SYMPTOMS

The symptoms of measles generally begin 10 to 14 days after exposure to the virus. Measles can be contagious 1 to 2 days before symptoms appear and up to 4 days after the rash appears. The complete course of symptoms generally lasts about 10 days. In children, measles usually causes only mild symptoms, but otitis media, inflammation of the middle ear, is a common complication.

Initial symptoms, which may include a runny nose, nasal congestion, and cough, are the result of the virus damaging the lining of the breathing passages. Fever, malaise, and possibly swollen glands (see GLANDS, SWOLLEN) are the result of the body's response to the infection. The gastrointestinal system may become involved because measles can cause diarrhea or vomiting. The eyes may become red and tear.

Within 2 to 4 days, tiny lesions called KOPLIK SPOTS develop on the inside of the cheeks near the back molars. At the same time or soon thereafter, the typical measles rash appears as very red eruptions that start on the forehead near the hairline and behind the ears, then spread over the trunk and to the extremities, including the palms of the hands and

the soles of the feet. The rash is not painful and does not itch. Within about 5 days, the rash begins to subside in the same sequence as it appeared, starting to fade first at the hairline and finally on the hands and feet. Areas of affected skin may temporarily retain a brownish discoloration or flaking as the rash fades.

People who become infected with measles and who also have HIV (human immunodeficiency virus) or certain leukemias or lymphomas tend to have severe, prolonged symptoms without the characteristic rash.

In adults, measles is a more severe illness, and older adults may develop bacterial PNEUMONIA, requiring hospitalization. Pneumonia and ENCEPHALITIS can develop in infants and in those who have weakened immune systems, as well as in older people. These severe complications are rare, but they can be extremely serious. Encephalitis presents an immediate risk of seizures, coma, and death, with a long-term risk of mental retardation, epilepsy, or very rarely, brain damage. In other rare instances, measles may directly attack the kidneys, the heart muscle, or the liver.

DIAGNOSIS AND TREATMENT

The doctor will take a clinical history to determine whether there has been recent exposure to a person who has measles or an unspecified rash and whether immunization to measles has been completed. A physical examination and evaluation of symptoms may be sufficient to diagnose measles. Blood tests may be ordered to detect antibodies to the measles virus, which can itself be detected in samples of urine or respiratory secretions.

Treatment of people who are otherwise healthy includes taking acetaminophen to reduce fever and relieve discomfort, bed rest, and the use of a cool-mist humidifier to alleviate cough and nasal congestion. Aspirin should not be given to children with measles because of the associated risk of REYE SYNDROME. Children and adults who are in good health generally make a complete recovery from measles.

In severe cases, particularly among children younger than 2 years, high doses of vitamin A may be prescribed. The antiviral medication ribavirin is used to treat some people with weakened immune systems.

M

Antibiotic therapy may be required to treat bacterial complications such as middle ear infections in children and bacterial pneumonia in older adults.

PREVENTION

There is an effective measles vaccine, which is generally given to children as part of the measles-mumps-rubella, or MMR, injection (see VACCINATIONS, CHILDHOOD). Women who are planning a pregnancy and who have never been immunized should be immunized before becoming pregnant. If measles occurs during a woman's pregnancy, there is an increased risk of premature labor, miscarriage, or low birth weight.

Infants younger than 12 months who are directly exposed to the measles virus may receive immunization therapy containing antibodies against the virus, which provides immediate immune protection. This treatment may also be used with people who have HIV or other conditions involving immune system suppression.

Meatus

An opening or passage through part of the body. The term usually refers to the external auditory meatus (ear canal), the passageway in the outer ear that leads from the outside to the eardrum.

Mebendazole

An antihelmintic drug used to treat worm infections. Mebendazole (Vermox) is used to treat roundworm, hookworm, pinworm, whipworm, and multiple worm infections. Mebendazole works by preventing the worm from absorbing glucose, or sugar, which depletes its energy supply and eventually leads to death of the worm.

Meckel diverticulum

A congenital malformation in which a pouch of tissue forms near the lower end of the small intestine. Often, a Meckel diverticulum causes no symptoms and requires no treatment. About one third of cases contain the same type of tissue that lines the stomach. In those cases, the gastric tissue may secrete acid and ulcerate, leading to bleeding. The pouch can also become infected or obstructed and cause bleeding, abdominal pain, vomiting, and fever.

Diagnosis of a Meckel diverticulum

is made by physical examination and tests such as radionuclide scans. Because their symptoms can be similar, it is important to distinguish a Meckel diverticulum from APPENDICITIS or a perforated DUODENAL ULCER. Severe symptoms often prompt an abdominal operation called an exploratory laparotomy (see LAPAROTOMY, EXPLORATORY). If a Meckel diverticulum is discovered during a laparotomy, surgeons remove it. Complications, such as peritonitis (an inflammation of the peritoneum, the membrane lining the abdominal cavity), can develop as a result of this condition and also require appropriate treatment.

Meclizine hydrochloride

An antihistamine; an antiemetic. Meclizine hydrochloride (Antivert, Bonine) is used to treat vomiting associated with motion sickness and vertigo. It is thought to work by affecting the central nervous system by decreasing stimulation to the body's balance centers in the middle ear, thereby managing motion sickness and controlling vomiting. Meclizine hydrochloride is available by prescription and over-the-counter.

Meconium

A newborn's first stool, consisting of a combination of swallowed AMNIOTIC FLUID and mucus from the baby's gastrointestinal tract. This dark, sticky material collects in the intestines of the fetus and makes up the first bowel movement of the newborn. Sometimes, meconium is released into the amniotic fluid before birth, which is usually considered a sign of fetal distress.

Medial

The center, or middle, of the body. Medial refers to the median of the body, the inner side of a body part, or any position or structure lying closest to the midline of the body. The medial side of a knee, for example, is the inner side of the knee. The opposite of medial is LATERAL.

Mediastinoscopy

An ENDOSCOPY of the chest in which the area between the lungs and above the heart is visually examined using a lighted instrument inserted through a

small incision. Often a tissue sample is removed for biopsy. A mediastinoscopy is performed in the hospital under general anesthesia and is used to diagnose diseases, such as lung cancer and tuberculosis.

Mediastinum

The central body cavity between the lungs, occupying the area between the breastbone and the spine, down to the diaphragm. Within the mediastinum are the heart and the major vessels leading in and out of it, the trachea, the esophagus, thymus gland, lymph nodes and vessels, and the vagus and phrenic nerves.

Medicaid

A federal- and state-funded health insurance program started in 1965 for low-income people of all ages. Medicaid money funds state programs that provide health services to people who qualify for welfare in their state. Individuals must meet income and resource guidelines. Medicaid is the major source of public funding for the long-term care of older people. However, the financial requirements are very strict. Older people cannot receive help from Medicaid until they have spent almost all of their own income and assets on care. Once this requirement has been met, Medicaid will pay for nursing home care, a limited amount of home and community-based care for those who would otherwise enter nursing homes, medications, eye examinations and eyeglasses, and transportation for medical care.

Medical examiner

A public office held by a physician whose responsibility it is to investigate sudden, unexpected, or violent deaths. The role of a medical examiner differs from that of a coroner in that a coroner is not necessarily a physician. A medical examiner brings medical expertise to the evaluation of the medical history and physical examination of the person who died. Medical examiners may be trained in any branch of medicine, but are often pathologists. Most physicians who are medical examiners obtain special training in death investigation.

A medical examiner may fulfill a number of public functions, including performing an AUTOPSY, a procedure used to study the body of the deceased. Autopsies are usually ordered to examine the bodies of people who have died by violence, suicide, or unknown circumstances to establish the cause of death. An autopsy may also be necessary when an individual is killed in the course of criminal activity, either to establish the cause of death or to initiate a legal proceeding, such as an inquest. See also FORENSIC MEDICINE.

Medical records

A detailed accounting of a person's health status over time. Medical records include information about vital signs, illnesses, injuries, test results, diagnoses, and treatments. Other pertinent information such as allergies to medications is also included. Medical records are useful tools in a physician's decisions about diagnosis and treatment. If a person changes doctors, he or she also transfers medical records. Medical records are confidential documents protected by federal law.

Medicare

A federal health insurance program started in 1965 for people over 65. Every American over age 65 is eligible for Medicare, regardless of income or assets. To receive Medicare, older adults file an enrollment application with the local Social Security office as they near age 65. Enrollment is automatic for someone who is already receiving Social Security benefits. The federal Center for Medicare and Medicaid Services (CMS) provides free volunteer counseling on Medicare.

TYPES OF COVERAGE

Medicare covers much of the cost of inpatient hospital care, skilled nursing facility care, some forms of home health care, and hospice care. However, strict conditions must be met. For example, Medicare pays nursing home bills only for older people who require skilled nursing or rehabilitation services. When an older person does not require skilled nursing care, Medicare does not cover general custodial care (help with daily activities including washing, dressing, and bathroom use) in nursing homes.

For home health care, Medicare

ITEMS THAT ARE NOT COVERED BY MEDICARE

Medicare does not cover all medical care required by older adults. Among the items not covered are:

- Acupuncture
- Cosmetic surgery
- Custodial care in a nursing facility
- Custodial care at home
- Most chiropractic services
- Care outside the United States
- Dental care
- Experimental procedures
- Eye examinations and eyeglasses
- Hearing aids
- Hospital telephones and televisions
- Private-duty nursing
- Most prescription drugs
- Routine preventive care, including physical examination, medical history, and preventive foot care

---

sometimes covers the services of a skilled nurse or a speech, physical, or occupational therapist. To receive benefits, a person must be considered homebound and receive care from a Medicare-certified home health agency. When skilled nursing is already being provided and covered, in some cases Medicare may also cover the cost of custodial care. This care includes help with bathing and hygiene, administered by a home health aide.

Many Medicare benefits are available only during a brief period of opportunity. For example, care in a skilled nursing facility is covered when it begins within 30 days of discharge from a hospital stay of at least 3 days. Home health care visits are covered when they begin within 14 days after a hospital stay of at least 3 days. Individuals are advised to check on what is and what is not covered. Older people should be aware of their own financial responsibilities, which generally include a deductible and 20 percent of the charges.

Doctors are called participating providers when they agree to accept Medicare's payment rates (assignment) for medical services. When doctors accept assignment, Medicare pays the doctor 80 percent of the

---

Medicare-approved charge, and the patient is responsible for paying the remaining 20 percent. When doctors do not accept assignment, by law they can only charge a maximum of 15 percent above the Medicare-approved charge.

Medication
See DRUG.

Meditation

A mind-body technique that uses quiet contemplation to induce a state of mental and physical tranquility. Meditation is used by conventional and alternative medical practitioners as a way to lower blood pressure, to help people with asthma breathe, to combat chronic chest pain, and generally to relax. Meditation is a safe, low-cost method of pain reduction and stress management.

Meditation has been called "mental fasting," meaning that it is a way of cleansing and purifying the mind and the spirit by withdrawing all distracting thoughts and disturbing emotions. Another way of describing meditation is as a way of emptying the body and mind of all input for a short time. Meditation is also a way of deliberately activating the parasympathetic nervous system, which is responsible for decreasing muscle tension, lowering blood pressure, lowering heart and breathing rates, and slowing bodily processes generally, following episodes of energetic activity. Researchers have found that meditating lowers levels of stress hormones, thereby supporting healthy immune function.

There are several methods of meditating, involving different techniques taught by experienced practitioners, but all involve controlled breathing. The goal of meditation is to achieve inner peace and relaxation. Practitioners usually recommend meditating in two sessions of 20 minutes each per day, usually before breakfast and before bedtime.

Meditation has been used effectively to treat hypertension, anxiety, headaches, irritable bowel syndrome, and insomnia.

Mediterranean diet

The diet typically consumed by Europeans who reside near the Mediterranean Sea. A widely known

1980 study comparing the cuisine of seven countries concluded that the Mediterranean diet was especially healthful. Its principal components are plentiful vegetables and fruits, seafood, dried peas and beans, and olive oil. Very little red meat and few fatty dairy products are consumed. For many years, it was believed that all fats were equally bad for one's health. However, although high in monounsaturated fat (olive oil), the Mediterranean diet is associated with low rates of heart disease. See also FATS AND OILS.

Medroxyprogesterone

A synthetic hormone. Medroxyprogesterone (Amen, Cycrin, Depo-Provera, and others) is chiefly used to treat breast cancer, although it is also used to treat cancers of the uterus, the kidney, and the prostate. It works by disrupting the process by which cancer cells divide and form tumors. Medroxyprogesterone is also given by injection as a long-acting contraceptive agent.

Medulla

The innermost portion of an organ. For example, the core tissue of the kidney is referred to as the medulla of the kidney. The term medulla is sometimes used to refer to the medulla oblongata, the part of the brain stem that joins the spinal cord.

Medulla oblongata

The lower portion of the BRAIN STEM just above the spinal cord. The medulla oblongata contains nerve centers that control breathing, heart rate, and blood pressure. See BRAIN.

Medulloblastoma

A cancerous brain tumor most often seen in children. A medulloblastoma is a rapidly growing GLIOMA that usually develops in the back of the brain. Symptoms associated with it include headaches, apathy, and unexplained vomiting, soon followed by difficulty in walking as the tumor grows larger. A medulloblastoma is an invasive tumor and the most common brain tumor of childhood.

Treatment starts with surgery to remove as much of the cancer as can be safely removed. After the surgery, tests are performed to see how many

cancer cells remain; these include MRI (magnetic resonance imaging), bone scans, and analysis of cerebral spinal fluid. Radiation therapy and chemo-therapy may be given. The 5-year survival rate for medulloblastoma is about 65 percant.

Mefloquine hydrochloride

An antimalarial drug. Mefloquine hydrochloride (Lariam) is used to prevent or treat malaria. It works in the bloodstream to poison the parasite that causes malaria. To avoid relapse after initial treatment with mefloquine hydrochloride, some people with malaria must take another antimalarial drug as well.

Megacolon

A distended colon. Symptoms of megacolon include severe constipation. In children, the condition is usually caused by Hirschsprung disease, a congenital defect in the function of the rectal muscle and anal sphincter. Psychological issues in toilet training may play a role in some cases. In older people, megacolon is linked with chronic constipation and

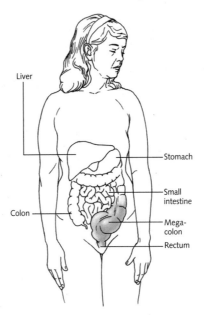

DISTENDED COLON
Severe distension of the colon, usually in the descending portion on the left side of the abdomen, may be caused by chronic constipation, long-term use of laxatives, or severe ulcerative colitis (an infection of the rectum that can involve parts of the colon).

the long-term use of laxatives. Toxic megacolon, an acute dilation of the colon, is a complication of a severe attack of ulcerative colitis. Diagnosis is made by X rays or a lower gastrointestinal (GI) series (also known as a barium enema). In severe cases, surgery is required.

Megestrol

Progestin; a hormone. Megestrol (Megace) is used to treat breast and endometrial cancers as well as to treat weight loss associated with anorexia (failure to eat) and wasting away that leaves a person thin and gaunt. Megestrol is effective in these conditions for reasons that are not entirely clear, although the drug is thought to stimulate the appetite by interfering with certain substances in the pituitary gland. It should never be used during pregnancy.

Meibomianitis

Inflammation of an oil-secreting gland in the eyelid. The meibomian gland is located between the eyelid's inner lining and the curved plate of connective tissue that forms its basic structure.

Meigs syndrome

A rare, benign tumor of the ovary that occurs in combination with excess abdominal fluid and PLEURAL EFFUSION, or excess fluid in the pleural cavity. The occurrence of the solid tumor and its related symptom of a swollen abdomen can be confused with cancer of the ovaries.

Meiosis

A type of cell division that takes place during germ cell formation and produces four daughter cells, each with half the number of chromosomes of the original cell. In meiosis, which occurs during the formation of gametes (mature male or female germ cells) in animals, the 46 chromosomes in the germ cell divide to make two new cells, each with 23 chromosomes that pair with corresponding chromosomes to exchange bits of genetic material. In women, X chromosomes inherited from both parents form a pair, while in men, one X chromosome inherited from the mother pairs with one Y chromosome inherited from the father. Once the genetic exchange is complete, meiosis continues. When the chromosomes of a cell duplicate in a single division to produce two new daughter cells each with the same number of chromosomes as the parent cell, the process is called MITOSIS.

Melanin

The pigment that normally determines the color of skin, hair, and eyes. Melanin functions as a sunscreen, protecting the skin from ultraviolet light. Skin that contains less melanin is more prone to sun damage and skin cancer. Melanin also has a role in susceptibility to other skin diseases.

Skin cells called melanocytes convert the amino acid tyrosine into melanin. Factors that can affect this process include heredity, injury, and radiation. Hormones in the body also influence pigmentation. Changes in any of these factors can result in hyperpigmentation (increased melanin production) or hypopigmentation (a decrease in melanin production). Changes in pigmentation can be temporary or permanent.

Skin conditions characterized by pigment changes include freckles, suntans, melasma, pityriasis alba, tinea versicolor, and vitiligo. In most cases, skin changes are cosmetic and do not affect general health but may be treated because they can cause extreme psychological stress. Treatments include topical corticosteroids, bleaching creams, and PHOTOTHERAPY (treatment with light).

Melanoma, eye

See EYE TUMORS.

Melanoma, juvenile

See SPITZ NEVUS.

Melanoma, malignant

A skin cancer that begins in the melanocytes, the cells that produce melanin. The pigment that gives skin its tan or brown color, melanin also protects its deeper layers from the sun. Generally, melanin and melanocytes are distributed evenly, making the color of the skin uniform. Concentrations of melanin form the flat, brown spots called freckles, or the darker raised spots called moles. Melanomas are usually dark brown or

black and can resemble dark freckles or moles. They are readily visible on the skin as unevenly colored irregular-shaped tumors that bleed easily.

DIAGNOSIS

Often, the first sign of malignant melanoma is a change in the size, shape, color, or feel of an existing mole. It can become larger or irregular in shape where one half does not match the other. The edges can become ragged, blurred, or irregular, and the pigment can spread into surrounding skin. The color of a mole can become uneven, incorporating shades of black, brown, tan, white, gray, red, pink, or blue. Melanomas are usually larger than healthy moles, exceeding ¼ inch in width. Malignant melanomas may also appear as new moles. Such new moles are usually black, abnormal in appearance, and unattractive.

Malignant melanoma is less common than other types of skin cancer, but it is much more serious. Early melanomas can be detected by having a doctor examine any changes in a mole or the skin in general. Tissue from the problematic area will be removed for biopsy to determine if it is malignant melanoma. If it is, blood tests, X rays, and scans may be recommended to determine if the melanoma has spread.

TREATMENT AND PREVENTION

Treatment includes surgery to remove the entire melanoma and some surrounding skin to prevent recurrence. Most malignant melanomas that are diagnosed at an early stage and have not spread can be cured by surgery. Sometimes, skin grafts or cosmetic surgery will be needed to restore the affected area after the melanoma is removed. Chemotherapy is used in some cases of advanced malignant melanoma; immunotherapy with interleukin 2 (IL-2) and interferon is also used.

Preventing malignant melanoma generally requires screening for abnormal moles and avoiding the direct rays of the sun. Many large medical centers offer clinics where moles can be photographed for examination by a dermatologist. Excessive exposure to sunlight, particularly in childhood, increases the risk for melanoma. For that reason, exposure to direct sunlight is not recommended between 10 AM and 2 PM standard

SKIN CANCER RISK

Developing malignant melanoma is more likely among individuals who have:

- **Fair skin and light eyes**
- **Many freckles**
- **More than 50 moles**
- **A family history of melanoma**
- **Had melanoma in the past**
- **Had severe, blistering sunburns, especially as a child or teenager**
- **Dysplastic nerve syndrome, a congenital condition characterized by many large, abnormal-appearing moles on the skin**

time (11 AM to 3 PM daylight savings time). Long sleeves and hats offer protection, as do sunscreens that block or absorb ultraviolet radiation and have a sun protection factor (SPF) of 15 or higher. See more on page 834.

Melanosis coli

A condition in which the colon's mucous membrane is abnormally pigmented with melanin (a dark brown or black pigment that normally occurs in the skin, hair, and other tissues), due to prolonged use of certain stimulant types of laxatives, such as senna and castor oil.

Melasma

A skin condition in which blotches of abnormally increased pigmentation appear on the face. In melasma, deposits of brown pigment may be noticed on the forehead, cheeks, or above the upper lip. The condition is referred to as the "mask of pregnancy" during pregnancy; skin usually returns to its normal color within a year. Melasma can also be caused by hormonal changes from oral contraceptives. Minimizing sun exposure and applying sunscreens are the usual treatments. Bleaching creams containing hydroquinone and tretinoin may be prescribed.

Melatonin

A hormone responsible for regulating the body's biological clock. Melatonin is produced in larger quantities at night than in the day by the pineal gland at the base of the brain. Because people produce less melatonin as they age, older people sometimes experience insomnia. Melatonin supple-

M

EARLY WARNING SIGNS: MOLES

A change in a mole may be the first sign of skin cancer. A doctor needs to look at any changing mole immediately. The ABCDs of skin cancer detection stand for Asymmetry, Border, Color, and Diameter.

NORMAL MOLE
Everyone has moles that are generally circular, brown, and constant in size.

ASYMMETRY
A mole can become asymmetrical. If an imaginary line is drawn down the middle of the mole, one half would be a different size or shape than the other.

COLOR
Most moles are a solid shade of brown or tan, but a melanoma may have more than one shade or color, such as black, blue, brown, red, or white.

BORDER
The border of the mole may be an irregular and blurred line, instead of the usual smooth, distinct circle.

DIAMETER
A mole that is growing should be checked—especially if it is larger than the tip of a typical pencil eraser.

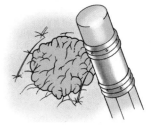

ments can help people sleep better, wake during the night less often, and cope with jet lag more effectively when traveling.

Melatonin supplements are available without prescription in the United States. They seem to be safe and effective when taken for sleep for short periods of time, although long-term safety has not been studied. Claims that melatonin can reduce normal aging processes and affect the outcome of a cancer diagnosis have not been clinically proven.

Melena
Partly digested blood in the stool. (See also FECES, BLOOD IN THE.) Melena, a sign of dangerous internal bleeding, is considered a medical emergency. Blood from internal bleeding passes into the intestines where it is digested and makes the stool loose, black, sticky, and strong-smelling. Internal bleeding may be a symptom of PEPTIC ULCER DISEASE, in which the membrane that lines the duodenum, stomach, lower esophagus, or small intestine becomes ulcerated; GASTRIC EROSION, a raw area in the surface of the membrane that lines the stomach; stomach cancer; or other disorders of the stomach, intestines, or esophagus. Black stools that may be mistaken for internal bleeding can also be caused by ingestion of iron or over-the-counter preparations for upset stomach that contain bismuth.

Membrane
A thin layer of tissue that covers a body surface, lines a cavity, divides a space or organ, lubricates joining parts, or anchors a body structure. There are two principal types of membranes. Mucous membranes are mucus-secreting tissue such as those that line the nose and mouth; they lubricate the cavity and protect against infection. Connective membranes cover bone or hold body parts in position. Examples are the synovial membrane which lines the cavities of the joints, and the eardrum, which separates the middle ear from the inner ear.

Memory
The process by which information, knowledge, and past events are recovered, reproduced, or recalled. Memory is thought to involve the storage of information through associative mechanisms. One hypothesis holds that memories are retained by changes made in nerve tissue in the brain, where they form engrams (memory traces).

Memory is often divided into short-term (recent) memory and long-term (remote) memory. Short-term memory involves the recall of information stored for just a few seconds, as is the case when a person remembers a phone number just long enough to dial it. Long-term memory involves the storage and retrieval of information over days, weeks, or years. Some disorders, such as Alzheimer's disease, damage the cognitive processes that control memory. As a general rule, long-term memory in such disorders is retained, while short-term memory is lost; memories can become jumbled, and the person can become confused, unable to remember where he or she lives or to recognize the people with whom he or she lives.

Memory loss, in older people

A common problem that ranges from mild difficulty in finding words and remembering names to an inability to recall recent events and/or function in unfamiliar circumstances. Mild memory loss is common and sometimes can be attributed to a poor diet, lack of sleep, medication, alcohol use, loneliness, or boredom. Correcting these underlying problems usually improves the memory loss, although some memory loss, or slowness in remembering, is a normal aspect of AGING. In other cases, memory problems are the sign of DELIRIUM (temporary confusion) or DEMENTIA (more persistent and progressively severe memory loss).

The most common cause of chronic memory loss is ALZHEIMER'S DISEASE. In this case, the loss of memory grows progressively worse over time and is not reversible. Memory loss can also be a sign of depression (persistent sadness and loss of interest in normal things).

DIAGNOSIS AND TREATMENT

Typically, a physician reviews a detailed medical history, conducts a physical examination, and conducts or orders various tests. The physician will ask when the memory problems began and how the memory loss interferes with daily living. Subsequent questions may focus on alcohol use, recent weight gain or loss, sleep disturbances, and recent illnesses. To determine whether drug reactions are involved, the doctor will review all medications being taken. Possible tests include neuropsychological testing, blood and urine tests, and imaging studies of the brain, such as CT (computed tomography) scanning or MRI (magnetic resonance imaging).

Once the diagnosis is made, the physician begins management of any potentially treatable problem. For example, because depression often responds well to psychotherapy, the physician would prescribe treatment for suspected cases of depression. When memory loss is suspected to be the side effect of a medication, the drug would be stopped or the dosage decreased. Reversible causes of dementia, such as thyroid disor-

ders, are also treatable. Alzheimer's disease is an irreversible form of dementia. However, the doctor can recommend medications to lessen some of its symptoms. See also DEPRESSION, IN OLDER PEOPLE; CONFUSION IN OLDER PEOPLE.

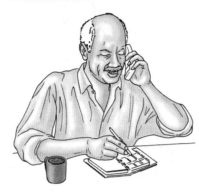

STIMULATING THE MEMORY
For many older people, loss of memory is manageable with simple memory aids such as taking thorough notes about telephone calls, faithfully updating a calendar, and placing reminder notes in prominent places. Research shows that mental stimulation—reading and writing, doing crossword puzzles, even doing simple math exercises—helps keep the memory healthy well into old age. Sometimes memory loss results from lack of sleep, medication, use of alcohol, or loneliness. Solving these problems will help improve a person's memory.

Memory, loss of

Forgetfulness that can result from brain damage or severe emotional trauma; amnesia. Pathological loss of memory can be caused by Alzheimer's disease, alcoholism, head injury, seizures, stroke, brain surgery, ECT (electroconvulsive therapy), the use of barbiturates or other tranquilizers, and other physical events or conditions. Depending on the cause, loss of memory can occur gradually or all at once, and it may be permanent or temporary.

A certain amount of forgetfulness is normal as people age. Normal aging is also associated with difficulty in learning new material—with age, it becomes harder to store and retrieve information and knowledge. Genuinely impaired memory is usually only associated with disease.

Menarche

The onset of MENSTRUATION, or a woman's first menstrual period.

Meniere disease

A disorder of the ear caused by an increase of fluid in the part of the inner ear called the labyrinth, which controls a person's sense of balance. The pressure of excess fluid against the membrane wall of the labyrinth distorts and sometimes ruptures the membrane. Periodic flare-ups produce severe disruption in a person's sense of balance and may also cause fluctuating impairment of hearing that tends to progress to a severe loss. The cause of Meniere disease is unknown.

Meniere disease occurs as discrete episodes, or attacks of VERTIGO, which may last a few hours or an entire day. The episodes may be preceded by a feeling of fullness in the ears. During attacks of the disorder, symptoms may include dizziness, nausea and vomiting, distorted hearing or hearing loss, ringing in the ears (see TINNITUS), and the feeling of pressure in one ear. The frequency and severity of attacks vary widely. The period between attacks of Meniere disease may last no longer than a few hours or as long as several years. For many people, the episodes occur rarely, and the disorder is no more than an inconvenience. Attacks generally become less severe over time, but some degree of hearing loss and ringing in the ears may linger between attacks. There is the danger that episodes of Meniere disease will become increasingly frequent and debilitating, producing profound deafness and disabling dizziness and nausea.

Several self-help strategies may be beneficial. When an attack occurs, lying still can ease the severity of symptoms. Reducing intake of caffeine, alcohol, and salt should decrease the frequency of the episodes, as well as the intensity of the symptoms. Reducing levels of stress and giving up cigarette smoking may also help lessen the severity of symptoms.

TREATMENT

A person experiencing symptoms of Meniere disease should see an ear, nose, and throat specialist (otolaryngologist). Tests including a CALORIC TEST (a balance test of the labyrinth), as well as MRI (magnetic resonance imaging), may help determine whether a person has this disorder. The physician may prescribe medication to con-

M

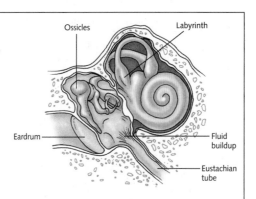

PRESSURE FROM FLUID BUILDUP
Meniere disease involves an excessive buildup of fluid in the labyrinth, a system of passageways in the inner ear that regulates balance. The excess fluid presses against the walls of the labyrinth and causes episodes of dizziness, loss of balance, distorted hearing, ringing in the ears, and nausea. The episodes are often preceded by a sense of fullness in the ears. The frequency and severity of attacks vary greatly among persons with the disease. Treatment may involve medication or surgery.

Labels: Ossicles, Labyrinth, Eardrum, Fluid buildup, Eustachian tube

trol nausea and vomiting and a diuretic to prevent excess fluid from accumulating in the labyrinth, thus helping to prevent further attacks.

If a person using the prescribed medication continues to be debilitated by the disorder or if there is sufficient extra fluid in the labyrinth to damage it, surgery may be an option. In one surgical procedure, a hole is made in the bone of the middle ear and a tiny silicone tube, called a shunt, is positioned to allow drainage of the excess fluid. This procedure is usually temporarily successful in relieving the symptom of dizziness and may prevent ongoing loss of hearing in the affected ear. However, Meniere disease usually returns after a year or more. There are two surgical procedures that may be considered when the disorder is severely disabling: one involves severing the nerve that is crucial to balance, called the vestibular nerve, and the other entails removing the membranous part of the labyrinth. Medications placed in the middle ear to control dizzy spells may help. The progressive hearing loss that usually accompanies Meniere disease has proven more difficult to prevent.

Meninges

The three, thin membranes that cover the BRAIN and SPINAL CORD. The innermost layer of tissue is called the pia mater, which lies against the surface of the brain and spinal cord. The middle layer, the arachnoid mater, is separated from the pia mater by the subarachnoid space, which is filled with cerebrospinal fluid. The dura mater is the tough outer layer that lines the inside of the skull and loosely encloses the spinal cord.

Meningioma

A benign tumor arising from the membranes, or meninges, that surround the brain and spinal cord. Meningiomas are rare tumors that can occur at any age, but most commonly they are diagnosed when the person is between age 50 and 70 years. Women are more often affected with meningiomas than men. Meningiomas develop from cells in the arachnoid, or middle layer of the meninges. Afterwards, the tumor typically becomes attached to the dura mater, or outer layer. Depending on size and location, meningiomas may cause symptoms such as headache, vomiting, impaired mental function, speech loss, and visual disturbances. However, many meningiomas do not cause any symptoms. If the tumor penetrates the overlying bone, thickening and bulging of the skull may occur. Meningiomas are detected through X rays, CT (computed tomography) scanning, or MRI (magnetic resonance imaging). Depending on the size and location of the meningioma, surgical removal may be required. When this is not possible, tumors are treated with radiation therapy. Asymptomatic meningiomas may not require treatment.

Meningitis

Inflammation of the membranes or meninges that surround the brain and spinal cord. Viral meningitis is a relatively mild disease; bacterial meningitis is life-threatening and requires immediate treatment. Meningitis is usually caused by infections that originate elsewhere in the body and travel in the bloodstream to the brain or spinal cord. Viral meningitis is far more common than the bacterial vari-

ety; it frequently occurs during the winter months and primarily affects people younger than 30 years. Bacteria that cause meningitis include *Streptococcus*, *Staphylococcus*, *Haemophilus influenzae* (*H. influenzae*), and *Meningococcus*. About 17,500 cases of bacterial meningitis occur in the United States each year. Although meningitis can occur at any age, it most commonly affects children.

SYMPTOMS
The symptoms of bacterial meningitis often come on suddenly and include fever, severe headache, nausea, vomiting, stiff neck, and sensitivity to light. There can also be changes in behavior, such as confusion, sleepiness, and difficulty waking up. These are important symptoms that indicate a need for emergency treatment. In infants, there may be irritability, tiredness, poor feeding, and fever. In viral meningitis, symptoms can be mild and resemble influenza.

DIAGNOSIS AND TREATMENT
Meningitis is diagnosed by LUMBAR PUNCTURE and examination of cerebrospinal fluid. Other useful tests include blood tests, X rays, and CT (computed tomography) scanning. Common viral meningitis is usually not serious, and symptoms typically disappear without treatment within 2 weeks. However, early diagnosis and treatment of bacterial meningitis are imperative to prevent neurological damage or death. Hospitalization is typically required. Large amounts of antibiotics are administered intravenously to control the infection. Secondary symptoms such as shock, brain swelling, and seizures must also be managed. Corticosteroids may be used to reduce brain swelling and inflammation. Anticonvulsants are given to prevent or treat seizures. Sometimes sedatives are prescribed for irritability and restlessness.

With early diagnosis and treatment, most people recover from bacterial meningitis. However, possible complications include hearing loss, brain damage, loss of vision, and deafness. Immunization with one of the three available *H. influenzae* type B vaccines makes children resistant to meningitis caused by the *H. influenzae* type B bacterium. (See VACCINATIONS, CHILDHOOD.) Since the introduction of the *H. influenzae* immuniza-

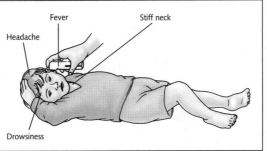

SYMPTOMS OF MENINGITIS
A child or adult with meningitis may have a severe headache, a high fever, stiffness in the neck, and drowsiness. Other symptoms include vomiting, seizures, confusion, a skin rash in the armpits or on the hands or feet, and sensitivity to light. Emergency medical attention is called for.

Fever

Stiff neck

Headache

Drowsiness

tion, the incidence of this type of meningitis has decreased dramatically in the United States.

Meningocele

A birth defect in which the membranes of the brain or spinal cord protrude through abnormal gaps in the skull or spinal column. See also NEURAL TUBE DEFECT.

Meningomyelocele

A severe form of SPINA BIFIDA, a neural tube defect. A birth defect in which the spinal canal does not close before birth, causing the spinal cord and the membranes that cover it to protrude from the baby's back. Meningomyelocele is one of the most common birth defects of the central nervous system, affecting as many as 1 of every 800 infants born. Meningomyelocele occasionally runs in families: children born to a family with a history of the disorder have a greater than average risk of having it.

Meningomyelocele occurs when the bones of the spine do not form completely, leaving the spinal canal incompletely closed. The protrusion of the spinal cord affects neurological function below the site of the defect. Most defects occur in the lowest areas of the back (lower lumbar or sacral areas), because in normal development they are the last parts of the spine to close. Symptoms of muscle weakness, paralysis, loss of sensation, and impaired bladder and bowel control are caused by damage to the spinal cord.

Symptoms include the presence of a sac protruding from the spinal cord on the back of a newborn baby. The exposed spinal cord is susceptible to infection, especially MENINGITIS. Neurological symptoms involve impairment of the body below the defect. These can range from weakness of the lower limbs to partial or complete paralysis. Impaired bladder and bowel function may also occur. Complications may also include meningitis, hydrocephalus, and other birth defects.

TREATMENT
Surgical repair of the defect is usually recommended and is generally successful. The surgery is sometimes performed within 24 hours of birth, although it can be postponed to help the newborn tolerate the procedure. Before surgery, the newborn must be handled with care to reduce damage to the exposed spinal cord. This involves modifications to normal methods of handling, feeding, bathing, and clothing the infant. Protective devices may be used. Antibiotics may be used to treat or to prevent infections, including meningitis and urinary tract infections. When bladder control is impaired by the defect, gentle downward pressure over the bladder can help to drain it, although in many cases urinary catheterization (see CATHETERIZATION, URINARY) may be needed. Impaired bowel function may be helped by a diet high in fiber and by bowel training programs. Physical therapy may be useful to reduce muscle weakness, but neurological damage is usually permanent and irreversible.

Some success has been reported in treating meningomyelocele with experimental fetal surgery (performed during pregnancy within the uterus). The meningomyelocele is closed, and the pregnancy continues. This procedure is performed in very few hospitals and carries a risk of inducing preterm labor. While fetal surgery can reduce continued damage caused during pregnancy and delivery, it cannot restore neurological function lost as a result of the original defect.

CAUSE AND PREVENTION
The root cause of meningomyelocele is not known. Both genes and environmental factors are thought to have a role. One possible cause is FOLIC ACID DEFICIENCY, thought to be involved in NEURAL TUBE DEFECT formation. Maternal use of valproic acid, a medication used to treat seizures and migraine headaches, increases the risk. Folic acid supplements may be effective in preventing meningomyelocele. Prospective mothers must begin taking supplements before becoming pregnant, because the defect develops very early in pregnancy.

Cases of meningomyelocele have decreased in recent years, in part because of prenatal testing. A large number of affected fetuses can be identified between 16 and 20 weeks of pregnancy with two tests: serum alpha-fetoprotein examination of the mother's blood with the AFP TEST; and ULTRASOUND SCANNING. Some parents may choose to interrupt the pregnancy if meningomyelocele is present, particularly in cases in which injury to the spinal cord is great and complications such as HYDROCEPHALUS are present.

Meniscal tears

A break or rupture in the crescent-shaped pad of cartilage, called the meniscus, located in the knee where the ends of the thighbone and lower leg bone meet to form the knee joint. Meniscal tears most commonly occur in the knee cartilage on the inner side of the leg but may also occur on the outer side. An impact injury or a rapid twisting motion from a squatting posi-

M

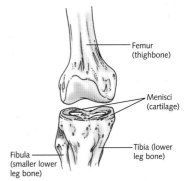

Femur (thighbone)

Menisci (cartilage)

Tibia (lower leg bone)

Fibula (smaller lower leg bone)

SHOCK ABSORBERS IN THE KNEE
A torn meniscus is a common sports injury, usually occurring when an athlete tries to pivot. In an older person, the meniscus is less resilient and can tear from even a minor misstep.

tion, which applies a rotational force on the knee when it is partially or completely flexed, is the usual cause of meniscal tears. Twisting movements with the knees bent may occur when a person is playing sports, such as tennis or football. In some cases, the person may feel a tearing sensation or hear a popping sound at the moment when the meniscus tears and may feel the knee collapse. In other cases, a person is able to continue with the activity that caused the meniscal tear without experiencing discomfort or weakness in the knee. A slight swelling typically occurs within several hours of the injury. There may be episodic, recurrent swelling, an inability to fully extend the knee ("locking"), and an instability of the knee such that it periodically gives way. The pain may become worse during weight-bearing activities.

Meniscal tears are diagnosed by physical examination, specifically by a swelling of the knee joint, a limited ability to fully extend the leg, and localized tenderness to the touch. Treatment may be easily remembered by the acronym RICE—rest, ice, compression, and elevation. Activities involving the knee should be stopped after injury to the joint. Ice and compression bandages may help limit swelling. Elevating the leg can help reduce pain and swelling. Physical therapy may be recommended to alleviate discomfort, promote healing, and help restore strength to the muscles that support the knee. Crutches may be used if there is swelling and pain with movement. Arthroscopic surgery may be considered to repair meniscal tears if they do not heal with more conservative treatments.

Meniscectomy

The surgical removal of a portion of one of the two pads of cartilage, called the menisci, which are located in the knee joint. The procedure is usually performed as ARTHROSCOPIC SURGERY under local or general anesthesia on an outpatient basis. Meniscectomy becomes necessary as a treatment for tears in the meniscus, which are generally caused by sports injuries, especially basketball, soccer, and football. Injuries requiring meniscectomy are usually diagnosed with MRI (magnetic resonance imaging).

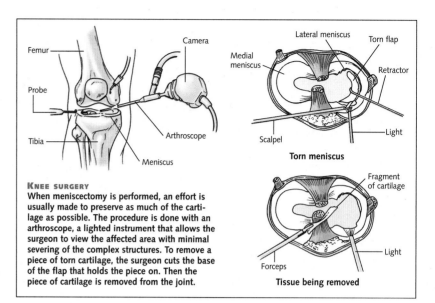

KNEE SURGERY
When meniscectomy is performed, an effort is usually made to preserve as much of the cartilage as possible. The procedure is done with an arthroscope, a lighted instrument that allows the surgeon to view the affected area with minimal severing of the complex structures. To remove a piece of torn cartilage, the surgeon cuts the base of the flap that holds the piece on. Then the piece of cartilage is removed from the joint.

Meniscus

A disk of loosely attached cartilage that helps protect the joint by absorbing shock and registering pressure against the joint. The knee joints contain menisci.

Menopause

The process during which a woman stops menstruating; literally, a woman's final menstrual period. Menopause, sometimes called the change of life, generally occurs between ages 40 and 55; the average age is 51. Menopause may occur as early as age 39 or as late as 58 and is considered premature when it occurs before age 40. Women will go through menopause early if they have had their ovaries (see OVARY) removed or if they have received radiation therapy to the ovaries. Smokers and underweight women tend to have an earlier menopause, while overweight women may have a later menopause. As a rule, a woman will tend to go through menopause at about the same age her mother did.

The process is lengthy and gradual, beginning during PERIMENOPAUSE, when the ovaries' production of ESTROGEN and other hormones slows down. Perimenopause can last for several years. Menopause has ended when a woman has not had a menstrual period for a minimum of 6 months. The most important hormonal change during menopause is a profound drop (by about 75 percent) in the production of estrogen. Changes in estrogen levels are responsible for the common physical complaints associated with menopause, such as hot flashes, vaginal dryness, night sweats, and urinary problems.

PHYSICAL CHANGES
Menopause is a gradual process that occurs slowly over time. Different women experience menopause in different ways. Most women experience some symptoms during perimenopause, whether mild or severe, with some of them lasting months or years. The earliest signs of approaching menopause occur in the menstrual cycle. The ovaries produce less estrogen, which may result in an occasional skipped period, lighter or heavier menstrual flow, or a period that is shorter or longer than usual. The menstrual periods become less and less regular, until eventually the ovaries stop making enough estrogen to thicken the lining of the uterus, and the menstrual periods stop. The most common symptom of menopause is hot flashes, experienced by 75 percent of menopausal women in the United States. Another common symptom is interrupted sleep, in particular REM SLEEP. Loss of sleep during menopause is most often caused by hot flashes, which can wake a woman from a deep sleep.

Loss of estrogen causes the lining of the vagina to become thinner and dryer, which makes the vagina more vulnerable to irritation and may cause pain during sexual intercourse. Loss of estrogen also causes the cells lining the urinary tract to deteriorate and the tissue around the urethra to weaken, which can result in some loss of bladder control. Some women experience stress incontinence, a sudden leaking of urine when they sneeze, cough, or strain physically.

Glandular tissue in the breasts is replaced by fat tissue, which causes them to sag. The risk of breast cancer increases with age, particularly after menopause. The hair and skin can also reflect changes in hormone production. Facial and body hair may darken and thicken, while hair on the scalp and in the pubic area may thin. Skin may also become thinner and less elastic, which can cause wrinkling and sagging.

EMOTIONAL CHANGES

During menopause women may experience sudden mood changes or depression. Many women feel nervous, irritable, or very tired beginning in perimenopause, either because of lack of sleep or because of the change in their hormone levels. While hormonal changes may explain some of the emotionalism associated with menopause, it can also be a response to aging or changing circumstances. Menopausal women may be mothers, grandmothers, widows, or caretakers of older parents— all circumstances that may contribute to their changing emotions.

LONG-TERM PROBLEMS

The hormonal changes involved in menopause are associated with an increase in the long-term risk of two life-threatening disorders, heart disease and OSTEOPOROSIS. More American women die of heart disease than of any other cause, including all cancers combined. For most of a woman's life, her estrogen levels place her at a lower risk than a man for heart disease, but by age 65, her risk equals that of a man. High blood pressure also occurs more frequently in women after menopause.

Some women going through menopause may consider HORMONE REPLACEMENT THERAPY, which may reduce the risk of osteoporosis but increase the risk of heart disease and breast cancer. During menopause, women should eat a low-fat, high-fiber diet; stop smoking; exercise regularly; maintain a healthy weight; and reduce stress to manageable levels.

Menopause, premature

The end of menstruation before age 40. One percent of all women stop menstruating before they turn 40, often for unknown reasons. In some cases, menstruation stops early because severe infections or tumors damage the ovaries and bring on menopause. Other possible causes include eating disorders, malnutrition, exposure to radiation, chemotherapy, and surgery that impair blood circulation to the ovaries.

Premature menopause also occurs when a woman's ovaries are surgically removed or are damaged by radiation therapy. The result in such cases is called induced menopause. Women whose ovaries suddenly stop working, for whatever reason, often experience menopausal symptoms that are particularly severe. For this reason, it is common practice when performing a HYSTERECTOMY on a premenopausal woman to leave the ovaries in place whenever possible. If the ovaries are removed, hormone replacement therapy may be prescribed to prevent menopausal symptoms and to reduce the risk of osteoporosis.

Menorrhagia

See MENSTRUATION, DISORDERS OF.

Menstruation

The monthly discharge of blood and other secretions from a woman's uterus and the beginning of the reproductive years in a woman's life. Most women have their first period (menarche) around age 12. Menstruation usually stops around age 50 (menopause). The length of the menstrual cycle for most women is 28 days. A woman's menstrual cycle is the time from the first day of one period to the first day of the next. Normal cycles can vary from 21 to 35 days. The number of days a woman menstruates also may vary. Most women have periods lasting from 3 to 7 days, with an average of about 5 days. Most women have monthly periods; others have irregular periods. Many different factors can change a woman's menstrual cycle, including weight gain or loss, an illness, stress, excessive exercise, pregnancy, or menopausal and adolescent transitions. See MENSTRUATION, DISORDERS OF.

THE CYCLE

Typically each month, the lining of the uterus thickens in response to the hormones estrogen and progesterone. During a 28-day menstrual cycle, ovulation (the release of an egg by an ovary into a fallopian tube) occurs about halfway through the cycle, on about day 14. Only at this point can pregnancy occur. As the egg moves into one of the fallopian tubes, a man's sperm can fertilize it. A fertilized egg will usually move into the uterus and attach to the uterine lining, where it begins developing into a fetus. An unfertilized egg will move into the uterus and eventually be absorbed or disintegrate. Estrogen and progesterone levels will then decrease, and the lining of the uterus will be shed during menstruation.

Birth control methods can affect a woman's cycle and period. Birth control pills help regulate menstruation, resulting in regular cycles with light bleeding. However, breakthrough bleeding (bleeding that occurs at a time in the cycle other than when it should), is a common side effect of birth control pills, especially if a woman forgets to take one or more. Intrauterine devices (IUDs) can cause heavy bleeding and severe cramps in some women. If the symptoms are severe enough, removing an IUD may be recommended. See The menstrual cycle on page 840.

Menstruation, disorders of

FOR SYMPTOM CHART
see Menstrual cramps or pain, page 16

Problems related to menstruation, including heavy bleeding, irregular cycles, halting of periods (amenorrhea), and premenstrual syndrome. A doctor can help identify the causes and suggest treatment options.

TYPES OF DISORDERS

Menstrual disorders are among the most common problems in women. Any abnormalities in the menstrual cycle can be symptoms of a problem in the pelvic area, including fibroids, endometriosis, or pelvic inflammaory disease. Disorders can include disruptions in the cycle itself, differences in the discharge, or other problems. Different disorders can be sympto-

M

THE MENSTRUAL CYCLE

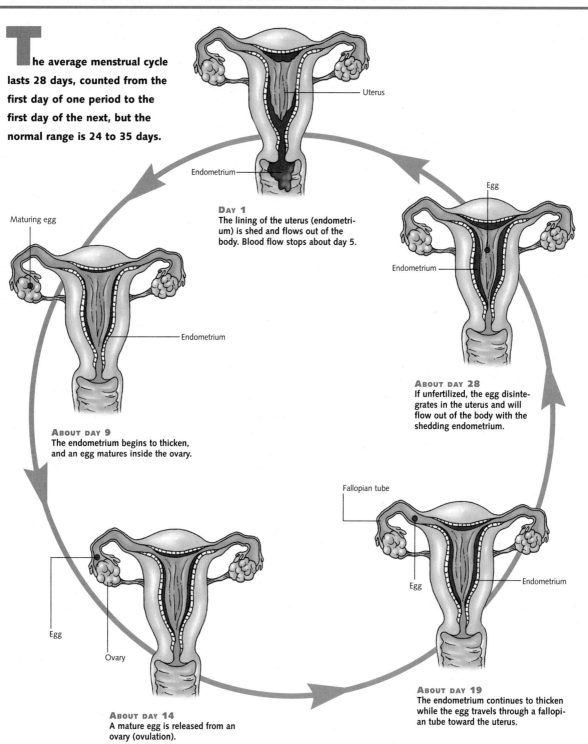

The average menstrual cycle lasts 28 days, counted from the first day of one period to the first day of the next, but the normal range is 24 to 35 days.

Uterus

Endometrium

DAY 1
The lining of the uterus (endometrium) is shed and flows out of the body. Blood flow stops about day 5.

Egg

Endometrium

ABOUT DAY 28
If unfertilized, the egg disintegrates in the uterus and will flow out of the body with the shedding endometrium.

Maturing egg

Endometrium

ABOUT DAY 9
The endometrium begins to thicken, and an egg matures inside the ovary.

Fallopian tube

Egg

Endometrium

ABOUT DAY 19
The endometrium continues to thicken while the egg travels through a fallopian tube toward the uterus.

Egg

Ovary

ABOUT DAY 14
A mature egg is released from an ovary (ovulation).

M

matic of different diseases or conditions.

■ *Heavy bleeding* Menstrual bleeding is abnormal if it lasts for more than a week or if it is different from a woman's usual menstrual pattern. Heavy bleeding can have many causes, including hormone imbalance, cancer of the uterus (see UTERUS, CANCER OF), MISCARRIAGE, infection of the uterus, or blood clotting problems. Heavy bleeding can result in deficient iron, causing anemia. An iron deficiency can be treated with iron supplements and a balanced diet. A woman who experiences heavy bleeding should contact her doctor.

■ *Irregular menstruation* A woman may experience a change in her regular pattern of menstruation for a number of reasons, especially when she first begins having periods and when she nears menopause. Irregular cycles can also occur because of illness, weight gain or loss, stress, heavy exercise, or other reasons. Since pregnancy can halt menstruation, a woman should see her doctor if she misses a period. A doctor can help determine the cause of periods that are irregular in the absence of pregnancy.

■ *Amenorrhea* Amenorrhea is the absence of a woman's menstrual periods. Primary amenorrhea is a condition in which a girl has not yet started menstruating by age 16. Secondary amenorrhea is the temporary or permanent absence of menstrual periods in a woman who has previously menstruated regularly; its most frequent cause is pregnancy. The primary type can occur when there is a delay in the onset of puberty. Such delays are usually not serious and resolve by age 16. In rare cases, a delay in puberty is caused by disorders of the endocrine system. In other rare cases, a congenital problem, such as having been born without a uterus, may be the cause. Secondary amenorrhea can occur in response to continued heavy exercise, an abrupt weight change, severe stress, hormonal abnormalities, or illness, in addition to pregnancy. A woman should see a doctor if she misses her period.

■ *Premenstrual syndrome (PMS)* Some women experience this specific type of physical and mental distress as the menstrual period approaches; it typically disappears during the cycle.

Common PMS symptoms include swollen and tender breasts, bloating (retention of water), headache, depression, mood swings, and irritability. The exact cause of PMS is unknown; however, most doctors believe it is related to hormonal changes that occur in a woman's body throughout her menstrual cycle. Most treatments are geared toward relieving the symptoms of PMS, which can be helped with lifestyle changes such as exercise and a healthy diet and several types of hormonal medications. The best response to treatment occurs with a class of drugs called serotonin reuptake inhibitors, or SRIs. Ibuprofen may be taken for headaches and cramping. Vitamin supplements and, in some situations, birth control pills, may be used to lessen symptoms.

■ *Dysmenorrhea* Severely painful menstruation is called dysmenorrhea. Most often, it is treated with analgesics (painkillers) such as ibuprofen. Sometimes, severe menstrual pain may be caused by a tumor, infection, or ENDOMETRIOSIS, a condition in which tissue that lines the uterus also grows outside the uterus. When a specific cause for the pain is diagnosed, treatment for the underlying problem may be needed.

Menstruation, irregular

A change in a woman's regular pattern of MENSTRUATION. See MENSTRUATION, DISORDERS OF.

Mental illness

Any of a number of disorders that disturb a person's thoughts, emotions, and behavior. Some mental illnesses cause relatively mild distress, while others result in severe impairment and may require hospitalization. Mental illness is also referred to as a psychiatric disorder, emotional disorder, or psychopathology. Common mental illnesses include DEPRESSION, ANXIETY DISORDERS, EATING DISORDERS (anorexia nervosa and bulimia), and PSYCHOSEXUAL DISORDERS (for example, arousal or orgasmic difficulties and exhibitionism). Treatment depends on the nature of the illness and the severity of the symptoms.

Mental retardation

A disorder characterized by below-average intellectual function accom-

panied by deficits in behavior that occurs before age 18 years. The cause of retardation in most children is not known. However, some of the most common causes include genetic disorders such as DOWN SYNDROME and FRAGILE X SYNDROME and environmental factors (such as maternal alcohol abuse during pregnancy). Other causes include BRAIN DAMAGE from head injury or infection, such as bacterial MENINGITIS.

SYMPTOMS
Parents are often the first to notice that an infant is not developing on schedule. He or she may lag in developmental milestones such as rolling over, sitting, crawling, smiling, or walking. This is usually known as DEVELOPMENTAL DELAY and is a sign of possible mental retardation.

There is a vast range in the degree of mental retardation. In a mild case, signs may not be recognizable until school age. Symptoms include lack of curiosity, decreased learning ability, failure to meet standard intellectual markers, persistence of infantile behavior, and inability to meet the requirements of school.

DIAGNOSIS AND TREATMENT
If mental retardation is suspected, an assessment of intellectual function and age-appropriate adaptive behavior must be made by a qualified professional. Indications of a problem are low scores (below 70) on a standard intelligence quotient (IQ) test. There is no cure for mental retardation. Treatment focuses on helping each individual reach his or her own maximum potential.

Mental status examinations

Careful examination by a physician, usually a psychiatrist or neurologist, to determine how well and how normally a person's mind is functioning. The physician checks the person's appearance and behavior, rapport, mood and emotional state, speech, thinking, content of thoughts, cognitive functions, and judgment.

Meralgia paresthetica

A condition caused by compression of a nerve that passes over the hip bone in the groin. When this nerve is compressed, it results in numbness and tingling in the thigh, predominantly

M

along the front and side. No weakness is associated with this condition, and it is more common among people who are obese or who wear tight belts or pants, which add to the compression. Pregnancy and diabetes mellitus, type 1 and type 2, may also be contributing factors. Meralgia paresthetica usually occurs only in one leg but can occur simultaneously in both. Most people with this condition require no treatment except weight loss and wearing of loose-fitting clothing. If burning pains are experienced (which are rare), medications may help. In severe cases, a nerve block can be performed; however, this will result in persistent numbness.

Mercury

A metallic element that is liquid at room temperature. Mercury was used widely in medications and as disinfectants for many years, but its use has been greatly reduced because of concerns about toxic effects. Mercury was formerly used in tooth powders, fungicides, and antiparasitic agents. Because it is nontoxic when combined with other metals, mercury is used as part of amalgam fillings in dentistry. Mercury may also be found in fireworks, hair dyes, and some paints.

Mercury poisoning occurs when metallic mercury is absorbed through the skin or its vapor taken in through the lungs. Acute poisoning causes vomiting, bloody diarrhea, and severe abdominal cramps in addition to the inability to produce urine. Chronic poisoning causes loose teeth, loss of appetite, sores in the mouth, tremors, anemia, and irritability. If someone is suspected of having consumed or absorbed metallic mercury, a POISON CENTER should be contacted immediately.

Mesalamine

A drug used to treat inflammatory bowel disease. Mesalamine (Asacol, Pentasa, Rowasa) is used to treat diseases such as ulcerative colitis. It works by reducing inflammation within the colon. Mesalamine is available as capsules, delayed-release tablets, rectal suppositories, and rectal enemas.

Mesentery

A supporting membrane that attaches various internal organs to the abdominal wall. The term is most frequently used to refer to the part of the peritoneum that enfolds most of the small intestine and attaches it to the rear wall of the abdominal cavity. The mesentery contains the arteries, veins, nerves, and lymphatic vessels that supply the large and small intestines.

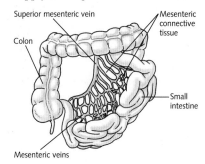

Superior mesenteric vein

Colon

Mesenteric connective tissue

Small intestine

Mesenteric veins

SUPPORTING AND CONNECTING
The mesentery is a heavily veined tissue that supports the organs in the abdomen and connects them to the abdominal wall. Behind the small intestine, the mesentery is supplied with blood by the superior mesenteric vein, and a network of veins branch throughout the connecting tissue to form a membrane.

Mesothelioma

A rare cancerous tumor of the membranes that line the abdominal and chest cavities and cover the lungs. Mesothelioma is strongly associated with long-term exposure to asbestos and can develop 30 to 40 years after exposure. Symptoms of mesothelioma of the lung can include shortness of breath, vague chest pain that may radiate to the shoulders or upper abdomen, loss of appetite and weight, fatigue, hoarseness, and general weakness. Symptoms of mesothelioma in the abdominal cavity can include nausea, vomiting, bowel and urinary obstruction, swelling of the legs and feet, and fever. Symptoms of pleural mesothelioma (in the chest cavity lining) may include pain in the lower back or the side of the chest or shortness of breath. Some individuals experience cough, fever, sweating, fatigue, and weight loss.

Diagnosis of mesothelioma involves chest X rays and CT (computed tomography) scans. Biopsy may require insertion of an ENDOSCOPE (fiberoptic tube used to view internal organs) through the chest into the lung (thoracoscopy), or making an incision in the chest wall (THORACOTO-MY). Biopsy of the abdominal cavity

lining is performed either by inserting an endoscope into the abdominal cavity (LAPAROSCOPY), or by making an incision in the abdomen (see LAPARO-TOMY, EXPLORATORY).

The choice of treatment depends on the extent of the disease. Mesothelioma is considered localized when it appears only in the membrane where it originates; advanced, when the tumor has spread to other parts of the chest or abdomen; or recurrent, when the tumor has returned after treatment. Surgery is the most common treatment of mesothelioma, although radiation therapy may also be used.

Mesothelium

A type of EPITHELIUM (surface cell layer) that lines the body cavities of the peritoneum (the membrane lining the abdominal cavity), the pleura (the membranes that cover the lungs), and the pericardium (the membrane surrounding the heart). Malignant tumors of this lining are often related to asbestos exposure.

Mestranol and norethindrone

A combination of hormones used in oral contraceptives (birth control pills). Mestranol and norethindrone (Necon, Norinyl, Ortho-Novum) are both female hormones involved in contraception; one is a form of estrogen and the other a form of progesterone. These hormones prevent pregnancy by causing the woman's cervical mucus to thicken, which makes it harder for sperm to reach the uterus and for an egg to implant in the uterus.

Metabolism

The entire range of biochemical processes by which living things transform substances into energy. Metabolism is commonly used to refer to the breakdown of food and its transformation into energy, but it incorporates all chemical and physical changes that take place within the body and enable it to grow and function.

Metabolism incorporates two component processes: catabolism and anabolism. Catabolism refers to the breakdown of nutrients or other organic constituents of the body by which energy is liberated and used for other physical processes. Anabolism refers to the building of complex substances from simple ones. The body uses these complex substances to make up tissues and organs.

Metabolism, inborn errors of

A group of inherited disorders of metabolism, many of which are associated with mental retardation. Inborn errors of metabolism usually involve deficiencies of enzymes needed to carry out an important chemical reaction. In most cases, affected infants appear normal at birth, but over time their development slows and symptoms emerge. These may include behavioral disorders, mental retardation, and muscular abnormalities. Inborn errors of metabolism vary in their symptoms and severity according to the specific deficiency involved.

A few are inherited as autosomal dominant traits, meaning that the defective gene is passed directly from an affected parent, while many others are inherited as autosomal recessive traits and must be inherited from both parents, who usually do not have the disease themselves. Individuals with the trait usually have one gene that can instruct the cell to produce enough of the normal enzyme to prevent the disease from expressing itself. Some metabolic errors are carried on the X chromosomes, making them a sex-linked trait. Since males have only one X chromosome, these sex-linked traits primarily affect males. Since women have two X chromosomes, they usually do not have the disease but may have the trait. Some progress has been made in the treatment of some metabolic disorders, whether by providing supplements to counteract the inborn deficiency or by regulating the diet to minimize the effect of the metabolic or enzyme deficiency. A genetic counselor can identify the risks of recurrence for parents who have a family history of metabolic disease.

Metabolite

Any substance produced by metabolism. A metabolite may be produced during metabolism, or it may be a constituent of food taken into the body.

Metaphysis

The end part of the long arm or leg bone, which contains the growth plate and is composed primarily of cartilage during bone development in children. If a fracture occurs in this area during childhood, complications with proper bone growth can occur.

Metaplasia

Cells that appear abnormal under a microscope yet do not show signs of malignancy. Metaplasia is an acquired condition, in which normal tissue is transformed into what may or may not be premalignant tissue. For example, squamous metaplasia of the cervix refers to a change in the cells on the surface of the cervix that is part of a normal repair process.

Metastasis

The spread of disease, usually cancer, from one part of the body to another; a cancer that has spread. When cancer spreads, it is still named after the part of the body where it first developed. If prostate cancer has spread to the lungs, for example, it is still considered prostate cancer. Meta-stasis involves the spread of cancer cells through the bloodstream or the lymphatic system. Lymph vessels are similar to blood vessels, except that they carry tissue waste products and immune system cells, called lymphocytes, instead of blood. Lymph vessels lead to lymph nodes, reservoirs of immune system cells that resist infections. Cancer cells can break off from tumors and enter either the bloodstream or the lymph vessels, to be carried to lymph nodes, where they may continue to grow. Surgeons removing cancerous tumors usually try to remove nearby lymph nodes as well.

Metastases are responsible for many cancer deaths. Most common cancers (prostate, breast, lung, and colon cancers) can be cured by surgery before the cancer has spread or metastasized. The more serious consequences of the common cancers are usually the direct result of metastasis, either because the disease has spread to an essential organ, such as the liver, or because it has spread to other organs and disrupted normal function. Early treatment of cancer helps prevent metastasis.

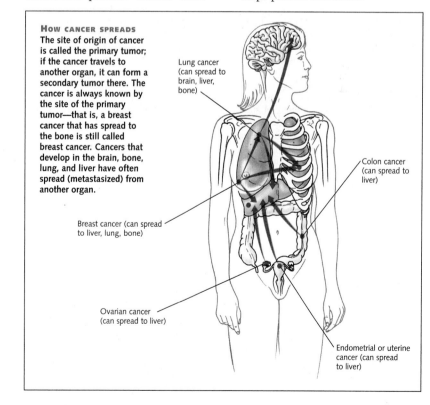

HOW CANCER SPREADS
The site of origin of cancer is called the primary tumor; if the cancer travels to another organ, it can form a secondary tumor there. The cancer is always known by the site of the primary tumor—that is, a breast cancer that has spread to the bone is still called breast cancer. Cancers that develop in the brain, bone, lung, and liver have often spread (metastasized) from another organ.

Lung cancer (can spread to brain, liver, bone)

Colon cancer (can spread to liver)

Breast cancer (can spread to liver, lung, bone)

Ovarian cancer (can spread to liver)

Endometrial or uterine cancer (can spread to liver)

Metatarsalgia

A pain in the metatarsal region of the foot. The metatarsal bones are the five long cylindrical bones that make up the central skeleton of the foot. They are located between the tarsal bones (which form the ankle and back of the foot) and the phalanges (the toes).

Metformin hydrochloride

An antihyperglycemic drug. Metformin hydrochloride (Glucophage) is used to treat type 2 diabetes mellitus. Metformin hydrochloride is used to lower the blood sugar level and to make it possible for the body to convert blood sugar to energy, which it does by decreasing the production of glucose by the liver and increasing tissue responsiveness to insulin. Metformin may be used alone, with another oral hypoglycemic medicine called a sulfonylurea, or with insulin, to lower blood sugar. This medication is not effective for type 1 diabetes, which requires insulin injections.

Methadone maintenance

Treatment of a person with heroin addiction to reduce withdrawal symptoms and a craving for the drug. Methadone is a long-acting synthetic narcotic painkiller developed in the 1960s. Methadone maintenance treatment is used throughout the world and is considered the most effective treatment available for heroin addiction. In methadone maintenance treatment, tolerance is deliberately induced to a stable dose of methadone that is high enough to block the narcotic and euphoric effects of morphine and other opiates, including heroin.

Methadone maintenance has been shown to reduce crime associated with addiction, to prevent the spread of HIV (human immunodeficiency virus) and AIDS (acquired immunodeficiency syndrome) by reducing the frequency of needle sharing, and to reduce and even eliminate heroin use among those addicted. Methadone maintenance has been extensively studied and has been shown to have almost no long-term negative health consequences, even when treatment continues for 20 or 30 years.

Methamphetamine hydrochloride

A central nervous system stimulant drug. Methamphetamine hydrochloride (Desoxyn) has limited medical uses, such as for the treatment of narcolepsy (sudden attacks of deep sleep), ATTENTION DEFICIT/HYPERACTIVITY DISORDER (ADHD), and obesity. Methamphetamine hydrochloride is powerfully addictive and affects the central nervous system, causing increased activity, decreased appetite, and a feeling of well-being that is often followed by a state of high agitation that can turn into violent behavior. Because it is easily prepared in illegal laboratories with inexpensive ingredients, methamphetamine hydrochloride has a high potential for drug abuse.

Methanol

Wood alcohol; also called methyl alcohol. Methanol is used as a solvent or fuel and is a clear, colorless, flammable liquid with a characteristic odor. Consumption of even a very small amount of methanol can produce permanent blindness, and 100 milliliters (about ½ cup) is likely to be fatal for an adult. Consuming as little as 2 tablespoons of methanol may be fatal for a child. Methanol is found in antifreeze, paint remover, shellac, and varnish.

The symptoms of poisoning from methanol include weakness, leg cramps, seizures, breathing difficulties, blurred vision, bluish lips and fingernails, nausea, headache, dizziness, and coma. Permanent blindness can occur after methanol ingestion. If a person is suspected of having consumed methanol, a POISON CENTER should be called immediately.

Methotrexate

An antimetabolite drug used to treat certain cancers, rheumatoid arthritis, and some forms of psoriasis. Methotrexate (Rheumatrex, Folex) works by blocking an enzyme needed by cells to live, thereby interfering with the growth of certain cells. Methotrexate is used to prevent the growth of certain cancer cells and skin cells that grow too fast in people with psoriasis. Methotrexate is also used to treat severe rheumatoid arthritis that has failed to respond to other therapies. The growth of nor-

mal body cells is also affected by methotrexate, causing hair loss and other side effects, some of which occur months or years after the drug is taken.

Methoxsalen

A drug used to treat skin conditions that increase the skin's sensitivity to sunlight. Methoxsalen (8-MOP, Oxsoralen) is a very strong medicine used along with ultraviolet light to treat vitiligo, a condition in which skin color is lost, and psoriasis, a skin disorder associated with red, scaly patches. It is also used with ultraviolet light to treat skin problems associated with a type of cancer called mycosis fungoides. Methoxsalen is capable of causing severe sunburn, premature aging of the skin, skin cancer, and cataracts. It should be used only as prescribed.

Methyl alcohol

See METHANOL.

Methylphenidate hydrochloride

A central nervous system stimulant drug. Methylphenidate (Methylin, Ritalin) is used to treat ATTENTION DEFICIT/HYPERACTIVITY DISORDER (ADHD), narcolepsy (sudden attacks of deep sleep), and other conditions. Methylphenidate is used to treat ADHD in combination with social, educational, and psychological therapies; the goal is to increase the attention span of a person while decreasing restlessness in children and adults who are hyperactive, impulsive, and easily distracted.

Methylprednisolone

See CORTICOSTEROIDS.

Metoclopramide

A drug that stimulates movements of the stomach and the first part of the small intestine; an antivomiting drug. Metoclopramide (Reglan and others) is used to treat a condition called diabetic gastroparesis by relieving symptoms of nausea, vomiting, loss of appetite, and a continued feeling of fullness after meals. Metoclopramide is given by injection to prevent nausea and vomiting that can occur following anticancer chemotherapy. It is also sometimes used to treat symptoms (such as heartburn) in people who have esophageal injury caused by the backward flow of gastric acid into the esophagus.

Metoprolol

An antihypertensive drug used to lower high blood pressure and decrease cardiac output. It is used to treat people who have had a heart attack by reducing heart rate and blood pressure. Metoprolol (Lopressor and Toprol-XL) works as a beta-adrenergic blocking agent. Like all BETA BLOCKERS, metoprolol works by decreasing the heart's need for oxygen and blood by reducing its workload and helping it to beat regularly. Metoprolol is also used to treat angina (chest pain) and to prevent migraine headaches.

Metronidazole

A drug used to treat infections. Metronidazole (Flagyl, Metro-Cream, MetroGel-Vaginal Gel) is used to treat various infections caused by bacteria or other microorganisms. Among the infections for which metronidazole may be prescribed are pelvic inflammatory disease (PID) and peptic ulcer disease. As a topical gel or cream, it may be used to treat acne, rosacea, or bacterial vaginosis. It is thought that metronidazole works by disrupting DNA and nucleic acid synthesis within the invading organism. It is available in many forms, including oral, injectable, and topical.

Metrorrhagia

Bleeding from the uterus that occurs between menstrual periods. Causes may include polyps or cancer of the endometrium (see ENDOMETRIAL CANCER), CERVICITIS, and cancer of the cervix (see CERVIX, CANCER OF). Spotty bleeding sometimes occurs during ovulation. Women who take estrogen therapy may experience metrorrhagia from the medication. See MENSTRUATION, DISORDERS OF.

Miconazole

An antifungal drug. Miconazole is used to treat certain types of fungus infections of the skin and the vagina. It is available by prescription for injection, as a vaginal suppository, and as a cream. Miconazole is also available without prescription in many brands as a cream, powder, spray, and vaginal suppository.

Microalbuminuria

A condition in which small amounts of the blood protein albumin leak into the urine. Microalbuminuria occurs during the early stages of KIDNEY FAILURE in people with diabetes. It is characterized by an elevated rate of filtration in the kidneys, with the glomeruli (filtering units of the kidneys) showing damage.

At first, microalbuminuria occurs only periodically. However, as the rate of albumin leakage into the urine increases, the condition becomes more constant. Normally, loss of albumin from the blood occurs at a rate of less than 30 milligrams during 24 hours. As microalbuminuria progresses, the loss may increase from 30 to 300 milligrams over 24 hours. When the loss of albumin is more than 300 milligrams over 24 hours, the condition is called ALBUMINURIA.

There is a special medical test (microalbuminuria test) to pinpoint the status of microalbuminuria. People who have type 1 or type 2 diabetes mellitus can remain in the early stages of kidney failure with microalbuminuria for a long time without further kidney damage. Maintaining normal blood pressure and controlling the blood sugar level help prevent rapid progression of the condition. Many doctors prescribe angiotensin-converting enzyme inhibitors (see ANTIHYPERTENSIVES) to help prevent kidney deterioration.

Microangiopathy

A disease of the very small blood vessels.

Microbe

Any living organism so small it can be viewed only under a microscope. Often, the word is used to describe disease-causing organisms, such as viruses, bacteria, protozoa, and fungi. The words microbe and microorganism have the same meaning.

Microbiology

The branch of medical science that studies organisms so small (microbes or microorganisms) they can be viewed only under a microscope. The organisms include disease-causing agents, such as bacteria, viruses, protozoa, and fungi.

Microcephaly

In a newborn, an abnormally small head. Microcephaly is associated with fetal alcohol syndrome and the rare disorder PKU, or phenylketonuria. It can have many other causes, including DOWN SYNDROME, RUBELLA, malnutrition, and exposure to radiation.

When a baby is born with a very small head, the head circumference will be measured at birth and laboratory tests will be used to identify any metabolic causes. Diagnostic tests, such as CT (computed tomography) scanning or MRI (magnetic resonance imaging), which identify abnormal brain structures, may be used. Once the cause is established, the doctor will provide GENETIC COUNSELING for the parents to help them understand the risk of microcephaly in any subsequent children. The doctor will help the family determine the appropriate care necessary to help the child develop, because many children born with microcephaly may be developmentally delayed.

Microorganism

Any living organism so small it can be viewed only under a microscope. Often, the word is use to describe disease-causing organisms, such as viruses, bacteria, protozoa, and fungi. The words microorganism and microbe have the same meaning. Microorganisms reside in humans, animals, and the environment.

Microscope

An instrument used to view an enlarged image of small objects, organisms, or structures and to see details that could not otherwise be seen. The most widely used microscopes are optical or light microscopes, which magnify the image with visible light. The specimen is placed on a thin rectangle of glass (a slide) and then positioned on the viewing stage of the microscope. Light from a source under the stage passes through the specimen and then travels up a closed tube with two lenses: one near the specimen, one near the eye of the viewer. Depending on the strength of the lenses, magnification 1,000 times or more is possible.

TYPES

Other types of optical microscopes are used for special purposes. The

M

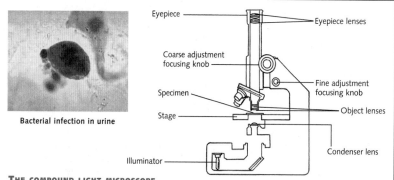

THE COMPOUND LIGHT MICROSCOPE
The specimen is placed on a glass slide, which is held on a stage. An optical condenser lens concentrates light from a built-in illuminator onto the specimen. The object lens magnifies the specimen, and the image is further magnified by the eyepiece, or viewing lenses. The user focuses by moving the object lens up or down to alter the distance from the specimen.

stereoscopic microscope uses two low-magnification microscopes that are arranged to provide a single three-dimensional image of a specimen. The phase microscope makes use of variations in the way light passes through different materials to view living cells.

Optical microscopes cannot allow the viewer to see objects or structures smaller than the wavelength of the light illuminating the specimen. To see smaller details, scientists use optical microscopes with different light sources, such as ultraviolet, which has a shorter wavelength and allows greater magnification, or electron microscopes. Electron microscopes illuminate the specimen with a beam of electrons that is focused on a fluorescent screen, a photographic plate, or a television screen. In a transmission electron microscope, the electrons pass through the specimen and provide a flat image that has been enlarged as much as 1 million times. In a scanning electron microscope, the electrons pass over the specimen to create a three-dimensional image of its surface enlarged 100,000 times or more. Electron microscopes are used to diagnose certain viral infections.

Microsurgery

Any delicate procedure in which a surgeon views the operation site through a special surgical microscope to operate on small structures within the body. Microsurgical techniques are used on the ear, brain, larynx, and reproductive system, in reconstruc-

tion of facial features, and in reattaching severed limbs.

The advantage of microsurgery is that it allows the surgeon accurate and precise access to very small structures. In RECONSTRUCTIVE SURGERY, for example, the surgeon can transplant tissue from one part of the body to another and then reconnect blood vessels that are only 1 to 2 millimeters in diameter. As a result, the transplant has a much better chance of succeeding.

Likewise, microsurgery has proved useful in restoring fertility to men and women with reproductive ducts damaged by venereal disease or prior

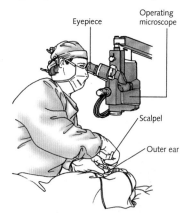

ADVANTAGES OF MICROSURGERY
A surgeon performing a microscopic procedure is able to work looking through a microscope that magnifies the operating site. The instruments used in microsurgery are also extraordinarily small and fine. The technique enables the surgeon to work on extremely small structures within the body (the middle ear in this case) that are not clearly visible to the eye.

sterilization surgery. In men, for example, successful reversal of VASECTOMY used to be limited by the small size of the vas deferens (see REPRODUCTIVE SYSTEM, MALE). With the use of a microscope of 10 to 40 times magnification, the surgeon can see the structure well, repair it, and insert tiny sutures to reconnect it precisely.

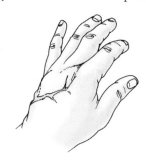

REATTACHED FINGER
Microsurgical technique enables the surgeon to reconnect tiny blood vessels and nerves that are only 1 to 2 millimeters in diameter, making it particularly useful for the reattachment of severed limbs and for organ transplant. For example, a finger severed from a hand can be reattached and very nearly normal function restored.

Micturition

The passing of urine; the act of urination. Micturition has been shown to occur in humans as early as 32 weeks' gestation, or about 2 months before birth.

Middle-ear effusion, persistent

See OTITIS MEDIA.

Midlife crisis

An intense, temporary pattern of disturbing feelings, usually anxiety and depression, that accompany the transition from early adulthood into middle age, particularly during the early 40s. The crisis consists of an emotional struggle within the self and with the external world about the meaning, purpose, and direction of the person's life. Individuals going through a midlife crisis question every aspect of their lives; often engage in self-recrimination over their choice of spouse, profession, or occupation; and may initiate major changes in relationships or work, such as a career change or a new partner. The midlife crisis is a developmental stage, not evidence of a psychiatric disorder. However, if the crisis remains unresolved, it can lead to disturbing emotional patterns that may require treatment.

Midwife

A person trained to assist women in CHILDBIRTH. Midwives typically provide care and education to women during the prenatal period (see PRENATAL CARE), through LABOR and delivery, and after the birth of the baby. They promote a noninterventional process of childbirth. While minimizing drug use, they use other approaches to labor pain management such as relaxation methods, breathing techniques, and suggesting various physical positions. Midwives often handle home deliveries and assist in birthing centers, where they work with a physician.

Midwives vary in levels of training and licensing. A certified nurse-midwife (CNM) is a registered nurse who has completed an accredited university program and passed national boards given by the American College of Nurse-Midwives. A CNM is licensed by the state both as a registered nurse and as a CNM. Some states license professional midwives who are not nurses but are trained in state-approved midwife programs. Some midwives are unlicensed; they may have extensive or very little training. Their practice is illegal in most states.

Well-educated midwives have appropriate clinical skills and can provide high-quality care in a normal birth. For serious complications of pregnancy and birth, a physician's skills are needed. Generally, midwives do not handle high-risk pregnancies, such as those in which the baby is in breech position (feet or bottom first) or the mother has diabetes or is carrying multiple fetuses. CNMs usually work closely with a physician to whom they refer problems beyond their training and expertise.

Migraine

A common form of primary HEADACHE. Migraine pain seems to run in families, and women are three times more likely than men to experience this type of headache. The onset is usually between age 10 and 46 years. Seventy to 80 percent of all migraine headaches are classified as common migraines (migraines without a preceding AURA, or an unusual sensation such as tingling or seeing zigzagging lights). Migraines that are preceded by an aura are known as classic migraines. Other forms of migraine include complicated migraine (with focal neurological symptoms), basilar migraine (with vertigo and occasionally loss of consciousness), and ophthalmic migraine (with eye pain and vision loss).

CAUSES

Migraine pain is typically associated with alternate constricting and relaxing of blood vessels in the brain. However, in recent years researchers have also focused attention on alterations in nerve pathways and imbalances in brain chemistry. The trigeminal nerve system is a major pain pathway; SEROTONIN, a neurotransmitter or nerve chemical, regulates pain messages passing through the trigeminal nerve system. A malfunction or chemical imbalance in this system is believed to be an underlying cause of headaches, including migraines.

There are many possible triggers of migraine pain. Triggers themselves do not cause pain; instead, they activate already existing brain chemical imbalances. Triggers vary from person to person, but may include hormonal fluctuations caused by birth control pill use (see CONTRACEPTION, HORMONAL METHODS), HORMONE REPLACEMENT THERAPY, and PREMENSTRUAL SYNDROME. In women who have migraines, more than half occur right before, during, or directly after their period. Migraines diminish in many women following menopause.

Other triggers include physical or mental stress, changes in sleep patterns, allergic reactions, smoking or exposure to secondhand smoke, bright lights, loud noises, alcohol, caffeine, and missed meals. Diet is widely implicated in migraine. Possible dietary triggers include foods that contain the amino acid tyramine (including red wine, aged cheese, figs, chicken livers, and smoked fish), chocolate, processed foods, food additives (such as monosodium glutamate [MSG]), meats containing nitrates (including hot dogs, bacon, and salami), nuts, peanut butter, dairy products, onions, and certain fruits (such as avocados and bananas).

SYMPTOMS

Migraine headaches are characterized by throbbing pain that most commonly begins on one side of the head. Pain may remain localized or spread to both sides. It can start on either side, beginning as a dull ache that gradually worsens into disabling pain, or it can begin abruptly with severe pain from the onset. Migraine attacks occur on a sporadic basis and can last from several hours to several days. Severe pain may be accompanied by other symptoms, such as nausea, vomiting, dizziness, chills, loss of appetite, irritability, fatigue, and extreme sensitivity to light and sound.

In some cases, migraine pain is preceded by fatigue, depression, or an aura. An aura may consist of dreamlike perceptions or visual disturbances. Possible preliminary or prodromal symptoms of migraine pain include tingling or numbness, strange tastes or odors, restlessness, confusion, eye pain, blurred vision, intolerance of bright light, zigzagging lights, flashing lights, and other visual hallucinations.

DIAGNOSIS

Diagnosis of a migraine is based on the nature of the pain, its frequency and duration, location, severity, and accompanying symptoms. In some cases, a migraine is a warning sign of a potentially serious problem. Tests such as CT (computed tomography) scanning, MRI (magnetic resonance imaging), electroencephalogram (EEG), and blood studies may be performed to rule out serious underlying causes of symptoms, such as a ruptured ANEURYSM, BRAIN TUMOR, STROKE, TRANSIENT ISCHEMIC ATTACK, or MENINGITIS. Doctors recommend immediate medical evaluation for those who experience migraines accompanied by a loss in consciousness; sudden, violent head pain; head pain that worsens over time and is accompanied by symptoms such as nausea, vomiting, fever, and a stiff neck; and head pain that is associated with abnormal neurological functions (including changes in speech, vision, balance, movement, and sensation).

TREATMENT

The management of migraine pain has improved dramatically during the last 10 years. Today doctors treat migraines with two categories of medications: abortive (to relieve pain and other symptoms) and prophylactic (to prevent migraines from developing). Abortive medications include triptans (such as sumatriptan and zolmitriptan), vasoconstrictors (such ergotamine tartrate), lidocaine nasal drops, muscle relaxants, narcotic analgesics, and aspirin and other nonsteroidal anti-inflammatory drugs (NSAIDs). Prophylactic medications include tricyclic antidepressants, serotonin antagonists, cardiovascular drugs (beta blockers and calcium channel blockers), antiseizure drugs (such as valproic acid), vitamin B2 (riboflavin), and magnesium. Preventive medication is usually recommended for people who have more than two migraine attacks a month and for people in whom pain is so severe that it prevents normal activity. Doctors advise people who experience typical warning symptoms (such as auras) to take medication at the first sign of an impending attack.

The mainstay of home care is rest in a dark, quiet room. Because poor lifestyle habits can contribute to migraines, many people benefit from regular sleep, exercise, a healthy diet, and avoidance of smoking, alcohol, and caffeine. Doctors also recommend strategies such as relaxation therapy and biofeedback. Whenever possible, it is important to identify and avoid the triggers of migraines (such as problem foods). Keeping a headache diary is a helpful way to do this. This entails maintaining a calendar record of headaches, associated symptoms, and environmental factors, such as diet, menstrual cycles, and sleep patterns. See Types of headaches on page 633.

Milia

Small, firm, superficial, benign (not cancerous), white bumps typically found on the cheeks and forehead. They are a common condition in newborns that generally disappear without treatment after several weeks. In adults, they may be removed by a dermatologist by making a small nick in the skin and expressing the contents of the cyst.

Milk-alkali syndrome

An imbalance of body chemistry that results from ingesting abnormally large quantities of antacids and milk over a long period. Milk-alkali syn-drome is rare and can be a potentially serious medical condition. It tends to occur in people who have chronic indigestion, which they attempt to treat with antacids and milk.

Mind-body medicine

A way of approaching health and illness that emphasizes the intricate relations among mind, body, and spirit and their mutual effects.

TYPES

Many conventional and alternative mind-body interventions exist.

■ *Psychotherapy* Psychotherapy is the treatment of a person's emotional and psychological health with medication, behavioral modification or re-education, and ongoing discussion of the person's concerns.

■ *Support groups* Groups such as Alcoholics Anonymous or groups for people who have the same disease help members form bonds with each other and promote sharing of information and experiences.

■ *Meditation* A self-directed practice for relaxing the body and calming the mind, meditation helps reduce pain, anxiety, high blood pressure, and cholesterol levels and provides useful techniques for coping with stress.

■ *Hypnosis* The induction of trance states and the power of suggestion can help a person manage pain, reduce bleeding in people with hemophilia, and lessen the severity of hay fever and asthma attacks, among other common ailments.

■ *Yoga* Yoga is way of life that seeks enlightenment and incorporates dietary practice, physical exercise, and ethical concerns. Yoga is used to reduce anxiety levels, lower blood pressure, reduce cholesterol levels, and help people stop smoking.

Mineral supplements

Dietary supplements containing essential minerals, usually in combination with vitamins. Together, minerals and vitamins are called "micronutrients," substances required in tiny amounts to promote essential biochemical reactions in the cells. The lack of a particular micronutrient for a prolonged period causes a deficiency disease or condition, which can generally be reversed by supplying the lacking micronutrients. While it is preferable to consume micronutrients from the diet, there are cases in which that is not possible, and supplements may be used. Minerals must come from either food or supplements; the body cannot manufacture them. Consulting a physician about dosages is prudent because large doses of some minerals can cause toxic effects.

MINERAL DEFICIENCY

A mineral deficiency may be caused by a person not getting enough of a mineral in his or her diet when ordinary nutritional needs increase or when a person is unable to absorb nutrients from consumed food. A mineral deficiency or a lack of a particular mineral in the diet can lead to a nutritional deficiency disease.

People at risk for nutritional deficiency include these groups:

- Children and pregnant or breast-feeding women, who have greater nutritional needs
- Teenagers who follow "fad" diets
- Poor or homeless people
- Older people who cannot or do not eat properly
- People who heavily abuse alcohol, tobacco, or drugs, all of which destroy minerals and vitamins
- People with chronic diseases
- People with limited, unvaried diets because of food allergies or intolerance
- People with intestinal disorders whose bodies cannot absorb nutrients
- People on strict weight-loss diets who consume fewer than 1,000 calories per day
- Vegetarians who do not obtain essential nutrients normally supplied by animal products

Mineralization, dental

The developmental stage of teeth when calcium and other minerals are acquired in the enamel, DENTIN, and CEMENTUM of the teeth. The enamel is almost entirely mineralized, or calcified, making it the hardest substance in the human body. To lesser degrees, the dentin and cementum are also mineralized. See also DECALCIFICATION, DENTAL; ENAMEL, DENTAL.

Mineralocorticoid

A corticosteroid hormone secreted by the adrenal cortex (the outer layer of the adrenal glands). Mineralocorticoids regulate the balance of water and electrolytes in the body, particularly sodium (salt) and potassium. They also have a role in normalizing blood pressure.

Three mineralocorticoids are released by the adrenal cortex. One of them, ALDOSTERONE, is responsible for most of the mineralocorticoid activity in the body. The function of aldosterone is to prevent the rapid depletion of sodium and water from the body and to promote the elimination of potassium. This is accomplished by stimulating the kidneys to reabsorb salt and water at an increased rate, which removes sodium ions from the urine and returns them to the blood. This makes the blood less acidic and prevents ACIDOSIS.

Minerals

Inorganic nutrients that are important for good health. Minerals help build structures such as red blood cells and bones.

ESSENTIAL MINERALS

The human body needs minerals to help regulate cell function and provide structure for cells. Major minerals include calcium, phosphorus, and magnesium. Lesser amounts of other minerals are needed, such as chromium, copper, fluoride, iodine, iron, manganese, molybdenum, selenium, zinc, potassium, and sodium.

■ *Calcium* is the most abundant mineral in the human body, with more than 99 percent of it found in the skeleton. Calcium is essential for blood clotting, contraction of muscles, enzyme activity, and neural transmission. Growing children, adolescents, and pregnant or breast-feeding women need large amounts of calcium.

The symptoms of calcium deficiency include brittle bones associated with old age and osteoporosis, a disease characterized by the loss of bone density. Muscle cramps may also indicate a lack of calcium.

Calcium is normally found in low-fat dairy products, green leafy vegetables, eggs, dried beans, nuts, seeds, and tofu.

■ *Phosphorus* works with calcium and vitamin D to build and maintain bones and teeth. It is also involved in enzyme activities related to metabolism. Deficiency of phosphorus is rare and is associated with disease.

The best sources of phosphorus are protein foods such as meat, fish, eggs, beans, and dairy products. Whole grains are also good sources.

■ *Magnesium* works with calcium to build bones and teeth and is involved in enzyme activities. It is essential for the functioning of the muscles, the nervous system, and the circulatory system, including the heart.

A deficiency of magnesium occurs when it is lost through alcohol abuse, kidney disease, diarrhea, or vomiting. Symptoms include muscle tremors or spasms, weakness, confusion, irregular heartbeat, and poor growth.

Good sources of magnesium include whole grains, legumes, nuts, and dark green, leafy vegetables, with smaller amounts found in meat, fish, and dairy products.

■ *Chromium* is essential in carbohydrate metabolism, part of the glucose tolerance factor that regulates blood sugar levels. It may also be a factor in prevention of high cholesterol levels and atherosclerosis. Deficiency is extremely rare and usually has been seen only in people being fed intravenously. Good sources include whole grains and molasses.

■ *Copper* is involved in the formation of red blood cells, bones, and hemoglobin. It is essential to many body processes, including metabolism of iron; pigmentation of hair, eyes, and skin; production of hormones; and, perhaps, cancer prevention. Deficiency is rare; symptoms include fragile bones, anemia, and diarrhea in infants.

Good sources are organ meats, shellfish, whole grains, and dried fruits.

■ *Fluoride* is important to bone and tooth formation; it is known to prevent tooth decay. The only known symptom of fluoride deficiency is tooth decay.

Good sources include seafood, tea, coffee, and soybeans. It is added to the water supply in most communities to prevent tooth decay.

■ *Iodine* is essential to the production of thyroid hormones, and adequate iodine intake during pregnancy is crucial to normal fetal development. The most common symptom of deficiency is goiter, in which an enlarged thyroid gland results in swelling of the neck and hypothyroidism.

Good sources of iodine are saltwater fish, shellfish, sea kelp, and iodized salt.

■ *Iron* is needed for production of hemoglobin and red blood cells, the delivery of oxygen to muscles and other body tissues, and protection against the effects of stress. Iron deficiency is common, particularly among women of childbearing age, who lose iron through menstruation. Symptoms of deficiency include anemia, fatigue, pale skin, brittle nails, lowered resistance to infection, and shortness of breath.

Iron is poorly absorbed through food; vitamin E can decrease iron absorption. The richest sources are red meat and organ meats. Other sources are whole wheat products, shellfish, nuts, and dried fruits.

■ *Manganese* is involved in enzyme production, sex hormone formation, and metabolism of fat, carbohydrate, and vitamin B1. It is essential for normal brain and bone development. Deficiency is extremely rare, usually appearing only in people unable to metabolize it.

Good sources include tea, green vegetables, rice, legumes, oats, dried beans, raisins, and pineapple.

■ *Molybdenum* is involved in enzyme activities, including several that involve uric acid. Deficiency is rare in humans. Good sources include milk, dairy products, whole-grain cereals, legumes, organ meats, leafy vegetables, and beans.

■ *Potassium* works with sodium to regulate bodily fluids and is essential to the healthy functioning of nerves and muscles, as well as to the proper regulation of cardiac rhythm. It is also involved in the metabolism of carbohydrates and protein and in the production of energy. A deficiency may occur whenever bodily fluids are lost, as in vomiting, diarrhea, kidney disease, or when taking drugs such as insulin and corticosteroids, which may affect the absorption of potassium. Symptoms include muscle weakness, fatigue, digestive disorders, loss of appetite, insomnia, and confusion.

The best sources include potatoes, dried fruits, bananas, legumes, raw carrots, avocados, and mushrooms. Lean meats, milk, fish, cantaloupe, spinach, and peanuts are also good sources.

■ *Selenium,* associated with vitamin E, helps protect cells and tissues from damage by free radicals. It may pro-

M

tect against some cancers. Deficiency has not been observed in humans, separate from vitamin E deficiency, although it is believed that people living in areas where the soil is low in selenium may have greater susceptibility to cancer.

Good sources include whole-grain cereals, fish, shellfish, meat, and egg products.

■ **Sodium** is essential to good health and works with potassium to maintain fluid balance in the body. It is also important for muscle contraction and control of cardiac rhythm. Deficiency is uncommon; symptoms include loss of appetite, muscle cramps, nausea, weakness, and dizziness.

Sodium is found in many foods and is added to many prepared foods.

■ **Zinc** is involved in enzymes, especially those involved with growth, skin, wound healing, reproductive organs, protein metabolism, and energy production. Children and older people are susceptible to zinc deficiency, and some people are unable to absorb zinc from food. Symptoms include poor wound healing, impaired growth in children, white spots on fingernails, loss of the sense of taste, night blindness, loss of hair, and frequent infections.

Rich sources include oysters, organ meats, lean red meat, yeast, whole-grain cereals, legumes, liver, and eggs.

Minilaparotomy

A procedure used in TUBAL LIGATION, a sterilization method for women. The doctor makes a small incision near the pubic bone and pulls the fallopian tubes (see FALLOPIAN TUBE) through the opening, ties them off with bands or surgical clips, and stitches the incision closed. This procedure is common in other countries but is rarely used in the United States, where LAPAROSCOPY is preferred. Minilaparotomy is generally used in the United States when laparoscopy is not technically possible.

Minipills

Birth control pills that contain only progestin. See CONTRACEPTION, HORMONAL METHODS.

Terms in small capital letters—for example, PHYSICAL THERAPY or PAGET DISEASE—indicate a cross-reference to another entry with more information.

Minocycline

An antibiotic. Minocycline (Dynacin, Minocin) is used to treat many bacterial infections, including urinary tract infections, acne, gonorrhea, and chlamydial infections. Minocycline is a tetracycline antibiotic. It should not be given to children younger than 8 years because it can discolor their teeth. The drug is not safe for pregnant women.

Minoxidil

A hair growth stimulant; also an antihypertensive drug. Minoxidil (Rogaine, Loniten) is applied to the scalp to stimulate hair growth in men and women with a particular type of baldness. The way in which minoxidil works is not entirely clear. When hair growth is achieved, it is usually noticed several months after the drug is first applied; hair growth continues only as long as the drug is used. Minoxidil is available without prescription as a hair growth stimulant.

Minoxidil is also used to treat high blood pressure. For this purpose, minoxidil comes in tablet form and requires a doctor's prescription.

Miosis

Constriction of the pupil in the eye. Miosis can result from changes in the muscle fibers of the iris (the colored portion of the eye) or be a sign of certain neurological diseases. Certain glaucoma drops, such as pilocarpine, cause miosis.

Miscarriage

Spontaneous abortion; loss of a pregnancy before the fetus is developed enough to survive outside the uterus, or before approximately 20 weeks of gestation. Fifteen to 20 percent of all pregnancies result in miscarriage. It is more common in women older than 35 years of age and in pregnancies with more than one fetus. A miscarriage often resembles an especially heavy menstrual period.

DIAGNOSIS

The most common symptom of a miscarriage is vaginal bleeding, with or without pain. The blood may be brown or bright red, and bleeding may occur repeatedly over several days. A pregnant woman who is bleeding should contact a doctor to find out if she is having a miscarriage. Typically, an ultrasound will be con-

ducted; symptoms will be monitored to control bleeding and pain and to confirm that the cervix remains closed. The woman will probably be advised to rest and to avoid intercourse. Normal activities or sex will not cause a miscarriage, but women who are bleeding during pregnancy should avoid vigorous exercise and get extra rest.

When bleeding and pain are accompanied by breaking of the amniotic sac surrounding the fetus and the opening of the cervix, a miscarriage is certain and the process is described as an inevitable miscarriage. In an incomplete miscarriage (also called an incomplete abortion), a miscarriage occurs, but some of the fetus remains in the uterus. In the condition called a missed miscarriage, or missed abortion, the uterus fails to expel the fetus after it has died. In both incomplete and missed miscarriages, symptoms of pregnancy may begin to disappear. In both situations, a procedure may be performed to remove the contents of the uterus. Most often, when a pregnancy has ended early, a D AND C (dilation and curettage) procedure is performed. If an incomplete miscarriage occurs late in a pregnancy, a doctor may induce labor to remove the fetus.

CAUSES AND RISKS

Fetal chromosome abnormalities frequently cause miscarriages. Miscarriage also is associated with anatomical problems in the mother, such as an abnormally shaped uterus, scar tissue on the lining of the uterus (the endometrium), fibroids in the uterus, or a hormonal imbalance. An abnormally shaped uterus is often a problem for daughters of women who took DES (diethylstilbestrol) when they were pregnant; DES is a synthetic hormone that was given to pregnant women in the 1960s to treat threatened abortion and premature labor. The condition often can be surgically corrected. Scar tissue in the lining of the uterus can result from fibroids or from a D and C procedure in which there were complications.

The risk for miscarriage is higher in women who smoke or have certain illnesses or conditions, including diabetes; lupus (a disorder of the connective tissue); a hormone imbalance;

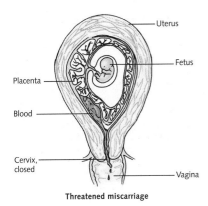

Threatened miscarriage

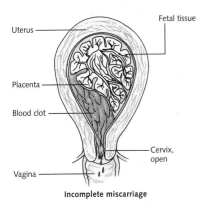

Incomplete miscarriage

LOSS OF A PREGNANCY
Bleeding from the vagina and cramping are the first signs of an impending, or threatened, miscarriage. If the cervix remains closed, the pregnancy may continue. However, if the amniotic sac containing the fetus breaks and the cervix opens, a miscarriage is in progress and cannot be halted. In some women, a miscarriage occurs, but some of the fetal tissue stays in the uterus and must be removed by a doctor.

high blood pressure; and certain infections, such as German measles (RUBELLA), herpes simplex (a sexually transmitted viral infection), and chlamydia (a sexually transmitted bacterial infection). Also, disturbances in certain antibody systems (anticardiolipin antibodies) are associated with an increased risk of miscarriage. Special monitoring and care are required when any of these illnesses or conditions affect a pregnant woman.

The vast majority of miscarriages are caused by factors that are beyond a woman's control. However, there are some steps that a woman can take to minimize her risk of losing a pregnancy. Smoking, drinking alcohol,

exposure to radiation and chemicals, use of illegal drugs, and interactions of over-the-counter or prescribed medications all can increase the risk of losing a pregnancy. A doctor can provide information on the risks of medications. Trauma to the abdomen also can induce a miscarriage, so participation in strenuous activities that could lead to falls or injuries in a pregnant woman should be avoided.

AFTER A MISCARRIAGE
Because miscarriages are common, a doctor may not consider them medically significant until a woman has had two or three in a row. Recurrent miscarriage can result from a variety of genetic, hormonal, infectious, structural, or immunological problems. The causes of some miscarriages cannot be identified. A doctor may recommend evaluation and testing to find out whether a problem exists that is contributing to the miscarriages. A family history may be taken to detect a history of miscarriage or of a disease that may be relevant to the pattern of miscarriage. Blood tests and screenings may be ordered to test a woman and her partner for a variety of problems. A special X ray may be done to analyze the shape of the uterus. With this information, a doctor may able to increase the woman's chances of having a normal pregnancy in the future. It is recommended that a woman not try to conceive until all evaluations are completed. A woman has a 70 to 80 percent chance of carrying a pregnancy to term after a miscarriage, unless there is a problem with autoimmune antibodies, chromosomal abnormalities, or a weak cervix. Sex can safely resume (after evaluation is complete) within 2 to 4 weeks following a miscarriage. A woman's body may be ready for another pregnancy after one or two menstrual cycles. However, grieving about a lost pregnancy must also be addressed before a couple attempts another pregnancy. Most women who experience a miscarriage have a healthy pregnancy later.

Misoprostol

An antiulcer drug. Misoprostol (Cytotec) is used to prevent stomach ulcers from developing in people who are taking anti-inflammatory drugs, including aspirin. Misoprostol helps the stomach protect itself

against damage from gastric acid, and it also decreases the amount of acid produced. It should not be taken by women who are pregnant.

Mitochondria

Small, spherical or rod-shaped components found in the cytoplasm of cells, the fluid in which most chemical changes take place. Mitochondria are the principal sites at which cells oxidize food, thereby generating energy in the form of ATP (adenosine triphosphate). Mitochondria contain enzymes used in the synthesis of proteins. They also contain RNA and DNA (see DEOXYRIBONUCLEIC ACID), which they can use to replicate and code their metabolic activities. On average, each cell contains between 500 and 2,000 mitochondria.

Mitochondrial diseases

Disorders caused by mutations affecting the MITOCHONDRIA in the cells of the body. Mitochondria generate energy from food by producing ATP (adenosine triphosphate). When genetic mutations affect the mitochondria, the available supply of ATP may be impaired, causing a disruption in energy supply that can be devastating. The most vulnerable cells are those requiring the most energy, such as those in the brain, heart, and skeletal muscles. Most mitochondrial diseases are inherited, and as many as one in 4,000 people are affected with a mitochondrial disease.

SYMPTOMS ASSOCIATED WITH MITOCHONDRIAL DISEASES
The chief problems associated with mitochondrial diseases are low energy, the production of free radicals (highly charged molecules that can damage DNA and cell membranes by oxidizing them), and a buildup of lactic acid. Because mitochondria are present in cells of all types, mitochondrial diseases can affect many organ systems.
■ *Symptoms of the cardiac system* Mitochondrial diseases can cause arrhythmias and heart failure.
■ *Symptoms of the digestive organs* When the digestive tract is affected, such symptoms as vomiting, chronic diarrhea, intestinal obstruction, and acid reflux (heartburn) appear. Liver failure can occur in babies born with depleted supplies of mitochondrial DNA. Altered kidney

M

function can result in loss of essential metabolites in the urine (Fanconi syndrome). Altered pancreatic funtion can result in diabetes and the inability to make digestive enzymes. Hypoglycemia, or low blood sugar, can also be present.

■ *Symptoms of the nervous system* When the nervous system is involved, symptoms may include seizures, tremors, developmental delays, dementia, early stroke (before age 40), deafness, migraine headaches, and poor balance.

■ *Symptoms of the eye* Visual problems range from drooping eyelids and the inability to move the eyes from side to side to blindness as a result of RETINITIS PIGMENTOSA (retinal degeneration).

■ *Symptoms of the skeletal system* People with mitochondrial diseases are subject to muscle weakness, exercise intolerance, and muscle cramps.

DIAGNOSIS AND TREATMENT
There is no simple diagnostic test or procedure for mitochondrial diseases. The process of identifying a disorder can be time-consuming and labor-intensive. Blood and urine tests, ECG (electrocardiogram, EKG) or audiogram (hearing test), and ophthalmologic examination may be helpful, as may MRI (magnetic resonance imaging) of the brain, electroencephalogram (EEG), and muscle biopsy.

Mitochondrial diseases cannot be cured but are managed by treating specific symptoms, both to alleviate them and to slow the progression of the disease. There are currently few treatments for the underlying diseases themselves. Some people may be helped with vitamin and enzyme therapies in addition to physical therapy. People with mild disorders tend to respond to treatment better than those with severe disorders.

Mitosis

The simplest type of cell division, mitosis is the process by which the body creates new cells. It is the normal division of cell nuclei, in which a cell divides to form two new, or daughter, cells, each of which contains the same complement of chromosomes as the parent cell. Unlike MEIOSIS, which is a type of cell division that takes place during germ cell formation and produces four daughter cells, each with half the number of chromosomes of the original cell, mitosis refers only to the division of cell nuclei. After mitosis is complete, the cytoplasm within the cell divides, in a process called cytokinesis.

Mitral insufficiency

Failure of the mitral valve of the HEART to close tightly, causing it to leak (regurgitate); also known as mitral incompetence and mitral regurgitation. The mitral valve connects the atrium (upper chamber) and the ventricle (lower chamber) on the left side of the heart. When the ventricle contracts, an incompletely closing valve allows some of the blood to leak back into the atrium, decreasing the flow of blood into the body. To compensate, the ventricle pumps harder, and over time it enlarges to compensate. Eventually, the ventricle begins to fail, and lung congestion can result from the pooling of blood in the left atrium. A type of rapid heartbeat known as ATRIAL FIBRILLATION can also develop, and a blood clot may form in the atrium, travel through the bloodstream, and lodge in a blood vessel (see EMBOLISM).

Mild forms of mitral insufficiency may not produce symptoms for years. As the condition worsens, symptoms including breathlessness (especially during mild exercise or at night), fatigue, and edema (the accumulation of fluid) in the ankles may develop.

Mitral insufficiency can be caused by any condition that weakens or damages the mitral valve. The valve can be affected by a heart attack, endocarditis (inflammation of the lining of the heart that often involves the heart valves), rheumatic fever, rupture of the chordae (cordlike structures that hold the valve to the wall of the heart), and cardiac ischemia (bouts of insufficient blood flow to the heart). In some cases, babies are born with mitral insufficiency.

The symptoms of mitral valve insufficiency can be lessened with medications. Diuretics are used to drain excess fluid from the lungs and lower extremities, cardiotonics can strengthen the heartbeat, anticoagulants can prevent blood clots, antibiotics can prevent infection, and angiotensin-converting enzyme (ACE) inhibitors can reduce the workload of the heart and prevent failure. Surgery to repair or replace the valve is also an option. See HEART VALVE SURGERY.

Mitral stenosis

Narrowing of the mitral valve in the HEART. The mitral valve connects the atrium (upper chamber) and the ventricle (lower chamber) on the left side of the heart. Since the narrowed valve keeps all the blood in the atrium from passing into the ventricle when the atrium contacts, blood pools in the atrium and backs up into the lungs. As the atrium stretches over time, a type of rapid heartbeat known as atrial fibrillation is likely to develop. A blood clot may form in the pooled blood in the atrium and then travel through the bloodstream and lodge in a blood vessel (see EMBOLISM), causing serious damage, particularly to the brain or lungs.

Mitral stenosis may develop before birth. It may also occur when a person reaches his or her 40s or 50s as a result of rheumatic fever earlier in life.

Mild forms of mitral stenosis produce no symptoms, but over time breathlessness with little or no exercise, constant fatigue, frequent bronchitis, chest pain, and palpitations (uncomfortably rapid heartbeat) may occur.

The severity of symptoms of mitral valve stenosis can be reduced with medications. Diuretics are used to drain excess fluid from the lungs, and digoxin is used to slow a rapid heartbeat. Surgery to repair or replace the valve may also be an option (see HEART VALVE SURGERY). Mitral balloon valvuloplasty is a common catheter-based technique used to open a mitral valve that is narrowed by rheumatic heart disease.

Mitral valve prolapse (MVP)

An abnormal bulging backward of the mitral valve when the HEART contracts. The mitral valve connects the atrium (upper chamber) and ventricle (lower chamber) on the left side of the heart. Normally, the two leaflets that make up the valve open when the atrium contracts, allowing blood to flow into the ventricle, and then close as the ventricle contracts to pump blood into the body. If the mitral valve is prolapsed, one or both leaflets balloon back into the atrium during ventricular contraction. In some cases of MVP, one leaflet is larger than the other; in other cases, the chordae (cordlike structures that

NARROWED MITRAL VALVE

When the mitral valve becomes diseased, the passage of blood through the narrowed valve is restricted. This condition, called mitral valve stenosis, frequently leads to atrial fibrillation, a rapid, highly irregular heartbeat. Mitral valve stenosis can be treated by mitral balloon valvuloplasty, a procedure in which a catheter (thin tube) with an inflatable balloon is threaded through a vein to widen the valve.

Left atrium

Mitral valve
Aortic valve

Left ventricle

HEALTHY HEART
When the mitral valves are free of disease, they close properly and blood is channeled normally through the heart to the rest of the body.

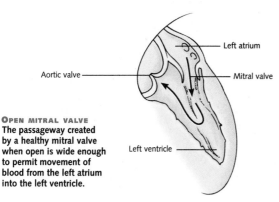

Left atrium

Aortic valve

Mitral valve

Left ventricle

OPEN MITRAL VALVE
The passageway created by a healthy mitral valve when open is wide enough to permit movement of blood from the left atrium into the left ventricle.

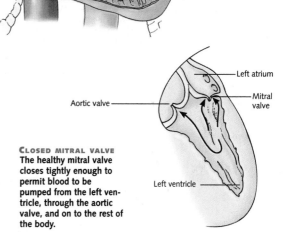

Left atrium

Aortic valve

Mitral valve

Left ventricle

CLOSED MITRAL VALVE
The healthy mitral valve closes tightly enough to permit blood to be pumped from the left ventricle, through the aortic valve, and on to the rest of the body.

M

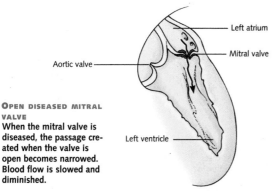

Left atrium

Mitral valve

Aortic valve

Left ventricle

OPEN DISEASED MITRAL VALVE
When the mitral valve is diseased, the passage created when the valve is open becomes narrowed. Blood flow is slowed and diminished.

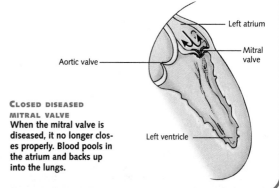

Left atrium

Mitral valve

Aortic valve

Left ventricle

CLOSED DISEASED MITRAL VALVE
When the mitral valve is diseased, it no longer closes properly. Blood pools in the atrium and backs up into the lungs.

FOCUS ON MVP

A mitral valve opens to let blood flow from the left atrium to the left ventricle, then closes when the ventricle contracts. When mitral valve prolapse (MVP) develops, the valve bulges into the atrium when closed, but it usually still closes. In a severe case, the valve does not close, and blood flows backward when the ventricle contracts.

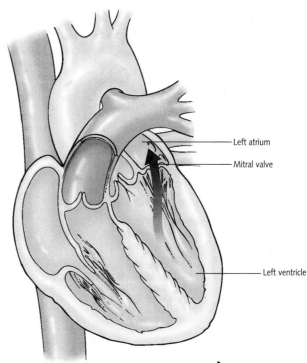

Left atrium

Mitral valve

Left ventricle

BACKWARD FLOW OF BLOOD
The mitral valve is located between the left atrium and left ventricle. With severe MVP, the valve cannot close well. When the left ventricle contracts, blood leaks back into the left atrium. This backward flow of blood is called regurgitation.

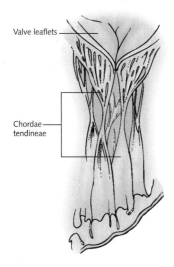

Valve leaflets

Chordae tendineae

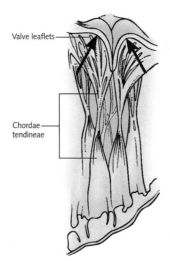

Valve leaflets

Chordae tendineae

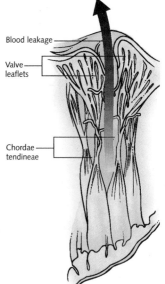

Blood leakage

Valve leaflets

Chordae tendineae

HEALTHY MITRAL VALVE
When a healthy mitral valve closes, the leaflets fit snugly together. The leaflets are secured to the wall of the heart by cordlike structures called chordae tendineae.

PROLAPSING MITRAL VALVE
When a prolapsed mitral valve closes, the leaflets bulge into the atrium. In most cases, the valve can still prevent blood from flowing backward.

SIGNIFICANT MVP
If the prolapsed valve goes untreated, some of the chordae tendineae may break. The valve leaflets cannot close properly, and blood leaks into the atrium when the ventricle contracts.

secure the leaflets to the heart wall) are stretched or, rarely, ruptured. MVP is sometimes referred to as click-murmur syndrome because of the distinctive sound the abnormal chorda makes as the valve opens and closes.

MVP is the most common heart valve problem, affecting approximately 1 person in 20. It is most likely to occur in women between the ages of 20 and 40 who are thin and have mild forms of back or chest deformities. MVP can also be a sign of MARFAN SYNDROME.

MVP is generally not serious and causes no symptoms; however, it must be monitored in case complications develop. In a small percentage of cases, MVP causes the mitral valve to regurgitate (leak) excessively. It can also lead to rapid heartbeat, chest pain, fatigue, pronounced anxiety and panic attacks, shortness of breath, syncope (fainting), and, rarely, heart failure or sudden death.

Since MVP increases the risk of endocarditis (inflammation of the lining of the heart, often involving the heart valves), people with MVP need to take antibiotics as a precaution before dental or medical procedures and surgery. Stimulants such as caffeine should be avoided. If symptoms develop, medications may be used. Beta blockers slow the heart and reduce the stretching of the mitral valve, which may alleviate chest pain. Antiarrhythmics regulate heart rhythms. In extreme cases involving major regurgitation or rupture of the chordae, surgery to repair or replace the valve is called for. See HEART VALVE SURGERY.

Mittelschmerz

Acute abdominal pain around the time of OVULATION.

Mobility

The ability of the body to put into movement or make mobile its various parts by use of the muscles, tendons, ligaments, bones, and joints. Fractures, arthritic changes in joints, and other ailments that affect the principal bone and muscle groups, including the hip, knee, ankle, and back, can impair the body's general mobilization. Also called mobilization, moving the body or its individual parts is sometimes as

important to healing as resting injured parts of the body. A doctor's directions regarding mobility should be followed.

With age, mobility slows down as a result of two normal components of aging: the gradual loss of strength and flexibility and a decrease in the rate of the metabolic system that supplies energy to the body's moving parts. The more active a person is throughout his or her life, the less dramatic this decrease in mobility functions will be. At the age of 60, a person who has exercised regularly may have lost little of his or her muscular strength. But, even an athlete may find his or her flexibility decreased, the reflexes slowed, and the coordination dulled by the sixth decade of life. However, being careful to avoid falls, doing strength training exercises such as weight training, and walking or getting other exercise regularly are the best ways to maintain mobilization as a person ages.

Mohs surgery

A type of surgery used in the treatment of SKIN CANCER; also known as microscopically controlled surgery. Mohs surgery is performed on an outpatient basis using a local anesthetic. In Mohs surgery, a cancerous tumor is removed one thin layer at a time. The surgeon slowly removes successive layers of skin until only healthy tissue remains. Afterward, the tissue is examined under a microscope.

Mohs surgery has the highest cure rates for both basal cell and squamous cell carcinomas. It is particularly useful for treating recurring tumors, large tumors, and tumors on

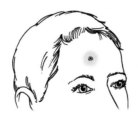

SURGERY IN MICROSCOPIC LAYERS
Some skin tumors send roots into surrounding tissue. To ensure removal, Mohs surgery traces and maps the roots microscopically. The tumor is removed in thin layers, and each layer is frozen and dyed to guide removal of the next layer. The technique enables thorough removal of the tumor, while preserving as much normal tissue as possible.

the face or the genitals. Although it is a slow, painstaking process, Mohs surgery results in a more pleasing cosmetic outcome by allowing normal skin near the tumor to be spared.

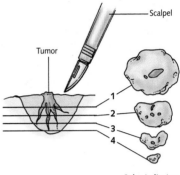

Color indicates extent of tumor

REVEALING BOUNDARIES OF A TUMOR
Mohs surgery enables the surgeon to see the full extent of a tumor as it grows under the skin. The technique is often used on tumors that have reoccurred after treatment. The rate of cure is excellent, and the preservation of normal skin around the tumor roots results in a better appearance after healing.

Molar pregnancy

An abnormal pregnancy that probably results from the fertilization of a so-called empty egg, an egg without chromosomes. In this condition, the fertilized egg degenerates, and the placenta grows into a mass of tissue resembling a cluster of grapes. Molar pregnancy is very rare, occurring in only one out of every 1,000 or 1,200 pregnancies. See HYDATIDIFORM MOLE.

Mold

A parasitic fungus that exists in multicellular colonies; the deposit or growth produced by molds. Molds and their spores are the cause of allergies for many people. Molds thrive in damp locations such as basements, bathrooms, upholstered furniture, wood, books, and wallpaper. Outdoor molds produce spores in summer and early autumn, or year-round in warm climates, while indoor molds produce and shed spores all year long.

Mold spores cannot be eliminated, but they can be minimized through use of air conditioners and dehumidifiers and by discarding moldy or mildewed articles. Mold-proof paint can be used

M

instead of wallpaper, and bathrooms can be cleaned with disinfectants.

Mole

A brown spot on the skin derived from cells that contain MELANIN, the pigment that gives skin its color; also known as a nevus. When a mole changes color or shape, it may indicate malignant melanoma (see MELANOMA, MALIGNANT), a serious form of SKIN CANCER. Risk factors for melanoma include having asymmetrical or unusually colored moles or more than 40 moles; a family or personal history of melanoma; having spent a lot of time outdoors; a tendency to burn or freckle easily when exposed to the sun; and overexposure to X rays or other forms of radiation.

ABNORMAL MOLES

Moles vary considerably. They may be brown, black, or blue; flat or raised; and hairless or hairy. Approximately one in every ten people has unusual or abnormal moles, including moles that are asymmetrical, have irregular borders, have variegated (mixed) colors, and are more than ¼ inch (about as big as a pencil eraser) in diameter. Unusual moles are more likely than typical ones to develop into malignant melanoma. Although not everyone who has abnormal moles develops melanoma, all abnormal moles must be closely monitored through regular self-examination and periodic appointments with a dermatologist. A physician should inspect the entire body

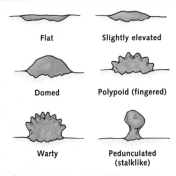

DEVELOPMENT OF COMMON MOLES
A common mole may change over a period of decades. Generally, a flat or slightly raised mole progresses into a more raised, irregularly shaped growth. The progression may stop at any time, and a person can develop new moles well into middle age.

> **MOLES: THE ABCD RULE**
>
> Unusual moles should be evaluated to rule out melanoma. People should be suspicious of moles that display any of the following traits:
>
> - **Asymmetry.** When divided in half by an imaginary line, one half of the mole does not match the other half.
> - **Border irregularity.** The edge of the mole is lopsided in any way.
> - **Color variations.** The mole seems to be a number of colors such as blue, gray, and black.
> - **Diameter greater than ¼ inch.** The mole is wider than a pencil eraser.

for skin changes, such as the appearance of a new mole or spot on the skin or variations in the surface or color of a mole. A common site for melanoma is on the back, where the disease may progress unnoticed. Some dermatologists use photography or computer imagery to help monitor changes in a mole. Early detection and removal offers the best chance for a cure.

Moles that develop into melanomas may grow on parts of the body not frequently exposed to direct sunlight. Theoretically, this may occur because these areas suffer the most severe burns when exposed. Statistically, experiencing even one or two sunburns as a child or teenager may double the chance of melanoma later in life. Doctors recommend seeking prompt medical attention when there is any change in a mole. Warning signs include variations in color, size, texture, or appearance, as well as pain, itching, or bleeding.

TREATMENT

Most moles are benign (not cancerous). However, if there are warning signs such as changes in size or shape or the presence of bleeding, itching, or pain, a physician should perform a skin biopsy. This entails removing a small tissue sample of the mole and examining it under a microscope.

Moles can be surgically removed by shaving the lesion off or by cutting it out and stitching the incision closed. Surgery is usually performed on an outpatient basis using a local anesthetic. If melanoma is diagnosed, nearby lymph nodes may be removed

---

for study to determine whether the cancer has spread. Most moles do not return after surgery.

Molecule

The smallest unit of a substance that can exist alone and that has all the chemical properties of that substance. A molecule is a collection of atoms bound tightly together by strong chemical bonds. Many of the Earth's substances are made of molecules. The nature of each molecule depends on the atoms it contains and how they are bound together.

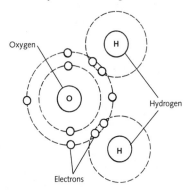

A WATER MOLECULE
Chemically, a water molecule (H_2O) is composed of one atom of oxygen with orbiting electrons and two molecules of hydrogen. The oxygen (negative electrical charge) attracts the hydrogen (positive charge), so the molecule is a V-shaped formation.

Molluscum contagiosum

A viral infection of the skin that produces multiple, firm eruptions that range in color from pearly pink to white and have a central, sunken opening that oozes a white, waxy substance. Molluscum contagiosum occurs when a virus invades the surface layers of the skin, infects the skin cells, and causes the cells to divide, producing numerous eruptions on the skin's surface.

The virus is transmitted by close physical contact and can occur almost anywhere on the body, especially in children. In adults, it is often one of the SEXUALLY TRANSMITTED DISEASES that produces the distinctive skin eruptions on the external genitalia and on the thighs and buttocks of both men and women. The virus may also be transmitted indirectly via contact with contaminated towels, massage, water in a swimming pool, or via contact sports such as wrestling.

The incubation period is usually 2 to 7 weeks but can be up to 6 months. The doughnut-shaped bumps may persist for as long as 6 to 9 months, then clear spontaneously as the result of the body's immune response. The infection can be treated to prevent its spread or if it presents a cosmetic problem. Treatment involves removal of the soft central tissue of the eruptions; the surrounding elevations of skin may be removed by freezing or by electrical or chemical burning.

Monarthritis

Inflammation, or osteoarthritis, of a single joint. It is rare for osteoarthritis to affect only one joint. While several joints are usually affected, pain is sometimes experienced in only one or two joints at a time. Causes of monarthritis include trauma and infection. See OSTEOARTHRITIS.

Moniliasis

An invasive fungal infection caused by *Candida* microorganisms, most frequently by *Candida albicans*. Moniliasis can cause lesions in the liver, spleen, kidneys, bone, skin, or more commonly the tissues of the mouth or vagina. When moniliasis affects the mouth, it may be referred to as oral THRUSH; when it affects the vagina, it may be called a vaginal yeast infection. Oral *Candida* infections can spread to the esophagus and cause *Candida* esophagitis.

Moniliasis is not a contagious infection. *Candida* fungi exist normally in the gastrointestinal tract, as well as in the mucous membranes of the mouth and vagina, where their growth is controlled by the presence of normally occurring bacteria. Uncontrolled overgrowth of the fungus may be caused by factors that reduce natural resistance, including illness or stress. Suppression of the immune system by disorders such as HIV (human immunodeficiency virus) infection or the long-term use of certain medications, including corticosteroids, may contribute to moniliasis.

Factors that disturb the normal balance of microorganisms in the gastrointestinal system, the mouth, and the vagina may also produce moniliasis. Antibiotic therapy, which destroys bacteria, can create an imbal-

ance that allows overgrowth of *Candida* fungi, as can uncontrolled diabetes mellitus (see DIABETES MELLITUS, TYPE 1; DIABETES MELLITUS, TYPE 2) and hormonal changes due to pregnancy and the use of birth control pills. Overuse of mouthwash and mouth spray can cause an imbalance in the mouth's microorganisms and may lead to moniliasis; overzealous douching or use of feminine hygiene sprays may have a similar effect in the vagina.

COMMON FORMS OF INFECTION
The oral form of moniliasis, or oral thrush, occurs most commonly in infants and young children, older people, and those with weakened immune systems due to disease or medical treatments, including cancer therapy. Xerostomia, a condition causing an abnormally dry mouth, increases the risk of infection. Symptoms of oral thrush include painful, raised sores in the mouth, usually on the tongue or inner cheeks, that have a creamy white appearance. It is diagnosed by evaluation of these characteristic signs; microscopic examination of the tissue from a sore in the mouth can confirm a diagnosis of moniliasis. Antifungal medications including nystatin, clotrimazole, and miconazole, used for 7 to 14 days, can successfully treat the infection. Improved oral hygiene techniques can aid in healing.

The symptoms of moniliasis in the vagina are local itching and irritation, as well as redness and swelling of the clitoris and labia. There may be a thick, white, odorous discharge and discomfort during vaginal intercourse. Frequent urination with stinging or burning and intense itching may occur. The infection is diagnosed by physical examination and may be confirmed by a culture of cells taken from the vaginal wall. Moniliasis is generally treated successfully with over-the-counter antifungal topical medications (creams or suppositories) for a period of about 7 days. Vaginal yeast infections may recur, in which case an oral antifungal medication may be prescribed and blood sugar testing for diabetes may be recommended.

Monoamine oxidase inhibitors

Antidepressant drugs. Monoamine oxidase inhibitors, also called MAOIs,

relieve depression by blocking the action of a chemical substance in the nervous system called monoamine oxidase. MAOIs are very effective for some people with certain types of depression.

People who take monoamine oxidase inhibitors must be very careful not to eat certain foods or drink certain beverages, because MAOIs interact with them and provoke dangerous reactions, including sudden high blood pressure and fast heart rate. The foods and drinks in question are all high in tyramine content and include aged cheeses, pickled herring, chocolate, fermented meats, sauerkraut, very ripe fruit, and some wines and beer.

There are currently only three MAOIs available orally for prescription in the United States: isocarboxazid (Marplan), phenelzine (Nardil), and tranylcypromine (Parnate).

Monoclonal antibody

See ANTIBODY, MONOCLONAL.

Monogamy

A pledged relationship in which neither partner has sex with anyone else. In a monogamous relationship, both partners make this promise. Unless or until it is certain that a monogamous relationship exists, doctors recommend using a condom as protection against SEXUALLY TRANSMITTED DISEASES.

Mononucleosis, infectious

An acute viral disease characterized by fever, sore throat, and swollen glands. Infectious mononucleosis is usually caused by the EPSTEIN-BARR VIRUS (EBV), but may also be caused by the CYTOMEGALOVIRUS (CMV). Both viruses are members of the herpes family. EBV is commonly transmitted in saliva, and because the disease is often spread through kissing, it is nicknamed the "kissing disease." Infectious mononucleosis, sometimes referred to as "mono," is also spread via airborne infectious droplets in the coughs and sneezes of an infected person. In rare cases, it may be spread via blood transfusion.

The infection occurs in people of all ages, but frequently affects young people between the ages of 15 and 25

M

years; as many as 2 out of 1,000 people in their teens and 20s may become infected. The illness is usually not serious, but the virus remains in the body for a lifetime. Most people build up antibodies to it and become immune.

SYMPTOMS

There are often no symptoms in children younger than 2 years who have infectious mononucleosis. Children between the ages of 4 and 15 years may have mild respiratory symptoms. In older teens and young adults, more severe and prolonged symptoms tend to occur, usually within 4 to 6 weeks of exposure. Typically, the first symptoms to appear include fever, headaches, night sweats, muscle aches, and severe fatigue that requires up to 16 hours of sleep a night. After several days, further symptoms may include sore throat and swollen tonsils, lack of appetite and weight loss, aching joints, abdominal pain, chills, swollen glands in the neck and armpits, and a red rash that generally appears on the chest. Less commonly, symptoms may include difficulty breathing, coughing, nausea, vomiting, yellowing of the skin and whites of the eyes (jaundice), irregular heartbeat, or sensitivity to light. Most symptoms tend to lessen in severity within 10 days but may persist for up to 4 weeks. Fatigue, in particular, may be prolonged. It can take 2 to 3 weeks before a person with mononucleosis is able to return to his or her regular activities, and it may take up to 3 months to regain normal energy and well-being. A person who has infectious mononucleosis should be careful to avoid strenuous activities, especially contact sports, for at least 4 weeks after the illness begins to prevent the risk of a ruptured spleen. Lifting heavy objects and drinking alcohol should also be avoided during this time.

People who have impaired immune systems as a result of having AIDS (acquired immunodeficiency syndrome) or taking certain medications following an organ transplant can have more severe symptoms and a more serious case of mononucleosis.

DIAGNOSIS AND TREATMENT

A clinical history and physical examination, including the possibility of exposure to mononucleosis, may lead to an initial suspicion of this disease. A physician is apt to look for fever, a reddened throat with tonsils that are swollen and coated with pus, swollen glands in the neck, a rash on the chest, and an enlarged spleen. To confirm a diagnosis, a doctor usually orders blood tests to detect unusual white blood cells and to measure the white blood cell and platelet counts. A blood test for antibodies to EBV and CMV, called the Monospot, is generally performed to confirm diagnosis of mononucleosis.

An antiviral medication to treat infectious mononucleosis is not available. If the tonsils are severely swollen, a corticosteroid medication such as PREDNISONE may be prescribed to reduce inflammation. If a streptococcal infection accompanies the sore throat of mononucleosis, antibiotics will be prescribed.

Bed rest and increased fluid intake are generally recommended for treatment of the illness. Drinking water and fruit juice are recommended to relieve fever and prevent dehydration. Associated discomfort and pain may be relieved by taking ibuprofen or acetaminophen for body aches and fever. Children younger than 18 years should not take aspirin because of the associated risk of REYE SYNDROME. Minor sore throat pain may be improved by gargling with salt water, drinking cold beverages, and eating frozen desserts.

RISKS AND COMPLICATIONS

Most people who contract infectious mononucleosis make a complete recovery within 3 weeks, but there are several complications of mononucleosis, including a form of hepatitis. A significant risk involves the spleen, an organ near the stomach that produces infection-fighting white blood cells. The spleen may become soft and enlarged, and in rare cases, the organ may rupture, causing sharp, sudden pain on the upper left side of the abdomen. A ruptured spleen can result in internal bleeding that is potentially fatal, so in those unlikely cases, a surgical procedure may be performed.

Another danger sign that may signal a complication includes difficult or noisy breathing, especially in young children. Swelling in the throat and tonsils may obstruct the airway. Corticosteroid medication can be prescribed to treat this condition, but hospitalization and surgery are sometimes required. Sinus or ear pain and symptoms that persist for longer than 4 weeks are also indications of more serious illness or conditions that require medical attention.

Complications involving the central nervous system are unusual but serious. These can include encephalitis, seizures, Guillain-Barré syndrome, damaged nerves, and aseptic meningitis.

Monoparesis

Motor weakness or partial PARALYSIS of a single part of the body.

Monosodium glutamate

See MSG.

Monounsaturated fats

A type of unsaturated fat that can lower levels of harmful LDL (low-density lipoprotein) cholesterol without also decreasing levels of HDL (high-density lipoprotein cholesterol). Mono-unsaturated fats may also help to maintain normal blood sugar levels. Olive and canola oils are good sources of monounsaturated fats. Avocados and nuts are also sources. See FATS AND OILS.

Monteggia fracture

An angulated break in the ulna, which is the longer of the two major bones in the forearm. Angulated breaks cause the bone segments to be at angles to each other and may cause the forearm to have a bent or deformed appearance. Monteggia fractures, although rare, are generally caused by a blow to the forearm or a fall onto the hand. Fractures of the ulna typically occur across the shaft of the bone and may involve a break in the other bone of the forearm, called the radius. Monteggia fracture is diagnosed by physical examination, pain and deformity of the forearm and elbow, and an X ray. Rotation of the forearm or elbow is painful. The forearm may be swollen and appear shortened. Treatment involves manipulating the bone segments into their proper position and immobilizing the forearm, usually with a cast or splint and sling, until the bone has healed in the correct position. Another treatment option is to surgically repair the ulna to promote healing.

Montelukast

An antiasthma drug. Montelukast (Singulair) is used to treat asthma. Leukotrienes are associated with the swelling of tissues and tightening of muscles in the throat that cause the airways to close during an asthma attack. Montelukast helps to prevent such attacks by blocking leukotrienes and their effects.

Mood

The pervasive, long-lasting emotional state that shapes how a person sees his or her life. Mood is usually used to describe elation, happiness, irritability, or depression, and it is the central aspect of such psychiatric disorders as BIPOLAR DISORDER and DEPRESSION.

Morbidity

Any type of disease or loss of physical and psychological health and wellbeing. Often morbidity is stated as a rate determined by dividing the total number of people in a group into the number of people who suffer illness or injury. For example, if a sample population of 1,000 people lives in a given city and 50 of them develop influenza (flu), the morbidity rate is 0.05.

Morning sickness

A common set of symptoms, including nausea, vomiting, and food and smell aversions, that affect many pregnant women in the mornings, although they can occur at any time of day. Most pregnant women experience morning sickness early in pregnancy, particularly in the first 3 months. For some women, morning sickness lasts throughout the pregnancy. Morning sickness becomes a serious problem if a woman is unable to keep food or fluids down and begins to lose weight or become dehydrated (see HYPEREMESIS GRAVIDARUM). If nausea and vomiting become severe, hospitalization or hydration and medication may be needed. Some women help reduce morning sickness by eating dry toast or crackers before rising and then getting up slowly. Sleeping with an open window for fresh air, eating several small meals instead of fewer large

ones, and drinking plenty of fluids have been found to help.

Morning-after pill

A series of hormonal pills that a woman can take to prevent pregnancy for up to 72 hours after having had unprotected sex or having been the victim of sexual assault. Hormones in the pills inhibit the development of a fertilized egg in the uterus. Taking a morning-after pill does not guarantee that a woman will not become pregnant. See CONTRACEPTION, EMERGENCY POSTCOITAL.

Morphea

A condition in which hard, oval, or irregularly shaped plaques (patches of thick raised skin) form in the skin; also known as localized SCLERODERMA. The plaques are usually white with lilac-colored rings around them. Most commonly they occur on the trunk but may also develop on the face, arms, legs, and other parts of the body. There is no effective treatment for morphea. Over time, morphea usually improves without treatment.

Morphine sulfate

A narcotic painkiller. Morphine sulfate is used to relieve severe pain. Morphine is often used to relieve the pain of cancer and the pain associated with surgery. Morphine is the drug of choice to relieve pain of myocardial infarction (heart attack). Morphine is thought to work in the central nervous system to alter the person's perception of pain.

If used consistently over time, morphine sulfate can cause physical and psychological dependence. Physical dependence may lead to withdrawal symptoms when the drug is stopped. Morphine sulfate is available by prescription in many different brands and formulations, including injection, capsules, suppository, and extended-release tablets. See NARCOTICS.

Mortality rate

A statistic that measures the frequency at which death occurs in a population within a given time. The mortality rate can be calculated in a number of ways. The crude mortality rate is determined by dividing the number of deaths within a population by the total number of people in that population, usu-

ally including everyone older than 1 year. With an age-adjusted mortality rate, the rate is modified mathematically to account for the number of people of different ages in the population. This allows researchers to compare mortality in different populations even if their age structures differ (for example, significantly more older people in one group than in another).

Age-specific mortality rates are limited to a particular age group, such as people in their 20s. The number of deaths in that age group is divided by the total number of people in the same age group. Cause-specific mortality rates are measured by dividing the number of deaths from a specific cause (for example, heart disease, gunshot wound, or cancer) during a period of time (for example, 1 year) by the number of people in the population at the midpoint of the time interval.

Morton neuroma

A benign, swollen enlargement of the sheath of nerve that runs across the bottom of the foot and out to the toes. Morton neuroma typically develops in the ball of the foot in the space between the third and fourth toes. A continual pinching of the nerve can cause the nerve sheath to enlarge. As it enlarges, it puts increased pressure on the nerve. The principal symptom is a burning pain in the ball of the foot, often occurring during weight-bearing activities such as walking, running, or using stairs. The pain may also be experienced as an aching, shooting, or tingling pain in the toes. In runners, the pain tends to occur in the middle of a run or at the end of a long run. Sometimes, wearing tight shoes causes pain early in running or other sports activities. The condition is usually caused by structural, functional, or mechanical irregularities in the foot. Improper movements of the foot, which may be caused by a bunion, for example, can put pressure on the nerve and irritate it. High-heeled or tight shoes, arthritis and other inflammatory conditions, trauma, and repetitive stress on the balls of the feet from sports activities may contribute to the development of Morton neuroma. The condition is diagnosed by physical examination. There is often tenderness between the base of the toes.

M

MRI (magnetic resonance imaging) or an ultrasound test may be used to pinpoint the irritated nerve, although those tests are rarely necessary. X rays are sometimes used to rule out other causes of the pain.

Nonsteroidal anti-inflammatory drugs (NSAIDs) such as aspirin or ibuprofen may be recommended. Icing the foot several times a day; wearing wider, low-heeled, and soft-soled shoes; and using a metatarsal pad may help relieve pressure on the nerve and diminish the pain. If these treatments are not successful, ORTHOTICS (specially designed shoe inserts) may be recommended, or a cortisone injection may be considered. In some cases, an outpatient surgical procedure performed under local anesthetic may become necessary to remove a Morton neuroma.

Mosaicism

An anomaly of chromosome division resulting in two or more types of cells containing different numbers of chromosomes; also, the occurrence of two or more genetically distinct cell lines in a single organism. Mosaicism may occur normally, as in the case of certain sex-linked genetic traits, or pathologically, as a result of gene mutation.

Motion sickness

A disorder brought on by certain kinds of motion such as being on a boat or ship during rough seas, traveling on an airplane when there is air turbulence, or riding in a car on curving or steep, hilly roads. Children may experience motion sickness on playground equipment or theme park rides. When motion sickness is mild, it produces a slight upset stomach. Bad odors often worsen motion sickness. When it is severe, there may be nausea, vomiting, dizziness, sweating, loss of balance, loss of coordination, and physical and mental exhaustion. The cause of motion sickness is excessive stimulation of the vestibular system in the labyrinth (part of the inner ear that controls balance). This system consists of three tiny semicircular tubes that record the body's position and transmit the information to the brain. Overstimulation of the system produces an abnormal perception of the body's movement and position in relation to

the environment, creating a sensation of disorientation that produces the symptoms. People who are prone to motion sickness may benefit from riding in the center of a moving vehicle and being seated over the wings when traveling by air. It may also be helpful for the person to keep his or her eyes on the horizon for orientation. Ginger or ginger root may also be effective for preventing and treating motion sickness. Medications containing meclizine, cyclizine, scopolamine, diphendydramine, or dimenhydrinate can often be effective for preventing motion sickness when taken before or during travel, but drowsiness is a frequent side effect. The scopolamine skin patch should not be used by children.

Motor

A term used to describe anything that brings about movement, such as a muscle or nerve. The word "motor" is commonly applied to nerves that carry impulses from the central nervous system to a muscle, producing movement.

Motor neuron disease

A group of rare, progressive disorders in which the nerves that control muscle activity degenerate within the brain and spinal cord. This results in muscle wasting (atrophy) and weakness. The cause of motor neuron disease is unknown.

TYPES OF MOTOR NEURON DISEASE
Amyotrophic lateral sclerosis, or ALS, is the most common form of motor neuron disease. ALS is also known as Lou Gehrig disease, after the baseball player who died of the disease in 1939. Other motor neuron diseases include PROGRESSIVE MUSCULAR ATROPHY and progressive bulbar palsy. In younger people, forms include infantile progressive spinal muscular atrophy (Werdnig-Hoffmann paralysis) and chronic spinal muscular atrophy.

SYMPTOMS
In ALS, muscle strength and coordination gradually decrease, while sensation and mental functioning remain unaffected. The eventual result is total paralysis. Nerves controlling the voluntary muscles of the arms or legs are often the first to shrink and disappear, causing weakness and muscle wast-

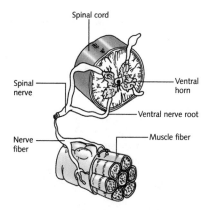

HEALTHY NEUROMUSCULAR ACTION
In the spinal cord, the ventral (front) horns of gray matter contain nerve cell bodies. Motor nerve fibers leave the ventral side of the spinal cord in bundles called motor nerve roots. The nerve fibers continue along the spinal nerves to activate individual muscle fibers. Degeneration of the nerves causes muscle wasting and weakness.

ing. Fasciculations (involuntary quivering of small areas of the muscles) may also occur. The loss of muscle control continues to progress, and more muscle groups become involved. Some people experience cramping and stiffness. Eventually all four limbs become involved. Deterioration progresses to speech impairment, difficulty swallowing, and trouble breathing. This typically leads to death from paralysis of respiratory muscles in 3 to 5 years. However, exceptions occur, and some people have lived 20 years or more following diagnosis.

DIAGNOSIS AND TREATMENT
Diagnosis of motor neuron disease is made through neuromuscular examination that indicates muscle weakness. Weakness often begins in a single limb or in the shoulders or hips. Examination may also reveal tremors, spasms, fasciculation, and atrophy. There may be abnormal reflexes and a clumsy gait (walk). Tests to confirm diagnosis and rule out other causes include electromyogram (EMG; measurement of muscle electrical activity), blood studies, CT (computed tomography) scanning, and MRI (magnetic resonance imaging).

As there is no cure, the goal of treatment is to control symptoms. Medication may be prescribed to manage spasticity and the ability to swallow. Helpful measures include physical therapy, rehabilitation, and orthopedic appliances (such as a wheelchair). To prevent choking, a tube must eventually be placed into the stomach for feeding. Because mental functioning remains intact, emotional support is vital for the person who is coping with one of the motor neuron diseases.

Mouth

The opening to the DIGESTIVE SYSTEM, where food is taken in and broken down into smaller pieces. The mouth, along with the nose, is also an entrance to the RESPIRATORY SYSTEM and has a role in speech production.

The PALATE forms the roof of the mouth and separates it from the nasal cavity. The palate is hard and bony in the front of the mouth and soft toward the rear. The TONGUE is anchored to the floor of the mouth and contains taste buds that are sensory receptors for taste. The TEETH, which surround the front and sides of the mouth, are anchored in the bones of the upper and lower jaw. The mucous membranes that line the mouth contain glands that secrete SALIVA to lubricate the mouth and help break down food. The lips (see LIP) form the outer rim of the mouth, helping to keep food in the mouth and to shape speech sounds.

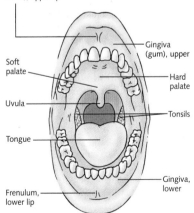

Frenulum (connecting tissue), upper lip

Gingiva (gum), upper

Soft palate

Hard palate

Uvula

Tonsils

Tongue

Gingiva, lower

Frenulum, lower lip

INTERIOR OF THE MOUTH
The lips, teeth, tongue, palate, and related structures of the mouth begin the digestive process by breaking down and swallowing food. The same structures participate in the final stage of speech production, by altering the sound waves emanating from the respiratory system to form specific sounds.

Mouth cancer
See ORAL CANCER.

Mouth guard
A flexible, removable, plastic device worn to protect the teeth, mouth, and head during sports and recreational activities. Mouth guards help to prevent the lower jaw from being forced into the upper jaw, which can cause a CONCUSSION, a cerebral hemorrhage (see HEMORRAGE, CEREBRAL), loss of consciousness, jaw fractures, and neck injuries. Mouth guards are especially recommended for young children who tend to damage or dislodge their teeth, fracture their jaws, or injure their lips during athletic play. Some schools require the use of mouth guards for children involved in contact sports, such as ice hockey, football, and boxing. Mouth guards are also recommended for noncontact sports, such as basketball, soccer, baseball, and gymnastics. Mouth guards are particularly important for preventing injuries in adults and children who are wearing ORTHODONTIC APPLIANCES, such as braces. They are effective in moving soft tissue in the mouth away from the teeth, which helps to prevent cuts and bruises of the lips and inner parts of the cheeks that are caused by metal braces.

There are several types of mouth guards. The most highly recommended is the custom-made mouth protector, which is custom-fit to a person's mouth by a dentist. Made from an impression (see IMPRESSION, DENTAL) to fit the teeth perfectly, they reduce bulk and discomfort and offer the best protection. Boil-and-bite mouth guards are adapted to the teeth when the acrylic or rubber lining of the device is immersed in boiling water and softened so that it will conform to the shape of the teeth and gums. Children need to be careful in order to prevent burning of the mouth. When placed in the mouth, the lining molds to the teeth and the material sets to the shape of the person's mouth. This type of mouth guard offers an acceptable level of protection. Stock mouth guards are the least expensive, but they offer the least protection because the fit is not customized and the jaw must be closed to hold them in place. This type of mouth guard may interfere with breathing and speaking.

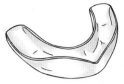

Mouth guard

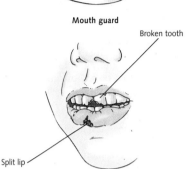

Broken tooth

Split lip

Injuries without guard

PROTECTIVE GEAR FOR THE MOUTH
A mouth guard, usually used in contact sports, cushions and shields the mouth and teeth from injury. Uncustomized mouth guards can be purchased at sporting goods stores, and some products can be immersed in boiling water and customized by the individual. The best guards are custom-made by a dentist to fit perfectly over the person's teeth.

Mouth guards must be regularly and properly cleaned with soap and warm water. They should be stored in a well-ventilated container and protected from extreme heat and sunlight. A mouth guard for a child may require replacement every year, depending on the child's growth rate.

Mouth ulcer
A break in the mucous membrane lining the mouth. Traumatic ulcers are those that occur due to injury (such as contact with a jagged tooth or denture). A canker sore, a common type of mouth ulcer, generally develops when a person is fatigued, under stress, or ill. Adolescents and premenstrual women are especially prone to canker sores. A cold sore in or around the mouth is a type of herpes infection. Most mouth ulcers heal spontaneously and do not require treatment. However, over-the-counter lozenges and applications may soothe pain and irritation. If a sore does not heal within 10 days, it is important to see the doctor. Rarely, a mouth ulcer is a symptom of a more serious underlying condition such as a tumor.

M

Mouth-to-mouth resuscitation

A technique used to restore oxygen to the lungs of someone who has stopped breathing; rescue breathing; also called ARTIFICIAL RESPIRATION. A part of CARDIOPULMONARY RESUSCITATION (CPR), mouth-to-mouth resuscitation is a first aid measure used when a person is unconscious and has stopped breathing. Mouth-to-mouth resuscitation, also known as rescue breathing or artificial respiration, is the quickest way to get oxygen into a person's lungs.

The person assisting should begin by tilting the person's head back and lifting the chin, both to open the airway and to move the tongue away from the back of the throat. The person's nose is pinched shut with the rescuer's fingers while a tight seal is made around the person's mouth by the rescuer's mouth. The rescuer will breathe slowly and gently into the person until the chest rises. A breath should be given approximately every 5 seconds, with pauses in between to let the air flow out. If the person remains unresponsive, not breathing or moving, then chest compressions should be started. Rescue breathing should continue until the person begins to breathe on his or her own, until another rescuer takes over, or until the rescuer is too tired to continue. See Helping a person breathe, page 863.

Movement

Muscles, bones, and joints provide the body with a supportive framework that permits flexibility of movement. All movement is carried out by muscles, which are composed of tissues that can contract.

VOLUNTARY MOVEMENT

The 206 bones of the skeleton provide a support system for the various parts of the body. Complex movements involve the coordination of many bones, joints, and muscles. Even a simple movement requires the activity of several muscles; some contract to initiate and maintain a movement, while others that oppose the movement contract to prevent sudden, uncontrolled movement. The shoulder (a ball-and-socket joint) allows movement in all directions. The knee, a hinge joint, permits movement in one plane only and in a limited range.

Voluntary skeletal movements are controlled by the part of the cerebrum (the largest and most developed part of the brain) called the motor cortex. This area of the brain sends instructions to muscles to permit voluntary movement, such as running, walking, speaking, or writing. The motor cortex is located in both halves (hemispheres) of the cerebrum. Motor cells in one hemisphere stimulate muscles on the other side of the body.

OTHER TYPES OF MOVEMENT

Movements of the internal organs are involuntary and are regulated by the AUTONOMIC NERVOUS SYSTEM. Involuntary movements include peristalsis (muscular contractions that propel food through the intestines) and the rhythmic contractions of the heart. Skeletal movements can also occur as involuntary reflexes to sensory warning signals, such as the blinking of an eye.

MOVEMENT DISORDERS

Disorders of the nervous system, muscles, joints, and bones may impair movement. There are many different types of movement disorders. For example, APRAXIA is a loss or impairment of the ability to perform purposeful movements. TREMOR is involuntary, rhythmic muscle movement caused by alternate contraction and relaxation of the muscles. In many cases, problems with movement are a symptom of an underlying medical problem, such as PARKINSON DISEASE, MULTIPLE SCLEROSIS, head injury, or emotional disorders.

Movement disorder

A disorder affecting the movement of the body. PARKINSON DISEASE is a type of movement disorder. Its four primary symptoms are tremor, rigidity, postural instability, and bradykinesia.

Moxibustion

The application of heat to specific points of the body to treat certain ailments; a form of ACUPUNCTURE. Moxibustion is a method of healing used in traditional CHINESE MEDICINE in which dried leaves of moxa, or Chinese mugwort, are burned at or near specific acupoints on the skin to treat such conditions as stiff neck, back problems, and fatigue. In some cases, moxa is formed into a pea-sized cone that is placed point up on the skin, lit, and left to smolder until the skin becomes warm. Sometimes pieces of smoldering moxa are placed on the handle of acupuncture needles so that the heat warms the skin and is drawn down into the body via the needle. Smoldering sticks of moxa may also be held near the skin. In no case is the skin itself burned.

MRA

Magnetic resonance angiography. See MRI.

MRCP

Magnetic resonance cholangiopancreatography. See MRI.

MRI

Magnetic resonance imaging; a diagnostic imaging technique that uses powerful magnetic fields and radio-frequency waves to produce computer-enhanced, cross-sectional images of internal organs and structures. MRI allows physicians to visualize interior body parts with great clarity and without exposure to the radiation involved in the use of X rays. The images created by MRI provide detailed pictures (for example, of the spine, brain, and soft tissues) that exceed previously available images.

A recent advance in MRI technology, called functional MRI, enables physicians to visualize the function of tissue and organs. Functional MRIs can provide measurements of nerve cell activity in the brain and locate areas of the brain activated in memory. Similarly, magnetic resonance angiography (MRA) offers detailed measurements of heart function and blood vessel flow. Magnetic resonance spectroscopy (MRS) uses magnetic fields and radio-frequency waves to assess the chemical changes caused by diseases such as tumors, strokes, and myocardial infarctions. Magnetic resonance cholangiopancreatography (MRCP) uses MRI to image the bile ducts, gallbladder, and pancreas in a noninvasive way.

WHY IT IS PERFORMED

An MRI is generally used to obtain two-dimensional views of an internal organ or structure. The technique is particularly helpful for visualizing internal areas of the nervous system, including the brain and spinal cord.

HELPING A PERSON BREATHE

The mouth-to-mouth method of artificial respiration is the forced introduction of air into the lungs of a person who has stopped breathing or is not breathing adequately. Mouth-to-mouth resuscitation must be started as soon as possible after the person has stopped breathing; a delay in breathing for more than 6 minutes can cause death.

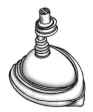

POCKET FACE MASK WITH ONE-WAY VALVE
An emergency worker may use a pocket face mask to prevent possible infection from the person who has stopped breathing.

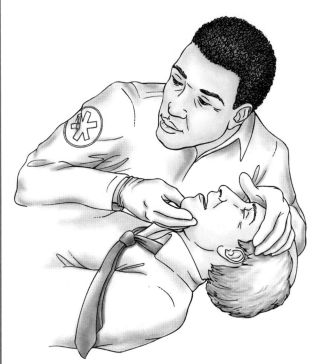

CLEARING THE AIRWAY
The first step in beginning mouth-to-mouth resuscitation is clearing the person's airway.

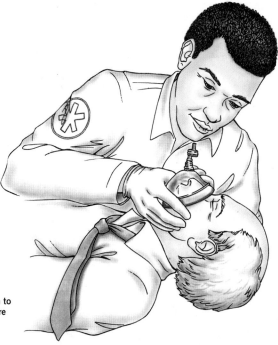

USING A FACE MASK FOR MOUTH-TO-MOUTH RESUSCITATION
The rescue worker places a face mask over the person to prevent infection from the person's bodily fluids before beginning mouth-to-mouth resuscitation.

M

GENERATING MOVEMENT

Movement begins in the cerebral cortex, where a coordinated motor plan is formed. Signals about the plan move to the motor cortex, then travel through motor nerve cells in the spinal cord to the peripheral nerves. The signals ultimately reach skeletal muscle fibers that contract or relax according to the motor plan.

M

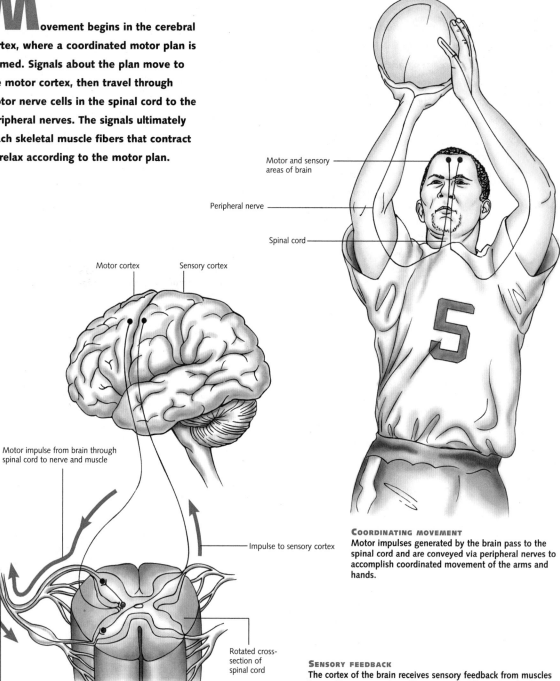

Motor and sensory areas of brain

Peripheral nerve

Spinal cord

Motor cortex

Sensory cortex

Motor impulse from brain through spinal cord to nerve and muscle

Impulse to sensory cortex

Rotated cross-section of spinal cord

Peripheral nerve

COORDINATING MOVEMENT
Motor impulses generated by the brain pass to the spinal cord and are conveyed via peripheral nerves to accomplish coordinated movement of the arms and hands.

SENSORY FEEDBACK
The cortex of the brain receives sensory feedback from muscles to monitor movements as they are made. The motor plan is continually altered to keep the movement going smoothly.

It may also be used to evaluate injuries to the bones and joints as a result of sports-related trauma. MRI is often used to monitor response to chemotherapy, radiation therapy, or other treatments for cancer and other diseases.

New uses for MRI include measuring brain volume to help diagnose Alzheimer's disease, specifically the volume of the hippocampus, which is the area of the brain that is important to memory function and is a site of the early development of the microscopic tangles of threadlike nerve fibers in the brain that are characteristic of Alzheimer's disease.

HOW IT WORKS

The strong magnetic field and radio-frequency waves transmitted by an MRI scanner alter the natural alignment of the nuclei of hydrogen atoms inside the body. The activity of the hydrogen nuclei is recorded and translated into tissue-slice images by computers. A magnetically active CONTRAST MEDIUM such as gadolinium may be injected into a vein to enhance the images of the parts of the body being evaluated. This contrast medium helps provide a better visualization of many disease processes.

HOW IT IS PERFORMED

MRI may be performed at a hospital unit, radiology laboratory, or diagnostic clinic. It takes between 15 and 60 minutes, depending on the area being examined. A contrast medium may be injected. During the MRI, the person must lie as still as possible on a narrow table that slides into a tube-like chamber. Because the chamber is only somewhat larger in diameter than the human body and encloses the person from head to toe, some people may need a mild sedative to calm them before the procedure, especially if they anticipate experiencing claustrophobia (an intense fear of enclosed spaces). The person being tested may be given a handheld device that will enable him or her to signal if he or she is claustrophobic or in distress, or for any other reason. Loud noises such as thumping or hammering sounds are heard intermittently during the procedure so the person being tested is usually given the option of using earplugs or listening to music with earphones. The health care professional administering the procedure may give instructions to the person in the chamber at various intervals.

Open MRI units do not enclose the entire body, and the person feels less confined. However, the images obtained by open units are often inferior and, thus, less accurate, than the images obtained by conventional closed MRI units. See Close-up on MRI, page 866.

RISKS

MRI is considered a safe procedure. The only known risks are for people who have cardiac pacemakers, aneurysm clips in the brain, or specific types of metal implants in the body. The radio-frequency waves of the magnet can cause a pacemaker to malfunction or an aneurysm clip to shift. It is generally safe to undergo an MRI if a person has orthopedic metal implants or surgical clips in the body, but it is important that the radiologist be notified.

MRS

Magnetic resonance spectroscopy. See MRI.

MS

See MULTIPLE SCLEROSIS.

MSG

Monosodium glutamate; a food additive that has been reported to cause adverse reactions in susceptible people. Reactions to MSG include headache, nausea, diarrhea, sweating, chest tightness, and a burning sensation at the back of the neck. Because MSG is best known for its role in Asian cooking, these symptoms are often referred to as "Chinese restaurant syndrome." However, MSG is also used to enhance flavor in a variety of restaurants and in many processed foods.

Mucocele

A swollen sac or cavity filled with mucus secreted from cells in its inner lining. Also known as mucus cysts, mucoceles consist of clear fluid trapped beneath a thin layer of mucous membrane. They usually appear on the inner surface of the lips and are caused by a sucking action drawing the mucous membranes between the teeth. Although mucoceles are harmless and usually painless, they can be bothersome. Treatment of serious cases may involve surgery.

Mucopoly-saccharidosis

A group of genetic disorders characterized by an accumulation of unwanted substances called mucopolysaccharides in body tissues. Under normal conditions, mucopolysaccharides form a gel-like substance found in mucous secretions as well as in body cells. Mucopolysaccharide disorders result in deposits of mucopolysaccharides in the arteries, skeleton, eyes, joints, ears, skin, and teeth. Deposits of mucopolysaccharides may also be found in the respiratory system, liver, spleen, central nervous system, and bone marrow. The buildup occurs because the underlying genetic disorder involves a deficiency of the enzymes necessary to break down mucopolysaccharides. Signs of the disorders include changes in facial appearance, mental retardation, heart failure, and shortened life expectancy. Examples of mucopolysaccharidosis-related disorders include Scheie syndrome, Hunter syndrome, Hurler syndrome, Sanfilippo syndrome, Maroteaux-Lamy syndrome, and Morquio disease.

Mucosa

See MUCOUS MEMBRANE.

Mucous membrane

A thin, soft tissue (found throughout the body) that lines a body cavity, passageway, or structure. A mucous membrane secretes mucus, a thick fluid that lubricates the tissue.

Mucus

A thick, viscous fluid produced by mucous glands. Mucus is secreted by glandular cells located within the moist mucous membranes that line many of the body's organs, cavities, and structures, where it functions as a protective barrier, a lubricant, and a carrier of enzymes. Mucus is secreted within the nasal sinuses, the respiratory tract, the gastrointestinal tract, and other structures.

Multi-infarct dementia

See VASCULAR DEMENTIA.

Multiple births

A pregnancy in which a woman is carrying more than one fetus. It occurs when two or more eggs are

M

CLOSE-UP ON MRI

A powerful electromagnetic field and radio waves are used in MRI (magnetic resonance imaging) to generate signals that are picked up by a computer and interpreted as two-dimensional images. Compared with CT (computed tomography) scanning, MRI can more clearly visualize the insides of organs and very fine soft-tissue details. In closed MRI, the person is enclosed in a hollow cylinder, which can be noisy and make some people uncomfortable. In open MRI, only the part of the body being scanned is positioned under the scanning mechanism.

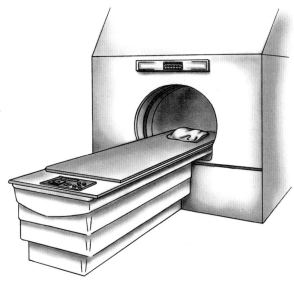

CLOSED MRI EQUIPMENT
In a closed MRI, the patient lies on a table that slides into the enclosed cylinder. If the person is uncomfortable with the confinement, he or she can be given a sedative before the procedure.

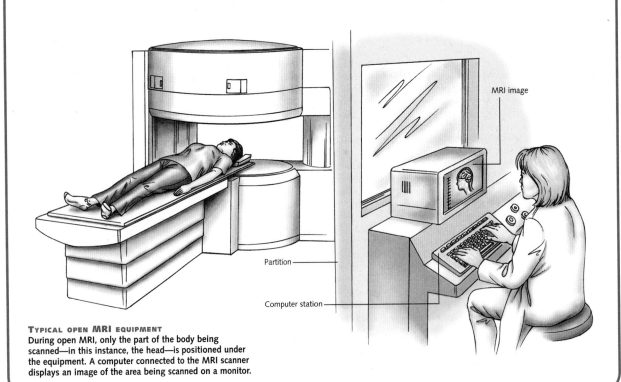

MRI image

Partition

Computer station

TYPICAL OPEN MRI EQUIPMENT
During open MRI, only the part of the body being scanned—in this instance, the head—is positioned under the equipment. A computer connected to the MRI scanner displays an image of the area being scanned on a monitor.

M

released simultaneously from the ovaries and are fertilized or when a single fertilized egg divides into two eggs early in development. A pregnancy with two or more fetuses is considered a higher risk pregnancy because multiple fetuses have greater nutritional needs than a single baby and place extra strain on the mother's body. Sleeping, eating, and physical comfort may become difficult earlier than in a one-baby pregnancy. Multiple births are more common now than formerly, because more women are taking fertility drugs, which increase the likelihood for multiple fetuses.

The risks of certain disorders, including high blood pressure, HYDRAMNIOS, and postpartum hemorrhage, are higher than in a one-baby pregnancy. Preterm labor is common in multiple births; about half of all multiple births are premature. Premature births usually occur before the 37th week of pregnancy (full term is considered to be around 40 weeks) because the fetuses grow too large for the uterus and trigger uterine contractions. Bed rest and abstinence from sexual intercourse may postpone early delivery. Bed rest helps the muscles in the uterus to relax and may improve blood flow to the uterus. Abstinence avoids stimulation of the cervix, which can cause the uterus to contract.

While TWINS may sometimes be delivered by vaginal delivery, triplets and quadruplets are usually delivered by CESAREAN SECTION. Labor may be slower and more difficult in a multiple birth. Multiple-birth babies are more likely to be of lower than average birth weight because there is less room in the uterus for them to grow. If there is a single placenta, there are increased demands on it for nutrients. Growth of multiple fetuses is monitored closely with ultrasound scanning.

Multiple chemical sensitivity

A syndrome in which a person reports multiple symptoms that he or she believes are due to low-level chemical exposure. A person with multiple chemical sensitivity (MCS) may have severe symptoms that interfere with daily life and work. People with this condition often report symptoms after they have been exposed to an environmental chemical, such as a pesticide or chemical used in a building remodeling. The exposure level is typically low enough that it should not cause symptoms, but after a suspected exposure, the person may have multiple symptoms in response to previously tolerated low-level exposures. Symptoms include fatigue, difficulty concentrating, a depressed mood, memory loss, weakness, taste disturbance, dizziness, headaches, and heat intolerance. In severe cases, people with MCS will alter their behavior and lifestyle to avoid what they presumed brought on their original symptoms. The condition, which affects women far more often than men, may cause or be associated with psychiatric conditions such as depression and anxiety.

Treatment of MCS focuses on helping the person control and manage symptoms, treating any psychiatric illness if appropriate, and encouraging the person to remain active and use relaxation exercises to help diminish the fear of perceived dangers.

Multiple myeloma

A cancer of the plasma cells. Normal plasma cells are found in the bone marrow and are the part of the body's immune system that produces antibodies. Abnormal plasma cells cause several problems. They compromise the ability to fight infections. By multiplying excessively, they reduce the ability of the bone marrow to function properly. Myeloma cells attack and weaken surrounding bone, causing pain and fractures, resulting in elevated calcium levels. The disease can also interfere with kidney function and cause renal failure.

When plasma cells grow out of control, they produce tumors, usually in the bone marrow. Plasma cell tumors can develop in several sites at once and then are called multiple myeloma. A common symptom of multiple myeloma is back pain, which can be mild or severe, caused by abnormal plasma cells in the bone marrow of the spine. Other symptoms include anemia, abnormal bleeding, infections, and poor kidney function. Diagnosis of multiple myeloma requires a blood test that identifies abnormal proteins produced by plasma cells. X rays of the back may show fractures or thinning of the bones. A bone marrow biopsy will be necessary to look for elevated numbers of plasma cells.

Multiple myeloma is usually treated with chemotherapy, which can often control the disease for several years but does not cure it. Individuals can be treated with medications that help to prevent bone fractures. Bone marrow transplantation is done on younger patients, who can survive for many years. Radiation therapy is also used to reduce bone pain associated with the disease. Pain is a particular feature of this disease, and many people take pain medication and wear neck or back braces. Multiple myeloma rarely occurs before age 40 and is more common in older men; it is twice as common in blacks as in whites. About a quarter of the people who have been diagnosed with this cancer survive for at least 5 years.

Multiple personality disorder

Another name for dissociative identity disorder, an emotional condition in which a person has two or more distinct identities that surface regularly, control the person's actions, and know little about the other identities; the identities are in conflict with one another. Multiple personality is considered one of the DISSOCIATIVE DISORDERS because the individual becomes detached, or dissociated, from fundamental aspects of reality.

When a person is under the control of one of his or her personalities, he or she cannot remember events that happened when another personality was in control. The personalities can be very distinct, with differences in speech patterns, names, mannerisms, thought processes, and such physical characteristics as gender, handedness, and prescription for vision correction. The change from one personality to another is often triggered by stress, and it usually occurs in a matter of seconds. The number of personalities varies from two to more than 100, with fewer than ten being most common.

Symptoms of multiple personality disorder include areas of missing memory, encounters with people who recognize the person yet whom the

M

individual does not recognize, coming to consciousness in an unknown place and not knowing how one got there, depressed feelings, discovery of items the individual does not remember purchasing, thoughts about suicide, self-mutilation, and hallucinations (for example, hearing voices, which may represent one personality speaking to another). In children the symptoms are less distinct. They include anxiety, conduct problems, and difficulty paying attention at school. Symptoms of POSTTRAUMATIC STRESS DISORDER, including flashbacks and nightmares, may also be present in both children and adults.

Multiple personality disorder usually emerges in early life, at approximately age 5 or 6, and is more common in females than males. Physical or sexual abuse is commonly associated with the disorder. The person creates another personality to receive the abuse as a way of defending against the pain and suffering. The diagnosis remains scientifically controversial. Treatment consists of psychotherapy to help break down the barriers between the different personalities and allow the person to create a single, unified identity.

Multiple sclerosis

Also known as MS, a chronic, often disabling disease of the central nervous system. The symptoms of MS range from mild (such as numbness in the limbs) to severe (including paralysis and loss of vision). Most people are diagnosed with MS between age 20 and 40 years. This disease is twice as common in women as in men.

CAUSES

Multiple sclerosis is an autoimmune disease (a disease caused by the reaction of a person's immune system against his or her own tissues). In most cases, the cause is unknown. In this disease, nerve impulses passing through the central nervous system are disrupted, causing potentially debilitating damage to the brain and spinal cord. A fatty substance called myelin normally protects and coats nerve fibers. In MS, the myelin becomes swollen and inflamed. Eventually, damaged myelin is detached from fibers and is destroyed (demyelination). When subsequent nerve impulses reach these damaged areas, they are blocked or

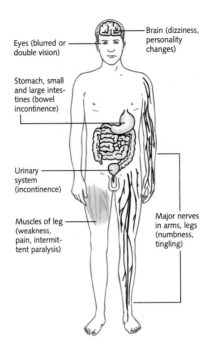

Eyes (blurred or double vision)

Brain (dizziness, personality changes)

Stomach, small and large intestines (bowel incontinence)

Urinary system (incontinence)

Muscles of leg (weakness, pain, intermittent paralysis)

Major nerves in arms, legs (numbness, tingling)

SYMPTOMS OF MULTIPLE SCLEROSIS
The symptoms of MS vary depending on the areas of the brain and spinal cord that are affected. The primary symptoms result from the impaired transmission of nerve impulses caused by the destruction of the myelin sheath on the nerves.

delayed, resulting in the symptoms of MS.

SYMPTOMS

Early signs of MS may be subtle. Symptoms range from mild to severe and from short-lived to long-lasting. The initial signs of MS are often abnormal sensations, such as pins and needles, and difficulty walking. Some people experience more serious pain and loss of vision as a result of optic neuritis (inflammation of the optic nerve). Less common initial symptoms include tremor, lack of coordination, slurred speech, the sudden onset of paralysis, and a decline in cognitive function (the ability to think, reason, and remember).

The primary symptoms of MS are a direct result of demyelination. This impairs the transmission of nerve impulses, leading to symptoms such as weakness, numbness, tremor, paralysis, pain, loss of vision, loss of balance, and bowel and bladder dysfunction.

The secondary symptoms of MS occur as complications of the primary symptoms. For example, inactivity

can lead to decreased bone density, poor posture and trunk control, and weakness from disuse. Paralysis can result in pressure sores.

The tertiary (third-level) symptoms of MS include the social and vocational consequences of the primary and secondary symptoms. For example, a person who can no longer walk or drive may lose his or her job. Depression is a common problem. Tertiary symptoms are managed by psychologists, social workers, physical and occupational therapists, and public health agencies.

DIAGNOSIS AND TREATMENT

Diagnosis is based on symptoms, medical history, and neurological examination. Tests such as lumbar puncture, EVOKED RESPONSES, and MRI (magnetic resonance imaging) may be performed to confirm the diagnosis. The progression of MS is variable and does not always result in complete disability. Flare-ups (attacks) are often self-limited in the early stages of MS. Some people with MS may have very few attacks and experience few problems. Because there is no cure, the goal of treatment is symptom relief. Corticosteroids are most often prescribed to relieve the inflammation of MS. However, because they have serious side effects, these drugs must be used with caution. Interferon beta and glatiramer acetate are used to decrease the frequency of flare-ups and ultimately decrease disability. These medications are given by injection on a daily, every other day, or weekly basis and are the first drugs

---

THE FOUR CLINICAL COURSES OF MULTIPLE SCLEROSIS

Multiple sclerosis (MS) takes one of four clinical courses, each of which can range from mild to moderate to severe:

- A relapsing-remitting course, characterized by partial or total recovery after attacks (the most common form of MS)
- A relapsing-remitting course that later becomes steadily more progressive (secondary-progressive MS)
- A progressive course from onset
- A rare, progressive course that is characterized by acute attacks from onset

available that alter the course of MS. These medications alleviate symptoms but do not provide a cure. Many new treatments are being tested to help treat more advanced and progressive disease.

Multivitamin

A dietary supplement that supplies the essential vitamins and minerals that people do not always obtain in sufficient amounts in their regular diets. Multivitamins, which often contain minerals, are usually taken daily. Taking a multivitamin does not compensate for poor food choices, and the health risks of high intakes of fat and refined sugars are not offset by multivitamin supplements. It is best to get necessary vitamins and minerals by eating a wide variety of foods. However, a multivitamin may be helpful for people who, for a variety of reasons, are not getting all the nutrients they need. Supplements may help individuals who are ill, older, vegetarian, or on low-calorie diets. Women who are breast-feeding, pregnant, or planning to be pregnant usually require multivitamins. For those who choose to take a multivitamin, doctors recommend products that provide no more than 100 percent of the Daily Value for vitamins and minerals. Too much of certain vitamins can pose health risks. See also FOOD GUIDE PYRAMID.

Mumps

A contagious viral infection that produces swelling in one or both of the two salivary glands located above the angle of the jaw in front of each ear and in the salivary gland located under the tongue.

The virus that causes mumps is spread from person to person via the coughs, sneezes, and saliva of a person who has mumps or by contact with surfaces contaminated with infectious respiratory secretions or saliva. Once it has entered the body, the virus spreads into the bloodstream and may migrate to many different glands, including the testes in a man, the ovaries in a woman, and in both sexes, the pancreas and the brain.

Mumps is no longer considered a serious health threat in the United States as a result of the effective vaccine against it, generally given as part of the MMR (measles-mumps-rubella)

vaccination to young children. The vaccine has essentially eradicated the disease, but rarely it can present a threat to a woman who is pregnant and in her first trimester, as it increases the risk of fetal death and miscarriage.

SYMPTOMS AND DIAGNOSIS

Mumps are contagious for 2 days before symptoms appear and up to 9 days after symptoms begin. After being exposed to someone who has mumps, a person who acquires the virus may or may not have symptoms. When symptoms occur, they tend to appear 2 to 4 weeks following exposure.

The symptoms of mumps tend to be vague but can include fever, headache, sore throat, muscle aches, poor appetite, and fatigue. Most people who have symptoms develop the characteristic painful swelling in one or more salivary glands, often producing tender fullness between the earlobe and the angle of the jaw. Chewing and swallowing can make eating uncomfortable. These symptoms may last for 10 days.

Some postpubertal males develop symptoms of inflammation and infection of the testes, including localized swelling, tenderness, and pain. If a woman's ovaries are involved, she may have pain in the lower abdomen.

Either sex may experience pain in the upper mid-abdomen, signaling a condition called mumps PANCREATITIS, an inflammation and infection of the pancreas. Headache, stiff neck, and sleepiness are symptoms of an associated condition called aseptic MENINGITIS, which is rare and produces mild illness with full recovery when it does occur. Very rarely, mumps travels to the brain, causing an infection and producing ENCEPHALITIS, which may begin with high fever and loss of consciousness. This can lead to long-term complications including deafness, seizures, and paralysis of facial muscles.

Mumps is diagnosed by taking a clinical history to determine possible exposure and by performing a physical examination, with particular attention given to the typical swelling of the salivary glands. The diagnosis can be confirmed by blood tests that measure specific antibodies to the mumps virus. Samples of urine, sali-

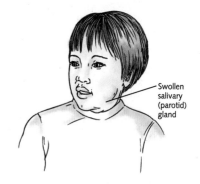

— Swollen salivary (parotid) gland

VIRUS IN SALIVARY GLANDS
The swelling associated with mumps is caused by enlarged salivary glands above the jaw and in front of the ears, as well as under the tongue. Depending on the extent of swelling, chewing and swallowing may be difficult. Treatment is focused on relieving symptoms.

va, or spinal fluid may be tested to detect the virus itself.

There is no antiviral medication to cure mumps. Treatment is based on easing symptoms. Acetaminophen may be taken to reduce fever and relieve body aches. (Aspirin should not be taken by children younger than 18 years because it is associated with REYE SYNDROME, a brain disorder in children with viral illness who have taken aspirin.) Warm or cold compresses may lessen any discomforts associated with tender, swollen salivary glands. Fruit juices and tart foods, such as grapefruit, which produces painful stimulation of the salivary glands, should be avoided; soft, bland foods are generally easiest for a person with mumps to chew and swallow. If the testes are affected, cool compresses and support of the scrotum are recommended. Severe testicular pain may require injection of a local anesthetic to ease discomfort.

Most healthy people who contract mumps recover completely. There is a small risk of sterility in males when both testicles are affected, but this is rare.

Munchausen syndrome

The intentional feigning or production of physical or psychological symptoms out of a deep-seated need to assume the sick role; a mental disorder also known as factitious disorder and pathomimicry. A person with Munchausen syndrome may make up the complaint and support it with lies or inflict injuries on his or her own body, such as injecting material under the skin to produce abscesses. In some cases, psychological complaints are primary; in others, physical complaints predominate; in yet others, both physical and psychological symptoms appear. The motivation behind Munchausen syndrome is not to gain some advantage, such as avoiding jury duty or military service. Rather, the person has an unconscious need to be cared for as a sick person. The disorder may result in unneeded medical tests and exploratory surgeries. Munchausen syndrome is thought to be rare, but it occurs equally in males and females.

In a related disorder known as Munchausen syndrome by proxy, an individual produces or feigns physical or emotional symptoms in another person under his or her care. Usually the victim is a young child, and the person producing the symptoms may be the child's parent or caretaker, most often the mother. The parent or caretaker has an unconscious psychological need to assume the role of a sick person and may have Munchausen syndrome, which is not expressed as long as she or he is able to make use of a victim. Munchausen syndrome by proxy usually involves symptoms in the digestive tract, urinary and reproductive systems, or central nervous system. The parent or caretaker may poison or inflict physical harm on the child victim, leading to criminal charges of child abuse and even murder.

Mupirocin

An antibacterial ointment. Mupirocin (Bactroban) is used to treat bacterial infections of the skin by killing bacteria or preventing their growth. It is often prescribed for the treatment of impetigo, a skin infection usually found in children.

Murmur

See HEART MURMUR.

Muscle

A fibrous structure in the body composed of cells that can contract or relax to generate movement. Different types of muscles can cause movement of the skeletal framework of the body (skeletal muscle), movement of the tissues of body organs (smooth muscle), or the specialized pumping action of the heart (cardiac muscle).

SKELETAL MUSCLE

The skeletal muscles, attached to bone, make up slightly less than half of the total body weight of an average person. These muscles vary widely in size and shape, from the large, long muscles that move the limbs, to sheets of muscles such as those in the chest, or the tiny circular muscles that move the eyeballs. But all skeletal muscles are similarly structured— they are bundles of varying numbers of muscle fibers. An individual fiber is composed of microscopically small filaments called myofibrils. A myofibril is further constructed of a repeating pattern of two dovetailed filaments; one contains a protein called actin, and the other contains a protein called myosin. When a signal from the nervous system directs movement, the actin filaments can actually slide into the myosin filaments, causing the entire filament to shorten, or contract. The microscopic protein filaments sliding out causes the opposing action of relaxing or lengthening the filament.

The skeletal muscles are controlled by the brain. Each muscle fiber contains a nerve ending that receives electrochemical signals from the brain, causing the protein sliding action and, thus, the shortening or lengthening of the muscle fibers. Nerve endings also monitor the degree of contraction or relaxation of the muscle fibers to appropriately limit the movement of the whole muscle. The movement of skeletal muscles is voluntary.

SMOOTH MUSCLE

Smooth muscle causes the movement of the internal organs such as the lungs and the intestinal system. This movement is not under conscious control; it is involuntary. The AUTONOMIC NERVOUS SYSTEM directs this movement to maintain the automatic functioning of the body. Smooth muscle is also affected by the secretion of hormones and other chemical balances in body tissue.

Smooth muscle tissue contracts and relaxes to cause movement, but the action is slower than in skeletal muscles. Smooth muscle fibers are constructed differently than skeletal or cardiac muscles, but the basic motion of the proteins actin and myosin occurs to generate muscle movement.

CARDIAC MUSCLE

Cardiac muscle, also called myocardium, is found only in the HEART. The structure of cardiac muscle fiber is somewhat similar to that of skeletal muscle, with bundles of myofibrils containing the dovetail pattern of actin and myosin filaments. But the muscle fibers branch in a unique way to form a network that can accomplish the rapid, rhythmic, continuous contractions of a regular heartbeat. This involuntary, vital muscle movement is controlled by the autonomic nervous system, in concert with hormonal activity. See also MUSCULAR SYSTEM.

Muscle relaxants

Drugs used to relieve pain caused by sprains, spasms, or injuries to skeletal muscles. Skeletal muscle relaxants work by relaxing muscles to relieve stiffness, pain, and discomfort. Most muscle relaxants work by acting on the central nervous system. Muscle relaxants are powerful drugs generally used in addition to rest, exercise, physical therapy, and other treatments. Muscle relaxants can impair a person's ability to drive.

CARISOPRODOL (SOMA)

This skeletal muscle relaxant has sedative effects. It may modify a person's perception of pain in the central nervous system. Carisoprodol is used to relieve discomfort in acutely painful musculoskeletal conditions. It is associated with many side effects, including drowsiness, dizziness, tremor, insomnia, rapid heartbeat, asthmatic episodes, skin rashes, fever, and others. Because carisoprodol increases the effects of alcohol, it should never be used with alcoholic beverages or cold remedies containing alcohol.

CHLORZOXAZONE (PARAFON FORTE)

Chlorzoxazone is a drug to reduce pain caused by acute, painful musculoskeletal conditions. It is associated with drowsiness, dizziness, lightheadedness, nausea, vomiting, heartburn, bruising of the skin, and many other side effects. It may turn urine orange or purple; it should never be taken with alcohol or cold remedies containing alcohol.

METHOCARBAMOL (ROBAXIN)

Methocarbamol is used to treat acute, painful musculoskeletal conditions

CLOSE-UP ON MUSCLES

There are three kinds of muscle tissue: skeletal, cardiac, and smooth. Under a microscope, the first two look striped, but the third does not. The skeletal muscles, which move bones, often work in pairs; when one muscle contracts, another relaxes.

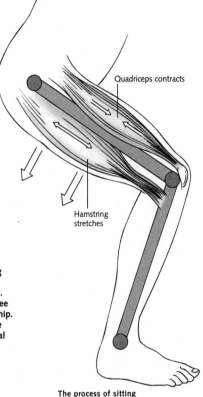

Quadriceps contracts

Hamstring
stretches

SITTING AND STANDING UP
When a person goes from a sitting to standing position, the hamstring muscle contracts, the knee bends, and the leg moves toward the hip. When the quadriceps muscle contracts, the knee straightens and the leg moves away from the hip. At the same time, the hamstring relaxes so the quadriceps can pull the limb back to its original length.

The process of sitting

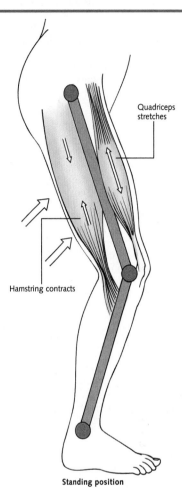

Quadriceps
stretches

Hamstring contracts

Standing position

M

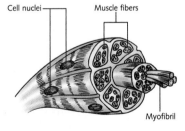

Cell nuclei — Muscle fibers

Myofibril

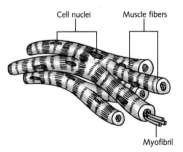

Cell nuclei — Muscle fibers

Myofibril

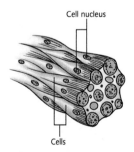

Cell nucleus

Cells

SKELETAL MUSCLE
Thick and thin muscle fibers permit a person to move when his or her brain tells them to. The skeletal muscles are under conscious, voluntary control. Skeletal muscles in a person's arms or legs, for example, stretch and contract rapidly and powerfully, but tire easily.

CARDIAC MUSCLE
Cardiac muscle, located only in the wall of the heart, is an involuntary muscle that works automatically. It is striped with branches connected end-to-end by membranes that allow for the flow of electrical current that helps the heart speed up or slow down, according to the body's needs.

SMOOTH MUSCLE
Smooth muscles are bundled together and are located in hollow organs that work automatically, such as in the stomach, where the muscles help move food along the intestines.

by sedating the person taking it, rather than by relaxing the muscles directly. It is associated with many side effects, including turning the urine various colors. Additional effects include drowsiness, dizziness, headache, light-headedness, blurred vision, skin rash, fever, and others. Because methocarbamol increases the effects of alcohol, it should not be used with alcohol or cold remedies containing alcohol.

Muscle spasm

Persistent involuntary tightening of one or more muscles, usually causing pain from excessive rigidity. Muscle spasm may be caused by a strain, injury, fracture of a related bone, or chronic overuse of a muscle. It may also be due to a muscle's protective action in the prevention of movement of a body part that is stressed. Examples of muscle spasms include what is called a "charley horse," as well as torticollis, or wryneck. Pain-relieving and antispasm medications may be prescribed; physical therapy may be helpful. Gentle moving and stretching of the area, especially in warm bath water, can help ease the pain of a muscle spasm. Immobilization of the area can help relieve the spasm, but prolonged immobilization will reduce muscle strength and create the risk of strains and sprains.

Muscle stimulants

Drugs used to stimulate muscular activity. Examples of muscle stimulants include LAXATIVES, which stimulate the smooth muscle of the bowel to promote defecation, and drugs such as METOCLOPRAMIDE that increase the movements or contractions of the stomach and first part of the small intestine to prevent nausea and vomiting.

Another example of a use of a muscle stimulant is a drug used to treat myasthenia gravis, a disease that causes muscle weakness.

Muscular dystrophy

A group of genetic diseases characterized by progressive muscle weakness and loss of muscle tissue, particularly of the muscles used to control movement. There are nine major forms of muscular dystrophy (MD). The type called Duchenne most com-monly affects children while the myotonic form most often occurs in adults. MD can occur at any age: some forms appear in infancy and childhood, but others may not appear until middle age or later. Duchenne MD is caused by an abnormal gene controlling the supply of the muscle protein dystrophin; dystrophin is missing or deficient in people with MD.

SYMPTOMS

The chief symptoms are related to progressive muscle weakness that gets worse over time. Depending on the type of MD, frequent falls, delayed development of motor skills, difficulty walking, drooping eyelids, drooling, and difficulty using specific muscle groups may all be symptoms. Other symptoms may include skeletal deformities, muscle deformities, clawfoot, clawhand, and HYPOTONIA, or decreased muscle tone. Muscle tightness is common and involves shortened muscle fibers around the joints, inhibiting joint mobility. Loss of muscle mass, or wasting, is also common. Some types of MD are associated with mental retardation.

DIAGNOSIS AND TREATMENT

The primary method by which MD is diagnosed is muscle biopsy. Other medical tests that may be used include electromyography (EMG), a test used to determine whether muscle weakness is caused by destruction of muscle tissue or by damage to nerves, and a blood test to determine the level of serum creatine kinase (CK), an enzyme found in muscle cells that may be elevated in people with the disease. People with MD may also have abnormal levels of other substances in the blood or urine, such as creatinine and myoglobin.

Because MD is inherited, there is usually a family history of the disorder. Diagnosis involves taking a detailed family history, which is important for distinguishing the type of MD. When Duchenne or Becker MD is suspected, DNA testing for the presence of an abnormality on the gene involved in producing dystrophin may be performed.

There is no known cure for MD. Treatment is intended to control symptoms to improve the person's quality of life. Various therapies are used. Physical therapy is used to prevent shortening of the muscles and to maintain muscle strength. Orthoses (orthopedic appliances), such as leg braces or wheelchairs, are used for support. Corrective orthopedic surgery can be performed. Medication can be given to treat myotonia (delayed relaxation of a muscle after a contraction) in myotonic MD, and a pacemaker can be used to treat cardiac problems associated with Emery-Dreifuss and myotonic MD.

TYPES OF MD

The outcome of the disease depends on the type of MD; while all types of MD worsen over time, some do so faster than others. Some cases can be very mild and progress slowly, with a nearly normal life span, while others progress rapidly with loss of the ability to walk and a reduced life expectancy.

■ *Duchenne muscular dystrophy (DMD)* DMD is the most common and most devastating of all the muscular dystrophies. It is an X-linked inherited disorder characterized by rapidly progressive muscle weakness, usually affecting only males. Females born with the gene for MD rarely have the disease but are carriers and may pass it on to their children. DMD occurs in 1 of 3,500 male births worldwide and in 1 of 5,000 male births in developed countries where genetic counseling is available to prospective parents. Prenatal testing for DMD is available.

The symptoms are usually noticed in the early years of life. Early signs of DMD include a tendency to fall, difficulty rising from a sitting position, and a waddling gait. The pelvic and leg muscles are usually affected first. Sometimes the calf muscles appear enlarged (pseudohypertrophy), and the child may walk on tiptoes. Gradually, strength diminishes in muscles throughout the body. Most individuals with DMD lose the ability to walk by late childhood or the early teens. The disease can progress until the child is virtually paralyzed, except for the fingers and toes. The heart muscle is also involved, leading to cardiac arrhythmias and heart failure. Males with DMD die in their late teens or early 20s. No current treatment is effective.

■ *Myotonic* This form of MD is the most common adult form of the disorder. Its characteristic symptom is myotonia, a muscle spasm or stiffen-

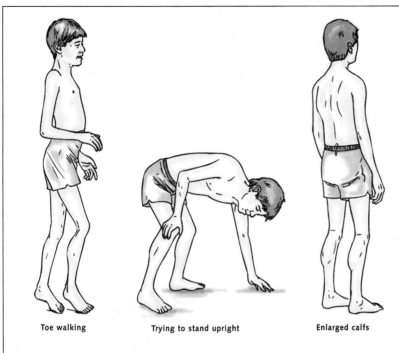

MUSCLE WEAKNESS AND MUSCLE LOSS
A person with muscular dystrophy may walk on his or her toes, because the muscles in the ankles have shortened and the ankle has become permanently flexed. In order to stand upright, a person with muscular dystrophy may "climb up" his or her own body by pushing on the thighs—a characteristic movement called the Gower sign. In addition, the calf muscles may look enlarged because fat and connective tissue have replaced muscle.

Toe walking

Trying to stand upright

Enlarged calfs

ing. Myotonic dystrophy progresses slowly, and symptoms can vary greatly. Congenital myotonic dystrophy is a severe form in the infants of affected parents. Cardiac problems and mild mental retardation are common features. Genetic testing is available, and genetic counseling is recommended.

■ *Becker* Similar to Duchenne, this type of MD usually appears later, as late as age 25, and progresses more slowly. People with Becker dystrophy are usually able to walk into their 30s. Only males are affected. Severity may vary, and life expectancy is longer than with DMD.

■ *Limb-girdle* This form of MD occurs in adolescence or early adulthood in both males and females. The disease causes progressive weakness starting in the hips and moving to the shoulders. After about 20 years, most affected individuals are unable to walk.

■ *Emery-Dreifuss* This type of MD affects only males in childhood or the early teens. The disease is character-ized by progressive weakness and wasting of shoulder, upper arm, and shin muscles, usually with joint deformities. The disease usually progresses slowly, although cardiac problems are common and need to be treated with pacemakers.

■ *Others* Facioscapulohumeral MD is a slowly progressive disorder that first affects the muscles of the face, the shoulders, and the upper arm. Congenital MD appears at birth and usually involves generalized muscle weakness and mental retardation. Oculopharyngeal MD occurs in late middle age and affects the eyelids and other facial muscles, and distal MD is a group of rare muscle diseases that involve weakness and wasting of the muscles of the forearms, hands, lower legs, and feet.

Muscular system
The more than 600 muscles that are attached to and supported by the bones of the skeleton. These muscles shorten or lengthen to move the bones to which they are attached.

These movements are voluntary, or under conscious control. Together, the muscles and bones form the moving framework of the body referred to as the musculoskeletal system.

Generally, an individual MUSCLE or set of muscles works in coordination with an opposing muscle or muscle set, perhaps with the support of other surrounding muscle groups, to accomplish movement. The movement usually takes place from the juncture of two bones called a JOINT. In the absence of movement, muscles are held in a state of partial contraction known as muscle tone. To initiate muscle movement, to bend the knee, for example, the brain sends a message for muscles in the back of the thigh to contract. The muscle fibers work to shorten the muscle to bend or close the knee joint. At the same time, the muscles on the top of the thigh lengthen to allow the movement to take place. To extend or open the knee joint, the brain directs the muscles in the top of the thigh to contract or shorten, while the muscles on the back of the thigh lengthen.

Muscles are attached to bones by straps of tough connective tissue called tendons. Usually a muscle has a stationary end, where the muscle is attached with a short tendon, and an insertion end, where the connecting tendon is longer and movement takes place.

Muscles vary widely in size and shape, ranging from large and powerful muscles of the hip and buttock, to tiny muscles that alter facial expression. In addition to the voluntary skeletal muscles, the body has other types of muscle involved with internal organs. See MUSCLE; The body's muscles, page 874.

Musculoskeletal system
The muscles, bones, and joints that form the moving structural frame of the body. See JOINT; MUSCULAR SYSTEM; and SKELETAL SYSTEM.

Musculoskeletal fitness
The overall health and function of the body's skeletal bones and the muscles attached to them. The skeleton provides a supporting framework for muscles to move and protects the organs in the body. The skeletal mus-

M

THE BODY'S MUSCLES

The human body has more than 600 major muscles; all are made up of tough, elastic tissue. Muscles account for about half of the body's weight, are more often injured than diseased, and are capable of self-repair. If part of a muscle is destroyed, the remaining part will grow larger and stronger in an effort to compensate.

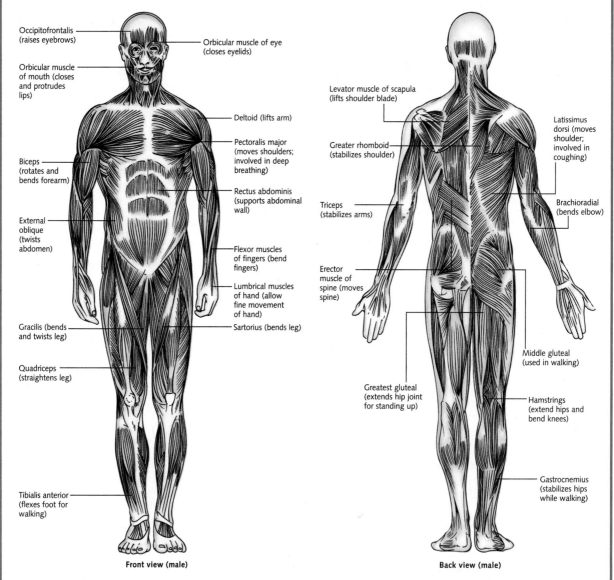

Occipitofrontalis (raises eyebrows)

Orbicular muscle of eye (closes eyelids)

Orbicular muscle of mouth (closes and protrudes lips)

Deltoid (lifts arm)

Pectoralis major (moves shoulders; involved in deep breathing)

Biceps (rotates and bends forearm)

Rectus abdominis (supports abdominal wall)

External oblique (twists abdomen)

Flexor muscles of fingers (bend fingers)

Lumbrical muscles of hand (allow fine movement of hand)

Gracilis (bends and twists leg)

Sartorius (bends leg)

Quadriceps (straightens leg)

Tibialis anterior (flexes foot for walking)

Front view (male)

Levator muscle of scapula (lifts shoulder blade)

Latissimus dorsi (moves shoulder; involved in coughing)

Greater rhomboid (stabilizes shoulder)

Triceps (stabilizes arms)

Brachioradial (bends elbow)

Erector muscle of spine (moves spine)

Middle gluteal (used in walking)

Greatest gluteal (extends hip joint for standing up)

Hamstrings (extend hips and bend knees)

Gastrocnemius (stabilizes hips while walking)

Back view (male)

SKELETAL MUSCLE MOVEMENT

The major muscles of the body act on the bones to which they are attached. Generally, one set of muscles shortens, or contracts, and an opposing set relaxes, or lengthens, to move bones at their joints. For example, to bend the arm at the elbow, the biceps muscle contracts while the triceps muscle lengthens. To straighten the arm, the triceps muscle contracts and the biceps relaxes.

cles are voluntary muscles that are controlled by nerve impulses from the brain; these muscles flex and extend joints and enable conscious movement throughout the body. A muscle's ability to perform well depends on the proper functioning of the nerves and the condition of the muscle tissue. Ligaments and tendons hold the body's joints together and keep the joints stable during movement.

Musculoskeletal fitness defines the ability of the bones and muscles to perform their roles properly. The strength of the musculoskeletal system is enhanced by physical activity that helps build healthy muscle and bone tissue. Muscle tissue is conditioned and increased by STRENGTH TRAINING exercises. Bone strength is increased by weight-bearing exercise (see EXERCISE, WEIGHT-BEARING). Both forms of exercise are essential to achieving and maintaining musculoskeletal fitness.

There are several categories of disorders that may impair musculoskeletal function. These include inflammatory disorders such as rheumatic or arthritic diseases; mechanical disorders caused by injuries such as fractured bones, torn ligaments, tendinitis, or slipped disks; the disintegration of cartilage in the joints, or osteoarthritis; metabolic bone diseases such as osteoporosis; and bone cancers.

Mutagen

An agent that can cause a change in a gene. Mutagens can alter the genetic makeup of cells by changing the structure of their DNA; these changes can increase the rate of mutation. Examples of mutagens include several kinds of radiation, X rays, ultraviolet light, many chemicals, and some viruses.

Some effects of mutagens are enhanced or suppressed by the presence of other, nonmutagenic substances. Oxygen, for instance, makes cells more sensitive to the mutagenic effects of X rays.

Mutation

A permanent structural change in the genetic material of a cell that can be passed on to subsequent generations. Mutations usually appear in single genes and result from changes in the DNA (deoxyribonucleic acid). However, mutations can also result in entire chromosomes being deleted or completely rearranged. Mutations can occur on any point of the DNA sequence. Most mutations either have no effect or are harmful, causing cancers, birth defects, and hereditary diseases. Some mutations can improve the survival chances of an organism.

A mutation can originate from a fault in the copying of a cell's DNA during cell division. Mutations can also occur from direct damage to the DNA by a MUTAGEN, an agent that increases the rate of mutation, such as X rays. An offspring cell inherits the faulty DNA, which is copied in subsequent cell divisions, giving rise to a population of cells containing the faulty DNA. Some physical and chemical agents make mutation more likely. High-energy radiation and carcinogenic compounds (cancer-inducing agents) are important mutagens.

Mutism

The persistent failure or refusal to speak in situations where speech is normal and expected. Complete mutism is a symptom of a type of SCHIZOPHRENIA. Selective mutism—silence in certain social situations, with speech in others—is found mostly in children. Children with this rare disorder may communicate with hand or body gestures or use short, single syllables.

Selective mutism is commonly associated with excessive shyness, fear of embarrassment, social isolation, clinging, compulsive behavior, negative attitudes, temper tantrums, manipulation, and obstinacy. Selectively mute children are commonly teased by other children and ridiculed. Language skills are usually normal, but in some cases the disorder arises in children who have a history of speech problems, such as stuttering, or who began to speak only at a late age. Selective mutism is often related to emotional problems at school or in the family. Treatment consists of counseling for the child and family. Antidepressant medication taken for 6 months sometimes reduces the shyness and anxiety about speech.

Myalgia

Muscle pain, often due to an overuse stress injury, that is generally caused by using the muscles in a new or unusual activity for a prolonged period of time. Myalgia is also common in people with a fever or viral infection.

Myasthenia gravis

Also known as MG, a chronic neuromuscular disease that affects the voluntary muscles of the body. Myasthenia gravis is an autoimmune disease (a disease caused by the reaction of a person's immune system against his or her own tissues). In most cases, the cause is unknown. In older men, MG may be associated with tumors of the thymus (part of the immune system).

SYMPTOMS

Myasthenia gravis can affect anyone, but is most common in young adult women and older men. In this disease, the voluntary muscles become weak and tire easily. Chronic weakness improves with rest and worsens with activity. Certain muscles are involved more often than others. These include the muscles that control eye movement, chewing, coughing, swallowing, and facial expression. Muscles that control the arms and legs may also be affected. Shortness of breath occurs when the breathing muscles become weakened. Other symptoms include double vision, trouble swallowing, drooping head, poor posture, difficulty chewing, and problems with talking. Weakness and paralysis tend to worsen with exertion while muscle function improves with rest.

DIAGNOSIS AND TREATMENT

Diagnosis is based on symptoms and medical history. The doctor may also order tests such as an electromyogram (EMG),which is a special test to evaluate muscle strength, nerve conduction studies, and blood tests for abnormal antibodies.

There is no known cure for myasthenia gravis. However, long-term remission is possible. Treatments include anticholinesterase medications and plasmapheresis (a blood-cleansing technique). If symptoms are severe, prednisone, a type of corticosteroid, may be prescribed. Lifestyle modifications such as scheduled naps and stress avoidance are helpful. In some cases, surgical removal of the thymus

M

is recommended. Hospitalization may be required when muscle weakness affects breathing. Pregnant women who have myasthenia gravis require special supervision.

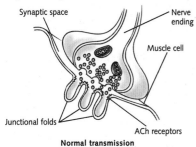

Normal transmission

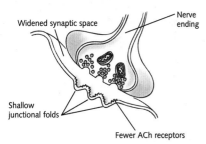

Myasthenia gravis

IMPAIRED NERVE AND MUSCLE SIGNALS
In a healthy person, nerve endings release a chemical called acetylcholine (ACh) into the space between the nerve and the muscle cell. ACh binds to a sufficient number of receptors on tiny folds on the muscle cells to cause the muscle to contract. In a person with myasthenia gravis, the body's immune system attacks the receptors, destroying them or impairing transmission.

Mycetoma

A localized infection of the tissues of the skin, muscles, and bone. Mycetoma appears as a swelling and distortion of the affected body part that progresses to an oozing abscess. Usually caused by fungi, it may be treated with antifungal medication, often in combination with surgery to remove the lesion. Treatment with KETOCONAZOLE over a long period of time has proven successful. Mycetoma is diagnosed by detecting the fungi via a microscopic examination of pus, secretions, or tissue taken from a lesion.

Mycology

The branch of biology that studies fungi. Mycology in medicine is the specialized study of fungi that are involved in causing disease in humans. These fungi are microorganisms that can be divided into two basic groups—yeasts and molds. Yeasts are formed of solitary cells that reproduce by budding. Molds grow in a threadlike form. Among the infections caused by fungi are various hair, nail, and skin diseases, as well as eye infections, mycetoma, candidiasis, blastomycosis, aspergillosis, sporotrichosis, and rhinosporidioisis.

Mycoplasma

A group of very small BACTERIA. Three types of *Mycoplasma* cause disease in humans. *Mycoplasma pneumoniae* is responsible for a mild type of bronchitis and pneumonia that is particularly common in adolescents and young adults. *Mycoplasma hominis* causes kidney disease, pelvic inflammatory disease, vaginal infections, and postpartum fever (after childbirth). *Ureaplasma urealyticum* infects the lower urinary tract, producing inflammation and a burning sensation upon urination. Mycoplasma infections are usually treated with antibiotics.

Mycosis

A system-wide fungal infection or disease. Mycosis infections may be caused by opportunistic fungi, particularly in people who are receiving corticosteroid therapy or immunosuppressant medications or in those with weakened immune systems, including AIDS (acquired immunodeficiency syndrome). In severely immunocompromised people, the infection can spread to the lungs, progressing rapidly to pneumonia. Other people who may be susceptible to mycosis include those with diabetes mellitus, emphysema, tuberculosis, lymphoma, or leukemia and people who have severe burns.

In people who are otherwise in good health, mycosis tends to be chronic, usually with mild symptoms, but sometimes produces fever, chills, night sweats, loss of appetite and weight, malaise, and psychological depression. When the fungus causing mycosis is inhaled into the lungs and spreads from there it can affect various organs of the body. The liver, spleen, and bone marrow may be involved; when the brain becomes involved, chronic meningitis develops; or a fungal disease called blastomycosis may produce one or more ulcers on the skin.

Blood tests can detect mycosis by isolating antibodies to the specific fungus involved. The causative fungus itself can be detect ed in samples of sputum, urine, blood, bone marrow, or infected tissues. Mycosis can be treated with systemic antifungal medications, including amphotericin B, flucytosine, fluconazole, and itraconazole. Surgery is sometimes necessary to remove sites of localized infection.

Mycosis fungoides

A rare cancer characterized by multiple scaly patches on the skin. Mycosis fungoides is a cancer of the T lymphocytes (a type of white blood cell) that affects the skin. Symptoms usually begin with generalized itching and the appearance of raised, reddened skin on any area of the body. The disease develops very slowly, and the raised patches on the skin may persist for years. A common treatment for mycosis fungoides is radiation therapy, although systemic chemotherapy and therapies designed to use the body's immune system to fight the cancer are also used. Individuals can be treated with a combination of ultraviolet (UV) light and medications that sensitize the cells to UV light.

Mydriasis

Widening of the pupil of the eye. Mydriasis may occur normally, as in dim light, or it may occur as a side effect of drug therapy. Mydriatic drugs, such as atropine, are deliberately used by ophthalmologists (eye doctors) to dilate the pupils of the eyes, so that the retina and optic disc can be examined more easily. Mydriatic drugs are also used to treat certain eye inflammations.

Myectomy

The surgical removal of all or a part of a muscle.

Myelin

The fatty substance covering and protecting nerves. Myelin is a layered tissue that surrounds nerve fibers, such as the axons. The sheath of myelin formed around the nerves speeds the transmission of electrical impulses along the nerve cells and acts as an electrical insulator.

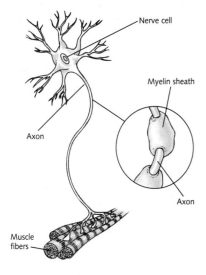

Nerve cell

Myelin sheath

Axon

Axon

Muscle fibers

INSULATING SHEATH
Myelin assists the function of a nerve cell by protecting and insulating the axon that carries the cell's electrical impulse. The so-called myelin sheath is composed of fatty cells surrounding the axon at intervals along its length. The myelin sheath speeds the conduction of the nerve impulse, which leaps across the intervals.

Myelitis

Inflammation of the spinal cord. Myelitis is often the result of a viral disease, such as polio, measles, or herpes. Transverse myelitis is a type of myelitis in which there is demyelination (loss of the fatty tissue around the nerves) of the spinal cord. It may be caused by viral infection, spinal cord injury, an immune reaction, or insufficient blood flow through the blood vessels in the spinal cord. Transverse myelitis may also occur as a complication of diseases, such as multiple sclerosis, smallpox, or chickenpox. Symptoms may include low back pain, spinal cord dysfunction, muscle spasms, discomfort, headache, loss of appetite, and numbness or tingling in the legs. Although there is no specific treatment for transverse myelitis, recovery usually begins within 2 to 12 weeks after its onset and may continue for up to 2 years. However, most people are left with considerable disability. Depending on the cause, the disabilities

include motor, sensory, and sphincter (bowel) deficits.

Myelocele

A developmental defect of the central nervous system in which a portion of the spinal cord protrudes through a congenital cleft in the vertebral column. See SPINA BIFIDA.

Myelodysplastic syndrome

A group of related, progressive disorders of the bone marrow characterized by low populations of abnormally developed blood cells. Since myelodysplastic syndrome precedes the development of acute leukemia in approximately one case in four, it is sometimes called preleukemia. This disease is most common in older people and rarely occurs in children and young adults.

The current understanding of this disease is that all blood cells (white, red, and platelets) develop from a single line of precursor cells, and this single line is abnormal. At about the time the abnormal cells are ready to enter the bloodstream, they self-destruct. Thus, the bone marrow is packed tight with abnormally developing blood cells, but the number of cells in the blood is unusually low. The cells that do appear in the bloodstream typically do not perform their functions as well as normal cells.

Exposure to radiation and benzene are known to increase the risk of developing myelodysplastic syndrome. In many cases, however, there is no clear-cut cause.

SYMPTOMS

All forms of myelodysplastic syndrome produce severe anemia (low number of red blood cells). Pallid skin, fatigue, and breathlessness after mild exertion are key symptoms. Leukopenia (low white blood cell count) increases susceptibility to infection, which often causes fever. The population of platelets, which have key roles in clotting the blood, is also low, leading to nosebleeds, unusually heavy bleeding after injury or surgery, or petechiae (small pinpoint hemorrhages under the skin). The spleen may also be slightly enlarged.

TYPES

Myelodysplastic syndrome is classified by the types of cells found in the

bone marrow and blood. In refractory anemia, the red blood cell count is low, and these red blood cells have the abnormal form known as blasts. The anemia is called refractory because it fails to respond to the usual treatments for anemia. If the red blood cells developing in the bone marrow contain rings of iron granules around the nucleus, the disease is known as refractory anemia with ringed sideroblasts. When refractory anemia occurs with higher than normal numbers of blasts in the bone marrow, it is called refractory anemia with excess blasts. If the number of bone marrow blasts is extremely high, the disease is classified as refractory anemia in transformation. The final type is known as chronic myelomonocytic leukemia, in which the number of blasts is not markedly increased, but the population of monocytes, a type of white blood cell, is greatly increased, and anemia is severe.

DIAGNOSIS, COURSE, AND TREATMENT

A significant number of cases are discovered before symptoms develop, usually as a result of routine blood tests during a medical examination. The diagnosis is confirmed by examination under a microscope of a small sample (biopsy) of bone marrow and bone.

Following diagnosis, myelodysplastic syndromes progress at different rates in different people. In some cases, the disease progresses only slowly, and treatment is not started until symptoms become pronounced. In other cases, the disease proceeds rapidly and quickly develops into acute leukemia.

The only cure for myelodysplastic syndrome is a bone marrow transplant (see BONE MARROW TRANSPLANT, ALLOGENEIC). Basically, abnormal bone marrow is destroyed by means of drugs and radiation, then replaced with bone marrow from a healthy donor. A bone marrow transplant is rigorous and difficult and is usually reserved for people who are younger than 50. Since myelodysplastic syndrome is unusual in younger persons, bone marrow transplant is not commonly used as a treatment.

In older people, treatment focuses on supportive therapy. Anemia can be treated with transfusions of red

M

blood cells, and platelet transfusions remedy bleeding. Treatment with corticosteroids and low doses of chemotherapy has proven successful in some cases. In younger people, myelodysplastic syndrome is treated in the same way as acute leukemia. See LEUKEMIA, ACUTE MYELOGENOUS for details.

Myelofibrosis with myeloid metaplasia

A disease in which normal bone marrow is replaced by scar tissue, and blood cell formation occurs outside the marrow. This disease is also known as agnogenic myeloid metaplasia, primary myelofibrosis, and idiopathic myelofibrosis. The word "myelofibrosis" indicates the presence of scar (fibro-) tissue in the bone marrow (myelo-), and the word "metaplasia" refers to blood cell formation in abnormal sites outside the bone marrow (also known as extramedullary hematopoiesis, or blood production outside the marrow). Most of this extramedullary blood cell formation occurs in the spleen and liver, and the spleen is usually enlarged. Myelofibrosis with myeloid metaplasia occurs primarily in middle-aged and older adults and rarely in children.

This disease causes anemia (an abnormally low red blood cell count), which leads to fatigue, weakness, pallid skin, and breathlessness after mild exertion. Enlargement of the spleen causes a feeling of fullness soon after eating, which in turn leads to decreased appetite and weight loss. Fever, lethargy, unusual bleeding and bruising, and night sweats are common symptoms.

Myelofibrosis with myeloid metaplasia is diagnosed with blood tests and a small sample (biopsy) of bone marrow and bone. The only cure for myelofibrosis with myeloid metaplasia is a bone marrow transplant (see BONE MARROW TRANSPLANT, ALLOGENEIC). Basically, abnormal bone marrow is destroyed by means of drugs and radiation, then replaced with bone marrow from a healthy donor. Bone marrow transplant is rigorous and difficult and is usually performed in people who are younger than 50.

Typically the disease progresses slowly after diagnosis; treatment depends on the severity of symptoms. Blood transfusions are used to combat anemia, and medications to stimulate red blood cell production, such as recombinant ERYTHROPOIETIN, may be prescribed. The spleen can be removed surgically (splenectomy) to relieve the symptoms an enlargement causes. Radiation and chemotherapy may also be used.

Without a bone marrow transplant, the disease invariably worsens over time, but often slowly, until death results from failure of the bone marrow. The average survival time is 5 years, although some people live as long as 20 years after diagnosis.

Myelography

X-ray examination of the spinal cord. In myelography, a dye or other contrast medium is injected into the space around the spine to clearly display the spinal cord on a series of X rays known as myelograms. Doctors perform myelography when more commonly used tests such as MRI (magnetic resonance imaging) and CT (computed tomography) scanning do not provide enough information to make a diagnosis of problems such as herniated disks.

Myeloma, multiple

See MULTIPLE MYELOMA.

Myelomeningocele

The most severe form of SPINA BIFIDA. In this developmental defect of the central nervous system, a portion of the spinal cord itself protrudes through the back. Tissues and nerves may be covered by skin or exposed. The term "myelomeningocele" is often used synonymously with spina bifida. This can be associated with a defect called Chiari malformation type II in which the base of the brain pushes down through the foramen magnum (the opening in the skull for the spinal cord).

Until recently, most children born with a myelomeningocele died shortly after birth. Today surgery is performed in the first 48 hours of life to drain spinal fluid and protect children against HYDROCEPHALUS, an accumulation of fluid in the brain. If hydrocephalus occurs, it is controlled by shunting (the implantation of a shunt or drain to relieve fluid buildup and prevent complications, such as brain damage, seizures, and blindness).

Myelopathy

Symptoms of spinal cord impairment from spinal cord disease. Types of myelopathy include syphilitic myelopathy (a form of NEUROSYPHILIS characterized by muscle weakness and abnormal sensations) and cervical spondylotic myelopathy (also known as CSM, a compression of the spinal cord in the neck).

SYPHILITIC MYELOPATHY

This is a rare form of neurosyphilis, which is a progressive, destructive, life-threatening infection of the brain and spinal cord that occurs in some cases of untreated SYPHILIS. Neurosyphilis, a complication that develops many years after primary infection, occurs more frequently in men than in women. Syphilitic myelopathy causes a progressive degeneration of the spinal cord and peripheral nerve tissue. There is increasing weakness of the arms and legs that may eventually lead to paralysis. Loss of coordination contributes to problems with walking.

Diagnosis of neurosyphilis is made with blood tests, such as a VDRL (Venereal Disease Research Laboratory) test or a rapid plasma reagin test, a cerebrospinal fluid VDRL test, lumbar puncture, CT (computed tomography) scanning or MRI (magnetic resonance imaging), and a cerebral angiogram. Treatment is with antibiotics such as penicillin. Follow-up blood tests are required to make certain that the infection has been eradicated. Although treatment can reduce progression of the disorder and reduce new nerve damage, it cannot cure existing damage.

CERVICAL SPONDYLOTIC MYELOPATHY

Compression of the spinal cord in the neck affects primarily older adults. Symptoms develop slowly and may include stiffness, numbness, pain, and weakness. Cervical spondylotic myelopathy causes problems with walking. Diagnosis is made through physical examination and tests such as MRI. Treatment of mild cases is with neck braces or traction; more serious cases may require surgery.

Myelopathy can also be caused by multiple sclerosis, transverse myelitis, spinal cord ischemia (loss of blood flow), or a tumor. When patients have symptoms of myelopathy, tests including MRI of the spinal cord, myelogram, and lumbar puncture should be performed.

Myeloproliferative disorders

A group of related and highly similar diseases that involve abnormally high production of certain kinds of blood cells because of malfunction of the bone marrow. The myeloproliferative diseases differ from one another in the primary type of blood cell affected. In some cases, one of the diseases changes into another as it progresses, an event that points to the close relationship among them. The myeloproliferative disorders primarily affect people older than 50, but can occur in younger people.

Normal bone marrow contains cells, known as hematopoietic cells or stem cells, that have the ability to reproduce themselves into what is known as a clone. Each clone can produce different cell lines that develop into red blood cells, several kinds of white blood cells, and platelets (cells that have key roles in blood clotting). In normal bone marrow, a number of clones are active in producing normal blood cells in normal proportions. In the myeloproliferative disorders, an abnormal clone takes over from the others, producing blood cells of one type that are essentially normal yet far too abundant, while the number of other blood cell types may be too low. Differences in the pattern of overproduction and underproduction distinguish one myeloproliferative disease from another.

All of the myeloproliferative disorders are diagnosed by means of blood tests to count the numbers of different types of blood cells and examination under a microscope of a small sample (biopsy) of bone and bone marrow.

POLYCYTHEMIA VERA

The distinguishing characteristic of polycythemia vera is an abnormally high number of red blood cells. In most cases, the numbers of granulocytes, which are a type of white blood cell, and platelets, which have key roles in blood clotting, are also too

high. The added mass of blood cells causes the blood to be thicker and stickier than normal and increases the blood volume. In a sense, a person with polycythemia vera has too much blood. Symptoms include headache, ringing in the ears, vertigo, blurred vision, hypertension (high blood pressure), nosebleeds, abnormally heavy menstrual periods in women, pain in the upper digestive system, gout, difficulty concentrating, inflamed veins because of blood clots (THROMBOPHLEBITIS, which principally affects the legs), numbness or tingling in the hands or feet, and enlargement of the spleen and liver. Polycythemia vera usually develops slowly and insidiously and is often present for 1 or 2 years before it is diagnosed.

The primary treatment for polycythemia vera is periodic removal (phlebotomy) of a limited amount blood. Phlebotomy reduces the volume of the blood and lowers the red blood cell count. Phlebotomy is repeated as often as needed to maintain a blood profile as close to normal as possible. The procedure is safe and usually produces few if any side effects. Drugs that suppress the bone marrow and slow blood cell production, such as hydroxyurea and INTERFERONS, are often used as well.

In many cases, these treatments are sufficient, and the person lives a normal life. In some people, however, the disease becomes more severe, entering what is known as the spent phase, when the bone marrow becomes heavily scarred and blood cell production falters and fails. If this occurs, a bone marrow transplant (see BONE MARROW TRANSPLANT, ALLOGENEIC) is a possible treatment. Basically, abnormal bone marrow is destroyed by means of drugs and radiation, then replaced with bone marrow from a healthy donor. Bone marrow transplant is rigorous and difficult and is therefore usually reserved to treat people younger than 50.

CHRONIC MYELOID LEUKEMIA

A myeloproliferative disease characterized by an abnormal increase in white blood cells. This disease is also known as chronic myelocytic leukemia, chronic myelogenous leukemia, and chronic granulocytic

leukemia. Chronic myeloid leukemia (see LEUKEMIA, CHRONIC MYELOID) is a progressive disease that can occur at any age but is most common among the middle-aged. It tends to remain in a long-lasting (chronic) phase that may extend for several years, followed by a sudden worsening known as a blast crisis, when the number of immature white blood cells (blasts) increases extremely rapidly. The blast crisis is very difficult to treat and usually results in death.

ESSENTIAL THROMBOCYTOSIS

An excessively high number of platelets is the identifying characteristic of this myeloproliferative disease. The disease is called essential because it appears on its own and not as a complication of another condition, such as surgical removal of the spleen (splenectomy) or some chronic infections. Because of their abnormally high number, the platelets tend to clump together in the blood. The result is both unusual bleeding, such as from the nose, gums, and digestive tract, and blood clots that can block blood vessels, causing blood clots in the legs, heart attack, or stroke. Other symptoms include visual disturbances, fatigue, heavy menstrual periods in women, enlargement of the liver and the spleen, numbness or tingling, skin itching, and ringing in the ears.

Medication is the primary treatment. Aspirin is used to lower the risk of clotting, while hydroxyurea and interferons suppress the bone marrow and reduce the number of platelets. Unless essential thrombocytosis progresses to acute leukemia, prospects for long-term survival are good with consistent monitoring and treatment.

MYELOFIBROSIS WITH MYELOID METAPLASIA

In this myeloproliferative disorder, the normal bone marrow is replaced by scar tissue, and blood cell formation occurs outside the marrow. MYELOFIBROSIS WITH MYELOID METAPLASIA is also known as agnogenic myeloid metaplasia, primary myelofibrosis, and idiopathic myelofibrosis.

M

Terms in small capital letters—for example, PHYSICAL THERAPY or PAGET DISEASE—indicate a cross-reference to another entry with more information.

The word "myelofibrosis" indicates the presence of scar (fibro-) tissue in the bone marrow (myelo-), and the word "metaplasia" refers to blood cell formation in abnormal sites outside the bone marrow (also known as extramedullary hematopoiesis, or blood production outside the marrow). Most of the extramedullary blood cell formation occurs in the spleen and liver; the spleen is usually enlarged. Myelofibrosis with myeloid metaplasia occurs primarily in middle-aged and older adults and rarely in children.

Myiasis

An infestation of living human tissue or organs by maggots, which are flies in an immature stage. Myiasis may be caused by the larvae of several different species of flies, called myiatic flies. Most of these flies exist in regions including central and tropical Africa, Central America, and South America. In most cases, the larvae of the flies penetrate the skin either when direct contact is made with infested soil or when an insect carrier, such as a mosquito, transmits the larvae by biting a person. Some females of a certain species of flies deposit eggs on the edges of a person's open wounds or sores and on healthy mucous membranes, such as those in the mouth or nose. Generally, the larvae feed on the host, mature to the next stage, and drop off.

Myiasis is not known to exist in the United States, but myiatic flies have been found in countries such as Australia where they have not been previously known to exist. It is believed that the flies may become more common with the increase in travel to Africa and Central and South America. Travelers may become infested with the larvae of myiatic flies and retain the infestation in deeper layers of the skin without awareness of it. By this means, the larvae can be carried into new regions of the world.

Myiasis begins with itchy sores that progress to form painful, oozing, boillike lesions, which are indications of the maggot's growth cycle. This maturation phase may be prolonged, and if the infestation is widespread, new lesions may appear intermittently. They are sometimes treated by applying petroleum jelly to the surface of the skin to cut off the maggot's air supply. This forces them to the skin's surface, where a portion of their bodies can be observed and they may be extracted. Maggots may also be removed with the use of a local anesthetic and surgical incision.

Myocardial infarction

The medical term for HEART ATTACK.

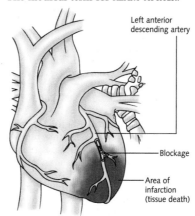

Left anterior descending artery

Blockage

Area of infarction (tissue death)

BLOCKING BLOOD AND OXYGEN
In a person having a heart attack (myocardial infarction), a blockage in one of the coronary arteries cuts off the flow of blood and oxygen to part of the heart muscle, and the tissue dies. Usually, the first symptom is chest pain that may radiate to the jaw, neck, back, or left arm. Immediate medical help is essential.

Myocarditis

Inflammation of the myocardium (the heart muscle). Myocarditis is uncommon and usually causes few or no symptoms, with recovery in several weeks. In a small percentage of cases, symptoms are severe enough to require hospitalization and treatment for heart failure and other complications, such as cardiac arrhythmia (irregular heart rhythm), cardiomyopathy (impaired heart muscle function), pulmonary embolism (a blood clot that can lodge in the lungs), or stroke. The disease is most common among middle-aged men, but can affect both sexes at any age.

Myocarditis is most often caused by common viruses, such as the COX-SACKIEVIRUS or the EPSTEIN-BARR VIRUS. It can also be caused by HIV (human immunodeficiency virus) and the viruses that cause influenza, hepati-tis, and the mumps. Other causes include autoimmune disorders (diseases in which the body is attacked by its own immune system), certain insect bites (such as those leading to CHAGAS DISEASE and LYME DISEASE), bacterial infections (for example, tuberculosis and bacterial endocardi-tis), illegal drug and excessive alcohol use, and exposure to radiation.

Mild myocarditis produces no symptoms. More severe cases produce symptoms similar to those brought on by influenza: fever, weakness, muscle aches, headache, or chest pain. People with myocarditis may develop the symptoms of congestive heart failure, which include shortness of breath, swelling in the legs, swollen neck veins, abdominal discomfort, mental confusion, and palpitations (uncomfortably rapid heartbeat).

In the absence of serious symptoms, myocarditis is treated with an anti-inflammatory medication, and persons with the disease are advised to rest for several days and to avoid alcohol, salt, and exercise. If symptoms are severe, treatment may include hospitalization and a variety of medications to stabilize the heart, reduce fluid accumulation in the lungs and legs, and prevent the formation of blood clots. Any underlying cause, such as Lyme disease, also must be treated.

Myoclonus

A spasm of a muscle or group of muscles. In EPILEPSY (a brain disorder in which clusters of nerve cells in the brain sometimes signal abnormally), myoclonic seizures cause twitches or jerks of the arms, legs, or upper body. In most people, seizures are controlled with antiepileptic drugs such as carbamazepine, valproate, and phenytoin.

Myofascial pain disorder

A group of conditions causing pain in or near the joint (called the temporomandibular joint, or TMJ) that connects the lower jaw to the skull and in the muscles that control chewing. Sometimes called temporomandibular joint disorder (TMD), myofascial pain disorder typically produces pain in the muscles and joints of the jaw, as well as in the bony region in front of the ear. Movement of the jaw may become partially or completely locked. The pain may become more severe when the jaw moves, and clicking or popping sounds may accompany movement of the jaw. Sometimes these noises occur without pain. The pain in the area of the jaw may spread to the shoulder and neck muscles and, in rare cases, may cause disturbances of vision and balance. Another symptom of the disorder is a sudden, noticeable change in the bite, or fit of the upper and lower teeth.

The causes of myofascial pain disorder are similar to causes of muscular pain elsewhere in the body. Severe injury to the jaw or the jaw joint can fracture the bones, disrupt the smooth movement of the lower jaw, and produce pain or locking. Other causes include grinding of the teeth (called bruxism) and arthritis. Stress is associated with the disorder, as it is with back pain, muscle tension headache, muscular neck pain, and other muscular pain problems.

TREATMENT

Periodic discomfort in the jaw joint and surrounding muscles is quite common and rarely serious. Usually it is temporary or sometimes occurs in cycles. In most cases, the pain disappears without treatment. However, people who have debilitating, ongoing symptoms should consult a doctor or dentist. Possible treatment options generally include the short-term use of muscle-relaxant, anti-inflammatory medications or antidepressants, which can help relieve muscular pain. The person with myofascial pain may also benefit from exercises to help relax the muscles of the jaw and from removable bite plate devices that can be fitted by a dentist. These devices cover the chewing surfaces of the upper teeth to reduce pressure on the jaw and discourage grinding or clenching of the teeth. Bite plates are usually worn at night. Rarely, surgery is recommended.

Self-help techniques for people with myofascial pain disorder include avoiding crunchy or chewy foods, alternately applying heat and ice packs, avoiding chewing gum, and not opening the mouth too wide when yawning or singing.

Myoglobin

A protein found in muscle cells containing iron. Myoglobin takes oxygen from the blood and releases it to muscles during strenuous exercise, where it generates energy by burning the blood sugar (glucose). Myoglobin closely resembles HEMOGLOBIN, a protein found in red blood cells. Too much myoglobin in the blood can cause kidney damage.

Myoma

See FIBROID, UTERINE.

Myomectomy

A surgical procedure for removing uterine fibroids (also called myomas). In this procedure, only the fibroids are removed, leaving the remaining uterus intact. A myomectomy is preferred to a HYSTERECTOMY when a woman wants to be able to have children, although it can be performed on women of any age (see FIBROID, UTERINE).

A myomectomy involves an incision into the abdomen, exposing the uterus. Fibroids on the surface of the uterus are cut off, while fibroids inside the uterus are removed after the surgeon cuts into the uterus. Some fibroids can be destroyed with LASER SURGERY performed through a HYSTEROSCOPY.

The procedure carries a risk of bleeding, and it can lead to the development of scars on the uterus that can cause pain or interfere with a woman's ability to bear children. Women who have had myomectomies are more likely to require delivery by CESAREAN SECTION if they become pregnant. Fibroids recur in about 20 percent of women who have undergone myomectomy.

Myopathy

Any primary disease or disorder of the muscle tissue, including FIBROMYALGIA, MUSCULAR DYSTROPHY, and MYOSITIS.

Myopia

See NEARSIGHTEDNESS.

Myositis

Inflammation of muscle.

Myositis ossificans

Abnormal bone formation in a muscle usually located near the elbow joint. It usually occurs from muscle damage or as a complication of a fracture. It can also be a common complication of thigh muscle injuries from activities such as soccer, wrestling, and football. Overaggressive rehabilitation may be a secondary cause. Proper rehabilitation with active range-of-motion exercises may be recommended to prevent this disorder. Treatment may include taking nonsteroidal anti-inflammatory drugs (NSAIDs), such as aspirin or ibuprofen, with a gradual return to range-of-motion exercises. Surgery is usually not considered unless conservative therapy fails to improve symptoms within 6 months.

Myotonia

A disorder of abnormally prolonged contractions of a muscle or group of muscles. For example, an affected person may have difficulty relaxing muscles after contracting them to grip an object. Myotonia is a symptom of disorders such as myotonic MUSCULAR DYSTROPHY.

Myringitis, bullous

An inflammation of the eardrum that produces small water or blood blisters on the eardrum and sudden, severe pain in the ear. There may be a yellowish or bloody discharge if the blisters rupture. Bullous myringitis is sometimes mistaken for a ruptured eardrum (see EARDRUM, PERFORATED). Also called infectious myringitis, the inflammation may be bacterial or viral. In many cases, the symptoms follow an infection of the respiratory tract, accompanied by a dry, nonproductive cough that is more severe at night. Bullous myringitis is generally treated with oral antibiotic medication or ear drops containing one of the CORTICOSTEROIDS and antibiotics. The goal of treatment is to prevent infection of the blisters as they break open. Painkillers may also be prescribed to treat severe discomfort. Although bullous myringitis can be extremely painful, it is not considered serious, and the eardrum usually heals within a week or two with proper treatment.

Myringoplasty

A surgical procedure to reconstruct a perforation in the eardrum's membrane when there is no middle ear

M

infection or disease of the ear bones. (Myringoplasty is similar to TYM-PANOPLASTY but is confined to repair of the eardrum.) The procedure seals the middle ear and usually improves hearing. The surgery is performed under local anesthesia through the ear canal. Tissue grafts from other parts of the ear may be used to close the perforation. Myringoplasty is usually performed on an outpatient basis. A person who has had the operation may return to normal activities within a week. Healing and a noticeable improvement in hearing generally occur within 6 weeks.

Myringotomy

A surgical procedure involving an incision into the eardrum to promote drainage of fluid from the middle ear to improve hearing and relieve pain. The eustachian tube acts as the drainage passage from the middle ear, and maintains hearing by opening to regulate air passage. Myringotomy is generally performed on children who have an accumulation of fluid in the middle ear, called middle ear effusion, which causes pain and impairs hearing. The fluid buildup in the middle ear is often caused by OTITIS MEDIA (inflammation of the middle ear). It may also be caused by a common cold (see COLD, COMMON), allergies, or a RESPIRATORY TRACT INFECTION. The buildup of pus and mucus puts pressure on the eardrum, causing pain, swelling, and redness. Because the eardrum does not vibrate properly, hearing is impaired. In some cases, the eardrum may rupture as a result of the pressure against it (see EARDRUM, PERFORATED).

THE PROCEDURE

A surgical procedure called myringotomy and tubes is the most commonly performed ear operation when antibiotic and decongestant treatment has not improved the condition. The procedure is safe and effective.

If myringotomy alone is performed, the incision made in the eardrum is likely to heal and close before the infection is gone and the fluid has drained. To prevent this, the surgeon usually inserts a tube, called a ventilation tube, into the middle ear. This tube will usually remain in place for the length of time necessary for the middle ear infection to clear and drain. The length of time varies from several weeks to several months, but is typically 7 to 9 months. In some cases, the tube may remain for years. Precautions must be taken while the tube is in place to prevent water from entering the ear, which can cause infection. Draining fluid from the middle ear improves hearing and relieves pain immediately. The incision usually heals within a few days, and there is rarely scarring or injury to the eardrum. Possible complications of the procedure are simple infections that are readily treated with antibiotics.

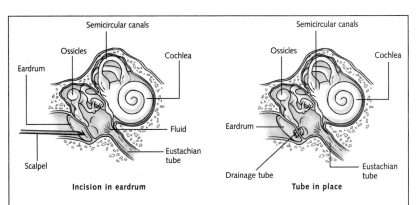

SURGERY FOR EAR INFECTIONS
The most common surgical procedure to correct middle ear infection (often caused by otitis media) is called myringotomy. First, a surgeon makes an incision in the eardrum to drain the excess fluid (pus) that has built up in the middle ear. Because the incision might heal before the drainage is complete, the surgeon usually inserts a tube through the eardrum to allow the fluid to drain until the infection is gone. The tubes can remain in place for several weeks or months.

Myxedema

A condition characterized by dry, puffy skin and swelling around the lips and nose. It is a feature of the most severe type of HYPOTHYROIDISM (a slowing of metabolism due to decreased activity of the thyroid gland). Other symptoms include intolerance of the cold, hair loss, decreased energy, hoarseness, muscle aches, constipation, weight gain, and memory loss. Left untreated, myxedema can lead to coma and death. Myxedema is diagnosed with thyroid function blood tests. Synthetic thyroid hormones are used to treat myxedema.

Myxoma

A noncancerous tumor occurring in soft tissue, such as muscles and ligaments. Myxoma is a jellylike tumor that usually develops under the skin. The uncommon tumors may also appear in the jaw bones or within muscles. Myxomas can grow very large.

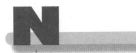

Nabumetone

See NONSTEROIDAL ANTI-INFLAMMATORY DRUGS.

Nafarelin acetate

A hormone similar to one released from the hypothalamus. Nafarelin acetate (Synarel) is used to treat endometriosis, a disease in which the tissue that forms the uterine lining in women grows outside the uterus, and premature puberty in both boys and girls. Nafarelin acetate works by decreasing the amount of estrogen and testosterone in the blood. It is available only as a nasal spray.

Nail

The hard, protective shield of protein on the top of each finger and toe tip. The protein of which the nail is composed is called keratin, the same substance that makes up hair and the outer portion of the skin. Like hair, the visible portion of the nail is dead, but it grows from a living nail root that extends back into a groove in the skin. The whitish, crescent-shaped area at the base of the nail is called the lunula. The cuticle, a piece of skin that lies just in front of the nail root, helps protect the new, emerging keratin cells. The nail protects the end of the finger or toe, and it also registers certain types of pressure involved in the sense of touch.

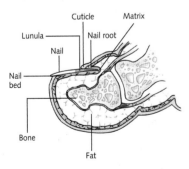

ANATOMY OF A NAIL
The nail matrix is the structure that produces the nail plate. The whitish lunula under the nail is the visible part of the matrix. The nail bed, which is visible as the pink part of the tissue under the nail, is rich in blood vessels and is grooved to fit tightly to the nail plate.

Naloxone

An antinarcotic drug. Naloxone (Narcan) is used to counteract the effects of narcotic-induced impaired breathing, sedation, and lowered blood pressure, whether caused by narcotics or methadone, a narcotic painkiller (often used to treat heroin addiction). Naloxone is also used to diagnose addiction to opiates such as heroin; it is given to a person suspected of being addicted to a drug to see whether the individual experiences withdrawal symptoms.

Naltrexone hydrochloride

An antinarcotic drug. Naltrexone hydrochloride (Trexan, ReVia) is used to help a person addicted to a narcotic or alcohol stay substance-free. Naltrexone works by blocking the effects of narcotics, particularly the enjoyable "high" associated with drug and alcohol use.

Naprapathy

A system of gentle therapeutic manipulations of the skeletal system, the ligaments, muscles, and other connective tissues; a form of APPLIED KINESIOLOGY. Naprapathy is based on the idea that many ailments and the pain associated with them are caused by a misalignment of the skeletal system. Naprapathic therapy focuses on areas of the body that have become stiff from tension, stress, bad posture, overwork, poor diet, and other environmental factors. The goal of naprapathic therapy is to restore energy and improve the circulatory system throughout the body, thereby aiming for a state of perfect health.

Naprapathy uses "stretchments," gentle but specific therapeutic manipulations of the ligaments, muscles, and other connective tissues to reduce pain and improve structural alignment. A naprapath may also teach relaxation techniques and train people in techniques to expand their range of motion. Nutritional counseling, exercise, and biofeedback are all part of naprapathic therapy as well.

Conditions that respond well to naprapathy include pain of the back, neck, hip, and joints; tension headaches; and digestive or menstrual disorders that have failed to respond to conventional medical treatment.

Naproxen

See NONSTEROIDAL ANTI-INFLAMMATORY DRUGS.

Narcissism

A personality pattern characterized by self-centeredness, grandiosity, a need for admiration, and a lack of empathy. In its extreme form, narcissism becomes a mental illness known as narcissistic personality disorder. Narcissistic individuals have a grandiosely inflated sense of their own importance and engage in fantasies of unlimited success, power, or beauty. They consider themselves superior and expect others to recognize them as such, demand excessive admiration, take advantage of or exploit others, and lack concern for the feelings or concerns of people around them. Often envious or believing themselves the objects of envy, narcissists behave in ways that are snobbish, arrogant, or patronizing. Narcissism may be a defense mechanism against vulnerability and low self-esteem. This personality pattern is named after Narcissus, a figure from classical mythology who fell in love with his own image reflected in a pool of water.

Narcolepsy

A disabling neurological sleep disorder characterized by overwhelming daytime drowsiness and sudden collapses into sleep. (See also SLEEP DISORDERS.) Narcolepsy is related to REM (rapid eye movement) sleep, the dreaming state of sleep. While its exact cause remains unknown, scientists have discovered that the brains of people with narcolepsy have dramatically fewer neurons containing a substance called hypocretin than the brains of people who do not have this disorder. Narcolepsy also seems to have a hereditary or genetic component.

SYMPTOMS

Symptoms generally develop after age 15. Narcolepsy has four classic symptoms: excessive daytime sleepiness, CATAPLEXY (sudden loss of voluntary muscle control), sleep paralysis, and hallucinations. Excessive daytime sleepiness, the primary characteristic of narcolepsy, is an overwhelming drowsiness and need to sleep during the day. Throughout the day, regardless of what he or she

N

is doing, an affected person may experience irresistible sleep attacks that last from 30 seconds to more than 30 minutes. Cataplexy, the second most common symptom, may cause a number of physical changes, ranging from slurred speech to total physical collapse. Sleep paralysis is a temporary inability to move or speak while sleeping or upon waking up. Hallucinations that occur as the person falls asleep are vivid, realistic, and sometimes frightening dreams.

DIAGNOSIS AND TREATMENT

Although early diagnosis and treatment are important, narcolepsy is often misdiagnosed. Diagnosis is made according to medical history and with tests such as an overnight polysomnogram (PSG) and the multiple sleep latency test (MSLT). These may be performed at a sleep center. In a PSG, various physiological functions are recorded while the person sleeps to evaluate sleep stages. An MSLT is a nap test in which people being tested are evaluated to see how quickly and deeply they fall asleep when given an opportunity to nap. Other possible tests include an ELEC-TROENCEPHALOGRAM (EEG).

There is no cure for narcolepsy. However, symptoms can be controlled through medications and lifestyle changes. The goal of treatment is to keep a person alert during the day and to minimize occurrences of cataplexy. Amphetamines and other stimulants have traditionally been used to treat excessive daytime sleepiness. However, these cause side effects and can be addictive. Today the new nonamphetamine drug modafinil is available to promote wakefulness. Antidepressants are prescribed to treat cataplexy. Proper diet, exercise, and short naps during the day are also helpful measures.

Narcotics

Analgesics (painkillers); sleep-inducing drugs. Narcotics act on the central nervous system to relieve pain. Doctors prescribe narcotics to help anesthetics work more effectively both before and during surgical operations. Other medical uses of narcotics are to relieve coughing and to control dependence on heroin and other drugs. Narcotics (opioids), such as heroin, are easily abused. No matter what the reason for their use, any

narcotics used for a long time can potentially cause physical and psychological dependence. Physical dependence can cause symptoms of withdrawal when the narcotic is stopped. Narcotics can impair the ability to drive.

CATEGORIES OF NARCOTICS USED IN MEDICINE

There are six types of narcotic drugs currently prescribed for medical purposes in the United States.

■ *Analgesic narcotics* Narcotics are used to relieve pain. They include buprenorphine (Buprenex), used for moderate to severe pain; butorphanol (Stadol), used for moderate to severe pain, including obstetric pain; codeine, used for mild to moderate pain and for cough suppression; hydromorphone (Dilaudid), used for moderate to severe pain; meperidine (Demerol), used for moderate to severe pain, including obstetric pain; methadone, used for severe, chronic pain and opiate addiction; morphine (Astramorph, Duramorph, Roxanol), used for severe pain; nalbuphine (Nubain), used for moderate to severe pain; oxymorphone (Numorphan), used for moderate to severe pain; pentazocine (Talwin), used for moderate to severe pain; and propoxyphene (Darvon), used for mild to moderate pain.

■ *Anesthesia aids* Narcotics are used to help anesthetics work more effectively. They include buprenorphine; butorphanol; meperidine; morphine; nalbuphine; oxycodone (Percodan); oxymorphone; and pentazocine.

■ *Antidiarrhea* Narcotics are sometimes used to treat diarrhea. Examples include codeine and morphine.

■ *Antitussive (cough relievers)* Narcotics are used as cough relievers; an example is codeine.

■ *Pulmonary edema therapy* Morphine is sometimes used to assist in the treatment of pulmonary edema (excess fluid in the lungs).

■ *Suppression of heroin dependence* Methadone is used to prevent symptoms of heroin withdrawal and to block the euphoric effects of heroin.

NARCOTICS USED FOR ILLICIT PURPOSES

The most widely used narcotic on the illegal market is the opioid heroin: 90 percent of all street drug narcotic abuse involves heroin. Other opiates that are abused include morphine,

codeine, and methadone. Narcotics are most often taken by injection, though they can be smoked in pipes or inhaled through the nose. Codeine, in the form of liquid cold medicines, is usually taken orally.

The short-term effects of narcotics include euphoria, drowsiness, loss of pain sensation, nausea, and constipation. Long-term effects include the loss of resistance to disease and infection, inflammation of veins, bronchial congestion, hepatitis, blood infection, and skin abscesses. Tolerance to narcotics develops faster than tolerance to almost any other drug. People typically feel cravings for heroin as soon as they come down from the narcotic-induced high. Withdrawal symptoms can start as soon as 12 hours after the narcotic is injected and can include shaking, vomiting, diarrhea, aches, chills, cramping, and stomach problems.

Nasal congestion

A symptom of the common cold or allergies produced by dilated, or expanded, blood vessels in the membranes of the nose and an increase and thickening of mucus in the nose. Nasal congestion, sometimes described as a stuffy nose or RHINITIS, narrows the air passages of the nose and respiratory system, making it difficult to breathe easily. Over-the-counter decongestants may help relieve the discomfort. If nasal congestion constantly recurs, a physician should be consulted. Also, tobacco smoke may be a cause of recurring nasal congestion in children. See also COLD, COMMON; COLD REMEDIES.

Nasal discharge
See RHINITIS.

Nasal obstruction
See RHINITIS.

Nasal polyps

Small saclike growths on the mucous membrane lining the inside of the nostrils. Nasal polyps protrude into the nasal cavity, appearing singly or in clusters, and are pearly gray. The polyps originate near the sinuses at the top of the nose and grow into the open areas of the nasal cavity. They are not true polyps because the growth is not new or abnormal tissue, but rather swollen tissue inside the nose. One-sided nasal polyps tend to be nonmalignant, while bilateral (two-sided) polyps may be malignant.

SYMPTOMS

The symptoms of nasal polyps include difficulty breathing, an impaired sense of smell and taste, and a runny nose. The nasal passages tend to feel blocked and never seem to clear completely. When polyps block the opening between the nasal cavity and one of sinuses, the condition may cause headaches, a feeling of pressure in the cheeks, and facial pain. Large polyps can obstruct the airways. Children who have nasal polyps sound congested and may have to breathe through the mouth. Nasal polyps can cause recurrent sinus infections. While antihistamines and decongestants may help prevent nasal polyps by keeping the nasal passages dry and clear, these medications will not relieve the symptoms when nasal polyps are already established.

CAUSES

Polyps are a consequence of chronic inflammation of the nasal lining. This inflammation may be related to asthma, hay fever, or other nasal allergies, but the specific cause may not be identifiable. Chronic sinus infections and, sometimes, CYSTIC FIBROSIS (a genetic disorder including persistent lung infections) can be associated with nasal polyps, especially in children. At times, the polyps occur following an infection of the respiratory tract or a common cold and may shrink and disappear by themselves as the infection clears.

TREATMENT

The doctor may look for polyps using a nasal speculum (tonglike instrument) to examine the inside of the nose. A CT (computed tomography) scan will always show increased density in the sinuses when polyps are present. Polyps will usually respond to one of the CORTICOSTEROIDS, which may be prescribed in the form of long-term nasal sprays or oral medication. Corticosteroid drugs may also be given by injection. Corticosteroid treatment usually shrinks the polyps and relieves symptoms.

When nasal polyps do not respond to medication, surgery becomes an option. The physician may make a referral to a specialist for surgery performed with an endoscope (lighted viewing instrument), usually performed in an outpatient operating room under local anesthesia. Sinus surgery may be indicated if polyps recur quickly after being removed. The polyp tissue is sent to a pathologist for examination under a microscope to rule out a malignant tumor, which is rare with nasal polyps. Polyps may recur, and additional surgery may be needed.

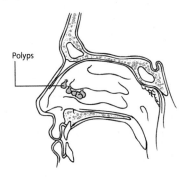

POLYPS IN THE NOSE
Nasal polyps are small growths, actually areas of swollen tissue, on the mucous membrane lining the inside of the nose. They can occur singly or in clusters, and they usually start at the top of the nose and grow down into the nasal cavity. They usually cause difficulty breathing, diminished senses of smell and taste, and a runny nose. The polyps are almost always noncancerous. Medication taken orally, in the form of a spray, or by injection usually shrinks the polyps enough to relieve the symptoms.

Nasal turbinates

Thin bone projections that subdivide each nasal cavity into a series of groovelike passageways and curve from the outer part of the nose in toward the septum (cartilage wall between the nostrils). The turbinates are covered by thick mucous membranes. Under the membrane, sensitive, spongy, erectile tissue causes the tissues in the area to fill with blood and swell when exposed to cold, dry, or contaminated air. This swelling narrows the nasal passages and slows the air coming in so that it can be warmed and humidified by MUCUS as the air is breathed in. The mucus also serves to trap dust particles. When the tissues lining the turbinates are exposed to cold air, mucus production increases, which results in a runny nose in cold weather.

NASH

See NONALCOHOLIC STEATOHEPATITIS.

Nasogastric tube

A thin, flexible, plastic tube that is passed through the nose down into the stomach. Its purpose is to provide a pathway for nourishment or to drain away secretions. Doctors may insert a nasogastric tube in cases such as a GASTRECTOMY, surgical removal of all or part of the stomach; intestinal PERFORATION, a hole or erosion most often caused by a peptic ulcer; or PYLORIC STENOSIS, partial or complete blockage of the outlet from the stomach to the duodenum.

Nasopharynx

The area connecting the nasal passages with the part of the pharynx (throat) that lies above the soft palate in the back of the mouth. The nasopharynx is part of the respiratory tract through which air passes into the lungs. When a person swallows, the soft palate moves back against the top of the throat to seal off the nasopharynx so that food does not enter it.

The eustachian tubes, which lead from the nose into the middle ear, open into the nasopharynx. In children, the adenoids (part of the immune system) are in the nasopharynx. As a child grows, the adenoids gradually shrink and generally disappear by puberty. See RESPIRATORY SYSTEM.

Nasopharynx, cancer of

A disease in which malignant cells are found in the tissues of the nasopharynx, which is the passage connecting the cavity behind the nose to the upper part of the throat. The airway passages in the nose lead into the nasopharynx, and two openings on the sides of the nasopharynx lead into the ears. The cause of this cancer is unknown. It occurs most commonly among people who are heavy cigarette smokers and is quite common in southern China. Cancer of the nasopharynx usually occurs after the age of 50 and is more common in men than in women. The principal known risk factor for this cancer is infection by the Epstein-Barr virus (a herpesvirus that causes mononucleosis; see VIRUSES).

N

SYMPTOMS AND DIAGNOSIS

There may be no symptoms, or they may be similar to the symptoms of the common cold, infections of the respiratory tract, or infections caused by other viruses. If these symptoms linger for 2 weeks or more, a physician should be consulted. Symptoms that may appear as the cancer progresses include difficulty with breathing or speaking, frequent headaches, a lump in the nose or neck, pain or ringing in the ear, recurrent blood in the saliva or nasal secretions, and impaired hearing. The doctor will examine the nose and throat using special equipment, possibly including a nasoscope (viewing instrument inserted into the nose). The neck may be examined for lumps. Diagnostic imaging procedures may be requested. A biopsy (a procedure to obtain cell samples for examination under a microscope) may also be required if abnormal tissue is suspected or detected. If cancer cells are found, more tests will be performed to determine whether the cancer has spread to other parts of the body.

TREATMENT

Cancer of the nasopharynx, also called nasopharyngeal cancer, is most effectively treated when diagnosed and treated in its early stages. There are four stages of nasopharyngeal cancer, based on the progress of the disease and the number of structures of the nasopharynx involved. The determination of the cancer's stage enables the physician to plan a course of treatment. Possible treatments for cancer of the nasopharynx include radiation therapy; surgery; chemotherapy; and participation in a clinical trial, possibly using biological therapy or immunotherapy (use of the body's immune system to fight the cancer). Radiation therapy to the site of the cancer and the lymph nodes in the neck is the most common treatment for cancer of the nasopharynx. If the cancer does not respond, surgery may be required. When large parts of the nasopharynx are removed, reconstructive surgery may be necessary. Chemotherapy may be combined with radiation therapy or surgery. Chances of recovery depend on the location of the cancer in the nasopharynx structure, the progress or stage of the cancer, and the person's age and general health.

National Institute of Occupational Safety and Health (NIOSH)

The federal agency responsible for conducting research and making recommendations about the prevention of work-related disease and injury. NIOSH is part of the CENTERS FOR DISEASE CONTROL AND PREVENTION (CDC). The institute conducts research into occupational diseases and injuries ranging from lung disease in miners to carpal tunnel syndrome in computer users; investigates potentially hazardous workplace conditions and recommends solutions when requested by employers, employees, or state or federal agencies. NIOSH also disseminates information and recommendations about preventing workplace disease, disability, and injury, and provides training to occupational safety and health professionals.

National Institutes of Health (NIH)

One of the eight health agencies of the Public Health Service, which is part of the US Department of Health and Human Services. Founded in 1887, the NIH is the focal point for medical research in the United States. The NIH goal is to acquire new knowledge to help prevent, detect, diagnose, and treat disease and disability. Research conducted or funded by NIH encompasses problems ranging from the common cold to the rarest genetic disorder.

Natural childbirth

Methods of vaginal delivery that emphasize pain management using relaxation and other techniques rather than pain-relieving drugs. Pain management techniques may include massage, changing of body positions, meditation, taking a warm shower, or breathing techniques. Part of natural childbirth includes eliminating fear and tension through preparation. It usually involves a partner or coach, usually the father, who provides emotional support and helps the mother use the various relaxation techniques in labor. Typically, a few months before the baby is born, the mother and partner attend childbirth classes where both learn what to expect during childbirth, as well as techniques

for breathing and relaxation intended to make labor more comfortable. Except in the case of an emergency cesarean section, the partner remains with the mother throughout labor and delivery.

Natural childbirth is sometimes wrongly assumed to be painless. In fact, it is based on the belief that women will find the normal pain of labor easier to handle if they are relaxed, cooperative, and know what to expect. Low doses of pain medication are sometimes used. Natural childbirth is particularly emphasized at BIRTHING CENTERS. Classes in natural childbirth are usually given through birthing centers and hospitals. Lamaze method and Bradley method classes are widely available.

Natural family planning

Prevention of pregnancy by abstaining from sexual intercourse when conception is likely to take place. The rhythm method is considered by some people to be a natural method of contraception because no drugs or devices are used. A couple practices the rhythm method by using one of a variety of methods to find out on which days during a woman's menstrual cycle she is likely to become pregnant and abstaining from intercourse on those days. Generally, the rhythm method requires abstaining from intercourse on days immediately before, after, or during ovulation.

Most women ovulate and are most fertile in the middle of the menstrual cycle. Complicating matters, the first half of the menstrual cycle is more variable than the second half, making it difficult to predict exactly when a woman will ovulate. Pregnancy is unlikely to result from having intercourse from about 10 to 11 days before the menstrual period, through the period, until about 2 days after the period. The span of 12 days that begins about 3 days after the period is considered unsafe to have intercourse, although the actual fertile time is only about 6 days. The risk of pregnancy is extended by the unpredictability of ovulation and the facts that sperm can live for up to 7 days in the female reproductive tract and an egg can be fertilized for up to 24 hours after it has been released.

Using the rhythm method successfully requires a couple's absolute ability to identify the fertile time and follow the rules of the method. Ideally, people who use a rhythm method, also called a fertility awareness method, should have low rates of conception. However, in reality, about 25 percent of typical users have an unintended pregnancy within a year.

In natural family planning, there are three methods commonly used to find out when a woman is ovulating and therefore likely to conceive. In one method, the woman takes her temperature every morning before getting out of bed and records it on a chart. She uses this information to detect the slight rise in temperature that occurs just after ovulation. Using this method, a couple will abstain from sexual intercourse from the end of the menstrual period until 3 days after the temperature rise was recorded.

A second method involves the woman's monitoring the changes in her vaginal secretions. Just before ovulation, the mucus (from the cervix) becomes wetter and more slippery, resembling raw egg white. Couples using this method will abstain from intercourse, beginning with the first signs of changes in cervical mucus and continuing until 4 days after the day of greatest wetness. This method is useful for women whose menstrual cycles are slightly irregular, but it requires considerable skill and experience to detect changes in mucus accurately.

The third method involves a combination of taking the woman's temperature every day and checking for signs of ovulation. Signs include breast tenderness, abdominal cramps, vaginal spotting, and changes in the firmness of the cervix. Couples will abstain from intercourse beginning at the first sign of increased vaginal wetness until the third day after the rise in temperature. This method can be more successful because it relies on more than one indicator, but it also requires skill and experience to detect subtle body changes. See CONTRACEPTION, OTHER METHODS.

Naturopathy

A philosophy of holistic health care that emphasizes the use of natural, noninvasive remedies. Naturopathy is a belief system based on the idea that the adoption of a healthy diet and lifestyle will lead to better health in general. Naturopathic practitioners include naturopathic physicians, massage therapists, chiropractors, herbalists, and others, all of whom believe in the wisdom of natural remedies whenever possible. These include the use of clinical nutrition, homeopathy, botanical medicine, and counseling. Naturopathy has long recommended that people eat a diet high in fruits, vegetables, and whole grains and that they take selected vitamins and food supplements. Such naturopathic practices are now often endorsed by conventional medicine.

Other naturopathic practices include natural childbirth, home birthing, acupuncture, and stress reduction. Naturopaths also use some methods that are controversial and possibly dangerous, such as detoxification by fasting or enemas to purify the body. The goal of naturopathy is always to cure disease by harnessing the body's own natural healing power. Naturopaths reject synthetic drugs and invasive procedures, preferring those that depend on the restorative properties of nature, seek the true underlying cause of disease, and treat the whole person.

Nausea

FOR SYMPTOM CHART
see Nausea or vomiting, page 46

A sensation of having an upset stomach or needing to vomit. Nausea can be a symptom of a wide variety of conditions ranging from the morning sickness of pregnancy to a stomach virus or indigestion. A general uneasiness in the stomach may also occur in response to stress or fear or as a side effect of certain drugs. If nausea is persistent or is accompanied by other symptoms, medical attention should be sought.

Navel

The scar on the abdomen that marks the site where the umbilical cord connecting mother to fetus during pregnancy was attached to the fetus. The medical word for the navel is the umbilicus.

Nearsightedness

A focusing (refractive) error of the eyes that makes it difficult to see distant objects clearly; also known as myopia. In most cases of nearsightedness, the eyeball is overly long from front to back. As a result, the distance is too great for the lens to focus incoming light rays on the retina (the thin, light-sensitive layer of nerve tissue at the back of the eye that relays visual information to the brain). Nearsightedness can also result from too much focusing power in the lens and cornea (the clear covering on the exposed surface of the eye). In both types of nearsightedness, distant objects are blurry while close ones are clear. Eyestrain and headaches can result. Nearsightedness affects one in four Americans.

Nearsightedness is generally present at birth and often detected during childhood. Nearsighted children tend to consistently squint, move closer to blackboards and televisions, hold books close while reading, and fail to notice distant objects. Nearsightedness usually worsens during childhood and adolescence and becomes stable only in the middle to late 20s. The condition affects men and women equally and tends to run in families.

Nearsightedness is most often treated with glasses or contact lenses that correct for the focusing error. People who do not wish to wear glasses or contact lenses may choose REFRACTIVE SURGERY, which permanently alters the shape of the eye to correct faulty vision. See Correcting nearsightedness, page 888.

Nebulizer

A device, such as a vaporizer, used to convert liquid medicine into a mist that can be inhaled. Nebulizers are used to deliver certain medicines to people with asthma, among other respiratory conditions. They are useful because of their ability to deliver medicine to areas deep within the lungs.

Neck

The narrow structure of the body that connects the trunk to the head. The neck is a complex structure of muscles, organs, blood vessels, and nerves surrounding the upper spine. Seven bones called the cervical vertebrae form the core of the neck and support the head. The cervical vertebrae fit together like a stack of rings, allowing them to rotate the head and

N

CORRECTING NEARSIGHTEDNESS

When the eye is too long or there is too much focusing power in the lens and cornea, light rays focus in front of the retina, causing nearsightedness (myopia).

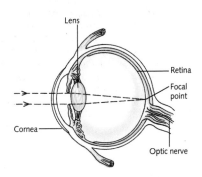

NORMAL EYE
In normal vision, light passes through the cornea and lens to its proper focal point on the retina.

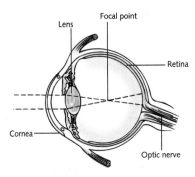

NEARSIGHTED (MYOPIC) EYE
Nearsightedness results when the focal point of light rays falls short of the retina.

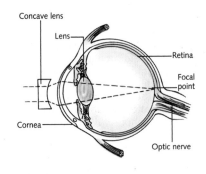

CONCAVE LENS CORRECTING NEARSIGHTEDNESS
Eyeglasses or contact lenses refocus light rays so that the focal point falls on the retina.

move it back and forth. The spinal cord passes through the cervical vertebrae and into the trunk. A number of nerves, such as those connecting with the arm, branch off the spine in the neck. Surrounding the vertebrae is a complex arrangement of straplike muscles that allows the various movements of the head and coordinates them with the actions of other parts of the trunk. Some of the muscles help maintain posture. Others in the back of

the neck run from the base of the skull through the neck to the vertebrae of the upper back, supporting the skull.

The vital passageways for food and air—the esophagus and the trachea, respectively—pass through the neck. The larynx (voice box), located between the pharynx (throat) and the trachea (windpipe), is the primary organ of the speech mechanism. Long blood vessels supplying the head and brain pass through the neck. The

principal arteries are the carotids, one on each side of the neck. The major veins of the neck, the jugular veins, also run up each side.

Neck dissection, radical

A surgical procedure to remove lymph nodes (see LYMPH NODE; small glands that act as a filter and as a barrier to infection) that may be involved in cancer of the head and neck. There are about 300 lymph nodes located in the head and neck; 75 are located on each side of the neck. Cancers in the head and neck may spread to the lymph nodes in the neck and have to be removed. The purpose of the procedure is to prevent further spread of cancer to other parts of the body. It is an effective method for controlling head and neck cancer in many cases. Complications of the surgery include injury to the nerves controlling the lower face, throat, shoulder, and tongue, as well as changes in skin sensation under the ear and jaw. Side effects may include weakness in the shoulder and pain in the neck. Radical neck dissection is sometimes combined with removal of parts of

STRUCTURES OF THE NECK
The neck contains the bones and muscles that support and move the head and connect it to the rest of the body and the major blood vessels that supply the brain. It also houses vital organs, such as portions of the esophagus and trachea and the larynx, and glands such as the thyroid and parathyroids.

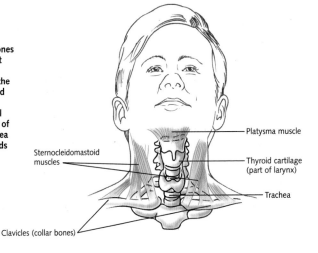

Platysma muscle

Sternocleidomastoid muscles

Thyroid cartilage (part of larynx)

Trachea

Clavicles (collar bones)

the jawbone and floor of the mouth, which may lead to disfigurement and loss of some of the nerves controlling the tongue and jaw.

Neck injuries

Injuries to the neck or cervical spinal cord. Symptoms of a neck injury include stiff neck, a head held in an unusual position, weakness, difficulty walking, paralysis of legs or arms, neck pain, loss of bladder or bowel control, or numbness or tingling in an arm or leg. Neck injuries can be the result of bullet or stab wounds or direct trauma to the head or neck in a fall, diving, motor vehicle collision, or contact sports such as football. Neck injuries can be extremely serious and can lead to loss of sensation and function in the parts of the body below the site of the injury. While neck and spine injuries make up only a small portion of all injuries, they are responsible for more than half the deaths caused by injury.

When someone has a spinal injury, any additional movement can cause further damage to the spine. The purpose of first aid for any neck injury is to prevent further harm to the person while emergency medical care is sought. The person should be kept absolutely immobile. Headgear, such as a helmet, should not be removed. The person should be kept warm to help prevent shock. Breathing should be checked and ARTIFICIAL RESPIRATION or CARDIOPULMONARY RESUSCITATION (CPR) administered if necessary. Any external bleeding should be stopped by applying pressure.

People can prevent neck injuries by wearing seat belts and helmets, by avoiding drinking and driving, and by not diving into lakes, rivers, surf, and pools where the depth of water is unknown.

Neck rigidity

Stiffness of the neck caused by spasm of the muscles in the neck and spine. Neck rigidity is an important symptom of MENINGITIS (inflammation of the membranes that surround the brain and spinal cord). Neck stiffness can also be caused by injuries such as whiplash.

Necrolysis, toxic epidermal

An extremely rare skin condition that causes large portions of the epidermis (the outer layer of skin) to fall off; also known as TEN syndrome or toxic EPIDERMOLYSIS BULLOSA. Toxic epidermal necrolysis is usually caused by a severe drug reaction to medications such as sulfonamides or seizure medications. In this condition, fever and cough are followed by the development of purple, targetlike lesions on the skin. The lesions merge and blister, and, eventually, the skin is shed.

Diagnosis of toxic epidermal necrolysis is made according to the appearance of the skin lesions and a medical history that includes the recent prescription of a new medication. Doctors generally consider toxic epidermal necrolysis to be a particularly severe form of erythema multiforme, a type of skin reaction in which targetlike lesions appear on the skin and sores develop on the mucous membranes.

People who have toxic epidermal necrolysis require hospitalization in an intensive care or burn unit. Treatment may include immunosuppressive medicines to manage inflammation, antibiotics to control secondary infections, and skin grafts. However, infection and shock due to loss of body fluids may cause death.

Necrophilia

Erotic or sexual interest in and activity with dead bodies.

Necrosis

The death or decay of tissue in a part of the body, such as a bone. Necrosis occurs when not enough blood is supplied to tissue. See also GANGRENE.

Necrotizing enterocolitis

A life-threatening intestinal disease in infants. Necrotizing enterocolitis can cause the death of intestinal tissue and can lead to scarring, narrowing, or rupture of the bowel. The disease is most common in low-birth-weight and premature infants. Its symptoms include intolerance to baby formula, a distended abdomen, and gas in the muscular layers of the intestinal wall. Some infants experience vomiting, diarrhea, blood in the stool, lethargy, and fluctuations in temperature. In low-birth-weight infants, these symptoms can take 2 months to develop. Severe enterocolitis can create a hole in the intestine. When that happens, an infant may develop peritonitis (a painful infection of the lining of the abdominal cavity), go into shock, and possibly die (see SHOCK, PHYSIOLOGICAL).

The exact cause of necrotizing enterocolitis remains unclear. It may be due to decreased blood flow to the intestine or a bacterial infection. Overly concentrated baby formula and stress have been implicated as possible causes. Outbreaks in hospital nurseries suggest that necrotizing enterocolitis may be contagious.

N

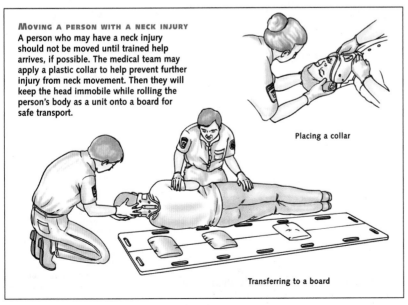

MOVING A PERSON WITH A NECK INJURY
A person who may have a neck injury should not be moved until trained help arrives, if possible. The medical team may apply a plastic collar to help prevent further injury from neck movement. Then they will keep the head immobile while rolling the person's body as a unit onto a board for safe transport.

Placing a collar

Transferring to a board

DIAGNOSIS AND TREATMENT

The typical infant diagnosed with necrotizing enterocolitis is a newborn who is still in the hospital. Diagnosis is based on the presence of symptoms. X rays, ultrasound scanning, and blood and stool tests are used in confirming the diagnosis. When the condition is suspected, feeding by mouth is stopped, and fluids are given intravenously. A small tube is inserted into the infant's nose, extending down into the stomach, to relieve trapped gas and to allow the bowel to rest. Antibiotic treatment is given intravenously. An infant may require the help of a mechanical ventilator to breathe. If shock occurs, additional intravenous medications and fluids may be necessary. In some cases, diseased intestines are surgically removed.

Necrotizing fasciitis group A

A severe, life-threatening infection caused by bacteria that attack the soft tissue beneath the top layers of skin, including the fibrous tissue that covers the muscles. Necrotizing fasciitis group A is usually caused by group A *Streptococcus* and other bacteria that enter the body via an infection or minor cut or lesion on the surface of the skin. It occurs most commonly on the arms and legs, but may also affect the perineum (the tissue between the external genitalia and the anus). The infection is sometimes a complication of surgery. People with diabetes mellitus may be particularly susceptible to necrotizing fasciitis group A, but it also affects people who are otherwise in good health.

The bacteria causing this infection are sometimes referred to as "flesh-eating bacteria" because they attack the body's soft tissue, moving very rapidly under the top layers of skin and killing the soft tissue they infect. Small blood vessels in this tissue may be blocked, and the loss of blood supply to the dead tissue causes GANGRENE of the skin.

SYMPTOMS, DIAGNOSIS, AND TREATMENT

Underlying tissues affected by the infection are usually severely painful, and the skin's surface is red, hot, and swollen. As it progresses, the skin becomes discolored, gangrene progresses, and the person has fever and low blood pressure.

Necrotizing fasciitis is diagnosed by observing the characteristic symptoms, principally swelling and dying of tissues under the skin, including the tissue that encloses the muscles and excluding muscle and bone. The metabolism of the bacteria may produce gases under the skin that can be detected on an X ray or a CT (computed tomography) scan.

In its early stages, the dead tissue, including outer layers of skin, underlying soft tissue, and fat, can be surgically removed. Cutting away of dead and infected tissue is performed during a surgical procedure. Cultures of pus from underlying tissue can determine the specific type of antibiotic required to treat the causative bacteria. Antibiotic therapy is generally begun immediately, pending culture results. Intravenous fluids are given to replace fluid lost from destroyed tissues.

Limb amputation is sometimes essential to prevent death, which is not uncommon with advanced stages of the condition. Insufficient removal of infected tissue can allow the infection to continue spreading. Repeated surgeries within 1 to 2 days may be necessary to make sure the bacteria and affected tissue have been removed. When the doctor is certain that no more tissue is being destroyed, the wound is closed and skin grafts are performed.

The decay of tissue with severe infection may progress to systemic shock, which causes respiratory failure, heart failure, low blood pressure, and kidney failure. Necrotizing fasciitis is one of the fastest spreading infections known. Prompt medical evaluation and treatment are essential to preventing death, which can happen within 24 hours if necrotizing fasciitis is untreated. Advanced age and other medical conditions decrease chances of survival. Usually, the progress of the infection occurs within hours to days from the time of initial exposure. The delay of an accurate diagnosis and appropriate treatment, in addition to surgery that does not remove all infected tissue, can contribute to a poor prognosis for survival.

Needle aspiration

Insertion of a hollow needle attached to a syringe into a cyst or lump in order to remove a sample of fluid for microscopic evaluation. In an aspiration BIOPSY, cells or tissue are suctioned into the syringe and examined for signs of malignancy (cancer).

Needle biopsy

Insertion of a special needle into a lump, cyst, or other area of concern in order to remove a specimen of tissue for microscopic evaluation. A needle BIOPSY is performed to determine whether or not a tumor is cancerous or to find the cause of infection or inflammation.

Needle localization

A procedure used to locate the place where a BIOPSY specimen will be taken from the breast. Using mammography (see MAMMOGRAM), the radiologist finds the precise area from which the biopsy sample will be taken and marks the skin directly above it. A thin, hollow needle containing a wire about the size of a strand of hair is inserted into the spot. Another mammogram is performed to make sure the needle is in the right place, after which the needle is removed, leaving the wire in the breast. The function of the wire is to show the surgeon performing the biopsy where the "suspicious" tissue is, because it cannot be seen with the naked eye. The surgeon will remove the wire along with the tissue to be examined.

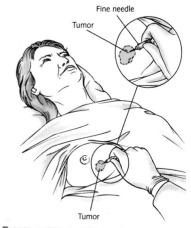

Fine needle

Tumor

Tumor

BIOPSY AFTER MAMMOGRAM
The doctor inserts a very fine, hollow needle into the breast at the site indicated on the mammogram and then threads a wire into the needle to mark the spot. The patient is moved to an operating room, where a surgeon removes the tissue as marked for biopsy, taking the wire along with the tissue sample.

Nefazodone

An antidepressant. Nefazodone (Serzone) is used to treat major depression. It works by increasing the amount of the hormone serotonin, which is known to improve a person's mood.

Nelfinavir mesylate

An antiviral drug. Nelfinavir mesylate (Viracept) is used along with other medicines to treat infection caused by HIV (human immunodeficiency virus). It works by preventing HIV from reproducing itself, thereby slowing the destruction of the human immune system and delaying the symptoms associated with AIDS (acquired immunodeficiency syndrome).

Nematodes

A group of worm organisms that are common parasites of humans and animals. Unlike other worm parasites, including flukes and tapeworms (see FLUKE; TAPEWORM INFESTATION), many species of nematodes are free-living, with life cycles that do not involve an intermediate host or vector, which is an insect or other organism that acts as a carrier. Infection is transmitted by these species from one host to another when the nematodes' eggs, which contain infective larvae, are ingested. Hookworm (see HOOKWORM INFESTATION), which is a nematode, is transmitted when the host's skin is penetrated by infective larvae that have hatched from the nematode's eggs. Several species of nematodes, including the filarial parasites that carry the infection FILARIASIS, have life cycles that require a vector.

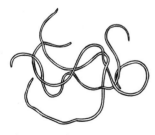

MULTICELLED WORMS
Nematodes are the most numerous multicelled animals in the world. Many species exist as parasites in other animals and insects, but some exist independently and feed on bacteria, fungi, and each other. A nematode is often described as a tube within a tube because the digestive tract runs the length of its body.

Neologism

A word invented by an individual; the meaning may be known only to him or her and is related to the underlying emotional conflict. Sometimes a neologism consists of a standard word given an unusual, emotionally relevant meaning by the individual.

Neomycin

An antibiotic. Neomycin (Mycifradin) is used to treat infectious diarrhea caused by *Escherichia coli* (E. COLI) bacteria, as well as to suppress intestinal bacteria in surgical patients and those with other bacterial infections. Neomycin works by stopping bacteria from making protein, a building block of bacteria. Neosporin is available as a tablet or liquid by prescription to treat intestinal infections and without prescription to treat skin infections, burns, wounds, and other minor injuries.

Neonatal intensive care

Hospital care that focuses on the problems of the distressed newborn. Neonatal intensive care units, or NICUs, are designed to meet the unique needs of immature and ill newborns. These include special fluid requirements, oxygen management (see OXYGEN, SUPPLEMENTAL), temperature control, and drug dosages. Located primarily in major medical centers, NICUs are staffed by teams of neonatologists and nurses who are specially trained in the care of newborns. Neonatal intensive care units contain a variety of sophisticated mechanical devices and equipment. The amount of physical contact a parent has with an infant in the NICU depends on the baby's condition and hospital policies.

INFANTS AT HIGH RISK
Infants at high risk for life-threatening conditions include those born prematurely (see PREMATURE BIRTH) or at a low birth weight, newborns who have birth injuries such as oxygen deprivation, and infants of multiple births such as twins. Babies born to mothers who were ill during pregnancy may also require special monitoring in the first few days of life. For example, gestational diabetes, in which the mother's blood sugar level is high, is a common complication of pregnancy. Infants of mothers who smoked, drank a significant amount of alcohol, or abused drugs during pregnancy all face higher risks than normal. Other infants in the neonatal intensive care unit may have severe congenital (present from birth) defects, which can be caused by genetic or chromosomal abnormalities.

PREMATURE INFANTS
The vast majority of infants in NICUs are premature newborns of low birth weight. Premature babies are those born before 37 weeks of pregnancy have elapsed. Normally, pregnancy lasts about 40 weeks. While full-term infants weigh about 7 pounds or more

N

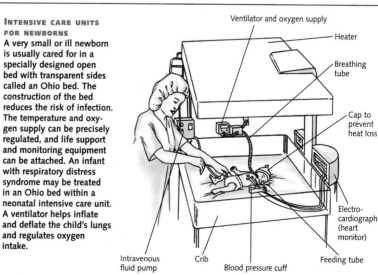

INTENSIVE CARE UNITS FOR NEWBORNS
A very small or ill newborn is usually cared for in a specially designed open bed with transparent sides called an Ohio bed. The construction of the bed reduces the risk of infection. The temperature and oxygen supply can be precisely regulated, and life support and monitoring equipment can be attached. An infant with respiratory distress syndrome may be treated in an Ohio bed within a neonatal intensive care unit. A ventilator helps inflate and deflate the child's lungs and regulates oxygen intake.

Ventilator and oxygen supply
Heater
Breathing tube
Cap to prevent heat loss
Electro-cardiograph (heart monitor)
Feeding tube
Blood pressure cuff
Crib
Intravenous fluid pump

at birth, premature babies usually weigh 5 pounds or less. After birth, premature infants face a greater risk of developing health problems. Their lungs are immature, which may lead to breathing difficulties. Very often they have trouble feeding and maintaining a stable body temperature. They also have a higher risk for infection and DEVELOPMENTAL DELAY.

NEONATAL CARE
Very small or ill newborns are cared for in incubators or on Ohio beds, special beds that provide for individualized temperature and oxygen needs and reduce the risk of infection. Infants may be connected to machines that help them breathe, provide food, or monitor vital signs. Because the lungs and other immature organs of a premature or ill baby do not always function correctly, a nurse will monitor them by taking regular blood samples from a catheter (tube) inserted through the navel or in the infant's arm or foot. Frequently, NICU patients are newborns with RESPIRATORY DISTRESS SYNDROME. To get enough oxygen, they require the assistance of a mechanical VENTILATOR. A ventilator controls their rate of breathing and amount of oxygen intake. Babies who do not suck well and have problems feeding may be fed through a tube inserted into the stomach. An infant who is very premature or has a digestive problem such as NECROTIZING ENTEROCOLITIS, can be given nutrients intravenously through a tube inserted into a vein.

Some infants, especially those born prematurely, become jaundiced. JAUNDICE is a yellowing of the skin and whites of the eyes. A surplus of the bile pigment called BILIRUBIN causes jaundice. Bilirubin is a normal by-product of the breakdown of red blood cells, but sometimes the immature liver and kidneys of a newborn cannot process a large amount of this substance. Left uncontrolled, very high bilirubin levels can lead to brain damage. (See also KERNICTERUS.) Phototherapy, which uses exposure to ultraviolet light, is the treatment most often used to bring high bilirubin levels under control.

Neonate

An infant from birth through 4 weeks of age. Neonates are closely monitored for growth and development in order to detect possible diseases and disorders present at birth. Prematurely born

neonates often are underweight, have immature organs, and need special care.

Neonatologist

A physician who specializes in the care of neonates (babies from birth to 4 weeks of age) and the diagnosis and treatment of their disorders. Neonatologists monitor, diagnose, and treat babies for conditions related to growth and development, food consumption and absorption, disease, and organ function. When a baby is born prematurely, a neonatologist will likely be consulted to help determine what special treatment is required.

Neonatology

The branch of pediatric medicine that focuses on the care of neonates, babies from birth to 4 weeks of age, and treatment of their disorders. Areas of interest include treatment of prematurely born infants, infants who have experienced birth trauma or are ill or underweight, and the early detection and treatment of congenital (present from birth) disorders such as spina bifida.

Neoplasia

An abnormal growth or tumor. Neoplasia is the result of a malfunction in the process of cell reproduction in which too many cells are created. The overgrowth of new cells may form a tumor, a type of neoplasm. Neoplasms can be benign or malignant, although the term is usually used to mean a malignant or cancerous tumor.

Nephrectomy

Surgical removal of a KIDNEY. Nephrectomy is generally undertaken only

if the person's other kidney is functioning normally. It is indicated when there is irreversible damage to a kidney. Cancer is the most common reason to perform a nephrectomy, but damage may be a result of traumatic injury to a kidney; chronic infection, obstruction, or pain caused by a large kidney stone; and KIDNEY FAILURE. Nephrectomy is also performed to obtain a kidney for a KIDNEY TRANSPLANT. It is sometimes indicated when there is an abnormality in the blood supply to the kidney or damage to the kidney caused by NEPHROSCLEROSIS, PYELONEPHRITIS, or congenital disease. Traditionally, the surgery is performed through an incision in the side, depending on several medical factors.

In many instances, a nephrectomy can be done through LAPAROSCOPY. Several dime-sized incisions are made in the abdomen; hollow tubes are inserted into the incisions. A fiberoptic camera placed in an incision transmits an image onto monitors that allow the surgeons to view the kidney. Surgical instruments for retrieving the kidney are placed in the other tubes. The kidney is encased in plastic and removed with a tool inserted into another incision about 2 inches wide. If the kidney was removed for donation, the donor usually stays in the hospital for 2 days.

Nephritis

Inflammation of one or both kidneys. Nephritis is among the most common of kidney diseases and occurs more frequently in childhood and adolescence than in middle age. It may result from an infection, particularly STREP-

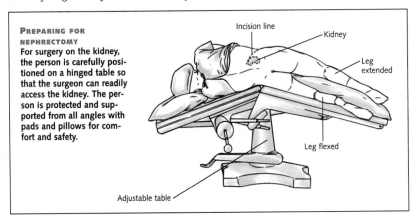

PREPARING FOR NEPHRECTOMY
For surgery on the kidney, the person is carefully positioned on a hinged table so that the surgeon can readily access the kidney. The person is protected and supported from all angles with pads and pillows for comfort and safety.

Incision line
Kidney
Leg extended
Leg flexed
Adjustable table

TOCOCCAL INFECTIONS, or an abnormal immune response. Disorders such as lupus erythematosus are associated with nephritis.

A urinalysis is used to diagnose nephritis. Examining the urine with a microscope reveals elevated levels of the protein albumin, indicating the condition ALBUMINURIA. Red and white blood cells and hyaline or granular casts are also present in the urine of people with nephritis.

There are two forms of nephritis: acute and chronic. People who have the acute form, especially children, usually recover. Symptoms include fatigue, appetite loss, facial swelling, pain in the abdomen or side, and a reduced quantity of dark urine. Acute kidney inflammation can progress to chronic nephritis, which can gradually destroy the kidney. Often there are no symptoms. When kidney function is severely impaired by chronic nephritis, high blood pressure may develop, possibly resulting in death caused by kidney or heart failure.

Interstitial nephritis is chronic inflammation of part of the kidney cells that surround the fluid-collecting units. It can lead to acute or chronic KIDNEY FAILURE. See also GLOMERULONEPHRITIS.

Nephrocalcinosis

A kidney disorder that is characterized by deposits of calcium oxalate or calcium phosphate in the tubules of the kidneys and the areas between the tubules. Nephrocalcinosis may result in KIDNEY STONES and reduced kidney function. Nephrocalcinosis may be caused by an excess excretion of calcium by the kidneys, acidosis of the tubules of the kidneys, a rare congenital condition called sponge kidney, an elevated calcium level in the blood, necrosis of the kidneys, and tuberculosis.

Nephrolithotomy

The surgical removal of KIDNEY STONES. Nephrolithotomy has been largely replaced by more technologically advanced and less invasive procedures for the treatment of kidney stones, but

Terms in small capital letters—for example, PHYSICAL THERAPY or PAGET DISEASE—indicate a cross-reference to another entry with more information.

it is still used in cases of very large kidney stones. See also LITHOTRIPSY.

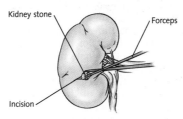

SURGICAL REMOVAL OF KIDNEY STONES
In the rare case that a kidney stone is removed surgically, an incision is made to the right or left of the spine. The surgeon enters the kidney at the junction between the kidney and the ureter, and the stone is removed with a forceps. The procedure may also be called pyelolithotomy.

Nephrologist

A physician specializing in the study and practice of the function, diseases, and disorders of the kidneys.

Nephrology

The branch of medical study and practice that specializes in the function, diseases, and disorders of the kidneys.

Nephron

Tiny structures of the kidneys that filter blood to remove waste products, regulate fluid and electrolyte content

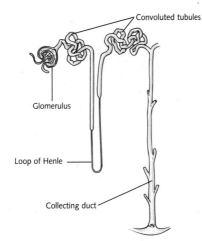

FILTERING UNIT
Each nephron contains a structure called the glomerulus, which filters waste substances from the blood and allows the filtered fluid to flow into the tubule. To prevent needed nutrients from being washed from the body, the tubules absorb water, proteins, and other substances back into the bloodstream. The loop of Henle regulates traffic of fluids within each nephron.

of the blood, and form urine. Nephrons are the working units of the kidneys. Each kidney is made up of approximately 1 million nephrons. The nephrons are composed of glomeruli (the filtering units of the kidneys), renal tubules, and their abundant supply of blood vessels.

Nephropathy, analgesic

Disease of the kidneys associated with excessive use of over-the-counter painkillers, or analgesics. Nonprescription analgesics—including aspirin, acetaminophen, ibuprofen, and naproxen—do not cause kidney damage in most people when the recommended dosage is taken. For people who have risk factors such as advanced age, systemic lupus erythematosus, or chronic kidney conditions, and for those who have recently binged on alcohol, analgesic nephropathy can result in acute KIDNEY FAILURE.

In rare cases, a single dose of analgesics or a recommended dosage taken over a 10-day period may be sufficient to damage the kidneys. Painkillers taken daily for several years have been known to cause analgesic nephropathy requiring DIALYSIS or a KIDNEY TRANSPLANT. The analgesic medications that can cause kidney damage are those that are excreted primarily through the kidneys.

Nephropathy, diabetic

Kidney disease caused by an elevated level of blood glucose, the primary characteristic of diabetes mellitus. Diabetic nephropathy eventually affects a significant proportion of people with type 1 or type 2 diabetes mellitus. It is produced by high levels of glucose in the blood, which damage the kidneys and increase the filtering of blood by the kidneys. If the damage is significant, it impairs the ability of the kidneys to remove waste products from the body.

Diabetic nephropathy may take many years to develop. It is one of the causes of glomerular nephropathy, or damage to the glomeruli. It is the leading cause of end-stage renal disease (see KIDNEY FAILURE) in the United States.

DECREASING THE RISKS
People who have diabetes can slow the pace of kidney damage by keep-

N

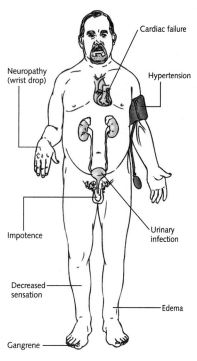

EFFECTS OF DIABETIC NEPHROPATHY
The possible long-term effects of kidney disease as a result of diabetes are profound: heart failure, high blood pressure (hypertension), impotence, urinary infections (with possible incontinence), nerve damage (neuropathy) that causes numbness or muscle weakness and a characteristic dropping of the wrist and foot, swelling (edema), and gangrene as a result of poor circulation.

ing their blood sugar level as close to normal as possible. Limiting protein intake, exercising regularly, and taking the right medications on the correct schedule are also beneficial.

People with diabetes should have periodic examinations of the urine for elevated albumin or protein levels. The person with diabetic nephropathy should seek medical treatment for urinary infections promptly and keep the blood pressure below 135/85 millimeters of mercury (mm Hg). Medications for lowering blood pressure such as the angiotensin-converting enzyme inhibitors (see ANTIHYPERTENSIVES) are especially effective at protecting the kidneys from damage. Pain medications containing phenacetin should be avoided as they can contribute to kidney damage. Exposure to any intravenous CONTRAST MEDIUM or other agent that might be harmful to the kidneys must be limited.

Nephropathy, IgA

A chronic, progressive kidney disorder that can lead to end-stage renal disease (see KIDNEY FAILURE). IgA (immunoglobulin A) nephropathy is caused by deposits of various composition inside the glomeruli (the filtering units of the kidneys). These units normally filter waste products and excess water out of the blood. The deposits associated with IgA nephropathy interfere with this filtering process, causing blood and protein to accumulate in the urine. Early symptoms include swelling of the hands and feet.

IgA nephropathy may progress over a period of up to 20 years. It is not known why deposits form, but it is believed that genetic factors may contribute to the disease. Treatment is based on slowing the progression of the underlying disorder and preventing complications such as high blood pressure, which contributes to more damage to the glomeruli. Recommended dietary restrictions for people who have nephropathy may include limiting protein to reduce the buildup of waste products in the blood. Cholesterol-lowering measures, including diet, medication, or a combination of the two, may help control the disorder.

Nephrosclerosis

A process that results in the replacement of healthy kidney structures by scar tissue. Nephrosclerosis is caused by hardening of the small arteries that supply the kidneys with blood. It is usually associated with chronically elevated high blood pressure. Nephrosclerosis can cause abnormalities such as excess albumin and white or red blood cells in the urine.

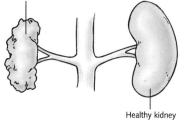

Kidney with nephrosclerosis

Healthy kidney

DAMAGED KIDNEY
If the kidney is not adequately supplied with blood, the healthy tissue will gradually be replaced by scar tissue (left). Ultimately, the opposite kidney may be affected as well.

Nephrosis

A condition produced by abnormalities in the glomerular membrane, the membranous part of the glomeruli (the filtering units of the kidneys). Nephrosis allows large amounts of protein in the blood to escape into the urine. It can occur in people of all ages but tends to be more common in children. Excessive protein loss can cause water and sodium to accumulate in the body, resulting in edema (swelling) around the ankles, feet, and eyes and in the abdomen. While nephrosis cannot always be cured, some forms of it can be suppressed by the use of corticosteroid hormones, specifically cortisone and prednisone.

Nephrostomy

Surgical formation of an opening that allows the introduction of a small tube into a kidney to drain urine to the surface of the abdomen. Nephrostomy allows urine to bypass a ureter (one of the two narrow tubes connecting a kidney and the bladder). The procedure may be performed after surgery to allow waste products to be removed through urine and to allow the ureter to heal.

Nephrotic syndrome

A combination of signs and symptoms caused by disorders that result in injury to the glomeruli (the filtering units of the kidneys). Damage to these structures results in abnormal excretion of protein in the urine.

Nephrotic syndrome may be the result of an infection, exposure to certain medications, a cancerous tumor, and autoimmune or hereditary disorders. The most common cause in adults is diabetes mellitus. Other diseases (including systemic lupus erythematosus, multiple myeloma, and amyloidosis) that affect multiple body systems can also cause nephrotic syndrome. Disorders of the kidneys, especially various forms of GLOMERULONEPHRITIS, are associated with nephrotic syndrome.

Nephrotic syndrome is diagnosed by blood and urine tests. The findings include abnormally high levels of protein in the urine, a decreased level of protein in the blood, and, in many cases, a high blood cholesterol level. Fat globules may be observed in the urine. Clinically, the loss of protein may cause fluid retention, resulting in edema (swelling) around the ankles and, in severe cases, ASCITES (accumulation of fluid in the abdominal cavity) and pulmonary edema.

Nerve

A cable of fibers that carries electrochemical impulses to and from the BRAIN or SPINAL CORD to a specific point in the body. The NERVOUS SYSTEM is a network of nerves passing throughout the body.

At a cellular level, a single nerve is composed of thousands of nerve fibers; each fiber is the tail (axon) of an individual nerve cell called a neuron. Each nerve fiber is insulated by a covering called the myelin sheath. The fibers are bundled together in groups called fascicles; a fascicle contains the types of nerve fibers—sensory, motor, and autonomic (involuntary)—needed to serve a particular site in the body. Most nerves contain all three types. Nerves may carry sensory information—from the sense organs or from the skin itself; they may carry motor information that causes the skeletal muscles to move; or they may communicate or direct internal body functions, such as heart rate or body temperature.

The brain and spinal cord (central nervous system) are linked to every area of the body via major nerves, known collectively as the peripheral nerves. Nerves are classified by where they originate: there are 12 pairs of cranial nerves originating in the brain and 31 spinal nerves, branching from the spinal cord. From the peripheral nerves, successively smaller nerve pathways travel to every part of the body.

Nerve block

A method of making an area of the body numb and pain-free by injecting medication around the nerves that control sensation in the area. A nerve block is performed when it is not possible to inject an anesthetic agent directly into the area being treated because of an inflammation or the risk of infection. One common type, the BRACHIAL PLEXUS BLOCK, is used for anesthesia during surgery on the hand, arm, or shoulder. Anesthesia of the legs and lower part of the body can be achieved by blocking the lower spinal nerves with spinal or epidural anesthesia (see ANESTHESIA, SPINAL; ANESTHESIA, EPIDURAL) or a CAUDAL BLOCK.

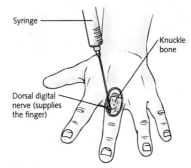

Syringe

Knuckle bone

Dorsal digital nerve (supplies the finger)

BLOCKING PAIN
If local anesthesia is not possible because the area is inflamed or infected, a nerve block can inject anesthetic into the nerves surrounding the area. A nerve to the finger is blocked so that surgery can be done on the finger.

Nerve entrapment

The compression of a nerve. Nerve entrapment causes symptoms such as numbness, tingling, and pain in the area supplied by the nerve. See PINCHED NERVE; CARPAL TUNNEL SYNDROME.

Nerve gas

A chemical warfare gas that is inhaled, ingested, or absorbed into the body through the skin. Nerve gas has paralyzing and other harmful effects, especially on the nervous and respiratory systems. Effects of poisoning depend on the type of gas, but can include immediate death or long-term disability.

Nerve growth factor

Also known as NGF, a substance that influences differentiation, growth, and maintenance of nerve cells. Studies are under way to try to synthesize nerve growth factor for use in treating many neurological conditions, including ALS (amyotrophic lateral sclerosis).

Nerve injuries

Crush or cut injuries to nerves that damage some or all of their conducting fibers. TINGLING is a symptom of damage or irritation to a nerve or nerves. NUMBNESS suggests that the affected nerve may be severed or dead. A brief tingling sensation, as when a person's hand or foot "falls asleep," is not a cause for concern. However, numbness or persistent tingling may indicate a significant nerve injury and requires medical attention.

In crush injuries, individual fibers within a peripheral nerve are damaged, but the nerve trunk remains intact. This means that new fibers can regenerate along the path left by degenerated fibers. However, when a nerve is completely severed, the fibers cannot regenerate, and there is no recovery of function. Surgical repair to reconnect the nerve is required to achieve some return of function.

N

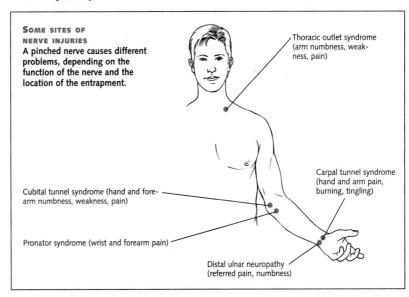

SOME SITES OF NERVE INJURIES
A pinched nerve causes different problems, depending on the function of the nerve and the location of the entrapment.

Thoracic outlet syndrome (arm numbness, weakness, pain)

Carpal tunnel syndrome (hand and arm pain, burning, tingling)

Cubital tunnel syndrome (hand and forearm numbness, weakness, pain)

Pronator syndrome (wrist and forearm pain)

Distal ulnar neuropathy (referred pain, numbness)

Nervous breakdown

A popular term for any psychiatric condition that leaves a person unable to function on a daily basis. It refers not to a specific disorder but to the effect a disorder has on a person's life.

Nervous habit

A repeated action used to alleviate stress, such as a cough, biting the nails, or pulling the hair.

Nervous system

The vast body system that gathers information, stores it, and controls the body's responses to it. The nervous system gathers data about both the external environment and the body's own internal state, analyzes the data, and initiates and directs the body's responses, ranging from automatic adjustment of body functions to complex motor movements and emotional or intellectual activity.

The basic unit of the nervous system is the NEURON, or nerve cell, that detects sensory information and conveys it in the form of an electrochemical impulse. Billions of neurons form nerves, which are bundles of fibers that transmit electrochemical messages back and forth between the brain and spinal cord and the rest of the body.

STRUCTURE AND ORGANIZATION
Anatomically, the overall nervous system includes both the CENTRAL NERVOUS SYSTEM (CNS), made up of the BRAIN and SPINAL CORD, and the peripheral nervous system, composed of all the nerves that branch out from the central nervous system and carry information between the brain and spinal cord and the rest of the body. Within the CNS, the brain is the body's computer and control center, constantly receiving sensory information, analyzing it, and deciding on reaction. The spinal cord is an extension of the brain, composed of two-way nerve tracts that can transmit signals both to and from the brain. The cord can also process some sensory input itself and initiate motor responses at an unconscious level. The peripheral nervous system provides the cabling that links the central nervous system to its input sites (sensory organs like the eyes and ears) and output sites (muscles and glands).

Within the peripheral nervous system, there are two important functional divisions: the AUTONOMIC NERVOUS SYSTEM and the somatic nervous system. The somatic system controls the skeletal muscles that perform voluntary movement. The autonomic system regulates the automatic, unconscious functioning of the internal body environment. The autonomic system is further broken down into the PARASYMPATHETIC NERVOUS SYSTEM that regulates internal body functions in a resting state and the SYMPATHETIC NERVOUS SYSTEM that takes over internal body responses to stress.

FUNCTION
The function of the nervous system is to detect changes in the internal and external environments of the body, to analyze the information, and to organize the body's response in the form of unconscious, involuntary activity and conscious, voluntary behavior. Higher areas of brain function include complex tasks of learning, memory, thought, emotional response, and language. These higher functions require that the brain constantly update, modify, and expand its own stored information. Much about how these extraordinary higher functions take place is not fully understood.

Neural tube defect

A birth defect that is the result of the failure of the spinal cord or brain to develop normally in an embryo. In a normal embryo, the neural tube eventually develops into the spinal cord and brain. When neural tube defects occur, the degree of deformity and disability depends on the level of neural involvement. Neural tube defects range from ANENCEPHALY (a fatal birth defect in which an infant's brain and skull fail to develop) to SPINA BIFIDA (a crippling but not fatal defect in which the backbones, or vertebrae, do not form a complete ring to protect the spinal cord). Spina bifida is much more common than anencephaly. Adequate folate levels in the first month after conception are important in the prevention of neural tube defects. As a result, doctors advise all women of childbearing age to take a daily multivitamin containing 400 micrograms of folic acid.

Neuralgia

Pain caused by irritation of or damage to a nerve. The pain of neuralgia occurs in brief bouts and may be severe, intense, burning, and stabbing. Neuralgia may be caused by nervous system disorders, such as SHINGLES (an infection of the nerves supplying the skin that is caused by the herpes zoster virus). The cause of neuralgia is often uncertain, or it can result from poor diet or systemic disease. There are a number of different types of neuralgia. One of the most common is TRIGEMINAL NEURALGIA, which is also known as tic douloureux. This is a disorder of the trigeminal nerve that causes severe pain on one side of the face. Other types are glossopharyngeal neuralgia (an intense pain that is felt in the throat, ear, and back of the tongue) and occipital neuralgia (in which there is pain, tingling, or numbness at the base of the back part of the skull). Treatment depends on diagnosis of the underlying disorder. Medications such as anticonvulsants, antidepressants, and topical painkillers may be helpful. In some cases, surgery is necessary.

Neurapraxia

A type of nerve injury in which the outward structure of a nerve appears normal, but in which some of the conducting fibers have degenerated or have been damaged. This results in a temporary loss of nerve conduction that may cause tingling, numbness, and weakness.

Neurasthenia

A 19th-century term for a disorder in which the individual lacks energy, feels lethargic, and has little or no appetite; often accompanied by weight loss, insomnia (difficulty falling or staying asleep), fatigue, and feelings of inadequacy. It can be a symptom of DEPRESSION, anxiety, or chronic illness. Treatment depends on the underlying cause.

Neuritis

A condition characterized by inflammation of a nerve. Nerve inflammation may be caused by an infection, such as the herpes zoster virus associated with SHINGLES. However, today the term "neuritis" typically refers to more general nerve damage and is

DEFECTS OF BRAIN AND SPINE

At an early point in fetal development, the flat strip of tissue along the back develops into a tube. For the spinal cord and brain to develop correctly, this tube must close. Most neural tube defects are caused by the incomplete closure of this tube, which creates openings in the skull or one or more sections of the spine.

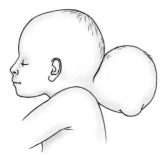

CRANIA BIFIDA
A defect in the skull during embryonic development allows the cranial meninges to herniate, or bulge.

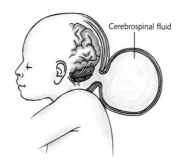

Cerebrospinal fluid

MENINGOCELE
A meningocele forms when the meninges protrude through an opening in the posterior part of the skull and fill with cerebrospinal fluid.

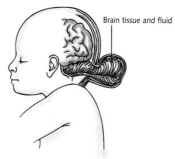

Brain tissue and fluid

ENCEPHALOCELE
An encephalocele forms when the meninges, brain tissue, and fluid protrude through an opening in the posterior part of the skull.

used synonymously with NEUROPATHY (disease, inflammation, or damage to any of the peripheral nerves that carry messages between the brain and spinal cord and the rest of the body).

Neuroblastoma

A cancerous tumor of the adrenal glands or sympathetic nervous system. Neuroblastoma, the fourth most common cancer in children, occurs most frequently in children younger than 5 years. Although the adrenal gland is the most common site, tumors may develop in the sympathetic nerve tissue located in the abdomen, pelvis, neck, or chest. Symptoms depend on the location of the tumor, but may include pain, paralysis, anemia, fever, and high blood pressure. Diagnosis of neuroblastoma is made through tests such as CT (computed tomography) scanning, MRI (magnetic resonance imaging), and biopsy. Additional tests may be performed to determine the stage of the cancer and its treatment. Options include surgical removal of the tumor, radiation therapy, chemother-

apy, and bone marrow transplantation. The outlook for recovery depends on factors such as the stage and location of the cancer and the age of the child. Infants younger than 1 year have the highest cure rate.

Neurodermatitis

Scaly plaques (patches of thick, raised skin) caused by vigorously scratching an itch. The skin becomes intensely irritated. Neurodermatitis is characterized by symptoms such as inflammation, itching, scaling, redness, blistering, oozing, and crusting. Chronic irritation leads to scratching, which causes further inflammation, scaling, and rawness. Eventually, skin may thicken and grow dry and leathery. Stress, environmental irritants, and dryness aggravate symptoms.

Diagnosis of neurodermatitis is based on the appearance of the skin. Very often the plaques are located in easily reached areas, such as the back of the neck and the outer part of the lower legs. Treatment depends on the severity of lesions and may include

avoiding irritants, using only mild soaps, and applying soothing lotions and topical corticosteroids.

Neuroendocrinology

The study of the interactions between the nervous system and the endocrine system. These two systems control many internal body functions and the manner in which the body responds to the external environ-

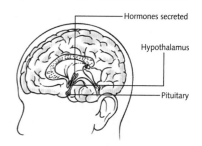

Hormones secreted

Hypothalamus

Pituitary

HORMONES AND NERVE ACTIVITY
The hypothalamus controls hormone secretion from the pituitary lobes. The brain organizes hormonal, behavioral, and involuntary responses to environment changes. Neuroendocrinologists study these functions and relationships with illness or aging.

N

ment. Hormones manufactured by the endocrine system affect many nervous system functions; special nerve cells called neurosecretory cells (located primarily in the hypothalamus) release hormones in response to stimulation by the nervous system. An example of the interaction between the two systems: stress is initially perceived by the nervous system, but it is the endocrine system that responds by releasing hormones from the pituitary and adrenal glands.

Neurofibromatosis

Genetic disorders characterized by changes in skin pigment, tumors growing on the nerves, and dysplasias (abnormal tissue development). Neurofibromatosis (NF) is known to exist in two forms, NF1 and NF2. Severity of symptoms can vary greatly, even between members of the same family. The disease can be severely disabling, be mildly disfiguring, or not cause any symptoms. NF is found in every racial and ethnic group and affects males and females equally. Both forms represent autosomal dominant genetic traits that can be inherited from one parent who has the disease. Both NF1 and NF2 can also appear in individuals without a family history of the disorder, as a result of spontaneous genetic mutations in either the sperm or egg cell. In the United States, one baby in every 4,000 is born with NF1; about 100,000 Americans have the disease at any given time. NF2, which is less common, occurs in one of every 40,000 births worldwide.

SYMPTOMS

A common early sign of NF1, also known as von Recklinghausen disease, is the presence of six or more tan spots on the skin, called café au lait (coffee with milk) spots. Often present at birth, the spots may increase in size and number with age, sometimes getting darker. Half of all affected children have signs of NF1 by age 2.

During adolescence, benign tumors begin to grow under the skin or deeper. Called neurofibromas, these tumors also grow on nerves and are made up of cells that normally surround the nerves. Neurofibromas can vary in size and may or may not be painful. An affected person can have anywhere from none to hundreds of neurofibromas. Tumors growing on the optic nerves can affect vision. Tiny tan tumors called Lisch nodules may appear on the iris of the eye beginning at age 6 to 10. These tumors usually cause no symptoms, but their presence suggests the diagnosis of NF1.

Most people with NF1 have mild symptoms and live a normal life. Some people have many neurofibromas on the face and body that appear as lumps, increasing in number during puberty and pregnancy as a result of hormonal changes. Scoliosis, or curvature of the spine, is common in NF. Children with NF1 may have learning disabilities, speech problems, and seizures; and they may have psychological problems related to their illness and deformities. Occasionally benign tumors may become malignant; regular examination by a physician is critical.

NF2 is associated with benign tumors that grow on the eighth cranial nerve (auditory nerve), one of 12 pairs of nerves serving the brain. The tumors, called schwannomas because they arise from Schwann cells, often put pressure on the auditory nerves, causing hearing loss, which is frequently the first symptom of the disease. Other symptoms include ringing in the ears, dizziness, or balance problems. Tumors may also develop in the brain or on the spinal cord, causing numbness, seizures, or headaches. Cataracts may develop at an early age.

People with NF2 rarely have café au lait spots or tumors under the skin; their symptoms may not emerge until after puberty. NF2 is also known as bilateral acoustic neurofibromatosis.

TREATMENT

There is no cure for NF. Treatment is directed at alleviating symptoms. Painful or disfiguring tumors on the skin can be removed surgically, although they may grow back. Tumors on the optic or auditory nerves that are causing symptoms can sometimes be removed or treated with chemotherapy or radiation. Scoliosis can be treated with surgery or by wearing a brace. The only treatments available for the tumors of NF2 are surgery and radiation therapy. Surgical removal of tumors on nerves in or near the brain or spinal cord may cause further injury to the nerves, with associated neurological problems. When surgery is not possible, radiation therapy is another option for treatment.

GENETIC TESTING

Genetic testing is available and can be used in some cases for prenatal diagnosis. It can also be used to help determine whether an individual with a family history of NF will develop the disease.

■ *Linkage analysis* This test is used for families with two or more affected members. The blood of all available family members is analyzed, tracking the chromosome that carries the relevant gene through two or more generations. Linkage testing is more than 95 percent accurate in predicting whether an individual will develop the disease.

■ *Direct gene mutation analysis* This test is used for one person and does not require the analysis of the blood of multiple family members. It is not useful in all cases, however, since it fails to detect one third of the mutations that cause NF1 and NF2. Genetic counseling may be helpful to people with NF who are thinking about having children.

Neurologist

A physician with specialized training in the diagnosis, treatment, and management of disorders of the brain and nervous system. In addition to 4 years of medical school and 1 year of an internship, neurologists have at least 3 more years of specialized training. Neurologists often act as principal care providers for people who have disorders such as epilepsy, multiple sclerosis, or Parkinson disease. In other cases, they act as consultants to primary care physicians. Neurologists do not perform surgery.

Neurology

The branch of medical science that deals with the diagnosis, treatment, and management of disorders of the brain and nervous system. Examples of neurological disorders include ALS (amyotrophic lateral sclerosis), Alzheimer's disease, brain tumors, epilepsy, headache, multiple sclerosis, Parkinson disease, peripheral nerve disorders, sleep disorders, spinal cord injuries, stroke, and tremor.

N

Neuroma

A noncancerous tumor composed of nerve cells and fibers. A neuroma may affect any nerve in the body. In most cases, the cause is unknown, but neuromas are often associated with neurofibromatosis (a rare genetic disorder characterized by noncancerous fibrous growths [neurofibromas] on the spinal cord and skin). Symptoms may include pain, numbness, and tingling in parts of the body supplied by the nerve. If the symptoms are troubling, the neuroma is surgically removed. See also ACOUSTIC NEUROMA.

Neuron

A nerve cell; the basic conducting cell of every structure in the NERVOUS SYSTEM. Neurons receive, interpret, and transmit information in the form of electrochemical impulses.

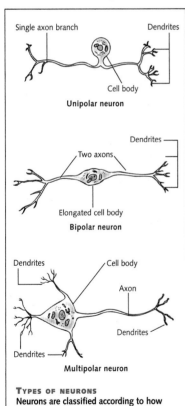

TYPES OF NEURONS
Neurons are classified according to how their dendrites (receiving signals) and axon (sending signals) are arranged. A unipolar neuron has one primary extension from the cell with an axon branch and dendrites. A bipolar cell has two axons extending from the cell with dendrites branching from one. Multipolar cells have one axon and multiple dendrites.

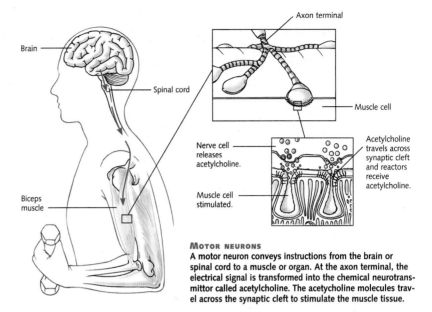

MOTOR NEURONS
A motor neuron conveys instructions from the brain or spinal cord to a muscle or organ. At the axon terminal, the electrical signal is transformed into the chemical neurotransmittor called acetylcholine. The acetycholine molecules travel across the synaptic cleft to stimulate the muscle tissue.

STRUCTURE

A typical neuron contains a nucleus and cytoplasm, contained within a cell membrane, where the basic functioning of the cell occurs. Extending from the body of the cell are branches called dendrites (from the Greek word for tree). These branches increase the surface area of the neuron to maximize the amount of information the cell can receive. A single long branch called the axon, actually an extension of the cell membrane, trails out from the main body of the cell. The axon carries signals from the neuron out to a particular site on an organ or tissue of the body. These axons bundle together to form nerve fibers, which are further bundled to form an individual NERVE.

The axon of many nerve cells is protected by the myelin sheath, which insulates the axon to promote faster, uninterrupted transmission. The end of the axon branches out into tiny filaments called terminal fibers. The end of each fiber is termed the synaptic knob.

FUNCTION

Each neuron receives input from many surrounding neurons through the dendrites, via chemicals called neurotransmitters. The neurotransmitters move from cell to cell across a tiny gap called a synapse. The neuron converts the chemical information into an electrical impulse that travels to the body of the cell. The neuron responds to this stimulus by firing an electrical charge down the length of its axon. At the end of the axon, the synaptic knobs release a chemical neurotransmitter to send the message to surrounding neurons. The response may be a signal to a muscle fiber or to a gland or organ.

An electrical charge can be transmitted because a resting neuron has a negative electrical charge. When it receives a stimulus, positively charged chemicals (neurotransmitters) emitted by other neurons enter the target neuron through the synaptic knobs. The positive charge moves along the dendrites to the cell body to cause the neuron to fire.

TYPES OF NEURONS

There are three types of neurons: motor neurons, sensory neurons, and interneurons. A motor neuron connects to a muscle or organ to convey instructions from the central nervous system (brain or spinal cord). A sensory neuron carries information about sensations such as heat, light, or sound waves to the central nervous system. An interneuron connects cells within the structures and pathways of the central nervous system.

Within the nervous system, there is another type of cell—not a nerve cell—that cannot transmit information. These so-called glial cells protect and nourish neurons, and they make proteins that stimulate the growth of neurons either during normal development or after injury. Glial cells form the myelin sheath that

N

insulates a nerve cell axon, and they help form scar tissue after injury.

Neurons do not divide and reproduce, so a dead nerve cell cannot be replaced. But glial cells help damaged neurons re-establish normal communication after injury, and nearby neurons can form alternative pathways to other nerve cells to maintain normal function after injury.

Neuropathic joint

Damage to the nerves of a joint, which may interfere with normal mobility and produce sensations of tingling, numbness, burning, or pain in the joint. A neuropathic joint may be the result of a sudden injury to the joint, prolonged pressure on a nerve of the joint, or the destruction of the nerve due to disease or poisoning. Because of loss of sensation, a neuropathic joint is easily damaged, and bony destruction can rapidly occur. Inherited disorders, nutritional deficiencies, alcoholism, syphilis, and diabetes mellitus may be associated with nerve damage.

Neuropathology

The study of disorders of the brain and nervous system. Neuropathology places a special emphasis on neurological causes and effects, especially the structural and functional changes caused by brain and nervous system disease. Neuropathologists are generally involved in research and diagnosis but not with treatment.

Neuropathy

Disease, inflammation, or damage to any of the peripheral nerves that carry messages between the brain and spinal cord and the rest of the body. The peripheral nervous system includes all nerves not in the brain or spinal cord. Neuropathy typically involves damage or injury to nerve cell axons (the conducting fibers that make up nerves) or the myelin sheaths that protect them. Neuropathy is not a specific disease, but a condition associated with many disorders, including vitamin and dietary deficiencies, diabetes, Friedreich ataxia, alcoholism, cancer, syphilis, thyroid disorders, and HIV (human immunodeficiency virus) infection.

Common symptoms of neuropathy include numbness, tingling, pain (NEURALGIA), abnormal or burning sen-

PERIPHERAL NERVE DAMAGE
In healthy nerve cells, transmission of a nerve impulse depends on the orderly interaction of the structures of the sending and receiving neurons. Injury, infection, toxic substances, hereditary disorders, or other problems can damage the nerve (neuropathy) and disrupt the connections.

Nucleus
Axon
Nissl substance
Glial cells
Cell body
Myelin sheath
Healthy nerve transmission

Cell breakdown
Damaged nerve
Transneuronal degeneration
Transneuronal degeneration
Terminal degeneration
Demyelination (myelin sheath breaks down)
Retraction of synaptic terminals
Nerve damage

sations, muscle weakness, and atrophy. There are different types of neuropathy. For example, entrapment neuropathy is characterized by compression of a single nerve where it passes through a narrow space. Polyneuropathy involves damage to multiple nerve endings as a result of a systemic illness. Diagnosis of neuropathy is made through neurological and muscular examination along with a detailed medical history. The doctor may also conduct tests such as an electromyogram (EMG), nerve conduction tests, a nerve biopsy, blood tests, and scans. Treatment depends on the underlying disease, but often includes pain medication, physical therapy, occupational therapy, and orthopedic surgery. Exercises may be helpful in increasing muscle strength and control, and some people benefit from devices such as splints, braces, or wheelchairs.

Neuropsychiatry

The branch of medicine that deals with the relationship between psychiatric symptoms and distinct neurological disorders. Typically, these are brain diseases such as infections, degenerative diseases, dementia, tumors, or temporal lobe epilepsy. Evidence indicates that subtle forms of brain damage may underlie certain psychotic illnesses. See also NEUROPSYCHOLOGICAL TESTING.

Neuropsychological testing

The administration of a set of standardized tests to examine the relationship between the brain and behavior. Neuropsychological testing measures brain dysfunction or damage. It focuses on higher cognitive functions than a regular neurological examination, which measures more elementary sensory and motor capacities. Neuropsychological testing may include tests of intelligence, mood, memory, organizational capacity, naming, and abstraction. It is a useful tool in the diagnosis and assessment of neurological disorders such as ALZHEIMER'S DISEASE, DEMENTIA, and LEARNING DISABILITIES and psychiatric disorders such as SCHIZOPHRENIA; however, it is important to note that neuropsychological testing alone is insufficient for diagnosis.

Neurosis

A term formerly used to describe mental disorders characterized by anxiety and avoidance. Typically, these disorders involve distressing symptoms, but the individual lives and functions normally and does not behave in a grotesque way. The person lacks a physical illness, such as brain damage, that causes the anxiety or avoidance.

In the psychoanalytic theory of Sigmund Freud, neurosis refers to any disorder in which unconscious emotional conflicts originating in childhood overwhelm the individual's mechanisms for defending the ego against them. The resulting anxiety expresses itself as abnormal fear (phobia), obsessive-compulsive disorder, anxiety disorder, depression, hysteria, or other illnesses.

Since the current classification of mental disorders uses symptoms rather than causes, neurosis no longer refers to one group of illnesses. The various neuroses are now known as ANXIETY DISORDERS, mood disorders (for example, depression), SOMATO-FORM DISORDERS, and DISSOCIATIVE DISORDERS.

Neurosurgery

Surgical treatment of the brain, spinal cord, or other parts of the nervous system. Conditions managed by neurosurgery include tumors of the brain, spinal cord, or meninges (the membranes that surround and protect the brain and spinal cord); an aneurysm (a weak point or bulge in an artery); brain abscess; hemorrhage; birth defects; or otherwise unmanageable pain.

Neurosyphilis

A progressive, destructive, life-threatening infection of the brain and spinal cord that occurs in some cases of untreated SYPHILIS. Neurosyphilis is a complication that develops many years after a primary syphilitic infection. It occurs more frequently in men than in women. There are four types of neurosyphilis: asymptomatic, meningovascular, tabes dorsalis, and general PARESIS. In asymptomatic neurosyphilis, there are abnormalities in cerebrospinal fluid, but no symptoms. Treatment at this time may prevent symptoms from developing.

Meningovascular neurosyphilis is characterized by pupillary abnormalities, cranial nerve palsies, and strokes. Blood vessels become inflamed by the infection and can narrow, causing stroke. In tabes dorsalis, there is syphilitic myelopathy (progressive degeneration of the spinal cord that can lead to an inability to walk) and additional symptoms of nerve damage. General paresis is characterized by dementia, tremors, seizures, and paralysis. This is caused by long-term brain damage from the infection.

Diagnosis of neurosyphilis is made through blood tests, such as a VDRL (Venereal Disease Research Laboratory) test or a rapid plasma reagin (RPR) test, lumbar puncture to analyze spinal fluid, CT (computed tomography) scanning or MRI (magnetic resonance imaging), and occasionally a cerebral angiogram. Treatment is with a long course of antibiotics, such as penicillin. Follow-up blood tests are required to make certain that the infection is gone.

Neurotoxin

A substance that damages nerve tissue. The principal effects of a neurotoxin are paralysis, numbness, or weakness in the part of the body supplied by the affected nerve. Neurotoxins are present in the venom of certain snakes and in shellfish that have eaten a poisonous dinoflagellate (a single-celled ocean algae). They are also released by certain types of bacteria, such as those that cause tetanus and diphtheria. Chemical poisons, such as arsenic and lead, are also neurotoxic.

Neurotransmitter

A nerve-signaling chemical in the brain. There are more than 50 different neurotransmitters. Their function is to carry nerve impulses across synapses (small gaps) between nerve cells (neurons). Neurotransmitters can either stimulate or inhibit electrical impulses. Examples of neurotransmitters include acetylcholine, dopamine, norepinephrine, and serotonin.

Nevirapine

An antiviral drug. Nevirapine (Viramune) is used alone or with other drugs to treat the infection caused by HIV (human immunodeficiency virus). Nevirapine helps to keep HIV from reproducing, thereby slowing its destruction of the immune system and delaying development of symptoms associated with AIDS (acquired immunodeficiency syndrome).

Nevus

See MOLE.

Newborn

A recently born infant.

NGU

See URETHRITIS, NONGONOCOCCAL.

Niacin

Also known as nicotinic acid or vitamin B3, a water-soluble vitamin of the B complex. (See VITAMIN B.) Niacin improves blood circulation by dilating arteries and is important for the skin, gastrointestinal tract, nervous system, and sex hormones. It is also a key element in the metabolism of nutrients such as carbohydrates and fats that create energy. Dietary sources of niacin include meats, poultry, fish, eggs, nuts, peanut butter, brewer's yeast, and wheat germ.

A deficiency of niacin can lead to symptoms such as weakness, fatigue, insomnia, irritability, tension, depression, nausea, vomiting, headaches, skin rashes, and tender gums. Severe deficiency causes pellagra, a disease characterized by dermatitis, diarrhea, and dementia. However, deficiency diseases such as pellagra are rare in the United States and other developed countries. In amounts available only by prescription, niacin lowers the levels of total and LDL (low-density lipoprotein) cholesterol and triglycerides. Some individuals are sensitive to high doses and respond with flushing of the skin. Niacin therapy is not recommended for individuals with diabetes because it may increase blood sugar levels.

Nicardipine hydrochloride

An antihypertensive drug. Nicardipine hydrochloride (Cardene) is used to treat high blood pressure and angina, chest pain caused by lack of oxygen to the heart. A calcium channel blocker, nicardipine hydrochloride reduces the workload of the heart by decreasing blood pressure and by widening the arteries to reduce the heart's workload.

Nickel

A metallic element that has a minor role in human nutrition. Nickel is a mineral of which people need only trace amounts for optimal health. It is thought to be involved in the body's use of fats and blood sugar (glucose). Nickel can be found in beans, vegetables, seafood, and grains. Nickel found in jewelry is one of the most common causes of a rash called CONTACT DER-

N

MATITIS. The amount of nickel found in a normal diet can vary, depending on the nickel content of the soil in which a person's food was grown.

A diet deficient in nickel produces few immediate symptoms, although it may aggravate anemia, a condition in which inadequate oxygen reaches the tissues. Too much nickel in the diet can be a serious problem, too. Toxic levels of nickel can cause headache, dizziness, vertigo, nausea, vomiting, chest pain, and coughing.

Nicotine gum

Smoking cessation chewing gum. Nicotine gum (Nicorette) is available without a prescription to help people quit smoking. As a person chews the gum, nicotine passes into the bloodstream through the lining of the mouth, reducing the withdrawal effects of not smoking.

Nicotine patch

A drug in patch form that helps people stop smoking. The nicotine in a nicotine patch passes through the skin into the bloodstream, taking the place of nicotine obtained by smoking in order to gradually reduce the physical withdrawal effects of not smoking. Nicotine patches (Nico-Derm, Nicotrol) are available with and without a prescription.

Nicotinic acid

See NIACIN.

Nifedipine

An antiangina, antihypertensive drug. Nifedipine (Adalat, Procardia) is used to treat high blood pressure and angina, chest pain caused by a lack of oxygen to the heart because of clogged arteries. Nifedipine is a calcium channel blocker that improves blood flow in the heart by dilating or widening the arteries to reduce the heart's workload.

Night blindness

Difficulty seeing in dim light. Night blindness primarily affects the person's ability to perform tasks such as driving a car after nightfall. The condition can be related to nearsightedness

Terms in small capital letters—for example, PHYSICAL THERAPY or PAGET DISEASE—indicate a cross-reference to another entry with more information.

or a birth defect, or it may be caused by a CATARACT (cloudiness in the lens of the eye), GLAUCOMA (an increase in fluid pressure within the eye causing damage to the optic nerve), or RETINITIS PIGMENTOSA (hereditary degeneration of the retina, the light-sensitive layer at the back of the eye). Night blindness can also be caused by a dietary deficiency in vitamin A (beta carotene), but this problem is rare in the United States. A person with night blindness should report the condition to his or her physician if it limits lifestyle or if it is accompanied by other unexplained symptoms.

Night sweats

HOT FLASHES that occur at night. Most women experience hot flashes, or sudden, brief increases in body temperature for about 1 to 2 years during MENOPAUSE. The effects of menopause are due to hormonal changes as the body begins to slow the production of estrogen. Hot flashes and night sweats vary greatly in intensity and frequency from woman to woman. In addition to an increase in the temperature of the skin, hot flashes cause a slight increase in the heart rate, which can lead to heart palpitations and dizziness. When night sweats occur, a woman may wake up drenched with sweat and have to change her nightclothes and bedding. Sweats may be followed by chills, and it may be difficult to get back to sleep. Estrogen or HORMONE REPLACEMENT THERAPY (HRT) is sometimes recommended for hot flashes and night sweats. For women who choose not to take HRT, other medications are available. In some cases, it is helpful to eliminate alcohol and beverages or foods containing caffeine. If anxiety is a trigger, stress reduction techniques may help.

Among the other causes of night sweats are tuberculosis, AIDS (acquired immunodeficiency syndrome), drug withdrawal, lymphomas, and bacterial and parasitic infections.

Night terror

An uncommon sleep disturbance experienced by children between ages 2 and 5. After an hour or two of sleep, a partially asleep child may sit up, scream, thrash about, kick, cry, or moan in fear and confusion. The physical signs of terror may include

sweating, shaking, a racing heart, bulging eyes, and heavy breathing. A child experiencing night terror may fail to recognize his or her parents and try to push them away. Night terrors may last from a few moments to 45 minutes. Parents are advised to remain calm, gently holding and comforting but not waking a child during a night terror. Afterward, the child will promptly return to sleep and have no later memory of the incident. A child who has frequent night terrors should be taken to see the family physician. Although frightening to parents, night terrors are not usually associated with severe problems and usually resolve as the child grows older. No treatment is typically needed.

Nightmare

A frightening dream that often causes the dreamer to awaken. Nightmares come during REM (rapid eye movement) sleep in the middle and later parts of the night. A nightmare can be a reaction to a medication, a scary movie, or a disturbing experience, such as a death of a loved one, accident, imprisonment, or war experiences. The nightmare will often clearly be remembered later if the dreamer has fully awakened. Nightmares are common for adults. A specific link between dreams and psychiatric illness has not been shown.

Children commonly experience nightmares, often as a result of a scary movie, television program, or story or in reaction to a disturbing event. Less frequently, a frightening dream occurs because a child is experiencing stress or abuse (see ABUSE, CHILD). Nightmares are most common in children younger than 6, although they can occur at any age. The child may wake up frightened, crying, and breathing rapidly. Unlike NIGHT TERROR (a sleep disturbance during which the child does not fully awaken), a child will usually remember a nightmare and may want to talk about it. He or she may be fearful and have trouble going back to sleep. Holding and comforting the child and providing reassurance of his or her safety will help overcome the effects of the nightmare. A nightlight may be helpful. Children who have frequent nightmares should see the family physician or pediatrician.

Nipple

The pigmented skin and tissue that projects from the middle of the BREAST. In women who are breast-feeding, the nipple is an outlet for milk ducts in the breast. The nipple has erectile tissue (meaning that it can fill with blood and become erect) and is sexually sensitive in women and in some men. The darker area of skin surrounding the nipple is called the areola.

Nit

The egg of a small insect, usually a louse. Head lice (see LICE, HEAD) live on the scalp and are spread through close contact, especially among school children. Nits are tiny lice eggs that look like small flakes of dandruff. However, unlike dandruff, they are firmly attached to hair shafts and do not flake off. Intense itching is the hallmark symptom of lice.

It is important to inspect the head of anyone who may have been exposed to lice. This is done by parting the hair into small sections and searching for moving insects and nits. Nits are commonly located around the nape of the neck and ears. Treatment is with over-the-counter or prescription shampoos and lotions. Nits must then be removed with a nit comb. If all nits are not removed, reinfestation can occur. To prevent reinfestation, it is also necessary to wash bed clothing, hats, combs, brushes, and other personal items in very hot water. Children should be encouraged to avoid sharing hats, combs, and brushes.

Nitrites

Food additives used to protect processed foods against bacterial growth and to preserve color and flavor. Nitrites are chemical salts of nitrous acid that are converted by the body into compounds called nitrosamines. Foods that contain nitrites include bacon, ham, and pickles. Because laboratory animals have developed tumors after consuming large amounts of nitrites, there has long been concern that nitrites may cause cancer in humans, especially stomach cancer. The evidence so far is inconclusive, although fresh foods are generally preferable to processed ones. The need for nitrites has been reduced over the years because of refrigeration.

An organic form of nitrite is used as a coronary vasodilator, a drug that increases blood flow by widening the arteries, and for the treatment of angina pectoris, which is chest pain caused when arteries are unable to deliver enough blood to the heart.

Nitrofurantoin

An anti-infective drug. Nitrofurantoin (Furadantin, Macrodantin) is used to treat infections of the urinary tract. It is thought to work by stopping bacterial cell wall formation and interfering with bacterial metabolism of carbohydrates.

Nitrogen

A colorless, gaseous element found in the air. Nitrogen forms about four fifths of the Earth's atmosphere. Nitrogen is a constituent of protein and nucleic acids and is therefore present in all living cells. Nitrogen is responsible for a serious condition (the bends, compressed air illness, or decompression sickness), which afflicts deep-sea divers and is caused when nitrogen dissolved in the bloodstream expands to form bubbles on return to normal atmospheric conditions.

Nitroglycerin

An antiangina drug. Nitroglycerin (Deponit, Nitro-Dur, Nitrolingual, Nitrostat, Minitran, and others) is used to treat the symptoms of angina (chest pain). Nitroglycerin is used in four ways. It relieves the pain of angina when it is taken at the beginning of an attack; prevents pain when taken before an attack is expected; reduces the number of episodes when taken on a regular basis; and treats congestive heart failure.

Nitroglycerin is available in different forms. It is sometimes placed under the tongue, under the lip, or in the cheek. In paste form it can be placed directly on the chest and covered. Nitroglycerin works by relaxing blood vessels to increase the supply of blood and oxygen to the heart and by reducing the heart's workload. Side effects include headache and low blood pressure.

Nitrosamines

Chemical compounds that may have a role in cancer cell formation. Nitrosamines are formed in the stomach and intestines through reactions of nitrites and proteins. Nitrites are produced from nitrates that are naturally present in vegetables or added as preservatives to meat, poultry, and fish. Antioxidants, which interfere with the formation of nitrosamines, can prevent this conversion from taking place and may offer protection against some cancers.

Nizatidine

An antiulcer drug. Nizatidine (Axid) is a histamine$_2$ (H$_2$)-receptor antagonist, or H$_2$-blocker, used to treat duodenal ulcers and prevent their return. It is also used for certain conditions in which the stomach produces too much acid.

Nocardiosis

An uncommon infection that may be acute or chronic and is caused by the bacterium *Nocardia asteroides*, which is found in the soil in areas of decaying plants. Nocardiosis is usually transmitted via inhalation of bacteria into the lungs. In rare instances, bacteria may enter the body through the gastrointestinal tract or the skin. Infection occurs worldwide, most often among older men. Underlying lung disease, organ transplantation, certain malignant tumors, and immunosuppressive therapies increase the risk of contracting nocardiosis. It can be an OPPORTUNISTIC INFECTION in people with advanced HIV (human immunodeficiency virus) infection or malignant tumors, in organ transplant recipients, and in people taking corticosteroids.

The disease generally begins as a lung infection, but may also occur initially as an abscess on the skin. When lesions form on the lungs, the symptoms can include cough, fever, chills, chest pain, weakness, loss of appetite, and weight loss. If abscesses form on the brain, they produce severe headache and cause nerve abnormalities. Nocardiosis is diagnosed by identifying the bacteria in tissues from lesions, which may be done by physical examination, X ray, or other imaging techniques.

Specific antibacterial antibiotics are used to treat the disease; this treatment is most successful with otherwise healthy people whose lesions have not spread beyond the lungs. Treatment is generally prolonged and

N

may last for several months. Surgery may be needed to drain abscesses. People who have a generalized, system-wide infection and receive antibiotic therapy have the poorest prognosis among infected people who are treated. Untreated, nocardiosis is usually fatal.

Nocturia

The need to urinate during the night. Nocturia is common in older people because as a person ages, the kidneys are less able to concentrate urine. Pregnant women urinate more often because the enlarged uterus presses on the bladder. Nocturia can also be caused by excessive fluid intake before bedtime, particularly alcohol, coffee, or caffeinated soft drinks. The condition may also be a symptom of other diseases, such as an enlarged prostate, infection of the bladder, kidney failure, or congestive heart failure.

Nocturnal emission

Involuntary ejaculation of semen (the sperm-containing fluid expelled from a man during sexual climax) during sleep. Nocturnal emissions are normal in adolescent boys and men who do not have sex. Since they are often accompanied by erotic dreams, nocturnal emissions are known as "wet dreams."

Node

A small mass of tissue that may feel or look like a swelling or knot; most commonly refers to a lymph node, which is part of a person's immune system. A mass of tissue that is abnormal is often called a nodule.

Nodule

A round, solid mass of tissue that may protrude from or be lodged deep within the skin.

Nodule, cold

A growth on the thyroid gland that does not absorb radioactive iodine during a DIAGNOSTIC IMAGING procedure called radioactive iodine uptake. A cold nodule does not absorb radioactive iodine because it is composed of nonfunctioning thyroid tissue, which does not attract or hold iodine. Nonfunctional nodules containing a gelatinous substance or consisting of cancer cells do not

absorb radioactive iodine and are not detected on the thyroid scan.

Radioactive iodine uptake is performed to determine if a thyroid nodule makes or does not make thyroid hormone. The person being tested drinks a small amount of radioactive iodine. He or she then reclines under a special camera that scans the thyroid gland and detects any areas of the thyroid gland that have absorbed the iodine.

Cold nodules can be further evaluated in a procedure called fine-needle aspiration, which permits the tissue that is withdrawn to be examined for cancer cells.

Nodule, hot

A growth on the thyroid gland that absorbs radioactive iodine during a DIAGNOSTIC IMAGING procedure called radioactive iodine uptake. A hot nodule absorbs radioactive iodine because it is composed of functioning thyroid tissue, which attracts and holds iodine. This generally indicates that the tissue is not cancerous.

Radioactive iodine uptake is performed to determine if a thyroid nodule makes or does not make thyroid hormone. The person being tested drinks a small amount of radioactive iodine. He or she then reclines under a special camera that scans the thyroid gland and detects any areas of the thyroid gland that have absorbed the iodine. Because hot nodules are made up of extra thyroid tissue that is functioning, they may produce excess amounts of the thyroid hormone THYROXINE, resulting in HYPERTHYROIDISM (overactivity of the thyroid gland).

Noise pollution

See POLLUTION, NOISE.

Nonalcoholic steatohepatitis

An inflammation of the liver that resembles alcoholic liver disease, but is not caused by alcohol. It may occur in a person with fatty liver, cirrhosis, and other forms of hepatitis. Nonalcoholic steatohepatitis (NASH) may be the most common liver disorder in the United States.

Nonconsensual sex

Sexual contact without mutual consent. Nonconsensual sex may range

from forced touching or fondling to RAPE.

Nongonococcal urethritis

See URETHRITIS, NONGONOCOCCAL.

Noninvasive

A term describing a medical procedure that does not involve penetration of the skin or entry into the body through one of the natural openings.

Nonnucleoside reverse transcriptase inhibitors (NNRTIs)

Anti-AIDS (acquired immunodeficiency syndrome) drugs. NNRTIs are a class of drugs being used in combination with nucleoside analogue drugs, such as zidovudine (AZT), ddI (didanosine), and others. NNRTIs work by blocking the ability of HIV (human immunodeficiency virus) to infect new cells; this is accomplished by preventing viruses from replicating.

NNRTIs are being used in combination with nucleoside analogues because the HIV develops resistance to the nucleoside analogue drugs in just a few weeks when they are used alone. NNRTIs are used to prevent resistance and limit side effects. The Food and Drug Administration has approved three NNRTIs for use in the treatment of HIV, always in combination with other antiretroviral drugs: delavirdine (Rescriptor), efavirenz (Sustiva), and nevirapine (Viramune).

Nonprescription drugs

Drugs that are available without a doctor's prescription. Nonprescription drugs, also called over-the-counter (OTC) drugs, tend to be medications that relieve minor symptoms at doses that are effective and safe. Nonprescription drugs are relatively inexpensive. Sixty percent of the medications purchased in the United States are nonprescription drugs.

Nonsteroidal anti-inflammatory drugs

Drugs used to relieve symptoms associated with arthritis and other painful conditions. Nonsteroidal anti-inflammatory drugs, or NSAIDs, are used to

> ### UNDERSTANDING NSAIDs
>
> Prostaglandins are substances produced by the body that can cause pain and inflammation. Nonsteroidal anti-inflammatory drugs (NSAIDs) work to block the formation of prostaglandins in the body, thus easing unpleasant symptoms. Most NSAIDs can also reduce temperature in a person with fever. Examples of over-the-counter NSAIDs include aspirin, ibuprofen (Advil, Motrin), and naproxen (Aleve).
>
> Not all NSAIDs work in the same way; the drugs also affect people differently. Benefits reported by one person may or may not be experienced by another person who takes the same medication. The same can be said for side effects experienced.
>
> Some side effects include stomach upset, easy bruising, high blood pressure, and water retention. A person taking NSAIDs may also feel drowsy and have a headache, but those side effects are usually mild. If symptoms are severe, the medication may need to be discontinued.
>
> Another common side effect from NSAIDs is stomach inflammation (gastritis) or gastric ulcers. Some NSAIDs may irritate the stomach, while other brands may not. Bleeding in the stomach from ulcers can lead to anemia, so it is important that the person take the medication with food. Sometimes, other medications may be prescribed to counteract the unpleasant side effects of the NSAIDs. People with peptic ulcers or duodenal ulcers should not take NSAIDs without first consulting a doctor.

relieve inflammation, swelling, stiffness, and joint pain. They are also used to treat attacks of gout; bursitis; tendinitis; sprains, strains, or other injuries; and menstrual cramps. In addition to their pain-relieving properties, some NSAIDs, including aspirin and ibuprofen, have fever-reducing properties. There are many brands of NSAIDs in both prescription and over-the-counter formulations.

Nonstress test

In pregnancy, external monitoring of a fetus, using ultrasound (see ULTRASOUND, OBSTETRICAL). A nonstress test is painless and requires no drugs or anesthesia. It can be performed in the doctor's office or in a hospital labor room and takes between 20 and 40 minutes. A belt with an electronic monitor is placed on the woman's abdomen for about 20 minutes, during which the fetal heart rate is measured and recorded on a long strip of paper. The nonstress test shows whether the baby is reactive, meaning that its heart speeds up in response to a uterine contraction or its own movements, or nonreactive, meaning the heart rate neither varies nor speeds up with a contraction or movement. Only about 20 percent of nonreactive babies are actually in danger. If a baby has a nonreactive nonstress test, the doctor may perform a CONTRACTION STRESS TEST, in which contractions are induced in the mother's uterus while the baby's heart is monitored.

The nonstress test is used to monitor the well-being of the fetus. Common indications for the test include a fetus that is more than 2 weeks past its due date, that is suspected to be of low birth weight, that is at risk for SICKLE CELL ANEMIA, or that has decreased its movements. A nonstress test may be given if twins or other multiple pregnancies are expected or when a woman has TOXEMIA OF PREGNANCY, high blood pressure, diabetes, heart or lung disease, lupus, or third-trimester bleeding. A woman who is over age 40 and pregnant for the first time or who has had a history of miscarriages, fertility problems, or other gynecological disorders will also be tested. Women with diabetes or heart disease may expect to have the test repeated weekly from 34 weeks until delivery. See also PRENATAL TESTING.

Nonunion

A condition in which a fractured bone fails to heal, preventing the fragments of bone from forming an uninterrupted, anatomically correct structure. Fracture nonunions are more common among adults and tend to occur more often among smokers. The bone of the upper arm and the shinbone are commonly affected. Open fractures, multiple crush fractures, and the removal of bone tumors may produce nonunion of bones. Nonunions may be treated surgically, with bone grafts, or with devices that encourage healing through electrical

stimulation of the bones. Clinical studies are underway on injectable compounds that could glue or paste the broken bone segments together.

Norepinephrine

One of the two principal hormones synthesized by the adrenal medulla (the inner layer of the adrenal glands). Norepinephrine and EPINEPHRINE regulate heart rate and blood pressure. They stimulate the sympathetic nervous system, the part of the autonomic nervous system that predominates at times of stress. The two hormones are largely responsible for the fight-or-flight response and help the body resist stress.

Nortriptyline

An antidepressant. Nortriptyline (Aventyl, Pamelor) is thought to work by increasing the amount of brain chemicals, particularly serotonin and norepinephrine, which improve a person's mood. Nortriptyline is one of the tricyclic antidepressants.

Nose

The facial structure that is the main organ of SMELL and the primary opening into the RESPIRATORY SYSTEM.

The supporting bones of the nose, the nasal bones, protrude from the skull. The nose is not actually a part of the skull, but is made up of a number of cartilages that attach to the nasal bones. The central piece of cartilage, called the nasal septum, splits the cavity inside the nose in half and contains arteries, nerves, and veins. The area immediately inside, lined with mucous membranes and nasal hair, is called the vestibule.

The two passages of the nose lead into the nasal cavity just inside the head. On the walls of the nasal cavity are the conchae, bony, shell-like protrusions that increase the surface area of the space and contain mucous glands. The nasal cavity is defined by the bones of the skull, upper jaw, and hard palate. The bones surrounding the nasal cavity contain membrane-lined spaces called the paranasal sinuses. At the back of the nasal cavity is the nasopharynx, which connects with the upper part of the throat and contains the openings of the eustachian tubes leading to the inner ear.

One of the principal functions of the nose is to cleanse inhaled air.

N

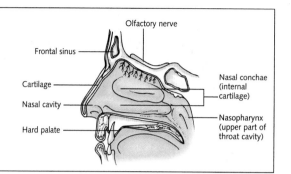

ANATOMY OF THE NOSE
The structures of the nose function in both the mechanical act of breathing and the sensory perception of smell. The sinus cavities of the nose are lined with mucous membranes to cleanse inhaled air. The olfactory nerve interprets specific sensations of smell to be carried to the brain.

Olfactory nerve
Frontal sinus
Cartilage
Nasal cavity
Hard palate
Nasal conchae (internal cartilage)
Nasopharynx (upper part of throat cavity)

Particles in the air entering the nose are trapped in the mucus and nasal hairs. The nasal conchae continue this filtering process. The air is warmed and moistened as it passes through the nasal cavity, and unwanted debris is sneezed or blown out of the nose, or it passes into the nasopharynx to be swallowed and neutralized in the digestive tract. From the nasopharynx, air passes into the pharynx and on into the trachea.

The air brought into the nose also stimulates the sense of smell. Nerve endings in the nasal cavity, called olfactory (pertaining to the sense of smell) receptors, lie just above the airstream in the upper part of each nostril. The tails of these receptors form a nerve pathway to the olfactory bulb in the brain. These receptors detect chemical vapors in the environment and pass the sensory input to the olfactory bulb, which interprets the stimuli as smells. The sense of smell is closely related to taste, the other sense that responds to chemical stimuli. The olfactory bulb is close to the area of the brain concerned with emotions and memory, so the sense of smell is evocative of past experiences.

The chambers of the nose, including the nasal sinuses, also function as resonating chambers for speech production. Air passing out of the nose during speech produces the nasal speech sounds.

Nose reshaping

A surgical procedure to change the shape and contour of the nose. Also known as a rhinoplasty, a nose reshaping can be performed to enhance the appearance of a person, to correct breathing problems, to repair damage from an injury or accident, or to correct a birth defect. A reshaping can make the nose larger or smaller, alter the shape of the bridge or tip, narrow the distance between the nostrils, or change its angle to the upper lip.

THE PROCEDURE
A nose reshaping is often done in the office of a physician or an outpatient surgery center as AMBULATORY SURGERY, with the patient returning home the same day. Complicated procedures may require a 1- or 2-night hospital stay. The surgery usually takes 1 to 2 hours, with complex reshapings requiring more time.

Anesthesia can be by either a local, combined with CONSCIOUS SEDATION, or a general anesthetic. With local anesthesia and conscious sedation, the patient is numb around the nose and awake but relaxed and insensitive to pain. General anesthesia puts the patient to sleep. The choice of anesthesia depends on the complexity of the procedure and the preferences of the surgeon and patient.

HOW IT IS DONE
The surgeon will elevate and then separate the skin of the nose from the bone and cartilage, which are then reshaped. The incision is made either inside the nostrils or through the strip of skin that separates the nostrils. The surgeon then chisels or files away bone and cartilage and then brings the nasal bones together. To narrow the bridge of the nose, the surgeon will trim cartilage from the tip of the nose. The skin is then draped over the reshaped bone and cartilage, and the incisions are closed with small sutures. A splint of plastic, metal, or plaster is taped onto the nose to hold it in shape. Nasal packing or soft plastic splints may be inserted into the nostrils to keep the SEPTUM (the wall that divides the nostrils) in place.

BEFORE AND AFTER SURGERY
As is true of all surgeries with anesthesia, the person may not eat or drink after midnight the night

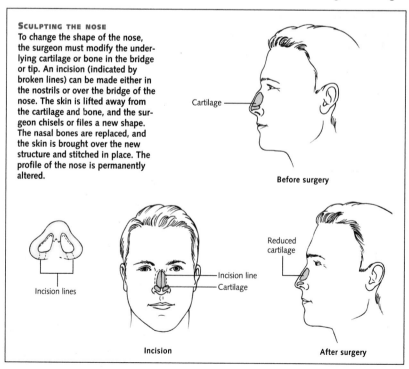

SCULPTING THE NOSE
To change the shape of the nose, the surgeon must modify the underlying cartilage or bone in the bridge or tip. An incision (indicated by broken lines) can be made either in the nostrils or over the bridge of the nose. The skin is lifted away from the cartilage and bone, and the surgeon chisels or files a new shape. The nasal bones are replaced, and the skin is brought over the new structure and stitched in place. The profile of the nose is permanently altered.

Cartilage

Before surgery

Incision lines

Incision line
Cartilage

Incision

Reduced cartilage

After surgery

N

before the procedure. The surgeon may also advise adding or avoiding certain medications or vitamins in advance of surgery. Blood and urine tests may be required before surgery to screen for undetected diseases that may affect safety and outcome, such as high blood pressure or diabetes.

For the first day after surgery, the face feels puffy and the nose is sore and achy. There may also be a dull headache. Oral pain medication, prescribed by the surgeon, should control this discomfort. Swelling and bruising peak after 2 or 3 days. Cold compresses or ice bags, applied to the nose, decrease the swelling and reduce pain. Most of the swelling disappears within 2 weeks, although a small amount, usually noticeable only to the surgeon and the patient, can remain for several months. Given the slowness of healing, the nose may not reach its final shape for up to a year.

Nasal packing is removed after a few days. Stitches and splints are removed after 1 week. If dissolvable sutures have been used, they will disappear in the same period.

The first day after surgery should be spent resting, with the head elevated. Most patients are up and around in 2 days, and they can return to sedentary work within several days. Any strenuous activity that raises blood pressure poses a risk for bleeding in the nose and should be avoided for 1 week. The patient also needs to protect the nose from being struck and to avoid sunburn and rubbing or blowing the nose for up to 8 weeks.

Contact lenses can be worn almost immediately after surgery, but eyeglasses pose a problem. After the splint is removed, glasses can be taped to the forehead or propped on the cheeks.

Infection following a nose reshaping is unusual. The procedure carries a small risk of NOSEBLEED. Scarring is rarely a problem when external incisions are used. Very small red spots caused by burst blood vessels may appear on the surface of the skin that covers the nose; sometimes, the spots are permanent. In a minority of cases, some cosmetic flaw remains, and follow-up surgery may be needed to correct it.

Nose, broken

A FRACTURE of the nose. A broken nose, the most common facial fracture, is usually caused by a blunt injury. Symptoms include pain, bleeding, swelling, bruising, signs of trauma, and a misshapen appearance. Ice packs should be placed over the bridge of the nose to help reduce swelling. Serious nose injuries require medical attention. A person who might have a broken nose should not try to straighten his or her own nose. Rhinoplasty, or NOSE RESHAPING, is often performed to repair damage that results from an injury.

Nosebleed

A flow of blood from the nose, a frequent occurrence in children between ages 2 and 10. Also called epistaxis, a nosebleed is commonly due to dryness caused by low humidity in the home or to nose picking. Other causes include inflammation of the nasal lining from a cold or allergies, a foreign object in the nose, blowing the nose too hard, or falling on or hitting the nose. Rarely, abnormal growths or a problem with blood clotting causes nosebleeds. Although nosebleeds may be frightening, they are usually not a serious cause for concern. When a child has a nosebleed, parents or caretakers should remain calm and avoid further alarming the child.

Minor nosebleeds can be treated at home. A person with a nosebleed should sit straight up and tip his or her head forward, so that blood will not flow down the throat. The individual should not lie down or tilt his or her head back. The sides of the nose should be pinched together for 10 to 15 minutes, while the person breathes through the mouth. Afterwards, an ice pack can be applied to the nose.

If bleeding continues despite these measures, a doctor should be consulted. The doctor may cauterize the problem-causing blood vessel with silver nitrate, a chemical substance (see CAUTERIZATION), or pack the nose with gauze to stop the bleeding. If the bleeding is coming from the back part of the nose, in either a child or adult, a posterior pack is needed. A posterior pack applies pressure to blood vessels deep in the nasal cavity. In this situation, hospitalization is generally required. A child or adult who has

very frequent nosebleeds or whose nosebleed was caused by an injury or is accompanied by dizziness should see a physician.

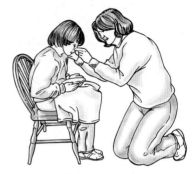

TREATING A NOSEBLEED
A person with a nosebleed should sit straight up and lean only the head forward, pinching the nostrils shut and breathing through his or her mouth. This posture prevents the blood from flowing into the throat. After 10 or 15 minutes, the nostrils can be opened slowly, and any accumulated blood can drain out into a bowl. The person should not lie down or tilt his or her head back.

Nosocomial infections

Infections that are acquired by people while they are hospitalized. To be categorized as nosocomial, the infection must not be present and the causative organisms must not be incubating at the time a person is admitted to the hospital. Symptoms of a nosocomial infection may not occur during hospitalization, but may appear after a person's discharge. When the incubation period of a disease is known, this time frame is used to determine whether symptoms that occur in a person during hospitalization were produced by a previous infection or one acquired in the hospital. When the incubation period is not known and symptoms occur during hospitalization, the infection is deemed to be nosocomial.

Nosocomial infections may include a wide range of infectious diseases. They may be transmitted directly or indirectly from one person to another. They may develop from microorganisms that routinely exist as part of the person's normal bacteria or as part of the hospital environment, and they are not usually disease-producing, but cause disease in the setting of illness and invasive procedures such as surgery and intravenous catheters.

Recent reports of infections occurring during hospitalization reveal that the greatest percentage of them involved the urinary tract, with lesser numbers involving the lower respiratory tract, surgical wounds, primary bacterial infections, and infections of the skin. Most reported nosocomial infections were caused by a single pathogen such as *Escherichia coli, Staphylococcus* bacteria, or *Pseudomonas aeruginosa.*

HOW THE INFECTIONS OCCUR

Certain features of the hospital environment may contribute to the occurrence of nosocomial infections. First, a large number and variety of microorganisms are likely to be found in a hospital setting. This is in part because people in varying stages of health are gathered into one small environment. Some of these people are apt to have infections acquired outside the hospital, with or without symptoms.

Care of hospitalized patients involves close contact with body fluids and excretions, which increases the risk of transmission of infectious agents from one person to another and to surfaces within the hospital environment. The increase in hospitals of strains of bacteria that resist antibiotics indicates that more virulent kinds of pathogens are developing in this environment. The large amounts of food, equipment, and biologic materials found in hospitals also provide many potential reservoirs where microorganisms can grow.

In addition, a person's immune system may be compromised as a result of disease or the treatments the person receives in the hospital. This makes the person more susceptible to infection by normally occurring microorganisms, opportunistic organisms in the environment, and pathogens. Many diagnostic and treatment procedures are invasive (for example, surgery or various forms of ENDOSCOPY), which enhances the opportunities for microorganisms to infect people who are hospitalized and receiving these procedures.

INFECTION CONTROL

The primary element in controlling nosocomial infections is preventing transmission as early as possible. How this is done depends on the disease process and the causative microorganism. Sterilization and disinfection are the standard tools for avoiding contamination and preventing infection. Limiting the exposure of hospitalized patients to visitors who may be infected is important, as is providing prompt antibiotic therapy for patients and hospital staff when bacterial infections occur.

Procedures to isolate patients with a contagious disease and to take precautions in handling patients' secretions and excretions are essential to controlling nosocomial infections. Hospital personnel must thoroughly wash hands between contacts with patients. Special care should be taken with medical devices such as intravenous catheters, urinary catheters, and endotracheal tubes, all of which have the capacity to introduce infection. Attention should be given to environmental air control, procedures involving sanitation and waste disposal, proper laundering procedures, and safe handling of specimens. In certain settings, medical workers should wear hospital gowns and use gloves when caring for patients.

People who have immunodeficiency diseases and conditions or are receiving immunosuppression treatments are at high risk for infection and require protective isolation. Sterile techniques and recommended procedures to minimize infection must be adhered to when treating these patients.

Other approaches to control infection include limited hospital stays before surgery, the use of preventative antibiotics when appropriate, the use of disposable equipment whenever possible, and the use of available vaccines against particular infections.

NSAIDs

See NONSTEROIDAL ANTI-INFLAMMATORY DRUGS.

Nuclear medicine

The branch of diagnostic and therapeutic RADIOLOGY that involves the use of very small amounts of radioactively tagged compounds, called radionuclides or radioisotopes, to create images of parts of the body and visualize biochemical processes within the body. These compounds

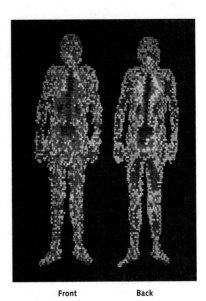

Front   Back

IMAGING BODY FUNCTION
These scans of a healthy man injected with a radioactive isotope demonstrate how the isotope concentrates in certain body structures. The way in which different organs and structures absorb the isotope reveals information about how the body functions and processes are working.

can be injected, ingested, or inhaled. Nuclear medicine enables physicians to obtain information about organ function, blood flow, and other physiologic activity. This form of relatively noninvasive imaging can be used as an initial procedure to determine the need for additional procedures that may be more invasive.

Specific radioactive compounds are administered according to the organ targeted for examination. For example, radioactive iodine localizes in the thyroid and radioactive thallium localizes in the heart. Once the radionuclide has been taken up by the organ to be examined, a gamma camera is used to measure and record the gamma rays emanating from that organ. This information is translated electronically into an image that is reproduced on film.

A nuclear imaging machine uses a scintillation camera that rotates around the body to pick up radiation given off by the radionuclide. A computer then produces a digitized image of the organ being examined. PET SCANNING (positron emission tomography scanning) uses radionuclides to allow visualization of the distribution of molecules so that real-time observations of biochemical processes can be made.

Nuclear medicine scans may be used to diagnose a wide variety of medical conditions. These include bone scans to diagnose injuries, fractures, tumors, or unexplained pain; heart scans to evaluate blood flow to the heart muscle, measure the function of the heart, or evaluate damage after a heart attack; renal imaging in children to evaluate kidney function; and brain imaging to investigate problems such as blood circulation to the brain. The thyroid gland and lungs may be evaluated, and gastrointestinal bleeding may be detected by means of nuclear medicine.

Nuclear medicine is sometimes used therapeutically; radioiodine is given as a treatment for thyroid disorders. Certain antibodies can be engineered to bind with a specific protein on malignant (cancerous) tumor cells and combined with radionuclides to be injected into the person with the tumor. When the antibodies bind with the tumor cells, the radionuclides destroy these cells without harming nearby normal cells. Radionuclides are also used in biomedical research to identify and learn how genes work.

Nucleic acids

The two organic acids found in all living cells. Nucleic acids include DNA (deoxyribonucleic acid) and RNA (ribonucleic acid), both of which are present in the NUCLEUS and in some cases in the cytoplasm (the fluid surrounding the nucleus) of every living cell. The chief functions of the nucleic acids are in protein synthesis (RNA) and heredity (DNA).

Nucleus

The portion of a living cell that contains DNA (deoxyribonucleic acid) and RNA (ribonucleic acid). The nucleus of a cell controls its metabolism, growth, and reproduction. The nucleus is separated from the surrounding cytoplasm by a double membrane called a nuclear envelope.

Numbness

Partial or total loss of sensation in part of the body that is caused by interference with the passage of impulses along sensory nerves. Numbness suggests that the affected nerve is damaged. It is a more serious condition than TINGLING or a PINS AND NEEDLES SENSATION, which suggest that a nerve is compressed but not damaged. Possible causes of numbness include nerve injury; lack of blood supply; diabetes mellitus, type 1 and type 2; thyroid problems; vitamin B12 (cyanocobalamin) deficiency; carpal tunnel syndrome; transient ischemic attack; stroke; and multiple sclerosis. Numbness may also be caused by damage to the spinal cord or sensory processing systems in the brain.

Nurse

A person trained in NURSING CARE. Nurses work in hospitals, nursing facilities, clinics, birth centers, physicians' offices, schools, workplaces, and home-care settings. Registered nurses (RNs) are licensed by the state to care for the sick and promote health. Other types of nurses include nurse practitioners, who usually provide health services under the supervision of a physician; nurse-midwives, who are specially trained in prenatal and postnatal care and delivery; and licensed practical nurses (LPNs), who provide basic care under the supervision of RNs and doctors. Nurses' aides assist nurses in the provision of care.

Nurse anesthetist

A nurse trained and qualified to administer anesthetic agents. Nurse anesthetists assess patients scheduled for anesthesia, develop treatment plans, administer and maintain anesthesia during surgery, and oversee the person's recovery following surgery. Nurse anesthetists, designated by CRNA (certified registered nurse anesthetist), have completed 2 to 3 years of training in anesthesia at the master's degree level. They must pass a national examination to become a CRNA. Under the laws of most states, nurse anesthetists practice under the supervision of a physician, usually an ANESTHESIOLOGIST.

Nurse practitioner

Also known as an NP, an advanced practice NURSE specially trained for a role in primary care. Types of nurse practitioners include family nurse practitioners, pediatric nurse practitioners, school nurse practitioners, adult nurse practitioners, women's health care nurse practitioners, and geriatric nurse practitioners. Most NPs today have graduate degrees from special nurse practitioner programs and work alongside physicians. However, regulations governing the profession vary from state to state. National certification is available through a number of nursing organizations, which usually require completion of an approved master's-level NP program before taking the certification examination.

Nursemaid elbow

Also known as pulled elbow, a painful injury in which nearby soft tissue slips into the elbow joint and is trapped there. Nursemaid elbow is most common among children under age 4. The injury can occur when a small child is lifted, yanked, or swung by the hand or wrist or falls on his or her outstretched arm. A suspected nursemaid elbow injury should promptly be supported by a sling and examined by a doctor. The doctor will check the area for pain, swelling, tenderness, and range of motion. X rays may be taken to rule out a fracture. If there is no fracture, the doctor will carefully manipulate the elbow joint to release the trapped tissue. While this procedure is

N

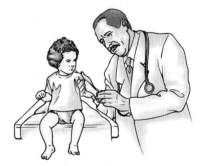

NURSEMAID OR PULLED ELBOW
A nursemaid elbow is a painful injury in which soft tissue is pinched in the elbow joint. The injury is so called because it most often occurs in children younger than 4 years who are lifted or yanked by the hand or arm. It can also result from a fall on an outstretched arm. If a child appears to have such an injury, the arm should be put in a sling, and the child should be taken to a doctor immediately.

painful, relief is immediate. If several hours have passed before the injured elbow is treated, the person may have to wear a sling for 2 or 3 days to allow the bruised tissue to heal.

Nurse-midwife

An advanced practice nurse specializing in women's health care needs, including prenatal care, labor and delivery, and postpartum care. Nurse-midwives work in health maintenance organizations, private practices, public health clinics, and birth centers. Some provide home birth services. Most nurse-midwives work in collaboration with doctors. Nurse-midwives usually work with women with low-risk pregnancies, while women at higher risk are more likely to see doctors. National certification is available through a number of nursing organizations, which usually require completion of an approved master's-level program before taking the certification examination. Certified nurse-midwives are known as CNMs.

Nursing

See BREAST-FEEDING.

Nursing care

The process by which a person is helped by a NURSE to recover from an illness or injury or to regain as much health and independence as possible. Nurses work closely with physicians and other health care professionals to care for the sick and promote health. Nursing care takes place in hospitals, nursing facilities, clinics, birth centers, physicians' offices, schools, workplaces, and home-care settings.

Nursing facility

Formerly known as a nursing home, a facility that offers a combination of housing, personal services, and health care to older or disabled people who are unable to care for themselves independently. Today a wide spectrum of nursing facilities is designed to fit different levels of needs. Assisted living and residential care models are geared toward people who must give up household chores but do not require continuous medical attention. The goal in these facilities is to provide maximum independence in a homelike environment.

Intermediate care facilities (ICFs) provide regular (but not around-the-clock) nursing care. As with assisted living, exercise and recreational opportunities may also be available at these facilities. Skilled nursing facilities (SNFs), which are overseen by doctors and provide around-the-clock nursing care, are meant for those who require more intensive medical and rehabilitative care. See also LONG-TERM CARE FACILITY.

Nursing home

See LONG-TERM CARE FACILITY.

Nursing home insurance

Private coverage for long-term custodial care. See LONG-TERM CARE INSURANCE.

Nutrient

A chemical substance in food that is essential to health maintenance, normal body function, growth, and reproduction. Nutrients must be supplied by food because the body cannot produce them independently or in enough quantities to meet the body's needs. VITAMINS, MINERALS, CARBOHYDRATES, fats, proteins, and water all are essential nutrients. Proteins are required for growth, muscle contractions, and other activities, and carbohydrates and fats for energy. Water, which makes up more than half of the body, carries nutrients and oxygen throughout the bloodstream and lymphatic system and is a vital component of the key enzyme reactions involved in digestion, absorption, and metabolism.

Nutrients are extracted from foods as they pass through the digestive system. More than 40 different nutrients are necessary for good health. Because no single food supplies them all, doctors advise eating a wide variety of nutrient-rich foods.

Nutrition

The study of the food people eat and its digestion and assimilation for growth, tissue repair, and physical activity. Areas of focus include diet, dietary deficiencies, and establishing minimum daily requirements for necessary nutrients (see DIETARY REFERENCE INTAKES and DIGESTION). No single food supplies all the nutrients

required for good health, so good nutrition consists of adequate and balanced amounts of seven groups of essential substances: proteins, CARBOHYDRATES, fats (see FATS AND OILS), fiber, VITAMINS, MINERALS, and water. In the daily diet, 50 to 60 percent of calories should derive from carbohydrates, no more than 30 percent (and preferably less) from fat, and 10 to 20 percent from protein. Complete daily food requirements are given in the US Department of Agriculture FOOD GUIDE PYRAMID.

Proper nutrition is necessary to health maintenance, normal body function, growth, reproduction, and the prevention of disease. A nutritionist or dietitian (see DIETITIAN, REGISTERED) may conduct a DIETARY ASSESSMENT to detect nutritional deficiencies. After a dietary assessment, a nutritionist may prescribe the use of a MULTIVITAMIN or the use of a WEIGHT LOSS diet or other type of special diet. Many common illnesses—including heart disease, high blood pressure, atherosclerosis, diabetes, and osteoporosis—are at least partially due to poor nutrition. Diseases such as anemia, scurvy, and pellagra are specifically attributable to vitamin deficiencies.

Nutrition Labeling and Education Act

Called the NLEA, federal legislation that requires most food products regulated by the Food and Drug Administration to be sold with a nutrition label containing specific information about nutrient content. The act defines the serving sizes that must be used for each food category and the amount of nutrient each serv-

---

FOOD LABELING CATEGORIES

The 14 label ingredients listed below are governed by the Nutrition Labeling and Education Act (10 additional components may be listed if they are contained in the food):

- Total calories
- Calories from fat
- Total fat
- Saturated fat
- Cholesterol
- Sodium
- Total carbohydrate
- Dietary fiber
- Sugars
- Protein
- Vitamin A
- Vitamin C
- Calcium
- Iron

ing must contain before it can make claims about amounts or health benefits. (NLEA does not apply to meat and poultry, which is regulated by the US Department of Agriculture.) The NLEA was signed in 1990 and became effective in 1994. It requires full nutritional labeling of 14 nutrients for most packaged products. Categories include iron, calcium, cholesterol, sodium, dietary fiber, and calories from fat.

The law was designed to discourage manufacturers from making misleading claims on labels such as "free" or "lite." In addition, only firmly established claims describing the relationship between a nutrient and a disease are allowed. For example, because scientific evidence shows that a lack of folate causes neural tube defects (a serious birth defect), this information can be included on labels of foods that contains folate. Less well-established relationships cannot be advertised.

Nutritional medicine

The use of diet to repair flaws in the body's response to disease. Nutritional medicine derives from the belief that all disease stems from a failure of the body to respond adequately to ward off outside forces. To correct this failure, nutritional medicine may use VITAMINS, MINERALS, ANTIOXIDANTS, HERBAL MEDICINE, and other nutritive elements to strengthen the body. A goal of nutritional medicine is to fortify and restore the immune system to achieve optimum

health. Advocates of nutritional medicine believe that by achieving optimum health, degenerative diseases associated with aging such as hypertension, arthritis, diabetes mellitus (type 2), and heart disease, can be delayed or avoided.

Among the common methods of practicing nutritional medicine is the use of vitamin and mineral supplements. As a general rule, a healthy diet containing a variety of foods can provide adequate amounts of nutrients, but nutritional deficiencies may occur in certain groups, including older people, pregnant women, and vegetarians. Vitamin and mineral supplements are helpful to these groups of people, who do not get adequate amounts of certain nutrients in their diets. Others who do not follow a healthy diet may not receive optimal levels of nutrients.

Nutritional medicine is also associated with the use of high doses of vitamins to treat disease, one of the therapies known as orthomolecular medicine. High doses of vitamin C, for example, are commonly used to ward off colds and other viral infections, and high doses of niacin have been used to lower cholesterol levels. In a controversial use of orthomolecular medicine, some doctors give high doses of vitamins to treat mental disorders, including schizophrenia. Extremely high doses of vitamins may be dangerous.

Some practitioners of nutritional medicine use a very strict diet called MACROBIOTICS to treat disease. In the

standard macrobiotic diet, whole cereal grains and vegetables are emphasized, with minimal consumption of animal products except fish. This diet is low in fat and high in fiber, factors that are associated with a reduced risk of cancer and heart disease. In traditional Asian macrobiotics, the choice of what foods to eat is based on the goal of achieving a balance between extremes, or yin and yang. People who eat macrobiotic diets are often deficient in vitamin B12 and other nutrients and should take supplements.

Nutritional supplements

Products intended to supplement the body's nutritional requirements. Nutritional supplements include vitamins, minerals, herbal products, and dietary aids. They are sold without prescription and are sometimes advertised as providing miraculous

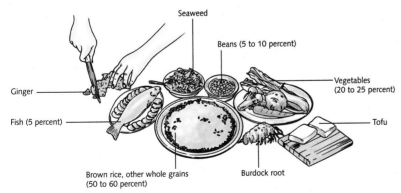

Seaweed
Beans (5 to 10 percent)
Vegetables (20 to 25 percent)
Ginger
Tofu
Fish (5 percent)
Brown rice, other whole grains (50 to 60 percent)
Burdock root

A MACROBIOTIC DIET
One approach to healthful eating is the macrobiotic diet, of Japanese origin. Whole grains make up the largest percentage of the diet, with vegetables, sea vegetables, some beans and bean products (such as tofu), and some fish making up the rest. This approach offers more protein than a strict vegetarian diet.

N

> **SAFETY AND NUTRITIONAL SUPPLEMENTS**
>
> The Food and Drug Administration (FDA) subjects food and drug products (prescription and nonprescription) to rigorous safety and effectiveness standards. But nutritional supplements—vitamins, minerals, herbal products, and dietary aids—are not similarly regulated.
>
> The FDA has the authority to intervene in the marketing of a nutritional supplement only when there is evidence that it is unsafe when taken as directed. However, since people rarely take nutritional supplements as directed and often take different types simultaneously, the harmful effects of nutritional supplements are extremely difficult to prove.
>
> Manufacturers of nutritional supplements are responsible for making sure that the information on the label is truthful and not misleading. But since these products are not subject to FDA regulation, there is no guarantee that all nutritional supplements are safe and effective. Furthermore, a person taking any type of nutritional supplement should share that information with his or her doctor(s) to make certain the substance will not interact adversely with other medications being taken.

SIDE EFFECTS OF NUTRITIONAL SUPPLEMENTS

Doctors generally agree that the best way to maintain nutritional health is with a well-balanced diet. If a nutritional supplement is used, it is important to be well-informed about the product before taking it. The following is a selected list of popular nutritional supplements and their possible side effects:

- **Gingko biloba,** a popular herbal product that may improve blood flow and circulation, can also cause gastrointestinal problems, headaches, and allergic skin reactions.
- **Glucosamine-chondroitin,** a natural remedy for osteoarthritis available in many health food stores, while not reported to produce serious side effects, may cause mild cases of diarrhea, heartburn, indigestion, and nausea.
- **Melatonin,** a natural hormone used to treat insomnia, jet lag, and seasonal affective disorder, may also cause headache, rash, and upset stomach and should be discontinued if normal sleeping patterns are disrupted.
- **Vitamin A,** if taken in daily doses of 25,000 IU or more, can cause birth defects, bone abnormalities, and severe liver disease.
- **Niacin,** if taken in slow-release doses of 500 mg or more a day or immediate-release doses of 750 mg or more a day, can cause stomach pain, vomiting, flushing, bloating, nausea, cramping, diarrhea, liver disease, muscle disease, eye damage, and heart injury.
- **Selenium,** an essential mineral, can cause tissue damage if taken in doses exceeding 800 micrograms a day.

---

benefits, such as curing disease or stopping the aging process. There is considerable debate as to whether people need to take nutritional supplements, and they are not without risk—especially when consumed in high doses. Problems have been associated with herbal supplements containing ephedrine, for example, because they can cause heart attacks, strokes, psychosis, and even death.

Most people can get all the nutrients they need through a well-balanced diet, but some people have genuine deficiencies in the nutrients they are able to consume. Those at risk of nutritional deficiencies include older people, smokers, people who drink alcohol to excess, people on diets of less than 1,000 calories per day, pregnant or breast-feeding women, and vegetarians.

Nystagmus

Involuntary, rapid, and repetitive movement of the eyes. Nystagmus usually involves both eyes, and it often increases when the person looks in a particular direction. The movement can be side to side (horizontal nystagmus), up and down (vertical), or circular (rotary). The condition may be present at birth or acquired later in life. Some forms of nystagmus accompany poor vision, as is found in albinos, people with extreme nearsightedness or farsightedness, or people who have scarred retinas (the light-sensitive tissue in the back of the eye) or optic nerves. Many people with good vision have horizontal nystagmus when looking far to one side. Nystagmus can also be caused by a brain tumor, Marfan syndrome, alcohol intoxication, overdose of drugs used to control seizures (for example, phenytoin), and multiple sclerosis.

In some cases, treating the cause of the nystagmus resolves the condition; often, however, it is permanent. Reduced vision can be improved with glasses that decrease eye movement and with low-vision aids. If vision is more stable when the person looks in a particular direction, glasses with prisms can be used to draw the eyes in that direction, or surgery can be performed on the eye muscles to position the eyes for best vision. With these corrections, many people with nystagmus are able to lead normal lives.

Nystatin

An antifungal drug. Nystatin (Mycostatin, Nilstat, Nystex) is used to treat infections caused by a fungus. This drug works by killing the fungus or preventing its growth. Nystatin is used to treat infections in the mouth, the vagina, and the intestines and on the skin.

Obesity

FOR SYMPTOM CHART
see Weight gain, page 60

A body weight 20 percent or more above an individual's ideal weight. Obesity is a condition that is a serious medical problem. Obesity is evaluated by calculating BODY MASS INDEX (BMI). Standard body mass index tables are based on calculations using an individual's height and weight. Obesity is defined as a BMI of higher than 30. When the BMI is above 40, a person is carrying approximately 100 pounds of excess weight and is considered morbidly obese. In morbid obesity, interventions such as surgery may be recommended. An operation may also be considered for people with a BMI between 35 and 40 who have obesity-related, life-threatening health problems such as heart disease or diabetes. Exceptions may be athletes, whose high BMI may be attributed to excess muscle rather than fat.

OBESITY AND HEALTH

Obese individuals face many increased health risks. Obesity is linked with serious weight-related problems such as high blood pressure (see HYPERTENSION), elevated CHOLESTEROL levels, coronary heart disease, cardiovascular disease, diabetes, stroke, and some cancers. It has been linked with colon and prostate cancer in men and with breast, uterine, and endometrial cancer in women. Other correlations include back pain, sleep apnea (a potentially life-threatening condition in which individuals stop breathing for short periods during sleep), gallstones, osteoarthritis, heartburn, gout, and varicose veins. Studies have shown that heavier people generally have a shorter life expectancy. Excess weight can also bring an increase in emotional and psychological problems. Although obesity often has a genetic component, very obese people are also likely to meet with social discrimination.

THE CAUSES OF OBESITY

Overeating is not always the cause of obesity. Regulation of body weight is complicated and involves genetic predisposition, nutrient intake, metabolism, and physical activity. Obesity is a growing problem in the United States, where more than half the population is either overweight or obese. An increasingly sedentary lifestyle, in which many people work at computers and sit down to watch television for relaxation, is at least partially responsible. Genes also have a clear role in obesity, since children of obese parents are 10 times more likely than other children to become obese. However, people who are genetically predisposed toward obesity can often make lifestyle choices that can prevent or control the problem. Poor eating and exercise habits are major contributing factors. Physical education has been eliminated from many schools, and obesity in children has been called an epidemic by major national health organizations.

CONTROLLING OBESITY

The best way to find a safe and healthy WEIGHT LOSS plan is to seek the advice of a doctor. A registered dietitian is also helpful. Instead of viewing dietary changes for weight loss as a temporary diet, it is preferable to think of it as a gradual change in eating and exercise habits that will result in a sustained lifestyle change. A sensible weight loss plan is one that emphasizes slow, gradual loss based on healthful eating and exercise choices. Specific dietary recommendations might include cutting back on total fat intake and replacing saturated fats with unsaturated ones, eliminating certain fatty foods or those that provide empty calories (energy without any additional nutritional value), opting for low-fat or skim milk dairy products, eating large amounts of vegetables and salads, choosing only small portions of fish and lean meats, distributing calories throughout the day instead of at one or two meals, and drinking eight glasses of water a day.

In order to shed pounds, doctors recommend that people who are obese subtract 500 calories from the amount that would maintain their ideal weight. Since one pound of fat equals 3,500 calories, eating 500 calories less than needed per day should result in about one pound of fat lost per week. Conversely, an extra 500 calories per day will result in a weight gain of 1 pound per week. Even smaller amounts of excess calories per day will result in gradual but significant weight gain over a long period of time. Consuming an extra 100 calories per day can cause a 10-pound weight gain over a year. Exercise is another influential factor in obesity. Weight loss takes place when calorie intake is less than calories burned, and exercise burns calories.

Obesity-hypoventilation syndrome

Also known as pickwickian syndrome; a group of symptoms that may accompany massive OBESITY. Obesity-hypoventilation syndrome is characterized by symptoms that often include shortness of breath, a flushed face, nighttime sleep disturbances such as SLEEP APNEA SYNDROME, and an irresistible urge to take short naps during the day. Because massive obesity interferes with breathing, people with this condition may also experience chronic HYPOXIA or decreased blood oxygen concentration. Obesity-hypoventilation syndrome can lead to serious complications such as pulmonary hypertension (see HYPERTENSION, PULMONARY), COR PULMONALE (right-sided heart failure), congestive heart failure, and CARDIOMYOPATHY. To lose weight, physicians recommend eating moderate amounts of nutrient-rich foods that are low in fat and calories, along with participating in a doctor-approved exercise program. See also WEIGHT LOSS.

Obsessive-compulsive disorder

A mental illness characterized by mild to severely persistent, intrusive, distressing thoughts, images, or impulses that occupy the mind uncontrollably (obsessions) or by repetitive actions the individual thinks he or she must perform (compulsions). Obsessive-compulsive disorder is commonly abbreviated as OCD. The obsessions cause the individual a disturbing level of anxiety, which the individual tries to alleviate with the compulsive acts. As a result, OCD is considered one of the ANXIETY DISORDERS.

O

SYMPTOMS

The obsessions and compulsions in OCD occur again and again, consume considerable amounts of the person's time, cause distress, and may make it difficult to handle social, occupational, or academic roles. The individual clearly knows that the obsessions and compulsions are extreme or unreasonable, but he or she cannot control or suppress them, despite recognizing that they originate in his or her own mind.

Obsessions are not simply excessive worries about real-life problems such as money, job, love, or illness, and they are not usually related to a real-life problem. The most common obsessions concern contamination (for example, from handling money or shaking hands); doubts (for example, about locking a door or turning off a stove); a need for objects to be ordered or arranged in a particular way; fear that a mistake will harm a loved one; repugnant religious or aggressive impulses (for example, the desire to shout obscenities in a church or torture the next-door neighbor); and repugnant sexual or violent imagery.

Compulsions are usually related to an obsession and performed to rid the individual of the anxiety that the obsession causes. An individual worried about contamination may wash his or her hands every few minutes; obsessions about doubt may lead to checking the same door lock or stove several dozen times during the day. In some cases, people develop personal rituals that seem unrelated to the obsession, such as counting backwards from 100 ten times whenever they feel the desire to shout an obscenity in church. The most common compulsions include washing (especially hand washing), cleaning, counting, checking, perfectionism, asking for reassurance, repeating the same action, and putting objects in order.

Many people with OCD avoid situations connected with their obsessions. Someone concerned about contamination may refuse to touch money or use a public restroom, for example. In extreme cases, the person may become housebound out of fear of encountering threatening situations outside. Obsessions can lead to extreme concern about health and illness, prompting repeated visits to the

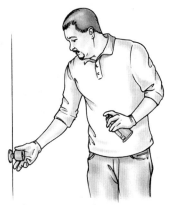

OBSESSIVE BEHAVIOR
An obsessive-compulsive person performs the same action extremely frequently and unnecessarily—often completely overdoing cleanliness or neatness. He or she anguishes over the perceived danger of not performing the act and becomes even more compulsive under stress.

doctor to seek reassurance. The person may feel guilty and responsible for actions beyond his or her control and have trouble sleeping. He or she may abuse drugs or alcohol in an attempt to suppress the obsessions or to sleep. In some cases, the obsessions or compulsions become the major focus of the person's life and result in major disability. OCD may be accompanied by depression, attention deficit/hyperactivity disorder, other anxiety disorders including panic attacks, eating disorders, or certain personality disorders. Suicide may be a risk in people with OCD and depression. The disease is particularly common in people with TOURETTE SYNDROME, a disease of the nervous system causing tics (jerkiness) of the face and voice.

COURSE AND CAUSES

OCD is equally common in males and females. The disease usually begins in adolescence (in males) or early adulthood (in females); onset in childhood or middle age is less common. Typically the disease starts earlier among men than women. In most cases, the condition begins gradually and develops slowly. Symptoms tend to worsen at times of stress, and they can improve markedly when the stress is removed. A pattern of flare-up and remission is common.

OCD appears to have an inherited biological cause. The disease is more common among siblings and children

of people with OCD, and studies of identical and fraternal twins also point to a pattern of inheritance. Research has shown that people with OCD have abnormal levels of activity in certain parts of the brain, which return to normal after they are treated and symptoms lessen.

TREATMENT

A number of medications have proven effective for treating OCD. These include antidepressants, anti-anxiety medications, and minor tranquilizers. Behavior therapies are also effective. They teach the person how to avoid the compulsive behavior associated with an obsession, use self-talk to suppress obsessive thoughts when they arise, and lessen the level of anxiety attached to feared objects, such as door knobs or open locks. In most cases, symptoms can be controlled to the point at which the individual is able to lead a normal life.

Obstetrician

A doctor who specializes in caring for women during pregnancy, labor, and childbirth. An obstetrician provides PRENATAL CARE, preconception counseling (see GENETIC COUNSELING), screening for BIRTH DEFECTS, ultrasound examinations (see ULTRASOUND, OBSTETRICAL), and childbirth education. Most obstetricians are also trained in GYNECOLOGY, and these specialists are referred to as obstetrician-gynecologists, or ob-gyns for short.

Obstetrics

The medical specialty involved in the care of pregnant women. Obstetrics includes care given during the period in which a woman is trying to conceive, pregnancy, labor and childbirth, and just after a baby is born. Family physicians, certified nurse-midwives, and obstetricians have all been trained in obstetrics. Most obstetricians are also gynecologists, doctors who specialize in caring for the female reproductive system.

Obstructive airways disease

A pathological process that involves narrowing of the bronchial airways. Obstructive airways disease may affect the windpipe, or trachea, as well as its smaller branches, the bronchi, which are connected to the lungs and supply air to them.

Obstructive airways diseases may be reversible or irreversible. ASTHMA, for example, is reversible, and CHRONIC OBSTRUCTIVE PULMONARY DISEASE caused by chronic BRONCHITIS, EMPHYSEMA, or a combination of the two is irreversible.

Occlusion

The closing or obstruction of a hollow organ or body part. Occlusion can occur in coronary arteries when a thrombus (blood clot) or sclerosis (hardening of tissue) blocks the artery, thereby preventing free flow of blood. Occlusion also happens in the vocal tract, when the act of producing sound causes the throat to close.

In dentistry, occlusion refers to the relationship between upper and lower teeth when the jaw is closed and the teeth come together.

Occult

A term meaning hidden or obscure. For example, an occult blood test is a chemical test performed to detect the presence of blood in the feces that is not visible to the naked eye.

Occult blood test, fecal

See FECAL-OCCULT BLOOD TEST.

Occupational health

A person's physical, mental, and social well-being as related to his or her job. Work-related diseases and injuries range from lung disease in miners to carpal tunnel syndrome in computer users. See also OCCUPATIONAL MEDICINE.

Occupational lung disease

Illness of the lungs caused by exposure to hazardous agents that exist in the workplace. Occupational lung diseases are usually caused by contact with irritants on a job site that are inhaled into the lungs repeatedly over time. This form of disease can also occur after a single exposure to an agent that is severely damaging to the lungs. The location, type of work performed, and environmental conditions surrounding a certain occupation are factors that can create greater risk for workers acquiring these diseases. Some examples of these occupations are coal mining, working in a car garage, and working in a manufacturing setting, where proximity to dangerous chemicals and fibers can cause lung disease. Exposure to dust in the workplace can cause susceptibility to DUST DISEASES.

Occupational lung diseases are leading work-related illnesses and include asbestosis, coal worker's pneumoconiosis, silicosis, byssinosis, hypersensitivity pneumonitis, and occupational asthma.

SYMPTOMS, DIAGNOSIS, AND TREATMENT
Individuals may experience the symptoms of these diseases in different ways, but the most common symptoms of these illnesses—regardless of the agents that have caused them—are cough, shortness of breath, chest pain, and chest tightness. These symptoms resemble those of other diseases and medical conditions and disorders, so it is important to inform a doctor of possible occupational exposures when giving a medical history.

A chest X ray and a pulmonary function test are generally required for a preliminary diagnosis. The X ray can usually provide sufficient information to determine which other tests may be needed to pursue a more complete diagnosis. Further tests may include an arterial blood gas analysis to measure the lungs' capacity for oxygen–carbon dioxide exchange, a biopsy of tissue or cells from the lungs to be examined microscopically, biochemical and cellular studies of lung fluids, measurements of respiratory or gas exchange functions, and an examination of airway or bronchial activity.

The first line of treatment is to reduce the person's exposure by removing the affected person from the work environment that is causing the illness or, in some cases, to ensure that proper protective equipment is used. Further treatment is determined by a person's age, general health status, and medical history, which all combine to affect his or her tolerance for certain medications, procedures, and therapies. The extent and type of lung disease involved is taken into account, as is a doctor's evaluation of what course the disease will follow, when determining the appropriate treatment options. The opinions and preferences of the person who has an occupational lung disease also have a role in the determination of treatment.

Occupational medicine

The branch of medicine that is concerned with the effects of a person's job on his or her health. Occupational medicine emphasizes the prevention of work-related disease and injury and the promotion of general health in workers. It encompasses problems ranging from lung disease in miners to carpal tunnel syndrome in computer users.

Occupational therapy

Treatment designed to help people disabled by an illness or injury to relearn physical skills and, when possible, to resume work. Occupational therapists work with people to restore, maintain, or increase their ability to perform daily tasks such as bathing, dressing, cooking, and eating. This may include the use of adaptive equipment such as special kitchen utensils, visual aids, and reaching tools. Occupational therapy, also called OT, often begins in the hospital and is continued on an outpatient basis or as home health care.

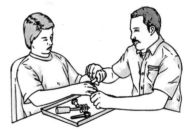

ACTIVITIES OF DAILY LIVING
Occupational therapy is goal-oriented, helping a person to relearn tasks that will enable him or her to return to work, perform daily activities, and live more independently. For example, a person who has lost hand-and-eye coordination as a result of injury or illness may need to learn again how to manipulate tools or household devices.

OCT

See OXYTOCIN CHALLENGE TEST.

Octreotide

An antidiarrhea drug. Octreotide (Sandostatin) is used to treat the severe diarrhea that is associated with some kinds of intestinal tumors, although the drug cannot treat the tumor. Octreotide is also used to treat acromegaly, a disorder of the growth hormone that causes large hands and feet in addition to arthritis and a low blood sugar level.

Oculogyric crisis

An abnormal condition in which the eyes are held in a fixed position for several minutes or hours. Oculogyric crises may occur in cases of postencephalitic parkinsonism (see PARKINSON DISEASE) or as a result of a medication reaction.

Oedipus complex

A possessive, romantic attachment of son to mother that, according to the theory developed by Sigmund Freud, is buried deep within the unconscious during childhood. The dilemma of attraction to the mother is resolved by the boy's subsequent identification with his father, from whom he learns moral values. This complex, an idea repressed into the subconscious, is named after a hero from ancient Greek drama who unknowingly killed his father and married his mother. The male equivalent of the Oedipus complex is the ELECTRA COMPLEX, an attachment of daughter to father.

Ofloxacin

See FLUOROQUINOLONES.

Olanzapine

An antipsychotic drug. Olanzapine (Zyprexa) is used to treat the symptoms of schizophrenia. It is unclear how olanzapine works, although it is known to have several effects on the neurotransmitters dopamine and serotonin, chemicals found in the central nervous system that affect a person's mood.

Older people, care of

See CAREGIVING FOR OLDER PEOPLE.

Oligodendroglioma

A rare type of brain tumor. Oligodendrogliomas grow very slowly and primarily affect young or middle-aged adults. Some of these tumors are cancerous, though most are benign. They can be present for years without being detected and diagnosed, and survival for many years after diagnosis is pos-

sible. Symptoms and treatment are the same as for other types of brain tumors.

Oligohydramnios

An abnormally small amount of AMNIOTIC FLUID encasing the fetus in a pregnancy. Oligohydramnios often signals the presence of an abnormality. It may mean that the woman has severe PREECLAMPSIA, or it may indicate kidney or urinary tract abnormalities in the fetus. Oligohydramnios in early pregnancy may result in a miscarriage; late in pregnancy, it can result in deformity or death of the fetus. It may be caused by premature rupture of the amniotic sac, obstruction of the fetal urinary tract, or extremely poor fetal growth. If oligohydramnios is suspected, the doctor will try to diagnose and treat the disorder causing it. If the pregnancy is advanced beyond the 37th week, the doctor may induce labor.

Oligomenorrhea

Irregular and infrequent menstrual periods that are more than 45 days apart. Reduced bleeding and lack of ovulation may occur. Irregular periods are associated with pregnancy, miscarriage, menopause, excessive weight loss, ENDOMETRIOSIS, disorders of the pituitary gland or hypothalamus, hypothyroidism, and estrogen-secreting tumors. Irregular periods may be a woman's normal pattern, but the abnormalities that may cause irregular bleeding should be ruled out by a doctor before making that assumption. Identifying and treating the cause of the oligomenorrhea should eliminate the condition. See MENSTRUATION, DISORDERS OF.

Oligospermia

An abnormally low concentration of sperm cells in semen, the thick, white fluid expelled from the penis at sexual climax. Men with oligospermia are generally infertile. The condition is caused by a disorder of the testicles or by an obstruction in the passageways leading from them. These disorders include hormonal imbalances and exposure to certain chemicals and medications, X rays, or radioactive materials. Obstructions can result from diseases that inflame and scar the reproductive tract, such as mumps in adolescent or adult men, or as a

complication of surgery. Treatment depends on the cause of the condition. Some types of hormonal imbalance can be treated with medication, and in some cases, obstructions can be repaired surgically.

Oliguria

Reduced ability to produce urine. Under normal circumstances, the body should produce at least 1 liter of urine a day. An amount less than this can be a sign of inadequate water intake and dehydration, kidney disease, infection, medication side effects, or other conditions. Diagnosis requires physical examination and may include blood tests and X rays of the kidneys.

Omentum

A double fold of the membrane lining the abdominal cavity. The greater omentum attaches to the stomach and hangs down over structures close to it, including the duodenum and colon. The lesser omentum covers the liver and parts of the stomach and small intestine. These folds store fat and may also prevent the spread of infection between abdominal organs. See PERITONEUM.

Omeprazole

An antiulcer drug; gastric acid pump inhibitor. Omeprazole (Prilosec) is used to treat conditions in which too much acid is present in the stomach, thereby causing injury to stomach tissue. It is one of a group of drugs called proton pump inhibitors (PPIs), drugs that block the formation of acid in the stomach. PPIs act at the sites within the stomach where hydrochloric acid is made and pumped into the stomach.

Omeprazole is used to treat peptic ulcers and gastroesophageal reflux disease (GERD), in which acid splashes back into the esophagus, causing injury. It is also used in combination with antibiotics to treat infections caused by the bacterium *Helicobacter pylori*, which is known to cause peptic ulcers. Omeprazole is used to treat a relatively rare disease, Zollinger-Ellison syndrome, in which too much stomach acid is produced.

Onchocerciasis

An infection spread by black flies that causes chronic skin disease and eye lesions, which may lead to vision impairment or blindness. Onchocerciasis is also referred to as "river blindness" because the black flies that cause it breed in rapidly flowing streams, most commonly in the Savannah regions of Africa, in Yemen and Saudi Arabia, in southern Mexico, and in certain countries of Central and South America.

When a black fly bites a person, its larvae reside in the skin and develop into adult worms during a period of 1 year. The female black fly worms can live in small, rounded masses of fibrous tissue, called nodules, located below the skin's surface, sometimes for as long as 15 years. The females are periodically inseminated by adult male worms as they migrate from one nodule to another and produce live microscopic offspring that migrate through the skin and invade the eyes. Some people who are infected may become visually impaired or blind as a result; onchocerciasis is the second leading cause of blindness worldwide. Blindness due to the infection is common in parts of Africa, but relatively rare in the Americas.

SYMPTOMS, DIAGNOSIS, AND TREATMENT

The principal symptom of onchocerciasis is the characteristic deep, firm lump. An associated skin inflammation called onchocercal dermatitis produces a severely itching rash of dark pimples and swollen glands in people with mild infections. This can progress to wrinkling, discoloration, scaling, and atrophy of the skin, in addition to massive swelling and possible obstruction in the lymph nodes of the groin, as well as leg lesions. If the black fly larvae invade the eyes, they can produce inflammatory lesions that cause temporary visual impairment without long-term damage or impairment. Or, the black fly larvae may produce inflammation and scar tissue in the blood vessels of the eye that dislocate the eye's lens and cause blindness or lead to conditions that deform the pupil of the eye, resulting in blindness.

Onchocerciasis is diagnosed by detecting the worm in the skin. Nodules that occur on the skin's surface may be excised and examined for adult worms; deeper nodules may be observed by ultrasound scanning or MRI (magnetic resonance imaging).

The medication ivermectin, which quickly destroys the black fly larvae in the skin and eyes, is used to treat the infection. This medication does not kill adult worms but obstructs reproduction for a period of several months. The medication suramin may be given intravenously over a period of several weeks. Surgical removal of nodules may be needed to rid the body of adult worms.

Oncogenes

Genes that contribute to the transformation of normal cells to cancerous ones; cancer-causing genes that can be passed from parent to offspring. CANCER occurs when the cells in a body tissue grow and differentiate in an uncontrolled, deranged manner. Normal cell growth can go wrong when a gene that stimulates cell growth becomes hyperactive; and that is what an oncogene does. As a rule, a single oncogene is not sufficient to change normal cells into cancer cells: many mutations in many different genes are usually required.

CANCERS INVOLVING ONCOGENES

Normal cell growth, which involves cell division, is strictly controlled, subject to a network of signals that together determine when a cell may divide, how often it may divide, and how errors are to be fixed. Mutations, or changes, in one or more of the elements that control growth can trigger cancer, in response to an environmental threat such as cigarette smoke, because of a genetic predisposition, or both. Rarely is a single trigger enough to produce a cancerous growth; malignant tumors generally develop only when several cancer-promoting factors are present. One of the chief mechanisms by which cancer is produced is the transformation of a normal gene into an oncogene.

Several types of cancer involve oncogenes, including the following examples.

■ *Breast cancer* Some women carry mutations in either of two genes, BRCA-1, found on chromosome 17, and BRCA-2, on chromosome 13. The presence of either mutation puts a woman at increased risk of developing breast or ovarian cancer. About 5 percent of breast cancers are genetically linked to a BRCA-1 or BRCA-2 mutation.

■ *Burkitt lymphoma* This rare form of cancer results from a broken chromosome 8, which changes the pattern of a gene by disrupting its usual function in controlling cell growth. Burkitt lymphoma is caused by a gene that has been changed into an oncogene.

■ *Chronic myeloid leukemia* In this cancer of the blood cells, normal bone marrow is replaced with malignant cells. Chronic myeloid leukemia is usually diagnosed by finding an abnormal Philadelphia chromosome, which is associated with a proto-oncogene on chromosome 9 called ABL (Abelson leukemia virus), combined with a gene from chromosome 22. The combined oncogene activates uncontrolled cell growth.

■ *Colon cancer* Colon cancer is one of the most common of the inherited cancer syndromes. The genes involved in colorectal cancer include MSH2 and MSH6, both found on chromosome 2, and MLH1, found on chromosome 3. If any of these genes have mutated and are therefore not working properly, DNA is damaged, which can result in cancer.

■ *Small cell lung carcinoma* In this type of lung cancer, part of chromosome 3 is absent, accounting for disruptions of cell growth and division.

■ *Malignant melanoma* In this aggressive skin cancer, mutation of the CDKN2 gene on chromosome 9 can account for a susceptibility to the disease that runs in families. The mutation stops skin cells from properly synthesizing DNA before they divide, which deprives the cells of a mechanism by which the normal cycle of cell division is controlled. When skin cells divide in an uncontrolled way, changes such as moles can suddenly appear on the skin.

Oncologist

A doctor who is trained in oncology, the medical specialty concerned with the diagnosis and treatment of cancer. Medical oncologists are internists with special knowledge of CHEMOTHERAPY and training in the treatment of cancer and its related problems. Radiation oncologists specialize in using RADIATION THERAPY to treat of people with cancer. Surgical oncologists specialize in cancer surgery, and pediatric oncologists treat children who have cancer. Often oncologists work with hematologists to treat cancer.

Oncology

The medical specialty concerned with the diagnosis, treatment, and study of cancer.

Oncology, surgical

The treatment of cancer with surgery. Surgical procedures are commonly used to cure cancer by removing it. Surgery to remove cancerous tissue, whether for biopsy or therapy, is generally performed by surgical oncologists.

Ondansetron hydrochloride

An antiemetic; an antinausea drug. Ondansetron hydrochloride (Zofran) is used to treat or prevent nausea and vomiting that may occur following chemotherapy or radiation therapy for a person with cancer, or following surgery.

Onlay, dental

A filling composed of gold or porcelain that is extended to cover the cusps (see CUSPS, DENTAL) or peaks of the teeth for greater protection of a tooth. An onlay fits into the space in a tooth that a dentist has prepared after removing decay and shaping the remaining hole. What differentiates an onlay is that it extends over the entire chewing surface, including the cusps of the tooth. This offers greater protection against the pressure caused by biting and chewing and helps to prevent possible fracture of the tooth. Dental onlays are most commonly used when a tooth has a large cavity or when the cusps of the tooth are chipped, fractured, or are very thin. The procedure for placing an onlay requires two dental visits. At the first visit, the tooth is prepared and impressions (see IMPRESSION, DENTAL) are taken. The impression is used to cast a model that can be used to fabricate an onlay that fits into the prepared space in the tooth. On the second visit, the onlay is adjusted and cemented into the cavity. See also INLAY, DENTAL.

Onycholysis

A condition in which the nail plate separates from the nail bed. The separated portion is white and opaque compared with the pink translucence of the attached portion. Onycholysis may be due to injury, psoriasis, drug PHOTOSENSITIVITY (heightened sensitivity to the sun), fungal disease, and thyroid problems.

Onychomycosis

Fungal disease affecting the nails of the fingers and toes in which the nails thicken and become opaque and brittle. See also ATHLETE'S FOOT.

Oocyte

A human egg; also called a female gametocyte or ovocyte. An oocyte carries the female half of the chromosomes that, when united with the complementary chromosomes from a sperm, form a zygote.

Oophorectomy

Surgical removal of the ovaries (see OVARY). Oophorectomy is usually performed as part of a HYSTERECTOMY, although it is sometimes performed alone. The procedure is used to treat cancer of the ovary, large ovarian cysts or tumors, and some cases of ENDOMETRIOSIS. When a woman has a very small benign tumor or cyst on an ovary, it can sometimes be removed while leaving the ovary intact in a procedure called a partial oophorectomy.

If only one ovary is removed during an oophorectomy, the woman can still get pregnant. Removal of both ovaries eliminates the primary source of estrogen and, consequently, produces menopause in any woman who has not yet had it. HORMONE REPLACEMENT THERAPY is sometimes used to relieve the symptoms associated with menopause, but it may not be used if the woman's history suggests heart problems.

Open-heart surgery

A procedure in which the HEART is operated on after it is exposed by means of a large opening in the chest wall. During the surgery, a heart-lung machine circulates and oxygenates the blood and takes over the work of the heart and lungs. The most common open-heart procedure is BYPASS SURGERY. Other types include procedures to replace heart valves (see HEART VALVE SURGERY) and HEART TRANSPLANT.

Operating room

The hospital room in which a surgical procedure is performed. The operating room is specially designed to be bacteria-free to reduce the risk of infecting open wounds; a ventilation system screens the air for impurities. The operating room is kept meticulously clean to avoid contamination of any kind that could endanger the health of the person undergoing the operation.

A holding room nurse receives patients and prepares them for surgery by presenting an informed consent form, inserting an intravenous line, administering presurgical medications, and usually cleaning and shaving the area to be operated on.

In the operating room itself, the primary surgeon is the lead medical practitioner. He or she may have an assisting, or second surgeon, plus a surgical assistant or technician, as well as a scrub nurse, all of whom help with the sterile and technical aspects of the surgical procedure. An anesthesiologist is responsible for the anesthesia, which is often administered by a specially trained nurse (usually a certified registered nurse anesthetist). After the surgery is complete, the patient is moved to a recovery room and monitored by the recovery room nurse until the anesthesia has worn off.

The central piece of equipment in the operating room is the table the patient lies on. It can be tilted, raised and lowered, and configured in a variety of ways, depending on the procedure being performed. The table is narrow to allow the surgeon easy access.

Inhaled anesthetics are pumped from an anesthesia machine into a mask over the patient's mouth and nose. The anesthesia machine regulates the amount of inhaled anesthetics, as well as the oxygen given during surgery.

The patient is connected to monitoring devices to keep track of vital signs as the procedure is being carried out. These devices register blood pressure, respiratory gases, adequacy of breathing, and heart rate. Monitors for muscle function, brain and spinal cord activity, and blood pressure may also be used.

OPERATING ROOM

A state-of-the-art hospital operating room is designed to reduce the risk of infections and to help the operating team perform surgery efficiently.

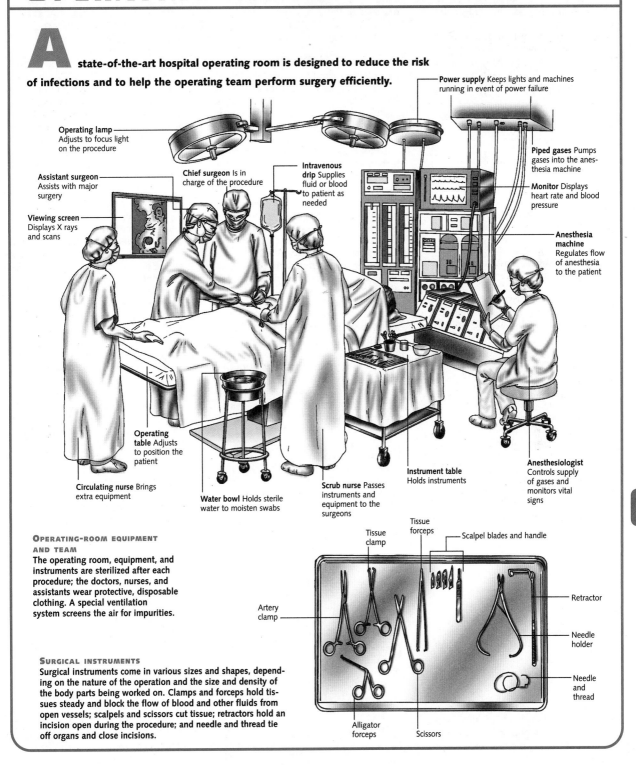

Power supply Keeps lights and machines running in event of power failure

Piped gases Pumps gases into the anesthesia machine

Monitor Displays heart rate and blood pressure

Anesthesia machine Regulates flow of anesthesia to the patient

Operating lamp Adjusts to focus light on the procedure

Intravenous drip Supplies fluid or blood to patient as needed

Assistant surgeon Assists with major surgery

Chief surgeon Is in charge of the procedure

Viewing screen Displays X rays and scans

Operating table Adjusts to position the patient

Anesthesiologist Controls supply of gases and monitors vital signs

Circulating nurse Brings extra equipment

Water bowl Holds sterile water to moisten swabs

Scrub nurse Passes instruments and equipment to the surgeons

Instrument table Holds instruments

OPERATING-ROOM EQUIPMENT AND TEAM

The operating room, equipment, and instruments are sterilized after each procedure; the doctors, nurses, and assistants wear protective, disposable clothing. A special ventilation system screens the air for impurities.

SURGICAL INSTRUMENTS

Surgical instruments come in various sizes and shapes, depending on the nature of the operation and the size and density of the body parts being worked on. Clamps and forceps hold tissues steady and block the flow of blood and other fluids from open vessels; scalpels and scissors cut tissue; retractors hold an incision open during the procedure; and needle and thread tie off organs and close incisions.

Tissue clamp

Tissue forceps

Scalpel blades and handle

Artery clamp

Retractor

Needle holder

Needle and thread

Alligator forceps

Scissors

O

Operation

A surgical procedure. The surgeon uses instruments that open, remove, or repair the part of the body being operated on.

Operations range from minor ones, such as a biopsy that can be performed in a doctor's office, to a surgical procedure lasting several hours, such as a heart transplant performed in a hospital.

HAVING AN OPERATION: WHAT TO EXPECT

These experiences are usual for most types of surgery:

- The surgeon will provide detailed information about the surgical procedure and answer any questions the patient may have.
- The patient will need to sign a consent form, authorizing the surgeon, anesthesiologist, and other medical staff to perform the procedure.
- The anesthesiologist will explain what kind of anesthesia he or she plans to use and what pain relief may be used following the operation.
- The patient will be given a sedative, either orally or by injection, to ease any anxiety about the procedure and to make the person sleepy before the anesthesia is given in the operating room.
- The patient may be shaved to remove hair from the area to be operated on.
- After the operation, the patient goes immediately into the recovery room for about half an hour to 2 hours (or more depending on the complexity of the surgery) to be monitored for any possible complications.
- If the person is very ill or the surgery extensive, he or she may be sent to an intensive care unit following surgery.

Ophthalmologist

A physician who specializes in treating eye conditions and diseases. An ophthalmologist has a medical degree (MD or DO) and at least 4 years of advanced specialized training in eye care.

Ophthalmologists diagnose and treat eye diseases and injuries, perform surgery on the eyes, and prescribe glasses and contact lenses.

Ophthalmology

The branch of medical science that studies the structure, function, and diseases of the eye. A physician who specializes in ophthalmology is an ophthalmologist.

Ophthalmoplegia

Paralysis of the eye muscles. There are three types of ophthalmoplegia: internuclear (affecting the structures in the central nervous system that coordinate eye movements), external, and internal. Internuclear ophthalmoplegia, a type of motor disturbance of the eye, results from damage to the area of the brain that coordinates eye movement and can be caused by multiple sclerosis, ischemic vascular disease, or brain stem tumor. External ophthalmoplegia involves dysfunction of extraocular muscles, the muscles that control the movement of the eye. Internal ophthalmoplegia involves disorders with associated dysfunction of the pupillary muscles.

Ophthalmoscope

A handheld device with a magnifier and a strong, focused light source that is used to examine the interior of the eye. During examination with an ophthalmoscope, the pupil may be dilated with drops to allow easier examination. The light shines in through the pupil to the back (fundus) of the eye and allows observation of the retina (the thin layer of nervous tissue that detects light and relays visual information to the brain), the retinal blood vessels, and the optic disc (the point where the optic nerve joins the retina). The fundus provides clues to the health of the eye and often of the whole body. Changes in blood vessels in the retina can indicate the severity of hypertension. Small particles in these same vessels signal the formation of plaques or clots containing cholesterol and indicate increased risk for heart attack or stroke. Changes caused by diabetes mellitus, type 1 and type 2, and tears or holes in the retina are visible through the ophthalmoscope. The shape and color of the optic disc can indicate eye disease.

Opioids

See NARCOTICS.

Opportunistic infection

Infections that occur in people with weakened immune systems. Opportunistic infections occur when organisms take advantage of the decreased efficiency of a person's immune system. When a person's immunity is functioning normally and he or she is exposed to potentially destructive organisms, the body's defense system attacks the infectious agents and routinely prevents infection. When the immune system is weakened or suppressed, organisms that would not normally produce infections or would result in localized infections with mild, treatable symptoms can become life-threatening. Without the body's immune system to control and combat them, these organisms flourish and spread, often producing serious infections, which are referred to as opportunistic infections.

CAUSES

A weakened or suppressed immune system may be caused by a number of factors, including long-term treatment with corticosteroids or antibiotics and anticancer treatments such as chemotherapy. Anticancer medications can hinder the normal defensive activity of white blood cells, which would otherwise attack infectious agents. Diseases such as leukemia, sickle cell disease, and diabetes mellitus can weaken a person's immune system, making that person more susceptible to infection. Human immunodeficiency virus, or HIV, eventually leads to acquired immunodeficiency syndrome, or AIDS, which is a fatal disease. HIV infection severely weakens the immune system and leads to a high risk of opportunistic infections gaining access and causing serious illness. A common infection such as a yeast infection, which would not endanger a person with a normally functioning immune system, can become dangerous to a person infected with HIV or AIDS. HIV also diminishes a person's resistance to certain cancers, including KAPOSI SARCOMA and LYMPHOMA of the brain.

The skin is an important barrier to infection that may be compromised by several conditions. Serious burns and severe eczema reduce the ability of the skin to act as a shield against infectious agents that exist in the external environment and internal tissues and structures of the body.

SPECIFIC DISEASES AND CONDITIONS

Common opportunistic infections include a variety of viruses, including those that produce several fungal infections and severe herpesviruses, including CYTOMEGALOVIRUS, or CMV. CMV is generally benign and not threatening to a person in good health, but the virus is a common life-threatening cause of viral opportunistic infection associated with severe immunodeficiency in people with AIDS. CRYPTOSPORIDIOSIS is an opportunistic infection that causes severe diarrhea in people who have AIDS. TOXOPLASMOSIS, which generally causes no symptoms or mild illness in healthy persons, can lead to serious complications and can cause brain abscesses in people with AIDS.

CRYPTOCOCCOSIS is a fungal infection that usually affects people with weakened immune systems; it can cause lung disease and may spread to the brain, producing MENINGITIS. The yeast infection candidiasis, or thrush, can occur as a result of long-term antibiotic therapy or in people with suppressed immune defenses. Aspergillosis is an opportunistic infection of the lungs.

The frequency and severity of tuberculosis are increased in people with AIDS. Food poisoning caused by *Salmonella* bacteria generally produces diarrhea and abdominal pain in otherwise healthy people, but in people who have AIDS, the lack of defensive immune activity fosters a speedy overgrowth of the bacteria. That overgrowth can lead to dangerous infections of the blood, which may spread the infection to other body organs, including the heart, lungs, and bones.

Optic atrophy

Wasting away of the optic disc, the area where the optic nerve joins the retina (the thin light-sensitive layer in the back of the eye). Optic atrophy indicates degeneration of the optic nerve. This is usually indicated by whitening (pallor) of the optic nerve.

Optic disc edema

Swelling of the region where the optic nerve joins the retina (the thin, light-sensitive area in the back of the eye). Because of swelling, the optic disc looks "angry" (inflamed and swollen), its margins become blurred and hard to distinguish, and the small cup in the center of the disc decreases in size. Optic disc edema is a sign of possible serious disease. If unilateral (in one eye only), possible causes include ischemic optic neuropathy, central retinal vein occlusion, and orbital optic nerve tumors. If caused by increased intracranial pressure and both eyes are involved, the condition is called PAPILLEDEMA. This can result from a brain tumor, bleeding into the brain tissue, and pseudotumor cerebri. Malignant hypertension may also cause bilateral disc swelling.

Optic neuritis

Inflammation of the optic nerve. If the inflammation affects the nerve where it connects with the back of the eye (papillitis), the sole symptom is usually gradual or sudden blurred vision or blindness of the affected eye. If the inflammation affects the optic nerve outside the eye (retrobulbar neuritis), pain as the eye is moved often accompanies blurred vision or blindness. Optic neuritis is caused by a viral infection, autoimmune disease, or multiple sclerosis. In most cases, optic neuritis disappears on its own within 2 to 8 weeks. Corticosteroid medications may be prescribed to hasten healing. In rare cases, surgery may be performed to relieve pressure on the nerve. Optic neuritis can recur, particularly in people with autoimmune disease or multiple sclerosis, and cause progressive visual impairment.

Optician

A technician trained to grind lenses for glasses and contacts. Opticians do not examine eyes for disease or focusing problems. Rather, they fill prescriptions for glasses and contact lenses written by ophthalmologists and optometrists.

Optometrist

A professional trained to diagnose and correct focusing errors of the eyes. Optometrists graduate from a school of optometry and hold a doctor of optometry (OD) degree. The scope of optometry practice is regulated by state law. In all states, optometrists examine eyes and prescribe glasses or contact lenses to correct focusing problems. In some states, optometrists can also use medications to treat certain eye diseases. Optometrists do not perform surgery.

Oral

Having to do with the mouth. An oral medication or solution is one that is given by mouth. An oral thermometer is one that is inserted into the mouth. The oral cavity refers to the mouth and its structures.

Oral and maxillofacial surgeon

A dental surgeon who specializes in diagnosing and surgically treating problems related to the jaw and related facial structures, including the teeth. A dental surgeon with this specialty extracts teeth, particularly when they are impacted (see IMPACTION, DENTAL) or when the removal is complicated by the location, abnormal formation, or attachment to the jawbone. An oral and maxillofacial surgeon also prepares the jaws for denture construction by specialized surgical techniques, including skin and bone grafts, and places implants (see IMPLANTS, DENTAL) to help stabilize DENTURES. The surgeon diagnoses and treats jaw abnormalities including temporomandibular joint disorder (TMJ; see CLICKING JAW), traumatic facial injuries, and local cancers, including cysts and tumors in the mouth. The surgeon may also perform RECONSTRUCTIVE SURGERY of facial malformations caused by growth disturbances of the jaws and for the correction of CLEFT LIP AND PALATE.

Oral cancer

Cancer developing in any of the components of the mouth and the oral cavity, including the lip, the tongue, the floor of the mouth, the lining of the cheeks, the tonsils, and the gums. Also known as mouth cancer, oral cancers are common and can be detected during examination of the mouth by a doctor or dentist. Early signs may be red, slightly raised areas with poorly defined borders; a lump that can be felt with the tongue; or a sore inside the mouth that does not heal.

A symptom of lip cancer may be a growth that forms a dry crust that bleeds when removed. Cancer of the gum may appear as toothache, loose teeth, or a sore on the gum that does not heal. Tongue cancer may involve a mild irritation, pain during eating or drinking, and difficulty speaking or swallowing. Cancer of the tonsils may appear as a persistent sore throat and an earache.

Because the symptoms of oral cancer can appear in many other disorders, a physical examination is essential. A doctor should be consulted if symptoms persist or get worse. A diagnostic workup of suspected oral cancer may include X rays, CT (computed tomography) scanning, MRI (magnetic resonance imaging), and biopsy.

Oral cancer typically affects adults older than age 40; men are twice as likely to develop it as women. The most frequent cause is tobacco use in all forms, including smoking cigarettes, pipes, or cigars and chewing tobacco. Oral cancer often appears at the precise spot at which the mouth is exposed to tobacco—the spot where the tip of a pipe makes contact with the mouth, for instance, or the place where chewing tobacco is held between the cheek and the gums. Alcohol consumption is also associated with oral cancers, possibly because alcohol contributes to the damage done to the lining of the mouth by smoking. People with broken teeth or ill-fitting dentures are also at risk for developing oral cancer. Exposure to excessive sunlight can cause lip cancer.

Treatment of oral cancer usually involves surgery and radiation therapy, sometimes in combination with chemotherapy. Laser therapy is sometimes used to treat oral cancer.

Approximately 90 percent of people who have lip cancer survive for 5 years after diagnosis, while 30 percent of people who have throat cancer survive for 5 years. Overall, about half of all people diagnosed with oral cancer survive 5 years or longer after diagnosis.

Oral contraceptives
See CONTRACEPTION, HORMONAL METHODS.

Oral hygiene
A group of procedures necessary for keeping the mouth and teeth clean and healthy. The primary aim of oral hygiene is to remove food particles and plaque (see PLAQUE, DENTAL) from the teeth daily to prevent TOOTH DECAY and gum disease (see PERIODONTAL DISEASE). The bacteria in the plaque can create acid and other substances that can cause cavities (see CAVITY, DENTAL), damage the gums, and harm the bone surrounding the teeth. Brushing the teeth thoroughly at least twice daily and using dental floss (see FLOSS, DENTAL) every day are the only ways to get rid of plaque. Generally, the brush should be moved from the gum area to the teeth, cleaning the teeth from the roots out to the tips of the teeth, and gently massaging the gums to stimulate circulation. The toothbrush should be replaced every 3 months.

Dental floss should also be used daily to remove food particles and plaque from crevices that cannot be reached with a toothbrush, especially the small spaces between the teeth and between the teeth and the gum line. Waxed or unwaxed floss should be moved up and down between the teeth, wrapping around the side of each tooth, especially near the gum line. A clean, 18-inch length of floss should be used for flossing. DISCLOSING AGENTS may be used to stain dental plaque temporarily so that it can be seen and removed with dental floss and a toothbrush. A dentist or dental hygienist can demonstrate proper brushing and flossing techniques.

The use of FLUORIDE to strengthen tooth enamel (see ENAMEL, DENTAL) is another component of good oral hygiene. A dentist can recommend or prescribe the use of fluoride in a mouthwash or tablet form. He or she may also apply a fluoride gel to the teeth if necessary. Children 13 years old and younger are in the stage of life when the tooth enamel is forming, and they should have fluoride applied to their teeth twice a year by a dentist.

Eating a well-balanced diet and restricting foods that contain sugar are also helpful in maintaining good oral hygiene.

Oral sex
Stimulation of the genitals with the partner's mouth and tongue. Cun-nilingus is oral stimulation of a woman's genitals with the partner's mouth and tongue; fellatio is oral stimulation of a man's penis with the partner's mouth and tongue. Partners stimulate each other simultaneously or take turns. For many women, oral stimulation of the clitoris by a partner is an effective way to achieve orgasm. Certain SEXUALLY TRANSMITTED DISEASES (such as herpes simplex and genital warts) can be transmitted through oral sex.

Oral surgery
A branch of dentistry that involves the diagnosis and surgical repair and treatment of disorders of the teeth, mouth, and jaws. These problems may include diseases, injuries, malformations, or structural deficiencies of the jaw and surrounding tissues in the mouth. The removal of teeth is an important part of the practice of oral surgery. See ORAL AND MAXILLOFACIAL SURGEON.

Orbit
One of the two bony cavities in the skull that contains the eyes as well as its associated nerves, blood vessels, muscles, and other structures. Each orbit is made up of seven bones (maxilla, zygomatic, frontal, lacrimal, palatine, ethmoid, and sphenoid) and lies just above the sinus cavities of the nose.

Orbital fracture
A break in any of the seven bones that form the eye socket (orbit). Orbital fractures commonly result from blunt trauma, such as a blow from a fist or impact against a dashboard in an automobile collision. The rim of the orbit breaks only with significant force, while the bones deeper within the orbit are thinner and break more easily.

Symptoms of an orbital fracture involve blood accumulating in the socket and pressing against the eye and optic nerve; impairment of the muscles that control the eyeball, causing double vision or difficulty in moving the eye; numbness in the upper teeth; protrusion of the eyeball from the socket; or collapse of the eye within the socket. When an orbital fracture is suspected, the physician will physically examine the eye and order X rays and CT (computed tomography) scans to determine the extent of the injury.

Minor orbital fractures that cause only temporary symptoms are allowed to heal on their own. Severe fractures require surgical repair. The surgeon puts the bones back in their proper position and secures them with small metal screws and plates. See page 258 for more on Blow-out fracture.

Orchiectomy

Surgical removal of one or both testicles. Removal of both testicles is known as castration. One testicle is usually removed because of cancer in the testicle (see TESTICLE, CANCER OF THE), dead testicle tissue (see TESTICLE, TORSION OF THE), or an undescended testicle (see TESTICLE, UNDESCENDED). Removal of one testicle usually does not affect sexual activity or fertility. Both testicles are sometimes removed as treatment for advanced prostate cancer. The procedure is done under spinal or local anesthesia. Full recovery takes about 3 weeks. Artificial testicles can be placed in the scrotum for cosmetic reasons, but this surgery is rarely performed today.

Orchiopexy

An operation performed to place an undescended testicle in the scrotum, the saclike pouch between the legs in a male, or to restore blood flow to a testicle that has twisted around its own blood vessels. The testicles develop in the abdomen and descend into the scrotum shortly before birth or, in some cases, during the first year of life (see TESTICLE, UNDESCENDED). If this does not occur, orchiopexy is performed to move the testicle out of the abdomen and into the scrotum, usually before age 2. Also, a normal testicle can become twisted and cut off its own blood supply (see TESTICLE, TORSION OF THE). Orchiopexy is performed to prevent the condition.

Orchitis

Inflammation of one or both testicles. Orchitis is most commonly caused by mumps, but it may also result from the spread of infection from elsewhere in the body, such as the bladder or prostate. The affected testicle becomes very large and painful. Fever, nausea, and vomiting may also occur. Anti-

biotics may be used to stop the infection, and painkillers can be prescribed to ease discomfort and lower fever. When the individual is in bed, ice packs and a rolled towel supporting the scrotum help to relieve pain. Wearing an athletic supporter can decrease pain when the person is mobile. Orchitis usually clears up within a few days to a couple of weeks.

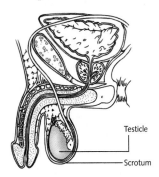

Testicle

Scrotum

Normal male reproductive organs

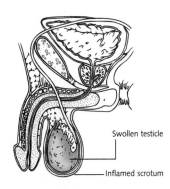

Swollen testicle

Inflamed scrotum

Inflamed testicle

SWOLLEN TESTICLE
Orchitis is usually caused by mumps or an infection in the bladder or prostate. Treatment with antibiotics and painkillers usually clears up the infection in a few days.

Order of protection

An injunction or court order issued to prohibit violent or threatening acts against a specific individual. An order of protection may be issued by a judge in cases when one person has a history of having threatened, harassed, or attacked another person. Orders of protection are often sought by victims of domestic or family violence to prevent further such acts. An order of protection may restrict a person's behavior very narrowly, or it may prohibit any contact, communi-

cation with, or proximity to another person. Orders of protection usually have expiration dates, although it is possible to have them extended or renewed.

An abused person who is granted an order of protection can call on police for protection at any time. The abuser can be arrested and charged with violating the order if he or she fails to comply with its terms. Failure to obey an order of protection is considered contempt of court, and violators risk fines or going to jail. See VIOLENCE, FAMILY.

Organ

A body part composed of more than one tissue that performs a specific function or functions. The specific function of an organ, such as the heart, lungs, and liver, is essential to the life or well-being of the whole. In animals, organs are usually made up of several tissues, one of which generally predominates and determines the chief function of the organ.

Organ donation

The agreement to take healthy organs or tissues from one person to replace damaged organs or tissues in another person. In most cases, the organ is taken from someone who has recently died. Kidneys are most often transplanted from a cadaver donor, but there are procedures for transplanting portions of the liver, lung, and pancreas from a living donor as well.

People who want to donate their organs upon death can sign a donor card (available with driver's licenses in some states) and carry it with them. They should tell their family members their wishes. Family members may also choose to donate the organs of a recently deceased person. There is no age limit on organ donation. The main criteria are the overall medical condition of the donor and the status of the organs at death.

Organs and tissues that can be donated include the kidneys, heart, liver, lungs, pancreas, intestine, corneas, skin, bone, the middle ear, bone marrow, connective tissues, and blood vessels. Organ donation is performed by surgeons in an operating room, and it does not disfigure the body. Donation does not rule out an open-casket funeral, for example.

O

Since organ donation requires a close match in blood type and genetic makeup between the donor and recipient, success is more likely if both come from the same ethnic group.

Organic

Any chemical compound containing carbon. Organic food is food grown without the use of chemical fertilizers or pesticides. Carbon-based organic compounds are found in or produced by all living systems. Organic foods are grown in soil that has been enriched with composting and mulching rather than with chemical fertilizers. In medicine, an organic disorder is one associated with changes in the structure of an organ or tissue.

Organic brain disorder

A term formerly used to describe mental illnesses due to a nonpsychiatric medical condition rather than a psychological cause. It is now known that all mental illnesses have at least some biological basis. Organic brain disorder is divided into three types of mental illness. The first is DELIRIUM—a state of mental confusion that develops over a few hours or days and tends to fluctuate, often rapidly. The second is DEMENTIA—a persistent state of cognitive deficit including impairment in memory. The third is amnestic disorder (see AMNESIA)—an impairment to memory alone that does not involve other cognitive functions. The causes of delirium, dementia, and amnestic disorder include various general medical conditions (for example, liver disease), diseases of the brain (for example, Alzheimer's disease, encephalitis, or a brain tumor), medications or toxins, abused substances (for example, alcohol or sedatives), poor circulation in the brain, stroke, and brain injury.

Organism

Any living thing. Organisms may be single-celled microorganisms or multicelled entities made up of differentiated but interdependent cells.

Terms in small capital letters—for example, PHYSICAL THERAPY or PAGET DISEASE—indicate a cross-reference to another entry with more information.

Complex organisms, such as human beings, are made up many different organs with separate functions that are mutually dependent on one another.

Orgasm

The climax stage of SEXUAL RESPONSE that follows the arousal and plateau stages in both men and women. It lasts for several seconds and consists of rhythmic muscular contractions, pleasurable sensations, and sometimes brief mental disorientation. Women experience muscular orgasmic contractions in the outer third of the vagina, the uterus, and the anal area. Men have orgasms in two stages that often are experienced simultaneously. First, the prostate and other glands contract, forcing semen (the fluid that carries sperm) into the base of the urethra; then, orgasmic contractions of the penis and urethra cause ejaculation of the fluid.

Orgasm, lack of

A persistent absence of the climax phase during sexual activity despite adequate stimulation. Lack of orgasm is also known as anorgasmia, and it can affect both men and women. The condition may be lifelong, or it may arise only in certain situations. Typically, lack of orgasm leads to dissatisfaction with sexual relationships and may affect body image and self-esteem.

Causes can be physical or psychological. Physical causes include diseases such as diabetes mellitus and multiple sclerosis, cancer in the pelvic region, tumors of the spinal cord, surgery to the genitals, drugs (alcohol and sedatives), chronic illnesses affecting energy level and sexual interest, and certain medications (such as those used to treat high blood pressure and depression). Psychological causes include negative attitudes about sexuality learned in childhood, anxiety about sexual performance, and discord or strife in the relationship.

Treatment depends on cause. If the cause is physical, treatment of the underlying condition or a change in medication may alleviate the problem. Psychological causes are best addressed in COUPLES THERAPY or SEX THERAPY.

Orlistat

A weight-loss aid. Orlistat (Xenical) prevents the digestion of some of the fat consumed in food. When fats are not digested, they cannot be absorbed by the body and so do not contribute calories. To work most effectively, Orlistat must be used in conjunction with a weight-reduction diet.

Orphan drugs

Drugs used to treat rare diseases. Orphan drugs are defined by the Food and Drug Administration (FDA) as those used to treat diseases or conditions affecting fewer than 200,000 people in the United States. Because so few people need them, the drugs are unlikely to prove profitable for manufacturers, and it sometimes is difficult to find sponsors for the drugs.

In 1983, the FDA created the Orphan Drug Act, which grants special privileges and marketing incentives to manufacturers who are willing to "adopt" orphan drugs. Research groups and pharmaceutical manufacturers now receive financial incentives or exclusive contracts to encourage them to develop drugs needed to treat rare diseases. The FDA also approves orphan drugs more quickly than products aimed at huge markets, since orphan drugs serve smaller populations and require smaller studies for quick approval. In 1993, for example, a drug to treat cystic fibrosis was approved in only 8 months.

Orthodontic appliances

Fixed or removable devices fitted on the teeth by an ORTHODONTIST to improve the position of the teeth in the jaw. Orthodontic appliances are generally made of metal and plastic; some may be gold-plated. Ceramic appliances are made of a tooth-colored material that is less noticeable than standard metallic braces; they are durable and may be the most appealing option for adults who need to wear braces. Orthodontic appliances may be used to improve the appearance of the teeth or to correct disorders and abnormalities that may cause dental and oral health problems. The most common orthodontic appliances are dental braces (see

STRAIGHTENING TEETH

Orthodontic appliances such as braces and retainers may be recommended to improve the appearance of teeth or to correct disorders or abnormalities that may cause dental problems or oral health problems. Over months or years, the appliances gently push the teeth into correct position and align the top and bottom jaws properly.

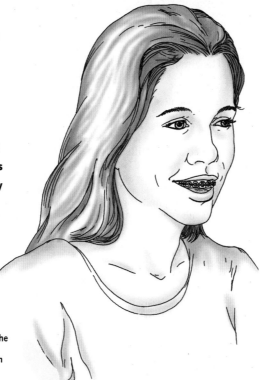

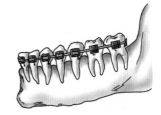

HOW BRACES WORK
Braces are made from metal or plastic brackets that are cemented over each tooth. Wires with tiny springs attach to the brackets so that the orthodontist can tighten the arch wires to help guide the teeth into correct alignment.

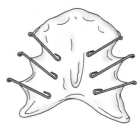

RETAINER
Once braces have been removed, a retainer may be worn for several months or years to keep the teeth from slipping out of position. The retainer can be removed before the person eats.

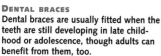

DENTAL BRACES
Dental braces are usually fitted when the teeth are still developing in late childhood or adolescence, though adults can benefit from them, too.

BRACES, DENTAL) and retainers (see RETAINER, DENTAL), typically worn after the braces have been removed. The general functions of these appliances are to push teeth into proper position, to stimulate the teeth and jaws to grow properly, to help teeth achieve a uniform length, and to align the top and bottom jaws properly. They are also used to separate teeth and provide more space for overcrowded teeth (see OVERCROWDING, DENTAL), to bring separated teeth closer together, to prevent molars from rotating, and to maintain spaces between PRIMARY TEETH so PERMANENT TEETH can grow. See also MALOCCLUSION.

Orthodontics

The branch of dentistry that involves the position of the teeth and the correction of MALOCCLUSION, or bite disorders. Orthodontics involves the detection, diagnosis, prevention, and treatment of irregular positions of the teeth and abnormal relationships between the upper and lower jaws in children and adults. The practice of orthodontics involves straightening the teeth and treating problems related to the growth and development of the jaws. Orthodontic treatment may include the use of corrective devices, TOOTH EXTRACTION, and ORAL SURGERY. See also BRACES, DENTAL; ORTHODONTIC APPLIANCES; and MALOCCLUSION.

Orthodontist

A dentist who specializes in ORTHODONTICS. Orthodontists have received special training in the design, application, and maintenance of orthodontic appliances. Their specialized skills are directed toward achieving proper alignment of the teeth, lips, and jaws. The clinical practice of an orthodontist is generally centered on using dental braces (see BRACES, DENTAL) to move the teeth into the proper position and improve the bite. Braces may be advised for children or adults.

Orthognathic surgery

An operation to change the position of the jawbone to help correct deformities or misalignments of the upper and lower teeth. Orthognathic surgery is often performed along with orthodontic treatment, which straightens the teeth.

Orthognathic surgery is not simply cosmetic. In many cases, it is the best remedy for serious dental problems, abnormalities of speech, impaired breathing, and related conditions. Orthognathic surgery is performed by an ORAL AND MAXILLO-

FACIAL SURGEON, a dental school graduate who has undergone extensive training in a surgery residency program.

HOW IT IS DONE

The procedure, performed with the patient under general anesthesia and asleep and pain-free, usually takes 3 to 4 hours. Incisions are made in the mouth to expose the jaws; then, the bones are surgically altered as needed to repair the defect. Miniature screws and plates hold the bones in place, and the incisions are closed with sutures. In some cases, rubber bands or wires are attached to the teeth to hold the jaws together during a healing period.

The hospital stay is usually 1 to 3 days. Activity should be limited during the first week after surgery, and strenuous, heavy exercise needs to be avoided for the first month. Swelling in the mouth and jaw is common. There may also be temporary discoloration of the face, which goes away within the first week or two. In most cases, recovery is complete in about 30 days.

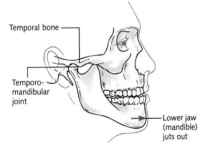

REPOSITIONING THE JAWS AND TEETH
Orthognathic procedures correct severe misalignments of the upper and lower jaw that, left untreated, would interfere with speech or breathing. Both the size and configuration of the mouth and palate, and the resulting alignment of the teeth, can be altered.

Labels: Temporal bone; Temporo-mandibular joint; Lower jaw (mandible) juts out

Orthopedic surgery

The medical specialty that studies, diagnoses, and treats disorders of the musculoskeletal system, including the bones, joints, muscles of the arms and legs, ligaments, tendons, nerves, the spine, and associated structures. Orthopedic surgery uses medical, surgical, and physical means to study and treat problems in the form and function of the body's bones, muscles, and joints that are inherited or have developed over a lifetime. These may include deformities, injuries, and degenerative diseases of the spine, hands, feet, ligaments, tendons, nerves, and joints in children and adults. See also JOINT REPLACEMENT; SPORTS MEDICINE.

Orthopedics

The branch of medicine that is involved with the correction or prevention of disease and disorders in the musculoskeletal system.

Orthopedist

A medical specialist who has been trained and qualified in the diagnosis and surgical and nonsurgical treatment of diseases and disorders of the musculoskeletal system, including the bones, joints, ligaments, tendons, muscles, nerves, and their associated structures.

Orthopnea

Difficulty breathing that occurs while lying down. People with orthopnea wake up at night feeling short of breath, and they find they can sleep restfully only when sitting upright or with several pillows under the head. Orthopnea is often a sign of heart failure, but it can be caused by other heart and lung problems or by anxiety.

Orthoptics

Exercises designed to bring the eyes into correct alignment. Orthoptics are sometimes used in the treatment of crossed eyes. See STRABISMUS.

Orthotics

Special devices that are used or worn to control, correct, or compensate for irregularities or injuries of the bones, muscles, or joints. Orthotics are sometimes called orthotic appliances and are often used to help treat sports injuries. They may be purchased commercially and sometimes are molded to improve fit, or they may be custom-made for an individual. An orthotic brace may be used to help straighten and support the spine in conditions such as scoliosis, or orthotics may be prescribed to be worn in the shoe for the treatment of foot disorders such as hammer toe. A foot orthotic is sometimes recommended to help correct irregularities in the mechanics of running or other

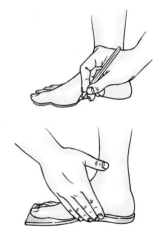

FITTING ORTHOTICS
Orthotics for the feet are worn inside the shoe. To custom-fit the orthotic, the person's foot is first carefully traced. Then a plastic material that is pliable until it sets is molded to the person's arch. The material comes in various densities that can be prescribed according to the person's activity level.

exercises. In this case, orthotics worn during the exercise may help prevent injuries.

Os

A Latin anatomical term meaning BONE. Os can also mean mouth and refer to an opening in the body, usually the cervical os (the opening in the CERVIX, the entrance to the uterus).

Oseltamivir

An antiviral drug. Oseltamivir (Tamiflu) is used to treat infections caused by viruses, particularly those caused by influenza A and influenza B viruses. Oseltamivir reduces the severity of flu symptoms, including fever, headache, cough, and sore throat, in a single day. It should be taken within 2 days of the start of flu symptoms to work best.

Osgood-Schlatter disease

An inflammation in the upper part of a child's shin bone that connects to the tendons around the kneecap. Although it can affect girls, Osgood-Schlatter disease is most common in very active boys between ages 9 and 14. Repeated stress or pulling on the thigh muscle and tendon attached to the tuberosity are responsible for the disorder.

O

Symptoms include pain, swelling, and tenderness in the shin, just below the knee. There may also be pain above the knee. Pain worsens when the child is physically active. Running, bicycling, and stair climbing, in particular, may cause pain. A doctor usually can diagnose Osgood-Schlatter disease after a medical history and a physical examination. X rays may be used to rule out other possible causes. With rest and limited activity, pain, swelling, and tenderness gradually subside. Ibuprofen (not aspirin) can also help control pain and swelling. Applying an ice pack after activity reduces the pain and inflammation. Other treatments include a temporary brace (see BRACE, ORTHOPEDIC) to support the knee and special exercises to strengthen the surrounding muscles. Children generally outgrow the problem by late adolescence.

Osmosis

Slow, gradual change in concentration of solutions through semipermeable membranes.

In osmosis, a solvent flows through a semipermeable membrane from a more concentrated solution to a less concentrated one by a process called DIFFUSION. Osmosis is essential in the regulation of the movement of water into and out of tissues in the bodies of living things.

Ossicle

A small bone. For example, the small bones known as the hammer (malleus), anvil (incus), and stirrup (stapes) in the middle ear are called the auditory ossicles.

Ossification

The process by which bone is developed from cartilage or fibrous tissue. The human skeleton is gradually transformed from cartilage to hard bone during infant and child development by ossification. As cartilage becomes bone, it is said to ossify.

Osteitis

Inflammation or infection of the bone.

Osteitis deformans

See PAGET DISEASE.

Osteoarthritis

FOR SYMPTOM CHARTS
see Ankle or foot problems, page 18
see Hip pain, page 42
see Knee pain, page 44

A condition caused by wear and tear on the joints accompanied by an erosion of their lubricated sliding surfaces, called the articular cartilage. Osteoarthritis is also called degenerative joint disease. As the cartilage flakes and cracks, the joint loses the cushioning that allows it to move smoothly. Cracking or popping of the joint often occurs. The bone of the joint becomes flattened, thickened, eroded, and distorted. Extra bone tissue develops at the joint margins. Typically, the weight-bearing larger joints, including those of the hips, knees, neck, and lower spine, are involved. The small joints of the fingers are also commonly affected. Although the cause is unknown, hereditary factors may have a role; aging seems to accelerate the process of degeneration. Osteoarthritis commonly occurs in middle-aged and older adults. See Osteoarthritic joints, page 928.

TREATMENT

Degenerative joint disease is often present to some degree in most adults older than 40. It may or may not cause pain. Often, the condition is discovered during a physical examination that includes X rays, and the disease does not usually require treatment. In many cases, the condition produces some amount of short-lived discomfort that disappears within a year. Limited and minor pain of osteoarthritis may occur at intervals of a few months or a year and can be treated by resting the joint, applying heat, and taking a nonsteroidal anti-inflammatory drug (NSAID) such as aspirin, ibuprofen, or naproxen.

When inflammation of the joint is involved, the condition causes pain and swelling. Several joints may be affected at the same time. In some instances slight discomfort may progress to severe pain that interrupts sleep and limits daily activities. Treatment at this point emphasizes control of the inflammation and swelling and relief of the pain. NSAIDs may be taken to ease symp-

toms and manage pain. Physical therapy, including exercise and massage, may be recommended to help control inflammation. The application of heat or ice may be part of physical therapy treatments; ultrasound or mild electrical currents may be used to reduce the inflammation in the joints.

The severe and persistent pain caused by osteoarthritis may be treated with prescription painkillers. Corticosteroid drugs can be injected into a painful joint to relieve discomfort, but this procedure carries the risk of damaging the joint cartilage if performed too frequently. Injectable joint fluid supplements are also available.

If more conservative treatment has not been effective and a person's general health is good, surgery may become an option. The doctor may recommend flushing the joint to remove chemicals or possibly an arthroscopic procedure to remove damaged tissue and debris. Surgical joint replacement is performed in cases that involve chronic, incapacitating pain or complete immobility of a joint. The hip and knee joints are most commonly and successfully replaced; ankle, shoulder, elbow, and finger joints may also be treated with this surgical procedure. The surgery involves replacing natural, damaged joints with artificial joints made of metal, plastic, or porcelain.

SELF-HELP MEASURES

Resting often, sleeping on a firm mattress, staying warm, and applying heat to a joint affected by osteoarthritis can help ease symptoms. Adequate nutrition, including vitamin supplements, is often advised. People with osteoarthritis who are overweight can relieve the extra stress on affected joints by losing weight. Strengthening the muscles surrounding diseased joints also helps to minimize symptoms. A physician or physical therapist can offer instructions in appropriate exercises. Using an assistive walking device, such as a cane for hip or knee pain, may be helpful.

Osteochondritis dissecans

A condition that develops from stress fractures of the underlying cartilage of a joint, often the knee, elbow, or

O

OSTEOARTHRITIC JOINTS

Osteoarthritis is a common joint disease and a major cause of disability in older people. The disease causes the cartilage at the end of the bones to erode. Without the cartilage, bone is rubbing on bone, causing pain and loss of mobility in the joint.

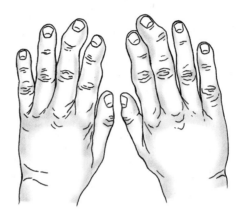

SWOLLEN FINGER JOINTS
Outwardly, joints affected by osteoarthritis often look swollen and bent. The appearance is caused by bony outgrowths called osteophytes on the ends of the bones in the joint.

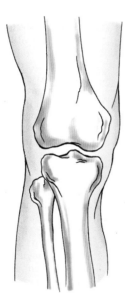

HEALTHY KNEE JOINT
Healthy cartilage is smooth and slippery, allowing the knee joints to move without friction.

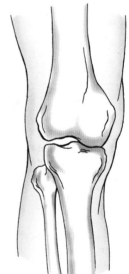

REDUCED JOINT SPACE
From within, the space between the bones in the knee joint is reduced because of the loss of protective cartilage.

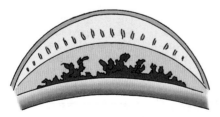

HEALTHY CARTILAGE
At a cellular level, the cells in healthy cartilage (called chondrocytes) are aligned perpendicular to the smooth surface on the bone end.

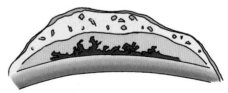

OSTEOARTHRITIC CARTILAGE
In osteoarthritic cartilage, the scaffolding of cells breaks down so that the surface is thin and eroded. Under the surface, the underlying layer thickens.

ankle joint. Osteochondritis dissecans (OCD) is caused by small fragments of cartilage and bone being separated and sometimes released into the interior of a joint, often the knee joint, followed by an interruption of blood supply to the fragment. Symptoms include an aching pain that becomes worse with activity. Range of motion of the joint is usually normal. OCD is generally diagnosed with X rays. MRI (magnetic resonance imaging) is sometimes recommended when it is necessary to evaluate the size and healing potential of the OCD lesion. When OCD is diagnosed in children, it is called juvenile osteochondritis dissecans. Juvenile OCD tends to heal in about half of all cases in which the fragment is not yet free in the joint and, when healed, does not lead to arthritic changes in the knee as the child becomes an adult.

When the condition does not heal independently, surgery becomes necessary to reposition or stabilize the fractured bone fragment. Standard knee surgery or arthroscopy (see ARTHROSCOPIC SURGERY), the use of a small viewing instrument to perform knee surgery, may be recommended to restore the knee joint to its original condition. In some cases, the fractured bone fragment may have to be pinned back into position.

Osteochondroma

A noncancerous, tumorlike lesion formed by a bony protrusion covered with cartilage. Osteochondroma, which is most common in people younger than 20, may form as a single lesion or as several lesions that are painless and slow growing. Sometimes the protrusions appear after an injury. They most commonly are found in tubular bones, including the thighbone, shinbone, or ribs, but may also occur in the pelvis. An osteochondroma generally stops growing when the bone is fully developed.

Osteochondrosis

A chronic condition in children involving inflammation and deformity of the ball-shaped bone of the ball-and-socket hip joint. Osteochondrosis is also called Calvé-Perthes, Perthes disease, and Legg-Calvé-Perthes disease. The disorder occurs most commonly in children, usually African American boys between the ages of 2 and 10. It is caused by an inadequate blood supply to the developing bone at the head of the thighbone (femur), which causes the bone to progressively deteriorate over a period of 2 to 3 years. The cause is unknown. Generally, only one hip joint is affected. Symptoms may include pain in the thigh and groin and a restriction of movement, sometimes resulting in a limp and muscle spasms. X rays are often used to make the diagnosis.

Treatment generally emphasizes containment of the hip with a reduction of pressure on the affected joint. A CALIPER SPLINT or other special brace may need to be worn for as long as 2 years while the bone heals naturally. Surgery is sometimes recommended. There is a more optimistic prognosis for children who develop osteochondrosis before the age of 6.

Osteodystrophy

The general term for any defective bone formation.

Osteogenesis imperfecta

See BRITTLE BONES.

Osteogenic sarcoma

See OSTEOSARCOMA.

Osteoid osteoma

A benign bone-forming tumor, which may occur anywhere but usually occurs in the legs, particularly the thighbone (femur). Osteoid osteoma is found most commonly in children older than 3 and in adults younger than 40. Symptoms include a dull aching pain that becomes progressively more severe over time. Discomfort tends to be more intense at night for most people. The pain can be felt when the body is at rest and is aggravated by activity, though movement itself does not necessarily cause the pain. The tumor can produce inflammation in surrounding soft tissues, creating the sensation of swelling or a lump in the area. Nonsteroidal anti-inflammatory drugs (NSAIDs), including aspirin and ibuprofen, can usually offer relief from the discomforts of osteoid osteoma.

Surgical removal provides definitive treatment.

Osteoma

A benign bone tumor that may be found in any bone in the body and that usually produces a painless swelling. A surgical procedure may be necessary to treat the condition.

Osteomalacia

A rare condition, usually due to a deficiency of vitamin D, which causes bones to demineralize and lose excessive amounts of calcium and phosphorus. The result is softened and weakened bones, which are more vulnerable to fracture under slight stress. Sometimes called adult rickets, osteomalacia most commonly affects the bones of the pelvis, legs, and spine. The symptoms of osteomalacia include deformity of the affected bones and tenderness and pain in the bones and joints, similar to the discomfort of RHEUMATOID ARTHRITIS. There may also be fatigue and stiffness, frequent cramping, and difficulty standing.

Osteomalacia is caused by the body's inability to absorb calcium and phosphorus or to deposit mineral salts in the protein structure of the bone. Calcium and phosphorus are essential to the development, calcification, and maintenance of strong bones. These dietary minerals are usually found in a healthy diet but cannot be absorbed by the body when vitamin D is deficient. An inability to absorb dietary fats may also contribute to the condition because vitamin D is a fat-soluble vitamin, and calcium must combine with dietary fat to be properly absorbed. Vitamin D is acquired from the diet and from the skin's exposure to sunlight. A deficiency of vitamin D that contributes to osteomalacia may be produced by chronic kidney failure, celiac disease, prolonged drug treatment for epilepsy, and certain digestive tract operations. The condition is usually diagnosed by blood and urine tests and X rays. Because X-ray images of bones affected by osteomalacia look identical to those affected by osteoporosis, a biopsy is sometimes the only way of distinguishing between the two disorders. In severe cases,

O

the disorder may be treated with a prescription for large doses of vitamin D supplements and treatment for any underlying disease.

Osteomyelitis

Inflammation of the bone marrow and adjacent bone. Also a medical term for all the infectious diseases of the bone, including the bone marrow. Osteomyelitis may be localized or widespread and may include the cartilage and the periosteum (a fibrous membrane that covers the surface of all bones, except at the joints). Bone infections may be caused by microorganisms, most commonly bacteria from a staphylococcal infection, that reach bone tissue via the bloodstream, a fracture, an injury, or a sinus infection or dental abscess. Symptoms include fever, pain, and redness and swelling of the affected area. X rays are not useful early in the course of this infection, but a bone scan can be useful in making the diagnosis. Antibiotics are prescribed for several weeks to treat osteomyelitis and prevent its spread through large areas of bone. Surgery may be needed to drain the pus or to stabilize the bone in cases of significant bone destruction. Left untreated, osteomyelitis may destroy bone extensively and spread to nearby joints. Rarely, it can cause abscesses that are ultimately fatal.

Osteonecrosis

The general medical term for the loss of tissue and destruction of bone structures in the knee, which may be caused by conditions or diseases including OSTEOCHONDROSIS and systemic lupus erythematosus (see LUPUS ERYTHEMATOSUS, SYSTEMIC). Osteonecrosis is generally diagnosed by MRI (magnetic resonance imaging) and possibly blood tests and is more common in women older than 50. Stiffness and knee swelling may occur. The blood tests can measure calcium levels to evaluate bone metabolism. These tests may also reveal improper levels of substances that can cause or contribute to osteonecrosis, including vitamin D deficiencies. Hormones and other substances in the blood may indicate disorders of other organs, such as the kidneys and parathyroid glands, that affect bone tissue. Anti-inflammatory

medications are useful. Rarely, knee replacement is necessary.

Osteopathic medicine

The branch of medicine that has historically focused on the interactive relationships among the many body systems and the shifting balance among them as it relates to a person's health. Doctors of osteopathic medicine, or DOs, have traditionally used musculoskeletal manipulations to treat a wide range of problems. However, over the years, the differences between osteopathic medicine and conventional medicine have narrowed. Today in all 50 states osteopaths receive the same medical license that physicians do, entitling them to full privileges in hospitals. Also, many DOs use more techniques of conventional medicine (such as prescribing medications or ordering laboratory work), while conventional medicine has given increased recognition to osteopathic tenets, such as the relationship between lifestyle and health.

Osteopenia

A thinning of the bones or low levels of bone calcium. A woman is diagnosed with osteopenia by having a bone density test (see DUAL-ENERGY X-RAY ABSORPTIOMETRY (DEXA); this typically means her bone density is below average. Treatment includes increasing calcium and vitamin D intake and performing regular weight-bearing and resistance exercises to prevent OSTEOPOROSIS.

Osteopetrosis

A rare hereditary disease characterized by abnormally dense bone. The dense bone tends to take up the space that normally is occupied by bone marrow, particularly in the long bones of the arms and legs, which results in the development of anemia. Osteopetrosis occurs in two forms. The more severe form appears in infancy or childhood. The other form appears in adolescence or adulthood. Osteopetrosis is sometimes called "ivory bones" or "marble bones." It is a recessive genetic disorder for which there is no cure and no test for detection. The infant form is always fatal.

Osteophyte

An outgrowth of bone tissue that forms at the edge of a joint that has

been affected by osteoarthritis. It is commonly known as a SPUR.

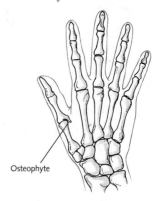

Osteophyte

BONY OUTGROWTH
Osteophytes frequently give the affected joint a knobby, swollen look.

Osteoporosis

A bone disease, usually diagnosed in postmenopausal women, which causes the bones to gradually lose protein structure and mineral content and eventually to deteriorate. Osteoporosis is the most common metabolic bone disease in the United States. The disease produces an imbalance in the ongoing breakdown and renewal cycle of normal healthy bone formation. This action prompts bone tissue to break down more quickly than it can be replaced. Osteoporosis causes a decrease of bone density and produces bone tissue that is thin, brittle, porous, and more vulnerable to fracture.

The disease is often present without pain or other symptoms until an affected bone breaks. Associated fractures are usually of the spine, hip, and wrist bones. When a spinal fracture occurs, the symptoms are a severe backache and a stooped, round-shouldered posture caused by the gradual compression of weakened vertebrae in the spine. As a result, normal height may become diminished.

CAUSES AND CONTRIBUTING FACTORS

All of the causes of osteoporosis are not known, but aging is suspected to be the most common cause. The loss of estrogen at menopause is one known risk factor for women because estrogen has a vital role in supplying calcium to the bone. Early menopause brought about by radiation therapy, hysterectomy, or removal of the ovaries also causes a lack of estrogen and makes a woman more susceptible to osteoporosis.

Contributing factors include a small body frame, alcohol abuse, cigarette smoking, a family history of the disease, an inadequate dietary intake of calcium and protein, and, in younger women, excessive exercise that causes a woman to stop having menstrual periods. Aging is an element in the disease; loss of bone mass tends to begin after the age of 35 and become progressively more severe with each passing year.

Certain medical conditions may make a person more susceptible to the development of osteoporosis. These include the use of corticosteroid medications such as prednisone; hyperthyroidism, hyperparathyroidism, Cushing disease, and other hormonal disorders; intestinal disorders such as malabsorption; and chronic liver disease. In men, chronic alcoholism and a decline in the male hormone testosterone can cause the disease. Other risk factors for osteoporosis include being Caucasian or Asian and reaching menopause before the age of 45. Osteoporosis may sometimes occur in association with OSTEOMALACIA.

DIAGNOSIS

Health care providers may recommend testing for the disease. People who think they are at risk should ask to be tested. X rays can reveal a thinning of bones and may be used as a preliminary diagnostic tool to rule out other bone disorders, including arthritic conditions. Bone density testing is more accurate for a definitive osteoporosis diagnosis.

DUAL ENERGY X-RAY ABSORPTIOMETRY (DEXA or DXA) is the most commonly used test and is considered the most accurate. DEXA is a painless bone density test that measures the bones' mineral content, which indicates the strength and density of bone tissue. These tests may be used to evaluate the loss of mineral content from the bones and, during treatment for osteoporosis, to measure the rate of increase in mineral content. Portable DEXA devices that can measure bone density in the finger or heel may be used at various locations on osteoporosis screening days. People whose test results indicate that they are at risk are referred to their physicians for further testing.

A device called a sonometer uses ultrasound (high-frequency sound waves) to measure bone density in the foot. This device can help a physician evaluate bone strength and predict future risk.

TREATMENT

Treatment options include prescription medications called antiresorptives, which can slow, and sometimes stop, the loss of bone minerals. The three most commonly approved medications in use today are estrogen, bisphosphonates such as alendronate, and calcitonin.

■ **Estrogen** Delivered in pill or patch form, estrogen is currently considered the most effective means of regaining lost bone mineral content, strengthening the spine, and preventing fractures. There are side effects and risks associated with taking estrogen. Beneficial side effects include a reduction in menopausal body temperature fluctuations and a reduction in the risks of heart disease and stroke. Side effects include uterine bleeding and breast soreness. Some studies have indicated a slightly increased risk of developing breast cancer with estrogen therapy.

For women who have their uterus, progestin may be prescribed along with estrogen to prevent possible increased risk of uterine cancer and to prevent uterine bleeding. This combined medication is called HORMONE REPLACEMENT THERAPY, or HRT.

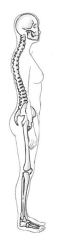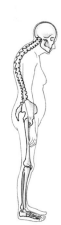

Healthy spine   Spine with osteoporosis

COMPRESSION FRACTURES IN SPINE
The bone-thinning effects of osteoporosis can cause a compression fracture, a type of fracture in which the front portion of the vertebra collapses. The result of compression fractures is a weakened and often abnormally curved spine—a condition commonly called dowager's hump.

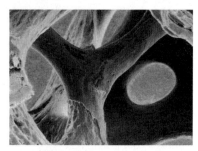

HEALTHY BONE TISSUE
Healthy bone has a layer of spongy tissue composed of minerals and the protein collagen, with a porous yet strong structure.

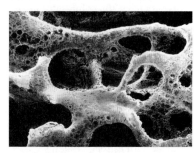

OSTEOPOROTIC BONE TISSUE
Osteoporosis weakens bone by reducing the mineral content, thinning the spongy layer and making the structure brittle.

■ *Bisphosphonate* Among bisphosphonates, alendronate is the only currently approved medication. It increases the bone mineral density, reduces bone loss, strengthens the spine and hipbones, and reduces the risks of spinal fracture. Bisphosphonates are not hormones and do not increase cancer risk or reduce the risk of heart disease. Side effects include nausea and abdominal pain. They are especially appropriate for men, young people, and people who have corticosteroid-induced osteoporosis.

■ *Calcitonin* This medication may be given by injection or nasal inhalation and is prescribed when estrogen and bisphosphonate are not appropriate. Calcitonin helps prevent bone loss, but it does not strengthen hipbones and has not been demonstrated to prevent bone fractures. Side effects may include nausea and skin rashes.

Osteosarcoma

A sarcoma or primary malignant tissue tumor in the bone. Found primarily in adolescents, bone tumors may be painful and weaken the bone tissue, making it vulnerable to fracture under slight pressure.

Cancerous bone tumors tend to spread rapidly to other parts of the body, especially to the lungs. If a lump develops on a bone, a doctor should be consulted. A physical examination and X rays are generally used to diagnose osteosarcoma. Removal of the tumor and a wide margin of normal tissue surrounding it may be necessary, along with other treatment.

Osteosclerosis

A rare hereditary disorder of bone formation characterized by an abnormal increase in bone density, which results in massive, fragile bones. With osteosclerosis, the long bones of the extremities are thickened and expand into trumpetlike shapes. In some cases, the increased thickness of the bones fills the spaces containing bone marrow, the tissue that produces red blood cells; this can cause severe anemia, which may prove fatal. Bone overgrowth at the base of the skull may cause pressure on certain structures of the eye and produce blindness. Pressure on the auditory nerves can result in deafness.

The cause is unknown but may be related to a defect in the function of bone cells during the ongoing breakdown and renewal cycle of bone tissue. One form of osteosclerosis, which can cause death when the fetus is in utero, during infancy, or during young adulthood, is due to destruction of bone marrow, severe anemia, or other related abnormalities. The main symptom of the other form is repeated bone fractures from slight trauma or pressure. In this form, life expectancy is normal. Osteosclerosis may also be called osteopetrosis or marble bone disease.

Osteotomy

An orthopedic surgical procedure for correcting deformed or diseased joints or bones. The bone may be cut, repositioned, or fractured to change its length or shape or to improve the stability of a joint. Osteotomy may be performed to straighten a severely bent spine caused by the fused vertebral bones of an inflammatory disease called ANKYLOSING SPONDYLITIS. The surgical procedure involves the risk of spinal cord damage and is usually performed only in extreme cases.

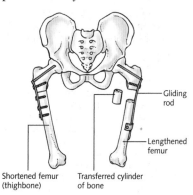

Gliding rod

Lengthened femur

Shortened femur (thighbone)

Transferred cylinder of bone

ADJUSTING LEG LENGTH
For a person whose legs are not of equal length, an osteotomy can lengthen one leg and shorten the other.

Ostomy

A surgical procedure that creates an opening, or STOMA. This opening may be in the wall of the abdomen to allow the discharge of bodily wastes. Or it may be in the windpipe to allow air to enter and leave the lungs without going through the nose or the mouth (tracheostomy). An ostomy is performed when a person has lost normal function of the bladder, bowel, or upper airway because of cancer or another serious disease, a birth defect, or an injury. Some ostomies are temporary, allowing the intestine or windpipe time to heal before it is reconnected. Others are permanent, particularly when a diseased or damaged organ, such as the bladder, rectum, or larynx, has to be removed.

An ostomy includes a number of different procedures, and the details, such as the number and placement of stomas, may vary with the particular surgery. In some ostomies of the urinary tract, a pouch is created inside the body, and accumulated urine is drained off by inserting a tube, or catheter, through the stoma. In a colostomy, for example—which connects the colon to the abdominal wall—the person wears a pouch that seals in place over the stoma, catches feces, and is emptied periodically. In a TRACHEOSTOMY, a permanent opening is created between the windpipe and the skin through a special tube.

THE PROCEDURE
An ostomy is performed with the

patient under general anesthesia, asleep, and pain-free. In the case of an ostomy in the abdomen, the area is opened, the diseased or damaged tissue is removed, and the healthy tissue is stitched to an opening in the abdomen to create the stoma before the abdominal incision is closed.

Most people spend 7 to 10 days in the hospital after an ostomy. Typically the person can resume eating within 2 to 3 days. Full healing takes from 1 to 2 months. During this time, the patient learns how to change the appliance and care for the stoma.

People who have received an ostomy are sometimes referred to as ostomates. Many people with ostomies find that they are able to return to most of the activities that they enjoyed before surgery. An exception is contact sports, since hard blows to the abdomen should be avoided. Heavy lifting should also be avoided. Other forms of exercise are encouraged because they strengthen the abdominal wall and help to maintain the health of the stoma. Some people with ostomies have to restrict their diets in certain ways. During the first 6 weeks after surgery, the person should avoid high-residue foods, such as fresh fruits, vegetables, and cereal, because those foods can plug up the colon and slow the transit time. People with an ostomy also need to eat slowly and chew their food well to avoid a stomal obstruction. A specially trained registered nurse, called an enterostomal therapist, may be called on to assist the person with stomal care.

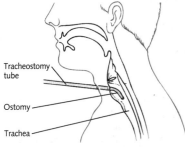

A SURGICAL OPENING
An ostomy is a term for any artificial hole in the body, created surgically to correct a serious condition. For example, a tracheostomy is an opening into the trachea (windpipe) that allows a person to breathe when the flow of air in the upper airway is blocked. A tube is inserted into the opening (stoma), and the person breathes through the tube.

Otalgia
See EARACHE.

Otic preparations
Drugs used to treat conditions inside the ear. Otic preparations, also known as ear drops, help provide relief from symptoms such as redness, irritation, and discomfort in the ear canal. For example, bacterial infections of the ear canal are sometimes treated with a combination of antibiotic and cortisonelike medications.

Otitis externa
See SWIMMER'S EAR.

Otitis externa, malignant
Inflammation due to a bacterial infection of the external ear canal that produces tenderness and severe pain in the ear, as well as a constant fluid discharge from the ear. It is caused by the bacteria that can lead to SWIMMER'S EAR, but the infection spreads to involve bone. Usually there is no fever. Malignant otitis externa does not mean the condition is cancerous; the term "malignant" refers to the infection's tendency to spread into surrounding tissue. It is more common in people whose immune systems are not effective, such as elderly people with diabetes. The diagnosis is usually confirmed by a bone scan. People who have symptoms should see an ear specialist for treatment. Large doses of the antibiotics may be prescribed for as long as 3 months, and surgery is rarely necessary. Left untreated, malignant otitis externa may result in damage to the facial nerves and other cranial nerves. It may also lead to a brain abscess. In severe cases, it may be fatal.

Otitis media
An inflammation of the middle ear resulting from infection, affecting one or both ears. Otitis media is most common in young children but may also affect older children and adults.
CAUSES
When the eustachian tube (which connects the middle ear cavity to the back of the nose and throat) becomes inflamed and swollen as the result of a common cold (see COLD, COMMON), allergies, or a respiratory tract infection, the passage-

way between the ear and the nose can become blocked. This condition is more common for young children because of the smaller size of the eustachian tubes. In response to the infection, pus and mucus accumulate behind the eardrum, increasing pressure in the middle ear and causing an earache, as well as swelling and redness of the eardrum. Because the pressure interferes with the vibrations of the eardrum, hearing may be impaired. The pressure may become sufficiently severe to rupture the eardrum and allow the fluid to drain out of the ear. More commonly, the pus becomes mucus and remains in the middle ear, trapped by the blocked eustachian tube. This condition is called middle ear effusion, or otitis media. The accumulated fluid can remain in the middle ear for weeks, months, or even years, causing recurring ear infections and difficulty hearing.

Children are at higher risk for otitis media if they have had an infection before 4 months of age, are in group child care, have frequent upper respiratory infections, or have siblings who have a history of recurrent ear infection. Children who are exposed to tobacco smoke and those who were bottle fed rather than breast-fed are also at higher risk.
SYMPTOMS
Symptoms of otitis media may include earache, problems with hearing, feelings of fullness or pressure in the ear, a discharge from the ear, dizziness and loss of balance, loss of appetite, nausea, vomiting, and fever. In young children, the difficulty hearing may delay speech development. In infants and preverbal toddlers, the symptoms can be recognized as pulling at the ear accompanied by difficulty hearing, crying, irritability, disturbed sleep, loss of appetite, fever, vomiting, and a discharge from the ear. Because ear infections can damage the hearing structures within the ear, a physician should be consulted for a checkup.
DIAGNOSIS AND TREATMENT
A physician will examine the ears using an OTOSCOPE (lighted viewing instrument inserted into the ear) to look for redness, swelling, and the presence of fluid behind the eardrum. Hearing tests may be performed if there is HEARING LOSS, and measure-

ments of air pressure in the middle ear may be performed to determine how well the eustachian tube is functioning and how well the eardrum moves.

If otitis media is diagnosed, one or more medications may be prescribed. These may include antibiotics to clear the infection, an antihistamine (to reduce mucus production), a decongestant (to relieve inflammation), and a painkiller. Because ear infections are often not bacterial, antibiotics are not used often. Analgesic ear drops may be given to relieve the pain of an earache. Follow-up visits to the doctor are very important to managing otitis media. If a child is younger than 15 months or if symptoms do not disappear with medication, the doctor should be seen again within 2 weeks. With older children and adults, once the symptoms clear up, follow-up within 6 weeks is recommended.

When fluid remains in the middle ear for 3 months or longer or when there is pronounced hearing loss, MYRINGOTOMY and tubes (a procedure that involves making a small opening in the eardrum and placing tubes in the ears to promote drainage of fluid and relieve pain) may be recommended. A ventilation tube may be placed in the opening for several months to promote ongoing drainage, improve hearing, and decrease the frequency of ear infections. If chronic infections of the adenoids or tonsils are involved in otitis media, the doctor may recommend removing them when the ventilation tube is inserted. See also ADHESIVE OTITIS MEDIA, CHRONIC.

Otolaryngologist

A physician who specializes in the medical and surgical treatment of people with diseases and disorders of the ear, nose, and throat and related structures of the head and neck. Otolaryngologists may also be called ENT (ear, nose, and throat) physicians.

Otolaryngology

The science, academic study, and medical practice of the field of diseases and disorders of the ears, nose, and throat and other structures of the head and neck.

Otoplasty

A cosmetic or reconstructive surgical procedure to improve the appearance of the outer ear. An otoplasty is usually done to flatten protruding ears; the surgery is known as pinning back the ears. The procedure is also used to reduce the size of overly large ears or, in the case of ears that have been damaged because of a severe injury or birth defect, to build a new outer ear. Abnormalities of ear shape, such as lop ears (the tip bends forward and down) or shell ears (the natural folds and creases of the outer ear are lacking), can also be repaired.

An otoplasty is usually done on children between the ages of 5 and 14 years. Before the age of 5 years, the ear is still growing rapidly so surgery is usually not performed. At 5 years, the ear has reached 90 percent of its adult size and can be repaired permanently. An otoplasty is often performed when children with overly large or protruding ears are young in order to minimize the emotional effects of teasing and ridicule as they grow up. An otoplasty can also be performed on adults.

The anesthesia used for an otoplasty depends on the extent of the procedure and the age of the patient. Young children usually find it difficult to lie still for the 2 or 3 hours that the procedure takes. As a result, general anesthesia, which puts them to sleep, is generally preferred. In older children, adolescents, and adults, local anesthesia with CONSCIOUS SEDATION (the person is drowsy but painfree and awake) is generally preferred. General anesthesia is used for complicated ear reconstruction, in which a short stay in the hospital may also be needed.

THE PROCEDURE

The outer ear consists of a framework of the tough, resilient tissue, known as cartilage, covered with skin. An otoplasty consists of reshaping this cartilage to give the ears the desired look.

In one common technique to bring protruding ears closer to the head, the surgeon makes an incision in the back of the ear to reveal the cartilage. Then the cartilage is sculpted, or a portion removed, to bend the ear back toward the head. In an alternative method, skin is removed rather than cartilage, which is stitched with permanent sutures to bend it back on itself and draw the ear close to the head. When the resculpting is finished, the incision is closed with fine sutures. The head is wrapped in bulky bandages to mold and heal the ears.

Reconstruction of a missing ear is a more complex process than a simple otoplasty, requiring more than one procedure. First, a pocket of skin is created where the ear should be, often by SKIN GRAFT. When this has healed, a section of cartilage is removed from a rib, shaped to resemble an ear, and then placed inside the pocket of skin and sutured. Again, the head is wrapped in bulky bandages during initial healing.

BEFORE AND AFTER SURGERY

As is true of all surgeries with anesthesia, the person should not eat or drink anything after midnight the day before the operation. The surgeon may also advise avoidance of certain medications or vitamins in advance of surgery. Blood and urine tests may be required before surgery, and the person may be screened for undetected conditions that may affect safety and outcome, such as high blood pressure or diabetes.

After a simple otoplasty, the person is usually up and around within a few hours. During the first days after surgery, the ears are likely to feel swollen and painful. Oral medication, prescribed by the surgeon, should control this discomfort. The bulky bandages are worn for several days; then, these bandages are replaced with a lighter bandage that looks like a headband and is worn for several weeks. Sutures are removed, or disappear on their own if they are dissolvable, within a week.

In most cases, adults can go back to work in 5 days after an otoplasty, and children can return to school in a week. Recovery is usually complete in 2 weeks. For a month, any activity that can bend the ear, such as sports or rigorous play, should be avoided. Scars are small, well hidden in the back of the ear, and usually fade to thin white lines within a year.

Recovery takes longer in the case of ear reconstruction. The bulky dressings are left in place for 10 to 14 days. The sutures are removed at this time, or they will disappear on their own if they are dissolvable.

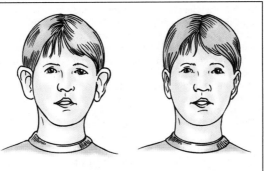

RESHAPING THE EAR
The most common reconstructive surgical procedure done on the ears is "pinning back" protruding ears. The operation is generally done on a child between the ages of 5 and 14, after the ear has grown to almost its full adult size. The procedure involves either cutting out a portion of cartilage or folding back a portion of skin behind the ear.

Before otoplasty   After otoplasty

OUTLOOK

Possible complications of an otoplasty include a blood clot on the ear that may disappear on its own or can be drawn out with a needle. If the cartilage becomes infected, it can be treated with antibiotics. Infection may form scar tissue that has to be removed later to preserve the appearance of the ear. Ears that have undergone a reconstruction or an otoplasty are often highly sensitive to cold, particularly in the first year after surgery.

Otorhinolaryngology

The longer name for OTOLARYNGOLOGY, derived from the Greek base words for ear, nose, and throat.

Otorrhea

See EAR, DISCHARGE FROM.

Otosclerosis

A disorder of the middle ear that involves the bone in the walls of the inner ear and causes progressive HEARING LOSS, generally affecting both ears. This disease usually develops during the teen or early adult years as a result of microscopic growth and changes in the composition of the sound-conducting bone in the inner ear. The usually hard, mineralized bone in this area becomes spongy, which leads to the immobilization of a bone of the ear that is normally movable. Specifically, the stapes bone (the tiniest bone in the body, located behind the eardrum and commonly called the stirrup because of its shape) becomes cemented to the surrounding bone and cannot vibrate. Because the vibrations of the stapes are essential to conducting sound waves to the inner ear fluids, hearing is impaired. If the nerves of the inner ear become involved, there is a distortion of sound that makes it difficult for a person to understand speech, no matter how loudly it is spoken. The cause of otosclerosis is unknown. The tendency to develop the condition is inherited.

DIAGNOSIS AND TREATMENT
Otosclerosis is generally diagnosed by means of hearing tests, including AUDIOMETRY, that can determine both the extent and the characteristics of hearing loss. The disease is most effectively and permanently treated

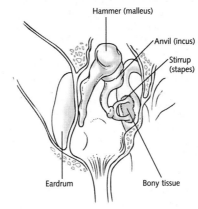

Hammer (malleus)

Anvil (incus)

Stirrup (stapes)

Eardrum   Bony tissue

AN IMMOBILIZED BONE IN THE EAR
In a person with otosclerosis, a tiny bone in the middle ear called the stirrup (stapes) becomes overgrown with spongy bone tissue and is immobilized. The stapes is one of three small bones (the hammer, anvil, and stirrup) that transmit sound waves between the eardrum and the inner ear. If the stapes bone cannot vibrate, hearing is impaired. The condition, which tends to be genetic, can be treated with a hearing aid or with a surgical procedure to replace the stapes with an artificial bone.

by a surgical procedure called a STAPEDECTOMY (a replacement of the stapes with an artificial bone), which usually restores normal functioning to the middle and inner ear. One ear is operated on at a time.

Stapedectomy is a well-established surgical procedure with a high rate of success. In most cases, functioning of the ear can be restored and hearing returns. A small number of people receive only partial restoration of hearing following a stapedectomy, and an even smaller number experience no improvement. Potential side effects of the procedure are rare but may include a change in the sense of taste, persistent ringing in the ears, an intolerance for loud noise, and VERTIGO, which is usually temporary. Not all people with otosclerosis are candidates for stapedectomy. When the procedure is not appropriate, HEARING AIDS will be recommended.

Otoscope

A lighted instrument inserted into the external ear canal to allow a physician to examine the ear and observe changes in the external ear canal and eardrum. The use of a pneumatic otoscope is considered the best method of testing for middle ear fluid, especially in children. This instrument blows a gentle puff of air through the external ear canal and onto the eardrum, enabling the doctor to determine how well the eardrum moves and to test for fluid behind the eardrum. The outer portion of the instrument, which goes into the ear,

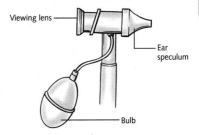

Viewing lens

Ear speculum

Bulb

PNEUMATIC OTOSCOPE
Doctors use an instrument called a pneumatic otoscope to detect fluid in the ear. The otoscope has a light and a magnifying lens. If the fluid is not visible through the semitransparent eardrum, the doctor can squeeze a bulb to direct a puff of air against the membrane. The movement of the eardrum tells the doctor whether fluid is present.

O

is usually a disposable speculum. An examination with an otoscope is usually not painful but requires the person being examined to remain still.

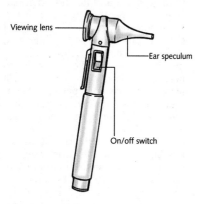

Viewing lens

Ear speculum

On/off switch

Otoscopy

The diagnostic process of observing the external ear canal and the eardrum using an OTOSCOPE. The physician pulls the top of the ear up and back to straighten the ear canal, which provides a clear view of the canal and eardrum when the curved tip of the otoscope is inserted into the canal. This examination may reveal a number of disorders and diseases of the external ear canal, the eardrum, and the middle ear. Otoscopy cannot measure a person's hearing level.

Ototoxicity

Poisoning of the ear caused by medications or chemicals that may damage organs of the inner ear, resulting in disturbances in hearing and balance. The organs affected by ototoxicity in some people are the COCHLEA (coiled structure in the inner ear responsible for hearing) and the cochlea's hair cells (sensory cells that transform sound waves into nerve impulses), as well as the vestibulocochlear nerve that sends balance and hearing information from the inner ear to the brain. Ototoxicity may be produced by a number of over-the-counter and prescription medications and by environmental chemicals. Specifically, the kinds of medications and chemicals documented to be toxic to the ear

include a class of antibiotics called aminoglycoside antibiotics; certain anticancer drugs; certain diuretics; aspirin and aspirin-containing compounds; certain quinines including tonic water; and environmental chemicals including arsenic, lead, and carbon monoxide.

SYMPTOMS

The symptoms of ototoxicity may range from mild to severe and from intermittent ringing in the ears to hearing loss in both ears. Hearing loss is often first experienced in the higher frequencies and can progress to difficulty comprehending speech. Noise injury may contribute to the chemical effects on the ears. Usually, job exposure to hazardous chemicals can cause hearing loss after about 2 to 3 years; it may occur sooner if there is significant noise exposure.

DIAGNOSIS AND TREATMENT

A person who experiences the symptoms of ototoxicity should see a doctor. The examination will include a complete medical history, a report of all symptoms, and testing to determine the degree of hearing impairment or disturbed balance function. There are no treatments at this time to reverse the damage caused by ototoxicity. The current goals of medical treatment are to reduce the effects of the damage and to rehabilitate hearing and balance function. HEARING AIDS may help people with hearing loss. A COCHLEAR IMPLANT may benefit people who have profound hearing loss in both ears. PHYSICAL THERAPY can aid people experiencing balance problems; physical conditioning and exercise may help reestablish coordination between vision and muscle function.

People who have been affected by ototoxicity are prone to repeated occurrences. They should avoid exposure to ototoxic substances and consider wearing a medical alert tag. Protecting vision is important for adjusting to problems with balance function. Annual eye examinations, including a GLAUCOMA test, are essential. Wearing protective eye gear in sun and wind conditions is also important.

Outpatient treatment

Medical or surgical care that may occur in a hospital facility but does not include an overnight stay.

Outpatient treatment may also be provided at a clinic or doctor's office.

Ovarian cyst

Small, fluid-filled areas that form on the ovaries. Very common in women during their childbearing years, ovarian cysts result from changes in hormone levels related to the menstrual cycle, as well as the production and release of eggs from the ovaries. Cysts can range in size from that of a pea to that of a grapefruit. Symptoms can include severe abdominal pain, irregular or delayed periods, a dull ache in the lower abdomen, or pain during sexual intercourse.

There are several different types of ovarian cysts. Functional cysts are formed from tissue that changes in the

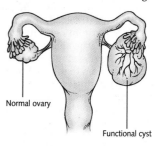

Normal ovary

Functional cyst

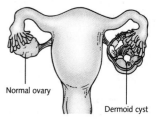

Normal ovary

Dermoid cyst

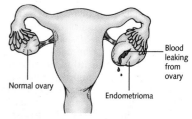

Normal ovary

Blood leaking from ovary

Endometrioma

COMMON GROWTHS ON THE OVARY
There are several types of ovarian cysts. A functional cyst forms from tissue within the ovary—usually from a structure called a follicle, from which an egg is released during ovulation. If the follicle does not release the egg, it can continue to grow into a fluid-filled cyst. Dermoid cysts are composed of different types of tissue, such as skin, hair, and teeth; they are usually benign. An endometrioma is made of blood-filled tissue similar to the endometrium (the lining of the uterus) that has attached to the outer surface of the ovary.

normal process of ovulation; these cysts usually cause minor symptoms at most and disappear within a few months. Dermoid cysts are made up of different kinds of tissue, including hair, skin, fat, and teeth; they can be small with no symptoms or large with symptoms and are usually benign. Cystadenomas develop from cells on the outer surface of the ovary and are usually benign; they can grow very large and cause pain. Other types of ovarian cysts include ENDOMETRIOMA and the cysts found in POLYCYSTIC OVARIAN SYNDROME.

Ovarian cysts are usually detected during a routine pelvic examination. Other methods used to diagnose the condition include ultrasound, laparoscopy, and blood tests. If a cyst is small and causing no symptoms, the doctor may simply monitor it for a few weeks, because most cysts go away by themselves over one or two menstrual cycles. Large or painful cysts can be treated with hormones or surgery, depending on the size and type of cyst, the woman's age and symptoms, and whether she wishes to have children. Oral contraceptives are often used to treat functional cysts. Surgical procedures used to remove ovarian cysts include OOPHORECTOMY, removal of the ovary.

Ovary

One of a pair of the female sex glands that contains eggs (female reproductive cells) and produces female sex hormones. It is a small organ, about 1 to 2 inches long and 1 inch thick, with an oblong shape. The ovaries are situated in the pelvis, one on either side of the uterus and below the openings of the fallopian tubes.

At birth, each ovary contains hundreds of thousands of eggs. At puberty, one of the ovaries release an egg approximately once a month, a process called OVULATION. This process begins when the pituitary gland in the brain releases a hormone called follicle-stimulating hormone (FSH), which signals the ovary to form a structure called a follicle. The follicle encircles an egg and nourishes it until the pituitary gland releases another hormone called luteinizing hormone (LH). At the direction of LH, the follicle releases the egg. The egg is channeled into the nearby fallopian

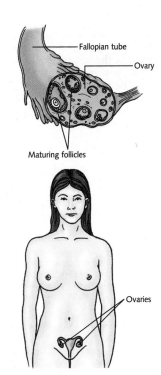

MONTHLY OVULATION
Within the ovaries of a mature woman, structures called follicles develop to nourish eggs (female sex cells). Once a month, one egg is released into the fallopian tubes to travel toward the uterus.

tube and travels toward the uterus. If sperm are present as a result of sexual intercourse, FERTILIZATION may occur in the tube.

Ovaries are also part of the ENDOCRINE SYSTEM because they release hormones directly into the bloodstream. They produce two sex hormones: estrogen and progesterone. Estrogen promotes the growth of female sexual characteristics like breasts and pubic hair, regulates MENSTRUATION, and prepares the wall of the uterus for pregnancy. Progesterone readies the uterus for a pregnancy and helps maintain pregnancy. The ovaries also produce a small amount of the male hormone androgen, which also has a role in the reproductive cycle. See REPRODUCTIVE SYSTEM, FEMALE.

Ovary, cancer of

A malignant tumor or abnormal growth of cells that begins in a woman's ovaries and can spread to other organs. Ovarian cancer is the sixth most common cancer in women. Because it is difficult to

detect at an early stage, ovarian cancer is more likely to be fatal than is cancer of the cervix or endometrium (the lining of the uterus). However, a woman's prognosis largely depends on the cellular type of ovarian cancer and how far the cancer has spread at the time of diagnosis.

The three types of ovarian cancer are classified according to the type of cells from which they develop. About 80 to 85 percent of ovarian cancers begin in the epithelial cells covering the lining of the ovaries. About 5 percent occur in the germ cells, the cells that form eggs. Less than 5 percent of ovarian cancers occur in the stromal cells, which both secrete hormones and hold the ovaries together.

DIAGNOSIS

Early stages of ovarian cancer usually have no symptoms. A tumor may first be detected when a doctor feels an enlarged ovary as part of a routine pelvic examination. At later stages of the disease, a woman may have vague intestinal problems, a feeling of fullness in her abdomen, or abdominal or pelvic pain or discomfort. A woman may notice that her waistline is expanding without an apparent cause. If ovarian cancer is suspected, a doctor may order an ultrasound or take a blood sample to screen for the protein CA-125, which becomes elevated in the blood of most women with ovarian cancer. However, neither test is completely reliable for detecting cancer. A doctor may use a laparoscope, a surgical device inserted through a small abdominal incision that allows viewing of the internal organs. A laparotomy, a procedure that requires a larger abdominal incision, may be performed to diagnose and find out if the cancer has spread to other organs or tissues.

Staging is the process by which doctors establish how widely the cancer has spread. In stage I, the cancer is contained within the ovary (the primary tumor site), in contrast to the more advanced stage IV, in which it has spread to other organs, such as the liver. Once the disease has been staged, a doctor will discuss a treatment plan with the woman.

TREATMENT

For most women with cancer of the ovaries, surgery is the recommended treatment. That may involve removal

O

of the uterus (HYSTERECTOMY) and removal of the fallopian tubes and ovaries (SALPINGO-OOPHORECTOMY). However, the extent of the surgery depends upon the stage of the cancer, the woman's age, and her general health. If cancer is confined to one ovary, the doctor may remove only that ovary, particularly if the woman is young and wants to have a family or add to her family. At times, some lymph nodes and parts of the bowel may be removed.

Surgery is usually followed by chemotherapy and, in rare cases, radiation therapy. Chemotherapy involves taking drugs that kill or halt the spread of cancer. The drugs cisplatin and carboplatin are often used in chemotherapy.

RISK FACTORS

A woman can develop ovarian cancer at any age; however, the risk increases with a woman's age. Ovarian cancer occurs most often in women who are between the ages of 50 and 75 years. Women who have had several children are less likely to develop ovarian cancer, as are women who have used or are now using birth control pills. Heredity plays a role in some cases. Established risk factors for ovarian cancer include having had few or no children or children later in life and extended use of fertility drugs. Other factors may contribute to ovarian cancer, such as a high-fat diet or the use of talc or baby powder in the genital area. However, a woman may have one or more risk factors and never develop ovarian cancer.

Overbite

Overlapping of the lower front teeth by the upper front teeth. A slight overbite is normal because the upper jaw is larger than the lower jaw. An overbite may be caused by tongue thrusting, when a person unknowingly and repeatedly pushes the tongue forward and applies pressure on the front teeth, or by thumb-sucking, which also pushes the top front teeth outward. It may also be caused by hereditary factors that determine the position of the teeth or result in a discrepancy between the length of the upper and lower jawbones. Overbites are treated with ORTHODONTIC APPLIANCES that bring the teeth into position or the jaws into alignment with

dental braces (see BRACES, DENTAL). If the condition is caused by an imbalance in the lengths of the upper and lower jawbones, orthopedic headgear may be worn to decrease the excess length of the upper jawbone or to develop the length of a shortened lower jawbone.

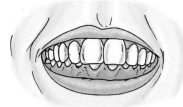

ALIGNMENT OF JAWS AND TEETH
Because the upper jaw is larger than the lower jaw, the upper front teeth slightly overlap the lower front teeth. In a person with an overbite, this overlap is greater than usual.

Overcrowding, dental

An ORTHODONTICS problem that involves too many teeth developing in a space that is inadequate in size. Overcrowded teeth may overlap each other and become difficult to clean properly. For this reason, the condition may lead to TOOTH DECAY and gum disease (see PERIODONTAL DISEASE). Dental overcrowding can also produce irregularities in the bite. Overcrowding may be hereditary. It is sometimes associated with FETAL ALCOHOL SYNDROME. Overcrowding of permanent teeth can be the result of premature loss of primary teeth. The permanent molars drift into the spaces vacated by lost primary molars. The result is a

lack of space for the permanent bicuspids, which are supposed to emerge in front of the first molars.

The condition can be treated by an ORTHODONTIST who may use dental braces (see BRACES, DENTAL) to help separate the teeth. TOOTH EXTRACTION may be necessary, in combination with braces, to provide sufficient space on the dental arch.

Dental retainers (see RETAINER, DENTAL) are often necessary after the braces have been removed. Some adults may require the placement of permanent retainers, worn behind the teeth, to prevent future crowding.

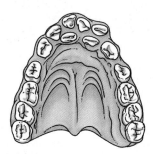

SEVERE CROWDING
Overlap or misalignment of permanent teeth, called crowding, may be inherited or caused by loss of primary teeth, emergence of wisdom teeth, or just shifting with age. Crowded teeth can be difficult to clean, cause chewing problems, or be cosmetically unappealing. The condition can be corrected with dental braces.

Overdose, drug

Consumption of excessive quantities of drugs. A drug dose that is large enough to be toxic is considered an overdose. An overdose may be acci-

SYMPTOMS OF OVERDOSE

Symptoms of a drug overdose will vary, depending on the drug involved, as follows:

TYPE OF DRUG	SYMPTOMS
Narcotic overdose	Sleepiness, slow breathing, unconsciousness
Uppers	Excitement, rapid breathing, increased heart rate
Downers	Slowed breathing and heart rate, depression
Mind-altering drugs	Paranoid thoughts, visual hallucinations, aggressive behavior, social withdrawal
Marijuana	Dilated pupils, red eyes
Alcohol	Drunkenness, staggering, slurred speech, unconsciousness

dental or deliberate, and it may involve one or more of the following types of drugs: narcotics, uppers (stimulants), downers (depressants), mind-altering drugs (LSD, PCP), alcohol, marijuana, or prescription drugs.

Emergency medical assistance should be sought for any suspected drug overdose. The local POISON CENTER can be called with any questions. Signs of a pending emergency include loss of consciousness; dangerously slow breathing; aggressive, hostile, or panicky behavior; or violence.

Overdose, medication

Excessive consumption of prescription or nonprescription medications. Medication overdoses occur both by accident and deliberately, involving even seemingly harmless drugs sold over-the-counter, such as aspirin, acetaminophen, iron, vitamins, antihistamines, and sleep aids, which in large enough doses can be lethal. Children and older people are at particular risk for harm from medication overdose, but any person who fails to read a drug label and follow a doctor's instructions may be at risk.

Overdoses may also occur if a child takes a drug of any kind under the assumption that it is candy. Any medication overdose requires a call to a POISON CENTER or a trip to the nearest hospital emergency department.

Overgrowth syndromes

Disorders of physical development, usually in the first years of life, characterized by overly rapid growth. Children with overgrowth syndromes usually demonstrate delayed motor, cognitive, and social development, in addition to reduced muscle tone and impaired speech development. Some syndromes are genetic disorders, and others are caused by tumors. Symptoms vary according to the disorder.

GIGANTISM

Excessive secretion of the growth hormone in childhood results in excessive growth of the long bones of the arms and legs. The increase in height is accompanied by overly large muscles and organs, and puberty may

be delayed as well. Pituitary gland tumors are often involved in this disorder, and surgery to remove the tumor usually limits the production of the growth hormone.

ACROMEGALY

Increased secretion of growth hormone after normal growth has been completed characterizes this disorder. A benign pituitary tumor is usually the cause. Symptoms include enlarged hands and feet, enlarged jaw and facial bones, headache, double vision, vomiting, excessive sweating, muscle weakness, joint pain, and carpal tunnel syndrome. Microsurgery to remove the pituitary tumor usually can correct the abnormal growth hormone secretion.

SOTOS SYNDROME

Children with Sotos syndrome are often taller and heavier and have larger heads than other children. While they look older than their peers, children with the disorder usually act younger and are at risk for poor self-esteem, poor peer relationships, and problems in school. Sotos syndrome, a genetic disorder, alters developmental timing, but any problems are usually resolved as the growth rate becomes normal after the first few years of life. In many cases, adults with Sotos syndrome are of normal height and intellect.

PROTEUS SYNDROME

This genetic disorder results in many abnormalities, including body asymmetry, multiple benign tumors of the skin and soft tissue, possible malignant tumors, large hands and feet, skull defects, eye defects, accelerated growth, and some heart problems. Severe SCOLIOSIS is often present.

BECKWITH-WIEDEMANN SYNDROME

In this disorder, babies are large at birth and many have umbilical defects and a large tongue that protrudes from the mouth. Many physical problems during infancy are associated with this syndrome, including severe hypoglycemia (lowered blood sugar) and increased risk of tumor development. Seizures and undescended testicles may also be present. Children who survive infancy generally develop satisfactorily.

Over-the-counter (OTC) drugs

See NONPRESCRIPTION DRUGS.

Overweight

Body weight that is 10 to 20 percent higher than the average for an individual who is a certain height and that represents an increased percentage of body fat. Being 20 percent or more overweight is considered OBESITY. A tool that correlates weight with body fat percentage is the BODY MASS INDEX (BMI). A person who has a BMI rating of 25 to 27 or higher is most likely overweight. Exceptions may be athletes, whose extra weight is more likely to be due to excess muscle than fat.

Overweight people are more likely to develop health problems such as high blood pressure, high cholesterol, cardiovascular disease, diabetes, osteoarthritis, and gout. Doctors advise people who are overweight to seek medical attention. See also WEIGHT LOSS.

Ovulation

The process by which a mature egg is released from an ovary into the fallopian tube. This stage of the female reproductive cycle takes place each month during a woman's reproductive years at around day 15 of the 28-day menstrual cycle. The egg, when fertilized by a sperm, implants itself in the uterus and eventually develops into a fetus.

MATURING EGGS

About 2 million immature eggs are present in the ovaries at birth. Only about 200 of them will ever mature and be released. A layer of cells surrounds each egg, and the entire structure is called a primary follicle. Most primary follicles degenerate before a girl reaches puberty, leaving most women with about 200,000 to 400,000 primary follicles at puberty. Each month after puberty, up to 25 primary follicles begin to mature into secondary follicles, stimulated by FSH (follicle-stimulating hormone). Only one secondary follicle or, occasionally, two will reach full maturation each month. It is from the mature follicle that the egg is released at ovulation. See more on ovulation on page 940. See also MENSTRUATION.

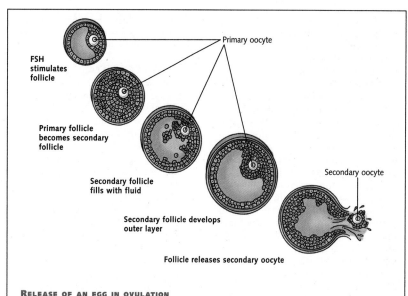

RELEASE OF AN EGG IN OVULATION
During a woman's monthly menstrual cycle, her reproductive system releases an egg that has the potential to be fertilized by a male sperm. The entire sequence of events that culminates in ovulation is stimulated by the interaction of hormones, orchestrated by the pituitary gland in the brain. At the start of the menstrual cycle, FSH (follicle-stimulating hormone) causes the enlargement of structures within the ovary called follicles, which contain primary oocytes (eggs).

Ovulation stimulants

Drugs used to cause more frequent ovulation; fertility drugs. Ovulation stimulants are prescribed when a woman has difficulty conceiving because she ovulates irregularly or not at all. The drugs do not improve fertility in women who ovulate regularly. Ovulation stimulants may be used to control the time of ovulation in a woman undergoing artificial insemination or other assisted reproductive technology.

Ovulation stimulants include CLOMIPHENE CITRATE, which is used to stimulate ovulation in women with infrequent periods and long menstrual cycles. Human chorionic gonadotropin, the most potent fertility drug, is used in women who are not ovulating and have not responded to clomiphene citrate. Bromocriptine is often recommended for women who ovulate irregularly because their pituitary gland secretes too much prolactin.

Ovulation, lack of

Anovulation; the inability of the ovaries (see OVARY) to produce mature eggs or to release mature eggs on a regular basis. Among the most common causes of infertility in women, these problems result from hormone imbalances, which may be caused by excessive weight loss, eating disorders, obesity, stress, strenuous exercise, or in some cases by POLYCYSTIC OVARIAN SYNDROME, a condition in which cysts develop in the ovaries.

TREATMENT
The most common cause of anovulation is excessive weight loss, which is sometimes the result of depression. Women who engage in extreme exercise regimens can also develop problems with ovulation. In many cases, restoring the woman's weight to normal and modifying her exercise routine will be enough to restore fertility. Sometimes, fertility drugs may be recommended after weight has been normalized. CLOMIPHENE CITRATE, the usual drug of choice to stimulate ovaries to produce eggs, is effective in most women. If clomiphene is not successful, the doctor may try stimulating the ovary with injections of GONADOTROPIN HORMONES or GNRH (gonadotropin-releasing hormone).

Some disorders of the pituitary gland lead to excess production of the hormone prolactin, which can suppress ovulation. High levels of prolactin can be reduced with a drug called bromocriptine, which inhibits secretion of prolactin. Occasionally, lack of ovulation is caused by hypothyroidism; when it is treated with thyroid hormone, ovulation resumes within a few months.

Ovum

The female reproductive cell—also known as an EGG—found in the ovaries. Typically, after puberty, a woman's body releases one ovum each month in the cycle known as OVULATION. See REPRODUCTIVE SYSTEM, FEMALE.

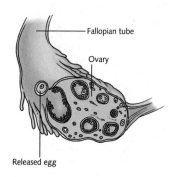

FEMALE REPRODUCTIVE CELL
The ovum, released each month from a female ovary, has the potential to be fertilized by a sperm (male reproductive cell) and develop into a fetus.

Oxaprozin

A nonsteroidal anti-inflammatory drug (NSAID). Oxaprozin (Daypro) is used to manage the symptoms of acute or chronic osteoarthritis or rheumatoid arthritis. Oxaprozin has pain-relieving, fever-reducing, and anti-inflammatory properties. It is available only by prescription.

Oxidation

The combination of a substance with oxygen. Chemical oxidation involves changes in the electrical charge of the atoms being combined with oxygen. Biological oxidation occurs when enzymes metabolize food, causing a release of energy. Most biological oxidations occur with the removal of a pair of hydrogen atoms from a molecule in a process called dehydrogenation.

Oximetry

A painless diagnostic test that measures the amount of oxygen in a person's blood. Oximetry, which measures oxygen saturation, is commonly performed on children and infants when there is concern that the child has insufficient oxygen in the blood. The test is also performed to test oxygen levels in an adult's blood. The test does not require a blood sample. Instead, a small device is placed on the finger, toe, or ear lobe. The device contains a sensor that is connected to a machine that displays the oxygen saturation and pulse rate of the person being tested.

Oxycodone

A narcotic pain reliever. Oxycodone (OxyContin, Percocet, Percodan, Roxicodone, Tylox, and others) is prescribed for moderate to severe pain. Oxycodone is more effective in episodes of acute rather than chronic pain. Like all narcotics, oxycodone has a high potential for abuse and can impair the ability to drive.

Oxygen

A colorless, odorless gas that is essential for all forms of life. Oxygen makes up about 21 percent of the Earth's atmosphere and about 90 percent (by weight) of water. Because oxygen combines readily with other elements, it is distributed throughout the solid matter of the Earth. Along with carbon and hydrogen, oxygen forms the chemical basis of much organic material. Every cell of the body requires oxygen; people obtain oxygen from the air and take it into the lungs through RESPIRATION.

The body's need for oxygen varies according to differing levels of activity. During strenuous exercise, for example, the oxygen needs of muscle cells are greater than the amount of oxygen the body can absorb, which leads to extended periods of labored breathing until normal balance is achieved and the muscles receive adequate oxygen. Such a temporary deficit is called "oxygen debt."

Severe reduction of the supply of oxygen to the body is called HYPOXIA and can occur during climbs to high altitudes or during some illnesses. Certain poisons, including cyanide and carbon monoxide, disrupt the distribution of oxygen to the body. Anemia and some diseases of the lungs, heart, kidney, and liver may also disrupt the oxygen supply, prompting the need for a person to receive supplemental oxygen by inhalation.

Oxygen, supplemental

Oxygen administered as a form of therapy when the oxygen level in the blood is significantly decreased. Supplemental oxygen may be helpful for people who have certain lung diseases, particularly end-stage illness. When such diseases reduce lung function, the body's oxygen needs are not met, and normal body functions cannot be supported. Supplemental oxygen can provide the oxygen that is essential to ongoing body functions and can help people be more active. It is most commonly prescribed to people who have CHRONIC OBSTRUCTIVE PULMONARY DISEASE (COPD), interstitial pulmonary fibrosis, dust diseases, and other occupational lung diseases.

Supplemental oxygen provides several benefits to people who do not get enough oxygen as the result of disease having damaged the lungs. It can improve their sleep patterns so they can get more rest, and it can benefit their mood, mental alertness, and stamina. Oxygen supplementation helps prevent heart failure in people with severe lung disease.

At abnormally high levels, oxygen may be harmful to general health and even toxic. For this reason, a doctor's supervision is essential for proper use of supplemental oxygen. However, it is no longer necessary for a person to be hospitalized to receive this form of oxygen therapy.

Oxygen supplementation can be prescribed by a doctor to those who need it, and there are several approaches to dispensing oxygen in the home. Oxygen gas can be dispensed in large steel or aluminum tanks for use at home and in smaller, portable tanks. Liquid oxygen is longer lasting and can be used by more active people because it can be stored in smaller tanks that are conveniently transported.

Oxygen concentrators are electrical devices that produce oxygen by concentrating the oxygen that is present in ambient air and eliminating other gases. These devices provide an easy method of oxygen supplementation in the home, are less expensive, and do not require refilling. Oxygen concentrators require electricity to operate, and backup strategies are necessary in case of power outages, but they are effective for many people who need extra oxygen.

Oxygen free radicals

Unstable particles formed as byproducts of the body's normal chemical processes. Oxygen free radicals are thought to increase the risk of disease and to hasten the aging process. Oxygen free radicals can damage cell membranes and disrupt the immune system, thereby possibly contributing to the development of diseases such as cancer, cataracts, and heart disease. Oxygen free radicals may interact with genetic material as well and may enhance the dangerous properties of LDL (low-density lipoprotein) cholesterol ("bad" cholesterol), thereby hastening the development of atherosclerosis (narrowing arteries). The supply of oxygen free radicals in the body is thought to be increased by smoking, stress, and air pollution.

Antioxidant vitamins such as vitamins A, E, and C are considered by some to be scavengers of oxygen free radicals, and some people believe that by consuming antioxidant vitamins, they reduce the risk of disease and thwart the normal aging process. The use of high-dose vitamin supplements is not necessarily risk-free, however, and people are better off altering their diet to include plenty of dark-colored fresh fruits and vegetables, which contain antioxidant vitamins and nutrients.

Oxytocin

A hormone released by the hypothalamus in large quantities in pregnant women who are about to give birth. Oxytocin stimulates the contraction of the smooth muscle cells in the uterus, preparing the uterus for labor. The hormone also prompts the contracting cells surrounding the ducts of the mammary glands to ready the glands for releasing milk.

At the beginning of labor, the cervix of the uterus becomes distended, triggering the hypothalamus to secrete more oxytocin, which is ultimately transported by the blood to the uterus where it reinforces contractions.

When a newborn begins nursing,

nerve impulses from the mother's nipples signal the hypothalamus to release oxytocin, which is carried by the blood to the mother's breasts. The oxytocin stimulates the smooth muscle cells in the breasts to contract and release milk from the mammary glands.

Oxytocin challenge test

External fetal monitoring performed on pregnant women to assess the health of the fetus in which the hormone oxytocin is used to stimulate uterine contractions. In the simpler NONSTRESS TEST, the baby's heart rate is monitored in response to normal movements. An oxytocin challenge test (OCT) is identical to a nonstress test, except that the mother is given an intravenous solution of oxytocin to stimulate mild contractions. The doctor observes the reaction of the fetus to the stress of the contractions. The doctor will assess how the baby will handle the stress of labor, in which contractions tend to cut down on the available supply of oxygen by compressing the placenta. A normal response to the OCT suggests that the fetus is healthy, is receiving enough oxygen, and will be able to withstand the stress of labor.

The doctor will look for signs of problems, such as a decreased fetal heart rate. A fetus that does not respond normally to the test may be experiencing difficulties that could worsen before labor begins, and the doctor may decide to deliver the baby early. To protect high-risk babies who might not be able to withstand contractions, the OCT is always performed in a hospital. The test is administered only after 34 weeks of pregnancy, when a baby could easily survive if the test itself were to induce labor prematurely.

The OCT is administered to women with conditions that are associated with impaired placental function, such as high blood pressure, toxemia, severe heart disease, and hyperthyroidism, and to women who are over age 40 or are more than 2 weeks past their due date. It may be given to women with diabetes. It is used when a baby is suspected of being a low birth weight or when amniotic fluid is stained with meconium (waste from the bowels of the fetus), a possible sign of fetal distress. The test is not given to women with third-trimester bleeding or those carrying more than one fetus because there is a risk of starting labor. It is also not given to women who have previously delivered by cesarean section or who are likely to have premature labor.

Ozena

See RHINITIS, ATROPHIC.

Ozone

A form of oxygen in which the molecules contain three atoms instead of the usual two. Ozone is formed when oxygen is exposed to the silent discharge of electricity, which accounts for the distinctive odor of the air following a thunderstorm and the air immediately surrounding high-voltage electrical equipment. Ozone occurs naturally in small amounts in the stratosphere (the ozone layer), where it protects life on earth by absorbing solar ultraviolet radiation.

On earth, ozone is irritating, particularly to the eyes, the lungs, and the mucous membranes, and it may even be toxic. Ozone is also explosive, even in small quantities. A chemical form of ozone is used to deodorize air, to purify water, and to treat industrial waste.

PABA

See PARA-AMINOBENZOIC ACID.

Pacemaker

An electronic device that causes the heart to beat by releasing small electrical discharges. A temporary pacemaker can be placed outside the body and used to regulate an abnormally slow heartbeat for a short time. It is connected to the heart by leads (wires) threaded through a narrow tube inserted into a vein in the neck, chest, or groin. An internal, or permanent, pacemaker is implanted in the chest wall to control the heartbeat for years. The pacemaker most commonly corrects bradycardia (an abnormally slow heartbeat) by electrically stimulating the heart to maintain a sufficient, predetermined heart rate. On occasion, pacemakers may also be used to correct tachycardia (an abnormally fast heartbeat). Modern pacemakers can increase the heartbeat automatically during increased physical activity.

An internal pacemaker consists of a waterproof metal box between 1 and 2 inches wide and weighing from ½ ounce to 3 ounces. It is powered by lithium batteries that have a life span of 5 to 10 years. The device is implanted during a minor surgical procedure that is performed under local anesthesia and takes approximately 1 hour. An incision is made in the skin below the collarbone, usually on the left side of the chest, and a small pocket made under the skin and fat. The pacemaker is placed in the pocket, and the leads are threaded through a vein in the upper chest until they reach the heart. The incision is closed with sutures, and it heals completely within 2 to 3 weeks. Complications from the procedure are rare and usually minor.

After a pacemaker is implanted, the person sees the doctor every 6 to 12 months to have the device checked with a special radio transmitter. Changes in the pacemaker's programming can be made at the same time. The internal pacemaker is replaced when the batteries show signs of weakening.

People with an internal pacemaker must avoid contact sports, such as football and rugby, and should also avoid firing a rifle or shotgun held against the shoulder closer to the pacemaker. They also need to be aware of strong electromagnetic fields that can interfere with the pacemaker's functioning. Caution should be exercised around metal detectors, MRI (magnetic resonance imaging) equipment, junkyards that use electromagnets, and running car engines. Microwave ovens do not pose a danger to people with pacemakers, nor do cellular phones if kept more than 6 inches away from the pacemaker. See Regulating the heart, page 944.

Paclitaxel

An antineoplastic drug. Paclitaxel (Taxol) is used to treat cancer of the ovaries and breast that has spread (metastasized), as well as certain types of lung cancer and a skin cancer associated with AIDS (acquired immunodeficiency syndrome). Paclitaxel works by interfering with the growth of cancer cells, which are eventually destroyed.

Paget disease

An irregular thickening and softening of the bones of the skull, the pelvis, and the extremities. It is most common in adults older than 50. The bones most commonly affected by Paget disease are the hip bones and shin bones. The thighbone, skull, spine, and collarbone are often involved as well. As a result of the disease, these bones become enlarged and deformed and are easily fractured. Bone pain is the most common symptom. The chronic aching sensation tends to worsen at night. The affected areas may feel warm and tender. When Paget disease affects the skull bones, it may cause deafness. Increased blood flow through the diseased bones may strain the heart, which can cause heart failure. Rarely, a bone tumor develops as a result of this disease.

The cause of Paget disease is unknown. The bone cells involved in the normal breakdown and renewal of bone tissue do not function normally in Paget disease. The usual

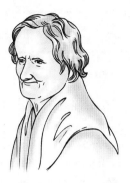

ENLARGED AND DEFORMED BONES
In a person with advanced Paget disease affecting the skull, the head looks enlarged and somewhat misshapen. The condition may cause bone pain, headaches, or hearing loss.

balance between bone formation and bone destruction is disrupted with the result that new bone tissue is produced faster than old bone tissue is broken down.

The disease is diagnosed by physical examination, X rays, and various blood tests. There is no cure, but symptoms may be treated by pain-relieving medication such as aspirin or ibuprofen. Injections of the thyroid hormone calcitonin may be given to relieve severe pain. Paget disease is also called osteitis deformans.

Paget disease of the breast

A rare malignant condition in which a tumor grows in the opening of the milk ducts in the nipple. Symptoms include itching and burning of the affected nipple and sometimes a sore on the nipple that will not heal. The disease resembles the skin condition eczema and mostly occurs in women after menopause. Diagnosis is made by biopsy, and treatment is similar to that for breast cancer.

Paget disease of the vulva

A form of skin cancer in the area of the vulva. Symptoms include recurrent severe itching and soreness. Red velvety lesions with clearly defined borders or white patches may appear on the vulva, anus, vagina, or the area between anus and vagina. Many women ignore the symptoms at first, and, consequently, the disease may not be diagnosed for a long time. The

P

REGULATING THE HEART

The heart's rhythm is regulated by signals from its built-in electrical system, which consists of the sinoatrial node (SA node) and the atrioventricular node (AV node). When problems occur that affect the heartbeat, a pacemaker may be used to track the heartbeat and, if necessary, send small electrical signals to the heart to keep it beating at the correct rhythm.

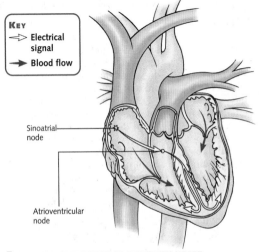

KEY
⇨ Electrical signal
➤ Blood flow

Sinoatrial node

Atrioventricular node

ELECTRICAL CONDUCTION IN A HEALTHY HEART
The sinoatrial node (SA node) and the atrioventricular node (AV node) produce electrical signals that start each heartbeat.

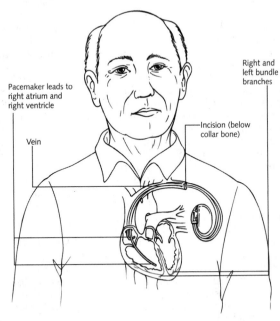

Pacemaker leads to right atrium and right ventricle

Vein

Right and left bundle branches

Incision (below collar bone)

PLACEMENT OF PACEMAKER
Although there are different types, a pacemaker is most commonly inserted in a procedure called endocardial implantation. The electrode wires, or leads, are threaded through an incision in a vein just below the collarbone and into the right atrium, the right ventricle, or both.

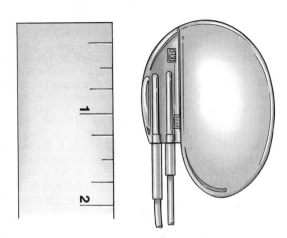

1

2

ACTUAL SIZE OF A PACEMAKER
A pacemaker is small enough to be implanted comfortably in the chest. The ruler measures in inches.

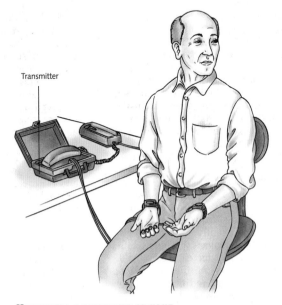

Transmitter

MONITORING A PACEMAKER AT HOME
A special telephone transmitter permits a doctor to monitor a pacemaker while the person is at home.

P

cause of Paget disease of the vulva is not known. It is diagnosed by biopsy, and surgical removal is usually required.

Pain

A sensation of hurting or strong discomfort in a part of the body, due to injury, disease, or functional disorder. Pain can sometimes be psychological in origin, and it can be acute or chronic. Acute pain, such as that following surgery, trauma, or heart attack, is severe. In the first 24 to 48 hours after surgery, it is difficult to relieve this type of intense discomfort, even with medication. Acute pain can also be a signal to seek emergency medical attention, as with acute ABDOMINAL PAIN or CHEST PAIN.

Chronic pain accompanies a number of conditions, including ARTHRITIS, FIBROMYALGIA, ENDOMETRIOSIS, BACK PAIN, and IRRITABLE BOWEL SYNDROME. This type of pain may be accompanied by physical disability, protective or guarding behavior, fatigue, irritability, restlessness, and depression. Medications such as analgesics can provide relief. Other measures include massage, exercise, rest, heat, cold, ACUPUNCTURE, BIOFEEDBACK, TENS, and RELAXATION TECHNIQUES. Oftentimes, a referral to a pain management clinic is required to aggressively treat chronic pain conditions.

Pain management

The treatment of pain. Pain may be acute or chronic. Acute pain is of a limited duration and is usually the result of an injury, surgery, or illness. As the body heals, acute pain normally diminishes. Chronic pain is more difficult to manage. This type of pain (which includes low back pain, arthritic pain, pain caused by shingles or headaches, and pain symptoms related to cancer and nerve problems) persists for long periods. Treatment options for pain management include medication (such as analgesics, anti-inflammatory drugs, antidepressants, and antiseizure medications), electrical stimulation, physical therapy, relaxation therapy, and surgery. Recently, there has been more interest in studying nontraditional methods of managing chronic pain, such as hypnosis and acupuncture.

Pain management, acute

Methods for controlling pain that has a limited duration (usually no more than 1 month), resulting from an injury, surgery, trauma, or illness. In most cases, acute pain resolves when the affected tissues heal. By contrast, chronic pain lasts for a significantly longer period and persists even after healing from injury, surgery, or illness (see PAIN MANAGEMENT, CHRONIC). Cancer pain is generally classified as acute pain, even though it may be long-lasting.

RATIONALE

Effective pain control after surgery, injury, or illness allows the person to recover his or her strength more rapidly and begin walking earlier. A prompt return to physical activity decreases the likelihood of serious problems that can arise from inactivity, such as pneumonia and blood clots.

Inadequate control of acute pain can slow recovery from surgery, illness, or injury and put the person at greater risk for developing chronic pain. The continued sensation of pain makes pain receptors even more sensitive to painful stimuli and may cause long-term changes in the pain pathway of the spinal cord. As a result, pain that persists over time becomes increasingly difficult to control.

MEDICATIONS

In most cases, acute pain responds well to medication. Three types of medication are available, depending on the type and the severity of pain to be controlled.

■ *Opioids* The most powerful anti-pain medications are the drugs derived from the poppy plant, such as codeine and morphine, as well as closely related synthetic compounds, such as OXYCODONE, hydromorphone, and hydrocodone. Called opioids or NARCOTICS, these medications may be subject to abuse as illegally obtained, addictive recreational drugs. When used correctly, they are highly effective at controlling even agonizing pain. Opioids block the transmission of pain signals through the spinal cord and stop the perception of pain in the brain. They also may provide a sense of diminished anxiety. When used for pain control under medical supervision, opioids rarely cause addiction.

Opioids are widely used for post-surgical pain. They are given as injections into the muscle or through a line into a vein, either by a nurse or in patient-controlled analgesia (see ANALGESIA, PATIENT-CONTROLLED). Opioids taken by mouth are slower and less reliable, but they are easy to take for home care patients with severe pain.

The drawback to the use of opioids relates to their side effects. They depress the respiratory system, may cause nausea and itching, and often result in constipation and inability to urinate. Adjusting doses to the right amount for the patient and taking other measures, such as increasing the amount of fiber in the diet, can alleviate or counter the side effects.

■ *Nonopioids* This group of medications includes aspirin, acetaminophen, and the NONSTEROIDAL ANTI-INFLAMMATORY DRUGS (NSAIDs), such as ibuprofen. Instead of affecting the pain receptors in the central nervous system, these medications block the synthesis of substances inside the cells involved in inflammation and tissue injury. They work well against mild, aching pain. Aspirin and NSAIDs are also effective against inflammation. They are slower to take effect, however, and work well against acute, postoperative pain.

The nonopioids also have some limiting side effects. NSAIDs and aspirin often can irritate the digestive system, sometimes leading to serious bleeding. They also interfere with blood clotting and, in large doses, may prove toxic to the liver and kidneys. New agents, however, do not pose clotting problems and still have a high degree of effectiveness.

■ *Combination drugs* These medications mix acetaminophen with an opioid, such as codeine. They are generally effective against relatively mild to moderate pain and are particularly useful for patients during their initial recovery at home after surgery.

ANESTHESIA

For moderate to severe pain of limited duration, local or regional anesthesia (see ANESTHESIA, LOCAL; ANESTHESIA, REGIONAL) can often provide excellent relief. After surgery, many surgeons inject local anesthetic agents into the area surrounding the incision. This blocks the sensation of pain as the surgical anesthesia wears

P

off and controls discomfort during the first few hours after surgery, when pain is likely to be the worst. A BRACHIAL PLEXUS block in the neck, for example, can alleviate the often severe pain that follows shoulder surgery.

For pain in the legs and lower portion of the body, a single dose of long-acting medication can be injected, along with the anesthetic medication, in spinal or epidural anesthesia (see also ANESTHESIA, SPINAL; ANESTHESIA, EPIDURAL). After the anesthetic wears off following surgery, the opioid continues to suppress pain for up to 24 hours, depending on the opioid used. The thin line, or catheter, for epidural anesthesia can also be left in place to allow opioids to be infused into the lower region of the spine with a small pump during postsurgical recovery of less than 48 hours. The drawback to these methods is that the opioid activity weakens control of the leg muscles, making walking difficult or impossible until the medication wears off. Most opioids cause constipation; a stool softener or mild laxative may be prescribed in addition to the pain medicine.

Pain management, chronic

Methods for controlling pain that continues after tissues injured by accident, disease, or surgery heal. Chronic pain often begins as acute pain (see PAIN MANAGEMENT, ACUTE) and continues after recovery. It can be caused by diseases such as shingles, osteoarthritis, diabetes, or cancer; traumatic injury, such as an automobile accident or a gunshot wound; or from surgery, such as the PHANTOM LIMB PAIN following amputation (see also PAIN).

Chronic pain harms overall health and often has serious psychological and emotional ramifications. If unrelieved, long-lasting pain produces feelings of helplessness, sadness, despair, anger, and rage. It can alter personality, disturb sleep, disrupt the person's career and work life, and damage close family relationships.

Every case of chronic pain is unique, so a treatment plan must be developed by a physician or a team of specialists, who, based on the medical characteristics of the case, chooses from several types of thera-

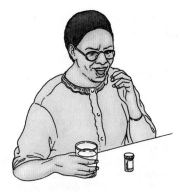

PAIN MEDICATION
Several different types of medications can help relieve pain. Nonsteroidal anti-inflammatory drugs (NSAIDs) such as aspirin, as well as some antidepressants and some anticonvulsants, are nonaddictive painkilling alternatives.

pies available. Sometimes, the person may be referred to a comprehensive pain center.

MEDICATIONS

Opioid medications, such as codeine and morphine, are highly effective at stopping acute pain, but the risk of chemical dependency may be counterproductive, except in some cases of chronic pain in people who are terminally ill. ACETAMINOPHEN and the NONSTEROIDAL ANTI-INFLAMMATORY DRUGS (NSAIDs) including ASPIRIN, which are not opioids (see NARCOTICS), are effective only against mild, aching pain. They do little to stop severe or sharp, lasting pain.

Some ANTIDEPRESSANTS help with chronic pain, even in people who are not depressed. AMITRIPTYLINE (Elavil), TRAZODONE (Desyrel), and IMIPRAMINE (Tofranil) can be combined with other analgesic medications, such as aspirin or NSAIDs, but unwanted side effects may include drowsiness, constipation, and dry mouth.

ANTICONVULSANTS, developed originally to treat epilepsy, are effective in controlling chronic nerve pain, such as TRIGEMINAL NEURALGIA. Examples include PHENYTOIN SODIUM (Dilantin) and CARBAMAZEPINE (Tegretol).

Other medications are used for specific kinds of pain. CORTICOSTEROIDS work well against pain caused by inflammation and swelling, such as osteoarthritis. Long-term use, however, can cause serious problems, such as bone thinning (see OSTEOPOROSIS), CATARACT, and high blood pressure. CAPSAICIN (Zostrix) is a cream that

works well against shingles pain in the skin, osteoarthritis, and NEUROPATHY caused by diabetes. TRAMADOL (Ultram) is used primarily for chronic pain and is available with acetaminophen for acute pain. Its mild dose-related side effects include some dizziness, drowsiness, nausea, and constipation.

OTHER APPROACHES

In some cases, local anesthetics can be injected around nerves or into joints to reduce the swelling, irritation, spasms in the muscles, or abnormal nerve transmissions causing pain. The anesthetic medication can be mixed with corticosteroids to amplify these benefits. However, local anesthetics last for a limited time and may provide only temporary relief. Dosage is limited because the absorption of large amounts of local anesthetics into the bloodstream can cause seizures and even cardiac arrest.

Transcutaneous electrical nerve stimulation (TENS) involves the use of a small battery-operated device that diminishes pain by stimulating nerve fibers through the skin with low-level electrical energy. This stimulation blocks the transmission of pain impulses along the nerves, through the spinal cord, and into the brain. The TENS devices, which are a little larger than a pager, can be carried on

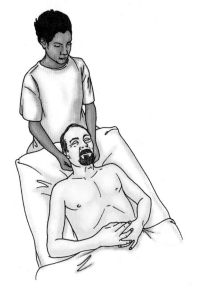

MASSAGE FOR PAIN RELIEF
Massage is a form of physical therapy for pain in the muscles and joints.

P

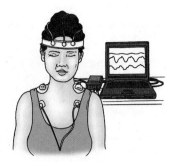

BIOFEEDBACK FOR PAIN
Biofeedback provides the person in pain with information about unconscious responses to pain, such as an increase in blood pressure or skin temperature. By becoming aware of these responses, a person can learn some degree of conscious control over them.

the belt or in a pocket and used for pain control over an extended time. The relief is often significant, except against severe pain. Risks are minimal. The electrodes can irritate the skin, and the electrical current may cause local discomfort.

ACUPUNCTURE and ACUPRESSURE are recommended by some physicians who treat chronic pain, but their effectiveness is not uniform for all pain conditions.

Physical therapy techniques, such as targeted exercises, whirlpool baths, ULTRASOUND TREATMENT, MASSAGE THERAPY, MANIPULATION, and the application of heat, can help to alleviate pain in the muscles and joints.

Chronic pain has major psychological consequences, and therapeutic approaches can help to manage the condition. Since stress makes pain worse, relaxation techniques, such as meditation and yoga, can lessen pain by decreasing stress. BIOFEEDBACK is useful for teaching the person how to be aware of, and learn to control, unconscious responses to pain, such as increases in blood pressure and skin temperature. OCCUPATIONAL THERAPY helps people with chronic pain learn how to perform ordinary tasks at home or work. Family therapy focuses on how chronic pain can affect intimate relationships

Painful arc syndrome

A painful condition of the shoulder; also called impingement syndrome. Painful arc syndrome is caused by repeated overhead movement of the arm, by abnormal anatomy of the

shoulder, or a combination of the two. If an anatomical abnormality of the shoulder bones is involved, it is typically due to a hooked shape at the outer portion of the shoulder blade. Symptoms of painful arc syndrome may include pain, stiffness, and a pinched feeling when the arm is raised. If BURSITIS (inflammation of the bursa in the shoulder) is involved, there may be pain at rest or during sleep.

Painful arc syndrome is diagnosed by physical examination and X rays. Preliminary treatments may include applying ice to the painful area, gentle massage, heat therapy, and physical therapy. A physical therapist can demonstrate proper techniques for using the affected arm and shoulder joint at work and when playing sports. Pain-relieving medications, including aspirin, ibuprofen, and other nonsteroidal anti-inflammatory drugs (NSAIDs), may be recommended to relieve pain and inflammation. If the problem persists, cortisone injections and ARTHROSCOPIC SURGERY may become necessary. Left untreated, painful arc syndrome can lead to ROTATOR CUFF DISEASE.

Palate

The roof of the mouth. The palate separates the oral cavity from the nasal cavity (see MOUTH; NOSE). The front portion of the palate is hard and bony (hard palate); the rear, soft and fleshy (soft palate.)

Palliative care

Any procedure or medication that is intended to ease pain and otherwise improve quality of life but does not cure disease. For example, a physician may perform palliative surgery on a person with advanced cancer in order to ease pain and treat other symptoms, even when it is not possible to cure the cancer.

Pallor

A lack of color or unusual paleness in the skin. Pale skin is not necessarily a sign of disease; a person may have inherited light skin, or pallor can be due to a lack of exposure to sunlight. However, doctors recommend medical attention if the pallor extends to the lips and tongue or is accompanied by other symptoms, such as shortness of breath or blood in the stool.

Palpate

To examine by means of touch during a physical examination. In palpation, the doctor's hands or fingertips are used to touch or feel a person's body to evaluate the health of an organ or body part.

Palpitations

The sensation of a strong, fast, irregular heartbeat. Palpitations can be unpleasant, but they usually last for only a few seconds. They may occur alone or with other symptoms, such as sweating, chest pain, dizziness, shortness of breath, nausea, and lightheadedness.

Palpitations may be related to an underlying heart condition. Possibile causes include hypertension (high blood pressure), cardiac arrhythmia (irregular heartbeat), mitral valve prolapse, hyperthyroidism (an overactive thyroid gland), anemia (a shortage of red blood cells), and coronary artery disease. They can also be brought on by stress, anxiety, panic attack, stimulants such as caffeine and nicotine, excessive alcohol, and medications (for example, some cold remedies, weight loss aids, and thyroid hormone replacements).

Treatment may include physical measures to alleviate or eliminate symptoms, such as deep breathing,

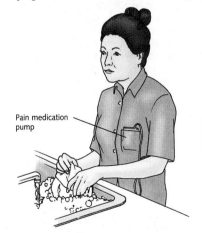

Pain medication pump

HELPING IMPROVE LIFE
Pain management is a form of palliative care because it helps a person control a debilitating symptom of disease—pain—rather than treating the disease itself. Now a person with chronic pain that does not respond to oral medication can get relief via a pocket-sized pump that delivers drugs through a tube inserted under the skin—a method called subcutaneous continuous infusion.

P

relaxation exercises, splashing cold water on the face, or drinking cold water. If a substance or medication is causing the problem, then the chemical can be reduced or eliminated. Palpitations caused by heart disease, anxiety, or stress often improve as that condition is treated. Medications to prevent or control palpitations are available.

Palsy

PARALYSIS in any part of the body that is sometimes accompanied by involuntary tremors.

Pancreas

A long, tapered gland located in the abdomen behind the stomach and beneath the liver. The pancreas has important roles in digestion and regulation of the blood sugar level. It contains both exocrine tissue, which secretes substances into ducts, and endocrine tissue, which secretes hormones directly into the blood.

The exocrine tissues that compose most of the pancreas secrete digestive enzymes into a network of ducts that lead to the main pancreatic duct. This main duct runs through the pancreas to join the common bile duct and enter the duodenum (the first part of the small intestine). The opening into the duodenum is called the ampulla of Vater. In the small intestine, these enzymes help break down proteins, fats, and carbohydrates. The secretions also include sodium bicarbonate that helps neutralize stomach acid.

The endocrine tissues in the pancreas secrete the hormones insulin, glucagon, and somatostatin into the blood to regulate the blood sugar level. This tissue is organized into groups of cells called islets of Langerhans, which are further organized into specialized cells that make each of the three hormones. If the blood sugar level gets too high, insulin takes glucose (a form of sugar) out of the blood and moves it into other body cells. If the blood sugar level gets too low, glucagon directs the release of glucose from the liver and stimulates the liver to manufacture more glucose. Somatostatin also has a regulatory role that is not fully understood. See BILIARY SYSTEM.

The passage of food from the stomach into the small intestine stimulates the pancreas to produce and release its enzymes. The powerful enzymes in pancreatic juice handle much of the digestive activity that occurs in the small intestine. They break down fats, carbohydrates, and proteins to be absorbed into the bloodstream. In a typical day, the pancreas produces a little over 2 quarts of digestive juices.

Other secretions from tissues in the pancreas are released into the blood, meaning that the pancreas functions as an endocrine gland. The pancreas produces two important hormones: glucagon and INSULIN. Glucagon increases the blood sugar level by prompting the liver to turn stored glycogen into glucose (simple sugar) and to make glucose from proteins called amino acids. Insulin promotes the absorption of blood-borne sugar by the cells and lowers the blood sugar level. Because of its effect on cellular activity, insulin has far-reaching effects. It influences the movement of nutrients and other key chemicals, helps cells to grow, and enhances metabolism in the liver, muscles, and fat tissues.

LOCATION OF THE PANCREAS
The pancreas is positioned under the liver between the stomach and the small intestine. It makes digestive enzymes that move into the small intestine through the common bile duct.

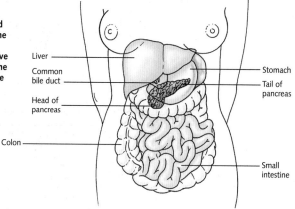

Liver

Common bile duct

Head of pancreas

Colon

Stomach

Tail of pancreas

Small intestine

Pancreas transplant

Replacing a diseased, nonfunctioning pancreas with a healthy organ from a donor. The pancreas, located in the upper abdomen near the stomach, produces insulin to regulate sugar levels in the blood. The organ works poorly or not at all in people with diabetes. Most recipients of pancreas transplants are people who are severely ill with diabetes who have no other prospect for extending their lives.

Even though diabetes can be controlled with insulin and sugar-lowering drugs, diabetes can cause severe complications. People with the disease are more at risk for kidney disease, gangrene of the feet or hands, and heart disease. For a person with serious diabetes and advancing kidney disease, for example, a pancreas transplant offers a way of producing a regular supply of insulin, rather than the intermittent doses provided by insulin injections.

The pancreas to be transplanted is taken from the cadaver of a person who has agreed to be an organ donor. In the most widely used technique, a portion of the duodenum attached to the pancreas is removed as well. After the recipient is given general anesthesia and is pain-free, an incision is made in the upper portion of the abdomen to expose the pancreas. The pancreatic artery from the donor is joined to that in the recipient, and the same is done for the pancreatic vein. The portion of the duodenum attached to the donor pancreas is joined to the bladder or to the small intestine so that pancreatic juice—which plays a role only in digestion and has nothing to do with controlling blood sugar levels—drains out with the urine or the feces.

Since many pancreas transplant candidates also have diabetes-related kidney disease, a kidney transplant is often performed at the same time.

OUTLOOK
Pancreatic transplant recipients usually have good outcomes. Within 24 hours, in most cases, the transplanted pancreas is producing insulin on its own, and the recipient no longer needs injected insulin. As with all transplants, drugs that suppress the immune system and prevent the body from rejecting the transplanted organ must be taken for life. The transplant will not reverse any disease, such as damage to the kidneys.

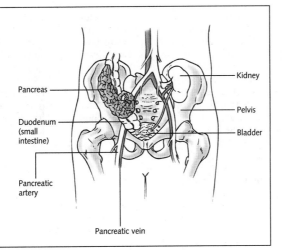

A NEW PANCREAS
A pancreas transplant, usually done with a kidney transplant as well, extends the life of a person with severe diabetes. The donor pancreas includes a length of the duodenum (upper portion of the small intestine), which is surgically attached to the recipient's bladder so that pancreatic digestive juices can be eliminated by the usual route. The transplanted kidney is similarly connected to the blood vessels and the bladder.

Pancreas
Kidney
Duodenum (small intestine)
Pelvis
Bladder
Pancreatic artery
Pancreatic vein

Surgery to replace a damaged pancreas with a healthy one from a donor. The pancreas is a large gland behind the stomach that manufactures digestive enzymes and powerful hormones such as insulin. In people who have diabetes, pancreas transplantation is often performed with a kidney transplant. In many cases, the pancreas transplant is less successful than the kidney transplant. However, the combination operation reduces the risk that diabetes will destroy the donor kidney and may save the individual from needing insulin injections. Because of the inherent risks in transplant surgery and because it is not essential to save an individual's life, transplanting the pancreas alone is considered more risky surgery. Donated organs are matched as closely as possible to the recipient's tissue type, but perfect matches are impossible.

The body's immune system would normally react to the new pancreas as an invader and try to attack it with white blood cells and antibodies. After a pancreas transplantation, drugs that suppress the immune system must be taken to help prevent rejection of the new organ. Although early immunosuppressive medications had many dangerous side effects, newer ones such as cyclosporine are much safer. However, cyclosporine requires close monitoring because it can harm the kidneys.

Pancreas, cancer of the

Cancer originating in the PANCREAS. Pancreatic cancer is the fourth most common cause of cancer deaths in the United States. Most cases occur in people older than age 60. In 10 percent of cases, cancer of the pancreas is hereditary. Long-term smokers have an increased risk of developing pancreatic cancer. Depending on which part of the pancreas (head, tail, or body) is affected, symptoms may include abdominal pain, loss of appetite, weight loss, nausea, vomiting, and jaundice (a yellowing of the skin and the whites of the eyes). Pain usually centers in the upper abdomen and may penetrate to the back. However, when cancer occurs in the head of the pancreas, there may be no

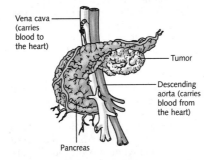

Vena cava (carries blood to the heart)
Tumor
Descending aorta (carries blood from the heart)
Pancreas

CANCER OF THE PANCREAS
Cancer of the pancreas (an elongated digestive organ located over the right kidney) can occur at different places on the organ, causing pain felt in different parts of the abdomen. Weight loss is another typical symptom. Treatment may involve surgery to remove the tumor or to relieve obstruction so that bile can flow into the small bowel.

pain. Other symptoms usually are not apparent until the cancer has advanced to an incurable stage.

Diagnosis of pancreatic cancer is made by blood tests and imaging procedures, such as CT (computed tomography) scanning and ENDOSCOPY. Early detection and pancreatectomy (surgical removal of all or part of the pancreas) provide the best chance of a cure. Pancreatectomy is generally used only in the early stages of the disease. Chemotherapy and radiation may also be recommended before or after surgery. Tumors confined to the area in the duodenum known as the ampulla of Vater (the passageway at the junction of the common bile duct and the pancreatic duct) have the best chance for a cure. Overall, the prognosis for pancreatic cancer is poor once it has spread to adjacent lymph nodes or other organs.

Pancreatectomy

Surgical removal of all or part of the PANCREAS. A pancreatectomy is the most effective treatment for pancreatic cancer. It is also performed in some cases of chronic pancreatitis, or long-term inflammation of the pancreas, and following severe traumatic injury to the pancreas. A total pancreatectomy is the removal of the entire organ, while a subtotal or distal pancreatectomy is the removal of the body and tail of the pancreas. The spleen is also sometimes removed in distal pancreatectomy. When the duodenum is removed along with all or part of the pancreas, the operation is known as a pancreatocduodenectomy or the Whipple procedure.

Prior to a pancreatectomy, imaging procedures, such as X rays, ultrasound and CT (computed tomographic) scanning, ERCP (endoscopic retrograde cholangiopancreatography), and angiography, may be conducted. A pancreatectomy requires a hospital stay of approximately 2 weeks. In cases of pancreatic cancer, CHEMOTHERAPY and RADIATION THERAPY may also be recommended before or after surgery.

Complications after a pancreatectomy can include postoperative bleed-

Terms in small capital letters— for example, PHYSICAL THERAPY or PAGET DISEASE—indicate a cross-reference to another entry with more information.

P

ing and delayed gastric emptying. Additional surgery or other procedures may be necessary to control bleeding. When food and liquids are slow to leave the stomach, nutrients are fed directly into the intestines through feeding tubes. Leaks that may develop between the pancreas and other organs are controlled by using drains that are inserted during surgery. Surgery also sometimes results in pancreatic insufficiency (a condition in which food can no longer be normally absorbed by the body) or inadequate insulin secretion. These problems are treated with pancreatic enzyme replacement therapy and insulin injections.

Pancreatitis

An inflammation of the PANCREAS. Pancreatitis may be sudden and acute or chronic and long-lasting. Most cases are associated with alcohol abuse or gallstones (hardened masses of cholesterol or bilirubin that develop in the gallbladder). Acute pancreatitis comes on suddenly and can result in life-threatening disease. Intense pain develops in the upper abdomen and can penetrate to the back. Other symptoms include nausea, vomiting, fever, and abdominal distension. Internal bleeding may cause bluish bruises on the abdomen.

Recurrent attacks of acute pancreatitis can lead to chronic inflammation of the pancreas. As the damaged organ gradually loses its ability to produce enzymes and hormones, complete recovery no longer occurs between attacks.

The primary symptom of acute or chronic pancreatitis is a dull, steady pain that is aggravated by alcohol and food. The pain often is diminished by sitting up and leaning forward. However, 10 percent of people with chronic pancreatitis experience no pain. Additional symptoms may include weight loss, indigestion, and JAUNDICE (a yellowing of the skin and the whites of the eyes). In severe cases, a deficiency of the fat-splitting enzyme lipase leads to excess fat in the feces, resulting in bulky, greasy, malodorous stools.

Chronic pancreatitis leads to a number of complications. An impaired pancreas can cause insulin deficiency, diabetes, and MALABSORPTION (impaired absorption of nutrients

through the small intestine). In some cases, pseudocysts (fluid-filled sacs in the pancreas) develop. As inflammation subsides, the cysts may disappear spontaneously. At other times, they must be surgically drained.

DIAGNOSIS AND TREATMENT
Pancreatitis is diagnosed by physical examination and tests, such as blood samples, X rays, ultrasound scanning, CT (computed tomography) scanning, and ENDOSCOPY (a procedure in which interior parts of the body are examined by using a slim, flexible, lighted tube). The pancreas produces insulin; therefore, the doctor usually orders a blood glucose test and may prescribe insulin if the blood glucose level is elevated. Cases of acute pancreatitis usually require hospitalization. Treatment may include pain relievers, drugs to control pancreatic juices, and possibly antibiotics. To allow the pancreas time to recover, there is no eating or drinking for at least several days. Fluids and pain relievers are given by vein. Surgery is sometimes necessary if there are complications such as bleeding, infection, or cysts. Severe cases of pancreatitis are life-threatening and may need to be treated in an intensive care unit.

Complete abstinence from alcohol is vital to recovery from both acute and chronic pancreatitis. In the chronic disease, the doctor may also prescribe drugs to relieve pain, along with digestive enzyme medication and insulin as needed. Adherence to a special low-fat diet is also essential. If gallstones are the underlying cause, their removal is generally indicated. In severe cases, a PANCREATECTOMY (surgical removal of all or part of the pancreas) can provide pain relief.

Pandemic

A disease that appears in abnormal proportions across a major geographical area, such as a region, a country, a continent, or the whole world. An example is the AIDS (acquired immunodeficiency syndrome) pandemic in Africa, which affects a large portion of the population south of the Sahara Desert. See EPIDEMIC.

Panic attack

A sudden, unexpected, overwhelming, and terrifying bout of anxiety in which the person feels as if he or she

is out of control and threatened with imminent death or destruction. Physical symptoms can include sensation of shortness of breath, dizziness or faintness, rapid pounding heartbeat, trembling, sweating, shakiness, chills, choking, nausea, heartburn, numbness or tingling in the hands or feet, chest pain or discomfort, flushed or clammy skin, paralysis of the face, and agitation. The symptoms come on rapidly, usually peak within seconds or minutes, and subside. Usually the whole episode peaks within 10 minutes and is over within 30 minutes. Panic attacks may recur. They can be a symptom of any of the ANXIETY DISORDERS, depression, and a number of physical conditions, including impaired breathing (asthma, emphysema, chronic obstructive pulmonary disease), heart disease, hormonal imbalances, metabolic disturbances (low blood sugar), inner ear malfunction, seizures, drug intoxication, and drug or alcohol withdrawal.

Panic disorder

A mental illness causing repeated, frequent, unexpected bouts of extreme anxiety called panic attacks and resulting in severe anxiety about further attacks. There are three key symptoms of panic disorder. The first is the presence of panic attacks. During a panic attack the individual feels out of control and in danger of dying or going insane. Physical symptoms can include shortness of breath, dizziness or faintness, rapid heartbeat, trembling, sweating, choking, nausea, heartburn, numbness or tingling in the hands or feet, chest pain or discomfort, flushed or clammy skin, paralysis of the face, and agitation. The symptoms come on rapidly, usually peak within seconds or minutes, and subside. Usually the whole episode lasts only 10 to 30 minutes. Frequency varies from individual to individual. The second indicator is the unexpectedness of the panic attacks. In other anxiety disorders, such as PHOBIA or POST-TRAUMATIC STRESS DISORDER, the attack has a clear, distinct cue, usually an encounter with the feared object or situation. In panic disorder, panic attacks seem to be random and occur "out of the blue." The third and final symptom is fear and anxiety over further panic attacks for at least 1 month

Psychiatrists list 13 physical and psychological symptoms of panic attack, of which at least four must be present for an incident to qualify as a true panic attack. The symptoms are:

- Palpitations, pounding heart, or accelerated heart rate
- Sweating
- Trembling or shaking
- Sensations of smothering or shortness of breath
- Feelings of choking
- Chest pain or discomfort
- Nausea or abdominal distress
- Feeling dizzy, lightheaded, faint, or unsteady
- Feelings of unreality ("This is a dream.") or depersonalization ("This is happening to someone else.")
- Fear of losing control or going crazy
- Fear of dying
- Numbness or tingling, usually in the hands or feet
- Chills or hot flashes

following an attack. This fear can lead the individual to change his or her lifestyle, particularly to avoid settings where escape may be difficult or help hard to find if an attack occurs. This often results in agoraphobia, a profound fear and avoidance of public places and crowds.

COURSE AND CAUSES

Panic disorder is two to three times as common in women as men. People with the disease usually experience their first panic attack between the late teens and the mid 30s. Onset in childhood or after age 45 is unusual but does occur. The severity of attacks tends to diminish in the 50s and 60s.

Panic disorder is often accompanied by other mental illnesses. Approximately one of eight people with the disease abuses alcohol or other drugs, usually in an attempt to self-medicate against the discomfort of panic attacks. Depression is likewise common. Anxiety disorder, obsessive-compulsive disorder, and phobia may also occur in people with panic disorder.

Panic disorder is more likely among the immediate family members of people with the disease than among the general population, indicating that inheritance has a role in developing the illness. No single cause of panic disorder has been identified; most likely a number of factors have a role. One theory is that a chemical abnormality in the nerve cells of the brain causes an overreaction to a perceived threat, leading to the panic attack. Another is that a metabolic imbalance sets off a false alarm about smothering that triggers a panic attack. Stress also has a role in bringing on the disease, as do thinking styles that overemphasize the danger of certain events.

Untreated panic disorder can cause serious harm. The disease may make it difficult for the individual to function in job, social, or family roles. Approximately one of five people with panic disorder attempts suicide. Repeated panic attacks may increase the risk of high blood pressure (hypertension), heart disease, and stroke.

TREATMENT

Panic disorder is highly treatable. The usual approach combines medication and psychotherapy. Medications effective against panic disorder include antidepressants and antianxiety drugs. Cognitive-behavioral therapy works well in identifying and changing thinking patterns that predispose the individual to panic and in helping the person learn how to deal with potentially threatening situations, such as crowded public places, without suffering a panic attack.

Pantothenic acid

Vitamin B5. A vitamin that aids the release of energy in cells and a number of other cellular reactions. See VITAMIN B.

Pap smear

A screening test for cancer of the cervix usually performed during a woman's annual health examination. To perform a Pap smear, a doctor inserts a speculum into a woman's vagina and, using a tiny brush or cotton swab and a narrow spatula, removes cells from the surface of the cervix. The cells are smeared onto a glass slide, dried, and fixed. Then, they are sent to a laboratory where they are examined microscopically for abnormalities, such as atypical cells, precancerous cells, and cancer-

ous cells. At times, the Pap smear can detect evidence of sexually transmitted diseases, such as herpes simplex, trichomoniasis, and human papillomavirus, which has been associated with cervical cancer.

A negative (normal) result from a Pap smear test means a woman's cervix is probably healthy. An abnormal result does not necessarily mean a woman has cancer. A Pap smear can detect precancerous cell changes that have not yet led to cancer. If a woman has a mildly abnormal Pap smear, the doctor may recommend retesting in 3 months to see if the abnormalities persist. If a woman has a moderately or severely abnormal Pap smear, her doctor will recommend further tests, such as a COLPOSCOPY or biopsy (removal of a small tissue sample for examination under a microscope), to confirm the presence of abnormal cells and to determine whether further treatment is necessary. See also CERVICAL DYSPLASIA; CERVIX, CANCER OF.

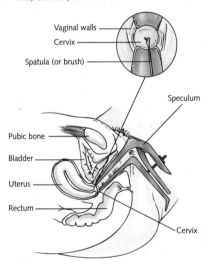

HOW A PAP SMEAR IS TAKEN
To take a Pap smear, the doctor opens the vagina by inserting a speculum. Then he or she uses a tiny brush or spatula to scrape cells off the surface of the cervix (the neck of the uterus) for laboratory analysis. The process takes only a few minutes.

Papilla

Any small structure that projects outward. For example, papillae on the front of the tongue—which look like tiny bumps about the size of a pin head—contain the taste buds, which are taste receptors for food.

Papilledema

Swelling of the region where the optic nerve joins the retina (the thin, light-sensitive area in the back of the EYE). Because of the swelling, the optic disc looks inflamed and swollen, its margins become blurred and hard to distinguish, and the small cup in the center of the disc decreases in size. Papilledema is caused by increased intracranial pressure, and both eyes are involved. Papilledema can result from a brain tumor, bleeding into the brain tissue, and PSEUDOTUMOR CEREBRI. Malignant hypertension, a medical emergency, may also cause disc swelling.

Papilloma

A small, soft, flesh-colored growth that protrudes from the skin. See also SKIN TAG.

Papule

A small, solid, superficial elevated bump on the skin that is red, white, or flesh-colored. Papules are a common feature of ACNE.

Para-aminobenzoic acid

The active ingredient in many sunscreens and sunblocks; also known as PABA. Products that contain para-aminobenzoic acid resist being diluted by sweat and water. However, people who have sensitive or allergy-prone skin are advised to choose PABA-free products.

Paracentesis

Also known as an abdominal tap; a procedure in which fluid is removed from the abdomen with a needle. The abdomen or peritoneal cavity normally contains little fluid. Paracentesis is performed to remove a sample of fluid to determine why it is present. The surgeon will also check for internal bleeding.

Paracentesis is performed under local anesthesia. During the procedure, a tap needle is inserted into the abdomen and a sample of fluid is withdrawn into a syringe. The anesthetic causes a slight stinging sensation, and there is a feeling of pressure when the needle is inserted. The procedure carries a slight risk of infection or puncture of the bladder, intestine, or blood vessels.

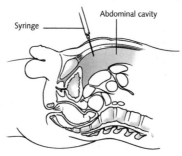

SAMPLING ABNORMAL FLUIDS
A person having paracentesis done receives a local anesthetic, and the abdominal area is shaved if necessary. Sometimes a small incision is made to help insert the needle. There may be a feeling of pressure as the needle goes in and some dizziness as the fluid is withdrawn. The puncture site will be bandaged.

Paraffin bath

Heated containers filled with melted paraffin and used as a treatment for soothing the pain of arthritis, stiff joints, inflammation, sports injuries, and muscle spasms. Paraffin baths offer a method for applying deep heat to the small joints in the hands or feet. The affected area is dipped into a bath of melted paraffin several times, then wrapped in plastic and covered with a towel. The warm wax holds heat on the area for about 15 minutes and is removed when it cools and hardens. Paraffin baths are available at medical supply stores.

Parainfluenza virus

Any one of three related viruses that cause a variety of respiratory infections ranging in severity from the common cold to croup to a type of pneumonia. Parainfluenza virus tends to cause illness, predominantly in young children. By adulthood, most people have established immunity to the virus and contract mild illness with infection. Different types of the virus cause different forms of disease. The most common infection in children is a respiratory illness with fever See COLD, COMMON.

SYMPTOMS, DIAGNOSIS, AND TREATMENT

Depending on the type of parainfluenza virus involved, the incubation period may range from 3 to 6 days. Associated fever may peak and subside quickly or persist for as long as 3 days. If the lower respiratory tract is involved, the fever may be prolonged, lasting a week or more.

Other symptoms may include a sore throat and dry cough, with hoarseness and CROUP that appear early in the infection. The croup may be severe in children and require hospitalization.

After the initial, acute phase of illness, an infection with parainfluenza virus can progress to BRONCHITIS and "walking" viral pneumonia in children and some adults. The virus is one of the more common causes of viral pneumonia in children.

With the exception of croup and viral pneumonia in children, the parainfluenza virus frequently causes illness, but the symptoms tend to be mild, localized, and of short duration. Bronchitis and pneumonia associated with one type of parainfluenza virus rarely cause disability or death. Secondary bacterial infections do not usually occur.

Infections caused by this virus are not clinically distinguishable from INFLUENZA, which is generally caused by other viruses, and specific identification of the parainfluenza virus by blood tests is not usually possible. Tissue cultures of infected cells from the respiratory tract may confirm the presence of the virus. Pneumonia may be diagnosed by chest X rays.

There is no medical treatment for the illness caused by parainfluenza viruses. Bed rest and treating symptoms with acetaminophen and cough medications are generally recommended. (Aspirin should not be given to children younger than 18 years because of the risk of REYE SYNDROME.)

Paralysis

The complete or partial loss of the power of motion or sensation, especially voluntary movement. Paralysis occurs when there is a loss of nerve impulses to a muscle, resulting in an inability to move that muscle. Sudden paralysis is usually the result of STROKE or trauma (such as a broken neck or back). Spinal cord injuries commonly result from car or motorcycle injuries, falls, sporting injuries, or gunshot wounds. Paralysis caused by this type of injury is often severe and can be irreversible. Other causes of paralysis include autoimmune diseases such as multiple sclerosis, genetic disease, premature birth, polio or other infectious disease, and toxic conditions such as botulism.

PATTERNS OF PARALYSIS
Depending on the location of nerve damage, muscles can be paralyzed in characteristic patterns. Injury to the lower spinal cord may affect the lower extremities on both sides; brain damage may affect one only side of the body; injury to the upper spinal cord may paralyze upper and lower extremities on both sides.

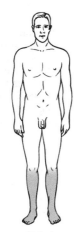

Diplegia

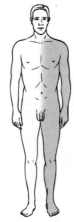

Hemiplegia

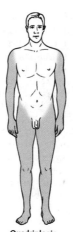

Quadriplegia

Paralysis occurs in a number of different forms. It can be temporary or permanent, localized or widespread, or sudden or spreading. PARAPLEGIA is paralysis that affects the lower extremities and most often occurs after injury to the lower spinal cord. Quadriplegia affects both the upper and lower extremities; it occurs as a result of damage to the upper spinal cord. Hemiplegia (paralysis of one side of the body) is usually caused by brain damage, often as the result of a stroke. Palsy is paralysis in any part of the body that is sometimes accompanied by involuntary tremors.

Other symptoms often accompany paralysis. These include numbness, tingling, pain, and problems with speech, vision, or balance. Spinal cord injuries frequently cause the loss of bladder and bowel control. Sexual dysfunction may also develop. Upper spinal cord injury can lead to problems with breathing. Paralysis is diagnosed according to physical examination and tests such as blood studies, CT (computed tomography) scanning, electromyogram (EMG), myelography, and X ray.

Treatment of paralysis is based on its underlying cause. A long-term rehabilitation program involves physical therapy and occupational therapy. The attention of other specialists—such as speech therapists, respiratory therapists, social workers, or psychiatrists—may also be required. Because prolonged immobility can lead to serious complications, doctors recommend frequent position changes and passive range-of-motion exercises for the person with paralysis. Good skin care and hygiene are also essential to prevent the development of PRESSURE SORES.

Paralysis, periodic

A group of inherited diseases characterized by recurring episodes of muscular weakness with apparent normal health and function between attacks. Periodic paralysis has been associated with potassium levels in the blood. When there is too much serum potassium present, attacks are frequent but mild (hyperkalemic periodic paralysis); when there are low levels of serum potassium involved, the attacks can last hours or days and can be triggered by exposure to cold or alcohol and carbohydrate consumption (hypokalemic periodic paralysis). Both diseases usually are inherited through an autosomal dominant pattern, although hypokalemic periodic paralysis is sometimes inherited as an X-linked trait.

Paramedic

A medical specialist trained in emergency medical procedures. Paramedics are able to perform many medical procedures at the scene of an accident or other emergency or in the ambulance on the way to a hospital. Paramedics are the most highly trained of all emergency medical technicians. See EMERGENCY MEDICAL TECHNICIAN (EMT).

Paraneoplastic syndrome

Symptoms related to a tumor that are not due to direct invasion by the tumor, but usually from substances secreted by the cancer cells. These substances usually produce symptoms in organs unrelated to the site of the tumor. An example of a paraneoplastic syndrome occurring in lung cancer involves a hormone called arginine vasopressin that is produced by SMALL CELL CARCINOMA cells. The hormone acts on the person's kidneys to cause a reduction in the level of sodium in the body. This can lead to confusion or even coma, symptoms not directly attributable to the tumor. In another example, hypercalcemia (increased blood calcium level) is a common paraneoplastic syndrome in breast cancer, lung cancer, and multiple myeloma.

Paraneoplastic syndromes can play a role in the diagnosis of cancer, because their appearance can be the first sign of disease, making it possible for the cancer to be detected early. The appearance of a paraneoplastic syndrome in a person who has had previous treatment of cancer may signal a recurrence of the disease.

Paranoia

A mental disorder characterized by extreme, pervasive, and unwarranted distrust of other people's actions and motivations. Individuals with paranoia assume that others want to deceive, harm, or exploit them, even in the absence of supporting evidence. They are preoccupied with doubts about the loyalty of friends, often pathologically jealous, and likely to assume that their spouses are unfaithful. People with paranoia are reluctant to confide in others or reveal personal information out of fear it will be used against them. They bear grudges and are unwilling to forgive injuries or insults, even minor ones, responding instead with extreme hostility. They often feel that their character has been under attack and thus attack in return, sometimes by filing lawsuits. Because paranoid individuals trust no one, they have an excessive need to be autonomous and self-sufficient. They often engage in grandiose fantasies, lack a sense of humor, are attuned to power and rank, and have negative opinions of racial and ethnic groups other than their own. A person with paranoia may seek out others with similar opinions and form groups or cults. In

P

some cases, paranoia may include hallucinations or delusions about conspiracy or persecution.

The cause of paranoia is unknown. There may be a connection to SCHIZOPHRENIA since paranoia is more common in the families of people with schizophrenia. Because paranoia undercuts the individual's ability to form a trusting relationship with a psychotherapist, treatment is difficult. Medications may be helpful, but a person with paranoia rarely trusts the doctor or the pills.

Paraparesis

Weakness but not total paralysis below the levels of the arms. Paraparesis refers to motor and sensory loss in the lower half of the body.

Paraphilia

A mental illness characterized by frequent, intense, sexual urges or fantasies involving nonhuman objects, humiliation of oneself or one's partner, or children or nonconsenting adults. Some individuals must engage in the paraphiliac fantasy or activity to become sexually aroused, while for others the fantasies or activities occur only from time to time. Paraphilia includes fetishism (undergarments, shoes, and other objects), exhibitionism (exposing the genitals to others without their consent), pedophilia (sex with children), masochism (receiving pain during sex), and sadism (inflicting pain on the partner). See also PSYCHOSEXUAL DISORDERS.

Paraphimosis

A condition in which the foreskin of the penis is retracted and will not return to its normal position. Paraphimosis results from long-term inflammation that decreases the size of the opening in the foreskin. This smaller opening tightens around the penis when the foreskin is pulled back. Left untreated, paraphimosis can cause severe swelling, pain, and even tissue death in the glans. Usually the foreskin can be returned to its normal position while the person is under sedation. Treatment includes antibiotics to resolve any infection that is present. In most cases, circumcision (removal of the foreskin of the penis) is advised to prevent recurrence.

Paraplegia

PARALYSIS of the legs. Paraplegia most often occurs after injury to the lower spinal cord, which may be the result of a car or motorcycle injury, fall, sporting injury, or gunshot wound. These injuries are often severe and can be irreversible. Less commonly, paraplegia is caused by a medical problem such as spina bifida or scoliosis. In addition to paralysis, other symptoms frequently include numbness, tingling, pain, and problems with speech, vision, or balance. There may be a loss of bladder and bowel control, as well as sexual dysfunction.

Paraplegia is diagnosed according to physical examination and tests such as blood studies, CT (computed tomography) scanning, electromyogram (EMG), myelography, and X ray. The immediate goals of treatment are to stabilize the injured spine, restore proper alignment, and decompress any affected neurological structures. Treatment thereafter consists of a long-term rehabilitation program involving physical and occupational therapy. The attention of other specialists (such as speech therapists, respiratory therapists, social workers, or psychiatrists) may also be required. Because prolonged immobility can lead to serious complications, doctors recommend frequent position changes and passive range-of-motion exercises. Good skin care and hygiene are also essential to prevent the development of pressure sores.

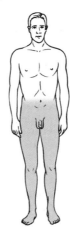

PARALYSIS OF THE LEGS
Usually as a result of injury, damage to the lower part of the spinal cord can result in complete paralysis of the lower body and legs (paraplegia).

Parapsychology

A branch of psychology that studies apparently supernatural phenomena, such as telepathy (the communication of thought from one person to another without the use of physical senses), clairvoyance (the ability to be aware of objects or events by means other than physical senses), extrasensory perception (also known as ESP; awareness or knowledge that is acquired without the use of physical senses), and telekinesis (the movement of objects simply by thinking). Paranormal experiences may be linked to brain disorders in some cases.

Parasite

An organism that obtains nourishment by living in or on other organisms, called hosts, producing disease in human or animal hosts. Parasites that cause infections in humans are most common in areas of the world where water safety standards are poor, for example, developing countries. In the United States, some forms of parasites have been found in well water, rivers, lakes, and streams, as well as in the public drinking water in some cities. The most common symptoms caused by parasitic infection include diarrhea, weight loss, loss of appetite, abdominal cramps, and mild fever. The parasites that live in or on people fall into three categories: protozoa; worms, also called helminths; and lice and mites, which are called ectoparasites (see ECTOPARASITE).

Protozoa are microscopic, single-celled organisms that ingest tiny food particles or absorb nutrients from their hosts; they may invade the cells of humans during different phases of their life cycle. MALARIA is the most prevalent of diseases caused by protozoa. SLEEPING SICKNESS is transmitted by tsetse flies; CHAGAS DISEASE (prevalent in South America) and LEISHMANIASIS are transmitted by sand flies. Some types of protozoa are transmitted from person to person, causing intestinal infections such as amebiasis and giardiasis and SEXUALLY TRANSMITTED DISEASES such as trichomoniasis. These protozoa may also cause an OPPORTUNISTIC INFECTION, such as toxoplasmosis or cryptosporidiosis, which primarily affects people with AIDS (acquired immunode-

TRANSMISSION OF PARASITES

Parasites that live in or on humans are common, but geographic conditions and social conditions affect what types of parasites are prevalent. Where sanitation is poor, parasites are easily spread via food and water that are contaminated with feces. Poor housing may promote parasitic insects. Even in parts of the world where sanitation and housing are good, parasites can be passed by direct human contact and flourish.

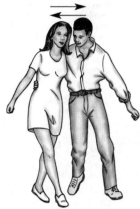

NO INTERMEDIATE HOST
Some diseases are spread by direct human contact—from breathing to sexual activity. The responsible virus completes its life cycle within one host (the organism in which the parasite resides).

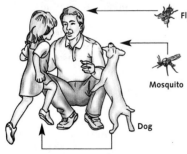

Fly

Mosquito

Dog

ONE INTERMEDIATE HOST
Some parasites develop in an animal or insect (the intermediate host) and then are passed to a human host to mature. An infected insect can bite a person, infecting him or her. An infected dog or cat can contaminate soil by defecating; a child playing in the soil can accidentally ingest the parasite's eggs.

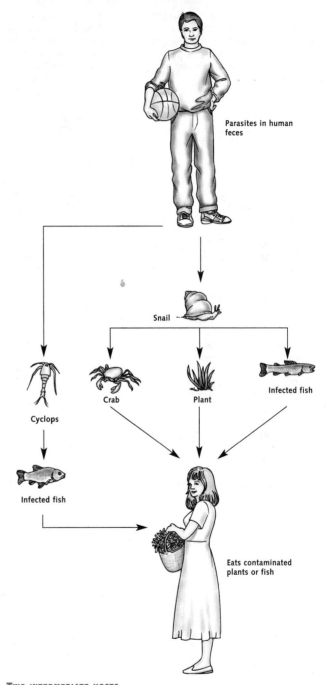

Parasites in human feces

Snail

Cyclops

Crab

Plant

Infected fish

Infected fish

Eats contaminated plants or fish

TWO INTERMEDIATE HOSTS
Some parasites live in contaminated water where they are eaten by a snail or other sea life (first intermediate host). The snails infest the skin and flesh of a fish or crab (second intermediate host), which is then eaten uncooked or undercooked by people. Plants can also be intermediate hosts.

P

ficiency syndrome). There are several medications to combat protozoa infestations and the diseases they cause.

Worms that are parasitic on human hosts are either in the nematode or roundworm group or the flatworm group. Those in the category of roundworms, which includes pinworms (see PINWORM INFESTATION), live in the intestines of humans and produce eggs that are eliminated from the body in feces. If food becomes contaminated by fecal matter and is ingested, the eggs hatch and develop into adult roundworms in a person's stomach, where they establish a new infestation. Some types of roundworm, such as those that cause TRICHINOSIS, occur in undercooked pork and may move through the body and settle in the muscles. A HOOKWORM INFESTATION, which can cause anemia, occurs by contact of the skin with contaminated soil in tropical areas.

The flatworm group includes tapeworms and flukes (see TAPEWORM INFESTATION; FLUKE), which are rare in the United States. Tapeworms spend part of their life cycle in animals and can infest people who ingest undercooked beef, pork, or fish. Flukes can invade the liver causing jaundice and can cause the illness SCHISTOSOMIASIS, which affects many people in tropical countries. Worm infestations are treated by antiparasite medications.

The third group of parasites that affect humans includes head lice, body lice, and CRAB LICE, all small insects without wings that feed on human blood. Scabies lice invade the skin and lay eggs, causing inflammation and itching. Lice parasites are treated with insecticidal shampoos or lotions.

Parasitology

The scientific study of parasitism; the existence and behavior of individual parasites and groups of parasites. A parasite is an organism that entirely lives off of another organism. In medicine, parasitology involves the study of parasitic diseases that affect humans. See PARASITE.

Parasomnia

A term that refers to a wide variety of sleep disruptions that occur during sleep or on arousal. Parasomnias are usually mild, infrequent, and occur more often in children than in adults. Sleepwalking, confusional arousals (in which a person appears awake, upset, and confused, but resists comfort), and teeth grinding are examples of parasomnias. In most cases, parasomnias are harmless and do not require treatment. However, when they occur frequently or become troubling, medical attention is required.

Parasympathetic nervous system

A division of the autonomic nervous system (part of the nervous system that controls unconscious body functions) that is dominant in the absence of stress (that is, the body's normal, resting state). The parasympathetic nervous system is designed to maintain body function and conserve the body's energy. (The other division, the sympathetic nervous system, activates during stress and uses the stored energy of the body.) Parasympathetic nerve activity includes narrowing the air passages in the lungs, constricting the pupils, decreasing the heart rate, lowering the blood pressure, maintaining normal digestive activity, and enabling the urinary bladder to empty. See NERVOUS SYSTEM.

Parathion

A widely used and highly toxic pesticide used in agriculture and horticulture. Ingestion, inhalation, or absorption through the skin of parathion causes nausea, vomiting, abdominal cramps, headache, confusion, loss of muscular control, salivation, diarrhea, weakness, seizures, and difficulty breathing. Doctors advise anyone who suspects he or she has been exposed to parathion to seek immediate medical attention.

Parathyroid glands

Four small glands located on either side of the thyroid gland; they are important in regulating the levels of calcium in the blood. The parathyroids are part of the ENDOCRINE SYSTEM because they release parathyroid hormone directly into the bloodstream. This hormone causes bone to release calcium and causes the small intestine to absorb more calcium from food consumed. To reduce the calcium level, the parathyroids decrease production of the hormone, and the bone tissue and small intestine respond accordingly. By adjusting hormone secretion, the parathyroid glands maintain the calcium level in the blood within a narrow range.

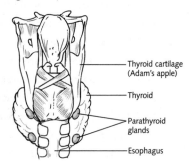

FOUR PARATHYROID GLANDS
Viewed from the back, the two pairs of parathyroid glands lie in the throat behind the thyroid gland. Although they are all parts of the endocrine system, the thyroid and parathyroids have unrelated functions. The parathyroids regulate calcium levels, while the thyroid is involved with growth and metabolism.

Parathyroid hormone

A hormone produced by the parathyroid glands that helps control the level of calcium in the blood; also known as PTH. Parathyroid hormone increases calcium in the blood when levels are too low by releasing calcium from the bones and decreasing calcium excretion from the kidneys. When blood calcium levels are elevated, the parathyroid gland is signaled to stop producing parathyroid hormone to reduce and normalize the amount of calcium in the blood. The kidney's production of biologically active vitamin D is stimulated by parathyroid hormone; the vitamin D helps increase intestinal absorption of calcium.

Parathyroid tumor

A growth on the parathyroid glands that usually results in excessive production of PARATHYROID HORMONE. Excess levels of parathyroid hormone produce elevated calcium in the blood and urine, which can lead to kidney damage and the formation of calcium-containing kidney stones. When the kidneys excrete large amounts of calcium, extreme thirst and frequent urination are often symptoms. Increased stomach acid secretion may cause heartburn or acid reflux.

Over time, calcium lost from the bones decreases the bone mineral density and may cause or worsen osteoporosis. Some people with a parathyroid tumor have no symptoms; in others, the condition may be detected during routine blood tests revealing elevated calcium levels.

Parathyroid tumors that secrete excess parathyroid hormone and produce abnormal conditions are generally surgically removed. If the tumor causes no problems, surgery may not be necessary. In this case, monitoring the blood calcium level, screening for kidney stones, and evaluating bone mineral density must be done periodically.

Parathyroidectomy

Surgical removal of parathyroid gland tissue for the treatment of HYPERPARATHYROIDISM, which is caused by the production of too much PARATHYROID HORMONE. For unknown reasons, the parathyroid glands may become enlarged and produce excessive amounts of parathyroid hormone.

Hyperparathyroidism is diagnosed by blood tests that reveal an elevated blood calcium level, usually followed by a test for an elevated parathyroid hormone level in the blood. To determine which of the glands are involved, DIAGNOSTIC IMAGING, including an ultrasound scan, an isotope scan, and possibly an ANGIOGRAM, may be performed. Parathyroidectomy usually cures the disorder.

Paratyphoid fever

An infectious disease caused by a specific strain of bacteria, *Salmonella paratyphi*, which causes illness in humans exclusively. Paratyphoid fever is caused by ingested food or water contaminated by human fecal matter; the incubation period is from 5 to 21 days. The disease affects the small intestine, causing severe diarrhea and abdominal cramping. The illness is sometimes referred to as enteric fever. Paratyphoid fever is uncommon but has been known to occur in India. It is treated with antibiotics. The disease is less severe than typhoid fever, which is caused by a related strain of bacteria,

Salmonella enterica typhi. It is usually treated with antibiotics.

Parenchyma

The essential or functional tissue of an organ, as distinguished from connective or supporting tissue.

Parenteral nutrition

The administration of a nutritional solution through a catheter. Total parenteral nutrition (TPN), also called hyperalimentation, is used in prolonged coma, severe malabsorption, burns, and other conditions in which feeding by mouth is not possible or does not provide adequate nutrition. Problems that may require parenteral nutrition in children include intestinal obstruction, structural abnormalities of the digestive tract, and severe chronic diarrhea.

The solutions that are used are composed of glucose, amino acids, lipids, vitamins, minerals, and other substances designed to meet the nutritional requirements of severely ill people, usually in hospital settings. In adults, the highly concentrated solution may be administered through a catheter inserted into the subclavian vein at the top of the chest and threaded into the superior vena cava (one of the two main veins conveying blood to the heart). In some cases, the catheter may be placed in a vein in the arm, although arm veins cannot tolerate as concentrated a solution as the subclavian vein. For infants and small children, catheters are placed beneath the scalp and threaded down through the jugular vein. Because there is a significant risk of infection with intravenous catheters, strict sanitary procedures are observed.

Paresis

Weakness; slight or partial paralysis. General paresis can also more specifically refer to a disease of the brain caused by SYPHILIS of the central nervous system. Its symptoms include mental and emotional instability and general weakness.

Paresthesia

An abnormal sensation of NUMBNESS, TINGLING, prickling, or pins and needles on the skin. Paresthesias are usually experienced in the extremities and can be an indication of nerve damage or poor circulation.

Parietal

Having to do with the walls of a body cavity, as opposed to its contents. The parietal bone is either of a pair of bones that form the top and sides of the cranium. The parietal lobe is one of the major divisions of the brain and is located just beneath the top of the skull. The word "parietal" comes from the Latin word "parietalis," which means "belonging to the wall."

Parkinson disease

A chronic, progressive disease characterized by tremors, rigidity, postural instability, and slowness of movement. Parkinson disease is the most common form of PARKINSONISM (the term for a group of disorders with these same four symptoms).

CAUSES
Parkinson disease occurs when nerve cells (neurons) in parts of the brain stem (particularly the substantia nigra) die or degenerate. These neurons normally produce dopamine, an important neurotransmitter that transmits signals about movement within the brain. In Parkinson disease, the loss of dopamine causes the corpus striatum part of the brain to fire out of control. This leaves affected persons unable to direct or control their movements in a normal manner. Free radicals, environmental toxins, genetic predisposition, and accelerated aging are mechanisms that scientists believe may have a role in causing nerve cell problems and, thus, Parkinson disease. Some medica-

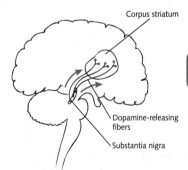

HOW PARKINSON DISEASE DEVELOPS
Deep within the brain, a chemical called dopamine carries signals about motor function from a structure called the substantia nigra to another called the corpus striatum. Loss of most of the dopamine-producing cells in the substantia nigra breaks down the communication and causes the symptoms of Parkinson disease.

P

tions, such as phenothiazines, can cause symptoms similar to those caused by Parkinson disease.

SYMPTOMS

The early symptoms of Parkinson disease are subtle and gradual. People may notice fatigue, malaise, irritability, or a slight shakiness. Handwriting may grow cramped, and an affected person might have trouble remembering a particular word or thought. These early symptoms are followed in time by the classic and obvious symptoms of Parkinson disease.

Family members may first notice a lack of expression and animation in a person's face (called the "masked face"). A person may appear rigid, stiff, unsteady, and slow and remain in one position for an unusually long time. As Parkinson disease progresses, shaking and tremor begin to interfere with daily activities. For example, it may be impossible for the person to hold a knife and fork steady enough to eat. Tremors may be worse with rest and improve with movement. Bradykinesia, or the slowing of automatic movement, may prevent a person from performing routine activities, such as washing and dressing. Postural instability can lead to suddenly freezing in place and toppling over. Other possible symptoms include depression, emotional changes, difficulty swallowing and chewing, speech changes, urinary problems, constipation, skin problems, and sleep problems.

DIAGNOSIS AND TREATMENT

Even for an experienced neurologist, Parkinson disease is difficult to diagnose in its early stages. As time goes on and symptoms become more evident, the diagnosis is made. The current "gold standard" of treatment for Parkinson disease is the drug levodopa. Nerve cells use levodopa to manufacture dopamine. Levodopa has serious side effects, however, including nausea, vomiting, low blood pressure, hallucinations, and restlessness. Involuntary movements may also develop, causing twitching, nodding, and jerking. In recent years, newer medications have become available to treat Parkinson disease, and research continues into new technologies and drug treatments. Surgery can now be done in some cases to decrease tremor and improve mobility.

Parkinsonism

A term referring to a group of disorders characterized by four primary symptoms: tremor, rigidity, postural instability, and slowness of movement (see also PARKINSON DISEASE). Parkinsonism also is the term usually used to describe the symptoms of Parkinson disease that are not caused by the degeneration of dopamine-producing cells in the substantia nigra, a part of the brain stem. People with parkinsonism produce enough dopamine but cannot seem to process it correctly. Strokes in the basal ganglia may damage nerve cells that use dopamine, resulting in parkinsonian symptoms, or parkinsonism.

Paronychia

An inflammation that affects the tissue surrounding a fingernail, sometimes extending to the tissue under the nail, and caused by a bacterium, virus, fungus, or a combination of several organisms. Paronychia, which can be acute or chronic, involves the skin through a sore or cut, possibly caused by a hangnail, as a result of other kinds of trauma to the nail bed, or from continuous irritation that may be caused by prolonged contact of the hand with water and detergents. Paronychia can also be caused by finger sucking.

SYMPTOMS, DIAGNOSIS, AND TREATMENT

Acute infections produce an abscess in the tissue surrounding the nail, often at the site of a hangnail or ingrown nail. The area quickly becomes painful, swollen, and reddened. When it occurs frequently, the infection eventually distorts the shape of the fingernail. In rare cases, paronychia penetrates deeper into the tissue surrounding the nail, infecting the finger's tendon and tendon sheath and causing tissue death.

Infections are treated with hot compresses or soaks and medication, such as an antibacterial or antiviral drug. The abscess may be surgically drained in an outpatient procedure. If the infection has extended into the tendon sheath, it requires surgical incision and drainage. Recurring and chronic infections may require partial or total removal of the fingernail and cultures to determine the organism that is causing the infection. Based on results, treatment may

include tincture of iodine or an antifungal lotion. Oral triazole antifungal medication may become necessary if the condition does not respond to initial treatments. When *Candida albicans* is involved, the gastrointestinal tract (and in women the vagina), may be tested for infection. Recurrences may be prevented by using gloves when hands are frequently in contact with water and detergents.

Parotid glands

One of two major salivary glands, located on either side of the mouth toward the back and under the rear of the jaw. (There are two other pairs of salivary glands called the sublinguals and submandibulars.) These glands produce a continuous flow of saliva into the mouth.

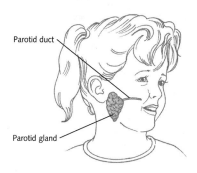

Parotid duct

Parotid gland

TWO SALIVARY GLANDS
A pair of salivary glands, the parotid glands are in the back of each cheek between the ear and the jaw. These glands can be infected by the virus that causes mumps.

Paroxetine

An antidepressant drug. Paroxetine (Paxil, Seroxat) is used to treat depression, obsessive-compulsive disorder, panic disorder, and social phobia, also known as social anxiety disorder. It is one of the new antidepressant drugs and it works by increasing the activity of the chemical serotonin in the brain, which is known to help improve a person's mood.

Paroxysm

An acute attack or intensification of the symptoms of a disease; also a sudden seizure or spasm.

Parturition

The birth process. Beginning with the softening and dilation, or opening, of the cervix, the process includes the contractions of labor and ends with delivery of the baby. Women who have given birth are called postparturients.

Parvovirus
See FIFTH DISEASE.

Passive smoking
Nonsmokers' exposure to smoke emitted by burning cigarettes or cigars and exhaled by cigarette or cigar smokers. Passive smoking, also referred to as secondhand smoke, puts people who do not smoke but live or work in the same indoor environment as smokers at risk of developing several health problems.

Secondhand smoke produced by cigarette and cigar smokers contains human lung carcinogens that can increase the risk of lung cancer in adult nonsmokers. It may also be associated with other cancers and with heart disease. Risks of lower respiratory tract infections, including bronchitis and pneumonia, are also greater to nonsmokers who are exposed to secondhand smoke, especially children. Children exposed to passive smoking have an increased prevalence of fluid in the middle ear, which is a symptom of chronic middle ear disease. They are also susceptible to irritation of the upper respiratory tract and may have significantly reduced lung function. Passive smoking can increase the frequency of

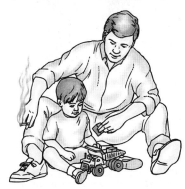

INVOLUNTARY SMOKERS
A child exposed to cigarette, pipe, or cigar smoke at home is more likely to get bronchitis, pneumonia, and other lung infections requiring hospitalization. The smoke can cause healthy children to develop asthma, and the attacks are more frequent and severe. Secondhand smoke also causes lung cancer and heart disease in thousands of nonsmokers.

episodes and the severity of symptoms in asthmatic children and may cause asthma in children who do not already have it.

Health professionals and government policymakers have taken appropriate steps to minimize people's exposure to tobacco smoke in the indoor environments of public and commercial establishments. People should take care to avoid passive smoking; smokers should protect their nonsmoking spouses and their children from the serious health risks of secondhand smoke by refraining from smoking in the home and family automobile.

Passive-aggressive personality disorder
See PERSONALITY DISORDERS.

Pasteurization
A process that uses heat to destroy harmful microbes in perishable food products without negatively affecting the food itself. Pasteurization was developed in the 19th century by the French scientist Louis Pasteur, who laid the foundation for the science of microbiology. Pasteur made his initial discovery by studying wine that had been contaminated by microorganisms. He demonstrated that these diseases could be destroyed by heating the wine to 55°C (131°F) for several minutes. The technique was also used on beer, milk, and milk products. Pasteurization came into use on these products throughout the world soon thereafter and continues to be the primary approach to preventing microbial contamination in perishable food and drink.

Patch test
A test used to detect hypersensitivity to a substance that comes in contact with the skin. There are so many substances that can cause allergic CONTACT DERMATITIS that it is impossible to test for all of them. A detailed medical history allows the dermatologist to select the most likely or the most common allergens. The patch test consists of applying a substance suspected to be the cause of a contact dermatitis to intact uninflamed skin. Test substances are applied to the upper back and removed after 48 hours. The substances causing the

allergies are identified when the skin reacts to them.

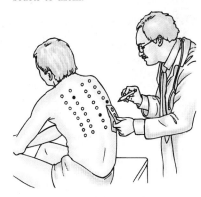

FINN CHAMBER TEST
The Finn chamber test is a patch skin test in which allergens contained in Finn chambers, or shallow aluminum cups, are taped to a person's back. After several days, the person is determined to be allergic to those substances for which a skin reaction is observed.

Patellar tendinitis
The inflammation of the tendon that connects the kneecap to the shinbone. Because it connects two bones, the patellar tendon functions as a ligament. The cause of patellar tendinitis is overuse, usually during athletic activity such as dancing, hiking, and jumping, all of which produce microscopic tears in the tiny fibers of the tissue. A number of these tears result in stretching the patellar tendon and causing painful inflammation. Symptoms include pain brought on by running or jogging and localized tenderness when pressure is applied to the point just below the kneecap, where the patellar tendon connects the kneecap to the shinbone. The condition is also known as "jumper's knee."

The initial discomforts of this inflammation are generally treated by resting the area, applying ice, and elevating the knee. The goal of treating patellar tendinitis is to allow healing by resting the area and strengthening the muscles that support the leg by performing gentle exercises that a physical therapist can demonstrate. If the muscles that support the legs become weak from inactivity, the tendinitis may become worse. Patellar tendinitis usually heals on its own within 3 weeks. If pain and discomfort persist for longer than that, a

P

physician should be consulted. See also TENDINITIS.

Paternity testing

Medical examinations designed to help determine the father of an infant or child. Most commonly, blood samples are taken from the infant soon after birth, the possible father, and sometimes the mother. These samples are then analyzed for compatibility.

DNA FINGERPRINTING is another form of paternity testing. It involves processing a person's DNA in a laboratory and interpreting the resulting pattern of bands on transparent film. A person's DNA is unique to that person and can be used to identify a particular man as the father of a particular child.

Very rarely, if a fetus needs to be tested for a chromosome abnormality or a genetic disorder, paternity testing may be done at the same time through amniocentesis. Amniocentesis is a procedure in which a fine needle passed through the woman's abdomen into the uterus is used to withdraw a small amount of the fluid that surrounds the fetus. The obtained fetal cells are then analyzed. But because amniocentesis is an invasive procedure and carries a slight risk of miscarriage, it is not solely for paternity testing.

Pathogen

Any agent that causes infection. A pathogen could be a virus, bacterium, microorganism, or any other substance that produces infectious disease.

Pathogenesis

The production or development of a disease.

Pathognomonic

Pertaining to the essential, characteristic symptoms specific to a disease, which permit diagnosis of that disease.

Pathologist

A doctor who specializes in PATHOLOGY, or the study of disease. Pathologists interpret and diagnose the changes made in tissues and body fluids by the presence of disease. For example, pathologists study tissue samples obtained by biopsy to find out whether the cells of the sample are cancerous. Tissue samples studied by pathologists may be taken from persons who are living or dead, either to establish the presence of disease or to identify the cause of a death.

Pathologist, forensic

A PATHOLOGIST who works in the area of FORENSIC MEDICINE. A forensic pathologist usually acts as a case coordinator for the medical and scientific assessment of a death. The pathologist studies the medical condition and history of the deceased, correlates all information, and reports the findings to law enforcement officials. A forensic pathologist may be subpoenaed to testify in criminal cases. See also PATHOLOGY, ANATOMICAL.

Pathology

The branch of medicine concerned with diagnosis of disease, its effects on bodily functions, and causes of death. Pathology can involve laboratory examination of bodily fluids (clinical pathology), cell samples (CYTOPATHOLOGY), and tissues (anatomical pathology). This specialty concerns all aspects of disease, particularly the nature, causes, and development of abnormal conditions in the body. Pathology also concerns itself with the structural and functional changes in the body that result from disease. Pathology can involve the study of DNA (genetic material) in fetal cells and identification of inherited genetic abnormalities. DNA testing is also used in pathology to establish the paternity of a child or to identify criminal suspects by the unique genetic pattern found in bodily fluids, hair, or skin left at the scene of a crime.

Pathology typically is concerned with disease-causing microorganisms, genetic material, poisonous chemicals, inflammation, degeneration, metabolic defects, nutritional disorders, and the effects of radiation and other carcinogens (substances that cause cancer). Hospital pathology departments are generally laboratories that specialize in clinical pathology, in which pathology is applied to solving clinical problems, such as diagnosing diseases.

Pathology, anatomical

A subspecialty of PATHOLOGY having to do with the examination of organs and tissues removed for biopsy. Anatomical pathologists, sometimes called surgical pathologists, examine tissues and organs from biopsies, surgical procedures, or autopsies, with and without using a microscope, to detect the presence of disease and its

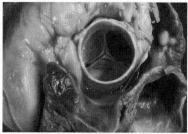

Healthy valve

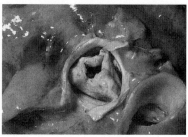

Aortic stenosis

ANATOMICAL EVIDENCE OF DISEASE
A healthy aortic valve contrasts with that of a heart with aortic stenosis as a result of rheumatic heart disease—the "leaflets" of the diseased aortic valve are thickened and fused.

causes. Tissue samples taken for biopsy can be examined microscopically to detect the presence of cancer cells or to find out whether cancer cells have spread from their site of origin. By using an electron microscope, the pathologist can see viruses and minute parts of individual cells, essential in classifying some kinds of tumors and illnesses. Anatomical pathologists also perform autopsies and examine tissue to determine the cause of a death. Anatomical pathologists present their findings in writing to the doctor who requested testing and provide a diagnosis based on those findings.

Pathology, surgical

See PATHOLOGY, ANATOMICAL.

Pathophysiology

The study of changes in body function caused by disease. Pathophysiology is concerned with changes in how organs function, rather than with disease-related changes in body structures.

Patient-controlled analgesia

See ANALGESIA, PATIENT-CONTROLLED.

PCB

Polychlorinated biphenyl; any of several substances in which chlorine replaces hydrogen in chemical compounds called biphenyls or diphenyls. PCBs are nonbiodegradable, toxic compounds used by industry in electrical insulators and as heat-transfer agents. PCBs are readily absorbed from the gastrointestinal tract and tend to accumulate in the tissues of humans and animals, where they can have toxic effects and may cause cancer. Because of their association with cancer, the use of PCBs has been considerably restricted in the United States.

PCOD

See POLYCYSTIC OVARIAN SYNDROME.

Peak flow meter

A device that measures airflow, called peak expiratory flow rate, one measure of lung function. Peak flow meters are commonly used to monitor and help manage asthma. The person being tested blows quickly and forcefully into the device, and a reading indicates how open the airways are.

Peak flow meters are used primarily to determine the severity of asthma and may be used as a diagnostic tool to detect an asthmatic condition before other symptoms appear. They are also used to check a person's response to treatment during an acute episode. Records of responses to using an inhalation bronchodilator, for example, can be helpful to the doctor treating a person's asthma. Because the meter monitors a person's progress during treatment of chronic asthma, it offers information to the doctor that may indicate the need for treatment adjustments.

Peak flow meters can detect a reduction in lung function and help avoid a potential flare-up. They can

also be used to monitor asthma induced by exercise, as well as other possible triggers. These triggers might include exposure to allergens, such as dust mites, and to irritants, such as cigarette smoke. Reactions to seasonal changes that involve exposure to different pollens, molds, and temperature changes, such as cold, dry air, can also be monitored.

The meters can be purchased over-the-counter but must be used under the supervision of a doctor who will demonstrate their proper use and explain how and when to record readings on a chart. A health care professional can also advise a person using a peak flow meter what should be done if readings fall below a certain level. The meter should be taken to a doctor's office at regular intervals so the readings can be checked for accuracy and proper use can be reviewed. See REACTIVE AIRWAY DISEASE.

Peau d'orange

Skin that is dimpled and thickened in appearance, resembling the skin of an orange. In peau d'orange skin, the openings of hair follicles and sweat glands are enlarged. Peau d'orange skin may occur over a breast tumor.

Pediatric rehabilitation

Treatment programs designed to help a child recover from a debilitating injury or illness. Pediatric rehabilitation helps a child cope with and compensate for disabling conditions that cannot be reversed with medical care. Rehabilitation may be prescribed for learning disabilities, head trauma, amputations, orthopedic or spinal injury, or congenital birth defects such as spina bifida. The goal is to restore a child's physical, sensory, and mental capabilities to as normal a state as possible.

Pediatric rehabilitation differs markedly from adult rehabilitation. A child is constantly growing and changing physically, emotionally, socially, and intellectually, and the various stages of development must be addressed throughout the rehabilitation process. That is especially true during adolescence, when factors such as body image and peer interactions increase in importance. The earlier or more gradual the onset of a disability or disease, the easier it is to

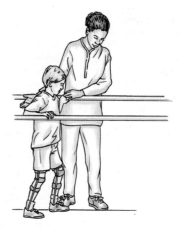

PEDIATRIC PHYSICAL THERAPY
Rehabilitation for a child recovering from a debilitating injury or illness differs from that for an adult because the child is still growing and changing physically, as well as emotionally and socially. Physical therapy usually involves some form of regular, graduated exercise to build up the child's muscles, bones, and joints. Therapists teach the child how to do the exercises correctly.

help a child cope with it. Older children and teens will need more assistance in coming to terms with an altered body image and the anger, fear of dependency, and loss of self-esteem that often come with it.

Pediatric rehabilitation usually involves a team approach, bringing parents, psychologists, and medical staff into the rehabilitation program. Counseling focuses on helping children and teens deal with social and emotional issues that accompany disability. Support groups for parents help them address their special needs. Parents are taught to be patient and understanding with disabled children and to resolve their sense of guilt when problems such as congenital (present from birth) defects are responsible. The main areas of pediatric rehabilitation are physical therapy, occupational therapy, and speech therapy. The approach to treatment is individualized to meet the needs of the child and the family. The duration of treatment depends both on the child's condition and his or her response to therapy.

PHYSICAL THERAPY
Physical therapy involves the use of exercise, heat, cold, massage, and whirlpool baths to help children function up to their physical potential. Therapy is generally prescribed

P

for children who have disorders affecting movements of the large muscles, such as those in the arms and legs. This type of treatment may be necessary after an injury or surgery or for children who experience severe swelling and joint pain from problems such as JUVENILE RHEUMATOID ARTHRITIS.

Exercise is the most widely used form of physical therapy. Therapists teach children how to correctly perform the exercises that, over time, will give them greater bone and muscular strength and increased joint flexibility. Depending on the nature of the problem, the therapist may begin by helping a child perform ankle, knee, hip, shoulder, elbow, or wrist movements. As time goes on, the child may be able to perform the exercises alone. Physical therapy encompasses a wide range of exercises. Range-of-motion or stretching exercises are designed to maintain or increase flexibility. Range of motion is the full extent to which any joint can normally move in different directions. Strengthening exercises can help a child regain muscle strength following an injury, such as a fracture. In some cases, exercises are performed in water to promote active movement without putting undue stress on injured muscles, bones, or joints. Exercise might also take place with the aid of equipment such as a stationary bike, WALKING AIDS, parallel bars, and pulleys and weights.

In addition to exercise, physical therapy includes treatments using heat, cold, massage, hydrotherapy

(water treatments such as whirlpool baths), and ultrasound equipment (the use of high-frequency sound waves). These techniques increase the flow of blood and oxygen to painful muscles and joints, generating heat and offering pain relief.

OCCUPATIONAL THERAPY

In occupational therapy, a therapist works with the child to perform day-to-day activities such as eating, dressing, and using the bathroom. Occupational therapy may be helpful for children following an injury or for those who have a chronic disease such as cerebral palsy. The goal is to allow children to function as independently as possible. A major objective is to enable the child to attend school with his or her peers. Occupational therapists are trained in ergonomics, or body mechanics, the science of moving the body in the proper way. Therapists teach a child how to sit, stand, lift, and move around without placing undue stress and strain on injured areas.

Occupational therapists can also fit a child with splints, braces (see BRACE, ORTHOPEDIC), walkers, artificial limbs, or other supportive devices designed to protect the body during therapeutic exercise or everyday tasks. Therapists will teach children how to correctly use adaptive equipment such as braces and a WHEELCHAIR. They visit children's homes and make suggestions about modifications such as rearranging furniture, widening doorways, or adding wheelchair ramps. For some children, the roles of physical and occupational therapists over-

lap. For example, either physical or occupational therapists can administer the pain-relieving technique known as transcutaneous electrical stimulation, or TENS. This therapy involves electrodes attached to the skin that transmit a painless, low-voltage current. As a result, the child feels a kind of tingling sensation. Stimulating nerves, it is believed, distracts the brain from noticing pain.

SPEECH THERAPY

Many speech problems can be corrected or improved with therapy. Children who experience difficulty communicating or with eating or swallowing are usually referred to a speech-language pathologist for evaluation and treatment. Because hearing deficits are often the cause, children who have speech difficulties should have their hearing evaluated. Speech problems also may be a sign of underlying learning disabilities. Ideally, speech therapy begins early in life, preferably before a child enters school. The process involves regular group or individual meetings, as well as home exercises. Physical exercises can strengthen muscles related to speech, while picture cards can reinforce memory and increase vocabulary. Computer programs are often used to sharpen speech and listening skills.

Pediatrician

A physician specializing in pediatrics, the medical specialty that concerns itself with children's physical and emotional development and the diagnosis and treatment of diseases and dis-orders in children and infants. Pediatricians advise on the care of the child, conduct periodic well-child examinations, and treat illness. Pediatricians also monitor the child's growth and development, give vaccinations, and watch for signs of child abuse.

Pediatrics

The medical specialty that concerns children's physical and emotional development, the diagnosis and treatment of diseases and disorders in children, and their growth and development from birth usually to age 21. Special areas of pediatrics include the care of newborn infants (see NEONATOLOGY) and disabled children.

PEDIATRIC OCCUPATIONAL THERAPY
One of the main goals of occupational therapy is to enable a child to go to school with other children. Therapists help a child learn to sit, stand, dress, and otherwise function as independently as possible. Occupational therapists can also fit a child with whatever supportive or adaptive equipment—such as braces or wheelchairs—is needed and help the child adjust to using it. For some children, the treatments in occupational therapy and physical therapy may overlap.

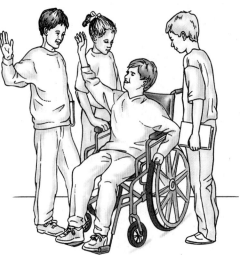

Pediculosis

An infestation with lice, which are ectoparasites (see ECTOPARASITE) that live on the human body. Pediculosis may affect the head, the body, or the pubic area (see CRAB LICE). It is transmitted via person-to-person close physical contact or by contact with infested surfaces, including clothing, towels, bed linens, combs, and hats. Head lice (see LICE, HEAD) infestation is common among school children. Overcrowded environments promote transmission.

The lice that cause pediculosis are equipped with claws on their legs that cling to hair or clothing and are adapted for feeding. Eggs, or nits, are laid, become attached to hair shafts close to the skin's surface, and incubate over a 1- to 4-week period. The lice and their eggs are visible to the naked eye, but the eggs are difficult to remove as they adhere to the hair shaft with a substance they emit called chitin.

Head lice cause intense itching of the scalp and inflammation of the skin, which may be particularly severe at the nape of the neck and behind the ears. They are treated with insecticidal shampoo or crème rinse, to be followed by combing out the dead lice and eggs using a fine-toothed comb. This treatment may need to be repeated. A doctor can recommend the appropriate product and offer instructions on its use. Pregnant women and infants should not use some insecticidal products. Following treatment, all hairbrushes, hair ornaments, and combs used by the affected person should be boiled in water. All bedding and clothing should be washed and dried at high temperatures. Hats and combs that cannot be cleaned should be discarded.

Body lice feed on a person's blood, but live in clothing and bedding. They are most prevalent in unsanitary environments where clothing and bedding are not washed regularly. Pediculosis caused by body lice is treated with the use of insecticidal lotion, followed by thorough washing and drying of clothing and bedding at high temperatures. Good hygiene is important in preventing infection.

Pedophilia

Repeated sexual activity by a person at least 16 years of age with children at least 5 years younger who have not yet reached puberty. Pedophilia is more common in males than females. Most pedophiles are attracted to females, but some are drawn to males or to both sexes. Typically those attracted to females prefer children in the 8- to 10-year-old range; those attracted to males usually prefer slightly older children. Some people with this disorder experience erotic sensations only toward children, while some are also attracted to adults. Pedophile sexual activity may be confined to undressing or fondling the child or masturbating in his or her presence, or it may extend to stimulating the child's genitals with the mouth or fingers or penetrating the anus, mouth, or vagina with fingers, objects, or the penis.

A person with pedophilia commonly rationalizes his or her sexual activity as having educational value for the child or claims that the child was sexually provocative and initiated the erotic encounter. People with this disorder may focus on their own children or stepchildren, or they may seek children outside the family. Some develop complicated methods of gaining access to potential victims, such as working with children, marrying a woman with young children, trading children with other pedophiles, or taking in foster children. Pedophilia usually begins in adolescence and continues throughout life, but in some rare cases the illness does not arise until middle age.

Peduncle

A term used to describe a narrow, stalklike piece of tissue. For example, the cerebellar peduncle is a narrow piece of tissue that connects the cerebellum with the brain stem.

Pellagra

A disorder resulting from a severe deficiency of niacin (vitamin B3). Symptoms include dermatitis, diarrhea, and dementia. If left untreated, pellagra usually causes death. Deficiency diseases such as pellagra are rare in the United States and other developed countries. See also VITAMIN B.

Pelvic examination

An examination of a woman's reproductive system. Pelvic examination is recommended for all women once a year, beginning at age 18 or when they become sexually active. The examination includes both an external and an internal review of the reproductive system. The external examination includes an inspection of the external genitalia, or the vulva, checking for redness, swelling, or signs of irritation or injury. The internal examination involves using a speculum to hold the walls of the vagina apart, permitting an inspection of the vaginal lining and cervix for redness, irritation, lesions, or discharge. The doctor collects specimens for tests, such as a PAP SMEAR and tests for various sexually transmitted diseases.

The doctor also examines the internal organs by palpation (touch and feel). Two fingers of one hand are inserted into the vagina while the other hand presses down on the abdomen. In this way, the doctor can determine the size, location, and shape of the uterus and check for pain and tenderness. The doctor will also examine the uterus and ovaries by inserting one finger in the rectum while the other remains in the vagina.

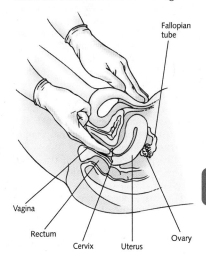

INTERNAL ORGAN EXAM
One part of a regular pelvic examination is called palpation—manually feeling the internal organs. The doctor inserts one or two gloved fingers into the vagina and feels the tip of the uterus. At the same time, he or she presses on the abdomen with the other hand to check the size, location, and shape of the uterus, ovaries, and fallopian tubes. The doctor will ask the woman if she feels pain or tenderness, apart from the mild discomfort of the examination.

Pelvic floor exercises

See KEGEL EXERCISES.

Pelvic inflammatory disease

A genital infection in women that has spread to the internal sexual organs, usually as a result of untreated GONORRHEA or CHLAMYDIA. Pelvic inflammatory disease (PID) is usually a complication of one of the SEXUALLY TRANSMITTED DISEASES (STDs). When these diseases are not treated, the bacteria that cause the diseases can affect the fallopian tubes, ovaries, and uterus, resulting in PID.

The infection may also be caused by the introduction of infecting organisms into the upper portions of the reproductive system as the result of procedures that generally carry the risk of infection, which may be increased if a woman also has an STD. These procedures may include an induced abortion, childbirth, or the insertion of an intrauterine device (IUD) for contraception.

Pelvic inflammatory disease is most common in women younger than 25 years who have multiple sex partners or whose one sex partner has multiple partners. It is currently considered the most common preventable cause of infertility in women in the United States, with the risk of infertility doubling with each episode of the disease. It is potentially one of the most serious common diseases that affect women. Untreated, PID can lead to ectopic pregnancy, infertility, and chronic pain in the woman's lower abdomen.

PID progresses through two stages. The organisms first infect the cervix, which is the opening to the uterus. Then, in some women, the infection spreads to the uterus, fallopian tubes, or ovaries.

SYMPTOMS, DIAGNOSIS, AND TREATMENT

There may be no symptoms at all, minor symptoms, or severe symptoms. When symptoms of PID occur, they may include mild aching in the lower abdomen, pain during intercourse, painful urination, discomfort during menstruation, irregular menstrual periods, breakthrough bleeding, and an abnormal vaginal discharge with a foul odor. There may

also be general malaise with fever or chills, nausea, vomiting, and weight loss. Symptoms may be difficult to differentiate from those associated with the diseases that cause PID, gonorrhea and chlamydia.

The specific site affected by PID may be detected during a pelvic examination performed by a GYNECOLOGIST or family doctor. The examination usually reveals tender or swollen reproductive organs. Because the site of infection is not always easily examined, a diagnosis may be difficult. Diagnosis may also be problematic because the symptoms mimic those of APPENDICITIS. A sexual history, including the type of birth control method used, may help in making a preliminary diagnosis.

Samples of cervical cells may be taken to be examined for the organisms that cause gonorrhea and chlamydia infections. Blood tests may also be performed. ULTRASOUND SCANNING may be used to examine the fallopian tubes for swelling or the presence of an abscess. The doctor may use LAPAROSCOPY, in which a thin viewing instrument is inserted through the navel or immediately below it, to examine the pelvic organs.

Treatment of milder cases is based on oral antibiotic therapy for 14 days. More than one type of antibiotic may be necessary when PID is caused by several different organisms. Bed rest and limited activity may be recommended. Over-the-counter or prescription pain medication and hot baths or heating pads placed on the abdomen or lower back may be used to control discomfort. Abstinence from sexual activity for the duration of the condition is essential. Sexual partners should be informed of possible infection and receive treatment whether symptoms have occurred or not.

If the diagnosis is uncertain and appendicitis cannot be ruled out or if the person has a severe infection, hospitalization may become necessary. Intravenous antibiotics and hospitalization may be necessary if there is high fever or severe nausea and vomiting. Scarring of tissues inside the fallopian tubes can damage the tubes or block them completely, resulting in infertility. This scarring or the possible rupturing of abscesses may require surgery. In a small num-

ber of severe cases, the disease causes death.

PREVENTION

Monogamous sexual relations are the first line of defense against PID and all STDs. Certain methods of contraception may offer some protection. These include vaginal spermicides and barrier methods used with spermicides, such as condoms, diaphragms, cervical caps, and sponges. Oral contraceptives can reduce the severity of PID, but barrier methods used with spermicides should also be used by women with multiple sex partners to prevent the infections that lead to PID. Following a diagnosis of PID, a woman should make sure that all sex partners receive treatment, even in the absence of symptoms.

Pelvic pain

FOR SYMPTOM CHART
see Abdominal pain, page 14

Pain in the pelvic region in women that may indicate severe illness. Pelvic pain can be acute, chronic, intermittent, or constant. Diagnosis will depend on the timing, severity, and location of the pain, along with symptoms. Sudden and severe pain in the lower abdomen or pelvis, accompanied by nausea, vomiting, faintness, and rapid pulse, is considered a medical emergency.

ACUTE PAIN

Sudden sharp pain in the pelvis can have several potentially serious causes. Possible sources of acute pelvic pain are an ectopic pregnancy, which occurs when a pregnancy grows outside of the uterus; pelvic inflammatory disease, an infection usually of the upper genital tract; and ovarian cysts, which can cause severe pain if they twist or rupture. Other causes of acute pelvic pain include actual or threatened miscarriage, vaginitis (vaginal inflammation), and cystitis (urinary tract inflammation). All of these causes of pelvic pain are potentially serious and should be diagnosed by a doctor. Acute pelvic pain is not always caused by disorders that involve the female reproductive system. Common diseases that can cause acute lower abdominal pain include appendicitis, inflammatory bowel disease, kidney stones, bladder infections, and gallstones.

CHRONIC PAIN

Chronic pelvic pain can come and go or it can be constant, and some illnesses begin with intermittent pain that later becomes constant. Intermittent or occasional chronic pelvic pain is associated with several common conditions, such as dysmenorrhea (menstrual cramps), endometriosis or adenomyosis, painful conditions associated with the menstrual period, and mittelschmerz (pain experienced during OVULATION).

Constant chronic pain may be experienced every day. It can disturb work, sleep, physical activities, and sexual relations, and it can cause considerable stress. Some causes of constant chronic pelvic pain include uterine fibroids or adhesions (scar tissue), formed between internal organs after surgery or severe infection. Endometrial polyps can cause pelvic pain, particularly if a very large polyp presses through the cervix. In rare cases, chronic pelvic pain is caused by ovarian, vaginal, or endometrial cancers, usually only in the later stages of the disease. Chronic pelvic pain may also be caused by gastrointestinal disorders, such as irritable bowel syndrome, or urinary tract problems, such as interstitial cystitis.

DIAGNOSIS AND TREATMENT

Diagnosing the cause of pelvic pain is based on the woman's medical history and a physical examination, followed by suitable laboratory tests, including tests of the blood and urine, a pregnancy test, Pap smear, and an ultrasound. If the pain is thought to involve the reproductive system but initial tests are not conclusive, exploratory surgery, such as a LAPAROSCOPY, may be necessary. When a diagnosis, such as an ectopic pregnancy or endometriosis, is made surgically, treatment can be performed at the same time.

Treatment depends on the underlying cause and can include medications, counseling and other nondrug treatments, or surgery. Women can learn to adapt to their symptoms with counseling; they can manage the symptoms by taking nonsteroidal anti-inflammatory drugs (aspirin or ibuprofen), antidepressant drugs, or oral contraceptives, if the episodes of pain are cyclical. Relaxation techniques are also helpful. Occasionally,

a hysterectomy (surgical removal of the uterus) is used for unexplained chronic pelvic pain, although between 5 and 20 percent of women still report persistent pain after the surgery.

Sometimes, no physical disorder can be found to explain pelvic pain, and psychological sources for the pain are suspected. Pain can represent a defense mechanism against emotional traumas like rape or incest, or it can be a symptom of depression. Psychotherapy may help resolve some of the pain and the stress associated with it.

Pelvimetry

Measurement of the pelvis, usually during labor, to ensure that the fetus will be able to pass through the birth canal safely. Most women can be assessed by the doctor and do not need pelvimetry studies. For those who do, several techniques are available: X ray, ultrasound (see ULTRASOUND, OBSTETRICAL), CT (computed tomography) scanning, and MRI (magnetic resonance imaging) are all used in pelvimetry. CT and MRI are particularly accurate, although predictions on the outcome of delivery have generally been unreliable.

Pelvis

The ringlike framework of bones in the lower portion of the trunk that supports the upper body and protects internal organs. The pelvis is constructed of the sacrum and the coccyx, which lie at the base of the spine, and two pelvic bones (hipbones), each of which is actually three fused bones (the ilium, ischium, and pubis). The two pelvic bones and the sacrum have rigid joints at the back of the body. The ilium flares out to form the hip. The ischium curves under and around, and the pubis leaves the ischium and extends forward. The two pubic bones meet at the front to form the pubic symphysis. The ring of bones encircles a central opening called the pelvic inlet. In women, the pelvic inlet is wider and shallower to ease childbirth. For the same reason, the fusion of the two pelvic bones is semirigid. In men, the bones of the pelvis are larger to support more body weight.

The muscles of the abdominal wall,

the buttocks, the back, and some of the thigh muscles are anchored to the pelvis. Within the pelvis are the bladder, the rectum, and some of the reproductive organs.

Pemoline

A drug that stimulates the central nervous system. Pemoline (Cylert) is used to treat children with ATTENTION DEFICIT/HYPERACTIVITY DISORDER, also known as (ADHD). Pemoline is used to decrease restlessness in overactive, easily distracted children and to increase their attention span. Pemoline is used as part of a total treatment plan that includes social, educational, and psychological therapies.

Pemphigoid, bullous

A blistering disease caused by an autoimmune reaction toward proteins in the skin. Bullous pemphigoid occurs mostly in people older than 60 years. Rigid, possibly tender or itchy blisters appear over multiple body areas. However, unlike PEMPHIGUS VULGARIS, another blistering disease, bullous pemphigoid does not usually cause lesions in the mouth. Diagnosis is made through biopsy and immunofluorescence studies. Treatment of bullous pemphigoid is with oral corticosteroids and other drugs that suppress the immune system.

Pemphigus vulgaris

A blistering disease caused by an autoimmune reaction toward proteins in the skin. Typically, men or women between 40 and 60 years old are affected. Painful and itchy blisters and sores may cover a significant portion of the body. Blisters may first appear in the mouth. Diagnosis is made through biopsy and blood tests. Treatment is with oral corticosteroids and drugs that suppress the immune system. Pemphigus vulgaris can lead to a life-threatening skin infection and is fatal if untreated.

Penicillamine

An antidote to certain heavy metals; a chelating agent. Penicillamine (Cuprimine, Depen) is used to treat Wilson disease, which is caused by too much copper in the body. Because it is a chelating agent, penicillamine forms stable compounds with cadmium, copper, iron, mercury, lead, and other heavy metals that can be excreted in the urine; it is particularly effective for chelating copper and mercury.

Penicillamine is also used to treat rheumatoid arthritis, although its mechanism of action in that disease is not clear. It is also used to prevent the formation of kidney stones and to treat cirrhosis of the liver.

Penicillins

Antibacterial drugs. The penicillins are used to treat bacterial infections. They work by killing bacteria or preventing their growth. There are many different kinds of penicillins, all of which share a common chemical makeup. There are four categories of penicillins.

NATURAL PENICILLINS
The natural penicillins are most active against gram-positive bacteria, defined as those with thick, rigid cell walls. Natural penicillins are used to treat infections caused by bacteria called pneumococci, also known as streptococci. Unfortunately, more than a third of these bacteria have become resistant to the natural penicillins. Examples of natural penicillins include penicillin G (Bicillin, Pfizerpen, and others), used to treat most infections caused by organisms sensitive to penicillin; and penicillin V, used to treat minor disorders, such as mild respiratory disorders, throat infections, and skin infections

EXTENDED-SPECTRUM PENICILLINS
The extended-spectrum penicillins include drugs that are effective against several types of microorganisms in addition to gram-positive bacteria. Examples of extended-spectrum penicillins include amoxicillin, used to treat minor infections, including chronic bronchitis, sinusitis, and ear infections. Amoxicillin is also used to prevent endocarditis, inflammation of the lining of the heart. Ampicillin is given to treat minor infections, pneumonia, meningitis, bacteremia (bacterial infection of the blood), and endocarditis.

PENICILLINS COMBINED WITH BETA-LACTAMASE INHIBITORS
Penicillins combined with beta-lactamase inhibitors are penicillins that have been combined with agents that can prevent bacteria from inactivating them with enzymes called beta-lactamases. These drugs are expensive and cause many unpleasant gastrointesti-

nal side effects. Examples include Augmentin, a combination of amoxicillin and clavulanate potassium, used to cure cases of hard to treat sinus and ear infections. Augmentin is also used to treat or prevent infections caused by animal bites. Other examples include Timentin, a combination of ticarcillin disodium and clavulanate potassium; Unasyn, a combination of ampicillin and sulbactam; and Zosyn, a combination of piperacillin and tazobactam. Timentin, Unasyn, and Zosyn are all used to treat complicated infections caused by many different bacteria, such as peritonitis caused by a ruptured appendix.

PENICILLINASE-RESISTANT PENICILLINS
This group of penicillins is resistant to destruction by penicillinase-producing bacteria. Penicillinase is the beta-lactamase enzyme produced by staphylococcal bacteria, and penicillinase-resistant penicillins are used only to treat infections caused by staphylococci. Examples include cloxacillin (Cloxapen and others), dicloxacillin (Pathocil and others), and nafcillin (Nafcil, Unipen).

Penile implant

Surgical insertion of semiflexible plastic bars or an inflatable prosthesis in the penis. A penile implant provides erections in men who have difficulty in obtaining or maintaining erections (see ERECTILE DYSFUNCTION). The semiflexible plastic bars provide a permanent semierection; the inflat-

able implant can be inflated temporarily to have sexual intercourse.

The surgery is performed under general or spinal anesthesia. For the plastic inserts, an incision is made in the underside of the penis. Tissue on both sides of the passageway in the penis (urethra) is expanded, and the inserts are placed inside the expanded tissue. For the inflatable implant, one incision is made in the underside of the penis, the tissue is stretched, and the implant is put in place. A reservoir containing fluid for the implant is positioned under the skin above the bladder, close to the base of the pubic bone. This can be done either through the same incision or through a separate one. Pressing on the pump mechanism inflates the implant.

Penile implant surgery requires a hospital stay of 1 day. Recovery takes approximately 4 weeks. Vigorous exercise should be avoided for 6 weeks. Sexual relations can be resumed as soon as the surgeon determines that healing is complete. Sensation in the penis and sexual arousal should be nearly normal. The principal complications are infection during recovery, damage to the urinary tract or skin, and malfunction of the implant.

Penile warts

Contagious, viral growths on a man's penis that first appear as cauliflower-like eruptions and increase rapidly in size. Penile warts usually cause itching and can spread from the tip of the

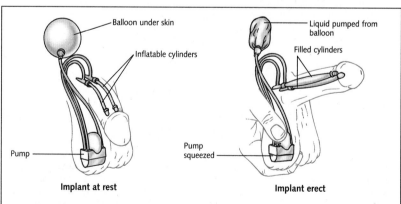

INFLATABLE IMPLANTS
To operate an inflatable penile implant and achieve an erection, the user squeezes the hand pump to send fluid from the fluid-filled balloon into the cylinders that extend the length of the penis. Then the pump deflates and returns the fluid to the balloon.

penis to the shaft and may also occur inside the urethral opening. They are one of the SEXUALLY TRANSMITTED DISEASES, produced by a local infection with a virus in the HUMAN PAPILLOMAVIRUS family.

Penile warts require medical evaluation to rule out more serious conditions, as the virus that causes them has been implicated in certain cancers of the genitals and the female reproductive system. A doctor can prescribe a special medication for removing penile warts, which should not be treated by over-the-counter wart removal preparations. Once a medical diagnosis is confirmed, sexual partners should be informed so that they can receive medical treatment. Without successful treatment, the warts can be transmitted among sexual partners indefinitely. Penile warts have been implicated in conditions that can lead to cervical cancer in women. See also CONDYLOMA ACUMINATUM; GENITAL WARTS.

Penis

The external male organ used for sexual intercourse and passing urine. The penis consists of three long cores of tissue that can engorge with blood and become erect (erectile tissue). The two larger such areas are at the base of the penis on either side and are called the corpora cavernosa. The smaller core, running the length of the front side, encircles the urethra (through which urine and semen pass) and is called the corpus spongiosum. It enlarges at the end to form the tip of the penis (glans). The three areas of erectile tissue are bound in sheets of connective tissue covered with skin. At the end of the penis, the gland is covered with a flap of skin called the foreskin, which is sometimes surgically removed. See CIRCUMCISION, MALE.

The penis matures at puberty. During sexual arousal, the penis engorges with blood, a state called an erection. Semen, a liquid containing sperm, pours into the urethra; muscles at the base of the penis contract and forcefully propel the semen out of the penis (EJACULATION). See REPRODUCTIVE SYSTEM, MALE.

For urination, urine flows out of the bladder into the urethra, which passes through the penis. The urethral opening is at the tip of the penis.

Although both semen and urine pass through the urethra, they cannot both be ejected simultaneously. During ejaculation, a reflex shuts an internal valve so that only semen can pass into the urethra.

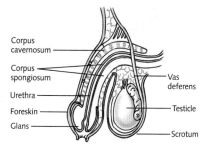

Side view of the penis

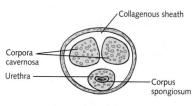

Cross section of the penis

ANATOMY OF THE MALE SEX ORGAN
The penis is made up of three masses of erectile tissue. Two of these masses are called the corpora cavernosa and are separated by a thin section called the collagenous sheath that goes along the top of the penis. Each corpus cavernosum surrounds a central artery. The other erectile mass, the corpus spongiosum, surrounds the urethra.

Penis, cancer of

A very rare cancerous tumor of the penis. The disease principally affects uncircumcised men older than age 50. The most common form of the disease begins as a persistent, painless, raised sore on the foreskin or the head (glans) of the penis. As the tumor invades, symptoms include pain, bleeding, discharge from the tumor, discomfort on urination, and enlarged lymph nodes in the groin. Cancer of the penis spreads quickly to the lymph nodes in the groin but slowly to distant organs.

The cause of the disease is unknown, but since cancer of the penis is rare in circumcised men, it may be associated with failing to keep the area under the foreskin clean. Risk increases with a history of recurrent infections of the foreskin and glans (balanitis), viral infections, and smoking.

Diagnosis involves the surgeon taking a sample of tissue (biopsy) from the tumor, careful evaluation of the lymph nodes, and a CT (computed tomography) scan to see if the cancer has spread. Treatment depends on how far the cancer has advanced when it is diagnosed. A tumor confined to the foreskin can be removed with circumcision, removal of the foreskin of the penis (see CIRCUMCISION, MALE).

More extensive tumors require removal of part or all of the penis; lymph nodes in the groin are removed if the cancer has spread or, sometimes, to check for possible spread of cancer. Radiation of the groin and pelvis may be recommended after surgery. Anticancer drugs (chemo-therapy) may be prescribed if the cancer has spread to other parts of the body.

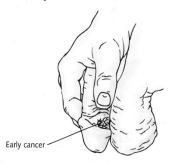

Early cancer

SYMPTOMS OF PENILE TUMOR
A cancer of the penis begins as a painless sore on the foreskin or the head (glans) of the penis. If the condition is not treated, the area may become painful, and there may be bleeding or discharge from the tumor, enlarged lymph nodes in the groin, and pain when urinating.

Pentamidine

An antiprotozoal drug. Pentamidine (Pentam 300 and others) is used to treat *Pneumocystis carinii* pneumonia (PCP), a very serious kind of pneumonia that frequently occurs in people with inadequate immune systems. Those susceptible to PCP include people with AIDS (acquired immunodeficiency syndrome), people who have cancer, and organ transplant recipients.

Pepsin

An enzyme that helps the body digest protein. Pepsin performs the first step in breaking down protein by splitting proteins in foods into smaller units

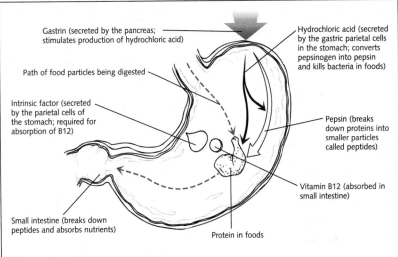

Gastrin (secreted by the pancreas; stimulates production of hydrochloric acid)

Path of food particles being digested

Intrinsic factor (secreted by the parietal cells of the stomach; required for absorption of B12)

Hydrochloric acid (secreted by the gastric parietal cells in the stomach; converts pepsinogen into pepsin and kills bacteria in foods)

Pepsin (breaks down proteins into smaller particles called peptides)

Vitamin B12 (absorbed in small intestine)

Small intestine (breaks down peptides and absorbs nutrients)

Protein in foods

THE ROLE OF PEPSIN IN DIGESTION
The all-important enzyme pepsin begins the breakdown of food proteins into strings of amino acids called peptides. The peptides travel into the small intestine to be further broken down into individual amino acids that can be absorbed. Other nutrients, such as vitamin B12, require a specific protein (called intrinsic factor) in order to be absorbed. The complex of intrinsic factor and vitamin B12 is absorbed in the small intestine.

called peptides. Pepsin functions only in acidic conditions. Hydrochloric acid (an acid produced by the stomach) converts pepsinogen in the stomach into pepsin, which helps break down protein into chemical components that enzymes can digest.

Peptic ulcer disease

A disease in which one or more raw areas develop in the membranes lining the duodenum, stomach, lower esophagus, or small intestine. The affected areas are damaged by strong acids and digestive enzymes secreted by stomach glands. The two main types of peptic ulcer disease are the DUODENAL ULCER and GASTRIC ULCER. Less frequently, stress ulcers develop following a major illness, serious injury, burn, or shock.

Duodenal ulcers occur primarily on the duodenal bulb, which is the first part of the duodenum, the part of the small intestine into which the stomach empties. Although gastric ulcers can occur anywhere in the stomach, they usually affect the lesser curve of the stomach between the main and lower portions. Although they vary in size, duodenal ulcers are usually less than a half-inch wide. Gastric ulcers are typically from one fifth of an inch to 3 inches wide.

Although the symptoms of duode-nal and gastric ulcers differ slightly, the disease processes are largely the same. Upper abdominal pain is the most common symptom of both. Burning, gnawing pain typically occurs after meals. Other possible symptoms, such as nausea, vomiting, and loss of appetite and weight, are more characteristic of gastric than duodenal ulcers. Men and women are equally susceptible to gastric ulcers, while men are more likely than women to develop duodenal ulcers.

Contrary to earlier belief, stress and diet are not the primary causes of ulcers. Evidence strongly suggests that infection with the bacterium *Helicobacter pylori* (H. PYLORI) is responsible for most cases of peptic ulcer disease. Other factors that play a role in ulcer development are the long-term use of nonsteroidal anti-inflammatory drugs (NSAIDs) such as aspirin and ibuprofen, heavy use of alcohol, and smoking. Like *H. pylori*, NSAIDs damage the protective lining of the duodenum, leaving it more vulnerable to attack by harsh stomach acids and enzymes. A family history of peptic ulcer disease also makes an individual more susceptible to ulcers, and stress may contribute to ulcer development.

DIAGNOSIS AND TREATMENT

Diagnosis is usually made through a careful medical history of symptoms and a variety of tests. Because ulcer pain and nausea tend to follow a pattern, the doctor will want to know when symptoms occur and how they are relieved. Pain and nausea are typically eased by food, milk, antacids, or vomiting.

Blood tests, breath tests, an upper GASTROINTESTINAL (GI) SERIES, and GASTROSCOPY are also useful for a diagnosis. Blood tests can detect the presence of antibodies to *H. pylori*, while a urea breath test determines the presence of the actual bacteria. In a gastroscopy, the doctor uses a slim, flexible, lighted tube called a gastroscope to view, photograph, videotape, and possibly take a sample of tissue from the esophagus, stomach, and duodenum.

Over-the-counter or prescription antacids often can provide relief. However, prolonged use of antacids can disrupt body chemistry. Therefore, many doctors prefer to prescribe drugs that reduce acid secretion: histamine blockers, anticholinergic agents, and proton pump inhibitors. A number of histamine blockers are now available over-the-counter, such as cimetidine (Tagamet) and ranitidine (Zantac). Other drugs coat the lining of the duodenum and stomach with a protective layer that prevents acid from reaching the ulcer. Although no single medication has proven effectiveness against *H. pylori*, a medical regimen called triple therapy (the use of three medications at once) can eradicate most cases of these bacteria. The three medications include two ANTIBIOTICS; the third is usually one of the PROTON PUMP INHIBITORS.

Lifestyle modifications can be useful. Doctors recommend avoiding excessive amounts of coffee and alcohol. Smokers should quit because smoking increases acidity in the stomach. Eating a number of small meals a day rather than two or three large ones may also be beneficial.

Possible complications of peptic ulcer disease include bleeding, rupture, scarring, and PYLORIC STENOSIS (a condition in which the outlet from the stomach to the duodenum, namely, the pylorus, becomes partly or completely blocked). Other risks vary according to the type of peptic ulcer disease a person has. There is a

P

> **STRESS AND PEPTIC ULCER DISEASE**
>
> It was once thought that stress caused peptic ulcers, but the impact of stress has come into question because eradicating *Helicobacter pylori* (H. PYLORI) bacteria has been found to eliminate ulcer recurrence. Yet, the role of the bacteria has not been entirely explained, since many people who are infected with it do not get ulcers. Doctors now believe that multiple factors, including *H. pylori* and psychological stress, contribute to ulcers. Some studies show an increased incidence of peptic ulcers in people facing war, natural disasters, or other stresses. Other studies show that stress causes ulcers in animals. There is no scientific evidence that relaxation, biofeedback, yoga, or other stress reducers can prevent peptic ulcer disease. But stress should not be ignored, and individuals should take steps to reduce it in their lives. People who have peptic ulcer disease should see a doctor for treatment of the *H. pylori* infection.

greater risk for cancer with gastric ulcers than with duodenal ulcers. However, duodenal ulcers are more likely to penetrate or perforate the wall of the stomach.

When peptic ulcer disease fails to respond to treatment or if complications develop, surgery may become necessary. The most frequently performed surgery for duodenal ulcers is VAGOTOMY, in which the vagus nerve is cut to reduce acid production. During the same procedure, the stomach outlet is often surgically widened (pyloroplasty). Less commonly, a surgeon performs a GASTROJEJUNOSTOMY to create a connection between the stomach and small intestine that bypasses the duodenum. In some cases, a GASTRECTOMY (surgical removal of part or all of the stomach) is required. The most frequently performed surgery for gastric ulcers is a

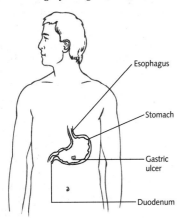

ULCERS OF THE DIGESTIVE TRACT
The most common types of peptic ulcers are gastric (in the stomach) and duodenal (in the duodenum, the part of the small intestine that joins the stomach). The cause may be a bacterial infection, but the ulcers are aggravated by the acidic digestive juices from the stomach.

partial gastrectomy, in which the lower part of the stomach is removed.

Perception

The process by which the body collects and analyzes information about the world. Perception consists of the conscious recognition and interpretation of sensory stimuli. It is the vehicle through which people know, understand, learn, or process data in order to make conscious or unconscious decisions about actions and reactions.

SENSORY RECEPTORS

It is the function of sensory receptors around the body to perceive stimuli and transmit data about them to the brain. Free nerve endings in the skin and taste buds on the tongue are examples of sensory receptors. In the skin, touch receptors perceive or detect touch, pressure, pain, temperature, and vibration. Elsewhere in the body, specialized receptors perceive odors, sounds, taste, and light. Internal receptors called proprioceptors collect and analyze information about the position of the body relative to its surroundings and of body parts in relation to each other. Sensory receptors transmit data about stimuli to the brain as nerve impulses. The brain interprets these impulses into meaningful sensory information.

THE FIVE SENSES

The SENSES receive sensory input from the environment, such as light, sound, odors, and vibrations. The body perceives sensory stimuli through five senses: TASTE, SMELL, TOUCH, HEARING, and VISION. The senses of taste and smell are closely related. There are approximately 9,000 taste buds (tiny clusters of cells that sense flavors from foods) on the surface of the tongue. Taste buds in dif-

ferent parts of the tongue sense the four basic tastes: salty, sweet, bitter, and sour.

The sense of smell is thousands of times more sensitive than the sense of taste. Flavors are recognized mainly through the sense of smell. Olfactory sensors in the nasal cavity are stimulated by odors. Nerve impulses travel to olfactory centers in the brain where this information is interpreted.

The skin, muscles, joints, tendons, and organs all have receptors that sense touch. The sense of touch relates to the body's ability to sense touch, vibration, pressure, temperature, and pain. These sensations are consciously perceived in the cerebrum, the largest and most developed part of the brain. The brain interprets these sensations variously as pleasing, displeasing, or neutral. See also SENSATION.

Hearing is dependent on a complex series of events that occur in the ear. Sound waves in the air are transmitted as vibrations that cross the eardrum to the inner ear. They are changed into nerve impulses and transmitted to the brain by the auditory nerve. Balance is also controlled in the inner ear.

Vision takes place when light is processed by the eye and interpreted by the brain. Light passes through the cornea. The retina converts light into a nerve impulse that is carried to the brain where impulses are translated into images and then interpreted.

Percussion

The tapping or striking of the chest, back, or other body part with a doc-

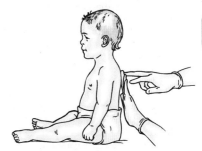

DIAGNOSIS OR TREATMENT
A doctor may use percussion to listen for sounds that indicate the presence of gas or mucus. On an infant, the doctor may tap the finger of one hand against the finger of another, to reduce the impact. Other forms of percussion can be used to loosen secretions in a person with a disease such as cystic fibrosis.

P

tor's fingers or small instruments in order to evaluate the condition of internal organs. For instance, when the lungs or abdomen are tapped, a hollow sound usually indicates the presence of gas.

Percutaneous umbilical cord blood sampling

A prenatal diagnostic test for genetic abnormalities and infection. Percutaneous umbilical cord blood sampling (PUBS) is one of the newest methods of sampling fetal blood for testing. The procedure is used only after the 17th week of pregnancy, and only when other diagnostic procedures have not yielded a definitive result. PUBS is exclusively performed by specially trained doctors because it is a complicated and difficult procedure. Guided by ultrasound, the doctor uses a sterile needle to take blood from the umbilical cord. PUBS is associated with more complications, such as injury to the umbilical cord, than either AMNIOCENTESIS or CHORIONIC VILLUS SAMPLING. PUBS is performed late in a pregnancy to diagnose conditions such as genetic abnormalities and to determine if a harmful infection has been passed from the mother to the fetus. It can also detect life-threatening anemia in the fetus that is caused by Rh incompatibility, and the same procedure can then be used to give the fetus a blood transfusion directly into the umbilical cord.

Perforation

An abnormal hole in an organ or tissue caused by disease or injury. For example, a DUODENAL ULCER may erode the wall of the duodenum or stomach, creating an opening. Perforation may permit fluid, air, or both to enter the abdominal cavity, which can result in contamination with bacteria and other substances. A perforation usually produces sudden and severe pain, shock, and inflammation.

Although perforation can occur anywhere, it is most common in the stomach, duodenum, sigmoid colon (the final S-shaped part of the colon that connects with the rectum), or the appendix. In the case of intestinal perforation, which is life-threatening, doctors treat the shock, administer antibiotics, and insert a tube to remove gas and fluid. A surgeon usually removes the affected area of the intestine, reattaches the remaining parts of the intestine, and performs a temporary COLOSTOMY (a surgically created opening or stoma in the abdominal wall to allow stool to pass into a bag).

Pergolide

An antidyskinetic drug; an ergot alkaloid used to treat Parkinson disease. In combination with levodopa or with the levodopa-carbidopa combination, pergolide (Celance, Permax) works by stimulating the specific parts of the central nervous system that are involved in Parkinson disease.

Pericarditis

Inflammation of the pericardium, the thin, fluid-filled sac that surrounds the heart. When the pericardium becomes inflamed, it may cause pain as the HEART moves against it. In addition, excess fluid can accumulate inside the pericardium and restrict the ability of the heart to beat. If fluid buildup prevents the heart from pumping sufficient blood to the body, an emergency situation known as tamponade results.

Pericarditis may be either acute (temporary) or chronic (persistent and recurring). Chronic pericarditis can stiffen and scar the pericardium and cause it to adhere to the heart, which may be prevented from filling completely with blood. This disease is known as constrictive pericarditis, and it can lead to heart failure.

Pericarditis occurs most often in men between ages 20 and 50. Symptoms include a characteristic sharp, piercing pain that begins behind the sternum (breastbone) and sometimes spreads to the neck and left shoulder. The pain worsens if the person takes a deep breath or lies down. Sitting up and leaning forward reduces the severity of the pain. Occasionally the pain is dull and persistent rather than sharp and piercing. Other symptoms can include shortness of breath, swollen abdomen, low fever, coughing, weakness, and pain when swallowing.

Pericarditis often has no identifiable cause. It can also result from viral infection (for example, mumps, influenza, or tuberculosis), bacterial

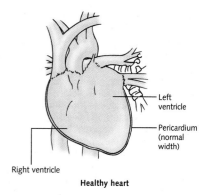

Left ventricle

Pericardium (normal width)

Right ventricle

Healthy heart

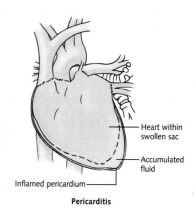

Heart within swollen sac

Accumulated fluid

Inflamed pericardium

Pericarditis

PRESSURE ON THE HEART
The fluid-filled pericardium is a thin, flexible cushion encasing the heart. In a person with pericarditis, excess fluid can build up and cause pain or restrict the muscular expanding movements of the heart. Some types of pericarditis cause the sac to stiffen, enclosing the heart in a rigid, constrictive container.

infection (for example, bacterial pneumonia), autoimmune disease (such as systemic lupus erythematosus or rheumatoid arthritis), cancer, injury, rheumatic fever, kidney failure, and a previous heart attack.

Treatment of pericarditis depends on its cause. Antibiotics are used for bacterial infection, and aspirin or ibuprofen is used to alleviate pain and reduce inflammation. Strenuous activity should be avoided during treatment. Tamponade, or the accumulation of fluid inside the pericardium that prevents the heart from pumping sufficient blood to the body, may result; if tamponade occurs, the fluid is drained by inserting a needle into the pericardium; sometimes a catheter (thin tube) is implanted to continue the drainage. In cases of

P

severe constrictive pericarditis, the pericardium may be removed surgically.

Pericardium

The sac that encloses the HEART and the origins of the large blood vessels leading into and out of it. The pericardium has a thick, protective outer bag called the fibrous pericardium that keeps the constantly moving heart in position. Within that is an inner sac of membrane—the serous pericardium—with two layers. The outer layer is separated from the inner layer by a cushion of lubricating fluid. The thin, inner layer secretes the fluid and is a smooth lining that allows the heart to move without friction as it beats.

Pericoronitis

An infection and inflammation of the gum tissue surrounding the natural crown of a tooth. Pericoronitis usually affects a partially impacted tooth (see IMPACTION, DENTAL), typically the third molar (WISDOM TOOTH). If there is an opposing tooth, it may be difficult and painful to close the jaw. The infection produces swelling of the gum and may result in fever and continual pain. When left untreated, pericoronitis can spread into surrounding gum and bone tissues, presenting serious complications. It is generally caused by the presence of food particles and the subsequent growth of bacteria in the spaces between the gum and the tooth. The infection can be treated with ANTIBIOTICS. If pericoronitis recurs and becomes chronic, an oral surgeon may be needed to remove some of the gum tissue and allow the tooth to emerge. If there is not adequate room for the tooth to develop and emerge normally, it may need to be extracted. Wisdom teeth are normally extracted when the tissue around them is infected. This is due to the difficulty in keeping the gums clean in that hard-to-reach location.

Perimenopause

A transition period leading up to MENOPAUSE, the cessation of menstruation. Symptoms of perimenopause usually begin in a woman's 40s, 2 to 3 years before her final menstrual period. The initial symptom is commonly an irregular menstrual cycle, which may include missed periods, longer intervals between periods, irregular bleeding, varying lengths of periods, or an increase or decrease in menstrual flow. Changes in MENSTRUATION may vary from month to month. Other symptoms include HOT FLASHES, NIGHT SWEATS, INSOMNIA, mood swings, and vaginal dryness, most of them the direct result of reduced levels of the hormone ESTROGEN.

Perimenopause typically lasts 4 to 6 years, although some women do not experience it. Oral contraceptives, which provide daily doses of estrogen and progesterone (a related hormone), may provide relief from the symptoms of perimenopause. Many of the symptoms of perimenopause are also associated with a variety of pelvic disorders. Any significant changes in the menstrual cycle should be reported to a doctor. See also MENSTRUATION, DISORDERS OF.

Perimetry

A diagnostic test to determine the extent of the visual field. In the simplest form of perimetry, the doctor sits in front of the person being examined, who covers one eye. The doctor moves his or her hand from the side to the center of the field of vision and asks the person being examined to report when he or she can first see the movement. The same test is repeated for the other eye. More formal testing is usually done under the direction of a specialist. In the automated test, the person being examined sits in front of a concave dome and focuses on an object or light in its center. One eye is covered. A computer program flashes small lights at various positions within the dome, and the person being examined presses a button whenever he or she sees a flash. The test is repeated for the other eye. The perimetry device prints out a chart that maps the visual field and reveals blind spots or other abnormalities.

Perimetry is useful for diagnosing and evaluating diseases that can limit or impair the field of vision, such as glaucoma, stroke, or a tumor in the brain. The test is painless and noninvasive.

Perinatal

Referring to the period beginning with the 20th week of pregnancy and ending after the first 28 days following delivery. Perinatal care, for example, is medical care provided during the first month of a baby's life, particularly immediately following birth. The medical care typically provided to a baby immediately after birth includes suction used to clear mucus from the infant's air passages and placement of an ointment, usually silver nitrate, in the baby's eyes. An APGAR SCORE is obtained immediately after delivery to help determine whether the baby needs special medical care. Circumcision may be performed on boys (see CIRCUMCISION, MALE).

Perinatologist

An OBSTETRICIAN or PEDIATRICIAN specializing in high-risk pregnancies. Perinatologists have been specially trained in the care of pregnant women who have diabetes or family histories of inherited genetic disorders. Other high-risk pregnancies occur among adolescents or in women who have high blood pressure or sexually transmitted diseases. A perinatologist may also treat women whose previous pregnancies have been problematic.

Perinatology

A subspecialty of OBSTETRICS and PEDIATRICS concerned with high-risk pregnancy. When the mother or fetus is at particular risk for complications, a PERINATOLOGIST may be involved in their care. Perinatology is a form of preventive medicine focused on the early detection of risks and subsequent intervention, before babies are born. This subspecialty, which combines the roles of obstetrician and pediatrician, is relatively new.

Perineum

The floor of the pelvic area. The perineum is the diamond-shaped area of skin and underlying muscle between the genital organs and the anus. In women, the perineum stretches during childbirth.

Period, menstrual

See MENSTRUATION.

Periodontal disease

Gum disease that produces inflammation and infection of the gums, ligaments, bone, and other tissues that surround and support the teeth.

Gingivitis and periodontitis are the two primary forms of periodontal disease, which is also called pyorrhea. Gingivitis is the result of plaque (see PLAQUE, DENTAL) and calculus (see CALCULUS, DENTAL) building up on the teeth. This buildup causes the gum to pull away from the teeth and leads to the formation of pockets, called periodontal pockets, between the gums and the teeth. If gingivitis is left untreated or is treated too late, the periodontal ligament and the bone of the jaw become involved. This condition is known as periodontitis. At this stage, the bacteria in the plaque begin to destroy the periodontal ligament that anchors the teeth to the bone. Eventually, the bone that surrounds and supports the teeth begins to demineralize and dissolve. As the bone erodes, the teeth become loose. They may fall out, or a TOOTH EXTRACTION may become necessary.

The accumulation of plaque and calculus on the teeth that causes periodontal disease is the result of poor ORAL HYGIENE in general and, specifically, inadequate or infrequent brushing and use of dental floss to clean the teeth. Poor oral hygiene may be exacerbated by other factors, such as an imbalance in the relationship between opposing cusps of the teeth, which can force food particles into the gums. Other causes include food debris left on and between the teeth, breathing through the mouth, irregularities in the position of the teeth, (causing BITE problems), hormonal changes, contraceptive medications, nutritional deficiencies, and tobacco smoking.

SYMPTOMS
Periodontal disease is associated with heart disease and stroke, and should be evaluated and treated by a dentist at the first sign. The symptoms include red, swollen, and sensitive gums that bleed easily when the teeth are brushed. Bleeding gums are an early sign of gingivitis and indicate the need for prompt dental attention.

When gingivitis persists, an infection of the tissues that help to anchor the teeth develops. This stage of gum disease is called periodontitis. The gums may appear to be separating from the bases of the teeth. Chronic BAD BREATH may be a symptom. There may be pus between the teeth and

gums. The teeth may become loose or pull apart. A change in the way the teeth come together when biting and chewing may be noticed.

TREATMENT
At an early stage, periodontal disease may be controlled by treating dental problems that cause plaque to form and build up on the teeth. A dentist or dental hygienist may offer special instructions on proper brushing of the teeth and the use of dental floss.

Crowded or crooked teeth may be especially vulnerable to plaque formation because they are difficult to clean. Orthodontic treatments, such as braces, may be used to correct dental overcrowding (see OVERCROWDING, DENTAL) or to reposition crooked teeth. If an improper bite is a contributing factor, this may be treated orthodontically, or the teeth may be selectively ground down to achieve a proper alignment.

Root planing is a procedure performed in a dental office that may be used to stop the progression of periodontal disease in its earlier stages. After the person is given local anesthesia, a dentist cleans below the gum line and smooths the roots so that the gum can reattach to the tooth.

In some cases, antibiotics that are effective against the specific bacteria involved in periodontal disease may be prescribed for short-term use, in combination with procedures to remove plaque and calculus. Because of the link between periodontal disease and cardiovascular disease, controlling the bacteria that cause gum disease may contribute to a reduction in the risks of heart disease and stroke.

If the periodontal pockets have become deep, a dentist uses a periodontal probe to measure the depth of the pockets and the extent of the disease. Minor surgical procedures,

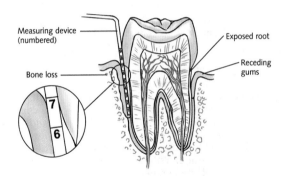

CHECKING FOR GUM DISEASE
In periodontitis or gum disease, bone and ligaments break down and pull away from the teeth, allowing pockets to hold infection-causing debris. If the dentist or periodontist suspects receding gums or an exposed root, a probe can be inserted alongside the tooth to see how deep the pocket is and the extent of the disease.

Measuring device (numbered)

Bone loss

Exposed root

Receding gums

such as flap surgery or GINGIVECTOMY, may be necessary to remove the soft tissue wall of the pocket. If the bone has become involved, surgical reshaping of the bone and gum may be required. Bone pockets must be removed because they harbor bacteria, which feed the disease.

If a root of the tooth has been exposed by periodontal disease, the covering of the root, called the CEMENTUM, may have been eroded. The cementum can be replaced by a synthetic material that is bonded to the tooth. A layer of sodium FLUORIDE, applied by a dentist to the eroded cementum, will protect it and prevent sensitivity. A special toothpaste that offers protection may be recommended. Procedures to anchor loose teeth may be recommended and loose teeth may be splinted together for support after gum surgery.

PREVENTION
Because periodontal disease can cause the loss of some or even all the teeth and is linked to serious diseases, preventing it is of primary importance. Gingivitis can be reversed within weeks by following good oral hygiene practice, including proper brushing at least twice a day and using dental floss at least once a day. (See ORAL HYGIENE.) A dentist should be visited every 6 months for a professional cleaning and evaluation.

Periodontics
The branch of dentistry that involves the study and treatment of diseases affecting the tissues that surround and support the teeth and their roots, including the bone, ligaments, and gums. See PERIODONTAL DISEASE.

Periodontist
A dentist who specializes in the diagnosis, treatment, and prevention of

diseases and disorders of the gums and underlying tissues. A periodontist has received specialized training in the treatment of inflammation and infection associated with gum diseases, such as gingivitis and periodontitis See PERIODONTAL DISEASE.

Periodontitis

See PERIODONTAL DISEASE.

Periosteum

A sheath of connective tissue that covers all BONE surfaces except the ends. Its rich supply of blood vessels delivers oxygen and nutrients to bone cells, it contains nerve pathways, and it has cells that can develop into bone.

Periostitis

An inflammation of the periosteum, which is the fibrous tissue layer that surrounds and covers bone. The causes of periostitis include infection, trauma to the area from an injury, or any abnormal growth in the tissue, including tumors. It is diagnosed by X rays and bone scanning. Symptoms include bone pain, localized tenderness and warmth, and swelling of the soft tissue. The pain may restrict movement. If infection is involved, there may be mild to moderate fever. Periostitis is generally treated by medication to relieve the pain and inflammation. When necessary, medication is prescribed to fight any associated infection.

Peripheral nervous system

The part of the nervous system that consists of all the nerves that emerge from the central nervous system and branch throughout the body. See NERVOUS SYSTEM.

Peripheral vascular disease

Any disorder of the blood vessels that lie outside the heart. Peripheral vascular disease can affect the arteries, which carry oxygen-rich blood from the heart to the body, or the veins, which carry oxygen-poor blood from the extremities to the heart.

The principal disease of the peripheral arteries is ATHEROSCLEROSIS, in which the arteries become narrowed and hardened by fatty deposits. Blood flow is restricted and may

even be blocked. This is most likely to occur in the arteries supplying blood to the brain, kidneys, lower abdomen, and legs (see CLAUDICATION). Peripheral arteries can also be affected by blood clots (see EMBOLISM; THROMBUS), VASCULITIS (inflammation of the blood vessels), or, in the case of the aorta, a tear between the inner and outer layers of the artery (aortic dissection), which can lead to a heart attack or stroke.

The principal diseases affecting the veins are THROMBOPHLEBITIS, VARICOSE VEINS, and chronic venous insufficiency, in which the veins permit the blood to flow backward. This causes swelling of the leg and both discoloration of and permanent damage to the skin.

A number of risk factors increase the risk of peripheral vascular disease of the arteries. These include smoking tobacco, a high-fat diet, uncontrolled hypertension (high blood pressure), uncontrolled diabetes mellitus, and obesity.

Peristalsis

Wavelike, rhythmic, muscular contractions that carry food through the digestive tract. Peristalsis occurs from the moment food enters the mouth until waste matter is expelled from the rectum. See also DIGESTION.

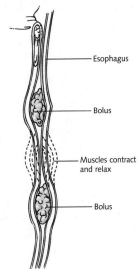

Esophagus

Bolus

Muscles contract and relax

Bolus

SWALLOWING FOOD
Food is moved through the esophagus by peristalsis. The muscles in front of the swallowed food (called a bolus) relax, and the muscles behind it contract, propelling the food down toward the stomach.

Peritoneal dialysis

A procedure that uses the lining of the abdomen, called the peritoneal membrane, and a cleansing solution, called dialysate, to filter the blood and remove excess water, waste products, and chemicals from the body.

HOW IT WORKS
A small, soft tube called a catheter is implanted into the abdomen, where it is left in place for as long as dialysis is necessary. Thin tubes connect the catheter to a bag of the dialysate solution, which is introduced through the catheter into the abdomen. The dialysate absorbs waste products and some excess fluid from the many tiny blood vessels in the peritoneal membrane. After several hours, the dialysate is drained from the abdomen. Fresh dialysate is then introduced into the abdomen again. The process of draining and replacing fluid is called exchange.

TYPES OF PERITONEAL DIALYSIS
There are two main types of peritoneal dialysis: continuous ambulatory peritoneal dialysis (CAPD) and continuous cycling peritoneal dialysis (CCPD).

CAPD is the most common type of peritoneal dialysis and involves the passage of dialysate from a plastic bag into the catheter where it enters the abdomen. The catheter is then sealed to retain the dialysate within the abdomen. The solution is drained into the bag after 4 to 6 hours; the draining process takes 30 to 40 minutes. The process is then repeated with fresh solution about four times a day. Because there is no machinery involved, a person can perform CAPD when it is most convenient. CAPD can be done at home in a variety of locations without help.

CCPD is similar to CAPD except that a machine is connected to the catheter to fill and drain the dialysate from the abdomen automatically. CCPD is generally done at night while a person is sleeping and lasts between 10 and 12 hours every night.

DIETARY CONSIDERATIONS
A person using peritoneal dialysis may be able to tolerate more salt, fluids, and protein in his or her diet than a person who uses HEMODIALYSIS. Potassium needs vary from person to person; potassium is necessary for good nutrition and health, but an excess of potassium can be dangerous

P

CLOSE-UP: PERITONEAL DIALYSIS

Several factors affect how much waste and excess fluid can be removed from the blood during peritoneal dialysis. The lining of the walls of each person's abdominal cavity (peritoneum) filters wastes at different rates. Whether peritoneal dialysis is effective also depends on the size of a person's abdominal cavity and how regularly the exchanges of the cleansing liquid (dialysate) are performed.

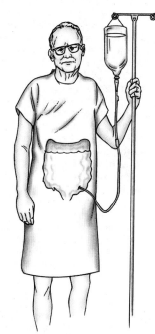

FILLING THE PERITONEAL CAVITY
Gravity is used to fill the peritoneal cavity with dialysate using a catheter.

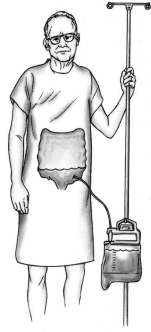

DRAINING DIALYSATE
After the dialysate remains in the peritoneal cavity for a sufficient length of time, gravity is again used to drain it, using the same catheter.

PREPARING FOR DIALYSIS
A flexible plastic tube (catheter) is inserted into the abdomen (peritoneal cavity), allowing dialysate to fill the abdomen or drain from it.

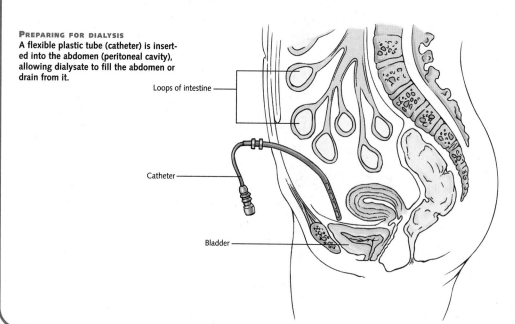

Loops of intestine

Catheter

Bladder

in a person with kidney failure. Because the sugar in the dialysate may cause weight gain, it may be necessary to reduce the number of calories in the diet.

RISKS AND COMPLICATIONS

An infection of the peritoneal membrane called PERITONITIS may occur if the area surrounding the catheter is infected or if there are problems with the connection of the catheter to the bag.

Peritoneum

The two-layered membrane that lines the interior of the abdominal cavity. It brings blood vessels, lymph vessels, and nerves to the organs. It supports the abdominal organs, anchors some of them to the abdominal wall, and completely surrounds some of them. It secretes a lubricating fluid so that organs can slide against each other, and it may help protect against infection. In some areas of the abdomen, the peritoneum forms multilayered membranes called the OMENTUM and the MESENTERY.

Peritonitis

Inflammation of the thin membrane, called the peritoneum, that lines the wall of the body's abdominal section, called the peritoneal cavity and surrounds the abdominal internal organs. Peritonitis occurs when bacteria or other substances contaminate the abdominal cavity. The resulting inflammation may be acute or chronic.

CAUSES AND SYMPTOMS

Acute peritonitis generally occurs as a secondary infection, most commonly caused by a perforation of structures in the gastrointestinal (GI) tract. This may be due to trauma to the abdomen, foreign bodies in the GI tract, severe intestinal obstruction, pancreatitis, pelvic inflammatory disease (PID), or severe vascular conditions such as a blood clot (embolism). Certain conditions, such as an ectopic pregnancy or ASCITES (excessive fluid in the abdominal cavity), and some medical procedures, including the insertion of abdominal shunts or drains, can lead to infections that cause peritonitis. Rarely, acute peritonitis is caused by an infection in the bloodstream.

Chronic peritonitis is caused by repeated infections or illnesses such as PID, certain postoperative infections, and chronic infections that affect the abdominal area of the body. The main cause of chronic peritonitis is TUBERCULOSIS. Fungal peritonitis usually occurs in people who had surgery or a bowel perforation and were treated with antibiotics or people who have weakened immune systems. Peritonitis may be a complication of dialysis involving long-standing catheters in the abdomen.

Symptoms of peritonitis vary in severity depending on the extent of the infection. Abdominal pain may be experienced suddenly over the entire abdominal region or in a localized area of the abdomen. There may be vomiting and high fever. Complications may include severe dehydration, respiratory distress syndrome, kidney failure, liver failure, and abscesses or adhesions.

DIAGNOSIS AND TREATMENT

X rays of the abdomen are taken, with a person lying down and in an upright position, to detect signs of perforation in the gastrointestinal tract. In some cases, fluid from the peritoneal cavity may be drawn out with a fine needle (aspirated), examined under a microscope, and cultured. An instrument for viewing internal organs of the abdomen, called a laparoscope, may be used, and abdominal surgery may be required to establish a diagnosis and cure the underlying problem.

Peritonitis is generally treated with antibiotics, the use of a nasogastric tube (a narrow, flexible tube that is passed through the nose, into the esophagus, and into the stomach) to remove fluids, treatment of respiratory symptoms if any, and replacement of fluids and electrolytes.

Peritonsillar abscess

An acute infection that occurs between the tonsil and the muscle at the back of the mouth. Peritonsillar abscess occurs most commonly in young adults and is usually caused by a *Streptococcus* infection (see STREPTOCOCCAL INFECTIONS), but may be due to other forms of bacteria. Symptoms include severe pain when swallowing, fever, and lockjaw. The soft palate becomes reddened and swollen, and the uvula (the appendage of the soft palate) is enlarged and repositioned to one side.

Treatment consists of antibiotic therapy, usually oral penicillin, taken for 12 days. Drainage of pus from the peritonsillar area may become necessary and is performed by surgical incision or aspiration. If abscesses recur, removal of the tonsils, or tonsillectomy, may be required.

Permanent teeth

The natural teeth that develop and emerge from the gums (see GUM) after the PRIMARY TEETH (or baby teeth) have fallen out. Each permanent tooth emerges individually in the space that is left when a primary tooth falls out, with the exception of the permanent molars, which erupt in the expanding area at the back of the growing jaw. There are 32 permanent teeth; each set of 16 includes four incisors (biting teeth) at the front; two canines (tearing teeth); four premolars; and six molars (grinding teeth) at the back of the mouth.

There are wide variations in the size of a person's teeth and jaws. Normally, the permanent teeth are larger and less white than the primary teeth, but the color, shape, position, and arrangement of the permanent teeth, as well as the BITE, may vary significantly from one person to another.

The appearance of permanent teeth begins at about age 6 years and is completed at the age of 23 years. Lower teeth usually appear sooner than the upper teeth, and appearance of the teeth in some people may vary by several years from the standard schedule.

The central incisors (top and bottom front teeth) are usually the first to appear, typically between the ages of 6 and 8 years. Lateral incisors (teeth to the sides of the front teeth) tend to emerge when a child is between 7 and 9 years old. Usually, the next teeth to appear are the canines, or cuspids (the eye teeth on the upper jaw and their opposing teeth on the lower jaw) between the ages of 9 and 12 years. The first bicuspids (teeth that normally have two peaks and are located next to the eye teeth on the upper jaw and the opposing teeth on

> Terms in small capital letters— for example, PHYSICAL THERAPY or PAGET DISEASE—indicate a cross-reference to another entry with more information.

P

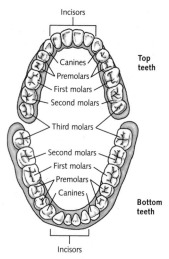

EMERGENCE OF PERMANENT TEETH
The permanent teeth appear in approximately the same order as the primary (or baby) teeth. The permanent teeth include three pairs of molars not present among the primary teeth. Often the four back molars (or wisdom teeth) do not emerge until a person is in his or her 20s. Sometimes some of the back molars never fully emerge.

the lower jaw) usually appear between 10 and 12 years of age. The second bicuspids (teeth next to the first bicuspids) tend to also emerge between the ages of 10 and 12 years. The first molars, also called the 6-year molars, are the most forward of the back teeth and may appear when a child is 6 or 7 years old. The second molars, called the 12-year molars, usually appear in back of the first molars between the ages of 11 and 13 years. The third molars, or the wisdom teeth (see WISDOM TOOTH), are the last teeth at the back of the jaw, and they tend to emerge when a person is 17 to 23 years old. There may not be sufficient room at the back of the jaw for these last four molars to erupt, and they may become impacted in the gum. A dentist or oral surgeon may need to remove any impacted teeth.

Permethrin
A lotion used externally to treat head lice and scabies infections. Permethrin (Acticin, Elimite, Nix) is available as a 1 percent lotion that acts by destroying lice and their eggs. In a 5 percent cream formulation, permethrin is used to kill the mites that cause scabies. It should not be used in infants.

Pernicious anemia
See ANEMIA, PERNICIOUS.

Pernio
Redness and swelling of the skin caused by overexposure to the cold; also known as chilblains. Pernio occurs chiefly on the hands, feet, and ears. Symptoms include blistering, burning, itching, and ulceration. Treatment is with protection from the cold and gentle warming. Smoking should be avoided because it constricts the blood vessels. Occasionally, medications are prescribed to expand the blood vessels and increase blood flow to the skin. See COLD INJURY.

Peroneal muscular atrophy
A group of inherited neuromuscular diseases characterized by wasting of the extremities, particularly the peroneal muscle groups of the lower legs. People with peroneal muscular atrophy are sometimes said to have "stork legs." See CHARCOT-MARIE-TOOTH DISEASE.

Personality
The consistent lifelong patterns of thought, action, emotion, and attitude that originate within an individual and are expressed in a wide variety of settings and situations. Personality accounts for individual differences in reactions to the same situation—for example, when two people are confronted by a mugger, one fights and the other flees.

The scientific study of personality investigates the characteristics that all humans share, the types of differences distinguishing individuals, and the patterns unique to some individuals. A number of theories have been advanced to explain personality. According to the psychoanalytic approach (see FREUDIAN THEORY), a person's unconscious mind is responsible for differences in personality. The trait approach holds that everyone lies somewhere along a continuum of various characteristics, such as aggression, talkativeness, shyness, and so forth. Personalities consist of individual deviations from the norm. In the biological approach, personality arises from inherited physiological predispositions from one's parents. The key to personality lies in the physical structure and chemical

processes of the brain determined by genetics. The humanistic theory identifies personal responsibility and feelings of self-acceptance as key to the development of personality. Behavioral-social learning theorists argue that personality is acquired as a habit produced by exposure to certain kinds of situations. Thus, talkative people become talkative because they have learned that their ease with words benefits them in social settings. In the cognitive approach, differences in the ways people process information accounts for differences in their personalities. People with a pessimistic personality, for example, interpret events negatively, while optimistic people see the same events positively.

Personality disorders
A group of mental illnesses that is characterized by persistent, inflexible, and dysfunctional patterns of thought, action, emotion, and attitude that cause significant distress in social roles, job performance, family relationships, and other key areas of day-to-day living. Individuals with a personality disorder differ markedly from the cultural norm in the ways they think, feel, relate to others, and control emotional impulses. This pattern begins in adolescence or early adulthood and holds true over time for a wide variety of personal and social situations.

TYPES
■ *Antisocial* People with this personality disorder have a complete disregard for the rights of others. Also known as sociopaths or psychopaths, they fail to conform to the law, engage in violence, and are often subject to arrest or imprisonment for their behavior. They manipulate or deceive others to gain money, power, or sexual pleasure; make decisions on the spur of the moment; exhibit a reckless disregard for their own safety and that of others; are consistently irresponsible; and show little remorse for the consequences of their actions.
■ *Avoidant* Social discomfort, fear of criticism, and timidity are the principal features of the disorder. People with avoidant personality disorder often stay away from interpersonal contact at work or in school because they fear criticism, disapproval, or

rejection. They commonly refuse to make new friends, have difficulty talking about themselves, and refrain from sharing intimate feelings because of a lack of self-esteem and feelings of inadequacy. They believe themselves to be socially inept, unappealing, or inferior.

■ *Borderline* The key features of this personality disorder are unstable personal relationships, shifting self-image, and impulsive behavior. Relationships are intense but unstable, reflecting sudden changes in how the individual perceives the other. The same sudden changes arise in self-perception; people with borderline personality disorder may change vocational plans, sexual identity, values, and types of friends almost on the spur of the moment. They take impulsive, dangerous risks such as driving recklessly, engaging in unsafe sex, or abusing alcohol or drugs. Suicide threats or attempts are common. A person with this disorder often feels empty inside, cannot control anger, and experiences periods of extreme mood, such as heightened anxiety or irritability.

■ *Dependent* People with this personality disorder have such an excessive need for others to take care of them that they submit and cling out of a pervasive fear of abandonment. They have great difficulty making everyday decisions and will allow others to tell them what they are to wear or which job to hold. Individuals with this disorder find it difficult to express disagreement with others for fear of losing the relationship. They often find it impossible to act independently, and they may make extreme self-sacrifices or submit to physical or sexual abuse to preserve the relationship with the person they depend on. Since they feel uncomfortable and helpless when alone, individuals with dependent personality disorder immediately seek out a new relationship if the former one ends. Even when the relationship is ongoing, they are often preoccupied with unrealistic, excessive fears of being left to care for themselves and feel utterly inadequate to do so.

■ *Histrionic* Extreme yet superficial emotions are the key feature of histrionic personality disorder. People with this disorder want to be the center of attention at all times, are often seductive or sexually provocative, and use physical appearance to draw attention to themselves. Their emotional expression is shallow and changes rapidly, and they talk in a manner that is full of emotional opinion yet short on detail. Histrionics are easily influenced by the opinions of others; they follow fads, play hunches, and often consider relationships more intimate than they are. Histrionics often have difficulty achieving emotional intimacy in sexual or romantic relationships.

■ *Narcissistic* This personality disorder is characterized by self-centeredness, grandiosity, a need for admiration, and a lack of empathy. People who are narcissistic have a grandiosely inflated sense of their own importance and engage in fantasies of unlimited success, power, or beauty. They consider themselves superior and expect others to recognize them as such, demand excessive admiration, take advantage of or exploit others, and lack concern for the feelings or concerns of people around them. Often envious or believing themselves the objects of envy, narcissists behave in ways that are snobbish, arrogant, or patronizing. They are hypersensitive to criticism. The disorder is named after Narcissus, a figure from classical mythology, who fell in love with his own image reflected in a pool of water.

■ *Obsessive-compulsive* The principal characteristic of this personality disorder is preoccupation with orderliness, perfectionism, and control of others, even when it undercuts efficiency, flexibility, and openness. Obsessive-compulsive individuals attempt to maintain control through extreme attention to details, rules, and procedures, sometimes to such an extent that projects are never finished. They are excessively devoted to work and often avoid leisure activities or friendships. Inflexibility about morals, ethics, and rules of the game often characterizes obsessive-compulsive people. They may be unable to discard old worn-out or worthless possessions, such as newspapers or junk mail, and are often stingy, stubbornly rigid, and reluctant to delegate to others.

■ *Paranoid* A person with this mental illness exhibits extreme, pervasive, and unwarranted distrust of other people's actions and motivations. Individuals suffering from paranoia assume that others want to deceive, harm, or exploit them, even in the absence of supporting evidence. They are preoccupied with doubts about the loyalty of friends, often pathologically jealous, and likely to assume that their spouse is unfaithful. People with paranoia are reluctant to confide in others or reveal personal information out of fear it will be used against them. They bear grudges and are unwilling to forgive injuries or insults, even minor ones, responding instead with extreme hostility. They often feel that their character has been attacked and attack in return, sometimes by filing lawsuits. Because paranoid individuals trust no one, they have an excessive need to be autonomous and self-sufficient. They often engage in grandiose fantasies, lack a sense of humor, are attuned to power and rank, and have negative opinions of racial and ethnic groups other than their own.

■ *Passive-aggressive* People with this personality disorder resent responsibility and express their resentment through forgetfulness, inefficiency, complaining, blaming others, procrastination, sullenness, and other behaviors rather than expressing how they feel. Passive-aggressive people scorn authority and resent helpful suggestions from others while being superficially compliant.

■ *Schizoid* The key feature of this personality disorder is detachment from social relationships and restricted emotions in social settings. People with the disorder avoid intimacy, lack interest in close relationships, and have little or no stake in being part of a family or a social group. They prefer being alone rather than spending time with others. Schizoid individuals experience reduced pleasure from physical or sensory experience, such as shared sexuality. They show few if any emotions and rarely reciprocate gestures like smiles or nods of the head.

■ *Schizotypal* Characterized by discomfort with, and reduced capacity for, close relationships, this personality disorder also involves eccentric or

P

superstitious ways of thinking and behaving. A person with this disorder is often highly suspicious of others, dresses in peculiar ways, and avoids social conventions, like making eye contact during conversation.

CAUSES, COURSE, AND TREATMENT
The causes of personality disorders remain unclear; most likely, several factors contribute to the development of these diseases. An inherited predisposition is likely since some personality disorders run in families. Psychological history may also have a role. Many individuals with borderline personality disorder, for example, were subjected to physical or sexual abuse or neglect during childhood, or they experienced the loss of a parent in their early years.

Personality disorders usually begin in adolescence and peak in early adulthood. In some cases, symptoms become less pronounced or troubling in middle age.

Treatment varies with the disorder. Counseling can help some individuals to understand their personality patterns and make efforts to improve them. Individuals with personality disorders often suffer from other mental illnesses, such as depression or anxiety, which can be treated with medication. Mood-stabilizing drugs such as lithium, carbamazepine, and antidepressants may be used when distressing symptoms such as anxiety or depression develop.

Personality tests

Pencil-and-paper tests used to determine the patterns of emotions, behaviors, and attitudes that make up a person's personality. Most personality tests ask the person taking the test a wide range of questions about their behavior, beliefs, and feelings. The typical inventory consists of a series of statements and asks the test-taker whether each statement holds true for himself or herself. A psychiatrist, psychologist, or mental health worker can draw conclusions about the person's personality from the responses.

The most widely used personality test is the Minnesota Multiphasic Personality Inventory (MMPI), which has been in use in various versions since 1945. The traditional MMPI contains more than 500 statements about personal functioning, mood,

morale, religious and sexual attitudes, social behavior, and symptoms of mental illness, such as hallucinations (hearing voices or seeing visions) or extreme fears (phobias). The person being tested answers each statement with "true," "false," or "cannot say." Statements in the test make up 10 scales such as masculinity and femininity, symptoms of mental illness, and shyness. A person's results are scored on the 10 scales from high to low, and the results are presented graphically. The MMPI is a valuable clinical tool, but alone it gives an incomplete picture of a person's emotional makeup. In addition, cultural differences can complicate the scoring. A response that could be considered normal in one culture, such as belief in possession by spirits, may be a sign of mental illness in another.

Other personality tests focus not on the whole personality but only on particular aspects of it, such as emotions, social skills, ways of thinking, learning difficulties, and sources of pleasure. Much research is being done to improve the usefulness of personality tests.

Perspiration

Secretion of fluid by the sweat glands to remove waste and cool the body; also called sweat. Perspiration is secreted by tiny tubular glands found throughout the skin and the tissue beneath it. Sweat is discharged through tiny openings in the surface of the skin, both to remove waste products, such as urea and ammonia, and to cool the body as the sweat evaporates. The characteristic odor of perspiration, or sweat, comes from the waste products being excreted.

Perthes disease

See OSTEOCHONDROSIS.

Pertussis

A serious bacterial infection of the lining of the breathing passages, particularly in the windpipe area. Pertussis, also called whooping cough, is extremely contagious. Symptoms of the infection include prolonged, violent, coughing spasms that often cause thick mucus and severe inhaling difficulties. The labored inhalation, or breathing in, of air causes the person to make a

high-pitched, crowing, or whooping sound. Pertussis can be fatal, but in the United States, widespread vaccination against the infection has made the disease rare.

Pertussis is usually caused by *Bordetella pertussis* bacteria and spread by infected respiratory droplets from the coughs and sneezes of people who have the infection. Infants younger than 1 year are most susceptible and have the most severe symptoms, but teenagers and adults may also contract milder cases of pertussis that are often mistaken for bronchitis. There is a danger that people with less severe, undiagnosed cases may spread the infection to infants who have not yet been immunized.

SYMPTOMS, DIAGNOSIS, AND TREATMENT
Symptoms of pertussis may begin within 3 to 12 days of exposure to an infected person. Initial symptoms can last as long as 2 weeks and mimic the common cold with nasal congestion, runny nose, sneezing, mild fever, and watery eyes. Following a 2-week course of illness, pertussis begins as a dry, hacking cough that progresses to prolonged coughing spasms. During these spasms, the tongue may protrude, the eyes may bulge, and the face may become discolored. Mucus may be produced, and vomiting may occur. Coughing spasms are often followed by noisy, whooping inhalations. Infants younger than 3 months and adults may not experience this characteristic sound when inhaling.

A history of symptoms and physical examination leads to a diagnosis, which may be confirmed by detecting the bacteria in cultures or smears of secretions from the nose and upper throat. Treatment is based on antibiotic therapy, which may also be prescribed to other members of an infected person's household to prevent the spread of infection. The infected person should be isolated for 5 days after antibiotic therapy has been started, and exposure to infants should be strictly avoided. Infants younger than 3 months who have pertussis are hospitalized; infants between 3 and 6 months may also need to be hospitalized.

Respiratory complications can be severe in infants and may include suffocation (asphyxiation.) Seizures can occur in infants who have pertussis. Middle ear inflammation, called OTITIS MEDIA, may occur. A form of pneumonia is a potentially fatal complication in an infected person of any age. EMPHYSEMA, cerebral hemorrhage, and encephalitis can occur.

Pervasive developmental disorders

A group of related mental illnesses affecting children and characterized by severely impaired social and communication skills or by repetitive, stereotypical interests or activities. These disorders are often associated with some degree of mental retardation. One pervasive developmental disorder is AUTISM, which severely limits communication and interaction with others and restricts the person's behavior and interest. Autistic children have little or no ability to communicate nonverbally (for example, with body language or facial expressions), make few if any friends, may fail to develop spoken language, are often preoccupied with movement (for example, the turning blades of a fan), and may move their bodies in strange, repetitive ways (for example, flicking the fingers or rocking the whole body for hours on end).

RETT SYNDROME is characterized by impairments that develop after a period of normal development as a newborn. Beginning at approximately 5 months, growth of the child's head slows and acquired skills in using the hands are gradually lost. Over the next few years, the child loses interest in social settings, develops few language skills, and has trouble with walking and moving the body.

In childhood disintegrative disorder, the child develops normally, then slips backward in language, social skills, toilet training, play, or motor skills between the ages of 2 and 10. Children with this disorder are similar to autistic children in their lack of nonverbal communication and their interest in repetitive movement.

ASPERGER DISORDER involves impaired social skills and interest in stereotypical repetitive movement similar to autism, but language, intellectual ability, self-help, and curiosity develop normally.

Pessary

A prosthesis placed in the vagina to support the uterus, cervix, or hernias of the pelvic floor. Pessaries are made of rubber or plastic, often with a metal band or spring frame, and come in several different shapes, including doughnut and cube. Their purposes are to tighten up the pelvic floor and to hold a prolapsed uterus, one that has dropped lower than normal, in place. Pessaries have existed for many years and were more widely used before surgery for uterine prolapse was as safe and available as it is now.

The pessary has several uses besides the support of a prolapsed uterus. It can be used by pregnant women to avert miscarriages due to structural problems in the uterus or an INCOMPETENT CERVIX, in which the cervical opening is too weak. A pessary can be used to relieve URINARY RETENTION or pain in midpregnancy, when it is caused by pressure from the uterus on the bladder. Pessaries are also used in nonpregnant women to treat conditions such as CYSTOCELE or RECTOCELE. Pessaries are sometimes used to aid conception when the cervix is displaced. Pessaries are fitted and inserted by a doctor and must be removed for cleaning every 1 to 2 weeks.

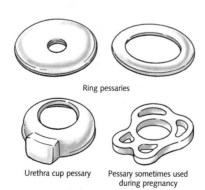

Ring pessaries

Urethra cup pessary   Pessary sometimes used during pregnancy

TYPES OF PESSARIES
Different types of pessaries are designed to provide varying levels of support as necessary. The ring pessary, which comes in a number of sizes, directly supports the uterus. The more sturdy urethra cup pessary combines the ring with a cup that is placed beneath the urethra. A less common model has extensions that branch out from the ring to provide extra support during pregnancy.

Pesticide poisoning

A chemical injury caused by exposure to substances intended to kill insects or vermin. Pesticide poisoning can occur in people who handle or are otherwise exposed to the chemicals used to kill insects. Exposure to pesticides can involve the skin, particularly of those who handle the chemicals while applying them to target areas; people may be exposed to pesticides by breathing the fumes; and exposure can occur when people smoke, eat, or drink around pesticides or do not wash their hands after using pesticides. Hands and forearms are most vulnerable to exposure, but the eyes, abdomen, and groin absorb pesticides most quickly.

Exposure to pesticides can be prevented by wearing unlined rubber gloves; waterproof clothing may be needed if the pesticide is sprayed. The greatest risk of exposure occurs when mixing concentrated chemicals, at which time a rubber apron should be worn.

Acute pesticide poisoning may involve flulike symptoms or a nervous system disorder. Chronic exposure to small amounts of pesticides over long periods may involve many parts of the body, although concerns that pesticides may cause cancer or birth defects have not been proved through research studies.

PET scanning

Positron emission tomography scanning; a scanning technique that combines NUCLEAR MEDICINE and chemical analysis to enable physicians to observe the function of certain organs of the body. At present, PET scanning is used more for research than for diagnostic purposes, but its clinical usefulness is growing. PET scans can be helpful for determining the stage of certain cancers and for evaluating Alzheimer's disease and other neurological diseases such as Parkinson disease and seizures. The procedure can detect mild, early changes in the brain before nerve damage, memory loss, or other symptoms occur. It may provide new information for research on medications for the treatment of Alzheimer's disease. It is used to evaluate heart function after a heart attack. It also helps to assess the effectiveness of certain drugs.

P

PET scanning works by introducing a special type of radioactive tracer, which includes a positron-emitting radioisotope, into molecules normally found in the body such as molecules of glucose or water. After injection of a radioactive compound, cross-sectional images are taken by a special camera to demonstrate how an organ or tissue is metabolizing the injected substance. This can be useful for identifying certain tumors and diseases that cannot be detected by CT SCANNING (computed tomography scanning) or MRI (magnetic resonance imaging).

Petechiae

Pinpoint, round, red spots in the skin caused by bleeding in the skin; a single spot is a petechia. Petechiae can be a sign of various blood diseases, such as LEUKEMIA, immune thrombocytopenic purpura, and MYELOPROLIFERATIVE DISORDERS.

Petit mal

An older term for an ABSENCE SEIZURE. See also SEIZURE.

Peutz-Jeghers syndrome

A rare inherited disease characterized by multiple benign polyps in the stomach, small bowel, and colon and by excessive freckling or spots on the skin. People with Peutz-Jeghers syndrome (PJS) develop dozens to thousands of polyps in their stomachs and small intestines. Spots on the skin are common diagnostic signs in childhood, and they are most likely to develop on the inner lining of the mouth, the gums, the lips, around the eyes and mouth, and on the fingers, toes, and genitals. The spots can vary from blue or blue-black to dark brown. In adulthood, the spots on the skin usually disappear, and gastrointestinal symptoms develop, including bleeding and pain from polyps.

PJS is usually diagnosed by endoscopy and microscopic examination of removed polyps. Treatment usually includes surgical removal of large polyps and part of the bowel. Although most polyps are benign, there is a risk that PJS may develop into colon cancer.

Peyronie disease

Severe curvature of the erect penis. A minor bend is normal and not a sign of disease. The curvature of Peyronie disease is pronounced; in severe cases, the penis can form a slight hook or corkscrew shape that makes sexual intercourse impossible. Peyronie disease is uncommon, affecting only about 2 percent of middle-aged and older men. The disease is caused by a scar or plaque, forming in the spongy tissue that fills with blood when the penis becomes erect. Because the plaque fails to stretch as the surrounding tissue expands during erection, the penis bends or curves. Peyronie disease begins as a small bump under the skin on the shaft of the penis. As the area grows in size, the bend or curve in the penis worsens. Some men with the disease report pain

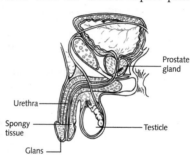

Healthy reproductive organs

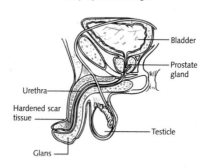

Penis with Peyronie disease

CURVED PENIS
In a healthy penis, spongy tissue fills the entire shaft and head. During an erection, this tissue fills with blood. In a man with Peyronie disease, plaque or scar tissue forms in this spongy tissue. As blood surges into the penis during an erection, the rigid tissue does not expand as the rest of the tissue does, and the penis curves. Sometimes the tissue beyond the curvature does not expand at all. The condition may be painful or make intercourse impossible.

during erections. Often, the portion of the penis beyond the scar tissue remains soft during erection. Occasionally, affected men cannot have intercourse because of the angle of the penis. There is no clear cause as to why the plaque forms. Some physicians believe that it results from injury to the penis during sex, but there is no conclusive evidence that this is the case.

In approximately half of the cases, Peyronie disease clears up on its own, usually within a year. If the disease lingers, medication can be prescribed for pain. Some physicians recommend vitamin E because it promotes healing and prevents scarring. Anti-inflammatory drugs may also be prescribed. In severe cases, surgery may be needed. In the simplest procedure, a stitch is sewn on the underside of the penis at the point of greatest curve. This tightens the penis and compensates for the curve, but it shortens the organ slightly. In more complex procedures, the plaque can be cut and then patched with a piece of vein. Sometimes, the plaque is cut away and tissue is grafted into its place. Both these procedures carry some risk of a change in sensation or of erectile dysfunction from injury to the penis. In the most extreme cases, the scar tissue can be removed completely, and surgery can be performed (PENILE IMPLANT) to allow erections.

pH

A measure of the degree to which a solution is either an ACID or an ALKALI. The pH measures the extent of hydrogen ion (H^+) concentration in a substance: the more acidic a substance is, the greater the concentration of hydrogen ions and the lower the pH. A pH of 7 is neutral; a pH of less than 7 indicates acidity; and a pH of more than 7 indicates alkalinity. The pH is used in medicine to measure the body's ACID-BASE BALANCE.

Phagocyte

A white blood cell that attacks foreign substances, such as microorganisms that have entered the body. Phagocytes are able to engulf and digest antigens (see ANTIGEN), and some may also be able to transfer antigens to the T LYMPHOCYTES, the white blood cells called T cells. This is an essential component of the body's IMMUNITY. The phagocytes are essential to regulating immune responses and developing the inflammatory response. They produce and distribute a wide variety of powerful chemicals, including enzymes, complement proteins, and regulatory factors. They also carry receptors that enable them to be activated to attack specific microorganisms and tumor cells.

The two major forms of phagocytes are monocytes and macrophages. The monocytes are present in the bloodstream and migrate into the body's tissues where they develop into macrophages. Macrophages are specialized cells that conform to characteristics of the tissues they inhabit. This may include the tissues of the lungs, the kidneys, the brain, and the liver. Macrophages are versatile and fulfill several roles. They are able to rid the body of worn-out cells and other debris, but their most important function is digesting and processing antigens, then giving them over to the T cells. This is essential to initiating the IMMUNE RESPONSE.

Phantom limb pain

A sensation of discomfort at the site of a missing limb. Pain in a phantom limb is a common phenomenon after an amputation (see AMPUTATION, SURGICAL). The majority of amputations in the United States take place as a result of circulation problems caused by diabetes (see DIABETES MELLITUS, TYPE 1; DIABETES MELLITUS, TYPE 2). Phantom pain usually begins within 24 hours following amputation. In some people, the pain is persistent and severe. Treatment is difficult. However, helpful measures include prosthetics that fit well, early rehabilitation, and addressing the emotional aspects of amputation.

Pharmacokinetics

The study of drug levels in the body over a period of time. Pharmacokinetics addresses several topics, including a drug's metabolism, the duration of its action, the time required for it to be absorbed, and how it is distributed throughout the body and then excreted or eliminated.

As a general rule, an oral drug dissolves quickly in the stomach and passes into the intestines. It is then absorbed into the blood by the blood vessels lining the intestines. Pharmacokinetics is concerned with the precise characteristics of this process, as applied to a particular drug.

Pharmacology

The study and science of drugs; the characteristics of a drug that make it medically effective. Pharmacology includes the study of the discovery, chemistry, effects, uses, and manufacture of drugs.

Pharyngitis

See SORE THROAT.

Pharyngoesophageal diverticulum

An abnormal pouch of tissue where the pharynx (the lower part of the throat) joins the esophagus (the muscular tube that connects the throat to the stomach). Diagnosis is usually made by an upper gastrointestinal (GI) series (an X-ray procedure).

When it does not cause symptoms, pharyngoesophageal diverticulum may not require treatment. However, because food can become trapped in the diverticulum and be inhaled, causing choking, doctors often recommend surgery to correct the problem. See also ESOPHAGEAL DIVERTICULUM; ZENKER DIVERTICULUM.

Pharynx

The passageway that connects the nose and mouth with the trachea (leading to the lungs) and the esophagus (leading to the stomach). The pharynx, also called the throat, is lined with mucous membrane. There are three areas of the pharynx. The NASOPHARYNX leads from the soft palate at the back of the mouth to the nasal cavity, a passage for air only. The oropharynx lies behind the nasopharynx and behind the base of the tongue; both air and food pass through it. The laryngopharynx is the lowest portion that connects with the esophagus, a passage for food only. Besides routing food and air into the body, the pharynx helps to protect against invading microorganisms and foreign matter. The adenoids in the upper pharynx and the tonsils in the lower pharynx contain lymphatic tissue and are part of the

IMMUNE SYSTEM. The pharynx also has a role in speaking (see SPEECH MECHANISM).

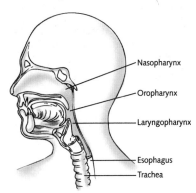

PASSAGE TO THE THROAT
The pharynx, the cavity between the back of the mouth and the esophagus, has three parts: the upper nasopharynx, between the nose and mouth; the oropharynx, behind the mouth; and the laryngopharynx, leading to the esophagus. The parts of the pharynx participate in breathing and swallowing.

Pharynx, cancer of

See THROAT CANCER.

Phenazopyridine

A drug that relieves pain caused by urinary infections. Phenazopyridine (Prodium, Pyridium, Urobiotic, and others) is used to relieve the pain, burning, and discomfort associated with infection or irritation of the urinary tract. It works by temporarily anesthetizing the urinary tract and relieving symptoms. Phenazopyridine is not an antibiotic and, thus, does not kill the bacteria.

Phenobarbital

An anticonvulsant drug; a sedative (see ANTICONVULSANTS; SEDATIVES). Phenobarbital (Barbilixir, Solfoton) is one of the BARBITURATES that is used to treat seizures associated with epilepsy. It works by suppressing the spread of seizure activity in the brain. Phenobarbital can also be used as a sedative because it acts throughout the central nervous system as a depressant.

Phenotype

The entire physical, biochemical, and physiological makeup of an individual, determined both genetically and environmentally. The phenotype is the physical manifestation resulting

P

from a specific genotype. A genetic trait can express itself in a range of phenotypes. For example, the gene for neurofibromatosis (an inherited disease of the skin and nerves) can result in a phenotype with multiple fibrous tumors or one with virtually none.

Phentermine

An appetite suppressant drug. Phentermine (Adipex-P, Fastin, and others) is used in the short-term treatment of obesity to reduce appetite. The appetite-suppressing effect of phentermine lasts only a few weeks and so is used temporarily while the person learns new ways to eat healthy food and to exercise. Phentermine is related to amphetamines and is a CONTROLLED SUBSTANCE.

Phenylalanine

An amino acid required for the normal growth and development of infants and children. Because it acts as an essential building block of protein, phenylalanine is also necessary for normal protein metabolism throughout life. This amino acid is also important to nitrogen balance. Good dietary sources of phenylalanine include meats, eggs, grains, and dairy products.

An excess accumulation of phenylalanine in the blood of infants is a sign of a serious enzyme deficiency and a condition known as PKU (phenylketonuria). An inherited disorder, PKU is treated by regulating the amount of phenylalanine in the diet. Left untreated, it can lead to mental retardation and other problems.

Phenylketonuria

See PKU.

Phenylpropanolamine

A drug used both as a nasal decongestant and an appetite suppressant. Phenylpropanolamine is marketed under many brand names, some of which were formerly available without prescription. As a nasal decongestant, it works by narrowing or constricting the blood vessels. As an appetite suppressant, phenypropanolamine works by stimulating the central nervous system, though only for a few weeks. Phenylpropanolamine has been associated with increased blood pressure and other serious side effects. At the recommendation of the Food and Drug Administration (FDA), phenylpropanolamine is no longer included in over-the-counter drugs.

Although phenylpropanolamine has been available in nonprescription products in the United States for many years, a recent study reported that taking phenylpropanolamine increases the risk of hemorrhagic stroke (bleeding into the brain or into tissue surrounding the brain) in women. Men may also be at risk. Although the risk of hemorrhagic stroke is very low, the FDA recommends that consumers not use products that contain phenylpropanolamine.

Phenytoin sodium

An anticonvulsant drug. Phenytoin sodium (Dilantin) is used to treat seizures associated with epilepsy and to prevent seizures during neurosurgery. Phenytoin sodium acts on the central nervous system to reduce the number and severity of seizures.

Pheochromocytoma

A tumor of the adrenal gland that causes the release of excessive amounts of the two medullary adrenal hormones EPINEPHRINE and NOREPINEPHRINE. One or more pheochromocytomas may develop, usually in the adrenal medulla (the inner layer of the adrenal glands). Pheochromocytomas may also develop outside the adrenal glands, usually in the abdomen. They occur with equal frequency in men and women and are more common in young adulthood to midlife. Only about 10 percent of all pheochromocytomas are malignant (cancerous).

SYMPTOMS

Symptoms may be frequent and sporadic and can increase in severity and duration over time. Headache and excessive perspiration are the most common symptoms. Blood pressure may be elevated or may fluctuate dramatically between highs and lows. Usually there is weight loss and weakness. Trembling, anxiety, and feelings of dread are sometimes experienced. There may be vision problems and shortness of breath. Some pheochromocytomas do not cause symptoms.

DIAGNOSIS AND TREATMENT

Pheochromocytomas may be difficult to diagnose because their symptoms mimic the symptoms of other conditions, including high blood pressure, psychological disorders, and heart disease. Diagnosis depends on the results of tests that detect excessive amounts of adrenal hormone or of breakdown products in blood or urine.

Once a biochemical diagnosis has been established, CT SCANNING (computed tomography scanning) or MRI (magnetic resonance imaging) may be used to locate the tumors. Scintigraphic scanning, which uses a radioactive substance that concentrates in the adrenal glands, can then make an image. Scintigraphic scanning is especially useful for diagnosing pheochromocytomas that are not located in the adrenal glands or that may be cancerous.

The majority of these tumors can be removed through surgery. Surgery to remove pheochromocytomas is considered a high-risk operation requiring complex monitoring procedures. Medication to control blood pressure may be necessary before surgery; postoperative disturbances in blood pressure may also require medication.

Pheromone

A substance secreted by the bodies of animals, including humans, which identifies them to members of the same species. Pheromones are often detected by smell. Specific instinctive behaviors, such as mating and aggression, are involved in the response to pheromones.

Phimosis

An abnormal condition in which the foreskin is too tight to be pulled back over the head (glans) of the penis. The condition can occur in adolescents and adults who fail to clean under the foreskin, which causes an infection called BALANITIS with swelling, tenderness, and discharge. The foreskin bulges during urination, and the urine stream is narrow and slow. In extreme cases, urination is blocked, and the backup of urine can cause kidney damage, called HYDRONEPHROSIS. If there is an infection, phimosis can be treated with antibiotics and corrected permanently by removing the foreskin surgically. See CIRCUMCISION, MALE.

Phlebitis

See THROMBOPHLEBITIS.

Phlebotomy

The act of using a syringe to collect a blood specimen through an incision or needle puncture. A phlebotomy may be performed to obtain a sample of blood for analysis, to remove blood for donation (see BLOOD DONATION), or as a treatment for blood disorders such as HEMOCHROMATOSIS (an inherited disorder that interferes with iron metabolism).

Phlegm

Thickened excess mucus that may accumulate in the throat or chest when the nose, sinus, and bronchi are inflamed, as occurs when a person has a common cold. Phlegm may also develop in response to exposure to chemicals, pollution, cigarette smoke, or the presence of a more severe infection. It can also occur with chronic bronchitis. The excess mucus can accumulate in the lungs and clog the smaller airways, called bronchial tubes, making breathing difficult and contributing to infections in the respiratory tract.

Phobia

A persistent, irrational, exaggerated, and involuntary fear of a specific object, place, activity, or situation. The fear results in an overwhelming desire to avoid the object, place, activity, or situation. In some cases, contact with the focus of the fear can prompt the severe anxiety reaction known as a PANIC ATTACK. Phobia is a form of an anxiety disorder. It is considered a mental illness requiring treatment only if it severely restricts or interferes with a person's life.

Simple phobias have a specific focus. Examples are fear of heights (acrophobia), snakes, spiders, closed spaces (claustrophobia), knives, and lightning and thunder. Social phobias include fears of meeting new people and of being embarrassed, humiliated, or ridiculed in front of others. Agoraphobia involves a fear of being trapped in physical settings, particularly crowded public spaces like churches or sports stadiums, where help is out of reach should a panic attack occur. Agoraphobia is often a feature of PANIC DISORDER.

Since a phobia is an extreme anxiety reaction, medications that control anxiety can help alleviate the symptoms of phobia. Antidepressants are useful in some cases as well. Behavior therapy techniques are also effective. Relaxation training can help individuals with a phobia limit physical symptoms such as increased heart rate, raised blood pressure, and shaking. Systematic desensitization (called exposure therapy) repeatedly exposes the person to the object of fear, either in imagination or in reality, until the fear diminishes. Often behavior therapy is combined with cognitive therapy, which teaches the person to recognize and change the mistaken beliefs that lead to the fear reaction.

Phocomelia

A pattern of congenital limb deformities producing severely shortened or missing arms and legs, resulting in the hands and feet forming close to the body's torso. Phocomelia can also cause an absence of the thumb and adjoining bone in the lower arm and similar abnormalities in the legs. Phocomelia is derived from the Greek words for "seal limbs." Phocomelia sometimes is related to other diseases or factors. In the past, the pattern was caused by the drug thalidomide, prescribed to treat a pregnant woman's morning sickness during the late 1950s and early 1960s. Thalidomide is currently unavailable for general use in the United States. A federal regulatory program called the System for Thalidomide Education and Prescribing Safety (STEPS) limits the prescription, dispensing, and use of the medication.

Phonological disorder

Formerly called developmental articulation disorder, this illness is characterized by a failure to articulate appropriate speech sounds for a person's age and dialect, which interferes with his or her communication. Speech onset may be delayed in young children. Lisping and misarticulation are common, along with errors of word or sound selection. Mild cases often improve without treatment, which consists of speech therapy.

Phosphates

Salts of phosphoric acid widely distributed in the body. Phosphates are particularly found in the bones and teeth. Inorganic phosphates are important in the maintenance of the ACID-BASE BALANCE in body fluids, including blood, saliva, and urine. Organic phosphates are involved in chemical reactions that provide the energy used in muscle contraction. Phosphates are also constantly being excreted in urine and feces and must be replaced in the diet by eating phosphate-rich foods, such as cereals, dairy products, eggs, and meat.

Phospholipids

A group of fatty substances that constitute an important component of the membranes that surround body cells.

Phosphorus

An essential mineral present in every cell of the body. Most of the phosphorus in the body (about 85 percent) is found in bones and teeth, and its main function is in their formation. Phosphorus also has a role in the breakdown of carbohydrates and fats, as well as in the synthesis of protein for growth, maintenance, and repair of cells and tissues. Phosphorus works with B vitamins and assists in muscle contraction, kidney function, nerve conduction, and heartbeat regulation.

Phosphorus is found in protein, principally in meat and milk. If a person's diet is adequate in calcium and protein, it is also adequate in phosphorus. Although phosphorus is present in whole-grain breads and cereals, it is found there in the form of phytin, which combines with calcium to form a salt that is unavailable for use by the body. Because phosphorus is so widely available in the food supply, there is no known deficiency.

Photocoagulation

A surgical technique that uses a laser to condense protein in the eye. Photocoagulation is used to reattach a detached retina (the thin layer of light-sensitive tissue at the back of the eye; see RETINAL DETACHMENT), seal or destroy abnormal blood vessels in the retina (see MACULAR DEGENERATION), or destroy EYE TUMORS.

P

Photophobia

Abnormal sensitivity to, and intolerance of, light. A small number of people have otherwise normal eyes that are very sensitive to light. In addition, photophobia can be a symptom of a variety of diseases and conditions, such as excessive wear of contact lenses, eye injury or infection, inflammation, migraine headache, meningitis (inflammation of the brain covering), and reaction to certain medications. Photophobia should be evaluated by a medical professional if it is unexplained, persistent, or accompanied by blurry vision or red eyes.

Photorefractive keratectomy

A laser-surgery operation on the clear surface (cornea) of the EYE to correct nearsightedness, farsightedness, or astigmatism; also known as PRK. PRK uses a kind of laser that vaporizes the outer layer of the cornea and reshapes it, thereby correcting the eye's focusing error. The procedure is performed with the person awake and the eye numbed with anesthetic drops. Unlike LASIK (laser in-situ keratomileusis), in which the laser removes tissue under a hinged flap cut in the surface of the cornea, PRK removes tissue from the corneal surface itself, which then regrows over the reshaped area. Because this regrowth requires a longer recovery period, PRK has largely been replaced by LASIK in recent years. PRK is also associated with more pain than LASIK.

PRK corrects nearsightedness, farsightedness, and astigmatism; most people who undergo the procedure no longer need glasses, or they require a weaker prescription. Side effects or complications can result from the procedure. These include undercorrection or overcorrection, difficulty with night vision, halos around lights, glare, and loss of best corrected vision (the person may see worse—even with glasses—after PRK than before).

Photosensitivity

Heightened sensitivity to the sun. Photosensitivity may occur as a result of disease, medications, or chemical components of the skin. After only brief exposure to both ultraviolet A (UVA) and ultraviolet B (UVB) light, the skin can become red, itchy, blistered, and swollen. UVA light from artificial sources, such as sun lamps or tanning beds, causes the same type of reaction.

Anyone, even dark-skinned people and those who tan easily, can develop a photosensitive reaction. Conditions that lead to photosensitivity include systemic lupus erythematosus, xeroderma pigmentosum, and a number of metabolic disorders. Photosensitizing medications include quinolone antibiotics, sulfonamides, tetracyclines, thiazide diuretics, tretinoin, tricyclic antidepressants, and some medications used to treat cancer, diabetes, and high blood pressure. In addition, many over-the-counter products, including perfumed soaps and sunscreens containing PARA-AMINOBENZOIC ACID, can lead to this type of photoreaction.

Degrees of photosensitivity vary. A photosensitizing medication may cause a mild reaction one time and a severe reaction the next. In addition, reactions vary from person to person. Diagnosis is made according to the appearance of the skin and a careful medical history. The doctor will want to know about any chemical exposure that has taken place and all drugs a person is taking. Goals of treatment are to identify and treat any underlying disorder and eliminate exposure to possible photosensitizing chemicals or medications. Photosensitive reactions are treated like sunburn. Home care includes cool baths or showers and over-the-counter analgesics. In severe cases, doctors can prescribe stronger medications.

Sometimes nonphotosensitizing drugs are prescribed to prevent photoreactions, but precautions must be taken. Doctors recommend avoiding exposure to the sun between the hours of 10 AM and 4 PM (when rays are at their most intense). The person should apply a broad-spectrum sunblock before going outdoors and wear a broad-brimmed hat, sunglasses, and protective clothing that covers most of the body.

Phototherapy

The treatment of disorders with the use of light. Phototherapy uses primarily ultraviolet A (UVA) and ultraviolet B (UVB) light to treat skin problems such as DERMATITIS, PSORIASIS, and VITILIGO. In photochemotherapy, phototherapy is used in combination with topical or systemic medications. Although phototherapy is often effective, in many cases long-term treatment is associated with an increased risk of skin cancer and premature skin aging.

TREATING SKIN DISORDERS

Phototherapy uses UVA and UVB light waves to treat certain skin disorders that are widespread or fail to respond to other treatments. People with psoriasis, vitiligo, or dermatitis typically benefit from three to five weekly phototherapy treatments for a month or more. Treatment continues until symptoms such as scaly, itchy, red plaques (patches of thick raised skin) are under control.

In some cases, phototherapy may involve the drug PUVA (psoralen plus UVA). Psoralen is a photosensitizing agent that maximizes the effect of ultraviolet light on the skin. Long-term treatment with PUVA is associated with an increased risk of skin cancer.

RISK FACTORS

Long-term exposure to ultraviolet light is known to increase the risks of skin cancer and premature skin aging. Consequently, long-term or high-dose treatment with many forms of phototherapy poses the same health risks. As a result, the potential benefits must be carefully weighed against the potential risks of treatment.

When other treatments fail and phototherapy is clearly required, doctors use the minimum possible exposure and monitor the skin closely.

JAUNDICE IN NEWBORNS

Phototherapy is an effective treatment for bringing down high bilirubin levels. Jaundice in newborns is usually due to HYPERBILIRUBINEMIA (elevated levels of bilirubin). Bilirubin, a by-product of the breakdown of red blood cells, is normally processed by the liver and eliminated in the urine. However, some newborns (especially those born prematurely) have more bilirubin in their bloodstreams than their immature livers can process. This is a potentially serious condition because high bilirubin levels are associated with problems such as mental retardation, cerebral palsy, delayed or abnormal motor development, deafness, problems with perception, and behavioral disorders. In the hospital, newborns are carefully exposed to blue fluorescent light, which accelerates the elimination of bilirubin.

Physiatrist

A physician who specializes in the field of PHYSICAL MEDICINE AND REHABILITATION. Physiatrists focus on restoring function in people who experience acute or chronic pain or who have musculoskeletal or neurological disorders. They treat a range of problems, from back pain to carpal tunnel syndrome to quadriplegia. In addition to 4 years of medical school, a physiatrist must successfully complete 4 years of residency training.

Physiatry

See PHYSICAL MEDICINE AND REHABILITATION.

Physical examination

See EXAMINATION, PHYSICAL.

Physical medicine and rehabilitation

Also known as physiatry, the field of medicine that focuses on restoring function in people with various musculoskeletal and neurological disorders. Physiatrists treat acute and chronic pain resulting from a wide range of problems, from back pain to carpal tunnel syndrome to quadriplegia. They may coordinate the long-

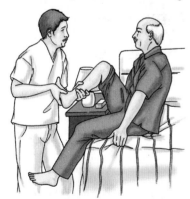

RESTORING FUNCTION
A specialist in physical medicine, or rehabilitation, coordinates efforts to help a person return to the highest possible level of function—physical, psychological, social, and occupational—after illness or disease. Often, he or she uses exercise, light, heat, or water instead of or in addition to medication.

term rehabilitation process of people who have experienced strokes, broken hips, or spinal cord injuries. In addition to graduating from medical school, a physiatrist must successfully complete 4 years of residency training.

Physical therapy

Specialized treatment for a person who has a disability, disease, or injury with the goal of achieving and maintaining functional rehabilitation or preventing malfunction or deformity. Physical therapy includes the evaluation, maintenance, and improvement of the functions of the body's various structures and systems, as well as the prevention of disability. Treatments by physical therapists are designed to complete or hasten convalescence, to increase comfort and well-being in the person being treated, and to minimize residual physical disability.

Physical therapy is achieved through the coordination and consultation of other health care professionals. A doctor may prescribe physical therapy to a person who has an orthopedic, neurological, vascular, or respiratory condition resulting from congenital disorders, an inherited dysfunction, or a disability caused by trauma or disease. The therapy is generally carried out under medical supervision.

Physical therapy services may be offered by a hospital, an industrial health program, a nursing home, or a clinic specializing in rehabilitation, sports medicine, pediatrics, or gerontology. Schools for handicapped children, as well as federal, state, and local health agencies, may offer physical therapy. The services are sometimes offered in private practice.

Physical therapy involves testing as well as treatment procedures and guidance in therapeutic exercise. The diagnostic tests may include muscle testing, electrical testing, perceptual and sensory testing, and measurements of the joints' range of motion. Functional activity tests evaluate a person's ability to carry out the everyday tasks required for self-care. Treatment procedures may include heat treatments using water, melted paraffin, or ultrasound devices that generate heat internally and the application of electric current to generate heat in body tissues.

Therapeutic exercise is a cornerstone of physical therapy and is used to increase strength and endurance, improve the coordination and functional movement that allow a person to engage in the activities of everyday life, and increase and maintain range of motion in joints. People who must use crutches, canes, walkers, braces, and artificial limbs are given gait training practice to improve their ability to walk comfortably with these devices. Physical therapy may also offer services such as massage, bandaging, strapping, and the fitting, application, and removal of splints and casts. People who receive physical therapy and their relatives may be instructed in exercise techniques to be practiced at home and in the use of orthotic devices for bracing injured areas.

Practitioners of physical therapy are called physical therapists. Physical therapists may be accredited by completing a bachelor's degree program, a certificate program, or a master's degree program. A practitioner with a bachelor's degree has completed a 4-year college course that includes clinical instruction and experience in providing physical therapy to patients. The certificate program is offered to college graduates who must complete a 12- to 16-month course of academic and clinical study in the fields of basic physical science, the health sciences, the clinical sciences, and the clinical arts. Physical therapists practice and their patients receive care in hospitals, nursing homes, doctors' offices, and clinics. Most US states and Puerto Rico require physical therapists to be licensed or registered in order to practice physical therapy.

Physician

A person licensed to practice medicine; a doctor of medicine. Physicians must successfully complete a rigorous course of instruction and training, including 4 years of graduate medical education. After graduating from medical school, all states require that a physician complete a residency in order to become eligible for licensure. Doctors who specialize in various fields (such as pediatrics, family medicine, or dermatology) receive additional postdoctoral residency training.

Physiology

The branch of biology dealing with the functions and vital processes of the human body.

Phytochemicals

A broad group of chemicals found in plants that is thought to provide considerable health benefits. There are hundreds of phytochemicals, such as flavonoids, isoflavones, indoles and other phenols, and protease inhibitors. Scientists are investigating the role these chemicals may have in the prevention and control of cancer, heart disease, and other diseases. Research suggests that phytochemicals may prevent cancer and slow its growth.

Flavonoids, chemicals that interfere with the reactions that promote cancer, are found in onions, apples, blueberries, and green tea. These chemicals function as antioxidants and help stop cells from mutating and becoming cancerous.

Isoflavones, like flavonoids, are a type of phenol that acts as an antioxidant with weak hormonelike activity. Laboratory tests have shown that an isoflavone in soybeans controls to some extent the growth of cancer cells. In Asia, where the soybean is a dietary staple, rates of breast and prostate cancer are much lower than in the United States. Many researchers believe that a high soy intake contributes significantly to the low risk of heart disease in Asia. Studies show that when soy protein replaces animal protein in the diet, the blood cholesterol level is lowered.

Many other phytochemicals may also have valuable roles in preventing and controlling cancer. Acids found in plant foods such as carrots and berries inhibit the formation of nitrosamines, chemical compounds that may have a role in cancer cell formation. Garlic and other members of the allium family (such as onions and leeks) contain allyl sulfides that appear to increase the production of cancer-fighting enzymes. Studies have indicated a link between garlic consumption and a reduced rate of colon cancer. Cruciferous vegetables such as broccoli and cabbage contain indoles that affect the way the body metabolizes estrogen, a hormone with a metabolism that has been associated with breast cancer.

INCORPORATING PHYTOCHEMICALS INTO THE DIET

Fruits and vegetables such as soybeans, garlic, onions, carrots, tomatoes, cruciferous vegetables, citrus fruits, berries, celery, barley, hot peppers, and green tea are rich sources of phytochemicals. Doctors recommend eating plenty of fruits, vegetables, legumes, and whole grains as the best way of including phytochemicals in the diet. Although many phytochemical supplements are sold, phytochemicals, like vitamins and minerals, can be toxic in large amounts. In addition, isolating one chemical from a nutritious plant food such as soy or broccoli is unlikely to provide the same health benefits as eating the whole food. Dietary supplements are subject to little regulation and vary widely in quality, dose of active ingredients, and composition.

Pica

An eating disorder in which there is an abnormal craving to consume substances that are inorganic, such as chalk, clay, paint chips, plaster, dirt, or coal. Pica is most common in children younger than age 6 who are hyperactive or who have behavior disorders. It typically develops in those living in poverty or without adequate emotional or intellectual stimulation; pica has been associated with AUTISM. Counseling can help change the behavior. Although most children outgrow pica, it can continue into adulthood.

Pick disease

A type of irreversible DEMENTIA in older people characterized by frontal lobe degeneration in the brain and the presence of distinctive Pick cells. Dementia is a brain disorder that eventually causes a progressive decline in memory and other intellectual functions. Symptoms of Pick disease include impaired speech, an inability to name objects, loss of insight, apathy, impulsiveness, dietary changes, and lack of inhibitions. As in ALZHEIMER'S DISEASE, over time people who have Pick disease grow unable to perform the usual activities of daily living. Eventually they become incapacitated. Pick disease differs from Alzheimer's disease in that the early stages of Pick disease have little effect on memory but are characterized by prominent personality changes and diminished executive function (coordinating the more complicated tasks of daily living, such as managing financial affairs).

PID

See PELVIC INFLAMMATORY DISEASE.

Pigeon toes

See INTOEING.

Pigmentation

Coloration of the skin, hair, and eyes with the pigment MELANIN. Melanin acts as a sunscreen, offering protection from the negative effects of ultraviolet light. The amount of pigment in the skin determines susceptibility to sun damage and skin cancer. Dark skin contains more pigment, which provides some protection from the sun. Pigmentation can be affected by many factors, including heredity, hormones, injury, and exposure to heat or radiation. The result may be hyperpigmentation (an increase in pigment production) or hypopigmentation (a decrease in pigment production). Pigment changes can be temporary or permanent.

Skin conditions characterized by altered pigmentation include freckles, melasma, pityriasis alba, suntans, tinea versicolor, and vitiligo. In most cases, skin changes are cosmetic and do not affect general health. Treatments for severe pigment disorders include bleaching creams, topical corticosteroids, and phototherapy (treatment with light).

Pill, birth control
See CONTRACEPTION, HORMONAL METHODS.

Pilocarpine
A cholinergic drug (Salagen) used to treat dryness of the mouth and throat caused by a decrease in the amount of saliva that can occur following radiation therapy for cancer of the head and neck. Pilocarpine, a drug that stimulates nerve fibers, can help people who have had radiation therapy speak without having to sip liquids, suck on hard candies, or chew sugarless gum. As eye drops, pilocarpine is used to treat glaucoma.

Pilonidal sinus
A hairy bump in the cleft of the buttocks in tissue near the tailbone; also known as a pilonidal cyst. A pilonidal sinus can become infected and form a painful abscess (pus-filled sac). Treatment is with antibiotics and, as necessary, either surgical incision and drainage or surgical excision (cutting out the cyst).

Pimple
A type of inflamed pustule (a small pus-filled blister) that is usually red at its base. A pimple may burst and form a yellow crust. Pimples are a common feature of skin conditions such as ACNE and IMPETIGO.

Pinched nerve
The compression or "trapping" of a nerve. A trapped nerve causes numbness, tingling, weakness, and pain in the area supplied by the nerve. A damaged nerve takes time to heal, causing symptoms to persist. In severe cases, surgery may be required. CARPAL TUNNEL SYNDROME is one of the most common examples of a trapped nerve. In this syndrome, numbness, tingling, and pain in the wrist and hand are caused by compression of the median nerve as it

passes between the bones and a ligament at the front of the wrist. Carpal tunnel syndrome is usually a REPETITIVE STRAIN INJURY. A pinched nerve is also caused by a lumbar disk pressing against the nerve following a back injury. See NERVE ENTRAPMENT.

Pineal gland
A small, hormone-producing organ located near the base of the brain. The pineal gland secretes MELATONIN, which has a role in daily biological cycles that are involved in sleep and mood. The secretion of the hormone varies during a 24-hour period and is heaviest at night. The gland also signals the onset of menstruation in girls and is involved in the menstrual cycle.

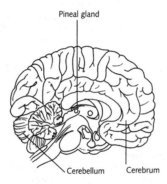

HORMONAL CLOCK
The tiny pineal gland, which secretes hormones that are involved in daily cyclical behavior, is located at the base of the brain.

Pinguecula
A soft, yellowish, noncancerous growth on the membrane covering the eye (conjunctiva). A pinguecula usually appears on the nasal side of the surface of the eye and is usually not painful. The growth is common among adults, particularly older people, and normally does not increase in size. The cause is uncertain, but sunlight exposure and eye irritation may have a role. In most cases treatment is unnecessary. A pinguecula can be removed surgically if it is cosmetically displeasing; if, as rarely happens, a pinguecula grows over the cornea, it is referred to as a PTERYGIUM.

Pinkeye
See CONJUNCTIVITIS.

Pinna
The portion of the ear that projects from the head; the external ear.

Pins and needles sensation
An abnormal prickling feeling in the skin. A pins and needles sensation may occur when a person's hand or foot "falls asleep." However, persistent pins and needles or TINGLING is a sign of damage or irritation to nerves or of poor circulation in the affected area. Possible causes of pins and needles include nerve injury, lack of blood supply, diabetes mellitus, thyroid problems, vitamin B12 (cyanocobalamin) deficiency, carpal tunnel syndrome, transient ischemic attack, stroke, and multiple sclerosis.

Pinworm infestation
An infection caused by the parasitic roundworm Enterobius vermicularis, which lays its eggs in the human intestines. Pinworm infestation is common in temperate zones and usually affects children between the ages of 2 and 12. The pinworm's eggs hatch and mature into adult worms in the intestines. Female adults usually travel at night to the area surrounding the anus (called the perianal area) and deposit their eggs there. The larvae inside the eggs develop within 6 hours. They remain alive and are usually infective for the following 7 to 10 days, but may remain infective for up to 20 days.

The infection is transmitted by the transfer of the eggs, which may be present on the hands or under the fingernails of an infected person or on clothing, bath towels, or bed linens. Self-infection can occur by the transfer of infective eggs to the mouth via fingers that have come in contact with the perianal area. After infective eggs have been ingested, the larvae hatch in the small intestine and the mature roundworms establish themselves in the colon.

Pinworm infestation frequently does not cause any symptoms, or there may be itching in the anal region, usually at night when the female roundworms migrate to that area. Other symptoms may include loss of appetite, irritability, and abdominal pain. Abrasions caused by scratching the area may lead to secondary bacterial infections. In

P

women, the infestation may sometimes invade the genital tract, producing vaginitis and scar tissue.

Pinworm infestation is diagnosed by the microscopic identification of eggs collected in the perianal area. The collection must take place first thing in the morning, before a person washes or has a bowel movement. Transparent, adhesive cellophane tape is pressed against the perianal skin, and then the tape is placed on a slide and examined under a microscope. This is called the "Scotch-tape test" or the cellulose-tape slide test. Anal swabs may also be used. Less frequently, the eggs may also be detected in samples of stool or urine or in vaginal smears.

Medications, including MEBENDA-ZOLE or albendazole, are generally used to treat pinworm infestations, but they cannot be taken by a woman during her pregnancy. Another medication, pyrantel pamoate (or pyrantel emboate), may be recommended for a woman who is pregnant and has a pinworm infestation. The infestation may require retreatment in 2 weeks. Measures to prevent reinfesta-

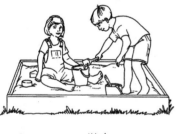

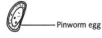

¼ inch

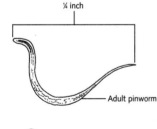

Adult pinworm

Pinworm egg

AN INTESTINAL PARASITE
Children pass pinworm eggs to each other by direct contact—sharing toys or using the same toilet seat. Pinworms lay eggs around a child's anus. The child passes the eggs on by scratching or touching the anus and releasing the eggs into the air, onto an object, or back into his or her own mouth. Adult pinworms are ¼ to ½ inch long; the eggs are tiny.

tion include strict personal hygiene, regular laundering of all bedding and underwear, examination of all family members and playmates of an infected child, and treatment when necessary.

Piroxicam

A nonsteroidal anti-inflammatory drug (NSAID). Piroxicam (Feldene) is one of a group of drugs used to relieve some symptoms caused by rheumatoid arthritis, osteoarthritis, and other conditions, including swelling, inflammation, stiffness, and joint pain.

Pituitary gland

A small, two-lobed gland at the base of the brain that secretes hormones that stimulate other glands throughout the body to produce hormones; a major part of the ENDOCRINE SYSTEM. The pituitary gland is itself directed by the HYPOTHALAMUS (a region of the brain close to the pituitary). Blood vessels and nerves connect the hypothalamus and the pituitary and coordinate their activities through both hormones and nerve signals. This connection helps ensure that the central nervous system and the endocrine system are working in coordination.

The secretions of the front lobe of the pituitary control hormone production by other endocrine glands, stimulate growth, and affect sexual maturity. Hormones released by the rear lobe help maintain blood pressure, initiate labor at the end of pregnancy, and cause the milk glands in the breast to release milk for breast-feeding.

The pituitary produces somatotropin, a growth hormone that stimulates bone and muscle development; ACTH (adrenocorticotropic hormone), which stimulates hormone production by the adrenal glands and affects metabolism; and TSH (thyroid-stimulating hormone), which causes the thyroid to secrete hormones that also influence body metabolism. The pituitary also produces FSH (follicle-stimulating hormone) and LH (luteinizing hormone), which regulate the function of male and female sex organs. The pituitary secretes a hormone that controls the darkening of the skin by stimulating pigment cells. Another pituitary hormone increases reabsorption of water into the blood-

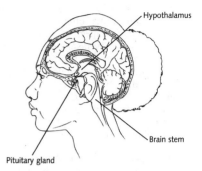

Hypothalamus

Brain stem

Pituitary gland

HORMONAL PROCESSES
To direct involuntary body processes hormonally, hormones from the hypothalamus pass into the pituitary gland, which in turn releases hormones directed at organs throughout the body. Feedback mechanisms among the hypothalamus, pituitary, and target organs maintain appropriate hormone levels.

stream by the kidneys and decreases urine production. Oxytocin stimulates contractions of the uterus during labor and the release of milk during breast-feeding.

Pituitary tumors

Abnormal growths that arise in the pea-sized PITUITARY GLAND located at the base of the brain. The pituitary gland is an endocrine gland that produces many hormones that regulate and control the activity of other glands in the endocrine system. Most pituitary tumors are not malignant. However, they can enlarge and damage nearby tissue.

Symptoms of a pituitary tumor include headache, seizures, personality changes, visual disturbances, drooping eyelids, weakness, lethargy, irritability, cold intolerance, skin changes, loss of body hair, breast development in males, nausea, vomiting, constipation, low blood pressure, and impaired sense of smell. Some pituitary tumors secrete an excess of hormones leading to gigantism or acromegaly (growth hormone excess), hyperthyroidism, or Cushing syndrome (a hormonal disorder characterized by muscle wasting, thin skin, and weakened bones).

A pituitary tumor is diagnosed through physical examination and tests, such as CT (computed tomography) scanning of the skull, MRI (magnetic resonance imaging), angiogram, spinal tap, and endocrine function tests. Examination of a person with a larger tumor often reveals abnormal

P

eye findings. Surgical removal is indicated if the tumor is large and pressing on the optic nerves. Radiation therapy may also be recommended.

Pityriasis alba

A common asymptomatic disorder characterized by round or oval, white, scaly patches on the skin. Patches most commonly occur on the cheeks but may also occur elsewhere on the face or on the upper arms, thighs, and neck. The patches may disappear and then return. Pityriasis alba occurs most often in young children and usually resolves by early adulthood.

Pityriasis rosea

A benign (not cancerous) skin rash that usually begins with a single oval patch ("herald" patch) and then spreads. The herald patch, which may be rosy pink, salmon, or tan, commonly appears on the trunk. Within a week or two after the emergence of the herald patch, smaller, similar plaques (patches of thick, raised skin) appear more generally over the trunk. Pityriasis rosea is most common in children and young adults and affects both sexes equally. It usually disappears on its own without treatment and usually leaves no permanent marks. Treatment with ultraviolet B light, antihistamines, and hydrocortisone cream may be prescribed to relieve itching. The exact cause of pityriasis rosea is unknown, although it may be linked to a virus.

PKU

Phenylketonuria; a rare genetic disorder characterized by the inability of the body to use the essential amino acid phenylalanine because of the absence or deficiency of an enzyme, phenylalanine hydroxylase. This deficiency leads to very high phenylalanine levels in the blood and tissues. Because excessive phenylalanine is toxic to the central nervous system, PKU, or phenylketonuria, results in mental retardation and neurological problems if not treated within the first few weeks of life. When treatment is begun shortly after birth and maintained consistently, children with the disease can expect normal development and a normal life span. Because treatment of PKU

is so effective, newborn screening for PKU is usually carried out routinely.

PKU affects 1 of every 10,000 newborns in the United States. Males and females are equally affected, but blacks are far less likely to be born with PKU than either whites or Asians. Since PKU is inherited through an autosomal recessive gene, a baby must inherit that gene from both parents to be affected. The parents will be carriers who do not have the disease themselves. One in 50 individuals is a carrier.

SCREENING AND DIAGNOSIS

The PKU test is a simple blood test administered before babies leave the hospital or birthing center—at least 24 hours after delivery, but within a week after birth. The baby's heel is pricked, and a few drops of blood are taken. The blood sample is sent to a laboratory, where it will be examined for signs of elevated levels of phenylalanine. When a baby's phenylalanine level is elevated, more tests will be performed to determine if the cause is PKU or some other disorder.

Infants with PKU appear normal at birth, although they may have fairer skin and hair than other family members. Untreated PKU may be associated with early symptoms of vomiting, irritability, a rash, and urine with an earthy odor, although most infants have no symptoms until brain damage has occurred. Later symptoms include seizures, mental retardation, small head, poor development of tooth enamel, and diminished body growth.

TREATMENT

The goal of treatment of PKU is to maintain a normal blood level of phenylalanine. This requires a very special diet, one that eliminates high protein foods, since all protein contains phenylalanine. Foods to be avoided include meats, eggs, fish, poultry, cheese, milk, dried beans, peas, and most baked goods. People with PKU are able to eat some starches, fruits, and vegetables in limited quantities. A special synthetic formula for all age groups is used as a substitute for most of the protein and vitamins needed in the diet.

Periodic blood tests to monitor levels of phenylalanine are required as part of an essential medical follow-up. The guidance of a nutritionist is advisable in the care of anyone with

PKU, particularly at times of fever and illness, when normal body proteins are liable to break down, which raises the level of phenylalanine in the blood. Women who have PKU are at high risk to have children with maternal PKU disease. High levels of phenylalanine affect the developing fetus, leading to mental retardation and severe birth defects. It is important for women with PKU who are of childbearing age to seek nutritional guidance.

Placebo

A substance used in medical research that resembles a drug but has no medical action. In clinical research, some participants are given the actual drug being tested, while others are given a placebo, usually a sugar pill that has no medicinal properties but—in what is called the placebo effect—may help provide relief in people who believe they are taking an actual medication. During a clinical trial, researchers can determine scientifically whether the drug has genuine effectiveness by comparing the response to the drug and to the placebo. The experimental drug must produce better results than the placebo to be considered an effective medication.

Placenta

The organ that links the blood supplies of the mother and fetus throughout a pregnancy. The placenta develops from the chorion, the outermost layer of cells on a fertilized egg. Also called the afterbirth, the placenta measures about 8 inches by 1 inch, weighs about 1½ pounds, and is connected to the placenta by the UMBILICAL CORD. Although the blood of the fetus and the blood of the mother do not actually mix, the placenta supplies the developing fetus with oxygen and nutrients from the mother's bloodstream and carries away waste products. The placenta also supplies the fetus with protective antibodies and essential hormones.

About 3 to 5 minutes after the baby has been delivered, the uterus begins contracting again to expel the placenta. With each contraction, the uterus shrinks further, squeezing the placenta, which begins to separate from the wall of the uterus. Once it is detached, the placenta is pushed out

P

of the uterus while the doctor or mid-wife applies abdominal pressure and pulls gently on the umbilical cord. Although the contractions are strong, they are not usually painful. Most women lose about 2 cups of blood during and after delivery, most of it from the placenta and the places where it separated from the wall of the uterus.

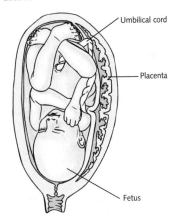

HOW A FETUS IS NOURISHED
The placenta provides vital nourishment—oxygen and nutrients—to the fetus from the mother's blood supply, and waste products from the fetus are carried away. The fetus is connected to the placenta (a separate organ) via the umbilical cord. Within the placenta, the woman's blood circulates into the tissue surrounding fetal blood vessels, and substances are exchanged at a cellular level through the walls of these vessels.

Placenta previa

In pregnancy, a placenta that has grown abnormally low in the uterus, partly or completely covering the cervix. Depending on how much of the cervix is covered by the placenta, this condition may cause problems toward the end of the pregnancy. Symptoms do not always occur, but if the placenta begins to separate from the uterus, the woman may experience sporadic, painless bleeding from the vagina, usually late in the pregnancy.

In most cases, a placenta that starts low in the uterus gradually migrates up the uterine wall as the pregnancy progresses without further complications. In severe cases, placenta previa may prevent the placenta from performing its normal function of linking the two blood supplies and may lead to severe vaginal bleeding or premature labor. If the placenta com-

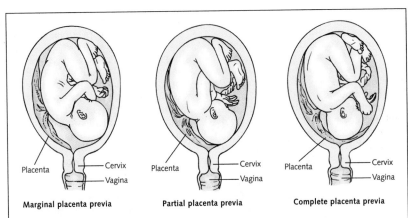

Marginal placenta previa

Partial placenta previa

Complete placenta previa

PROBLEMS WITH THE PLACENTA
In placenta previa, the placenta is attached to the uterus at the wrong place—near the bottom of the uterus instead of on the side or nearer the top. As a result, the placenta covers or nearly covers the cervix, blocking the passage into the vagina to some extent. At the time of delivery, as the cervix begins to widen, parts of the placenta may tear away and cause bleeding. If the placenta becomes entirely detached, the fetus will be without an oxygen supply and immediate delivery is necessary. If the blockage is only partial, the condition may not affect the pregnancy at all.

pletely covers the cervix, a CESAREAN SECTION will be required. Placenta previa is unusual, occurring in only one of every 200 pregnancies, and its cause is unknown. It occurs more often among women who have had five or more children and women carrying twins. Other women at risk are those older than 35 years, those who have had a previous cesarean section, and those who have had placenta previa before. Treatment usually includes bed rest to prevent excessive bleeding.

Placenta, retained

A placenta that has become trapped in the uterus after birth. A retained placenta is one that has not been pushed out of the uterus and delivered within 30 minutes of the baby's birth. Retained placentas generally have not separated entirely from the wall of the uterus. To remove the placenta, the doctor usually administers an anesthetic to the mother, reaches inside the uterus, and removes the placenta. The mother is then given a drug to encourage the uterus to contract to prevent excessive bleeding.

Placental abruption

A condition in which the placenta becomes detached from the wall of the uterus during pregnancy. This very rare condition is considered a life-threatening emergency, because it can cut off the blood circulation of the fetus. The chief symptom is sudden abdominal pain, caused when the placenta detaches from the uterus. Some women also experience nausea and vomiting. Vaginal bleeding may or may not occur, because the blood may remain trapped between the placenta and the uterus.

The cause of placental abruption is not known, although it is more common in women with a deficiency of the vitamin folic acid. It is most common among women with high blood pressure or PREECLAMPSIA or who have had many previous pregnancies. Although many times a fetus can be delivered vaginally, an emergency CESAREAN SECTION is performed when there are signs of fetal distress.

Plague

A bacterial disease that is transmitted among rodents by the bites of infected fleas. Plague may be contracted by humans when they are bitten by a flea that has acquired the infection from a rodent or when people have contact (direct handling or inhalation of tissue or fluid) with living or dead animals that have the disease. Plague is more common in animals than in humans. In the United States, plague is extremely rare.

There are three forms of plague. Bubonic plague, the most common form, may cause very painful, tender swellings called buboes in the neck, under the arm, or in the groin. Septicemic plague is a more severe form of plague that occurs when the bacteria get into the bloodstream, usually through an open sore on the skin. Pneumonic plague is the most dangerous and the least common form. It occurs when the plague bacteria infect the lungs and is highly contagious because it is transmitted to others via respiratory droplets from an infected person's coughs and sneezes. See also BUBONIC PLAGUE.

Planned Parenthood

Planned Parenthood Federation of America; a national organization founded in 1916 that provides education about reproduction and counseling and medical care for sexually active individuals. It also acts as an advocate for reproductive rights related to birth control, pregnancy, patients' rights, and sexuality and promotes research into reproductive health.

Plantar wart

A hard, rough-surfaced area on the sole of the foot that is caused by a virus. See WART.

Plants, poisonous

Plants that cause an allergic or direct chemical reaction on the skin. POISON IVY, oak, and sumac are three of the most common causes of allergic reactions from plants. Most people develop an allergic reaction or allergic CONTACT DERMATITIS when they are exposed to these plants. The cause of the resulting rash, blisters, and itch is urushiol, an oily substance in the sap of the plant that sticks to almost all surfaces and can be carried in the wind if burned in a fire.

Itching and discomfort can be relieved by applying cool compresses, soothing lotions (such as calamine lotion), and prescription topical corticosteroids, and by taking oatmeal baths and oral antihistamines. Although fluid in the blisters will not spread the rash, fingernails may carry germs that could cause an infection, so scratching should be avoided. If reaction to the plant is severe, or if the rash develops on the face or in the genital region, it is important to seek medical attention. Prescription corticosteroid drugs may be necessary. To prevent a rash and blisters from developing after contact with the plant, doctors recommend rinsing the exposed skin with cold water within 5 minutes of exposure. Washing with soap is not necessary and may spread the oil. Contaminated clothing should be laundered. Wearing long pants, long sleeves, gloves, and boots is recommended in areas where poisonous plants are likely to grow.

Plaque

Deposits of fatty substances, cholesterol, calcium, and other materials on the inner walls of an artery. Plaque formation begins when fats in the bloodstream damage the inner lining of the artery walls. Fatty materials such as cholesterol collect at the injury sites, build up, and accumulate in the artery walls, causing scar tissue to develop and calcium to accumulate. White blood cells also rush to the injury sites, where they release chemicals that make the artery lining sticky and allow further accumulation of fats. Clot-producing platelets collect over the site, trapping even more white blood cells and fat particles. As the plaque builds, it may develop a thick covering of calcium, which causes the characteristic hardening of the artery in ATHEROSCLEROSIS.

In addition, the growing plaque narrows the opening in the artery and restricts blood flow, sometimes causing blood to pool behind the restriction and ballooning the artery into an ANEURYSM. Over time, the artery may close completely, or a piece of the plaque can break free, travel through the bloodstream, and cause blood clots that can lodge in a smaller artery and block it, resulting in an EMBOLISM.

The term plaque also refers to deposits on the teeth and gums See PLAQUE, DENTAL.

Plaque, dental

A sticky deposit of bacteria, saliva, and food debris that forms on the teeth, particularly in the spaces between the teeth and gums. When plaque accumulates and hardens on the teeth, it forms calculus (see CALCULUS, DENTAL). Plaque is the primary cause of tooth decay and periodontal disease, which can lead to losing the teeth. It must be removed every day by brushing the teeth and using dental floss (see FLOSS, DENTAL) to prevent it from building up. Because plaque is colorless and odorless, it can be detected only when it is stained with DISCLOSING AGENTS. The agents temporarily stain the teeth where plaque has formed so that a person can see where the plaque needs to be removed. Good ORAL HYGIENE is the best approach to preventing the damage that plaque can cause.

Plasma

The liquid portion of the BLOOD. A straw-colored fluid, plasma represents a little over half of the body's total volume of blood. Mostly water, plasma serves as the medium that transports the blood cells. It also contains proteins (see PLASMA PROTEINS), hormones, acids, salts, nutrients, oxygen, carbon dioxide, and cellular waste products.

Plasma cells

Small round or oval cells that circulate in the bloodstream and produce antibodies to fight invading microorganisms and foreign substances. Plasma cells are also known as plasmacytes (from Greek roots meaning "plasma cells").

Plasma proteins

A protein compound occurring in plasma, the liquid component of BLOOD. There are hundreds of different types of proteins in plasma. These proteins have a number of important roles. Some are carrier proteins that bind with other substances and transport them through the blood. Coagulation proteins, also called clotting factors, help the blood clot around injuries and wounds. Antibodies and related proteins attack and destroy invading microorganisms and foreign matter. Still other proteins make up enzymes, which accelerate chemical reactions, or serve as precursors to other substances.

Plasmapheresis

A process for collecting plasma, the liquid portion of the blood. Blood is drawn, and the plasma is separated from the blood cells in a centrifuge. The cells are then returned to the donor, and the plasma is replaced with fresh frozen plasma (see TRANSFUSION). Plasmapheresis is performed to collect components from the plasma or to treat certain blood diseases.

P

Plasminogen activator

Any of a group of substances able to divide plasminogen and convert it to plasmin. Plasminogen is a substance normally present in blood plasma, and plasmin is an enzyme that digests the protein fibrin and is necessary for the dissolving of blood clots.

Tissue plasminogen activator, or TPA (also t-PA), is a naturally occurring enzyme used in thrombolytic therapy to dissolve blood clots. Because TPA acts directly on clots, it rarely causes body-wide or systemic bleeding.

Plastic surgeon

A physician who specializes in plastic surgery, the technique of repairing visible defects that result from injuries, burns, or disease. Plastic surgeons also operate on healthy people to improve their appearance or to minimize the effects of aging.

Plastic surgery

Any operation that repairs, restores, or improves parts of the body that have been lost, injured, or altered by disease or aging. The surgical specialty includes both COSMETIC SURGERY and RECONSTRUCTIVE SURGERY.

CHOOSING A PLASTIC SURGEON

To find a skilled plastic surgeon, begin by asking a trusted doctor for a recommendation and make sure the surgeon chosen is skilled in the particular procedure under consideration.

- Find a surgeon who is specially trained in reconstructive surgery and is certified by the American Board of Plastic Surgery.
- Choose a doctor who has performed the particular procedure many times—at least several times a month and no longer than 6 months ago.
- Ask if the doctor has hospital privileges, even if the surgery will be done in an office setting or as an outpatient. Doctors with operating room privileges have to meet certain medical staff requirements at the hospital that could provide the patient peace of mind in the event of an emergency.

Platelets

Blood cells that help repair injured blood vessels. Also known as thrombocytes, platelets stop the loss of BLOOD by plugging holes in blood vessels, the first step in the formation of a clot. Coagulation proteins carried in the blood complete the process. Platelets are colorless oval disks with an average life span of 9 to 14 days. Like most blood cells, they form in the bone marrow from large cells called megakaryocytes and then migrate into the blood. Similar to a red blood cell, a platelet cell does not contain a nucleus, so it cannot replicate.

Play therapy

A technique for dealing with emotional problems in children that uses play materials, such as a sandbox, toys, musical instruments, and picture books, to help children express thoughts and feelings in the presence of a therapist.

Pleura

The double-walled membrane that covers the surface of and encases the LUNG and lines the wall of the chest cavity. The space between the two layers is filled with a lubricating fluid that helps the lungs move readily and without friction as they expand and contract.

Pleural effusion

A collection of fluid between the two membrane layers, called the pleural membranes, that cover the lungs and line the chest cavity. Normally, there is a small amount of lubricating fluid between the two thin, flexible membranes. When blood or other fluids accumulate in the pleural space, the space between the two membranes, lung volume is reduced. The effusion may be caused by any of several conditions. In some cases, despite numerous tests, the cause of pleural effusion is not determined.

Blood in the pleural space is generally the result of a physical injury from trauma to the lungs. Other causes of a bloody pleural effusion include a spontaneous collapsed lung, a pulmonary embolism, tuberculosis, a ruptured aortic aneurysm that bleeds into the pleural space, and cancer. When the pleural effusion is the result of an infection, the fluid

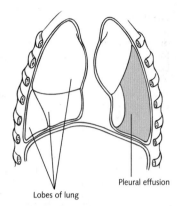

FLUID BETWEEN MEMBRANES
The outer (parietal) pleura lines the chest cavity, while the inner (visceral) pleura encases each lung, even between the individual lobes of the lungs. When fluid collects in part of the space between these two membranes, they can no longer glide smoothly over each other, restricting lung expansion.

becomes thickened into pus, and the condition is referred to as EMPYEMA. The presence of a pleural effusion containing cholesterol is rare and generally caused by long-standing, underlying disease.

Heart failure, cirrhosis, and pneumonia are among the most common causes of fluid collection in the pleural space. Malignant tumors, usually those of the lung or breast, can metastasize to the pleural membranes and produce pleural effusion. Rheumatoid disease can cause small to moderate pleural effusions, usually in older men who have had the disease for several years. Inflammation of the pancreas and cysts on the pancreas sometimes result in pleural effusion. A small number of people who are continually exposed to asbestos over a period of 5 years or more have pleural effusions; rarely, the condition occurs as a result of diseases acquired by people who have AIDS (acquired immunodeficiency syndrome).

SYMPTOMS, DIAGNOSIS, AND TREATMENT

Chest pain and breathing difficulties are the most common signs of pleural effusion. However, the condition may be asymptomatic and discovered during a physical examination or diagnostic testing. Chest X rays are considered the most accurate method for confirming the presence of pleural effusion.

CT (computed tomography) scanning may be indicated in some cases because it is helpful for evaluating underlying lung disease associated with pleural effusions. Ultrasound scanning, either alone or with THORACENTESIS, may be used to confirm the presence of pleural effusion. Thoracentesis, a procedure in which fluid is withdrawn from the pleural space, is usually performed to evaluate the various characteristics of the fluid, which provide clues to its cause. Removal of some of the pleural effusion can relieve the labored breathing caused by large pleural effusions.

If the cause of the effusion is a bacterial infection, antibiotic therapy is the first line of treatment. As the infection clears, the excess fluid is generally reabsorbed, and the condition resolves spontaneously. If there is pus in the pleural effusion (empyema), it is treated with antibiotics and chest tube drainage. Alternatively, a surgical procedure to open the chest, either thoracoscopy or THORACOTOMY, may be used to drain the pus-filled fluid. When the pleural effusion is composed of blood or pus, a procedure known as water-sealed tube drainage is performed.

Pleurisy

An inflammation of the two thin, transparent membranes, called the pleura or pleural membranes, that cover the lungs and line the chest wall. Pleurisy most commonly occurs when a virus or bacterium infects the membranes and produces inflammation. Fluid may accumulate in the space between the two membranes, producing the condition PLEURAL EFFUSION. If there is no fluid accumulation, the inflammation is termed dry pleurisy.

The primary causes of pleurisy are pneumonia, tissue death produced by a pulmonary embolism, cancer, tuberculosis, rheumatoid arthritis, and systemic lupus erythematosus. Other causes may include parasitic infection, pancreatitis, physical injury to the chest area (for example, a fractured rib), inhaled irritants (such as asbestos), and allergic reactions to certain prescription medications.

SYMPTOMS, DIAGNOSIS, AND TREATMENT

Sudden chest pain is the most common symptom of pleurisy. This may be experienced as discomfort or as severe, stabbing pain that occurs continually or only when a person breathes deeply or coughs. Pain may be localized at the site of inflammation or felt as referred pain in the abdomen or neck and shoulder area. Labored breathing may be experienced, and breaths may be rapid and shallow in an attempt to avoid the deep breathing that intensifies pain.

Pleurisy is considered relatively easy to diagnose because the chest pain is distinctive. During a physical examination with a stethoscope, a rubbing sound known as a pleural rub may be detected. A chest X ray does not reveal pleurisy but can show underlying causes of the inflammation, including rib fracture, lung disease, and pleural effusion.

Treatment is based on the cause of pleurisy. Antibiotics are prescribed to treat a bacterial infection. No treatment is required for a viral infection, and if an autoimmune disease is present, treatment of the disease will usually help resolve the pleurisy. Symptoms such as chest pain may be treated with over-the-counter acetaminophen or ibuprofen. Stronger pain-relieving narcotics, such as codeine, should be used cautiously for the pain associated with pleurisy because these pain relievers suppress coughing, and coughing can help prevent pneumonia. A person with pleurisy is advised to try to breathe deeply and cough as the condition becomes less painful. Coughing may be less painful if a pillow is held firmly against the chest during the cough.

Plexus

A tightly organized network of veins, lymphatic vessels, or nerves. For example, the brachial plexus refers to a series of closely spaced nerves that originate from the spine in the neck, travel under the collarbone, and radiate into the chest wall and arm.

Plication

A surgical procedure in which an organ is shortened by making folds or tucks in it before it is sutured in place. Plication is used to reduce the size of a hollow organ or to tighten weakened or stretched tissues, such as the neck of the urinary bladder in a person with a leaky bladder. A pli-

cation procedure called ANTIREFLUX SURGERY is used to remedy chronic severe heartburn. See FUNDOPLICATION.

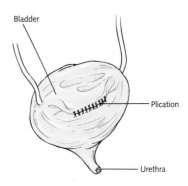

MAKING AN ORGAN SMALLER
Plication can reduce the size of any organ. For example, a plication can make a leaky bladder smaller or tighter so that it does not overextend when it fills with urine.

Plummer-Vinson syndrome

A rare syndrome characterized by dysphagia (difficulty swallowing), iron-deficiency anemia, and esophageal webs (thin mucous membranes in the upper part of the esophagus). Plummer-Vinson syndrome primarily affects women and usually occurs between ages 40 and 70. Diagnosis is made through physical examination, blood tests, esopha-goscopy (internal examination of the esophagus with a lighted viewing tube), and an upper gastrointestinal (GI) series (an X-ray procedure also called a barium swallow).

Treatment of iron deficiency is required. Sometimes, ESOPHAGEAL DILATION (widening of the esophagus) is needed to relieve dysphagia. The passageway can be enlarged with a flexible rod called a bougie or a water-filled rubber bag. A laser is used to relieve blockages and to destroy cancerous tissue if it is present. Because Plummer-Vinson syndrome is a precancerous condition, doctors recommend follow-up esophagoscopies.

PMS

See PREMENSTRUAL SYNDROME.

Pneumaturia

The passage of gas in the urine. Pneumaturia occurs because of an abnormal opening (fistula) between the bladder and the intestine caused by birth defect, injury, or disease. It can be a complication of disorders such as Crohn disease, cancer, and diverticular disease.

Pneumoconiosis

Diseases produced by the inhalation of and lung tissue reaction to naturally occurring or synthetic mineral dusts. Pneumoconiosis in coal miners is also known as black lung disease or coal worker's pneumoconiosis. This form of the disease occurs as a result of continuous inhalation of coal dust over long periods, usually 10 years or more. The coal dust accumulates around the small airways, or bronchioles, in the lungs and spreads throughout the lungs, showing up as small dots on a chest X ray. When workers are exposed to silica dust, the pneumoconiosis may progress in a few cases to a more serious disease called progressive massive pulmonary fibrosis, which scars large areas of the lungs. The tissue and blood vessels in the lungs can be destroyed by this scarring. Caplan syndrome, a rare disorder in which pneumoconiosis is associated with rheumatoid arthritis, causes large nodules of inflammation in the lungs.

SYMPTOMS, DIAGNOSIS, AND TREATMENT

There may be no symptoms, or there may be coughing and shortness of breath. If the disease becomes severe and progressive, massive pulmonary fibrosis results, coughing is intense, and shortness of breath can be disabling.

A clinical history of a person who has worked underground in a coal mine over a long period and a chest X ray that reveals the characteristic spots on the lungs are the principal elements of a diagnosis of pneumoconiosis. There is no cure for this disease. Medications that keep airways open and free of secretions, such as those used to treat chronic obstructive pulmonary disease (COPD), may offer help in breathing freely. Some people with advanced disease are treated with oral corticosteroids.

PREVENTION

Prevention is important because there is no effective treatment for pneumoconiosis. It is recommended that people who work in coal mines have chest X rays every 4 to 5 years to diagnose the disease at an early stage. If detected, pneumoconiosis can be prevented from developing into progressive, massive pulmonary fibrosis by transferring the worker to an area in which mineral or coal dust levels are low or by eliminating the exposure to coal dust entirely.

Pneumocystis pneumonia

An infection caused by a one-celled organism believed to be a fungus, called *Pneumocystis carinii*. This fungus, which is found in the environment and in the lungs of healthy humans and animals, becomes a dangerous and aggressive pathogen in people who have weakened immune systems. Pneumocystis pneumonia is the resulting disease that occurs in these people, including people who have AIDS (acquired immunodeficiency syndrome), people who are malnourished, and premature infants. The pathogenic organism invades both lungs and multiplies, obstructing the tiny sacs (called alveoli) that enable the exchange of oxygen and carbon dioxide between the bloodstream and the lungs. The vital role of the alveoli is impaired as they become thickened and enlarged.

Symptoms of this form of pneumonia include difficult and labored breathing, dry cough, and fever. A chest X ray generally reveals involvement of both lungs. Diagnosis can be confirmed by identification of the causative organism in sputum or other respiratory secretions. In some cases, a biopsy of the bronchial tubes or the lungs may be necessary to establish a diagnosis of pneumocystis pneumonia.

The disease is treated with medications, including trimethoprim-sulfamethoxazole, pentamidine, trimetrexate plus folinic acid, atovaquone, primaquine plus clindamycin, and trimethoprim plus dapsone. If untreated, the disease can progress to life-threatening respiratory troubles and even cause a collapsed lung.

Pneumonectomy

The surgical removal of a lung, usually performed as a treatment for LUNG CANCER. Pneumonectomy may also be performed when irreparable damage to a lung has occurred as a result of severe trauma to the chest, especially if the wound has caused irreversible injury to the lung's principal airway or major blood vessels.

Pneumonectomy is generally the only option when a malignant tumor is located in the central area of the lung and when a significant part of the pulmonary artery or pulmonary veins are involved. Because pneumonectomy reduces breathing capacity by half, surgeons often attempt to perform more localized surgeries, such as LOBECTOMY, on the diseased lobe of the lung if the location and extent of the cancer permit this lung-sparing approach.

Some people may be eligible for less invasive, alternative treatments that have been more recently developed. These include video-assisted laparoscopic thoracic surgery, which reduces postoperative convalescence and the length of the hospital stay.

PREPARATION

Preparation for pneumonectomy involves extensive testing of the lungs to ensure that the unaffected lung is strong enough to assume the entire breathing workload. Cardiac screening is performed to confirm that the heart is sufficiently healthy to undergo the stresses of major surgery. In people with lung cancer, blood tests and scans, including a bone scan and CT (computed tomography) scans of the head and abdomen, may be performed to determine if the cancer has metastasized, or spread, from the lungs to other areas of the body. Cigarette smoking must be stopped before the surgery can be performed, and all medications that thin the blood or prevent blood clots (including aspirin) must not be taken for about a week before the date of pneumonectomy. Food and beverages are withheld the night before surgery to reduce the risk of vomiting during the procedure.

HOW IT IS PERFORMED

Pneumonectomy is performed under general anesthesia with an intravenous tube inserted into the arm to deliver fluids and medications. A large surgical incision is made on the side of the chest in which the diseased lung is located. This incision extends from below the shoulder blade on the back, around the side of the body along the curve of the ribs,

INCISION FOR LUNG REMOVAL

For pneumonectomy, the person is positioned on the side opposite the diseased lung, and an incision is made from beneath the shoulder blade around to the front of the chest. At the level of the fifth rib, the membrane over the ribs is opened, and part of the rib may be removed to expose the lung.

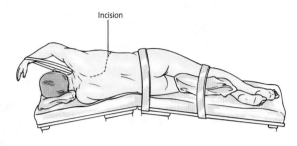

Incision

to the front of the chest. A portion of the fifth rib may need to be removed to provide the surgeon with adequate room to remove the lung.

The diseased lung is then collapsed, and its major blood vessels are tied off. The lung's main airway is clamped and cut off as near to the trachea as possible and sealed with staples or stitches to ensure that no air is leaking out. The lung is then removed, and the incision is stitched closed with sutures, leaving a temporary drain placed in the space between the two membranes covering the lungs and lining the chest.

EXTRAPLEURAL PNEUMONECTOMY

A particular form of the surgery called extrapleural pneumonectomy may be used as a treatment for certain people who have a form of cancer associated with asbestos exposure, malignant pleural MESOTHELIOMA, which is a cancer of the pleural membrane, the membrane that covers the lungs and lines the chest cavity. Extrapleural pneumonectomy involves removing the diseased lung, part of the membrane from the chest wall, portions of the lining surrounding the heart, and part of the diaphragm on the affected side. The surgeon replaces the removed tissue with a safe, synthetic material.

The surgery is followed by observation in the surgical intensive care unit (ICU) for a few days, where breathing is often assisted with a ventilator. In most cases, a person who has undergone pneumonectomy is transferred to a hospital room and remains there for about 10 days or until the sutures and drain are removed. Hospitalization and recovery for extrapleural pneumonectomy may require a few more days.

RECOVERY AND RISKS

Follow-up visits are scheduled before release from the hospital, and normal daily activities may be gradually resumed as the remaining lung slowly adjusts in compensating for the removed lung. Recovery from pneumonectomy tends to be slow, and tolerance for exercise tends to remain significantly limited by shortness of breath for up to 6 months or longer after surgery.

Survival rates following pneumonectomy depend on the underlying condition and are generally good. Temporary postoperative complications may include a prolonged need for a ventilator; heart problems, such as cardiac arrhythmia and myocardial infarction; pneumonia; infection of the surgical site; PULMONARY EMBOLISM (a blood clot in an artery in the lungs); problems with the severed airway; EMPYEMA (a collection of pus in the pleural space); accumulated fluid in the lungs; and kidney failure. The development of postpneumonectomy syndrome, in which the organs in the chest shift toward the side from which the lung was removed, is a long-term risk. This is corrected by surgically implanting a fluid-filled prosthesis in the area from which the lung was removed.

Pneumonia

FOR SYMPTOM CHART
see Coughing, page 28

A serious infection of the lungs that causes inflammation of the lung tissue. Pneumonia causes the air sacs in the lungs to fill with pus and other fluid, obstructing the flow of oxygen into the bloodstream. The depletion of oxygen in the blood interferes with normal functioning of the body's cells. If this occurs in combination with the infection's spread throughout the body, pneumonia can cause death. The use of antibiotics in the United States has greatly reduced the life-threatening potential of pneumonia.

When pneumonia affects one section or lobe of a lung, it is called lobar pneumonia. When areas throughout both lungs are affected, the disease is referred to as bronchial pneumonia, or bronchopneumonia. The term pneumonia may refer to any one of 50 different diseases that range from a mildly uncomfortable respiratory infection to a potentially fatal condition. The range in severity is due in part to the many different causes of pneumonia, which may be due to infection by one of more than 30 different pathogens. The three most common of these are bacteria, viruses, and MYCOPLASMA, a group of microorganisms that are similar to bacteria. Other causes include various chemicals and other infectious agents, such as the fungus that causes PNEUMOCYSTIS PNEUMONIA.

Pneumonia may also be caused by inhaling food, liquid, gases, foreign bodies, or dust. Bronchial obstructions, including the presence of a tumor, are not causes of pneumonia, but may promote its development. Diseases that have effects on the lungs can also lead to pneumonia; these include Rocky Mountain spotted fever, typhus, Q fever, psittacosis, and tuberculosis. Tuberculosis pneumonia is extremely serious and requires immediate medical treatment.

The way in which a person acquires pneumonia offers another set of criteria for categorizing the various forms of the general illness. When pneumonia is contracted from exposure to infected persons during the course of everyday life, it is called community-acquired pneumonia and is commonly due to pneumococci, *Mycoplasma*, or the influenza virus. The illness may also occur as the result of exposure to pathogens during a hospital stay, which may involve a wider variety of infecting agents with the potential to cause more severe infections. This category of pneumonia is called a nosocomial infection (see NOSOCOMIAL INFECTIONS), meaning it was contracted in a hospital setting. Aspiration pneumonia occurs when foreign material is breathed into the lungs, most commonly when stomach contents enter the lungs after vomiting.

P

TYPES OF PNEUMONIA

Most cases of pneumonia are caused by viral or bacterial infection, which inflames the lungs. Pneumonia can affect one or both lungs, and it can follow a common cold or flu.

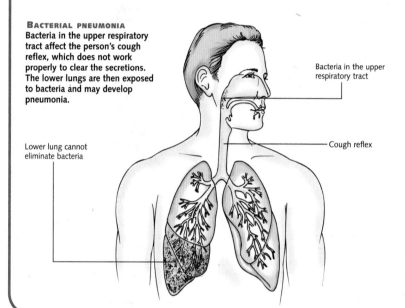

BACTERIAL PNEUMONIA
Bacteria in the upper respiratory tract affect the person's cough reflex, which does not work properly to clear the secretions. The lower lungs are then exposed to bacteria and may develop pneumonia.

Bacteria in the upper respiratory tract

Lower lung cannot eliminate bacteria

Cough reflex

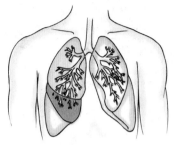

LOBAR PNEUMONIA
Lobar pneumonia affects one lobe of the lungs.

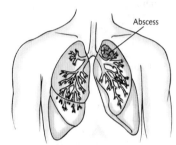

Abscess

NECROTIZING PNEUMONIA
Necrotizing pneumonia, the death of lung tissue caused by bacterial pneumonia, occurs when an inflammation of the bronchial tubes and lungs forms pus-filled abscesses in the lungs.

BACTERIAL PNEUMONIA

The bacterium *Streptococcus pneumoniae* is the most common cause of bacterial pneumonia; there is a vaccine available for some forms of the disease. While it can occur in any age group, risk factors for bacterial pneumonia include cigarette smoking, alcoholism, disabilities, respiratory diseases, viral infections, postsurgical infections, and compromised immunity (as occurs in people with AIDS [acquired immunodeficiency syndrome] or those who have had transplant surgery). The bacteria that cause this form of pneumonia may sometimes be present in the throats of healthy people. When the body's defenses against infection are diminished by factors including illness, advanced age, poor nutrition, or impaired immunity, the bacteria can multiply, invade the lungs, and produce inflammation in the alveoli, or air sacs, of the lungs.

Symptoms of bacterial pneumonia may come on suddenly or gradually. They include a fever as high as 105°F, profuse perspiration, chills, severe chest pain, and coughing that produces mucus that is green or rust-colored. Other symptoms may include an increase in pulse rate and breathing, bluish discoloration of the lips and nail beds, and confusion or delirium.

VIRAL PNEUMONIA

Viral pneumonia is rarely serious or prolonged in healthy people. It is estimated that as many as half of all cases of pneumonia are caused by viruses. Most viruses that cause respiratory infections affect the upper respiratory tract, but some affect the lungs and cause pneumonia, particularly in children. When the influenza virus attacks the lungs, the disease is severe and can be fatal; risk factors for this form of pneumonia include pre-existing heart or lung disease and pregnancy.

Symptoms of this infection are similar to those of the flu, including fever, dry cough, headache, muscle pain, and weakness. The symptoms generally escalate within 12 to 36 hours, progressing to difficulty breathing, a more severe cough with mucus, and possible bluish discoloration of the lips. Viral pneumonia can be complicated by bacterial invasion, which adds on the characteristic symptoms of bacterial pneumonia.

MYCOPLASMAL PNEUMONIA

Mycoplasma are microscopic, free-living pathogens that are neither bacteria nor viruses, but are similar to both, and can cause a mild form of pneumonia. All age groups are susceptible, with older children and young adults most commonly affected. Mycoplasma pneumonia rarely causes death, even when untreated.

The principal symptom is violent, sporadic coughing that produces a small amount of pale mucus. Fever and chills may be the first symptoms, and there may be nausea or vomiting, but rarely. Recovery may be prolonged with feelings of extreme weakness that linger.

DIAGNOSIS

When there is a suspicion of pneumonia, a physical examination by the doctor includes listening to the person's chest with a stethoscope to detect distorted breathing sounds. Bronchial and other forms of pneumonia are detected by chest X rays. Further diagnostic testing depends on the suspected pathogen causing the infection. A sample of sputum may be tested to try to identify the pathogen causing the infection. It may be necessary to insert a bronchoscopy tube into the windpipe to collect secretions for a diagnosis. Other tests can detect viral antigens in secretions and may lead to a diagnosis of viral pneumonia.

TREATMENT

Factors that promote a rapid recovery from pneumonia include youth, good health, early detection and treatment, and a well-functioning immune system. Early treatment with antibiotics generally cures bacterial infection and speeds recovery from mycoplasmal pneumonia. Antiviral medications may be used to treat certain kinds of viral pneumonia, but there is no specific treatment for this form of the disease.

The specific medication chosen to treat pneumonia is determined by the pathogen that has caused the illness and the doctor's judgment. It is important to continue medical therapy after symptoms improve and a person feels better in order to prevent recurrence. Relapses of pneumonia can be more serious than the initial episode of illness.

In severe cases, hospitalization is sometimes required. Supportive treatment for pneumonia may include bed rest, good nutrition, and giving the person oxygen to increase the supply of oxygen in the blood. Medications to relieve the discomforts of chest pain and violent coughing may be prescribed. Some people, especially younger people in good health, can expect to feel well within a week of recovery. Others may have prolonged weakness and fatigue following recovery, particularly after mycoplasmal pneumonia.

Pneumonitis

Inflammation of the lungs generally caused by hypersensitivity to inhalation of natural or chemical agents. Pneumonitis usually occurs with repeated and prolonged exposure to an irritant to which a person is sensitive, and the inflammation can persist for a few weeks to as long as many years. Diseases that produce pneumonitis include FARMER'S LUNG, BAGASSOSIS, and HUMIDIFIER LUNG.

In its acute form, the symptoms resemble those of a flulike illness with a cough. It may also take the form of recurrent PNEUMONIA or be experienced chronically with shortness of breath, a productive cough, and weight loss. These symptoms may appear within 4 to 12 hours following exposure to the causative irritant.

Pneumonitis can improve or resolve completely within a few days when the exposure causing it is promptly terminated. When exposure is continued, the inflammation may progress to PULMONARY FIBROSIS. See also DUST DISEASES; OCCUPATIONAL LUNG DISEASE.

Pneumothorax

The presence of air between the pleural membranes, the two membranes that cover the lungs and line the chest cavity. Pneumothorax occurs when air leaks from inside a lung to the space between the lung and the chest wall. The air in this space increases pressure on the lung, resulting in a collapsed lung (see LUNG, COLLAPSED). Traumatic pneumothorax is caused by something puncturing the lung. Spontaneous pneumothorax occurs when air enters the pleural space, the space between the two membranes, without previous trauma to the lungs.

Spontaneous pneumothorax is not usually associated with exertion but may worsen as a result of pressure changes, such as those that may occur during scuba diving or high-altitude flying. It can occur in healthy people or in those with extensive underlying lung disease, such as people who have emphysema, asthma, lung abscess, or cystic fibrosis.

Pneumothorax may also occur as a result of procedures in which air is used to replace fluid before thoracoscopy (a visual examination of the lung surfaces and pleural space performed with a viewing tube) or to enhance X-ray visualization of growths or structures in the chest.

Rarely, in infants, pneumothorax may result when MECONIUM is inhaled in the womb before birth or when the infant makes strenuous efforts to breathe. If oxygen is administered through a mask or tube to the baby, a hole in a baby's lung may result from excessive pressure. A small hole producing a minimal leak of air generally heals spontaneously without treatment. A larger hole requires surgical treatment.

SYMPTOMS, DIAGNOSIS, AND TREATMENT

A small pneumothorax may cause only mild discomfort. Initial symptoms are usually a sudden sharp chest pain, shortness of breath, and sometimes a nonproductive, hacking cough. Referred pain can occur in the chest or the shoulder and abdomen on the affected side. Intense shortness of breath, shock, and life-threatening conditions, such as respiratory failure and circulatory collapse, can occur when pneumothorax is more severe.

Pneumothorax may be suspected if

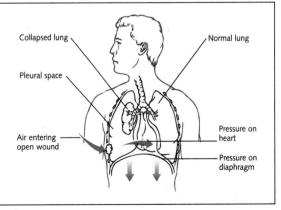

COMPRESSING THE LUNG
In a person with pneumothorax, inhaling causes air to leak (from a weakened lung or from injury) into the pleural space between the two membranes surrounding the lung. As air collects in the space, it compresses the lung and "collapses" it. Pneumothorax may also put pressure on other organs, including the heart.

Collapsed lung

Normal lung

Pleural space

Air entering open wound

Pressure on heart

Pressure on diaphragm

P

breath sounds heard through the stethoscope are diminished. When a large pneumothorax occurs, the movement of the chest wall on the affected side may be decreased and breathing sounds are significantly diminished or inaudible. Blood tests may reveal a lack of adequate oxygen supply in the blood. A chest X ray can reveal a collapsed lung and the presence of air outside structural outlines, especially if the person being examined exhales before the X ray is taken.

If a spontaneous pneumothorax is small, the air is generally reabsorbed within a few days and no treatment is needed. If the air space is larger, there is a risk of complications, including PLEURAL EFFUSION (a collection of fluid in the pleural space), and the condition is generally treated by placement of a CHEST TUBE to aspirate the air and to reexpand the collapsed lung.

In newborns, pneumothorax resulting in a collapsed lung requires immediate emergency treatment under a local anesthetic. A chest tube is inserted to draw off the air filling the chest cavity on the side in which the lung has collapsed so the lung can reexpand during inhalation. The tube is left in place, and the infant is treated and observed in an intensive care unit for several days.

If pneumothorax recurs, it can cause considerable disability and may require surgical treatment with the use of a thoracoscope (a device for viewing the membranes covering the lungs), including THORACOTOMY (surgery to open the chest wall) and pleurectomy (removal of portions of the two membranes covering the lungs and lining the chest).

Pocket, gingival

A deep opening between a tooth and the gum tissue that surrounds it. Gingival pockets are caused by the toxin-producing bacteria in plaque (see PLAQUE, DENTAL), which also contains a mix of saliva and food deposits. If plaque remains on the surface of a tooth too long, the toxins released by the bacteria in the plaque destroy the fibers that anchor the tooth to the gum. When the fibers are destroyed, an opening, or pocket, is created in the area where the tooth is normally attached to the gum. As the pockets extend deeper, they can erode the underlying bone that sur-

rounds and supports the tooth. The tooth may be loosened and eventually fall out. Gingival pockets are an indicator of PERIODONTAL DISEASE.

Podiatrist

A health care provider who specializes in the care of the feet, especially foot disorders. Podiatrists must complete 4 years of podiatry school involving rigorous instruction in general medicine with a focus on diseases and problems related to the feet. Podiatrists treat problems such as bunions, calluses, and corns. They also treat foot sores and examine feet preventively for people with diabetes mellitus.

Podiatry

The branch of medicine concerned with the care of the feet, especially foot disorders.

Poison

FOR FIRST AID

see Food poisoning, page 1322
see Poisoning, page 1327

Any substance that irritates, damages, or impairs the activity of the body's tissues. In large enough amounts, nearly any substance can act as a poison, although the term is usually reserved for substances that are harmful in relatively small quantities, such as ARSENIC and CYANIDE. Poison can be swallowed, inhaled, injected by a stinging insect, or absorbed by skin contact.

Some poisons have a specific antidote that can neutralize or counteract their effect. If a person is suspected of having come in contact with a poison, the wisest action is to call the local POISON CENTER.

Poison center

A center staffed by health professionals trained to deal with the prevention and treatment of poisonings. Most communities have a poison center whose phone number is listed on the inside cover of the community phone book. In the event of a poisoning or suspected poisoning, a telephone call to the poison center will elicit instructions from a trained health professional (usually a nurse or pharmacist) on how to handle the emergency at home. When appropriate, the poison center will also direct persons who have been poisoned to the hospital emergency room.

Poison ivy

A type of allergic CONTACT DERMATITIS that is caused by contact with an oily substance in the sap from the poison ivy plant. Poison ivy is characterized by red, intensely itchy patches of skin that soon begin to swell and blister. A rash can also develop if a person touches clothing, shoes, or a pet that has been exposed to poison ivy. In addition, smoke from the burning plants may cause a rash. See PLANTS, POISONOUS.

Poison ivy develops within 12 to 48 hours after exposure to the sap; the rash peaks after 5 days and generally disappears within 14 to 20 days without treatment. Itching and discomfort can be relieved by applying cool compresses, soothing lotions (such as calamine lotion), and prescription topical corticosteroids; taking oatmeal baths; and taking oral antihistamines. While scratching will not spread the rash, germs in fingernails can lead to infection, so scratching should be avoided. If poison ivy is severe or located on the face or in the

---

PREVENTING POISONING

Accidental poisoning is one of the leading causes of unexpected trips to the hospital emergency department. To help prevent poisoning, people should:

- Keep all medicines, chemicals, and other poisonous substances locked up.
- Never place poisonous substances in unmarked containers.
- Never store poisonous substances in juice or soda bottles.
- Never reuse containers of chemical products.
- Never store poisonous substances with food or in a refrigerator.
- Never leave discarded medicines where children or pets can reach them. It is best to pour liquids down the drain and rinse the container.
- Read the label before using any chemical product.
- Never give or take medicines in the dark.
- Never tell a child that medicine is candy or tastes like candy.

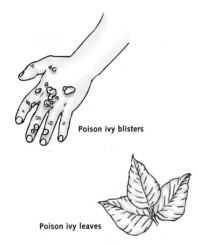

Poison ivy blisters

Poison ivy leaves

BLISTERING RASH
The skin rash and blisters from poison ivy are a reaction to a toxic substance found in all parts of the plant. The rash often appears as lines of bumps or blisters. Poison ivy leaves are bright green and glossy and grow in three-part formations.

genital region, it is important to seek medical attention. Doctors advise people who have had serious reactions in the past to see a physician as soon as possible after exposure to poison ivy. Severe cases are treated with oral cortico-steroids.

The best defense against poison ivy is learning to recognize the characteristic three-leaved plant and avoiding contact with it. Even after exposure to poison ivy, immediate action can prevent a rash from developing. Doctors recommend rinsing the exposed skin thoroughly with cold water within 5 minutes of contact. Washing with soap is not necessary and may spread the oil. Contaminated clothing should be laundered. The rash of poison ivy cannot be passed from person to person.

Poisoning, carbon monoxide

FOR FIRST AID
see Resuscitation (CPR), page 1328
see Poisoning, carbon monoxide, page 1327

Poisoning from the inhalation of carbon monoxide. Carbon monoxide, also known as CO, is a tasteless, nonirritating, odorless, colorless gas produced by the incomplete burning of any carbon-based fuel. Many cookstoves, barbecue grills, lamps, space heaters, hot water heaters, furnaces, and engines

PREVENTING CARBON MONOXIDE POISONING

Inhaling poisonous fumes can cause breathing trouble, unconsciousness, and even death. Carbon monoxide is a colorless, odorless, tasteless gas. Here are some guidelines to prevent poisonings:

- All heaters, stoves, fireplaces, and flame-burning appliances must be properly installed, operated, and ventilated.
- Ovens and gas ranges should never be used for heat.
- Gas-powered vehicles should never be operated in enclosed spaces, such as garages or basements.
- Charcoal should never be burned inside a house, tent, or recreational vehicle.
- Electronic carbon monoxide detectors should be placed on every floor in a person's home.

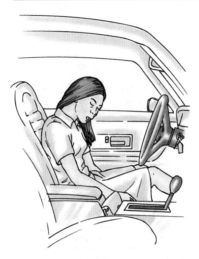

EFFECTS OF CARBON MONOXIDE
A person who sits in a closed car for a long time with the motor running could show signs of carbon monoxide poisoning, such as loss of consciousness, headache or dizziness, or respiratory difficulties.

produce carbon monoxide. The symptoms of carbon monoxide poisoning include headache, fainting, confusion, unconsciousness, chest pain, breathing difficulties, bluish color of lips and fingernails, pale skin, nausea and vomiting, low blood pressure, abnormal heartbeat, hyperactivity, seizures, coma, and shock.

When levels of carbon monoxide are too high, it will take the place of oxygen in the blood. When the concentration of carbon monoxide is very high, muscle paralysis, seizures, coma, and death can occur. If carbon monoxide poisoning is suspected, the person should be moved out into the fresh air immediately and the suspected area ventilated. Emergency medical assistance should be sought, and the local POISON CENTER should be

called. ARTIFICIAL RESPIRATION may be required.

Electronic carbon monoxide detectors can alert the homeowner or resident when an excessive amount of carbon monoxide is present.

Poisoning, chemical

FOR FIRST AID
see Poisoning, page 1327

Ingestion, inhalation, or absorption of toxic chemicals. Chemical poisoning can occur when children swallow cleaning or petroleum products, when chemicals are sniffed or "huffed" by people seeking a drug "high," or as a result of industrial accidents.

The signs of poisoning from swallowed chemicals include burns around the lips and mouth, excessive salivation, and difficulty swallowing. When cleaning or petroleum products have been swallowed, the breath could have an odor resembling the offending chemical. Signs of chemical poisoning by inhalation include choking, coughing, and headache. Signs of chemical absorption poisoning include itching and burning at the site of absorption. In all cases of chemical poisoning it is essential to follow the instructions of a poison center professional and to seek emergency medical assistance.

Poisoning, hydrogen sulfide

Excessive or prolonged exposure to hydrogen sulfide, a highly toxic gas produced naturally by decaying organic matter. Hydrogen sulfide is sometimes called "sewer gas" or "stink damp." It is a colorless, flammable, very toxic gas with a characteristic rotten egg odor. Hydrogen sulfide poisoning chiefly occurs through inhalation of the gas, although it can occur through direct contact with the liquefied gas used in certain industrial processes. The gas is naturally produced and released from sewage sludge, liquid manure, sulfur hot springs, and natural gas.

Hydrogen sulfide poisoning is rare and occurs mostly in industrial settings. The gas is absorbed rapidly by the lungs and, because it is heavier than air, can accumulate in enclosed, poorly ventilated, and low-lying areas. Even the rotten egg odor is not a reliable indicator of its presence, because people who are inhaling hydrogen sulfide may experience paralysis of the olfactory nerve (sense of smell) and so may not receive adequate warning of the presence of the gas. Low-level exposures usually produce irritation of the eyes and mucous membranes. However by paralyzing the respiratory control center in the brain stem, breathing can stop, and high-level exposures to hydrogen sulfide can be rapidly fatal. There is no proven antidote for hydrogen sulfide poisoning, and aggressive emergency treatment by specially trained rescue workers should be sought immediately.

Poisoning, mushroom

FOR FIRST AID

see Food poisoning: mushroom poisoning, page 1323

Consumption of inedible, poisonous mushrooms or "toadstools." Of the thousands of kinds of mushrooms native to North America, only about 100 are poisonous to humans. Poisonous mushrooms contain organic toxins that destroy cells in the central nervous system, kidneys, liver, blood vessels, and muscles.

The symptoms of mushroom poisoning include severe abdominal cramps, nausea, vomiting, and violent diarrhea. These symptoms usually appear 8 to 12 hours after the mushroom is eaten. If untreated, coma and death will follow in 2 to 3 days. Any suspected mushroom poisoning should be referred to a specialist at a poison center immediately.

Mushrooms growing in the wild can sometimes be tough, woody, bitter, or tasteless. While there is no simple rule for distinguishing edible and poisonous mushrooms, common edible species do have identifiable characteristics and any collecting of wild mushrooms for cooking should be limited to those species. Caps of edible mushrooms are white or slightly brownish on top, with a pink or dark brown color underneath. A plant handbook or botany book may have more information on the characteristics of edible mushrooms. When in doubt, the only safe procedure is to discard all suspect mushrooms. Commercially grown mushrooms are always edible.

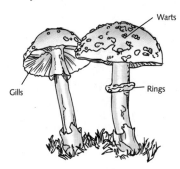

POISONOUS MUSHROOMS
The Amanita type of mushroom is poisonous, causing severe abdominal pain; diarrhea; and ultimately, fatal kidney, liver, and heart failure. Amanita mushrooms have telltale characteristics of toxic mushrooms: white gills, evident rings, and perhaps warts on the cap.

Poisoning, plant

Consumption of or contact with poisonous plants. Many plants, both cultivated and wild, are poisonous and should not be eaten, including many berries, mushrooms, flowers, flower bulbs, and leaves of otherwise edible plants, such as the leaves of tomatoes and rhubarb.

Symptoms of plant poisoning include a burning pain in the mouth and throat; swelling in the throat that may make breathing difficult; vomiting and abdominal pain; and hallucinations, seizures, and unconsciousness. Emergency assistance must be sought by calling a POISON CENTER specialist for instructions.

Some plants, including POISON IVY, poison oak, and poison sumac, produce an itchy rash and blisters in sensitive people who come in contact with the sap from bruised parts of the plant. The contact may be indirect—

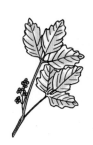
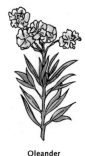

Poison oak   Oleander

POISON ON CONTACT
Poisonous American plants include poison oak, a bush or vine; and oleander, a yellow-flowering shrub. These plants contain a toxic chemical that can cause irritation on contact with the skin. The best way to prevent plant poisoning is to learn to identify common poisonous plants and avoid them.

coming in contact with an animal who came in contact with the plant, for example—or it may involve contact with sap on garden tools, clothing, and sports equipment. Some people are allergic to the pollen of poisonous plants. Symptoms include itching, burning, redness, blisters, and swelling of the skin. At the worst, the person will be uncomfortable for a while, unless exposed areas of the skin are not kept clean, in which case a secondary skin infection may occur. First aid measures that should be taken include washing the affected area with cold water and applying cortisone cream to help relieve the itching. If the reaction is severe, emergency medical assistance should be sought.

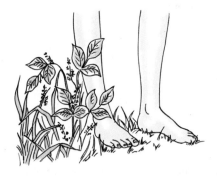

RINSING OFF TOXINS
A person who may have handled or walked through poison ivy should wash the hands or feet with cold running water as soon as possible. This may help to minimize skin irritation and avoid spreading the plant oil to other parts of the body.

Poisoning, swallowed caustics

FOR FIRST AID
see Poisoning, page 1327

Consumption of strong cleansers containing acidic or alkaline substances that cause tissue damage. Swallowed caustic poisoning, or caustic ingestion, can occur when children drink strong household cleansers containing substances such as lye. Signs of caustic ingestion include burns or swelling of the lips or tongue, drooling, and breathing problems, although many children with caustic burns show no symptoms at first. Emergency medical assistance should be sought immediately in cases of suspected swallowed caustic poisoning. Vomiting should not be forced because the esophagus could be damaged.

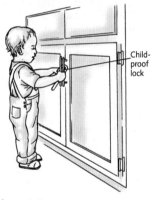

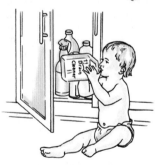

CHILD-PROOFING THE HOME
Many types of devices are available to lock cabinet doors. But it is a better idea to keep hazardous substances above the child's reach instead of in floor-level cabinets. Otherwise, a child may drink a poisonous liquid, mistakenly thinking it is juice.

Polarity therapy

A system developed in the 1920s based on a view of health as a reflection of the condition of people's so-called energy fields. Polarity therapy assumes that health is achieved when energy systems are fully functional and energy can flow smoothly within the body. When energy is unbalanced or blocked because of stress, pain, or disease, polarity therapy seeks to find ways of releasing energy and restoring normal flow patterns.

Diet, stretching exercises, YOGA, and BODYWORK are used by polarity therapists to restore energy flow. Counseling to enhance a positive attitude and increase self-awareness may also be used to treat blockages in energy flow thought to be caused by negative thoughts or emotional shock. Polarity therapy is a form of alternative medicine and has not been validated by clinical research.

Polio

An acute viral infection that can affect the nervous system and the skeletal muscles. Polio, which is a shortened term for poliomyelitis, has become a rare disease since polio immunization has become widespread in developed countries. The infection is caused by an enterovirus, called poliovirus, and occurs more commonly in infants and young children, particularly in environments in which hygiene is poor.

Polio is highly contagious, spreading via direct contact with an infected person or with their respiratory secretions or feces. An infected person is most contagious from 7 to 10 days before and after symptoms begin, but the virus can be transmitted as long as it is present in the throat and feces. Poliovirus may persist in the throat for up to 1 week and is excreted in the feces for as long as several weeks. The poliovirus enters the body through the nose or mouth and spreads into the throat and intestines where it multiplies. Ultimately, the virus spreads into the bloodstream and lymph system.

SYMPTOMS AND DIAGNOSIS

The symptoms of polio are related to the pattern of infection. In some infections, there may be no symptoms or mild symptoms that last for 72 hours or less and include mild fever, headache, malaise, reddened and sore throat, abdominal pain, and vomiting. Nonparalytic polio causes symptoms that persist for 1 to 2 weeks and may include moderate fever, headache, stiff neck, vomiting, diarrhea, fatigue, muscle tenderness and spasm, and pain or stiffness in the torso, neck, back, and extremities. Paralytic polio causes fever occurring 2 to 7 days before other symptoms, headache, stiff neck and back, general sensitivity to touch, difficult urination, constipation, difficulty swallowing and breathing, drooling, and muscle contractions or spasms, especially in the calf, neck, or back. With the paralytic pattern of infection, there is also a sudden muscle weakness in one arm or leg that progresses to paralysis in the area of the spinal cord affected.

A physical examination reveals inflexibility of the neck and back that makes it difficult to move the head forward and backward. There may be difficulty lifting the head or the legs from a lying position. Reflexes may be abnormal, and testing may reveal an abnormality in the nerve tracts originating in the brain. If the cranial nerves are affected, there may be abnormal facial expressions, choking, and difficulty with swallowing, chewing, and breathing. Some polio symptoms may mimic MENINGITIS or ENCEPHALITIS. Cultures of throat secretions, stool, or cerebrospinal fluid that reveal the presence of the poliovirus can confirm the diagnosis.

TREATMENT AND PROGNOSIS

In severe cases when paralysis affects the muscles involved in breathing and swallowing, emergency breathing assistance in a hospital may be a lifesaving measure. Symptoms are treated depending on their severity. Associated urinary tract infections are treated with antibiotics, and medications may be given to reduce retention of urine. Painkilling medications and the use of moist heat may be recommended to reduce discomforts and muscle spasms; narcotic painkillers cannot be given in most cases because they may promote breathing difficulties. When muscle function or strength are lost or impaired, treatment may include physical therapy, using braces or corrective shoes, and orthopedic surgery.

The prognosis for people who have contracted polio depends on the pattern of infection—subclinical, nonparalytic, or paralytic—and the body area that has been affected. In the

P

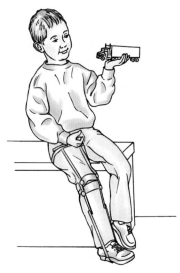

A RARE FORM OF PARALYSIS
If the poliovirus invades the brain or spinal cord, it can cause paralysis. This complication is rare, affecting only 4 percent of the people who contract the virus. A paralyzed limb will be treated with corrective devices, such as braces, or with physical therapy or surgery, depending on the nature of the damage.

great majority of cases, the spinal cord and brain are not affected, and complete recovery can be expected. In the small number of cases that involve the brain or spinal cord, disability caused by paralysis or, more rarely, death can occur. Paralysis is more common and tends to be more severe when older people contract polio.

Lifelong immunity to polio depends on the type of poliovirus a person has contracted. It is rare for a person who has been infected to acquire the disease a second time, and second infections are often caused by a different type of the virus. Postpolio syndrome is a condition that can affect people who were infected with the poliovirus many years or even decades after their initial infection. This syndrome can occur even in the absence of paralysis and may include symptoms such as diminished strength and endurance.

Poliomyelitis

See POLIO.

Pollen

An airborne, fertilizing agent that carries a plant's male genetic material to a female plant. Pollen is produced by trees, shrubs, grasses, and weeds and can be inhaled, producing the symptoms of allergies, such as HAY FEVER, and asthma. Many plants produce as many as 1 million tiny pollen particles, and as few as 20 particles per cubic yard can produce an allergic reaction. Pollens of different plants may appear identical to the naked eye, but under a microscope the differences between the pollens produced by different plants can be easily distinguished.

Some pollens consist of relatively large grains that have a waxy texture. These pollens are generally carried from plant to plant by bees and rarely produce allergic reactions. Other pollens, such as ragweed, are so light that they can be carried through the air as far as 400 miles out to sea and as high as 2 miles up into the air. For this reason, it is difficult for people who have pollen allergies to avoid pollen completely. Many pollen particles that cause allergic reactions are tiny or invisible, so they can easily enter a home through open windows, doors, and screens without being noticed.

The pollens that are most powerful at producing allergic symptoms are those of the grass family, ragweeds, and birch and oak trees. Pollination periods for the same plants differ in different regions of the country and may be affected by daily weather fluctuations, especially wind. Hot, dry winds stir up pollen, while rain washes pollen into the ground. Different plant species have different cycles. Pollen allergens from several different plants with different pollination cycles may be present year-round in some areas of the country.

In warmer climates with long growing seasons, pollen may be airborne for 8 or 9 months of the year. In more temperate zones, the presence of pollen is more predictable. In the spring, deciduous and evergreen trees produce pollen. Grasses and flowers produce pollen in early summer, usually June and July. Early autumn is when late blooming plants, such as ragweed, produce pollen.

Ragweed is the pollen that most people are susceptible to among the plants growing east of the Rocky Mountains in the United States. Sagebrush, tumbleweed, redroot pig-weed, spiny amaranth, burning bush, and English plantain are other pollen-producers that may cause allergy symptoms.

The grass varieties that produce pollen allergens include rye, timothy, redtop, Bermuda, orchard, sweet vernal, and the bluegrasses. Most species of trees produce allergenic pollens, including maple, oak, ash, birch, poplar, elm, pecan, juniper, and cottonwood.

Pollution, air

Harmful substances in the atmosphere. Air pollution causes damage to the environment and to human health and quality of life. Air pollution makes people sick by causing breathing problems, and it harms animals, plants, and the ecosystems in which they live. Air pollution has altered the atmosphere by letting in increased amounts of radiation from the sun, thereby increasing people's risk of developing skin cancer. At the same time, air pollution traps heat in the atmosphere, which leads to GLOBAL WARMING. Scientists warn that global warming caused by air pollution will eventually affect the world's food supply, the sea level, weather, and the spread of tropical disease.

The chief cause of air pollution is the burning of natural gas, coal, and oil to fuel industrial processes and motor vehicles. The burning of fuels puts CARBON DIOXIDE, carbon monoxide, nitrogen oxides, sulfur dioxide, and tiny particles of lead into the atmosphere. Nitrogen oxides from car exhaust and sulfur oxides are air pollutants that return to Earth in the form of acid rain. Decomposing garbage in landfills and other disposal sites also contributes to air pollution in the form of methane gas.

Air pollution can cause or exacerbate several diseases. Adult asthma can be worsened by increased levels of nitrogen oxides, while childhood asthma can be worsened by increased exposure to sulfur dioxide. Air pollution also predisposes people to pneumonia, congestive heart failure, ear infections, and sinusitis. Cigarette smoke can also make asthma and bronchitis worse.

Pollution, noise

Unwanted sounds intruding into daily life. Noise pollution is associated with urban development and includes noise caused by air, road, and rail transport; industrial activities; and recreational events such as loud parties or concerts. Many common sounds contribute to noise pollution, including jackhammers, jet planes, car alarms, and excessively loud music, all of which are likely to exceed 90 decibels (the measure of the intensity of sound). Repeated exposure to noise in excess of 90 decibels can cause permanent hearing loss. See ACOUSTIC TRAUMA.

Pollution, water

Contamination of streams, lakes, underground water, bays, and oceans by substances harmful to living things. Water pollution is particularly dangerous for living things, all of which require water to survive, either because their bodies contain it or because they live in it. Polluted water can kill large numbers of fish, birds, and other animals, and in some areas, pollution has destroyed entire species. People who drink polluted water can become sick, develop cancer, or give birth to children with birth defects.

Water pollutants can be chemical, biological, or physical materials. Landfills in which hazardous wastes have been discarded are potential sources of contamination. Tanks at gas stations that are not properly maintained can cause groundwater to become contaminated. Runoff from farmlands treated with chemical fertilizers or pesticides can contaminate groundwater, lakes, rivers, and streams, as can runoff from industrial sites. Septic tanks in rural and semi-

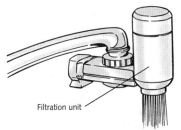

Filtration unit

FILTERING TAP WATER
Running water through an activated-carbon filter, which can be mounted on any faucet, removes traces of chemicals that might be present in some water systems. Tap water can be tested for contaminants by a state-certified laboratory, and if necessary, an appropriate home water treatment system can be installed.

rural areas can contribute to groundwater pollution. Asbestos from water pipes and heavy metals can pollute water supplies as well.

Polyarthritis

An inflammatory condition that affects several joints at the same time. Polyarthritis is characterized by pain in the joints, with possible swelling, redness, and localized sensations of heat.

Polychondritis, relapsing

An inflammatory disorder in the cartilage and other connective tissues of the joints, as well as the ears, nose, larynx, trachea, eye, heart valves, kidney, and blood vessels. The cause of relapsing polychondritis may be related to defects in the function of the immune system; it is often associated with connective tissue diseases.

When the disorder affects the joints, the symptoms include pain and arthritis in large and small joints on both sides of the body. Relapsing polychondritis is diagnosed by clinical history and laboratory tests. Mild cases of the disorder are generally treated with nonsteroidal anti-inflammatory drugs (NSAIDs), such as aspirin and ibuprofen, to relieve pain and inflammation. More severe cases may be treated with a corticosteroid drug, such as prednisone, and the most severe cases, with immunosuppressive agents, such as cyclophosphamide.

Polycystic kidney disease

An inherited disorder in which the kidneys are enlarged and contain clusters of fluid-filled cysts (see KIDNEY CYST; KIDNEY, POLYCYSTIC). Polycystic kidney disease may produce only a few small cysts or many cysts. The cysts can range from the size of a pinhead to the size of a grapefruit. When there are many cysts or when the cysts are very large, a kidney, which is usually about the size of a fist, can grow as large as a football. Some have weighed up to 38 pounds. In time, the cysts tend to destroy working kidney tissue so that the kidneys of individuals with polycystic kidney disease gradually fail. See KIDNEY FAILURE.

The two forms of polycystic kidney disease are hereditary. Autosomal dominant polycystic kidney disease is the most common of all life-threatening genetic diseases. Most individuals with polycystic kidney disease inherit the disease from a parent who has the disease. A small percentage of people acquire autosomal dominant polycystic kidney disease through spontaneous mutation rather than through an inherited gene. Another form of polycystic kidney disease called autosomal recessive polycystic kidney disease is a relatively rare condition that can cause death in the first month of life.

SYMPTOMS
There may be no symptoms early in the disease. For this reason, polycystic kidney disease may go undiagnosed in many people. One of the first signs is likely to be high blood pressure (which can be caused by enlarging cysts that compress blood vessels) and production by cysts of hormones that increase blood pressure. Other symptoms may include blood in the urine, called HEMATURIA, or feelings of heaviness or pain in the back, sides, or abdomen. The discomfort may be mild and intermittent; in rare cases, it may be severe and constant. URINARY TRACT INFECTIONS or KIDNEY STONES may also be among the initial signs of the disease.

DIAGNOSIS AND TREATMENT
Indications that a person may have polycystic kidney disease include a family history of the disease, certain signs and symptoms, and the discovery of cysts in the kidneys during medical testing for other conditions. Three imaging tests may be used for diagnosis: ULTRASOUND SCANNING, CT SCANNING (computed tomography scanning), and MRI (magnetic resonance imaging). A gene linkage study is the most accurate test because it provides a 99 percent probability even when cysts cannot be observed by means of imaging tests. A gene linkage study is expensive and requires family members to provide blood samples.

There is no known treatment or cure for polycystic kidney disease. LAPAROSCOPIC SURGERY may be indicated

P

Terms in small capital letters—for example, PHYSICAL THERAPY or PAGET DISEASE—indicate a cross-reference to another entry with more information.

for people who have severe pain from cysts larger than 5 centimeters in diameter. Laparoscopic surgery offers relief from pain but does not preserve kidney function.

Diet and exercise are known to help control the development of polycystic kidney disease. A low-protein diet, with avoidance of red meat, is generally recommended, as is limiting salt intake and alcohol consumption. Drinking lots of water to allow the kidneys to produce more urine is beneficial. It is currently believed that caffeine may contribute to kidney enlargement. Drinking caffeine-containing beverages is generally discouraged for people who have polycystic kidney disease.

Polycystic ovarian syndrome

A condition in which the ovaries become enlarged and contain multiple cysts. Polycystic ovarian syndrome (PCOS) is caused by a hormone imbalance that affects a woman's menstrual periods and her abilities to ovulate and get pregnant; PCOS typically appears in young women who have not yet established a normal monthly cycle. Because these women rarely or never ovulate, their menstrual periods are irregular, often separated by several months. When they have periods, they are often very heavy. Other symptoms include hirsutism (excess hair on the face and body), acne, and obesity. The cysts are usually painless, and diagnosis is often made during a search for the cause of a woman's infertility.

CAUSE

Polycystic ovarian syndrome results from an increase in the production of androgen hormones by the ovaries and the adrenal glands. The increase in these male hormones causes irregular menstrual periods and interferes with OVULATION by causing the persistent growth of cysts on the follicles in the ovaries. Follicles are cavities where eggs develop. Cysts develop when a follicle has failed to release a mature egg during ovulation and grows larger instead. As a result of their failure to ovulate, women with PCOS continue to make estrogen, but they do not produce progesterone. The result is an imbalance in normal hormone production that increases the risk that the endometrium, which

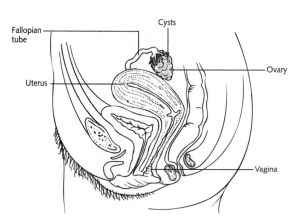

MULTIPLE CYSTS

In a woman with polycystic ovarian syndrome, the ovaries enlarge and contain numerous cysts. The cysts develop when structures within the ovary called follicles—each of which holds a single egg—fail to release the eggs as a part of the normal process of ovulation. Instead the follicles grow and distend the ovary. The condition results from a hormonal imbalance. The cysts are not associated with ovarian cancer.

Fallopian tube
Cysts
Ovary
Uterus
Vagina

lines the uterus, will grow too much. See ENDOMETRIAL HYPERPLASIA.

DIAGNOSIS AND TREATMENT

During a pelvic examination, a doctor may note that the ovaries are enlarged. Blood tests can confirm the hormone imbalance, showing abnormal quantities of the relevant hormones. The choice of treatment depends on whether the woman wishes to become pregnant. Fertility drugs, such as clomiphene, may be prescribed to stimulate ovulation in a woman who wants to become pregnant.

For women who do not want to become pregnant, either progesterone or birth control pills may be prescribed to regulate the menstrual periods. Taking progesterone, in natural or synthetic form, compensates for the failure of the body to produce it naturally after ovulation, which permits menstruation to take place. The restoration of regular menstruation is essential in the treatment of PCOS, because the overgrowth of the uterine lining, if untreated, can increase the risk of cancer.

Polycythemia

An increase in the number of red blood cells circulating in the bloodstream; also known as erythrocytosis (from erythrocyte, the medical term for red blood cell). The added mass of blood cells causes the blood to be thicker than normal and increases blood volume. In a sense, a person with polycythemia has too much blood, a condition that increases the risk of blood clots and can lead to heart attack, stroke, or thrombophlebitis (inflammation of the veins because of blood clots), particularly in the legs.

Polycythemia can be an appropriate physiological response to conditions in which the body faces a higher than normal demand for oxygen, and increased production of red blood cells compensates by allowing for more oxygen transport. This is the case for people who live at high altitudes or who have respiratory diseases such as chronic obstructive pulmonary disease, which impairs the oxygen levels in the blood. Smoking is also a common cause of polycythemia. The carbon monoxide in tobacco smoke displaces oxygen in the red blood cells and deprives the body of oxygen, stimulating the creation of more red blood cells.

Polycythemia can also arise as a result of disease that increases production of red blood cells. The form known as polycythemia vera is caused by a defect in the bone marrow (see MYELOPROLIFERATIVE DISORDERS). Kidney tumors or kidney disease may increase synthesis of the substance that stimulates red blood cell production. Similar effects can arise from tumors of the brain, liver, ovary, uterus, prostate, thymus, and adrenal glands.

Polycythemia can also occur when a person loses a significant portion of plasma (the liquid portion of the blood), increasing the relative proportion of red blood cells in the bloodstream. This can happen as a result of severe burns, dehydration, hyperemesis (repeated vomiting), or diuretic medications (which increase urine production).

Polydactyly

A birth defect characterized by the presence of more than five fingers or

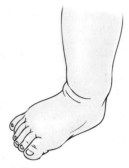

EXTRA DIGITS
A person with polydactyly, which tends to run in families, is born with an extra toe or finger. The defect can be a single-gene disorder; that is, the trait is determined by a single pair of genes and is transmitted by basic laws of heredity, just like hair or eye color.

toes on a hand or foot. Polydactyly can be an inherited trait.

Polydipsia

Intense and constant thirst over extended periods. Polydipsia is often one of the first signs of type 1 or type 2 diabetes (see DIABETES MELLITUS, TYPE 1; DIABETES MELLITUS, TYPE 2). When associated with diabetes, polydipsia is caused by the spillover of excess glucose into the urine, which prompts more frequent urination. When the body loses fluid at this increased rate, a person experiences thirst as the signal to replace fluid loss.

Psychogenic polydipsia is an excessive thirst that originates from psychological or emotional causes rather than from a physical disorder. This form of polydipsia most commonly occurs in women older than 50 years.

Polyhidrosis

Heavy perspiration; also called hyperhidrosis. Polyhidrosis is a condition in which intense sweating on the palms, soles of the feet, and underarms occurs whenever the person is under stress. As many as 1 percent of people experience polyhidrosis, which is not a harmful condition but one that can be embarrassing. In some cases, polyhidrosis is the result of a genetic disorder called emotional hyperhidrosis.

Polyhidrosis can be treated with the use of antiperspirants, either over-the-counter preparations or stronger preparations available by prescription. Other rarely used therapeutic options to treat polyhidrosis include

surgery to remove sweat glands, the injection of drugs that block sweat glands, and the application of electrical current to block the sweat glands in the affected area.

Polyhydramnios

In pregnancy, an excess amount of amniotic fluid. Sometimes the amount of fluid increases either gradually or suddenly. Maternal symptoms of polyhydramnios include a larger than expected abdominal size, abdominal discomfort, breathlessness, nausea, or swelling of the legs.

Polyhydramnios is diagnosed by physical examination and ultrasound. Tests may be done to check for fetal abnormalities, such as a defect that prevents the fetus from swallowing, or certain types of neural tube defects in which spinal fluid spills into the amniotic fluid. In most cases, the fetus is normal and no treatment is required. Sometimes, excess fluid is removed from the amniotic sac in order to relieve symptoms, using a procedure similar to AMNIOCENTESIS. If symptoms are severe and occur in late pregnancy, the doctor may recommend inducing labor.

Polymyxin B sulfate

An antibiotic. Polymyxin B sulfate (Betadine, Cortisporin, Neosporin, Polytrim, Terramycin solution) is an antibacterial drug used in many forms to treat eye and skin infections. Polymyxin B sulfate is available both with and without prescription.

Polymyalgia rheumatica

An inflammatory disorder that causes widespread aching and stiffness in the muscles and joints. Polymyalgia rheumatica (PMR) is the most common inflammatory joint disorder among older people, typically affecting people older than the age of 50. PMR may be caused by an immune system malfunction. Heredity also seems to be involved as it occurs more often in people of northern European origin. Women are affected twice as often as men. The symptoms of muscular aching and pain may come on slowly, or the disorder may at first resemble the flu with joint and body aches, fatigue, low-grade fever, and sometimes a diminished appetite. These symptoms remain for

longer than a few weeks or even a month, which distinguishes them from flu symptoms. The pain, which tends to affect the shoulders and hips, may vary from moderate to severe. Typically, pain is most severe in the morning but may also continue throughout the day and disturb sleep at night.

There is no known cure for PMR, which generally improves on its own within a year or two. Treatment of the symptoms, however, can provide relief. Diagnosis of PMR is made by a doctor taking a history of symptoms and a blood test to measure the degree of inflammation. If symptoms are mild, nonsteroidal anti-inflammatory drugs (NSAIDs) may be recommended. In more severe cases, the doctor might prescribe PREDNISONE to reduce the inflammation causing the pain. The effects of this medication may be experienced within 24 hours, but long-term use raises concern because of potentially serious side effects.

Polymyositis

A rare neuromuscular disease of children and adults that produces inflammatory swelling, irritation, and weakness in the voluntary muscles, such as those of the arms and legs that normally govern movement. The cause is a disturbance in the body's IMMUNE SYSTEM. Symptoms of polymyositis include muscular weakness in the hips or shoulders and discomfort in the small joints, including possible pain, swelling, and localized redness and sensation of heat. When severe, the disease may make it difficult to climb stairs or perform daily tasks, and it may become necessary for a person to use a wheelchair and to require assistance with everyday activities. Polymyositis may be associated with certain malignant tumors.

Polymyositis is diagnosed by a physical examination and a history of symptoms. Other diagnostic tools may include blood tests, electromyography to measure the electrical patterns of the muscles, and a biopsy of the affected muscles to obtain a tissue sample for laboratory study. The disease is primarily treated with the corticosteroid drug prednisone; other medications may be used if this does not relieve symptoms. When the medication has taken effect, physical therapy or a special exercise program may be prescribed by the doctor.

Polymyositis may improve on its own within a few months of first appearing. However, the disease can prove fatal if the throat muscles are affected, making swallowing difficult or if the lungs become involved.

Polyp

A mass of tissue that develops on the inside wall of a hollow organ. Polyps are usually benign and are commonly found in the nose or sinuses, where they are associated with obstruction, chronic infection, and nasal discharge. Other sites where polyps may occur include the ear, the stomach, and the colon. Over time, some types of polyps found in the colon may become malignant.

Polypectomy

The removal of polyps, abnormal tissue growths that typically grow in the linings of the nose, cervix, intestine, or any other mucous membrane. Polyps protrude stalklike from the organs on which they grow. They can be benign (noncancerous) or malignant (cancerous). Some benign polyps pose no risk. Adenomas are benign polyps that may become malignant and should be removed. Most often, they are discovered during a routine ENDOSCOPY (a procedure in which interior parts of the body are examined by using a slim, flexible, lighted tube). SIGMOIDOSCOPY and COLONOSCOPY are two types of endoscopy commonly used in the detection and removal of polyps in the colon. Through a sigmoidoscope or colonoscope, it is possible to see abnormal growths and remove them by using a wire snare, ultrasound, or laser beam. After they are removed, a pathologist examines polyps under a microscope to determine whether they are cancerous or benign. If there is a malignancy, further surgery may be necessary.

Polypharmacy

The administration of many drugs at the same time. Polypharmacy can create problems, particularly if more than one doctor is treating a person without realizing other medications have been prescribed. Polypharmacy is a particular concern in older people who take many drugs and are known to experience reactions and interactions among the medications. It has been reported that 10 percent of all hospital admissions are directly related to drug reactions when a person is taking more than one medication.

Polyposis, familial

An inherited condition in which 100 or more polyps can form in the large intestine. A polyp is a collection of cells that form a tissue mass that hangs from a stalk; polyps can be benign or precancerous. In familial polyposis, the polyps begin as precancerous adenomas that often become cancerous by age 40.

ADENOMAS

Adenomas are a category of polyps, classified into three varieties: tubular, villous, and tubulovillous. Adenomatous polyps all have the potential to become malignant, particularly when villous characteristics are present. Tubular adenomas are usually less than one-half inch in diameter; they are the most common type of adenoma. Villous adenomas are less common but are often at least 1 inch in diameter and are associated with a mucus-like discharge in the stool. Tubulovillous adenomas combine characteristics of both.

As a rule, adenomas begin to develop in people with familial polyposis beginning at puberty. Over time, adenomas associated with familial polyposis increase in size and number. They can occur without symptoms or may cause rectal bleeding. In 5 to 10 years, adenomas can become cancerous, especially without treatment.

SYMPTOMS

The warning signs of familial polyposis include blood or mucus in the stool, diarrhea, and occasional abdominal cramps, with or without weight loss. By the time such symptoms have developed, cancer may already be present, so it is particularly important that people with family histories of familial polyposis be examined for the condition early in childhood or adolescence.

Early symptoms of familial polyposis include tiny eye freckles at the back of the retina. Harmless cysts may also appear on the skin of the scalp, face, arms, or legs. Bony growths in the jaw or on the skull sometimes appear, as do tiny extra sets of incomplete teeth. All of these early symptoms provide clues to the presence of familial polyposis and should lead to tests of the colon.

DIAGNOSIS

Familial polyposis is diagnosed by direct examination of the bowel. There are two ways to do this: sigmoidoscopy and colonoscopy.

■ *Sigmoidoscopy* In children at risk for familial polyposis, examination of the lower bowel is sufficient to make the diagnosis, beginning at about age 10. The examination is performed by inserting a fiberoptic tube called a flexible sigmoidoscope through the rectum into the lower bowel. The sigmoidoscope carries a light source and provides a magnifying eyepiece for the doctor to look through. Children at risk for familial polyposis can expect to have this procedure repeated every 2 years until age 40.

■ *Colonoscopy* A more extensive view of the entire large bowel is possible with the use of a longer tube, called a colonoscope. The colonoscope is a fiberoptic tube, similar to a sigmoidoscope, but because of its length, it can be used to examine the entire colon. A biopsy sample can be taken or polyps can be removed through a colonoscope. This procedure is recommended for people in families with atypical polyposis, such as attenuated familial polyposis, a condition in which adenomas tend to predominate in the upper part of the colon.

TREATMENT AND PREVENTION

There is no cure for familial polyposis. Surgery is usually required, because the condition is associated with large numbers of adenomas and a virtual 100 percent risk of colon cancer over time. Surgical removal of the colon, or COLECTOMY, is standard treatment and is the only certain way to prevent the development of more adenomas in the colon. The procedure usually performed is a colectomy with ILEOSTOMY, in which an opening, or STOMA, from the intestine to the outside is created in the abdomen and pouches are worn to collect waste products. After surgery, nutritional counseling is recommended to help plan a diet suitable for the altered digestive tract. Regular examinations of the rectum throughout the person's life are essential.

Familial polyposis is an inherited condition. Each child of a parent with the condition has a 50 percent risk of inheriting the altered gene, which has been named the adenomatous polyposis coli, or APC, gene, which is located on chromosome 5. A blood test has been developed to determine which family members have inherited the altered gene and can be expected to develop the disease. In this test, the blood sample is analyzed to identify the altered APC gene.

Polyuria

The passing of an abnormally large volume of urine. Polyuria is medically defined as excreting more than 2½ liters of urine a day. It is one of the first signs of type 1 or type 2 diabetes (see DIABETES MELLITUS, TYPE 1; DIABETES MELLITUS, TYPE 2). Polyuria tends to be most noticeable when it occurs during the night. The usual causes are drinking large amounts of fluid, drinking too many caffeine-containing or alcoholic beverages, increased salt in the diet, psychogenic POLYDIPSIA, and taking diuretics or other medications that stimulate urination.

Polyuria may be associated with a number of diseases or disorders including KIDNEY FAILURE and SICKLE CELL ANEMIA. It is also a sign of excess glucose in the blood in people with diabetes mellitus. There may be a temporary increase in urine volume for up to 24 hours after diagnostic procedures that use a contrast medium.

Polyuria requires medical attention if it persists over several days and does not have an apparent cause such as an increased intake of fluids or taking certain medications that stimulate thirst or urination.

Pore

A small opening, particularly in the skin. Sweat glands secrete through one kind of pore, and hairs emerge from another. Pores in the tongue have a role in the sense of taste. Small sacs in the lungs also have pores that allow air to pass from one to another.

Porphyria

A group of rare inherited blood disorders characterized by defective production of heme, the oxygen-carrying component of hemoglobin in the red blood cells, and by accumulation of substances called porphyrins in the blood and body fluids. Porphyrias are associated with three sets of symptoms: photodermatitis, a sensitivity to light that results in skin rashes or blistering; neuropsychiatric problems, such as personality changes during acute attacks of the disease including confusion, hallucinations, and seizures; and abdominal pain and cramps.

Porphyrias can develop during childhood, adolescence, or adulthood. Some forms involve acute attacks characterized by severe abdominal pain followed by vomiting, constipation, personality changes, numbness and tingling, weakness, paralysis, sensory changes, and muscle pain. Acute attacks can be life-threatening, producing severe imbalances of electrolytes in the blood, low blood pressure, and shock.

Porphyrias are lifelong illnesses. Treatment of acute episodes involves careful monitoring of electrolytes and blood gases in addition to intravenous glucose and medication for the blood disorder. Long-term management between episodes will include avoiding alcohol, nicotine, and medications that can precipitate an attack; a high carbohydrate diet; avoiding sunlight by wearing clothing that covers the skin; and sometimes removal of the spleen. Some forms of porphyria affect the skin and teeth only. In most forms, particularly those primarily involving the skin, the urine may turn red or brown.

Port-wine stain

A type of vascular BIRTHMARK or blood vessel malformation. Port-wine stains appear at birth. They may be pink, red, or purple and can be of any size. Port-wine stains occur most frequently on the face, neck, arms, and legs. Although this type of birthmark is flat, over time it can thicken and grow bumps or ridges. Port-wine stains are considered a type of arteriovenous malformation. However, unlike a capillary HEMANGIOMA, another type of vascular birthmark, port-wine stains increase in size as a child grows and do not disappear on their own.

It is essential for a doctor to diagnose this type of birthmark and monitor its growth. This is particularly important when port-wine stains are located on the forehead, eyelids, or sides of the face. Large port-wine stains at these sites are associated with an increased risk of glaucoma or seizures (see STURGE-WEBER SYNDROME). Port-wine stains may also develop a PYOGENIC GRANULOMA (a small, inflamed bump on the skin that bleeds easily). In most cases, pyogenic granulomas must be surgically removed.

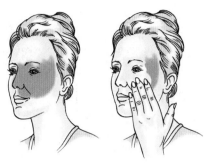

TREATMENT FOR PORT-WINE STAINS
Full-coverage makeup can hide a port-wine stain and relieve some emotional or social distress caused by its appearance. Laser surgery is the most promising treatment because it destroys the involved capillaries without damaging the outer skin. Laser treatment of infants can be successful, but older stains may be difficult to remove.

Emotional stress is the most common complication of port-wine stains, particularly when they are located on the face. Special makeup is often used to cover up the blemish. Now, many port-wine stains can be removed with LASER SURGERY, which destroys the blood vessels. However, laser surgery is not successful in all cases, and possible complications include pigmentation changes, bleeding, swelling, crusting, and discomfort that young children may not tolerate well.

Positron emission tomography scanning

See PET SCANNING.

Postcoital contraception

Birth control methods used after sex has taken place. Historically, ineffective folk remedies, such as cola soft-drink or vinegar-water douches, have been used for postcoital contraception. However, certain types of birth

P

control pills and intrauterine devices can be used with some success to prevent pregnancy after unprotected sex. See CONTRACEPTION, EMERGENCY POSTCOITAL.

Posterior

In anatomy, the back part of the body or an organ. The opposite of posterior is anterior, or the front part of the body or an organ.

Postmaturity

A condition in which pregnancy lasts longer than 42 weeks. After 40 weeks, the amount of oxygen and nutrients delivered to a fetus begins to decline, because the placenta becomes less efficient. As the fetus continues to grow, the amount of amniotic fluid may decrease, which can cause the umbilical cord to become pinched as the baby moves or the uterus contracts. If a baby grows too large, the mother may be unable to complete a normal vaginal delivery. A postmature baby is also more likely to experience fetal distress during labor, especially if the mother is age 35 or older.

About 10 percent of all pregnancies extend past their projected due dates. Ultrasound and electronic fetal monitoring may be used to determine whether the fetus is healthy and can wait for delivery. The tests may be performed twice each week until the baby is born. Often, labor is induced 2 weeks beyond the due date.

Although risks to the health of mother and baby increase after 42 weeks of pregnancy, 95 percent of postmature babies are born without incident.

Postmortem examination

See AUTOPSY.

Postnasal drip

The sensation of mucus dripping down the throat from the back of the nose and accumulating in the throat. It is associated with the common cold (see COLD, COMMON), ALLERGIES, and other conditions causing inflammation of the mucous membranes of the nose. Symptoms include clearing the throat often, along with mild and unproductive cough (usually at night). Therapy may involve decongestants, nasal sprays, and avoiding known allergens. Antibiotics are rarely required unless the sinuses are involved. See RHINITIS.

Postoperative care

A period during which a person is closely monitored for possible complications following surgery. Immediately following an operation, the person is wheeled from the operating room to the postanesthesia care unit; also called the recovery room. The person is given oxygen, and cardiac and pulse monitors are used so that the nursing staff may observe vital signs. The anesthesiologist and surgeon will tell the recovery room nurses what to watch for in the way of possible complications that may result from the surgical procedure and about any special needs. Blood samples may be obtained, and X rays may be taken. Pain or other prescribed medications may be given to make the person feel more comfortable. When the person becomes awake and alert, he or she is transferred back to his or her hospital room.

SPECIALIZED CARE IN THE HOSPITAL

Many hospitals provide units for patients who have special needs. These units usually provide close nursing support with the capacity for intensive monitoring of vital signs, organ function, and powerful medications.

- **Intensive care unit (ICU):** A hospital unit that provides round-the-clock monitoring and care of seriously ill patients. The medical staff is trained to intervene whenever necessary to save a person's life. A surgical ICU (SICU) is usually reserved for trauma or postoperative patients.
- **Coronary care unit (CCU):** An ICU to care specifically for people who have had a heart attack or other serious, life-threatening heart condition.
- **Neonatal intensive care unit (NICU):** Another type of ICU to care for seriously ill newborns and premature babies.

Postpartum cardiomyopathy

Heart failure after pregnancy caused by a disorder of the heart muscle. This serious and sometimes critical condition occurs mostly in women over age 30 who have had many pregnancies without previous evidence of heart disease or in women who have had preeclampsia, eclampsia, or a multiple pregnancy. Symptoms include moderate respiratory distress and left-sided chest pain.

Postpartum cardiomyopathy usually occurs in the first month after childbirth, but it can occur as much as 5 months later, and it can also occur in women who have had a stillbirth or even an early abortion. In a small number of cases, the disorder occurs in the last month of pregnancy. The cause is unknown.

Treatment includes standard care for pulmonary edema (fluid in the lungs) and the use of digitalis drugs, which make the heart work more efficiently. The doctor may prescribe anticoagulant drugs. Extended bed rest speeds recovery. If imaging tests show that a woman's heart size has returned to normal within 6 months, she has a good prognosis and can resume normal activities, including subsequent pregnancies.

Postpartum depression

FOR SYMPTOM CHART
see Depression, page 32

A depressed mental condition after childbirth that does not resolve within a few weeks. Up to 80 percent of women experience transient moodiness and depression, or postpartum blues, for a short period following childbirth due to rapid hormonal changes and exhaustion. Other women develop a more serious, longer-lasting condition called postpartum depression. A woman with severe postpartum depression may experience symptoms that interfere with normal activities. Postpartum depression may be caused by the sudden change in hormone levels that occurs with the end of pregnancy. A lack of sleep, breast engorgement pain, and difficulty in adjusting to new responsibilities may contribute to postpartum depression.

Signs of this form of severe depression in a woman may include feelings of guilt, anxiety, or hopelessness that do not go away after 2 weeks; inability to sleep; sleeping too much; anxiety or panic attacks; lack of interest in the baby or other family members; fear of harming the baby or herself; suicidal thoughts; changes in appetite; concentration problems; or extreme fatigue.

Emotional support from family, friends, and a woman's partner may help her cope with many of the stresses contributing to the depression. Help with household chores and child care can also give a woman the time she may need to adjust to motherhood. When depression persists, though, or interferes with her ability to function, a woman should see her doctor. A doctor can prescribe ANTIDEPRESSANTS, or recommend a psychiatrist or counselor for treatment.

Postpartum hemorrhage

In childbirth, an excessive loss of blood from the uterus or vagina after delivery. Postpartum hemorrhage often occurs when the muscles of the uterus do not contract firmly enough to cause it to shrink and compress the blood vessels inside. As a result, the bleeding produced when the placenta separates from the uterus is not controlled adequately. Very long labor or the birth of multiple babies can also cause hemorrhage. When more than about a pint of blood has been lost after delivery, postpartum hemorrhage is said to have occurred.

Postpartum hemorrhage can also occur if bits of the placenta remain inside the uterus and prevent it from tightening up sufficiently. Treatment includes the use of medications that help the uterus contract. Fragments of placenta must be removed from the uterus, when that is the cause of bleeding. Cervical or vaginal tissue is sometimes torn during delivery, which can lead to hemorrhage. Tears can be stitched up after the woman is given an anesthetic.

Postpolio syndrome

Also known as PPS, a condition that affects some people who have previously had POLIO. Postpolio syndrome, which occurs 20 to 30 years after the original disease, causes slow, progressive weakening of the muscles. Other symptoms include fatigue, lack of energy, decrease in muscle size (called atrophy), involuntary twitching of muscles, muscle and joint pain, respiratory and sleep problems, trouble swallowing, and cold intolerance. The diagnosis is made primarily through medical history. When a person who has had polio experiences muscle weakness years later, doctors strongly suspect PPS.

There is no cure for postpolio syndrome. However, there are many treatments available to relieve symptoms. These include anti-inflammatory medications, rest, heat treatments, ice packs, TENS (transcutaneous electrical nerve stimulation), massage, stretching, assistive devices, household adaptive equipment, lifestyle modifications, and avoidance of stress. Some people require braces to support weakened muscles, while others benefit from wheelchairs or motorized scooters. Respiratory difficulties may lead to a need for oxygen supplementation or a machine to aid breathing.

Posttraumatic stress disorder

A mental illness involving the re-experiencing of a traumatic event evoking intense fear, helplessness, and horror through hallucinations, flashbacks, or nightmares. Commonly abbreviated PTSD and classified as one of the ANXIETY DISORDERS, posttraumatic stress disorder also involves avoidance of all things associated with the event and a state of increased vigilance and arousal, such as extreme alertness and difficulty sleeping (insomnia). Feelings of detachment from others and a sense that the future is short, bleak, and hopeless are also common. PTSD can arise after accidents involving maiming or death, natural disasters, a fire, war, physical abuse, assault, rape, and torture. PTSD usually develops within 3 months of the trauma, but can begin years later. The disorder may arise at any age. It may be associated with depression and alcohol or drug abuse.

The causes of PTSD are uncertain. Most likely, various predisposing psychological, genetic, physical, and social factors are involved. Antianxiety and antidepressant medications are often used in treatment to alleviate the symptoms of anxiety. Hypnosis has been used with some success. Psychotherapy that aims to aid the person in expressing grief over the traumatic event is also helpful, as are support groups made up of other people who have been through similar experiences.

Postural drainage

A form of RESPIRATORY THERAPY in which special positioning of the body allows mucus to drain from the lungs. Postural drainage involves tilting a person at an angle that helps drain lung secretions. Chest percussion, or clapping a person on the chest or back with a cupped hand, may be performed by a therapist. A mechanical vibrator may also be used to help loosen secretions during postural drainage.

Postural drainage is used at various intervals to provide relief to people

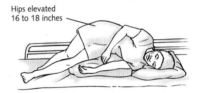

Draining the right lower lung

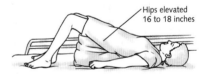

Draining lower lungs

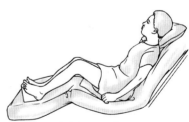

Draining upper lungs

DRAINING THE LUNGS
Assuming certain postures can help drain phlegm from specific areas of the lungs or help a person cough up phlegm more effectively. The person usually stays in the position for 5 to 15 minutes at a time. Percussion (tapping or clapping), vibration, or suctioning the lungs may be part of the therapy.

who produce excessive sputum as a result of conditions including cystic fibrosis, bronchiectasis, and lung abscess. It may also be used when sputum cannot be coughed up effectively by people who are older or disabled by conditions causing muscular weakness. The technique is also effective for draining mucus from the lungs of people who are recovering from surgery, injuries, or severe illnesses.

Postural hypotension

See HYPOTENSION.

Posture

Position of the limbs or carriage of the body as a whole. Posture is usually taken to refer to the manner in which a person carries his or her body, particularly when standing.

Potassium

A mineral involved in both electrical and cellular functions in the body. Potassium is important to the body as an ELECTROLYTE involved in the regulation of both water and ACID-BASE BALANCE. Potassium also helps in protein synthesis from amino acids, in carbohydrate metabolism, in the building of muscle, and in normal growth processes.

Potassium is acquired from fish such as salmon, cod, flounder, and sardines. Some meats contain potassium, as do citrus fruits, apples, bananas, and apricots, particularly dried apricots. Many vegetables contribute potassium to the diet, such as broccoli, peas, lima beans, tomatoes, potatoes and their skins, spinach, lettuce, and parsley. The average American diet provides between 2 and 6 grams of potassium per day, more than the minimum of 2 to 2.5 grams recommended by experts.

Some people experience potassium deficiency, usually because of aging or chronic disease. The most common problems associated with potassium deficiency are hypertension, congestive heart failure, cardiac arrhythmias, depression, and fatigue. Potassium supplements should be taken only by prescription, because increased levels of potassium (hyperkalemia) can occur, particularly in people with reduced kidney function or severe infection.

Pott fracture

A break at the lower end of the more slender bone of the lower leg (fibula) where it meets the outer portion of the ankle bone. A Pott fracture can also involve, although rarely, injury to the larger bone of the lower leg, the shinbone, or tibia. See also FRACTURE.

Power of attorney

A signed, dated, and witnessed legal document that sets up a surrogate for making decisions See ADVANCE DIRECTIVES.

PPO

Also known as a preferred provider organization, a group of physicians, pharmacists, and hospitals that offers services to subscribers at a discount. PPOs may be organized by insurance companies, companies with self-insurance plans, or groups of individual physicians.

Prader-Willi syndrome

A genetic disorder that causes incomplete sexual development, short stature, cognitive disabilities, and an insatiable appetite that leads to obesity. Prader-Willi syndrome (PWS) is caused by a spontaneous genetic error occurring near the time of conception for unknown reasons. One in 12,000 to 15,000 people has PWS.

Characteristics of PWS may include infantile hypotonia (muscle weakness and low muscle tone) that improves with age; feeding problems and poor weight gain in infancy; rapid and excessive weight gain between ages 1 and 6; narrow face with almond-shaped eyes and a small mouth with down-turned corners; undescended testicles and small penis in males; scant or no menstrual periods in females; delayed puberty; overall developmental delay before age 6, including mild to moderate mental retardation or learning problems; and compulsive eating and preoccupation with food.

PWS is known to involve the absence of active genetic material on chromosome 15. Chromosome analysis can confirm the diagnosis of PWS through genetic testing. Since the condition can recur within an affected family, genetic testing is recommended to determine whether such a family is at risk for recurrence.

COMPLICATIONS

PWS is associated with overeating that leads inevitably to obesity. The cause of this problem is a flaw in the hypothalamus in the brain, which normally registers feelings of hunger and being "full." People with PWS evidently never feel full, but have a continuous urge to eat that they are unable to learn to control. They actually need less food than other children their age, because their bodies have reduced muscle and tend to burn fewer calories.

Infants with PWS are often underweight, because their low muscle tone makes it hard for them to suck. By school age, however, children with PWS have developed an intense interest in food and will become obese if calories are not rigorously restricted.

Although small children with PWS are usually happy and loving, older children and adults with the disorder frequently have behavior problems, often beginning at the same time as their preoccupation with food. Difficulties in behavior management usually peak at adolescence. Depression is common among adults, who also tend to exhibit obsessive-compulsive symptoms and mood swings See OBSESSIVE-COMPULSIVE DISORDER.

TREATMENT

The most challenging aspect of treating a child with PWS is weight management. To date, no medication or surgical intervention has been identified that could eliminate the need for rigorous dieting. Most people with PWS must follow an extremely low-calorie diet all their lives and must live in an environment that severely limits their access to food. Some families have to lock the kitchen or the refrigerator and cabinets to prevent overeating by a child with PWS.

Adults with PWS function best in group-home settings with other people with PWS, where food access can be restricted. If weight can be controlled, life expectancy can be normal and general health can be good.

Pravastatin

A drug used to lower cholesterol and other fats in the blood. Pravastatin (Pravachol) is an antilipemic drug that lowers cholesterol and lipoprotein by inhibiting a liver enzyme involved in the production of cholesterol. Pravastatin works by reducing the amount of cholesterol created by the body. The drug should be used as an adjunct to a proper low cholesterol diet.

Precancerous

The term used to describe a condition that may become cancerous if left untreated. This term is used whether or not the condition eventually becomes cancerous.

Preconception counseling

See GENETIC COUNSELING.

Predisposing factors

Influences that make a person susceptible to a particular medical condition.

Prednisolone

An anti-inflammatory and immunosuppressant drug. Prednisolone (Prelone, Pediapred) is a corticosteroid, a cortisonelike drug that is used to treat severe inflammation in various parts of the body. Prednisolone lessens the inflammation and itching associated with allergic reactions. It is used to treat adrenocortical insufficiency as well as severe allergies, skin disorders, asthma, eye irritations, and arthritis. Prednisolone also helps to modify the body's immune response to disease.

Prednisone

An anti-inflammatory and immunosuppressant drug. Prednisone (Sterapred) is a corticosteroid, a cortisonelike drug that is used to treat severe inflammation (redness and swelling) in various parts of the body. Prednisone lessens the inflammation and itching associated with allergic reactions. It is used to treat severe allergies, skin disorders, asthma, arthritis, acute episodes of multiple sclerosis, and some forms of cancer. Prednisone also helps to modify the body's immune response to disease.

Preeclampsia

A complication of pregnancy, also known as toxemia of pregnancy, in which the woman's blood pressure rises to an abnormal level. Swelling and abnormal amounts of protein are associated with preeclampsia. Symptoms of preeclampsia include a severe, continuous headache, abdominal pain, nausea, and vision problems, such as blurred vision and blind spots. Sudden weight gain (more than 2.2 pounds in a week) due to swelling or fluid retention can also be a symptom. One in 10 pregnant women develops preeclampsia, typically after the 20th week of a first pregnancy.

The cause of preeclampsia is not known. Some scientists think that preeclampsia results from the pregnant woman's immune system reacting abnormally to the presence of the fetus and producing chemicals that cause the woman's blood vessels to narrow. The narrowing, combined with a complicated sequence of immunological responses, can contribute to increased blood pressure.

DIAGNOSIS

As part of routine PRENATAL CARE, the woman's blood pressure is monitored and her urine is checked for the presence of a protein called albumin, a sign of the condition. A sign of a possible problem in a pregnant woman is a blood pressure reading of higher than 140/90. Other causes for concern include a rise in her systolic pressure (the top number of the reading) of more than 30 points since her first trimester of pregnancy or a rise in her diastolic pressure (the bottom number) of more than 15 points. If blood pressure readings are elevated, they should be confirmed by a second test at least 6 hours later. A simple urine test can detect the presence of albumin in the woman's urine.

TREATMENT AND RISK FACTORS

The only cure for preeclampsia is delivery of the baby. When the condition is mild, doctors often recommend rest and allow the pregnancy to continue with careful monitoring of both the woman and the baby. Doctors often recommend that the woman lie on her left side to avoid having the uterus rest on a major vein, which restricts placental blood flow. Because preeclampsia usually develops late in pregnancy when the fetus is mature, doctors sometimes advise early delivery. Various tests, such as a nonstress test, may be performed to evaluate the health of the fetus and to determine whether an early delivery is required.

Preeclampsia is more likely to occur in a female in her teens, older than age 45, or one who has a history of high blood pressure, diabetes, or kidney disease. Women pregnant with more than one fetus are also at increased risk for developing preeclampsia. Doctors rely on providing good prenatal care, including frequent blood pressure and urine checks, to detect preeclampsia early. Some obstetricians use low doses of aspirin to help prevent preeclampsia for women at high risk. In about one pregnancy in 1,000, preeclampsia can progress to a more serious condition, called ECLAMPSIA, in which seizures and coma may occur. Eclampsia must be treated in a hospital to protect the lives of both the woman and the fetus.

Preferred provider organization

See PPO.

Pregnancy

FOR FIRST AID
see Childbirth, page 1317

The process of carrying a developing embryo or fetus in the uterus from conception on. Birth typically takes place around the 40th week. Pregnancy causes numerous physiological changes in a woman, including cessation of the menstrual period, enlargement of the breasts, pigmentation changes (nipples and sometimes elsewhere), and progressive enlargement of the abdomen as the fetus grows. Many over-the-counter products are available to test for pregnancy. However, if used incorrectly, the home tests can be misleading. If a woman tests negative but believes she may be pregnant, she should see a doctor for more accurate testing. A doctor may perform a urine test and blood tests, along with a pelvic examination to detect a pregnancy, and will ask a woman the date of the first day of her last period. This information is used to calculate the delivery date.

STAGES OF PREGNANCY

Each of the three stages of pregnancy, or trimesters, lasts about 3 months. Throughout a pregnancy, a woman's body changes in predictable ways as the uterus enlarges and the fetus grows.

■ *First trimester* This is the most critical time in the development of the

P

TRIMESTERS OF PREGNANCY

A normal pregnancy is about 40 weeks long and is divided into three 3-month periods called trimesters. During each stage there are dramatic changes in the woman's body and in the fetus.

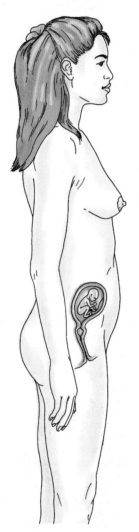

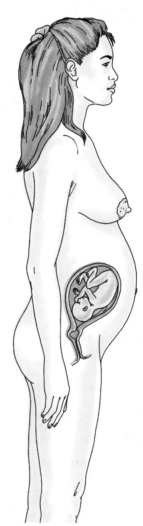

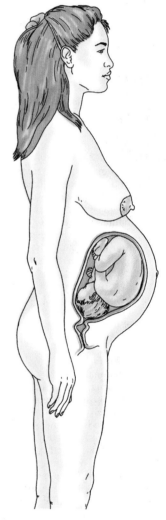

END OF FIRST TRIMESTER

After 3 months, the fetus's limbs and major organs are fully formed, the heart beats, and fingers, toes, and teeth buds have developed. During the first trimester, the woman's breasts grow fuller and are tender, and she may feel tired or nauseous. She may have the urge to urinate more often as the uterus presses on her bladder.

END OF SECOND TRIMESTER

By 6 months, the fetus sleeps and wakes, moves and kicks, urinates, and hears. The woman's abdomen protrudes, and she may have back pain. Her breasts continue to enlarge, and the nipples are darker and larger.

FULL TERM

Toward the end of the ninth month, the fetus is growing to birth weight and is fully developed. It usually moves into the normal birth position. In the third trimester, the increasing size of the fetus can make movement more difficult and can cause shortness of breath.

embryo, or fetus, as it is called after the eighth week of pregnancy. The fetus grows rapidly and is most vulnerable to damage from substances that can cause birth defects or death, including bacteria, viruses, drugs (legal and illegal), alcohol, and environmental agents, such as chemicals. By the end of the trimester, the arms, legs, and major organs of the fetus are fully formed, and it measures about 4 inches and weighs about an ounce. The mother may feel tired and have bouts of nausea and vomiting, or so-called morning sickness, during this period. Her breasts may swell and become tender.

■ *Second trimester* This is usually the most comfortable trimester for a pregnant woman. The nausea common to the first trimester has subsided, and the uterus is not yet large enough to cause the discomforts that are part of the final trimester. Women in this stage may experience low back pain, heartburn, indigestion, flatulence, and constipation. Hormones may cause the nipples to darken and may cause a line, the linea nigra, to form from a woman's navel to her pubic hair. Around the 16th week of pregnancy, a woman may begin to feel the fetus moving. It sleeps, awakens, and passes urine into the amniotic fluid. It also can hear sounds. By the end of the sixth month, a fetus is 11 to 14 inches long and weighs 1 to 1.5 pounds. A fetus this small may survive outside the womb with highly specialized medical care.

■ *Third trimester* During the third trimester, the mother's discomfort may increase as the fetus grows to its

birth weight. Moving around, sitting, and sleeping may be more difficult, and stretch marks may appear on the skin. A woman's breasts may leak a small amount of colostrum in preparation for breast-feeding. Colostrum is the yellowish, milky liquid that precedes true breast milk. By the end of the trimester, the uterus expands to the lower diaphragm. Eating large meals may make a woman uncomfortable, and breathing may be difficult. Once the fetus descends into the pelvic cavity, breathing and eating may be more comfortable. Common during the last month of pregnancy are Braxton Hicks contractions. These mild, irregular contractions last from 30 seconds to 2 minutes, but are not true labor pains, which grow progressively stronger and more frequent. Labor usually begins in weeks 37 to 42 of pregnancy. The fetus grows to its final birth weight and may kick, suck its thumb, open and close its eyes, and even hiccup. In the final month, the fetus shifts into the birth position—typically head down and facing toward the mother's back with its arms and legs flexed. See also LABOR.

Pregnancy tests

Tests that use a woman's blood or urine to detect a pregnancy. Doctors check for pregnancy by testing the woman's blood or urine. Over-the-counter HOME PREGNANCY TESTS that evaluate a urine sample are available at drug stores; if used correctly, they are nearly as accurate as those performed by a doctor. All of these tests involve the detection of a hormone called HUMAN CHORIONIC GONADOTROPIN (HCG) in the woman's urine or blood. HCG is produced in large quantities by the developing placenta during the first few weeks of pregnancy.

Urine pregnancy tests are most accurate when the urine sample is taken first thing in the morning. A first-of-the-morning urine sample is more concentrated than one taken later in the day, making it easier to detect HCG. Urine tests can detect pregnancy as soon as 14 days after conception, or on approximately the first day of a missed menstrual period. Serum pregnancy tests, which use a blood sample, are even more sensitive than urine tests. Blood tests can

detect a pregnancy even before the woman has missed a menstrual period because HCG shows up in the blood earlier than in the urine.

All pregnancy tests give results that are either positive or negative. A positive result almost always means that the woman is pregnant. A negative result may mean that the woman is not pregnant. However, a pregnant woman can get a negative result if the test is performed incorrectly or, in a urine test, if the urine tested was not a first-of-the-morning sample, or if the test was conducted too early in the pregnancy for the HCG to show up.

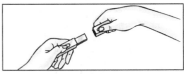

Remove cap from test strip.

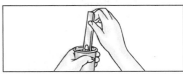

Insert strip in urine.

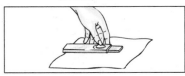

Lay test strip flat.

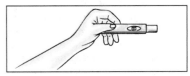

Read results on color indicator.

OVER-THE-COUNTER PREGNANCY TESTS
Commercial home pregnancy tests are highly accurate, inexpensive, and convenient. To use the test at home, the woman collects a sample of her urine, then dips the test strip into the urine. After a designated waiting period, the color of an indicator on the test strip tells the woman if she is pregnant.

Pregnancy, multiple

A pregnancy in which there is more than one fetus. Women are more likely to have multiple pregnancies if they are black, are between the ages of 35 and 40, have had many pregnancies, are taking fertility drugs, or have a family history of twins. Multiple pregnancy is suspected if the uterus grows at an unusually

P

rapid pace, the doctor detects more than one fetal heartbeat, or there is more fetal movement than in previous pregnancies. Sometimes, multiple pregnancies are discovered incidentally during an ultrasound done for another purpose.

Multiple pregnancies carry an increased risk of complications. High blood pressure, PREECLAMPSIA, and POLYHYDRAMNIOS are more common during multiple pregnancies. Bed rest, or in severe cases, early delivery may be recommended. Preterm labor is common; about half of all multiple births occur before the 37th week of pregnancy because the fetuses grow too large for the uterus, which triggers uterine contractions. Labor may be slower and more difficult. A cesarean section may be needed.

Babies in multiple births are more likely to be of low birth weight, because of decreased space within the uterus and increased demands on the placenta for oxygen and nutrition. Women pregnant with multiple fetuses will undergo frequent ultrasound examinations to monitor fetal growth and to watch for changes in their positions. A NONSTRESS TEST may be used if one or more of the fetuses are not growing at a normal rate. See also TWINS.

Prehypertension

A condition that puts a person at risk for the long-term complications of HYPERTENSION. A blood pressure reading of 120 over 80 (120/80 mm HG) or lower was once considered normal, but national guidelines now say a person is considered to have prehypertension if readings are consistently from 120/80 up to 139/89. People with prehypertension are urged to get regular exercise, maintain a healthy body weight, limit alcohol to two drinks a day, and avoid a salty diet. See also BLOOD PRESSURE; HYPERTENSION.

Preleukemia

See MYELODYSPLASTIC SYNDROME.

Premature birth

The delivery of a baby before or during the 37th week of pregnancy. Approximately 10 percent of all babies are born prematurely. Smaller and more fragile than full-term babies, premature infants, (preemies), must be closely monitored in neonatal centers. They sleep in incubators,

where oxygen, temperature, and humidity are controlled. At increased risk of injury during birth, they may have breathing and liver problems and low blood sugar levels, and they are at particular risk for infection and bleeding.

CAUSES
Poor maternal health and nutrition, stress, and heavy smoking during pregnancy can increase a mother's chances of having a premature baby. Many low-income women and young teenagers receive inadequate prenatal care, which increases the chance that they will deliver prematurely.

Specific causes of premature birth include TOXEMIA OF PREGNANCY, diabetes, thyroid disturbances, PLACENTA PREVIA, fetal abnormalities, multiple pregnancies (twins, triplets), and infectious diseases, such as syphilis. Sometimes labor is induced before a pregnancy is full term because the mother's health makes it safer for the baby to be born than to continue in the womb. Maternal diabetes and high blood pressure are examples of medical disorders that sometimes dictate deliberate preterm delivery.

CARING FOR PREMATURE BABIES
Once delivered, premature babies have very particular needs. Because their lungs may not have manufactured SURFACTANT, a substance necessary to keep air sacs (ALVEOLI) open, they are at great risk of developing RESPIRATORY DISTRESS SYNDROME, which can be fatal. Intensive care nurseries have developed special methods of helping premature babies breathe by keeping the alveoli open with oxygen and the use of artificial surfactant administered through a tube in the baby's windpipe. Premature babies are monitored constantly for temperature changes, low blood sugar levels, sudden hemorrhages within the skull, and intestinal rupture or necrotizing enterocolitis, a life-threatening intestinal disease. Despite being at risk for numerous diseases and disorders, most premature babies grow up to be normal and healthy. See PRETERM LABOR.

Premature ejaculation

Discharge of semen (the thick, white fluid expelled from the penis) soon after sexual stimulation begins and before the partner experiences a satis-

fying level of arousal. Premature ejaculation can occur at any age after sexual maturity. The problem is almost always caused by psychological factors and only rarely arises from a physical condition, such as inflammation of the prostate. Premature ejaculation is common in the first sexual interactions between a couple. It also develops in relationships characterized by anxiety over sexual performance, pregnancy, or sexually transmitted disease; by guilt over breaking religious or social taboos; or by poor communication between partners.

Premature ejaculation can be treated to gain better control over an orgasm. Sensate focus exercises aim to give sensual pleasure in ways other than intercourse. In the start-and-stop technique, the man is stimulated until he feels an ejaculation is about to happen. The stimulation is withdrawn for 30 seconds, and then resumed. In the squeeze technique, the man or his partner squeezes the ridge below the tip (glans) of the penis between the thumb and forefinger when he feels he is about to ejaculate. The pressure is continued until the urge to ejaculate passes. The man teaches himself to control ejaculation until both partners are satisfied. Medication may also be effective.

Premature ovarian failure

The end of OVULATION and the menstrual cycle before age 40. See MENOPAUSE, PREMATURE.

Premenstrual syndrome

Physical and mental changes that some women experience each month as their menstrual periods approach. Also called PMS. See MENSTRUATION, DISORDERS OF.

Prenatal care

Health care provided to pregnant women. Prenatal care also involves education about pregnancy, labor, delivery, and parenting and the promotion of adequate nutritional support. Prenatal care ideally begins before the woman becomes pregnant. It continues with monthly visits until 28 weeks of gestation, then every 2 to 3 weeks until 36 weeks' gestation, and then weekly until the baby is born. Prenatal care makes possible the early detection and treatment of problems. A variety of diagnostic tests are available. Prenatal care also includes regular monitoring of the mother's weight and diet to ensure good nutrition, essential for the growth and development of the baby.

When pregnancy is confirmed, the doctor or midwife establishes the baby's due date and takes a detailed medical history, including a gynecological and obstetrical history. Such information will focus on previous pregnancies (including abortions and miscarriages), infertility tests and treatments, surgery on reproductive organs, and any gynecological problems, such as an abnormal PAP SMEAR result or abnormal discharge from the vagina, or any infections. A family medical history will illuminate any inherited disorders, such as hemophilia or sickle cell anemia, to which the baby may be subject. The obstetrical care provider will ask about any drugs that the woman takes regularly, including prescription and over-the-counter medications, alcohol, and illegal narcotics. Alcohol, drugs, and medication taken by the woman are likely to affect the developing fetus.

A complete physical examination, including a pelvic examination, should be done in all pregnant women. Checking the blood pressure and the heart, legs, and abdomen are important. Examining the uterus is critical because it provides vital information about fetal growth and age. A pelvic examination is important, and a Pap smear and cultures for sexually transmitted diseases are usually done. The doctor also estimates the size of the pelvis to predict whether the delivery will be difficult or whether a cesarean section may be required.

Prenatal tests that are usually performed only if necessary include AMNIOCENTESIS, CHORIONIC VILLUS SAMPLING, ultrasound (see ULTRASOUND, OBSTETRICAL), and fetal blood sampling, which is used when RH INCOMPATIBILITY is anticipated.

Prenatal testing

Tests and procedures to help ensure that a pregnancy produces a healthy baby while maintaining the mother's health. Several routine tests are recommended for all pregnancies, while more specialized testing is generally reserved for high-risk pregnancies, such as those involving mothers with heart disease or diabetes. Pregnancies that last longer than 42 weeks may also merit special testing.

Routine maternal blood tests are used to check blood type, Rh factor, and immunity to hepatitis B and German measles (rubella) and to rule out the presence of anemia and syphilis. Urine tests are given regularly to detect diabetes and the protein albumin, a sign of PREECLAMPSIA (a condition of pregnancy in which blood pressure is raised).

MONITORING HEART RATE

Two tests commonly used to monitor a baby's heart rate for possible problems are the CONTRACTION STRESS TEST and the NONSTRESS TEST. Both tests involve monitoring the fetal heart rate and the frequency and duration of any contractions in the uterus. A reactive nonstress test is one in which the baby has an increased heart rate in response to movement or contractions and is a sign of a healthy fetus. In a contraction stress test, the uterus is made to contract with the hormone oxytocin, which is either administered as a medication or produced naturally by gently stimulating the mother's nipples. A negative response to a contraction stress test is a good sign of a healthy baby, while a positive response may indicate potential problems. However, this test is associated with a high percentage of misleading results, and about 25 percent of babies with positive results are actually healthy. The doctor may repeat the test or use other tests to confirm positive results.

OTHER TESTS

Ultrasound (see ULTRASOUND, OBSTETRICAL) is an imaging procedure that helps a doctor evaluate the size, health, and position of the fetus. It can be used when the uterus appears to be either too small or too large, depending on the date of conception. Ultrasound is required to perform a test called a biophysical profile, which evaluates fetal muscle tone, breathing, heart rate, movement, and the quantity of amniotic fluid. Screening for suspected genetic disorders is conducted when a fetus is at risk for them. In CHORIONIC VILLUS SAMPLING (CVS), a tiny piece of tissue is removed from the placenta to test for genetic abnormalities in the fetus as early as the 10th week of pregnancy.

AMNIOCENTESIS is used to find chromosomal abnormalities in the amniotic fluid that may indicate Down syndrome or Tay-Sachs disease.

Depending on the circumstances, a doctor may order an AFP TEST (alphafetoprotein test) to screen for neural problems, as well as tests for sickle cell anemia, human immunodeficiency virus, tuberculosis and sexually transmitted diseases.

HIGH-RISK PREGNANCIES

Pregnant women who have diabetes, high blood pressure, or preeclampsia often need to have increased fetal surveillance. This may require nonstress tests, contraction stress tests, and a biophysical profile. Late in their pregnancy, women with diabetes may be required to undergo daily tests, because sharp changes in blood chemistry may signal immediate danger to the unborn baby.

Continuous surveillance of both fetal heart rate and uterine contractions is used in complicated and high-risk deliveries. Electronic FETAL MONITORING may be external or internal. External monitors are strapped around the mother's abdomen, while internal monitors are attached to the baby's scalp after amniotic membranes have ruptured and the cervix has opened to at least 1 centimeter. In high-risk situations, doctors considering early delivery need to find out whether fetal lung development is adequate to enable the baby to breathe on his or her own after birth. They may use amniocentesis to measure the quantity of certain fats present in the amniotic fluid that are associated with lung development. Also, if there is a deficiency of SURFACTANT, a liquid chemical produced by the lungs to facilitate breathing, steps can be taken to prevent RESPIRATORY DISTRESS SYNDROME in the fetus.

If a pregnancy has lasted more than 42 weeks, it is considered late, or postdate. A postdate pregnancy places the fetus at increased risk, and the doctor needs to test whether the fetus is healthy enough to remain in the uterus. Many doctors will check a baby's amniotic fluid during amniocentesis for the presence of MECONIUM, a sign of fetal distress.

Preoperative care

On the day of surgery, the patient is admitted into the hospital or the

P

same-day surgery center before being directed to the preoperative holding area. Before the person is sent to the operating room, the nurse checks to make sure that the patient has signed a surgical consent form and has had nothing to eat or drink for at least 6 hours, depending on the physicians' orders. In the preoperative area, vital signs will be monitored; sometimes the person being operated on will need a chest X ray, an electrocardiogram, or blood work, depending on the procedure. Often, the person's blood has been previously typed and cross-matched in case a blood transfusion becomes necessary during surgery. The anesthesiologist, surgeon, and nursing staff will discuss the procedure with the patient and answer any questions that the person may have. An intravenous catheter to provide a balanced salt solution will be inserted into the hand or arm to hydrate the patient during the surgery. The intravenous catheter can also be used to deliver a preoperative sedative or other appropriate medication before the patient is wheeled into the operating room where the surgery will take place.

Prepuce
A covering of skin, usually referring to the FORESKIN on the penis.

Presbycusis
See HEARING LOSS, IN OLDER PEOPLE.

Presbyopia
Age-related, progressive loss of the ability to focus on close objects. Close-up focusing depends on the lens of the eye changing shape (see ACCOMMODATION). As people age, the lens loses elasticity and becomes increasingly rigid. Presbyopia occurs to some degree in everyone and cannot be prevented. See Correcting farsightedness on page 550. Most people first notice difficulty with close vision at approximately age 40 to 45 years, when they need to hold reading material farther away in order to focus on it. Eyestrain, fatigue in the eyes, and headache may occur after close work. Presbyopia worsens gradually until approximately age 65 years, when the eyes have lost almost all of their ability to focus on close-up objects.

Presbyopia is usually treated with glasses. The degree of correction is prescribed by an eye specialist following an examination. People who also need correction for distance vision commonly use bifocals, which contain the distance correction in the upper half of the lens and a reading correction in the bottom half. People who need no distance correction may use only half glasses or reading glasses. Because presbyopia worsens gradually until age 65 years, the prescription for close vision typically needs to be changed every few years between ages 45 and 65 years.

Preservatives
Chemicals added to food to keep it from spoiling or rotting. Preservatives are used in the processing of many foods, including baked goods, dressings, hot dogs, bologna, salami, canned vegetables, dried fruit, fruit juices, jams and jellies, relishes, teas, and processed seafood products. Although preservatives are generally safe, certain ones (notably sulfites, benzoates, parabens, nitrates, and nitrites) cause adverse reactions in susceptible individuals. Signs of a problem include headaches, hives, abdominal cramps, diarrhea, chest tightness, light-headedness, lowered blood pressure, and weakness. Rarely, sulfites may also trigger asthma attacks. An allergist can help individuals identify the preservatives to which they are sensitive. Individuals can identify and avoid foods with preservatives by reading labels on processed foods.

Pressure points
Points on the body at which arteries can be compressed with a finger. Pressure points are spots on the body at which relatively slight pressure can be used to press an artery against an underlying bone, thereby stemming or slowing blood flow to the part of the body served by that artery. Such compression can reduce bleeding from a wound. For example, the femoral artery can be compressed against the pelvic bone in the groin.

Pressure sores
Open sores that develop on the skin from sustained pressure on a small

part of the body; also known as bedsores or decubitus ulcers. Pressure sores occur when a person sits or lies in the same position for an extended time. The pressure causes blood vessels to squeeze shut, stopping the flow of blood and inhibiting proper nourishment to the skin. Pressure sores most often occur on the buttocks, tailbone, shoulder blades, heels, and ankles. If left untreated or if they become infected, pressure

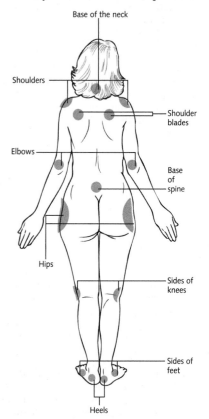

SENSITIVE AREAS ON THE BODY
Older people or those with chronic diseases who need caregiving are prone to pressure sores, often called bedsores. Areas in color are sensitive and most likely to develop pressure sores if the person is not moved frequently.

sores can even be life-threatening. They are most common in older people who are confined to bed in nursing homes and in disabled people who regularly use wheelchairs and are unable to shift position.

Pressure sores progress through four stages of severity. In stage 1, the skin over a bony area becomes pink or red and warm to the touch. In stage 2, a small break in the skin develops, and the area becomes blistered and ulcerated. In stage 3, the pressure sore penetrates the layer of fat under the skin. At this point, there is increasing likelihood of pain and drainage. In stage 4, the pressure sore extends all the way down to muscle or bone. It may turn white or black and have a foul odor. There is a risk of BACTEREMIA (bacteria in the bloodstream) or SEPSIS, a potentially fatal condition.

The first step in the treatment of pressure sores is to relieve the pressure. Open sores must be kept clean, rinsed, and covered with a dressing. Antibiotics may be required to combat infection. Severe pressure sores require surgery to remove dead tissue and encourage healing. Pressure sores can be prevented by regularly changing the position of people who use wheelchairs or are confined to bed. Those at risk of developing pressure sores require regular monitoring since a pressure sore can develop within hours. Good hygiene is essential; specially designed beds, mattresses, and cushions can also be helpful in prevention.

Preterm labor

Labor that occurs before or during the 37th week of pregnancy. Preterm labor can threaten the life of the fetus. Women at greatest risk for preterm labor are those who have delivered prematurely before, are carrying more than one fetus, have an infection during pregnancy, have an abnormality of the uterus or the cervix, have bleeding after the first trimester, or use cocaine. The warning signs of preterm labor include vaginal bleeding, watery vaginal discharge, abdominal cramps that may be accompanied by diarrhea and fever, pressure in the pelvis, low backache, and uterine contractions or tightening. Any of these signs should be reported to the doctor or midwife immediately.

The diagnosis of preterm labor is made by examining the cervix. If it has begun to open or shorten, the doctor may order an ultrasound to estimate the size and age of the fetus and determine its position in the uterus. The mother may be asked to monitor the contractions for a few days, noting any increase in frequency or severity. The cervix will be examined frequently to detect changes that indicate labor has begun, such as dilation (opening) or effacement (thinning).

TREATMENT
The doctor may try to stop labor if it is detected early enough and if neither mother nor baby is in danger from infection, bleeding, or other medical complications. Bed rest and extra fluids given by mouth or by intravenous drip are sometimes enough to stop contractions, and if labor can be stopped, the mother may be able to remain at home. Medications, such as terbutaline and ritodrine, may be used to prevent labor. Some women may need to stop certain physical activities, such as climbing stairs, while others may require partial or total bed rest for the balance of the pregnancy. The doctor may recommend cervical cerclage, a surgical procedure intended to hold the cervix closed. See CERCLAGE, CERVICAL.

If labor is established, hospitalization becomes necessary. In some cases, preterm labor has advanced too far to be stopped, while in others, medical problems for either the mother or fetus make premature birth preferable to leaving the baby in the uterus. See PREMATURE BIRTH.

Prevalence

The number of people in a population who have a given disease or characteristic within a particular time. Prevalence is usually expressed as a rate, which is determined by dividing the number of people with the disease (for example, 10,000) by the total population (200,000) in 1 year. In this example, the prevalence would be 0.05.

Priapism

Persistent, painful erection of the penis without sexual desire or arousal. Priapism is a rare but serious condition caused by blood trapped in the penis. The condition primarily affects young men. Priapism can result from prolonged sexual activity, injury or infection in the genitals, certain medications, blood disease (leukemia, sickle cell anemia), cancer in the pelvis, a pool of clotted blood in the pelvis, or a tumor on the spine affecting the nerves that control erections. Prompt treatment is necessary to prevent severe, permanent injury to the penis. Immediate treatment consists of pain medication, drugs to reduce blood pressure or thin the blood, drawing blood from the penis through a needle, or injecting medication into the penis. In rare cases, surgery may be necessary. In addition, any underlying condition causing the problem has to be treated.

Primary

A term denoting a disease or disorder that originates within the affected organ or tissue and is not derived from any other cause or source. For example, primary lung cancer arises from the tissues of the lung, whereas metastatic lung cancer is caused by the spread of a cancer originating elsewhere and spreading to the lung.

Primary care physician

The doctor who is usually the first contact for a patient experiencing a health problem. A primary care physician provides comprehensive and continuing care to people with any undiagnosed symptoms or health concerns. The area of primary care encompasses health promotion, disease prevention, patient education, and the diagnosis and treatment of acute and chronic illnesses. Primary care physicians coordinate consultation with or referrals to other doctors as appropriate. Primary care specialties include general internal medicine, family medicine, and pediatrics.

Primary teeth

The first set of teeth to appear, also called DECIDUOUS TEETH or baby teeth. The first primary teeth usually break through the gums when an infant is 6 months old, although it is not uncommon for them to appear sooner or later. The first primary teeth may appear at an earlier age in girls than in boys. Primary teeth are normally small and bright white; their roots are short and not firmly anchored in the jawbone. The enamel covering the crowns of the primary teeth is relatively thin and vulnerable to tooth decay. See BABY BOTTLE TOOTH DECAY.

Between the ages of 4 and 12 years, the primary teeth begin to come out, as they become crowded from below the gum line by the larger and heavier PERMANENT TEETH. The primary teeth are important for guiding the perma-

P

nent teeth into position. If a primary tooth is lost too early, the adjacent teeth can shift inward toward the empty space, blocking the emergence of the permanent tooth below. Primary teeth must be cleaned regularly to keep them healthy. If a primary tooth becomes decayed, infection in the gum and jawbone may cause the permanent teeth to become damaged.

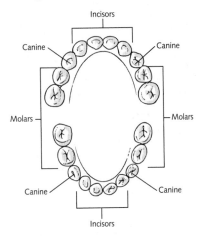

APPEARANCE OF FIRST TEETH
Generally, the primary teeth emerge from the front to the back of the jaws, starting with the lower front teeth. By the age of 2 to 3 years, all 20 of the primary teeth have usually emerged. Although the primary teeth begin to fall out between the ages of 4 and 7 years, they are just as important as the permanent teeth. The first teeth promote the development of the jaw bones and muscles, and they make space for the permanent teeth and guide them into position.

PRK

See PHOTOREFRACTIVE KERATECTOMY.

Procainamide hydrochloride

A drug used to treat cardiac arrhythmias. Procainamide hydrochloride (Procanbid, Pronestyl) is used to treat life-threatening disorders affecting the rhythm of the heart, including ventricular tachycardia (rapid heartbeat). Procainamide hydrochloride works by slowing nerve impulses in the heart and reducing the excitability of cardiac tissue.

Procaine

A medication used as a local anesthetic before surgical or dental treatment. Since procaine is short-acting

and relatively weak in its anesthetic effect, it is used for minor surgical procedures that require limited pain control.

Prochlorperazine

A drug used to control severe nausea, vomiting, and vertigo. Prochlorperazine (Compazine) is an antiemetic drug used to treat nausea before a surgical operation or any episode of severe nausea, vomiting, or vertigo. Prochlorperazine also has antipsychotic and antianxiety properties and is one of a group of drugs used to treat schizophrenia.

Procidentia

The PROLAPSE or slipping out of place of an organ. The term procidentia usually refers to a prolapsed uterus. See UTERUS, PROLAPSE OF.

Proctitis

Inflammation of the rectum. In some cases, proctitis is related to ulcerative colitis (inflammation of the lining of the colon). Sometimes, when the rectum is the only part of the colon to become inflamed, proctitis is more likely to be the result of a sexually transmitted disease, or STD (see SEXUALLY TRANSMITTED DISEASES). Proctitis due to SYPHILIS causes an open sore in the rectal area; GONORRHEA leads to a puslike or cloudy mucus discharge from the rectum; and herpes causes blistering ulcers. All can lead to itching and pain in the rectum and around the anus.

Sexually transmitted diseases, which are readily spread through vaginal or anal intercourse, can have grave consequences and require a prompt diagnosis. The treatment of proctitis depends on its underlying cause. Doctors generally prescribe anti-inflammatory drugs for colitis. Appropriate treatment of an STD depends on the type of infection.

Proctoscopy

Examination of the anus and rectum by using a rigid, cylindrical tube called a proctoscope. Proctoscopy enables the doctor to locate the source of bloody discharge from the anus. However, today proctoscopy has been largely superseded by flexible SIGMOIDOSCOPY. In contrast with proctoscopy, flexible sigmoidoscopy allows the physician to see upward

from the rectum into the sigmoid colon by using a slim, flexible, lighted tube called an endoscope. A flexible endoscope is usually more comfortable and easily passes further up the colon. An even more extensive alternative is COLONOSCOPY (examination of the large intestine from the rectum up through the colon, to the lower end of the small intestine, with a special endoscope).

Prodrome

An indication or symptom of the impending outbreak of a condition or disease. For example, a tingling or burning sensation is a prodrome or warning sign of a COLD SORE. Many infectious diseases are most contagious during their prodromal phase.

Progeria

A rare genetic disease that causes premature aging in young children. Symptoms include severe growth retardation in infancy, baldness, a widened face, large head for face size, small jaw, loss of eyebrows and eyelashes, limited range of motion, skeletal abnormalities such as osteoporosis, and thin, dry skin. Intelligence is unaffected. There is no treatment for progeria, and death usually occurs in the early teenage years because of severe arteriosclerosis of the coronary arteries, a disorder that causes thickening and loss of elasticity in the heart's arterial walls.

Progesterone

A female sex hormone produced by the ovaries. Progesterone secretion increases after ovulation and the second half of the menstrual cycle. Progesterone prepares the endometrium (lining of the uterus) for a fertilized egg. It is vital to a successful pregnancy as it promotes the normal growth and functioning of the placenta (the organ that develops in the uterus and links the mother's and fetus's blood supplies). The role of progesterone in placental development and function is essential to sustaining a healthy fetus. Progesterone is also produced in small amounts by the adrenal glands in men and women and in the testicles in men.

Synthetic progesterone is useful for treating various disorders. Inadequate production of progesterone may affect menstrual periods. This may be remedied by normalizing the balance of estrogen and progesterone with HORMONE REPLACEMENT THERAPY. Women with premenstrual syndrome sometimes obtain relief from symptoms with monthly injections of progesterone. The mini-pill is a form of birth control that contains only progesterone and is considered safer than estrogen for women with high blood pressure, diabetes, or a history of blood clots. A form of progesterone is included with estrogen in hormone replacement therapy occasionally prescribed to treat problems linked to a decreased estrogen level. Progesterone is included because it reduces the risk of endometrial cancer.

Progestin

A natural or synthetic hormone with effects similar to PROGESTERONE, an essential hormone of the female reproductive system. A woman with an intact uterus who takes HORMONE REPLACEMENT THERAPY should use a combination of estrogen and progestin to reduce the risk of ENDOMETRIAL CANCER associated with estrogen alone. Taken with estrogen, progestin limits the growth and buildup of the lining of the uterus, which is associated with cancer. Progestin is usually administered as a tablet. Some women who are receiving hormone replacement therapy take progestin along with estrogen every day, while others take it for only the first 12 to 14 days of the month. Women who take progestin for only part of the month are likely to have vaginal bleeding once the progestin has been withdrawn. Women who take progestin every day can take smaller doses. They may still have irregular bleeding for the first 6 months.

Progestin is also used as a contraceptive. Its advantages include lower risks for cardiovascular complications, endometrial and ovarian cancers, and pelvic inflammatory disease. Some women experience irregular vaginal bleeding, weight gain, breast tenderness, and depression when they use progestin alone without estrogen.

Prognathism

An abnormally projecting lower jaw. Prognathism may cause malocclusion (misalignment of the biting surfaces of the teeth). This condition may simply be an inherited facial shape, or it can be a symptom of an underlying disorder.

Prognosis

A prediction concerning the probable course of a disease and the chances of recovery. Based on the usual course of an illness and the special features of each individual case, doctors make a prognosis regarding a person's prospects of survival and recovery.

Progressive muscular atrophy

A type of MOTOR NEURON DISEASE in which the muscles of the hands, arms, and legs weaken and waste or atrophy. Involuntary twitching is another symptom. There is no cure for progressive muscular atrophy. This progressively debilitating condition eventually spreads to other muscles in the body.

Progressive systemic sclerosis

A form of chronic autoimmune disease involving the skin and connective tissue of the internal organs. Progressive systemic sclerosis (PSS) is a relatively rare disease that is a form of SCLERODERMA. It is also known as systemic sclerosis (SS) and the CREST SYNDROME and results in inflammation of the connective tissue surrounding the capillaries (tiny blood vessels). Internal scarring occurs as the inflammation heals; this shrinks and hardens the tissue. The disease may involve body organs and systems, including the esophagus, which tends to stiffen, as well as the intestines, lungs, heart, and kidneys. Gastrointestinal bleeding can occur. PSS can occur in both men and women, but usually affects women in their 30s and 40s. Individual incidents of disease are different from one another, and severity may vary widely from one person to another.

Typically, PSS causes an irreversible skin condition in which the skin becomes uncomfortably tight and glossy over the trunk and upper arms, in addition to areas of the face, chest, and extremities. Shortness of breath is often experienced as a result of scarring or fibrosis of the lungs. General symptoms such as a pro-longed, low-grade fever, malaise, and a loss of appetite resulting in weight loss are often experienced with PSS. Carpal tunnel syndrome can also occur. Several complications are involved, including gastrointestinal damage, lung damage, kidney failure, heart failure, and joint problems.

Diagnostic procedures for PSS may include blood tests and a barium swallow. If a diagnosis is confirmed, medication may be prescribed to help manage symptoms. Rehabilitation, including physical therapy and occupational therapy, may be recommended to help an affected person maintain a more independent life.

Prolactin

A hormone made in the pituitary gland that stimulates production of breast milk. Prolactin stimulates a pregnant woman's mammary glands to begin producing breast milk a few days before childbirth and to continue doing so as long as she breastfeeds her baby. Throughout pregnancy, high levels of ESTROGEN prevent production of milk, but once the baby is born, prolactin begins to stimulate the mammary glands (see BREAST) to start producing milk. Milk is not produced when women are not pregnant because the hypothalamus inhibits production of prolactin. When a mother begins to breast-feed her newborn, the act of sucking causes her hypothalamus to stop inhibiting prolactin and her breasts begin to produce milk.

Prolactin is produced on demand. When a baby empties his or her mother's breasts, the hypothalamus reduces its production of prolactin-inhibiting factor, and more milk is produced. When a mother's breasts are full of milk, the hypothalamus secretes prolactin-inhibiting factor in order to slow production. A mother with twins will produce twice as much milk as a mother with a single baby. If a mother stops breast-feeding for 2 to 3 weeks, prolactin production will stop altogether.

Nonpregnant women sometimes have high levels of prolactin that cause their breasts to secrete a milky discharge. Elevated prolactin levels can also cause a woman to have infrequent periods or no periods at all. Drugs such as tranquilizers, oral contraceptives, narcotics, antidepres-

P

sants, and some antihypertensive agents can induce high prolactin levels. The most common cause of excess prolactin is an abnormality in the pituitary gland. See BREAST-FEED-ING.

Prolactinoma

A noncancerous tumor of the pituitary gland that causes it to produce too much prolactin, the hormone that stimulates breast milk production. The chief symptom of prolactinoma is fluid leaking from the nipple of a woman who is neither pregnant nor breast-feeding. A doctor will examine the breast and test the fluid in a laboratory examination. If there are no abnormal cells in the fluid and the level of prolactin in the blood is normal, abnormal milk production is not a serious threat. However, if the level of prolactin in the blood is high enough, it can reduce production of ESTROGEN by the ovaries. Lack of estrogen can cause irregular or absent menstrual periods, infertility, and bone loss. The tumor can also cause headaches or put pressure on the optic nerves, limiting side vision. Prolactinoma can occur in men as well as women.

Prolapse

Displacement of all or part of an organ from its normal position. There are various types of prolapse. In uterine prolapse (see UTERUS, PROLAPSE OF), the uterus falls or slides from its normal position in the pelvic cavity into the vaginal canal. RECTAL PROLAPSE is the abnormal movement of the rectal mucosa down to or through the anal opening. MITRAL VALVE PROLAPSE (MVP) is a disorder in which the mitral heart valve bulges into the atrium, which may allow blood to leak back into the atrium from the ventricle. These conditions require medical evaluation and occasionally treatment, which varies according to the type of prolapse involved.

Prolotherapy

Treatment for chronic joint pain involving nonsurgical reconstruction of the ligament. Prolotherapy refers to the proliferation, or growth, of new ligament tissue holding bones to one another in the joints. Prolotherapy seeks to restore blood supply and nutrients to weakened ligaments and tendons (tissue holding bones to muscles), thereby stimulating the tissue to repair itself. To accomplish this goal, prolotherapists inject sugar water into the ligament or tendon at the point of attachment to bone. This causes localized inflammation that increases the blood supply to the affected area. Once ligaments or tendons have been treated by prolotherapy, the theory is that nerves in the area are no longer irritated, and chronic pain decreases.

Promethazine

A drug used to treat motion sickness, nausea, and allergies. Promethazine (Mepergan, Phenergan) is a drug that has antiemetic (antinausea), antivertigo, and antihistamine properties. In addition to being used to treat motion sickness, nausea, and allergies, promethazine is used to sedate a person before surgery or during labor and delivery.

Pronation

A prone position in which the body lies face downward or the arm rotates so that the palm of the hand faces downward and backward.

Prophylactic

A drug, procedure, or device used to prevent disease. The term "prophylactic" is also used to refer to a CONDOM.

Propoxyphene

A narcotic painkiller. Propoxyphene (Darvon) is used to relieve mild to moderate pain, providing pain relief equivalent to that from aspirin. Propoxyphene works by altering the person's response to painful stimuli. Although it is considered a mild narcotic, propoxyphene is nevertheless a controlled substance and can impair a person's ability to drive.

Propranolol

A beta blocker used to treat high blood pressure. Propranolol (Inderal, Inderide) has many properties and is used to treat other conditions besides high blood pressure. These include angina pectoris (chest pain), cardiac arrhythmias (irregular heartbeat), migraine headache, and tremors. Propranolol is also given to people who have had heart attacks to help increase survival rates.

Proprietary name

The brand name of a drug. As long as a pharmaceutical company holds a patent on a drug, it alone will produce and sell that drug, which will have a brand name in addition to its generic (established) name. The generic name is associated with the class of medicine and the chemical composition of the drug. The brand name belongs to a specific company and can be used only by that company as part of a promotional or marketing strategy for the drug.

Proprioception

The process by which the body collects and analyzes information about its position relative to its surroundings and of the body parts in relation to each other.

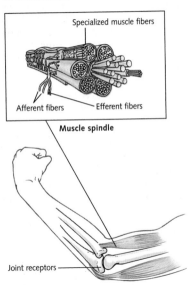

SENSE OF LIMB POSITION
Information about the position of an arm comes from different types of receptors. Joint receptors in the connective tissue control movement of the joint. Muscle spindle receptors are specialized muscle fibers entwined in nerve fibers. When a muscle is stretched, afferent (incoming) nerve fibers are activated. Efferent (outgoing) fibers are similarly activated when the muscle fiber is contracted.

Proprioceptive training

The instruction and practice of physical exercises designed to aid an athlete's perception of his or her body's position in space. Proprioceptive training is especially important to gymnasts who perform multiple turns in the air and must land upright on their feet. Balance and the ability to change directions of movements rapidly and smoothly are some components that are challenged in proprioceptive training.

Proptosis

See EXOPHTHALMOS.

Prostaglandins

Hormonelike substances manufactured in the body that produce a wide range of effects, including pain and inflammation in damaged tissue.

Prostate gland

A walnut-sized organ located just below the bladder and in front of the rectum in a man. The gland produces fluids that form part of semen, the substance released during EJACULATION. Sperm (male sex cells) pass through a duct in the prostate, and the fluids produced there nourish them and make them more active. Muscular tissue in the prostate also has a role in ejaculation. During ejaculation, the fluids are forced out of the prostate into the urethra and then out of the body.

The prostate gland consists of two main parts; the inner part produces the secretions that keep the lining of the urethra moist, and the outer part produces the secretions that mix with sperm.

The prostate gland matures and enlarges during puberty and may continue to grow slowly in men even after the age of 50.

Prostate, cancer of the

A malignant tumor of the prostate gland, which is part of the male reproductive system. The prostate is located under the bladder and surrounds the urethra, the tube that carries urine and semen out of the body through the penis. The prostate produces much of the fluid that makes up semen, the thick, white fluid expelled from the penis at sexual climax. Prostate cancer is the second most common cancer among men, exceeded only by skin cancer; it affects about one man out of eight over the course of a lifetime. Prostate cancer is also the second most common cause of cancer deaths among men, exceeded only by lung cancer.

SYMPTOMS AND DETECTION

In most cases, prostate cancer progresses slowly. As a result, prompt detection greatly increases chances for long-term survival. In its early stages, when the tumor is small and confined to the prostate, prostate cancer causes no symptoms. The symptoms appear only as the tumor enlarges and spreads outside the prostate, first to nearby organs (bladder, urethra, seminal vesicles), and

later to distant parts of the body, particularly the bones. Symptoms can include blood in the urine; pain or difficulty in urination; the need to urinate frequently, particularly at night (NOCTURIA); inability to achieve or maintain erections (ERECTILE DYSFUNCTION); and persistent pain in the pelvis, lower back, or upper legs. These symptoms are not unique to prostate cancer and can be caused by other noncancerous conditions.

CAUSES AND RISK FACTORS

The cause of prostate cancer is not known for sure, but a number of factors are suspected to increase risk. One is age. Prostate cancer is rare in men younger than age 50 and most common in men older than age 65. Heredity plays a role. Men whose fathers or brothers have had the disease, particularly when young, are at higher risk. Nationality is another risk factor. The disease is much more common in North America and northwestern Europe than in Africa, Asia, and Latin America. Among Americans, prostate cancer is twice as common among black men than among white men. Diet (increased fat consumption from dairy and red meat) and environmental factors may also play a role, since men of racially similar backgrounds living in different environments have varying rates of prostate cancer.

DETECTION AND DIAGNOSIS

Because prostate cancer causes no symptoms until it is advanced, the disease in its early stages is usually detected during routine medical examination. Physicians use two basic methods to screen for prostate cancer. One is the digital rectal examination. The physician inserts a gloved, lubricated finger into the rectum and feels the prostate to check for abnormalities. The exam is uncomfortable, but it causes no pain and takes only a few minutes. The second method is the PSA (PROSTATE-SPECIFIC ANTIGEN [PSA] TEST). This test checks the blood for PSA, a protein released by prostate cells. High levels of this protein can indicate prostate cancer. If an abnormality is found by the exam or PSA, a sample (biopsy) of prostate tissue is needed to determine whether cancer is present. The most common method is a core needle biopsy, a surgical procedure in which a physician uses an ultrasound image to guide a needle

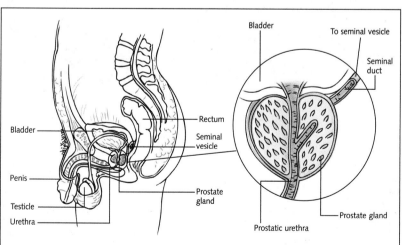

Bladder
To seminal vesicle
Seminal duct
Rectum
Seminal vesicle
Bladder
Penis
Testicle
Urethra
Prostate gland
Prostatic urethra
Prostate gland

ANATOMY OF THE PROSTATE
The prostate gland surrounds part of the urethra, just beneath the bladder. Sperm formed in the testicles go to the prostate gland, which bathes them with fluids, then stores and nourishes them in sacs called the seminal vesicles (at the base of the prostate) before releasing them into the urethra during ejaculation.

P

FOCUS ON PROSTATE CANCER

Prostate cancer is a malignant growth of the cells of the prostate gland that generally develops slowly over a period of years. As the tumor grows, the cancer may spread to the bladder and seminal vesicles or to the lymph nodes of the pelvis and the bones of the spine. Black men have a higher risk of getting prostate cancer than do Asian or white men.

A DIGITAL RECTAL EXAM
In a digital rectal exam, the physician inserts a gloved finger into the rectum and feels for lumps within the prostate gland and in the rectal wall. Men should start yearly rectal exams at the age of 40, and yearly PSA (prostate-specific antigen) blood tests at the age of 50. Men with family histories of prostate cancer and black men should consider starting these tests earlier. If either the digital rectal exam or the PSA test result suggests cancer, a prostate ultrasound and biopsy may be recommended.

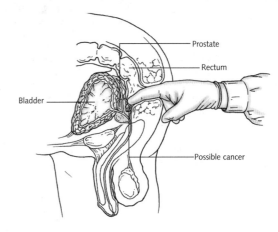

Prostate
Rectum
Bladder
Possible cancer

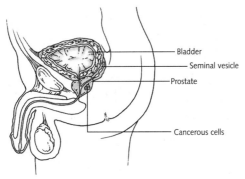

Bladder
Seminal vesicle
Prostate
Cancerous cells

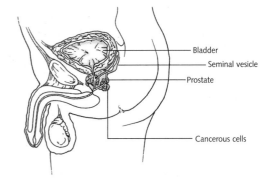

Bladder
Seminal vesicle
Prostate
Cancerous cells

STAGE II PROSTATE CANCER
In stage II prostate cancer, the cancer is still contained within the prostate capsule and is confined to one lobe of the prostate. However, the lump is large enough for the doctor to feel in a digital exam.

STAGE III PROSTATE CANCER
In stage III prostate cancer, the cancer has grown through the prostate capsule and has begun to invade surrounding organs. Biopsies of the rectum and bladder and imaging tests such as CT scan and MRI are used to determine whether the cancer has reached this stage.

BRACHYTHERAPY
Brachytherapy is a newer treatment for dealing with prostate cancer in which radiation is targeted directly into the prostate tissue. The goal is to shrink the tumors, while minimizing radiation damage to the surrounding organs, and to prevent a prostatectomy. By using a fine needle, and with ultrasound as a guide, the physician implants 60 to 120 radioactive pellets (each about the size of a grain of rice) into the prostate gland. Pellet placement is usually accomplished within an hour; spinal anesthesia is used.

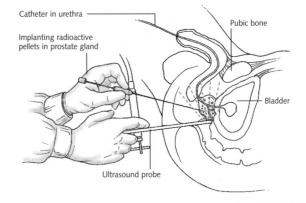

Catheter in urethra
Pubic bone
Implanting radioactive pellets in prostate gland
Bladder
Ultrasound probe

P

through the wall of the rectum to take thin cylinders of tissue from the prostate. Usually six or more samples are removed: upper, middle, and lower from each side. A biopsy is performed in the office of a doctor and takes about 10 minutes. The doctor uses a special instrument to insert and withdraw the needle in a fraction of a second to minimize pain and discomfort.

If cancerous cells are found in the biopsy specimen, further tests are performed to determine the stage of the disease. A radionuclide bone scan may be ordered to look for prostate cancer that may have spread to the bones. The man is injected with a low-level radioactive substance that is attracted to diseased bone cells throughout the skeleton. These areas appear in the scan as dense, gray areas called hot spots, which may be due to the spread of cancer. Hot spots can also be caused by other diseases, including arthritis, and follow-up tests may be needed to determine their exact nature. Another nuclear medicine test uses injected radioactive material attached to a monoclonal antibody that is attracted to prostate cells, both normal and cancerous. The monoclonal antibody scan can detect cancer in enlarged lymph nodes and bone; the amount of radiation used in radionuclide and monoclonal antibody scans is very low and poses little risk.

TREATMENT

The choice of therapy for prostate cancer varies greatly from case to case, depending on the stage of the disease, the age and general health of the man, and his preferences regarding long-term survival versus tolerating the side effects of treatment. A number of options are available. The type of treatment should be chosen by the individual in consultation with his physician.

■ *Watchful waiting* Since prostate cancer progresses slowly, some men opt for no immediate treatment. This option is well suited to older men who are experiencing no symptoms or who may have other serious or more immediate health problems. The cancer is checked regularly, usually by DRE and PSA tests every 6 months and prostate biopsies every year. If the cancer begins to grow or symptoms become troublesome, treatment can begin.

MONITORING PROSTATE SYMPTOMS

Most prostate cancers are discovered during a man's routine rectal examination; there usually are no symptoms. Bothersome symptoms, however, are usually caused by an enlarged prostate, not cancer. Watch for any of the following symptoms and report them to a doctor:

- **The urge to urinate frequently, especially at night**
- **A weak or interrupted stream of urine**
- **Difficulty starting or stopping urination**
- **Pain or burning while urinating**
- **Blood in the urine**
- **Stiffness or pain in the lower back, hips, or upper thighs**
- **Painful or blood-tinged ejaculation**
- **Inability to urinate**

■ *Surgery* The goal of radical PROSTATECTOMY is to eliminate the cancer by removing the prostate and surrounding lymph nodes. Radical prostatectomy is major surgery requiring general or regional anesthesia, a hospital stay of about 3 days, and an at-home recovery period of 3 to 5 weeks. Possible complications include difficulty in retaining urine (see INCONTINENCE, URINARY), failure to achieve or maintain erections (ERECTILE DYSFUNCTION), abnormal bleeding, and injury to the rectum, bladder, or the tube connecting the kidney and bladder (ureter).

If the man is troubled by urinary blockage and other symptoms, a transurethral resection of the prostate (TURP) may be performed. This surgery is not intended to cure the disease or remove all of the cancer, but to alleviate symptoms. After administration of general or spinal anesthesia, a tool with a small loop of wire at the end (electrocautery) is inserted through the opening in the penis and into the prostate. Electricity passing through the wire cuts away the excess prostate tissue and seals cut blood vessels. A hospital stay, typically 1 or 2 days, is required. Complications can include ejaculation into the bladder rather than out through the penis (retrograde ejaculation), erectile dysfunction, and, rarely, incontinence.

■ *Radiation* Radiation therapy involves the use of high-energy rays or particles to kill cancer cells. It can be used in place of surgery for cancer that is localized in the prostate or has spread to nearby tissue. Radiation is as effective as surgery in stopping early-stage prostate cancer. It may also be used to shrink the tumor and alleviate symptoms in instances of more advanced disease.

There are two types of radiation therapy. In external-beam radiation, rays or particles from a source outside the body are focused on the cancerous area. Men are usually treated 5 days a week for 7 or 8 weeks. Treatment takes place in an outpatient clinic, lasts a few minutes, and is painless. External-beam radiation can cause damage to the rectum and the bladder. In most cases, these problems clear up within a few months of treatment. Erectile dysfunction may also appear as long as 1 to 2 years after treatment. Fatigue often develops during radiation therapy and then clears up within 1 or 2 months after treatment ends.

The second type of radiation therapy is brachytherapy, also known as internal or interstitial radiation therapy. Small radioactive iodine pellets about the size of rice grains are placed directly in the prostate. The pellets are arranged inside thin needles that are inserted through the skin of the perineum. An imaging device, such as ultrasound, is used to guide the needles accurately. Sometimes, pellets that give off low doses of radiation for weeks or months are used; they are left inside the prostate. Since the pellets are small, they cause little or no discomfort. High-dose pellets may also be used; they are left in place for less than a day and then removed. For approximately 1 week after therapy, the perineum may be sore, and urine may have a red-brown color. Brachytherapy can cause significant rectal problems (burning, diarrhea, pain) that are difficult to treat, but it has a lower risk of causing erectile dysfunction than does prostatectomy or external-beam radiation.

Men with advanced, metastatic prostate cancer affecting the bones

---

📖 Terms in small capital letters—for example, PHYSICAL THERAPY or PAGET DISEASE—indicate a cross-reference to another entry with more information.

P

may be treated with injections of strontium-89, a radioactive substance that binds to areas of bone cancer. Sometimes strontium-89 injections are combined with external-source radiation aimed at the worst bone metastases. These treatments do not cure the cancer, but they reduce pain and other symptoms.

■*Hormone therapy* Male hormones, or androgens, cause prostate cancer cells to grow. Lowering the level of androgens can slow the growth of the tumor or shrink it. Hormone therapy is used for patients whose cancer has spread to other parts of the body or has returned after surgery or radiation. Testosterone, which is produced in the testicles, is the primary androgen; surgically removing the testicles (orchiectomy) is sometimes recommended as the most direct mode of hormone therapy. An orchiectomy reduces or eliminates sexual desire (libido) and often causes erectile dysfunction. In addition, breast tissue may become tender and grow. Medications can also be used to decrease the amount of testosterone produced by the testicles and to block the ability of the body to use androgens. These medications may be given continuously or intermittently, whenever a rising PSA level indicates that the cancer is growing. They may also be combined with orchiectomy. Complications of hormone therapy medications may include reduced or nonexistent libido, hot flashes, breast tenderness or growth, nausea, diarrhea, and fatigue.

■*Chemotherapy* Cancer-killing medications are used for patients whose disease has spread outside the prostate and who are no longer helped by hormone therapy. Chemotherapy does not eliminate the cancer, but can slow its progression and often alleviates pain. It is not used for men with early-stage prostate cancer. Side effects include hair loss, nausea and vomiting, loss of appetite, fatigue, and increased risk of infection and bleeding caused by changes in the blood. These side effects are temporary, ceasing when the therapy ends. Many men can be treated with other medications to counter the negative side effects caused by chemotherapy.

PREVENTION
Since the causes of prostate cancer remain unclear, no preventive strategy has yet been developed. Diet may play a role in the development of this disease, so many physicians advocate a diet rich in fruits, vegetables (especially tomatoes), and grains and low in fats, particularly from dairy or animal sources. Regular exercise is also advised. Early detection of prostate cancer before it has spread outside the gland offers the best chance for successful treatment. Current guidelines suggest that all men older than age 50 in otherwise good health have a rectal exam and PSA test as part of their annual physical examination. High-risk men, including blacks and those whose fathers or brothers have had prostate cancer, are commonly advised to begin screening between ages 40 and 45.

Prostate, enlarged
Noncancerous swelling of the PROSTATE GLAND. The prostate, located at the base of the bladder and surrounding the tube (urethra) that transports urine to the outside, helps to produce semen. An enlarged prostate is also known as benign prostatic hyperplasia (BPH), which is usually a result of aging. The disease is rare before age 40 but affects more than half of all men by age 60. However, only about half of the men with enlarged prostates experience symptoms that require medical attention.

SYMPTOMS AND DIAGNOSIS
Benign prostatic hyperplasia develops first in the portion of the prostate surrounding the urethra, narrowing this urinary passage. Signs include slowed or delayed start of urination, a weak urine stream, pain during urination, blood in the urine, difficulty emptying the bladder, frequent urination, repeated urinary tract infections, increased urination at night, a strong sudden desire to urinate, and leaking of urine (see INCONTINENCE, URINARY). Sexual functioning is usually not affected. In severe cases, the ability to urinate may be lost because of blockage to the urinary tract by the enlarged prostate or by a loss of muscle tone and strength in the bladder as a result of the disease. The inability to urinate may develop slowly, leading to kidney damage and kidney failure, or it can occur suddenly and be very painful. Complete blockage is a medical emergency.

An enlarged prostate is usually diagnosed with a digital rectal examination; the physician inserts a finger into the rectum to examine the prostate. Additional tests may be performed, for example, to determine the rate of urine flow or the amount of urine left in the bladder after urination or to visually inspect the prostate and bladder (cystoscopy). Although an enlarged prostate does not cause or lead to cancer, the two conditions may occur together. A blood test for prostate cancer, the PSA (prostate-specific antigen) test, is often recommended.

TREATMENT
Severity of symptoms and the inconvenience and difficulty they pose for the person are key criteria in choosing a treatment option.

■*Annual monitoring* For men with no or minor symptoms, the condition may be monitored annually to see if it

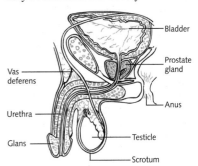

Healthy male reproductive system

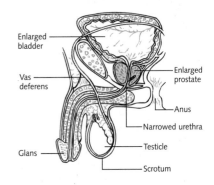

Enlarged prostate gland

NONCANCEROUS PROSTATE SWELLING
Because the prostate gland wraps around the first part of the urethra, an enlarged prostate constricts the urethra. Urination is slow or painful; emptying the bladder is difficult so the bladder becomes distended. Sexual function is generally not affected.

worsens. In a significant number of cases, BPH does not worsen or it improves without treatment. Self-help measures can be successful with minor symptoms. These include moderating alcohol and fluid intake, particularly in the evening, and urinating at first urge.

■ *Medication* Alpha-1 blockers, usually used to treat high blood pressure (HYPERTENSION), relax the muscles of the bladder for easier urination. A medication called finasteride lowers prostate hormone levels, reducing the size of the gland and decreasing BPH symptoms. In a small number of people, finasteride decreases sex drive or causes impotence. Antibiotics are given to individuals with chronic infections of the prostate and bladder because eliminating the infection may alleviate symptoms.

■ *Surgery* Surgery is recommended for men with incontinence, blood in the urine, long-standing inability to empty the bladder, or severe, repeated infections. The type of surgery depends on the severity of symptoms and the size and shape of the prostate.

Transurethral incision of the prostate (TUIP) is a surgical procedure used when the prostate is relatively small. After anesthesia is given, an incision is made in the prostate to enlarge the outlet of the bladder and the opening of the urethra and to allow easier passage of urine. The procedure is performed as same-day or ambulatory surgery and does not require an overnight hospital stay. Complications can include excessive bleeding, infection, damage to the urethra, and ejaculation into the bladder rather than through the penis, which is called retrograde ejacula-

tion. Inability to achieve or maintain erections (ERECTILE DYSFUNCTION) is an uncommon complication.

Transurethral resection of the prostate (TURP) is the most common type of surgery for BPH. After the person receives spinal or epidural anesthesia, a surgical tool with a small loop of wire at the end (electrocautery) is inserted through the opening in the penis and into the prostate. Electricity passing through the wire cuts through the excess prostate tissue and seals cut blood vessels. A hospital stay of 1 or 2 days is required. Complications can include retrograde ejaculation, erectile dysfunction, and, rarely, incontinence.

Open PROSTATECTOMY involves the removal of the prostate through a surgical incision, but only the middle of the prostate is removed. Prostatectomy is a procedure involving a hospital stay of 5 to 7 days, and it is used only for severe cases with massively enlarged prostate glands. Complete removal of the prostate (radical prostatectomy) is performed for prostate cancer. Complications include erectile dysfunction and incontinence.

Prostatectomy

Surgical removal of all or part of the PROSTATE GLAND, which produces much of the fluid in semen. The prostate is positioned below the bladder and surrounds the tube (urethra) that carries urine and semen out of the body through the penis. Prostatectomy is performed to eliminate the symptoms of an enlarged prostate (see PROSTATE, ENLARGED) or to treat cancer of the prostate (see PROSTATE, CANCER OF THE), particularly in its early stages. Different procedures are used, depending

on the health of the man, the size and condition of the prostate, and the reason for surgery.

TRANSURETHRAL INCISION OF THE PROSTATE (TUIP)

The least extensive and invasive form of prostatectomy, TUIP is used to treat urinary difficulties in men whose prostate is enlarged but still relatively small or normal-sized. It is not used to treat cancer. The procedure is performed on an outpatient basis, after the man has been given general or regional anesthesia, and does not require a hospital stay. A viewing instrument is inserted into the opening of the penis to allow the surgeon to see inside the prostate, and a small incision is made where the prostate joins the bladder. The incision serves to enlarge the opening between the bladder and urethra and improve the flow of urine. A rubber tube (catheter) is often placed in the urethra to drain the bladder after surgery; it is removed after a few days. Complications from TUIP include urinary difficulties, erectile dysfunction, and ejaculation into the bladder rather than through the penis (retrograde ejaculation).

TRANSURETHRAL RESECTION OF THE PROSTATE (TURP)

The TURP is similar to TUIP, but the procedure is more extensive, with more of the prostate being removed. The procedure is performed after the man has been given general or spinal anesthesia. A hospital stay of 1 or 2 days is required. A viewing instrument is inserted into the prostate via the penis and used to guide a tool with a small loop of wire at the end (electrocautery). Electricity passing through the wire cuts away the tissue and seals cut blood vessels. A catheter is often placed in the urethra to drain the bladder for several days after surgery. At first, the urine appears very bloody and contains shreds of tissue. Fluid may be introduced into the bladder through the catheter to flush it out and prevent clogging. The bleeding decreases and the catheter is removed within a few days. Complications can include excessive bleeding, retrograde ejaculation, erectile dysfunction, and, rarely, incontinence.

RADICAL PROSTATECTOMY

An incision is made and the prostate is taken out as a single unit along with some surrounding tissue, partic-

P

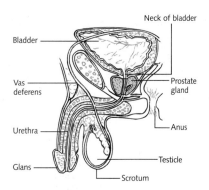

Neck of bladder
Bladder
Vas deferens
Prostate gland
Urethra
Anus
Glans
Testicle
Scrotum

Before radical prostatectomy

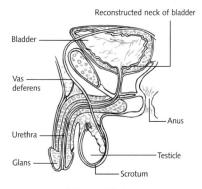

Reconstructed neck of bladder
Bladder
Vas deferens
Urethra
Anus
Glans
Testicle
Scrotum

After prostatectomy

RADICAL PROSTATECTOMY
If a man has prostate cancer that has not spread to other organs, the recommended treatment may be a radical prostatectomy to remove the prostate and, generally, the neck (lower portion) of the bladder and the seminal vesicles. The neck of the bladder is then reconstructed and reattached to the urethra.

ularly the seminal vesicles (which produce secretions that mix with prostate fluids to make the liquid portion of semen). Radical prostatectomy is a major surgery performed after the man has been given general or spinal anesthesia, lasting 1 to 4 hours on average, and requiring a hospital stay of approximately 3 days and from 3 to 5 weeks off work. The operation generally serves as treatment for prostate cancer in its early stages.

There are two main types of radical prostatectomy. In the retropubic procedure, the surgeon makes an incision in the lower abdomen below the navel to expose the prostate. Lymph nodes can also be removed and examined for spread of cancer from the prostate. In a nerve-sparing retropubic radical prostatectomy, the sur-

geon checks the nerve bundles that lie close to each side of the prostate; if no cancer is present, the nerves are left in place. Since these nerves are responsible for erection of the penis, leaving them intact lowers the risk of erectile dysfunction following surgery. In the perineal procedure, the surgeon reaches the prostate through an incision in the skin between the scrotum and the anus (perineum). If lymph nodes are needed for examination, they are removed through a thin tube (laparoscope) inserted through a small incision in the abdomen. Nerve sparing is more difficult with the perineal procedure than the retropubic.

Following a radical prostatectomy, a catheter is usually placed in the urethra (the tube that carries urine out of the body from the bladder). The catheter remains in place for 2 to 3

weeks following surgery to aid in healing. After it is removed, the man can urinate on his own.

Radical prostatectomy, like all abdominal surgery, carries a risk of blood clots that can block major blood vessels. Stockings to prevent clotting are often worn after the surgery, and men are encouraged to get out of bed and begin walking as soon as possible. Other postsurgical complications include infection of the wound or the urinary tract and excessive bleeding. Long-term problems include difficulty in holding urine (incontinence) and erectile dysfunction.

Prostate-specific antigen (PSA) test
A blood test used to detect and monitor prostate cancer (see PROSTATE, CANCER OF THE). Prostate-specific anti-

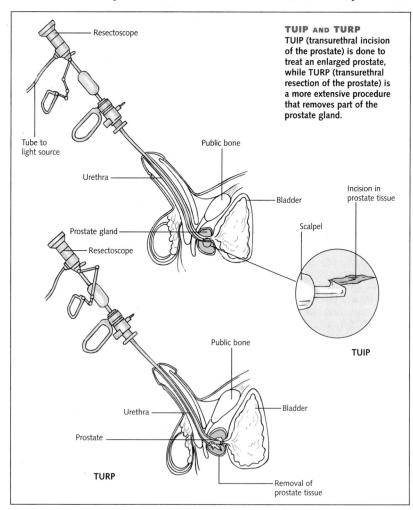

Resectoscope
Tube to light source
Urethra
Prostate gland
Resectoscope

TUIP AND TURP
TUIP (transurethral incision of the prostate) is done to treat an enlarged prostate, while TURP (transurethral resection of the prostate) is a more extensive procedure that removes part of the prostate gland.

Public bone
Bladder
Incision in prostate tissue
Scalpel
TUIP

Public bone
Urethra
Prostate
Bladder
Removal of prostate tissue
TURP

gen is a protein normally found in the blood of adult men. Its level increases with prostate disorders, and it can rise substantially with cancer of the prostate. Monitoring the PSA level over time may be of help in detecting prostate cancer in its early stages, when the chances of successful treatment are highest. The test can also be used after prostate cancer treatment to determine the effectiveness of that treatment.

The test is performed by drawing blood with a needle from a vein in the back of the hand or the inside of the elbow. The blood is then analyzed by a medical laboratory for the PSA concentration. The PSA results are reported in nanograms of PSA per milliliter of blood (ng/mL). A normal PSA level is below 4 ng/mL, while a level above 4 ng/mL increases the risk of prostate cancer.

The difficulty in interpreting PSA results is that high values do not necessarily indicate cancer, nor do low values mean that a patient is cancer-free. Noncancerous enlargement of the prostate (see PROSTATE, ENLARGED) raises PSA values, while PSA results do not increase with some cancers. In addition, PSA values rise with age. As a result, a normal value in an 80-year-old man would be an abnormal reading in a 40-year-old man. The physician must combine PSA results with other tests and examinations to determine the health of the prostate.

If a man younger than 70 has elevated PSA results and examination of a sample (biopsy) of his prostate detects no cancer, doctors use two other PSA measurements as a follow-up. One is PSA velocity. If PSA results rise at an annual rate equaling or exceeding 0.75 ng/mL in the years following the biopsy, the biopsy may be repeated. The second is PSA density, which helps to distinguish PSA values increased by benign disease as opposed to cancer. The physician divides the PSA result numbers by the prostate's volume. If the result exceeds a certain number, the biopsy will most likely be repeated.

The PSA testing is also used to monitor the success of treatments for prostate cancer. After complete surgical removal of the prostate (radical prostatectomy), the PSA value should fall to 0. If it fails to do so, some cancer remains. If it falls to 0 and then rises, the cancer has probably recurred. Likewise, dropping PSA values after treatment for advanced cancer indicate success in slowing the progression of the disease.

Guidelines on PSA testing to screen for prostate cancer differ among various groups of physicians. Each man should decide whether to be tested and how often in consultation with his physician, based on his concern about prostate cancer, the side effects of treatment, and his individual risk.

Prostatitis

Inflammation of the prostate, a gland in the male reproductive system that is located under the bladder. The prostate produces much of the fluid in semen, the thick, white fluid expelled from the penis at sexual climax, and the prostate surrounds the tube (urethra) that carries semen and urine out of the body through the penis.

Prostatitis can be caused by any of a number of microorganisms, such as bacteria normally found in the intestinal tract, those that cause certain sexually transmitted diseases, and those that cause bladder and urinary tract infections. In some cases, the microorganism cannot be identified.

Symptoms may come on suddenly and severely (acute prostatitis), or they may be long-standing and only mildly bothersome, with periodic flare-ups (called chronic prostatitis). Symptoms can include fever and chills, along with pain in the lower back, abdomen, testicle, or the area between the scrotum and anus. Other symptoms include pain or burning upon urination, ejaculation, or bowel movement; increased urge to urinate; blood in the urine or semen; and aches in the muscles and joints. The infection may also involve the bladder, testicles, or epididymis. In severe cases, the man cannot urinate, and urine must be drained from the bladder through a thin rubber tube (catheter) placed surgically through the skin of the lower abdomen and left in place until the infection is brought under control.

Bacterial prostatitis is treated with antibiotic medication during a 4- to 16-week period. Nonbacterial prostatitis may require only a 2-week course of medication. Stool softeners may be used to prevent pain during bowel movements. Sitting in a tub of warm water can help to alleviate pain and aching in the lower abdomen and pelvis. Men with prostatitis are also advised to drink large amounts of fluid to help clear the urinary tract of infectious microorganisms and to avoid foods and beverages that irritate the urethra, such as caffeine, alcohol, spicy food, chocolate, tomatoes, and citrus juices. Treatment is generally successful, but recurrence of the infection is common and requires additional treatment.

Prosthesis

An artificial or manufactured substitute for a missing or nonfunctioning body part. Prostheses can include artificial legs, arms, teeth, eyes, joints, dentures, hearing aids, pacemakers, and many other substitutes for body parts. Prostheses can replace body parts that are nonfunctional or have been amputated, as in the case of a person's leg. Advances in the field of surgical amputation and the art of designing artificial limbs have made it possible for people who have lost a limb to receive a prosthesis that closely resembles the original and works nearly as efficiently. People are usually fitted with a prosthesis immediately after surgical amputation of a body part so that they can resume movement right away without risking the complications of inactivity.

Prostheses are made of various materials, including wood, aluminum, and plastic, all of which can

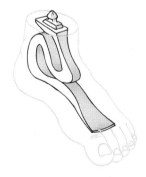

ARTIFICIAL FOOT
One type of foot prosthesis, attached at the ankle, provides the support and balance of the missing foot (shown in outline). Many modern prostheses are cosmetically and functionally realistic. Computer-controlled prostheses simulate natural movements, programmed to accommodate an individual's needs.

P

be used to construct artificial limbs. Muscle power may be reinforced by means of various mechanical devices. The most common artificial limb is the knee-jointed leg, fitted on people who have had a leg amputated above the knee. Artificial arms are available, designed in various ways according to the occupational needs of the person. A person who does heavy work will require a purely functional artificial arm, while others will prefer a cosmetic arm meant to look as natural as possible. A great many different types of hand prostheses are available, including mechanical hands.

Prosthodontics

The specialized branch of dentistry that involves the replacement of missing teeth and their supporting structures. This field includes COSMETIC DENTISTRY, as well as the evaluation and treatment of MALOCCLUSION, an irregular alignment of the teeth. Dentists who specialize in prosthodontics are called prosthodontists. They are trained in the design, construction, and fitting of artificial substitutes for the teeth, including DENTURES, crowns, bridges, and dental implants (see CROWN, DENTAL; BRIDGE, DENTAL; and IMPLANTS, DENTAL). Prosthodontists evaluate the health of the existing teeth and the supporting structures to determine the appropriate replacements for teeth that may have been lost due to tooth decay, periodontal disease, or physical trauma.

Protease inhibitors

A drug class used to treat AIDS (acquired immunodeficiency syndrome). Protease inhibitors work by suppressing the ability of the HIV (human immunodeficiency virus) to reproduce. Protease inhibitors are always used in combination with other AIDS drugs and sometimes with other protease inhibitors. There are four protease inhibitors currently on the market: indinavir (Crixivan), nelfinavir (Viracept), ritonavir (Norvir), and saquinavir (Invirase).

It is important for protease inhibitors to be taken exactly as prescribed, because drug resistance can develop very quickly in the virus that causes HIV. People with AIDS should never use protease inhibitors alone, and they should never miss doses or days of therapy.

Protein synthesis

The process by which molecules of protein are broken down into AMINO ACIDS. Protein synthesis is a necessary part of digestion that takes place in the stomach and small intestine. Giant molecules of protein must be digested by enzymes before they can be used to build and repair body tissues. For the most part this process takes place in the small intestine, where enzymes from the pancreas and intestinal lining break the large molecules down into small ones called amino acids. Amino acids can be absorbed into the blood and carried throughout the body to build and repair tissues.

Proteins

Complex organic compounds found in every living cell. Proteins are made up of chains of AMINO ACIDS containing carbon, hydrogen, oxygen, and nitrogen. Protein is necessary in the diet to provide the body with adequate amino acids for PROTEIN SYNTHESIS. Protein is the main component of muscles, organs, and glands. The cells of muscles, tendons, and ligaments are maintained with protein. A nutritionally balanced diet will contain adequate protein, whether from animal or plant products.

Proteinuria

The presence of protein in the urine. Proteinuria indicates that the kidneys are not functioning properly. It may be discovered by a urine dipstick test taken in the doctor's office. In a dipstick test, a strip of cellulose is dipped into a sample of urine. The strip will change color to indicate the presence of protein in the urine. A more precise measurement of protein in the urine involves collecting urine for 24 hours and then testing the urine for protein.

One function of healthy kidneys is separating protein from waste products in the blood. Healthy kidneys remove waste products while leaving protein in the blood. When protein is passed into the urine, it indicates that the kidneys are not working properly. Very foamy urine may be a sign of high protein levels.

Proton pump inhibitors

Antiulcer drugs; called proton pump inhibitors and used to treat peptic ulcers; gastroesophageal reflux disease (GERD), in which stomach acid backs up into the esophagus, causing painful heartburn; and diseases such as Zollinger-Ellison syndrome, in which too much acid is released into the stomach. Proton pump inhibitors work by blocking the production of stomach acid. The drugs do this by inhibiting the proton pump, an enzyme system responsible for making stomach acid.

The proton pump inhibitors include lansoprazole (Prevacid) and omeprazole (Prilosec). Proton pump inhibitors are usually taken before meals.

Protozoa

The simplest single-celled organisms classified as animals; the smallest type of life. The word protozoa means "primitive animals" in Greek. Certain protozoa can infect the body and cause disease, such as dysentery and sleeping sickness.

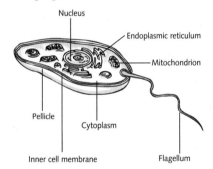

SINGLE-CELLED ORGANISM
Structural components of protozoa include a nucleus that contains the cell's genetic material; the endoplasmic reticulum that makes proteins for the cell's maintenance; cytoplasm, the fluid that contains dissolved food and chemicals and waste products of the cell's activity; mitochondria that produce energy; the pellicle that is the cell's outermost membrane; and the flagellum, which propels the cell.

Proximal

In anatomy, the portion of a body part located nearest its point of origin or attachment, or close to the median line (center) of the body. For example, the proximal end of the femur, or thighbone, forms part of the hip joint. The opposite of proximal is DISTAL.

Prurigo

A chronic mild to severe inflammatory skin condition characterized by intense itching. Prurigo consists of very itchy papules (small superficial bumps on the skin) and nodules (solid masses of tissue) on skin areas that are easily reached. The small, dome-shaped bumps are caused by repeated scratching and picking. The lesions may become infected and crust over, and skin can grow thick. Itching can be relieved to some extent by applying cool compresses and prescription topical corticosteroids and by taking over-the-counter or prescription antihistamines. Corticosteroid injections into the bumps and phototherapy (treatment with light) are sometimes successful treatments.

Pruritus

The medical term for itching. Pruritus ranges from a mild urge to scratch to an overwhelming, unbearable itch. Common causes of pruritus include insect bites; allergic contact dermatitis (such as poison ivy); irritants such as chemicals, detergents, soaps, or wool; dry skin; ALLERGIC REACTION to food or drugs; hives; lichen planus; and parasites (such as lice or scabies). Pruritus that occurs all over the body without skin lesions can be a sign of diabetes, liver disease, kidney failure, thyroid disorders, cancer, or psychological problems. Whatever its underlying cause, stress can worsen itching.

In most cases, pruritus responds to treatment. Scratching should be avoided. Lukewarm showers are less drying than long, hot baths; however, an oatmeal bath may be soothing. Mild, soapless cleansers should be used. Especially in winter, it is helpful to use a moisturizer, particularly after showering or bathing when the skin is still damp. It is helpful to wear loose clothing. In cases of persistent or severe pruritus, it is important to consult a dermatologist for diagnosis and treatment. A complete physical examination and medical history will help determine the nature of the problem. Doctors may prescribe medications such as topical corticosteroids or antihistamines.

Pseudarthrosis

An abnormal joint formed at the site of an incomplete fracture healing.

The condition affects the shinbone (tibia), which may create an inequality in leg length, a foot deformity, or an outward bowing of the lower leg. These features usually become apparent within the first 2 years of life and generally affect only one leg. Pseudarthrosis may be treated with orthotic devices or by surgical treatment, which includes bone-grafting and limb-lengthening procedures. See also NEUROFIBROMATOSIS.

Pseudo-obstruction

Dilation or enlargement of the colon that mimics a mechanical obstruction in the absence of an actual blockage. This condition typically develops after abdominal surgery or in people who are otherwise severely ill. (See also ILEUS, PARALYTIC.) Most people with pseudo-obstruction are successfully treated with bed rest, insertion of a NASOGASTRIC TUBE for suction, and administration of intravenous fluids to prevent dehydration and shock. If the enlargement continues, potentially life-threatening PERFORATION (a hole or erosion in the intestine) is a risk. Sometimes the pseudo-obstruction can be relieved by colonoscopy. Surgery is also sometimes required. See SMALL-BOWEL TRANSPLANT.

Pseudodementia

A disorder that is caused by depression and resembles DEMENTIA—a widespread loss of intellectual function, including memory, due to a disease affecting the brain. Pseudodementia is not caused by a physical illness and usually can be reversed by time or treatment. It also refers to extreme apathy and indifference in someone who is not suffering from a mental disorder.

Pseudoephedrine

A nasal decongestant. Pseudoephedrine is used to relieve the nasal or sinus congestion caused by the common cold, sinusitis, hay fever, and other respiratory allergies. It is also used to relieve ear congestion caused by an ear infection. Pseudoephedrine is available in dozens of products, with and without prescription.

Pseudofolliculitis

See SHAVE BUMPS.

Pseudogout

A form of arthritis caused by crystals of calcium pyrophosphate dihydrate (CPPD) in one or more joints. Pseudogout, or false gout, is distinguished from true gout by the difference in the composition of the crystals. Pseudogout usually involves large joints such as the knees, wrist, and ankles. Gout developed from uric acid typically involves the first joint of the big toe. In pseudogout, the CPPD crystals in the joint cause severe inflammation and produce symptoms such as pain, swelling, and localized redness.

Diagnosis is accomplished by X rays and removing fluid from the involved joint to be analyzed in a laboratory. The fluid is observed under a polarized light with a microscope to identify the crystals and confirm a diagnosis of pseudogout. There is no effective treatment for this form of arthritis. Symptoms may be relieved with nonsteroidal anti-inflammatory drugs (NSAIDs) or corticosteroid injections into the joint.

Pseudo-hermaphroditism

A condition in which a baby's genitals are ambiguous and the sex of the baby is not clearly identifiable. Pseudohermaphroditism is distinguished from HERMAPHRODITISM in that individuals with pseudohermaphroditism have the genitals of one sex and not both.

Males with pseudohermaphroditism have normal 46,XY chromosomes but have ambiguous genitals or even femalelike genitals. This can be caused by incomplete development of the genitals in the fetus, abnormal hormone levels, and genetic mutations. Females with the condition have normal 46,XX chromosomes but have ambiguous or male-appearing genitals. This is usually due to a genetic disorder causing abnormal cell growth but can also result from abnormal hormone levels.

A priority in the early care of a child with pseudohermaphroditism is accurately determining the gender as soon after birth as possible. A specialist in hormonal problems in infancy, such as an endocrinologist, should be consulted and thorough testing and evaluation undertaken to make the correct assignment of sex.

P

Once the sex is identified, hormones may be used to treat the child. Reconstructive surgery can also be performed. Genetic counseling is recommended for the parents.

Pseudomembranous colitis

Inflammation of the mucous lining of the colon that develops as a complication of antibiotic use. Overuse of antibiotics results in the death of bacteria that normally reside in the colon and control the growth of other organisms. When these protective bacteria are no longer present, infection with the bacterium *Clostridium difficile* (*C. difficile*) may develop. The *C. difficile* bacteria produce a toxin that causes the pain and inflammation of pseudomembranous colitis. Severe watery diarrhea, NECROSIS (death of tissue cells), and TOXEMIA (the presence of poisons in the bloodstream) can occur in pseudomembranous colitis. An antibiotic, vancomycin or metronidazole, is given to combat the *C. difficile* infection. Severe pseudomembranous colitis can be a life-threatening disorder that normally requires hospitalization.

Pseudotumor cerebri

Also known as benign intracranial hypertension, a syndrome caused by increased pressure within the brain. Symptoms of pseudotumor cerebri can mimic those of a tumor and include headache, vomiting, double vision, and papilledema (swelling of the first part of the optic nerve), but no tumor is found on cerebral imaging. The condition is most common in obese young women and may resolve on its own. However, treatment may be necessary to protect vision. Diagnosis is made by measuring the spinal fluid pressure during a lumbar puncture. Treatments include diuretics, optic nerve fenestration (opening a small slit in the optic nerve to allow the fluid pressure to be released), and surgical placement of a shunt (with the shunt tip in the ventricle of the brain and the draining end in the peritoneal cavity).

Psittacosis

A rare bacterial disease that infects the lungs and is transmitted from birds to humans. Psittacosis is also referred to as "parrot fever" or ornithosis. The infection is caused by a *Chlamydia* strain of parasitic bacterium and is carried by parrots, pigeons, poultry, and other birds. Infected birds may not have any symptoms, or they may show symptoms such as diarrhea, respiratory distress, and weakness. They are generally treated with antibiotics in their feed or water.

Humans become infected with psittacosis by inhaling dust particles or feathers contaminated with infected birds' droppings, by handling infected live birds or carcasses, and by bite wounds from infected birds. Well-cooked poultry does not transmit the disease.

In humans, the symptoms may resemble mild influenza, or they may vary in severity and include high fever, chills, sore throat, severe headache, loss of appetite, nausea, and vomiting. The infection can progress to severe pneumonia with fever as high as 105°F. Psittacosis is diagnosed after a physical examination, a history of contact with birds, and by laboratory evaluation of respiratory secretions. It is usually treated successfully with antibiotics for 10 to 14 days.

The infection occurs most commonly among poultry farmers, pigeon breeders, veterinarians, workers in poultry-processing plants, pet store employees, and owners of pet birds, particularly parrots, parakeets, and cockatiels.

Psoriasis

A chronic, noncontagious skin disorder characterized by scaling. Scaling occurs when cells in the epidermis (outer layer of skin) form too rapidly and pile up on the surface of the skin. Psoriasis appears most often on the scalp, elbows, knees, and lower back. Psoriasis can also affect the toenails and fingernails.

The most common type of psoriasis is psoriasis vulgaris, consisting of red plaques (patches of thick raised skin) with silvery scales. Other varieties include pustular psoriasis (in which there are puslike bumps); erythrodermic psoriasis (red scaly areas involving the entire body); guttate psoriasis (characterized by red, teardroplike spots); and inverse psoriasis (in

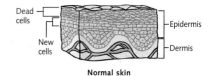

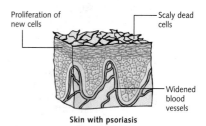

A COMMON SKIN DISORDER
In normal skin, new skin cells continually replace the largely dead cells on the surface. In skin with psoriasis, new cells are produced too rapidly, the process becomes disordered, and the outer dead cells pile up in a thick, scaly covering. Widened blood vessels in the dermis cause inflammation.

which there are smooth red plaques in the skin folds). In one in ten people, PSORIATIC ARTHRITIS (a painful form of arthritis affecting the fingers, toes, and spine) precedes or follows psoriasis of the skin.

While the exact cause of psoriasis remains unknown, genetic predisposition is thought to have a role. A person with a parent or close relative with psoriasis is more likely to develop it. When someone has a genetic tendency to develop psoriasis, it can be "triggered" by a number of factors that signal the immune system to cause inflammation in the skin. This causes the skin to shed too rapidly. Consequently, the thick, scaly lesions of psoriasis develop. Common triggers include systemic infections such as strep throat, emotional stress, injuries to the skin, and certain medications.

DIAGNOSIS

Usually psoriasis is characterized by raised red or pink plaques covered by thick, silvery scales. While psoriasis can affect any skin area, lesions most commonly appear on the scalp, elbows, knees, lower back, palms, soles, armpits, and genitals. The onset varies widely, from gradual and mild to swift and severe. Lesions vary from small patches of dandrufflike scaling to major eruptions covering large areas of skin. Moderate to severe cases lead to painful cracking or splitting of the skin. Other complications include itching, bleeding, soreness, and aching joints. Widespread psoriasis often causes emotional discomfort and embarrassment. It affects women and men equally and occurs in varying degrees of severity throughout an affected person's life.

Psoriasis is diagnosed through a thorough examination of the skin and nails. A skin biopsy (taking a small sample from the lesion and examining it under a microscope) may also be necessary. This distinguishes psoriasis from seemingly similar diseases, such as DERMATITIS.

TREATMENT

Treatment is based on the type of psoriasis, its severity, the extent of skin areas involved, and a person's responsiveness to initial treatments. Bath treatments and moisturizers are soothing but must be combined with more potent remedies. Prescription treatments may need to be switched periodically as individuals become resistant to them or experience adverse reactions.

The first line of treatment is topical medication applied to the skin. Topical treatments for psoriasis include corticosteroid creams, lotions, and ointments; synthetic forms of vitamin D3; coal tar; anthralin; topical retinoids; and salicylic acid. Side effects of these treatments must be carefully taken into account. Long-term use of corticosteroids can lead to thinning of the skin and dilated blood vessels. After many months of treatment, the psoriasis may become resistant to the topical corticosteroid. Topical retinoids can be irritating to the skin, and women of childbearing age should use topical retinoids cautiously and discontinue use if they are pregnant or breast-feeding.

If topical medications do not work, PHOTOTHERAPY (treatment with light) is tried. Ultraviolet light slows the rapid growth of skin cells and is used when psoriasis has not responded to topical treatments or is extensive. Ultraviolet B (UVB) light is used to treat psoriasis. The drug PUVA (psoralen plus ultraviolet A) is also used. Treatment with UVB light is considered safer than PUVA. Long-term use of PUVA is associated with an increased risk of skin cancer. In general, two to three treatments a week for 2 to 3 months are required.

In severe forms of psoriasis, dermatologists prescribe oral medications including cyclosporine, methotrexate, and retinoids. These are powerful medications with significant side effects. Retinoids must be avoided by women who are pregnant or planning to become pregnant. Possible side effects include high blood pressure with cyclosporine, liver damage and a decrease in the white blood cell count with methotrexate, and elevation of fat levels in the blood with retinoids.

Psoriatic arthritis

A specific type of ARTHRITIS that develops in the joints of some people who have psoriasis. Psoriatic arthritis tends to occur between the ages of 30 and 50 years. A person is likely to inherit this condition; there is some evidence that the immune system is involved. Trauma to a joint and the presence of bacteria are possible triggers for development of the condition.

SYMPTOMS AND DIAGNOSIS

Symptoms may be mild and appear gradually, or they may come on suddenly. They may include restricted range of motion and discomfort in one or more joints, stiffness, pain, throbbing, swelling, or tenderness. The joints closest to the ends of the fingers and toes and the knees and elbows are most often affected. Other joints, including those of the lower spine and the wrists or ankles, may be involved. Joints may be affected singly or in pairs. There may be morning stiffness and tiredness. The nails of the fingers and toes may become separated from the nail bed and become pitted. Eye inflammation, including conjunctivitis, may occur.

Diagnosis is made on the basis of clinical history, physical examination, blood tests, X rays, and laboratory study of fluid drawn from the affected joints. Other forms of arthritis, RHEUMATOID ARTHRITIS, GOUT, and REITER SYNDROME, are ruled out by clinical findings and laboratory examination of the person's blood. Treatment of mild psoriatic arthritis may include residing in a year-round warm climate and the use of aspirin, ibuprofen, or other nonsteroidal anti-inflammatory drugs or (NSAIDs). Physical therapy, exercise programs, applying heat, soaking in warm

water, and the use of splints may also be recommended. In severe cases, medications including METHOTREXATE, SULFASALAZINE, ETRETINATE, PUVA, and GOLD COMPOUNDS, by injection or taken orally as capsules, may be prescribed.

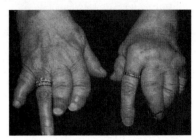

ARTHRITIS AND PSORIASIS
People with psoriasis sometimes develop an associated form of arthritis in which the joints of the fingers and wrists are affected, with typical thickening of joints and gnarling of fingers.

Psyche

The conscious and unconscious aspects of the mind, including thought, judgment, and emotion.

Psychiatric hospital

An inpatient medical institution that specializes in the treatment of people with severe mental illness. In most cases, people with mental illness are first treated in an outpatient setting. If this approach is not effective, the person is hospitalized for a short period to monitor, diagnose, and stabilize the condition, then released back to the community. Some psychiatric hospitals are state funded, and others are privately owned.

Psychiatrist

A physician who specializes in the treatment of mental illnesses and emotional disorders. Psychiatrists attend medical school for 4 years to earn an MD degree, then receive advanced training in psychiatry during a residency that lasts 4 years. Since psychiatrists are physicians, they can diagnose mental disorders and separate them from other diseases and conditions (for example, diabetes mellitus, Tourette syndrome, stroke), prescribe medications, and use psychotherapeutic techniques to treat patients.

Psychiatry

The branch of medicine that studies, treats, and prevents mental illness.

P

Psychoanalysis

A theory of psychological development and a method for treating mental illness originally devised by Sigmund Freud (see FREUDIAN THEORY). Although there are various approaches to psychoanalysis, all focus on understanding the relationship between the conscious and unconscious mind. Emphasis is put on childhood experiences, particularly repressed emotional conflicts, as central to the development of adult behavior and emotions. Various techniques are used to explore the unconscious and its conflicts, including free association and dreams. The psychoanalyst's role is to help the person understand these conflicts and their sources rather than simply eliminate distressing behaviors or feelings. Traditionally, the person lies or sits on a couch and the therapist takes notes.

Psychoanalyst

A psychotherapist who specializes in the use of PSYCHOANALYSIS. Most psychoanalysts are psychiatrists, psychologists, or social workers who have received 6 to 10 years of advanced training and undergone psychoanalysis themselves.

Psychoanalytic theory

The ideas that underlie PSYCHOANALYSIS, a theory of psychological development and an approach to treating mental illness first developed by Sigmund Freud. See FREUDIAN THEORY.

Psychogenic

A symptom or illness that arises from psychological causes, such as stress, interpersonal conflicts, or family issues, rather than a physical disease.

Psychological counseling

See COUNSELING, PSYCHOLOGICAL.

Psychological testing

Devices for assessing aspects of mental and emotional functioning. Psychiatrists, psychologists, and other mental health workers use psychological tests to learn information that may not emerge from interviewing or observing people and to compare them with others. The more than 500 tests in current use fall into five basic categories. Projective tests ask people to respond to purposely ambiguous or unstructured material. An example is the inkblot or RORSCHACH TEST. Projective tests are so vague that people reveal information about themselves in responding. Self-report tests consist of statements that people judge as characteristic or uncharacteristic of themselves, thereby revealing their emotions, beliefs, and personalities (see PERSONALITY TESTS). Psychophysiological tests measure physical responses such as heart rate, blood pressure, and muscle tension as indicators of psychological state, such as anxiety or sexual arousal. Neuropsychological tests reveal possible impairment of mental processes, such as memory loss, that may not be discovered in physical examination, X rays, or similar tests. INTELLIGENCE TESTS measure a person's intellectual capacity.

Psychologist

A nonphysician professional who specializes in the study of human behavior. Clinical psychologists, who treat emotional disorders in private practice, psychiatric hospitals, mental health settings, and schools, have a PhD or PsyD degree, which requires 4 to 6 years of graduate study beyond an undergraduate degree. The licensing requirements in most states also require clinical psychologists to complete a postdoctoral internship. Since psychologists are not physicians, they generally cannot prescribe medications unless they have additional training in pharmacology. Some professionals in the field are seeking changes in state laws to allow them to prescribe medications. Psychologists use various techniques of psychotherapy to treat mental illness and also consult to businesses on time and anger management.

Psychology

The branch of science that studies the mind, mental and emotional processes, and behavior. Psychology investigates learning, memory, sensation, perception, motivation, emotion, thinking, language, personality, social behavior, intelligence, development during infancy and childhood, and mental illness. Among the subspecialties of psychology are clinical psychology (diagnosing and treating mental illness), child or educational psychology (the mental, intellectual, and emotional development of children), and analytical psychology (study of the human mind through PSYCHOANALYSIS). Animal behavior has also been studied for more than a century by psychology researchers.

Psychometry

The scientific discipline that specializes in measuring mental processes and behavior. Examples of psychometry are PERSONALITY TESTS and INTELLIGENCE TESTS.

Psychoneuroimmunology (PNI)

The study of ways in which the mind and neurological system influence physical health. Psychoneuroimmunology is a term coined in 1975 by a US scientist interested in relationships among neurological pathways, the immune system, and the brain. PNI research investigates connections among the mind and neuroendocrine and immune systems, seeking better understanding of interactions among mental and emotional states, immune system function, and physical well-being.

RESEARCH TOPICS

PNI researchers are interested in various factors integrating the mind and the body to understand how the mind can influence physical phenomena. One such scientist researched the complex network through which chemicals communicate between the brain and the mind, discovering the neural receptor directly involved in addiction to opiate drugs, such as heroin. Other PNI researchers have studied the effects of stress on different people, finding that some thrive on stress, while others respond to stress by becoming physically sick. For some vulnerable people, chronic low-grade stress can undermine immune system functioning, which can ultimately lead to serious disease.

The goal of PNI research is to expand research beyond traditional concepts and theories of conventional medicine to make the art of healing more holistic. PNI is not based on any single system of healing but incorporates techniques and therapies developed by many disciplines. PNI assumes that there is no single answer to the question of human wellness.

PNI AND THE IMMUNE SYSTEM

The body's immune system is of particular interest to PNI researchers. It is assumed that the activity of the immune system varies in strength at different times, which means that each person's susceptibility to disease varies at different times. PNI researchers are interested in learning what phenomena in the environment, the diet, or people's emotional attitudes have direct or indirect effects on modulating the immune system.

A study of women with breast cancer has found, for example, that women who feel supported by family and friends have greater immune activity and survive longer than those who do not. Similarly, women in the study who were in emotional distress had measurably diminished immune systems, based on the number of "natural killer cells" in their bodies. PNI tries to identify and decipher such instances of interplay among mind, body, and the immune system, in hopes of developing new disease-fighting approaches able to harmonize and balance the mind and body.

Psychoneurosis

An obsolete term used by Sigmund Freud to describe emotional disorders in which unconscious emotional conflicts originating in childhood overwhelm the individual's mechanisms for defending the ego against them. The resulting anxiety expresses itself as abnormal fear (phobia), obsessive-compulsive disorder, anxiety disorder, depression, hysteria, or other illnesses.

Psychopathology

The signs, symptoms, and other physical and emotional manifestations of mental illness. Psychopathology also describes the branch of medical science that studies the nature and causes of mental illness.

Psychopharmacology

The study and use of medications to control psychological states, particularly in the treatment of mental illness. Most psychopharmacological agents affect chemicals in the brain known as neurotransmitters, which convey signals from one brain cell to another. By raising or lowering the levels of certain neurotransmitters, sometimes in specific portions of the brain, medications can change how the brain reacts, often eliminating or reducing the symptoms of mental illness.

Psychopharmacological agents that act in similar ways are grouped into broad categories. Antidepressants are used to treat depression; antipsychotics (also known as neuroleptics), in the treatment of schizophrenia and other severe mental illnesses in which the individual loses touch with reality; stimulants, for attention deficit/hyperactivity disorder and for depression in medically ill individuals; antimanics, for manic-depressive illness; antianxiety medications (anxiolytics), for anxiety and phobias; and cholinesterase inhibitors, for Alzheimer's disease.

The first psychopharmacological agents were used in the 1950s, and they revolutionized the treatment of mental illness. Before that time, people with severe disorders had to be hospitalized, often for years. The advent of psychopharmacology meant that a person with mental illness could be treated as an outpatient. Increasing research in the intervening decades has led to the development of drugs that are more selective, have fewer side effects, and are focused in their action.

Psychosexual disorders

Mental illnesses that often involve changes or abnormalities in sexual function, behavior, and identity.

SEXUAL DYSFUNCTIONS

The principal characteristic of a sexual dysfunction is a persistent problem with desire, completion of the sexual act, or sex that distresses the person emotionally and may result in relationship difficulties. The disturbance in normal sexuality can occur at any point in the cycle from arousal to orgasm. Desire for sex may itself be absent (hypoactive sexual desire disorder). Some people avoid sex and are repulsed or disgusted by sexual activity (sexual aversion disorder).

Both males and females may fail to become aroused enough to experience enjoyable sexual relations. In women, the vagina fails to lubricate; in men, the penis remains flaccid or loses erection before orgasm (ERECTILE DYSFUNCTION, also known as impotence). Both men and women may fail to reach orgasm after sufficient stimulation. In men, orgasm and ejaculation may occur sooner or later than is desired (premature or delayed ejaculation). For both sexes, sexual relations may be painful (dyspareunia). In women, the vagina may constrict so tightly that it cannot be entered (vaginismus).

Sexual dysfunctions have a number of possible causes. Lack of sexual knowledge is a frequent cause. Psychological issues can be a factor. For example, fear of pregnancy, performance anxiety, embarrassment, inhibitions, or guilt can inhibit arousal or prevent orgasm. Rape or physical trauma is sometimes the cause of vaginismus. Physical factors can also have a role. Certain diseases, such as diabetes mellitus and multiple sclerosis, may lead to sexual dysfunction. General medical conditions, such as cancer, may leave an individual too fatigued to be interested in sex or to become aroused. Sexual dysfunction can also follow surgery or radiation treatment, particularly on the sexual organs themselves or nearby body parts. Substances can also be responsible for dysfunction. These include abused drugs, such as alcohol and heroin, and certain medications, such as chemotherapy or those used to treat depression and high blood pressure (hypertension). Treatment for sexual dysfunction depends on the nature and cause of the problem.

PARAPHILIA

This psychosexual disorder is characterized by frequent, intense, sexual urges or fantasies about completing the sex act with nonhuman objects (such as an animal), suffering or humiliation of oneself or one's partner during sex, or having sexual relations with children (PEDOPHILIA) or nonconsenting adults (rape). Some individuals need the paraphiliac fantasy or activity to become sexually aroused, while for others the fantasies or activities occur only from

P

time to time. Paraphilia includes fetishism (undergarments, shoes, and other objects), exhibitionism (exposing one's genitals to others without their consent), pedophilia, voyeurism (watching unsuspecting individuals disrobe or make love), sexual masochism (receiving pain), and sadism (inflicting pain) for sexual arousal. Some types violate the law and are considered criminal (exhibitionism, pedophilia).

The causes of paraphilia are unclear. Treatment is difficult, usually because individuals with these disorders may not wish to change and therefore resist therapy. Some are jailed.

GENDER-IDENTITY DISORDER

This disorder involves persistently acting and presenting oneself as a member of the opposite sex, combined with strong feelings of discomfort in one's own physical gender, it is also called gender dysphoria. Children with the disorder want to be the opposite sex, express revulsion at their own genitals, cross-dress (dress in the clothes of the opposite sex), play games and pursue pastimes typical of the opposite sex, and prefer the company of the opposite sex. Adults with the disorder (transsexuals) typically want to be rid of their genitals, desire to live as a member of the opposite sex, and believe their emotions and feelings are more like those of the opposite sex than their own. They may be erotically oriented to same-sex or opposite-sex relationships and seek to rid themselves of the obvious characteristics of their sex by taking hormones, having facial hair removed or added, or undergoing SEX CHANGE surgery. Both children and adults tend to be socially isolated by peer pressure and rejection. Some experience depression and anxiety.

The course of the disorder depends on when it begins. In boys, the disorder may begin between 2 and 4 years of age. Sometimes, the disorder improves by the time the boy is an adolescent. However, in other cases the disorder continues into adulthood. Some cross-dress in private (transvestites) and are aroused in this way to complete the sex act. Others (transsexuals) seek sex change surgery as adults. Each unique individual will differ in the intensity, expression, comfort, or distress related to

the condition. Some seek psychiatric help, while others do not. Self-help and internet information has become available. The disorder occurs less frequently in girls, and the course remains unclear.

The cause of gender-identity disorder is not fully understood. Theories linking the disorder to inherited abnormalities, imbalances in hormones, and defective bonding to parents in early childhood have been proposed. Some physicians have been perceived as insensitive in this area. Intersex groups seek political assistance or legal changes to declare a third "intersex" for those who struggle with gender differences. Treatment consists of family, individual, and group therapy. Sex change surgery is an option for some people, but emotional problems may continue after the operation. Changing the genitals does not always relieve the emotional distress.

Psychosis

Any severe mental illness characterized by a disruption with reality, perception, and organized thoughts. Typically, people with a psychosis may act, communicate, or think in bizarre or incomprehensible ways, yet not realize their actions are abnormal. They lose contact with reality. Some perceive things that do not exist, such as hearing voices or seeing visions (hallucinations), or hold to mistaken beliefs (illusions, such as perceiving shadows on the wall as invading hordes of ants) or false ideas (delusions, such as considering themselves reincarnations of Jesus or Napoleon). Psychosis may be due to psychiatric or medical causes.

Psychoses may include SCHIZOPHRENIA (an illness involving delusions, hallucinations, abnormal speech, and strange behavior), BIPOLAR DISORDER (characterized by swings in mood from extreme elation and energy, or mania with delusions, to abnormal sadness and lethargy, or depression), dementia (such as ALZHEIMER'S DISEASE), and PARANOIA (extreme, pervasive, and unwarranted distrust of another person's actions and motivations, often accompanied by delusions about conspiracy or persecution).

Psychosomatic

Pertaining to a physical symptom or illness that originates in, or is worsened by, emotional factors. Examples include ulcers, migraine headaches, irritable bowel syndrome, and lower back pain. In the psychosomatic illness known as CONVERSION DISORDER, a distressed person develops physical symptoms that mimic a disease of the nervous system or a general medical condition but are in fact not due to any physical cause. Symptoms can include frequent urination, difficulty walking, paralysis or localized weakness, inability to speak, difficulty swallowing (lump-in-the-throat feeling), inability to urinate, loss of sense of pain or touch, blindness, double vision, deafness, hallucinations, and seizures.

Another psychosomatic illness, known as SOMATIZATION DISORDER, involves a history of symptoms that lack a physical cause, usually affecting the gastrointestinal system, the heart and lungs, the central nervous system, or the genitals.

Psychosurgery

Surgery on the brain performed to treat a psychiatric disorder or mental illness. Psychosurgery in the past consisted principally of the prefrontal lobotomy, a procedure designed to sever the nerves connecting the frontal lobe to the rest of the brain. The procedure gained popularity in the mid-1930s through the work of the Portuguese neurologist António Egas Moniz, who won the 1949 Nobel Prize in medicine for developing the surgery. At the time, prefrontal lobotomy was hailed as a major step forward in treating people with severe mental disease that kept them in an asylum for more than 20 years, such as schizophrenia and obsessive-compulsive disorder. The surgery often mitigated the disease, but it also had severe side effects, blunting the person's emotions and leaving the person with little or no initiative. As a result, the procedure became less and less common after the late 1940s and when psychotropic medications became available after the 1950s.

Prefrontal lobotomy today is a treatment of last resort, used only with extremely severe disease that has failed to respond to any other treat-

P

ment. The operation is now rare, subject to review by state-appointed boards, and illegal in some parts of the United States.

Psychotherapist

A professional who uses psychological techniques, such as re-education, suggestion, retraining, and exploration of the emotions, to treat emotional problems and mental illness. Psychiatrists, psychologists, social workers, mental health counselors, and trained members of the clergy may all be psychotherapists. Under the laws of some states, the term "psychotherapist" can be used by anyone, even someone without professional training, and is not a guarantee of credentials. A person seeking a psychotherapist should inquire about whether the specialist is licensed in his or her state.

Psychotherapy

The treatment of emotional problems, behavioral issues, or mental illnesses primarily through verbal communication. Most psychotherapy is done on a one-to-one basis, but it may also be used with couples, groups, and families. Sometimes the word "psychotherapy" describes the treatment of severe disturbance, while "counseling" refers to the treatment of people with mild problems. However, the words are often used interchangeably. Psychotherapy is also known as talk therapy.

There are three fundamental approaches to psychotherapy. The first, psychodynamic psychotherapy, was developed originally from the ideas of Sigmund Freud (see FREUDIAN THEORY). It is based on the theory that understanding the self, particularly the emotional past and the hidden feelings of the unconscious mind, is key to resolving EMOTIONAL PROBLEMS or illnesses. Behavior therapy, the second approach, focuses on current actions, not emotions rooted in the past, and aims to improve the person's functioning whether the origin of the problem is understood or not. Increasingly, behavior therapists also work with the thoughts, or cognitions, that influence a person's actions, following an approach known as COGNITIVE-BEHAVIORAL THERAPY.

The third approach, humanistic therapy (also known as existential therapy or GESTALT THEORY), focuses on the person's immediate feelings, rather than thoughts or behaviors, and works toward increasing the person's self-awareness. Many psychotherapists combine elements from all three approaches, either to fit their own professional styles or to meet the differing needs of people they treat.

Psychotropic drugs

See ANTIPSYCHOTIC DRUGS.

Psyllium

A bulk-forming laxative. Psyllium is derived from the seed of a plant called *Plantago indica*. It is a mild natural laxative that acts by absorbing water and providing indigestible bulk in the intestines. The bowel is stimulated by the presence of the mass formed by psyllium. More than a dozen products containing psyllium, can be purchased without a prescription. See LAXATIVES.

Pterygium

A pinkish, triangular growth on the clear outer layer of the EYE (cornea) to the nasal side. A pterygium occurs in the membrane that covers the eyelids and eye (conjunctiva) and attaches to the cornea as it grows. Some pterygia continue to grow throughout a person's life, while others stop growing once they reach a certain size. Only rarely does a pterygium become large enough to cover the pupil of the eye. Pterygia are most common in people between ages 20 and 40 years who live in sunny climates. The cause is not known, but the increased incidence of pterygia in warmer climate regions points toward exposure to sunlight as a likely cause. Dust and air pollution can irritate a pterygium, making it red

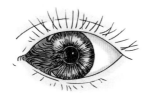

ACCUMULATED TISSUE
Thickening of tissue on the conjunctiva (outer membrane covering the eye), called pterygium, may become red and inflamed, or it may interfere with tearing, causing dry eye. Rarely, it moves across the cornea (a focusing structure) and can harm vision.

and swollen and more apparent. The growth can be removed surgically for cosmetic reasons, because of discomfort, or if vision is obscured.

PTH

See PARATHYROID HORMONE.

Ptosis

A drooping of one or both upper eyelids. See EYELID, DROOPING.

Puberty

The period of life in which a child makes the transition into adulthood. Sexual characteristics develop, and sexual organs mature, making reproduction possible. Puberty is triggered when the pituitary gland and hypothalamus in the brain signal the body to begin producing sex hormones. In girls, the ovaries begin to produce estrogen (the female hormone) and other hormones; in boys, the testicles begin to produce testosterone (the male hormone) and other hormones. Girls generally reach sexual maturity by age 16 and boys, by age 17 or 18. Puberty is also characterized by dramatic growth (see GROWTH, CHILDHOOD). The hormonal changes of puberty provoke strong sexual feelings and urges. Two out of three teenagers become sexually active by their senior year in high school. See ADOLESCENCE; SEX EDUCATION.

THE ONSET OF PUBERTY

Sexual changes usually begin between ages 8 and 13 in girls and between 9 and 14 in boys. Heredity is an important factor in the timing of sexual development. For example, a girl will begin menstruating around the same age her mother did. Sexual development before age 8 in girls and age 9 in boys is called precocious puberty. Children who develop early or late may be teased by their peers; however, such differences are normal and temporary. Puberty with an exceptionally early or late onset should be evaluated by the child's pediatrician. A commonly used method to identify the stages of puberty is the Tanner system, which classifies sexual maturation of adolescents into 5 stages. Sexual maturation normally proceeds in a regular order. When the order is disturbed, a doctor should be consulted.

P

STAGES OF PUBERTY IN GIRLS

Spurred by growth and sex hormones, girls begin a dramatic growth spurt at about age 10. By age 16 to 18, they achieve adult height and weigh twice what they weighed at age 10. Estrogen causes girls to develop a higher ratio of fat to muscle and bone than that for boys. Girls usually start their growth spurt earlier than boys and so, are heavier and taller than boys the same age. Puberty in girls usually proceeds in five specific stages.

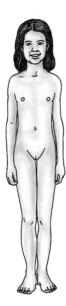 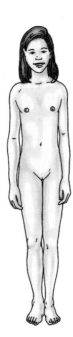 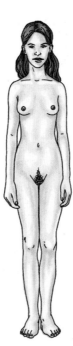 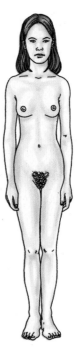 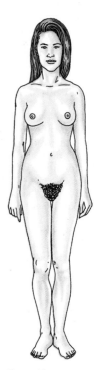

STAGE 1
This period, called prepuberty, immediately precedes the onset of puberty. Ovaries are preparing to produce hormones, but no visible sexual development has occurred.

STAGE 2
Puberty begins when the pituitary gland and hypothalamus in the brain signal the ovaries to start producing hormones. The first outward sign of puberty is the enlargement of the nipples and the appearance of breast buds. Sparse pubic hair starts to grow, and height and weight increase rapidly.

STAGE 3
Breasts gradually grow fuller. Pubic hair fills in and starts to curl. Underarm hair sprouts about a year later, and sweat glands in the underarms increase their perspiration. Skin, particularly on the face, produces more oil.

STAGE 4
Height and weight increase steadily. Breasts and nipples develop. Pubic hair grows in. A white creamy vaginal discharge is emitted 6 to 12 months before the first menstrual cycle, which starts during stage 4. Ovulation (release of egg cells) begins in some, but typically not in a monthly routine until the fifth stage. Once this process begins, a girl can become pregnant.

STAGE 5
Girls reach full physical and sexual maturity around age 18. Periods and ovulation become regular. Breasts and internal organs reach adult size.

P

STAGES OF PUBERTY IN BOYS

Puberty in boys can begin anytime after about age 12. Production of the male hormone testosterone increases boys' proportion of muscle and bone to fat. Because boys start their growth spurt later than girls, they are temporarily smaller and shorter than girls the same age. Puberty in boys starts at different ages and can progress at varying rates. However, it generally progresses in five predictable stages.

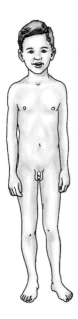
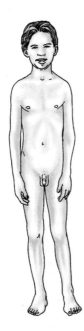
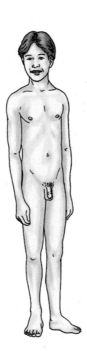
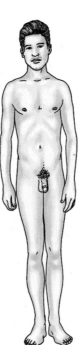
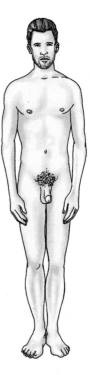

STAGE 1
In the first stage, called prepuberty, no visible signs of sexual maturation appear. However, the testicles are preparing to release more hormones.

STAGE 2
Puberty begins when the pituitary gland and hypothalamus in the brain start producing hormones that signal the testicles to begin producing testosterone and other male hormones. The first visible sign of puberty is enlargement of the testicles and scrotum, the sac that covers the testicles. Perspiration increases, producing a stronger body odor.

STAGE 3
Sparse pubic hair begins to grow. The penis grows longer, and ejaculation begins, either during sleep or masturbation. The voice deepens noticeably as the vocal cords grow. For a few months, the voice suddenly may change pitch uncontrollably.

STAGE 4
The testicles continue to grow, and the penis becomes longer and thicker. The skin of the penis and scrotum darkens. Pubic hair fills in, curls, and coarsens. Underarm hair appears; hair may also grow in on the upper lip and chin. A great spurt in height may occur.

STAGE 5
Boys reach physical and sexual maturity. Pubic hair now grows on the inner thighs, and hair may start growing on the chest. Growth in height starts to slow until adult height is achieved around age 18, although some boys do not stop growing until age 21.

P

PUBERTY IN GIRLS

After age 10, girls begin a period of rapid growth. Girls normally double their 10-year-old weight by age 18. Because estrogen adds body fat, while testosterone builds muscle, girls acquire a larger proportion of fat to muscle and bone than do boys. The earliest visible sign of female puberty is the appearance of breast buds. Soon afterward, pubic hairs start to sprout. Two to 2½ years normally elapse between the start of puberty and a girl's first period. During this time, breasts grow fuller, and more pubic hair appears. Underarm hair begins to grow, and sweat glands under the arms cause an increase in perspiration and body odor. Surging hormone production can lead to outbreaks of acne on the face. Six to 12 months before a girl's first period, a white, creamy vaginal discharge appears. The nipples of the breasts may become more apparent, and the pubic hair is almost fully grown. Ovaries start to produce an egg each month, and girls can become pregnant. A girl usually gets her first menstrual period between the ages of 11 and 14. MENSTRUATION is the cyclical shedding of blood from the lining of the uterus. Thin or athletic girls may start menstruating later because their bodies produce less estrogen. Periods are usually irregular for the first 2 to 3 years of menstruation. Girls should be given information about their periods and the necessary supplies before they actually begin menstruating.

PUBERTY IN BOYS

Because puberty is later in boys, they are temporarily smaller than girls the same age. Because testosterone builds muscle while estrogen adds fat, boys have a larger proportion of muscle and bone to fat. The enlargement of the testicles and scrotum is the first visible sign of puberty in boys. Soon afterward, sweat glands under the arms cause an increase in perspiration and body odor.

Puberty progresses at different rates from boy to boy. However, its next manifestations are usually the appearance of pubic hair, a deepening voice, and the boy's first ejaculation. Testicles continue to grow, and the penis becomes thicker and longer. The pubic hair eventually begins filling in, and the penis and scrotum darken.

Hair sprouts on the chin and under the arms. Boys normally experience a great gain in height at this time.

Pubes

Hairs on the genitals. Also called pubic hair. Unlike scalp hair, most pubic hair does not grow after puberty.

Pubic lice

Parasitic insects found in the human genital areas; infestation with pubic lice is one of the SEXUALLY TRANSMITTED DISEASES. See CRAB LICE; PEDICULOSIS.

Public health

A specific area of medicine concerned with assessing, safeguarding, and improving the health of entire populations or communities. The public health discipline seeks to prevent epidemics and the spread of disease; protect against environmental hazards such as air and water pollution and toxic waste; and prevent injuries through such measures as automobile seat belt laws and workplace safety regulations. The discipline also promotes healthy behaviors and mental health; responds to disasters; and ensures that health services are available to the people who need them.

Public health agencies and professionals engage in a variety of activities. They monitor the health status of the community in order to identify and solve problems. Public health professionals are heavily involved in identifying emerging health threats, such as winter influenza (flu) epidemics, and orchestrating the response to them, such as alerting physicians, hospitals, and medical laboratories about the presence of disease. Public health workers inform and educate people about health issues such as smoking and the spread of sexually transmitted infections. Often public health agencies and professionals organize community partnerships and mobilize actions to address health issues. The making of policy that benefits community health, such as setting air pollution standards or sanitation requirements for public accommodations, also falls within the area of public health, as does the enforcement of health and safety regulations

(for example, food preparation practices in restaurants). Many public health agencies have a role in providing individuals, particularly those in poverty or in high-risk populations, with the health care services they need and in evaluating the effectiveness of these services. Finally, public health often includes research into issues relevant to community health, such as the spread of disease and the economic factors affecting the availability and quality of health care.

PUBS

See PERCUTANEOUS UMBILICAL CORD BLOOD SAMPLING.

Pudendal block

An injection of anesthesia given in the vagina that relieves pain during childbirth. The injection is given shortly before delivery to block pain in the perineum, the area between the vaginal opening and the anus. The drug usually given is the anesthetic lidocaine, which is injected into the tissues surrounding the pudendal nerves, one on either side of the vagina. A pudendal block does not relieve the pain of labor and is given only to block pain that is associated with the baby's passage through the birth canal.

A block is usually given to women who have had very long or complicated labors or if pain interferes with a woman's ability to push the baby through the birth canal. It may be used in breech and forceps deliveries. The pudendal block takes effect very quickly and has no serious side effects. It is one of the safest forms of anesthesia. See also ANESTHESIA, EPIDURAL.

Puerperal sepsis

An infection of the uterus following childbirth. The term puerperal refers to the PUERPERIUM, or the time just after a baby is born. Puerperal sepsis was once a major cause of death in women after childbirth, and it can sometimes still prove fatal.

Puerperium

Medical term for the 6 weeks following childbirth. During this period, a woman's body begins to return to normal after having experienced the significant physical and emotional changes that accompany pregnancy and childbirth. Internal organs, including the uterus and the cervix, must shrink back to normal size, and hormone levels change.

Pulling teeth

See TOOTH EXTRACTION.

Pulmonary

The medical term that describes diseases, conditions, disorders, or structures related to the lungs.

Pulmonary disease, chronic obstructive

See CHRONIC OBSTRUCTIVE PULMONARY DISEASE.

Pulmonary edema

A life-threatening condition involving the accumulation of fluid in the lungs caused by increased pressure in the lungs' capillaries or leakage of fluid from damage to the tissue lining the capillaries and airways. In pulmonary edema, the fluid pressure in the veins of the lungs builds up, and the resulting increased pressure in the veins forces fluid from the capillaries into the alveoli (air sacs of the lungs). The excess fluid in the air sacs interferes with their normal function of exchanging oxygen and carbon dioxide.

Pulmonary edema may be caused by or may be a complication of heart conditions, including a heart attack, disease of the mitral or aortic valves, and cardiac dysfunction. Other associated disorders include kidney failure, infection, toxic inhalation, pulmonary embolism, aspiration of water into the lungs in near-drowning incidents, and abuse of medications or illegal drugs, especially narcotics such as heroin. Rarely, it is caused by exposure to high altitude. In infants, pulmonary edema may be caused by fluid overload.

SYMPTOMS, DIAGNOSIS, AND TREATMENT

The symptoms may include shortness of breath with severe difficulty breathing and a sensation of being unable to take in enough air. Wheezing, flaring nostrils, and coughing that sometimes brings up blood may be accompanied by feelings of anxiety and restlessness. Perspiration may be excessive, and the skin may be pale.

During a physical examination using a stethoscope, a doctor can detect a crackling sound in the lungs or abnormal heart sounds that indicate pulmonary edema. Chest X rays can reveal fluid in the lung space.

Pulmonary edema is a medical emergency requiring immediate hospitalization and treatment. Diuretic medications are given to remove excess fluid, and morphine is given to relieve congestion and anxiety. If a heart disorder is involved, appropriate treatment and medication are given. In severe cases, oxygen is given by mask to restore the blood oxygen level. Pulmonary edema can usually be cured with proper medical treatment and management of the underlying disorder.

Pulmonary embolism

The sudden blockage of an artery in the lung by a blood clot or by fat, tumor tissue, bone marrow, or an air bubble that has traveled through the bloodstream. Pulmonary embolism may be caused in pregnancy by amniotic fluid. In most cases, other unblocked arteries can deliver sufficient blood to the affected area of the lung to prevent death of lung tissue. When a large vessel is blocked or when there is underlying lung disease, the amount of blood may be inadequate to prevent lung tissue death, a condition called PULMONARY INFARCTION.

CAUSES AND RISK FACTORS

The most common cause of pulmonary embolism is a blood clot that has originated in a vein of the leg or pelvis, a condition called deep vein thrombosis (DVT; see THROMBOSIS, DEEP VEIN). These clots tend to form when a person is stationary and blood flow is slow or stopped; these clots can break loose and travel to the lung. Leg exercises and elastic support stockings can help prevent clots from forming. Less commonly, blood clots from the right side of the heart or from tumors in the circulatory system can cause pulmonary embolism.

When a bone fractures, fat can escape into the blood from the bone marrow and be carried by the bloodstream into the lungs. Amniotic fluid that enters the system during childbirth can also form an embolus that travels to the lungs. These materials usually lodge in small blood vessels of the lungs and rarely form obstructions large enough to block the central lung arteries.

Risk factors for pulmonary embolism include the use of oral contraceptives, childbirth, cancer, stroke, immobility, heart attack, fractures of the hip or thighbones, and major surgery. Walking and other activities soon after surgical procedures can decrease this risk. Prolonged bed rest and physical inactivity are risk factors that may be decreased by the use of low doses of HEPARIN, an anticoagulant, injected under the skin. Other risk factors include obesity and a hereditary deficiency of a blood clotting factor.

SYMPTOMS

If the arterial blockage in the lungs is small, there may be no symptoms, but there is usually some degree of shortness of breath and chest pain. A pulmonary infarction can cause a cough that begins suddenly and sometimes produces blood or blood streaks in the sputum. Light-headedness, fainting, dizziness, and seizures are experienced as initial symptoms by some people and are caused by the sudden decrease in the heart's ability to deliver sufficient amounts of well-oxygenated blood to the brain. Irregular heart rate can also occur with these symptoms.

A person with pulmonary embolism may experience a sudden shortness of breath. Associated chest pain may be experienced as sharp, stabbing, burning, and aching or as a dull, heavy sensation. It can occur under the breastbone or on one side of the body. Chest pain may be worse when breathing deeply or coughing. Referred pain may occur in the shoulder, arm, neck, jaw, or other areas of the body.

Other symptoms may include anxiety, sweating, wheezing, rapid breathing, and a fast heart rate. The skin can become clammy and take on a bluish discoloration. The pulse may be irregular, weak, or temporarily absent, and breathing may stop temporarily. Blood pressure may drop. If the source of the pulmonary embolism is a clot in the lower extremities, there may be pain and swelling in one or both legs.

DIAGNOSIS AND TREATMENT

A lung perfusion scan involves a small amount of radioactive material

P

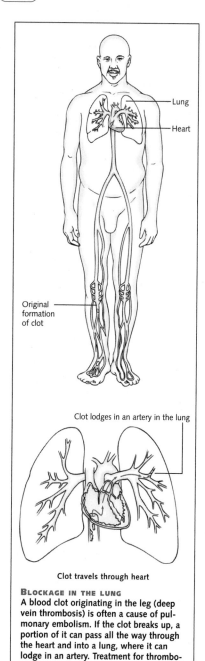

Original formation of clot

Lung

Heart

Clot lodges in an artery in the lung

Clot travels through heart

BLOCKAGE IN THE LUNG
A blood clot originating in the leg (deep vein thrombosis) is often a cause of pulmonary embolism. If the clot breaks up, a portion of it can pass all the way through the heart and into a lung, where it can lodge in an artery. Treatment for thrombosis aims to dissolve the clot at its origin, to prevent it from breaking off.

that is injected into a vein and travels to the lungs, where it outlines the blood supply of the lung and can reveal an obstruction of a blood vessel. Lung ventilation scans, performed with the perfusion scan, reveal the areas in which air is being exchanged, and these areas are then compared with the pattern of blood supply to the lung. With these combined scans, a pulmonary embolism will show normal ventilation with decreased blood supply.

A type of CT (computed tomography) scan called a spiral or helical CT is also useful for diagnosing a pulmonary embolism. In addition, ANGIOGRAPHY images the blood supply to the lungs and may be used to diagnose pulmonary embolism. However, since angiography is a more invasive procedure requiring the threading of a catheter into the pulmonary artery, it is reserved for cases in which the diagnosis is uncertain after performing less invasive tests.

Pulmonary function tests and analysis of arterial blood gases can be used to evaluate the functional state of the lungs. An electrocardiogram can reveal abnormalities and may support the diagnosis of pulmonary embolism. The definitive diagnostic test for pulmonary embolism is pulmonary arteriography, in which a contrast dye is injected into an artery and flows into the arteries of the lung. When an X ray of the chest is performed, the embolism blocking an artery is clearly revealed. Other tests may be conducted to determine the cause of a pulmonary embolism. To detect a deep vein thrombosis, a doctor may order venography of the legs, blood flow studies, ultrasound scanning of a particular extremity, and other examinations of the legs.

Pulmonary embolism requires emergency medical treatment and hospitalization. Treatment requires anticoagulant therapy, which is done to inhibit the formation of more clots. Thrombolytic therapy may be used to dissolve a large, life-threatening embolism (see THROMBOLYTIC DRUGS). It consists of using medication such as streptokinase or tissue plasminogen activator (TPA), which dissolves clots. Anticoagulant therapy includes intravenous infusions of heparin or injections of low-molecular-weight heparin followed by warfarin taken orally. Oxygen therapy is used to maintain a normal concentration of oxygen in the body while the injury to the lungs heals.

Ongoing anticoagulant therapy with medications that inhibit blood clotting can reduce the rate of recurrence substantially. Surgery to insert a filter to prevent clots from traveling to the lungs may be recommended for people who are at high risk for recurrent pulmonary embolism or for people unable to take anticoagulants.

Pulmonary fibrosis

A disease in which LUNG tissue has become scarred and thickened from inflammation of the lung tissue. Pulmonary fibrosis can be the result of any of several diseases and conditions, particularly those that involve abnormalities of the immune system. Other causes include infection with viruses, rickettsia, or mycoplasma; disseminated tuberculosis; and exposure to mineral dusts (such as silica, carbon, metal, and asbestos) or organic dusts (such as molds and bird droppings). Exposure to gases, fumes, or vapors (such as chlorine and sulfur dioxide) and to radiation in the workplace or radiation administered for therapeutic reasons is sometimes associated with pulmonary fibrosis. Certain medications and toxic materials can also cause pulmonary fibrosis. When the cause is unknown, it is referred to as idiopathic pulmonary fibrosis, which is the case in about half the people who have the disease. Pulmonary fibrosis is also known as interstitial lung disease or interstitial fibrosis of the lung.

SYMPTOMS AND DIAGNOSIS

Some forms of pulmonary fibrosis have a known cause, while others occur for unknown reasons. The known causes include occupational and environmental exposure to irritants that cause DUST DISEASES, including ASBESTOSIS and SILICOSIS, and other inflammatory lung conditions. The inflammation may be a side effect of certain medications. Rheumatoid arthritis, systemic sclerosis, systemic lupus erythematosis, and connective tissue or collagen diseases may result in pulmonary fibrosis. Genetic factors are possible but are the least common causes of the condition.

Specific diseases that cause pulmonary fibrosis include sarcoidosis, a disease of unknown cause that is characterized by inflammatory cells, and histiocytosis, a disease that attacks the small airways of the lungs and associated arteries and veins.

If no definite cause can be determined, the condition is called idiopathic (of unknown origin) pulmonary fibrosis. Although the cause is uncertain, many experts believe that it is probably a type of autoimmune disease.

All forms of pulmonary fibrosis begin with inflammation in some area of the lung. When this occurs in the walls of the small airways called bronchioles, it is called BRONCHIOLITIS. If the air spaces and alveoli (air sacs) are affected, it is called ALVEOLITIS. Inflammation of the small blood vessels or capillaries of the lungs is called VASCULITIS.

SYMPTOMS

Pulmonary fibrosis causes the permanent loss of the affected lung tissue's capacity to absorb oxygen into the blood. The extent of the scarred tissue determines the level of disability experienced by the person who has the disease.

People who have pulmonary fibrosis have the same kind of symptoms, although the symptoms may range from very mild to moderate to extremely severe. In the early stages, the symptoms may be barely noticeable and would not necessarily prompt a person to seek medical care. One of the earliest symptoms is a dry cough and breathlessness during exercise.

The course of pulmonary fibrosis is unpredictable. Symptoms can develop gradually or follow a rapidly progressive course. If the disease is detected in its initial stages when the inflammation occurs, medication may prove beneficial. As scarring progresses, the normally soft lung tissue stiffens, which also contributes to a person's shortness of breath.

DIAGNOSIS AND TREATMENT

A complete medical history is an important diagnostic tool for this disease. Pulmonary fibrosis may be diagnosed by evaluating blood test and chest X-ray findings and with the use of pulmonary function tests during rest and exercise. These evaluations can help determine the extent of disease and help rule out other possible lung conditions. BRONCHOSCOPY, lung biopsy, and CT (computed tomography) scans may also be used in the diagnostic evaluation of idiopathic pulmonary fibrosis. Bronchoalveolar lavage is a test performed during bronchoscopy that removes some cells from the lower respiratory tract for microscopic examination and may have a diagnostic role in identifying inflammatory processes in the lung tissue.

CORTICOSTEROIDS may be administered, sometimes in combination with other medications, to treat inflammation associated with pulmonary fibrosis and can reverse the disease in certain cases. Oxygen therapy may be prescribed to help with breathing. Vaccination against influenza and pneumococcal pneumonia is recommended to prevent infections. In severe cases or if other lung diseases are present, lung transplantation may be recommended.

Specially designed exercise programs, support groups, and programs aimed at rehabilitation and education are sometimes helpful to people who have pulmonary fibrosis and to their families. Although disease progression varies with the cause, the mean period of survival after diagnosis is approximately 5 years.

Pulmonary function tests

A series of tests that measure the lungs' capacity to hold air, their ability to move air in and out, and their ability to exchange oxygen and carbon dioxide. Pulmonary function tests are commonly used to determine the type and severity of lung disorders, rather than the specific cause of lung problems. They may be used to evaluate the symptom shortness of breath and to diagnose asthma. The results of the tests are compared with normal standards based on a person's age, height, weight, and sex and are expressed as a percentage of the predicted value for an average, healthy person.

Pulmonary function tests include several different forms of measuring lung function. SPIROMETRY measures vital capacity, or the amount of air exhaled by a maximum effort on the part of the person being tested. This test also measures how fast the air is expelled and compares this flow of air with normal standards. These measurements do not generally provide a specific diagnosis. OXIMETRY, also called an oxygen saturation test, measures the amount of oxygen in the blood.

Lung volume and flow rates provide a measurement of how air is distributed in the lungs. The amount of air that is exchanged with each breath is called the tidal volume. The residual volume is the amount of air that is retained in the air sacs continuously. A change in the distribution of air may reveal a pattern of disease that may suggest certain diagnoses. Total lung volume is tested by two methods. In one, a person breathes in a special gas mixture containing oxygen for a few minutes, and lung volume is calculated by the amount of nitrogen the person exhales. In another method, the person sits in a glass booth called a body box and breathes against a mouthpiece. The pressure changes in the body box are analyzed while the person breathes, and the volume of gas in the lungs is determined.

Diffusion capacity is a pulmonary function test that determines how well gas is exchanged or transferred from the air sacs in the lungs to the blood vessels. It is commonly used as a sensitive test for evaluating breathing disorders such as EMPHYSEMA and PULMONARY FIBROSIS. The person being tested breathes a special gas mixture containing carbon monoxide, and the air that is exhaled is analyzed to compare the amount of carbon monoxide that is inhaled with the amount that is exhaled and that is transferred to the blood.

Exercise testing is different from the other pulmonary function tests because it is not conducted when a person is at rest but rather during exertion. The person being tested exercises on a stationary bicycle or a treadmill, slowly increasing the level of intensity until a certain heart rate is attained or until shortness of breath occurs. During the test, blood pressure, oxygen levels, and breathing rate are monitored, and an electrocardiogram traces the heart's electrical activity. Spirometry is performed after the exercise, and a measurement of maximum oxygen uptake is evaluated by contrasting it with normal standards. This allows doctors to determine whether the source of

P

breathlessness is related to heart or lung disease or to a lack of conditioning. Exercise testing is especially useful for people who experience shortness of breath when exerting themselves, such as people with exercise-induced asthma. In these people, the bronchial tubes constrict and impair airflow only during physical activity.

Measurements of blood gases (the levels of oxygen and carbon dioxide in the blood) can indicate the presence of a breathing disorder and its severity. In this form of pulmonary function testing, blood is obtained from an artery, because arterial blood has undergone gas exchange in the lungs. The blood is usually taken from the radial artery located at the wrist, and the levels of oxygen and carbon dioxide in the arterial blood are measured.

Pulmonary hypertension

See HYPERTENSION, PULMONARY.

Pulmonary hypertension, primary

Abnormally high blood pressure in the pulmonary artery that may occur for no apparent reason or can be caused by diseases or conditions of the heart or lungs. Primary pulmonary hypertension is a rare disorder of unknown cause; moreover, preventive methods are not known. The disorder develops in response to increased resistance to blood flow in the lung's arterial blood vessels. The increased workload of pumping blood against this resistance causes the right side of the heart to become enlarged, and progressive heart failure and respiratory failure eventually develop. Pulmonary hypertension affects people of all ages and both sexes, but primary pulmonary hypertension usually affects women between 20 and 40 years.

SYMPTOMS, DIAGNOSIS, AND TREATMENT
Progressive shortness of breath on exertion is the primary symptom. Other symptoms include hyperventilation, chest pain under the sternum, sensations of weakness and fatigue, dizziness, light-headedness when standing upright, fainting, and coughing up blood.

Primary pulmonary hypertension may cause distension (enlargement from internal pressure) of neck veins, liver enlargement, and general swelling caused by fluid retention in the body's tissues. Diagnostic tests may include an electrocardiogram, a chest X ray, an echocardiogram, cardiac catheterization, a lung scan, and a pulmonary arteriogram.

Because there is no known cure, the goal of treatment is to control the symptoms. Vasodilators may be beneficial to some people with primary pulmonary hypertension. Diuretics and calcium channel blockers may be prescribed to help relieve symptoms. Oxygen therapy may be needed to treat shortness of breath and improve the quality of life as the disease progresses. When available donors are found for suitable candidates, heart-lung transplantation is a treatment option.

The prognosis for primary pulmonary hypertension is usually poor. Progressive heart failure usually develops, and death ensues within 2 to 8 years. See also CHRONIC OBSTRUCTIVE PULMONARY DISEASE.

Pulmonary infarction

A disorder produced by the death of lung tissue that occurs when there is insufficient blood supply to a part of the lungs (see LUNG) and the tissue dies. Pulmonary infarction may be associated with PULMONARY EMBOLISM. The disorder can also be caused by congenital heart disease associated with severe pulmonary hypertension or sickle cell disease.

The symptoms develop over a period of several hours and include coughing, blood-stained sputum, sharp chest pain with breathing, and fever. They may be experienced for several days, becoming milder with the passage of time.

Pulmonary infarction can be diagnosed with evaluation of a chest X ray or other scanning technique that reveals a lesion on the lung and a collection of fluid, or PLEURAL EFFUSION, on the side in which the infarction has occurred. Blood test results may reveal abnormalities that indicate tissue death in the lungs.

Small areas of dead tissue may heal spontaneously by absorption, leaving

narrow scars, or they may reabsorb entirely, leaving normal lung tissue.

Larger areas of dead tissue may be irreversible.

Pulmonary insufficiency

A condition of breathing dysfunction resulting in impairment of oxygen and carbon dioxide exchange so that the exchange is insufficient to support body functions; also referred to as respiratory insufficiency. Pulmonary insufficiency results in reduced oxygen levels or elevated levels of carbon dioxide, which cause respiratory acidosis, a condition affecting acid-base balance of the body. Pulmonary insufficiency can progress to respiratory failure, in which the function of vital organs is impaired or threatened.

The condition is associated with lung diseases including CHRONIC OBSTRUCTIVE PULMONARY DISEASE (COPD), EMPHYSEMA, chronic BRONCHITIS, and PULMONARY FIBROSIS. The leading cause is cigarette smoking. Smoking cessation and early detection and treatment of diseases of the small airways may help prevent progression of pulmonary insufficiency. Acute conditions such as PULMONARY EDEMA (fluid in the lungs) and PNEUMONIA can also cause pulmonary insufficiency.

SYMPTOMS, DIAGNOSIS, AND TREATMENT
The primary symptom is shortness of breath that occurs when a person is at rest and persists for a period ranging from several months to years. A respiratory rate faster than 20 breaths per minute is another sign of pulmonary insufficiency.

A physical examination by a doctor can reveal rapid, labored breathing and the excessive use of chest muscles during inhalation. An examination of the chest with a stethoscope can detect abnormal breath sounds or inadequate air exchange.

Treatment is based on supportive care, smoking cessation, and low-flow oxygen therapy if needed. Complications include enlargement of the heart and heart failure. Lung disease support groups may be recommended. Acute pulmonary insufficiency requires aggressive treatment of the precipitating cause and respiratory support with supplemental oxygen. In severe cases, mechanical respiration may be required.

Pulmonary rehabilitation

Programs designed to offer education, therapeutic exercise, and functional activities for people with lung disorders and diseases. Pulmonary rehabilitation may be recommended to people who have emphysema, chronic bronchitis, pulmonary fibrosis, and other conditions. The goals of the program are to improve understanding of the lung condition and to offer help with coping with the disease so a person can function more comfortably and independently in his or her everyday life.

A doctor may refer a person who has a lung disorder or is recovering from lung disease to a pulmonary rehabilitation program. The person will be evaluated for his or her current level of functioning, including pulmonary function tests and studies, laboratory tests, an electrocardiogram, and a pulmonary stress test, as well as a consultation with a doctor who specializes in pulmonary medicine.

Individualized programs of educational activities, progressive exercise regimens, and support group participation are designed to meet personal needs and abilities. People are usually grouped with others who share similar breathing problems. Pulmonary rehabilitation programs usually require two to three weekly visits to the facility for 8 to 12 weeks, with each visit lasting several hours. Often a home exercise program is designed combining aerobic conditioning activities and routines to improve strength and endurance. The costs are usually covered by health insurance plans when pulmonary rehabilitation has been prescribed by a doctor.

Pulp, dental

The soft inner structure of a tooth (see TEETH). Dental pulp is sometimes referred to as the nerve of the tooth. The pulp is contained within the part of the tooth called the pulp chamber, which occupies the space in the center of the crown (see CROWN, DENTAL) and extends through the root canal to the small opening at the end of the

root. It is through this opening at the root tip that the nerves and vessels in the dental pulp are connected to arteries, veins, and nerves in the jaws. This connection offers blood supply to the tooth. The blood supply of the pulp is essential to the continual formation of the DENTIN, which surrounds and protects the pulp. The dentin also supports the structure of the tooth. If the pulp is destroyed, the tooth becomes weaker and more brittle, and the dead pulp tissue tends to darken teeth to gray or black shades. The dead tissue is removed and the health of the tooth improved by ROOT CANAL TREATMENT.

Pulpectomy

The removal of the entire dental pulp (see PULP, DENTAL) from a tooth, usually by an ENDODONTIST as part of ROOT CANAL TREATMENT. The pulp is the soft tissue inside the tooth that contains blood vessels and nerves.

Pulpitis

Inflammation of the dental pulp (see PULP, DENTAL), or the nerve of the tooth, due to acute infection. When tooth decay is untreated and penetrates through the enamel (see ENAMEL, DENTAL) and dentin to the dental pulp, bacteria invade the nerve cells in the pulp tissue. The bacteria may eventually destroy the bone at the tip of the root, producing a TOOTH ABSCESS. If the periodontal ligament that holds the root in the gum becomes infected and swells, the tooth is pushed outward from the gum and becomes highly sensitive. This causes severe pain in the tooth, especially with the pressure of biting or even lightly closing the teeth. Pressure from within the pulp chamber will also cause the tooth to ache. Often, the jaw will swell. Treatment involves a root canal or extracting the tooth.

Pulpotomy

A partial removal of pulp, the soft tissue that is located in the crown (see CROWN, DENTAL) section of the tooth. A pulpotomy is generally performed on the primary tooth of a child to save the tooth until it falls out naturally. In this procedure, the entire nerve is not removed; only the dental pulp within the pulp chamber is taken out. The ends of the nerves that lead to the

root canals are covered with a capping material, and the tooth is filled or fitted with a preformed stainless steel crown to restore function until it comes out and is replaced with a healthy, permanent tooth.

A pulpotomy may be performed on a permanent tooth as a temporary measure, but there is a greater risk that the nerve left in the root canal will degenerate. This can cause an infection in the root that eventually requires full ROOT CANAL TREATMENT or TOOTH EXTRACTION.

Pulse

The rhythmic dilation of an artery that results from the beating of the heart. The pulse is made up of a series of pressure waves within an artery caused by contractions of the left ventricle of the heart. The waves correspond with the heart rate, or

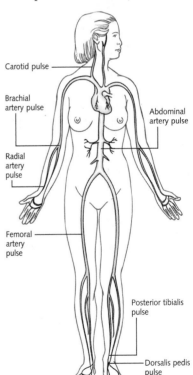

Carotid pulse

Brachial artery pulse

Radial artery pulse

Femoral artery pulse

Abdominal artery pulse

Posterior tibialis pulse

Dorsalis pedis pulse

PULSE POINTS
The pulse can be felt at various points on the body—with varying degrees of difficulty—where the blood vessel lies close under the skin. Usually the carotid pulse in the neck is the easiest to detect. The thumb often has a pulse of its own, so the index and middle fingers should be used to feel for a pulse.

P

number of heartbeats per minute. The pulse is usually measured by feeling radial arteries in the wrist, although it is also easily detected within the carotid artery in the neck.

The normal adult pulse rate at rest ranges from 60 to 80 beats per minute, although exercise, illness, injury, and emotion can produce much faster rates. Pulse rates lower than 60 beats per minute are referred to as BRADYCARDIA, and rates higher than 100 beats per minute are referred to as TACHYCARDIA.

Puncture wounds

Injuries in which an object penetrates through the skin or a body part. Puncture wounds can include such injuries as stepping on a nail or being stabbed, shot, or impaled on a stick or railing. Puncture wounds often do not bleed heavily, and sometimes the wound appears to close up right away, but in this case appearance may be deceptive, because puncture wounds are susceptible to infection and so can be very dangerous. A puncture wound through a shoe is particularly prone to serious bacterial infection. Medical care should be sought for puncture wounds to prevent infection and to protect against tetanus. If a person has been impaled on an object, it should be left in place until medical help has arrived.

Pupil

The opening in the center of the EYE though which light passes. The iris, the colored area encircling the pupil, contains muscles that adjust the size of the pupil in response to the amount of light and focusing needed. The iris opens (dilates) the pupil to allow more light to enter or to focus on far objects. The pupil contracts to restrict light coming in and to focus on near objects.

Purpura

Red, black and blue, or purple hemorrhages due to leakage of blood into the skin. Purpura is common in older people (especially on the arms and legs) because skin grows thinner with age and the loss of fat and connective tissue around blood vessels makes the blood vessels more susceptible to injury. Older people who sunbathe

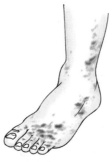

REDDISH SPOTS AND DISCOLORATION
Purpura generally appears on the legs and feet, for reasons that are not clear. Various treatments, such as medication, vitamins, or support hose, have been tried without much success. The condition may fade in a few weeks or months or may last for years.

are more likely to develop purpura because their skin has been weakened by sun damage. There are also vascular causes of purpura, such as drug-induced inflammation of blood vessel walls. Medications such as aspirin and warfarin make people more susceptible to bruising and purpura.

Purulent

Conditions that discharge pus or cause the production of pus; also, human secretions that consist of pus or contain pus. Purulent may describe an inflammation, a wound, or an infection that produces pus. See also PUS.

Pus

A thick, yellow-to-white opaque fluid that consists of white blood cells, cellular debris, and dead tissue cells. Pus forms in infected tissue of body structures and is produced by the inflammatory process of SUPPURATION.

Pustules

Superficial elevations of the skin containing pus, which are the result of inflamed hair follicles. Pustules, also called "pimples," are formed when hair follicles or sweat pores become blocked and the body oil called sebum is trapped in the follicles. This promotes the multiplication of bacteria that are normally present in the hair follicles. The increase in bacteria attracts infection-fighting cells that release substances that create inflammation in the skin, causing irritation

and redness at the site of the affected follicle. When the follicle ruptures, its contents are spread into surrounding skin, which causes the inflammation to spread. See also ACNE.

PUVA

A type of PHOTOTHERAPY (treatment with light) that combines the drug psoralen with exposure to a carefully measured amount of ultraviolet A (UVA) light. Psoralen promotes PHOTOSENSITIVITY (heightened sensitivity to the sun) by maximizing the effect of ultraviolet light on the skin. PUVA is often an effective treatment for skin disorders such as psoriasis and vitiligo. However, long-term treatment is associated with an increased risk of skin cancer. Treatment must be carefully monitored by a dermatologist. Because psoralen remains in the lens of the eye, eyeglasses that block UVA rays must be worn on the day of treatment.

Pyelography

An X ray of the urinary system made with a special dye that highlights the kidneys and ureters (the urine tubes that carry urine from the kidneys to the bladder). The test is performed when a person has symptoms that may indicate abnormalities, infection, tumors, injury, or disease in the urinary system. There are three ways of introducing the dye into the kidneys. In the simplest test, intravenous pyelography (IVP), a thin needle is inserted into a vein, usually on the inside of the elbow or the back of the hand, and the dye is injected through it. X rays are taken as the dye passes through the kidneys, the ureters, and the bladder. In retrograde pyelography, a small tube

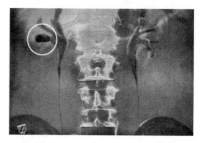

IMAGE OF A KIDNEY STONE
Dye inserted during intravenous pyelography is a contrast medium that highlights the presence of a kidney stone.

is inserted into the urinary tract and through the bladder into the ureters. The dye is then sent up the tube into the ureters and kidneys, and X rays are taken. For antegrade pyelography, the dye is injected into the kidney through a needle inserted through the skin. X rays are taken as the dye moves through the kidneys and down the ureters into the bladder. Pyelography allows the physician to see any birth defects, tumors, disease, or damage that may be present.

Before pyelography, the person must not drink or eat anything for a specified number of hours. A laxative is often given to rid the intestine of gas or feces that can obscure the findings of the X rays. During IVP, a few individuals experience nausea, vomiting, or headaches after the dye is injected. There is also a small chance of an allergic reaction. The amount of radiation used in the X rays is low and poses little risk, except for pregnant women and small children who are more sensitive to X rays.

Pyelolithotomy

A surgical procedure to remove one or more KIDNEY STONES. Pyelolithotomy is major surgery and requires a 4- to 6-week recovery period. This open surgical technique was once performed routinely but now is performed in less than 2 percent of people who require the removal of kidney stones. Pyelolithotomy may become necessary if LITHOTRIPSY is not appropriate or has failed. It may also be implemented in people who are obese or have physical abnormalities such as obstructions in the pelvis.

Pyelonephritis

FOR SYMPTOM CHARTS
see Abdominal pain, page 14
see Backache, page 20

An inflammation of the kidney caused by a bacterial infection. Pyelonephritis is usually associated with a urinary tract infection (see URINARY TRACT INFECTIONS) that has spread to the kidneys. The spread of infec-tion may be promoted by any condition that inhibits or obstructs the flow of urine through the ureters, which are tubes that carry urine from

the kidneys to the bladder. A reflux of infected urine up the ureters and into the kidneys also contributes to pyelonephritis. The condition is uncommon in men who have normal urinary tracts. Women may be predisposed to pyelonephritis by physical changes that occur during pregnancy or by catheter use. In men or women, diabetes mellitus, sickle cell disease, or kidney damage due to overuse of analgesics may sometimes be associated with pyelonephritis.

SYMPTOMS, DIAGNOSIS, AND TREATMENT

Initial symptoms of acute pyelonephritis begin suddenly and may include backache (especially tenderness in the middle and lower areas of the back), a high fever with shaking chills, side pain, nausea, and vomiting. Some people may also experience frequent urges to urinate and find it difficult and painful to urinate. These symptoms require immediate medical attention as the infection can spread from the kidneys to the bloodstream and cause a person to collapse. There is also a risk of permanent kidney damage if the condition is not treated promptly.

Chronic pyelonephritis may cause symptoms that are mild and transitory, including side pain or abdominal pain. In cases affecting children, the inflammation may produce masses of fatty deposits in the kidneys, and symptoms may include side pain, fever, fatigue, anorexia, and weight loss.

Diagnosis is made after a physical examination. The person's urine may be tested for the presence of pus and bacteria. The doctor may perform a CYSTOSCOPY, examining the ureter through a viewing instrument. In some cases, blood tests may be performed, and CT (computed tomography) scanning may be ordered to rule out other causes of symptoms.

Pyelonephritis is generally treated with oral antibiotics. In severe cases, hospitalization and treatment with intravenous fluids and antibiotics may become necessary.

Pyloric stenosis

A rare disorder in which the pylorus, the outlet from the stomach to the duodenum, becomes partially

or completely blocked. Pyloric stenosis is usually the result of a chronic peptic ulcer (see PEPTIC ULCER DISEASE), which causes scarring and deformity of the outlet. Damage and blockage result from strong acids and digestive enzymes secreted by stomach glands. Less commonly, this condition is due to STOMACH CANCER. Pyloric stenosis blocks the passage of food and secretions from the stomach to the duodenum. This often results in a bloated, uncomfortable feeling. Because the stomach is never fully emptied, the abdomen becomes distended. Vomiting may occur several hours or more after eating. Total blockage of the pylorus results in repeated vomiting, weight loss, dehydration, malnutrition, and chemical imbalances.

Diagnosis of pyloric stenosis is usually made by GASTROSCOPY (internal examination of the esophagus, stomach, and duodenum with a flexible viewing tube). To treat abdominal distension, doctors insert a nasogastric tube through the nose down into the stomach to drain away secretions. Surgery is necessary if scarring is extensive, if there are recurring ulcers, or in cases of stomach cancer.

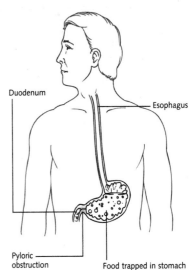

Duodenum

Esophagus

Pyloric obstruction

Food trapped in stomach

BLOCKAGE OF THE PYLORUS
Scarring from ulcers, or sometimes cancer, can cause a thickening of the pylorus, the outlet from the stomach into the small intestine (duodenum). The thickening can partially or completely block the movement of partially digested food out of the stomach.

P

Pyloroplasty

See VAGOTOMY.

Pyoderma gangrenosum

A noninfectious ulcerative disease of the skin. Pyoderma gangrenosum does not involve gangrene, despite its name. It most often affects young to middle-aged adults and most commonly occurs on the legs. Lesions begin as tender, pus-filled papules (small superficial bumps on the skin) and blisters. The lesions develop into painful ulcers with ragged purple edges that heal with scarring. Pyoderma gangrenosum is sometimes associated with other conditions, including inflammatory bowel disease, leukemia, and rheumatoid arthritis. Diagnosis is based on clinical impression and ruling out other skin diseases through a biopsy. Because treatment differs, it is important to distinguish pyoderma gangrenosum from other types of ulcers. Treatment includes prescribed corticosteroids and other immunosuppressant medications, including cyclosporine.

Pyogenic granuloma

An inflamed papule (small superficial bump on the skin) that bleeds easily. Pyogenic granulomas often appear at the site of an injury or irritation but can also occur as a complication of a PORT-WINE STAIN. They are most common on the face, arms, and hands and are seen most frequently in children and in pregnant women. Lesions tend to persist without treatment and must be removed using cauterization, surgery, or laser. To prevent recurrence, it is important to eliminate the entire lesion.

Pyorrhea

See PERIODONTAL DISEASE.

Pyramidal system

A complex pathway of brain tissue and nerves that controls fine, skilled movements, so called because the nerve tracts look like pyramids under a microscope. The tracts of the pyramidal system begin in the areas of the cerebrum that control movement. They travel down through the cerebrum into the cerebellum, then into the portion of the brain stem known as the medulla oblongata, and finally into the spinal cord. Nerves leaving the spine connect with muscles such as those in the hands and fingers that coordinate precise skills like writing.

Pyrexia

An abnormal elevation in body temperature. See FEVER.

Pyrogen

Any substance or agent that tends to cause a rise in body temperature and produces FEVER.

Pyromania

An abnormal, compulsive desire to start fires. The fires are not set for economic gain, such as collecting on an insurance policy, or for reasons of revenge. Rather, the person experiences a buildup of tension that is released when the fire is set. Often he or she remains in the area of the fire to watch it burn. A person with pyromania usually has a low or borderline IQ (intelligence quotient) and chronic stress. The prevalence of alcoholism is higher among people with pyromania than among the general population. Typically this disorder begins in childhood, and it sometimes leads people to seek work as firefighters. Since they have a compulsion to repeatedly set fires, they may endanger the family or community. Psychiatric evaluation and treatment are needed.

Pyuria

The presence of white blood cells or pus in the urine. Pyuria is usually the sign of a urinary tract infection (see URINARY TRACT INFECTIONS) or an infection of the kidney, such as PYELONEPHRITIS.

P

Q fever

A ZOONOSIS, or disease transmitted by animals, that is caused by an organism. Q fever occurs in domestic and farm animals without symptoms. Sheep, cattle, goats, and ticks are primarily responsible for its transmission to humans. Rodents, birds, and other animals may also have a role in spreading the disease to humans. The infective organism is present in these animals' feces, urine, milk, and body tissues, particularly the placenta. Humans can contract the disease by handling infected animal parts and products and by inhaling airborne particles and dust that are contaminated. Inhalation of a single organism can be enough to cause an infection in a person.

SYMPTOMS, DIAGNOSIS, AND TREATMENT

In humans, Q fever is characterized by a sudden high fever, chills, severe headache and fatique, loss of appetite, and muscle pain. Infection of the connective tissue that surrounds the lungs' air sacs often causes chest pains. The fever may be as high as 104°F and last for as long as 3 weeks. Other possible symptoms include sore throat, abdominal pain, vomiting, or diarrhea. During the second week of infection, there may be a dry cough. At this stage, chest X rays may reveal inflammation of the lungs. Q fever is almost never fatal, but prolonged infections can progress to HEPATITIS or ENDOCARDITIS, especially in people with previously existing heart abnormalities.

Q fever may be misdiagnosed as the flu. An evaluation of the symptoms typical of the disease, a history that includes contact with animals, and a physical examination that may reveal an enlarged liver or spleen may lead to a suspicion of Q fever. Blood tests that include specific complement fix-ation (CF) and agglutination testing can detect antibodies to the organism.

Treatment includes oral antibiotics such as tetracycline in adults and chloramphenicol in young children. In acute cases, antibiotics are usually continued for 5 days after the fever has subsided.

Qigong

Ancient Chinese system of healing; a form of ENERGY MEDICINE. Qigong, pronounced "chee gung," uses breathing, meditation, visualization, and repetitive physical exercises to cleanse and strengthen the body. Qigong literally means "working with energy." It is an element of CHINESE MEDICINE that promotes health by strengthening the flow of qi, or vital energy. The exercises associated with qigong are designed to teach improved breathing and to positively affect heart rate and circulation of the blood. Qigong exercises involve relaxation, concentration, and controlled breathing. The martial arts T'AI CHI and kung fu developed from qigong.

Quackery

Fraudulent actions, claims, or methods in medicine. A person practices quackery when he or she recommends a treatment or nonprescription medicine with no known value—for example, the old patent medicine "tonics" that were mainly alcohol.

Quadriparesis

Weakness, slight paralysis, or motor and sensory malfunction that involves both the upper and lower extremities.

Quadriplegia

See PARALYSIS.

Quarantine

The isolation of a person or persons for the purpose of preventing the spread of a known or suspected infection with a contagious disease. Quarantine is a medical strategy for limiting a large or small community's exposure to infectious pathogens. It may be imposed on people who have been exposed to serious contagious diseases, as well as on those who have acquired a contagious infection or who are believed to have been infected.

Quickening

The first movements of a fetus that a pregnant woman feels. The woman usually feels quickening for the first time during the 16th week of her first pregnancy. In subsequent pregnancies, quickening can occur as early as the 14th week. Quickening is usually felt as a flutter, while later in the pregnancy, the woman will feel distinct kicks that are sometimes visible on her abdomen.

Quinapril

A drug used to treat high blood pressure and congestive heart failure. Quinapril (Accupril, Accuretic) is an angiotensin-converting enzyme (ACE) inhibitor, one of a class of drugs that lowers blood pressure by blocking the formation of a substance that contracts blood vessels. Quinapril works by relaxing blood vessels, thereby lowering blood pressure and increasing the supply of blood and oxygen to the heart.

Quinidine

A drug used to treat abnormal heart rhythms; an antimalarial drug. Quinidine (Quinaglute) is effective in the treatment of abnormal heart rhythms because it slows cardiac activities in all parts of the heart. Quinidine is also used to treat malaria when QUININE is unavailable, although the two drugs are not the same and should not be confused with one another.

Quinine

An antimalarial drug. Quinine works by disrupting the parasite's ability to reproduce itself in red blood cells. The drug is also useful for treating leg muscle cramps that occur at night when a person is in bed.

Q

Rabies

FOR FIRST AID
see Bites and stings: animal bites,
page 1314

A life-threatening disease that affects the central nervous system. Rabies is caused by a virus that is found in the saliva of infected warm-blooded animals and is usually transmitted to humans and domestic pets by the bites of infected animals. Less commonly, the illness may be spread by contamination of an open skin wound or exposure of mucous membranes to the saliva from an animal that has rabies, called a rabid animal. The virus in the animal's saliva initially affects the nerve nearest the site of the animal bite or point of entry, then travels along nerve pathways to the brain. Untreated, the disease is almost always fatal.

The group of animals in the wild that are most at risk for rabies infection includes bats, raccoons, foxes, coyotes, and skunks. Weasels and other wild carnivores may also become infected and spread the disease to people. Groundhogs can become infected with rabies by inhabiting dens previously used by infected animals. Other rodents, including squirrels and rabbits, are rarely infected with rabies. Domestic dogs, cats, and farm animals can acquire rabies by being bitten by wild, rabid animals. Rabies occurs less frequently in pets and farm animals, but these domestic animals present a greater risk to humans since they are more closely associated with people. All dogs, cats, and livestock that come into contact with wild animals should be vaccinated against rabies.

COURSE OF INFECTION IN ANIMALS

The incubation period in an animal is usually 3 to 8 weeks, but it can be as long as 18 months. The wide range in time between an animal's exposure and the development of the characteristic signs of rabies depends on the species of animal, the amount of rabies virus the animal was exposed to, the virulence of the virus, the age of the animal bitten, and the location of the bite on the animal's body.

Symptoms in animals vary. An infected animal may become irritable and snap or bite constantly, running long distances and attacking everything in its path. The animal's personality may become vicious and violent. Paralysis occurs soon after the first signs of disease and usually affects the animal's hind legs first. An infected animal usually dies within 4 to 7 days of the first signs of rabies. In another pattern of infection, the affected animal may become drowsy and sluggish, but snap at nearby movement. In some cases, the lower jaw may become immobilized. Animals showing these signs tend to become comatose and die within 3 to 10 days after symptoms begin.

HUMAN SYMPTOMS AND DIAGNOSIS

Whenever a person has been bitten by a warm-blooded animal, there is a possibility of exposure to rabies. As an immediate first-aid procedure, the site of the animal bite should be thoroughly washed with soap and hot water as soon as possible. A doctor should be notified, or the person who has been bitten should visit the nearest hospital emergency department at once; prompt medical attention is essential to preventing death from the infection. If a person has been bitten by a wild animal, the local animal control officer should be notified. If a domestic animal was responsible for the bite, information should be obtained regarding the animal's rabies vaccination status.

The time between the biting incident and the appearance of the first signs of rabies is usually 3 to 7 weeks, but the range extends from 4 days to 2 years. The first symptoms of rabies are often similar to those of any viral infection, including high fever and general malaise. Within 2 to 3 days of these symptoms, rabies infection causes pain followed by tingling at the site of an animal bite. The skin becomes sensitive to changes in temperature, there is excessive production of saliva with drooling, and there are severe muscle spasms in the mouth and throat. The infected person also experiences dramatic mood swings between rage and calm and, ultimately, has seizures. The symptoms, including extreme thirst and choking caused by an inability to swallow liquids, has given rabies the name "hydrophobia," which means fear of water. Untreated, rabies causes complete paralysis, as well as heart or respiratory failure within 7 to 25 days following the start of symptoms

Rabies can be quickly and accurately diagnosed by a fluorescent antibody test done on tissue from biopsy of the nape of the neck. The course of treatment involves the use of a passive antibody injected directly into the wound. A vaccine is also injected, usually at five intervals, over a 28-day period. Treatment is usually effective if started promptly. See Protection against rabies, page 1049.

Rabies immune globulin, human

An immunizing agent. Rabies immune globulin (BayRab, Imogam Rabies-HT) is used along with rabies vaccine to prevent infection caused by the rabies virus. It works by providing antibodies needed to neutralize the rabies virus. The effects of rabies immune globulin will last long enough to provide protection until the body can produce its own antibodies against the rabies virus.

Rabies immune globulin is given to people who have been bitten, scratched, or licked by an animal known or suspected to have rabies. Because its purpose is to prompt the body to create its own antibodies, rabies immune globulin is given only once. The animals most likely to have rabies are wild and include raccoons, skunks, and bats. Cats, dogs, and foxes are also susceptible to rabies, but it is rare for domestic dogs or cats to be rabid.

Rad

The unit used to measure the amount of ionizing radiation absorbed during X-ray procedures. See X RAYS.

Radial keratotomy

A surgical procedure to correct near-sightedness by making small incisions in the clear outer covering (cornea) of the eye in a spokelike (radial) pattern. The incisions penetrate almost all the way through the cornea, which flattens in the center and becomes steeper in its outer, downward-sloping portion. This change shifts the way light rays are

PROTECTION AGAINST RABIES

Rabies is a potentially fatal but preventable viral disease of the central nervous system. It is carried in the saliva of an infected animal that spreads the disease by biting or licking an open wound on another animal or a person. Any person who is bitten by an animal should wash the bite immediately with soap and water and get medical advice.

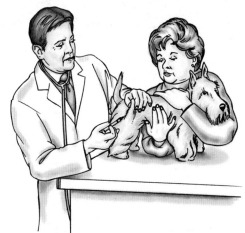

VACCINATION OF PETS
Pets in the United States must be vaccinated against the rabies virus. Today, thanks to vaccination, dogs do not spread the disease to people in the United States, but travelers still get rabies from encounters with dogs in other countries.

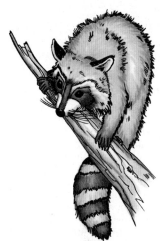

WILD ANIMAL CARRIERS
In the wild, animals such as raccoons, skunks, bats, and wolves are the primary carriers of rabies, but other mammals can also be infected.

bent as they pass through the cornea, allowing them to focus on the retina (the light-sensitive nerve layer at the back of the eye) and correcting the nearsightedness. The number of incisions (from 4 to 16) depends on the person.

Only one eye is operated on at a time. Radial keratotomy is usually performed on the nondominant eye first and on the other eye a week later.

Radial keratotomy is performed as an outpatient procedure in a physician's office or an ambulatory (same-day) surgical facility. The person undergoing the procedure is given a mild sedative to help him or her relax, and the eye is numbed with anesthetic drops. Working through a microscope, the surgeon cuts the incisions with a very small, very sharp diamond blade. When all the incisions are made, the eye is rinsed, treated with antibiotic drops, and patched for 2 hours. The procedure takes approximately 20 minutes.

For the first 24 hours following surgery, sensitivity to light, a scratchy sensation, and redness in the eye are likely. Pain is usually mild and can be controlled with medication.

Radial keratotomy is generally effective in reducing mild to moderate amounts of nearsightedness; most people who undergo the procedure no longer need glasses or they require a weaker prescription. A number of side effects and complications may follow the procedure. These include glare in night vision, sensitivity to light, fluctuation of vision during the day, overcorrection or undercorrection, severe scarring of the cornea, infection, the growth of blood vessels in the incisions, perforation of the cornea, and an increased risk of rupture of the cornea. Radial keratotomy has become a less popular procedure in recent years, particularly since the introduction of LASIK (laser in-situ keratomileusis), which uses a laser to reshape the cornea.

Radiation

The emission of high-energy, penetrating waves used to diagnose and treat various medical conditions. In medicine, radiation generally refers to ionizing radiation, which produces immediate chemical effects on human tissue. Ionizing radiation includes X rays, gamma rays, and parti-

cle bombardment such as neutron beams, electron beams, and protons. Radiation is used as a diagnostic tool in the form of X rays. It is also used therapeutically to treat cancer in the form of X rays, cobalt, and radium.

Background radiation is ionizing radiation that occurs naturally in the environment of the earth. On average, diagnostic X rays emit a much lower dose of ionizing radiation than what is absorbed from background radiation. RADIATION THERAPY, which is targeted to specific tissues being treated, uses much higher levels of ionizing radiation.

Radiation is also used in NUCLEAR MEDICINE. The diagnostic uses of radiation include newer X-ray technologies such as CT SCANNING (computed tomography scanning) and PET SCANNING (positron emission tomography scanning).

Radiation sickness

Also known as radiation poisoning; symptoms and illness that result from exposure to excessive doses of ionizing radiation. Radiation sickness may be caused by a single exposure to radiation at a very high level or by

R

ongoing exposure to lower levels over time. Radiation sickness caused by long-term exposure is generally delayed and can result in cancer and premature aging. The severity of radiation sickness depends on the amount of radiation, the type of radiation, the duration of the exposure, and the areas of the body that have been exposed.

Radiation therapy

Also known as radiotherapy; treatment of malignant (cancerous) tumors and benign (not cancerous) conditions using X rays or radionuclides. Radiation therapy is the use of high-energy radiation to destroy malignant or benign cells by carefully regulating the dose and by targeting to the treatment site. Radiation therapy is usually well tolerated and the organs treated are usually preserved.

WHY IT IS PERFORMED

Radiation therapy may be the primary treatment, or it may be combined with other treatments before or after surgery. When it is used before surgery, the goal is to shrink a cancerous tumor. After surgery, radiation may be used to stop the growth of remaining cancer cells. It may be part of a treatment plan that includes CHEMOTHERAPY or other anticancer medications. Radiation therapy may be used to treat cancers of the head and neck, skin cancer, tumors of the central nervous system, bladder cancer, prostate cancer, cervical cancer, endometrial cancer, ovarian cancer, cancers of the vagina and vulva, breast cancer, gastrointestinal tumors, lung cancer, sarcomas, lymphomas, and most pediatric cancers. Even when a cure is not probable, radiation can be used to shrink tumors (to decrease pain and relieve pressure) or to stop tumors from bleeding.

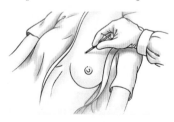

MARKING AREA BEFORE RADIATION
A woman having radiation therapy receives a tiny tattoo on her breast so that the therapist can precisely pinpoint the area needing treatment.

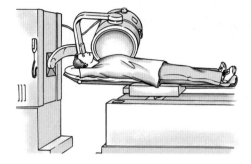

RADIATION TREATMENTS
External radiation treatments are painless and brief—usually about 5 minutes long. The person is positioned on a table and the X-ray beams are directed at the area affected by cancer. External radiation works best on small, isolated areas of cancer.

In cases of cancer that has spread, radiation therapy can improve the quality of life and increase survival rates. Bone metastases may be treated with radiation to provide pain relief and help prevent fractures. Medical emergencies resulting from cancer, such as compression of the spinal cord or airway, often respond quickly and well to radiation therapy.

Certain benign diseases may be treated with radiation therapy. It can prevent the recurrence of certain eye conditions after surgical treatment. Keloids, which are scars on the skin produced by an abnormal healing process, may be treated with low-dose radiation to help prevent local recurrence. Radiation therapy may also be used to treat pituitary adenomas. Low-dose radiation sometimes improves conditions that have not responded successfully to other treatment. These conditions include eye disorders such as Graves ophthalmopathy and skin disorders such as HEMANGIOMA and KERATOACANTHOMA. It may be used to prevent abnormal bone formation after orthopedic surgery. A certain kind of radiation therapy may be used to eliminate malformations in the blood vessels of the central nervous system that cannot be treated surgically.

HOW IT WORKS

Radiation is a local treatment that works by damaging the DNA of malignant cells. Because normal cells have a better ability to repair DNA damage than cancer cells have, radiation therapy is able to destroy the cells of tumors while minimizing damage to normal cells.

HOW IT IS PERFORMED

Radiation is commonly delivered through a linear accelerator, which accelerates electrons (to be used as a treatment beam) or generates X rays (to be used as a treatment beam). The procedure is painless and generally lasts about 5 minutes. The course of radiation therapy may be given in a single session or multiple sessions. The treatment is given over a period between 2 and 7 weeks, with five treatments per week. The frequency and dosage of radiation therapy depend on the goals of treatment and possible side effects. When the goal is to cure, the course of treatment is usually longer and tends to consist of smaller daily doses (which minimizes side effects). If cure is not possible and the goal is to relieve symptoms, larger daily doses over a shorter time may be given.

Some types of cancer are treated with a radioactive isotope that is ingested, injected, or inserted into the body. The radioactive substance, such as iodine, is chosen with the goal of destroying abnormal cells in the part of the body to be treated and preventing the malignant tumor from spreading.

RISKS OR SIDE EFFECTS

While radiation therapy is not physically disfiguring (as radical surgery can be), there may be unpleasant side effects that occur during or immediately after treatment. These side effects are usually mild but may be severe for some people. Typically, the symptoms are temporary and usually improve within 3 to 6 weeks. Fatigue is a commonly experienced temporary side effect.

Some side effects are associated with the damage X rays can do to normal tissue. Because the treatment is localized, these effects tend to be limited to the area that received radiation, including irritated or thickened skin, swallowing difficulties, dry mouth, nausea, diarrhea, and hair loss. The severity of the side effects is generally related to the site and amount of radiation used.

R

Serious side effects (which are the result of injury to tissue cells) usually occur—if they happen—months or years after radiation therapy and are more likely to be permanent. They can lead to scarring or death of the tissue cells.

Radiation therapy, interstitial
See BRACHYTHERAPY.

Radiculopathy
Damage to the nerve roots that enter or leave the spinal cord. Radiculopathy may be caused by problems such as disk prolapse (see SLIPPED DISK), spinal ARTHRITIS, or thickening of the meninges (the membranes that cover the brain and spinal cord). Symptoms include severe pain and sometimes loss of feeling in the area supplied by the affected nerves. There may also be weakness, paralysis, and wasting of the muscles supplied by the nerves. Treatment of the underlying disease is required. Analgesics and physical therapy provide some relief of symptoms.

Radioactivity
The spontaneous emission of radiation. Radioactivity is caused by the disintegration of the nuclei of atoms when they emit electromagnetic rays called X rays and gamma rays. There are three components present in the radiation of radioactivity: alpha particles, beta particles (which are electrons and penetrate 100 times more than alpha particles), and gamma rays (which penetrate much more than beta particles and consist of electromagnetic radiation of the same nature as X rays but of substantially greater energy). Radioactivity was discovered in 1896 by the French physicist Antoine Henri Becquerel as he was studying uranium. Around the same time, Marie Curie and Pierre Curie made further studies of radioactivity, measuring the heat associated with the decay of radium.

Radiograph
Also known as a radiogram; formerly known as a roentgenogram. A radiograph is a film image made by means of X rays. See also RADIOGRAPHY.

Radiography
Formerly known as roentgenography; the making of images of internal structures of the body by passing X rays through the body to act on specially sensitized film. The image results from the varying amounts of radiation absorbed by tissues of different density.

Radioisotope scanning
A NUCLEAR MEDICINE technique that uses injected radioactive isotopes injected into the bloodstream to visualize internal organs. Radioactive isotopes are substances that give off beta or gamma rays, which are similar to X rays. Radioisotope scanning allows the observation and study of the size, shape, and location of organs or bones. The procedure can be used to evaluate organ function or to locate sites of disease, structural abnormalities, abscesses, or tumors. Radioisotope scanning may also be used to monitor and evaluate ongoing treatment for a disease or condition.

HOW IT WORKS
A radioactive isotope is introduced into the body through a catheter into a vein. After the isotope has accumulated in the organ to be studied, a scanner is positioned above the person being tested. The scanning device detects the gamma rays that are emitted by the isotope and transmits the information to a computer. The computer displays an image of the organ or body area being scanned, which may be reproduced onto X-ray film. The amount of radioactivity or the intensity of radioactivity may be recorded.

Normally, bones and organs absorb the isotopes uniformly. A number of conditions can produce abnormal accumulations of the isotope, including trauma, cancer, arthritis, intrauterine bleeding, leakage of spinal fluid, bone fractures, acute infections, abscesses, blood clots, and embolisms.

Radiologist
A physician who is trained in the use of radiant energy, specifically X rays and radionuclides, radiation physics, and biology. Diagnostic radiologists are also trained in ULTRASOUND SCANNING and MRI (magnetic resonance imaging). They assess and interpret the results of these diagnostic tests as well as the results shown on X-ray film. Therapeutic radiologists, also known as radiation oncologists, treat tumors with various forms of radiant energy.

Radiology
A branch of medicine concerned with the use of radiant energy in the diagnosis and treatment of disease. Radiology is the scientific discipline of medical imaging with the use of X rays, NUCLEAR MEDICINE, MRI (magnetic resonance imaging), and ULTRASOUND SCANNING.

Interventional radiology is a subspecialty of radiology that includes both diagnosis and treatment. The related procedures use all available imaging techniques for guidance in providing treatment options including angiography, angioplasty, certain catheter placements, infusions of chemotherapeutic medications, and implanting ports in the person for regular infusions of medication.

Radiolucent
The characteristic of being partially or completely able to be penetrated by radiation, especially by X rays. Radiolucent areas of the body are less dense than surrounding tissues and structures, which makes them appear darker on X-ray film. For example, air within the lungs is radiolucent, which makes the lungs appear dark or black on the film. Radiolucent is the opposite of radiopaque. Radiopaque is the characteristic of not allowing X rays to penetrate completely, making these areas appear white on X-ray film.

Radionics
The use of extrasensory perception (ESP) to heal disease by identifying and correcting disturbances in energy flow. Radionics assumes that a trained practitioner can identify and modify energy patterns, or vibrations, that have been unbalanced or disrupted by illness, injury, stress, malnutrition, pollution, or poor hygiene. By using radionic instruments, the altered energy pattern is "read," or identified, from any part or element of the body and treated with messages that enable the body to heal itself with restored energy flow. Radionic instruments are believed

R

capable of reading energy patterns from such samples as blood spots, fingernail clippings, or locks of hair, which means that it is not necessary for the person to be anywhere near the instrument to be treated. The reading of energy patterns is sometimes known as radiesthesia and is based on the belief that each living thing has a unique energy "signature" that can be detected by a trained and sensitive observer. Used in conjunction with HOMEOPATHY (the treatment of disease with remedies that cause similar symptoms), radiesthesia is sometimes called psionic medicine. Such treatments remain unproven.

Radionuclide scanning

See NUCLEAR MEDICINE.

Radiopharmaceuticals

Drugs used to diagnose or to treat certain medical conditions. Radiopharmaceuticals are used by nuclear medicine specialists to study how a particular organ is working and to detect tumors or cancer that may be present. Radiopharmaceuticals are radioactive, given in very tiny, safe amounts—about the same or less than the radiation received from an X ray. When used to diagnose disease, a radiopharmaceutical passes through a targeted organ of the body; the radioactivity can then be detected, and the suspect organ can be clearly pictured using special imaging equipment.

Some radiopharmaceuticals are used in larger amounts to treat certain kinds of cancer or other diseases. The radiopharmaceuticals are taken up in the cancerous area of an organ, where they destroy the cancerous tissue. Many types of radiopharmaceuticals are available; selection of a radiopharmaceutical depends on the organ that is to be studied or treated.

Radon

A colorless, gaseous, radioactive element produced by the disintegration of radium, uranium, lead, zinc, and iron ore. Radon is thought to cause an increase in lung cancer when found in microscopic particles in environmental airborne dust. It is odorless, colorless, tasteless, and not irritating to the lungs, which is why it is important for people to get their homes tested for radon. It is believed that 11 percent of lung cancer cases are related to radon. Radon is used in RADIATION THERAPY.

Raloxifene

A drug used to prevent osteoporosis in postmenopausal women. Raloxifene (Evista) is a drug that works like an estrogen (female hormone) to stop bone loss in women after menopause. Raloxifene does not treat symptoms of menopause, such as hot flashes. The drug is also being studied for the prevention of breast cancer.

Ramipril

A drug used to treat high blood pressure and congestive heart failure. Ramipril (Altace) is an angiotensin-converting enzyme (ACE) inhibitor, one of a class of drugs that lowers blood pressure by blocking formation of a component that constricts blood vessels. Ramipril works by relaxing blood vessels, thereby lowering blood pressure and increasing the supply of blood and oxygen to the heart. Ramipril is also used in some people after a heart attack to help slow the weakening of the heart muscle.

Range-of-motion exercises

Physical motion that involves extending and flexing a joint by the degrees of a circle. Range-of-motion exercises may involve the spine, neck, shoulder, elbow, wrist, hand, fingers, hip, or foot. The exercises may be performed with the help of a physical therapist as part of a preliminary evaluation. The therapist may guide a person's joint through a series of range-of-motion movements to determine the extent of a joint's impairment. Range-of-motion exercises may also be practiced to increase and maintain the mobility of a joint that has been impaired by disease or injury. For people who have OSTEOARTHRITIS, range-of-motion exercises can help avoid stiffness and prevent future problems.

Ranitidine

An antiulcer drug used in the long-term treatment of gastric ulcers. Ranitidine (Zantac) is also used in the short-term treatment of duodenal and gastric ulcers and to prevent ulcers caused by stress. Ranitidine is used to treat gastroesophageal reflux disease (GERD), in which stomach acid leaks back into the esophagus, causing painful heartburn and other stomach conditions from oversecretion of gastric acid.

Ranitidine comes in many forms. As a prescription drug, it is available in tablets, capsules, syrup, effervescent granules, and injections. As a nonprescription drug, ranitidine is available in tablet form for the relief of heartburn, acid indigestion, and sour stomach.

Rape

FOR FIRST AID
see Rape/sexual assault, page 1327

Any form of sexual intercourse that is forced on a person without consent. Although most frequently men commit rape against women, it can be committed by men or women against men or by women against women. Rape is a crime of aggression and violence and is not a form of healthy sexual relations. It is usually committed by someone who feels anger and sexual urges simultaneously. Abnormal brain chemistry and abnormal early sexual experiences are each thought to play a role in the behavior of rapists.

Rapists often take advantage of the smaller size, younger age, or lack of experience of their victims. They may also take advantage of a victim's impaired mental capacity, whether due to consumption of drugs and alcohol or mental illness or mental retardation. The rapist can be a stranger, although in about half of all rapes, the victim knows him or her. A rapist is often a family member, friend (SEE DATE RAPE), or even the victim's spouse. Victims can be of all ages, from infants to older adults.

Being treated for rape is complicated because rape is a crime. Injuries must be treated at the same time that evidence is collected. Someone who has been raped should be examined by a physician before washing, so that samples of the rapist's blood, hair, or SEMEN can be obtained for use as evidence of the crime. In addition to injuries due to physical force, the physical effects of rape can include a sexually transmitted disease or, for women, pregnancy.

The doctor can prescribe hormones that reduce the risk of pregnancy. Medications are also available to reduce the risk of acquiring a sexually transmitted disease.

Rape has profound psychological effects on victims. Some victims wrongly assume that they are responsible for having been raped because they did not resist effectively. Some victims feel ashamed of having been raped and find it difficult to tell police, family, or friends about the experience. Insensitive responses on the part of police or defense attorneys can be very difficult for victims. They may need to seek psychological counseling for help in dealing with these effects.

Rash

A flat or raised skin eruption characterized by changes in skin color or texture. Symptoms of rashes vary widely. Redness is common, and many are crusted or blistered. While some rashes cause no physical pain, many cause itching, swelling, and inflammation. Even otherwise symptom-free rashes can be cosmetically disturbing and lead to emotional distress. Rashes are due to a wide variety of causes, including allergic reactions (commonly to drugs or poisonous plants) and bacterial or viral infections. Rashes usually respond well to simple home remedies such as applying cool compresses and soothing lotions and taking over-the-counter antihistamines. However, when rashes are persistent, cause severe discomfort, or are accompanied by fever, it is important to consult a doctor.

Raynaud disease

A condition in which the arteries carrying blood to the fingers or toes constrict on exposure to cold or during emotional upset. The fingers or toes turn chalky white, and they may also sting or feel cold and numb. The skin may turn blue or red while normal blood flow is restored. Unlike Raynaud phenomenon, which is caused by underlying conditions, including hormone imbalances (such as HYPOTHYROIDISM) and rheumatic diseases (such as RHEUMATOID ARTHRITIS and SCLERODERMA), Raynaud disease exists on its own as an exaggerated version of a normal reflex that restricts blood flow to the extremities. It affects four to five times as many women as men and is most likely to begin between the ages of 15 and 40. Long-term consequences such as gangrene or skin ulcers are rare, and the disease is usually more of a nuisance than a disability.

Prevention is the best approach to Raynaud disease. This includes protection against the cold, avoiding tobacco use (nicotine constricts blood vessels in the hands and feet), using insulated glasses for cold drinks, adopting a contraceptive method other than birth control pills (which affect circulation), avoiding cold remedies that may include phenylpropanolamine, and using mittens to handle frozen foods. Medications may also be prescribed to prevent blood vessel spasms.

Raynaud phenomenon

A condition in which the arteries carrying blood to the fingers or toes constrict on exposure to cold or during emotional upset. The nose and ears may also be affected. The phenomenon is an exaggerated version of a normal reflex that restricts blood flow to the extremities. The fingers or toes turn chalky white, and they may also sting or feel cold and numb. The skin may turn blue or red while normal blood flow is restored. The entire episode can last from less than a minute to several hours.

The difference between Raynaud phenomenon and Raynaud disease is that Raynaud phenomenon occurs as a result of an underlying condition, such as SCLERODERMA, exposure to certain chemicals (for example, vinyl chloride), or long-term use of vibrating equipment, such as pneumatic drills or jackhammers. Raynaud disease is independent of any underlying condition.

RDIs

See REFERENCE DAILY INTAKES.

Reactive airway disease

A group of lung and lower airway disorders characterized by wheezing, a high-pitched whistling sound. Causes of reactive airway disease include the chronic condition asthma, bronchial infections such as BRONCHIOLITIS and BRONCHITIS, colds (see COLD, COMMON), congenital lung defects, a tumor, cystic fibrosis, inhalation of a foreign object, and pneumonia. Wheezing is the hallmark symptom of reactive airway disease. It occurs when airways inside the lungs become inflamed (reddened) and irritated. This irritation may trigger spasms in the muscles lining the airway, which narrows the passage for air. Airways that have already been narrowed by swelling and spasms can also become clogged with mucus, which makes breathing increasingly difficult. Other characteristics of reactive airway disease include chest tightness or pain, straining of chest muscles while breathing, and rapid breathing. In severe reactive airway disease, a lack of oxygen may cause the skin to grow bluish or gray.

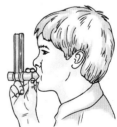

USING A PEAK FLOW METER
A peak flow meter measures the rate at which air flows out of the lungs, an indicator of the severity of reactive airway disease. The child takes a deep breath and then blows as hard as possible into the mouthpiece. The higher the measurement, the more easily air moves through the lungs.

RASH ALERT

Most rashes are not serious. However, in some cases they are a symptom of a severe underlying problem, such as meningitis, Rocky Mountain spotted fever, or a drug reaction. **Warning:** Immediate medical attention is needed if one or more of these danger signs accompanies a rash:

- A fever of 102°F or higher
- Abnormally rapid breathing
- Noisy or difficult breathing
- Severe headache
- Seizures
- Drowsiness or confusion
- Severe sore throat
- Neck pain when bending the head forward
- Sensitivity to bright light
- Nausea or vomiting

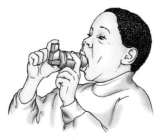

A child with a reactive airway disease such as asthma may use an inhaler to take bronchodilators to open clogged passageways in the lungs or corticosteroids to fight inflammation. These drugs are often taken with a device called an inhaler. Some inhalers have a spacer, which makes the device easier to use properly. The child needs to learn to shake the inhaler, exhale, and close the lips around the spacer.

DIAGNOSIS

To diagnose the condition, the physician will ask about any history of breathing problems and conduct a thorough physical examination. Although wheezing is sometimes clearly audible, most often, the physician must listen to the lungs with a stethoscope to detect wheezing. The doctor may also order blood tests, chest X rays, and sputum or phlegm cultures. Devices such as a spirometer or a peak flow meter may be used to measure lung function. The spiro meter records the rate at which a patient exhales air from the lungs and the total volume exhaled. A peak flow meter assesses the degree of obstruction to airflow and monitors treatment. If an attack is severe, the physician may measure the oxygen level in the bloodstream.

TREATMENT

Treatment of reactive airway disease varies according to its underlying cause. If wheezing is caused by a foreign body, the object must be removed. An ear, nose, and throat specialist or a pulmonologist (a lung specialist) can do this using a device called a bronchoscope. If the cause is a congenital lung defect or tumor, surgery may be necessary. Several types of medication commonly are prescribed to treat reactive airway disease. They are bronchodilator drugs, CORTICOSTEROIDS, and allergy medications. Bronchodilators relax the muscles around airways and open bronchial tubes. Taken by mouth or inhaled, bronchodilators allow air to move more freely in and out of the lungs. Corticosteroid are anti-inflam-

matory drugs that reduce swelling and inflammation in the airways. They can be taken by mouth, inhaled, or given as an injection. Inhaling a corticosteroid drug is considered safest.

In some people, reactive airway disease is triggered by allergies. An allergy is an overreaction of the immune system to a substance that is harmless to other people. Allergy testing can confirm whether allergies are the problem. Using medications and avoiding known allergens, such as cat dander, often alleviate allergy symptoms. People with more severe allergies may benefit from a series of allergy shots. See also ALLERGIES; ASTHMA.

Reagent

A substance used to produce a chemical reaction to detect, measure, or produce other substances. For example, one reagent (Ilosvay reagent) is used to test for the presence of nitrites: several substances are mixed together to produce a sediment that is then dissolved in acetic acid. It is then combined with the substance suspected of containing nitrites. If present, the nitrites will cause the solution to turn red when heated.

Receptor

A nerve cell that responds to a stimulus in the environment by producing nerve impulses. The term "receptor" may also refer to the area on the surface of a cell to which a chemical must bind to have its effect.

Recombinant DNA

Altered DNA (DEOXYRIBONUCLEIC ACID) created by the insertion of a portion of DNA from another source. Recombinant DNA has been altered by chemical,

biological, or enzymatic means to enable the foreign DNA that is placed in the host DNA to be replicated along with the host DNA.

Genetic traits can be transferred from one organism to another by recombining the DNA of one organism with that of another. The process of inserting a portion of DNA into another strand of DNA is similar to editing text, or "cutting and pasting." Recombinant DNA technology currently uses a number of techniques for cutting apart and splicing together different pieces of DNA. In one of them, a single gene is spliced into the DNA of a bacterium. When the bacteria divide, they will very shortly create billions of copies of themselves, each carrying within its DNA a perfect copy of the gene pasted into the original host cell. The genetically altered cells can then produce the protein associated with the inserted DNA.

CLONING A DESIRABLE GENE

Recombinant DNA is currently used to develop substances of medical value, as in GENE THERAPY, or of economic value, as in the GENETIC ENGINEERING of food plants. A desirable gene is introduced into a host in the hope of providing a desirable trait or inducing the production of a valuable protein. In one example, the human gene that controls the production of human insulin is transferred and cloned in bacteria.

First, the appropriate gene is cut from human DNA and spliced, or pasted, into a special kind of DNA called plasmid DNA, which is circular and is a useful vehicle for splicing. The cutting of DNA is performed by enzymes known as restriction enzymes, which cut DNA very precisely at specific points. When the gene to be spliced into host DNA is ready for transfer, it

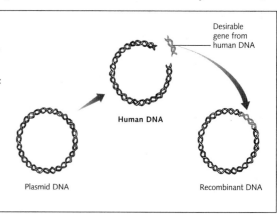

SPLICING DESIRABLE GENES
Desirable DNA can be artificially produced in a laboratory. The process begins with a tiny packet of genetic information in a circular form (plasmid DNA). A desirable gene (such as the gene for resistance to a certain microorganism) from human DNA is cut out and new DNA is inserted into the plasmid DNA ring to make recombinant DNA.

Desirable gene from human DNA

Human DNA

Plasmid DNA

Recombinant DNA

is pasted into place with another enzyme, one called DNA ligase. The result is a recombinant DNA molecule. The recombinant DNA molecule can be inserted into a bacterium, and the cell becomes a factory that produces a protein such as human insulin. The cells can also pass the information about insulin production along to all subsequent generations, creating billions of cells capable of creating insulin.

Reconstructive surgery

Any surgical operation to restore function to body structures that are defective or damaged. Reconstructive surgery focuses on congenital defects, such as CLEFT LIP AND PALATE, and deformities caused by injury, disease (for example, the loss of a breast to cancer surgery), or aging.

Recovery

Also known as sobriety; the physical and mental state of an individual who has been dependent on alcohol or drugs and is now living without the addictive substance. A person in recovery has accepted treatment and is happy living a lifestyle marked by abstinence. See ALCOHOL DEPENDENCE.

Recovery room

See POSTOPERATIVE CARE.

Rectal bleeding

Bleeding from the rectum can be a sign of a digestive system disease. Often, rectal bleeding results from a minor problem such as HEMORRHOIDS. But it may be caused by a more serious disorder such as COLITIS, CROHN DISEASE, or cancer. Any rectal bleeding requires prompt medical attention. Regular screening tests are also recommended to detect rectal bleeding that may not be visible. A rectal examination should be conducted annually at age 40 and older. A fecal-occult blood test to detect hidden traces of blood in the feces should be done yearly after age 50. GASTROSCOPY, PROCTOSCOPY, SIGMOIDOSCOPY, and COLONOSCOPY are the typical procedures used to determine the cause of rectal bleeding.

Rectal examination

A digital examination of the rectum to check for cancer. In the examina-

tion, the doctor inserts a gloved finger into the rectum to check for growths and to evaluate the prostate gland in men. Doctors recommend annual rectal examinations for everyone age 40 or older. Those at high risk due to a personal history of colitis or polyps or having an immediate family member who has colon or rectal cancer are advised to be tested annually at an earlier age.

Rectal prolapse

A condition in which the end of the rectum bulges or protrudes out of the anal canal. Rectal prolapse occurs when the muscles supporting the perineum (the area between the anus and genital organs) become stretched or weakened. This condition is most common in older people and is usually the result of straining to defecate. Other causes may include weakness of the pelvic muscles, loss of control of the anal sphincter, a neurological condition, or a genetic predisposition. When rectal prolapse develops in children, it is normally due to constipation that can be relieved with a high-fiber diet.

In its early stages, poor sphincter control may be the only sign of rectal prolapse. Often, the condition is temporary, and the end of the rectum can be pushed back into the canal with a finger. However, as time goes on, straining may cause the rectum to protrude further. The condition may become permanent, resulting in constant leaking of stool and mucus. Prolapse is usually diagnosed through

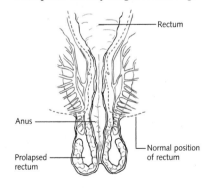

A FALLEN RECTUM
Rectal prolapse may be caused by straining to defecate or may result from aging. The rectum may descend out of the anus altogether. Sometimes it can be pushed back in with a finger, but the prolapse can become permanent. Surgery can correct the problem.

sigmoidoscopy (a visual examination of the rectum and the sigmoid colon using a flexible, lighted tube). In permanent cases, surgery may be recommended. Surgeons can use wire or nylon to tighten the anal sphincter or reposition the rectum. However, surgery is not always successful.

Rectocele

A weakness in the back wall of the vagina causing a woman's RECTUM to bulge into the vagina. Rectoceles are usually caused during childbirth by the stretching of the pelvic muscles that support the vagina, rectum, and bladder.

Symptoms may include pressure or aching in the vagina and a feeling of pressure or discomfort during a bowel movement. Constipation can also occur, because stool can collect in the area where the rectum presses into the vaginal wall.

A doctor can easily diagnose a rectocele during a routine pelvic examination. Minor symptoms can be relieved by practicing KEGEL EXERCISES —alternately contracting and relaxing pelvic floor muscles. In severe cases, surgery may be recommended, in which the surgeon makes an incision along the back wall of the vagina, pushes the rectum back and up, and stitches it in its normal position.

Rectum

The last segment of the large intestine, or COLON, which connects with the anus. Food that has been fully processed in the small and large intestines is stored as stool, or feces, in the colon, then moved into the rectum by muscular contractions.

Three folds of membrane extending across the rectum (transverse folds) act like valves to control the movement of feces through the rectum until the urge to defecate occurs. When feces distend the walls of the rectum, the pressure causes nerve impulses to pass to the brain, which sends messages to the muscles in the ANUS to relax and allow passage of the stool. See also DIGESTIVE SYSTEM.

Rectum, cancer of the

Cancer that originates in the rectum, the lower part of the large intestine just below the colon. Colon and rectal

R

cancers are often jointly called colorectal cancer. Most cancers of the large intestine grow slowly; therefore, colorectal cancer can often be cured with early detection and treatment. Men and women are equally susceptible to this disease; the risk increases with age and is most common after age 60. Rectal cancer is more common in countries where people consume a diet low in fiber and high in refined foods. Colon disorders, such as COLITIS, can also increase the risk of its occurrence.

SYMPTOMS

Warning signs include blood in the stool or a sudden change in bowel habits. Any abrupt or persistent, unexplained constipation or diarrhea after years of regularity is cause for concern. Any blood in the stool or changes in bowel habits require immediate medical attention. Rectal discomfort, bloating, rumbling, and an urgency to pass stool are other symptoms. There may be a feeling that the bowel has not emptied completely and, sometimes, tenderness or a lump in the lower part of the abdomen. There may be no symptoms until the cancer causes an intestinal obstruction (see INTESTINE, OBSTRUCTION OF) or the intestine ruptures. Rupture can lead to peritonitis (a life-threatening inflammation of the peritoneum, the lining of the abdominal cavity). As cancer cells multiply, the intestinal lining grows rough and hard. The lining may enlarge, often becoming bloody and ulcerated. Cancer in the rectum may narrow the passageway for stool, causing bowel movements to be thinner in shape or potentially blocking the passage of stools. Left untreated, cancer can spread to nearby organs.

DIAGNOSIS AND TREATMENT

Tests commonly ordered to determine the cause of symptoms include a lower gastrointestinal (GI) series (an X-ray procedure also called a barium enema) and sigmoidoscopy or colonoscopy (examinations of the rectum and colon using flexible viewing tubes passed through the anus). Other tests include a rectal examination, fecal-occult blood test (a test for traces of hidden blood in the stool), and stool sample analysis.

When cancer is not advanced, surgery is the best treatment. If the tumor is located in the upper part of the rec-

tum, the surgeon cuts out the diseased portion of the rectum and rejoins the colon to the remaining healthy rectal tissue. When cancer occurs lower in the rectum, it may be necessary to remove the rectum and anus. In these cases, a permanent COLOSTOMY is created to form an artificial exit for feces. Following surgery, doctors may recommend CHEMOTHERAPY and RADIATION THERAPY. Surgery is less likely to be successful when cancer has spread to adjacent organs. Nonsurgical treatments include laser and electrocautery (burning) removal.

Because most cancers of the large intestine develop and spread slowly, early detection is the key to successful treatment. The American Cancer Society recommends regular screening tests, including an annual fecal-occult blood test and a sigmoidoscopy every 3 to 5 years for everyone older than age 50. Colonoscopy is recommended for those at high risk because of prior cancer, a family history of cancer, or a history of chronic digestive problems. Some doctors recommend colonoscopy every 10 years for those older than age 50 instead of sigmoidoscopy.

Red eye

A term used to describe inflammation of the eye that causes the eye to have a red appearance. Depending on its cause, red eye may be accompanied by pain, tearing, tenderness, or changes in vision. Since red eye can have a variety of causes, the eye needs to be examined by a medical professional to determine the underlying disease. Possible causes include infection in the membrane covering the eye and eyelid (CONJUNCTIVITIS), inflammation and infection in the eyelid (styes, CHALAZION, or BLEPHARITIS), infection of the tear sac (DACRYOCYSTITIS), injury (EYE INJURY), a foreign body, glaucoma, allergy, or inflammation of the eyeball.

Reduction

A manipulative procedure for realigning displaced broken bone ends or "reducing" the dislocated bones of a joint to normal angles. Reduction is the technical term for the repositioning of bones. When surgery is required to treat a fracture or joint, the technique is called open

reduction. An incision is made to gain access to the broken bone so it can be repositioned and secured. After reduction, sometimes a rod, pins, a plate, screws, or special bone cement is used to hold the reduced bone fragments in place. If a hip, shoulder, or other joint becomes dislocated as a result of trauma, reduction involves setting the displaced bones by manipulating them into their proper position without surgery. This is called closed reduction.

Reference daily intakes

RDIs; a set of dietary references for protein, vitamin, and mineral intakes used to identify amounts per serving on food labels. RDIs, which replaced the term "US RDAs" (recommended daily allowances), have been used by the US government since 1996. Intakes for all other nutrients are referred to as Daily Reference Values (DRVs).

Referred pain

Pain felt in a part of the body other than its original source. Referred pain occurs because at times different parts of the body are supplied by the same nerve or nerve root. When nerve impulses reach the brain, they are misinterpreted as coming from the other area. For example, heart disorders may be felt as pain in the left

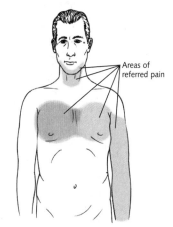

Areas of referred pain

PATTERNS OF PAIN

Pain from heart attack, angina, or coronary artery disease usually occurs in a fist-sized area in the center of the chest (as shown), or it may be felt on the left side of the chest, down the left (or more rarely, the right) arm, or in the throat and jaw area. The site of the referred pain is a good indicator of its cause.

shoulder or arm or in the jaw, while the pain of gallbladder disease may be experienced in the shoulder region.

Reflex

An automatic or involuntary response to a sensory stimulus, generally without a person's awareness. A reflex action usually occurs before the brain has had time to send a mes-

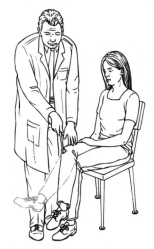

KNEE-JERK REACTION
The familiar knee-jerk reflex occurs because a tap on the knee stretches the knee ligament, which in turn yanks on the thigh muscle. Stretch receptors in the muscle send a message to the spinal cord, which stimulates the thigh muscle to contract in response, and the lower leg jerks upward. The reflex helps maintain balance and posture.

sage to the muscles involved, as happens when a finger is pricked with a pin or a needle. In response, the finger is automatically withdrawn from the source of pain in less time than the brain needs to send its message to the muscles. Examples of reflexes include the following:

• Gag reflex—automatic contraction of the throat muscles following stimulation of the pharynx, or inside of the throat

• Patellar (knee-jerk) reflex—involuntary jerk or kick caused by a light blow on the patellar ligament of the knee joint that results in automatic contraction of the quadriceps muscle

• Corneal reflex—the blink that automatically occurs when the eye is irritated

• Nasal reflex—sneezing, which happens automatically when something irritates the mucous membrane that lines the interior of the nose.

Reflex sympathetic dystrophy

Also known as reflex sympathetic dystrophy syndrome or RSDS, a chronic condition characterized by severe burning pain accompanied by swelling, excessive sweating, and extreme sensitivity to touch, pressure, motion, or temperature change.

CAUSES AND SYMPTOMS
Reflex sympathetic dystrophy syndrome is a nerve disorder that most commonly follows an injury or an illness, such as a heart attack. It is especially common after trauma, such as a high-velocity gunshot wound. However, sometimes RSDS occurs for no known reason. This condition can develop at any age, but most often strikes people between the ages of 40 and 60 years. Reflex sympathetic dystrophy syndrome is also growing more common among young adults and adolescents.

Reflex sympathetic dystrophy most commonly affects the arms or legs. The pain described by people with this condition is typically severe and out of proportion to any original injury. Pain continues to worsen over time. A visible symptom of RSDS is warm, red, dry skin that later turns bluish, cold, and sweaty. There may also be muscle cramps, stiffness, localized swelling, and muscle wasting (atrophy). Some people experience tremors, depression, and sleep problems.

DIAGNOSIS AND TREATMENT
Diagnosis of reflex sympathetic dystrophy is based mainly on observation of symptoms. Doctors may also conduct a test to detect the temperature changes that are typical of this condition. X rays or bone scans are also useful in making the diagnosis.

Early treatment gives the best results. If treatment is started within 3 months, complete recovery is possible. A variety of drugs are prescribed for RSDS, including anti-inflammatory drugs, corticosteroids, antidepressants, anticonvulsants, calcitonin, and opioids. Most people also require at least one sympathetic NERVE BLOCK, in which doctors inject numbing

anesthetic into nerves. In severe cases, doctors recommend SYMPATHEC-TOMY (using chemicals or surgery to kill the sympathetic nerves leading to the painful body part). Other options include TENS (transcutaneous electrical nerve stimulation) and physical or occupational therapy.

Reflex, primitive

Involuntary muscular responses to sensory stimuli seen in infants. Primitive reflexes govern the infant's movements and disappear as the baby's neurological system matures. Physical examination of newborn babies includes the attempt to elicit various reflexes, because the absence of normal primitive reflexes can indicate neurological disorders.

Examples of normal primitive reflexes include the Moro (startle) reflex in which the baby, in response to a loud noise or rough handling, arches its back, throws its head back, and throws its arms and legs out and brings them back. This reflex usually disappears by 3 months. In the grasp reflex, when a baby's palm is stroked, he or she automatically grasps the finger doing the stroking; this reflex disappears at about 6 months. Another type of reflex is the rooting reflex, in which—if a baby's cheek or lips are stroked—he or she will turn toward the stroking object and root for a nipple; this reflex usually disappears at about 4 months.

In adults, primitive reflexes can occur as a result of diseases that affect brain function, such as Alzheimer's disease, stroke, or brain damage from trauma. See A baby's reflexes, page 1058.

Reflexology

A form of massage therapy in which pressure is applied to specific points on the feet and hands to relieve symptoms throughout the body; a form of ZONE THERAPY. Reflexology is used to alleviate stress-related problems and symptoms of other disorders, although no claims are made for its ability to address underlying causes of any disorders. Advocates of

R

Terms in small capital letters—for example, PHYSICAL THERAPY or PAGET DISEASE—indicate a cross-reference to another entry with more information.

A BABY'S REFLEXES

In the first 3 to 6 months of life, a baby has automatic reflexes, probably related to feeding or protecting himself or herself, even before neurological development is complete. These reflexes will gradually disappear as the child gains conscious control over muscle movements.

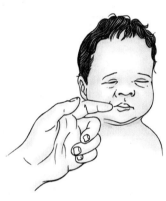

ROOTING REFLEX
Stroking a baby's cheek causes him or her to turn toward the finger and open his or her mouth, searching for a breast or bottle.

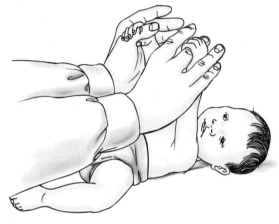

GRASPING REFLEX
Pressing a finger or an object into a baby's palm causes him or her to grasp it and hang on tightly. This reflex is so strong that it can support the baby's entire weight.

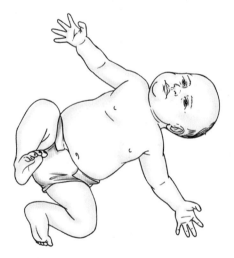

STARTLE REFLEX
A loud noise or the sensation of falling stimulates the startle (or Moro) reflex, in which the baby arches the back and stretches out the arms, legs, fingers, and neck. Then he or she quickly brings the arms and legs back in toward the chest and clenches the fists.

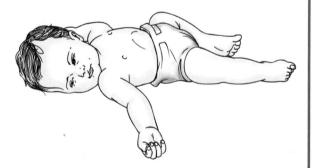

TONIC NECK REFLEX
In the first week or so of life, when a newborn turns the head to one side, the arm and leg on that side will extend, while the arm and leg on the other side will flex. This reflex lasts longer in premature infants.

R

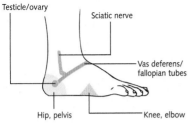

Testicle/ovary
Sciatic nerve
Vas deferens/ fallopian tubes
Hip, pelvis
Knee, elbow

Right foot, outer side

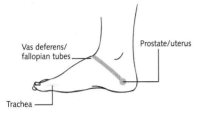

Vas deferens/ fallopian tubes
Prostate/uterus
Trachea

Right foot, inner side

REFLEX POINTS IN THE FEET
Reflexologists claim that massage to specific areas of the feet restores healthful energy balance in other parts of the body. On either foot, a certain reflex point represents only half of the body or one side of an organ, so manipulation of both feet is thought to be imperative.

reflexology believe that reflex points on the foot correspond to such health problems as headache, premenstrual tension, asthma, acne, and chronic pain from arthritis and sciatica. The toes, for example, represent the head, while the arch of the foot corresponds to the internal organs in the center of the body.

The idea behind reflexology is that by applying pressure to specific points on the feet and sometimes the hands, reflexologists can relax, normalize, and bring balance to the body. It is thought that pressure placed on points on the foot triggers the body's own healing energy, opening up energy channels and stimulating the circulatory and nervous systems. Pressure on the soles of the feet is also believed to break down materials called "crystals" that impair normal foot function. Relexology is practiced by professional reflexologists and as self-care by some people, but it has not been clinically proven to be effective.

Reflux
See ESOPHAGEAL REFLUX.

Refraction
An eye test that determines the type and degree of focusing errors in vision and is used to prescribe corrective lenses. The test is conducted in the office of an eye specialist, either an optometrist or an ophthalmologist. Sitting in a chair, the person undergoing this test looks through a special device (Phoroptor) at an eye chart about 20 feet away. The Phoroptor contains lenses of various strengths that can be moved into the person's line of view. As the specialist tries different lenses, the person undergoing the test is asked whether the eye chart is more or less clear. Information from the refraction test identifies the type of refractive error and allows the eye specialist to prescribe glasses or contact lenses to correct the vision error.

Refractive surgery
An operation that can improve or correct the ability of the eye to focus by permanently changing the shape of the cornea (the clear outer layer of the EYE). Refractive surgery may eliminate the need to wear glasses or contact lenses or reduce the strength of the correction. Various types of refractive surgery can be used to correct nearsightedness (difficulty seeing distant objects), farsightedness (difficulty seeing close objects), and astigmatism (tilted, distorted vision due to an irregularly shaped cornea). In RADIAL KERATOTOMY, which is used to correct nearsightedness, small incisions are made in the cornea in a spokelike (radial) pattern to flatten the cornea and reduce its focusing power. A similar surgery is used to correct astigmatism. LASIK (laser in-situ keratomileusis) uses a laser to change the shape of the cornea; a hinged flap is cut in the surface of the cornea, and the laser is applied to the tissue underneath to reshape it. LASIK can correct nearsightedness, farsightedness, and astigmatism. PHOTOREFRACTIVE KERATECTOMY (PRK) also uses a laser, but the beam is focused on the surface of the cornea and no flap is cut. PRK corrects nearsightedness, farsightedness, and astigmatism. An INTRACORNEAL RING is a small semicircle of plastic inserted in the cornea to change its shape and correct nearsightedness.

Regional anesthesia
See ANESTHESIA, REGIONAL.

Regional enteritis
See CROHN DISEASE.

Regression
A return to an earlier, less mature developmental stage in the face of stress. For example, an adult who sucks his or her thumb on hearing bad news is experiencing regression. Regression helps provide comfort during stress and conflict and is considered one of the DEFENSE MECHANISMS.

Regurgitation
The forceful, involuntary ejection of stomach or esophageal contents through the mouth. (See also VOMITING.) The backflow of blood through a defective heart valve is also known as regurgitation.

Rehabilitation
The process of using therapeutic measures and education to physically restore the health or ability of a person who is disabled, has undergone surgery, or has been injured or ill. Rehabilitation focuses on helping a person regain the physical abilities that have been lost or impaired. Doctors may refer patients to rehabilitation or physical therapy centers, sometimes as an alternative to more surgery or more invasive medical procedures. Services at a rehabilitation center are generally given by a physical or occupational therapist and monitored by the referring doctor or specialist. The therapist may aid in restoring or strengthening muscles and other parts of the body by applying heat or cold, by giving massage, or by using ultrasound equipment. Instructions for restorative exercises may be given, assistive devices prescribed, and instructions for all tasks of daily living supervised.

Rehabilitation may be offered by a hospital as an outpatient service, or a hospital can recommend rehabilitation centers or physical therapists. Therapists offering rehabilitation services may have a clinical practice or a private office-based practice, or they may be associated with an HMO (health maintenance organization). These therapists sometimes make home visits to persons unable to travel from their homes. Rehabilitation for athletes, as well as for people who need to regain or improve the use of

R

> **HOW TO FIND A REHABILITATION CENTER**
>
> Finding a reputable rehabilitation center may take some detective work. Here are some guidelines that stress acceptable standards that a person inquiring about such a facility should be seeking. Finding a good rehabilitation center should be based on:
>
> - The credentials of the director, who should be a board-certified physician with a specialty in physical medicine and rehabilitation
> - Accreditation of the doctor and the staff by the American Physical Therapy Association or American Occupational Therapy Association
> - A close working relationship between the rehabilitation center doctor and staff and the referring physician
> - A good match between the center's specialization and the specific goals, needs, condition, age, and lifestyle of the person seeking rehabilitation
> - A good therapist-to-client ratio, ideally 1 to 2
> - A program geared toward teaching a long-term commitment to exercise and muscle strengthening

their limbs and muscles, is offered at sports medicine clinics, which may be independent or run by a hospital as a separate department.

Rehabilitation services may be recommended before surgical treatments for help with learning how to use crutches or walkers or after surgery for strengthening the upper body.

Rehydration fluid, oral

A preparation designed to treat dehydration due to DIARRHEA. Watery diarrhea can rapidly cause a loss of body fluids and crucial body salts. Left untreated, this depletion can lead to shock. Young children and older people are particularly at risk. Oral rehydration fluid is available over-the-counter at pharmacies. It contains water, salts, and glucose. Homemade preparations can also be used. Doctors advise drinking rehydration fluid at half-hour intervals until pale-colored urine is passed. In cases of severe diarrhea, it may be necessary to drink several quarts of solution

> **REHYDRATION SOLUTION**
>
> Watery diarrhea can cause dehydration. Symptoms that persist for longer than 2 days should be reported to a doctor. Drinking a rehydration solution can help. Two or 3 pints of the (cooled) mixture should be drunk every day until diarrhea stops. Mix:
>
> ½ teaspoon salt
> 2 teaspoons sugar
> ½ teaspoon baking soda
> 1 pint boiled water

before this occurs. Once diarrhea begins to subside, other types of fluid (such as clear broth or unsweetened fruit juice) can be consumed. Most diarrhea lasts for no longer than 48 hours. Medical attention is necessary if diarrhea continues longer than 2 days or if it is especially severe.

Reiki

A Japanese form of spiritual healing and form of ENERGY MEDICINE. Reiki literally means "universal life force" and refers to the energy flow thought to permeate and surround living things. Energy flow, called "ki" in reiki, is known as "qi" ("chee") in CHINESE MEDICINE. The theory behind reiki is that all living things are connected with a universal life-force energy, which can be used to heal disease. A practitioner of reiki uses his or her healing ki to strengthen the ki of others. To heal blocked or weakened ki, a practitioner channels his or her own self-healing energy to the person, using specific techniques that address all levels of the person—body, mind, and spirit. Most reiki treatments do not involve touching; the healer usually places his or her hands above the body part to direct energy into it. The goal of reiki is to support the body's natural ability to heal itself. This form of healing has not been clinically proven as effective.

Reimplantation, dental

Replacing a tooth torn from its socket in an injury to the mouth. If the tooth is properly preserved until a dentist

can be seen, the tooth can often be saved by being reimplanted into the gum by the dentist. It is recommended that the tooth be kept in milk. If milk is not available, it may be placed in cool water or wrapped in a clean wet cloth or gauze until the dentist can reimplant the tooth. A blood clot will form in the socket of the tooth within 24 hours, so the tooth must be reimplanted well before that time elapses. The dentist can replace the tooth into the original socket under sterile conditions and may also attach the tooth to the adjacent teeth until it becomes reattached to the gum. It is important not to remove any fibers that are attached to the root of the tooth before the dentist reimplants it because this connective tissue may be essential to the tooth reattaching itself to the socket.

Dental reimplantation is performed on primary teeth and permanent teeth. In the case of a primary tooth, the procedure is performed to assure the development and positioning of the permanent tooth below it.

Reiter syndrome

A form of inflammatory arthritis transmitted by sexual contact and the organisms that cause dysentery; it occurrs in people who have a genetic susceptibility to it. Typically, the first symptom in men is a penile discharge. Subsequent symptoms for men or women include painful joints, often in the knee, heel, or fingers. An eye inflammation called CONJUNCTIVITIS and a skin rash similar in appearance to psoriasis may follow. An episode of Reiter syndrome may last a few weeks or several months. The symptoms may appear once or return. The joints are rarely damaged permanently. When severe, Reiter syndrome can cause tenderness and pain in the joints and is generally treated with pain-relieving medication such as nonsteroidal anti-inflammatory drugs (NSAIDs), including aspirin and ibuprofen.

Relapse

Return of symptoms and signs of disease after a period of improvement or good health. Relapse also describes a situation in which a person's condition that had been improving gets worse during an illness.

Relapsing fever

A disease that is transmitted to humans when they are bitten by ticks or lice. Relapsing fever is characterized by a high fever that recurs intermittently and lasts 3 to 5 days each time it occurs. Between bouts of illness, there are intervals of recovery varying in length from several days to more than a week. The disease is also referred to as tick fever, recurrent fever, and famine fever. In the United States, the disease is always tick-borne and is generally limited to the western regions of the country, where people are infected most often between the months of May and September. Ticks in the western United States acquire the infection from infected rodents and carry it in their saliva and excrement. Relapsing fever is carried by lice only in areas of Africa and South America; the lice become carriers when they feed on infected people.

SYMPTOMS, DIAGNOSIS, AND TREATMENT

The parasites that cause relapsing fever are called *Borrelia* spirochetes. Carried in insect vectors and transmitted to humans, these parasites enter the bloodstream and travel to internal organs, particularly the spleen, liver, and brain. The most prominent symptoms occur within 3 to 11 days after exposure and include sudden chills with high fever, rapid heartbeat, severe headache, vomiting, muscle and joint pain, and delirium. The high fever persists for 3 to 5 days, then suddenly clears, followed by a lack of symptoms for up to a week. A phase without symptoms is followed by a relapse of illness that occurs with a sudden return of fever. JAUNDICE may occur with relapse. Again the illness abates, usually followed by two to ten relapses at 1- to 2-week intervals. The relapses are progressively diminished in severity and eventually cease to occur as a person develops immunity to the parasite. Because there can be possible complications, medical attention should be obtained if there is a suspicion of relapsing fever.

Complications include the possibility of abortion (miscarriage) in a woman who is pregnant, exacerbated asthma, inflammatory rashes on the skin and mucous membranes, and severe inflammation of the eyes that may lead to blindness. Heart failure may also occur. Death from relapsing fever is rare, but young children, pregnant women, older people, and people who are malnourished or debilitated are more vulnerable to severe disease. Mortality is higher when the illness is carried by lice.

Relapsing fever is diagnosed by an evaluation of the recurring fever and by blood tests taken during an episode of illness. It is treated with oral tetracycline or erythromycin for 5 to 10 days. Intravenous medication may be given in severe cases or when vomiting precludes a person from being able to take oral medication. Supportive treatment may include replacing fluids and restoring electrolyte balance, prescription narcotic painkillers to relieve severe headache, and medical treatments for nausea and vomiting.

Relaxation techniques

Methods of reducing the symptoms of stress and anxiety by eliminating tension held in the body. Relaxation techniques lower heart and breathing rate, decrease oxygen consumption, and reduce the levels of chemicals in the blood that rise in response to stress.

Most relaxation techniques share two components: repeating a word, phrase, sound, muscular activity, or prayer over and over; and disregarding distracting thoughts in order to return to the repeated word, phrase, sound, muscular activity, or prayer. Some relaxation techniques are similar to meditation as practiced in Eastern and Western spiritual traditions. The person sits in a quiet place, relaxes the muscles, breathes slowly and naturally, repeats a single word or phrase on every exhalation, and disregards distracting thoughts for 10 to 20 minutes. Deep-breathing techniques deliberately slow the increased breathing rate that accompanies tension and anxiety. The individual inhales slowly through the nose and expands the abdomen with the inhalation, then exhales through the mouth, contracting the abdominal muscles to push the air out. This pattern is repeated until it becomes natural and the rate of breathing slows. In progressive muscle relaxation, the person lies in a quiet place with the arms at the side. He or she alternately tenses and relaxes each group of muscles, working downward from head to toe. Exercise disciplines such as T'ai chi, an ancient Chinese method of harmonizing mind and body, and yoga, a system of postures and stretches, are also used for relaxation.

Research has shown that relaxation techniques, combined with medication, are effective for treating stress-related diseases, such as migraine headaches, high blood pressure (hypertension), ulcers, irregular heartbeat, and asthma.

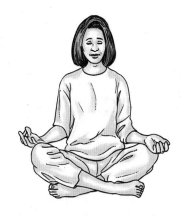

RELAXING BODY AND MIND
Yoga and meditation are popular forms of relaxation exercises that can help lessen the discomfort and symptoms of stress such as headaches, anxiety, high blood pressure, and sleeping difficulties. Yoga emphasizes body flexibility and breathing exercises to achieve mental and physical control.

REM sleep

Rapid eye movement sleep. Throughout the night, people move through different stages of sleep. These stages include the activity of REM sleep, as well as the four stages of NREM (nonrapid eye movement) sleep: transitional sleep, light sleep, and two stages of deep or delta sleep. Dreams occur during REM sleep, when the body becomes still except for eye movement and brain activity speeds up. Brain functions slow during more restful NREM sleep.

Remission

Disappearance of the signs and symptoms of a disease. For example, cancer is in remission when there is a reduction in the size of a tumor and in the symptoms it causes. A remission may be temporary or permanent.

R

Renal

Pertaining to or around the kidneys.

Renal biopsy

See KIDNEY BIOPSY.

Renal cell carcinoma

A type of malignant kidney tumor that occurs only in adults; also known as hypernephroma. Renal cell carcinoma is the most common form of cancer of the kidney and affects men more than women, especially men over the age of 55. Renal cell carcinoma forms on the edge of the kidneys.

SYMPTOMS

As the tumor enlarges, it grows into healthy kidney tissue, causing symptoms such as persistent fever, loss of appetite, and weight loss. Renal cell carcinoma spreads much more slowly than many other kinds of cancer. It is unusual for the cancer to result in kidney failure before it is diagnosed. If some of the cells enter the bloodstream and metastasize, or spread, to a bone, the affected person may have pain in the bones. If the cells spread to the lungs, the affected person may cough. Bleeding from the tumor may produce red or cloudy urine.

DIAGNOSIS AND TREATMENT

Early detection of renal cell carcinoma is crucial. It can be cured if the tumor is discovered and removed at

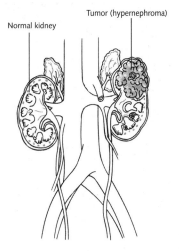

Normal kidney

Tumor (hypernephroma)

KIDNEY TUMOR
A hypernephroma is a slow-growing kidney tumor that often gives no early warning signs. Symptoms may include pain between the ribs and hip, weight loss, fatigue, or a mass on the kidneys that a doctor discovers. As the tumor grows, it may cause blood in the urine.

an early stage. Urine samples will be obtained for analysis. Diagnostic tests may include INTRAVENOUS PYELOGRAPHY, ULTRASOUND SCANNING, CT SCANNING (computed tomography scanning), and MRI (magnetic resonance imaging) of the kidney.

If renal cell carcinoma is diagnosed, the affected kidney is removed. The remaining healthy kidney can usually compensate for the missing one. Regular checkups are essential to monitor possible recurrence of the cancer. See KIDNEY CANCER.

RISK FACTORS

A history of smoking increases risk substantially. There may be a hereditary factor involved because a history of kidney cancer in the family increases the risk. Renal cell carcinoma is associated with the hereditary disorder called von Hippel-Lindau disease, which affects the capillaries of the brain. Dialysis treatment also increases the risk.

Renal colic

Painful, intermittent, and severe spasms on one side of the back usually caused by one or more KIDNEY STONES.

Renal diet

A diet prescribed in cases of chronic kidney (renal) failure. In individuals with kidney damage, the kidney may be less efficient at eliminating waste in the urine. Consequently, these waste products, normally cleared by the kidneys, build up in the blood. In such cases, doctors recommend a renal diet, which limits the intake of protein, potassium, sodium, phosphorus, and fluids.

Bread, cereal, pasta, and rice are the main sources of calories in a renal diet. Special flours and bread that are protein-free and low in potassium and phosphorus are used. Protein intake is restricted, and usually milk, meat, and eggs supply the limited amount needed. Depending on potassium and phosphorus restrictions, a small amount of vegetables and fruits are permitted. Because renal diets may not provide all the necessary nutrients, doctors may recommend supplementation with electrolytes and vitamins.

Renal failure

See KIDNEY FAILURE.

Renal transplant

See KIDNEY TRANSPLANT.

Renal tubular acidosis

A condition that produces an acidic imbalance as the result of the inability of the kidneys to excrete adequate amounts of the acid normally generated by chemical processes in the body. The normal pH balance of the body is slightly alkaline, with the acidic substances, such as carbon dioxide and hydrogen-containing molecules, being buffered by the alkaline ones, primarily bicarbonate. In renal tubular acidosis, there is a partial defect in the secretion of hydrogen ions in the renal tubule, which produces a reduction in the reabsorption of bicarbonate from the tubule back into the bloodstream. This tips the pH balance toward acidic. Acidity causes problems such as calcium loss from the bones. The dissolved calcium accumulates in the bloodstream and is excreted by the kidneys, resulting in abnormal bone structure (called OSTEOMALACIA), impaired growth in children, skeletal deformities, and muscle weakness. The incidence of kidney stones is also increased by renal tubular acidosis.

CAUSES AND SYMPTOMS

Renal tubular acidosis may be caused by several factors including autoimmune disorders; a condition called hypercalciuria, which is an excess of calcium in the urine; recreational drug use; genetic disorders; and heredity, which is the most common cause in children.

There may be no symptoms, or symptoms may include fatigue, weakness, confusion, diminished alertness, an increased respiratory rate, dehydration, nausea, and muscle pain.

DIAGNOSIS AND TREATMENT

Blood tests and urinalysis are used to diagnose renal tubular acidosis. Alkaline medications, including sodium bicarbonate and potassium citrate, may be given to correct the acidic pH in the body and to increase lowered potassium levels. Thiazide diuretics may also be necessary to increase the reabsorption of bicarbonate. Vitamin D and calcium supplements may be beneficial for reducing possible bone deformities.

R

Renal vascular hypertension

High blood pressure caused by disorders of the blood vessels that supply the kidneys with blood. About 20 percent of the blood pumped from the heart passes through the kidneys. The blood enters through the renal artery (a major branch of the aorta), is filtered by the kidneys, and returns to the heart via the renal vein. Impairment of the renal artery or the renal vein disrupts kidney function and is a major cause of secondary high blood pressure.

CAUSES

Renal vascular hypertension may be caused by renal artery stenosis, a narrowing of the renal artery that usually blocks blood flow. In older people, renal artery stenosis is most commonly the result of ATHEROSCLEROSIS. PREECLAMPSIA and ECLAMPSIA, conditions that can occur in pregnant women shortly before giving birth, can contribute to problems with the blood vessels within the kidneys. VASCULITIS, which is an inflammation of the arteries, is also associated with renal vascular hypertension. Another condition, called fibromuscular dysplasia, is seen primarily in women between the ages of 20 and 40 and is a thickening of the artery wall that narrows the renal artery.

DIAGNOSIS AND TREATMENT

The first indication that the renal artery has been severely narrowed or blocked may be a loud noise or murmur heard through a doctor's stethoscope placed over the kidneys. INTRAVENOUS PYELOGRAPHY can reveal a decrease in the size of the affected kidney, and ULTRASOUND SCANNING will measure the flow of blood through the artery (see KIDNEY IMAGING). An arteriogram (an X ray of an artery) can locate the precise position of the narrowing or blockage.

Medication may be prescribed to control high blood pressure in people who have renal vascular hypertension. To prevent progressive KIDNEY FAILURE and to improve high blood pressure conditions, surgery may be indicated in some cases.

A more recently developed treatment called percutaneous transluminal angioplasty has been successful in treating renal artery stenosis and improving high blood pressure. In this procedure, a catheter with a

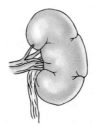 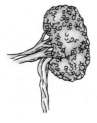

Normal kidney   Kidney with renal vascular hypertension

EFFECTS OF RENAL HYPERTENSION
If an artery to the kidney (renal artery) is blocked or narrowed, high blood pressure results. The effect on kidney tissue is gradual wasting and shrinking, as well as the formation of scar tissue that gives the kidney a granular texture.

deflated balloon at its tip is threaded through an artery in the thigh, then guided upward into the narrowed renal artery. When the catheter reaches the renal artery, the balloon is inflated to dilate the artery, and the catheter is removed, leaving the artery open. Percutaneous transluminal angioplasty has been particularly effective for treating people whose condition is caused by fibromuscular dysplasia.

Renin

An enzyme released into the blood by the kidney in response to stress. Renin reacts with the liver to produce angiotensin, which eventually causes constriction of the blood vessels and an increase in blood pressure. It is estimated that 10 to 15 percent of people with high blood pressure have too much renin in their blood. The overproduction of renin can occur from a condition called renal (kidney) hypertension. See RENAL VASCULAR HYPERTENSION.

Repetitive strain injury

An injury that occurs when repeated movements of one part of the body damage the tendons, nerves, muscles, and other soft tissues. Rapid and forceful movements that are repeated create the greatest risk of repetitive strain injury (RSI), which may also be called overuse injury, repetitive stress injury, or cumulative trauma disorder. The muscles and tendons in the arms are most commonly affected by the condition. People who engage daily in jobs requiring repetitive

movements of the fingers, hands, arms, and shoulders are particularly vulnerable to RSI. Those jobs include typing on a keyboard, using a computer mouse, playing a musical instrument, and working on an assembly line. CARPAL TUNNEL SYNDROME, TENDINITIS, TENOSYNOVITIS, and certain other disorders that cause muscle and tendon pain are sometimes included in the classification of repetitive strain injuries.

SYMPTOMS

Typically, the symptoms of RSI develop gradually and may be experienced only when a person is performing repetitive movements. Pain, aching, tingling, coldness, numbness, tightness, burning, or restricted movement may be felt. Sometimes, there is swelling in the affected area. Clumsiness or loss of strength and coordination in the hands may be another symptom. At first, these symptoms tend to disappear when the repeated movements are stopped and the body part involved is rested. As the condition progresses, there may be symptoms when at rest, including pain that disturbs sleep. Early symptoms should be evaluated by a doctor, as RSI becomes more difficult to treat when it is chronic.

DIAGNOSIS AND TREATMENT

A physician can diagnose RSI by taking a medical history, including asking the person about lifestyle factors that may contribute to the condition, and by physical examination. X rays and blood tests may be necessary to rule out RHEUMATOID ARTHRITIS and other similar disorders. Nonsteroidal anti-inflammatory drugs (NSAIDs)

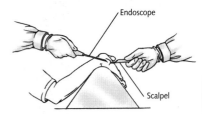

Endoscope

Scalpel

R

ENDOSCOPIC SURGERY
A procedure called carpal tunnel release takes pressure off the median nerve in the wrist so that nerve function can resume. The procedure, which involves dividing the transverse carpal ligament, can be done with an endoscope (a hollow, lighted instrument inserted through small incisions). The endoscopic surgery leaves muscles and connective tissues intact to help support the divided ligament.

are often recommended to relieve pain and reduce swelling. Physical therapy and splinting of the affected parts may help relieve pain.

When symptoms are apparently related to a person's job, an occupational doctor or nurse can offer advice about posture changes and special equipment to help prevent RSI. Adjustable seating, a properly arranged work station, and regular breaks from repetitive tasks can help avoid unnecessary stress on muscles and tendons. When RSI is diagnosed early and a person makes an effort to avoid its cause, a complete recovery can be expected. Sometimes, people may be severely affected and become unable to perform certain tasks or activities without discomfort.

Reportable diseases

Diseases reported to the CENTERS FOR DISEASE CONTROL AND PREVENTION (CDC) on a timely basis so that epidemiologists can identify and attempt to control outbreaks to protect public health. Reportable diseases, also called notifiable diseases, are those the CDC seeks to gather information about on a regular basis as a way to control and prevent them. Other reasons may include the need to measure the impact of immunizations or established therapies, as well as the need to study and understand current epidemic trends and disease-prevention policies.

The list of reportable diseases in the United States is constantly being revised as new pathogens emerge and as the prevalence of certain diseases diminishes. Through collaboration, the US Public Health Service, the Council of State and Territorial Epidemiologists, and the CDC determine which diseases should be reportable on a national basis. Reporting is mandated at state and local levels, so reportable diseases may vary within the United States. International diseases requiring quarantine, which include cholera, plague, and yellow fever, are reported by all localities in the United States to comply with the international health regulations of the World Health Organization.

Among the infectious diseases currently designated as reportable at the national level are AIDS (acquired immunodeficiency syndrome) and HIV (human immunodeficiency virus) infection, botulism, diphtheria, various forms of encephalitis and hepatitis, *Escherichia coli* infections, and most of the major SEXUALLY TRANSMITTED DISEASES. Lyme disease, malaria, measles, mumps, pertussis, polio, rabies, German measles, some streptococcal diseases, tetanus, toxic shock syndrome, trichinosis, tuberculosis, and typhoid fever are also reportable diseases.

Reproduction, sexual

Production of a child through the FERTILIZATION of a woman's egg with a man's sperm (see illustration below). In SEXUAL INTERCOURSE, a woman's vagina is penetrated by a man's penis. Once inside, the penis ejaculates, or releases a thick fluid called semen. This fluid contains millions of sperm, which then may travel through the uterus into a fallopian tube, find and fertilize an egg, and result in an embryo and PREGNANCY. Sexual reproduction can also take place through ARTIFICIAL INSEMINATION (the introduction of semen via an artificial method).

Reproductive system, female

The group of organs and structures, both internal and external, involved in a woman's capacity to have sexual intercourse, produce eggs (reproductive cells), become pregnant, and give birth.

EXTERNAL ORGANS
A woman's external genital area is called the vulva, located between her thighs and encompassing all the structures that surround and protect the entrance to her internal reproductive organs.

The mons pubis is the hairy mound of tissue that covers the pubic bone of the pelvis. Under the mons pubis there are two sets of labia (or lips) that cover the opening into her body. The outer labia majora are covered with hair; the inner labia minora are hairless. The CLITORIS, a small button of tissue that lies at the point where the two labia minora meet at the top, is extremely sensitive and can become erect during sexual arousal. The urethral opening, from which urine leaves a woman's body, lies just below the clitoris. Below the urethral opening is the opening to the vagina, the entrance into the internal reproductive organs. Immediately inside is a thin, elastic membrane called the HYMEN that surrounds the vaginal opening.

INTERNAL ORGANS
The VAGINA is the muscular canal that leads into the uterus from the outside of the body. It accommodates the male penis during sexual intercourse, and it is the birth canal during CHILDBIRTH. At the point where the vagina enters the uterus, a hard, round organ called the CERVIX forms the lower end (or neck) of the uterus. The cervix is actually doughnut shaped, with an opening in the middle through which menstrual fluids can pass and that can widen to permit childbirth.

The UTERUS is the central organ of the reproductive system, lying inside the protective framework of the pelvis. It is a hollow organ with muscular walls; the inner walls are lined with tissue (endometrial tissue) rich-

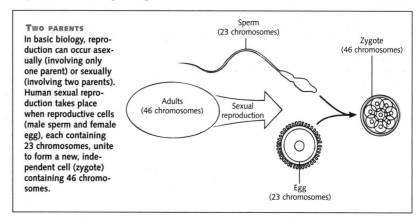

TWO PARENTS
In basic biology, reproduction can occur asexually (involving only one parent) or sexually (involving two parents). Human sexual reproduction takes place when reproductive cells (male sperm and female egg), each containing 23 chromosomes, unite to form a new, independent cell (zygote) containing 46 chromosomes.

Sperm (23 chromosomes)

Zygote (46 chromosomes)

Adults (46 chromosomes)

Sexual reproduction

Egg (23 chromosomes)

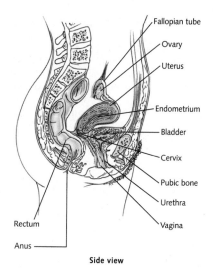

Side view

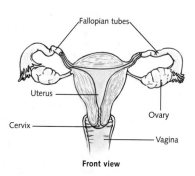

Front view

FEMALE REPRODUCTIVE ORGANS
The internal organs of a woman's reproductive system are located in the lower abdomen. The processes that take place in these organs are orchestrated from the brain by the carefully balanced and timed release of sex hormones.

ly supplied with blood vessels. In the event of pregnancy, a fertilized egg will develop into a fetus inside the uterus, nourished by the endometrial tissue.

Extending from either side of the uterus are two fallopian tubes. These passages carry eggs from the ovaries to the uterus. At the end closest to the ovary, the tube opens out to enable it to receive an egg from the ovary. The ovaries contain hundreds of thousands of eggs, present in a woman's body from birth. Each of these eggs lies in a tiny cavity called a follicle. Within the follicle, the female hormones ESTROGEN and PROGESTERONE are produced. These hormones, together with hormones produced in the brain, regulate the reproductive cycle that

releases one egg each month for possible fertilization.

DEVELOPMENT AND FUNCTION

At PUBERTY, a process that takes place any time from age 8 to 15 years, a girl's reproductive organs mature. The menstrual cycle begins—the monthly process by which the woman's body prepares for the possibility of fertilization and pregnancy. She can release eggs (a process called OVULATION), can have SEXUAL INTERCOURSE, can accommodate the fertilization process, can become pregnant and carry a fertilized egg throughout a pregnancy, and can give birth.

The reproduction process is triggered by hormones as one of the ovaries releases an egg that travels down a fallopian tube toward the uterus. If sperm (male reproductive cells) are present, the sperm and the egg can combine in a process called FERTILIZATION. The fertilized egg travels into the uterus, where it implants on the thickened walls and can develop into a fetus. If fertilization does not occur, the thickened walls flow out of the body (along with the egg) through the vagina in a process called MENSTRUATION.

A woman's reproductive (or fertile) years continue until sometime between the ages of 40 and 60, when MENOPAUSE—the end of the menstrual cycle—occurs. At this time, the ovaries stop producing estrogen, eggs are no longer released each month, and fertilization can no longer take place.

Reproductive system, male

The group of organs involved in a man's capacity to produce SPERM (male reproductive cells), have sexual intercourse, and fertilize an egg (female reproductive cell) to produce offspring.

ORGANS

The penis and the testicles are the visible male reproductive organs. The testicles, also known as testes, are two glands lying in a pouch of skin (called the scrotum) between a man's thighs. Each TESTICLE produces sperm (male reproductive cells) and secretes the male hormones called androgens, including testosterone. The testicles continually produce millions of sperm in densely packed tubules. These tubules lead to another struc-

ture called the EPIDIDYMIS, located on the back of each testicle. Sperm move from the testicles into the epididymis, where they mature in 10 to 20 days.

During sexual arousal, sperm travel from the epididymis into a long tube called the vas deferens, which passes up into the body into the seminal vesicles—two sacs that lie just behind the bladder. In the seminal vesicles, fluid (called seminal fluid) is added to the sperm to produce the liquid called semen. The seminal vesicles also produce a lubricating secretion in the urethra. Semen moves into the urethra, a tube that leads from the bladder to the outside of the body. (The urethra can carry both semen and urine.)

As the semen passes into the urethra, it receives additional fluids from the prostate gland, a small gland that surrounds the urethra just under the bladder. Muscular tissue in the prostate also has a role in the ejaculation of semen from the body.

The penis, extending from between the testicles, is composed of tissue that can become engorged with blood during sexual arousal; the engorgement causes the penis to lengthen and become erect. Semen passes through the urethra in the erect penis and is propelled out of the body by strong contractions during a sexual orgasm, a process called ejaculation.

During sexual intercourse, when a man's penis is inserted into a woman's vagina, an individual sperm in the semen can unite with a female egg—a process called FERTILIZATION—and the fertilized egg can develop into a fetus within the woman's body.

DEVELOPMENT AND FUNCTION

At PUBERTY, around the age of 9 to 14, a boy's reproductive organs mature. The first change is in the testicles and scrotum, which enlarge. Next, the testicles continue growing and the penis becomes longer and thicker. Pubic hair then fills in and the genitals darken. At this point he can have sexual intercourse and ejaculate seminal fluid, or semen.

Sperm and male sex hormones are produced in the testicles. Sperm pass from the testicles into the epididymis (a long narrow tube) where they mature and are stored. Sperm are then carried along in the semen, which

R

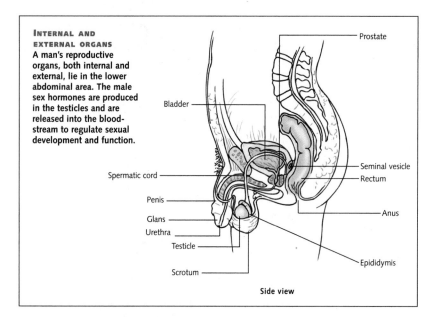

INTERNAL AND EXTERNAL ORGANS
A man's reproductive organs, both internal and external, lie in the lower abdominal area. The male sex hormones are produced in the testicles and are released into the bloodstream to regulate sexual development and function.

Labels: Prostate, Bladder, Spermatic cord, Penis, Glans, Urethra, Testicle, Scrotum, Seminal vesicle, Rectum, Anus, Epididymis

Side view

also contains other hormones from glands, such as the PROSTATE GLAND.

When a man reaches orgasm, semen is released from the erect penis through the urethra. The semen then enters the woman's vagina during sexual intercourse. Sperm, if present, can combine with an egg to cause fertilization.

A man's reproductive years continue indefinitely, in contrast with a woman's. However, biological changes due to aging or erectile dysfunction can affect a man's performance. By the age of 40 men may experience reduced sexual sensation and difficulty having or maintaining an erection. Hormone levels may have a role in age-related changes in sexuality, and testosterone production declines throughout life in men. As a man ages, various medical problems can also affect the ability to complete sexual intercourse.

Research study
See CLINICAL TRIAL.

Resection
Surgical removal of all or part of an injured or diseased organ. For example, the removal of a portion of the small intestine is called a small-bowel resection.

Resident
A medical school graduate who is undergoing postgraduate training in a supervised training program. In a teaching hospital, residents are overseen by an ATTENDING PHYSICIAN.

Residential care facility
A NURSING FACILITY that offers a combination of housing, personal services, and health care to older or disabled people who are unable to take care of themselves independently. Residential care or assisted living facilities are geared toward people who can no longer maintain a household without assistance but do not require continuous medical attention. The goal in these facilities is to provide maximum independence in a homelike environment. Exercise and recreational opportunities may also be available.

Resistance exercises
See EXERCISE, RESISTANCE.

Resistance, drug
The capacity of disease-causing pathogens to withstand drugs previously toxic to them. Over time, multiple generations of disease-causing bacteria and viruses mutate to compensate for the threat posed to them by drugs. Drug resistance is a serious threat to medical progress against infectious diseases such as tuberculosis, malaria, diarrhea, sexually transmitted diseases (STDs), and various tropical diseases. The effectiveness of drugs intended to fight these infections is diminishing as drug-resistant microbes develop and spread.

Drug resistance is a worldwide problem, and international health organizations have begun to collaborate on systems to collect data about drug-resistant organisms in order to manage infectious disease more effectively. Drug resistance is caused by many things, including the use of antibiotics to treat low-level diseases such as colds and the widespread use of them to prevent disease in livestock. People can help prevent drug resistance by not asking their doctors for antibiotics to treat colds and other viral illnesses and by taking prescription drugs exactly as directed.

Resorption, dental
A condition in which the roots of a tooth dissolve and the structure of the roots is broken down, resulting in loosened teeth. Dental resorption of the roots in the primary teeth allows the deciduous teeth to shed, and this is a normal stage in the development of permanent teeth. But dental resorption of the roots of the permanent teeth is usually caused by excessive pressure on the tooth or by certain disorders. Resorption of a tooth may be caused by ongoing pressure of orthodontic appliances, irregularities in the bite, or dental impaction of adjacent teeth. The following factors also can lead to dental resorption: lesions, tumors, or cysts in the gums near the roots of the teeth; inflammation caused by infection, such as PULPITIS; or physical trauma. Sometimes, the causes of dental resorption are unknown. The condition is diagnosed by X rays. Underlying causes must be treated to prevent further loss of structure in the roots of the teeth.

Respiration
The total process by which the body takes in oxygen from the environment, transports it in the blood to body cells, uses it to create energy, and gets rid of the waste products of cell function in the form of carbon dioxide in exhaled air. Respiration is often thought to be synonymous with BREATHING, but breathing is only the mechanical, or external, part of the respiratory function.

Internal respiration begins in lung tissue, where oxygen from inhaled air passes through the walls of air sacs called alveoli, then through the walls of capillaries to enter the bloodstream. The blood carries it to body tissues, where the oxygen passes into body cells, and is used to metabolize glucose into energy. At the same time, carbon dioxide—a waste product of metabolism—passes from the cells into the capillaries to be carried back to the lungs. In the lung tissue, the carbon dioxide is absorbed by the blood and is exhaled into the environment.

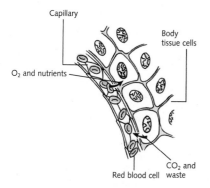

Respiration in any cell

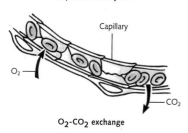

O_2-CO_2 exchange

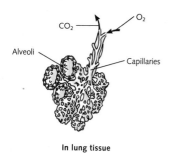

In lung tissue

INTERNAL RESPIRATION
Within lung tissue, tiny capillaries entwine minute air sacs called alveoli. Energy-giving oxygen molecules (O_2) from inhaled air pass from an alveolus into a capillary, while waste-carrying carbon dioxide molecules (CO_2) pass the other way to be exhaled. The capillaries interface with tissue throughout the body to distribute oxygen and pick up carbon dioxide.

Respirator

An apparatus that modifies the air inhaled through it. A respirator may be a face mask worn by a firefighter, for example, to block the inhalation of dust particles or other undesirable items, such as smoke. A respirator may also be a life-supporting device (ventilator) that supplies oxygen or a mixture of oxygen and carbon dioxide given to someone who cannot breathe independently.

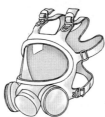

FACE MASK RESPIRATOR
Firefighters and other people in occupations that expose them to airborne hazardous substances can wear respirators that filter air through a resistant barrier. The respirator may be designed to filter solids, liquids, or oily substances. Some equipment contains an air-purifying unit.

Respiratory arrest

FOR FIRST AID
see Resuscitation, page 1328

The cessation of spontaneous breathing usually caused by some airway obstruction. Respiratory arrest may also be associated with weakness in the muscles involved in breathing. Respiratory arrest is a life-threatening emergency. If respiratory arrest is prolonged, cardiac arrest soon follows as oxygen deprivation in the blood interferes with the heart's function.

Respiratory arrest can be caused by an airway that is completely or partially blocked. In a person who is unconscious, the tongue can obstruct breathing as a result of a loss of the use of the muscles that control the tongue's movement. Obstruction of an upper airway may be caused by the presence of blood, mucus, vomit, or a foreign body in the throat. Spasms or swelling of the vocal cords can also result in a blocked airway. The presence of severe inflammation of the throat's lining, a tumor, or an injury resulting from trauma to the neck may also obstruct airflow and cause respiratory arrest. The obstruction of lower airways positioned closer to the lungs

can be caused by aspiration of food particles from the stomach, severe spasms of the bronchial tubes, or lung conditions such as pneumonia and pulmonary edema.

Respiratory distress syndrome

FOR FIRST AID
see Resuscitation, page 1328

Respiratory failure produced by an illness or injury that produces an accumulation of fluid in the lungs, a condition called PULMONARY EDEMA. Respiratory distress syndrome is a medical emergency that can progress to extreme difficulty in breathing and results in a life-threatening deficiency of oxygen in the blood.

Respiratory distress syndrome is caused by diseases that injure the lungs directly or indirectly. It is sometimes caused by SEPSIS (severe, widespread infection in the body). The syndrome occurs when the lungs' small air sacs and capillaries are damaged, which allows blood and fluid to leak into the spaces between the air sacs and ultimately into the air sacs themselves. This causes inflammation and the formation of scar tissue that interferes with the normal functioning of the lungs.

SYMPTOMS AND DIAGNOSIS
Symptoms develop rapidly, generally within 24 to 48 hours of the illness or injury. Shortness of breath and shallow breathing are the primary symptoms. The skin may develop a mottled appearance or a bluish coloration, and the person may be disoriented or unconscious as the brain is deprived of oxygen.

A doctor can detect wheezing or crackling sounds in the lungs when examining the chest with a stethoscope. Analysis of blood gases usually reveals a decreased oxygen level in the blood. Chest X rays may indicate fluid accumulating in lung and airway spaces normally filled with air. Other tests may be performed to differentiate respiratory distress syndrome from heart failure.

TREATMENT AND COMPLICATIONS
Immediate medical attention is essential to preserve life. A person who has respiratory distress syndrome must be treated promptly in a hospital's intensive care unit. Low oxygen levels are treated with oxygen

R

therapy provided by a face mask or administered with the use of a ventilator, which delivers oxygen under pressure via a tube inserted into the mouth, nose, or throat. The gas from a ventilator may be delivered with extra pressure to keep the lung tissue from collapsing. Pressure is adjusted to ensure that the small airways and air sacs are kept open and allow oxygen to enter the blood.

Supportive care includes providing intravenous fluid and intravenous feedings to prevent dehydration and malnutrition. Lung infections, such as bacterial pneumonia, commonly occur at some point during the syndrome. If this or other underlying infections are present, antibiotic therapy is given.

Complications, such as scarring of lung tissue, can occur if treatment involves use of a ventilator for a long period. Complications can also occur shortly after the onset of respiratory distress syndrome as a result of oxygen deprivation in the bloodstream that affects vital organs. When oxygen levels are severely reduced over longer periods, kidney failure and brain damage can occur.

When respiratory distress syndrome responds to treatment, complete recovery is possible with minimal or no long-term residual abnormalities to the lungs.

Respiratory failure

A condition in which failure of the lungs results in an increase in carbon dioxide and a decrease of oxygen in the blood. Respiratory failure may be chronic or acute and can be caused by any of a number of lung diseases and disorders of the lung, including respiratory distress syndrome, lung infections, and structural injuries or abnormalities of the lungs and chest wall. The condition results in an inadequate amount of oxygen to meet the vital needs of organs. This deprivation of oxygen can cause a range of symptoms, including personality changes, headache, confusion, cardiac arrhythmia, loss of consciousness, and coma. Pulmonary hypertension (see HYPERTENSION, PULMONARY) and heart failure (see HEART FAILURE, CONGESTIVE) may eventually occur.

An arterial blood test to measure the oxygen, carbon dioxide, and pH levels in the blood can diagnose and determine the severity of respiratory failure. PULMONARY FUNCTION TESTS can be used to evaluate nerve and muscle function in the lungs.

The goal of treatment is to maintain sufficient delivery of oxygen to the lungs, usually by means of oxygen therapy, and to restore the normal exchange of oxygen and carbon dioxide in the bloodstream. Corticosteroid therapy may be administered to some people with certain conditions. Regularly changing the body position to upright can increase lung volume, and strategies to clear secretions from the upper and lower airways may be beneficial. Bronchodilators may be used when bronchospasm is a factor in respiratory failure, and antibiotics may be necessary to treat associated infections.

Respiratory function tests

See PULMONARY FUNCTION TESTS.

Respiratory system

The group of organs that brings oxygen from the air into the bloodstream and expels the waste products, including carbon dioxide. The organs of the respiratory system accomplish the physical process of breathing to bring air into the body and then expel it, as well as the more complex biochemical process of RESPIRATION to fuel the cells of the body with oxygen.

The respiratory tract begins at the NOSE, where air is drawn into the body and filtered. (Air can also be taken in by mouth.) Hairs inside the nostrils trap the largest particles of dirt, and smaller particles stick to the mucous membrane that lines the nostrils. The mucous membrane secretes mucus, the substance that catches the dirt, and also has tiny hairs called cilia that move the dirt particles along into the throat to be swallowed and expelled. From the nose the air moves into the throat, or PHARYNX, that is similarly lined with mucous membrane to continue the filtering. Air, fluids, and food all pass through the mouth and throat, but the passageway divides at the LARYNX (voice box). Food and fluids pass into the digestive tract by way of the esophagus, while the filtered air follows the respiratory tract into the larynx. The air passes through the vocal cords, which are involved in speech production (see SPEECH MECHANISM), and into the TRACHEA (windpipe). The trachea (also lined with mucous membrane) divides into two large branches called bronchi, which carry the air directly into the lungs.

The lungs lie within the chest cavity, protected by the rib cage. In the lungs, the bronchi subdivide into a vast, branching network of successively smaller passageways for air. Deep within LUNG tissues, the small-

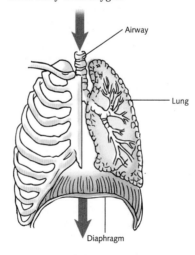
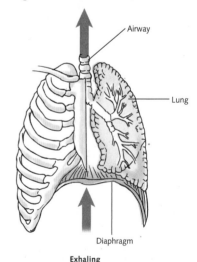

Inhaling   **Exhaling**

INHALING AND EXHALING
As a person breathes in, the diaphragm contracts and moves toward the abdomen, pulling oxygen-rich air through the airway into the lungs. As a person exhales, the diaphragm relaxes and air is compressed in the lungs and expelled.

R

est branches called bronchioles end in clusters of tiny elastic air sacs called alveoli; the air inhaled into the lungs finally enters these sacs.

Parallel to these branching airways in the lungs, a network of blood vessels brings blood into the lungs. Through the walls of tiny capillaries that cover the surface of the alveoli, oxygen passes from the alveoli into the blood. Carbon dioxide, a waste product of body metabolism carried in the blood, passes into the alveoli. The oxygen-enriched blood then flows back to the heart to be pumped throughout the body, while the carbon dioxide is exhaled back into the air through the respiratory tract. See also CARDIOVASCULAR SYSTEM.

Respiratory therapy

A program of evaluation, treatment, and care for people with breathing problems. Respiratory therapy is conducted with the supervision of a doctor who prescribes this course of treatment to people with chronic lung conditions, including asthma and emphysema. The therapy is provided in hospitals and is usually associated with the hospital's department of pulmonary medicine. Respiratory therapy may also provide life-support treatment in emergency medical situations to treat heart failure, drowning, or shock. This form of therapy includes the use of devices that provide oxygen or medication that is inhaled as a mist or gas. The equipment includes mechanical ventilators and aerosol generators.

Respiratory therapists are trained in a 2-year associate degree program or in a 4-year university course that leads to a bachelor's degree. The therapists pass a certification examination and are licensed by the state in which they practice. They can teach breathing exercises, operate equipment such as mechanical ventilators, and monitor physiological responses to various breathing therapies.

Respiratory tract infection

A viral infectious disease of any of the organs or structures involved in breathing. Respiratory tract infections occur when viruses invade and destroy cells in a person's breathing passages. When the infections affect the upper area of the RESPIRATORY SYS-TEM, they are generally referred to as common colds (see COLD, COMMON). Lower respiratory tract infections may involve the larger airways in the lungs, causing BRONCHITIS, or the smaller airways in the lungs, producing BRONCHIOLITIS. Viral infections of the deeper parts of the lungs can cause viral PNEUMONIA.

Individual respiratory tract infections are diagnosed on the basis of a complete history including all symptoms, physical examination, and blood tests. Since there are no effective antiviral medications currently available to treat these infections, treatment is usually based on supportive therapies to ease discomforts.

Respite care

A variety of services that offer caregivers temporary relief from their responsibilities. Caring for disabled or older people can be rewarding but is also demanding. Many caregivers consequently experience INSOMNIA, fatigue, or other physical or emotional problems. Respite care addresses problems arising from the stresses of providing care. (See also CAREGIVING FOR OLDER PEOPLE.) Respite care is offered through in-home and community services, such as home health care, adult day care (see DAY CARE, ADULT), and temporary, short-term institutional care. Available services may include transportation, home-delivered meals, home health services, and adult day care programs. Nursing homes and board-and-care facilities often accept a resident for a short period of time. Home health agencies can arrange for care assistance in the home. Older adults can spend part of each day in an adult day care program.

Restless leg syndrome

Also known as RLS or Ekbom syndrome, a rare condition characterized by unpleasant, restless sensations in the legs and an irresistible impulse to move them. People with RLS may experience tingling, twitching, fidgeting, aching, prickling, or burning of the legs when they lie in bed or sometimes even when they sit down. These sensations are usually worse at night and can lead to INSOMNIA. Sensations are relieved by activity, such as walking. Many people with RLS also experience periodic limb movements in sleep (PLMS), and affected people are likely to have daytime fatigue. Although its exact cause remains unknown, RLS has been linked with medical problems such as alcoholism; iron deficiency; anemia; diabetes mellitus, type 1 and type 2; and rheumatoid arthritis. Diagnosis is made through a detailed medical history and tests, such as sleep studies. Treatment includes care for any pre-existing underlying condition and sometimes use of medications, such as anticonvulsants, benzodiazepines, opioids, levodopa, and dopamine agonists. See also SLEEP DISORDERS.

Restoration, dental

A filling or appliance that replaces part or all of the structure of a tooth. A dental restoration is also the process of reconstructing a damaged or missing tooth. Restoration materials include amalgam (see AMALGAM, DENTAL) and composite fillings (see BONDING, DENTAL), inlays, onlays, crowns, dental veneers, bridges (see INLAY, DENTAL; ONLAY, DENTAL; CROWN, DENTAL; VENEERS, DENTAL; and BRIDGE, DENTAL), and partial or complete DENTURES. Restorations serve the general purpose of making existing teeth stronger and adding support to the teeth in areas adjacent to missing teeth. They are used for preventing further damage to the teeth and surrounding structures, improving or normalizing the appearance of the teeth, reinstating the proper function of the teeth, and eliminating sensitivity of the teeth.

The type of restoration that a dentist chooses may depend on the size of the area to be restored in a single tooth, the number of teeth to be replaced, or the location in the mouth of the tooth or teeth to be restored. Financial considerations, aesthetic concerns, and a person's age may also be factors in the decision.

In most small- to moderate-sized cavities, the material for restoring a prepared tooth is either silver amalgam or composite resin. While amalgam restorations may last longer, the use of composite filling material is more aesthetically pleasing and more effective at conserving the tooth structure. Amalgam is stronger and more appropriate for restoring the

R

chewing surfaces of teeth. It is also the less costly of the two restoration materials. Either amalgam or composite may be used to repair cavities in PRIMARY TEETH and PERMANENT TEETH.

The other types of dental restorations repair or replace only the permanent teeth. Inlays and onlays are used to restore larger losses of tooth structure from decay or breakage. Crowns restore teeth that do not have enough structure remaining to be treated with amalgam or composite fillings or with inlays or onlays. Dental veneers can be applied only to nonchewing surfaces of the teeth and are generally used for cosmetic improvement. Bridges fill in spaces left by missing teeth in areas where there is sufficient support from adjacent teeth. Dentures are used to replace some or all of the teeth.

Resuscitation

The process of restoring breathing to an injured person. Resuscitation is used as first aid to help people who have stopped breathing because they are choking, have heart disease, or were rescued while drowning, and for other causes. Resuscitation of a person who is choking usually involves using the HEIMLICH MANEUVER; a person who has stopped breathing because of heart problems is usually resuscitated through CARDIOPULMONARY RESUSCITATION (CPR); and a person drowning may be resus-

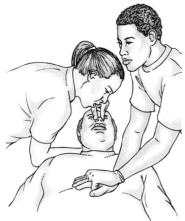

CPR WITH TWO RESCUERS
Cardiopulmonary resuscitation can be performed by two trained people. One rescuer does timed chest compressions, while the second rescuer performs mouth-to-mouth rescue breathing at intervals and checks frequently for a pulse.

citated with rescue breathing. See Resuscitation steps, page 1328.

Retainer, dental

An appliance that is worn after the removal of braces or other orthodontic appliances to stabilize the teeth that have been moved into proper position. The dental retainer is generally used on the upper teeth during an important stage of orthodontic treatment called retention. During this stage, the teeth, which have been repositioned by the braces must be held in place for a period to establish permanently the corrected alignment and bite. The retainer holds the teeth in place as the jaw hardens and the teeth become strongly attached to the jaw. Some removable retainers are constructed of plastic and wire. Others are made entirely of metal wire. The orthodontist who fits the retainer offers individualized instructions on how often and for how long the retainer must be worn, depending on factors including age and the condition of the gums and teeth. Usually, the retainer is worn only at night. If a child who has worn braces is still growing and if all of his or her permanent teeth have not yet erupted, fixed retainers may be bonded inside the lower teeth or cemented to the back teeth.

Reticulocyte

An immature red blood cell that has developed beyond the stage in which a nucleus is present.

Retina

The light-sensitive membrane that forms the inner layer of the back of the EYE and contains the nerve receptors for VISION. Light that has passed into the eye reaches the retina as an inverted image. The retina is a complex structure, a ten-layered membrane lined with two kinds of light-sensitive cells. Rod cells—so-called because of their shape—perceive shape and movement. Cone cells are sensitive to both light and color and have a role in visual acuity, or sharpness of perception. Because the retina has many more rods than cones, the eye can perceive light in darkness, but it sees color best in bright light. Rods and cones—also called photoreceptors—respond to light focused on the retina by translating

the stimulus into electrochemical nerve signals.

Nerve fibers from each retina join to form the optic nerves, and the two optic nerves meet to send information about the image to the visual cortex in the brain. Some input from the right eye goes to the left side of the brain, and vice versa, so that the two eyes together produce a three-dimensional image. The brain automatically rights the inverted image from the retina.

Retinal artery occlusion

Blockage of a blood vessel that carries blood to the retina (the light-sensitive tissue at the back of the eye). The blockage results from a fat deposit or a blood clot. The blockage cuts off the blood supply to the retina, and the affected portion stops working. The principal symptom of retinal artery occlusion is sudden blurring or blindness in one eye. Since the retina is made up of nerve tissue, its light-sensitive cells begin to die in the absence of a blood supply. Emergency treatment consists of massaging the eyeball, with the hope of dislodging the blockage. Carbon dioxide gas may be given to widen the artery and move the clot or fat deposit, thereby reducing the size of the affected area of the retina. Anticoagulant drugs are given to dissolve blood clots and restore normal blood flow. Even with treatment, some or all vision in the eye may be lost because of irreversible damage to the retina.

Retinal artery occlusion can be a sign of increased risk of stroke. The condition is most likely to occur in older people as a result of underlying disease, such as diabetes mellitus, type 1 and type 2; high blood pressure (hypertension); abnormally high pressure within the eye (glaucoma); coagulation disorders; abnormally high fat levels in the blood (hyperlipidemia); and artery disease (atherosclerosis). Measures used to reduce the risk of coronary artery disease, such as regular exercise and a low-fat diet, are thought to help prevent retinal artery occlusion.

Retinal detachment

Separation of the retina (the light-sensitive layer at the back of the eye)

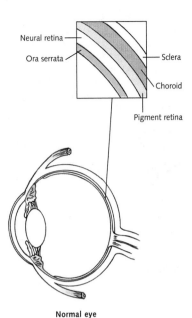

LAYERS OF RETINA
The retina is a multilayered, light-sensitive membrane surrounding the back part of the eye. The vitreous body, a jellylike shock absorber inside the central cavity of the eye, helps support the retina.

from the underlying tissues. Retinal detachments are usually caused by a tear or hole in the retina. Eye fluids leak through the opening and accumulate under the retina, lifting it off the tissues that support it. A retinal detachment is painless, but it causes major changes in vision. These include bright flashes of light, particularly off to the sides of the visual field; a sudden increase in floaters (translucent shapes that move through the field of vision); blurred vision; or the sensation that a thick curtain is being pulled across the eye. Retinal detachment is an emergency condition that requires immediate medical attention.

Treatment depends on the extent of detachment. If the retina has a scar or hole but is not completely detached, it can be repaired in one of two ways. The first is to use a laser (photocoagulation) to form microscopic scars that seal the retina from detaching. The other method (cryopexy) uses an intensely cold probe that causes an inflammation in the area of a hole or small detachment. A scar results from the inflammation, and the retina seals or reattaches. Both photocoagulation

and cryopexy can be performed in the doctor's office under local anesthesia.

If the retina has a large detachment, more extensive surgery is needed. One method (scleral buckling) involves pushing the surface (sclera) of the eye against the retina to hold it in place and allow it to heal. A soft piece of silicone is stitched to the sclera to maintain the indentation until the retina reattaches. Another procedure (pneumatic retinopexy) entails injecting a gas bubble into the fluid (vitreous) in the back of the eye to push the retina into place and allow it to heal. In very severe cases, the vitreous may be removed completely and replaced with air or fluid to move the retina to its correct position. Over time, the cavity naturally refills with fluid.

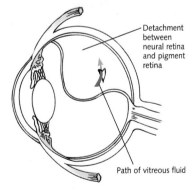

Retinal detachment

LEAKING FLUID
As a result of aging or trauma, the neural retina can break and the vitreous body can become more liquid. The vitreous fluid passes under the neural retina and separates it from the adjacent pigment retina, causing the serious condition called retinal detachment.

Repair of retinal detachment is highly successful. In a minority of cases, a second surgery is required.

Retinal detachment can result from trauma, aging, a tumor in the eye, severe nearsightedness, and inflammation. In some cases, it occurs for no apparent reason. The condition is most common among people who are male, white, and nearsighted and those who have had surgery for cataracts. A genetic factor may be involved since retinal detachment often affects more than one member of the same family.

Retinal hemorrhage
Bleeding from small blood vessels in the surface of the retina (the light-sensitive layer at the back of the eye). Retinal hemorrhage is usually caused by extremely violent force to the eye; it is a common sign of SHAKEN BABY SYNDROME, a type of severe child abuse. The condition can also result from falls from at least 50 feet, serious motor vehicle accidents, certain abnormalities of the nervous system and blood vessels, infection, and high-altitude mountaineering and, rarely, as a complication of normal childbirth and general anesthesia.

Retinal tear
See RETINAL DETACHMENT.

Retinal vein occlusion
Blockage of a blood vessel that carries blood away from the retina (the light-sensitive tissue at the back of the eye). The blockage is usually caused by a diseased arterial wall compressing the venous wall at a crossing point or by a blood clot. Retinal vein occlusion impairs sight if swelling or ischemia (poor blood flow) occurs in the center of the retina. Often the blood and fluid are absorbed naturally, and vision may return to normal. If the blood persists, the change in vision may be permanent. Laser therapy may treat any persistent swelling of the retina. Retinal vein occlusion is most likely in older people as a result of disease, such as diabetes mellitus, high blood pressure (hypertension), abnormally high pressure within the eye (glaucoma), coagulation disorders, vasculitis, and atherosclerosis (hardening of the arteries).

R

Retinitis

Inflammation of the retina (the light-sensitive tissue at the back of the eye). See RETINOPATHY.

Retinitis pigmentosa

Progressive degeneration of the retina (the light-sensitive tissue at the back of the eye) leading to poor vision in dim light, loss of vision to the sides, and reduced central vision. The disease takes its name from the darkly pigmented appearance of the retina in an eye examination. Retinitis pigmentosa is rare, and it is thought to be hereditary. The disease is often detected during childhood, but visual impairment does not begin until early adulthood. In many cases, blindness eventually results. No treatment is known. Wearing sunglasses to block ultraviolet light and taking antioxidants such as vitamin E may delay progression of the disease.

Retinoblastoma

See EYE TUMORS.

Retinoic acid

An antiacne skin cream. Retinoic acid, also known as tretinoin (Retin-A), is a derivative of vitamin A that prevents the spread of acne by preventing the formation of pimples. It is applied to the skin and is available as a cream, a gel, and a liquid. Retinoic acid should not be taken or used by pregnant women because the drug can cause birth defects in fetuses.

Retinoids

A group of compounds that are structurally related to retinol and function like VITAMIN A. Retinoids are used in the treatment of various skin diseases and digestive ailments.

Retinol

See VITAMIN A.

Retinopathy

Abnormality of the retina (the light-sensitive tissue at the back of the eye), which can be caused by many different conditions. Retinopathy of prematurity occurs in sick infants who are born prematurely. In its most severe form, blood vessels grow abnormally in the retina and scar, pulling the retina away from the inner surface of the eye causing a reti-

nal detachment and resulting in extreme distortion of vision or blindness. Less severe forms of the disease can be treated surgically. Retinopathy can also occur with high blood pressure (hypertension). The arteries in the eyes narrow and may bleed; visual disturbances and headaches can result. This type of retinopathy is treated by controlling blood pressure. Retinopathy can also be caused by diabetes mellitus, type 1 and type 2 (see RETINOPATHY, DIABETIC).

Retinopathy of prematurity

An eye disease in extremely premature infants. In the past, retinopathy of prematurity arose when excessive oxygen was given to manage respiratory problems and vitamin deficiencies. But now it is seen mostly in very premature infants.

In this disorder, the developing blood vessels of the light-sensitive retina become damaged. Vision problems ranging from nearsightedness to blindness can result. Retinopathy of prematurity is most common in extremely low-birth-weight babies who were born at 28 weeks of pregnancy or less.

Retinopathy of prematurity develops when there is an initial lack of blood flow to the premature infant's retina, followed by a compensatory growth of blood vessels. The new growth of blood vessels is often excessive and fragile. Consequently, blood may leak into the eyeball, the retina may buckle, and retinal detachment (the tearing away of the retina from the eye) may result. Only an OPHTHALMOLOGIST (a doctor who specializes in eye disorders) can diagnose and manage retinopathy of prematurity. Diagnosis is made by examination with an OPHTHALMOSCOPE (a medical instrument designed to examine the interior of the eye). After the baby's pupils are dilated, the ophthalmologist uses the ophthalmoscope to detect any abnormal blood vessel growth in the eyes.

TREATMENT AND PREVENTION

In many infants, retinopathy heals on its own. Other times, surgery is necessary. Damaged blood vessels can be repaired with either CRYOTHERAPY (freezing) or LASER SURGERY. Surgery does not always completely correct the problem. After treatment, a

child's vision is closely monitored to determine whether eyeglasses or therapy for the visually impaired may be required. Premature infants must be examined regularly by an ophthalmologist throughout the first year. If abnormal blood vessel growth continues unchecked, retinal detachment can result, causing a wide range of potentially serious vision problems.

Retinopathy, diabetic

Progressive damage to the retina (the light-sensitive layer at the back of the eye) as a result of diabetes. Diabetic retinopathy develops as a long-term complication of both type 1 (insulin-dependent) and type 2 (non–insulin-dependent) diabetes (see DIABETES MELLITUS, TYPE 1; DIABETES MELLITUS, TYPE 2). About half of those who have had diabetes for 10 years or longer develop some degree of diabetic retinopathy. The disease can lead to severe or complete vision loss, and it is the leading cause of blindness in the United States and the other developed nations for those between ages 20 and 65 years.

SYMPTOMS AND STAGES

It is believed that diabetic retinopathy arises from metabolic changes that damage blood vessels in the retina and reduce delivery of oxygen and nutrients to the retina. Small retinal blood vessels (capillaries) leak protein and fluid, which form deposits (exudates) on the retina. The capillaries tend to close off, decreasing the supply of oxygen to the retina. Diabetes can weaken the walls of the larger blood vessels, resulting in a ballooning out of the blood vessel that appears as small round dots on the back surface of the eye known as microaneurysms. Then, the microaneurysms can rupture and bleed.

This initial stage of the disease is known as background (or nonproliferative) diabetic retinopathy. It causes no pain, and, although the changes in the retina are visible to a specialist during an eye examination, they lead to only subtle changes in vision. Vision changes noticeably if bleeding and fluid leakage occur in the macula, the central portion of the retina, which is responsible for sharp, central vision. This macular edema, as it is known, causes blurred vision.

Vision also changes noticeably if

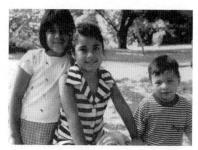

Normal vision

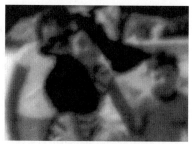

Diabetic retinopathy

BLURRED VISION AND BLACK SPOTS
In a person with the early stages of diabetic retinopathy, a clear scene might appear blurry. The blurred image is the result of macular edema (leaking fluid on the retina), and the black spots are caused by floating specks of blood.

proliferative diabetic retinopathy develops. The lack of oxygen in the retina from the closed capillaries prompts the growth of new blood vessels, which are abnormally weak and rupture easily. Blood leaking into the vitreous (the clear jellylike substance in the center of the eye) blocks the passage of light and impairs vision. The formation of scar tissue may pull the retina away from the back of the eye and cause RETINAL DETACHMENT, which can lead to blindness.

Diabetic retinopathy is compounded by the fact that many people with diabetes have high blood pressure or hypertension, which often worsens diabetic retinopathy. Hypertension also causes swelling of the retina and bleeding and adds to the overall deterioration of the eye. Nonproliferative diabetic retinopathy affects many people who have had diabetes for 20 years or longer. The proliferative form of the disease is less common, affecting approximately 5 percent of people with diabetes.

PREVENTION AND TREATMENT
Controlling the blood sugar level and the hypertension that often accompanies diabetes are the best measures for delaying or preventing the start of diabetic retinopathy. Avoiding tobacco, exercising regularly, and reducing fats in the diet may also help. In addition, every person who has diabetes should undergo a thorough eye examination at least once a year to detect any retinal changes in the earliest stages. Women with diabetes who are pregnant are at increased risk for retinopathy and should have their eyes examined during each trimester of the pregnancy.

If macular edema develops, it is treated with laser photocoagulation. This technique uses a tightly focused laser in the area of leakage to help the retina resorb (soak up) the residual fluid. If new blood vessels develop and lead to proliferative diabetic retinopathy, photocoagulation can be used on the peripheral retina to help shrink the abnormal blood vessels. This treatment seems to eliminate the low oxygen state on the retina. It results in some loss of peripheral vision in order to preserve the critical central vision. Photocoagulation is performed in a doctor's office or outpatient surgery facility using a topical anesthetic applied to the eye with drops.

In cases in which bleeding into the vitreous has clouded vision, a vitrectomy is needed. The surgeon makes a small incision in the white (sclera) of the eye and inserts an instrument that draws out the cloudy vitreous and replaces it with a clear salt solution. This surgery can be performed under a local or a general anesthetic and may require an overnight hospital stay. The eye is red and irritated for a few days to weeks following the surgery, and a protective covering may be worn to shield the eye until healing is complete. Vision following a vitrectomy can be greatly improved.

If the retina pulls away from the wall of the eye, it has to be put back in place to prevent vision loss or blindness. Treatment ranges from photocoagulation to surgery.

Retractor

An instrument used to hold the sides of a surgical incision open or hold back the surrounding organs and tissues so that the surgeon has access to the area being operated on. Retractors come in various shapes and sizes, depending on the type of surgery being done.

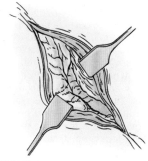

ACCESS TO A SURGICAL SITE
Instruments called retractors hold an incision open or hold back organs and body tissue and fat, so that the surgeon can reach the area to be operated on.

Retrobulbar optic neuritis

See OPTIC NEURITIS.

Retroperitoneal fibrosis

A noncancerous mass of fibrous tissue that grows in the back of the abdomen and may block the tubes (ureters) connecting the kidneys and bladder. The disease occurs mostly in men and is rare. Symptoms include pain in the abdomen, back, testicles, or side under the ribs; nausea or vomiting; general weakness; decreased output of urine; difficulty retaining urine (incontinence); or difficulty urinating. Diagnosis is usually made with X rays or CT (computed tomography) scans of the person's abdomen. Treatment consists of surgery to relieve the obstruction of the kidneys and a biopsy of the removed mass.

Retropubic suspension

A surgical procedure for women to correct stress incontinence (urine leakage when coughing or sneezing) caused by a CYSTOURETHROCELE, a weakness in the tissues supporting the bladder and urethra. In this procedure, an incision is made in the abdomen, and the supporting tissue around the upper urethra is lifted to its normal position behind the pubic bone and stitched in place. Surgery is indicated only when KEGEL EXERCISES, HORMONE REPLACEMENT THERAPY, and other treatments have not been effective in correcting the pelvic support problems that cause urine leakage.

Retrovirus

An infectious particle that consists of RNA (ribonucleic acid) genetic material, instead of DNA (see DEOXYRIBONUCLEIC ACID). Retroviruses contains proteins, which can attach to cell membranes and produce infection. The virus that causes AIDS (acquired immunodeficiency syndrome) is a retrovirus, as is the virus that causes T-cell leukemia (see LEUKEMIA; T CELL).

Rett syndrome

A rare, pervasive developmental disorder in children. Rett syndrome, which is most likely caused by genetic mutation, occurs primarily in girls. An affected child's head is of normal circumference at birth, followed by a gradual slowing of head growth. Rett syndrome occurs in four stages. In stage one, children appear to develop normally for their first 6 to 18 months. Development slows and eventually comes to a halt in stage two. In stage three (between 9 months and 3 years), the child begins to lose previously acquired speech and motor skills. There may also be a loss of interest in social activities. Stage four sees a gradual return of learning, but at a slower rate. Most children with Rett syndrome are mentally retarded. They may also experience problems with coordination and walking; difficulties with breathing, chewing, or swallowing; constipation; seizures; repetitive hand movements; and poor circulation in the extremities. Treatment options are limited, but psychotherapy, social skills training, and physical or occupational therapy are helpful to some children. Most people with Rett syndrome will need some degree of custodial care.

Reversible ischemic neurological deficit

See RIND.

Reye syndrome

A very rare childhood disorder that is potentially fatal to children under 18; it is strongly associated with taking aspirin, but the exact cause remains unknown. In Reye syndrome, a child's brain and liver swell, following a viral infection (such as influenza or chickenpox) or an upper respiratory tract infection. A third of cases occur in children who have chickenpox. Most cases occur in children between ages 4 and 16. Like viral infections, Reye syndrome most frequently occurs in winter. Educating parents about the association of aspirin with the disease has greatly reduced the number of cases seen in the United States. To avoid risk, children should be treated for fever with ibuprofen or acetaminophen instead of aspirin.

SYMPTOMS

Three to 7 days after the start of a viral illness, an affected child begins to vomit forcefully every 1 to 2 hours over a 24- to 36-hour period. There may be a headache and changes in consciousness from lethargy and sleepiness to agitation and anger. Additional symptoms include confusion, disorientation, delirium, hallucinations, and a rapid heartbeat. If the disorder progresses, brain swelling and injury can eventually lead to a seizure or coma.

DIAGNOSIS AND TREATMENT

A child showing the symptoms of Reye syndrome should be brought immediately to a hospital emergency department. A prompt diagnosis is important to avoid risk of brain damage and death. A physical examination should then be performed. Blood and spinal fluid (see SPINAL TAP) may be tested to detect chemical disturbances. A liver biopsy and imaging studies such as CT (computed tomography) scanning or MRI (magnetic resonance imaging) may also be used to check for liver and brain damage.

Hospitalization is mandatory for children diagnosed with Reye syndrome. Fluids lost during vomiting need to be replaced intravenously. Children must be monitored for brain swelling, and medications may be administered to control it. By increasing a child's breathing rate, a VENTILATOR (mechanical breathing device) can also help control pressure on the brain. A blood transfusion or kidney dialysis may be required. In some cases, surgery may be performed to reduce pressure on the brain.

There is no cure for Reye syndrome. Prospects for recovery often depend on the seriousness of the case and the effectiveness of the treatments. If the disorder is treated promptly, a child can recover completely in 5 to 10 days. In some cases, however, the syndrome causes brain damage. Because of earlier intervention and the more effective treatments available today, Reye syndrome is far less often fatal than it was in the past.

Rh immune globulin

A blood protein used as a treatment if a person with Rh-negative blood is exposed to Rh-positive blood; also known as RhoGAM. (See RH INCOMPATIBILITY.) Rh immune globulin is also used to treat a bleeding disorder known as immune thrombocytopenic purpura.

Rh incompatibility

A potentially life-threatening condition that develops when a mother with Rh-negative blood has a baby with Rh-positive blood. Rh-positive and Rh-negative indicate the presence or absence of an inherited blood characteristic known as the Rh factor (named after the rhesus monkey, the species in which the factor was originally identified). If Rh-positive blood mixes with Rh-negative blood, the Rh-negative blood develops antibodies to the Rh factor and attacks it. Such a situation can arise when a woman with Rh-negative blood is carrying a fetus with Rh-positive blood. Small amounts of blood from the fetus leak across the placenta during pregnancy and birth and stimulate an antibody response (Rh isoimmunization) in the mother. Usually the incompatibility poses little or no problem the first time it occurs, but in the woman's subsequent pregnancies with fetuses who have Rh-positive blood, the mother makes antibodies on reexposure to Rh factor that attack the baby's blood cells. This risk increases with each Rh-positive pregnancy. Consequences in the newborn range from mild to very severe. Only 10 to 20 percent of infants with severe disease survive, and the survivors are likely to have major impairment.

Rh incompatibility is now almost entirely preventable. Early in pregnancy the mother's Rh blood group is established with a simple blood test (see BLOOD GROUPS). If she has Rh-negative blood, she is given an injection of Rh immune globulin during the 28th week of pregnancy to destroy any Rh-positive fetal red blood cells in her bloodstream and prevent the formation of antibodies. This injection has no risk, even if the fetus proves to have Rh-negative blood. If the newborn has Rh-positive blood, another injection of Rh immune globulin is given within 72 hours of birth to eliminate any fetal blood cells that entered the mother during labor.

In rare cases in which antibody sensitization in the mother has already occurred, the fetus is given blood transfusions in the uterus to replace the Rh-positive blood with Rh-negative blood. The baby is then delivered before it reaches full term.

Rh isoimmunization
See RH INCOMPATIBILITY.

Rhabdomyolysis
A skeletal muscle injury that can result in kidney damage. The condition is caused by toxic effects from the pigment myoglobin when it is released by muscle cells damaged by trauma or other events. When damaged muscle tissue releases myoglobin into the bloodstream, it is filtered through the kidneys, where it breaks down into potentially toxic compounds and may block the organ, damaging it and causing kidney failure. Rhabdomyolysis may also be caused by severe exertion during physical activities such as marathon running, especially during hot and humid weather. Other causes include seizures; the abuse or overdose of drugs such as cocaine, amphetamines, heroin, and PCP (phencyclidine or "angel dust"); trauma; heat intolerance or heatstroke; or alcoholism that produces muscle tremors.

Symptoms include urine that is dark, red, or cola-colored and tenderness, stiffness, aching, and weakness in the muscles, as well as overall weakness. Unintentional weight gain, seizures, pain in the joints, and fatigue may be associated with rhabdomyolysis. The condition is diagnosed by urine and blood tests. Intravenous hydration can stabilize the condition. Diuretics may be pre-

scribed to flush the myoglobin out of the kidneys, and bicarbonate may be used to help prevent the myoglobin from forming toxic compounds. The condition should be treated as soon as possible to limit the extent of kidney damage and prevent the serious complication of kidney failure.

Rhabdomyosarcoma
A soft-tissue malignant tumor originating in the muscles of the head and neck area, in the genital or urinary tract, or in the extremities. This type of cancer, found most often in children, can also be found in the chest area, in the gastrointestinal tract, and in the anal region. Diagnosis is made by a biopsy of the tumor and evaluation of the tissue sample. Surgery, chemotherapy, and radiation therapy are the treatments. Rhabdomyosarcoma is considered a curable disease with early, aggressive treatment.

Rheumatic fever
An inflammatory illness that occurs as a delayed complication of group A *Streptococcus* infection of the upper respiratory tract. Rheumatic fever results in a small percentage of people who have had strep throat and is thought to be produced by an abnormal immune response to the *Streptococcus* organism. The illness, which is not contagious, can occur within 3 to 35 days after a person has had strep throat without medical treatment. Rheumatic fever can usually be prevented from developing by treating strep throat with antibiotics. A mild sore throat condition in which the throat appears reddened and inflamed should be evaluated by a physician so that a throat swab can be taken to detect streptococcal infection.

Rheumatic fever occurs more commonly in temperate regions of the world, including large portions of the United States and Canada, and particularly in the late winter or spring. It tends to affect children aged 3 to 15, and there is evidence that a genetic predisposition to the disease exists.

The infection produces inflammatory lesions in the connective tissue of the heart, joints, tissues below the skin, and central nervous system. Complications of rheumatic fever following a single episode of the illness

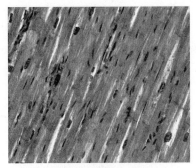

NORMAL HEART MUSCLE
The texture of normal human cardiac muscle (above) differs markedly from tissue affected by rheumatic fever.

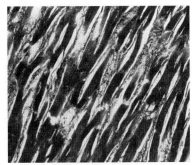

INFLAMED HEART MUSCLE
A person with rheumatic fever, which is rare today, may develop myocarditis, or an inflammation of the heart muscle.

are unusual, but they may include valvular heart disease, congestive heart failure, and persistent arthritis. The infection may recur, producing several episodes of illness that may increase the risk of complications, especially heart disease.

SYMPTOMS
A child with rheumatic fever has a high temperature, a lack of appetite, and general malaise. He or she is often pale and sweaty. Symptoms may include painful joint swelling and the joints may become reddened and hot to the touch. The swelling tends to migrate from one joint to another, usually affecting the wrists, elbows, knees, and ankles initially, then disappearing within 24 hours. Pain and swelling of the joints may return later and involve the hips, shoulders, fingers, and toes. Another symptom of rheumatic fever is chorea, a condition characterized by uncontrolled jerking movements that indicate nerve damage.

R

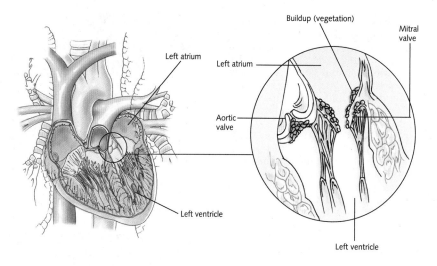

Buildup (vegetation)

Left atrium

Mitral valve

Left atrium

Aortic valve

Left ventricle

Left ventricle

INTERFERENCE WITH VALVE
As a result of rheumatic fever, a buildup of bacteria and blood clots can accumulate on the mitral valve and the pulmonary valve of the heart. The buildup, called vegetation, can interfere with the valve's action, causing leakage and reducing the heart's ability to pump blood.

If the heart is affected without involvement of the joints and the infection is mild, there may be only mild symptoms including fatigue, poor coloring, and general malaise.

In severe infections, the principal symptom is breathlessness, especially with exertion or when the person is in a lying position. This requires emergency medical attention because without treatment heart failure can occur. Another symptom of serious infection with rheumatic fever is an accumulation of fluid under the skin that produces swelling, particularly in the legs and on the back. Also, a rash of reddish circles with pale centers may appear on the front and back of the trunk. Individual lesions of the rash, which does not itch, can become as large as 2 inches across and may continually change in shape. Small, round swellings or nodules that are firm and painless may appear below the skin over joints of the elbows, knees, and fingers and at the back of the head.

DIAGNOSIS AND TREATMENT
Rheumatic fever may be suspected in a person with the typical symptoms combined with a history of strep throat. Blood samples and a culture of the throat are generally taken for analysis in a laboratory. The results can confirm a diagnosis of rheumatic fever. An examination of the heart is performed to determine if the heart has been affected by the infection.

All cases of rheumatic fever are treated with antibiotics to combat any remaining bacteria from the original strep throat infection and to prevent ongoing or recurrent infection. In mild cases of the illness, complete bed rest is required until tests reveal that the infection has passed. Hospitalization may be necessary in more severe cases so that the pain and swelling of joints and the effects on the heart can be medically treated. Anti-inflammatory corticosteroid medication may be necessary to treat very severe cases in which the heart is seriously affected. In rare cases in which heart failure occurs, medication such as digitalis-based drugs (for example, digoxin or digitoxin) to strengthen the heart's capacity to pump blood may be prescribed, along with diuretics to promote urination so the body can eliminate excess fluid that has accumulated.

Rheumatism

A common term, now considered medically obsolete, that may be used to indicate a variety of conditions characterized by soreness, stiffness, or pain in the muscles or joints. Specific diseases that may be referred to as rheumatism are RHEUMATIC FEVER, OSTEOARTHRITIS, MYOSITIS, BURSITIS, and RHEUMATOID ARTHRITIS.

Rheumatoid arthritis

FOR SYMPTOM CHARTS
see Ankle or foot problems, page 18
see Hip pain, page 42
see Knee pain, page 44

A type of joint inflammation in which several parts of the body may be affected. In this more serious, systemic form of ARTHRITIS, the immune system develops antibodies that create a gradual and chronic inflammation of the thin membrane lining the joints. The inflammation eventually spreads to other parts of the joints and weakens the bones that are linked together by the joints.

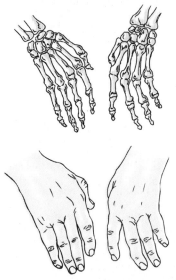

ARTHRITIC JOINTS
Rheumatoid arthritis commonly affects the joints of the fingers. Inflammation swells the cartilage, muscles, tendons, and ligaments in the joint. The ends of swollen, eroded bones and inflamed soft tissues inside the joint cause fingers to look lumpy and bent.

Sometimes the symptoms of rheumatoid arthritis may not appear in the joints until several weeks or months, during which time a person may feel generally ill, have no appetite, lose weight, experience muscular aches, and have a low-grade fever. In other instances, the painful joint inflammation may come on suddenly. Usually the small joints are affected, primarily the knuckles and toe joints of the hands and feet. Other joints, including the wrists, knees, ankles, and neck, are sometimes

R

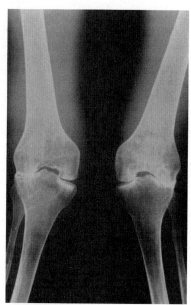

ARTHRITIC KNEES
A person with rheumatoid arthritis may develop a deformation of the knees, which causes the bones to bend toward each other (knock-knee).

affected. The inflammation may also involve the eyes, heart, lungs, blood vessels, and other tissues just beneath the skin. Rheumatoid arthritis is characterized by morning joint stiffness for several hours, fatigue, muscle aches, low-grade fever, and weight loss. Small joints of the fingers, wrists, elbows, hips, knees, ankles, and feet are usually involved. The neck can also be affected.

Rheumatoid arthritis is diagnosed by a rheumatoid arthritis screening test or by blood tests called the erythrocyte sedimentation rate (ESR) and the rheumatoid factor (RF), both of which indicate a generalized inflammation in the body. A biopsy or monitoring over a period of several weeks or months may also be necessary. This type of arthritis can occur in a single mild episode followed by complete recovery. Or, it may occur in a series of episodes that become increasingly debilitating and leave a person completely arthritic and disabled. In the latter case, a person may have to learn to deal with a permanent condition.

The use of nonsteroidal anti-inflammatory drugs (NSAIDs), such as aspirin, ibuprofen, and naproxen, and heat applications may help control pain. Removable splints made by

occupational therapists may be used when painful joints need support and rest. Exercises may be recommended by a physical therapist. In active cases of rheumatoid arthritis, medications that interrupt the process that produces the disease may be prescribed. These include penicillamine, gold compounds, sulfasalazine, and methotrexate. Chemotherapy drugs may be given to reduce the blood levels of antibodies. In early stages, surgical removal of the inflamed membrane covering the joint (a procedure called a synovectomy), may be considered. In later stages, joint replacement surgery may become necessary.

Rheumatoid arthritis, juvenile

See JUVENILE RHEUMATOID ARTHRITIS.

Rheumatoid nodules

Painless lumps under the skin that are a prominent feature of RHEUMATOID ARTHRITIS and other rheumatoid diseases. Rheumatoid nodules usually are found on the bony part of the forearms, around the ankles, or on the fingers. They may be caused by inflammation around small blood vessels. Rheumatoid nodules typically last only a few months and are rarely a significant medical problem.

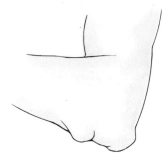

LUMPS ON BONES AND JOINTS
People with rheumatoid arthritis sometime develop nodules on the joints or bones that are visible under the skin. They may be fixed or movable, and they may fluctuate in size.

Rheumatoid spondylitis

An inflammation of the vertebral joints. See ANKYLOSING SPONDYLITIS.

Rheumatologist

An internist or pediatrician who has received additional training and

experience in the diagnosis and treatment of arthritis and other diseases of the joints, muscles, bones, and associated fibrous tissues. Rheumatologists have an additional 2 to 3 years in specialized rheumatology training after completing 4 years of medical school and 3 years of training in internal medicine or pediatrics. Most rheumatologists who treat patients in a medical practice have passed an examination to become board certified. A rheumatologist may conduct research into the causes of rheumatoid diseases and improved methods of treatment.

Rheumatology

The medical science that is concerned with rheumatoid diseases, or diseases that affect the joints, muscles, bones, and associated fibrous tissues.

Rhinitis

Inflammation of the mucous membrane lining the nose that may result from a number of causes, including the common cold (see COLD, COMMON), ALLERGIES, irritation of the nose from air pollutants, and the side effects of medications such as over-the-counter nasal decongestant sprays.

SYMPTOMS AND CAUSES
The most common symptom of rhinitis is a stuffy nose. Nasal obstruction (blockage of nasal passageways) is another typical symptom, causing the person to breathe through the mouth, which dries the tissues of the mouth and throat. Postnasal drip (the sensation of mucus dripping from the back of the nose into the throat) is another common symptom. The cause is often an infection with a virus (see VIRUSES), such as the one that causes a cold.

Chronic rhinitis may be caused by continual exposure to chemicals in the workplace (such as house paint or photo-developing solutions), environmental pollutants, or ongoing contact with irritants such as chlorine in a swimming pool. It may also be due to allergies, an anatomic obstruction, adenoid enlargements, or other diseases. With sufficient exposure, any chemical substance can cause irritation and inflammation of the nasal membranes.

Allergic rhinitis (hay fever) is the result of an exaggerated defensive response to inhaling (breathing in) a foreign substance such as pollen, mold, tobacco smoke, animal dander, or components of household dust, specifically dust mites. The allergic response causes a release of many chemicals, including histamine (a

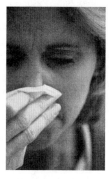

STUFFY NOSE
Rhinitis is an inflammation of the mucous membrane lining the nose; it often stems from a cold, allergy, or other irritant.

body chemical released during an allergic reaction), which increases blood flow to the nasal membranes, causing nasal congestion and an excess production of mucus.

Vasomotor rhinitis is nasal inflammation caused by the expansion of the abundant supply of blood vessels in the nose. The expansion may be from sensitivity to temperature changes, stress, or environmental irritants such as smoke or smog. As a result of the expanded blood vessels, the nasal membranes swell, producing nasal congestion and nasal obstruction. These symptoms tend to go away when a person is no longer exposed to the cause of the inflammation. If the symptoms persist over a long time, the blood vessels may lose their capacity to constrict and, therefore, remain in an expanded state. The continual expansion of the blood vessels narrows the nasal passageways and causes ongoing obstruction, congestion, and the feeling of stuffiness in the nose, especially when a person lies down.

DIAGNOSIS AND TREATMENT
Rhinitis is diagnosed by examination and evaluation by a doctor. The treatment depends on the cause of rhinitis. If the condition is caused by the common cold, the doctor may recommend one or more medications and lifestyle suggestions. Over-the-counter or prescription antihista-

Terms in small capital letters—for example, PHYSICAL THERAPY or PAGET DISEASE—indicate a cross-reference to another entry with more information.

mines may help reduce the sneezing, itching, and mucus production. Decongestants can decrease the swelling and congestion (see COLD REMEDIES). Treatment on the inside of the nose, possibly with injections of one of the CORTICOSTEROIDS, and efforts to eliminate possible irritants, may be recommended to relieve chronic rhinitis and vasomotor rhinitis. Allergic rhinitis is most effectively treated by an allergist. Over-the-counter or prescription antihistamines may help reduce the flow of nasal discharge and relieve the itch and sneezing associated with allergies. Certain prescription nasal sprays may be helpful.

Avoidance of allergens is an effective approach. Such allergens may include grass, cat dander, and tobacco smoke. Weekly allergy injections (immunotherapy) may also be helpful when other measures fail. The injections work by forming antibodies in the bloodstream to block histamines and create interference with the allergic reaction.

RISK FACTORS
Rhinitis caused by a virus makes the nasal area more susceptible to a bacterial infection; the condition may evolve into a bacterial sinus infection. When this occurs, the nasal discharge generally takes on a yellow or green color. Pain and tenderness in the cheeks and upper teeth, between and behind the eyes, or above the eyes and in the forehead, may occur. These infections generally respond to antibiotic medication. When the condition is chronic, surgery may be recommended. If rhinitis persists, it may lead to abnormal function of nasal structures; the most effective treatment is surgical removal of part of the affected structures. See SINUSITIS.

Rhinitis, allergic
An allergy-related inflammation of the membranes lining the nasal passages, throat, and eyes caused by sensitivity to airborne pollens, molds, and other allergens. Seasonal allergic rhinitis is also known as HAY FEVER.

The allergens that cause allergic rhinitis combine in the body with antibodies, causing the release of histamine and other chemical substances into the bloodstream. This process produces the symptoms of the allergy.

Perennial allergic rhinitis is a reaction that occurs year-round to allergens that occur primarily indoors. Animal dander, DUST MITES, feathers, mold spores, or cockroaches are usually responsible for the symptoms produced by this form of allergic rhinitis, which include sneezing, itchy and runny nose, stuffy nose, red and watery eyes, and itchy throat. This group of allergic symptoms occurs most commonly in people who have a family history of allergies or a personal history of allergy-related conditions, including eczema and childhood asthma.

Perennial allergic rhinitis may be difficult to diagnose because the symptoms resemble those of the common cold (see COLD, COMMON), and there is no clear pattern of illness. Blood and skin scratch tests may be performed to determine the causative allergen. Treatment generally consists of over-the-counter or prescribed antihistamines, decongestants, prescribed corticosteroid nasal sprays, and immunotherapy, or allergy shots.

Prevention of seasonal allergic rhinitis involves lifestyle changes. These include moving all unnecessary furniture and carpeting out of the bedroom, keeping the bedroom and bed linens clean, enclosing the box spring and mattress in dust mite–proof plastic coverings, storing clothing in dust-free closets, covering or filtering all vents, using pillows and comforters stuffed with synthetic materials rather than feathers or down, using a vacuum cleaner instead of sweeping, and using a HEPA (high-efficiency particle-arresting) filter. The intensity of allergic reactions may be reduced by following certain health habits, including maintaining a healthy diet, drinking adequate fluids to loosen secretions in the nose and throat, exercising regularly, and elevating the head during sleep to prevent nasal congestion at night. See ALLERGIES.

Rhinitis, atrophic
An atrophy or shrinking away of the soft tissue just under the membrane lining the nose, producing a thick crust of dried material that may eventually decompose and cause a foul odor. The condition can impair the sense of smell and cause nosebleeds. Atrophic rhinitis may result from a

R

lack of activity of the mucous glands in the mucous membrane of the nose or from extensive nasal surgery. It may also be caused by a thinning of the membrane or by a structural abnormality, such as excessively large nasal chambers. It may be caused or aggravated by overuse of over-the-counter nasal decongestant sprays. An otolaryngologist (ear, nose, and throat specialist) can diagnose the condition. Treatment is not always effective but may involve saline irrigation (a procedure in which the doctor flushes a salt water solution through the nasal cavities) and physical removal of any crusts. The use of a vaporizer in the home and workplace may help relieve discomfort.

Rhinophyma

A swollen, bright red nose associated with a skin condition called ROSACEA. In rhinophyma, oil glands enlarge, leading to a buildup of excess tissue on the nose. Treatment includes avoiding factors that aggravate rosacea such as spicy foods, hot beverages, and alcohol; limiting exposure to sunlight and extreme temperatures; and using green-tinted make-up to conceal redness. Doctors can also prescribe topical or oral antibiotics. In severe cases, excess tissue may be removed from the nose with laser surgery.

Rhinoplasty

See NOSE RESHAPING.

Rhinorrhea

The symptom of a runny nose that may be caused by allergies or an infection. Rhinorrhea occurs when the immune system responds to an ALLERGEN or an infectious agent, such as a virus or bacterium. The immune response produces inflammation of the nasal membranes, which promotes excess mucus secretion. When the mucus is clear, the cause of a runny nose is usually an allergy or a virus. Yellow or green mucus generally indicates an infection.

Rhythm method

See NATURAL FAMILY PLANNING.

Rib

Any one of the oval, curved bones that form most of the skeleton of the chest. There are 12 pairs of ribs, each of which joins a vertebra in the spine. The upper seven pairs of ribs join the sternum (breastbone) in the front of the body and are called true ribs. They form a protective cage around the heart, lungs, major blood vessels, and other chest organs. Three pairs of so-called false ribs branch from the true ribs above them. The lower two pairs of ribs, called floating ribs, are attached only to the spine. The intercostal muscles between the ribs expand and contract the rib cage so that the lungs can inflate and deflate for breathing. See SKELETAL SYSTEM.

Rib, fractured

A broken rib bone that may be caused by forceful trauma, such as a fall or a blow to the chest, or by the pressure of intense coughing or sneezing. A fractured rib, which tends to occur more often in older adults, may be broken in more than one place. Symptoms include pain that intensifies when a breath is taken, tenderness and shallow breathing, and bruising at the site of the injury. In most cases, a fractured rib will heal naturally within 3 to 8 weeks. A physician should be notified if the

---

SELF-HELP GUIDELINES FOR A FRACTURED RIB

In most rib fractures, the bone ends remain in alignment, and healing is spontaneous and straightforward. Here are some guidelines to speed healing of a fractured rib:

- Strenuous activity should be avoided.
- The injured rib should be protected from further pressure or trauma.
- The lungs must be kept free of infection by taking several deep breaths at intervals throughout the day.
- The area of the rib should not be tightly belted or bound.
- To help relieve pain, heat may be applied using a heating pad, whirlpool bath, or warm, moist towels.
- Over-the-counter painkillers, including acetaminophen, and nonsteroidal anti-inflammatory drugs (NSAIDs) such as ibuprofen and aspirin may relieve discomfort.

---

person has a high temperature, a cough develops, or thick or bloody sputum is coughed up. Emergency medical care should be sought when there is difficulty breathing or an increase in pain or if the person has nausea, vomiting, or abdominal pain.

Ribavirin

One type of antiviral drug. Ribavirin (Rebetron, Virazole) is used to treat severe viral pneumonia in infants and young children. It is given by oral inhalation and breathed in as a fine mist by the child. Ribavirin is sprayed into a hood, tent, or face mask by a special machine called a NEBULIZER.

Riboflavin

Vitamin B2, an important nutrient in the metabolism of carbohydrates, fats, and protein. See VITAMIN B.

Ribonucleic acid

A macromolecule consisting of a nucleic acid found in all cells and in many viruses. Ribonucleic acid, or RNA, is the nucleic acid that translates genetic information and directs the cell's activities. Ribonucleic acid occurs in many different forms, such as messenger RNA, transfer RNA, and complementary RNA.

RICE (first aid)

FOR FIRST AID
see Strains and sprains, page 1331

First aid techniques used to minimize bleeding and swelling. RICE stands for:
- **Rest** The person should lie quietly while medical assistance is sought.
- **Ice** An ice pack or cold compress may be used to minimize swelling of the injured area.
- **Compression** A tight bandage may be used to reduce swelling and bleeding.
- **Elevation** The person's feet should be elevated about 12 inches higher than the head, to keep blood flowing to the brain.

Rickets

A disease affecting the bones in the skeleton, characterized by inadequate calcium and phosphate in the bones. Rickets is usually caused by a severe deficiency of vitamin D; it occurs mainly in infancy and childhood if

R

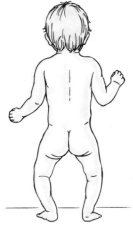

ALTERED BONE STRUCTURE
Rickets causes weakening of the bone structure with resulting skeletal deformities—most typically bowed legs.

milk or vitamin D–fortified beverages are not consumed and exposure to sunlight is limited. Symptoms include bowlegs and knock-knees, nodular enlargements on the bones, muscle pain, profuse sweating, chest deformities, spinal curvature, and enlargement of the skull, liver, and spleen. The bones may be tender when touched. Treatment is with a diet rich in calcium, vitamin D, and phosphorus. Adequate exposure to sunlight is also beneficial.

Rifampin

An antimycobacterial drug. Rifampin (Rifadin) is used to treat active tuberculosis (TB). It works by impairing the synthesis of the RNA (ribonucleic acid) of bacteria responsible for TB. It is usually prescribed with other anti-TB drugs. Rifampin is used by itself to treat carriers of meningitis who are not infected but who can carry the bacteria to others.

Rifampin is a powerful antibiotic that is very susceptible to drug resistance—resistance to rifampin by TB, for example, can develop rapidly. Rifampin is generally prescribed in combination with other anti-TB drugs to prevent or delay resistance. Rifampin is not effective for the treatment of colds, flu, or other viral infections.

Rigidity, muscle

A condition in which muscles become immobilized. Rigidity of the facial muscles and generalized body rigidity are characteristics of PARKINSON DISEASE.

Rigor

A rigidity of muscle tissue that prevents the muscle from responding to stimulation.

Rigor mortis

The temporary stiffening of the muscles of the body after death. Rigor mortis typically sets in from 3 to 7 hours after death, and it generally disappears between 3 and 4 days later, when decomposition begins. Pathologists study rigor mortis to assess the time of a death and the amount of exertion by the body preceding death.

Riluzole

A drug used to treat people who have Lou Gehrig disease, or amyotrophic lateral sclerosis (ALS). Riluzole (Rilutek) will not cure ALS, but it can extend survival in the early stages of the disease.

Rimantadine hydrochloride

An antiviral drug. Rimantadine hydrochloride (Flumadine, Roflual) is used to prevent or treat influenza type A. Rimantadine hydrochloride may be given alone or in combination with flu shots. Rimantadine hydrochloride is not effective against the common cold, other types of flu, or some viral infections.

RIND

An acronym for reversible ischemic neurological deficit; a strokelike episode from which the person can recover in a week or less. ISCHEMIA (reduced blood flow) may be caused by ATHEROSCLEROSIS (narrowing of the arteries).

A TRANSIENT ISCHEMIC ATTACK (TIA) results in a temporary loss in brain functions that may last from several minutes to several hours. A RIND usually lasts longer than 24 hours but resolves in less than 1 week.

Ringing in the ears

See TINNITUS.

Ringworm

A fungal skin infection characterized by ring-shaped, red, scaly patches. See also TINEA.

Risk factors

Influences that contribute to a person's likelihood of developing a particular disease or condition. For example, heredity and being overweight are two important risk factors for type 2 diabetes mellitus. Risk factors such as alcohol use, drug consumption, smoking, and poor diet can adversely affect pregnancy. Some risk factors (such as genes) are beyond a person's control. However, doctors advise people to manage other significant risk factors, such as lifestyle choices about diet, exercise, smoking, drinking, and sexual activity.

Risperidone

An antipsychotic drug. Risperidone (Risperdal) is used to treat the symptoms of schizophrenia and other psychotic disorders.

Ritodrine

A drug used to stop premature labor. Ritodrine (Yutopar) is given intravenously to women who are experiencing premature labor after the 20th week of pregnancy. Ritodrine works by suppressing uterine contractions.

Rituximab

An anticancer drug; a monoclonal antibody. Rituximab (Rituxan) is used to treat non-Hodgkin lymphoma, a type of cancer. Rituximab works by destroying cancer cells.

RNA

Ribonucleic acid. A molecule consisting of a nucleic acid found in all living cells and in many viruses. RNA is the nucleic acid that carries the flow of genetic instructions from the DNA (deoxyribonucleic acid) to the rest of the cell.

RNA occurs in several forms defined by their functions, including messenger RNA, transfer RNA, and chromosomal RNA. RNA reads the chemical genetic code of the DNA that defines each gene. In order for a cell to make a protein, the DNA dictates the genetic code to a strand of messenger RNA, which then moves outside the cell nucleus to the cytoplasm where RNA directs the production of protein according to the genetic code. See also GENETIC CODE.

R

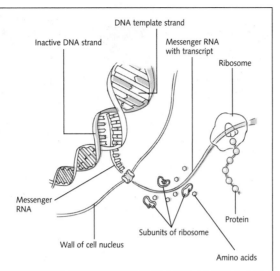

PROTEIN PRODUCTION VIA RNA
DNA in a cell nucleus makes a protein by first splitting open to make two strands. One strand becomes a template that pairs up with an RNA molecule to make a new structure called messenger RNA, which moves into the body of the cell and attaches to a structure called a ribosome, where proteins are produced. Amino acids already in the cell recognize and link with amino acid codes on the messenger RNA. The assembled chain of amino acids forms a specific protein.

DNA template strand

Inactive DNA strand

Messenger RNA with transcript

Ribosome

Messenger RNA

Protein

Subunits of ribosome

Wall of cell nucleus

Amino acids

Rocky Mountain spotted fever

An infection in humans that is transmitted by microscopic parasites called rickettsiae; also known as tick fever. Wood or dog ticks are the vector of infection, transmitting the disease from rodents to humans. *Rickettsia rickettsii,* the bacteria that cause Rocky Mountain spotted fever, attack the endothelium (cells that line the walls of small blood vessels). Occurring primarily in the Rocky Mountain regions, Rocky Mountain spotted fever is also common in Long Island, Cape Cod, and the southeastern coastal states. Four states (North Carolina, Oklahoma, Tennessee, and South Carolina) account for about half of the cases. Ninety percent of cases occur between April and September.

The parasites that cause Rocky Mountain spotted fever usually incubate for 2 to 14 days before symptoms appear. Within 1 to 2 days of being bitten by an infected tick, a person may experience a loss of appetite and general malaise. The actual start of Rocky Mountain spotted fever is evident with symptoms such as fever, headache, chills, muscle and joint pain, light sensitivity, and pain at the back of the eyes. Abdominal pain, nausea and vomiting, a sore throat, irritability, and delirium may also occur. A rash of small red spots typically appears on the ankles and wrists 2 to 3 days after the fever begins. The rash

then spreads to the limbs, trunk, and occasionally the face. As the rash progresses to large sores, Rocky Mountain spotted fever is easily distinguishable from the other diseases it resembles (HUMAN GRANULOCYTIC EHRLICHIOSIS, MEASLES, TYPHUS, and TYPHOID FEVER).

If not treated, Rocky Mountain spotted fever can be fatal. Prompt treatment with chloramphenicol and tetracyclines for a minimum of 10 days is usually effective. With treatment, fever usually resolves within 3 days.

Rofecoxib

A drug used to relieve arthritis symptoms. Rofecoxib (Vioxx) is used to treat some symptoms of arthritis, including joint pain, swelling, stiffness, and inflammation. Rofecoxib does not cure arthritis. It is also used to relieve the pain of moderate menstrual cramps and pain following surgery.

Rolfing

A system of manipulation of connective tissues to relieve physical misalignment. Rolfing, which is also called structural integration, bodywork, and Hellerwork, was invented by a biochemist who believed that physical and emotional stress, as well as gravity, can throw the body out of vertical alignment, thereby causing connective tissue to become rigid and inflexible. By using intense pressure and stroking to stretch the

rigid connective tissue back into shape, rolfers and hellerworkers restore flexibility and resilience to muscles, tendons, and bones. Rolfing, which can involve ten sessions, is chiefly used to help reduce stress and improve mobility, address posture problems, and reduce back pain. Rolfing is sometimes included in sports medicine treatment programs and may be used for those whose activities lead to repetitive stress injuries.

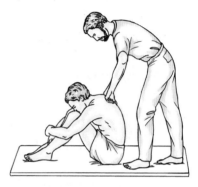

VIGOROUS MASSAGE
A practitioner of Rolfing examines the person's posture and body structure and then applies pressure on specific areas to realign muscle and bone. The rolfer uses his or her hands, fingers, knuckles, or elbows to focus the pressure; the experience can be painful.

Root canal treatment

A therapeutic procedure to treat an infection of the soft inner core (the dental pulp) in the tooth. The pulp or nerve is the soft tissue inside the natural crown and root portions of the tooth. The pulp contains the nerves, blood vessels, and lymph vessels and is contained within a structure of the tooth called the pulp chamber. Root canals are thin tunnels that extend from the pulp chamber in the natural crown of a tooth down into the bottom tip of the root where a small opening connects the small nerves and blood vessels to the larger structures in the gum. All teeth have at least one root canal, and some larger teeth may have as many as four root canals. Each root will have at least one canal and some will have two or more.

Deep tooth decay or a dental fracture that penetrates the hard outer layers of the teeth can injure the pulp by exposing this soft, fragile

R

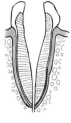

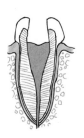

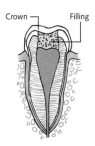

| Cavity extending into root | Decay and infected pulp removed | Pulp chamber filled with antibiotic paste | Filling and crown completed |

REMOVING DEEP TOOTH DECAY
When tooth decay penetrates into the pulp, the nerves and vessels that extend through the root canal into the gum can become infected. A dentist or endodontist performs root canal treatment to remove the decay and infected pulp. The cleaned-out root canal is medicated to destroy any remaining infection, and a temporary filling is usually put in place. Finally, the root canal is permanently filled and sealed. If large portions of the crown of the tooth need to be removed, an artificial crown will be placed over the natural tooth.

tissue to bacteria in the saliva. If untreated, this can cause the nerves and vessels inside the tooth to become infected and die. The infection may spread through the opening of the root canal at the tip of the root of the tooth, causing the surrounding bone to erode. A small sac of pus, called an abscess, can form at the root. An abscess can cause a severe toothache.

The purpose of root canal treatment is to remove the infected pulp from the tooth before the damage spreads and results in bone damage or an abscess. The treatment saves the remaining tooth structures from dying and prevents the infection from spreading, which precludes the need for a TOOTH EXTRACTION.

HOW IT IS PERFORMED
The procedure is performed by a dentist in general practice or an endodontist (a root canal specialist) with the use of local anesthesia to prevent discomfort or pain. A small rubber sheet is placed around the affected tooth to prevent contamination. A dental drill is used to create an opening in the tooth through the enamel (see ENAMEL, DENTAL) and DENTIN and into the pulp chamber. The infected pulp is removed with small instruments. The root canals are cleaned and shaped. Medication may be placed in the pulp chamber and root canals to prevent reinfection. If the treatment will require more than one visit, the crown of the tooth is temporarily filled to protect the tooth from recontamination. In

some cases, the tooth may be left open to drain. Antibiotics may be prescribed to control an infection that has spread beyond the tooth. The final step of root canal treatment is to fill and seal the root canals. If the tooth needs to be reinforced, a metal post may be cemented above the canal, filling in the top half of the canal. The post helps to hold the filling material that is needed to replace the lost tooth structure.

Even though the pulp, or nerve, of a tooth has been removed, the tissue surrounding the tooth that has been treated may be inflamed and cause discomfort for several days afterward. This discomfort is generally remedied with over-the-counter painkillers recommended by the dentist or endodontist.

Root canal treatments involve the removal of relatively large portions of the crown of the tooth. Because of this, the structure of the tooth must be restored, usually with a dental crown (see CROWN, DENTAL). A person who has had root canal therapy may consult his or her dentist for this restoration or may be referred to a prosthodontist (a specialist in creating and fitting crowns). With good oral hygiene, a restored tooth that has received root canal treatment can remain healthy for a lifetime.

Rorschach test
A psychological examination in which a person is asked to describe the images he or she sees in a series of ten inkblots. The Rorschach test is

also known as the inkblot test. The inkblots in the Rorschach test are purposely vague and ambiguous. In describing the images the inkblots suggest, the individual reveals information about his or her personality, particularly its unconscious aspects. The Rorschach test has been used extensively since it was developed in the early 20th century by Hermann Rorschach, a Swiss psychiatrist.

Rosacea
A skin disease characterized by varying degrees of facial redness due to enlargement and dilation of blood vessels beneath the skin surface; also known as adult acne. Rosacea appears more frequently in women than men, but the symptoms are usually more severe in men. It is common in fair-skinned people who flush or blush easily, but the exact cause is unknown.

SYMPTOMS
Common signs of rosacea are redness, pimples, and the appearance of spidery small blood vessels on the face. Often people have only one or two symptoms. Usually, chronic inflammation and redness affect the forehead, cheeks, chin, and nose. Redness first appears to be a blush or sunburn but gradually becomes more noticeable and does not go away. Eventually, small, red, solid or pus-filled pimples may begin to appear. Dilated small blood vessels occur on the nose and cheeks.

A serious complication of rosacea is RHINOPHYMA, a swollen, bright red nose caused by oil glands that enlarge and lead to a buildup of excess tissue. Eye problems are another possible complication. In about half of the people affected, there may be redness, burning, tearing, and irritation of the eyes. The eyelids can become swollen and infected. Although some people experience blurred vision, serious vision impairment is rare.

DIAGNOSIS AND TREATMENT
Rosacea is a treatable (but not curable) disorder that often goes undiagnosed. It may be mistaken for acne or sunburn. A dermatologist can diagnose rosacea by observing the appearance of the skin. Early diagnosis is essential because rosacea can become progressively worse without treatment. Doctors recommend identifying and avoiding the triggers of

R

rosacea including foods, hot beverages, alcohol, stress, anger, embarrassment, strenuous exercise, exposure to the sun, or extreme temperatures. These factors can increase blood flow, causing small blood vessels in the face to expand. Irritating cosmetics and facial products, such as facial scrubs and alpha-hydroxy lotions, should be avoided. Hydrocortisone-containing creams may also cause or aggravate rosacea.

Treatment is tailored to the individual. Using sunscreen and green-tinted makeup is recommended. When topical antibiotics such as metronidazole prove ineffective, oral antibiotics including tetracycline, minocycline, erythromycin, or doxycycline may be prescribed. Improvement is usually seen within 1 to 2 months. Isotretinoin is an option in treatment-resistant rosacea. But because isotretinoin can cause serious side effects, including birth defects, women who take isotretinoin must use effective birth control. In severe cases of rosacea, laser surgery is used to remove excess tissue from the nose.

Roseola infantum

A benign infectious disease, usually caused by human herpesvirus 6 (HHV-6), that typically affects infants and young children between the ages of 6 months and 3 years. Roseola infantum is characterized by a high fever and a rash, which occurs as the fever lessens. There are no other symptoms, and the infant or child is generally alert and active during the illness. The high temperature begins abruptly and may rise to as high as 105°F. In some cases, there may be seizures as the temperature increases. The fever rapidly declines by the third or fourth day of illness, and a rash then appears, most commonly on the chest and abdomen, but also sometimes on the face, arms, and legs. The rash is short-lived and may disappear after a few hours to a few days. Body temperature, at this point, returns to normal.

Diagnosis of roseola infantum is generally made by ruling out other possible causes of the fever and rash. The symptoms are treated to make the infant or child more comfortable, but there is no medical treatment for the illness, which improves on its own within a week.

Rosiglitazone maleate

An antidiabetic drug. Rosiglitazone (Avandia) is an oral medication used to treat type 2 diabetes mellitus when diet and exercise alone are not sufficient. The drug may be used alone or in combination with another type of oral antidiabetic drug, METFORMIN HYDROCHLORIDE.

Rotator cuff disease

A defect in the muscles at the back of the shoulder; also called supraspinatus syndrome. The rotator cuff is the muscle group attached to the shoulder blade. It activates circular motions of the shoulder and aids in lifting the arm. Defects in the rotator cuff may be due to injury, strain, or overuse that causes tears in the muscle. PAINFUL ARC SYNDROME, left untreated, can lead to rotator cuff disease.

The symptoms of rotator cuff disease are stiffness, pain with movement, and restriction of movement. Left untreated, the tears may cause muscle tissue loss. In some cases, gentle stretching and strengthening exercises may help restore normal use of the muscle. In more severe cases, surgery may be recommended to improve the strength and muscular balance of the shoulder.

Rotator cuff tendinitis

Inflammation of the muscles and tendons that connect the upper arm bone to the shoulder blade. These muscles

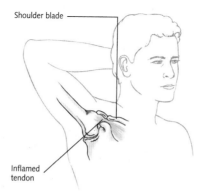

Shoulder blade

Inflamed tendon

SHOULDER INFLAMMATION
A tendon in the rotator cuff area may become inflamed when it rubs against the long end of the shoulder blade, which projects over the shoulder joint.

and tendons are called the rotator cuff. Rotator cuff tendinitis may be caused by repetitive stress on the muscles. It may also occur if the tendons become pinched under the shoulder bones, which may occur when inflammation or bone spurs narrow the tendon space. It can occur with repetitive elevation of the affected arm. See also TENDINITIS.

Rotavirus

An infectious virus that is the most common cause of diarrhea in children. Prevalent in the winter, rotavirus quickly spreads among children in facilities such as child care centers and preschools. Almost all children have had a rotavirus infection before age 3 or 4. Most develop symptoms such as nausea, vomiting, diarrhea, and low-grade fever. Although fever and vomiting disappear after a few days, diarrhea may continue for several more days. Diarrhea and vomiting can make the body lose too much fluid, leading to dehydration, a potentially serious problem that may require hospitalization. A child suspected of being dehydrated should be seen by a doctor. Warning signs include dry lips, tongue, and skin; sunken eyes; fewer tears when a child cries; a sunken soft spot on a baby's head; and less frequent urination.

TREATMENT
Although a vaccine to prevent rotavirus was briefly in use, it was temporarily removed from the market in 1999 to be evaluated. A child who has rotavirus should drink adequate fluids. Commercially prepared electrolyte solutions can be used to speed up the rehydration process. The solutions usually contain salt, sugar, and water. If the dehydration is severe, hospitalization may be necessary to give the child fluids intravenously. See also VIRUSES.

Roundworms

A type of worm that lives in the intestines of humans and other mammals. Roundworms, along with pinworms, infest people in the United States more frequently than other worms. In the adult stage, a roundworm can be almost 10 inches long, and thickness varies; sometimes the roundworm is as thick as a pencil. The females produce eggs in the intestines, which pass out of the body in the feces.

R

Infestations generally occur via the fecal-oral route, such as when a person ingests food that has been contaminated with fecal material containing roundworm eggs. Infestation may also occur among children who handle an infested dog or have contact with contaminated soil, then put their fingers in their mouths. Once the eggs have been ingested, they hatch into larvae and mature to the adult stage in the intestines, establishing a new infestation. The worms are sometimes eliminated in feces or vomit.

A light infestation of roundworms can cause mild abdominal pain. In more severe infestations, the larvae can migrate to organs including the liver, lungs, and eyes, where they may cause allergic reactions, including asthma, and serious complications, including vision loss. Diagnosis is made by identifying the roundworm eggs under microscopic examination of fecal cultures. The infestations are cured by medications that destroy or paralyze the worms or break down the roundworms' attachment to the intestinal wall so they can be eliminated in the feces. These worm-combating medications are also referred to as anthelmintic medications.

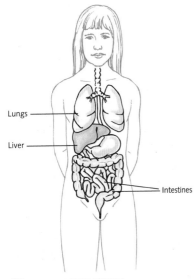

WHERE PARASITES THRIVE
Roundworms most typically live in the intestine, but they can travel to other organs, including the lungs and liver. If they lodge in the lungs, they can cause symptoms of reactive airway disease, such as wheezing and coughing up blood.

Lungs

Liver

Intestines

Rubella

FOR SYMPTOM CHART
see Rashes in infants and children, page 50
see Rashes in adults, page 52

A contagious viral infection, also called German measles. Rubella is caused by a virus and spread from person to person via contact with airborne, infected respiratory droplets that may occur when a person who has the illness sneezes or coughs. The infection may also be spread by direct contact with the nasal or throat secretions of an infected person.

SYMPTOMS AND DIAGNOSIS
Symptoms of rubella usually appear within 16 to 18 days after exposure. About half the people who become infected get a rash. The rash generally appears first on the face and neck, which may become flushed, then spreads to the trunk and extremities. The disease in an infected person is contagious from 10 days before the rash appears up to 15 days after the rash appears. Other symptoms may include mild fever, aching joints, headaches, general malaise, runny nose, and reddened eyes. There may be swelling, tenderness, and pain in the lymph nodes behind the ears and at the back of the neck. The throat may become red but not sore.

Sometimes rubella is mild and the person has no symptoms. Fatigue, swollen glands, and soreness in the joints may occur in children. These symptoms may or may not appear in adolescents and adults. Adults may become aware of the infection when a rash appears on the chest, arms, or forehead or when lymph glands behind the ears become swollen and tender.

Symptoms of rubella must be clinically differentiated from other infections, including measles and scarlet fever. Blood tests are generally used to identify antibodies to the virus and confirm a diagnosis of rubella. Because rubella is usually mild and self-limiting, symptoms are treated to make the infected child or person more comfortable; there is no medical cure for rubella. The rash commonly lasts up to 3 days, and the fever lasts from 1 to 5 days.

PREVENTION AND RISK FACTORS
A safe and effective vaccine can prevent rubella. The rubella vaccination is commonly given in combination with vaccines against measles and

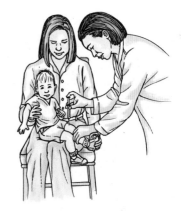

MMR VACCINE
The safe, effective MMR (measles-mumps-rubella) vaccine is routinely given to infants between the ages of 12 and 15 months, providing lifelong immunity to these diseases. An injection for a baby is usually done so quickly that the infant is barely aware of it. A quick cuddle will usually soothe the child.

mumps, and is called the MMR (measles-mumps-rubella) vaccine. The MMR vaccine is routinely given to children, but may also be administered to adults who have not received it previously. General guidelines for the MMR vaccination include adults who have not been vaccinated and children who do not have conditions that would preclude them from getting the vaccine. It is also recommended that certain groups of people be vaccinated, including college and university students, health care personnel, women of childbearing age who are not currently pregnant, child care workers, teachers, and people who travel internationally.

Complications of rubella are rare but may include arthritis, bleeding, ENCEPHALITIS, and middle ear infections. Rubella is most dangerous when it occurs in a woman who is pregnant, especially if she becomes infected during the early phases of pregnancy when the virus can cause abortion, stillbirth, or congenital defects in the infant.

Rubeola
See MEASLES.

Runner's knee

FOR SYMPTOM CHART
see Knee pain, page 44

A sports injury (see SPORTS INJURIES) caused by mechanical malfunctions

R

of the knee during running activities, resulting in a softening of the cartilage in the kneecap. It can also be caused by repetitive stair climbing or performing squats with heavy weights. Runner's knee is known medically as CHONDROMALACIA of the kneecap (patella.) The cartilage of the kneecap relies on intermittent compression to release waste products and receive nutrients from the knee joint's synovial fluid. If the kneecap shifts to the side or does not track smoothly in its thighbone groove during running, portions of its cartilage may not be able to release waste and receive nutrients normally. The result is a deterioration of the cartilage. Symptoms include pain around and under the kneecap, which may be experienced after sitting for some time with the knees bent. The pain may also be felt while running downhill or descending stairs. Bending the knee produces increased pressure between the surface of the kneecap and the thighbone. In this position, the injured area is stressed, and the joint does not receive sufficient cushioning from the damaged cartilage; the result is pain.

Runner's knee may originate with weakened muscles in the thigh or an imbalance of strength among the thigh muscles, all of which attach to the knee and may cause a pulling on the kneecap. Some physical characteristics that may contribute to this situation include wide hips, knock knees, a dislocated kneecap, a high kneecap, and flat feet.

When runner's knee is first detected, running or stair climbing should be decreased to rest the knee area and allow healing. Activities involving bending the knee and downhill running should be strictly avoided. Exercises to build strength in the hip and thigh muscles will not stress the kneecap and may help recondition the knee. Running shoes that provide extra support may be helpful. In some cases, special shoe inserts (called orthotics) may be helpful.

A physical examination by a doctor specializing in sports medicine should rule out other possible knee, hip, ankle, and foot problems. If more conservative measures are not successful, injections of corticosteroids or arthroscopic surgery may be considered.

Running injuries

The group of physical disorders produced by running, usually occurring as a result of overloading musculoskeletal structures of the lower limbs. Running injuries may result from running too hard or too soon after beginning an exercise program. A progressive and relentless weekly increase in mileage distance, the amount depending on the fitness of the athlete, may also be responsible for many running injuries. Running on surfaces that are too hard or wearing worn-out shoes can cause injuries as well.

Sports medicine specialists often recommend keeping a runner's diary in which details of distance and track conditions may be noted. The diary can help trace the origin of running-related injuries.

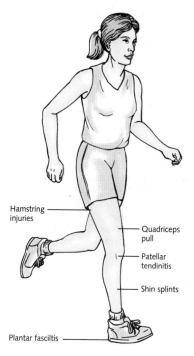

COMMON RUNNING INJURIES
Five common running injuries include hamstring injuries (pulling or tearing of the hamstring muscle in the back of the thigh); quadriceps pulls (pulling of the large muscle in front of the thigh); patellar tendinitis (inflammation of a tendon in the knee); shin splints (pain from a muscle pull, bone stress fracture, or inflammation of the membrane covering the bone in the shin); and plantar fasciitis (small tears and inflammation of the plantar fascia, a protective band of tissue that runs under the foot).

PREVENTING RUNNING INJURIES

Preventive strategies are the best approach to avoiding painful injuries caused by running. Here are some helpful guidelines for runners who want to keep their bodies in top form:

- Runners who seek the goal of increasing speed should incorporate a few short-distance sprints into regular runs and ease into a faster pace gradually and incrementally.
- Running shoes should be replaced at regular intervals to make sure they are providing adequate support. Runners who average 20 miles per week should replace their shoes every 4 to 6 months, depending on conditions and shock absorption needs.
- Certain exercises, including stretching, can help prevent injuries. The hamstrings at the back of the thighs and the calf muscles should be stretched regularly. Exercises to strengthen the hip and thigh muscles and the shin muscles should be performed often. Abdominal muscles that support the back should be exercised for added strength.
- A trainer or physical therapist can demonstrate proper techniques for stretching and strengthening muscles that help prevent running injuries.
- Most runners should take 1 or 2 days off from running every week to allow the body time to recover and build up strength again.
- Maintaining a healthy body weight is essential to preventing excessive load on muscles and tendons during running. Beginning runners who are overweight should take special care to increase speed and distance gradually in direct proportion to progressive weight loss.

R

Rupture

A break or tear in an organ or tissue. A rupture in the muscles of the groin can cause a hernia, which may require surgery. When inflammation causes a rupture in an intestine, it is a life-threatening emergency.

S

Sac

Any structure or body organ shaped like a bag or pouch. An example is the fluid-filled amniotic sac that surrounds the fetus during pregnancy.

Saccharin

One of the low-calorie ARTIFICIAL SWEETENERS. Saccharin has been widely used as a sugar substitute for more than a century. In the 1970s, research suggested that saccharin, when ingested in large amounts, caused bladder cancer in laboratory animals. As a result, the US Food and Drug Administration (FDA) in 1977 proposed banning it. The public strongly opposed the ban, and as a result, Congress instead imposed a moratorium on saccharin. The moratorium remains in place today, and products that contain saccharin—including soft drinks and sugarless gum—must bear labels that warn that saccharin causes cancer in laboratory animals. However, there is no research to indicate that saccharin causes cancer in human beings.

Sacralization

A congenital abnormality involving fusion of a vertebra in the lower spine with the triangular bone at the base of the spine.

Sacroiliitis

An inflammation of the sacroiliac joint, which is one of a pair of joints in the lower back near the pelvis. Sacroiliitis produces an aching pain in the lower back and may be a symptom of a variety of conditions or diseases. When the pain occurs on both sides of the lower back, it can be caused by ANKYLOSING SPONDYLITIS, REITER SYNDROME, PSORIATIC ARTHRITIS, RHEUMATOID ARTHRITIS, or JUVENILE RHEUMATOID ARTHRITIS. When there is pain on one side, sacroiliitis may be due to GOUT, OSTEOARTHRITIS, or an infection. Sacroiliitis is diagnosed by X rays and blood tests. Treatment is with nonsteroidal anti-inflammatory drugs (NSAIDs), such as ibuprofen and aspirin, or if the joint is infected, antibiotics.

Sacrum

A triangular bone in the lower SPINE. The sacrum lies just above the last bone of the spine, the coccyx or tailbone, and below the lumbar spine. The sacrum joins with the hip bones at the sacroiliac joints to form the rear of the PELVIS.

SAD

See SEASONAL AFFECTIVE DISORDER.

Saddle block

See ANESTHESIA, SPINAL.

Sadomasochism

A mental illness characterized by sexual arousal and pleasure in receiving humiliation, pain, or suffering (masochism) or inflicting humiliation, pain, or suffering (sadism). Sadomasochism involves actual acts, not just fantasies. People with masochism may inflict pain on themselves (for example, using electrical shock, mutilating the body, or sticking pins or needles into the flesh), or they may endure pain inflicted by a dominating partner, who is likely to be afflicted with sadism. Sadomasochistic acts can involve binding or restraint (bondage), blindfolding, cutting, electrical shock, paddling, spanking, piercing and pinning, and humiliation, such as defecating or urinating, crawling around and barking like a dog, or licking shoes. In some cases, people with sadism use nonconsenting victims, who may be seriously injured or killed. In most cases, sadism and masochism begin in adolescence or early adulthood and continue throughout life; the severity increases over time. Sadomasochism is more common among men than women. Psychiatric counseling may help.

Safer sex

Also called safe sex; the exercise of precautions while participating in sexual activity in order to decrease the risk of transmitting or acquiring SEXUALLY TRANSMITTED DISEASES (STDs). Safer sex behaviors may also include precautions to avoid undesired pregnancy (see CONTRACEPTION). To prevent both pregnancy and STDs, physicians recommend the use of male or female condoms during SEXUAL INTERCOURSE. In order to be effective, condoms must be in place before the beginning and until the end of sexual activity and must be used during every encounter. When a male condom is used, it must be placed on the penis before it touches any part of the female genital area; this is because the penis may release small drops of fluid called pre-ejaculate, which can contain disease-causing organisms and sperm. Other safer sex measures include abstinence and a faithful, monogamous sexual relationship. To practice safer sex, it is important to know one's partner, including his or her sexual history, and to stay sober.

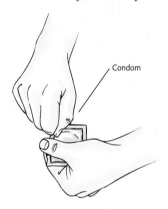

Condom

EFFECTIVE PROTECTION
A latex or polyurethane condom (male or female) protects against both pregnancy and sexually transmitted diseases (STDs). Condoms made of other materials (such as lambskin) do not protect against STDs, nor do any other methods of contraception. Package inserts show how to use a condom corrcetly.

Saline

A solution of salt in purified water. Saline is 0.9 percent sodium chloride in water that can be mixed with medication for injection or administered intravenously to replace lost sodium and chloride to the blood. Saline can also be used as a plasma substitute for the temporary maintenance of living cells. A knocked-out tooth, for example, should be kept in milk or a saline solution until medical help has been obtained. It can also be used as eye or nasal drops for treatment of dry or inflamed eyes or nasal membranes.

Saliva

The watery mixture of secretions from glands in the mouth. Saliva is a clear, alkaline, somewhat sticky fluid secreted by the parotid, submaxillary, and sublingual salivary glands. Saliva is made up of water, mucus, and enzymes. The functions of saliva are to keep the mouth moist, to help in the swallowing of food, to digest starch, and to minimize changes of acidity in the mouth.

The major salivary glands are in pairs. The parotid glands are located below and in front of each ear, secreting saliva through openings in the cheeks on each side, opposite the upper teeth. The submaxillary glands, located inside the lower jaw, discharge saliva upward through openings in the floor of the mouth. The sublingual glands, located below the tongue, also discharge saliva through the floor of the mouth. Together, the salivary glands secrete about 3 pints of saliva each day.

Salivary gland stones

One or more tiny, hard particles that form in the duct of one of the SALIVARY GLANDS when chemicals and salts in the saliva become encrusted around a speck of mucus or other solid material. About 80 percent of these stones are found in the salivary glands in the floor of the mouth. When salivary gland stones obstruct the duct, the large amount of saliva produced when food is eaten cannot flow freely into the mouth. The blocked saliva causes the salivary gland to swell and become painful, especially when a person is eating. The pain and swelling may be experienced in front of the ear or under the chin. Salivary gland stones may also contribute to inflammation of the gland (see SIALADENITIS).

DIAGNOSIS AND TREATMENT

It may be possible to see or feel the stones. The doctor may recommend an X ray of the mouth and the salivary gland. Ultrasound scanning or CT (computed tomography) scans may also be necessary to help diagnose the condition. The stone may need to be removed surgically. If the condition recurs, a permanent opening can be made along the duct to permit saliva to be released into the mouth. These procedures are usually performed under local anesthesia. If salivary gland stones are persistent or severe or if the stone is lodged inside the salivary gland, the gland may be removed.

Salivary gland tumors

Abnormal growths in the salivary glands located in the neck or in the parotid glands located above the sides of the jaw. Most salivary gland tumors grow slowly and are benign. Swelling of the affected gland is usually the only symptom, although there may be slight pain. Salivary gland tumors are diagnosed through imaging studies, such as ultrasound and CT (computed tomography) scanning. A sample of tissue is taken to confirm the diagnosis. In most cases, tumors are surgically removed. Although surgery carries a small risk of damage to the nerves that control facial movements, the damage can usually be surgically repaired. If there is a malignant tumor, doctors recommend radiation therapy following removal of the tumor.

Salivary glands

Three pairs of glands in the mouth that secrete saliva into the mouth. Saliva is a clear fluid that helps clean the teeth and gums, moistens food for swallowing, and adds an enzyme (chemical accelerator) to chewed food that converts complex starches into sugars. There are three major pairs of salivary glands: the submandibular glands lie toward the back of the mouth close to the sides of the jaw; the sublingual glands are located at the base of the tongue; and the parotid glands are in the back of the mouth. The parotid glands are the largest of the three pairs. From the salivary glands, which contain tiny saliva-secreting sacs, a network of ducts carry the saliva into the mouth.

Salivation, excessive

The production and release of excessive SALIVA into the mouth, which may cause a person to drool. Excessive salivation may occur more frequently during dental procedures known to stimulate the SALIVARY GLANDS that produce saliva. Dentists clear the mouth of saliva to examine and treat dental patients. The mouth must be dry for certain procedures to be performed and for the effective use of certain adhesives, fillings, and bonding materials.

Dental tools for drying excess saliva include cotton rolls, rubber dams, or suction devices. If these are not adequate to control excessive salivation, short-term medication may be given while the person receives dental treatment. Since the saliva carries important digestive enzymes, as well as substances that help to mineralize and protect the teeth, excessive salivation outside the dental office may be a cosmetic problem rather than a health risk.

Salmeterol

An antisthma drug and a long-acting bronchodilator. Salmeterol (Serevent) is used with anti-inflammatory drugs to prevent asthma attacks. Salmeterol is unlike other drugs in its class (adrenergic bronchodilators), because it does not act quickly enough to relieve an attack of asthma that has already begun. The person with asthma uses an inhaler to breathe in salmeterol through the mouth to open up the airways in the lungs; it can be used to prevent exercise-induced asthma.

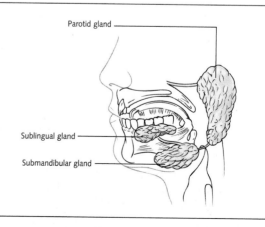

THREE PAIRS OF GLANDS
Three major pairs of salivary glands lubricate the mouth and help begin the digestive process: the parotid, the sublingual, and the submandibular glands. Each gland has a duct to carry the saliva into the mouth. Other small salivary glands lie in the mucous membranes lining the mouth and tongue.

Parotid gland

Sublingual gland

Submandibular gland

S

Salmonella

FOR FIRST AID

see Food poisoning: *Salmonella* poisoning, page 1323.

A strain of microscopic bacteria that can be present in food or water without affecting the appearance, smell, or taste. *Salmonella* is the most frequently reported cause of food-borne illness in the United States and has been known to exist for more than 100 years. The bacteria was discovered and named after the American scientist, Dr. Daniel E. Salmon. Infections with *Salmonella* may involve only the intestinal tract, or they may spread to the bloodstream and to other areas of the body. The bacteria are usually transmitted by the oral-fecal route, and the source of infection is usually the ingestion of food or water contaminated by fecal matter.

Salmonella bacteria live in the intestinal tracts of humans and other animals, including birds, and can grow on most foods that have been contaminated by infected fecal matter. With time, the bacteria grow and multiply under the right conditions, which include nourishment, moisture, and warm temperatures, ideally 40°F to 140°F. Bacteria survive on raw foods and may be present in the juices of raw poultry and beef. If these juices are not completely removed from kitchen cutting utensils and boards, the bacteria may be spread to other foods that come into contact with these items. Raw foods, such as vegetable salads that become contaminated in this way, are particularly vulnerable because *Salmonella* can multiply to dangerous levels on these foods when they are left at room temperature for extended periods. For this reason, proper cleaning of kitchen equipment used when preparing meat, vegetables, and fruits is essential to preventing *Salmonella* infections. The bacteria are destroyed when foods are thoroughly cooked.

Foods of animal origin are often the carriers of the bacteria, and these may include beef, poultry, seafood, dairy products, and eggs. All foods, particularly raw vegetables and fruits, may be potential carriers.

Close contact with infected persons can also spread *Salmonella* infection. Person-to-person transmission may occur when a person who is carrying the infection in his or her intestines does not follow good personal hygiene, such as hand washing following toilet use. Food handling and preparation by an infected person whose personal hygiene is poor may also transmit the infection. *Salmonella* infection may also occur in the course of handling animals that carry the bacteria in their intestines, including pet turtles and other reptiles, baby chicks, frogs, and snails.

SYMPTOMS, DIAGNOSIS, AND TREATMENT

The symptoms of *Salmonella* infection can occur within 8 to 72 hours of ingesting contaminated food or water. These symptoms, which may persist from 4 to 7 days, include severe headaches, chills, abdominal cramps, diarrhea, nausea, vomiting, mild fever, and muscle aches. The bacteria may be harbored in the intestines without symptoms, increasing the risk of transmission to others. *Salmonella* infection is diagnosed by testing a stool specimen for the presence of the bacteria.

When severe, the infection may spread to the bloodstream and cause serious conditions, including menin-

---

PREVENTING SALMONELLA INFECTIONS

Salmonella bacteria present on food do not have to cause infection. Preventing the bacteria from multiplying to dangerously high levels is key to avoiding illness. This can be accomplished by following safe food handling guidelines:

- Special care should be taken to wash hands with hot soapy water after using the bathroom, changing diapers, or handling pets.
- Cutting boards, dishes, utensils, and countertops should be cleaned with hot, soapy water after each use. Cutting boards that can be washed in the dishwasher are best for preparing raw animal products, such as meat.
- The use of disposable paper towels instead of cloth towels can help prevent the spread of bacteria in the kitchen; if cloth towels are used, they should be washed frequently in the washing machine's hot cycle.
- Raw meat, poultry, and seafood should be stored separately to avoid contact with other food items when packed in grocery bags or kept in the refrigerator. Special care should be taken to prevent possible contamination of foods that are usually eaten raw.
- Raw animal products should be cut and prepared on a different cutting board from the one used for other foods, particularly foods such as salad vegetables that are not normally cooked.
- Cooked food should never be placed on a dish or platter on which raw meat, poultry, or seafood was previously placed.
- A cooking thermometer, thoroughly cleaned between uses, should be used to ensure that meat and casseroles are completely cooked throughout. Roasts and steaks should be cooked to at least 145°F; ground beef should be well cooked to at least 160°F; poultry should be heated to 170°F; and whole poultry, such as a chicken, must reach a temperature of 180°F.
- Eggs with cracked or dirty shells should be discarded. All eggs should be cooked until both the white and yolk are firm; recipes that include raw or partially cooked eggs as ingredients should be avoided. (This is important even if eggshells appear whole and clean; a strain of *Salmonella* can infect the ovaries of hens and contaminate eggs before the shells form.)
- Fish should be cooked through until the flesh is opaque and flakes easily with a fork.
- Foods cooked in a microwave oven should be covered, stirred, and turned frequently during cooking to prevent cold spots where bacteria can survive.
- When reheating, sauces, soups, and gravies should be heated to boiling, and leftovers should be heated through to at least 165°F.
- Perishables should be refrigerated or frozen within 2 hours. Food should never be defrosted at room temperature; longer thaws in the refrigerator are preferable. Or, frozen food may be thawed under cold running water or in the microwave.
- Foods should be marinated in the refrigerator, and marinades used on raw meat, poultry, or seafood should not be used as sauces for cooked foods.
- Large quantities of warm leftovers should be divided into smaller containers before refrigerating to ensure quick cooling. Refrigerators should not be overloaded, as this interferes with proper cooling temperatures.

S

gitis and even death, if antibiotics are not taken promptly. Such cases require hospitalization, ISOLATION, and supportive medical care. Young children, older people, and people with impaired immune systems are most at risk for severe infections. Milder infections generally improve without treatment within a week, during which time the treatment usually recommended includes rest, a diet of clear liquids, applying warmth to the abdomen to relieve cramps, and the use of acetaminophen for pain and fever while the bacteria are being eliminated from the intestines. The use of antibiotics in mild cases may interfere with the necessary shedding of the bacteria from the intestines.

Some people who have been infected with *Salmonella* bacteria may recover completely, but bowel habits may be abnormal for several months. In rare cases, *Salmonella* infections can cause REITER SYNDROME, a condition involving painful joints, eye irritation, and painful urination. This syndrome may persist for months or even years and can cause chronic arthritis.

Salpingectomy

Surgery in which one or both fallopian tubes (the tubes that transport an egg from an ovary toward the uterus) are removed. Salpingectomy is usually performed to treat an ectopic pregnancy (one that develops outside the uterus) or a chronic pelvic inflammation that has damaged a fallopian tube. This treatment is usually used only when a fallopian tube is hopelessly destroyed by disease. See PELVIC INFLAMMATORY DISEASE.

The procedure may be done with a laparoscope, a viewing tube that is inserted through a small incision in the abdomen. Regional or general anesthesia is used, and the hospital stay is 1 or 2 days. Surgery done to treat chronic pelvic infection may require a laparotomy, in which the incision is larger, to allow the surgeon to see and remove all scar tissue. Most women are up and walking by the third day after surgery, gradually resuming all normal activity over the next 2 months.

Salpingitis

A condition occurring when infectious agents invade the uterus and spread to the fallopian tubes, ovaries, and surrounding tissues. Acute salpingitis, which is a type of PELVIC INFLAMMATORY DISEASE, causes pain and tenderness in the lower abdomen and often a high fever. Chronic salpingitis causes recurring mild pain in the lower abdomen, sometimes with a low-grade fever and a backache. Menstrual periods may be heavy in both acute and chronic infections, and the woman may have an abnormally heavy, foul-smelling vaginal discharge.

Salpingitis is most commonly caused by sexually transmitted infections. The infection begins in the vagina and cervix and spreads to the uterus, fallopian tubes, and sometimes into the abdominal cavity. Salpingitis can also occur after an intrauterine device (see IUD) is inserted, or after a miscarriage, abortion, D and C, endometrial biopsy, hysterectomy, or other procedure that requires inserting instruments into the uterine cavity. It is most common among young, sexually active women. Treatment usually includes antibiotics for the infection and aspirin or acetaminophen to relieve the abdominal pain.

Salpingo-oophorectomy

Surgical removal of the ovaries and fallopian tubes. This procedure is used to treat cancer of the ovary and some cases of PELVIC INFLAMMATORY DISEASE. The fallopian tube is usually removed with its adjacent ovary, because the tube is typically damaged by the same condition that affects the ovary. The surgery involves an incision into the abdomen.

In menstruating women, the removal of both ovaries dramatically reduces hormone levels and induces menopause immediately. Surgery-induced menopause can involve symptoms that are much more severe than those associated with menopause occurring naturally, because hormone levels are altered suddenly, not gradually. HORMONE REPLACEMENT THERAPY may be recommended.

Salpingostomy

A surgical procedure used to treat fallopian tubes (see FALLOPIAN TUBE) that have become blocked at the end nearest the ovary. In this procedure, the fingerlike projections at the end of the tube are opened outward. The edges of the opening of the tube are turned slightly down and stitched to keep the tube from closing up again. Salpingostomy is usually performed after an ectopic pregnancy, a pregnancy in which the fertilized egg has attached outside of the uterus.

Salsalate

One of the nonsteroidal anti-inflammatory drugs (NSAIDs). Salsalate (Disalcid, Salflex) is a pain-relieving, fever-reducing, anti-inflammatory medication in the same category as aspirin. It is used to relieve pain, to reduce fever, and to ease some symptoms of arthritis, including joint pain, swelling, and stiffness.

Salt

Any compound of a base and an acid; sodium chloride (common salt). Common salt, or table salt, is only one of many salts; others include magnesium sulfate or Epsom salt; sodium sulfate or Glauber salt, and potassium sodium tartrate or Preston salt.

Common salt is a necessary part of the diet, because sodium is essential to the regulation of blood pressure and fluid volume and is needed to help carry nutrients into the cells. However, only a small amount of salt need be consumed in the diet.

Excessive amounts of salt can be harmful, and the consumption of too much salt has been associated with health problems such as high blood pressure, heart disease, asthma, gastric cancer, kidney stones, osteoporosis, and other conditions.

About 75 percent of the sodium consumed by Americans is found in processed foods. Restaurant food is also high in salt. Excessive salt intake can be reduced by avoiding convenience or "junk" foods and salt-based condiments. The consumption of salt should be balanced by the regular consumption of foods rich in POTASSIUM, such as fresh fruits and vegetables.

Saquinavir mesylate

An antiviral drug; a protease inhibitor. Saquinavir (Fortovase) and saquinavir mesylate (Invirase) are AIDS (acquired immunodeficiency syndrome) in combination with other drugs to treat the infection caused by HIV (human immunodeficiency virus). Saquinavir and saquinavir mesylate cannot cure HIV or AIDS, but they can help keep HIV from reproducing itself. The drugs seems to slow the destruction of the immune system.

Sarcoidosis

A chronic, multisystem, autoimmune disorder that can affect many body systems, but most commonly involves the lungs or lymph nodes. Sarcoidosis is characterized by the appearance in affected tissues of small, round lumps of dead tissue. These lumps, called granulomas, usually heal and disappear on their own, even without medical treatment. When the granulomas do not resolve, the affected tissues remain inflamed, and scarring develops.

The disease is caused by an immune system disorder that occurs for no known reason. There may be a genetic predisposition, and it is known to be most common among African Americans and people of northern European background. It occurs at a higher rate in Sweden and in the southeast section of the United States. Incidence is significantly higher in women than in men, and it usually occurs before age 40.

SYMPTOMS AND DIAGNOSIS

Sarcoidosis varies in severity and may affect any part of the person's body. Individual cases may be quite different from one another. Sometimes there are no symptoms or only a few, while some people experience many symptoms, or the condition may develop gradually and produce intermittent symptoms throughout a person's lifetime. Fatigue and general malaise are the most common initial symptoms. Pulmonary symptoms include cough and shortness of breath. A skin rash may also suddenly appear on the face, arms, or shins. Inflammation of the eyes occurs in about 15 percent of cases. The disorder can cause an irregular heart rate, and lead to the implanting of a pacemaker. Sarcoidosis may be complicated by a high calcium level.

Sarcoidosis is difficult to diagnose and is sometimes misdiagnosed as tuberculosis (TB). A preliminary diagnosis is generally based on a medical history, a physical examination, and a chest X ray, which reveals abnormalities in about 90 percent of cases. Angiotensin-converting enzyme levels are often elevated, as they are in active pulmonary diseases. The diagnosis may be confirmed by ruling out other possible conditions and diseases, including berylliosis, farmer's lung, fungal infections, rheumatoid arthritis, rheumatic fever, multiple sclerosis, and lymphoma.

There is presently no cure for sarcoidosis, and there is a small risk of death. Prevention and treatment possibilities are currently under investigation by medical researchers. The disease can be managed with proper self-care. An affected person should avoid cigarette smoke and exposure to dust and chemical irritants that might cause further damage to the lungs. Regular physical examinations, including an eye examination, are important for people with sarcoidosis, even if no symptoms of the disease have been apparent for a year or more. Corticosteroids may be useful for those with active symptoms.

Sarcoma

A type of cancerous tumor arising in a number of tissues, including bones, cartilage, connective tissues, muscles, the inner layer of the skin, fibrous tissues, fat, blood vessels, nerves, the linings of the chest and abdominal cavities, and the coverings of the lungs, abdominal organs, and heart. Sarcomas, which are relatively uncommon, can arise almost anywhere in the body, often beginning in fat or muscle or in an arm or leg. The most common symptom is a swelling that is sore and becomes progressively larger.

The diagnosis of sarcoma is usually made by physical examination, X ray, CT (computed tomography) scanning, MRI (magnetic resonance imaging), and biopsy. Treatment may include surgery, radiation therapy, and chemotherapy. Some sarcomas may be very aggressive, with a strong tendency to spread elsewhere in the body, particularly to the lungs. Because of this tendency to metastasize (spread), surgery to remove the primary cancer completely is performed whenever possible. In many cases, successful surgical removal of a sarcoma can restore normal functioning. About half of all people with sarcomas achieve long-term survival. Sarcoma of the arm or legs can be eliminated without removing the entire limb.

Sarcoma risk factors include exposure to radiation and certain chemicals used in the plastics industry. Genetic abnormalities, such as NEUROFIBROMATOSIS, increase the risk for a type of sarcoma called neurofibrosarcoma, a malignant tumor of the fibrous covering of the nerves.

SARS

See SEVERE ACUTE RESPIRATORY SYNDROME (SARS).

Saturated fats

Fats that come from meats, poultry, dairy products, and solid vegetable fats that are mostly hard at room temperature. The exceptions are coconut and palm kernel oils, which remain liquid at room temperature. Saturated fats (along with trans-fatty acids) are the fats most responsible for high cholesterol levels and an increased risk of heart disease. See FATS AND OILS.

Saw palmetto

An herbal remedy used to treat prostate disease. The berries of the saw palmetto tree have been used to treat prostate disorders for many years, first by Native Americans, who also used it to treat stomachache and dysentery. It reportedly helps increase urinary flow through the prostate without affecting prostate size, although this has not been proven scientifically. Saw palmetto is used today in France and Germany to treat prostate disorders, and it is available over-the-counter in the United States.

Scabicides

Drugs used to treat scabies, a parasitic infection. Scabicides are available as shampoos, creams, or lotions to be rubbed into the affected skin, where scabies mites have burrowed into the skin. Scabies is usually found between the fingers, on the buttocks, on the male genitalia, and elsewhere. Scabicides work by killing the mites, which absorb the drug through their outer covering.

To treat scabies, a scabicide cream or lotion is usually applied in a thin layer to clean skin and rubbed in thoroughly, then washed off after 8 to 12 hours. The treatment can be repeated after 1 week if needed. An example of a scabicide is lindane, also called gamma benzene hexachloride.

Scabies

A parasitic infestation that causes intense itching and a rash. In scabies, small mites burrow into the skin to lay eggs. Scabies is usually spread through close contact with an infested person. Although anyone can have scabies, it is most frequently seen in people living in crowded conditions. Children and elderly people in nursing homes are particularly susceptible.

The first symptom of scabies is intense itching, especially at night. The early rash may be composed of small red bumps, like pimples. Eventually, the burrows made by the mites appear as thin red marks on the skin. In severe cases, the skin becomes crusty, scaly, and thickened. Scabies is most common between the fingers; in the armpits; on the waist, elbows, wrists, ankles, and feet; and in the areas around the breasts, buttocks, and genitals.

Scabies is usually diagnosed through a physical examination, taking special care to inspect skin crevices. Diagnosis can be confirmed by removing a mite from its burrow and identifying it under a microscope. Scabies is treated with prescription creams containing ingredients such as permethrin or lindane. The creams are applied all over the

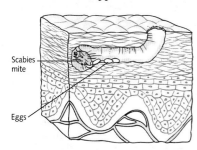

A BURROWING MITE
Scabies is caused by a mite that burrows under the skin, especially around the hands, feet, and male genitals, to lay eggs. The first symptom is itching, especially at night, followed by a rash. Sometimes the burrows are visible, but the rash and itching typically spread beyond the location of the mites.

body at bedtime and should be washed off 8 to 12 hours later. Topical treatment should be repeated in a week. Ivermectin, an oral antiparasitic agent, is also effective. Itching is controlled with lotions and antihistamines. Family members and others in close contact with the affected person must also be treated. To prevent reinfestation, clothes and bedding should be washed in hot water. Upholstered furniture and carpets should be vacuumed and the vacuum bag thrown away.

Scalds

Burns caused by hot liquids or hot vapors. Scalds are burns that result from contact with moist heat. Scalds are usually not as deep as those created by contact with flames, but they can produce deep burns. Hot beverages usually produce injuries to the uppermost layers of skin, while hot grease and hot soup can sometimes cause injuries that penetrate all the layers of the skin. Scalds are the leading cause of accidental death in the home for children from birth to age 4, and they account for almost half of the burn injuries for children up to age 14. Scalds are also common accidents for older adults.

If the clothing of a person is saturated with scalding, hot liquid, the clothes should be removed quickly but carefully. In the case of small scalds, cold water will stop further tissue damage and lessen pain, but ice should never be placed directly on the wound. If the person is scalded over a large area of his or her body, the person may be in a state of shock, and emergency medical care must be sought at once.

Scaling, dental

A procedure to remove the hard deposit of calcified plaque, called calculus, from the surface of the crown or the roots of the teeth. The purpose of dental scaling is to eliminate deposits on the teeth that cannot be removed by routine brushing and dental flossing. Calculus releases toxins that cause TOOTH DECAY. Deposits of calculus that adhere to the surface of the teeth contribute to the formation of pockets between the gum and the tooth (see POCKET, GINGIVAL) and can cause PERIODONTAL DIS-

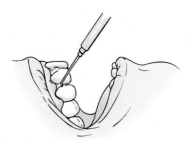

REMOVING TARTAR
A dental hygienist scales the teeth to remove tartar (calculus) from the teeth that is too hard to be removed by regular brushing and flossing. The hygienist uses a handheld or ultrasonic instrument to loosen and scrape away the deposits. Left on the tooth, tartar can release toxins that cause tooth decay.

EASE. Dental scaling is one of several procedures referred to as dental prophylaxes, which are treatments designed to prevent more serious dental conditions.

Dental scaling is accomplished by firmly scraping the surfaces of the teeth with a handheld instrument called a scaler, or by an ultrasonic instrument that produces vibrations to loosen the calculus deposits. The procedure is performed in a dental office by a dentist or dental hygienist.

The calculus to be removed on the tooth may be located at the base of the crown near the gum line or below the gum line on the surface of the root where it meets the natural crown. In this case, the scaling instrument is gently inserted between the surface of the root and the gum. Local or topical anesthesia may be required to numb the gums during this procedure. The instrument is scraped toward the top of the crown to dislodge the calculus adhering to the surface. The scraping movements may be repeated if the deposits are particularly resistant. The surface of the root may then need to be planed smooth to discourage plaque from adhering to it.

Scalp

The tough skin that covers the skull above the face and ears that is usually covered with hair. The scalp has five layers of tissue with an extensive blood supply. Scalp hair, which helps prevent heat from leaving the body, grows faster than any other hair on the body—an average of about ½ inch every month. Underlying muscles loosely attach the scalp to the skull.

Scalpel

A very precise surgical knife used to cut tissue in operations. A plasma scalpel is a device that uses a high-temperature gas jet for cutting rather than a blade.

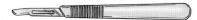

A SURGICAL KNIFE
A scalpel is a specialized straight-handled knife used in all types of surgery.

Scaphoid

A bone in the wrist shaped like a peanut that acts as a block to prevent the wrist from bending too far. The scaphoid is vulnerable to injury from falls and collisions, particularly among athletes such as gymnasts, skaters, and football players who are likely to fall on outstretched wrists.

Scar

A mark left on the skin or other tissue after a wound, burn, ulcer, lesion, or other injury has healed. The degree of scarring depends on the nature of the injury, as well as a person's age, heredity, and skin type. Scars tend to shrink and become less noticeable as they age. However, some individuals undergo surgery to improve the appearance of scars. A KELOID is a raised, firm irregularly shaped scar caused by abnormal healing; it has a tendency to return.

Scarlet fever

An infection caused by group A *Streptococcus* bacteria (see GROUP A STREPTOCOCCUS INFECTION) that occurs in a small number of people following an initial streptococcal infection of the throat (strep throat) or skin. Scarlet fever was once considered serious, and it commonly occurred in children between the ages of 2 and 10 years. For unknown reasons, scarlet fever is less common at the current time, despite a constant level in the number of streptococcal infections. The bacteria that cause scarlet fever are spread by direct contact with infected persons or by airborne droplets in the coughs, sneezes, and exhalations of an infected person.

SYMPTOMS, DIAGNOSIS, AND TREATMENT
Scarlet fever causes a characteristic bright red rash that begins under the arms and on the neck, chest, armpit, inner thighs, and groin area as small red spots that gradually become elevated and spread over the body. Within a few days, the redness fades and a finely textured rash, sometimes referred to as a sandpaper rash, develops. The rash is caused by toxins produced by the streptococcal bacteria. In addition to the rash, symptoms of scarlet fever may include sore throat, fever, vomiting, a red and swollen tongue, chills, headache, and general malaise. A bright red coloration of the creases under the arm, in the crook of the arm, and in the groin (called the Pastia sign) may appear while the rash is still red. The rash and skin discoloration usually last for about 3 to 7 days, at which time there may be peeling of skin around the fingertips and toes and in the groin area.

The illness is diagnosed by a physical examination combined with a throat culture that tests positive for group A *Streptococcus*. The infection is treated with antibiotics, usually penicillin, and acetaminophen for fever and discomfort. Bed rest and increased fluid intake are also recommended. Given proper treatment, scarlet fever is usually easily cured within a week or less. Complications are rare if the illness is treated, but the bacteria may spread to other parts of the body causing ear infections, sinusitis, rheumatic fever, or GLOMERULONEPHRITIS, an acute kidney inflammation.

Schistosome

A parasite of birds and mammals that is released by infected snails into natural bodies of water, including those used for recreational swimming. Schistosomes can cause a skin rash that is also called schistosome dermatitis, or "swimmer's itch," and often affects children. The skin irritation is acquired by swimming or wading in water infested with schistosomes and then allowing the water to evaporate from the skin, rather than using a towel to dry the skin. As the water evaporates from the skin, a tingling sensation may be experienced as the schistosome parasite penetrates into the skin. This mild itching generally subsides within 10 to 15 hours and then resumes as an extremely intense itch, which may persist for a week. Initial exposure to infested water may not cause schistosome dermatitis, but repeated episodes of exposure thereafter increase sensitivity to the parasite. The rash is treated with creams and lotions containing specific antiparasite ingredients.

Schistosomiasis

A parasitic disease (also known as bilharziasis) that is a major health problem in many tropical countries, affecting more than 200 million people worldwide. Schistosomiasis is caused by a flat-bodied worm, or FLUKE, called a schistosome, which is carried by snails and migrates through water to penetrate a person's skin. The disease can be acquired by swimming or bathing in natural bodies of water that are infested, such as rivers and lakes, but not by contact with bodies of salt water. The infestation producing schistosomiasis can cause bleeding and the formation of scar tissue inside the bladder, intestines, or other organs, including the liver and lungs.

The disease may occur 4 to 6 weeks after an initial infection, and symptoms can include fever, cough, abdominal pain, diarrhea, and allergic reactions. When the infection persists untreated, complications may include colon polyps with bloody diarrhea, increased blood pressure in a large blood vessel of the liver with bloody vomit, inflammation of structures of the urinary system with blood in the urine, inflammation of the kidneys' filtering units, and lesions in the central nervous system. Schistosomiasis is diagnosed by microscopic identification of parasite eggs in the stool or urine. The disease is treated with worm-combating medications.

Schizophrenia

A severe mental illness characterized by persistent, bizarre disturbances in thought, communication, perceptions, emotions, and behavior. Schizophrenia is considered a psychosis because people with the disease become detached from reality.

SYMPTOMS AND TYPES
The symptoms of schizophrenia fall into three groups. The so-called positive symptoms, or abnormalities not present in healthy people, include false beliefs that the person continues to hold despite evidence to the con-

trary (delusions) and false sensory perceptions, such as hearing voices or seeing visions that do not exist (hallucinations). Delusions commonly focus on persecution. The person believes that he or she is being spied upon, tormented, tricked, or beset by powerful outside forces. The delusions may also be grandiose, such as the belief that one has amazing magical powers. Hallucinations can affect any sense, most commonly hearing. The person hears voices that he or she perceives as coming from an outside source. The voices are often threatening or critical.

The second group, called the disorganized symptoms, includes thinking, speech, and behavior that do not make sense. People with the disease may talk senselessly. They speak in an apparently normal manner, but their words carry little or no meaning. Behavior can range from silly and childlike to extremely agitated. The individual may appear disheveled and strange (for example, wearing two overcoats on a hot day), engage in inappropriate sexual behavior such as masturbating in public, or shout and swear for no reason. In some cases, people with schizophrenia become physically rigid, holding the same pose for hours or days or moving repetitively in an unusual way (called catatonia).

The so-called negative symptoms refer to the lack of normal characteristics present. They include emotional flatness, absence of facial expression, speaking only in single words or short sentences, and a lack of pleasure in living.

Schizophrenia is classified into subtypes depending on the prominence of symptoms. For a person with paranoid schizophrenia, delusions or hallucinations, usually about persecution or grandiosity, are central. Anger, aloofness, and argumentativeness are often associated with this subtype of the disease. Disorganized schizophrenia is characterized by disordered thinking, speech, and behavior and by a lack of normal emotion. People with this form of the disease may show little emotion or laugh at inappropriate times. They have difficulty with simple, day-to-day activities such as brushing their teeth or dressing. Delusions and hallucinations are also common. In catatonic schizophrenia, motor disturbance is most prominent. Individuals immobilized by catatonia may hold a bizarre posture for hours or resist being moved; those who are hyperactive engage in frantic behavior that has no apparent purpose. Symptoms may also include resistance to all instructions, inability to talk (mutism), stupor, strange gestures or grimaces, unusual mannerisms, purposeless repetition of a word just spoken by someone else (echolalia), and repeated imitation of someone else's movements (echopraxia). Undifferentiated schizophrenia refers to disease in which no one set of symptoms is central. In residual schizophrenia, the person has experienced an episode of the disease but is not currently detached from reality.

COURSE AND CAUSES

In most cases, schizophrenia develops between late adolescence and the 30s. Usually the disease begins earlier in men (the early 20s) than in women (the late 20s). Symptoms may start suddenly, or they can develop gradually over an extended time. How well the individual can function depends on the disease subtype. People with paranoid schizophrenia are usually the least severely ill and those with disorganized schizophrenia, the most severely ill. Most people with schizophrenia do not marry and are socially isolated and withdrawn. The disease continues throughout life. In some cases, schizophrenia alternates between flare-ups and remissions, and in others it is chronic. Symptoms may worsen over time, or they can remain stable. About half of all people with schizophrenia have a substance abuse problem and attempt suicide.

Although the exact cause of schizophrenia remains unclear and is the subject of ongoing research, the disease clearly has an inherited component. Schizophrenia occurs at the same incidence in all racial and cultural groups throughout the world, indicating a genetic basis rather than a social one. The siblings and children of people with schizophrenia have a greater risk of developing the disease than do people from families without a history of schizophrenia. Studies of schizophrenia in twins also point to a genetic link. If one twin has the disease, the other is many times more likely to have it if he or she is an identical rather than a fraternal (nonidentical) twin. Since identical twins have exactly the same inheritance, the genetic link is clear. Research, as yet, has failed to find a single schizophrenia gene, however. Apparently the disease results from abnormalities in several genes, and environmental influences may also have some role. The fundamental mechanism of the disease is thought to be an abnormality of brain structure and chemistry.

TREATMENT

Because schizophrenia is a severe illness that often leaves the individual incapable of functioning, hospitalization may be required to prevent harm to the person during disease episodes. Medications known as antipsychotics or neuroleptics are used to control symptoms. Usually the drugs are used continuously, since stopping medication can result in a return of symptoms. In some cases, BEHAVIOR THERAPY or PSYCHOTHERAPY can be helpful. Family therapy can help teach those close to the person with schizophrenia how to cope with the disease.

Schuessler biochemic system

See TISSUE SALTS THERAPY.

Sciatica

Pain that radiates along the sciatic nerve that extends from the lower back down into the buttocks and down along the back of the leg past the knee. Sciatica is usually caused by pressure on the nerve from a herniated or ruptured disk. Often sciatica is diagnosed as a radiculopathy (a protruding disk that is putting pressure on the nerve). Pain ranges from merely irritating to severe and debilitating. It usually affects only one side. Treatment includes physical therapy and medication, such as NSAIDs (nonsteroidal anti-inflammatory drugs), oral corticosteroids, or epidural corticosteroid injections. In some cases, surgery is necessary.

Scirrhous

A term for cancers that have a firm and hard structure. Also called hard cancers, scirrhous cancers often are formed in the muscle wall of internal organs, such as the stomach. The cancerous cells infiltrate the muscle wall and turn it into rigid, leatherlike scar tissue that cannot stretch or move.

Sclera

The tough, white, fibrous covering of the eyeball. In the front of the eyeball, the sclera is continuous with the CORNEA, which is clear and admits light. In the back, the sclera is continuous with the sheath (meninges) covering the optic nerve. The sclera is formed from collagen, a protein, and is strong enough to protect the inner structures of the eye from injury.

Scleritis

Inflammation of the white (sclera) of the eye. Symptoms can include severe eye pain, red or purple patches in the eye, blurred vision, sensitivity to light, excessive tearing, or rarely, a protrusion of the eyeball. Scleritis is relatively uncommon and occurs in adults between 30 and 60 years. Fifty percent of patients with scleritis have an associated systemic disease—frequently one of the chronic diseases affecting the immune system, such as rheumatoid arthritis, lupus, or inflammatory bowel disease. Less commonly, scleritis is the result of infection, such as from tuberculosis or Lyme disease. Scleritis is a serious condition that can lead to perforation of the eyeball. Treatment usually consists of oral corticosteroid or nonsteroidal anti-inflammatory drugs and medical management of any underlying disease.

Scleroderma

A chronic autoimmune disease of the connective tissue. Scleroderma is a relatively rare disease that involves symptoms that are apparent when they affect the skin. If the skin is unaffected, the person may have internal organ abnormalities affecting the heart, lungs, gastrointestinal tract, and kidneys. The disease process involves overproduction of collagen, but the precise cause or causes are not known. It affects women more commonly than men.

There are two classifications of scleroderma. The localized form occurs more frequently in children and generally affects only a few areas of skin

or muscle tissue. This rarely develops into the systemic form of the disease. PROGRESSIVE SYSTEMIC SCLEROSIS can involve many body tissues and organs. The skin, esophagus, gastrointestinal tract, blood vessels, muscles, joints, lungs, kidneys, heart, and other internal organs may be affected.

SYMPTOMS, DIAGNOSIS, AND TREATMENT
One or more of the following symptoms may be experienced with scleroderma: swelling of the hands and feet; extreme sensitivity to cold in the extremities; stiff, aching joints and possible structural abnormalities of the joints; thickening and hardening of the skin; dry mucous membranes; and problems involving the digestive system, gastrointestinal tract, the mouth, the face, or the teeth. There may also be generalized symptoms including weakness and severe fatigue, weight loss, and mild sensations of soreness in the muscles, joints, and bones.

Diagnosis might involve medical specialists including rheumatologists (arthritis experts) and dermatologists (skin specialists). Diagnostic blood studies and other specialized tests are determined based on the organs affected. It may be difficult to confirm a diagnosis as many symptoms of scleroderma are the same or similar to those associated with other connective tissue diseases, including rheumatoid arthritis, lupus, and polymyositis. A program of treatment for scleroderma is entirely dependent on the symptoms and their severity. Corticosteroids, immunosuppressive drugs, and medications to treat high blood pressure may be prescribed. A physical therapy regimen and special nutritional programs may be recommended as well.

Scleromalacia

Severe thinning of the white of the eye (sclera). Scleromalacia occurs in people with rheumatoid arthritis. The eye is not inflamed and not painful. Rarely, perforation can occur without trauma.

Sclerosis

The hardening of a body part, often as a result of inflammation. Sclerosis is often used to describe changes in the circulatory system (such as those that occur in ATHEROSCLEROSIS, the medical

term for hardening of the arteries by fat deposits, or aortic valve sclerosis, in which the aortic valve hardens and calcifies over time).

Scoliosis

An abnormal curvature of the spine found in infants, young children, adolescents, and some adults. The spinal curve in scoliosis may have an "S" or a "C" shape. What causes scoliosis in most young people is unknown. Genetic, hormonal, and metabolic factors may have a role. The curvature becomes more apparent as it becomes more pronounced in the early teen years, when there may also be uneven levels of the shoulders and hips. Most cases of scoliosis are mild and painless and have no apparent symptoms. In severe cases, the spine rotates in addition to curving so that the ribs on one side of the body become prominent. There may be constant back pain and breathing problems. Adolescent girls are more likely than boys to have serious scoliosis.

SYMPTOMS
Pediatricians examine the child's back and spine during regular check-

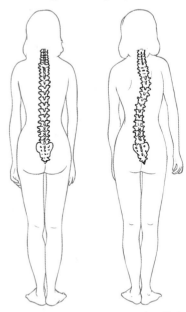

Healthy spine   Spine with scoliosis

SPINAL CURVATURE
Scoliosis may involve twisting of the vertebrae in the area of the curve. There may also be two areas of curvature (an "S" shape) or a single curve (a "C" shape).

ups. Parents should watch for symptoms of scoliosis, including uneven shoulders, prominence of one or both shoulder blades, an uneven waist, elevated hips, or a tendency to lean to one side. If signs of scoliosis are noted, the child should see the doctor. Diagnosis is based on a physical examination and sometimes X rays. The X rays reveal the size of the curve, which may help the doctor determine treatment. At a certain level of curvature, bracing of the back may be recommended to prevent a worsening of the condition in a child who is still growing.

TREATMENT

When the curve is most severe, surgical treatment may become necessary. The most common surgical procedure connects the vertebrae in the curve with solid bone and holds them there with metal devices. The surgery takes 4 to 5 hours followed by up to a week of hospitalization. The child's activities are then restricted for the 3 to 12 months it takes for the bones to fuse together.

Scopolamine

A drug with many uses and often used as an eye drop to dilate (enlarge) the pupil. Scopolamine (Isopto Hyoscine) is used to dilate the pupil before eye examinations and before and after eye surgery and to treat eye conditions such as UVEITIS. It is also used to prevent motion sickness. Scopolamine is also used preoperatively to help produce amnesia and to decrease lung secretions.

Scorpion stings

Painful wounds made by a scorpion, a type of arachnid with a venomous stinger in its tail. Most scorpion bites cause local reactions similar to a bee sting and are not life-threatening. However, the sting of the bark scorpion (Centruroides sculpturatus) of the southwestern United States can be fatal, especially to children. Several hours after the sting, symptoms include seizures, labored breathing, muscle spasms, nausea, tingling, and numbness. Treatments include applying cold packs to the sting area and taking mild painkillers. People with more severe symptoms may require hospitalization and treatment to maintain blood pressure and respiration.

Scotoma

An area of lost or diminished vision within a person's visual field.

Scratch test

An approach to allergy testing performed to identify the allergen that produces symptoms in an affected person. Scratch tests are also called skin prick testing and involve introducing a drop of allergen extract into the skin using a small sharp instrument that causes a small break in the skin. Either the back or the forearm may be chosen. Antihistamine use should be discontinued 3 to 7 days before a skin scratch testing date because this medication can alter results. Some antidepressants may also affect test results, and their use may be stopped before testing in consultation with the physician conducting the test.

Placing the allergen extract on the skin produces a reaction within 20 minutes. If the reaction is negative, there is no change in the skin's surface. A positive reaction produces a small red welt at the site of the skin scratch test. Positive results may only indicate possible allergies. Improper technique may result in false-positive results due to skin irritation. A false-negative result can occur if the allergen extract is not sufficiently potent. A medical history and physical examination along with skin scratch testing are important for confirming and identifying allergens.

Screening

The testing of apparently healthy people to detect a specific disease or disorder at an early, treatable stage. Screening is the cornerstone of preventive medicine and includes testing for problems such as high blood pressure, high cholesterol, and certain types of cancer. Doctors recommend periodic blood pressure measurements, cholesterol tests, dental checkups, eye examinations, and skin examinations. In addition, women are advised to have Papanicolaou (Pap) smears, clinical breast examinations, and mammograms. Prostate and testicular examinations are recommended for men. Other screening tests a doctor may order include blood tests, bone density measurements, urinalysis, electro-cardiograms, and tests for sexually transmitted diseases.

The ages and intervals at which screening should take place vary from test to test and from person to person. For example, dental examinations are recommended every 6 months throughout life, while many other tests (such as bone density measurement, prostate-specific antigen tests, sigmoidoscopy, and colonoscopy) are more important as people grow older. People who have a personal or family history of a medical problem (such as cancer or hypertension) merit earlier and more frequent screening.

Screening tests for newborns

Tests for specific disorders in newborn infants, in which symptoms may not be seen before irreversible damage has been done and for which effective treatments are available. These tests are performed on all babies born in most states within the United States. The baby's heel is pricked to obtain blood for laboratory analysis, and the same blood sample can be used to screen for several diseases. Findings are sent to the doctor responsible for the baby's care.

Babies in all 50 states are routinely screened for PKU (phenylketonuria), a digestive disorder that can cause brain damage and mental retardation, and HYPOTHYROIDISM, a hormone deficiency that can retard growth and mental development. Most states screen for GALACTOSEMIA, a metabolic disorder that can cause death or blindness and mental retardation. Screening can also be done for SICKLE CELL ANEMIA, an inherited blood disease that can cause severe pain and even death; CYSTIC FIBROSIS, a chronic respiratory disease; congenital adrenal hyperplasia, a disease in which certain hormones are deficient; and biotinidase deficiency, an enzyme deficiency that can cause death. Screening tests are currently being developed for many other disorders.

Scrofula

The name formerly applied to TUBERCULOSIS. Scrofula, in current terminology, refers to a specific form of tuberculosis of the bones and lymphatic glands, seen especially in children.

S

Scrotum

The pouch of delicate skin and connective tissue that hangs below the penis and contains the testicles. The scrotum has oil-secreting glands and fine pubic hairs on its surface. See REPRODUCTIVE SYSTEM, MALE.

Scuba-diving medicine

See DIVING MEDICINE.

Scurvy

A condition caused by a prolonged lack of VITAMIN C (ascorbic acid) in the diet. Foods rich in vitamin C include citrus fruits, such as oranges and lemons, sweet peppers, and leafy green vegetables. This nutrient is an important antioxidant involved in lipid and vitamin metabolism, the development of connective tissue, brain activity, immune function, and wound healing. The symptoms of scurvy include fatigue, muscle weakness, joint and muscle aches, and a rash on the legs. Gums swell and bleed easily, and teeth eventually loosen. In children, painful swelling in the legs is accompanied by fever, diarrhea, and vomiting.

Scurvy was once a common disease among sailors and others who went without fresh fruits and vegetables for extended periods. British sailors later carried limes on long voyages to prevent scurvy, earning the nickname limeys. Today scurvy is rare in the United States and other countries where fresh produce is readily available. However, it can also develop as a result of an extremely restricted diet, severe stress, or alcoholism. Smoking tobacco raises a person's requirement for vitamin C. When infants are weaned from breast milk to cow's milk without supplementation from vitamin C, scurvy may develop. Treatment of this disease is with supplements of vitamin C.

Sealants, dental

A plastic resin applied to the pits and grooves of the chewing surfaces of the premolars (the teeth in front of the molars) and molars at the back of the jaw. Dental sealants bond to the enamel on the surface of the teeth and act as a physical barrier to protect the teeth from the plaque (see PLAQUE, DENTAL) and acids that cause TOOTH DECAY. The treatment is especially recommended for children whose PERMANENT TEETH are newly emerged, because these new teeth are particularly susceptible to cavities. Dental sealants are also appropriate for teenagers and adults. People who have DRY MOUTH, or xerostomia, can benefit from sealants because they lack the protective qualities of adequate salivation and, consequently, are more susceptible to tooth decay.

HOW SEALANTS ARE APPLIED

Sealants are applied by a dentist. The office treatment is painless and takes about 5 to 45 minutes to complete, depending on the number of teeth to be treated. The teeth are first cleaned and then rinsed well to remove all the cleaning solution. An acid solution or etching gel is applied to the chewing surfaces to make them rough and help the sealant to adhere. The solution is rinsed off with water after 15 seconds. After the surfaces have dried, the thin, plastic sealant material is painted onto the chewing surface of the tooth, one at a time, where it bonds to the enamel. A special curing light may be used to help the sealant harden. Sealants generally last for several years and may need to be reapplied. Regular dental checkups should be scheduled to make sure the sealant remains bonded to the surfaces of the teeth. As long as the protective barrier remains intact, sealants are highly effective at preventing cavities. Many sealants also release fluoride, which also prevents tooth decay.

Seasickness

A form of motion sickness resulting from being in a boat or on a ship during rolling, heaving, or rough seas (see MOTION SICKNESS). The person affected may experience a range of symptoms from mild nausea to severe vomiting. Like other forms of motion sickness, seasickness is caused by a disturbance in the relationship among the balance system of the inner ear, the visual system of the brain, and the proprioception system of the brain (a person's sense of his or her position in surrounding space). With seasickness, the changing and unsteady horizon line may have a part in this disturbance. Some people find that being in a closed environment on a boat or ship intensifies seasickness; others find that focusing their eyes on close work causes or worsens the symptoms. Psychological stimuli, such as the smell of diesel or chlorine fumes, sometimes can exacerbate seasickness. Over-the-counter oral medications for seasickness are helpful to some people, although they tend to cause sleepiness. Medicated patches containing scopolamine, which are attached to the skin with adhesive, are considered effective. Getting fresh air and drinking plenty of nonalcoholic fluids is often recommended for relieving the symptoms of seasickness. Eating various forms of ginger may be helpful. Some people find relief with seasickness bands worn on the wrist.

Seasonal affective disorder

A form of recurring depression that begins in the fall or winter and resolves in the spring or summer. Seasonal affective disorder is commonly abbreviated SAD. In addition to the fall or winter onset of low mood, symptoms include lack of energy, loss of interest in work and other important activities, declining sexual interest, craving for carbohydrate foods (such as pasta, rice, potatoes, and pastry), increased appetite and weight gain, lengthened sleep time, and movement that is slow, sluggish, and lethargic. The cause of SAD is thought to be connected to changes in body temperature and hormone regulation under low-light conditions. Light therapy is an effective treatment. The individual sits or works nears bright lights (special portable light boxes are available) each day and increases the amount of time spent outdoors on sunny days. Antidepressant medication can also be effective.

Seat belts

Safety belts worn in vehicles to protect drivers and passengers in case of accidents. Seat belts are designed to hold the driver and passengers in place during an accident, preventing them from being hurled forward and injured by the force of the crash. When properly used, seat belts include both lap and shoulder belts. The shoulder belt must cross the collarbone, and the lap belt should fit low and snugly. The use of seat belts is required by law in virtually all states within the United States. See CAR RESTRAINTS.

Sebaceous cyst

See EPIDERMAL CYST.

Sebaceous glands

Oil-producing glands in the skin. The sebaceous glands secrete sebum, the fatty acid that lubricates the skin. In teenagers, hormonal changes stimulate the sebaceous glands to produce excess sebum, which can lead to clogged pores and ACNE. As a person grows older, the sebaceous glands become less active, and the skin becomes drier.

Seborrheic dermatitis

A chronic, benign (not cancerous) skin condition characterized by red, greasy skin covered with yellowish or white flaky scales. Inflammation occurs in areas having the greatest number of sebaceous (oil-producing) glands in the skin. Seborrheic dermatitis may begin in infancy as CRADLE CAP, return in adolescence when the sebaceous glands become more active, and persist throughout life. Seborrheic dermatitis commonly affects the scalp (see DANDRUFF), the area between the eyebrows, the sides of the nose, the area behind or just inside the ears, the chest, and the groin. A yeastlike organism normally found in healthy skin may contribute to the cause.

Diagnosis of seborrheic dermatitis is made through physical examination. Treatment is with over-the-counter dandruff shampoos containing ingredients such as coal tar, salicylic acid, selenium sulfide, sulfur, and zinc pyrithione. Shampoo is massaged into the scalp and other affected areas, left in place for several minutes, and rinsed thoroughly. Individuals may need to try several shampoos before finding one that works. A doctor may prescribe a stronger shampoo that contains ketoconazole. Because shampoos may lose effectiveness over time, they should be alternated. If the problem persists, the doctor may recommend an over-the-counter or prescription hydrocortisone lotion or an overnight coal tar preparation for the scalp. Topical NONSTEROIDAL ANTI-INFLAMMATORY DRUGS in cream form, such as ketoconazole or ciclopirox, may be prescribed if skin on the face is involved.

Seborrheic keratosis

A brown, black, or flesh-colored benign (not cancerous) skin lesion that has a waxy, wartlike appearance. Seborrheic keratoses are most common in people older than 30 years. They are a common feature of aging. Although they can occur anywhere on the body, these growths are most common on the chest or back. Seborrheic keratoses are not a serious health problem and are not related to skin cancer, warts, or moles. However, if growths become large or irritated, bleed easily, or are cosmetically disturbing, they can be removed surgically through CRYOSURGERY (freezing with liquid nitrogen), CURETTAGE (scraping), or electrodesiccation (burning with an electric current delivered through a probe).

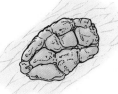

HARMLESS GROWTHS
A seborrheic keratosis is usually darkly colored with a raised, rough surface and clearly defined edges. These growths may change in color and size, but the changes are harmless. The tendency to develop seborrheic keratoses is inherited.

Sebum

Secretions from SEBACEOUS GLANDS in the dermis (the inner layer of skin). Sebum is an oily substance composed of fatty acids that lubricates the skin and prevents it from drying out.

Secondary

Pertaining to a disease, disorder, or complication that occurs during or after treatment for a PRIMARY disease. Secondary prevention refers to delaying, preventing, or moderating the effects of an established disease.

Secondhand smoke

See PASSIVE SMOKING.

Secretion

The body's release of chemical substances, such as estrogen or adrenaline, into the bloodstream.

Sedation

The use of a drug to calm and relax a patient. Sedation is used to control excessive anxiety and aggressive behavior. It is also sometimes used as a premedication for a person who is about to undergo an uncomfortable surgical procedure.

Sedation, conscious

See CONSCIOUS SEDATION.

Sedatives

Drugs used to cause drowsiness or sleep; ANTIANXIETY DRUGS. Sedatives are intended to cause various degrees of relaxation. Sedatives can reduce anxiety in doses that do not promote sleep. Sedatives include several classes of drugs and are used to treat insomnia, anxiety, and epilepsy. All sedatives affect the central nervous system and can create a euphoric state of mild intoxication if taken in too large a dose, which makes them vulnerable to abuse. Sedatives usually impair a person's ability to drive.

Examples of classes of sedatives include BENZODIAZEPINES, used to reduce anxiety; BARBITURATES, used to treat epilepsy; and HYPNOTIC DRUGS, used to induce sleep.

Seizure

FOR FIRST AID
see Seizures, page 1329

A sudden episode of uncontrolled electrical activity in the brain. Seizures may cause a series of involuntary muscle contractions, behavioral changes, sensory abnormalities, or a temporary lapse in consciousness. Seizures are often but not always a sign of EPILEPSY, a neurological disorder characterized by repeated seizures, caused by abnormal electrical activity in the brain.

CAUSES
Clusters of nerve cells (neurons) sometimes signal or fire abnormally. When normal neuronal activity is disturbed, there may be unusual sensations, emotions, or behavior, or convulsions, muscle spasms, and loss

S

of consciousness. The normal rate at which neurons signal is 80 times a second. In a seizure, they fire as many as 500 times a second. Not all seizures are epileptic seizures. For example, a child may have a single febrile seizure (see SEIZURE, FEBRILE) as a result of a high fever, and this does not mean that he or she has epilepsy. A person has to have two or more seizures before he or she is considered to have epilepsy.

About half of all seizures have no known cause. In other cases, seizures are linked to infection, trauma, substance abuse, or other medical problems. Epilepsy may also run in families. In children, seizures are frequently associated with CEREBRAL PALSY and other neurological abnormalities. In people with epilepsy, seizures can be triggered by lack of sleep, alcohol consumption, stress, smoking, and hormonal changes associated with the menstrual cycle.

TYPES OF SEIZURES

There are more than 30 different types of seizures. Seizures are divided into two main categories: partial seizures and generalized seizures.

■ *Partial seizures* Partial seizures start in just one part of the brain. Frequently these seizures are identified by the part of the brain with which they are associated (for example, partial frontal lobe seizures). In a simple partial seizure, a person remains conscious but experiences symptoms related to the part of the brain in which the abnormal impulses develop. In temporal lobe epilepsy, these may include unexplainable sensations of joy or anger or unusual thoughts or feelings. In a complex partial seizure, a person experiences a change in or loss of consciousness. People who have this type of seizure may engage in unusual repetitive behavior (such as blinks or twitches) called automatisms.

Partial seizures (especially complex partial seizures) are often preceded by auras. An AURA is an unusual sensation that is a warning sign of an impending seizure. An aura may consist of a strange feeling, abnormal perceptions, or visual disturbances such as seeing stars or flashes. When there is no loss of consciousness, an aura is actually a simple partial seizure in which a person maintains consciousness.

■ *Generalized seizures* Unlike partial seizures, generalized seizures are caused by abnormal neuronal activity in multiple parts of the brain. These seizures may cause convulsions, massive muscle spasms, falls, and loss of consciousness. There are many different kinds of generalized seizures. In absence seizures (formerly called petit mal), a person seems to be staring into space and may have jerking or twitching muscles. Tonic seizures cause stiffening of the muscles, and clonic seizures cause repeated jerking movements. A person having an atonic seizure loses muscle tone and may fall down. Tonic-clonic seizures (formerly called grand mal seizures) cause stiffening, jerking, and a loss of consciousness.

DIAGNOSIS

Many different techniques are used to diagnose the cause of seizures. These include medical history, blood tests, an electroencephalogram (EEG), and neuropsychological testing. A number of imaging techniques are also used to detect any anatomical abnormalities that may be causing the seizures.

The most commonly used brain scans are CT SCANNING (computed tomography scanning), MRI (magnetic resonance imaging), and PET SCANNING (positron emission tomography scanning); CT scanning and MRI reveal the structure of the brain, while PET scanning and a special type of MRI known as a functional MRI are used to monitor the brain's activity and possible abnormalities. A relatively new brain scan called SPECT (single-photon emission computed tomography) may be used to locate problems in the brain.

TREATMENT

Correct treatment depends on the accurate diagnosis of the underlying cause of seizures. Mild seizures, such as absence seizures, require no immediate first aid treatment. However, it is important to see the doctor for medical evaluation. First aid for tonic-clonic seizures involves laying an affected person on his or her side, loosening their clothing, removing any sharp and hard objects, and not restraining the person or putting anything in his or her mouth. Anyone who has this type of seizure must be evaluated by a physician as soon as possible. If the seizure lasts for longer than 5 minutes or if there are repeated seizures, emergency medical attention is required.

Antiepileptic drugs are the first line of treatment for epileptic seizures. Medications include traditional alternatives, such as carbamazepine, valproate, and phenytoin. Most people with seizures are able to lead relatively normal and productive lives. Occasionally seizures are not controlled with the more traditional medications and one of the new medications is needed. For example, special drugs, such as fosphenytoin, are administered in hospital settings to treat STATUS EPILEPTICUS (a life-threatening occurrence of repeated or prolonged epileptic seizures). When seizures cannot be adequately controlled with medication, doctors consider surgical alternatives.

Seizure, febrile

A SEIZURE experienced by a child with a high fever. A febrile seizure generally follows a rapid rise in body temperature. The affected child experiences a tonic-clonic (or grand mal) seizure, characterized by jerking of the arms and legs, stiffening of the body, and a loss of consciousness that lasts from 30 seconds to 5 minutes.

Other possible symptoms of a febrile seizure include incontinence, clenched teeth or biting of the cheek or tongue, difficulty or absence of breathing, and bluish skin color. Following the seizure, the child usually goes to sleep. He or she usually has little or no memory of the event and afterwards may feel drowsy, and have mild confusion and a headache.

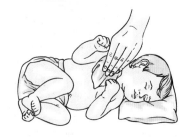

BRINGING DOWN A FEVER
After a child has had a febrile seizure, gently sponging him or her with lukewarm water may help reduce the fever. Water should not be thrown in the child's face, and the child should not be put in a tub of water during the seizure because he or she might inhale the water.

Although their symptoms appear alarming to parents, most febrile seizures have no lasting effect on a child and are rarely associated with epilepsy. In fact, epilepsy in children is defined as seizures that recur in the absence of fever (although it is also true that children with epilepsy are more likely to have seizures when they have a fever). Febrile seizures do not lead to brain damage, and the majority of children outgrow them by age 5 years. In addition, most children who experience one febrile seizure will never have another.

DIAGNOSIS AND TREATMENT

Febrile seizures are diagnosed when children with no history of epilepsy experience a tonic-clonic seizure during the course of an illness accompanied by fever. When first-time febrile seizures occur, the child should be evaluated by a doctor as soon as possible. The physician will conduct tests to make sure that a first-time seizure does not have a more serious underlying cause, such as meningitis or encephalitis. Tests may include an electroencephalogram (EEG), lumbar puncture (spinal tap), and blood and urine tests.

In the past, children who experienced febrile seizures were treated with anticonvulsant drugs to prevent epilepsy. Today, this is no longer the case. Doctors have discovered that in most instances the long-term risks of anticonvulsants, such as possible damage to the developing brain, outweigh any benefits. Consequently, treatment with anticonvulsants is now recommended only when the febrile seizure is prolonged or complicated, when there is a family history of epilepsy, or when signs of nervous system impairment occur before the seizure.

Selective serotonin reuptake inhibitor drugs

Selective serotonin reuptake inhibitor (SSRI) drugs are antidepressants that work by blocking the reuptake of a chemical transmitter called serotonin into nerve cell endings. This activity keeps the concentration of serotonin in the brain higher, which reduces symptoms of depression and other psychological disorders.

Selective serotonin reuptake inhibitor drugs first came on the market in 1988. In addition to the treatment of depression, SSRIs are now used to treat obsessive-compulsive disorder, generalized anxiety disorder, panic disorder, social anxiety disorder, and bulimia nervosa, an eating disorder. SSRIs are widely prescribed in the United States, although some critics say that they are overprescribed and should be reserved only for people who are truly disabled by their mental illness.

Selegiline

A drug used to treat the very early stages of Parkinson disease. Mostly, selegiline (Eldepryl) is used in combination with levodopa or the levodopa-carbidopa combination to treat Parkinson disease. Selegiline works to increase and prolong the effects of levodopa and may help slow the progression of the disease.

Selenium

A trace mineral found in soil and food. Selenium is an essential mineral believed to be closely associated with vitamin E. Selenium is also one of the ANTIOXIDANTS that protect cells from certain chemical reactions associated with aging, heart disease, and cancer. It is thought to stimulate the formation of antibodies in response to vaccines, and it improves the production of sperm and sperm motility.

Selenium is available in brewer's yeast, wheat germ, red meat, chicken, liver, butter, fish, shellfish, garlic, grains, sunflower seeds, and Brazil nuts. Selenium is destroyed when foods are processed or refined, so to obtain adequate amounts in the diet, it is important to eat fresh foods. The amount of selenium in vegetables depends on the amount present in the soil in which they were grown. Selenium is included in vitamin-mineral supplements and should be taken with vitamin E for best results.

Although selenium is usually not toxic, very high doses (more than 1,000 milligrams per day) can cause fatigue, arthritis, hair or fingernail

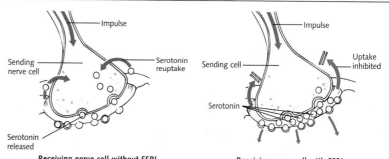

MEDICATION FOR DEPRESSION
In the brain of a person with untreated depression, the transmission of serotonin from one nerve cell to the next does not occur properly, and the sending cell reabsorbs some of the serotonin. As a result, the receiving cell is deprived of serotonin. When the person takes a selective serotonin reuptake inhibitor (SSRI), the drug slows down that reabsorption, so the receiving cell is adequately supplied.

loss, garlicky breath or body odor, irritability, gastrointestinal disorders, and behavior problems in children. People who are considering the use of selenium supplements should first check with their doctor.

Self-esteem

The value an individual places on himself or herself. Individuals with high self-esteem are motivated to understand themselves, judge themselves competent in dealing with life's challenges, and consider themselves worthy of happiness. Individuals with low self-esteem move away from self-understanding, judge themselves to be poorly equipped to deal with challenges, and consider themselves unworthy of happiness.

Encouragement to acknowledge strengths and achievements is part of individual therapy. A positive yet realistic level of self-esteem is essential to living an emotionally healthy life.

Self-image

The way in which an individual perceives himself or herself.

Self-mutilation

A mental illness in which a person feels, for emotional reasons, compelled to cut, burn, or do other forms of painful harm to his or her body. Self-mutilation is also known as cutting and burning. The most common injuries in self-mutilation are cuts inflicted with knives, razors, broken glass, nails, paper clips, scissors, tacks, and other sharp objects. Cigarette burns are also common. Self-mutilators may hit hard objects until their hands are bloody, swallow pins or other sharp objects, strike themselves, or break bones. Most self-mutilators are women between adolescence and age 30. Some were victims of sexual or physical abuse in childhood. Self-mutilation is not a suicide attempt, but people who mutilate themselves are at greater risk for suicide. The disorder also carries the risk of infection from using dirty instruments.

A number of theories may explain self-mutilation. One is that people who self-mutilate regain control of their bodies, which have been treated like the personal property of the person or persons who abused them and

have had pain inflicted at the whim of the abuser. Some people who self-mutilate associate stress with pain, and when they are under stress turn to self-inflicted, self-controlled pain as a way of alleviating anxiety and taking control of themselves. Others say the pain makes them feel alive rather than detached. Another hypothesis is that a person who self-mutilates believes he or she is a bad person deserving punishment. One theory is that self-mutilation is a strategy for the individual to become unattractive, thereby decreasing the possibility that other people will be sexually interested in him or her.

Self-mutilation is often accompanied by mood disorders such as depression and anxiety. Medication may be useful for controlling mood. Alleviating the desire to self-mutilate requires psychotherapy or group therapy to uncover and treat the underlying emotional issues.

Self-screening test

A questionnaire that a person can use to determine whether he or she is at risk of developing, or has developed, dependence on alcohol or drugs. Self-screening tests are not foolproof, but research has shown that they are more accurate in assessing abuse or dependence than are laboratory tests on blood, urine, or liver function. Research indicates that most people are honest in their responses about drug and alcohol use on a questionnaire.

A number of self-screening tests exist. The shortest is the CAGE test, which has just four questions. The longer Self-Administered Alcoholism Screening Test (SAAST) exists in both long (35-question) and short (9-question) forms. Complementing the SAAST is the SAAST-II, which has 9 questions to be completed by someone close to the individual, such as a spouse, roommate, or partner. The Michigan Alcoholism Screening Test (MAST) consists of 25 weighted questions. It also comes in an abbreviated form known as the Short Michigan Alcoholism Screening Test (SMAST), which has 13 questions. Alcoholics Anonymous (AA) uses a 12-question test known as the Twelve Questions. Narcotics Anonymous provides a related but longer questionnaire on the use of drugs. Of all these tests,

> ### THE CAGE
> #### SELF-ADMINISTERED SCREENING TEST
>
> The CAGE test consists of four questions, each of which assesses an important aspect of alcohol dependence. The letters in the word CAGE stand for the terms "Cut back," "Annoyed," "Guilty," and "Eye-Opener."
>
> 1. Have you ever felt the need to cut back your level of alcohol consumption?
> 2. Have people ever annoyed you with their criticisms of your drinking habits?
> 3. Have you ever felt guilty while you were drinking?
> 4. Have you ever started the day with a drink, either to wake yourself up or to cure a hangover?
>
> Two or more yes answers may indicate a problem with alcohol and suggest the need for professional evaluation.

research has shown the CAGE, the SAAST, and the MAST to be the most valid and reliable.

Semen

The thick fluid that is internally secreted and discharged from the penis upon ejaculation. Semen contains millions of sperm, which can travel from the vagina and within the uterus into a fallopian tube and fertilize an egg. When semen is released by the penis into the vagina during SEXUAL INTERCOURSE, PREGNANCY may result. If pregnancy is not desired, it is important for either partner to use an effective means of CONTRACEPTION. Many SEXUALLY TRANSMITTED DISEASES are transmitted via semen, so barrier methods of contraception, such as a condom, should be used.

Semen analysis

A laboratory test to determine the fertility of a man. Semen is the thick, white fluid containing sperm cells that is expelled from the penis during orgasm. Semen analysis is performed to determine whether an abnormality in the semen is the reason a couple cannot conceive a child or to check on the effectiveness of male sterilization surgery (vasecto-

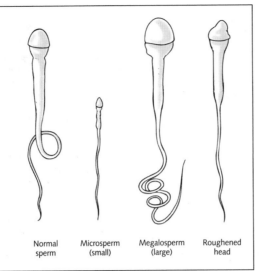

THE APPEARANCE OF SPERM
When a semen sample is examined in a laboratory, the sperm are analyzed for quantity, movement (motility), and chemical factors. The appearance of the sperm under a microscope is another indicator of health. Compared with a normal, healthy sperm, some sperm can be too small, too large, or have a roughened head. There is no clearly defined standard for fertility, but fertility tends to be adversely affected by some problem with the above factors.

| Normal sperm | Microsperm (small) | Megalosperm (large) | Roughened head |

my). A sample of semen is obtained either by self-stimulation (masturbation) and ejaculation into a sterile container or by sexual intercourse using a special condom. The semen is then analyzed for its quantity, the number of sperm cells it contains, the movement of sperm cells (motility), and its chemistry, such as the presence of the sugar fructose or the time it takes the semen to coagulate. This analysis can tell the physician whether the man is producing enough healthy sperm cells to make pregnancy possible. In some cases, semen chemistry may indicate whether certain structures that help to produce and transport semen inside the body are blocked or damaged. Usually a man giving a semen sample for analysis is instructed to refrain from ejaculating for 2 to 5 days beforehand. If the sample is collected away from the laboratory, it must be kept out of direct sunlight and delivered to the laboratory within 1 hour. Since semen content varies each time a man ejaculates, semen analysis is usually performed on at least three samples during a 2-month period to obtain accurate results. See FERTILITY.

Semen, blood in the
See HEMATOSPERMIA.

Seminoma
The most common form of testicular cancer. See TESTICLE, CANCER OF THE.

Sensate focus technique
A relaxing behavioral method of treating sexual disorders, such as erectile dysfunction or lack of orgasm that have psychological causes. The couple is instructed to refrain from intercourse and to focus instead on hugging, kissing, total body massage, and other forms of nongenital stimulation. By reducing the pressure to have intercourse, the couple can learn how to better communicate their sensual needs and build a foundation for improved lovemaking. It is also a term for extended foreplay.

Sensation
The power or process of receiving conscious sense impressions through direct stimulation of the body or through the sense organs. Sensation can refer to an immediate reaction to external stimulation of a sense organ. For example, when it snows in the winter, there is a sensation of cold. The five SENSES (TASTE, SMELL, TOUCH, HEARING, and VISION) are also known as sensations. See also SENSATION, ABNORMAL.

PERCEPTION
PERCEPTION consists of the conscious recognition and interpretation of sensations or sensory stimuli. It is the process by which the body collects and analyzes information about the world. Sensory receptors around the body perceive stimuli and transmit data about them to the brain. Free nerve endings in the skin and taste buds on the tongue are examples of sensory receptors. In the skin, touch receptors perceive or detect sensations, including touch, pressure, pain, temperature, and vibration. Elsewhere in the body, specialized receptors perceive odors, sounds, taste, and light. Internal receptors called proprioceptors collect and analyze information about the position of the body relative to its surroundings and of the body parts in relation to each other. Sensory receptors transmit data about stimuli to the brain as nerve impulses. The brain interprets these impulses into meaningful sensory information.

THE FIVE SENSES
The senses receive sensory material from the environment such as light, sound, odors, and vibrations. The sense of touch relates to the body's ability to sense touch, vibration, pressure, temperature, and pain. The skin, muscles, joints, tendons, and organs all have receptors that sense touch. These sensations are consciously perceived in the cerebrum, the largest and most developed part of the brain. The brain interprets these sensations variously as pleasing, displeasing, or neutral. Factors such as medication and brain injury can affect how a person interprets sensations.

The senses of taste and smell are closely related. There are approximately 9,000 taste buds (tiny clusters of cells that sense flavors from foods) on the surface of the tongue. Taste buds in different parts of the tongue sense the four basic tastes: salty, sweet, bitter, and sour. However, the sense of smell is thousands of times more sensitive than the sense of taste, and flavors are recognized mainly through smell rather than taste. Olfactory sensors in the nasal cavity are stimulated by odors. Nerve impulses travel to olfactory centers in the brain where this information is interpreted.

Hearing is dependent on a complex series of events that occur in the ear. Sound waves in the air are transmitted as vibrations that cross the eardrum to the inner ear. They are changed into nerve impulses and transmitted to the brain by the auditory nerve. Balance is also controlled in the inner ear.

S

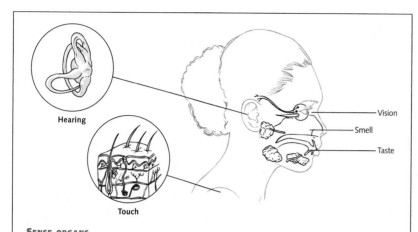

SENSE ORGANS
Sensory impulses travel from the sense organs to specialized sensory areas of the brain, where they are precisely interpreted as sight, smell, taste, sound, or touch. Major sense organs include the eyes (vision); the nose (smell); the tongue, salivary glands, and nose (taste); the ear (hearing); and skin (touch).

Vision takes place when light is processed by the eye and interpreted by the brain. Light passes through the cornea. The retina converts light into a nerve impulse that is carried to the brain and then interpreted.

Sensation, abnormal

An unusual feeling. There are a variety of abnormal sensations. TINGLING, an abnormal, prickling feeling in the skin, can be a sign of damage or irritation to nerves in the affected area. It is a different problem than NUMBNESS, which suggests instead that a nerve is damaged. A brief tingling sensation, as when a person's hand or foot "falls asleep," is not a cause for concern. However, a persistent tingling or PINS AND NEEDLES SENSATION may be caused by medical problems such as nerve injury; lack of blood supply; diabetes mellitus, type 1 and type 2; thyroid problems; vitamin B12 (cyanocobalamin) deficiency; carpal tunnel syndrome; transient ischemic attack; stroke; or multiple sclerosis. People with epilepsy may experience auras of unusual smells, unusual visual perceptions, or unusual tastes, all of which are also abnormal sensations.

Senses

TASTE, SMELL, TOUCH, HEARING, and VISION. Senses provide people with information about the world around them. The senses receive sensory material from the environment, such as light, sound, odors, and vibrations. Sensory receptors, such as free nerve endings and taste buds, respond to these stimuli and transmit data about them to the brain as nerve impulses. The brain interprets these impulses into meaningful sensory information.

The senses of taste and smell are closely related. There are approximately 9,000 taste buds (tiny clusters of cells that sense flavors from foods) on the surface of the tongue. Taste buds in different parts of the tongue sense the four basic tastes: salty, sweet, bitter, and sour.

The sense of smell is thousands of times more sensitive than the sense of taste. Flavors are recognized mainly through the sense of smell. Olfactory sensors in the nasal cavity are stimulated by odors. Nerve impulses travel to olfactory centers in the brain where this information is interpreted.

The skin, muscles, joints, tendons, and organs all have receptors that sense touch. The sense of touch also relates to the body's ability to sense vibration, pressure, temperature, and pain. These sensations are consciously perceived in the cerebrum, the largest and most developed part of the brain. The brain interprets these sensations variously as pleasing, displeasing, or neutral. See also SENSATION.

Hearing is dependent on a complex series of events that occur in the ear. Sound waves in the air are transmitted as vibrations that cross the eardrum to the inner ear. They are changed into nerve impulses and transmitted to the brain by the auditory nerve where the brain interprets the impulses as sounds. Balance is also controlled in the inner ear.

Vision takes place when light is processed by the eye and interpreted by the brain. Light passes through the cornea. The retina converts light into a nerve impulse that is carried to the brain where it is translated into images and then interpreted.

Sensitive teeth

See DENTIN.

Sensitization

A person's first exposure to an ALLERGEN or other foreign substance, such as an infectious agent. Sensitization leads to an immune response that can produce the symptoms of allergies, a process also called allergic sensitization. When the sensitized person is exposed to the same allergen subsequently, he or she will have a more immediate and stronger allergic reaction to it.

During the period of sensitization, the immune system produces antibodies, which are chemicals normally produced by white blood cells to fight infections and other foreign invaders of the body. Allergic sensitization involves a mistaken response to substances such as pollen, animal dander, dust mites, drugs, or certain foods that are not actually harmful to the body. Once the immune response is in place, physical and chemical changes take place in the body that produce the symptoms associated with allergies.

Sensitization may also refer to the body process that is mimicked by IMMUNIZATION, which involves exposing a person to an ANTIGEN that provokes an immune response. The goal is to increase immunity and set the stage for a more vigorous secondary immune response when a person is later exposed to the same antigen.

Sensory cortex

An area on the outer surface of the cerebrum, the main body of the brain, that processes sensory information at a conscious level. The primary somatic sensory cortex receives information from the skin about temperature, pressure, and pain. The primary visual cortex interprets aspects of vision such as light and dark and borders. The primary auditory cortex interprets aspects of sound such as volume and pitch. The gustatory area receives signals relating to taste.

Sensory deprivation

The absence of stimulation to the senses, particularly hearing, vision, and touch. Complete sensory deprivation, which has been researched experimentally as a form of torture, causes severe anxiety, a loss of intelligence and memory, hallucinations (such as hearing nonexistent voices), and changes in personality, including withdrawal. These effects can be reversed if the deprivation is stopped and stimulation returns to normal. Partial sensory deprivation over an extended time causes similar effects, which can be seen in prisoners held in solitary confinement and sometimes in patients living in nursing homes or similar institutions.

Separation anxiety

Profound distress experienced by a child or adolescent when apart from parents, family, or familiar surroundings. The distress lasts for more than 4 weeks and begins before the child is 18. The anxiety can be severe enough to cause a PANIC ATTACK. Children or adolescents with separation anxiety may develop physical complaints to stay at home and may exhibit multiple fears, one being a phobia about school. In addition, children with this disorder may exhibit excessive fears at bedtime, often demanding that an adult stay in their room until they fall asleep or frequently awakening at night to go to their parent's bedroom. Older children often complain of their heart racing, dizziness, or feeling faint. School phobia sometimes reflects problems in the family, such as alcoholism or marital difficulties, as well as depression or anxiety in the individual. Often a home visit from the school social worker can reveal problems at home causing the child's unwillingness to separate from a parent.

Sepsis

A system-wide response to bacterial infection of a wound or tissues, which may lead to the rapid multiplication of bacteria and an accumulation of bacterial toxins in the bloodstream. See also SEPTIC SHOCK.

Septal defect, atrial

A hole in the septum (wall) between the atria (two upper chambers of the heart). Atrial septal defect can be congenital (present at birth), and it occurs in three times as many girls as boys, particularly in children with Down syndrome. Because of the defect, blood is shunted from the left atrium to the right when the heart fills with blood. This increases blood flow to the lungs, forcing the right ventricle (a lower chamber) of the heart and the lungs to work harder. Over time this can lead to abnormal enlargement of the right ventricle and pulmonary hypertension (high blood pressure in the lungs). Lung congestion, an unusually large number of respiratory infections, blood clots that may cause a stroke, and cardiac

HOLES IN THE HEART

Depending on their size, atrial (upper chamber) and ventricular (lower chamber) septal defects, or holes in the walls of the heart, can be serious medical conditions requiring surgery. When atrial septal defects are recognized between 1 and 6 years of age, they are usually closed surgically. However, ventricular septal defects, if small, may close on their own.

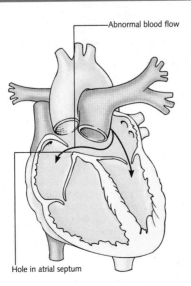

Abnormal blood flow

Hole in atrial septum

ATRIAL SEPTAL DEFECT
A hole in the septum (wall) between the two atria allows oxygenated and deoxygenated blood to mix.

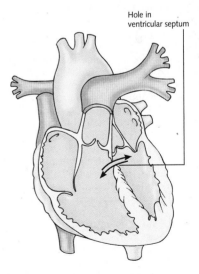

Hole in ventricular septum

VENTRICULAR SEPTAL DEFECT
A hole in the septum between the two ventricles also allows deoxygenated blood to mix with oxygenated blood.

S

arrhythmia (abnormal heartbeat) may also follow.

The majority of people with atrial septal defect show no symptoms early in life. Often the problem is detected by a doctor who hears a murmur (the sound of abnormal blood flow).

As a rule, it is best to repair an atrial septal defect sooner rather than later, before permanent damage occurs. The repair is made surgically. Small defects can be stitched shut; larger ones can be closed with a patch of synthetic material or a small piece of the person's own tissue. Repair of an atrial septal defect without other complications has an excellent outcome, and life expectancy is normal. If the defect is not repaired, however, the person is unlikely to live past age 50. A catheter technique has recently been developed and approved in which a closure device is inserted into the atrial septal defect.

Septal defect, ventricular

A hole in the septum (wall) between the ventricles (two lower chambers) of the heart. Ventricular septal defect can be congenital (present at birth) and is the most common congenital heart defect. Because of the defect, blood that does not normally flow between the ventricles can flow from the left ventricle to the right as the ventricle contracts, increasing blood flow in the right side of the heart. If the hole is large enough to substantially increase blood flow, the right ventricle and the lungs must work harder to compensate. Over time this can lead to abnormal enlargement of the right ventricle and pulmonary hypertension (high blood pressure in the lungs). Lung congestion, an unusually large number of respiratory infections, blood clots that may cause a stroke, and cardiac arrhythmia (abnormal heartbeat) may also follow.

Many small ventricular septal defects close on their own before age 18 and cause no symptoms except for a murmur (the sound of abnormal blood flow). If the defect is large or fails to close, it can be repaired surgically, ideally before any permanent damage has been done to the heart or lungs. Repair of a ventricular septal defect without other complications

has an excellent outcome, but long-term follow-up by a doctor is required.

Septic shock

FOR FIRST AID
see Septic shock, page 1330

An inflammatory response that is caused by toxins produced by bacteria, which damage tissues and trigger a dramatic drop in blood pressure. Septic shock is a life-threatening condition that occurs when bacterial infections get into the blood, multiply rapidly, and produce bacterial toxins. The condition requires immediate medical treatment, including intravenous antibiotic drugs and medical procedures to maintain blood pressure and blood volume. In some cases an infected organ or structure, such as the gallbladder or appendix, may need to be removed to eliminate the infection.

Septic shock is commonly associated with infections caused by staphylococci, meningococci, or *Candida* organisms. When the cause is staphylococcal toxins, septic shock may be referred to as TOXIC SHOCK SYNDROME, which occurs most frequently among young women. The condition may be caused by NOSOCOMIAL INFECTIONS (those acquired in a hospital) caused by bacteria, particularly when invasive medical devices such as catheters are used. Newborns, older people, and pregnant women are also more susceptible to septic shock. It occurs more often in people with weakened immune systems and in those with chronic diseases. Conditions that may predispose a person to septic shock include having diabetes mellitus, cirrhosis, or conditions in which white blood cell counts are diminished, especially when associated with tumors and cancer-fighting medications. Other factors include previous infections of the urinary tract, gastrointestinal tract, and the organs and ducts in which bile is transported to the small intestine.

CAUSES AND SYMPTOMS
The initial cause of septic shock is not fully understood. When bacterial toxins are produced by the organisms causing the infection, the immune system responds in a number of complex ways that are influenced by

other conditions in the body at the time. Septic shock develops from the condition called bacteremia, in which bacteria enter the bloodstream. The first symptom is usually a decrease in mental alertness. Blood pressure drops, and the skin and extremities become warm to the touch, which is the opposite of the anticipated effect of lowered blood pressure. The heart beats at an abnormally rapid rate, and breathing rate increases dramatically. Fever or even low body temperature often develops.

As septic shock progresses, the extremities become cool and pale. Organ failure can occur involving the kidney, lungs, and liver. Blood clots may form in the blood vessels, and heart failure may occur.

DIAGNOSIS AND TREATMENT
Diagnosis of septic shock is begun by differentiating the condition from other serious conditions. What characterizes septic shock is an increase in the heart's output of blood combined with decreased blood pressure and warm, dry skin. Significantly lowered or elevated white blood cell and platelet counts may be revealed in blood tests. Urinalysis may indicate the source of infection in the urinary tract; blood cultures will test positive for the bacteria.

Septic shock must be diagnosed and treated early to prevent death. Once a high concentration of acid in the blood has become established, especially when coupled with the failure of several organs, the condition can become irreversible even with treatment. When septic shock is identified, the person requires care in an intensive care unit of a hospital where vital signs can be monitored and treatment can be given. Early antibiotic therapy is essential to preventing death. Other treatment generally includes intravenous fluid replacement, respiratory support, and medications to normalize blood pressure and urination. Surgical procedures are often necessary to drain pus and remove infected tissues, structures, and organs.

Septicemia

A systemic illness caused by the spread of bacteria or their toxins into the bloodstream; also known as blood poisoning. The bacteria may come from a local, severe infection of the respiratory system (for example, pneumonia), urinary tract, digestive system, bone (osteomyelitis), or brain and spinal cord (meningitis). The bacteria move quickly through the blood to other organs, causing spiking fevers and chills, fast heartbeat, rapid breathing, a seriously ill appearance, and a feeling of impending doom.

If the septicemia is untreated, the result is septic shock, which causes low blood pressure and body temperature and mental confusion. Widespread blood clotting, kidney failure, and respiratory failure may occur. Death occurs in more than half of the people who develop septic shock, even with antibiotic therapy.

Hospitalization, usually in an intensive care unit, is required to treat septicemia. Fluids and medications are given through a vein to maintain blood pressure, and antibiotics are administered against the infectious organism. The individual is given oxygen to raise the oxygen content of the blood.

Appropriate care of local bacterial infections, such as strep throat or an infected cut, is important to prevent the infection from spreading into the bloodstream. Children should be immunized against HAEMOPHILUS INFLUENZAE type B, which is a common cause of septicemia. Those whose spleens have been removed surgically or damaged (for example, by sickle cell anemia) are susceptible to pneumococcal infection and should receive the vaccine against it.

Septum

A wall or partition that divides one section of a body part or cavity from another. An example is the septum in the nose, a piece of cartilage that divides the nasal passages.

Septum, deviated

A deformity of the septum, the structure that separates the nostrils and is composed of bone and cartilage covered by a layer of mucous membrane. Although no septum is perfectly straight or centered, a deviated septum is the condition in which a portion of this bone is crooked or curves to one side. People may be born with a deviated septum, or more commonly, it is the result of injury.

SYMPTOMS

A deviation in the septum is rarely severe enough to cause symptoms that require treatment. However, air flow may be obstructed, and breathing through the affected nostril can be difficult. The reduced flow of air can encourage growth of bacteria and trap pollen. People who have asthma, hay fever, and other allergies may experience more severe symptoms as a result of a deviated septum. The breathing difficulty can lead to mouth breathing, dry mouth, and snoring.

DIAGNOSIS AND TREATMENT

A deviated septum is diagnosed by a physical examination of the nose. If the deviation causes health problems or recurrent disease, surgery may be recommended. This operation, called septoplasty, is performed by an otolaryngologist and involves the removal of the bent or excess cartilage from the septum. The procedure is usually done in a hospital-based ambulatory surgery unit, using local or general anesthesia. Rhinoplasty to reshape the nose is sometimes performed at the same time.

Septum, perforated

An opening or hole in the surface of the septum, the wall inside the nose that separates the two nostrils. The mucous membrane, cartilage, and bone of the septum may be perforated by several means. Occupational hazards include prolonged exposure to arsenic and other elements of fuel. Long-term use of one of the nasal CORTICOSTEROIDS for the treatment of allergies and RHINITIS, and long-term use of cocaine, inhaled through the nose in powdered form, can perforate the septum. The condition can cause bleeding, crusting, and whistling in the nose. If the perforation is severe and causes health problems, the hole may be surgically repaired.

Sequela

A disease condition resulting from a previous disease.

Sequestration

The formation of a fragment or fragments of dead bone, which have lost their blood supply and become detached from adjoining sound bone.

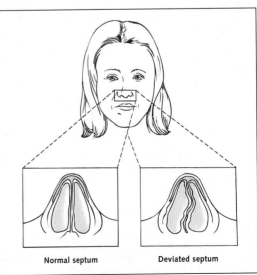

ALIGNING THE SEPTUM
The septum is the narrow wall of bone and cartilage that separates the nostrils. The structure usually divides the nose into two fairly symmetrical spaces (left). A deviated septum (right), which may or may not be visible, can obstruct the flow of air through one or both nostrils, making breathing more difficult—especially if the person has asthma or other allergies. A deviated septum sometimes causes snoring.

Normal septum   Deviated septum

Serology

Laboratory tests of the blood used to determine the amount of a specific antibody, measure the effectiveness of medical treatment, and detect certain kinds of microorganisms and other infectious agents. Antibodies react with specific antigens and can help doctors identify the presence of specific microorganisms. Depending on the type of suspected antibodies, there are various serology tests that can be used to identify disease.

Serotonin

A chemical that functions primarily to transmit signals between the nerve cells of the human brain. Recent research has indicated that abnormally low levels of serotonin are associated with depression, obsessive-compulsive disorder, and eating disorders. Antidepressant medications increase the supply of serotonin, which is thought to be effective in helping to alleviate depression. Serotonin is also known as 5-hydroxytryptamine (5-HT).

Sertraline

An antidepressant and antiobsessional drug. Sertraline (Zoloft) is one of the SELECTIVE SEROTONIN REUPTAKE INHIBITOR DRUGS used to treat major depression, obsessive-compulsive disorder, and panic disorder. It works by increasing the amount of serotonin in the brain, which helps improve a person's mood.

Serum

The clear fluid portion of blood. Serum does not contain blood cells. It is essentially similar in composition to blood plasma, but lacks fibrinogen and other substances used in the coagulation (clotting) process. Serum contains many proteins, including antibodies formed as part of the immune response to protect against infection.

Serum sickness

A severe immune response to a foreign protein that occurs most frequently as a reaction to antibiotic medications or vaccinations, particularly those containing animal serum. Serum sickness occurs when the immune system's response to the medication or vaccine is so intense that it results in substantial inflammation and tissue damage. Symptoms may include low-grade fever, fatigue, headache, joint pain, fluid retention and swelling in the arms and legs, enlarged lymph nodes, and hives. The symptoms usually appear within 5 to 21 days of having taken the medication or receiving the vaccine, and they persist for 2 to 3 weeks.

Treatment for serum sickness includes withdrawing the medication causing the reaction. Fever may be treated with acetaminophen, pain may be managed with ibuprofen or corticosteroids, and antihistamines may be given for allergy symptoms.

Severe Acute Respiratory Syndrome (SARS)

A serious form of pneumonia that does not respond to standard antibiotic treatment. Symptoms of severe acute respiratory syndrome (SARS) include high fever, shortness of breath, a dry cough, and difficulty breathing. The illness, which was first reported in Hong Kong, can be fatal. Deaths have also been reported in China and Toronto, Canada. Many of those initially infected by the disease were health care workers who had close contact with infected people. The fatality rate was about 9 percent in 2003. ISOLATION is recommended for those with SARS symptoms; QUARANTINE, for those who have been exposed to SARS.

Sex

Another term for male or female gender; also a commonly used synonym for SEXUAL INTERCOURSE and many other forms of sexual activity. See also SEXUALITY.

Sex change

The surgical and medical process used to change a person's sex from male to female or female to male. The surgical aspect of sex change is known as sex-reassignment surgery. Sex change is performed as treatment for gender-identity disorder, in which an individual acts and presents himself or herself as a member of the opposite sex and feels profoundly uncomfortable with his or her physical sex. Before surgery, an individual must live for a period of time (2 years) as a member of the opposite sex to be sure that reassignment will be successful. In addition, the person takes opposite-sex hormones and may begin the transition to the opposite sex by having unwanted hair removed, the breasts enlarged or removed surgically, or facial structure altered. In the actual sex-reassignment surgery, the genitals are reconstructed into the organs of the opposite sex. After the individual recovers from surgery, hormone treatment is continued.

Sex chromosomes

Chromosomes associated with the determination of sex and gender.

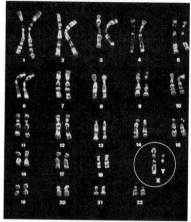

Male chromosomes

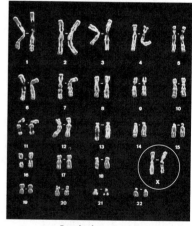

Female chromosomes

DETERMINING GENDER
All human cells (except eggs and sperm) contain 46 chromosomes arranged in 23 pairs. The 23rd pair consists of the sex chromosomes that determine gender. In a man, this pair consists of an X chromosome and a Y chromosome, the latter of which confers maleness. In a woman, the pair contains two X chromosomes.

In mammals, the sex chromosomes consist of the female X chromosome and the male Y chromosome. Females have two X chromosomes; males have an X and a Y.

Sex determination

The sex of humans and other mammals, as regulated by the presence or absence of the Y chromosome. Humans have 22 sets of non–sex chromosomes and one set of sex chromosomes. Females have two X chromosomes, while males have one X and a small Y chromosome. The sex chromosomes, X and Y, though paired in males, are different from each other, and the presence of a Y chromosome is necessary for male sexual characteristics to develop.

Sex drive

The desire to seek sexual gratification; also known as libido. Sex drive is thought to peak in the early 20s, and decline slowly thereafter. However, it varies from person to person and with environmental factors such as stress, opportunity to be sexual, and religious and cultural factors.

Sex education

Also called sexuality education. Courses given to children and adolescents by a school or community group to provide an opportunity for young people to learn about sexuality and how it can affect their lives. A comprehensive sex education curriculum typically incorporates topics related to human sexuality including growth and development, human reproduction, anatomy, physiology, masturbation, sexual response, sexual orientation, contraception, and abstinence. Sex education may also include topics on abortion, family life, pregnancy, childbirth, parenthood, sexual abuse, HIV and AIDS (human immunodeficiency virus and acquired immunodeficiency syndrome), and other sexually transmitted diseases. Courses emphasize the personal and social responsibilities that sexual activity demands. The goals of sex education include reducing incidences of teen pregnancy and sexually transmitted diseases and promoting adult sexual health. Sex educators believe that parents should begin educating their children about reproduction and sexually transmitted diseases long before they are likely to think about having sex.

A majority of children in the United States receive some form of formal sex education. Quality and content vary widely, and most programs are not presented until junior high or high school. Until age 14, fewer than 10 percent of US children have had a comprehensive sex education course. In many communities, social and religious influences can affect the content of programs. Research has shown that sex education courses can significantly reduce teen pregnancy. The programs are not known to have any impact on rates of sexual activity or sexually transmitted diseases among teenagers. Educators suggest that providing the programs at earlier ages may more effectively combat spread of sexually transmitted diseases. The United States has one of the world's highest teen pregnancy rates. In European countries, where sex education is commonly provided in the lower grades, teen pregnancy rates are consistently lower.

Sex hormones

The hormones that influence sexual differentiation and development and enable the reproductive cycles to function properly. Sex hormones are secreted by the ovaries in females and the testicles in males at an early stage of fetal development. They trigger the hypothalamus to secrete the hormones appropriate to the sex of the fetus, which produce the sex-appropriate sexual characteristics, including the genitals that make males and females physically different. The hypothalamus initiates and maintains the cycle of female hormones in girls and women and sustains a constant pattern of male sex hormone secretion in boys and men.

The major female sex hormones, ESTROGEN and PROGESTERONE, are produced mainly by the ovaries. These hormones have vital roles in a woman's menstrual cycle, her ability to conceive a child, and the ability of her body to support a healthy pregnancy. The male sex hormones, ANDROGEN HORMONES, include TESTOSTERONE, which is produced by the testicles. Testosterone is important to a man's bone and muscle growth and sexual development. It is also involved in the male sex drive. Testosterone is also produced in small amounts in a woman's ovaries and adrenal glands and has a role in female sex drive.

Follicle-stimulating hormone (FSH) and luteinizing hormone (LH) are sex hormones produced by the pituitary gland in both men and women. In women, they stimulate ovulation and regulate the menstrual cycle. In men, they regulate the production of sperm in the testicles.

COMMON MISBELIEFS ABOUT SEX

Sexual difficulties are often rooted in mistaken information drawn from inaccurate popular beliefs. Some examples:

- "Men always want sex and are ready for it all the time." Sexual desire rises and falls in men just as in women. Believing that they are always ready puts men in the situation of trying to make love in situations where they are not feeling well or not emotionally prepared. Sexual difficulties can result.
- "Men should guide sex." A man who thinks this way is not allowing himself to hear how the woman wants to be pleasured. He may think more of what he wants without considering the woman's needs and responses.
- "Sex has to be spontaneous and natural." This idea prevents couples from telling each other what they find pleasurable. Time pressures may necessitate scheduling opportunities for sex in order to achieve a satisfying love life, with humor included to diffuse tension.
- "Sex equals vaginal intercourse." In fact, there are many ways of giving and receiving sexual pleasure. None counts less than any other; a climax is a climax.
- "Pregnancy and childbirth make a woman less sexually responsive." Except for discomfort in the last weeks before delivery, pregnancy actually makes many women more interested in sex and more responsive because of the increased blood supply in the pelvis.
- "Menopause ends a woman's sex life." Since they no longer have to worry about conception, many women find menopause sexually freeing rather than inhibiting.

S

Sex therapy

A directive approach to treating sexual problems that focuses on the problems themselves rather than only on their roots in the individual's personality. Problems treated in sex therapy may include erectile dysfunction (impotence), premature ejaculation, and lack of orgasm. Sex therapy is most often conducted with both partners, not only with the person who is perceived as having the sexual problem.

Treatment begins with assessing and conceptualizing the problem and with teaching the couple that they both share the sexual issue. The therapist provides accurate information about sex to correct misbeliefs the couple may have and helps the couple identify and change destructive attitudes about sex, particularly emotional reactions that obstruct sexual arousal.

Sensate focus home exercises are key to sex therapy. The couple initially refrains from sexual intercourse and engages instead in teaching each other how to hug, kiss, and give whole-body massage, at first avoiding the genitals and breasts to learn sensual pleasure. At the same time, the partners learn how to tell each other honestly what they find stimulating and to experiment with different types of stimulation and positions.

Over time the couple progresses to full sexual intercourse. Also, the couple is helped to identify the interactions that make sex difficult (for example, making love only late at night, when fatigue is a major issue) and to create new sexual patterns.

Sexual abuse

See ABUSE, SEXUAL.

Sexual addiction

A condition characterized by a preoccupying desire to repeatedly engage in sex that is driven by a deep-seated, compulsive need, with only brief tension release after orgasm.

The person with sexual "addiction" may feel out of control and experience shame, pain, and self-loathing

Terms in small capital letters—for example, PHYSICAL THERAPY or PAGET DISEASE—indicate a cross-reference to another entry with more information.

as a result of the behavior. The addiction can involve any number of sexual practices and may be directed toward same-sex or opposite-sex partners. Over time, some people with sexual addiction tend to engage in increasingly dangerous behaviors (especially unprotected sex with prostitutes) and become highly preoccupied with sexual activities and rituals. Typically the behavior disrupts romantic, love, and family relationships, and it can lead to blackmail, arrest, financial trouble, despair, and low self-esteem. The person often tries repeatedly to stop the maladaptive behavior, only to return to it and experience another wave of self-loathing. Sexual compulsions may be associated with alcohol or substance-abuse and eating disorders or with mood disorders, including depression and anxiety. The term addiction has been challenged as an inaccurate analogy to substance abuse. However, the use of the treatment model of Alcoholics Anonymous, and the TWELVE-STEP PROGRAM steps of self-help, may be helpful.

Sexual assault

See ASSAULT, SEXUAL.

Sexual characteristics, secondary

Signs of a young person's development. PUBERTY is the start of physical and sexual changes in the body, which usually begin soon after age 10 or 11 years in girls and shortly after age 12 or 13 years in boys. The development of breast buds is the first secondary sexual characteristic in girls. This is followed by the appearance of pubic hair several months later and a rounding of the hips. About a year later, underarm hair begins to grow, and sweat glands under the arms cause an increase in perspiration and body odor. Shortly before a girl's first period, nipples of breasts may protrude and the pubic hair is almost fully grown.

The enlargement of the testicles and scrotum is the first visible sign of puberty in boys. Soon afterwards, chest muscles enlarge and sweat glands under the arms cause an increase in perspiration and body odor. This is followed by the appear-

ance of pubic hair, a deepening voice, and the boy's first ejaculation. Testicles continue to grow, and the penis becomes thicker and longer. The pubic hair eventually begins filling in, and the penis and scrotum darken. Hair sprouts on the chin and under the arms.

Sexual desire, inhibited

An absence of normal sexual fantasies and desire for sexual activity that causes significant distress or difficulty in relationships. Inhibited sexual desire is also known as hypoactive sexual desire disorder. The lack of desire may be lifelong (primary), or it may appear after a period of normal sexual activity (secondary). The inhibition may apply to all forms of sexual expression with all partners, or it may hold true for only one particular activity or for one partner.

This disorder is often associated with difficulty in achieving sexual satisfaction, and it can arise from feelings of failure, lack of sexual knowledge, or low expectations surrounding sex. In some cases, what appears to be inhibited sexual desire is actually a marked disparity in sexual interest between the two partners.

Inhibited sexual desire is the most common sexual dysfunction. The cause can be physical, such as low hormone levels or certain medication side effects, but it is more often a psychological issue, particularly difficulties in the relationship, such as a lack of emotional closeness, power struggles between the partners, or a lack of time alone. Insomnia, fatigue, general medical conditions (for example, cancer or heart disease), and psychological disorders that inhibit desire, particularly DEPRESSION, may also have a role. Inhibited sexual desire can also appear in persons who were abused sexually or raped as children. Treatment consists of SEX THERAPY to resolve relationship difficulties. Medication and psychotherapy can also be helpful for individuals with depression or for resolving the emotional effects of abuse or rape.

Sexual dysfunction

Any impairment in sexual response that causes emotional distress and prevents an individual or couple from experiencing satisfaction as a result of sexual activity. Sexual dysfunction can be present throughout life or develop after a period of normal responsiveness. The problem may develop gradually or suddenly. Sometimes both partners are aware that conflict is the cause, but they have not found a way to make peace so they can make love again.

TYPES
Sexual dysfunctions are classified into four groups. In sexual desire disorders (see SEXUAL DESIRE, INHIBITED), there is an abnormal absence of sexual fantasies and desire for sexual activity.

Disorders of sexual arousal are commonly referred to as frigidity in women and impotence in men (see ERECTILE DYSFUNCTION). Some women with this type of dysfunction experience revulsion to sex and avoid lovemaking. In men, the dysfunction appears as the inability to achieve or maintain an erection. In both women and men, the result is a lack of pleasure and excitement surrounding sex.

Sexual pain disorders consist of pain during intercourse (dyspareunia; see INTERCOURSE, PAINFUL) and an involuntary spasm of the vagina that prevents entry (see VAGINISMUS). Orgasm disorders refer to the inability to reach climax following sufficient foreplay or stimulation (see ORGASM, LACK OF). In some men, orgasm may occur too soon, before either partner is satisfied, a dysfunction known as PREMATURE EJACULATION. In other men, ejaculation may be difficult (delayed or absent ejaculation), but the difficulty is not caused by medication, alcohol, or street drugs.

CAUSES AND TREATMENT
The causes of sexual dysfunction can be physical, psychological, or a combination of both. Physical causes include general medical conditions causing fatigue (for example, cancer, diabetes mellitus, or heart disease), lack of sleep (insomnia), certain diseases (for example, diabetes mellitus, multiple sclerosis, and tumors of the spinal cord), injury to the spinal cord or pelvic nerves, surgery on the genitals (such as removal of the prostate or ovaries), and radiation of the genitals or pelvis in the treatment of cancer. Sexual dysfunction can also be caused by drugs (including tobacco, alcohol, and cocaine), medications (for example, those used to control high blood pressure and depression), circulation problems and artery disease, and abnormally low sexual hormone levels. Psychological causes include guilt or fear surrounding sex and emotional trauma from sexual abuse or rape. Treatment of sexual dysfunction depends on the cause. It can include changing medications, addressing underlying medical conditions, and counseling that focuses on sexuality (see SEX THERAPY).

Sexual intercourse
The penetration of a woman's vagina by a man's penis. The penis must be erect or semierect to enter the vagina. Once inside, the penis ejaculates or releases a thick fluid called semen. This fluid contains millions of sperm, which may travel from the vagina through the uterus into a fallopian tube and fertilize or unite with an egg. In order to prevent pregnancy, it is important for either partner to use effective means of CONTRACEPTION during sexual intercourse.

Intercourse is also the most common way for SEXUALLY TRANSMITTED DISEASES to spread. If a person is not in a mutually monogamous relationship, doctors recommend the practice of SAFER SEX, such as the use of male or female condoms. If using a male condom to prevent pregnancy and sexually transmitted diseases (STDs), it must be placed on the penis before it touches any part of the female genital area; this is because the penis may release small drops of fluid called pre-ejaculate, which can contain sperm and disease-causing organisms. See also CONTRACEPTION, BARRIER METHODS.

There are many different positions for sexual intercourse. The partners can face one another, or the woman's back can rest against the partner's chest. Sexual intercourse can be practiced lying down, sitting, or standing. Alternatively, couples may engage in anal intercourse. Safer sex is also essential in the practice of this type of intercourse, in order to prevent the transmission of STDs.

Sexual orientation
Persistent emotional, affectionate, romantic, or erotic attraction to persons of a particular sex. Three sexual orientations are recognized. HETEROSEXUALITY refers to attraction to members of the opposite sex; HOMOSEXUALITY, to members of the same sex; and BISEXUALITY, to members of both sexes. Homosexual people are also referred to as "gay" and homosexual women as "lesbian." Heterosexual people may be known as "straight."

The development of sexual orientation is not well understood. Most scientists believe that sexual orientation arises at an early age as a result of a number of interacting biological, social, and psychological factors. Sexual orientation is not a matter of choice. Sexual identity confusion is not uncommon; a teen may benefit from a psychiatric evaluation and a few visits to a therapist to discuss any questions. There is no medical evidence that sexual orientation can be changed through psychotherapy or so-called transformational ministry (also known as reparative therapy).

Sexual response
A sequence of physiological changes that occur in men and women during sexual intercourse (or other sexual activities) in four stages over an average of 14 minutes. Arousal, the first stage, involves several physical changes, including swelling of the breasts in women and the penis in men; increased heart rate, blood pressure, and body temperature; and flushing of the skin and increased sweating.

Plateau, the second stage, involves an intensification of the physiological changes occurring in the arousal stage: heart rate and blood pressure further increase and breathing becomes heavy. In women, the VULVA reddens, the CLITORIS enlarges, and the VAGINA opens and widens. In men, the penis is fully erect. Involuntary movements occur as muscle tension increases.

Orgasm, or climax, the third stage, is a series of pleasurable contractions. In women they are centered in the muscles surrounding the vagina and the area between the vulva and the anus. In men, the muscles at the base of the penis and the anus contract. Contractions lasting about one-eighth of a second can be felt in other parts of the body. Blood pressure, heart

5

rate, and breathing rate reach their peaks. Men have orgasms in two stages that often are experienced simultaneously. First, the prostate and other glands contract, forcing semen (the fluid that carries sperm) into the base of the urethra; then, orgasmic contractions of the penis and urethra cause ejaculation of the fluid.

In resolution, the fourth stage, the body returns gradually to its unaroused state. Muscles relax; blood pressure, heart rate and breathing decrease; and individuals usually experience a sense of deep relaxation.

Sexuality

All aspects of a person's life related to sex, including physical and psychological development, as well as sexual thoughts, fantasy, behavior and activity, attitudes, relationships, gender identity, selection of partners, and reproduction. Sexuality changes throughout life.

BEFORE BIRTH

During the first 6 weeks after fertilization, male and female human embryos are identical except for their chromosomes. The male has an X and a Y chromosome, and the female has two X chromosomes. When no Y chromosome is present, the gonads develop into ovaries. In the presence of a Y chromosome, they develop into testicles, which begin producing male hormones (androgens, mainly testosterone) by the eighth week. The androgens promote the development of the penis, scrotum, and other male genital structures. Without androgens, these tissues develop into the female reproductive and genital organs. The different hormones in two sexes also make for differences in the development of the brain. The significance of these differences for variations between men and women in later life is unclear and the subject of research and debate.

CHILDHOOD

Beginning at birth, a baby is treated in a manner considered culturally appropriate to its gender. This sex-role socialization applies to such areas as expected behavior, toys, and play. From birth, boys can achieve erections and girls can become vaginally lubricated. Many small children masturbate simply because the stimulation feels good. Young chil-

dren are also curious about their parents' bodies, may want to touch or explore, and sometimes engage in exploratory games with playmates. These behaviors are seen as normal. However, by age 6 or 7 most children in a nonnudist culture develop a sense of privacy and do not like to be seen unclothed or to see their parents or other adults exposed.

PUBERTY AND ADOLESCENCE

This stage is marked by the development of the genitals, the appearance of secondary sexual characteristics such as increased height, muscles, and a deeper voice in boys and a rounder body shape and breasts in girls, and the development of reproductive capacity in both sexes (see PUBERTY). As puberty progresses, interest in sex surges. At some point during adolescence, if not before, most individuals become aware of their SEXUAL ORIENTATION as homosexual, heterosexual, or bisexual. Fears and worries about sexual orientation are common, particularly among homosexual and bisexual adolescents, who may be subjected to ridicule, ostracism, or even violence from their peers, teachers, parents, and others.

ADULTHOOD

From the 20s on, sexuality is expressed principally in longer-term relationships, such as dating, marriage, or living-together arrangements. The frequency of sexual activity varies from individual to individual. In most cases, couples make love less the longer they are together. Sexuality, however, continues well into old age.

Research has shown that the majority of married people past age 70 still engage in lovemaking, even though physical changes that accompany aging can lead to a decline in the frequency of sexual activity. After menopause, the walls of the woman's vagina thin, and the amount of lubrication lessens.

In men, testosterone production decreases with age, leading to less force and lower volume in ejaculation, adding to the time needed to achieve erection, and increasing the period between erections. Erectile dysfunction (impotence) is more common in older men because of medications, vascular diseases (which may impede blood flow into

the penis), diabetes mellitus, and other diseases. Erection therapy has become a subspecialty of many urologists because of the millions of older men seeking help.

Sexually transmitted diseases

A large group of disease syndromes that are transmitted by sexual contact and sexual activities. Sexually transmitted diseases include more than 25 different infectious diseases that are spread from one person to another via behavior involving the genitals, with or without apparent symptoms and signs in the genital area. The term sexually transmitted diseases, or STDs, includes a wider range of illnesses and infectious syndromes than the previously used and outdated term, "venereal disease."

Although the incidence of STDs increased steadily between the 1950s and the 1970s, the numbers of new cases generally stabilized in the 1980s, with the exception in the rise of HIV (human immunodeficiency virus) cases and of AIDS (acquired immunodeficiency syndrome). SYPHILIS and GONORRHEA showed decreased growth from the mid-1980s to the mid-1990s in the United States and elsewhere. Nevertheless, certain STDs remain widespread in the United States, and STD incidence rates remain high in most of the world, even with new advances in diagnosis and treatment. It is estimated that more than 40 million people have chronic genital herpes (see HERPES, GENITAL), for example, and that there are 4 million new cases of CHLAMYDIA each year.

Some bacterial STDs, including syphilis, gonorrhea, and chlamydia, can have long-term consequences, including PELVIC INFLAMMATORY DISEASE, which may cause INFERTILITY in women. HUMAN PAPILLOMAVIRUS (HPV) is the cause of genital warts and is known to be associated with cervical cancer (see CERVIX, CANCER OF) in women. STDs can make a person more susceptible to infection with HIV, the virus that causes AIDS.

Teenagers are at the highest risk for contracting STDs of any segment of the population in the United States.

This is partially due to teenagers' tendency toward more risk-prone behavior and also to this age group's greater biological vulnerability to certain infections. Chlamydia and gonorrhea infections occur more readily in the cervix of a teenage girl, for example.

Women in general have a higher risk than men of acquiring STDs during heterosexual intercourse, and women are at great risk of sustaining long-term consequences as a result of STDs. For example, a woman is twice as likely as a man to be infected with chlamydia in a single act of unprotected intercourse with an infected partner. Women may also undergo more severe and persistent complications of STDs because the anatomy of their genitalia can obscure early signs and symptoms of infection. As a result, their STDs may not receive the early medical treatment that can prevent disease progression and long-term consequences. Also, during pregnancy, STDs can cause complications and may produce disease or abnormalities in the fetus.

CAUSES, SYMPTOMS, AND DIAGNOSIS

Any person who is sexually active is susceptible to STDs, and it is estimated that 1 in 5 people in the United States is a carrier. These diseases are transmitted by contact with infected body secretions, including semen, blood, and vaginal fluids. Several pathogens can infect these secretions and be sexually transmitted to cause STDs. These include bacteria, including those that cause gonorrhea, syphilis, and chlamydia among other STDs; viruses, which are responsible for STDs including herpes simplex, human papillomavirus, strains of HEPATITIS, MOLLUSCUM CONTAGIOSUM, CYTOMEGALOVIRUS, and HIV and AIDS; protozoa, such as those causing TRICHOMONIASIS; fungi; and ectoparasite infestations, including CRAB LICE. Some STD syndromes may be caused by more than one pathogen, and a single pathogen can result in multiple STD syndromes. Multiple bacterial and viral infections, and parasitic infestations, may be frequent in people who engage in oral-genital or oral-anal sexual behavior with many partners.

An infected person may not have symptoms of an STD. Most people

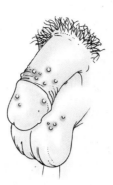

SYMPTOMS OF HERPES
The symptoms of genital herpes in a man may start as a swollen, reddened, itchy spot on the penis and then become a group of small blisters. However, many STDs do not have obvious symptoms at all in men or women—which is why prevention is so important.

who are infected with HIV have no symptoms. If there are STD symptoms, they may include sores, pain, and itching in the genital area for both men and women. In addition, men may experience a discharge from the penis, painful urination, and swelling and pain in the testicles. Women may notice a vaginal discharge or change in usual vaginal secretions. If an STD has progressed to pelvic inflammatory disease, there may be lower abdominal pain and painful sexual intercourse.

STDs are often difficult to diagnose. In some cases, there are identifiable symptoms, such as a discharge or genital warts. However, genital warts may not appear for 2 to 5 months after infection with the human papillomavirus, and very small warts inside the opening of the penis may be detected only by a doctor. Many people with STDs do not have symptoms. Gonorrhea symptoms, for example, may not appear in women until 60 days after the infection has occurred.

Clinical examinations and laboratory testing can identify characteristic symptoms and infective pathogens, but for many STDs, there is no completely accurate test that can confirm the diagnosis. An infection may be present without being identified with medical testing for several days, or even several years. Also, a person who has an early or mild infection may have negative test results despite the presence of an STD.

TREATMENT AND PREVENTION

Treatment of STDs depends on the infective pathogen involved. Bacterial STDs, including gonorrhea, chlamydia, syphilis, and CHANCROID, are treated with antibiotic therapy and can be cured with treatment.

There are no available treatments for some viral STDs such as herpes, which tends to become a lifelong infection, but there are methods for minimizing some of their symptoms, including using prescribed medications such as acyclovir, famciclovir, or valaciclovir to help speed the healing process. Outpatient surgery may be recommended to treat genital warts and sometimes provides an effective cure. There are new medical approaches to controlling the progress of HIV and AIDS, and there is increased success with treating associated illnesses, but there is no cure for hepatitis. Treatment is based on medical strategies for treating related illnesses and symptoms. STDs caused by fungi and parasites may be treated with oral medications and topical preparations.

An important aspect of medical treatment for STDs involves locating and treating the sexual contacts of infected persons. Medical monitoring of people who have been treated is also essential to assure that the infections have been cured and will not continue to be spread. Public education on SAFER SEX techniques and the prevention of STDs is another vital element in reducing the incidence.

Abstinence from all forms of sexual activity is the only completely effective way to prevent infection with STDs. This approach may not be an option for many people, and avoidance of direct oral, genital, or anal contact with sexual partners is the first line of defense for sexually active people. It is also helpful to limit the number of sexual partners. Any strategy or barrier device that limits a person's exposure to a sexual partner's bodily secretions, including semen, vaginal fluid, and blood, can help to reduce the risk of infection with an STD. The proper use of condoms or other latex barriers during sexual contact has been proven to reduce risks, but does not guarantee absolute protection, espe-

5

cially against viruses. Incorrect and sporadic use of barriers decreases their risk-reduction capacity.

Seeking immediate medical treatment when an STD is suspected can prevent severe infection and long-term consequences. Abstaining from sexual activity until a doctor has determined that the infection is no longer contagious helps prevent reinfection and halts the spread of STDs. Informing all sexual partners so they can be treated is also essential to preventing further transmission.

Clinical trials of STD vaccines are currently underway, but at present, there is no effective vaccine available for prevention of STDs.

Sézary syndrome

A rare condition caused by lymph node abnormalities, skin rashes, and abnormally circulating T cells (see T CELL). Sézary syndrome is a form of the primary cutaneous T-cell LYMPHOMA (cancer of the lymph nodes). In this syndrome, there is an abnormal overgrowth of lymphoid cells (lymphocytes) in the skin, liver, spleen, and lymph nodes. Immunosuppression may result in an increased incidence of SQUAMOUS CELL CARCINOMA (a form of SKIN CANCER) and internal malignant neoplasms (cancerous tumors). The first signs of Sézary syndrome are often red, scaly patches on the skin that spread to form a severe, flaky, itchy rash over the entire body. Other symptoms include an accumulation of fluid beneath the skin, baldness, and distorted nail growth. Treatment is with anticancer drugs and RADIATION THERAPY. However, Sézary syndrome is an aggressive disease with a median survival rate of less than 3 years.

Shaken baby syndrome

A severe and potentially fatal form of child abuse in which the abuser violently shakes a baby. An infant's head is heavy in relation to the rest of his or her body. Because the neck is not strong enough to support the head, shaking a baby strains the neck muscles and upper spine severely. Shaking or throwing down the baby in anger can cause blindness, eye injury, brain damage, and death. It most often involves babies younger than 6 months of age. Caregivers sometimes shake a baby when excessive crying perturbs

them. Doctors are required by law to report all cases of this and other forms of child abuse to legal authorities.

SYMPTOMS AND DIAGNOSIS

The signs of shaken baby syndrome range from subtle to severe. A shaken infant may exhibit symptoms such as poor feeding, vomiting, lethargy, or irritability. These signs can be mistaken for those of a mild virus or colic. In some children, there may be telltale marks on the upper arms or whatever part of the body was grasped when the baby was shaken. Severe shaking can lead immediately to respiratory difficulty, a seizure, or loss of consciousness.

Shaken baby syndrome can be difficult to diagnose. Often there are no visible external injuries. Violently shaking a baby can cause serious damage to the interior of a baby's eyes and to the brain, injuries that are hard to detect in their less extreme forms and sometimes are detected inadvertently. A regular physical examination may reveal unexplained bruising on a baby's body. X rays, typically used to investigate respiratory difficulties, sometimes show unexplained rib fractures. Once abuse is suspected, CT (computed tomography) scanning may be used to evaluate the nature and extent of a suspected brain injury. Sometimes MRI (magnetic resonance imaging) is also used. A SPINAL TAP may yield bloody fluid, also evidence of brain injury. The results of an eye examination in which the pupils are dilated can reveal the retinal hemorrhage that is typical of shaken baby syndrome.

TREATMENT

In addition to the care of a pediatrician or family physician, a shaken baby may require treatment by a neurologist, neurosurgeon, or ophthalmologist. A neurologist can evaluate an infant's head injury and refer the child to a neurosurgeon if necessary. An ophthalmologist can treat injuries to the eyes. In addition to treatment of the original injury, follow-up care is necessary. The long-term consequences of shaken baby syndrome include mental retardation, severe motor dysfunction, seizure, and blindness. Because shaken baby syndrome is a form of abuse, assessing the home situation and reporting the case to the local child protective agency is mandatory (see ABUSE, CHILD).

Shave bumps

Papules (small superficial bumps on the skin) or pustules (small pus-filled blisters) that commonly occur in the beard, on the legs, or in the groin; also known as pseudofolliculitis. (See also HAIR REMOVAL.) Shave bumps are a common skin condition in the beard area of black men and others who have curly hair. Shave bumps often result as a foreign-body reaction to a hair. A sharp, tapered hair reenters the skin as it matures. Inflammation of the hair follicles may also occur from razors harboring bacteria. Pustules can develop when shaving nicks become infected or when hair follicles become clogged with debris. Treatment of shave bumps caused by a bacterial infection is with prescription antibiotics.

To prevent shave bumps, doctors recommend avoiding close shaves. The skin should be dampened and lubricated with a shaving gel or cream and should not be stretched before shaving. People with a tendency to have shave bumps should shave in the direction of hair growth and should pat (rather than rub) the skin dry, and use a moisturizing lotion after shaving.

Shiatsu

Japanese massage therapy. Shiatsu, which literally means "finger pressure," is used to release energy ("ki") in the body at points where it is blocked. Shiatsu practitioners use knuckles, fingers, thumbs, palms, elbows, knees, and feet to apply pressure to specific points on the body thought to correspond to energy channels, known as meridians. Shiatsu is similar to ACUPRESSURE, particularly in its emphasis on unblocking the flow of energy. However, in shiatsu it is common to massage the entire length of a meridian, rather than specific points, to maximize the flow of ki. Shiatsu is used to maintain health and prevent disease rather than to treat specific ailments. Followers believe blocked ki is thought to cause pain, emotional distress, fatigue, depression, and eventually, disease.

Shigellosis

An infectious disease caused by a genus of bacteria called *Shigella* that causes diarrhea in humans.

S

Shigellosis, also known as dysentery, is transmitted by contact with an infected person's diarrheal stools and occurs most commonly when basic personal hygiene, including hand washing, is not practiced. The infection tends to occur among toddlers who are not fully toilet-trained and is often spread in child care settings. Family members who are in contact with toddlers between the ages of 2 and 4 are also more likely to contract the disease.

Shigellosis can also be acquired by ingesting food that has become contaminated by infected food handlers. Food contamination may also occur when vegetables are exposed to sewage during growing or harvesting. Flies that breed in infected feces may also contaminate food. A natural body of water can be contaminated with sewage or by an infected person swimming in the water. Swimming in or drinking contaminated water can cause shigellosis. The disease is more common in developing countries than in the United States, and in many of those communities, the infection is present most of the time.

SYMPTOMS, DIAGNOSIS, AND TREATMENT

Infected people develop diarrhea, fever, and stomach cramps within 1 or 2 days of exposure. The diarrhea may be bloody and become so severe that hospitalization becomes necessary, especially when young children, people who are older, or people with impaired immune systems have severe diarrhea. Children younger than 2 years may have high fever and seizures. In some cases, a person infected with shigellosis has no symptoms but can still transmit the disease.

The infection is diagnosed by laboratory tests that identify the *Shigella* bacteria in a stool specimen of an infected person. More specialized tests may be required to identify the specific type of *Shigella* bacteria causing the infection. These tests can help determine the appropriate antibiotic for treating shigellosis. Correct antibiotic therapy kills the *Shigella* bacteria in an infected person's stools and shortens the length of the illness. Some of these bacteria have become resistant to antibiotics, and the continuing use of antibiotics can increase the bacteria's resistance

to this therapy in the future. Mild infections generally improve without treatment in 5 to 7 days, but it may take several months for bowel habits to become normal again. In rare cases, REITER SYNDROME is a complication of shigellosis.

Shin splints

An injury common to runners that involves one of the muscles in the lower leg pulling on the shinbone (tibia), which sometimes results in tiny tears in the muscle. Usually the anterior tibial muscle located on the front of the shin is affected. Shin splints cause pain along the front or inner side of the shin, depending on the muscle involved. Anterior tibial stress syndrome is the term for shin splints that appear at the front of the shin, and medial tibial stress syndrome is the medical name given to shin splints on the side of the shin. Stretching can make the pain worse.

SYMPTOMS

The pain of shin splints may be felt at the start of a run or jog and decrease gradually as the workout continues, or it may be felt throughout the activity. Runners may have a tendency to roll the foot inward, called overpronation (see PRONATION), or roll the foot outward, called oversupina-

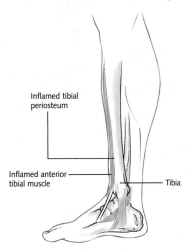

Inflamed tibial periosteum

Inflamed anterior tibial muscle

Tibia

PAIN IN THE LOWER LEG
The pain of shin splints can occur on different parts of the shin, depending on the structure affected. Many injuries involve the anterior tibial muscle, located on the front of the shin, just next to the shin bone (tibia). Another common site of injury is the tibial periosteum (outer covering of bone). These injuries can occur in athletes at all levels of fitness.

tion (see SUPINATION). An improper shoe fit or wearing shoes that are worn out and have lost their support may contribute to shin splints. The fit and support of footgear is especially important when running or jogging on hard indoor surfaces or on outdoor streets. A sudden and dramatic increase in training time or intensity or a change in running surface can cause shin splints. A person who has one leg even slightly longer than the other or who has an improper running form can also be a candidate for shin splints.

When the pain is intense and localized on the shin bone, medical attention should be sought to rule out the possibility of a stress fracture or other bone or muscle lesions. A doctor may diagnose the source of pain by using an X ray, a bone scan, MRI (magnetic resonance imaging), or a CT (computed tomography) scan. If shin splints are found to be the basis for the pain, the doctor may pinpoint the specific cause by taking a detailed history of the person's athletic activity.

TREATMENT

Stopping the exercise that caused the pain is generally recommended the first 2 to 3 days after symptoms appear, depending on the individual. The pain may be treated by applying ice before and after training. Nonsteroidal anti-inflammatory drugs (NSAIDs), such as aspirin and ibuprofen, may help. Taping or splinting the affected area is sometimes beneficial. Physical therapy, including whirlpool, ultrasound massage, and exercises to strengthen and stretch the muscles, may be prescribed.

In some cases, the pain disappears without treatment and then suddenly recurs. Pain without direct trauma during any athletic activity is almost always a sign of excessive training and should be observed as a signal that the affected leg requires rest and care. When the pain of shin splints is persistent and prolonged, consultation with a sports medicine specialist is recommended.

Shingles

A painful rash that is a second outbreak of the varicella-zoster virus, the virus that causes CHICKENPOX; also known as herpes zoster. Shingles is due to reactivation of the virus that remains dormant in the body after

S

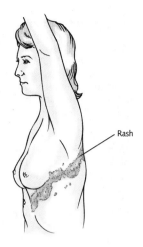

Rash

A VIRUS IN THE NERVES
The painful rash of shingles often wraps around the body, along the strip of skin supplied by one pair of spinal nerves (which exit from the spinal cord). The rash may be intermittent along the pathway, or the entire path may be involved. The shingles virus lives in the nerves throughout the person's lifetime.

S

causing the initial chickenpox infection. Most adults have had chickenpox and are at risk for developing shingles. However, individuals who have never had chickenpox should be immunized with the varicella vaccine.

Shingles is characterized by a rash and blisters that typically occur on one side of the body following the path of a nerve. The rash often wraps around part of the chest or back. Blisters near an eye require evaluation by an ophthalmologist because permanent eye damage can result.

Shingles usually heal within a few weeks. However, in some older people or those people with weakened immune systems, an agonizing condition called postherpetic neuralgia can result.

Postherpetic neuralgia is caused by nerve damage. In this condition, a person continues to experience severe pain in the areas where blisters occurred, even after the skin has healed. The pain can be sharp, burning, or aching. The skin may become hypersensitive to changes in temperature or to the slightest touch.

Doctors recommend seeking medical treatment at the first sign of itching, burning, and tingling. The virus that causes shingles can be passed on only to people who have not had chickenpox. Primary treatment of

shingles, with antiviral drugs such as acyclovir, is most effective when begun within 3 days of developing the rash. Applying cool compresses and soothing lotions may help relieve the itching and burning. Other treatments include anti-inflammatory drugs and pain medications. Sometimes antidepressants, capsaicin cream, and certain antiseizure medicines are prescribed to relieve the painful symptoms of postherpetic neuralgia.

Shivering

Involuntary contraction of muscles in the skin in response to low temperatures or the start of a fever.

Shock

See SHOCK, PHYSIOLOGICAL.

Shock therapy

See ECT (electroconvulsive shock therapy).

Shock, anaphylactic

A life-threatening type of allergic reaction affecting the entire body. Anaphylactic shock occurs when a person has been sensitized to a substance and the immune system has been triggered to recognize that substance as a threat. If the sensitized person encounters the substance again, the body reacts with a sudden, severe reaction affecting all body systems. Symptoms include hives; itching; swelling of the eyes, lips, tongue, hands, and feet; wheezing, coughing, and breathing problems; blue or red skin; and dizziness, confusion, rapid pulse, nausea and vomiting, diarrhea, and abdominal cramps. Symptoms usually develop rapidly, within seconds or minutes.

Anaphylactic shock can occur in response to any allergen. Common causes include insect bites or stings, horse serum used in some vaccinations, food allergies, and drug allergies. Pollens and other inhaled allergens rarely cause anaphylactic shock. Although anaphylactic shock occurs infrequently, it is life-threatening and can occur at any time. To prevent it, people with known allergies should avoid the suspect allergens, and people with histories of allergic reactions to insect bites or stings may be instructed to carry an emergency kit containing injectable epinephrine to

use in an episode of anaphylactic shock.

Shock, electric

Injury caused by exposure of skin or internal organs to electric current. The human body is a conductor of electricity, and direct contact with electrical current can be fatal. Electric current can cause injury in three ways: by causing cardiac arrest, by damaging muscle tissue, or by burning the skin.

While some electrical burns look minor, serious internal damage may have occurred, especially to the heart or the brain. Symptoms of electric shock may include fatigue, broken bones, headache, impaired hearing, heart attack, hyperventilation, muscle pain, breathing problems, vision loss, and unconsciousness.

First aid for electric shock includes shutting off the electric current, if possible. If turning off the power source is not possible, a dry, nonconducting object such as a broom, wooden chair, rubber doormat, or rug can be used to push the person away from the source of the electrical current. A person should never touch an individual who is still in contact with the electrical source. Once away from the source of the current, the person's breathing should be checked, and rescue breathing or cardiopulmonary resuscitation (CPR) should be started if necessary. Any burned skin should be bathed in cool running water to help relieve pain. Emergency medical

---

PREVENTING ELECTRIC SHOCK

Receiving an electric shock can cause a person to stop breathing or the heart to stop beating. Here are ways to prevent a serious electric shock:

- Child safety plugs should be placed in electrical outlets.
- Electrical cords must be kept out of the reach of children.
- Children should be taught the dangers of electricity.
- Electrical appliances should never be used in the tub or shower or while wet.
- Electrical kitchen appliances should not be used while touching faucets or cold water pipes.

care should be sought, to make sure no internal injury has occurred. See CPR steps on page 1328.

Shock, insulin

A condition in which an abnormally low blood sugar (glucose) level results in unconsciousness; also called hypoglycemia. Insulin shock occurs when excessive insulin is released into the bloodstream by the pancreas; it is most likely to occur in a person who takes insulin for diabetes. Insulin shock is most likely to occur several hours after eating or after exercise. Symptoms are progressive: over a period of less than an hour, a person experiencing an insulin reaction can progress from feeling nervous, hungry, apprehensive, and confused to sweating profusely to loss of consciousness or seizure.

First aid measures for insulin shock include providing the person with some kind of carbohydrate or sugar, such as orange juice, candy, or carbonated drinks made with sugar. Symptoms usually disappear within 15 to 30 minutes from the time the sugar is consumed, although sometimes it takes longer for full mental function to be restored. If the person does not recover promptly, emergency medical assistance should be sought.

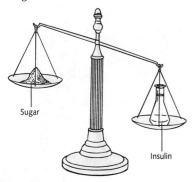

IMBALANCE OF GLUCOSE AND INSULIN
Insulin shock, or hypoglycemia, occurs when the body's level of insulin (a hormone that increases the use of glucose by the body) is too high and the level of blood glucose (sugar) is too low. Providing the person with a carbohydrate or sugar helps bring the level of glucose back up.

Shock, physiological

A condition occurring when insufficient blood flows through the body. Physiological shock is characterized by very low blood pressure, a decreased amount of urine, and cell or tissue damage. Physiological shock is a common complication of injury, infection, and burns, and it can also be caused by any condition that reduces blood flow, such as acute heart failure, bleeding, vomiting, diarrhea, inadequate fluid intake or DEHYDRATION, or kidney disease. Symptoms of physiological shock include irritability or lethargy; bluish lips and fingernails; chest pain; cool, clammy skin; cold hands and feet; dizziness or feeling faint; nausea and vomiting; rapid pulse; shallow breathing; excessive thirst; unconsciousness; weakness; and confusion.

If physiological shock is suspected, emergency medical aid should be sought immediately. Physiological shock is a life-threatening condition, and it can get worse very suddenly. Immediate first aid measures that should be taken while waiting for medical assistance include placing the person on his or her back with feet elevated higher than the head to maintain blood flow to the brain. Tight clothing should be loosened, and the person should be covered with a blanket if the weather is cool. If the weather is hot, the person should be shaded from the sun, if possible.

Shock, septic

See SEPTIC SHOCK.

Shock, spinal

Type of shock caused by a failure of the vascular system to respond to stimuli as a result of neurological damage to the spinal cord. Spinal shock occurs in response to neurological trauma. Symptoms include very low blood pressure and rapid heartbeat. Traumatic spinal shock is a medical emergency, and medical assistance must be sought. While awaiting medical assistance, the person should be kept lying down on his or her back, with the feet higher than the head, to maintain blood flow to the brain. Blankets should be used to keep the person warm.

Short stature

A term applied to individuals who are among the shortest 5 percent of people of their age and sex. Short stature may be a symptom of a medical condition, such as delayed or precocious puberty, HYPOTHYROIDISM, or SKELETAL DYSPLASIA, among others, or it may represent a normal inherited trait. People of short stature can sometimes benefit from growth hormone medication.

Shortness of breath

See BREATH, SHORTNESS OF.

Shoulder separation

A severe sports injury caused by a strong force powerful enough to tear the ligaments that connect the bones of the shoulder joint. Shoulder separation most commonly occurs in young adults who are involved in contact sports such as football, hockey, and soccer. The injury may also occur as a result of a hard fall during sports activities. See also SHOULDER, DISLOCATED.

Shoulder, dislocated

An injury in which the ends of the bones that form the shoulder joint are forced from their normal positions. A dislocated shoulder is usually caused by a blow, a fall, or other trauma. The shoulder has the greatest range of motion of any joint in the body, which makes it particularly prone to dislocation. An injured shoulder that is visibly out of position, misshapen, swollen, difficult to move, and intensely painful probably has been dislocated or broken. Numbness can indicate nerve damage. Medical attention should be sought immediately. A dislocated shoulder is diagnosed by physical examination and X ray and treated by a procedure called REDUCTION, followed by at least 2 weeks of arm immobilization in a sling.

Shoulder-hand syndrome

A chronic, painful condition that most commonly affects the arm or leg, but may develop in any part of the body. Shoulder-hand syndrome is most commonly seen in people who have had a stroke. Treatment includes reducing pain with medications, such as anti-inflammatory drugs, and providing the person with active range-of-motion exercises. See REFLEX SYMPATHETIC DYSTROPHY.

S

Shunt

An abnormal or surgically created passage between two usually unconnected body channels or cavities. Shunting is surgical creation of a passage that is commonly performed to relieve HYDROCEPHALUS, an accumulation of fluid in the brain. In this procedure, a drain or shunt is implanted from the ventricle in the brain to the abdominal cavity to drain obstructed spinal fluid. The procedure prevents pressure buildup and consequent complications, such as brain damage, seizures, or blindness.

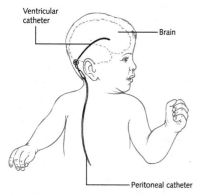

Ventricular catheter

Brain

Peritoneal catheter

INTRACRANIAL SHUNT
In a child with hydrocephalus (excess cerebrospinal fluid in the brain), an intracranial shunt drains excess fluid. The shunt consists of a ventricular catheter (tube into the ventricles, or spaces, in the brain) and a peritoneal catheter (tube into the peritoneal, or abdominal, cavity). The lining of the peritoneal cavity absorbs the fluid. The shunt lies entirely inside the body.

There are many other types of shunts. For example, an arteriovenous (or AV) shunt permits blood to flow from an artery to a vein without passing through a capillary network, a cardiovascular shunt is an abnormal passage between heart chambers or between systemic and pulmonary circulatory systems, a dialysis shunt is an external link in the arm or leg between a peripheral artery and a vein to permit hemodialysis, and an external shunt is a device that allows the passage of body fluid between different body cavities.

Shy-Drager syndrome

A progressive disorder of the central and autonomic nervous systems. Shy-Drager syndrome is also known as multiple system atrophy with autonomic failure. Its hallmark symptom is postural hypotension, a condition in which a person experiences a drop in blood pressure upon standing or sitting up. This causes dizziness and blackouts.

There are three types of Shy-Drager syndrome: the parkinsonian type, the cerebellar type, and the combination type. Symptoms of the parkinsonian type include slow movement, stiff muscles, and mild tremors. The cerebellar type is characterized by loss of balance and a tendency to fall. In the combination type, there are symptoms of both the parkinsonian and cerebellar varieties. Other signs of Shy-Drager syndrome include constipation, sexual impotence in men, generalized weakness, vision disturbances, speech impairment, difficulty breathing and swallowing, sensory changes, heartbeat irregularities, an inability to sweat, and diarrhea. Unstable blood pressure typically leads to severe headaches.

Shy-Drager syndrome is usually diagnosed by a neurologist after a careful assessment of symptoms. Treatment is difficult because of the fluctuations in blood pressure. Antiparkinsonian medication such as levodopa may be helpful, but must be used with care because it can lower blood pressure. Corticosteroids can relieve low blood pressure, but are associated with many side effects. Dietary increases of fluid and salt can help elevate blood pressure, and it may be useful to sleep in a head-up position at night. Some people eventually require an artificial feeding or breathing tube.

Sialadenitis

Inflammation of the salivary gland, which is a symptom of an infection, often caused by bacteria, that develops in the gland as the result of an obstruction of the duct, or tube, that carries saliva from the gland into the mouth. The obstruction may be due to SALIVARY GLAND STONES in the duct or to abnormalities in the duct system of the major salivary glands; the ducts may have small constrictions or narrowings that interfere with the normal flow of saliva. Infections of the salivary glands may also be caused by a virus (see MUMPS).

SYMPTOMS
Bacterial infections and obstructions of saliva flow most often affect the glands in the neck near the angle of the jaw. The saliva that cannot pass freely through the duct pools in the gland and becomes infected, causing swelling and pain.

These symptoms may become more severe when the glands are actively producing saliva, such as when a person is eating. Over time and if infected salivary glands are not treated properly, they may become abscessed.

DIAGNOSIS AND TREATMENT
A person with swelling in the mouth, under the chin, or around the jaw, with or without fever, should consult a physician or dentist. Sialadenitis is generally diagnosed with laboratory tests.

If the condition is due to a bacterial infection, antibiotics will probably be prescribed. If obstruction is the suspected cause of the infection, it may be necessary to anesthetize the openings of the ducts in order to probe and open them. If the infection persists, a doctor may recommend a sialogram (X ray of the salivary gland) or a CT (computed tomography) scan. If there is irreversible damage to the gland, it might have to be surgically removed. Other salivary glands can compensate for the one removed.

Sibling rivalry

Competition, resentment, or jealousy among brothers and sisters in the same family. Sibling rivalry exists in

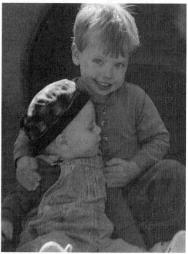

SIBLINGS' NATURAL FEELINGS
An older child feels important and needed when parents ask for help with a younger brother or sister.

S

nearly any family with more than one child. The typical scenario emerges when a new baby arrives. Older children are no longer the center of attention and consequently feel jealous and resentful. This dynamic is especially true when there are close age differences of 1½ to 3 years. Because preschool children have difficulty in sharing their parents' attention, they feel the most intense jealousy toward a newborn brother or sister. As children grow up together, they gradually become friends. However, some degree of competition and squabbling over toys or privileges are likely to remain. Intense sibling rivalry rarely lasts into adulthood.

THE NEW SIBLING

An older child can be made ready for the arrival of a new sibling. Involving an older child in the preparations for the new baby's arrival can help address feelings of insecurity. An older child might help pick out baby clothes or fix up the baby's room. Reading books about infant care with the parents can be helpful. Changes such as moving a child from a crib to a bed or into a new room should be made several months before a new baby is born. In this way, an older sibling is less likely to associate the change with the baby or feel resentment toward him or her.

The older sibling's involvement should continue once a new baby is born. For example, he or she might hold or feed the infant. A preschool child may regress at this time by sucking a thumb or wanting his or her bottle back. School-age children may react to a new sibling with pleas for attention in the form of aggression or misbehavior. Parents should respond with patience and understanding. Older siblings need reassurance that they are still loved and have not been replaced. Despite their natural feelings, older children need to recognize that aggression toward a baby is unacceptable. If an older sibling is dangerously aggressive toward a new baby, parents should consult the pediatrician or family physician. In some cases, the doctor may refer the family to a mental health professional for counseling.

Sibutramine

An appetite suppressant. Sibutramine (Meridia) is used with a reduced-calorie diet and exercise to help very overweight (obese) people lose weight and maintain weight loss. Sibutramine is thought to work by increasing the levels of the neurotransmitters norepinephrine and serotonin in the brain, which causes a feeling of fullness after a person begins to eat.

Sick building syndrome

A set of symptoms characterized by fatigue, headaches, eye irritation, dizziness, and respiratory complaints that affect people who work in modern airtight office buildings.

Although the exact cause of the syndrome remains unknown, it is believed to be caused by long-term exposure to low concentrations of airborne pollutants such as mold, formaldehyde fumes from the furniture and dry wall, carpet glues, latex caulking, and pesticides. Sick building syndrome became a problem once building design focused on the use of windows that do not open.

Modifications to buildings, such as an improvement in ventilation, may be beneficial. Doctors may recommend antihistamines, analgesics, and other medications to control symptoms.

Sick sinus syndrome

A group of signs and symptoms caused by inadequate function of the heart's natural pacemaker. In the healthy HEART, a region known as the sinus node initiates the heartbeat. If the sinus node malfunctions, it may initiate the heartbeat too slowly, pause for too long between beats, skip beats, or fire too rapidly. If it stops functioning altogether, another part of the heart's electrical system takes over the sinus node's role, but usually at a heart rate that is substantially lower than normal.

The leading sign of sick sinus syndrome is bradycardia, a slow heartbeat, less than 60 beats per minute. Palpitations (uncomfortably rapid heartbeats) may also occur, or the person may sense both fast and slow heartbeats.

Sick sinus syndrome may develop slowly over years, and its signs often pass unnoticed until the heartbeat drops below 50 beats per minute and the condition is advanced. At that point, fainting spells, chest pain from insufficient blood supply to the heart, dizziness, shortness of breath, unusual fatigue, disturbed sleep, muscle aches, or confusion may arise. If sick sinus syndrome continues untreated, it may lead to heart failure as the heart cannot supply sufficient blood to the body.

Sick sinus syndrome may develop as a result of other diseases. Possible causes include cardiac ischemia (insufficient blood flow to the heart), heart attack, kidney failure, certain medications (antiarrhythmics, beta blockers, and cardiotonics), hypothyroidism (an underactive thyroid), hypoglycemia (abnormally low blood sugar levels), sleep apnea (breathing disturbances during sleep), cardiomyopathy (impaired heart muscle function), diphtheria, hemochromatosis (an abnormal accumulation of iron in the tissues), muscular dystrophy, and amyloidosis (abnormal accumulation of the body protein amyloid in the tissues). Sick sinus syndrome is often associated with coronary artery disease, hypertension (high blood pressure), or diseased heart valves. It is not known, however, whether these three diseases actually cause the syndrome or whether they are simply likely to occur along with it.

Sick sinus syndrome is relatively uncommon and particularly rare among those younger than 50. In children, the syndrome occurs principally among those who have undergone open-heart surgery.

In its mild form with no symptoms, sick sinus syndrome requires no treatment. Treatment begins only when the syndrome becomes advanced and symptoms are distressing or dangerous. The usual treatment consists of surgically implanting a pacemaker, an electronic device that controls heartbeat, and prescribing antiarrhythmic medications to prevent abnormal heartbeat rhythms. If the person has coronary artery disease, BALLOON ANGIOPLASTY may be performed to improve blood flow to the heart muscle.

Sickle cell anemia

An inherited, chronic blood disorder that alters the shape of red blood cells and causes them to function abnor-

5

mally; also known as sickle cell disease. The cause of the disease is an abnormality in hemoglobin, the pigment in red blood cells that transports oxygen. After they give up their oxygen, molecules of the abnormal hemoglobin, called hemoglobin S, tend to clump into rods that deform the normally round red blood cells into sickle shapes. Unable to squeeze through small blood vessels because of their shape, the sickle cells block blood flow, causing tissue and organ damage and pain. In addition, the sickle cells have a life span of only 10 to 12 days versus 120 days for normal red blood cells. The body cannot replace them fast enough, resulting in anemia, an ongoing decline in red blood cells.

CAUSE AND INCIDENCE
Sickle cell anemia results from a defect in the gene that codes for the hemoglobin protein. If a child inherits this gene from only one parent, he or she is said to have SICKLE CELL TRAIT. Sickle cell anemia occurs only in those who inherit the gene from both parents.

Sickle cell trait and sickle cell anemia occur primarily in people whose ancestry can be traced to sub-Saharan Africa, parts of the Middle East, India, and the Mediterranean. In the United States, the disease occurs in approximately 1 of every 500 blacks and in 1 of every 1,000 to 1,400 Hispanic Americans. One in 12 blacks carries the sickle cell trait.

SYMPTOMS AND COMPLICATIONS
The clinical manifestation of sickle cell anemia varies from one person to another. Some people have mild symptoms, while others have severe manifestations of the disease. Blockage of blood vessels by sickle cells cause many of the symptoms.

Children with sickle cell anemia do not usually show evidence of the disease until they reach 4 months of age. One of the first signs results from blockage of small blood vessels in the hands and feet, which causes them to swell painfully. Growth and development tend to be slower than normal, and puberty is delayed. Chronic anemia causes fatigue, pale skin, weakness, and breathlessness after mild exercise. Because the bone marrow expands to increase red blood cell production, the bones thin, making them vulnerable to fracture. The

rapid breakdown of red blood cells may cause the skin and sclera (whites of the eyes) to take on a yellow color (jaundice). Vision deteriorates if the retinas (light-sensitive tissue at the back of the eyes) receive too little oxygen, and visual impairment can result. Some children have strokes when sickle cells clog blood vessels in the brain, leading in some cases to serious injury or death. Sickle cells can collect in the lungs, producing an illness resembling pneumonia called acute chest syndrome that can be life-threatening.

Many with the disease experience crises when sickle cells cut off blood flow to a part of the body. Practically any organ or joint can be affected. Crises cause severe pain that lasts from a few hours to several weeks. They can be brought on by any situation that increases the demand for oxygen, such as extremely high altitudes, infection, strenuous exercise, delivering a baby, and stress.

Over time, sickle cell anemia can harm the internal organs. The liver and the spleen are commonly affected. The liver may malfunction, and the spleen may become scarred, cease to function, and have to be removed surgically. The heart often enlarges as a way of compensating for the decrease in oxygen flowing into the body and may set the stage for heart failure later in life. Areas of lung tissues can die from lack of blood supply. In addition, ulcers may appear on the legs.

People with sickle cell anemia are more susceptible to infection because of damage to the spleen, which then fails to filter bacteria from the bloodstream. Infants and young children in particular are subject to bacterial diseases, such as pneumonia, that can kill them in a matter of hours.

TREATMENT AND PREVENTION
There is no cure for sickle cell anemia. In the past, the disease resulted in premature death. With current therapies, however, approximately 50 percent of people with sickle cell anemia survive to their mid-40s, although fewer than 10 percent live beyond 60.

The goal of treatment is to prevent crises and reduce symptoms when they occur. People with the disease are advised to avoid extremely high altitudes (for example, flying in

unpressurized airplanes or mountaineering), stress, extreme fatigue, strenuous exercise, dehydration (for example, from long-term exposure to the sun), and sources of infection (such as crowded public spaces during flu season). Folic acid supplements are usually advised since sickle cell anemia increases the need for this nutrient. Infants and young children are commonly prescribed penicillin to prevent infection. Older people should be vaccinated against pneumonia, particularly if the spleen has been removed. When a crisis occurs, the person may require hospitalization for pain management and intravenous liquids to dilute the blood and restore normal flow. Transfusions are given in some cases. In some people with sickle cell anemia, a chemotherapy drug called hydroxyurea may reduce the rate of painful crises, although it is unknown whether treatment with hydroxyurea will prevent the development of chronic organ damage.

People who carry the trait and are considering having children should seek GENETIC COUNSELING to assess their risk of passing on the disease.

Sickle cell trait
Inheritance of one copy from one parent of the gene that causes sickle cell anemia. Inheritance from both parents is required for full-blown sickle cell anemia. In the United States, 1 in 12 blacks are carriers of the sickle cell trait. Most experience no symptoms, but conditions that greatly increase the oxygen demands on the body, such as extremely high altitudes or extreme cold, may produce a crisis. Life span is usually normal for people with sickle cell trait, and no treatment, except for crises, is required. Genetic counseling may be helpful for persons with sickle cell trait who are planning a pregnancy. If two carriers of the trait have children together, they have a 25 percent chance of having a child with the disease and a 50 percent chance of having a child who is a carrier. See SICKLE CELL ANEMIA.

Side effect
An unwanted drug effect; an adverse drug reaction. Most drugs produce unintended effects in addition to the

FOCUS ON SICKLE CELL ANEMIA

Normal red blood cells are round. In people with sickle cell anemia, however, the red blood cells are sickle shaped, a defect that is caused by the accumulation of an abnormal hemoglobin molecule inside the cells. Rarely, bone marrow transplants from healthy siblings can be effective in curing children with this disease.

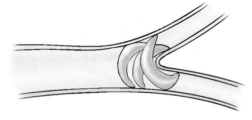

SICKLE CELL OBSTRUCTION
Because of their unique shape, sickle cells may accumulate in a small arteriole and create an obstruction.

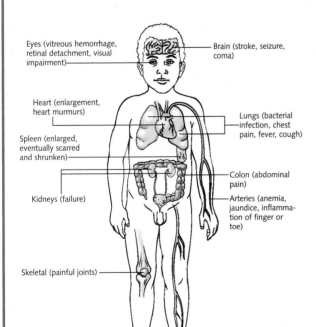

Eyes (vitreous hemorrhage, retinal detachment, visual impairment)

Brain (stroke, seizure, coma)

Heart (enlargement, heart murmurs)

Lungs (bacterial infection, chest pain, fever, cough)

Spleen (enlarged, eventually scarred and shrunken)

Colon (abdominal pain)

Kidneys (failure)

Arteries (anemia, jaundice, inflammation of finger or toe)

Skeletal (painful joints)

ORGANS OR SYSTEMS AFFECTED
Blockage of blood flow to organs and parts of the body causes varying symptoms.

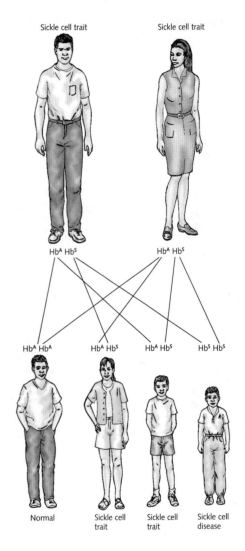

Sickle cell trait

Sickle cell trait

Hb^A Hb^S

Hb^A Hb^S

Hb^A Hb^A

Hb^A Hb^S

Hb^A Hb^S

Hb^S Hb^S

Normal

Sickle cell trait

Sickle cell trait

Sickle cell disease

INHERITANCE PATTERN
If both parents have the sickle cell trait, then each of their children has a 25 percent chance of being disease-free, a 25 percent chance of having sickle cell anemia, and a 50 percent chance of having the sickle cell trait. (Note: Hb^A refers to the normal hemoglobin gene; Hb^S refers to the sickle cell hemoglobin gene.)

S

intended action. Most side effects are predictable and range from mild to very serious. For example, hair loss is a common side effect of anticancer chemotherapy, and fatigue is a common side effect of radiation therapy.

Some side effects are serious and, rarely, can even be life-threatening; such side effects are usually referred to as adverse effects or an ADVERSE DRUG REACTION. About 10 percent of all hospital admissions in the United States are estimated to be for treatment of adverse drug reactions.

SIDS

See SUDDEN INFANT DEATH SYNDROME.

DRUG FACTS LABEL FOR OVER-THE-COUNTER DRUGS

All over-the-counter medications sold in the United States are required to print a Drug Facts label on their packaging. This label prominently features a "Warnings" section listing the most common side effects that can be expected while taking a particular drug. Serious side effects, if any, are also listed, indicating instances in which the individual taking the medication should stop using it and contact his or her doctor immediately. In addition, it includes information on possible interactions with food and with other medications.

- **Active ingredient** gives the name of any drug(s) in the medicine
- **Uses** describes what symptoms the drug is intended to treat
- **Warnings** describes circumstances when a person should not take the drug, warns about interactions with other medications or with foods, describes common and potentially serious side effects, and warns about potential problems for women who are pregnant or breast-feeding, or what to do if a child accidently swallows the medicine.
- **Directions** gives dosage instructions based on age
- **Other information** describes how the medicine should be stored to stay fresh
- **Inactive ingredients** tells a person what substances are in the drug to color or bind the ingredients

This example from the Food and Drug Administration (FDA) is for an over-the-counter antihistamine product.

Drug Facts

Active Ingredient (in each tablet)	Purpose
Chlorpheniramine maleate 2mg	Antihistamine

Uses
Temporarily relieves these symptoms due to hay fever or upper respiratory allergies: ■ sneezing ■ runny nose ■ itchy, watery eyes ■ itchy throat

Warnings
Ask a doctor before use if you have:
■ glaucoma ■ a breathing problem such as emphysema or chronic bronchitis ■ trouble urinating due to an enlarged prostate gland

Ask a doctor or pharmacist before use if you are taking tranquilizers or sedatives

When using this product
■ you may get drowsy ■ avoid alcoholic drinks ■ alcohol, sedatives, and tranquilizers may increase drowsiness ■ be careful when driving a motor vehicle or operating machinery ■ excitability may occur, especially in children

If pregnant or breast-feeding, ask a health professional before use.

Keep out of reach of children. In case of overdose, get medical help or contact a Poison Center right away.

Directions

Adults and children 12 years and over	take 2 tablets every 4 to 6 hours; not more than 12 tablets in 24 hours
Children 6 years to under 12 years	take 1 tablet every 4 to 6 hours; not more than 6 tablets in 24 hours
Children under 6 years	ask a doctor

Other information ■ store at 20-25°C (68-77°F) ■ protect from excessive moisture

Inactive Ingredients D&C yellow no. 10, lactose, magnesium stearate, microcrystalline cellulose, pregelatinized starch

---

Sight

The act of seeing. VISION is one of the five SENSES. The eye acts as a sophisticated camera, providing valuable information about a person's environment.

Sigmoid colon

The lowest section of the colon, or large INTESTINE, before the rectum. This section of the colon gets its name from its S shape. The sigmoid colon connects to the descending colon above and the rectum below. See DIGESTIVE SYSTEM.

Sigmoidoscopy

A procedure in which the interior of the large intestine is examined by using a flexible, lighted tube called a sigmoidoscope. Sigmoidoscopy is a type of ENDOSCOPY that allows a doctor to view, photograph, and videotape the inside of the lower part of the large intestine without surgery. This procedure is used to look for early signs of cancer and other abnormalities in the rectum and sigmoid colon (the last part of the colon). The American Cancer Society recommends a screening sigmoidoscopy every 3 to 5 years for all Americans older than age 50.

A liquid diet for 12 to 24 hours or an enema is usually necessary before the procedure. During the examina-

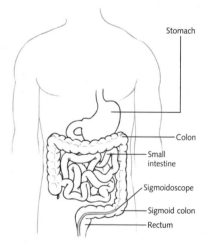

FLEXIBLE FIBEROPTIC SIGMOIDOSCOPY
Flexible fiberoptic sigmoidoscopy is far more comfortable for the patient than older rigid instruments. The sigmoidoscope is advanced through the intestine as far as is comfortable. If necessary, a sample of tissue for analysis can be obtained through the sigmoidoscope.

tion, the individual wears a hospital gown and lies on an examination table. The doctor slowly guides the sigmoidoscope into the colon. If a polyp or inflamed tissue is detected, tiny instruments are passed through the sigmoidoscope to remove a sample of tissue for microscopic inspection by a pathologist. Slight pressure and cramping may occur in the lower abdomen during the procedure. Complications, though uncommon, may include bleeding and puncture of the colon. Sigmoidoscopy generally takes 10 to 20 minutes.

SIL

Squamous intraepithelial lesion. A system for classifying CERVICAL DYS-PLASIA, abnormal cells on the cervix. Squamous intraepithelial lesion refers to abnormalities in the squamous cell layer that covers the cervix. The classification system is used to describe abnormal Pap smear results by differentiating them on a continuous spectrum among low-grade, moderate, or high-grade dysplasia (abnormalities).

SIL 1 describes mild cellular change. This classification includes both mild dysplasia and changes seen in women infected with HUMAN PAPILLOMAVIRUS, a sexually transmitted disease that can cause venereal warts and is often a precursor of cancerous cells. Moderate or severe dysplasia and carcinoma in situ of the cervix (where the cancer has not penetrated beyond the surface layer of the cells) are classified as high-grade or severe, or SIL 3 or 4.

Sildenafil citrate

An anti-impotence drug. Sildenafil citrate (Viagra) is prescribed for men who have difficulty obtaining or maintaining an erection during sexual intercourse, a condition called erectile dysfunction, or impotence. Sildenafil citrate works by blocking the action of an enzyme that causes a reduction in blood flow to the penis, thus increasing the blood supply. Sildenafil citrate works only in men whose erectile dysfunction is caused by poor blood flow to the penis.

Silicone

Any of a group of compounds in which some or all of the carbon has been replaced by silicon. Silicone is unusually stable over a wide range of temperatures, it is extremely water-repellent, and it does not react chemically with other substances. Silicone is used extensively in adhesives, lubricants, protective coatings, paints, ceramics, and electrical insulation. In the past, silicone was used to make a prosthesis for a person who had a nonfunctioning or amputated body part, including breast replacement for women after a mastectomy, and for breast enlargements. Because of safety and leakage problems, most plastic surgeons now use saline-filled implants almost exclusively.

Silicosis

Permanent scarring of the lungs that is caused by long-term exposure to and inhalation of silica (quartz) dust. Silicosis is an OCCUPATIONAL LUNG DISEASE that is caused by inhaling the primary constituent of sand, which is silica. It occurs among miners who work in coal, lead, copper, silver, and gold mines. Some coal miners are also affected, as are foundry workers, people who work with pottery, sandstone and granite cutters, sandblasters, and people who work in tunnels or in the abrasive cleanser industry.

SYMPTOMS, DIAGNOSIS, AND TREATMENT

Symptoms usually appear after 20 to 30 years of working in an environment in which there is continual exposure to the dust. In certain workplaces, including those that involve sandblasting, tunneling, and the manufacture of abrasive cleansers, high levels of silica dust are produced, and symptoms tend to develop within 10 years of exposure. Inhalation of silica dust causes scarring of lung tissue, which decreases the lungs' flexibility and produces difficulty with breathing. This eventually interferes with the normal ability of the lungs to transfer oxygen into the blood.

Mild cases of silicosis do not cause breathing difficulties. Coughing that produces sputum is a common early symptom. More severe silicosis results in severe shortness of breath, which initially occurs only on exertion but eventually occurs when a person is at rest. Breathing problems can continue for 2 to 5 years even if the person is no longer exposed to silica dust.

Lung damage associated with silicosis adds strain to the heart and may lead to heart failure (see HEART FAILURE, CONGESTIVE), a potentially fatal condition. People who have silicosis are also more susceptible to TUBERCULOSIS.

The disease is diagnosed with a chest X ray that reveals scarring and the presence of small round nodules that are characteristic of silicosis. The illness cannot be cured, but elimination of exposure to silica dust can halt its progress in some cases. Breathing problems may be improved with treatments used for CHRONIC OBSTRUCTIVE PULMONARY DISEASE (COPD), including courses of medications that keep airways open and free of secretions.

People with silicosis should have regular chest X rays and skin tests for tuberculosis because they are at high risk for contracting tuberculosis. Sandblasters should have X rays every 6 months, and other workers should have X rays every 2 to 5 years to detect conditions early. Exposure to silica dust should be discontinued if possible or controlled in the workplace. Sandblasters should wear protective gear that filters out tiny particles of silica dust or hoods that supply clean external air. Whenever possible, workers should avoid sand as an industrial abrasive.

Simethicone

An antigas drug; an antiflatulent. Simethicone is used to relieve painful symptoms associated with the presence of too much gas in the stomach and intestines. It works by enabling bubbles of gas in the stomach and intestines to come together, thus permitting easier passage of gas. Gas can occur for several reasons, including swallowing air, indigestion, ulcers, irritable bowel syndrome, diverticulosis, and surgery. Simethicone is a nonprescription drug. Simethicone products include Imodium Advanced, Maximum Strength Maalox, Mylanta Gas Relief, Gas-X, and Mylicon Infants' Drops.

Simvastatin

A drug used to lower cholesterol and other fats in the blood. Simvastatin (Zocor) is an antilipemic drug that lowers cholesterol and lipoprotein by inhibiting a liver enzyme involved in the production of cholesterol. Simvastatin works by reducing the amount of cholesterol created by the body and is usually prescribed when diet, exercise, and weight loss have failed to reduce an elevated cholesterol level.

Simvastatin is used to reduce the total amounts of cholesterol in the blood including LDL (low-density lipoprotein) or "bad" cholesterol, triglycerides (fat), and apolipoprotein B, a protein needed to produce cholesterol. Simvastatin is also used to increase the level of HDL (high-density lipoprotein) or "good" cholesterol in the blood. Taken together, these actions can reduce the risk of hardening of the arteries, which can lead to heart attack, stroke, and other diseases. This drug should not be taken by a woman who is pregnant or breast-feeding.

Sinew
See TENDON.

Single-photon emission computed tomography
See SPECT.

Sinus
A cavity or channel, usually within a bone, such as the air-containing spaces in the bones of the nose, lined with mucous membranes. There are numerous sinuses in the bones of the skull.

Sinus, facial
Any of the air-containing spaces in the bones of the face. There are four pairs of facial sinuses: the frontal sinuses in the bone of the forehead, just over the eye sockets; the maxillary sinuses in the cheekbones under the eyes; the ethmoid sinuses on either side of the bridge of the nose; and the sphenoidal sinuses directly over the bridge of the nose. The sinuses are lined with mucous membrane that helps trap particles in the air inhaled through the nose; the mucus drains into the nose.

Sinus bradycardia
An unusually slow heartbeat brought on by normal causes, such as deep relaxation or excellent fitness, or by abnormalities of the conduction systems, such as sick sinus syndrome.

Sinus bradycardia requires no treatment unless it causes symptoms.

Sinus tachycardia
A fast heartbeat originating in the sinus node, the heart's own pacemaker. Sinus tachycardia is normal during exercise or when a person experiences anxiety. It may also be caused by shock, hypotension (low blood pressure), hypoxia (insufficient oxygen supply), congestive heart failure, or fever.

Sinusitis

FOR SYMPTOM CHART
see Headache, page 38

An inflammation and infection of the moist air cavities, called sinuses, located around the nose, behind the cheeks, and in the forehead above the eyes. Sinusitis is considered acute when it lasts for fewer than 30 days and chronic when it persists for more than 30 days. The infection may be caused by bacteria, such as streptococcal bacteria or by viruses including rhinovirus, influenza, and parainfluenza. The infection is sometimes due to fungal infections or allergic reactions. In rare instances, a dental infection is associated with sinusitis. An upper respiratory tract infection sometimes precedes sinusitis and is often associated with it.

Sinusitis occurs when the mucous membrane of the nose becomes swollen and obstructed. Secretions from the mucous membrane may

then fill the affected sinus, and this accumulated fluid becomes a medium for bacteria or other infective agents. Children most commonly acquire infections that involve the sinuses around the nose and behind the cheeks, while teens and adults generally find that their sinuses in the forehead are more commonly involved.

SYMPTOMS, DIAGNOSIS, AND TREATMENT
Swelling and tenderness in the affected sinus or sinuses is usually the first sign of sinusitis. Headache is a common symptom, and there may be a discharge of yellow or green mucus from the nose. Pain behind and between the eyes accompanied by a severe headache may also occur. Fever, chills, and malaise may indicate spread of the infection.

In children, sinusitis causes a runny nose or nasal congestion. A fever and discharge of a thick, green or yellow mucus from the nose then develop. There may be swelling around the eyes, bad breath, and tenderness or a heavy sensation in the cheeks or around the nose. When sinusitis is chronic, a child may snore during sleep or have a persistent cough that interrupts sleep. Pain around the upper teeth may be mistaken for a dental problem, but in the presence of other symptoms, is usually produced by infection in the sinuses in the cheeks.

Sinusitis may be diagnosed by an evaluation of physical symptoms. CT

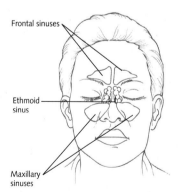

Frontal sinuses

Ethmoid sinus

Maxillary sinuses

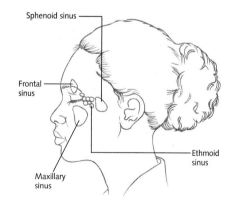

Sphenoid sinus

Frontal sinus

Ethmoid sinus

Maxillary sinus

SINUS INFECTION
The nasal bones of the skull contain air chambers that surround and drain into the nose. When infection swells the mucous membranes in the nose and causes an increased accumulation of fluid, drainage may be slow and the sinuses may become congested. Pressure from the swelling and congestion may be painful.

(computed tomography) scans or X rays of the sinuses may be performed to determine the extent and degree of the infection. Dental X rays may be necessary to exclude the possibility of a dental abscess. In children, if fluid has accumulated in the sinuses, the fluid may be gently suctioned out through the nose. In cases of chronic sinusitis, the doctor may suggest an examination to detect nasal polyps or enlarged adenoids.

Adults are treated for sinusitis by methods to improve nasal drainage and control infection. Steam inhalation and saline nasal washes may be used to promote drainage of the sinuses. Medications to constrict swollen membranes and open up the sinuses may be prescribed or recommended, either in topical form or to be taken orally. A course of oral antibiotic therapy of at least 10 to 12 days' duration is generally prescribed to control infection. In some cases of chronic sinusitis, antibiotic therapy may be prolonged over a period of 4 to 6 weeks. When sinusitis does not respond to antibiotics, functional endoscopic sinus surgery (see FESS) may be necessary.

Children are treated for sinusitis with a 2- to 3-week course of oral antibiotics, usually amoxicillin (see PENICILLINS), which may be changed to another antibiotic if symptoms do not improve within 2 days. Chronic sinusitis may require antibiotic therapy lasting as long as 6 weeks. Decongestants may also be prescribed in some cases. Acetaminophen may be recommended to reduce fever and relieve pain associated with sinusitis. A cool-mist vaporizer may be used to help open clogged nasal passages. Increased fluid intake is generally recommended. Older children may be more comfortable with an extra pillow to elevate the head when in bed. Decongestant nose drops and sprays are usually not advised as they can make symptoms worse if used too frequently or over long periods.

Situs inversus

A right and left reversal or transposition of the abdominal organs. The condition seems to be related to a gene mutation, and a person with situs inversus will often also have congenital heart disease. Surgery will not entirely correct the disease.

Sitz bath

A bath in which only the hips and buttocks are immersed in warm water for 15 to 20 minutes several times daily; also a bathtub shaped like a chair. Sitz baths are used to relieve pain and discomfort after rectal or vaginal surgery. They may also be recommended for people with cystitis, hemorrhoids, or pelvic cavity infections.

Sjögren syndrome

A disease in which the salivary glands and the lacrimal glands (which produce tears) are progressively destroyed by malfunction of lymphocytes (white blood cells that fight infection) and plasma cells (white blood cells that produce antibodies). The glands producing moisture in the vagina may also be involved. Tissues and structures of the skin, respiratory tract, gastrointestinal tract, the sweat glands, liver, kidneys, lungs, and thyroid glands may also be affected. Sjögren syndrome more commonly affects middle-aged women but may also occur in men. Rarely, this disease occurs in children. This syndrome may be involved in RHEUMATOID ARTHRITIS, systemic lupus erythematosus (see LUPUS ERYTHEMATOSUS, SYSTEMIC), POLYMYOSITIS, or SCLERODERMA.

SYMPTOMS AND TREATMENT

While there is currently no cure for Sjögren syndrome, there may be relief for most of its major symptoms. DRY MOUTH is sometimes the first symptom to appear, making it difficult for a person to chew, swallow, or talk. There may be a burning sensation in the mouth and throat, and the voice may become hoarse and weak. Cracks may develop on the tongue and lips, especially at the corners of the mouth. Swelling of the salivary glands can give the appearance of mumps. Smell and taste may be diminished. Yeast infections and dental decay can result. Drinking fluids frequently, especially when eating, may help keep the mouth moist. Using sugarless gum and hard candy can be helpful for stimulating the salivary glands. Spicy, dry, or sugared foods and alcohol and tobacco should be avoided because they irritate or dry the tissues of the mouth. Over-the-counter artificial salivas in spray form may also be beneficial. Good

dental hygiene and regular visits to the dentist can help control problems with the teeth.

Sjögren syndrome can cause the eyes to become dry, red, and painful; they may also feel gritty or sandy or as if a foreign body has become lodged in them. The eyes may be fatigued and sensitive to light, and the eyelids may swell. Many people with the syndrome cannot produce tears. These symptoms may be made worse by dry environmental conditions and can be improved by the use of humidifiers. Over-the-counter artificial tears may be used with a doctor's supervision. A prescription medication in the form of a small pellet, which is positioned inside the lower eyelid, may be used to disperse a lubricant over the eyes continually for several hours. A procedure called punctal occlusion that temporarily or permanently blocks the tiny drainage canals at the inner corner of the eyelids may help retain natural or artificial tears on the eye's surface for a longer time. Wearing protective eye wear can help reduce moisture loss from the eyes.

Other symptoms may include a dry and crusty feeling in the nose and dryness of the throat. These problems may be helped by over-the-counter saline sprays and humidifiers. Vaginal dryness may be lessened with the use of over-the-counter sterile lubricants. Overwhelming fatigue and feelings of depression may be present and can be relieved with prescription antidepressant medication. While most people who have this syndrome may already be under a physician's care for treatment of associated diseases, early diagnosis and treatment of the symptoms are important for avoiding complications.

Skeletal dysplasia

The medical term for dwarfism. A group of genetic disorders characterized by abnormal tissue development involving the bones. Most skeletal dysplasias are associated with short stature, though the causes and symptoms vary among individual disorders.

SHORT-LIMB DWARFISM

The most common form of short-limb dwarfism is ACHONDROPLASIA. It is caused by an abnormal gene and is characterized by short arms and legs

5

and an enlarged head. Another form, hypochondroplasia, is characterized by mild shortening of the limbs and short stature. Diagnosis is usually made between ages 2 and 4 and may be confused with familial short stature. Final adult height is usually between 50 and 54 inches. Other symptoms include prominent forehead, short fingers, and mild bowlegs that disappear as the child matures.

Pseudoachondroplasia begins with normal growth, but growth slows when the child is 2 or 3 years old. At about the same time, a characteristic waddling style of walking is noted, due to deformities of the hips. Bowlegs and knock-knees are common, and osteoarthritis occurs in early adulthood. Corrective surgery for the knees and hips is usually performed. The final adult height is usually 32 to 50 inches.

Cartilage-hair hypoplasia is a rare form of dwarfism that is characterized by short stature, fine, sparse hair, impaired immunity, and anemia. Orthopedic problems are rare in people with cartilage-hair hypoplasia; although occasionally surgery is necessary to correct bowlegs. Adult height ranges from 41 to 59 inches. This condition was first noticed among the Old Order Amish in the United States, where it is common. It is also found in Finland.

A person who has Ellis-van Creveld syndrome has short limbs, knock-knees, and an extra finger next to the "pinkie." An additional toe is found in 10 to 25 percent of cases, and half of the people with this disorder also have congenital heart defects, usually correctable with surgery. Adult height ranges between 42 and 60 inches.

Diastrophic dysplasia is a rare condition except in Finland. It is characterized by clubfeet (see TALIPES), cleft palate (see CLEFT LIP AND PALATE), cauliflower ears, scoliosis, or curvature of the spine, and respiratory problems in infancy. Average adult height is 40½ inches, depending on the degree of scoliosis and foot deformities present.

TYPE II COLLAGEN CONDITIONS

Several skeletal dysplasias are caused by changes in collagen, a protein that is present in bone, cartilage, and connective tissue. Type II collagen is the principal type of collagen found in the spine, cartilage, and part of the

eye. Changes in type II collagen are involved in short-trunked dwarfism, myopia (nearsightedness), and retinal degeneration.

Hypochondrogenesis is characterized by short trunk and short limbs at birth. Babies with the condition will have a characteristically puffy appearance and large, oval-shaped heads. Clubfeet and cleft palates are common as well. These babies frequently die soon after birth because they are born with very small rib cages and have great difficulty breathing.

Congenital spondyloepiphyseal dysplasia is a condition involving nearsightedness, retinal detachment, a waddling gait, sway-backed spine, and a very short neck. Adult height is between 34 and 52 inches.

Kniest syndrome is usually diagnosed at birth. Cleft palate is present in 50 percent of cases, and nearsightedness, retinal detachment, cataracts, and glaucoma may also be present. Hearing loss can occur. Clubfoot and severe curvature of the spine are possible. Adult height is between 40 and 58 inches.

Skeletal system

The bones of the body that together form a structural framework and protect internal organs and soft tissues. Bones are attached to one another at a juncture called a JOINT, with tough fibrous bands known as ligaments. The skeletal muscles are attached to bone with connective bands called tendons. Together, the bones, muscles, and joints form a moving structural system known as the musculoskeletal system.

The typical human body has 206 individual bones forming the skeleton. Male and female skeletons are structurally similar, although a woman's skeleton has slightly smaller and lighter bones, particularly in the arms and legs, and the female pelvis is wider and more open to allow for childbirth. The skeleton is organized into two parts: the axial skeleton, which includes the skull, vertebrae, rib cage, and breastbone, and the appendicular skeleton, which consists of the bones of the limbs and the bones that attach the limbs to the axial skeleton.

AXIAL SKELETON

The SKULL, at the top of the axial skeleton, contains 22 individual

bones. Among them are the eight immovable bones that form the cranial vault, in which the brain lies, and the 14 bones of the face, including the movable lower jaw bone. Within the skull are the three tiny bones of the two middle ears and the single bone suspended at the back of the tongue.

The spinal column includes 33 individual bones called vertebrae that encircle the spinal column. The vertebrae are classified according to the region of the spine they occupy: there are seven cervical, 12 thoracic, and five lumbar vertebrae that form the flexible length of the spine; then there are five fused sacral vertebrae, and four fused vertebrae that form the coccyx. Also included in the axial skeleton are the 12 pairs of ribs enclosing the torso and the breastbone.

APPENDICULAR SKELETON

Two sets of bones—called the shoulder girdle and the pelvic girdle—attach the bones of the limbs to the axial skeleton. The shoulder girdle includes the collarbone and the shoulder blades; the pelvic girdle includes a pair of pelvic bones that are actually three fused bones.

Suspended from the shoulder girdle are the bones of arms, one in each upper arm and two in the forearms. The radius is the shorter of the two long bones of the forearm; the other is the ulna. Each wrist contains eight bones, each hand has five bones, and each set of fingers has 14 bones (two in the thumb and three in each finger).

The pelvic girdle protects the organs of the reproductive, intestinal, and urinary systems in the lower part of the body, supports the upper part of the body, and connects the lower limbs to the axial skeleton. There are four bones in each leg, including the thighbone, the kneecap, and two bones in each lower leg. The tibia is the supporting bone of the lower leg; the fibula is narrower and runs parallel to the tibia. Each ankle contains seven individual bones, each foot has five bones, and each set of toes contains 14 bones (two in the big toe and three in the others).

FUNCTION

The skeleton is the strong, movable, and flexible supportive framework for the entire body. Parts of the frame-

THE BODY'S FRAMEWORK

The human skeletal system is usually made up of 206 bones that support and shape the body as well as hold the bones together with joints. The skeleton, accounting for about 20 percent of a person's body mass, also protects internal organs and helps to store minerals needed by the body.

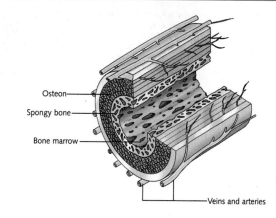

Osteon
Spongy bone
Bone marrow
Veins and arteries

CROSS-SECTION VIEW OF LIVING BONE
Bone is a type of connective tissue that is strong but also lightweight. Made up of cells, fibers, and a gel-like mix of water, mineral salts, and carbohydrates, bone tissue is not completely rigid. It breaks down and rebuilds during a person's growth and after an injury.

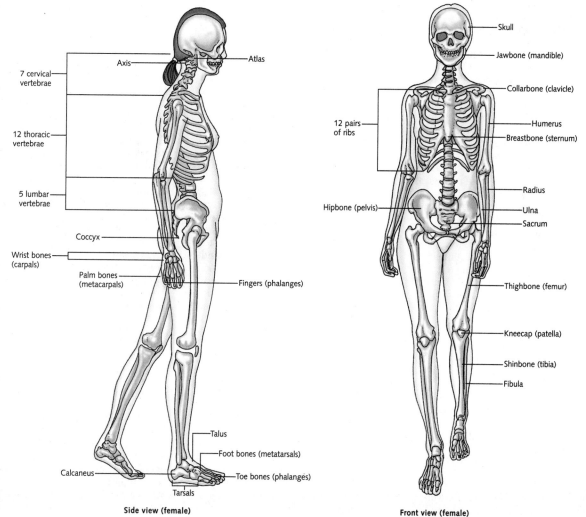

Axis
Atlas
7 cervical vertebrae
12 thoracic vertebrae
5 lumbar vertebrae
Coccyx
Wrist bones (carpals)
Palm bones (metacarpals)
Fingers (phalanges)
Talus
Foot bones (metatarsals)
Toe bones (phalanges)
Calcaneus
Tarsals

Side view (female)

Skull
Jawbone (mandible)
Collarbone (clavicle)
12 pairs of ribs
Humerus
Breastbone (sternum)
Radius
Hipbone (pelvis)
Ulna
Sacrum
Thighbone (femur)
Kneecap (patella)
Shinbone (tibia)
Fibula

Front view (female)

S

work provide rigid or semirigid protection for the fragile tissues and organs that lie within. The relative rigidity of different parts of the skeleton is determined by the relative range of motion of the joints between bones. But the bones of the skeleton are living structures. Within a bone, in the bone marrow, blood cells are produced. The bones also store calcium and other minerals that can be released into the body's blood supply when needed.

Skeleton

The bones of the body. See SKELETAL SYSTEM.

Skier's thumb

A sprain of the ligament that is attached to the joint of the thumb and controls the bending and straightening motions as well as side-to-side movements of the thumb. Skier's thumb results in instability of the thumb and a loss of function. There may be pain and swelling in the area. The ability to bring together the ends of the thumb and forefinger may be limited. It is common among snow skiers because they tend to stretch their thumbs backward while grasping their ski poles during a fall. It may also occur among football and basketball players. A person with this condition often complains of pain while opening jars or car doors. The injury is also known as "gamekeeper's thumb," because gamekeepers used to acquire a chronic strain of the thumb ligament from skinning rabbits. Skier's thumb is diagnosed by physical examination and possibly an X ray to rule out fractures. X rays may indicate a complete rupture of the ligament. If the thumb joint is sufficiently stable, a thumb cast or brace may be worn for 3 to 6 weeks to immobilize the joint and allow healing. If the ligament is completely ruptured, surgery is usually necessary to reconnect the torn ends of the ligament. The thumb must remain in a cast for 6 weeks following surgery to assure complete healing.

Skilled nursing facility

See LONG-TERM CARE FACILITY.

Skin

The protective outer tissue covering the body. The skin holds in body flu-

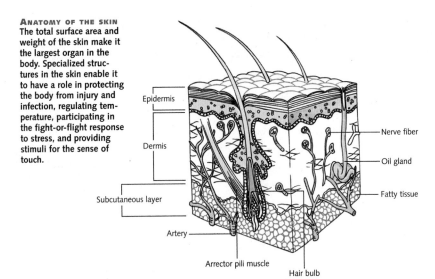

ANATOMY OF THE SKIN
The total surface area and weight of the skin make it the largest organ in the body. Specialized structures in the skin enable it to have a role in protecting the body from injury and infection, regulating temperature, participating in the fight-or-flight response to stress, and providing stimuli for the sense of touch.

Epidermis
Dermis
Subcutaneous layer
Artery
Arrector pili muscle
Hair bulb
Nerve fiber
Oil gland
Fatty tissue

ids, helps regulate body temperature, and forms the first line of defense against infection and injury to internal body structures and tissues. The skin is also a vast sensory organ, filled with nerve endings that register touch, pressure, heat, and cold. Skin averages about one-tenth of an inch in thickness but varies by location on the body—from thin on the eyelids to thick on the palms and soles. The skin has three distinct layers: the epidermis, the dermis, and the subcutaneous layer.

EPIDERMIS

The epidermis is the thin outer layer of the skin. A covering of dead cells on the surface helps protect the living cells underneath. The surface of the epidermis varies in texture depending on the part of the body it covers; for instance, the grooved surface of the fingertips provides a better grip. The cells of the epidermis manufacture keratin, a protein that gives skin its toughness and durability. The epidermis has a fatty component that keeps in water to maintain resiliency and keeps out water from the environment. The surface of the skin is covered with sweat and oil (sebum) and a covering of fine hair, all of which help to resist against germs. As dead cells are sloughed off, many microbes are shed with them. In addition to these passive germ-fighting mechanisms, specialized cells called the cells of Langerhans actively provide information to the immune system about what type of microorgan-

ism is entering the body. At the bottom (base) of the epidermis are the basal cells, which are the rapidly multiplying new cells. As the new cells are pushed up toward the surface, they increase the amounts of keratin to maximize the toughness. Toward the bottom of the epidermis are melanocytes, cells that produce the pigment melanin to help limit damage from sun light.

DERMIS

Under the epidermis is the thicker layer called the dermis. The dermis is connective tissue made of the proteins collagen and elastin, which give skin its strength and elasticity. The dermis contains blood vessels, lymph vessels, oil (sebaceous) glands, and sweat glands. The skin contains two kinds of sweat glands. Eccrine glands cover the whole body, except for the lips and external genitalia, and are most numerous on the palms, soles, forehead, and underarms. The apocrine glands, particularly abundant under the arms and around the nipples and genitals, produce sweat with a strong scent. Apocrine glands secrete in response to body temperature and emotion. Sweating is primarily controlled by the hypothalamus in the brain. The hair follicles, which contain the roots of the HAIR, are also in the dermis; in fact hair cells (and nail cells) are a differentiated type of skin cell. Small involuntary muscles attached to the hair follicles cause the hair to stand up in response to certain emotions, such as fear—leading to the tingling sensation known as goose bumps.

SUBCUTANEOUS LAYER

The deep underlying layer of the skin is composed of fat cells that act as a shock absorber between the skin and more delicate internal tissues and organs.

Skin allergy

A skin reaction that is caused by exposure to an allergy-causing substance. (See also CONTACT DERMATITIS.) Skin allergy occurs in response to a substance that may cause no apparent rash or inflammation the first time a person is exposed to it. However, on subsequent occasions, after the skin has become allergic to the substance, further exposure produces an eruption. An allergic skin reaction is different from a skin reaction brought on by irritants, which is caused by contact with substances that will cause inflammation on anyone's skin. However, many substances can act as both irritants and allergens.

Symptoms of skin allergy vary from person to person but often include redness, itching, inflammation, or scaling. Diagnosis is made through a detailed medical history and examination of the skin. A PATCH TEST may be performed to test a person's sensitivity to commonly encountered substances. In patch testing, traces of possible allergens are briefly applied to the skin. Some materials—such as cosmetics, feminine deodorants, hair dyes, latex, nickel, perfumes, poison ivy, and wool—are more likely than others to be allergens.

A dermatologist can help people avoid allergens by identifying the substances that cause reactions. Treat-ments to control symptoms may include applying cool compresses, soothing lotions, and topical corticosteroids and taking antihistamines. Taking oatmeal baths may relieve itching. Scratching should be avoided to allow a rash to heal. The affected person should wear loose clothing and avoid excessive heat and humidity.

Skin and muscle flap

A section of skin and tissue, including muscle, that is surgically moved to cover another area in which the skin and tissue have been damaged.

Skin and muscle flaps offer an alternative to skin grafting for certain kinds of RECONSTRUCTIVE SURGERY. Generally, they maintain better color and texture than skin grafts, prove more durable, and at least partly preserve hair growth nerve endings that relate to sensation and sweat glands. In skin and muscle flap surgery, the blood supply for the tissue that is surgically moved remains intact.

Skin biopsy

A procedure in which a small sample of skin is removed for examination after a local anesthetic is applied. A skin biopsy may be performed to determine whether a growth is benign (not cancerous) or malignant (cancerous) or to evaluate a skin rash.

There are several different methods of skin biopsy. In a shave biopsy, a superficial to deep layer of skin is removed with a scalpel. No stitches are required. A punch biopsy involves removing a plug of tissue with a small cylindrical punch that comes in various sizes. A stitch or two is necessary to close the wound. In an excisional biopsy, the doctor removes an entire skin lesion with a scalpel. Stitches are required to close this wound. Larger excisions may require skin grafts. Aluminum chloride or electrocautery is applied to control bleeding. Stitches must be kept clean and dry. Facial stitches are removed in 5 to 7 days, while stitches elsewhere remain in place 7 to 14 days. Biopsy sites may be treated with antibiotic ointment and covered with adhesive strips. Pain medication may be necessary.

Skin cancer

The most common form of cancer in the United States. Skin cancer is linked to cumulative exposure or chronic exposure to the ultraviolet rays of the sun. While the risk of nonmelanoma skin cancers increases with cumulative exposure to the sun, melanoma—the most serious type because it spreads to other organs—is linked to intermittent intense sun exposure, genetic factors, and moles. People who have one or two severe sunburns in childhood may double their risk of developing melanoma later in life. Ultraviolet radiation from tanning booths or sunlamps is equally dangerous. Individuals must be especially vigilant about sun exposure when taking medications that promote PHOTOSENSITIVITY (heightened sensitivity to the sun). These medications include NONSTEROIDAL ANTI-INFLAMMATORY DRUGS, sulfa drugs, tetracycline, thiazide diuretics, and tricyclic antidepressants.

Fair-skinned people with red or blond hair and blue or green eyes are at an especially high risk of skin cancer. Other risk factors include a family or personal history of skin cancer; a tendency to burn or freckle easily when exposed to the sun; having many moles; having spent a lot of time outdoors; a history of sunburns; repeated exposure to X rays or other forms of radiation; and exposure to arsenic, coal, industrial tar, paraffin, and certain types of heavy oils.

To detect skin cancer, doctors recommend regular self-examination. It is important to consult a doctor upon finding any new skin growth; a change in the surface or color of a MOLE; a spot or bump that is getting larger, scaling, oozing, or bleeding; a sore that does not heal within 3 months; or itchiness or pain in a lesion. Diagnosis is made through physical examination. The doctor will examine the size, shape, color, and texture of the lesion in question; ask about the history of the growth, such as when it first appeared and how it has changed in size or appearance; check the rest of the body; inquire about any personal or family history of skin cancer; and perform a skin biopsy (take a small sample from the lesion and examine it under a microscope).

TYPES OF SKIN CANCER

There are three main types of skin cancer: BASAL CELL CARCINOMA, SQUAMOUS CELL CARCINOMA, and malignant melanoma (see MELANOMA, MALIGNANT). Basal cell and squamous cell carcinomas are often referred to as nonmelanoma skin cancers to differentiate them from melanoma, which is by far the most serious of the three. Most skin cancers occur on areas of the skin that are frequently exposed to sunlight.

■ ***Basal cell carcinoma*** Basal cell carcinoma is the most common form of skin cancer in the United States, accounting for three of every four cases of skin cancer. Basal cell carci-

S

noma has a cure rate of more than 95 percent and rarely spreads to other parts of the body. As with other forms of cancer, early diagnosis and treatment are essential. Left untreated, basal cell tumors will continue to enlarge and can eventually extend below the skin and invade nearby nerves.

Basal cell carcinomas most commonly develop on sun-exposed areas of the body, such as the head, neck, and chest. They first appear either as small, shiny, pink bumps or as flat, scaly, red areas. Lesions vary from light pink to flesh colored. Blood vessels may be visible in the carcinomas themselves or in surrounding skin. These tumors grow slowly, taking months or even years to expand to a diameter of half an inch. Basal cell cancers bleed easily after a minor injury and may bleed and crust over in repeated cycles.

Most basal cell carcinomas are completely cured by fairly minor surgery. The type of procedure depends on factors such as the size, type, depth, and location of the cancer. Surgical options include simple EXCISION (cutting), CURETTAGE (scraping), electrodesiccation (burning with an electric current delivered through a probe), and MOHS SURGERY (microscopically controlled surgery removing one layer of skin at a time). Radiation may be helpful for tumors that are difficult to treat surgically and for people unable to tolerate surgery. Less frequently, CRYOSURGERY (freezing with liquid nitrogen) may be used. In most cases, surgery is performed on an outpatient basis using a local anesthetic. In the removal of large cancers, skin grafting and reconstructive surgery may be necessary.

■ *Squamous cell carcinoma* This is a more serious type of skin cancer. Left untreated, squamous cell carcinoma may spread into lymph nodes and become incurable. However, with early treatment, this type of cancer has a high cure rate.

Any new growth that ulcerates or bleeds can be an indication of squamous cell or another type of skin cancer. Squamous cell carcinoma usually develops from a red, scaly, precancerous skin lesion known as an ACTINIC KERATOSIS. Actinic keratoses typically occur on parts of the body that expe-

rience the most exposure to ultraviolet light, such as the face, ears, and backs of the hands. They are rough, pink, and scaly. There is a significant risk that actinic keratoses will become squamous cell carcinomas.

Early diagnosis and treatment of both actinic keratoses and squamous cell carcinomas are critical. It is important to have a doctor examine any new skin lesion that grows or bleeds. Diagnosis of squamous cell carcinoma is usually confirmed through skin biopsy. In their early stages (BOWEN DISEASE), growths can be removed by topical chemotherapy, cryosurgery, or electrodesiccation and curettage. Most squamous cell carcinomas, however, must be removed through surgical excision or Mohs surgery. These are minor procedures that take place on an outpatient basis using a local anesthetic.

■ *Malignant melanoma* A serious form of skin cancer, melanoma may spread to other parts of the body, often the liver and lungs, resulting in the vast majority of deaths from skin cancer. It is potentially curable with early detection and treatment. While still relatively uncommon in comparison with nonmelanoma skin cancers, the number of people who develop melanoma is growing each year. This type of cancer is most common in fair-skinned people who live where sunlight is most intense. However, unlike nonmelanoma skin cancer, it is not as rare for people with dark brown or black skin to develop melanoma. Also in contrast with nonmelanoma skin cancers, which are caused by cumulative exposure to the sun over a lifetime, melanomas appear to be more closely

linked to intermittent intense sun exposure. Malignant melanoma is an aggressive cancer that originates in the melanocytes, the cells in the epidermis that contain and produce melanin (the pigment that gives skin its color). A MOLE occurs when melanocyte-derived nevus cells form a cluster. When a mole changes color or shape, medical attention must be sought at once. Moles range in color from brown to black to blue and are not necessarily located in sun-exposed areas. In fact, moles that develop into melanomas may appear on parts of the body not frequently exposed to direct sunlight, such as the buttocks or inside the mouth.

Risk factors for melanoma include irregular moles; a large number of moles (the normal range is between 10 and 40); a personal history of melanoma; a close relative who has had melanoma; a history of one or more severe sunburns as a child; fair skin that burns or freckles easily; and living in an area with a high level of ultraviolet radiation. About one in ten people have unusual moles. Abnormal moles are more likely than normal ones to develop into malignant melanoma. Although not everyone who has an abnormal mole develops melanoma, it is important that all moles be closely monitored.

Even more than with nonmelanoma skin cancers, early diagnosis and treatment of melanoma is essential since early diagnosis provides the best chance of a cure. To detect melanoma, doctors recommend regular skin self-examination. It is essential to seek medical attention when confronted with any new skin growth or change in a mole. In whole body

5

examinations, dermatologists periodically inspect the entire body for changes, such as a new mole or blemish or variations in the surface or color of a mole. Lesions that could be skin cancer can be detected in these examinations and a skin biopsy performed to confirm if there are cancerous cells. If a melanoma is detected, lymph nodes in the area are also removed and examined under a microscope to see if the cancer has spread. Other tests, such as a chest X ray, can also help determine if the cancer has spread. Once the stage of melanoma has been assessed, the doctor can plan the appropriate treatment. Treatment usually involves surgical excision of the melanoma and surrounding tissue and depends on the depth and location of the melanoma. Other options include chemotherapy and immunotherapy if the melanoma has spread.

Skin graft

A plastic surgery technique to repair damaged skin, usually as a result of a serious burn or in RECONSTRUCTIVE SURGERY. In a skin graft, a portion of skin is separated surgically from its original place on the body and moved to a new location. Skin grafts are commonly taken from an inconspicuous area, like the buttocks or upper part of the thigh, and transplanted to a site on the same individual (called an autograft). The graft can also be made between different individuals (allograft) or between different species (XENOGRAFT). After the graft is made, the transplanted skin receives its blood supply from the new site. During healing, the blood vessels in the graft connect or penetrate the graft and nourish it.

Skin patch

A small, adhesive device applied to the skin like a bandage that releases a measured dose of nicotine (when the goal is smoking cessation; patches containing other drugs are used for other purposes) into the bloodstream over 24 hours. Skin patches, also called transdermal patches, help overcome the symptoms of withdrawing from nicotine and are used to aid people who want to stop smoking. Skin patches are used daily over a 6- to 12-week period. Side effects may include headache, insomnia,

HOW A NICOTINE SKIN PATCH WORKS
Under a plastic backing, a nicotine skin patch contains a reservoir of nicotine that adheres to the skin and controls the rate at which nicotine is delivered (see inset). The wearer stops smoking completely, and the patch delivers just enough nicotine to reduce symptoms of withdrawal. The patch is replaced periodically with gradually decreasing doses of nicotine.

dizziness, anxiety, irritability, fatigue, stomach upset, local skin irritation, diarrhea, or constipation. Skin patches are effective but may not work for all people trying to end nicotine dependency. See SMOKING CESSATION.

Skin tag

A small, soft, flesh-colored growth that protrudes from the skin; also known as a cutaneous papilloma. Although their cause is unknown, skin tags are most common during pregnancy and in obese individuals. These harmless growths usually appear on the neck and armpits but may also occur under the breasts and on the chest, inner

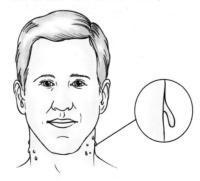

SKIN GROWTH
Skin tags are benign and harmless. They generally appear in middle age or later life. They can vary quite a bit in appearance, but typically hang from the surface of the skin on a loose stalk of tissue.

thighs, or face. If they are irritated by clothing or cosmetically disturbing, skin tags can be snipped off by a doctor with special scissors or removed by CRYOSURGERY (freezing with liquid nitrogen) or electrodesiccation (burning with an electric current delivered through a probe).

Skin tests

Tests in which an antigen, an allergy-causing substance, is applied to the skin in order to observe the response of the person being tested. Skin tests are commonly performed to determine whether a person is capable of having an immune response, to identify whether a person has allergic reactions to specific allergens, and to determine whether a person has been exposed to or is immune to an infectious disease. Common skin tests include the PATCH TEST, the SCRATCH TEST, and intradermal tests, in which a small amount of antigen is injected under the skin. In intradermal tests, if redness and swelling develop within 20 minutes, the skin test result is positive. Skin tests are useful in detecting ALLERGIES to insect bites, penicillin, and foods; respiratory allergies; and infectious diseases, such as tuberculosis.

Skull

The bony framework of the head. The skull contains 22 separate bones.

CRANIUM AND FACE
The bones of the skull comprise the cranium, which houses the brain, and the facial skeleton, which provides the structure for the face. These bones interlock to form a strong, yet somewhat flexible framework.

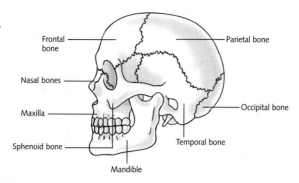

- Frontal bone
- Nasal bones
- Maxilla
- Sphenoid bone
- Mandible
- Parietal bone
- Occipital bone
- Temporal bone

Eight bones form the cranium, which houses the brain. These curved plates of bone have interlocking edges that are a type of immovable joint called a suture. The structure of the skull is able to withstand heavy blows without damage to its contents. Openings in the bottom of the skull, called foramens, allow nerves and blood vessels to pass through. The largest such hole, the foramen magnum, is in the occipital bone at the base of the skull. The brain stem goes through this opening, and the spinal cord emerges from the brain stem. The skull rests on the first cervical vertebra (called the atlas).

Fourteen bones form the facial skull. The facial bones also have immovable joints, except for the two temporomandibular joints on either side of the lower jaw. Many of the bones in the face—particularly those around the nose—contain spaces called sinuses, making the skull lighter and creating resonant chambers for speech production.

There are four tiny bones that are not part of the skull itself, but are within it. The hyoid bone, sometimes called the hyoid cartilage, is suspended by ligaments from the skull at the back of the tongue. It anchors the muscles of the tongue. Three small bones, also called the auditory ossicles, are in the middle ear. Named for their shapes—the hammer (malleus), anvil (incus), and stirrup (stapes)—these bones conduct sound waves into the inner ear.

When a baby is born, the bones of the cranium are not yet fully fused in order to ease passage through the vagina during the birth process. The gaps (fontanelles) between some of the bones will close and harden within 18 months or less. The cranium and facial bones grow at different rates. The cranium reaches its mature size first, but the facial bones continue to grow throughout childhood.

Skull, fractured

A break in the cranial (skull) bones. Skull fractures can occur in head injuries in which a severe impact or blow damages the cranial bones. A fractured skull may involve visible damage to the cranial bones, including heavy bleeding; but a skull fracture can be hidden by the hair. Symptoms of a skull fracture can include bruising or discoloration behind the ear or around the eyes; blood or clear fluid leaking from the ears or nose; unequal sized pupils; or deformity of the skull, including swelling or depressions. Other symptoms may include loss of consciousness, memory lapses or amnesia (loss of memory), blurred vision, confusion, irritability, and headache.

A fractured skull is a medical emergency, and medical assistance must be sought to prevent brain damage or death. Risk factors for skull fracture include playing contact sports or those involving equipment that can cause injury, such as baseball bats or golf clubs. Skull fractures can occur as a result of sports in which it is possible to fall on the head, including gymnastics, basketball, diving, and cycling. Preventive measures include the wearing of suitable helmets or other headgear during athletic activity in which head injury is possible.

SLE

See LUPUS ERYTHEMATOSUS, SYSTEMIC.

Sleep

The body's rest cycle, including a state of natural unconsciousness. Sleep is characterized by a mostly unmoving body posture and diminished sensitivity to external stimuli. Sleep is triggered by complex hormonal activity that responds to cues from the body and the environment. The sleep-wake cycle is controlled by the body's internal clock.

Most sleep—about 80 percent—is dreamless and is known as nonrapid eye movement (NREM) sleep. During NREM sleep, breathing and heart rate are slow and regular, blood pressure is low, and the sleeper is relatively still. Rapid eye movement (REM) sleep is associated with dreaming, which occurs during three to five periods of REM sleep each night at intervals of 1 to 2 hours. REM sleep is characterized by irregular breathing and heart rate, as well as by involuntary muscle jerks. Periods of REM sleep are variable in length.

As a general rule, adults require about 8 hours of sleep per night to function well, although some people need more and others need less. Men tend to require about 1 hour less

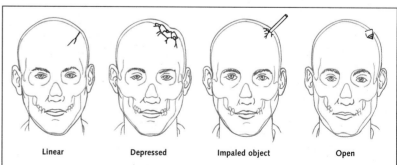

Linear   Depressed   Impaled object   Open

FOUR TYPES OF SKULL FRACTURE
Four types of skull fracture include linear, a simple break in the bone; depressed, a dent that displaces the bone; impaled, in which an object penetrates the bone; and open, in which part of the bone is displaced and the brain is exposed.

S

sleep than women. Children, particularly teenagers, require 9 to 10 hours of sleep per night.

Sleep apnea syndrome

A group of sleep disorders involving repeated episodes when a person stops breathing while asleep. Sleep apnea syndrome, which is also referred to as sleep-disordered breathing, may be caused by a momentary blockage or obstruction in the throat or upper airway, or it may occur as the result of a dysfunction in the area of the brain that controls breathing.

Sleep apnea is more common in men than in women. Several factors increase the risk of developing the syndrome or tend to make it worse, including obesity, age, tobacco smoking, alcohol use, and lung diseases (such as emphysema). Having a narrowed throat and upper airways, which predisposes a person to sleep apnea syndrome, can be an inherited characteristic that affects members of the same family.

SYMPTOMS AND DIAGNOSIS

The symptoms of sleep apnea syndrome occur primarily when a person is sleeping. For this reason, they must be observed and described by another person who is with the sleeping person and awake. Snoring is the most common symptom and may be associated with intermittent gasping, choking, and absence of breathing that awaken the person in a state of anxiety. Episodes when breathing stops during sleep can last more than 10 seconds and may occur as many as 60 times per hour. These events may be experienced 30 to 300 times during a single night and can be serious if the oxygen supply to the blood and brain decreases while the level of carbon dioxide in the body increases. Over time, severe sleep apnea may result in headaches, debilitating sleepiness during daytime hours, and diminished mental ability. Heart failure (see HEART FAILURE, CONGESTIVE) and PULMONARY INSUFFICIENCY can eventually develop.

A person who has sleep apnea syndrome may describe severe daytime drowsiness as the primary symptom, but the other symptoms of the disorder, such as loud snoring and abnormal sleep patterns, are usually reported by the sleep partner of the affected person. An otolaryngologist (ear, nose, and throat specialist) can perform a complete examination of the nose, mouth, throat, palate, and neck to investigate possible causes and rule out certain diseases. The person who has the syndrome may be referred to a sleep study laboratory to confirm the diagnosis, evaluate the severity of the disorder, and analyze the possible causes.

TREATMENT

When the syndrome is determined to be caused by blockage in the throat and upper airways, the first line of approach to treatment involves lifestyle changes. If the affected person smokes, he or she must quit. Excessive alcohol intake must be avoided, and excess weight must be lost. If heavy snoring and episodes of choking occur, the affected person should avoid tranquilizers, sleeping pills, and other sedating medication.

If sleep apnea is caused by a dysfunction in the section of the brain that controls breathing, the affected person may need to use an artificial breathing device while sleeping. A change of sleep position may also be helpful; sleeping on the side of the body or face down can improve symptoms. Also, a dentist can design a custom device worn during sleep that reduces sleep apnea and snoring.

If these lifestyle changes and procedures do not eliminate the risks associated with sleep apnea, a treatment technique called continuous positive airway pressure (CPAP) may become necessary. Most people find they can quickly adapt to the use of this device. It is worn like a small oxygen mask over the nose and delivers a mixture of air under pressure through the nose. CPAP maintains regular breathing during sleep by keeping the airway open.

In rare and severe cases, a person with sleep apnea syndrome may require a surgical procedure, called a TRACHEOSTOMY, in which a permanent opening in the windpipe through the neck is created. Other surgical procedures may be performed in cases in which the upper airway needs to be widened to alleviate obstruction to breathing.

Sleep deprivation

A condition caused by lack of sleep. Sleep deprivation is very common in the United States, according to research findings. Most American adults sleep only about 6 hours per night, even though most need 8 or more hours of sleep. Sleep deprivation promotes excessive sleepiness during the day and interferes with daily activities, including driving. Sleep deprivation also affects mood and emotional well-being.

Sleep deprivation can also result from a number of sleep disorders, such as persistent insomnia, snoring, and sleep APNEA. Psychological disorders, medical problems, drug use, and medications can all interrupt sleep patterns.

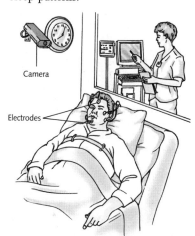

Camera

Electrodes

EVALUATING SLEEP PROBLEMS
To diagnose and treat sleep disorders, a doctor may prescribe laboratory evaluation—a procedure called polysomnography. In the laboratory, electrodes are placed on the person's scalp and perhaps other areas of the body to monitor brain waves and other physical functions during sleep. The data are recorded and analyzed.

Sleep disorders

FOR SYMPTOM CHART
see Sleep problems, page 54

A host of disorders including INSOMNIA, NARCOLEPSY, RESTLESS LEG SYNDROME, parasomnias, and SLEEP APNEA SYNDROME. Problems sleeping can affect a person's energy level, and his or her overall health. Difficulty getting to sleep or remaining asleep are symptoms of this common problem, which can be short and self-limiting or persist for years. Narcolepsy is characterized by overwhelming daytime drowsiness and sudden, irresistible collapses into sleep. Restless

5

GETTING ENOUGH SLEEP

Knowing good sleep hygiene is useful for coping with sleep disorders. Doctors recommend the following tips:

- Getting up at a regular time every morning, even on weekends.
- Trying not to nap during the daytime. If sleepiness is overwhelming, limiting the nap to no longer than 30 minutes is helpful.
- Avoiding caffeine, alcoholic beverages, nicotine, and strenuous exercise for 4 to 6 hours before bedtime.
- A light snack before retiring can be beneficial. However, heavy meals before bedtime should be avoided.
- Minimizing noise, light, and extreme temperatures in the bedroom.
- Trying to sleep when drowsy.
- If unable to sleep, leaving the bedroom, engaging in a quiet activity elsewhere, and returning to bed only when drowsy.
- Seeking professional help if sleeplessness persists.

leg syndrome is a rare condition characterized by unpleasant, restless sensations in the legs and an irresistible impulse to move them. Breathing that stops for varying amounts of time during sleep is a sign of sleep apnea syndrome. This is a potentially serious medical condition that can become life-threatening. Sleep disorders may be diagnosed and treated either by general practitioners or by doctors who specialize in this type of problem. Parasomnias are abnormal behaviors that occur during sleep, such as sleepwalking, talking in one's sleep, and teeth grinding.

Sleep paralysis

A temporary inability to speak or move while falling asleep or waking. Sleep paralysis is a classic characteristic of NARCOLEPSY (a sleep disorder characterized by overwhelming daytime drowsiness and sudden, irresistible collapses into sleep).

Sleep problems in older people

Circadian rhythms, the 24-hour cycles that govern many of a person's biological processes, change with age. As a result, sleeping problems such as INSOMNIA increase in older people. It is a myth that the need for sleep decreases with age. Various disturbances, such as the need to urinate, often prevent older adults from getting a good night's sleep; however, older people continue to need as

much sleep as they did when they were younger adults. An older person might have trouble falling asleep, waken frequently during the night, wake up too early in the morning, or feel sleepy during the day and, consequently, need to nap. Severe SNORING is a symptom of some sleep disorders and often wakens partners.

CAUSES

Sleep problems may arise from underlying illness, DEPRESSION, medications, alcohol, caffeine, or poor sleep hygiene, such as taking daytime naps. Some older people are prone to developing SLEEP APNEA SYNDROME, a condition characterized by temporary pauses in breathing during sleep. Sleep apnea leads to nonrestorative sleep and sleepiness during the waking hours. Periodic limb movements in sleep (PLMS) is a sleep disorder, common in older people, in which uncontrollable leg kicks occur 20 to 30 seconds apart, on and off throughout the night. The resulting partial awakenings disrupt sleep. See also RESTLESS LEG SYNDROME.

DIAGNOSIS AND TREATMENT

Diagnosis of sleeping disorders is based on a detailed medical history and a complete physical examination. Use of substances such as caffeine, alcohol, tobacco, and medications is evaluated. When the normal sleeping cycle has been disrupted by a change in circadian rhythm, daytime exposure to bright sunlight is recommended. If problems such as sleep apnea or abnormal muscular movements can be ruled out, the physician may prescribe sleeping medications to temporarily reduce brain cell activity for sleep. Usually these medications are used only briefly until the sleep cycle can be reestablished. Weight loss often helps control sleep apnea by reducing the fatty tissue that can obstruct breathing. Physicians may refer some older people for further evaluation and treatment by a sleep specialist. More aggressive treatment such as supplemental oxygen or surgery to remove breathing obstructions may be necessary.

Establishing good sleep habits can help prevent sleep disorders. These habits include going to bed at the same time every night, getting regular exercise, and spending time outdoors to increase exposure to light. Naps during the day should be limited to 30 minutes or less. Alcohol, caffeine, and tobacco should be avoided in the evening. Limiting the amount of liquid drunk near bedtime can help diminish the need for bathroom trips.

AGING AND SLEEP
Aging often leads to sleep disturbances that make it difficult for an older person to get a good night's rest—and older people need just as much sleep as younger people. Sleep disorders are much better understood than they once were. A doctor will diagnose sleep problems by taking a detailed medical history and physical examination. He or she can also offer suggestions about good sleep habits to help resolve any problems.

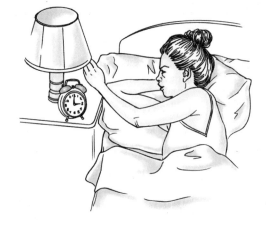

📖 Terms in small capital letters—for example, PHYSICAL THERAPY or PAGET DISEASE—indicate a cross-reference to another entry with more information.

Sleeping sickness

An illness that is caused by parasitic protozoa that are carried by tsetse flies. Symptoms of sleeping sickness include high fever and swollen glands. After a latency period of 4 to 6 months, the illness causes extreme sleepiness and inflammation of the brain, the membrane covering the brain (called the meninges), and the spinal cord. The disease is common in tropical Africa.

Sleeping sickness is acquired when a person is bitten by an infected tsetse fly. The site of the insect bite becomes red, painful, and swollen, and the parasites enter the bloodstream, where they multiply in the blood and the lymph nodes, causing fever, headache, profuse sweating, and swollen lymph nodes.

Eventually, after a period of latency, the parasites invade the central nervous system and the brain, producing extreme behavior changes, anxiety, and mood swings. These symptoms are followed by headache, fever, and general fatigue. One strain of the protozoa causes an inflammation of the heart muscle and, ultimately, complete heart failure within 6 months. Another type of the parasite has a 2-year period of latency before the central nervous system becomes involved. Symptoms of this form of sleeping sickness include daytime drowsiness that progresses to a complete comatose state.

Sleeping sickness is diagnosed by blood tests, lymph node aspiration, and other tests to identify the protozoa causing the illness. Physical examination may show signs of inflammation of the meninges, the brain, and the spinal cord. Antiprotozoal medications used to treat sleeping sickness include suramin, melarsoprol, and pentamidine. Early diagnosis and treatment, before the nervous system and brain are involved, can be life-saving. Untreated, sleeping sickness is almost always fatal. Insect control can help prevent the spread of sleeping sickness.

Sleepwalking

A disorder characterized by periods of sitting up, moving about, or engaging in other complex activities (such as dressing or eating) while still asleep. Episodes of sleepwalking can include a variety of actions. In mild cases, the individual may simply sit up in bed and lift the sheets or blankets. More commonly, sleepwalkers get out of bed and move about, sometimes even leaving the room or building. In some cases people eat, use the bathroom, or talk, although usually nonsensically and with poor articulation. Occasionally individuals with the disorder try to escape some apparent threat by running or engaging in frantic action. Most episodes last fewer than 30 minutes, but they range from only a few seconds to several hours. During the sleepwalking episode, the individual looks blank, is unresponsive, and stares. If awakened during sleepwalking, the individual appears confused, but returns to normal consciousness in a few minutes. Often the person returns to bed on his or her own and awakens in the morning with little or no memory of sleepwalking.

Injury from a fall, walking through a window, wandering outside, or bumping into obstacles is a serious risk of sleepwalking. This risk is heightened if sleepwalking includes frantic actions such as running. Contrary to popular belief, a sleepwalker may be awakened without risk. However, since the individual will feel confused and disoriented for a few minutes, it is often better to simply lead him or her back to bed.

Sleepwalking is most common in children from 6 to 12 years of age; it affects more boys than girls and also appears in adults. Since the disorder is associated with the nondreaming stage of sleep, it occurs most frequently during the first third of the night. Sleepwalking may be related to fatigue, previous sleeplessness, or anxiety. In adults, sleepwalking can be a sign of a mental or brain disorder. It can also be caused by alcohol and some medications.

Sleepwalking is treated by ensuring a safe environment to prevent injuries and avoiding alcohol or other suspect medications. In some cases, tranquilizers are prescribed.

Sling

A cloth bandage suspended from the neck to support and immobilize an injured shoulder, arm, or hand. A sling is generally used, with or without other supports, to treat sprains or fractures of the arm or elbow.

Slipped disk

A common back disorder in which the rupture of the backbone disk through its protective cartilage covering creates painful pressure on spinal nerves. A slipped disk may also be called a herniated disk or disk prolapse. It usually occurs in the lower back but may also take place in other areas of the back including the cervical, or neck, region. The soft pads of cartilage that lie between and cushion the vertebral bones of the spine have a highly elastic, jellylike center that helps the disk absorb the shock of the back's normal movements.

CAUSES

There are several possible causes of the displacement of the disk's center that may produce a slipped disk. The aging process, improper posture, or an injury may result in the outer fibrous rings of cartilage becoming worn and cause the soft, jellylike center of the disk to bulge out into the cartilage surrounding it. Sudden movements or overuse of the back may cause the disk's pulpy center to herniate through the cartilage. Typically, the disk's center protrudes toward the spinal cord and the spinal nerves. When the herniated, or slipped, disk exerts pressure, irritates, or pinches the spinal nerves, it produces sudden, severe, and often disabling lower back pain. Numbness and restriction of movement may also be felt with a slipped disk. If the sciatic nerve is pinched, the pain and numbness can radiate down into the buttocks, into the back of the thigh and calf, and even into the foot. This type of pain is called SCIATICA. If the bulging center of the disk puts pressure on the spinal cord, nerve tissue may be damaged. If left untreated, a slipped disk can cause the destruction of spinal nerves by constant pressure on the nerve root.

DIAGNOSIS AND TREATMENT

The condition of the disks is evaluated by X ray, CT (computed tomography) scan, myelogram, MRI (magnetic resonance imaging), a diskogram, or a combination of these diagnostic aids. The first line of treatment for a slipped disk may include bed rest and taking nonsteroidal anti-inflammatory drugs (NSAIDs) such as aspirin or ibuprofen. Prescriptions for muscle relaxant and painkilling medications may be given. It may be

S

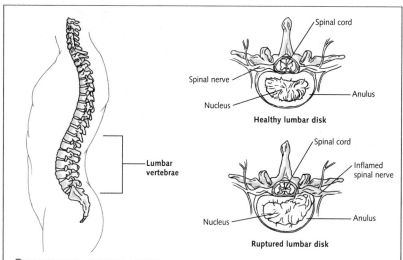

DISK PRESSURE ON SPINAL NERVES
A slipped disk most often occurs in the lower (lumbar) area of the spine. A healthy interverte-bral disk has a ring of tough cartilage (anulus) surrounding a jellylike inner core (nucleus). If the nucleus protrudes through the cartilage as a result of wear or injury, it may press on a spinal nerve, causing pain, numbness, or loss of mobility.

necessary to wear a back brace or a cervical collar. Traction may be used to open intervertebral spaces. Applications of heat or cold may be advised. When the pain subsides, physical therapy, including exercise, may be prescribed to help strengthen weakened back muscles and restore mobility of the back. If pain, numbness, and disability persist, surgery to remove the herniated disk to relieve pressure on the spinal nerves may become necessary.

Slit lamp

An instrument for eye examination using a high-intensity light source that can be shaped into a slit. The slit lamp is used with a twin-eyepiece microscope to give the eye specialist a close look at the various structures in the eye.

The person undergoing the exami-nation rests his or her chin on a rest in front of the slit lamp to hold the head steady while the light is focused into the eye and examined through the microscope.

In some cases, a dye (fluorescein) is placed in the eye to improve visuali-zation of the cornea (the clear outer covering of the eye). The pupil may also be dilated with eye drops to allow better examination of struc-tures in the back of the eye. See EYE, EXAMINATION OF.

Slow virus diseases

Infections that are caused by viruses and characterized by a lengthy peri-od of incubation or a prolonged dura-tion of illness. Slow virus diseases can be caused by a conventional virus, such as a RETROVIRUS, and by infectious agents that cause degener-ative brain disease. The illnesses they cause develop slowly and tend to progress relentlessly. Their distin-guishable signs and symptoms may not appear for months or years after the initial exposure to the infectious agent.

Slow virus diseases caused by a conventional virus include progres-sive multifocal leukoencephalopa-thy, an opportunistic infection that produces a progressive disorder of the central nervous system, usually in people with impaired immune systems. Tropical spastic parapare-sis, also known as HTLV-I–associated myelopathy, is a slow virus disease that affects the spinal cord and is caused by a retrovirus; the infection is characterized by spastic weakness in the legs.

The slow virus diseases that are caused by encephalopathy agents are generally rare but they include CREUTZFELDT-JAKOB DISEASE, kuru, Gerstmann-Sträussler-Scheinker dis-ease, and the inherited condition called fatal familial insomnia. These diseases are characterized by changes in certain parts of the brain.

Illnesses similar to Creutzfeldt-Jakob disease in humans have been linked to ingestion of meat from cows infected with mad cow disease, or bovine spongiform encephalopathy. However, a confirmed connection has not been determined. It is believed that mad cow disease may be the result of using cattle feed containing sheep parts infected with the slow virus animal disease called scrapie. Creutzfeldt-Jakob disease tends to occur in North Africa, where the brains and eyes of sheep are elements of the typical diet. Kuru, a degenera-tive nerve disease, is an infection that was once prevalent among natives in New Guinea who practiced cannibal-ism. With the abandonment of this practice, incidents of kuru have become rare.

There are no known medical cures for slow virus diseases; the prognosis for people infected with them is poor.

Small cell carcinoma

A form of LUNG CANCER. Small cell carcinoma, also known as oat cell carcinoma, is characterized by cells that are small and round or oval and look like oat grains when seen under a microscope. It is the most aggres-sive type of lung cancer and is usual-ly found in people who smoke or used to smoke. Small cell carcinoma often has no noticeable symptoms until it is fairly advanced. Common symptoms include a chronic cough, blood in the sputum, wheezing, repeated episodes of pneumonia, fever, weakness, weight loss, and chest pain. Advanced disease may also include hoarseness, shortness of breath, enlarged lymph nodes in the neck, pain in the arm and shoulder, difficulty swallowing, and drooping eyelids.

A diagnostic workup of small cell carcinoma may include a chest X ray, CT (computed tomography) scan, biopsy, and visual examina-tion of the lung through endoscopy, a procedure in which a fiberoptic tube is used to view the inside of the lungs and chest cavity. Examples of such procedures include BRON-CHOSCOPY, THORACOTOMY, and MEDI-ASTINOSCOPY. Treatment will depend on the stage of the disease, the gen-eral health of the person, and other factors. Chemotherapy and radiation therapy are commonly used to treat the disease. Surgery is rarely recommended in cases of small cell lung cancer because the tumor typically spreads throughout the body even at an early stage. Although most cases of small cell carcinoma are not curable, radiation combined with chemotherapy may cure a small cell carcinoma that is diagnosed while the tumor is small and limited to the lungs.

Small-bowel resection

A surgical procedure in which part of the small intestine is removed. A small-bowel resection is performed to treat serious intestinal disorders, such as cancer, obstruction, or inflammatory bowel disease. To prepare for the procedure, blood and urine studies, X rays, an electrocardiogram, and other tests may be ordered. A light or liquid diet may be prescribed for several days before surgery. Bowel-cleansing enemas and antibiotics may be administered to cleanse the intestine and rid it of bacteria.

In a small-bowel resection, which is done after the person has been given general anesthesia, an incision is made in the abdominal wall, and the tumor or diseased part of the intestine is removed. When possible, only part of the intestine is excised, allowing the healthy remaining sections to be joined, maintaining a passageway for stools. Some cases require an ILEOSTOMY, the creation of an opening or STOMA in the small intestine that allows the discharge of feces into an exterior bag. An ileostomy may be temporary or permanent.

After surgery, nutrients are given intravenously while fluid is drained from the abdomen. The person is encouraged to get out of bed as soon as possible after 8 hours. In 2 to 3 days, a special diet is prescribed, beginning with liquids alone. Weight loss commonly follows a bowel resection. However, over a period of months, weight and strength slowly return. Possible complications of small-bowel resection include bleeding, infection, pneumonia, and pulmonary embolism (passage of a blood clot to the lungs).

Small-bowel series

A series of X rays using the contrast medium barium to examine the small bowel (intestine). A small-bowel series can reveal the causes of malabsorption syndrome or detect the presence of Crohn disease or a tumor. The test is typically performed, as necessary, in conjunction with an upper GASTROINTESTINAL (GI) SERIES.

Before a small-bowel series, the individual fasts for 6 to 12 hours and then, just before the test, drinks a chalky barium solution, which coats and outlines the walls of the small intestine. Barium makes organs show more clearly on X rays. During the test, the individual is placed in different positions on a tilting table to spread the contrast material and scan the intestine for a series of images, which appear on an X-ray machine called a fluoroscope. The series takes about 6 hours, or until the ingested barium travels throughout the intestine. There is little discomfort, although barium may cause constipation and white stools for a few days after the procedure.

Small-bowel transplant

Surgical procedure to treat chronic intestinal failure. Small-bowel transplantation is considered for people who have intestinal failure and cannot tolerate tube feeding. Immunosuppressive drugs increase the chances for survival and the return to normal eating after a transplant. Serious risks include infection and organ rejection. Because of the risks, the procedure is performed less frequently than kidney, heart, or liver transplants.

Smallpox

An acute infectious disease that is caused by a virus. Smallpox has not existed as a naturally acquired infection since 1977. The last case of the disease occurred in Somalia in 1977. The World Health Organization declared the disease officially eradicated throughout the world in 1980. The only cases that have occurred since that time took place in laboratory settings where workers were infected by exposure to the smallpox virus or one closely related to it, which was under study.

The possibility of use of the smallpox virus as a biological weapon by terrorists has led to a renewed interest in improving the vaccine. Many health care workers and military personnel have been vaccinated to better protect the public against the threat of a smallpox attack by terrorists. Adverse reactions to the vaccine can be treated with vaccinia immune globulin (VIG).

When smallpox existed as a significant health threat, it was a contagious infection for those in very close quarters, characterized by a rash of small blisters filled with clear fluid. The virus causing smallpox was readily transmitted via exposure to the respiratory secretions of infected people, through direct contact with the lesions of the skin and mucous membranes, or by contact with materials such as clothing and bed linens that had been contaminated by an infected person's open lesions or scabs.

The symptoms of smallpox included fever, chills, headache, nausea, vomiting, and severe muscle aches. By the fourth day of illness, the fever decreased and the characteristic rash appeared. The fluid-filled blisters, called vesicles, enlarged and filled with an opaque, puslike fluid. Fever reoccurred with the appearance of these pustules, which formed scabs and fell off.

The incubation period of smallpox was usually 10 to 12 days, but the first symptoms sometimes appeared between 6 and 22 days after exposure. The rash generally occurred within 2 to 4 days of the first symptoms. The disease, also called variola, generally lasted 3 to 4 weeks. Some strains of smallpox infection caused permanent scarring; others had a high rate of mortality.

A smallpox diagnosis could be confirmed by blood tests or cultures of material from the lesions in which the virus could be isolated. Antibodies to the virus could be identified in blood tests. There were no medications to treat the disease. Antiviral medication was sometimes used to treat people immediately after they had been exposed to the infection. The primary course of treatment was supportive nursing care of the symptoms of smallpox.

S

Smart drugs

Drugs designed to maximize the working of the brain; cognition-enhancing drugs. Smart drugs include supplements, food additives, or other cerebroactive chemicals intended to enhance mental performance, either by increasing blood flow to the brain or by boosting the levels of neurotransmitters thought to have a part in learning and memory. Smart drugs are sometimes called "nootropics," drugs thought to enhance learning and memory, facilitate the flow of information between the cerebral hemispheres (right brain and left brain), and enhance the resistance of the brain to injury, whether physical or chemical.

Smart drugs developed out of research directed toward improving the memory of individuals with Alzheimer's disease or those who had strokes. The drugs are controversial among neuroscientists. Advocates of smart drugs contend that 140 chemicals, food additives, and drugs that may improve memory are already in existence, although scientific evidence supporting their claims is not convincing.

Smear

A small amount of body tissue or fluid spread on a glass slide for examination under a microscope. Common examples are a blood smear or a cervical Pap smear test. When infection is suspected, a smear can help to identify the microorganism and allow the physician to prescribe the right medication.

Smell

The perception of odors and scents through stimulation of the olfactory (pertaining to smell) nerve in the upper portion of the nose. When special sensory cells in the nose are stimulated by tiny molecules in substances in the environment, the thin, sensitive fibers in the olfactory nerve convey these smell sensations to the olfactory bulb, located at the front of the brain, behind the nose. These smell sensation messages are then identified by the brain as specific odors, scents, and fragrances. The sense of smell belongs to the body's chemical sensing system. The sensory cells responsible for smell are regularly replaced throughout life; how-

ever, the sense of smell tends to decline with age because the cells are replaced more slowly. When the nerves and fibers in the olfactory area are damaged or destroyed or when the olfactory bulb is damaged, the loss of smell may be permanent.

Viral infections like the common cold (see COLD, COMMON), an infection of the upper respiratory tract, sinus infections, and other sources of inflammation of the nasal tissues may cause temporary disturbances in the ability to smell. Persistent difficulties may be caused by an obstruction in

the nose. The obstruction can be caused by NASAL POLYPS, swelling and inflammation of the mucous membrane lining the nasal passages, or a tumor. Other possible causes include ALLERGIES, an injury to the head, psychological factors, or hormonal disturbances. Problems with the sense of smell may also be side effects of certain medications (painkillers, antibiotics, or sedatives) or associated with radiation therapy for cancer of the head and neck. Exposure to certain chemicals, such as insecticides, paint, or metals, may be involved.

CAUTION ON "SMART DRUGS"

Any person considering taking any type of supplement needs to make sure the herb or drug does not adversely interact with other over-the-counter medicines or prescription drugs the person may be taking.

Here are just a few examples: The herb Ashwagandha cannot be taken by a person taking sedatives. DHA (docosahexaenoic acid) can cause problems for a person taking hormones, and gingko biloba should not be taken by a person who is taking prescription blood-thinning medication. Here is a list of common "smart drugs" and what they purport to do:

- Ashwagandha ("Indian ginseng"): thought to clear the mind, strengthen the nervous system, and rejuvenate tissues throughout the body
- Choline: precursor to the neurotransmitter acetylcholine that is essential for memory and cognition
- DHA: polyunsaturated omega-3 fatty acid, a building block of brain tissue crucial for communication between neurons
- DHEA: steroid hormone found in the blood thought to preserve youthfulness and prevent brain cell degeneration
- Gingko biloba: herbal remedy thought to improve blood circulation in the brain
- Phosphatidyl serine: a form of fat abundant in the brain that enables nutrients to enter brain cells
- Piracetam: drug used to improve verbal learning and enhance mental powers
- Pregnenolone: natural precursor to steroid hormones, thought to enhance cognition and intellectual performance
- Pyroglutamate: amino acid found in the brain whose function is not well understood; thought to improve learning and memory
- Vinpocetine: vasodilator drug used to improve blood flow and raise energy levels in the brain

---

THE SENSE OF SMELL
The nose is the portal for the sense of smell. Molecules in the substances a person inhales are detected by sensory receptor cells in hairlike projections (cilia) on the roof of the nasal cavity. The sensory signals are carried by nerve fibers through the surrounding bone to the olfactory bulbs. These bulbs are actually swellings at the ends of the olfactory nerves that enter the lower side of the brain and carry sensory signals to the smell centers in the brain.

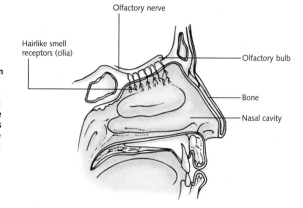

Olfactory nerve

Hairlike smell receptors (cilia)

Olfactory bulb

Bone

Nasal cavity

SMELL CENTERS IN THE BRAIN
SMELL CENTERS IN THE BRAIN
The smell centers in the brain are in areas of the frontal lobe and involve the limbic system—part of the brain that governs instinctual behavior and emotion. The olfactory bulbs, which carry sensory nerve impulses to the brain via the olfactory nerve, are part of the limbic system. The connections between the olfactory bulbs and other parts of the limbic system explain why the sense of smell has a major role in emotionally charged responses such as sexual behavior and certain kinds of memories.

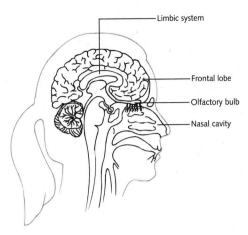

Limbic system
Frontal lobe
Olfactory bulb
Nasal cavity

Disorders may be present at birth. Abnormalities in the sense of smell may be associated with obesity, diabetes mellitus, hypertension, malnutrition, and certain diseases of the central nervous system such as Parkinson disease, Alzheimer's disease, and Korsakoff psychosis. In some cases, a changed or decreased sense of smell can signal the beginnings of a disease.

AGING can also cause loss of smell, with older men being more affected than older women. Diagnosis of smell disorders may include a test involving comparisons of different intensities and kinds of chemical odors and a scratch-and-sniff test. Internal structures of the head may be examined by use of CT (computed tomography) scanning or MRI (magnetic resonance imaging). A short course of treatment with one of the topical CORTICOSTEROIDS may clear up persistent inflammation of the nasal passages. Determining the cause of smell disorders can lead to treatment of an underlying cause of the problem. If the olfactory nerves are torn as a result of head injury or damaged by serious viral infections, the loss of smell may be irreversible, but many smell disorders are curable. Common treatments include surgery to open the nasal passages or medications to reduce nasal inflammation. Psychological or psychiatric treatments may be of benefit in situations involving emotional or psychological issues. When loss of smell or disturbances in the sense of smell cannot be cured, counseling may help a person adjust to the disorder. In rare instances when there is no associated nasal condition and the sense of smell is distorted such that people experience brief episodes of unusual or foul odors, an examination by a neurologist may be recommended.

Smoke inhalation
See INHALATION, SMOKE.

Smoking cessation
A process of ending dependence on nicotine, the addictive drug in tobacco products. Since nicotine is highly addictive, withdrawal from it is often unpleasant, causing an intense craving for cigarettes (or other tobacco products,) difficulty concentrating, irritability, hunger, constipation, and trouble sleeping. Because tobacco use is the single greatest cause of disease and premature death in America today (over 430,000 deaths a year), doctors strongly encourage quitting smoking. Research has shown that fewer than 3 in 100 people who smoke can stop using tobacco products on their own.

People who smoke often need help to quit. Brief tobacco dependence counseling by health care professionals is effective, and increases in effectiveness with more intense therapy. Individual, group, and telephone counseling ("quit-lines") are all effective. Numerous medications for smoking cessation now exist, and should be tried since they can dramatically increase success rates. The "first-line" products include a variety of nicotine-replacement products ("gum," skin patches, inhaler, nasal spray, and lozenge) and oral medication. Some are available without prescription. Persons using nicotine replacement therapy must not smoke while using the medication, and should continue treatment at least 6 to 8 weeks for optimal success. Relapse is most common in the first few days or weeks after quitting, but relapse should not be considered a failure. The person should learn from the attempt, and try again. Abstinence that lasts 3 months or more strongly indicates success. See Aids to stopping smoking, page 1138.

Smoking, tobacco
Puffing or inhaling the smoke of cigarettes, cigars, or pipes. The primary active substance in tobacco smoke is nicotine, a highly addictive drug that has both stimulant and depressant effects. Smoking is the leading cause of preventable death and disability in the United States, and it results in more deaths annually than all other drugs combined. One in 5 deaths in the United States every year is caused by tobacco.

When tobacco smoke is inhaled, nicotine enters the bloodstream and reaches the brain. There it stimulates the release of the hormone EPINEPHRINE (adrenaline), resulting in increased insulin production, a sudden release of sugar into the blood, and a quick burst of energy. Nicotine promotes memory and alertness, enhances certain cognitive skills, reduces appetite, and decreases stress. As the nicotine level in the blood drops and the epinephrine and sugar subside, the person feels depressed and fatigued. This effect induces the smoker to smoke again.

Nicotine prompts the release of the brain chemical dopamine, which affects the nerve pathways controlling pleasure and reward. A similar action is seen in cocaine, marijuana, alcohol, narcotics, and other abused drugs, and it explains nicotine's powerful potential for addiction. Nicotine also produces tolerance (the need to smoke more to achieve a desired effect) and unpleasant withdrawal symptoms, as do other addictive substances. Because of nicotine's addictiveness, people find it difficult to stop smoking even if they understand the serious health consequences.

SMOKING AND HEALTH
While a smoker is smoking, the heart rate increases from 10 to 20 beats per minute, and blood pressure rises from 5 to 10 millimeters of mercury as blood vessels constrict, causing the heart to work harder. Smoke also con-

S

AIDS TO STOPPING SMOKING

The most successful programs to stop smoking typically involve the person gradually giving up tobacco to reduce the addiction to nicotine; receiving counseling and education; and developing substitute behaviors, such as exercise.

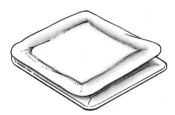

NICOTINE PATCH
Skin patches are applied to the skin like a bandage to release a measured dose of nicotine into the person's bloodstream and help overcome the symptoms of withdrawal.

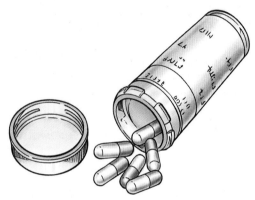

DRUGS TO HELP STOP SMOKING
Medications are often used in smoking cessation programs to help prevent or reduce withdrawal symptoms and make it easier for a person to quit smoking.

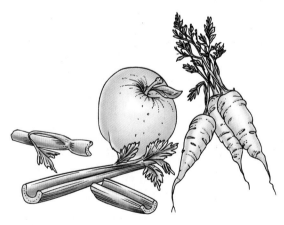

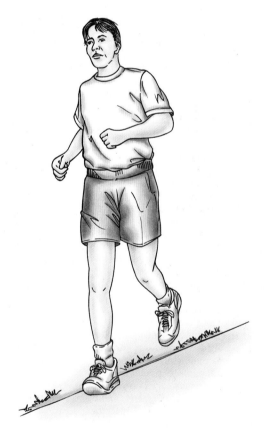

HEALTHY SNACKS
Many former smokers enjoy low-calorie, high-fiber snacks such as apples, celery, or carrots. These snacks help satisfy oral urges without adding pounds.

EXERCISE
Part of a successful smoking cessation program includes exercising, which can improve circulation, increase lung function, and give a person stamina and energy.

tains carbon monoxide, which displaces oxygen in the blood and reduces the oxygen supply to the heart and other organs. These effects result in severe damage to the heart and circula-tory system from chronic smoking. Smoking causes one of every four deaths from coronary artery disease, and it also contributes to artery damage (see ATHEROSCLEROSIS) throughout the body. In addition, smoking increases the tendency of blood to clot, which contributes to the two to three times increased risk of stroke found in smokers and also makes certain kinds of heart attacks more likely.

Of the more than 4,000 chemicals in tobacco smoke, at least 63 are cancer-causing (carcinogenic). These chemicals are found principally in the tar, a thick, sticky, brownish substance that forms when tobacco burns. Tar accumulates in the respiratory tract as smoke passes through and exposes the surfaces to carcinogenic chemicals. Smoking is the leading cause of cancer of the mouth, pharynx (throat), larynx (voice box), and lungs. Some of the tar chemicals also penetrate the walls of the respiratory system and enter the bloodstream, where they affect other organs, or they mix with saliva and enter the digestive system. As a result, smoking is also linked with cancer of the stomach, urinary bladder, esophagus, cervix, and kidney.

Smoking has a role, too, in the development of 85 percent of EMPHYSEMA and chronic bronchitis cases. Women who smoke enter menopause earlier than nonsmokers, and smokers who are pregnant increase the risk of stillbirth and low birth weight in their newborns. Reduced circulation of oxygen in the body results in slower wound healing (for example, after surgery or an accident) and increased wrinkling of the skin, which can make smokers look older than they are. Smoking contributes to the development of ulcers in the stomach and upper intestine and can prevent them from healing. Smoking may also cause sexual problems, particularly erectile dysfunction (impotence) in men, because of impaired blood flow to the genitals, and it can contribute to high blood pressure (hypertension). Smoking also impairs the senses of smell and taste.

Secondhand or passive smoke also poses serious health risks. In fact, the noninhaled, or sidestream, smoke from a cigarette contains more tar, carbon monoxide, and certain carcinogens than the inhaled smoke. Secondhand smoke causes lung cancer and heart disease in people exposed to it. Infants whose mothers smoked during pregnancy and are exposed repeatedly to tobacco smoke after birth are more likely to die of SUDDEN INFANT DEATH SYNDROME (SIDS). Children raised in households with smokers are at higher risk of asthma, ear infections, pneumonia, bronchitis, and tonsillitis than children in nonsmoking families.

So-called smokeless tobacco (chewing tobacco and snuff) is addictive and has health risks, as does cigar smoking, which can increase a person's risk of lip and mouth cancer. See TOBACCO CHEWING.

TREATMENT

When a person stops smoking, the negative health consequences of the addiction begin to reverse themselves. Within as little as 2 or 3 days, ex-smokers notice a sharpening of taste and smell, for example. Within a few months, lung function increases and shortness of breath eases, circulation improves, walking and exercise become easier, and the risk of respiratory infections drops. Over the next several years, the increased chance of cancer and heart disease from smoking decreases. After 5 years of non-smoking, the risk of heart disease falls to that of a person who has never smoked. After 10 to 15 years of non-smoking, the risk of lung cancer and heart disease, the two biggest killers, is no higher in an ex-smoker than in someone who has never smoked.

Despite the obvious health benefits, smoking can be difficult to quit because of the powerful addictive effect of nicotine. Withdrawal from nicotine causes intense, unpleasant craving for cigarettes, irritability, hunger, constipation, difficulty concentrating, and trouble sleeping (insomnia). Research has shown that fewer than 3 smokers in 100 can quit smoking entirely on their own. The most successful programs, which have success rates of 20 to 40 of every 100 participants, involve gradual reduction of tobacco use leading up to the quit date, psychological counseling, peer support, and education on developing substitute behaviors and handling possible relapse situations. Such programs, available through health care organizations, the American Cancer Society, and the American Lung Association, last 4 to 8 weeks and provide 1 or 2 hours of support per week. Nicotine substitutes, such as nicotine chewing gum or skin patches (see SKIN PATCH), are often used in smoking cessation pro-

LIFE-THREATENING EFFECTS OF SMOKING
Lung cancer is the most widely known health hazard from smoking, but by no means the only one. Smoking also contributes to or causes stroke, heart disease, ulcers, childbirth complications, bladder cancer, pancreatic cancer, and cancers of the throat, mouth, and larynx. Not smoking is the single most important step to take toward good health.

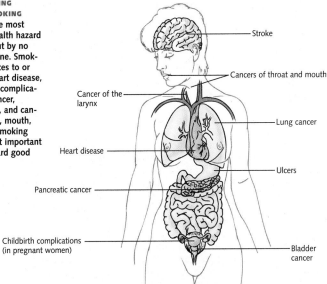

Stroke

Cancers of throat and mouth

Cancer of the larynx

Lung cancer

Heart disease

Ulcers

Pancreatic cancer

Childbirth complications (in pregnant women)

Bladder cancer

S

grams to prevent or reduce withdrawal symptoms and make it easier to quit.

Snails and disease

The association between snails carrying parasites or their larvae and the infections they cause in humans, who are usually exposed to the snails in natural bodies of water. Clonorchiasis is a chronic parasitic infestation of the liver in humans that is caused by the ingestion of freshwater fish containing the larvae of the liver FLUKE, which have undergone a stage of their development in the liver glands of water snails. Swimmer's itch is caused by parasites of birds and mammals that are carried by infected snails and released into natural bodies of fresh water by the snails.

Snakebite

Injury caused when the flesh is pierced by the fangs of a snake; reptile bite (see BITES, REPTILE). Most snakes are not poisonous, and their bites are not particularly dangerous. Although thousands of people are bitten by snakes each year, fewer than 10 percent die of their injuries. Poisonous snakes in the United States include rattlesnakes, copperheads, water moccasins, and coral snakes. In the United States, most poisonous snakebites involve rattlesnakes. Depending on the species of snake, the venom either destroys tissue and blood or causes neurological damage that leads to cardiac and respiratory arrest.

First aid for a nonpoisonous snakebite includes thorough washing of the area of the bite and the application of antibiotic cream and a bandage. If the area of the bite changes color, swells, or is painful, the snake was probably poisonous, in which case, it is essential to obtain emergency medical assistance. The person should lie as quietly as possible to limit circulation of the venom. The part of the body that has been bitten should be kept as still as possible.

Sneezing

An explosive, involuntary expulsion of air brought on by irritation in the nose or a tickling sensation deep in the nasal passages. People sneeze for several different reasons. Sneezing may be a way to clear the nose when a person has a cold. People who have allergic rhinitis (see RHINITIS, ALLERGIC; also called hay fever) may sneeze to expel allergens (allergy-causing particles) from the nasal passages. People with a constantly running nose may sneeze from time to time as a result of blood vessels in the nose overreacting to humidity and temperature changes. Some people who do not have ALLERGIES release histamine (a chemical that produces allergy symptoms), which causes sneezing. When sneezing is a symptom of a cold, it goes away when the cold is over. If sneezing persists and is accompanied by other allergy symptoms, such as a congested nose, excess mucus from the nose, a SORE THROAT, and/or irritated eyes, an allergist or immunologist should be consulted.

Sneezing may be alleviated with over-the-counter or prescription antihistamines to dry mucous membranes in the nose or decongestants to shrink swollen blood vessels blocking the nose. Nasal sprays containing CROMOLYN SODIUM may help control sneezing by preventing the release of histamine. Cortisone nasal sprays may be prescribed to reduce inflammation that causes sneezing. Sneezes should never be stifled because mucus could be forced into the middle ear or sinuses and cause infection. In some instances, a stifled sneeze can cause backed-up air pressure in the ear sufficient to rupture an eardrum.

Snellen chart

A display showing letters arranged in lines of increasingly smaller size and used to test sharpness of vision. Typically the person is asked to read the letters on the line that can be seen by people with perfect vision from 20 feet away. If the person can do this, he or she is said to have 20/20 vision. If vision is less sharp—if, for example, the person can read at 20 feet that which a person with normal vision can read at 60 feet—he or she has 20/60 vision. Testing with the Snellen chart is part of a standard eye examination. See VISION TESTS.

Snoring

Noisy sounds produced during sleep because of an obstruction to the free flow of air through the passages at the back of the mouth. Snoring affects up to 60 percent of the adult population.

The sound of snoring is produced when the structures at the back of the mouth and throat collapse against one another and vibrate as air is breathed in and out. Snoring is more frequent in men and in people who are overweight and may become more pronounced with age.

CAUSES

Snoring may be caused by poor muscle tone in the tongue and throat or by overly relaxed muscles resulting from deep sleep, alcohol intake, narcotics, or SEDATIVES. The relaxed muscles cause the back of the tongue or the top of the throat to collapse and obstruct the airway. An extended soft palate or a long uvula can intensify snoring. Colds, sinus infections, and allergies can block the nasal passages and contribute to the mouth breathing that often causes snoring. Deformities of the nose, such as a deviated septum, may also have a role. Children with large tonsils or adenoids and children with asthma may be more prone to snoring.

Snoring may be most disturbing to a person attempting to sleep within hearing distance of the person snoring. It may also disrupt the normal sleeping patterns of the person who snores, causing daytime fatigue. Corrective techniques that may help include sleeping on the side rather than on the back and elevating the head with an extra pillow.

Extremely loud snoring can be a symptom of obstructive sleep apnea (see SLEEP APNEA SYNDROME), a disorder in which there are recurrent episodes of interrupted breathing during deep levels of sleep. It is caused by an obstruction of air move-

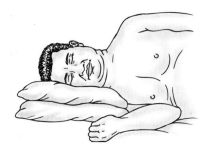

SLEEP POSITION FOR A PERSON WHO SNORES
Sleeping on the side with extra pillows to elevate the head may help alleviate snoring. A person is more likely to snore lying on his or her back because the jaw tends to fall open.

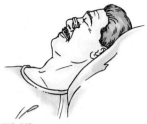

SNORING AID
Over-the-counter snoring strips may hold the nostrils open during sleep to keep the airway unobstructed. When the ends are affixed to each nostril, the strip holds the sides of the nostrils out as well. The strips help some people, but most need to see a doctor for snoring problems.

ment in the upper respiratory passages. The person may experience extreme sleepiness during the day and headaches in the morning.

A person who experiences these symptoms and whose breath stoppage during sleep has been observed should consult a physician. If the person is overweight, diet and exercise changes may provide significant relief from severe snoring and sleep apnea. The doctor may also refer a person with symptoms of sleep apnea to a sleep laboratory to confirm diagnosis of the condition. A sleep disorder specialist may recommend the use of continuous positive airway pressure (CPAP). This treatment involves a mask being placed over the nose during sleeping hours while a device delivers air at slightly increased pressure. The small increase in air pressure may be sufficient to open the upper airway passages of the person sleeping, which can prevent the occurrence of sleep apnea and snoring. Surgical procedures to increase the size of the throat are generally only partially effective for treating sleep apnea.

Sobriety

The state of being free from addiction to a drug or substance. In a person who has been drug or alcohol dependent, sobriety is also known as recovery. The two terms are used to describe a person who has changed his or her lifestyle and is happy living a sober life.

Sodium

A mineral needed by the body for normal function. Sodium controls the volume of fluid outside the cells and helps to maintain ACID-BASE BALANCE. Sodium helps to maintain the electrical system within the nervous tissue, thereby maintaining function of nerves and muscles. The amount of sodium in the body is controlled by the kidneys.

Sodium occurs naturally in most foods and drinking water, and it is easily absorbed. Sodium is also added to many food products as baking soda, monosodium glutamate, sodium nitrite, sodium saccharin, and sodium benzoate. Processed meats, including bacon and ham, canned soups and vegetables, and fast foods are all very high in sodium. Adults should consume a maximum of between 1,100 and 3,300 milligrams of sodium per day; but since a single teaspoon of table salt contains 2,300 milligrams of sodium, it is easy to consume too much.

Too much sodium can cause a condition known as hypernatremia in which the blood carries excessive sodium. An excessive level of sodium in the blood in turn can lead to EDEMA or swelling of the body tissues. A high-sodium diet can also worsen HYPERTENSION (high blood pressure).

Soft spot, infant

Soft area on the top of an infant's head where the skull bones have not yet joined (see FONTANELLE).

Soft-tissue injury

Any injury to the muscles, tendons, or ligaments generally caused by overuse or physical trauma. Soft-tissue injuries include muscle strains and sprains, bruises, pulled muscles, TENDINITIS, fibrositis, and CARPAL TUNNEL SYNDROME. A soft-tissue sprain of the back muscles may be caused by minor injury, increased athletic activity, poor posture, or improper body position during sleep. This type of sprain can cause strong muscle spasms and severe back pain. Back pain caused by soft-tissue strain is generally treated with anti-inflammatory or muscle relaxant medication. The condition can be prevented with regular exercises to stretch and strengthen the back muscles and the abdominal muscles that help support the back.

Soiling

See ENCOPRESIS.

Solar plexus

A network of interconnected nerves in the abdomen that lies behind the stomach and between the adrenal glands. Also called the celiac plexus, the solar plexus sends out nerve branches to the stomach, intestines, and most other abdominal organs.

Soluble fiber

See FIBER, DIETARY.

Solvent abuse

See INHALANTS.

Somatic

Having to do with the body. Somatic is an adjective referring to the body as distinct from the mind.

Somatization disorder

A mental illness characterized by frequent complaints about physical symptoms that have no discernible physical cause and that arise from emotional conflict or anxiety. The symptoms and complaints can affect any body system and often persist for years. Common symptoms include painful menstruation, pain during

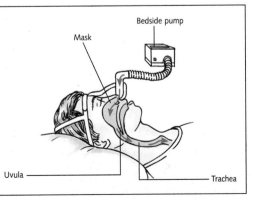

SNORING AND SLEEP APNEA
Snoring may be caused by sleep apnea, a condition in which tissues at the back of the throat temporarily block breathing during deep sleep. Doctors may prescribe continuous positive airway pressure (CPAP). To be treated with CPAP, the person wears a mask to bed that pumps air into the nose during sleep. The force of the air opens the airway so that air can enter the trachea (windpipe) and lungs.

Bedside pump
Mask
Uvula
Trachea

5

intercourse (dyspareunia), lack of sexual desire, distress in the gastro-intestinal tract (nausea, vomiting, bloating, or diarrhea), paralysis or weakness of muscles, temporary blindness, and pain in the chest or joints. Symptoms tend to begin or worsen during the period of grief during or following a loss and often intensify under stress. Somatization disorder usually begins before age 30 and is most common in adolescent and young-adult females.

Somatization disorder can lead to serious complications, in addition to the pain and discomfort the individual feels from the symptoms. Repeated diagnostic tests to determine the cause of the complaints can be risky and expensive. Because people with the disorder have a history of unsubstantiated complaints without physical evidence, physicians may miss the appearance of a real disease. Family and work life can be seriously disturbed.

Treatment consists of developing a relationship with one doctor to prevent repeated unnecessary testing, reassuring the patient that follow-up will control symptoms, encouraging discussion about causes of stress, and teaching new ways of dealing with stress.

Somatoform disorders

A group of closely related mental illnesses characterized by distressing physical symptoms that lack a physical cause and arise instead from emotional conflict or anxiety. Examples include HYPOCHONDRIASIS (an excessive concern with the possible symptoms and signs of illness), body dysmorphic disorder (a disabling preoccupation with an imagined or exaggerated physical defect), pain disorder (frequent, persistent complaints about pain lacking a physical cause), SOMATIZATION DISORDER (frequent, persistent complaints about symptoms with no physical cause), and conversion disorder (symptoms affecting voluntary motor or sensory neurologic function).

Somatotype

Classification of body shape and type of physique. The three somatotypes are ectomorph, endomorph, and mesomorph. Ectomorphs are thin and angular, endomorphs are round and tend to be overweight, and mesomorphs are muscular and athletic.

Somnoplasty

Surgical treatment to eliminate snoring. Somnoplasty uses heat energy to remove tissue of the soft palate and the uvula, the flap found at the back of the throat. The procedure is usually performed in the surgeon's office with local anesthesia. It is not used to treat sleep apnea syndrome.

Sonohysterogram

A diagnostic technique used to evaluate abnormal vaginal bleeding. This relatively new technique involves filling the uterus with saline (sterile salt water) during a vaginal ultrasound. A sonohysterogram is considered particularly useful in helping the doctor visualize intrauterine polyps (see POLYP) and differentiate benign polyps from malignant lesions.

Sore throat

Pain in the throat caused by inflammation of the tissue lining the throat passage. The medical term for sore throat is pharyngitis. A sore throat can become more painful when a person speaks or swallows. It is sometimes a symptom of infection that may have originated elsewhere in the body.

CAUSES

The cause of a sore throat may be a viral infection, such as flu, common cold (see COLD, COMMON), or mononucleosis. The cause may also be bacterial, such as *Streptococcus* (the bacterium that causes strep throat), or *Staphylococcus* (a common bacterium that can release toxins into the bloodstream). Infectious mononucleosis (see MONONUCLEOSIS, INFECTIOUS; an acute viral infection) can cause a sore throat, as can oral GONORRHEA (a bacterial sexually transmitted disease). Irritation of the throat's lining from air pollution, smoking or other tobacco use, or excessive alcohol intake can cause a sore throat.

DIAGNOSIS AND TREATMENT

A doctor can identify and evaluate a sore throat by observing the red, swollen tissue lining the throat. If the condition has persisted for more than a few days, the doctor may also use a swab to collect a sample of throat cells and secretions to be examined in a laboratory. A culture is performed primarily to distinguish between viral infections, which tend to be less serious, and bacterial infections, which if untreated may lead to more serious complications.

Sore throats caused by a cold or flu or by localized irritation usually pass when the infection disappears or when the irritants are avoided. A sore throat that persists needs medical attention. Home remedies to ease the discomfort of a sore throat include gargling with warm salt water or a small amount of hydrogen peroxide diluted in water, sucking over-the-counter anesthetic throat lozenges, and drinking hot fluids such as tea and clear broth.

Sound therapy

The use of sound vibrations to cure disease and achieve higher levels of conscious awareness. Sound therapy uses sound waves for many purposes, especially to reduce the pain and inflammation of muscle, joint, tendon, and ligament disorders. Sound vibration therapy can be administered to sore muscles through a hand-held machine that emits inaudible sound waves through the skin. Ultrasound vibrations, which are very high-frequency sounds inaudible to the human ear, are used to shatter kidney stones without surgery; and ULTRASOUND SCANNING is a standard diagnostic aid.

Music therapy is a form of sound therapy used to relieve pain, improve a person's mood, calm or sedate an anxious person, and boost a person's level of physical, mental, and social functioning. Music therapy uses tuning forks, chanting, singing, and other musical instruments to create harmonic resonance that may help promote health and well-being.

Sound therapy is often used with imagery to promote relaxation and exploration of the unconsciousness. It has been successfully used preoperatively for pain management, and also to calm women during high-risk childbirth.

Soy

A type of bean that may have significant health benefits. In laboratory tests, a chemical in soybeans has been of benefit in limiting the growth of cancer cells. Rates of breast and prostate cancer in Asia, where soybeans are a staple of the diet, are much lower than in the United States. A number of studies in humans have demonstrated that soy protein lowers total cholesterol and LDL (low-density lipoprotein) cholesterol without lowering HDL (high-density lipoprotein) cholesterol, the "good" cholesterol. Soy has also been associated with estrogen production in women. See PHYTOCHEMICALS.

Soy preparations

Soybean products believed to have medicinal properties and the ability to prevent certain diseases. Soy isoflavones, naturally occurring plant chemicals found in soy, have mild estrogenlike effects and are taken by many women to relieve symptoms of menopause, such as hot flashes. Soy isoflavones are also thought by some people to have the ability to prevent hormone-related cancers, such as breast and prostate cancer. There are no definitive studies to verify these claims.

Soy protein is one of the few plant proteins comparable to animal protein, containing all the amino acids essential for the building and maintenance of body tissues. Soy protein contains no cholesterol, is high in fiber, and may be effective in preventing atherosclerosis (hardening of the arteries).

The Food and Drug Administration (FDA) has authorized a nutrition label for soy products that states that

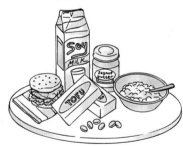

POPULAR SOY PRODUCTS
A variety of soy products are available in the United States. Soy milk, derived from the soy plant, can be used like dairy milk. Tofu is a cheeselike food made from soy milk. Soy butter is made from roasted soy beans and soybean oil. Textured soy protein is made from compressed soy flour; when rehydrated, it can be used like ground meat.

at least 25 grams of soy protein consumed per day as part of a low-fat diet can lower high blood cholesterol levels. Soy protein is used as meat and milk substitutes and as an ingredient in baby formula.

Space medicine

See AEROSPACE MEDICINE.

Sparfloxacin

See FLUOROQUINOLONES.

Spasm

An involuntary muscle contraction. Muscle cramps (see CRAMP) are sudden, painful spasms caused by an excessive and prolonged contraction of the muscle fibers. Spasms may be due to overuse, muscle stress, or dehydration. Exercise-related cramps usually occur during or immediately after workouts, due to muscle fiber damage and a buildup of chemicals such as lactic acid.

Other types of spasms include hiccups, stuttering, and tics. A SEIZURE (a sudden episode of uncontrolled electrical activity in the brain) can also cause a series of involuntary muscle contractions. Internal spasms can affect the blood vessels, bronchi, esophagus, pylorus, or other hollow organs. Minor spasms do not require treatment. However, a person with an unexplained, persistent, or painful spasm should seek a doctor's care.

Spastic colon

See IRRITABLE BOWEL SYNDROME.

Spastic paralysis

Also known as spastic paraplegia, a neurological disorder characterized by increased rigidity of the muscles (spasticity) and weakness or paralysis of the lower body. The progress of spastic paralysis, which can be caused by a genetic disorder, varies from person to person. In some cases, there is only mild stiffness, weakness, and heaviness in the legs. Other people may eventually require a wheelchair. Children with this disorder can experience difficulty learning to walk, or they may gradually lose the ability to walk. Although some medications may reduce spasticity, there is no specific treatment to slow degeneration of affected nerves. Supportive measures include physical therapy and walking aids. Other

causes of spastic paralysis include infections, multiple sclerosis, and spinal cord tumors.

Spasticity

A condition characterized by stiff or rigid muscles. In spasticity, certain muscles are continuously contracted. This can interfere with movement, gait, or speech. Spasticity is usually caused by damage to part of the brain or spinal cord that controls voluntary movement. Possible causes of damage include stroke, cerebral palsy, multiple sclerosis, and spinal cord or brain injury. Spasticity can manifest itself in a number of different ways. Symptoms include clonus (a series of rapid muscle contractions), hypertonicity (increased muscle tone), exaggerated deep tendon reflexes, fixed joints, muscle spasms, and scissoring (involuntary crossing of the legs). Treatment includes medication (such as baclofen, clonazepam, and diazepam) and physical therapy (for example, range-of-motion exercises and muscle stretching). In some cases, surgery is necessary. Injections of botulinum toxin type A (Botox) into the muscles can also relieve spasticity.

Spatulate

A surgical instrument with a flat, blunt, spoonlike end. Spatulate also refers to a procedure in which the opening of a tubular structure of the body, such as a blood vessel, is widened before it is joined to another such structure to make the joined area more secure and less likely to narrow.

Specialist

A doctor who focuses on a certain part of the body or on specific diseases. For example, cardiologists are specialists in heart disorders, oncologists are specialists in cancer, and gastroenterologists are specialists in digestive system disorders. Specialists have many years of training in their areas of specialty or subspecialty.

Specimen

A sample of a body fluid or tissue for laboratory analysis. Doctors may order the collection of tissue or blood, urine, or other body fluid samples in order to diagnose and treat disease.

S

SPECT

Single-photon emission computed tomography. SPECT is a nuclear scanning technique that is similar to CT SCANNING (computed tomography scanning) because a specialized cameralike device receives signals and feeds them into a computer. The computer then transmits the results to a monitor that displays cross-sectional or two-dimensional images.

SPECT uses some of the same radionuclides as NUCLEAR MEDICINE but with a more sophisticated camera to detect the radiation. SPECT is used to evaluate brain disease and abdominal disease.

Speculum

An instrument used to hold open the vagina for a pelvic examination or a procedure. Before insertion, the speculum usually is warmed with lukewarm water. When inserted, the speculum allows the doctor a clear view of the cervix and permits a PAP SMEAR to be done easily. A smaller speculum is available to accommodate small vaginal openings; larger ones are used for procedures that require more exploration than usual.

Speech

Oral communication. Speech is one of the most important ways in which people relate to their environment. SPEECH DISORDERS in children may be the result of problems such as mental retardation, cerebral palsy, hearing loss, or cleft palate. In older people, difficulties with speech are commonly caused by injury, stroke, or brain tumor. People who experience speaking problems can benefit from SPEECH THERAPY.

Speech disorders

A group of disorders that result in ineffective or impaired communication due to difficulty speaking. Speech is one of the primary ways in which people relate to their environment. The most common cause of speech problems in children is MENTAL RETARDATION. Other potential causes include ATTENTION DEFICIT/HYPERACTIVITY DISORDER (ADHD), AUTISM, CEREBRAL PALSY, cleft palate (see CLEFT LIP AND PALATE), dental problems, HEARING LOSS, LEARNING DISABILITIES, palate disorders, TOURETTE SYNDROME, and

vocal cord injuries. Adults can also develop speech disorders as a result of STROKE, ALS (amyotrophic lateral sclerosis), PARKINSON DISEASE, or MULTIPLE SCLEROSIS.

TYPES OF SPEECH DISORDERS

There are many different types of speech disorders. Voice disorders entail differences in the quality, loudness, and pitch of sound. Articulation is the process by which sounds, syllables, and words are formed; in articulation deficiencies, sounds are made inappropriately or incorrectly. For example, "rabbit" may be pronounced as "wabbit." An articulation problem sometimes sounds like "baby talk," and this speech pattern is common in preschool years. However, children should make all the normal sounds of English by age 8 years. Like many speech disorders, articulation problems in older children and adults may impact negatively on social, emotional, educational, or vocational status.

Dysfluencies are rhythm disorders characterized by the repetition of a sound, word, or phrase. STUTTERING is a type of dysfluency. It is a disturbance in the normal fluency and time patterning of speech. Developmental stuttering is the most common form of stuttering. It includes all cases of gradual-onset childhood stuttering that are not the result of brain damage. A second type of stuttering is persistent developmental stuttering; this is developmental stuttering that has not gone into remission spontaneously or as a result of speech therapy.

DIAGNOSIS AND TREATMENT

Early evaluation and treatment of speech disorders are best. A child can quickly fall behind if speech and language development is delayed. It is especially important to evaluate children who are at high risk because of problems such as cerebral palsy or chronic ear infections. Treatment of a speech disorder depends on its underlying cause. In many cases, primary care doctors refer people with speech disorders to speech-language pathologists. A speech-language pathologist is a professional who is trained at the master's or doctoral level to evaluate speech disorders and prepare plans to improve speech.

SPEECH THERAPY is the primary treatment for many types of speech disorders, such as stuttering and articulation deficiencies. Depending on the results of evaluation, different services may be recommended. For children, play may be used to teach communication, language models, or rules of conversation (such as turn-taking). Responses are consistently stimulated, and correct responses are rewarded. In the case of stuttering, antidepressants have also proven useful.

Cleft palate is a common cause of speech disorders. Surgery to repair a cleft palate generally takes place when a child is aged 6 to 12 months. About one in five children will benefit from a second operation on the palate to obtain better speech. A procedure called an alveolar bone graft may be done between ages 6 and 10 years to put extra bone in the gum and allow the permanent teeth to come in better.

Speech mechanism

The structures involved in the production of sound that is modified into spoken language.

SPEECH PRODUCTION

The production of speech sounds begins with air that is pushed out of the lungs and passes up through the trachea into the LARYNX (voice box). The larynx is a hollow organ, located between the pharynx and the trachea, and constructed of several pieces of cartilage. The largest of these is the thyroid cartilage, commonly called the Adam's apple, which lies at the front of the throat and projects slightly outward. The cricoid cartilage is just below it, connecting the thyroid cartilage to the trachea. At the back, on top of the cricoid cartilage, are two projections called the arytenoid cartilages. The VOCAL CORDS (also called vocal folds) stretch across the larynx, suspended from the thyroid cartilage in front and the arytenoid cartilages at the back. At rest, the vocal cords lie apart, forming an opening (called the glottis) through which air passes for breathing.

For speech production, the vocal cords contract and become taut, so that they vibrate as air passes between them to produce sound. The

THE ANATOMY OF SPEECH

The production of speech requires the precise coordination of muscles in the head, neck, chest, and abdomen. Speech is generated when exhaled air passes across the vocal cords, two fibrous bands of tissue located in the larynx. Vowel sounds begin in the throat and are given their distinctive "shapes" by adjustments of the mouth and tongue; consonants are formed by controlled interruptions of exhaled air.

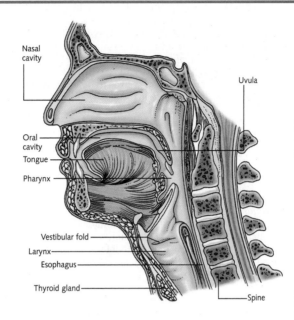

Nasal cavity
Uvula
Oral cavity
Tongue
Pharynx
Vestibular fold
Larynx
Esophagus
Thyroid gland
Spine

HOW SPEECH IS PRODUCED
The larynx and the vocal cords are primarily responsible for the production of voice, but exhaled air must cross the vocal cords to produce sounds, which are articulated by the mouth and tongue to produce meaningful speech.

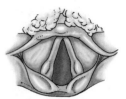

OPEN VOCAL CORDS
The vocal cords remain open while air is inhaled and exhaled.

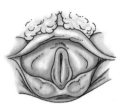

CLOSED VOCAL CORDS
The vocal cords close on exhalation, and sounds are produced when air vibrates through the folds.

cords can be opened, closed, and vibrated to modify the air stream. Changes in the tightness of the cords produce changes in the pitch of the sound, and changes in the size of the larynx and other chambers in the throat and head alter the volume. From the larynx, the sound passes into the pharynx (upper throat) and mouth and is modified by positioning and moving the palate, tongue, teeth, and lips to produce different speech sounds. Air can also be channeled through the nose to produce nasal sounds.

SPEECH AND LANGUAGE

Speech is only one form of communication by language, a broader term that encompasses the comprehension and expression of ideas through the use of symbols that form words. Two areas of the brain that control speech and language are in the cerebral cortex (the top layer of the cerebrum). The Wernicke area (located close to the auditory cortex

that interprets sound stimuli) is involved in recognizing and understanding spoken words and choosing words to be spoken. It sends this information to the Broca area, which receives information about what is to be spoken and coordinates the learned movements that produce speech that is used to express thought. Based on direction from the Broca area, the motor cortex sends signals to the muscles in the throat and face that are involved in speech production.

The complex language function is generally located on one side of the brain, in the so-called dominant hemisphere. In right-handed people, the left side of the brain almost always controls language. In left-handed people, the language function is not always confined to either hemisphere; the language area tends to be on the left side, but may be on the right side or shared by both sides.

Speech therapy

Treatment to help people overcome problems with oral communication. Speech is one of the most important ways in which people relate to their environment. Speech therapy is the primary treatment for many types of SPEECH DISORDERS, such as stuttering and articulation deficiencies. Different types of speech therapy are recommended for different problems. For children, play is commonly used to teach communication, language models, or rules of conversation (such as turn-taking). Responses are consistently stimulated, and correct responses are rewarded.

Speech therapy is usually conducted by a speech-language pathologist, a professional who is trained at the master's or doctoral level to evaluate speech disorders and prepare plans to improve speech. Early evaluation and treatment of speech disorders are best. A child can quickly fall behind if speech and language development is

S

delayed. It is especially important to evaluate and treat children who are at high risk as a result of problems such as MENTAL RETARDATION, CEREBRAL PALSY, HEARING LOSS, or cleft palate (see CLEFT LIP AND PALATE). In older people, speech problems may be the result of various causes such as injury, STROKE, or BRAIN TUMOR. People of any age can benefit from speech therapy. Speech therapy can be helpful for people who are having trouble either speaking or expressing their thoughts. Speech therapists also work with those who have trouble swallowing.

Sperm

The male reproductive cell, maturing and multiplying in the testicles beginning at puberty. The production of sperm is triggered by the male sex hormone testosterone and gonadotropin hormones produced in the pituitary gland. A single sperm has an enlarged head, which contains the cell nucleus and genetic material. A tail on the cell propels the highly mobile sperm. Sperm cells exit a man's body in a fluid called semen, during the process of EJACULATION. An ejaculation can contain 500 million sperm. (See REPRODUCTIVE SYSTEM, MALE.) As a result of sexual intercourse, a single sperm may join with an egg in the process of FERTILIZATION, which may result in pregnancy. Because of the unique way that both sperm and egg cells divide (MEIOSIS), a single sperm contains only half as much genetic information as any other cell in the body. When a sperm and egg unite, the genetic material from each parent is mixed in the new cell that is formed.

Sperm bank

A place that holds a collection of donor sperm (male sex cells) in order to fertilize female eggs. If a male partner cannot produce a sufficient number of normal sperm, or if a single woman chooses to become pregnant without a male partner, ARTIFICIAL INSEMINATION with semen from a sperm bank is a fertilization option. All sperm donors are carefully screened for medical problems and sexually transmitted diseases. They are registered according to age, race, hair and eye color, and body build. See also INFERTILITY.

Sperm count

A laboratory test to determine the number of sperm cells in a sample of semen (the thick, white fluid expelled from the penis at sexual climax). A sperm count varies from 20 to 250 million sperm cells per milliliter of semen. A sperm count is performed as part of SEMEN ANALYSIS, a series of related tests to determine the fertility of a man. It is also used after surgical sterilization (vasectomy). If the semen contains no sperm cells, the operation was successful.

Sperm extraction

A surgical procedure used to collect sperm from a man when ejaculation is not possible or when sperm does not reach the ejaculate. Sperm extraction is used in men who have a structural abnormality or an obstruction of the vas deferens, the tube through which sperm move during ejaculation. It is sometimes performed after a vasectomy or after a failure to reverse a vasectomy. Before the procedure, the man may have general anesthesia, but usually a local anesthetic is used. Seminal fluid containing sperm is removed either with a tube or a needle through an incision. Alternatively, a needle biopsy directly from the testicles is obtained, and sperm cells are recovered. The sperm is then treated and prepared for ICSI (intracytoplasmic sperm injection) and IN VITRO FERTILIZATION.

Sperm motility

A laboratory test to determine the ability of sperm cells to move (motility) or be motile. Normally, about 50 percent of sperm are motile. Sperm cells that move poorly or not at all are generally incapable of fertilizing a female egg cell and causing pregnancy. Sperm motility is performed as part of SEMEN ANALYSIS, a test repeated several times to determine fertility in a man.

Spermatocele

A noncancerous mass that develops in the small coiled tubules (epididymis) on the back of the testicle. A spermatocele is filled with fluid and dead sperm cells and is usually painless. It requires medical treatment only if it grows large enough to cause discomfort or difficulty.

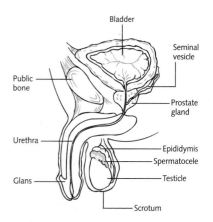

A FLUID-FILLED CYST
A spermatocele feels soft and will give slightly when squeezed. It requires removal only if it grows large enough to cause pain.

Spermatozoa

Also known as SPERM, the male sex cells that fertilize female eggs. Sperm is found in SEMEN, the thick fluid that is secreted by the male reproductive organs and is discharged from the penis upon ejaculation during SEXUAL INTERCOURSE. Semen contains millions of sperm, which have well-defined heads, midsections, and tails and move with swimming motion. Whenever sperm are released by the penis into the vagina, they can travel through the uterus into a fallopian tube, where they can fertilize an egg, resulting in PREGNANCY. To prevent pregnancy, it is important for partners to use an effective means of CONTRACEPTION.

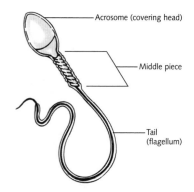

MALE REPRODUCTIVE CELL
Seen under a microscope, the head of a sperm cell, which contains the nucleus, is covered by the acrosome, which contains enzymes that enable the sperm to penetrate an egg. In the middle piece of the sperm, energy is generated. The tail, or flagellum, propels the cell through a fluid environment.

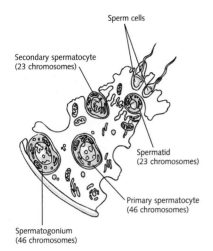

Sperm cells

Secondary spermatocyte
(23 chromosomes)

Spermatid
(23 chromosomes)

Primary spermatocyte
(46 chromosomes)

Spermatogonium
(46 chromosomes)

SPERM PRODUCTION
Spermatogenesis, or sperm production, involves the mitosis (division) of spermatogonia to become primary spermatocytes. These undergo the first division to form secondary spermatocytes. These undergo the second division resulting in four spermatids, which subsequently become sperm. Overall, it takes approximately 2 months for sperm to reach maturity.

Spermicides

Chemical agents that kill sperm or make them unable to fertilize an egg. Spermicides are used as a form of birth control and are most effective when combined with another birth control method, such as a condom, diaphragm, or cervical cap. See CONTRACEPTION, OTHER METHODS.

SPF

See SUN PROTECTION FACTOR.

Spherocytosis, hereditary

An inherited abnormality of the proteins that normally stabilize the membranes of red blood cells. Hereditary spherocytosis is a common cause of hemolytic anemia among people of northern European descent; it is found infrequently among blacks and members of other ethnic groups. In some cases, the defect appears spontaneously, with neither parent affected by the disease. About 1 in 5,000 people in the United States has the condition.

Symptoms can vary widely but may first appear at birth with JAUNDICE. The clinical expression of hereditary spherocytosis can range from no symptoms to life-threatening anemia,

either from the abnormal cells breaking apart (hemolysis) or from an aplastic crisis, in which the bone marrow stops making new cells. An aplastic crisis is sometimes caused by a folic acid deficiency. Blood transfusions may be required. Surgical removal of the spleen, which usually must be postponed until the child is at least 5 years old, can correct the hemolytic anemia. The indications for removal of the spleen are controversial but include severe hemolytic anemia or a milder anemia associated with gallstones. Until the spleen can be removed, folic acid (usually in the form of folate) must be given, and transfusions may be needed if aplastic anemia develops. Affected individuals have a 50 percent chance of passing the disease on to their children.

Sphincter

A ring of muscle fibers that narrows a passage or closes an orifice. For example, sphincters control the opening and closing of the bladder and anus. A sphincter acts as a valve, regulating inflow or outflow. A sphincter can function automatically or can be partly under voluntary control, as with the bladder.

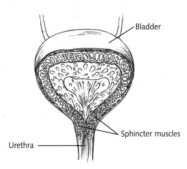

Bladder

Sphincter muscles

Urethra

BLADDER MUSCLE
At the base of the bladder, a sphincter controls the flow of urine into the urethra. When the muscle is contracted, the urine remains in the bladder; when the muscle is voluntarily relaxed, the urine is released into the urethra.

Sphincter, artificial

An artificial device designed to correct incontinence. Sphincters are the rings of muscle that narrow or close off a passageway by contracting. Two common sphincters are located at the anus and at the opening from the bladder to the urethra. Because the efficiency of muscle sphincters

declines with age, the inability to control the passage of urine (see INCONTINENCE, URINARY) or feces (see INCONTINENCE, FECAL) most frequently occurs in older people. Artificial urinary sphincters have been successfully used to treat urinary incontinence since the 1970s. More recently, artificial anal sphincters have been used to control fecal incontinence.

Older people usually have urinary incontinence only, which may be linked to urinary tract infections or prostate problems. Of cases involving artificial urinary sphincters, about 90 percent have been successful in controlling urinary incontinence. FECAL IMPACTION (an accumulated hard mass of feces in the rectum) and constipation are common causes of fecal incontinence. As with the urinary variety, implantation of the anal sphincter is an alternative to more complicated surgery. With an implanted device, muscles are stimulated with implanted neural stimulators. Individuals can exercise voluntary control over their artificial sphincters by using radio frequency controllers. Ordinary urinary sphincters were originally applied in cases of fecal incontinence. However, anal devices have since been modified to take specific anal anatomy into account. The artificial anal sphincter works by increasing pressure within the rectum and raising the volume of feces a person can hold.

Sphincterotomy

Surgical cutting of a sphincter muscle, typically the one that is located at the junction of the intestine with the bile and pancreatic ducts. Since the 1970s, endoscopic sphincterotomy (also known as endoscopic retrograde sphincterotomy, or ERS) has been a useful treatment for abnormalities of the bile ducts, pancreas, and gallbladder. Until then, open surgery was required to diagnose and treat most problems in these organs. ERS developed as an extension of the diagnostic procedure ERCP (endoscopic retrograde cholangiopancreatography). ERCP combines the use of X rays and ENDOSCOPY to examine the stomach, duodenum, bile ducts, and pancreas. In endoscopy, a slim, flexible, lighted tube is used to view, photograph, videotape, and take a sample of tissue for study. ERS permits the treatment

S

of problems diagnosed through ERCP. Many times, the term ERCP is also used to refer to the treatments performed in ERS.

Before ERS, an individual fasts for 6 to 12 hours because the upper intestinal tract must be empty. Shortly before an ERS, the individual's throat is sprayed with a local anesthetic to reduce discomfort, and additional pain medication or a sedative helps the person to relax during the procedure. Antibiotics may be required before and after the procedure.

In ERS, tiny instruments are passed through the endoscope to cut or stretch the sphincter. Once this is accomplished, additional instruments can be inserted to remove gallstones and stretch strictures (areas of the ducts that have narrowed). Drains (stents) can be used to prevent further strictures. Rest, for at least several hours after the procedure, is required to be sure that there are no complications. Complications may include perforation, CHOLANGITIS (inflammation of the bile ducts), PANCREATITIS (inflammation of the pancreas), and bacteremia (the passage of bacteria into the bloodstream).

Another type of sphincterotomy is used for anal fissures (ulcers in the anal lining) that do not respond to topical therapy. The surgeon cuts the internal anal sphincter, which decreases sphincter spasms, reducing the tendency for anal fissures.

Sphygmomanometer

An instrument used to measure blood pressure in the arteries. A sphygmomanometer consists of an inflatable BLOOD PRESSURE CUFF connected by a rubber tube to a measurement panel with a graduated scale. The cuff is applied to the person's arm and then inflated to exert pressure on a large artery until the blood flow stops. The pressure is then slowly released, and by listening to the pulse through a STETHOSCOPE, a doctor or nurse can determine both the systolic and diastolic pressures, which can be read on the scale.

Systolic pressure represents the amount of pressure in the artery when blood is pumped into it with each heartbeat, while diastolic pressure is the amount of pressure in the artery between heartbeats. These two readings are recorded as a numerical frac-

tion representing systolic (the upper figure) and diastolic (the lower figure). The average blood pressure measurement for a healthy adult is 120/80 millimeters of mercury, referring to the height blood in the artery would spurt if it weighed as much as mercury.

Spider veins

An unsightly pattern of bluish blood vessels that can have a spiderlike appearance and are visible in the skin of the legs. Spider veins are a mild form of VARICOSE VEINS. They are common and medically insignificant, but some people seek treatment for cosmetic reasons. One type of treatment, known as sclerotherapy, involves injecting a saltwater solution into a visible vein. This scars the vein and prevents blood from flowing into it. In most cases, the treated vein loses color in 2 months or less. Some people develop a yellow-brown discoloration at the treatment site that may not fade for several months.

Spina bifida

A birth defect in which there is incomplete closure in the spinal column. (See also BIRTH DEFECTS; NEURAL

CLOSE-UP ON SPINA BIFIDA

Spina bifida ("divided spine") is one of the most commonly occurring severe birth defects in the United States. In 1992, the US Public Health Service issued its recommendation that all women of childbearing age (15-44 years) who are capable of becoming pregnant take 400 micrograms of folic acid daily. Since then, the risk of infants acquiring spina bifida and other neural tube defects has dropped by 50 to 70 percent.

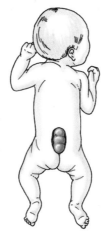

BABY WITH SPINA BIFIDA
A flattened mass of nervous tissue along the spine is exposed in spina bifida.

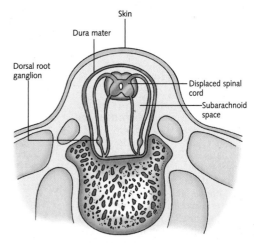

SPINA BIFIDA WITH MYELOMENINGOCELE
Incomplete closure of the lower end of the neural tube and the vertebral column can result in a portion of the spinal cord protruding through the back.

S

TUBE DEFECT.) There are three major types of spina bifida: spina bifida occulta, meningocele, and myelomeningocele. In spina bifida occulta, the mildest form, there is an opening in the vertebrae of the spinal column but no apparent damage to the spinal cord. Meningocele, the rarest form, is the presence of a cyst protruding through the open part of the spine; this can be removed by surgery, allowing for normal development.

The term "myelomeningocele" is often used synonymously with spina bifida. In this most severe form, a portion of the spinal cord itself protrudes through the back. Tissues and nerves may be covered by skin or exposed. Until recently, most children born with a myelomeningocele died shortly after birth. Today surgery is performed in the first 48 hours of life to drain spinal fluid and protect children against HYDROCEPHALUS, an accumulation of fluid in the brain. If hydrocephalus occurs, it is controlled by shunting (the implantation of a shunt or drain to relieve fluid buildup and prevent complications, such as brain damage, seizures, and blindness).

Children with myelomeningocele may continue to need operations throughout childhood. They may also need training to manage bowel and bladder function and help with mobility skills. Crutches, braces, or wheelchairs may be required. Children who also have a history of hydrocephalus can experience learning problems. Adequate folic acid intake in women of childbearing age and during the first month after conception is important in the prevention of neural tube defects, such as spina bifida. As a result, doctors advise all women of childbearing age to take 400 micrograms of folic acid daily.

Spinal anesthesia

See ANESTHESIA, SPINAL.

Spinal cord

A ropelike elongation of nerve tissue that extends down the back from the BRAIN and is enclosed within the bones of the spine. The brain and spinal cord are the two main structures of the CENTRAL NERVOUS SYSTEM. Together, these two structures receive and send signals throughout the body to control and coordinate all functions and activities. The spinal cord is primarily the

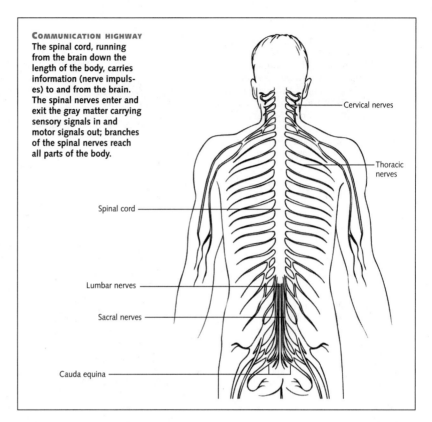

COMMUNICATION HIGHWAY
The spinal cord, running from the brain down the length of the body, carries information (nerve impulses) to and from the brain. The spinal nerves enter and exit the gray matter carrying sensory signals in and motor signals out; branches of the spinal nerves reach all parts of the body.

Cervical nerves

Thoracic nerves

Spinal cord

Lumbar nerves

Sacral nerves

Cauda equina

information highway between the brain and rest of the body.

The spinal cord extends downward from the medulla in the lower back of the brain, emerging from the skull through an opening called the foramen magnum. Running about 18 inches down the back, the cord is housed in the column of individual bones called vertebrae. Within this bony spinal column, the nerve tissue is further protected by an extension of the meninges, the three layers of membrane that protect the brain, and a cushioning layer of cerebrospinal fluid between the inner two layers.

Also like the brain, the spinal cord is constructed of gray matter and white matter. The gray matter lies in the center of the cord, with two "butterfly wings" extending outward. The gray matter is composed entirely of the bodies of nerve cells (neurons) and supporting cells called glial cells. In different areas of the gray matter, there are specialized types of neurons. Interneurons carry impulses between the cells of the brain and spinal cord. Motor neurons conduct signals to muscle fibers throughout

the body to initiate movement; the signals travel along the tails (called axons) of the neurons that extend into the spinal nerves branching out from the spinal cord. The axons of sensory neurons enter the gray matter of the spinal cord, bringing sensory information from body organs and tissues.

The inner core of gray matter is surrounded by white matter, composed of nerve fibers that carry messages up and down the spinal cord. Ascending tracts of fibers bring messages to the brain; descending tracts carry instructions from the brain to the rest of the body.

The spinal cord can receive, interpret, and initiate response to some kinds of sensory information independently of the brain. For example, many reflex actions are governed by the spinal cord alone. Most of these reflexes are aimed at protecting against injury. To carry information beyond the spinal cord, pairs of spinal nerves project out of the cord from between each of the vertebrae. These spinal nerves then continue to branch to form a network throughout the body. See also NERVOUS SYSTEM; NEURON.

S

Spinal fusion

A major surgical procedure sometimes considered to treat severe, persistent back pain, such as that caused
by a slipped disk. Spinal fusion is
accomplished by joining two or more
adjacent bones of the spine, or vertebrae; by using bone fragments
obtained from the person undergoing
the surgery; or by using bone tissue
from a bone bank or a synthetic bone
material.

Spinal injury

Injuries affecting the bone or cartilage
that make up the spine, as well as
injuries that damage or destroy the
spinal cord, which is made up of
nerve pathways that transmit impulses between the brain and the body.
See BACK PAIN; SLIPPED DISK.

Spinal cord injuries are caused by
severe trauma to the back, such as
from motor vehicle collisions, industrial injuries, falls, gunshot wounds,
and sports injuries. They usually lead
to some degree of permanent disability. When the spinal cord is injured in
the cervical, or neck area, the injury
may cause death if the nerves that
control breathing are damaged.
Spinal cord injuries in the neck area
can also result in complete paralysis
and general numbness in both the
arms and the legs (quadriplegia).

The symptoms of spinal cord damage in a person who has been injured
include an inability to move the legs
and a lack of physical sensation, or
numbness. The person should not be
moved, and emergency medical
attention should be sought immediately. Spinal cord injuries are diagnosed by X rays. Myelograms, CT
(computed tomography) scans, or
MRI (magnetic resonance imaging)
may also be used to observe defects,
breaks, and obstructions in the
spinal cord and evaluate the potential outcome of surgery. A severely
damaged spinal cord cannot heal
independently and may not always
be significantly improved by medical
or surgical treatment. Several months
of testing and observation may be
required to assess the degree of disability and the potential for possible
recovery. REHABILITATION, counseling,
and guidance are recommended for
the person to learn to use any remaining muscle strength and for coping
and adjusting to disabilities. New

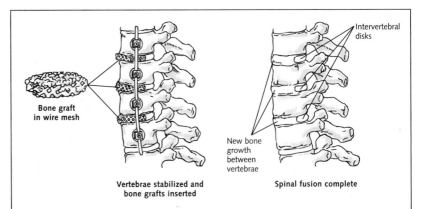

Vertebrae stabilized and
bone grafts inserted

Spinal fusion complete

SURGERY TO LIMIT PAINFUL MOVEMENT
Spinal fusion stops movement in a painful area of the vertebral column by inserting a bone
graft that grows between the vertebrae and makes the area rigid. First, vertebrae are stabilized
with a system of rods and screws, and then bone graft material is inserted between vertebrae.
New bone growth fuses the vertebrae into position to stop movement and decrease pain.

treatment techniques, including functional electrical stimulation implants,
are currently making advances in
restoring some physical function to
people who have spinal cord injuries.

Spinal stenosis

A narrowing of the bony spinal canal
formed by the vertebrae and the intervertebral disks. Spinal stenosis is
caused by arthritis in the joints of the
spine, which enlarges the joints and
diminishes the openings of the spinal
canal. This condition compresses
and pinches the nerves that travel
through the lower spine into the legs.
Symptoms include aching in the
lower back and sometimes a sharp
pain that extends into both buttocks,
the thighs, and, at times, the calves
and feet. Pain may be felt in one or
both legs and may become more
severe with walking. Rest usually
relieves the discomfort. A forward-
leaning posture also tends to relieve
the pain of spinal stenosis and causes
people who have the condition to
bend forward when standing and
walking. Spinal stenosis tends to
appear with episodes of achiness,
numbness, and possibly weakness in
both legs. The symptoms tend to
increase progressively as the spinal
arthritis continues to narrow the
spinal canal.

X rays may be used as a preliminary
diagnostic tool to reveal arthritis in
the spine, which is typically a precursor to spinal stenosis. A myelogram of the lower back and MRI (mag-

netic resonance imaging) will show
details of nerves, soft tissue such as
disks, and the bones of the spine.
These tests can reveal the pinched
nerve roots that are characteristic of
the condition and will also rule out
other possible causes of back pain,
such as a SLIPPED DISK or a tumor.
Electromyogram (EMG) nerve testing
may be used to evaluate nerve

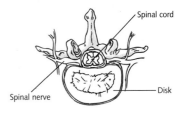

Healthy vertebra

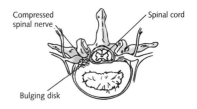

Vertebra with stenosis

ARTHRITIS IN SPINAL JOINTS
When arthritis affects the joints between vertebrae, the enlarged joints narrow the spaces
through which the spinal cord and nerves pass.
In a healthy vertebra, the spinal cord runs
through a central canal, and branching nerves
pass through spaces within and between the
vertebrae. Inflammation and bony outgrowths
on the joints disrupt the normal relationships
between structures and put pressure on nerves.

involvement and the degree of damage to nerves.

Anti-inflammatory medication and physical therapy are usually the initial treatments offered for spinal stenosis. Physical therapy may include swimming pool exercises and training that emphasizes forward flexing of the spine to help decompress the affected nerve roots. Low-impact activities, such as walking and swimming, are also often recommended. Reducing excess body weight and maintaining an ideal weight are recommended to relieve the pressure on the spine's joints and lessen the symptoms of spinal stenosis. A back support brace, such as a lumbar corset, may be beneficial. Stopping smoking can improve blood flow and oxygen to the pinched nerves in the spinal canal and help them heal. Epidural injections of corticosteroids may be tried to relieve the inflammation and pain caused by pinched nerves. In severe and persistent cases, surgical decompression of the lower back area, called lumbar LAMINECTOMY, may be considered.

Spinal tap

A diagnostic procedure that involves inserting a needle into the spinal canal to remove a sample of cerebrospinal fluid for analysis. See LUMBAR PUNCTURE.

Spine

The column of bones and cartilage that extends down the back, supporting the head and torso and enclosing the spinal cord.

Each of the individual bones of the spine is called a vertebra. Altogether, the spine contains 33 vertebrae: seven in the neck (cervical vertebrae), 12 in the upper back (thoracic vertebrae), five below the ribs in the lower back (lumbar vertebrae), five fused into a single unit called the sacrum, and four fused into a single unit called the coccyx (tailbone). Each vertebra is a uniquely shaped, asymmetrical bone. It is a ring enclosing a central canal. Winglike projections extend from the back of the ring. The spinal cord passes through the canal. Nerves branching off of the spinal cord pass between the vertebrae.

A cushion of fibrous cartilage with a gelatinous center lies between all the vertebrae except the first two below

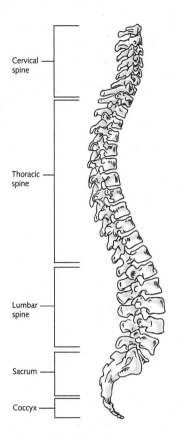

AREAS OF THE SPINE
The spine is composed of 24 individual bones, the vertebrae, plus fused vertebrae in the lower parts. The first seven vertebrae are called the cervical spine; the next 12 are called the thoracic spine; the next five are the lumbar spine; five fused bones form the sacrum; and four fused bones form the tailbone, or coccyx.

Cervical spine

Thoracic spine

Lumbar spine

Sacrum

Coccyx

the skull and those in the sacrum and coccyx. These flexible cushions, called disks, allow the spine a range of movement and flexibility, even as it bears much of the body's weight and protects the spinal cord. Ligaments running the length of the spine and smaller ones between the vertebrae hold the spine together.

The seven cervical (neck) vertebrae allow the head to move backward, forward, sideways, and around. The 12 thoracic (chest) vertebrae each support a pair of ribs. The ribs help stabilize the spine and protect it from injury. The five lumbar vertebrae, between the lowest ribs and the pelvis, are quite mobile and bear the weight of the upper body. The sacrum, together with the hipbones, forms an arch that transfers the

weight of the upper body to the bones of the leg. Together with the sacrum, the tailbone (coccyx) forms the back of the pelvis, the bony structure that protects the internal organs of the lower body. Seen from the back, the spine looks straight, but viewed from the side it gently curves in the shape of an S. This curve helps carry the considerable weight of the head in an upright posture.

Spinocerebellar degeneration

An inherited disease characterized by progressive dysfunction of the cerebellum, spinal cord, and peripheral nerves. See FRIEDREICH ATAXIA.

Spirituality and healing

The use of divine energy channeled from a spiritual source through a healer to heal the sick. Spirituality can involve the acceptance of a higher power or refer to a person's individual belief. Healing involves the transmission of energy through, not by, a healer. Spiritual healers believe that the mind, body, and spirit make up a single interdependent unit that must be in a state of harmony for a person to achieve and maintain good health. In this view, much physical and emotional illness is thought to derive from spiritual disharmony.

The process of healing through spirituality begins with the belief that all people have a healing mechanism, or energy force, available to keep body, spirit, and mind in balance. Stress, poor diet, negative attitude, or personal crisis may interfere with this healing mechanism, leading to illness. Spiritual healing provides energy needed to restore a person's blocked or disrupted healing mechanism. By laying his or her hand on the person, a spiritual healer believes he or she is a conductor of divine energy to aid the healing.

Because research has shown that prayer can promote relaxation and reduce stress, spiritual healing is currently being studied in an effort to integrate aspects of spirituality into conventional medical practice to benefit general health. Prayer intended to heal the sick is practiced in almost all societies, many of which recognize a universal force or life energy that is considered central to general health.

S

Spirochete

A member of a group of spiral-shaped, elongated bacteria. Spirochetes are long, slender, and tightly coiled like tiny springs. They can cause serious disease in humans, principally infections of the genital, urinary, and gastrointestinal tracts. Among the diseases caused by spirochetes are syphilis, relapsing fever, and Lyme disease. The characteristic environment of spirochetes is liquid; this includes mud and water in the natural environment and blood and lymph fluid in the bodies of humans and animals. The bacteria can survive with or without oxygen and may be free-living or parasitic. In some cases, the parasitic spirochetes may be beneficial to their hosts. A type of spirochete that lives in a part of a cow's stomach, for example, breaks down cellulose and other components in the cow's diet to aid in the animal's digestion.

Spirometry

A test that measures the function of the lungs. Spirometry helps doctors evaluate the lungs' capacity to take in air, the amount of air the lungs can hold, the amount of air exhaled by the lungs, and the rate of speed (airflow) of exhalations. The results of this test, usually in combination with measurements taken in other pulmonary function tests, may be useful for determining the cause of or diagnosing certain breathing problems and lung disorders, including asthma, bronchitis, emphysema, and occupational lung diseases. Spirometry may also be helpful for evaluating the effectiveness of medications and for monitoring progress during treatment of lung diseases or disorders.

Preparation for spirometry involves avoiding a heavy meal and refraining from cigarette smoking for 4 to 6 hours before the test session. In some cases, the person to be tested will be asked not to use bronchodilators or other inhaled medications before testing. In other cases, certain medications may be inhaled as part of the test to see how they affect breathing.

The person being tested with spirometry breathes through a mouthpiece while nose clips are applied to the nostrils to prevent nasal breathing. The spirometer records the amount of air inhaled and exhaled and the rate of airflow within a specified period. The person is requested to breathe normally for some parts of spirometry testing, to breathe rapidly at other times, and to forcefully inhale and exhale for certain sections of the test, which can result in shortness of breath.

The measurements produced by spirometry are based on specific age, height, weight, and sex categories. Results of the test are expressed as a percentage of what is predicted for the person being tested. A test result is considered abnormal if it falls below 80 percent of the predicted value for a person's category.

For most people, the risks involved in spirometry are minimal. Rarely, people with certain types of lung disease may be at risk and should not be given the test. The physical effort required for spirometry may also present risks to people who have recently had a heart attack or have certain types of heart disease.

Spironolactone

A diuretic drug used in combination with other medications to treat high blood pressure and swelling due to liver cirrhosis or congestive heart failure. Spironolactone (Aldactone) is a potassium-sparing diuretic that helps to reduce the amount of the water in the body by acting on the kidneys to increase the flow of urine. This helps lower blood pressure. Unlike other diuretics, spironolactone does not take potassium from the body. Spironolactone is also sometimes prescribed to treat people who have inadequate levels of potassium. It is also used to treat congestive heart failure and excess hair growth in women taking anabolic steroids.

Spitz nevus

A benign (not cancerous) growth characterized by the appearance of a papule (a small superficial bump on the skin) with a smooth surface; also known as juvenile melanoma. Most commonly, the papule develops on the face or scalp of a child. Although harmless, it may be mistaken for a malignant melanoma (see MELANOMA, MALIGNANT). Spitz nevi are most common in children between the ages of 9 and 13.

Spleen

An organ in the upper left side of the abdomen, next to the stomach and pancreas, that filters old or damaged red blood cells out of the bloodstream and produces some infection-fighting agents.

The largest structure in the LYMPHATIC SYSTEM, the spleen is composed of lymph tissue that produces antibodies (proteins that can destroy certain foreign microorganisms), phagocytes (cells that can ingest some microorganisms), and lymphocytes (a type of white blood cell).

The spleen also keeps the bloodstream healthy by screening the blood for old, damaged, or dead red blood cells and removing them. Blood is brought to the spleen by a large artery that branches throughout the organ. In a fetus, the spleen produces red blood cells; at birth the bone marrow assumes this function.

The spleen is soft and spongy, which makes it vulnerable to injury, especially when it enlarges. It can be removed, because other organs in the lymphatic system can take over its many activities. However, the body may be more susceptible to certain infections as a result.

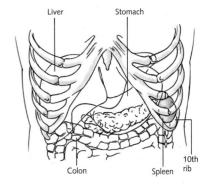

LOCATION OF THE SPLEEN
The spongy, purple spleen lies in the upper part of the abdominal cavity, just under the rib cage on the left side of the body.

Splenectomy

The surgical removal of the SPLEEN, a large organ in the upper left part of the abdomen that plays a major role in maintaining and filtering the blood supply. A splenectomy is performed in patients whose spleen has been injured in an accident or when a person is bleeding internally or has leukemia or lymphoma, diseases that cause the spleen to enlarge beyond its normal size. Because the spleen is important in removing infectious microorganisms from the blood, people who have undergone a splenectomy are at increased risk for severe infection.

Splenomegaly

An abnormal enlargement of the spleen, an organ in the upper left part of the abdomen that removes and destroys aging red blood cells and helps to fight infection. Causes may include portal hypertension (increased blood pressure in the portal vein, which carries blood from the intestines to the liver); CIRRHOSIS (a severe liver disease); hemolytic anemia (see ANEMIA, HEMOLYTIC); malignant lymphoma; leukemia; systemic lupus erythematosus; malaria; infections (such as mononucleosis); and hypersplenism (a condition in which the activity of the spleen accelerates abnormally and it removes red blood cells that are still functioning normally). Hypersplenism may occur as a primary disorder or secondary to other problems such as malaria or tumors.

The signs of splenomegaly are pain in the upper left side of the abdomen and a feeling of abdominal fullness. An enlarged spleen is diagnosed by a physical examination, palpation (careful feeling) of the spleen, a complete medical history, and tests that may include a complete blood cell (CBC) count, liver function tests, and imaging studies such as ultrasound or CT (computed tomography) scanning. Treatment depends on the underlying cause of splenomegaly. In severe cases, removal of the spleen (see SPLENECTOMY) may be necessary.

Splint

A support device made of a rigid material that is strapped onto an injured or diseased joint or a fractured bone to keep the area temporarily stable and immobilized. Splints help relieve pain, promote healing, and protect a body part from further injury. A splint may be made of plastic, wood, fiberglass, or metal; it should be lightweight and comfortably fitted. There are splints for use on the wrist, neck, hand, elbow, back, knee, ankle, and finger. They may be available ready-made or can be cus-

tom-fitted by an orthotist or a physical or occupational therapist.

When a splint is worn to rest and protect a joint that has become inflamed by arthritis, it should be used only during painful flare-ups. Incorrect or extended use may increase the stiffness in joints, decrease their strength, and limit flexibility. Splints worn to help manage arthritic joints should be removed several times daily to permit gentle range-of-motion movements.

A splint may be made and used to support an injured limb when medical attention is not immediately available. A temporary splint can help minimize discomfort and the risk of further injury. A first-aid splint can be made of any rigid material—for example, an oar, a broom handle, a board—and should immobilize the joint movement below the bone it is intended to support. It can be fastened to the injured limb by using strips of any soft material and should be wrapped from the outermost end of the extremity in toward the torso. The wrapping should prevent movement, but not be so tight as to impair blood flow or nerve activity.

Splinters

FOR FIRST AID
see Splinters, page 1331

Sharply pointed fragments that enter the skin. Most splinters can be removed with tweezers and a needle. Instruments must first be sterilized by cleaning them in rubbing alcohol. If a splinter protrudes from the skin, it should be pulled out with tweezers at the same angle it entered the skin. If a splinter is not protruding from the skin but can be seen beneath it, a sterilized needle can be used to first loosen the skin around and over it before removing the splinter with tweezers. Deeply embedded splinters require removal by a physician. After removal, the area should be cleansed with soap and water and covered with an antibiotic ointment and a bandage.

A splinter in an eye should not be removed by anyone other than a physician. Instead, both eyes should be covered loosely and the person with the injury should be taken to an ophthalmologist or hospital emergency department.

Splinting, dental

Reinforcement for loose teeth, or the joining together of adjacent teeth to support a wide dental bridge (see BRIDGE, DENTAL). Dental splinting may be a temporary measure to strengthen teeth and maintain their position during healing or following orthodontic treatment. Splinting may also be a permanent technique for reinforcing teeth that are supporting partial DENTURES. The purpose of dental splinting is to reduce the stresses of chewing on weakened teeth or to buttress the teeth that are essential to securing a bridge. Fiber-reinforced composite is generally the material used to construct dental splints.

Split personality

A common name for MULTIPLE PERSONALITY DISORDER, an emotional condition in which a person feels two or more distinct identities that surface regularly, control the individual's actions, and know little about the other identities. The identities are in conflict with one another. Split or multiple personality is known medically as dissociative identity disorder. It is one of the DISSOCIATIVE DISORDERS, a group of related mental illnesses in which an individual becomes detached from fundamental aspects of waking consciousness, such as personal identity, memory, or awareness of self and body. Dissociative disorders are thought to originate in overwhelming traumatic experiences, such as wartime combat, physical or sexual assault, or severe accidents. When unable to integrate the trauma into his or her normal consciousness, the individual detaches from the disturbing experience as a way of coping with it.

Spondylarthropathy

A term describing the group of arthritic diseases that involve the spine, including ANKYLOSING SPONDYLITIS. REITER SYNDROME, PSORIATIC ARTHRITIS, SCLERODERMA, and CROHN DISEASE are other conditions that may affect the spine.

Spondylitis

A condition involving inflammation of one or more vertebrae. Spondylitis is another term for the chronic inflammatory disease called ANKYLOSING SPONDYLITIS, which affects the vertebral joints of the spine and the joints between the spine and the pelvis, eventually causing them to fuse together.

Spondylolisthesis

A condition in which one vertebra in the spine slips forward on the vertebra below it and becomes out of alignment with the other spinal vertebrae. The misaligned vertebra puts pressure on nearby spinal nerves. Spondylolisthesis is usually caused by a defect in a part of the vertebra located directly above, a condition called SPONDYLOLYSIS. The defective top vertebra becomes unable to hold the vertebra below it in proper position. This puts increased pressure on the intervertebral disk between the two vertebrae and causes the disk to stretch, which allows the upper vertebra to slide forward.

In most cases involving adults, the forward movement of the upper vertebra is minimal and there is no risk of continual slippage that would cause the upper vertebra to become disconnected from the vertebra below it. A rare severe form of the condition, in which the upper vertebra almost completely slips off the lower vertebra, may sometimes occur in teenagers.

Spondylolisthesis increases the risk of chronic lower back pain. The forward movement of the vertebra makes the spinal canal smaller and may put pressure on the nerve roots, causing back pain. Common symptoms include stiffness and pain across the small of the back that extends into the buttocks and possibly into the leg and foot. Numbness and weakness of the foot may also be experienced. The condition is aggravated with activity and relieved with rest. Tightness of the hamstrings is common.

DIAGNOSIS AND TREATMENT

The condition is diagnosed with X rays, CT (computed tomography) or MRI (magnetic resonance imaging), or a bone scan. Treatment involves reducing symptoms by strengthening the back muscles. Physical therapy exercises to strengthen the back and abdominal muscles may help stabilize the spine. Medication may be prescribed to control pain and ease associated muscle spasms. Bed rest at short intervals may be beneficial for acute, painful episodes, and a brace, or lumbar corset, may be used to help relieve pain. Surgery becomes necessary only if more conservative treatment fails to control severe pain. In such cases, a LAMINECTOMY may be considered to relieve pressure and irritation of spinal nerves. Spinal fusion, a major surgery to join two or more adjacent vertebrae, is usually performed following the laminectomy to stabilize the spine.

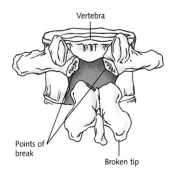

Vertebra

Points of break

Broken tip

AN INJURED VERTEBRA
If the protruding tip of a vertebra breaks, it can slip down onto the vertebra below it and compress spinal nerves and the disk between the vertebrae. It also no longer helps hold the lower vertebra in position. As the body tries to contain the unstable segment of the spine, the joints enlarge and cause further pressure.

Spondylolysis

A defect in a vertebra in the lower back, typically the last vertebra at the bottom of the spine, an area called the lumbar spine. The defective area of this vertebra is the bony ring that protects the spinal cord and connects the vertebral bone to the facet joints at the top and bottom of each vertebra. In spondylolysis, the back part of the vertebra and the facet joints are connected only by soft tissue. It is believed that this can be caused by an incompletely healed STRESS FRACTURE of the vertebra affected. There is usually a lump of hardened tissue in the area where the stress fracture did not completely heal. This tissue may press on the nerve roots at the bottom of the spine, causing pain that extends down into the legs. The condition first appears in childhood and is common among young football players and girls who are gymnasts or ballet dancers.

Spondylolysis can result in a condition called SPONDYLOLISTHESIS, in which one vertebra slips forward on the vertebra below it. Symptoms and treatment options for the two conditions are the same.

Spondylosis

A term referring to various degenerative diseases of the spine.

Sporotrichosis

A chronic fungal infection caused by a mold that is found on rose or barberry bushes and on sphagnum moss or other mulches, as well as in the soil. Sporotrichosis most commonly affects horticulturists, florists, and garden, farm, or timber workers. Often called "gardener's disease," it occurs when open cuts or sores on the skin make contact with the mold, which is spread via lymphatic fluid and forms small, round masses of tissue on the skin's surface or deep within the skin. If the infection is not treated, these nodules break down into inflamed, pus-filled cavities in the skin or become open sores. These painless, red lesions typically occur on one hand and arm, but may also form on exposed skin of the face or feet. In some instances, there may be no outbreak on the skin, but the lungs may become infected. If the infection spreads through the bloodstream, other areas of the body may be affected, particularly the joints.

The lesions caused by sporotrichosis may be easily misdiagnosed as spider bites. A swabbed culture from an active lesion offers a definitive diagnosis. The oral antifungal medication itraconazole is generally used to treat the infection when the skin is affected. If the lungs or bloodstream are involved, amphotericin B is administered intravenously. Relapses often occur, but with treatment, sporotrichosis can be successfully cured. It is potentially fatal only if the skin lesions become infected with bacteria, causing SEPSIS.

Sports injuries

The group of conditions and disorders of the musculoskeletal system that are caused by participation in athletics or other forms of exercise. Sports injuries may involve injury to the bones, joints, muscles, ligaments, and tendons. They are generally caused by overtraining, overuse, or trauma that occurs while a

SELF-CARE FOR SPORTS INJURIES

The acronym RICE is helpful for remembering the first line of treatment for avoiding further injury and promoting recovery from sports injuries:

- **R** stands for **resting** the injured area or extremity for a period of 24 to 48 hours.
- **I** stands for applying **ice** to the area for 5 to 20 minutes every hour for the first 24 to 48 hours, if possible, or until swelling and localized heat subside.
- **C** stands for **compression** of the area. Compression controls initial swelling and is done by wrapping at the point farthest from the heart and continuing toward the center of the body. Compression is done for the first 24 to 48 hours after an injury.
- **E** stands for **elevating** the area by propping it up during the day and during sleep, which helps reduce swelling.

In addition to RICE, over-the-counter nonsteroidal anti-inflammatory drugs (NSAIDs) may help relieve pain and reduce swelling. Aspirin, ibuprofen, or naproxen sodium may be taken according to package dosage directions; they should be taken only by adults 19 years of age and older, unless directed by a physician. NSAIDs should be taken with a full glass of milk or water to prevent stomach irritation.

When pain and swelling have decreased, exercises as recommended by a physical therapist can aid further healing and restoration of function. The acronym MSA represents a series of techniques that are helpful for promoting complete recovery:

- **M** stands for **movement** of the injured area to establish a full range of motion, help maintain flexibility as the area heals, and prevent scar tissue from impairing future activity.
- **S** stands for **strengthening** an injured area gradually by means of exercises that may be performed when inflammation has abated and range of motion has been reestablished.
- **A** stands for **alternative** activities that involve movements to avoid strain or pressure on the injured body part; these activities may be started while the injury is still healing and should be begun as soon as possible to maintain muscle tone and flexibility throughout the body.

person is engaged in athletic activities. The injuries may include twisted ankles, painful joints, side stitches, shin splints, blisters, and stiff, sore muscles. Muscular discomfort is usually a sign of a person exerting himself or herself too strenuously or over too long a period. It can be prevented by doing warm-up exercises to stretch the muscles before an activity, by avoiding overtraining, and by slowing the pace for 5 minutes at the end of an activity to cool down.

Specific sports injuries include BASEBALL ELBOW, BASEBALL FINGER, GOLFER'S ELBOW, JUMPER'S KNEE, RUNNER'S KNEE, SKIER'S THUMB, SURFER'S NODULES, SWIMMER'S SHOULDER, and TENNIS ELBOW. If a person suspects he or she has such an injury and experiences numbness, an inability to move, or a noticeable deformity in the injured area, emergency medical care should be sought. If the pain is severe or if there is swelling and bruised discoloration, then a doctor should be consulted. If none of these symptoms are present, most minor sports injuries may be helped by self-care procedures. See box above.

Sports medicine
The field of medical study and practice that involves injuries to the body from sports and athletic activities that usually involve musculoskeletal injuries. Physicians from a variety of areas of training may specialize in sports medicine.

Sports, drugs and
The use of certain chemicals and substances to enhance athletic performance and gain a competitive advantage; commonly referred to as doping and often illegal. Athletes whose use of these substances is detected, usually by blood or urine testing, are disqualified from competition and may face lengthy suspensions from their sports or loss of amateur or professional status. In addition, sports drugs involve health risks. A number of types of drugs are outlawed under current athletic regulations.

STEROIDS
The class of drugs known as anabolic steroids, called androgenic-anabolic steroids, and the type most widely abused by athletes. The word "anabolic" refers to the muscle-building effects of these drugs and the word "androgenic" to their masculinizing effects. They are used legally as prescription medications to treat conditions in which the body produces abnormally low levels of the male hormone testosterone, such as certain kinds of erectile dysfunction (impotence) and delayed puberty, and to prevent body wasting and weight loss in people with AIDS (acquired immunodeficiency syndrome).

Athletes use steroids illegally to increase lean muscle mass, gain strength, and endure longer workouts. Steroids are particularly popular in weightlifting, bodybuilding, football, wrestling, swimming, bicycling, and track and field. Anabolic steroids are taken by mouth or injected, typically for weeks or months, then discontinued for a time, a practice known as cycling. Some users combine several kinds of steroids at once to maximize the effect, a practice called stacking.

In spite of their athletic benefits, steroids produce a number of health hazards. The principal dangers include tumors and cancer of the liver, jaundice (yellowish discoloration of the skin, eyes, and body fluids), swelling from fluid retention, high blood pressure, and an increase in the low-density lipoprotein cholesterol level, along with a decrease in the high-density lipoprotein cholesterol level, changes that contribute to heart disease. Other health problems can include kidney tumors, severe acne, and tremors. Among adolescents, particularly those who have not gone through the growth spurt typical of the teenage years, anabolic steroids can halt growth by causing the skeleton to mature prematurely and accelerate puberty. In addition, because they work much like male sex hormones, anabolic steroids produce certain sex-specific effects. In men, steroids can cause

5

Terms in small capital letters—for example, PHYSICAL THERAPY or PAGET DISEASE—indicate a cross-reference to another entry with more information.

AN ARTIFICIAL ADVANTAGE
Athletes may turn to drugs in an effort to temporarily improve their endurance or performance. These drugs are illegal in competition—and they are physically devastating over time.

Painkillers (mask pain from injury or stress)

Stimulants (increase alertness and create a "high")

Anabolic steroids (build muscle mass)

Erythropoietin (builds red blood cells)

Diuretics (reduce weight)

Creatine (may promote muscle growth)

Anti-inflammatory drugs (reduce discomfort from inflammation)

shrinking of the testicles, reduced sperm count, infertility, baldness, development of breasts, and increased risk of prostate cancer. In women, the changes can include growth of facial hair, baldness, altered or suspended menstrual cycle, deepened voice, and enlarged clitoris. There are also psychiatric side effects. Most users say they feel good while taking anabolic steroids, but extreme mood swings, outbursts of violence, paranoid jealousy, extreme irritability, delusions (false beliefs), and poor judgment have also been reported.

SYMPATHOMIMETIC AMINES
This class of stimulant drugs imitates the natural effects of stimulation to the sympathetic nervous system, which increases alertness and endurance and suppresses fatigue. Sympathomimetic drugs include ephedrine (derived from ephedra) and pseudoephedrine, which are commonly used in medications for colds and hay fever; also included is phenylpropanolamine, formerly used in non-prescription medications. All the sympathomimetic medications are banned under the rules of the International Olympic Committee (IOC) and most other governing bodies and may not be used by competing athletes.

PSYCHOMOTOR STIMULANTS
Drugs that accelerate body functions, such as amphetamine, dextroamphetamine, methamphetamine, and methylphenidate hydrochloride (Ritalin), have been banned because they can give athletes a competitive edge, both physically and psychologically. These stimulants increase heart rate, blood pressure, and respiration, and they lead to alertness, confidence, and even euphoria. Some of these drugs are used in medicine to treat attention deficit/hyperactivity disorder (severe difficulty in concentrating, often compounded by constant movement; found mostly in children) and narcolepsy (a disease in which an individual falls asleep suddenly and unpredictably). Abusers usually take stimulants orally, but some inject them for a faster, stronger effect. Side effects include dizziness, heart palpitations, insomnia (inability to sleep), erectile dysfunction (impotence), and psychotic reactions. In a few cases, death has resulted from extreme physical activity under the influence of stimulants.

BETA₂-ANTAGONISTS
Used to treat asthma, these drugs have a stimulantlike effect. Examples include metaproterenol (Alupent and Metaprel); albuterol, also called albutamol (Ventolin and Proventil); and terbutaline (Brethaire). Under current rules, these medications are banned in their oral forms but permitted as aerosols or inhalants.

NARCOTICS
Painkilling narcotics, such as heroin, morphine, and codeine, raise the pain threshold and may produce a feeling of euphoria. They raise the risk of injury by masking pain, and they can be highly addictive.

BETA BLOCKERS
In medicine, beta blockers are used to treat heart disease and high blood pressure by slowing heart rate and decreasing the amount of blood the heart pumps with each beat. They also reduce the body's reaction to stimulation. Archers and target shooters have used them illegally to achieve greater steadiness and accuracy.

GROWTH HORMONE
Like anabolic steroids, growth hormone has been used, usually as an injection, to promote muscle growth and endurance. Such use is banned by the IOC and most other governing bodies.

DIURETICS
These drugs eliminate fluid from the body as urine. Some athletes in weight-class sports, such as wrestling and boxing, have used them to lose pounds before competition. Others have used them to lower the blood concentration of other banned drugs and escape detection. Diuretics affect the balance of minerals such as sodium and potassium in the body. Misuse can lead to irregular heartbeat and even sudden death.

CORTICOSTEROIDS
These drugs, which have a powerful anti-inflammatory effect, are legal in topical applications, such as creams and ointments; as injections into the joints; or as inhaled preparations for treating asthma. They are illegal if an athlete takes them by mouth or injects them into a vein.

Sprain

FOR SYMPTOM CHART
see Ankle or foot problems, page 18

FOR FIRST AID
see Strains and sprains, page 1331

A forcible wrenching or twisting of a joint that may involve severe stretching or tearing of attached ligaments. A sprain does not involve dislocation of the joint, but may cause injury to surrounding blood vessels, muscles, tendons, or nerves. A sprain is a more serious injury than a STRAIN, which is an overstretched muscle, ligament, or tendon. Sprains generally produce significant swelling and pain, as well as bruising if blood vessels are ruptured. The pain may prevent joint movement. Sprains occur most frequently in the ankle joint or in the lower back area and are treated initially by cold compresses (with heat later), wrapping with a compression bandage, resting, and, when possible, elevating the injured area. After the pain subsides, exercises are prescribed to regain function.

Sprue

See CELIAC DISEASE.

Sprue, tropical

Chronic DIARRHEA in a person who has recently visited a tropical area. In tropical sprue, there are no signs of parasites or other infection. Diarrhea results from malabsorption (impaired absorption of nutrients through the small intestine). Because fat passes through the intestine unabsorbed, stools are bulky and strong smelling. Although the exact cause of tropical sprue remains unknown, in most cases it can be successfully treated with antibiotics.

Spur

An abnormal, spike-shaped outgrowth of bone tissue, often found on the bottom of the back of the heel. Bone spurs may be tender when gentle pressure is applied and usually cause sharp pain when weight is placed on the foot. Over time, if a protective bursa develops over the spur, the bursa (a fluid-filled sac that acts as a cushion) may become inflamed, causing swelling and increased pain. Favoring the sore

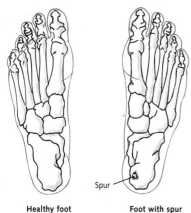

Healthy foot   Foot with spur

HEEL BONE SPUR
In response to repetitive stresses and inflammation, bony deposits may form in the soft tissue over the heel bone (the plantar fascia). The so-called heel spur may or may not cause pain.

heel may alter the gait and contribute to back pain. When bursitis is associated with a heel spur, the foot should be rested and protected from pressure by a special pad. Nonsteroidal anti-inflammatory drugs (NSAIDs) may be recommended. Localized corticosteroid injections are sometimes considered, and surgery may become necessary if the condition persists and pain makes walking difficult or impossible. See OSTEOARTHRITIS.

Sputum

Mucus and other matter coughed up and expectorated (spat) from the mouth. Sputum is coughed up from the lungs, the airways, and the throat and can be collected for analysis. The analysis of sputum is an important component in the diagnosis of certain diseases, especially tuberculosis. Sputum can be cultured for the purpose of identifying bacteria or analyzed with the microscope to detect bacteria or abnormal cells. Doctors use sputum cultures to select appropriate antibiotic therapy for the treatment of tuberculosis, pneumonia, and bronchitis.

Squamous cell carcinoma

The second most common type of SKIN CANCER. The two other types are BASAL CELL CARCINOMA and malignant melanoma (see MELANOMA, MALIGNANT). Squamous cell carcinoma arises from the epidermis (the outer layer of skin). It is more aggressive than basal cell cancer and more likely to spread to other locations such as nearby lymph nodes. Left untreated, tumors may even spread into internal organs and become incurable. Squamous cell carcinoma is slow growing and, when properly treated, has a very high cure rate (more than 95 percent). The principal risk factor for developing squamous cell cancer is chronic sun exposure. Other causes are exposure to arsenic, coal, industrial tar, paraffin, and certain types of heavy oils.

SYMPTOMS AND DIAGNOSIS

Any new growth that ulcerates or bleeds can be an indication of squamous cell carcinoma. Squamous cell carcinoma usually develops from a red, scaly, precancerous skin lesion known as ACTINIC KERATOSIS. Actinic keratoses usually occur on sun-dam-

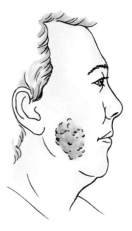

AGGRESSIVE SKIN CANCER
Squamous cell carcinoma appears as a scaly, crusty growth and can enlarge slowly and steadily. It starts on the outer layer of skin (epidermis) and invades the deeper layer (dermis). It can invade nearby tissue, such as the eye.

aged parts of the body, such as the face, scalp, ears, and backs of the hands. Lesions are typically rough, pink, and scaly. Squamous cell carcinomas may also develop in an old burn or scar.

For early detection, doctors recommend regular skin self-examination. Doctors advise medical attention for any new skin growth; changes in the surface or color of a mole; a spot or bump that is getting larger, scaling, oozing, or bleeding; a sore that does not heal within 3 weeks; or itchiness or pain in a lesion.

If a doctor suspects skin cancer, he or she will take a complete personal and family medical history; examine the size, shape, color, and texture of the lesion in question; ask about the history of the growth, such as when it first appeared and how it has changed in size or appearance; check the rest of the body; and perform a skin biopsy. Diagnosis is made through biopsy (taking a small sample and examining it under a microscope for malignant cells).

TREATMENT

In the early stage of the disease, squamous cell carcinoma in situ (BOWEN DISEASE) can be removed by topical chemotherapy, CRYOSURGERY (freezing with liquid nitrogen), or electrodesiccation (burning with an electric current delivered through a probe) and

S

curettage (scraping). However, most squamous cell carcinomas must be surgically removed. Surgery is usually performed on an outpatient basis using a local anesthetic. Factors such as the size, type, depth, and location of the cancer determine choice of treatment. Surgical options include simple excision (cutting out the tumor) and MOHS SURGERY (microscopically controlled surgery removing one layer of skin at a time). If there is a suspicion that the cancer has spread, nearby lymph nodes are removed and studied under a microscope. For large cancers, skin grafting and reconstructive surgery are often necessary. Radiation therapy may be considered when surgical removal is not feasible.

RISK FACTORS AND PREVENTION

Squamous cell carcinoma is most common in fair-skinned people with blond or red hair and blue or green eyes. Other risk factors are a family or personal history of skin cancer; a tendency to burn easily when exposed to the sun; having spent a lot of time outdoors as a child; overexposure to X rays or other forms of radiation; and exposure to arsenic, coal, industrial tar, paraffin, and certain types of heavy oils.

It is common for people who have experienced one squamous cell cancer to develop another within 5 years. Tumors can recur in the same site or in new locations. Consequently, doc-

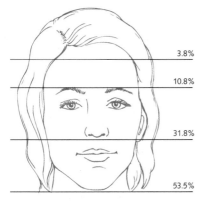

3.8%

10.8%

31.8%

53.5%

LOCATION OF SKIN CANCERS
Of the squamous tumors that develop on the face and head, more than 50 percent occur on the lower part of the face and jaw, and more than 30 percent occur across the nose and cheeks. Less frequently, the tumors appear on the forehead and scalp.

tors recommend both monthly self-examination and regular examination by a health care provider every 6 to 12 months.

Squamous intraepithelial lesion
See SIL.

SSRI drugs
See SELECTIVE SEROTONIN REUPTAKE INHIBITOR DRUGS.

St. John's wort
An herbal remedy used to treat mild to moderate depression, anxiety, seasonal affective disorder, and sleep disorders. St. John's wort is a wild flowering herb that has been used for centuries to treat mental disorders and nerve pain. St. John's wort is thought to work by reducing the rate at which brain cells reabsorb the neurotransmitter serotonin, low levels of which are associated with depression.

St. John's wort is most widely used in Germany, but it has become popular in the United States in recent years and is widely available in capsule, tea, and other forms. Although some clinical studies have been performed that suggest that St. John's wort is effective for the treatment of mild to moderate depression, the Food and Drug Administration has approved it for sale only as a dietary supplement, noting that it is not yet a proven therapy for clinical depression. St. John's wort can cause a fast heart rate and stomach pains.

Stable
A term describing a state of health or disease from which little imminent change is expected.

Stage
A period or phase of a disease or condition. For example, cancer is said to progress through various stages of severity.

Staining
Adding artificial color to tissues, microorganisms, or cells to make them visible under a microscope. One of the most common techniques involves using the GRAM STAIN, which makes normally colorless bacteria visible. Other types of stains can be

used to highlight particular kinds of tissue or cells in a larger sample. For example, an acid-fast stain is used to identify the bacteria that causes tuberculosis.

Stammering
See STUTTERING.

Stapedectomy
A surgical procedure to treat hearing loss caused by OTOSCLEROSIS, an inherited disorder of the middle ear. Stapedectomy is performed through the ear canal under local anesthesia. Using a high-powered operating microscope, the surgeon turns the back half of the eardrum forward to gain access to the stapes (a bone in the inner ear that is essential to conducting sound waves to the inner ear fluids). The stapes, which has become cemented to surrounding bone because of the disease, is partially or completely removed. This procedure may be done using instruments, a drill, or possibly a laser. An artificial bone is inserted to replace the stapes, and the eardrum is returned to its normal position. The artificial stapes allows sound vibrations to pass from the eardrum membrane to the inner ear fluids. The resulting hearing improvement is usually permanent and may become apparent 3 weeks after a stapedectomy. A person who has undergone this operation may return to normal activities within 7 to 10 days; air travel is generally permissible within 2 days. The maximum improvement in hearing takes about 4 months. Sometimes the improvement is only partial or temporary, and the ear may require a second operation.

Stapedectomy is a well-established surgical procedure with a high rate of success, but improvement in hearing may vary from one person to another. Rarely, following the operation, the development of scar tissue, infection, spasms of the blood vessels, inner ear irritation, or a leak of fluid in the inner ear (through a fistula) can further decrease hearing. More rarely, severe complications in the healing process can cause complete hearing loss. In these unusual cases the person may have ringing in the ears or head and an impairment of balance.

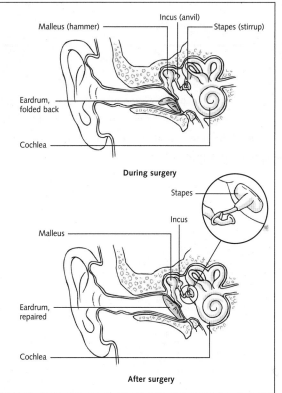

ARTIFICIAL BONE IN THE EAR
A surgical procedure called stapedectomy is done to replace a small bone in the ear (the stapes, or stirrup) that has been immobilized by otosclerosis, causing hearing loss. The stapes is the third of three tiny bones (the other two are the hammer, or malleus; and the anvil, or incus) that vibrate to carry sound waves from the eardrum to the oval window, a membrane of the inner ear. To do the procedure, the surgeon folds back the eardrum, removes the stapes that has become fixed to surrounding bone, and inserts an artificial bone or wire. The insert is positioned as the stapes was, connected to the adjoining bone, the incus. The eardrum is put back in place, and hearing is restored.

Malleus (hammer) — Incus (anvil) — Stapes (stirrup)
Eardrum, folded back
Cochlea

During surgery

Stapes
Incus
Malleus
Eardrum, repaired
Cochlea

After surgery

Staphylococcal infections

FOR FIRST AID

see Food poisoning: *Staphylococcus* poisoning, page 1323

The group of infections caused by bacteria of the *Staphylococcus* genus, commonly known as staph. Staphylococcal bacteria produce illness directly by causing infection or indirectly by making products, such as toxins, that are responsible for food poisoning and toxic shock syndrome. Under the microscope, the bacteria resemble clusters of tiny round berries or grapes. Some species of staphylococcal bacteria can be present on the skin and in the nose of a healthy person without causing problems; others can cause fatal illness. People who have diabetes or weakened immune systems are particularly vulnerable to staph infections.

Staphylococcal bacteria that live harmlessly on skin surfaces, particularly in the area of the nose, mouth, genitals, and rectum, can cause an infection when the skin is broken and the bacteria enter the wound. Scalded skin syndrome, or Ritter disease, an infection that affects newborns and young children, may begin with a localized staph skin infection. Folliculitis, boils, and impetigo are caused by the bacteria. Potentially scarring skin eruptions, such as acne pustules, may also be due to staph infection. Abscesses that form almost anywhere on the body may be caused by staph infections. Keeping the skin clean is a good preventative measure to combat staph infections. Other measures to prevent staph infections include keeping cuts, rashes, and all skin wounds clean and covered and using antibiotic ointments as recommended by a doctor.

Staphylococcal bacteria can cause serious infections such as bacterial endocarditis, an inflammation of the heart valve. Bone infections, joint infections, and some forms of pneumonia may be caused by staphylococcal bacteria. Staph food poisoning can occur when these bacteria release a toxin into contaminated food, which causes severe gastroenteritis with nausea, vomiting, and diarrhea. It is usually associated with custard-filled bakery goods, canned foods, processed meats, potato salad, and ice creams.

Staph infections are treated with antibiotics, but the bacteria have the capacity to develop resistance to these medications. Staphylococcal bacteria can produce substances that break down antibiotics such as penicillin and tetracycline. For this reason, it is important not to use these antibiotics when they are not clearly needed. It is also important to take the recommended dosage for the prescribed length of time. Inadequate amounts or an incomplete course of antibiotics encourages the development of bacterial resistance to the medication. See Preventing staph infections, page 1160.

Staples, surgical

Metal devices used to connect surgically severed tissue and close incisions. Staples are made of a variety of materials, including titanium, stainless steel, and silver. They are particularly advantageous in situations where ordinary SUTURING (stitches) is difficult or when time is of the essence and the surgeon must work quickly for safety reasons. Some staples are used to close incisions and are removed after healing is complete. Others are left in place permanently. An example would be the staples that are used in reducing stomach size during bariatric surgery.

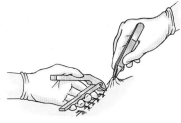

STAPLING A WOUND OR INCISION
To close a wound with staples, the surgeon holds the edges of the wound together with a forceps and evenly spaces the staples over the length of the wound.

Starch

See CARBOHYDRATES.

Starvation

Suffering extremely or dying of a lack of food. Starvation occurs primarily during famine conditions in developing countries. However, the eating

PREVENTING STAPH INFECTIONS

The term staph infection covers all infections caused by a type of bacteria normally present on a person's skin in a hramless form. But some forms of staph can lead to serious disorders or even death. In addition to causing infections, some staph organisms release a toxin into contaminated food that causes severe nausea, vomiting, and diarrhea.

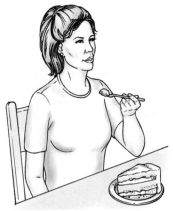

STAPH CAUSES FOOD POISONING
Staph food poisoning can occur when bacteria release a toxin into contaminated food, such as custard-filled cake that has not been properly refrigerated.

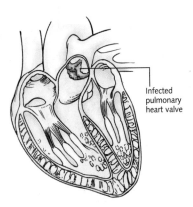

Infected pulmonary heart valve

STAPH INFECTS THE HEART
In endocarditis, clumps of bacteria form on heart valves and cause leaking that can be fatal. Infection develops when aggressive bacteria enter the bloodstream and settle on the valves.

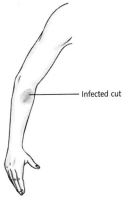

Infected cut

STAPH INFECTS A WOUND
Skin is a barrier against many infections, but broken skin or a wound can be contaminated by air, contact with contaminated surfaces, or a person's fingers. Washing hands frequently and cleaning and covering a wound are important to prevent staph infections.

disorder anorexia nervosa and prolonged malabsorption of nutrients due to intestinal diseases, cancer, infections such as HIV (human immunodeficiency virus), or abdominal surgery (see MALABSORPTION SYNDROME) can also lead to starvation and wasting. Weight loss and fatigue are common symptoms. Starvation may also be accompanied by iron-deficiency anemia (see ANEMIA, IRON-DEFICIENCY), vitamin B12–deficiency anemia, vitamin D deficiency, and KETOSIS (an abnormal accumulation of ketones in the body caused by a deficiency or inefficient use of carbohydrates). In individuals in whom there is an underlying cause, treatment requires addressing that health problem.

Stasis
Stagnation or stoppage of a flow of liquid. Stasis may refer to a slow-down of the flow of blood, lymph, or intestinal contents during digestion. A stasis ulcer, for example, is one that develops in an area of poor circulation, such as the ankle. Stasis often appears as a suffix, or word ending, as in hemostasis (slowing or stopping of blood flow).

Statistics, medical
Clinical data used to demonstrate trends in disease or treatment. For example, the statistical results of two surgical treatments may be compared with the option of not operating. A statistician may advise how to analyze medical statistical results. In addition, medical statistics may be analyzed for the incidence and prevalence of various disorders and disease, infection rates following surgery, and the frequency of side effects from drugs.

Statistics, vital
Systematic data on births, deaths, marriages, and divorces. In the United States, such information is recorded by government agencies from birth and death certificates, marriage licenses, and divorce decrees.

Status asthmaticus
An intense and continuous asthmatic state. Status asthmaticus produces severe shortness of breath that results in exhaustion and collapse and does not respond to the usual treatments for ASTHMA.

This extreme asthmatic state, which has become increasingly prevalent in children, requires aggressive treatment, including the use of beta agonists, ANTICHOLINERGIC AGENTS, and CORTICOSTEROIDS to quickly reduce bronchospasms and inflammatory conditions. Oxygen therapy with the use of mechanical ventilation may become necessary, but steps should be taken to reduce the risks of BAROTRAUMA and HYPOTENSION that can accompany mechanical ventilation used to treat asthma.

Status epilepticus

The occurrence of repeated or prolonged seizures without periods of awakening. Status epilepticus is a severe, life-threatening condition that may occur as a result of tumors, trauma, or other problems that affect the brain. People with epilepsy are also at increased risk for this condition.

It is essential to treat a person with status epilepticus as quickly as possible. The sooner medication is administered, the better the chance of recovery. Anyone who has a prolonged seizure lasting for more than 5 minutes requires emergency medical treatment. This applies not only to convulsive seizures, but also to repeated or prolonged nonconvulsive seizures. In a nonconvulsive seizure, symptoms such as confusion and agitation appear in a person who does not usually have this kind of impairment. Benzodiazepines, phenytoin, and phenobarbital given intravenously are commonly used to treat status epilepticus.

Stavudine (d4T)

An antiviral drug used along with other medications to treat the infection caused by HIV (human immunodeficiency virus). Stavudine, also known as d4T (Zerit), helps to keep HIV from reproducing, thereby slowing the destruction of the immune system. Stavudine is not a cure for AIDS (acquired immunodeficiency syndrome) or HIV, but it helps to delay the development of problems associated with the disease.

STDs

See SEXUALLY TRANSMITTED DISEASES.

Steatorrhea

Excess fat in the feces. Steatorrhea is characterized by loose, greasy, strong-smelling stools that result from fat passing through the intestine unabsorbed. Steatorrhea can be caused by malabsorption, the impaired absorption of nutrients through the small intestine, and by CELIAC DISEASE, a disorder in which the lining of the small intestine is damaged by an allergic reaction to gluten.

Steele-Richardson-Olszewski syndrome

Also known as progressive supranuclear palsy, a rare progressive neurological disorder. Steele-Richardson-Olszewski syndrome is characterized by eye muscle paralysis, muscle rigidity, palsy, and ataxia (an inability to coordinate the muscles, which can affect balance, gait, movement, or speech). There may also be dementia (a progressive deterioration of mental ability) and an expressionless or masklike face as in Parkinson disease, a progressive, degenerative disease of the nervous system characterized by muscle rigidity, weakness, and tremor. Treatment is with the antiparkinsonian drug levodopa.

Stem cell

A cell with the ability to divide indefinitely and give rise to the specialized cells that make up tissues and organs. Stem cells are found in humans at every stage from embryo to adult. In the embryo, they occur as the inner mass of cells in the early developmental stage known as the blastocyst. Since these cells eventually develop into every tissue and organ in the human body, they are called pluripotent (from Latin and meaning "many-powered"). Found mostly in the bone marrow and in smaller numbers in the bloodstream, stem cells in infants, children, and adults have the ability to develop into any of the many kinds of blood cells.

Pluripotent cells taken from human embryos may have the potential to grow into cell lines in the laboratory, which could then be used for cell therapy (methods of treating disease by replacing diseased cells with healthy ones grown from stem cells). An example is diabetes mellitus, which results from malfunction in cells in the pancreas. Researchers are looking into ways of producing healthy pancreas cells from stem cells that could be transplanted into people with diabetes mellitus. However, the use of cells taken from embryos has been the subject of controversy and of regulations.

Bone marrow transplant (see BONE MARROW TRANSPLANT, ALLOGENEIC; BONE MARROW TRANSPLANT, AUTOLOGOUS) is a way of replacing pluripotent stem cells that have been killed by high doses of chemotherapy and radiation during cancer treatment. The transplant restores the ability of the bone marrow to produce blood cells. Increasingly, stem cells filtered from the blood are being used as a substitute for bone marrow in transplantation.

Stenosis, valvular

A narrowing, stiffening, or obstruction, particularly of one or more heart valves. In the healthy HEART, four valves act like gates that open to allow blood to flow from one area to another, then close to prevent backward movement. Valvular stenosis limits blood flow. Symptoms depend on which valve is affected.

AORTIC STENOSIS

Aortic stenosis affects the valve connecting the heart to the aorta (the body's main artery). Because the narrowing partially blocks the aortic valve, blood flow to the body is reduced, and the heart must work harder to compensate. The greater workload can enlarge the left ventricle, the heart chamber in which the aortic valve is located. Over time, the left ventricle becomes thickened and enlarged, resulting in a condition known as ventricular hypertrophy. Congestive heart failure (see HEART FAILURE, CONGESTIVE), which is life-threatening, can also result. Aortic stenosis is more severe if CORONARY ARTERY DISEASE is also present because it deprives the enlarged heart of the blood supply it needs.

Aortic stenosis may exist in a mild form for years before symptoms appear. Symptoms include fatigue, abrupt fainting spells, shortness of breath with exercise or at night, angina (chest pain), and swelling in the ankles. The disease may be caused by damage to the valve from rheumatic fever, congenital valve defects (those present at birth), or the buildup of calcium deposits on the aortic valve because of aging. The condition can appear at any age but is most common in those between ages 30 and 60. Aortic stenosis is three times more likely to occur in men than in women.

Medications may be used to treat

the symptoms of aortic stenosis. These include angiotensin-converting enzyme (ACE) inhibitors, which lower blood pressure and decrease the workload of the heart; anticoagulants, which discourage the formation of blood clots; and diuretics, which remove salt and fluid from the body. Once symptoms of aortic stenosis become severe, surgery to repair or replace the valve (see HEART VALVE SURGERY) is the preferred treatment. If coronary artery disease is also present, valve replacement surgery may be combined with coronary bypass surgery in a single procedure.

MITRAL STENOSIS

The mitral valve connects the atrium (upper chamber) and the ventricle (lower chamber) on the left side of the heart. Stenosis of the mitral valve impairs blood flow from the atrium to the ventricle when the atrium contacts. As a result, blood can pool in the atrium and back up into the lungs, causing pulmonary congestion. A type of rapid heartbeat known as atrial fibrillation is likely to develop. A blood clot may form in the pooled blood in the atrium, then travel through the bloodstream and lodge in a blood vessel (see EMBOLISM).

Mitral stenosis may develop before birth. It can also arise, usually when a person reaches his or her 40s or 50s, as a result of RHEUMATIC FEVER earlier in life.

Mild forms of mitral stenosis produce no symptoms or symptoms that become noticeable only as the disease worsens with age. Symptoms include breathlessness with little or no exercise, constant fatigue, frequent bronchitis, chest pain, and palpitations (uncomfortably rapid heartbeat).

The symptoms of mitral valve stenosis can be treated with medications. Diuretics are used to drain excess fluid from the lungs, and digoxin is used to slow a rapid heartbeat. Surgery to repair or replace the valve is also an option.

PULMONARY STENOSIS

Blood flows from the right ventricle through the pulmonic valve to the pulmonary artery, which leads to the lungs. Pulmonary stenosis limits the flow of blood into the lungs. As the heart works harder to compensate for the loss of pumping efficiency and the body's need for oxygen, the right ventricle enlarges over time,

turns flabby, and finally fails. Possible symptoms include fatigue, shortness of breath with exercise, light-headedness, and loss of consciousness. In severe cases, pulmonary stenosis leads to swelling in the arms, legs, and abdomen and to an enlarged liver.

Pulmonary stenosis is usually congenital (present at birth). In rare cases, it is caused by rheumatic fever or a cancerous tumor.

Untreated pulmonary stenosis usually causes death before age 30. The traditional cure has been open-heart surgery to replace the pulmonic valve. Increasingly, a procedure known as balloon valvotomy is used. This is a minimally invasive procedure that involves threading a catheter (thin tube) through a blood vessel into the heart to the mitral valve. The catheter is tipped with a balloonlike device that is inflated in the pulmonary valve to force it open and restore normal blood flow.

TRICUSPID STENOSIS

Blood returning from the body flows into the right atrium, through the tricuspid valve, and into the right ventricle. Tricuspid stenosis limits the blood flow from the right atrium to the right ventricle. Possible symptoms include general weakness and pain in the upper right abdomen. Shortness of breath, fluid retention, and fatigue may also occur when disease in the aortic or mitral valve is also present.

Tricuspid stenosis that causes symptoms is rare, commonly occurs in conjunction with other valve problems, and is usually caused by congenital heart disease or rheumatic fever. Treatment often depends on the severity of the associated valve disease. Surgery may be needed to repair the damaged valve.

RISK OF ENDOCARDITIS

A person with valvular stenosis is at increased risk of developing endocarditis (inflammation of the lining of the heart and usually the heart valves), which can worsen the valve disease and be life-threatening. As a precaution, those with valvular stenosis should take antibiotics before dental, medical, or surgical procedures.

Stent

A small, cylindrical tube of wire mesh inserted into a section of diseased artery to hold it open. The stent

is put into place with a catheter, a thin tube threaded into a vein and guided to the site of the diseased artery. Stenting is performed primarily in the coronary arteries (the arteries that supply the heart with blood) and in conjunction with BALLOON ANGIOPLASTY, a catheter-based procedure for opening arteries closed by fatty deposits (plaque). The stent serves to preserve the widening of the artery created by balloon angioplasty. Within a month of insertion, the stent is covered with the cells that make up the inner lining of the artery, and it becomes a permanent part of the artery. After receiving a stent, anticoagulant medications are prescribed temporarily to prevent the formation of a blood clot at the site of the stent. In some cases, plaque again develops in a stented artery within 6 months, narrowing it once more. Stents are not affected by mechanical equipment, nor do they set off metal detectors.

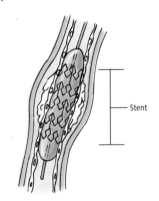

PLACING A STENT
To place a stent in a narrowed artery, the surgeon puts the device on a balloon-tipped catheter and guides it to the site of the blockage. The balloon is inflated to fully widen the half-inch long stent and compress the plaque against the artery wall. The catheter is removed, leaving the stent.

Stereotactic breast biopsy

Also known as stereotactic localization biopsy; a technique that uses X rays to guide the needle for a biopsy of a mass in the breast that cannot be felt. Stereotactic breast biopsy takes X rays of the breast from two different angles. A computer plots the exact location of the area where there is a suspected lesion. When the target area is clearly identified, a radiologist can position the apparatus that holds the needle and advance the biopsy needle into the lesion.

This procedure may be performed in one of two ways. Specialized stereotactic equipment can be attached to a standard mammography machine to locate the lesion. Or the X-ray machine and maneuverable biopsy needle device can be set up underneath an examining table that has an opening in it to allow the breast to protrude downward.

An important advantage of stereotactic breast biopsy is that a smaller area of the breast is exposed to radiation, in doses similar to those of standard mammography.

Stereotactic surgery

Also known as stereotaxic surgery; guided brain surgery. Stereotactic surgery is performed through a tiny hole in the skull and guided by CT SCANNING (computed tomography scanning). This procedure may be performed in people with advanced PARKINSON DISEASE (a progressive, degenerative disease of the nervous system characterized by muscle rigidity, weakness, and tremor), for whom medications are no longer effective. It can also be used to remove deep brain tumors or abscesses that are not accessible with standard surgical techniques. Recent advances in stereotactic surgery have created a new resurgence of interest in this technique. See Focus: stereotactic surgery, page 1164.

Sterility

The condition of being free from live bacteria or other pathological microorganisms. Sterility in medicine applies to maintaining a state of cleanliness in medical settings that prevents the transmission of infectious agents, either directly or indirectly. Achieving sterility in a health care environment involves using a variety of methods and strategies to ensure that people being cared for are not exposed to microorganisms that may cause infection or disease. See also STERILIZATION.

In popular language, the terms sterility or being sterile are sometimes used to refer to people who are unable to conceive or deliver a child; the medical term for this condition is INFERTILITY.

Sterilization

The use of physical or chemical procedures for the purpose of destroying all disease-causing microorganism life, including bacterial endospores (organisms that reproduce asexually) that may be resistant to such procedures. In health care settings, sterilization generally involves all reusable medical devices and patient-care equipment that have contact with normally sterile body tissues or with any structure involved in the vascular system. These devices and this equipment are sterilized before each use.

In hospitals, the primary sterilizing agents used are moist heat, ethylene oxide gas, and dry heat. Medical instruments and devices that are in contact with the bloodstream or normally sterile body tissues are always reprocessed by these methods of sterilization. Heat-sensitive medical devices that are used on or near mucous membranes, such as flexible fiberoptic endoscopes (see ENDOSCOPE), endotracheal tubes, and respiratory therapy equipment, may receive high-level disinfection with chemical germicides, called sterilants; accessories to this equipment that are heat-stable are sterilized with heat-based methods. Disinfection differs from sterilization in that it destroys all identified disease-causing microorganisms, though not necessarily all microbial forms, such as the bacterial endospores, of these microorganisms.

Sterilization, female

See TUBAL LIGATION.

Sterilization, male

See VASECTOMY.

Sternum

The breastbone; the long bone in the front wall of the chest. The sternum joins with the collarbones (clavicles) at the top, and seven pairs of ribs are attached to it. The sternum is extremely strong to protect the heart from injury.

The sternum has three sections (from the top down): the manubrium, body of the sternum, and the xyphoid process. The ribs are attached by the costal cartilages, which are flexible enough to allow the rib cage to expand and contract for breathing, without compromising the protection for the heart. The xyphoid process is joined to the rest of the sternum by cartilage, also to provide some movement for breathing.

Steroids

See ANABOLIC STEROIDS; ANDROGENS; CORTICOSTEROIDS; and SPORTS, DRUGS AND.

Stethoscope

An instrument used to hear and amplify sounds produced within the body. The stethoscope is used to hear the sounds produced by the heart, lungs, and other internal organs. A simple stethoscope consists of an open bell-shaped structure and a disk called a diaphragm, which is connected by rubber or plastic tubes to earpieces worn by the doctor or nurse. More complicated stethoscopes may include electronic amplification systems to help in diagnosis.

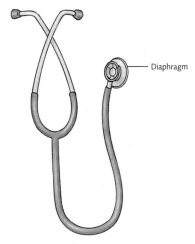

Diaphragm

LISTENING TO THE BODY
Doctors commonly use a stethoscope to listen to the heart, lungs and airways, and the stomach and intestines. The instrument helps the doctor locate a possible problem and determine whether further testing is necessary.

Stevens-Johnson syndrome

See DRUG ERUPTION.

Stiff neck

Limited mobility of the neck, often because of a simple muscle spasm. A more chronic and serious stiff neck may be caused by osteoarthritis, osteoporosis, or slipped or degenera-

S

FOCUS: STEREOTACTIC SURGERY

Stereotactic surgery was created so that surgery could be performed on lesions in the spinal cord and brain without injuring nearby structures. Three-dimensional images help surgeons to access specific sites in the spinal cord or brain. Effective uses of stereotactic surgery include the removal and precision radiation of hard to reach tumors.

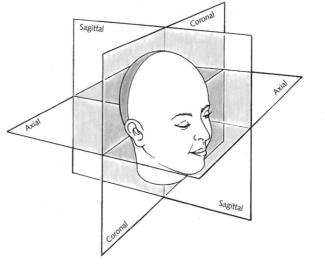

Monitor

Display screen

Video control unit

Video camera

Probe
(entering
brain)

Arc radius device
(halo apparatus)

Electromagnetic
transmitter

STEREOTACTIC SURGICAL EQUIPMENT
Neurosurgeons use precision stereotactic equipment to locate precisely areas of the brain that control specific functions.

DEFINING STEREOTACTIC SPACE
Any point in the head can be defined during stereotactic surgery by three coordinates, each corresponding to the distance between the point and the axial, coronal, or sagittal plane.

Sagittal

Coronal

Axial

Axial

Sagittal

Coronal

tive disks in the cervical spine. Stiffness upon waking or exposure to extremes of cold can also contribute to a stiff neck. Possible trauma to the neck includes whiplash injuries that occur when the neck is jerked too hard from impact during a rear-ended motor vehicle collision and sports injuries.

Muscle spasms in the neck can also produce stiffness in the area. A stiff neck can be a symptom of meningitis when fever, headache, sensitivity to light, and vomiting are also present.

It is important to have a stiff neck evaluated and diagnosed by a doctor before self-help treatment is attempted. Recommended treatment may depend on the cause of the condition. If an injury is the cause, heat, massage, traction, and the use of a supportive neck collar may be recommended. Medications to control pain and swelling may also be given.

Stiffness

Loss of suppleness and flexibility in the muscles and joints. Stiffness may be caused by an injury or an inflammatory or degenerative disease such as OSTEOARTHRITIS. Persistent, prolonged, and disabling stiffness in muscles and joints should be evaluated by a doctor.

Still disease

A rare disease, also known as JUVENILE RHEUMATOID ARTHRITIS (JRA), that affects children from 2 to 5 years of age and produces inflammation in the joints, organs, and other parts of the body. Still disease may be caused by an autoimmune disorder. The symptoms usually flare up in intermittent episodes that last for a few weeks and decrease in severity with time. They usually disappear by puberty.

Adult-onset Still disease is a disorder that is characterized by intermittent high fever, rash, and arthritis. Adult-onset Still disease is diagnosed by physical examination in combination with blood tests. It is generally treated with corticosteroid therapy to reduce the inflammation.

Stillbirth

The birth of a dead baby after the 28th week of pregnancy. Stillbirths can have many causes, the most common being severe birth defects. Other causes include a lack of oxygen to the fetus as a result of PLACENTAL ABRUPTION or a knot in the umbilical cord. Hemorrhage, high blood pressure, diabetes, Rh incompatibility, and maternal smoking can cause stillbirth. Infections, including measles, chickenpox, influenza, toxoplasmosis, rubella, genital herpes, syphilis, and malaria, can also cause stillbirth. In about a third of all stillbirths, the cause is unknown.

The death of a fetus is usually diagnosed with fetal monitoring and ultrasound. When a fetus dies during pregnancy, labor may start spontaneously soon afterwards. If it does not start, the doctor may arrange for induction of labor. Stillbirths are rare, but they are emotionally difficult for both parents. Psychological counseling or supportive group therapy is often recommended.

Stimulants

Drugs that temporarily increase the rate of activity or function of all or part of the body. Some stimulants affect specific organs, such as the heart, lungs, or brain. Doxapram hydrochloride, for example, is a stimulant that increases the activity of the respiratory system, usually after anesthesia has been administered.

Most stimulants, however, help to activate the central nervous system. Examples include caffeine, which is found in food and beverages such as coffee, chocolate, and tea, or in medication used to restore alertness when drowsiness occurs. Other central nervous system stimulants include the amphetamines, such as METHAMPHETAMINE HYDROCHLORIDE, and drugs used to treat attention deficit/hyperactivity disorder such as METHYLPHENIDATE HYDROCHLORIDE.

Stimulus

An action or agent that causes or changes an activity in an organ or other part of the body. The body responds to stimuli, such as temperature, touch, and pain.

Stings, bee

See BEE STINGS.

Stings, marine

Injury caused by a marine animal. Marine stings can be very painful and quite toxic. Marine animals known to sting include the jellyfish, sea anemone, Portuguese man-of-war, stingray, sea urchin, and spiny fish, some of which, even after they are dead, can inject venom through their tentacles into the skin of swimmers. Marine stings can cause an acute stinging or burning sensation, rash, blistering, physiological shock, and allergic reactions. Death rarely occurs except when the person drowns as a result of shock.

First aid measures include the removal of all tentacles by someone who is wearing gloves, to prevent being stung themselves. The area of the sting should be washed with seawater followed by vinegar or rubbing alcohol. Hydrocortisone cream should be applied, and medical attention should be sought.

In the case of a sting from a jellyfish, sea anemone, or Portuguese man-of-war, fresh water should not be used to wash the area because it will increase pain. Stings from stingrays, sea urchins, and spiny fish may be washed with fresh water. It is not recommended that meat tenderizer be applied to the area, as some believe. See Marine animal stings, page 1166.

Stokes-Adams syndrome

Fainting, sometimes accompanied by a seizure, caused by a heart rhythm disorder. Stokes-Adams syndrome occurs when there is a temporary interruption in the normal heartbeat as it passes from the upper to the lower chambers of the heart, a condition known as HEART BLOCK. The heart rate falls so low that the body and brain receive insufficient oxygen. Stokes-Adam syndrome can be caused by some heart medications (for example, beta blockers, calcium channel blockers, and digoxin), heart disease, certain neuromuscular conditions (such as muscular dystrophy), and connective tissue diseases that affect the heart, including systemic lupus erythematosus. To treat Stokes-Adams syndrome, medications that affect the heart rhythm should be stopped. A PACEMAKER, an electronic device that controls heartbeat, can also be implanted in the chest to maintain a normal heart rate.

S

MARINE ANIMAL STINGS

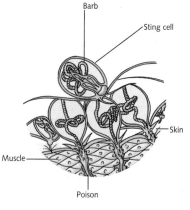

Barb
Sting cell
Skin
Muscle
Poison

Marine stings can be painful and dangerous, depending on the animal and severity of the sting. If a person is stung, first aid should be sought immediately.

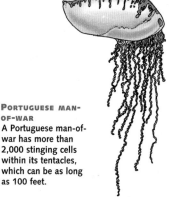

PORTUGUESE MAN-OF-WAR
A Portuguese man-of-war has more than 2,000 stinging cells within its tentacles, which can be as long as 100 feet.

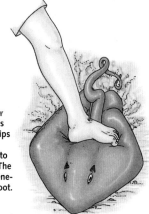

STINGRAY INJURY
When a stingray is stepped on, it whips its tail to inject venom, usually into the person's leg. The spine can even penetrate a person's boot.

HOW JELLYFISH STING
The stinger is triggered when it touches the person's skin. The cell bursts open, pushing the stinger into the skin. The stinger shoots a long tube into the wound and injects poison into the person's skin.

Stoma

A surgically created opening in the body. A stoma is commonly made in the abdominal wall to allow stool to pass from the body into a bag. Stomas are used in the treatment of digestive diseases, such as ulcerative COLITIS, CROHN DISEASE, or colorectal cancer. (See COLON, CANCER OF THE.) In a colostomy, the stoma opens from the large intestine. In an ileostomy, the stoma opens from the lower part of the small intestine (the ileum). Colostomies and ileostomies can be temporary or permanent. When they are temporary, the stoma is surgically closed after the intestine has recovered from inflammation or surgery.

Stomach

A major organ of the DIGESTIVE SYSTEM, located in the upper left side of the abdomen. The stomach receives swallowed food from the esophagus and breaks it down further by means of acidic secretions and churning action. From the stomach, the food passes into the small INTESTINE.

Rhythmic waves of muscular con-tractions (called PERISTALSIS) bring food down the esophagus to the gas-troesophageal junction, which opens to allow entrance to the stomach. The walls of the stomach have three layers of smooth muscle, arranged to make the hollow organ very flexible. Peristalsis continues in the stomach to help to break down food and mix it with digestive secretions. The stomach expands when food is eaten, with a capacity of about 3 pints in the average person. As a result, the stomach can store food for hours at a time.

Specialized cells in the lining of the stomach walls chemically promote digestion in several ways. Some cells secrete hydrochloric acid, which pro-vides the right chemical environment for another secretion called pepsin and kills microorganisms that may be in the food. Other cells secrete pepsinogen, a chemical that is con-verted into pepsin by the hydrochlo-ric acid. Pepsin starts the digestion of protein in food by breaking it down into smaller units called peptides. The peptides in turn cause the release of a stomach hormone called gastrin.

Other cells in the stomach wall secrete the gastrin into the blood-stream. The gastrin in the blood returns to the stomach to stimulate production of more hydrochloric acid. Still other cells produce lipase, which starts to break down fats in food. Finally, mucus-secreting cells in the stomach walls protect it from its own acid secretions.

Processing in the stomach turns the now partially digested food into a liq-uid called chyme. Chyme passes into the duodenum, the first part of the small intestine, through an exit valve called the pyloric sphincter.

Stomach cancer

Cancer that originates in the STOMACH. The incidence of stomach cancer has dramatically declined in the United States. It is now one fourth as com-mon as it was in 1930. The decline may be due to increased use of refrig-eration for food storage and conse-quent drops in the use of foods pre-served with salt and smoking, which have been associated with stomach cancer. Stomach cancer is twice as common in men as in women, and the chances of developing it increase with age. Risk factors include consumption of smoked or nitrate-cured foods, low intake of fruits and vegetables, and infection of the stomach by *Helicobacter pylori*, a bacterium.

SYMPTOMS

At first, the symptoms of stomach cancer may mimic those of PEPTIC ULCER DISEASE. These include vague indigestion, loss of appetite, and discomfort after eating. In more advanced cases, there may be abdominal pain, weight loss, difficulty swallowing, frequent vomiting, and abdominal swelling. Signs of internal bleeding can appear. These include anemia, vomiting with blood, and MELENA (blood in the stool). Melena makes the stool black, sticky, and strong-smelling.

If a person older than age 45 has a sudden case of indigestion, it is important to see a doctor. Early diagnosis and treatment of stomach cancer offer the best chance for a cure. Stomach cancer can spread to other parts of the body, including the liver, lungs, or bones. More obvious symptoms may not appear until the cancer has spread so widely that it is incurable.

DIAGNOSIS AND TREATMENT

Diagnosis of stomach cancer is made through tests, such as GASTROSCOPY (visual examination of the esophagus, stomach, and duodenum using a lighted viewing tube called a gastroscope) and an upper GASTROINTESTINAL (GI) SERIES (an X-ray procedure also called a barium swallow). In a gastroscopy, a tissue sample can also be taken for examination under a microscope. A CT (computed tomography) scan is used to determine how far the disease has advanced. When stomach cancer is diagnosed at an early stage, it can be surgically removed. A GASTRECTOMY (surgical removal of all or part of the stomach) is performed to treat some cases. When stomach cancer is advanced, surgery may still be recommended to relieve symptoms and prevent obstruction. CHEMOTHERAPY and RADIATION THERAPY may also alleviate symptoms and slow the course of the disease.

Stomach imaging

A noninvasive examination of the stomach to diagnose problems such as tumors or ulcers. Stomach imaging is generally done as part of an upper GASTROINTESTINAL (GI) SERIES. In this procedure, a series of X rays is taken using the contrast medium barium, which coats the lining of the stomach, making it visible.

Stomach pumping

FOR FIRST AID
see Poisoning, page 1327

Also known as gastric lavage or stomach flushing, the washing out of the stomach. In the past, people who swallowed poisons routinely had their stomachs pumped. Today, doctors may recommend this treatment only when a life-threatening amount of poison has been ingested within the preceding 60 minutes. Stomach pumping is not used when a person is having seizures or when a corrosive substance, such as acid, lye, or ammonia, has been swallowed.

Stomach pumping is usually done in a hospital emergency department. In the procedure, the doctor repeatedly introduces water or saline into the stomach through a tube and then suctions the fluids out along with poisonous substances. In addition to removing poisons, the procedure is occasionally performed to control stomach bleeding. Possible complications include inhaling any liquids or poisons, pneumonia, and bleeding.

Stomach stapling

A common type of surgery for obesity. Its purpose is to reduce stomach size and slow the rate at which the stomach empties. Stapling is performed only on people who are at least twice their ideal body weight who have been unable to lose weight in supervised weight loss programs. This severe level of obesity is associated with a higher risk of many health problems, including coronary heart disease, diabetes, and certain types of cancer.

Stomach stapling is performed in a hospital under general anesthesia and takes 2 to 3 hours. In the procedure, the surgeon reduces the volume of the stomach using four rows of stainless steel staples. A small pouch is created, attached at one end to the esophagus and at the other to the small intestine. Following surgery, food bypasses the major portion of the stomach and flows through the pouch. Stapling reduces the volume of food that the stomach can hold. The opening into the small intestine is purposely made small to slow the movement of the food.

A hospital stay of about a week is necessary after stomach stapling. A liquid diet is required for 2 to 3 weeks and, in some cases, longer. This is followed by a month of pureed food. Most people can tolerate solid foods after 2 months. However, high-fat foods are difficult to digest and must be avoided. It is also necessary to eat slowly and to consume only small meals. After surgery, doctors recommend changes in diet and exercise that will facilitate weight loss. Risks of stomach stapling include bleeding, infection, leaking or stretching of the pouch, and loosening of staples. Other possible complications are diarrhea, intestinal discomfort, vomiting, and lactose intolerance. See also BARIATRIC SURGERY.

Stomach ulcer

A sore or wound in the mucous membrane lining the stomach. See GASTRIC ULCER.

Stomatitis

Any viral infection of the mouth that causes inflammation of the gums and ulcerations. Frequent causes of stomatitis include certain medications for which dry mouth is a side effect and AIDS (acquired immunodeficiency syndrome). See COLD SORE; CANKER SORE.

Stool

Excrement passed from the anus in a bowel movement. See FECES.

Stool softeners

Drugs used to treat constipation. Stool softeners are a type of laxative (see LAXATIVES) used to promote the formation and passage of soft, formed stools without straining. Doctors sometimes recommend the use of stool softeners to people who have hemorrhoids because softer stools make it easier to empty the bowels without putting pressure on the veins. Stool softeners are also useful for people who have had recent rectal surgery; people with heart conditions, including high blood pressure;

S

people with hernias; and women who have just had babies.

Stool softeners are typically available without prescription. Stool softeners are sometimes sold in combination with stimulant laxatives. Examples of stool softeners and stool softener/stimulant laxatives include docusate sodium (Colace), docusate sodium and casanthranol (Peri-Colace), docusate sodium and senna (Senokot, Gentlax), and docusate sodium and phenolphthalein (Ex-Lax, Feen-a-Mint, Correctol).

Strabismus

Misalignment of the eyes so that they point in different directions; also known as crossed eyes. In esotropia, the most common form of strabismus in infants, one eye turns inward. Accommodative esotropia mostly affects children who are farsighted (have difficulty focusing on close objects). Trying to focus the eyes for vision at short distances causes the eyes to cross. In exotropia one eye turns outward. Exotropia is most likely to be obvious when a person is trying to focus on a distant object or when he or she is tired, ill, or daydreaming.

In normal vision, with both eyes aimed at the same point, the brain combines input from each eye into a single image that offers depth perception. When strabismus develops in a young child, the brain may ignore the input of the misaligned eye and see primarily through the better-performing eye. The resulting image is flat and lacks depth. In addition, the nerve pathways between the misaligned eye and the brain fail to develop properly. Vision in the misaligned eye does not develop completely and may be severely reduced, a condition known as amblyopia. Prompt treatment is needed to prevent amblyopia from becoming permanent.

Occasionally strabismus arises in adults. Since the nerve pathways between the eye and brain have already developed, double vision (seeing the same image twice) rather than amblyopia is the likely outcome.

INCIDENCE AND CAUSES

Strabismus is a common disorder, affecting 4 of every 100 American children. The disease occurs equally in males and females and may run in families, although many people with strabismus have no relatives with the disorder. In children, the disease is most common in the presence of other disorders affecting the brain, such as cerebral palsy, Down syndrome, hydrocephalus, and brain tumors. Injury to the eyes can also cause strabismus. In adults, strabismus can result from brain and systemic diseases (for example, Guillain-Barré syndrome or Apert syndrome) or certain nerve poisons (for example, botulism or paralytic shellfish poisoning).

TREATMENT

Strabismus in children often needs to be treated very early, even in infancy, in order to reduce the risk of permanent vision loss in the misaligned eye. For accommodative esotropia, eyeglasses may be sufficient to solve the problem. The power in the glasses allows the accommodative reflex to relax, resulting in less turning in of the eyes. Sometimes a prism is ground into eyeglass lenses to help realign the eyes.

Exercises have been used to strengthen eye muscles and bring the eyes into alignment, but they are generally thought to be of little value. In some cases, botulinum toxin type A (Botox) is injected into an eye muscle. Botox paralyzes the muscle temporarily and allows the opposite muscle to strengthen and realign the eye. Botox wears off in a few weeks, but the change in alignment may be permanent.

Many cases of strabismus require

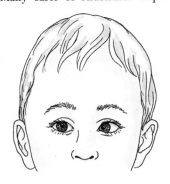

CONVERGENT STRABISMUS
The most common form of strabismus is for one eye to turn in. A newborn infant's eyes may move independently at first. But by 3 or 4 months, the eyes are usually aligned, and by 6 months, the child can usually focus both eyes on near and distant objects.

surgical repair. In children, the operation is done under general anesthesia in a hospital; in adults, local anesthesia in an outpatient clinic may be an option. The surgeon makes a small incision in the tissue covering the eye to reach the muscles that control movement of the eyeball, then repositions them to change the alignment of the eye. Depending on the individual case, surgery may be performed on one or both eyes. Recovery from strabismus surgery is rapid; most people can resume normal activities in a few days. Glasses may be prescribed after the operation. In some cases, two or more surgeries are needed to keep the eyes straight.

Treatment for strabismus is effective. As long as the condition is detected and treated early, a child with strabismus is likely to have normal vision.

Strain

FOR SYMPTOM CHART
see Ankle or foot problems, page 18

FOR FIRST AID
see Strains and sprains, page 1331

A modestly pulled or stretched muscle. Strains are usually confined to muscle but may also involve tendons or ligaments. Some muscle fibers may be damaged by a strain. Sudden, strenuous movements, often occurring during sports activities, are most frequently the cause. Muscles in the back and abdomen may be strained by heavy lifting.

The symptoms of a strain are not usually as intense as those of a SPRAIN, but, depending on the degree of the injury, may include pain, swelling, and bruising, as well as some loss of function or strength. Severe strains may produce painful muscle spasms. Strains usually heal independently within 2 to 3 days. Resting, applying ice, and taking over-the-counter nonsteroidal anti-inflammatory drugs (NSAIDs) may relieve discomfort and speed healing. If a strain persists for more than a few days, a doctor should be consulted to rule out the possibility of a more serious injury.

Strangulation

Interruption of blood supply to a loop of intestine trapped inside a HERNIA (a protrusion of soft tissue through the muscle wall that normally contains it). Symptoms include abdominal pain, nausea, and vomiting. A strangulated hernia often requires emergency surgery (see HERNIORRHAPHY). Otherwise, gangrene (death of tissue) may develop.

Strangury

Slow urination or difficult urination with pain, caused by a muscular spasm of the bladder and the tube (urethra) through which urine passes out of the body.

Strapping

A preliminary treatment for heel pain that has been diagnosed as caused by a mechanical problem in the foot. Strapping, or wrapping adhesive tape to exert pressure and hold the heel in place, for example, is considered an effective approach to testing the potential of ORTHOTICS therapy (the use of custom-made shoe inserts) for individual cases of foot pain. Generally, if strapping reduces foot pain significantly within the first 24 to 72 hours, an orthotic device is prescribed for ongoing treatment. Joints can also be strapped.

Strawberry nevus

See HEMANGIOMA.

Strength training

The activities and exercises devoted to building muscle by challenging muscle tissue and forcing it to adapt to stress. Weight lifting and resistance training, often using machines that can be adjusted to an individual's needs and requirements, are the basic elements of strength training. Strength training offers the benefit of stimulating and strengthening bones as well as muscles. With age, muscle fibers shrink in number and size and become less responsive to signals from the central nervous system. This aging process can cause an overall reduction in lean muscle tissue, strength, balance, and coordination. Strength training can combat these changes that normally occur with aging. Strength training can also aid in weight control. When lean muscle tissue develops to replace fat tissue, the body requires more calories to maintain routine functioning, even at rest. A recommended strength training program works all the major mus-

cle groups including the arms, shoulders, abdomen, chest, back, and legs for 20 to 30 minutes per session, two to three times a week. Muscle groups should be rested for a full 24 hours between strength training routines to prevent the risk of injury. A fitness professional or trainer should be consulted to give demonstrations in proper form as strength training can result in injuries if not performed correctly.

Strengthening exercises

See EXERCISE, STRENGTHENING.

Strep throat

An inflammation of the section of the throat located between the tonsils and the larynx, or voice box. Strep throat is usually caused by an infection with group A streptococcal bacteria. The illness is spread via direct person-to-person contact with infected nasal secretions or saliva. It is most prevalent in children 5 to 10 years old and tends to occur most commonly between the months of October and April. Strep bacteria can exist in the throat of a healthy person without producing symptoms, and small children often have such mild symptoms that a diagnosis cannot be made.

When symptoms of strep throat appear, they may include a sore, reddened throat, difficulty swallowing, a fever that comes on suddenly, tender and swollen glands in the neck, malaise, nausea, loss of appetite, and sometimes a rash. Less commonly, symptoms that may be associated with the infection include neck pain, nasal congestion or discharge, difficulties with the tongue, muscle pain, stiffness in the joints, headache, and an abnormal sense of taste.

DIAGNOSIS AND TREATMENT

Diagnosis is generally based on the finding of streptococcal bacteria in a throat culture. Most symptoms improve within a week when antibiotics are used to treat strep throat. Treatment can prevent serious associated complications including middle ear infection, sinusitis, abscesses on the tonsils, rheumatic fever, scarlet fever, impairment of kidney function, and mastoiditis (inflammation of the bone behind the middle ear).

Self-care methods may help to

relieve symptoms. These include gargling with warm salt water several times a day and taking acetaminophen for a sore throat. Also, if someone in the household has strep throat, family members should wash their hands frequently in hot water and should not share cups or eating utensils.

Streptococcal infections

Infections caused by the *Streptococcus* genus of bacteria. There are several classified groups within this genus, each one responsible for a different group of infections: group A *Streptococcus* and group B *Streptococcus* are the two principal groups responsible for many common infections, as well as severe illnesses. Group D *Streptococcus*, *Streptococcus pneumoniae*, and the *viridans* group of streptococci are three other groups within this genus of bacteria that can cause infection.

A GROUP A STREPTOCOCCUS INFECTION is frequently found in the throat or on the skin of healthy people who have no symptoms of infection. This group usually causes mild illness and is responsible for the skin infection impetigo and most cases of pharyngitis, an inflammation of the part of the throat between the tonsils and the voice box. STREP THROAT is a common form of pharyngitis.

Infections that are termed invasive group A streptococcal disease include two potentially fatal infections. Streptococcal toxic shock syndrome causes a dramatic drop in blood pressure and organ failure. The second,

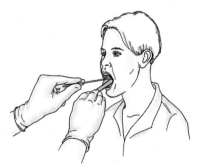

THROAT CULTURE
Many group A *Streptococcus* infections occur in the mouth and throat, causing a sore throat, mild fever, and fatigue. To diagnose the infection, a doctor will take a sample of phlegm from the throat for analysis.

S

necrotizing fasciitis (also known as "flesh-eating disease"), is a severe, painful inflammation of the fibrous sheath that encloses and connects the muscles, causing tissue death in surrounding muscle, fat, and skin. The invasive group A streptococcal diseases can be treated with many different antibiotics. Supportive care in an intensive care unit of a hospital is sometimes necessary to treat severe illness, and surgery may be required to treat necrotizing fasciitis. Early treatment may reduce the risk of death.

Group B streptococcal bacteria can cause infections in newborns, in pregnant women, in people who are older, and in adults with chronic illnesses, including those with diabetes and liver disease. These bacteria are the most common cause of life-threatening infections in newborns, including sepsis and meningitis. They are also a common cause of newborn pneumonia. Group B bacteria cause SEXUALLY TRANSMITTED DISEASES in women that affect the urinary and genital tracts. Diagnosis of these infections is especially important to pregnant women because the infection can spread to the newborn during childbirth. Bladder infections, womb infections, and stillbirth can also occur in pregnant women with group B streptococcal infections. Among adults, blood infections, skin or soft tissue infections, and pneumonia are the most common diseases caused by group B streptococcal bacteria. Cultures of blood or spinal fluid are taken to identify these bacteria, and the infections are successfully treated with antibiotics, usually penicillin.

Group D streptococcal bacteria

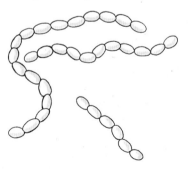

DISEASE-CAUSING BACTERIA
Under a microscope, the *Streptococcus* group of bacteria usually appears in long chains of round organisms.

cause a number of infections. Many of the strains of these bacteria are harmless, and some are normally found in human feces. However, there are pathogenic forms in this group that can produce complications in the human digestive tract. Bacteria in this group are also associated with diseases or conditions including septicemia, endocarditis, and appendicitis. There are two divisions of group D streptococcal bacteria: one is a cause of urinary tract infections, and the other has proven to be resistant to many common antibiotics. Most group D streptococcal infections are successfully treated with antibiotics, usually ampicillin alone or in combination with gentamicin.

Streptococcus pneumoniae bacteria cause pneumonia, meningitis, and middle ear infections. *Streptococcus viridans* bacteria inhabit the mouth and are responsible for a significant percentage of tooth decay.

Streptokinase

One of the original THROMBOLYTIC DRUGS. Streptokinase (Streptase) is used to dissolve blood clots that have formed in blood vessels. Streptokinase is usually prescribed when a blood clot threatens the flow of blood to certain areas of the body. It is given by injection.

Streptokinase is also used to dissolve blood clots that form in tubes that are placed in the body to make it possible to carry out treatments, such as during dialysis or for some long-term intravenous injections.

Stress

The physical and psychological reaction to a challenging or adverse stimulus. Stress is part of life, and some degree of it is necessary to maintain normal alertness. Excessive stress, however, can be highly damaging and may contribute to physical or mental illness. There are two basic types of stress: a short, intense experience known as the FIGHT-OR-FLIGHT RESPONSE, and a less intense, longer-term response mobilizing the body's resources for endurance in meeting a challenge.

The symptoms of stress and the degree of challenge needed to cause these symptoms vary greatly among individuals. Symptoms include anxi-

ety (a general feeling of uneasiness, dread, uncertainty, and fear in response to, or in anticipation of, a real or imagined threat), rapid heartbeat, fainting, hot flashes, or chills. A person with stress may also have intestinal distress, difficulty sleeping, nightmares, poor concentration, heavy or absent menstrual periods, sexual disturbances, chest pain, and tearfulness. Stress also leads to distortions in thinking, such as feelings of unreal weakness or assessing a situation as hopeless when in fact remedies are available.

CAUSES
Stress can have a physical cause. An overactive thyroid gland (hyperthyroidism) may produce anxiety symptoms. Drugs, including caffeine, oral decongestants, asthma inhalers (bronchodilators), thyroid supplements, tricyclic antidepressants, and certain cold remedies, can lead to the signs of stress. Withdrawal from certain drugs and medications may cause stress symptoms as well. In addition, any physical illness, from the flu to cancer, adds to the burden on the body and is likely to produce symptoms. Working too hard, drinking too much alcohol, eating a poor diet, and sleeping too little can also contribute to a person's stress.

Stress may arise from psychological causes. Examples include a boring or demanding job, grief over the death of a loved one, strain or conflict in a marital or love relationship, and financial difficulties.

STRESS AND DISEASE
Stress can trigger, exacerbate, or worsen a variety of physical diseases. Asthma and migraine headaches occur more often during periods of stress. Stress also contributes to ulcers, irritable bowel syndrome, ulcerative colitis, neurodermatitis (a skin disorder accompanied by intense irritation), menstrual disorders, and high blood pressure (hypertension). In addition, stress can lead to mental illness, particularly one of the ANXIETY DISORDERS (for example, posttraumatic stress disorder or panic disorder) or depression.

TREATMENT
Treatment begins with identifying the cause of the stress. Once the cause is known, steps can be taken to reduce or manage it. For stress rooted in psychological causes, RELAXATION TECH-

NIQUES (training that focuses the mind on recognizing and reducing the reaction to stress symptoms) and changing one's mental attitude toward the source of stress are helpful. In some cases, psychotherapy and medication are also recommended.

Stress fracture

A small crack or break in a bone that is caused by repeated jarring or pressure to the bone. Stress fractures may occur in the feet and upper part of the shinbones as a result of overuse, improper form, or repetitive impact during running, dancing, or aerobic exercise. Long-distance running or repetitive jumping may cause a stress fracture. They are common in young women who exercise excessively, are underweight, and have stopped menstruating. The symptoms include gradually increasing pain and localized tenderness that are relieved with rest. Stress fractures are not usually visible on X rays, though they can be seen on a bone scan. Diagnosis may be made after a doctor's physical examination and the taking of a medical history that includes details of athletic or aerobic activities. The only treatment for stress fractures is a period of rest, usually for about 6 to 8 weeks, sufficient to allow complete healing.

Stress testing

See CARDIAC STRESS TESTING.

Stress ulcer

A type of peptic ulcer that may develop following a major illness, serious injury, burn, or shock. See PEPTIC ULCER DISEASE.

Stretch marks

Streaks or lines in the skin that are associated with rapid growth, certain diseases, and long-term use of corticosteroid creams; also known as striae atrophicae. At first the lines appear red and glossy but over time become whitish and scarlike. Stretch marks most frequently appear on the abdomen, breasts, hips, thighs, and buttocks. They are due to thinning of the skin. Common causes include rapid growth, pregnancy, obesity, diseases such as diabetes or Cushing disease, and medications that cause swelling, including corticosteroids. There is no effective treatment for stretch marks. Tretinoin cream and laser surgery have been tried with mixed success.

Stretcher

A framelike cot for carrying sick or injured persons. A stretcher usually consists of a sheet of canvas stretched between two poles. A stretcher may also be used to carry the disabled.

Striae atrophicae

See STRETCH MARKS.

Stricture

Narrowing or closure of a tubular body part, such as the esophagus, bowel, or urethra. Strictures are usually caused by tumors, inflammation, injury, or scar tissue.

Stridor

Shrill wheezing and noisy, hoarse breathing that is most common in young children with a respiratory infection. Stridor occurs when their upper airways narrow, usually due to swelling and an increase in mucus from a respiratory tract infection. (However, narrowing can also occur without stridor.) Very often, the cause of stridor is CROUP, an inflammation of the larynx and trachea that makes breathing noisy and difficult. Other times, the symptoms could be due to a congenital abnormality or an obstruction from inhaling a foreign object. Less commonly, an allergic reaction can cause swelling of the airway and stridor. Difficulty breathing accompanied by drooling and high fever can be a sign of the rare but potentially fatal inflammation called EPIGLOTTITIS.

TREATMENT

A physician should see any young child with stridor as soon as possible. A child whose stridor is caused by croup has a distinctive cough that sounds like the bark of a seal. A vaporizer or steam from a shower can help relieve the congestion of croup, and the pediatrician may prescribe antibiotics to cure an underlying bacterial infection. In epiglottitis, which mainly affects children from ages 2 to 6, the valve at the top of the windpipe, or trachea, becomes swollen due to infection. This emergency requires immediate medical care. To permit the child to breathe comfortably, it may be necessary to bypass the swelling by inserting a tube through the nose into the trachea. Very severe cases may require a tracheostomy, in which a breathing tube is placed into the trachea through a small incision in the neck. When a child develops stridor but does not have a respiratory infection, he or she may have inhaled a foreign object. Because this can block the air passage, a child who has sudden difficulty breathing should be taken to the hospital emergency room. Stridor may also occur with a congenital problem known as laryngomalacia. This condition is usually not serious and is attributed to immaturity of the tissues of the larynx. Although breathing is noisy, children typically grow out of the problem by age 12 to 18 months.

Stroke

FOR FIRST AID
see Stroke, page 1332

Damage to part of the brain caused by an interruption to its blood supply or leakage of blood outside of vessel walls. Stroke, a type of brain injury, is the third leading cause of death in the United States. Risk factors for stroke include HYPERTENSION (high blood pressure), cigarette smoking, heart disease (see HEART DISEASE, ISCHEMIC; HEART DISEASE, CONGENITAL), TRANSIENT ISCHEMIC ATTACK, warning signs or history of stroke, and diabetes (see DIABETES MELLITUS, TYPE 1; DIABETES MELLITUS, TYPE 2).

CAUSES

There are several different causes of stroke. Most strokes are ischemic; that is, they are caused by reduced blood flow to the brain when blood vessels are blocked by a clot or become too narrow for blood to pass through. Brain cells are consequently deprived of oxygen and die. The most common causes of an ischemic stroke are ATHEROSCLEROSIS or CEREBRAL THROMBOSIS, which are most common in older people. Clots rarely form in healthy arteries. However, in atherosclerosis, there is a thickening and loss of elasticity in artery walls. The arteries narrow and become lined with PLAQUE. Blood flow slows, and clots are more likely to form. When a clot becomes lodged in an artery in the brain, the result is a stroke. It is possible for a wandering clot to be carried through the bloodstream until it plugs up a brain artery and cuts off

S

FOCUS ON STROKE

Strokes occur when blood clots obstruct an artery or blood vessel or when blood vessels rupture, interrupting blood flow to areas of the brain. Without blood to supply oxygen, brain cells in the immediate area die, usually within minutes to a few hours. For this reason, doctors call strokes "brain attacks" in order to urge the public to react to the symptoms of stroke with the same urgency as heart attacks.

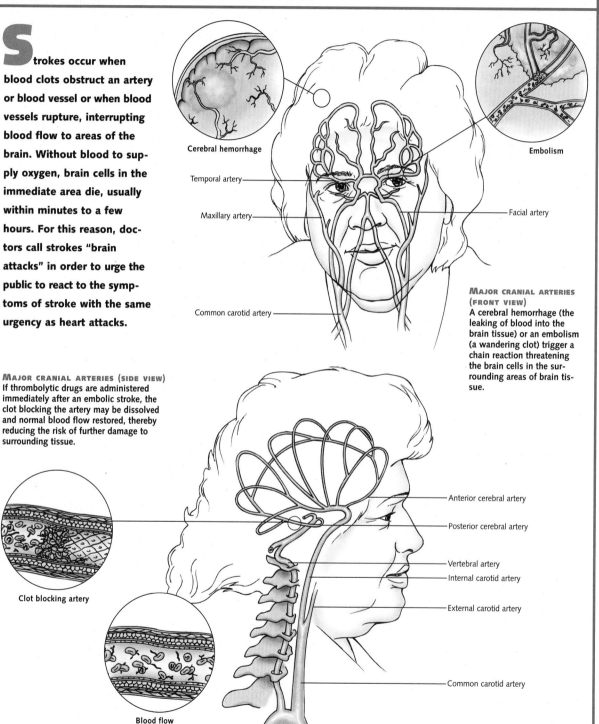

Cerebral hemorrhage

Embolism

Temporal artery

Maxillary artery

Facial artery

Common carotid artery

MAJOR CRANIAL ARTERIES (FRONT VIEW)
A cerebral hemorrhage (the leaking of blood into the brain tissue) or an embolism (a wandering clot) trigger a chain reaction threatening the brain cells in the surrounding areas of brain tissue.

MAJOR CRANIAL ARTERIES (SIDE VIEW)
If thrombolytic drugs are administered immediately after an embolic stroke, the clot blocking the artery may be dissolved and normal blood flow restored, thereby reducing the risk of further damage to surrounding tissue.

Clot blocking artery

Blood flow restored to artery

Anterior cerebral artery

Posterior cerebral artery

Vertebral artery

Internal carotid artery

External carotid artery

Common carotid artery

blood flow; this is called a cerebral EMBOLISM.

A hemorrhagic stroke occurs when blood vessels are damaged or ruptured. Rupture of a blood vessel in or near the brain can cause a cerebral hemorrhage or subarachnoid hemorrhage (see HEMORRHAGE, CEREBRAL; HEMORRHAGE, SUBARACHNOID). A subarachnoid hemorrhage is most often caused by a cerebral ANEURYSM (abnormal ballooning or widening caused by a weakening of an artery wall) that has ruptured or burst. Aneurysms may occur as a congenital defect or when there is a weakened wall in a blood vessel. Hemorrhages can also be caused by other blood vessel abnormalities (such as an ARTERIOVENOUS MALFORMATION) or trauma.

SYMPTOMS

Stroke symptoms most commonly affect only one side of the body. Changes in brain function depend on the location and extent of injury to the brain. Common symptoms of a stroke are paralysis, weakness, numbness, tingling, decreased sensation, cognitive decline, impaired vision, an inability to recognize or identify stimuli, problems with swallowing, loss of coordination, loss of memory, vertigo, personality changes, depression, changes in consciousness (such as sleepiness, apathy, stupor, or loss of consciousness), and lack of control over the bladder or bowels. Language difficulties following a stroke may include difficulty speaking or under-

---

TREATABLE RISK FACTORS FOR STROKE

A risk factor is a condition or behavior that occurs more frequently in people who have, or are at a greater risk of getting, a disease than in those who do not. Many risk factors for stroke can be successfully managed. These include:

- High blood pressure
- Cigarette smoking
- Heart disease
- Warning signs or history of stroke
- Diabetes mellitus, type 1 and type 2
- Hyperlipidemia (elevated concentrations of lipids in the blood)

STROKE WARNING SIGNS

Any or all of the following can be symptoms of a major stroke:

- **Sudden weakness or numbness of the face, arm, or leg, especially on one side of the body**
- **Sudden confusion, trouble speaking, or difficulty understanding**
- **Sudden trouble with vision in one or both eyes**
- **Sudden trouble walking, dizziness, loss of balance, or loss of coordination**
- **Sudden severe headache of unknown cause**

---

standing speech, slurred speech, and problems with reading or writing. When the symptoms of a stroke last for less than 24 hours and are followed by complete recovery, the episode is known as a TRANSIENT ISCHEMIC ATTACK. This can be a warning signal of a future stroke.

DIAGNOSIS AND TREATMENT

Immediate medical attention is required to diagnose and treat a stroke. Diagnostic tests may include MRI (magnetic resonance imaging), CT (computed tomography) scanning, angiography, ultrasound, functional MRI, and magnetic resonance angiography (MRA). (See BRAIN IMAGING.) An electrocardiogram (ECG) or echocardiogram may be used to detect any heart problem that may have contributed to the development of a stroke. Blood tests are also important, and examination may include neurological, sensory, and motor evaluation.

A stroke is a life-threatening condition for which immediate emergency treatment is required. Hospitalization is necessary and usually includes lifesaving interventions and supportive measures. There is no cure for a stroke. The goal of treatment is to prevent the spread of the stroke, control symptoms, and maximize an affected person's ability to function. Surgery may be required to remove a blood clot or to repair damage. Possible medications include corticosteroids, diuretics, anticonvulsants, and analgesics. Blood products and intravenous fluids may be necessary to counteract loss of blood. Outcomes vary widely. Even with

prompt treatment, death may occur. A person may also recover completely or suffer permanent brain damage. People who have had strokes can be given a medication that breaks up the clot and restores blood flow back to the damaged area. Unfortunately, this is only helpful if given within 3 hours from the start of symptoms. Otherwise, the brain may sustain irreversible damage and there may be an increased risk of bleeding once the clot is broken up.

Strongyloidiasis

An infection caused by the roundworm *Strongyloides stercoralis*. Strongyloidiasis occurs when human skin is penetrated by larvae of this roundworm that exists in contaminated soil. The larvae migrate through the bloodstream to the lungs and are transported through the bronchial tree to the throat, where they are swallowed and move down into the small intestine. They mature into females in the small intestine, where the females live in the lining of the intestinal walls and produce eggs, which yield larvae. These larvae are either eliminated in the stool or remain in the body and penetrate the mucosal lining of the intestines or the skin of the area surrounding the anus. These larvae then follow the route from the lungs to the small intestines where they mature into adults and begin their life cycle again. This ongoing cycle causes persistent infection and reinfection in the human host.

SYMPTOMS, DIAGNOSIS, AND TREATMENT

A person with strongyloidiasis may not have any symptoms, or the infection may cause gastrointestinal symptoms that include abdominal pain and diarrhea. There may be pulmonary symptoms, including Löffler syndrome (a benign, self-limiting disease in which infiltrations of the lungs cause cough, fever, and shortness of breath). An itching, hiveslike rash may appear on the buttocks and near the waist.

In people with weakened immune systems (for example, those with AIDS [acquired immunodeficiency syndrome] or those who recently had transplant surgery), strongyloidiasis causes pain and distension of the

S

abdomen, shock, abnormalities of the lungs and nervous system, and septicemia. It is potentially fatal for this group of people.

Strongyloidiasis is diagnosed by identifying the larvae microscopically in the stool or in fluid taken from the duodenum, the uppermost section of the small intestines. In severe cases, the larvae may be detected in the sputum. A series of samples may need to be examined to confirm diagnosis. Treatment is accomplished with antiworm medications including ivermectin, thiabendazole, and albendazole.

Structural integration
See ROLFING.

Stuffy nose
See RHINITIS.

Stump
The end portion of the limb that remains after amputation. If the stump is large enough, an artificial limb, or PROSTHESIS, can be attached to it and controlled by the brain impulses that continue after amputation.

Stupor
A state of reduced consciousness from which a person can be aroused only briefly and only by vigorous external stimulation. See also UNCONSCIOUSNESS; COMA.

Sturge-Weber syndrome
A congenital disease characterized by a PORT-WINE STAIN that follows the distribution of the trigeminal nerve of the face in association with vascular malformations in the eye and brain. Sturge-Weber syndrome may lead to calcification of the cerebral cortex, seizures, glaucoma, or optic atrophy. There is no known cure. Treatment of symptoms includes antiseizure medications and treatment of glaucoma.

Stuttering
A speech disorder characterized by speech that is interrupted by stopping and frequent repetition or prolongation of sounds. Ninety-eight percent of the time, stuttering begins before age 10 and usually resolves by age 16. It occurs in about 1 percent of the adult population. The problem is most intense when the person who stutters is feeling anxious or using the telephone. Stuttering usually is not present while the individual sings or talks to pets or inanimate objects. Tics, eye-blinks, or tremors of the lips and face may accompany stuttering. Stuttering primarily has psychological causes, although a popular unproven theory suggests that it is due to a brain abnormality.

Between the ages of 2 and 4, many children normally appear to stutter as they develop complex language skills. Most outgrow the trait around age 5 when they begin school. A child who continues to stutter after age 5 or a younger child whose stuttering significantly interferes with his or her speech should see a doctor. A hearing test may be recommended. A speech therapist may be asked to do an evaluation and recommend possible treatment. Reducing stress is a key goal of therapy in eliminating a stutter. The stuttering child should not have to speak in stressful situations or compete with others, such as siblings, to be heard. It is harmful to correct children who stutter, tell them to slow down, or finish their sentences for them. See also SPEECH DISORDERS.

Stye
A small abscess occurring on the edge of the upper or lower eyelid or in the eye's corner. A stye, also called a hordeolum, is caused by a bacterial infection, which is usually due to staphylococcal bacteria, of the glands at the base of the eyelid. The surrounding area may be red and swollen and painful or itching. The stye may range from the size of a pinhead to the size of a pea. Styes usually drain without treatment; they may drain internally or externally.

Self-care of a stye may include applying warm, moist compresses held gently against the area for 10 to 15 minutes, three or more times daily. The compress should be clean and changed daily. The moist heat can bring the pus in the stye closer to the skin surface and promote efficient draining. Once the stye has begun to drain, frequent washing of the area with warm water will help prevent crusting, which may block further draining. Eye makeup should not be used as long as the stye remains. To prevent spreading a stye, the person who has it should not share towels, pillowcases, or other items that come into contact with the eyes with others. Styes can be prevented by keeping the hands clean, not sharing eye makeup, and avoiding contact with the eyes when the hands are not well-washed.

If a stye forms a whitehead without opening up or gets worse over time, it may need to be drained by a doctor. Antibiotic ointment or drops may be prescribed to help speed recovery.

Subacute
A term describing the stage of a disease or condition that is between ACUTE (short-lived and relatively severe) and CHRONIC (persisting for a long period).

Subacute nursing facility
A facility that offers a combination of housing, personal services, and health care to older or disabled people with diseases or conditions that lie between the ACUTE (short-lived and relatively severe) and CHRONIC (persisting for a long period) stages.

Subarachnoid hemorrhage
See HEMORRHAGE, SUBARACHNOID.

Subclinical
A term describing a disease or condition that is in its early stages and is so mild that it produces no symptoms.

Subconjunctival hemorrhage
Bleeding under the external membrane of the eye (conjunctiva). A subconjunctival hemorrhage looks like a bright red patch on the white of the eye and produces no pain. Forceful sneezing or coughing can be a cause. Subconjunctival hemorrhages can also appear without warning or injury and are often noticed when looking in the mirror first thing in the morning. Subconjunctival hemorrhages disappear on their own in 1 to 2 weeks and require no treatment unless bleeding elsewhere in the body is present.

People may have an increased risk for developing subconjunctival hemorrhage if they are taking aspirin or other blood thinners. Persons who develop subconjunctival hemorrhages without an identifiable cause should be checked for high blood pressure and possible bleeding disorders.

Subconscious

Mental activity that occurs just below the level of normal conscious awareness. In the psychoanalytic theory of Sigmund Freud (see FREUDIAN THEORY), the subconscious level lies between the conscious and the unconscious.

Subcutaneous

A medical term meaning beneath the skin. An example would be a subcutaneous injection, meaning an injection of medication into the tissue under the skin.

Subdural hemorrhage

Bleeding into the space between the two outer membranes (called the dura mater and the arachnoid) of the three membranes covering the brain. Blood leaking from the outermost membrane, the dura mater, is caused by ruptured blood vessels, usually small veins. The blood seeps slowly into the space between the two membranes and collects there, forming a blood clot, or subdural hematoma. Subdural hemorrhage is usually caused by a blow to the head or other head injury. It sometimes occurs in older people who may have fallen. Concussion, or a brief loss of consciousness, may follow a blow to the head that results in subdural hemorrhage. Symptoms may include drowsiness, confusion, persistent headache, listlessness, imbalance, vomiting, and weakness or numbness on one side of the body. Over a few days or several weeks, these symptoms may appear intermittently, then become progressively more severe. Prompt medical attention is essential. The doctor should be informed of any recent accidents, falls, or other injuries to the head.

DIAGNOSIS AND TREATMENT

Diagnostic tests may include a CT (computed tomography) scan or MRI (magnetic resonance imaging). If a subdural hematoma is detected, surgery to remove the clot may be recommended, depending on the size. If the clot is small, the blood is usually gradually absorbed and does not present further problems. Ongoing medical monitoring is important. REHABILITATION therapy may prove beneficial.

Subglottic stenosis

A condition produced by lesions that narrow the channel in the area of the lower throat directly below the VOCAL CORDS. The lesions may be present at birth or appear later in life. When the condition is congenital, the symptoms may include noisy breathing, hoarseness, a barking cough, or a weak or unusual cry. If the lesion causes minimal obstruction, there may be no symptoms until an infection of the respiratory tract causes inflammation in the area and further narrows the air passage. If the obstruction is severe at birth, the newborn may breathe noisily in the delivery room. Diagnostic imaging techniques, such as X rays of the neck, and LARYNGOSCOPY (examination of the vocal cords with a mirror or viewing tube) may be used to evaluate the condition. Some young children outgrow the condition by the time they reach 3 or 4 years of age. Others may require periodic dilation of the trachea with tracheal dilators. In some instances, TRACHEOTOMY (a surgical opening to insert a tube into the trachea to keep the airway open) may be necessary.

When subglottic stenosis is acquired, it is considered a more serious medical condition. It may be caused by infection, chemical irritation, or a foreign body in the throat, but it is most often caused by prolonged intubation beginning at birth or shortly thereafter. Tracheotomy and other surgical treatments are more often required when subglottic stenosis is acquired.

Sublimation

The unconscious diversion of unacceptable or repressed instinctual drives into a channel that is personally or socially permissible. For example, a person who channeled rage at a childhood sexual abuser into a career as a social worker helping children would be practicing sublimation. Sublimation, one of the DEFENSE MECH-ANISMS, is an automatic, unconscious psychological process that protects a person against anxiety or impulsive actions in response to stress and internal emotional conflict.

Subluxation

The partial dislocation of a joint. The most common joints affected by subluxation include the shoulder, elbow, kneecap, and the neck. See DISLOCATION, JOINT; SHOULDER, DISLOCATED.

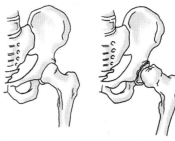

Healthy hip joint   Subluxation

PARTIAL DISLOCATION
Subluxation refers to the partial dislocation of a joint—that is, the head of the bone has moved partly out of the socket into which it fits. (In a true dislocation, the head is completely out of the socket.)

Subphrenic abscess

A pus-filled sac that develops on or near the diaphragm. A subphrenic abscess is usually the result of PERITONITIS (inflammation of the peritoneum, the membrane that lines the abdominal cavity and covers the stomach, intestines, and other abdominal organs).

Substrate

The substance on which a given enzyme acts. Enzymes are very specific in their activity and catalyze specific chemical reactions between a few very closely related compounds, which are known as the substrates of that enzyme.

For example, the substrate for an enzyme in the saliva is starch, while the substrate for the enzyme ribonuclease is RNA (ribonucleic acid).

Sucralfate

An antiulcer drug (Carafate) used to treat duodenal ulcers. Sucralfate works by forming a coating over the ulcer, protecting it from stomach acid and giving it time to heal.

Sucrose

A disaccharide SUGAR composed of two simple sugars (monosaccharides). Sucrose is made of fructose and glucose and is the compound in white table sugar. Sucrose occurs naturally in sugar beets and sugar cane, from which it is extracted to produce table sugar. It is also found in fruits and vegetables. Molasses is its least refined form. Like other sugars, sucrose is a carbohydrate that serves as a source of energy for the body. Whether eaten as pure sugar or as an additive to foods such as breakfast cereal or desserts, sucrose provides empty calories, meaning calories with no other nutrients.

Suction

The aspiration of a gas, liquid, or solid by reducing air pressure over its surface. Pressure then forces the material into the vacuum. Suction has a number of uses in medicine. For example, nasogastric suction is the removal of a gas, liquid, or solid from the stomach or small intestine by insertion of a tube through the nose. This procedure is performed in situations such as the removal of toxic substances, decompression of the stomach or small intestine, and preparation for gastrointestinal operations.

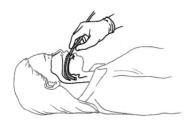

SUCTIONING THE THROAT
To remove mucus from the trachea (windpipe), a nurse or doctor will insert a tube against the roof of the mouth, gently push the tip of the tube to the beginning of the throat, and apply suction.

Sudden death

An unexpected death occurring from any cause other than violence or trauma. Sudden deaths may be instantaneous or may happen over a period of minutes or hours. Examples include sudden death from a cardiac arrhythmia and SUDDEN INFANT DEATH SYNDROME (SIDS), in which a baby dies unexpectedly for reasons that cannot be explained, even following an AUTOPSY.

Sudden infant death syndrome

The sudden and unexpected death of an apparently healthy infant while asleep, reported since Biblical times. Once called crib death, sudden infant death syndrome (SIDS) is the leading cause of death of infants in the first year; the highest incidence comes between ages 1 and 4 months. Sudden infant death syndrome occurs most frequently in the winter and affects slightly more boys than girls.

Doctors suspect that SIDS may have a number of causes. They include a delay in the maturation of arousal centers in the brain, abnormal regulation of breathing and heart rates, and insufficient airway control. Probable risk factors include premature birth; low birth weight; babies sleeping on their stomachs; a family history of SIDS; poor prenatal care; smoking, drinking alcohol, or use of narcotics by pregnant women; and birth to a very young mother. Many other suspected causes—such as infection, milk allergy, and pneumonia—have been dismissed.

PREVENTION
Placing a sleeping infant on his or her back is of primary importance, especially in the first 6 months of life when SIDS is most common. Contrary to popular belief, choking is no more common in infants lying on their backs than in those lying in another position. Tight-fitting, firm mattresses in cribs that meet current safety standards are recommended. A baby's head should not be covered while sleeping.

Other prevention methods focus on observing and responding to changes in a healthy infant's breathing. Home monitors are sometimes used by parents to monitor any sounds of choking or labored breathing, but medical research has not confirmed that monitors help prevent SIDS. Some parents train in cardiopulmonary resuscitation (CPR) for emergencies. An infant who stops breathing or turns blue requires immediate medical care. A physician will assess the severity of the problem and search for treatable causes.

For premature infants, the doctor may prescribe caffeine or theo-phylline to stimulate respiration. Although prematurity is often beyond an individual's control, pregnant women can help ensure the health of a developing fetus by getting regular checkups, following a healthy diet and not smoking, drinking alcohol, or using narcotics.

IMPACT ON PARENTS
Parents of an infant lost to SIDS experience unique feelings of pain, grief, and guilt. Psychiatric or family counseling and the aid of relatives, friends, and support groups often are used by the grieving parents of infants who die of SIDS. Mental health professionals have observed a particular devastation to such parents and can provide specific therapies for them. Local and national SIDS groups also offer assistance to the parents.

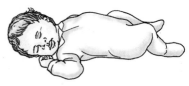

SAFEST SLEEP POSITION
Placing an infant on his or her back to sleep significantly reduces the risk of sudden infant death syndrome. The baby needs plenty of time on his or her stomach during the day, so that he or she can learn to push with the arms and legs. The baby should have a firm crib mattress that fills the frame completely, without gaps between the mattress and the sides of the crib. A child's head should not be covered while sleeping.

Sudeck atrophy

A disorder of the sympathetic nervous system, which involves the network of nerves located along the spinal cord. These nerves control certain functions including those associated with the working of the blood vessels and sweat glands. Sudeck atrophy is also called posttraumatic osteoporosis, which is part of reflex sympathetic dystrophy. The disorder most commonly affects women older than 50, but may affect anyone. Sudeck atrophy often occurs following an injury (such as a forearm fracture) or heart attack or stroke, but in many cases, the cause is unknown. The symptoms include swelling and severe pain that may be experienced as a burning sensation usually in the hand or foot, but also possibly in the knee, hip, shoulder, or other area of the body. The skin in the affected area may become thin or shiny, and there may be a localized increase in perspiring and hair growth. As Sudeck atrophy progresses, the pain may be accompanied by weakness and wasting, or dystrophy, in the affected region. There may also be contracture, which is when the muscle becomes shortened and immobilized.

Diagnosis of the disorder is made by physical examination, clinical history, and evaluation of the symptoms of pain and dysfunction. X rays will reveal that the bones have been thinned by a loss of minerals, so-called posttraumatic osteoporosis. Sudeck atrophy is treated with pain-relieving medication, applications of hot and cold, local or regional nerve blocks of the sympathetic nerve, physical therapy, vigorous exercise, and, in some cases, prescribed medications.

Suffocation

FOR FIRST AID
see Resuscitation, page 1328

Severe oxygen deprivation that leads to a life-threatening deficiency of oxygen in the blood. Suffocation may be caused by accidental events that prevent air from being breathed in, such as foreign objects or food lodged in the throat or upper airways or near-drowning events that occur when a person is under water for a long time but survives. Deprivation of oxygen may also be caused by RESPIRATORY FAILURE and other severe lung or heart disorders. Absence of breathing is the primary symptom.

Episodes involving suffocation may injure the lungs and reduce the amount of oxygen delivered to vital organs. Permanent damage to the brain and heart may also occur. Survival generally depends on how quickly breathing and lung function are restored and how soon oxygen reaches the vital organs of the person who is suffocating.

TREATMENT
Visible foreign objects obstructing airflow should be removed from the mouth or throat if possible. MOUTH-TO-MOUTH RESUSCITATION should be started immediately for a person who does not appear to be breathing. If the person does not have a heartbeat, CARDIOPULMONARY RESUSCITATION (CPR) should be given.

CHOKING ON FOOD
When a person swallows, involuntary reflexes cause the epiglottis to seal off the trachea momentarily so that food does not enter it. If these reflexes are disrupted, food can either enter the trachea or lodge against the epiglottis, preventing it from opening again. The Heimlich maneuver is one technique to remove a foreign object from the trachea.

Esophagus

Trachea

Food

Epiglottis

A person who is suffocating should be taken to a hospital emergency department by trained emergency personnel. Resuscitation efforts should continue during travel to the hospital. Hospitalization is essential to evaluate and monitor the effects of oxygen deprivation, even after a person who has had an episode of suffocation regains consciousness. In a hospital setting, the person may be placed in an intensive care unit where efforts will be made to provide oxygen to the bloodstream with the use of a face mask or a mechanical ventilator. Oxygen delivered in a high-pressure, or hyperbaric, chamber may be required.

Strategies such as mechanical hyperventilation to reduce cerebral swelling are used to prevent or minimize brain damage in a person who has survived an episode of suffocation. In some cases of prolonged oxygen deprivation, the person may have permanent brain damage.

Sugar

A carbohydrate that serves as a major source of energy for the body. Sugars may be refined to produce table sugar. When consumed in their natural forms, sugars are consumed along with fiber, minerals, and vitamins. (See also CARBOHYDRATES.) Refined sugar provides calories with no other nutrients. Excess sugar in the diet may lead to decay in the teeth. As a result, unrefined simple sugars and complex carbohydrates are a healthier choice of fuel for the body. There are many different types of sugars. Ordinary white table sugar is SUCROSE, which is made from fructose

OTHER NAMES FOR SUGAR

Avoiding refined sugar is necessary for health reasons such as weight control and preventing or controlling diabetes. It is important to know that sugars have many different names, such as:

- High-fructose corn syrup
- Dextrose
- Fructose
- Glucose
- Honey
- Lactose
- Malt syrup
- Maltodextrin
- Maltose
- Mannitol
- Maple syrup
- Molasses
- Sorbitol
- Sucrose

and glucose. Other types of sugar include honey, lactose, and corn syrup. The US Department of Agriculture Food Guide Pyramid advises individuals to derive the smallest proportion of their diet from fats, oils, and sugars. Naturally occurring unrefined sugars consumed in fruits and vegetables do not usually need to be restricted because they also provide other nutrients.

Suicide

A self-inflicted death that results from a person's intended, direct, and conscious effort to kill himself or herself. Women make three times more suicide attempts than men, but men are three times more likely to complete suicide. The apparent reason for this difference is that men use more violent methods, particularly firearms. Suicide is least common among married adults with children and most common among divorced individuals. Whites have a higher suicide

5

rate than racial and ethnic minority groups, except for American Indians, who kill themselves at a rate four times higher than the national average. The risk of suicide increases with age among whites and is highest among older white men. In recent decades, however, suicide among adolescents and young adults has increased dramatically, becoming the third leading cause of death after accidents and homicides.

A pregnant teen-ager who fears rejection from her partner or parents is a major suicide risk.

FACTORS ASSOCIATED WITH SUICIDE

Suicidal acts often result from current events or conditions profoundly affecting a person's life. Chief among these are stressful situations, such as the loss of a loved one (divorce, romantic breakup, or death), loss of a job, academic or occupational pressure, serious illness, and abusive or violent environments. Increased feelings of sadness and helplessness typically precede suicide and may be accompanied by anxiety, shame, or anger. Alcohol use often rises before suicide, and other drugs can also have a role. Suicide is particularly common among people with mental or emotional disorders, particularly depression, manic-depressive illness, schizophrenia, and substance-abuse disorders. Suicide rates also tend to rise after the highly publicized suicides of celebrities.

CAUSES

The exact cause of suicide remains unclear. While it is true that various factors are associated with suicide, many people with the same situations and disorders do not commit suicide. Researchers who have studied suicide follow three basic schools of thought.

One theory takes the biological view that suicide is the result of a person with an abnormal or malfunctioning brain. Research has shown that the brains of people who commit suicide have abnormally low levels of the transmitter chemical serotonin. Low serotonin levels have been linked to depression and an increase in strong aggressive impulses.

The psychodynamic theory of suicide, identified principally with the work of Sigmund Freud, holds that self-destruction results from depression and anger directed at the self. Research has shown that suicidal people are likely to have endured a significant loss, such as the death of a parent, as children. There is also some evidence that aggression directed at the self has a role. Suicide rates fall during wartime, presumably because aggression flows outward toward a common enemy rather than at oneself.

The third theory, called the sociocultural, holds that suicide is most common among individuals who are least connected to the principal social institutions, such as family and church. Evidence supports this point of view. People who are actively religious are the least likely to commit suicide, and suicide rates rise when societies undergo changes, such as economic depression or high unemployment rates.

TREATMENT

When an individual survives a suicide attempt, the initial need is for immediate medical care to treat the physical consequences. A suicide attempt can leave a person with a brain injury, damage to organs, broken bones, cuts, or poisoning. Once the person's physical condition is stable, psychotherapy can begin. The goal of treatment is to keep the person alive and help him or her find a state of mind in which suicide is no longer a solution to distress and develop better ways of solving problems.

Suicide prevention programs aim to help people who are contemplating suicide before they actually commit a lethal act. Suicide prevention hotlines, for example, are 24-hour telephone services in which trained volunteer counselors answer calls from people thinking about killing themselves. The counselor attempts to establish a positive relationship with the caller, helps the individual see his or her situation realistically, assesses the threat of suicide in the situation, and motivates the caller to take advantage of the available resources he or she has and to formulate a plan of action.

Suicide, threatened

Direct or indirect threats or attempts to commit suicide. Many people who commit suicide talk about it before making an attempt. Suicidal behaviors occur as a response to situations that the suicidal person finds over-

SUICIDE WARNING SIGNS

Although no two people are alike, there are some common signs and behaviors of possible suicide. Medical help should be obtained promptly for the following:

- **Withdrawal and isolation from friends and family**
- **Use of alcohol and drugs**
- **Decline in school or job performance**
- **Irritability**
- **Dramatic change in appearance, activities, or friends**
- **Giving away possessions**
- **Talking about suicide**
- **Depression**
- **Aggressive and dangerous behavior, such as reckless driving, that suggests a loss of respect for his or her own life and that of others**

whelming, such as social isolation, death of a loved one, drug or alcohol abuse, physical illness, financial problems, and aging. Because most suicides are preventable, suicide threats or attempts should always be taken seriously (see also DEPRESSION).

Any attempted suicide must be treated as a medical emergency; help must be sought as quickly as possible. If the person has stopped breathing, CARDIOPULMONARY RESUSCITATION (CPR) should begin. If the person is bleeding, first aid should be used to stop it.

Sulfa drugs

Antibiotics used to treat bacterial and some fungal infections. Sulfa drugs are medically known as sulfonamides. Sulfa drugs work by interfering with the metabolism of bacteria and fungi, thereby killing them. Sulfa drugs were considered "wonder drugs" before penicillin was discovered, and they are still used today. Because sulfa drugs concentrate in the urine before being excreted, they are often used to treat urinary tract infections. Sulfa drugs are not effective for the treatment of colds, flu, or other viral infections.

OPHTHALMIC SULFA DRUGS

Ophthalmic sulfa drugs are used to treat infections of the eye. They are available as eye drops or ointments. Examples include sulfacetamide (Blephamide, Klaron) and sulfisoxazole (Gantrisin).

SULFONAMIDES AND PHENAZOPYRIDINE

Sulfonamides and phenazopyridine are combination drugs made up of sulfa drugs and a urinary pain reliever, used to treat infections of the urinary tract and to relieve the associated pain, burning, and irritation.

SULFONAMIDES AND TRIMETHOPRIM

Sulfonamides and trimethoprim are found in a combination used to treat several infections. Sulfadiazine and trimethoprim are used to treat urinary tract infections; the combination is also used to treat bronchitis, middle ear infection, and traveler's diarrhea.

ERYTHROMYCIN AND SULFISOXAZOLE

Erythromycin and sulfisoxazole (Pediazole) is a combination antibiotic used to treat ear infections in children.

Sulfamethoxazole

See CO-TRIMOXAZOLE.

Sulfasalazine

Sulfasalazine (Alzulfidine) is a sulfa drug used to treat and prevent inflammatory bowel disease, such as ulcerative colitis or Crohn disease. It works inside the bowel to reduce inflammation and other symptoms of the disease. Sulfasalazine is also used to treat rheumatoid arthritis for people who experience side effects from other arthritis drugs.

Sulfonamides

See SULFA DRUGS.

Sulfonylurea

An oral hypoglycemic (blood glucose–lowering) medication widely used to treat hyperglycemia (high blood sugar) in type 2 diabetes. Sulfonylurea must be used carefully in combination with blood sugar monitoring to help avoid the side effect of hypoglycemia (low blood sugar), which can result in coma and possibly death.

Sulfur

A mineral that occurs either freely or combined with hydrogen or oxygen in the form of sulfides and sulfates. Sulfur has been used medically in the treatment of diseases such as rheumatism and gout. Sulfur normally is obtained by consuming protein, since sulfur-containing sulfates from protein are sufficient to meet the body's needs. Sulfonamides, or sulfa drugs, which contain sulfur, continue to be an important treatment for bacterial infections.

Sulindac

A drug used to treat arthritis; one of the non-steroidal anti-inflammatory drugs (NSAID). Sulindac (Clinoril) is used to relieve inflammation, swelling, stiffness, joint pain from rheumatoid arthritis, osteoarthritis, and ankylosing spondylitis, a progressive arthritis of the spine. Sulindac is also used to treat bursitis, tendinitis, gouty arthritis, and other conditions. Sulindac reduces pain and inflammation.

Sumatriptan

A drug used to treat migraine. Sumatriptan (Imitrex) is used to treat acute migraine and cluster headaches. Sumatriptan is thought to work by constricting or narrowing the blood vessels in the brain that dilate during a migraine attack. Sumatriptan cannot prevent migraine or cluster headaches; it is used to treat a headache that has already begun.

The sooner the drug is used in an attack, the better it works.

Sun exposure, adverse effects of

The adverse effects of sun exposure are numerous and include SUNBURN, an increased risk of SKIN CANCER, premature aging of the skin, suppression of the immune system, and eye damage such as cataracts. Extended exposure to ultraviolet light from the sun first causes an increase in skin pigment, or a tan. Although a suntan may not seem to be an injury, it is the first sign that skin damage has taken place. The red and blistering skin of sunburn is a more obvious sign of injury. In addition to their immediate pain and discomfort, repeated sunburns are linked with a greater long-term risk of malignant melanoma (see MELANOMA, MALIGNANT). Repeated exposure to the sun is also associated with an increased risk of other types of skin cancers, such as basal cell carcinoma and squamous cell carcinoma. In addition, cumulative sun exposure can cause premature aging of the skin, leading to wrinkles, sagging, and brown spots.

The most effective way to prevent adverse effects is to avoid exposure to the sun. To protect skin from harmful ultraviolet radiation, doctors recommend applying a sunscreen with a sun protection factor (SPF) of at least 15 before going outdoors; using a broad-spectrum sunscreen that provides protection not only from ultraviolet B (UVB) rays, which cause sunburn and skin damage, but also from ultraviolet A (UVA) rays, which enhance the harmful effects of UVB; reapplying sunscreen every 2 hours, especially if swimming or sweating; avoiding exposure to the sun between the hours of 10 AM and 4 PM when rays are at their most intense; wearing a broad-brimmed hat and protective clothing that covers most of the body; using sunglasses that provide UVA and UVB protection; and, when possible, staying in the shade.

Sun protection factor

A measurement of the effectiveness of sunscreen in blocking ultraviolet B (UVB) light. Protection from the sun is essential in the prevention of skin cancer and other skin damage. (See also SUN EXPOSURE, ADVERSE EFFECTS OF.) Doctors recommend sunscreens with a sun protection factor (SPF) of at least 15. They are available in sprays, gels, creams, and wax sticks. Fair-skinned people require sunscreens with higher SPFs. A high SPF indicates better protection from the effects of UVB light, which causes sunburn and an increased risk of skin cancer. However, SPF does not refer to the level of protection against the effects of ultraviolet A (UVA) light, which enhances the damaging effects of UVB. Consequently, it is best to choose a broad-spectrum sunscreen that also offers UVA protection. Sunscreens must be reapplied every 2 hours, especially if a person is swimming or sweating.

Sunburn

Tender, red, swollen skin due to overexposure to the ultraviolet rays of the sun. Sunburns can also be caused by sun lamps or tanning beds. Initial symptoms of pain and redness are often followed by itching and blistering. In addition to their immediate discomfort, scientists believe that repeated sunburns are linked with a greater risk of malignant melanoma (see MELANOMA, MALIGNANT) later in life. Chronic exposure to the sun is also associated with an increased risk of other types of SKIN CANCER, premature aging of the skin (such as brown spots, wrinkles, and sagging), suppression of the immune system, and cataracts.

Symptoms generally develop 2 to 4 hours after sun exposure. Minor sunburn consists of a first-degree burn that reddens skin. Second-degree burns lead to blistering. Sensations of pain and heat usually peak after 24 hours and last 48 hours.

Most sunburns respond to treatment. Applying cool compresses and taking cool baths can relieve some of the heat and discomfort. Helpful medications include over-the-counter oral ibuprofen for discomfort and 1 percent topical hydrocortisone cream. The person with sunburn must drink enough fluid to prevent dehydration. If blisters break, torn skin should be carefully cleansed with soap and water and an antibiotic ointment applied to prevent infection. If sunburn is severe or accompanied by fever, or if the skin becomes infected, medical attention is necessary.

To prevent sunburn, doctors recommend applying a sunscreen with a SUN PROTECTION FACTOR (SPF) of at least 15 before going outdoors, using a broad-spectrum sunscreen that provides ultraviolet A (UVA) and ultraviolet B (UVB) protection, and wearing protective clothing. People who are taking medications (such as many commonly prescribed antibiotics) that increase sun sensitivity must stay out of the sun or use a sunblock. See also SUN EXPOSURE, ADVERSE EFFECTS OF; PHOTOSENSITIVITY.

Sunscreens

Substances that block the effects of harmful rays from the sun. Sunscreens are lotions or oils spread on the skin to prevent SUNBURN, a cause of early wrinkling and SKIN CANCER. Chemical sunscreens protect against sunburn by absorbing damaging ultraviolet (UV) light, while physical sunscreens protect against sunburn by reflecting, scattering, or blocking the UV rays.

CHOOSING A SUNSCREEN

A sunscreen product is appropriate for a person with a certain skin type if it has an SPF (sun protection factor) rating in the range given or higher.

SKIN TYPE	DESCRIPTION	SPF
Very fair	Always burns; rarely tans	20 to 30
Fair	Always burns easily; tans minimally	12 to 20
Light brown	Burns moderately; tans gradually	8 to 12
Medium brown	Burns minimally; always tans without sunscreen	4 to 8
Dark brown	Rarely burns; tans profusely	2 to 4

The choice of a sunscreen involves selecting a product with a suitable SPF (sun protection factor) rating. The number of the rating is a comparison of the amount of time it takes to produce sunburn on protected skin to the amount of time needed to cause sunburn on unprotected skin. SPF 2 means that if it takes 10 minutes to produce sunburn on unprotected skin, it will take 20 minutes on skin protected with a lotion rated SPF 2. If the same person uses a product rated SPF 15, it will take 150 minutes, or 2½ hours, to develop that sunburn. Sunscreens rated SPF 15 or higher are recommended as effective protection, but people should limit their exposure to the sun even when using sunscreen protection.

Sunstroke
See HEAT STROKE.

Superego
In the psychodynamic or FREUDIAN THEORY of the psyche, the part of the self that contains the sum total of exterior rules, moral values, and expectations taught by parents and parentlike figures, such as teachers and members of the clergy. The individual typically experiences his or her failure to meet the demands of the superego as shame or guilt. The superego is in part unconscious, and it can cause feelings of guilt not justified by any wrongdoing.

Superficial
In anatomy, situated at or near a surface; shallow. Superficial blood vessels, for example, are those close to the surface of the skin. A shallow cut is referred to as a superficial injury.

Superinfection
A second infection that occurs in addition to a previous infection. Superinfections are often caused by a different microbial agent than the one that caused the first infection. This new infectious agent may have originated from a source outside the body or from within the body. If the initial infection was medically treated, the microorganism causing the superinfection may be resistant to the treatment used.

Superinfections can produce life-threatening illness. Influenza, for example, can progress to pneumonia with a superinfection of a more virulent strain of bacterial pneumonia, such as *Pseudomonas* pneumonia.

Supernumerary teeth
Extra teeth located in the dental arch. Supernumerary teeth may be present anywhere along the jaw where the 32 PERMANENT TEETH are normally positioned. They most commonly appear among the top teeth, between the two front teeth, or behind the third molar (wisdom tooth). When supernumerary teeth are located between the two front teeth, there may be one or two of them and they may be fully erupted (grown out from the gum), impacted, inverted, or fused to one of the front teeth. When they are impacted, they are detected with the use of X rays. Supernumerary teeth are usually surgically removed, especially when they interfere with the positioning of the permanent teeth. There are rarely additional teeth among the 20 PRIMARY TEETH; when this occurs, it is usually in the area of the upper incisors (the teeth between the central front teeth and the eye teeth) and

S

the cuspids (the eye teeth). A dentist can evaluate the need for intervention when there are supernumerary teeth among the primary teeth.

Supernumerary teeth may develop from an extra tooth bud in the jaw or from the division of a single permanent bud. The condition is believed to be hereditary.

Supination

The position of lying on the back (face up) or the outward rotation of the arm (palm upward).

Suppository

A cylinder-shaped capsule containing a drug and an inactive material, such as cocoa butter, that dissolves once inside the body. Tiny suppositories are inserted into body cavities such as the rectum or vagina. Drugs administered by suppository include antifungal drugs, local anesthetics, laxatives, corticosteroids, antibiotics, and drugs to prevent vomiting and nausea.

Suppuration

The formation of PUS. Suppuration is a term that describes the accumulation of material into pus and the process of discharging pus. The process occurs at the site of a bacterial infection where dead white blood cells collect and combine with other body fluids.

Suprarenal glands

Another name for the ADRENAL GLANDS.

Supraspinatus syndrome

See ROTATOR CUFF DISEASE.

Surfactant

A fatty substance that is secreted by cells lining the alveoli (the lungs' air sacs) that coats the alveoli. Surfactant helps the air sacs expand, stretch, and maintain flexibility as a person inhales and exhales air. It also lowers the surface tension in the air sacs so pressure is evenly distributed.

When there is an insufficient supply of surfactant, a great deal more pressure is required to inflate each individual air sac. Pressure throughout the lungs is not equalized if the surfactant coating is not evenly distributed. This can cause the air sacs

to completely collapse in on themselves.

Several diseases and disorders may contribute to inadequate production of surfactant and the consequent loss of elasticity in the lungs. In a person with EMPHYSEMA, for example, habitual smoking dissolves the elastic fibers that make up the walls of the air sacs. This damages the cells that produce surfactant and causes the air sacs to lose elasticity, enlarge, and possibly rupture. The exchange of oxygen and carbon dioxide in the blood is decreased when this occurs.

The immature lungs of premature infants may not make enough surfactant to prevent collapse of the alveoli. This can lead to respiratory distress in the newborn. Coricosteroid therapy may be given to the mother during labor before delivery to increase the infant's surfactant levels. Surfactant may also be given directly to infants to reduce the risk of respiratory distress.

Surfer's nodules

Knobby lumps that form just below the knees of surfers or on the upper surface of their feet. Surfer's nodules are caused by the repeated or constant friction and pressure of the hard, rough surfboard on these areas. Surfers who may spend many hours in a kneeling position on their surfboards tend to develop these characteristic nodules, which are also called surfer's knobs, surfer's lumps, and surfer's knots. The nodules appear as firm, fluid-filled cysts or as hematomas. They improve when the surfer stops kneeling for long periods. In

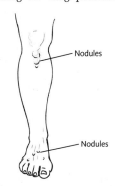

— Nodules

— Nodules

SKIN NODULES
Regular kneeling on a moving surfboard may cause the development of fluid-filled cysts just below the knees and on the tops of the feet. They are usually harmless.

some cases, the nodules may need to be treated by a physician. Surgical removal is sometimes necessary.

Surgeon

A physician specially trained to perform operations that involve the cutting of body tissue. General surgeons perform operations on various parts of the body, while some surgeons operate only on particular parts of the body within their specialty.

Surgery

The specialty in medicine that focuses on diseases, injuries, or conditions best managed or treated by procedures that involve opening, manipulating, and repairing a part of the body. Also, the word "surgery" is used to refer to a specific procedure or operation, such as bypass surgery.

Surgicenter

See AMBULATORY SURGERY.

Surrogate motherhood

An agreement between an infertile couple and a woman who agrees to bear the couple's baby and give it to them at birth. Surrogate mothers are sought by some women who are unable to become pregnant because they have had hysterectomies or repeated miscarriages or because their reproductive systems are otherwise unable to produce a pregnancy. The infertile woman's egg can be fertilized by her partner's sperm in a laboratory and surgically implanted into the surrogate mother, who then carries it to term. In other cases, the surrogate mother's egg can be fertilized by the man's sperm, using ARTIFICIAL INSEMINATION. Homosexual couples who want to have children also use surrogate motherhood. Surrogate mothers usually are paid for their services and all their expenses. This approach is very controversial ethically and is illegal in some states.

Susceptibility

A person's receptivity to disease or infection. Susceptibility is influenced by several general human characteristics, such as the ability of the person's immune system to respond to specific pathogens that a person may make or be exposed to. Age, sex, ethnic group, and heredity also have

S

important roles in a person's susceptibility. Diet, personal hygiene, and other cultural behaviors can be involved, as can geographic and environmental conditions. The general health status of a person, including his or her level of nutrition, amount of physical activity, and the state of hormonal balance (for example, not having any hormonal abnormalities), can influence susceptibility to disease. The presence of disease or other debilitating conditions, including impaired immunity, is also a factor.

Suture

A surgical stitch to repair an incision, tear, or wound. Various materials are used for sutures, including silk, wire, and synthetic materials. Some sutures must be removed; others dissolve. Types of sutures include the chain stitch, which is a continuous stitch; an interrupted suture, which is a single suture tied separately; an apposition suture that holds the margins of an incision close together; and buried sutures, which draw together soft tissues beneath the outer layer of skin.

Suturing

The closing of a wound, whether from surgery or an accident, with a surgical needle and thread. The type selected for a given procedure depends on the nature and placement of the wound or surgical incision to be closed. Some types of sutures are removed after surgery, while others dissolve after the incision is healed. In a few surgeries, such as an otoplasty, sutures are left in place permanently.

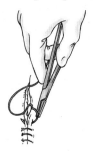

STITCHING A WOUND OR INCISION
To close a wound or incision with sutures, the surgeon uses a curved needle, held in the hand or in a needle-holder (above). The needle is passed through the skin, down through the full depth of the wound, up through the skin on the other side, and then tied off with an individual square knot.

Swab

A wad of absorbent material, cotton, or gauze wrapped around the end of a thin stick or clamp. Swabs are used to apply medication, remove matter from a site on the body, such as the ear canal, or take a sample of cells for laboratory testing, such as for strep throat.

Swallowing

The process by which food is transferred from the mouth to the esophagus; deglutition. In swallowing, the tongue is raised within the mouth to push the food back toward the throat, thus stimulating reflex actions in which the larynx at the top of the throat and the nasal passages are closed, so the food will not enter the trachea (windpipe). The process of swallowing is completed by the passage of the food through the esophagus to the stomach.

Swallowing difficulty

Problems with passing food or liquid from the mouth to the stomach, a condition medically termed dysphagia. Normally, when a person eats or drinks, the chewed food or liquid is swallowed by means of several mechanical events. The tongue pushes the material to the back of the throat where muscle contractions quickly move it along. It passes from the back of the throat to the esophagus, the tube connecting to the stomach. Muscles at the top and bottom of the esophagus open and close quickly to propel food into the stomach. Difficulty swallowing can be painful and disturbing. The causes of the condition vary; most are not medically serious and can usually be treated effectively.

CAUSES AND SYMPTOMS

There are generally two categories of conditions that may cause difficulty swallowing. The most common category, called esophageal dysphagia, is produced by a narrowing of the lower esophagus. It is often caused by stomach acid that backs up into the esophagus (SEE ESOPHAGEAL REFLUX), which can cause inflammation and scarring of the lower esophagus. Tumors or an abnormal band of tissue constricting the lower esophagus may also narrow the channel. The person has the sensation of food being lodged in the base of the throat, maybe accompanied by pressure or pain in the chest. Another condition, called oropharyngeal dysphagia, is the weakening of throat muscles that may be caused by age or by a stroke or neuromuscular disorder. The weak muscles in the throat make it difficult to pass food from the mouth into the throat, resulting in coughing or a choking sensation or the feeling that food is going down the windpipe. Other possible causes of difficulty swallowing

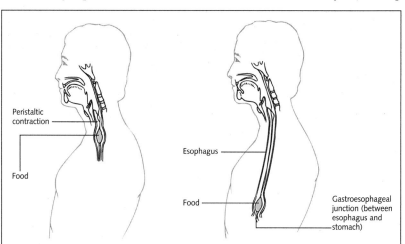

MOVING FOOD TO THE STOMACH
Once food has entered the esophagus, wavelike muscular contractions called peristalsis move the food along. Esophageal muscles above the food contract, while the muscles in front of it relax, pushing it toward the stomach. Finally, the muscles at the entrance to the stomach relax to allow the food to enter.

Labels on diagram: Peristaltic contraction, Food, Esophagus, Food, Gastroesophageal junction (between esophagus and stomach)

include the formation of a small pouch, called a diverticulum, in the back of the throat or esophagus and radiation burns from treatments for cancer. Difficulty swallowing may also result from an inflammation of the tongue, called glossitis.

For some people, difficulty swallowing is not based on any structural impediments and may be triggered only by specific kinds of swallowing—such as attempts to swallow pills, tablets, or capsules. Stress can trigger muscle spasms or the sensation of a lump in the throat. Frequent clearing of the throat can increase irritation of the throat's lining and result in difficulty swallowing. Intermittent, mild difficulty swallowing is not cause for concern. If it is experienced continually and severely, however, it can be a symptom of a serious medical problem, such as esophageal cancer, and should be evaluated medically. The presence of other symptoms—including HEART-BURN, pain, a backup of stomach acid or food into the throat, and weight loss—also indicate the need to consult a physician.

DIAGNOSIS AND TREATMENT
Tests to evaluate the condition may include a BARIUM SWALLOW, which involves drinking a barium solution to coat the inside of the esophagus so changes in its shape can be imaged and observed. Endoscopy is a procedure for viewing the esophagus, which involves passing a thin, flexible tube called an endoscope down the throat. MANOMETRY can measure the muscle contractions of the esophagus by recording the pressure produced when swallowing occurs.

If difficulty swallowing is determined to be caused by gastroesophageal reflux, medications to reduce stomach acid may be prescribed. If there are spasms of the esophagus, tranquilizers or muscle relaxants may also be prescribed. If the condition is caused by a narrowing of the esophagus, a procedure called ESOPHAGEAL DILATATION may be performed. This procedure involves the use of an endoscope with a balloon attached to its end; the balloon is gradually inflated to gently expand the width of the esophagus. If difficulty swallowing is interfering with healthy eating patterns, special liquid diets or tube feeding may become

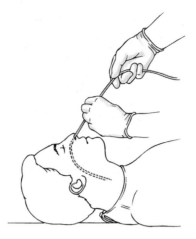

MANOMETRY TO TEST SWALLOWING
A test called esophageal manometry measures the "squeeze pressure" in the esophagus—that is, the force of the normal muscular contractions that move food through the digestive tract. For the test, a local anesthetic is applied to the esophagus, and a tube is passed down the nose or mouth, through the esophagus, and into the stomach. Pressure recordings are taken to test the function of the muscular sphincter at the top of the esophagus, throughout the length of the esophagus and at the lower sphincter between the esophagus and the stomach. The person is asked to inhale and exhale and to swallow to see how the esophagus reacts. The test takes 15 or 20 minutes. Afterward, the person can return to normal activities.

necessary. Surgery can remove a tumor or diverticulum. A person who experiences difficulty swallowing may be referred to an otolaryngologist (throat specialist) or a neurologist for further evaluation. A speech pathologist or a program of exercise therapy may be recommended in some cases.

Sweat glands
A structure in the skin that produces sweat, a salt solution. Sweat glands are located in the dermis layer of the skin. There are two kinds of sweat glands. Eccrine glands, the more common type, are found in much of the skin, except for the lips and external genitals. The eccrine glands release sweat onto the surface of the skin for cooling by evaporation. Apocrine glands secrete strongly scented sweat onto hair follicles instead of onto the skin surface. These glands, found in the underarms close to the nipples and around the genitals, secrete sweat in response to emotion or stress.

Sweating is regulated by the hypothalamus in the brain, as part of the autonomic nervous system (which controls involuntary body functions).

Sweating
The secretion of fluid by the sweat glands; perspiration. Sweating occurs naturally when the sweat glands (sudoriferous glands) situated in the top layers of the skin discharge sweat through tiny openings in the surface. Sweating is necessary to remove certain waste products from the body, including urea; it is also essential in the regulation of body temperature, because as sweat dries, it has a cooling effect. Sweat is a transparent, colorless, acidic fluid with a characteristic odor caused by waste products.

Increased sweating (called diaphoresis) is often caused by pain, nervousness, nausea, and certain drugs. Sweating may be reduced by diarrhea, colds, and some drugs.

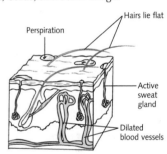

Cooling off skin

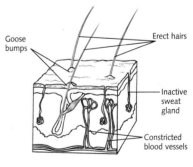

Warming up skin

TEMPERATURE CONTROL
When body temperature climbs above normal, the brain directs the blood vessels to dilate (widen) to dissipate heat, hairs to lie flat, and the sweat glands to produce moisture so that evaporation of sweat on the skin will have a cooling effect. When body temperature drops, the opposite actions take place to conserve heat.

S

Swedish massage

A widely practiced form of MASSAGE THERAPY. Swedish, or European-style massage features long, soothing strokes, kneading, pressing, and light pounding movements as a method to get blood moving and to loosen tight muscles. Swedish massage was invented by a Swedish fencing master who blended elements of European folk massage with Asian techniques and a knowledge of anatomy and physiology. It is used to promote relaxation, relieve stress, ease joints, and for physical therapy and general well-being. It is practiced by physical therapists and massage therapists to flush the tissues of lactic acid, uric acid, and other metabolic wastes and to keep ligaments and tendons supple. Swedish massage stimulates the skin and soothes the nerves simultaneously, thereby reducing both emotional and physical stress.

Sweeteners, artificial

See ARTIFICIAL SWEETENERS.

Swimmer's ear

An infection in the ear canal, often caused by swimming in polluted water. The medical term for the condition is otitis externa. This condition usually begins with a blocked feeling and itching of the ear. These feelings may progress to intense pain caused by swelling of the tissue in the ear canal pressing against surrounding bone. There may also be tenderness just outside the ear canal. There is often a discharge from the ear, which may be a yellow, foul-smelling pus or a milky liquid. The discharge may block the ear canal and impair hearing. Glands in the neck may become swollen.

CAUSES

Swimmer's ear may begin with the development of eczema, an inflammation of the skin inside the ear canal that causes itching and flaking; people with eczema tend to develop swimmer's ear more readily. The eczema causes breaks and openings in the skin's surface that allow bacterial or fungal infections to invade the tissues of the canal. Often bacteria that thrive

> Terms in small capital letters—for example, PHYSICAL THERAPY or PAGET DISEASE—indicate a cross-reference to another entry with more information.

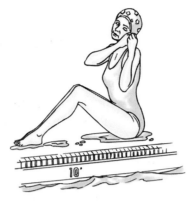

PREVENTING SWIMMER'S EAR
Using a swimming cap and ear plugs may help prevent swimmer's ear, an infection in the ear canal. The condition is often the result of swimming in polluted water or inadequately chlorinated swimming pools where bacteria can thrive.

in inadequately chlorinated public pools cause the infection. Exposure to a hot, humid environment can help cause swimmer's ear. Rarely, the infection is caused by a fungus (a condition called otomycosis). A specific fungus that produces black spores deep in the ear canal is difficult to treat and may persist after the eczema has cleared. Swimmer's ear can also be caused by hair spray or hair coloring dye that enters the ear canal.

DIAGNOSIS AND TREATMENT

A physician can diagnose swimmer's ear by physically examining the ear and evaluating the symptoms. A culture may be taken to identify the bacteria or fungus causing the infection. Ear drops containing one of the CORTICOSTEROIDS are usually prescribed to treat swimmer's ear. Antibiotics are also applied in the ear to cure the infection. When swelling is severe, a cotton wick may be placed in the ear for 1 or 2 days to allow the corticosteroid and antibiotic drops to reach the ear canal skin. Fungus infections are generally treated with thorough, repeated cleaning and medications; rarely are antibiotics prescribed. People with AIDS (acquired immunodeficiency syndrome) or DIABETES MELLITUS, TYPE 1, or DIABETES MELLITUS, TYPE 2, should be treated promptly for swimmer's ear.

The ears should be kept dry while the infection is being treated. A heating pad may help diminish the pain. After the condition has healed, the

use of ear plugs when swimming may help avoid a recurrence; soft silicone earplugs that fit into the shell of the ear tend to remain in place best, especially when used with a swimming cap. When hair sprays or dyes are used, balls of water-repellent lamb's wool in the ear may help prevent recurrence.

A preventive strategy for swimmers involves combining equal, small amounts of rubbing alcohol and white vinegar in a dropper and placing a few drops into each ear canal if water remains in the ears after swimming. The alcohol and acidic vinegar help dry out the ear and may also destroy some bacteria or fungi.

Swimmer's shoulder

Tendinitis or tears of the rotator cuff muscle caused by a strain on the shoulder joint produced by the constant motion of a person swimming. Swimmer's shoulder can be prevented by resting the shoulder regularly between swims and stopping a swim at the first sign of shoulder pain. Proper swimming technique may help prevent swimmer's shoulder. The swimmer should vary strokes when practicing, keep the body high in the water and evenly balanced while stroking, engage the hip and abdomen muscles to take some of the load off the shoulders, and keep the head low in the water. Weight lifting with lighter weights and increased repetitions may help condition the shoulders. Physical therapy is generally recommended for treating swimmer's shoulder. Cortisone injections into the area may be recommended if other measures fail. See also ROTATOR CUFF TENDINITIS; TENDINITIS.

Sympathectomy

The use of chemicals or surgery to deaden sympathetic nerves leading to a painful body part. The surgical division of sympathetic nerve pathways is most often performed to improve circulation for those with diseases such as atherosclerosis, claudication, Buerger disease, and Raynaud phenomenon. Less commonly, sympathectomy is used for other purposes, such as to relieve severe, chronic pain or to inhibit excess sweating. The goal of a sympathectomy is to minimize the effects of sympathetic nerve activity. Before performing sur-

S

gery, the doctor will usually assess the operation's potential benefits by injecting the person with a local anesthetic to temporarily block sympathetic nerve impulses and monitor for improvement in symptoms.

Sympathetic nervous system

The division of the AUTONOMIC NERVOUS SYSTEM (which controls unconscious, automatic body functions) that directs the body's responses to stress or danger (the so-called fight-or-flight response). This activity consumes stored energy in the body. Typical sympathetic activity includes widening the air passages in the lungs, increasing heart rate, opening the pupils wider, decreasing saliva production, slowing down digestive activity, filling the urinary bladder, and stimulating the production of the hormones epinephrine and norepinephrine.

Symptom

An indication of a disorder, disease, or condition that is felt by a person before seeking medical evaluation or advice. Symptoms help a doctor to identify and diagnose a condition or disease.

Synapse

The microscopic gap between two neurons, or nerve cells. To send a nerve impulse across this gap, the sending NEURON releases chemicals known as neurotransmitters from a structure called the synaptic bulb. The neurotransmitters bind with receptors on the neighboring nerve cell. The receptors open channels on the target cell that allow electrochemical activity in the target cell. The neurotransmitters then excite or inhibit the receiving cell.

Syncope

A loss of consciousness caused by a temporary deficiency of blood supply to the brain. See FAINTING.

Syndactyly

An inherited condition of the feet and hands in which webs appear between fingers and toes. Variations of syndactyly include webbing that extends from the base of the fingers or toes to the tip (complete syndactyly) and complicated syndactyly, in which the bones or nails of the fingers or toes

are fused. Syndactyly can affect one, two, or three pairs of fingers or toes.

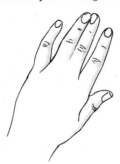

WEBBED FINGERS OR TOES
Syndactyly can take the form of partial or complete webbing between fingers or toes. In more severe cases, the bones of the digits are fused.

Syndrome

A number of symptoms occurring together that characterize a specific disease. Examples include CARPAL TUNNEL SYNDROME, DOWN SYNDROME, and REYE SYNDROME.

Synovectomy

The surgical removal of the membrane, called the synovial membrane, that lines the inside of a movable joint. Synovectomy is performed, usually through an arthroscope, to treat recurrent SYNOVITIS, which is an inflammation of the synovial membrane. The surgery may be performed to treat the early stages of RHEUMATOID ARTHRITIS when the synovial membrane of only one joint is badly inflamed.

Synovitis

An inflammation of the synovial membrane, a condition that often accompanies RHEUMATOID ARTHRITIS. The synovial membrane is a layer of cells that lines the inner surfaces of movable joints. The membrane produces the viscous fluid that bathes and lubricates the joint as it moves, thus helping the joint remain limber and flexible. The synovial membrane is essential to the health of the joint tissues because it provides nutrients and oxygen and removes waste. When disease causes inflammation and swelling of the synovial membrane producing synovitis, the function of the joint is severely impaired.

A transient form of synovitis may occur in the hip of children, more commonly boys, between the ages of 1 and 5. The child may complain of a

groin or knee pain and walk with a limp for up to 2 weeks. There may be a low-grade fever. Ultrasound can usually help diagnose the condition. Treatment consists of bed rest, acetaminophen for pain, crutches, and possible traction.

Synovitis, toxic

A childhood disorder that causes inflammation in the hip joint. Toxic synovitis is most common between the ages of 3 and 6 and more frequently affects boys than girls. Although its exact cause remains unknown, toxic synovitis is most likely connected to a viral infection. A limp and hip pain (usually on one side of the body) are the most common symptoms of toxic synovitis. Often an affected child has a viral illness, such as a cold or flu. There may also be a low-grade fever of up to 101°F and associated pain in the knee or thigh of the affected leg. Symptoms usually disappear within 1 to 4 weeks.

Diagnosis is based on a physical examination and a number of tests. The pediatrician will check the range of motion in the affected hip. If a decreased range of motion or a limp raises further questions, blood tests and various types of imaging such as an ultrasound scanning, radionuclide scanning, MRI (magnetic resonance imaging), or X rays may be performed. The doctor may also insert a needle into the child's hip joint and draw a sample of fluid to look for inflammatory changes that might suggest an infection or inflammatory arthritis. The primary treatment for toxic synovitis is bed rest. The child must avoid placing pressure on his or her hip until the condition is resolved. A family physician or pediatrician may also prescribe anti-inflammatory drugs.

Synovium

A layer of cells that form a membrane to line the inner surfaces of a joint. The synovial membrane secretes synovial fluid that fills and lubricates the joint space. This fluid is essential to proper functioning of the joint. Articular cartilage aids in the movement of joints, supplies nutrients and oxygen to the joint tissues, destroys foreign matter in the blood and tissues of a joint, and fights infection to protect the health of a joint.

S

Syphilis

A serious bacterial infection and usually one of the SEXUALLY TRANSMITTED DISEASES (STDs) or, infrequently, a nonvenereal infection that may be transmitted to the newborn by the infected mother or acquired through a contaminated blood transfusion. Both forms of syphilis are spread by direct contact with the skin sore that usually occurs as a result of the infection. Endemic syphilis occurs mostly in arid countries of the eastern Mediterranean region and in western Africa. This form of the disease is transmitted by mouth-to-mouth contact with an infected person or the sharing of eating and drinking utensils with an infected person.

Sexually transmitted syphilis is found throughout the world and is acquired by direct contact with a syphilis sore on the external genitals, vagina, anus, or the inner rectum. The sores may also occur on the lips or in the mouth. The infectious organism is most commonly transmitted by vaginal, anal, or oral sex. This form can also be transmitted, though rarely, by sharing needles with an infected intravenous drug user. It is estimated that more than 120,000 new sexually transmitted cases occur in the United States each year. Most of these cases occur in 15- to 30-year-olds, who tend to be most sexually active. Syphilis can be debilitating and potentially fatal if not medically treated.

SYMPTOMS AND DIAGNOSIS

There are three stages to syphilis. The primary stage can occur within 10 to 90 days of exposure; the average incubation period is 21 days. The first symptom of this stage is a single small sore called a CHANCRE that is firm, round, and painless. The sore appears at the site where the bacterium entered the body and lasts 1 to 5 weeks before healing. If the person does not get medical treatment during this stage, the infection progresses to a second stage.

Secondary stage syphilis occurs as a rash on one or more areas of the skin that appears when the chancre is fading or several weeks thereafter. This rash typically lasts 2 to 6 weeks before clearing up on its own and can take any one of a number of different forms. It often erupts as rough spots on the palms of the hands and the soles of the feet. It may also appear to be a prickly heat rash or occur in small blotches or scales all over the body. It can resemble a bad case of acne or chickenpox with pus-filled bumps. Other skin problems may include moist warts in the groin area, slimy white patches in the mouth, or sunken dark circles the size of penny, usually on the palms of the hands or the soles of the feet. The rash may be so mild and faint that it is not noticed. Other possible symptoms during the second stage include fever, swollen lymph glands, sore throat, patchy hair loss, headaches, weight loss, muscle aches, and fatigue. A person in the second stage of syphilis continues to be able to transmit the disease to others.

The latent stage of untreated syphilis begins when the symptoms of the secondary stage disappear. There are no symptoms or signs of infection, but at this stage, the bacteria can remain active in the body and begin to damage internal organs, including the brain, nerves, eyes, heart, blood vessels, liver, bones, and joints. In rare cases, internal damage becomes apparent years later as the third, or tertiary, stage of syphilis in about one third of persons who have the infection and have not received medical treatment for it. Symptoms of this stage may include an inability to coordinate muscle movements, paralysis, numbness to pain, progressive blindness, dementia or other psychological changes, impotency, intense pain, blockage or irregular expansion of heart vessels, severe abdominal pain, repeated vomiting, damaged knee joints, deep sores on the feet or toes, and tumors on the skin, bones, liver, or other organs.

A pregnant woman who has untreated syphilis has an increased risk of stillbirth, or the newborn has an increased risk of death shortly after birth. There is an increased potential for the baby to be born with congenital syphilis, with symptoms that usually develop within a few weeks.

First- and second-stage syphilis infections are diagnosed by microscopic detection of the bacterium in infectious sores. An accurate and inexpensive blood test can also identify antibodies to the bacteria soon after the infection occurs. If a suspected infection has occurred 2 to 3 weeks before the blood test and test results are negative, retesting may be recommended. It is recommended that all pregnant women have this blood test. A person who has tested positive should refrain from sexual activity until the results of at least two follow-up blood tests are negative. Diagnosis of third-stage syphilis may require an examination of spinal fluid.

A baby's symptoms of syphilis may include skin sores, profuse nasal discharge that may be bloody, slimy patches in the mouth, inflammation of the bones in the arms and legs, a swollen liver, anemia, jaundice, or a small head. If untreated, an infected baby may have seizures and is at risk for retardation. The infection can also cause the baby's death.

TREATMENT AND RISK FACTORS

If a person has had syphilis for less than a year, a single injection of penicillin will completely cure the infec-

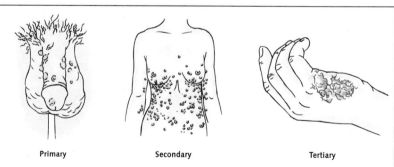

Primary   Secondary   Tertiary

THREE STAGES OF SYPHILIS
The primary stage of syphilis involves a chancre sore at the point of infection—usually the genitals. Secondary syphilis, characterized by a rash with sores about the size and color of a penny, occurs 3 to 6 weeks after the first chancre. The tertiary, or late stage, involves a rubbery, grayish tumor (gumma) anywhere in or on the body, including vital organs.

S

tion. Repeated doses are required when a person has had the disease for longer than a year. Babies born with congenital syphilis require daily penicillin treatment for 10 days. Penicillin therapy destroys the bacterium that causes syphilis and prevents further damage, but it cannot reverse damage that has already occurred.

People who have been diagnosed with primary stage syphilis and are receiving medical treatment for the infection must abstain from sexual contact until the sores have healed. The person should also notify all sex partners to seek medical attention, including treatment if necessary. A person who has had syphilis and has been treated successfully for it remains susceptible to infection.

Following safer sex practices, including the use of a latex condom throughout sexual encounters, is a good defense against becoming infected. It is not always apparent that a sexual partner has syphilis since the characteristic sores may be located inside the vagina, rectum, or mouth. An abnormal discharge, sore, or rash, particularly when located in the groin area, should prompt a person to refrain from sexual activity and obtain a medical evaluation.

Complications of untreated syphilis for adults and newborns are serious and can be life-threatening. Long-term effects of the infection include increased susceptibility to hepatitis, meningitis, and diseases of the bones, joints, heart, blood vessels, and central nervous system. Having syphilis also increases the risk of acquiring HIV (human immunodeficiency virus) sexually. The risk of HIV is increased as much as fivefold in a person who has a syphilis infection.

Syringe

A medical instrument used to inject fluids into the body or to remove fluids from it. A syringe is a small hand pump, consisting of a small cylindrical barrel and piston or a barrel and a soft rubber bulb. Many types of syringes are available, including hypodermic syringes, which usually have a narrow barrel and end in a hollow, small-bore needle. Syringes are used to inject drugs into the tissues. Dentists use water syringes designed to permit controlled sprays of water

into specific areas of the mouth. Syringes that have rubber bulbs are used to create a vacuum for the gentle suction of small amounts of body fluids, such as nasal or oral secretions.

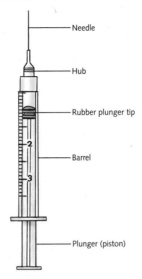

Needle

Hub

Rubber plunger tip

Barrel

Plunger (piston)

HOW A SYRINGE WORKS
The syringe operates like a hand pump that can inject or suction out small, measured amounts of fluid. The development of the disposable syringe greatly diminished the risk of infection.

Syringing of the ears

A technique used by a physician to remove earwax. A syringe is used to gently squirt warm water into the ear canal. The water flows along the canal until it bounces off the eardrum. As the water flows back along the bottom of the ear canal, it carries out earwax.

Syrinx

An abnormal, growing, longitudinal cavity that forms within the spinal cord, most frequently in the cervical or neck region. A syrinx may extend into the gray matter (as in syringomyelia) or into the lower brain stem (as in syringobulbia). A common symptom of an invading syrinx is loss of pain and temperature sensations. There may also be weakness of the hands or arms and serious respiratory abnormalities, including hoarseness, stridor (harsh, obstructed breathing), hypoventilation (breathing at an abnormally slow rate, which increases

the amount of carbon dioxide in the blood), and apnea (a total cessation of breathing, either momentarily or for a prolonged period). Sudden death as a result of SLEEP APNEA SYNDROME is a risk of syrinx. Neurological examination and tests such as myelography, MRI (magnetic resonance imaging), and CT (computed tomography) scanning are useful in the diagnosis of a syrinx. Management of sleep apnea syndrome (such as the use of a mask over the nose or a dental device to force the jaw forward) is vital. The only specific treatment for the syrinx itself is surgery. However, the results of surgery are varied and unpredictable. A syrinx is often seen in association with a Chiari malformation, trauma, and spinal cord or skull-based abnormalities.

System

A group of organs and tissues associated with a particular physiological function. The members of a body system function together in a common purpose to produce results that no single member of the system could achieve alone. Examples include the central nervous system, consisting of the brain and spinal cord; the cardiovascular system, made up of the heart and blood vessels; and the endocrine system, including glands and organs that release hormones into the circulatory system.

Systemic

Affecting organs and tissues throughout the body rather than a specific organ or body part. For example, systemic disorders such as diabetes mellitus or hypertension can affect the entire body.

Systemic lupus erythematosus (SLE)

See LUPUS ERYTHEMATOSUS, SYSTEMIC.

Systolic blood pressure

The force blood exerts against the arteries when the heart is contracting. Systolic blood pressure is the first of two numbers in a blood pressure measurement, for example, 120/80. The lower number is a measurement of DIASTOLIC BLOOD PRESSURE. See BLOOD PRESSURE.

S

T cell

A variety of white blood cell that orchestrates the immune system's response to infected or malignant cells; also known as a T lymphocyte. The T cell is a type of white blood cell that develops in the thymus and is part of the immune system. T cells act directly to fight diseases or organisms, such as bacteria; to stimulate B lymphocytes or helper T cells; and to suppress some B lymphocyte functions.

T cells that have been activated by an antigen, or substance considered foreign by the body, differentiate into different types of cells including memory cells and various types of regulatory cells. Cytotoxic T cells, for example, which are also called "killer cells," are responsible for the destruction of cells carrying certain antigens, the mechanism involved in cell-mediated immunity.

A count of a person's T cells can be helpful in the diagnosis of immunodeficiency or lymphocytic diseases. The test requires that blood be drawn from a vein and examined under a microscope in a laboratory. B or T lymphocytes can be counted under an electron microscope or by other methods, including flow cytometry. Some diseases may be indicated by greater than normal T-cell levels, while others are indicated by lower than normal T-cell levels, such as in AIDS (acquired immunodeficiency syndrome).

Tabes dorsalis

An infectious disease of the central nervous system caused by *Treponema pallidum*, the same bacterium that causes SYPHILIS. Tabes dorsalis, also known as Duchenne disease, is a sexually transmitted disease that occurs as a complication of third-stage syphilis, which is rare because earlier stages of syphilis can successfully be treated with pencillin. The disease causes a breakdown of the fatty sheaths that surround and insulate nerve cells and involves the brain, cranial nerves, and spinal cord. This damage to nerve cells causes a progressive condition in which an infected person is unable to control muscle coordination. The sense of balance and the ability to walk are impaired. Movements of the limbs may be affected, and there may be speech irregularities. Abnormalities in a person's vision are common. Damage to cranial nerves can cause a drooping eyelid and poor tone in the facial muscles. Loss of reflexes in the legs, sphincter dysfunction, and sexual dysfunction also occur. A lack of sensation in the legs may lead to the condition called CHARCOT JOINT.

Tabes dorsalis is diagnosed by blood tests, and the infection can be halted with penicillin. Many complications of the disease are irreversible, however, so recovery is limited.

Tachycardia

An abnormally rapid heartbeat. In an adult, tachycardia refers to a heartbeat higher than 100 beats per minute. Symptoms include palpitations (uncomfortably rapid heartbeat), shortness of breath, chest pain, light-headedness, and fainting. Tachycardia is classified and treated by its point of origin in the heart (see TACHYCARDIA, PAROXYSMAL SUPRAVENTRICULAR; TACHYCARDIA, VENTRICULAR). Tachycardia may be caused by exercise, stress, congenital heart defects (those present at birth), cardiomyopathy (impaired heart muscle function), myocarditis (inflammation of the heart muscle), or kidney failure.

Tachycardia, paroxysmal supraventricular

An abnormally rapid heartbeat (higher than 100 beats per minute) that begins in the upper region of the heart and occurs sporadically. Paroxysmal supraventricular tachycardia is not usually life-threatening, but it can be very uncomfortable and distressing. In adults the heartbeat can rise to between 150 and 250 beats per minute; in children it may go even higher. The person is aware of an uncomfortably rapid heartbeat and may experience feelings of anxiety and doom, shortness of breath, chest tightness, fainting, and dizziness and may appear pale. Symptoms may start and stop suddenly, and an attack may last from a few minutes to 1 or 2 days.

Paroxysmal supraventricular tachycardia is most common in young people and infants with healthy hearts. Smoking tobacco, excessive alcohol use, and caffeine intake increase the risk of attacks.

If symptoms are mild, using a technique called the Valsalva maneuver may interrupt the attack. This consists of holding the breath and straining or coughing while leaning the upper body forward. Splashing cold water on the face is helpful in some cases. Medications may be prescribed to control heart rhythm.

In some cases, applying an electric shock to the heart (see CARDIOVERSION) restores a normal heartbeat. A minimally invasive technique called radiofrequency ablation (see ABLATION THERAPY) can be used to alter the heart's electrical pathway permanently and prevent future episodes. An alternative is to implant a PACEMAKER, an electronic device that controls the heartbeat.

Tachycardia, ventricular

An abnormally fast heartbeat that originates in the ventricles (lower chambers) of the heart. Ventricular tachycardia requires urgent medical attention and may be life-threatening. Sustained ventricular tachycardia tends to deteriorate into ventricular fibrillation, in which the heart flutters rapidly and inefficiently rather than pumping. Ventricular fibrillation results in death within minutes unless a normal heart rhythm is restored.

In most cases ventricular tachycardia is associated with heart disease, and it is particularly likely to occur in the first few days following a heart attack. It can also be caused by congenital heart defects (those present at birth), cardiomyopathy (impaired heart muscle function), myocarditis (inflammation of the heart muscle), and kidney failure. Symptoms include shortness of breath, dizziness, fainting, chest pain, and palpitations (uncomfortably rapid heartbeat). In some cases, the heart will stop beating suddenly (cardiac arrest), and the person collapses.

The most common treatment for ventricular tachycardia is medication with drugs known as antiarrhythmics. If this approach fails, a normal heartbeat may be restored with cardioversion (an electrical shock to the chest). If episodes of ventricular tachycardia continue after cardioversion, a device called an implantable cardioverter defibrillator (ICD) can be placed surgically in the chest. The ICD monitors the heartbeat and corrects it if it becomes abnormally fast. Alternatively, the heart's abnormal rhythm may be corrected using a minimally invasive technique called radiofrequency ablation (see ABLATION THERAPY). This may also be used to treat areas of the heart that fire irregular impulses, triggering ventricular tachycardia.

Tachypnea

Abnormally fast, deep breathing. Tachypnea can upset the balance of gases in the blood by decreasing the levels of carbon dioxide in the bloodstream. It is slightly more common in women than in men and typically occurs in people who are tense or anxious. Tachypnea can also be a symptom of many diseases and disorders.

CAUSES

Stress, anxiety, and nervousness are common causes of tachypnea. Alcohol use may be associated with its occurrence. Diseases and conditions including asthma, croup, pneumonia, pulmonary embolism, ketoacidosis, pulmonary fibrosis, chronic obstructive pulmonary disease (COPD), interstitial pneumonia, bronchiolitis, pneumonitis caused by exposure to chemicals, pulmonary edema, and respiratory distress syndrome all can produce tachypnea.

In children, tachypnea may be caused by croup; in newborns it may be caused by aspiration of feces in the uterus or by blood poisoning caused by group B streptococci.

Severe pain or fear may produce tachypnea. It is sometimes associated with an overdose of medications, such as aspirin. Psychological causes may include a person's perception of being in a situation in which there is an advantage to having a sudden episode of dramatic disability.

DIAGNOSIS AND TREATMENT

A complete history and physical examination may reveal the cause of recurrent tachypnea. Diagnostic tests may include an electrocardiogram, X rays of the chest, and blood tests to measure arterial blood gas levels.

Treatment is generally aimed at controlling the cause of the symptom, since treating the symptom itself will not solve the problem over the longterm. In some cases in which tachypnea is caused by anxiety, tranquilizing medications may be prescribed.

When deep, fast breathing is caused by fear or anxiety, it generally passes when the emotions subside, but if it persists and does not improve with self-care techniques, it may be a medical condition called HYPERVENTILATION. If there is a question as to what is causing tachypnea or if there is severe pain, medical attention should be promptly sought. The symptoms of hyperventilation are reduced by replacing carbon dioxide in the lungs. This can be accomplished by breathing into a small paper bag held loosely over both the nose and mouth while breathing for about 5 to 15 minutes.

Tacrine

A drug used to treat Alzheimer's disease. Tacrine (Cognex) cannot cure Alzheimer's disease or prevent it from getting worse, but it can slow the progression of the disease and may improve the thinking ability of some people. Tacrine works by inhibiting the breakdown of the neurotransmitter involved in Alzheimer's disease.

Tacrolimus

An immunosuppressant drug, Tacrolimus (Prograf) is used to impair the body's natural immune system function in a person who has received an organ transplant, such as a liver, kidney, pancreas, lung, or heart. Tacrolimus works by preventing white blood cells from rejecting the transplanted organ.

Tag, skin

See SKIN TAG.

T'ai chi

An ancient Chinese discipline integrating mind, body, and spirit to reduce stress, promote balance and flexibility, and ease pain. T'ai chi originated in China in the 13th century as a martial art but today is used as a preventive health therapy, using exercises that incorporate Taoist philosophy to harmonize opposing forces of yin and yang in order to maintain health and vigor.

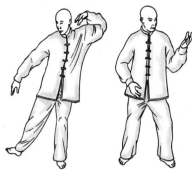

Cloud hand posture   **Brush sparrow's tail**

SLOW, GENTLE MOVEMENT
T'ai chi is a series of postures based on the movements of animals. The movements are slow and graceful, and the practice has been called "meditation in motion."

T'ai chi is a form of energy medicine and a component of CHINESE MEDICINE. It is believed to increase strength and promote calm and harmony by improving the flow of internal energy, or qi (pronounced "chee") in the body. T'ai chi has a calming, meditative aspect that makes it useful for reducing anxiety and stress. At the same time, T'ai chi is an aerobic exercise that benefits the entire body by increasing muscle strength and flexibility. T'ai chi involves meditation and deep breathing to calm the mind, and it requires focus and concentration to achieve unity of body, mind, and spirit. Its exercises involve a series of slow, flowing movements that require regular practice.

T'ai chi as a fitness regimen can be used as a complement to conventional medicine. Its low-intensity, low-impact exercise is well suited to people recovering from injury. T'ai chi is helpful for people with arthritis and older people and is thought to help prevent brittle bone disease (osteoporosis) and help reduce the risk of falls in older people. It also has been shown to improve hypertension and heart disease.

Talipes

The name for clubfoot. A congenital deformity in which the foot is twisted out of shape or position. Clubfoot may take many forms. A heel that is turned inward or outward can cause an individual to walk on the side of the foot; or a raised heel may cause a person to walk on his or her toes. The classic clubfoot is a deformity in

T

which the heel is both raised and twisted. Treatment may include special shoes, braces, physical therapy, or surgery.

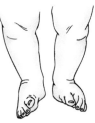

CLUBFOOT
In a child with clubfoot, the bones in the front part of the foot are misaligned. Usually, the front part of the foot turns in. Treatment, including casting, can begin immediately after birth. Most children can be treated successfully and can lead fully active lives.

Talk therapy

Any method for treating mental or emotional problems that relies principally on verbal interaction between the person and a professional therapist. Many varieties of talk therapy are available. See COGNITIVE-BEHAVIORAL THERAPY; GROUP THERAPY; and PSYCHOTHERAPY.

Tall stature

Extreme growth in height that begins in childhood or adolescence; also known as gigantism. Unusually tall stature is caused by the pituitary gland overproducing GROWTH HORMONE, usually due to a pituitary tumor. The excess pituitary hormone causes all parts of the body to grow extremely large. The condition differs from ACROMEGALY in that it occurs before full maturation and the bones of the arms and legs are affected.

If a child or adolescent seems to be growing at an exceptional rate, a doctor should be consulted. CT SCANNING (computed tomography scanning) or MRI (magnetic resonance imaging) can detect and locate the presence of a pituitary tumor. Radiation therapy or surgery may be recommended to eliminate the tumor. Medications such as bromocriptine are sometimes prescribed to control a pituitary tumor. The medication somatostatin stops the growth of pituitary tumors by inhibiting growth hormone. In most cases, treatment can reverse this disorder.

Tamoxifen

An anticancer drug. Tamoxifen (Nolvadex) is used to treat and prevent some kinds of breast cancer that require the hormone estrogen in order to grow. Tamoxifen works by blocking the actions of estrogen on the breast. Tamoxifen is used to treat breast cancer in women and men.

Tamoxifen is also used to reduce the risk of developing breast cancer in women who are at increased risk of developing the disease. These include women who are at least 35 years old and have a combination of risk factors, including a family history of breast cancer, early menstruation, late pregnancy or no pregnancy, and a history of breast biopsy.

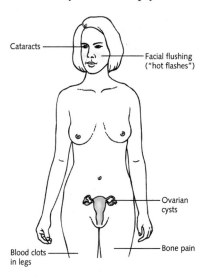

Cataracts

Facial flushing ("hot flashes")

Ovarian cysts

Bone pain

Blood clots in legs

POSSIBLE SIDE EFFECTS OF TAMOXIFEN
Tamoxifen has been proven to substantially reduce the occurrence of breast cancer in women who are at high risk. But as with many drugs, tamoxifen use involves risk of side effects. A doctor will carefully monitor the state of a woman's health as she takes the drug, and a woman who experiences any side effects should discuss them with her doctor.

Tampon

Small absorbent packing that is placed in the vagina to absorb blood during the menstrual period. Tampons have been used during menstruation since ancient Egypt, when they were made from papyrus (a plant used to make paper). Tampons today are made of absorbent cotton or rayon material and are cylindrical, with a string attached to one end for removal. They are available over the counter in different absorbencies to accommodate different levels of menstrual flow. Tampons should be removed when soaked with blood, or at least every 4 to 6 hours. Following these guidelines can reduce the risk of TOXIC SHOCK SYNDROME, a potentially severe bacterial infection associated with the prolonged use of highly absorbent tampons. The most highly absorbent tampons have been removed from the market. Tampons can be used by menstruating women of any age. Using a tampon does not affect a woman's virginity, although women with intact hymens may need to use narrower designs to bypass the hymen comfortably.

Tamponade

Accumulation of so much fluid inside the pericardium (sac surrounding the heart) that it prevents the heart from pumping sufficient blood to the body. Tamponade is caused by pericarditis (inflammation of the pericardium), which can be caused by tuberculosis, a tumor, an aneurysm (ballooning) of the major artery that carries blood into the body, injury to the pericardium in surgery or in an accident, hypothyroidism (an underactive thyroid gland), radiation therapy of the chest, systemic lupus erythematosus, or a viral infection.

Tamponade is a medical emergency that requires immediate attention. The excess fluid can be removed by means of a needle inserted through the chest wall into the pericardium. In some cases surgery to repair or remove the pericardium is required.

Tamsulosin

A drug used to treat noncancerous enlargement of the prostate (benign prostatic hyperplasia, or BPH). Tamsulosin (Flomax) is used to treat the symptoms of BPH, a condition that can occur in men as they age. BPH can cause problems urinating, including the need to urinate frequently and the feeling of not being able to empty the bladder completely. Tamsulosin works by relaxing the muscles in the prostate and the opening of the bladder, helping to increase the flow of urine. Tamsulosin cannot shrink the prostate.

T

Tannin

A substance found in certain plants or teas that was formerly used in medicine as an astringent; also called tannic acid. Tannin, a substance found in oak bark, can be absorbed through the mucous membranes of burned or scraped skin. If too much is absorbed, liver damage can result.

Tantrum

A sudden outbreak of rage or unruly behavior. In an adult who is out of control, it may be a sign of a psychiatric disorder. Tantrums are common among small children, who sometimes use crying, screaming, and kicking to express frustration, anger, or disappointment. Tantrums are a normal part of development between the ages of 1 and 3. As children learn greater self-control, they ordinarily outgrow tantrums by age 4 or 5.

The frustration that preschool children feel often produces tantrums as children separate from their parents and begin to enter the larger world. During this significant period of child development, safety dictates setting definite rules and limits that often require compromise, self-discipline, and restraint on the part of the child. Frustration results from these restrictions, and children do not always have the vocabulary to describe those feelings. Consequently, they may express anger and frustration by crying or screaming loudly and flailing their arms and legs. Some children hold their breath until they become blue or faint.

TREATMENT

Because they are a temporary developmental problem, minor tantrums are best ignored by parents. Intervention is necessary if a child is hitting or kicking others, throwing objects at others, or screaming for a prolonged period of time. A child who holds his or her breath and faints should see a pediatrician. The doctor should also be consulted if tantrums persist past age 4, if a child causes injury during tantrums, or if tantrums are accompanied by other problems such as frequent nightmares or extreme anxiety. If the doctor thinks that tantrums may indicate an underlying emotional disturbance, the child will be referred to a psychiatrist or another mental health professional.

RISK FACTORS AND PREVENTION

Although most young children have an occasional tantrum, certain circumstances increase their likelihood. Children who are ill, overtired, hungry, or anxious are more likely to have tantrums. Children of parents who are either overly strict or overly permissive are more likely to have more frequent and severe tantrums. Parents can help prevent tantrums by making sure children are well rested and fed. They can create a good model by controlling their own tempers and maintaining calm in the home. When the child is not having a tantrum, parents should be generous with their affection.

Tapeworm infestation

Infestation by worms that are carried in immature forms by animals, especially cattle, pigs, and fish. Tapeworm infestation occurs in humans after eating undercooked, infested animal products, such as beef, pork, and fish. The animals become infested after eating the eggs of tapeworms, which are found in soil, grass, and water. Larvae hatch from the eggs in the animals' digestive tracts, and the larvae migrate throughout the animals' bodies. When the infested meat is not sufficiently heated, the larvae survive and are acquired by people who eat it. The larvae enter a person's intestines and within 2 months grow into adult tapeworms that attach to the intestinal wall. Mature tapeworms can survive in the human intestines for more than 30 years.

Symptoms of tapeworm infestation are generally mild. In some cases, segments of a tapeworm may detach and be eliminated in the feces. Rarely, fish tapeworms cause anemia. APPENDICITIS and inflammation of the bile duct, called CHOLANGITIS, can be complications of tapeworm infestation.

Diagnosis is accomplished by microscopic identification of the tapeworms' eggs from a stool culture. The eggs are not produced until the tapeworms have reached maturity, about 3 months following the initial infestation. Blood tests for the detection of antibodies may be useful in the first stage of infestation before any eggs have been produced.

Anthelmintic medications, including mebendazole, thiabendazole, ivermectin, pyrantel, and niclosamide, can destroy or paralyze the worms, loosening their attachment to the intestinal wall and allowing them to be passed out of the body in the stool.

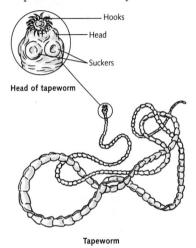

Head of tapeworm

Hooks
Head
Suckers

Tapeworm

SEGMENTED FLATWORM

A mature tapeworm is a flat (tapelike), segmented worm that latches onto the wall of the intestine with the suckers on its head. It reproduces by detaching a segment, which contains 80,000 to 100,000 eggs. The segment migrates to the anus and is passed in fecal matter; the eggs can exist for years before hatching in a host animal.

Tarsal tunnel syndrome

A condition produced by compression of a nerve that passes through a narrow passage behind the ankle bone located on the inner side, running down into the heel and foot. The cause may be an injury to the ankle, including a sprain or fracture, or a growth such as a cyst or tumor that presses against the nerve. Symptoms may include pain, numbness, tingling, or burning sensations anywhere along the bottom of the foot. Pain and other symptoms may be more commonly experienced at night.

Diagnosis is made on the basis of physical examination and possibly imaging, such as X rays. The discomforts of tarsal tunnel syndrome can be relieved by the use of ORTHOTICS, special shoe inserts, to aid in the redistribution of body weight and to take pressure off the affected nerve. Corticosteroid injections may be

T

considered. Surgery to release the compressed nerve is sometimes recommended.

Tarsalgia

The general medical term for pain in the ankle or the foot.

Tarsorrhaphy

A surgical procedure to narrow the opening between the upper and lower eyelids. Tarsorrhaphy is used to treat various conditions of the eye, especially those of the cornea caused by too much exposure to air (if the eyelids do not close properly) or by irritation from contact lenses. After the person is given a local anesthetic, a thin slice of the underlying framework (tarsus) of the upper eyelid and its membrane (conjunctiva) is removed, then a matching portion of the lower lid is stitched into its place. After the incision heals, the sutures are removed.

Tartar

The calcified bacterial plaque (see PLAQUE, DENTAL) that forms from mineral salts in the saliva and accumulates on and adheres to the surfaces of the crowns and roots of the teeth. Tartar is another word for calculus. Once plaque has built up on the teeth and hardened into tartar, it cannot be removed with routine brushing and dental flossing at home. It must be removed by a dentist in an office procedure called dental scaling (see SCALING, DENTAL). Left untreated, tartar can lead to PERIODONTAL DISEASE.

Taste

One of the five SENSES. Taste belongs to the body's chemical sensing system. It is closely related to smell, for flavors are recognized mainly through the sense of smell. There are approximately 9,000 taste buds (tiny clusters of cells that sense flavors from foods) on the surface of the tongue. Taste buds in different parts of the tongue sense the four basic tastes: salty, sweet, bitter, and sour. The sides of the tongue are more sensitive to sour and salty substances; the back of the tongue is more sensitive to bitter substances. Scientists also suspect there are more taste sensations than just these four. In addition, the texture and temperature of foods contribute to how they taste.

When food or drink comes in touch with certain areas of the tongue, nerve impulses are generated and travel along nerve fibers to a special sensory area of the brain.

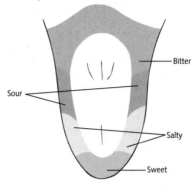

TASTE BUD SITES
The taste buds in the tongue are specialized cells with receptors that are stimulated by chemicals found in saliva. The taste buds located on certain areas of the tongue respond best to one of four basic categories of taste: bitter, sour, salty, and sweet.

Taste, loss of in older people

A gradual decline of intensity in the sense of taste that commonly occurs in older people. Like vision and hearing, the sense of taste grows less acute with age. Food may taste and smell less appealing than it once did. This in turn can lead to a loss of interest in food and a reduced appetite. See also APPETITE, LOSS OF IN OLDER PEOPLE.

In some cases, a loss of taste is due to factors other than aging. It may be the result of an illness or a medication. Drinking alcohol and smoking cigarettes can dull the sense of taste. Even if food no longer tastes as flavorful as it once did, proper nutrition is important throughout life. To avoid health problems, older people should make an effort to continue to eat a sensible and varied diet. Some people find adding additional seasonings to food to be helpful.

However, increased use of salt is not recommended because it can contribute to high blood pressure and other conditions. An underlying condition that contributes to a loss of taste—such as an illness, alcohol abuse, smoking, or depression—can be treated. When loss of taste is related to a medication, a physician is sometimes able to adjust the dosage. In many cases, proper management of underlying problems will spark a renewed interest in food.

Tattooing

Permanent discoloration and inscriptions from pigment applied to the skin and then forced into the skin with needles. Tattoos are a form of body decoration drawn by professional artists who use electrically powered instruments to inject pigment into the skin. Other times tattoos are self-administered or drawn by amateurs with instruments such as pencils, pens, or needles using materials such as India ink or charcoal.

Many health-related risks are associated with unsanitary tattooing methods, including both localized infection and blood-borne illnesses such as hepatitis and HIV (human immunodeficiency virus). Eventually, some individuals may regret getting

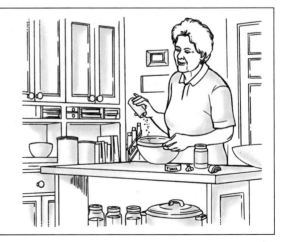

OVERCOMING DIMINISHED SENSE OF TASTE
An older person may find that his or her sense of taste has become less acute with age—but good nutrition and a varied diet are as important as ever. Adding extra seasoning to foods may help increase appetizing flavors and smells. Some bottled seasoning mixes are available that enhance flavor without adding excess salt (sodium). People need to read labels carefully to check salt content.

T

tattoos. Formerly, tattoos were removed using techniques such as EXCISION (cutting out the tattoo) or DERMABRASION (removal of the surface layer of skin by high-speed sanding), which left scars. Today the preferred method of tattoo removal is LASER SURGERY, which removes tattoos without scarring.

Tay-Sachs disease

A progressive neurological genetic disorder characterized by the accumulation of a fatty substance in the nerve cells of the brain. The most common form of the disease affects infants, who appear healthy at birth and seem to develop normally for the first few months of life. However, they lack the enzyme hexosaminidase A (hex A), which is necessary for the ongoing breakdown of a substance called ganglioside GM2 and other fatty substances in the brain and nerve cells. In babies with Tay-Sachs disease, these substances accumulate in nerve tissue, gradually destroying brain and nerve cells until the damage to the central nervous system leads to death. Children with Tay-Sachs disease usually die by age 5.

As their nerve cells gradually become clogged with fatty material, babies with Tay-Sachs disease gradually become unable to smile, crawl, or turn over, and they lose the ability to grasp or reach with their hands. Eventually they become deaf, blind, and unable to swallow. Their muscles weaken and become paralyzed. There is no cure for Tay-Sachs disease. Treatment is limited to making the child as comfortable as possible.

FORMS OF THE DISEASE

Tay-Sachs disease is most common in infants, but other rare deficiencies of hex A, including juvenile and late-onset forms, are sometimes categorized as Tay-Sachs disease. Symptoms are milder and begin much later in life. In juvenile Tay-Sachs disease, for example, symptoms develop between the ages of 2 and 5. Mental abilities, vision, and hearing are unaffected, but speech may be slurred, muscles may be weak, and mental illness may be present. Death usually occurs by age 15.

In late-onset Tay-Sachs disease, symptoms usually appear between adolescence and a person's mid-30s.

> ### CHANCES OF INHERITING TAY-SACHS DISEASE
>
> If both parents are carriers, their children have:
>
> - A 25 percent chance of inheriting the disease
> - A 25 percent chance of being free of the disease
> - A 50 percent chance of being a carrier
>
> If only one parent is a carrier, his or her children have:
>
> - Zero risk of having the disease
> - A 50 percent chance of being a carrier

Symptoms may include clumsiness, tremors, falls, mood alterations, and abnormal behaviors. Memory may be impaired, and attention span may be shortened. Psychotic episodes, in which the person loses contact with reality, seizures, or depression may be present. Treatment is aimed at symptoms and may include psychoactive medications.

RISK FACTORS AND DETECTION

Tay-Sachs disease occurs most frequently among descendents of central and eastern European (Ashkenazi) Jews. Approximately one of every 30 Jews in the United States carries the gene for Tay-Sachs. Two other ethnic groups that are at risk for the disease are non-Jewish French Canadians from the East St. Lawrence River Valley of Quebec and Cajuns from Louisiana.

A Tay-Sachs carrier has one normal gene for hex A and one gene for Tay-Sachs. When two carriers become parents, each of their children has a one in four chance of having the disease, a one in four chance of being free of the disease, and a two in four chance of becoming a carrier. When only one parent is a carrier, none of the children can have the disease, but each child has a 50 percent chance of being a carrier.

Potential parents can have a blood test to measure the quantity of hex A in their blood. Tay-Sachs carriers will have about half as much hex A as noncarriers. DNA testing of the blood can also be performed to identify known mutations of the hex A gene that are implicated in the dis-

---

ease. Potential parents who may be carriers of Tay-Sachs disease are encouraged to seek GENETIC COUNSELING. Prenatal diagnosis of Tay-Sachs disease can be accomplished using either amniocentesis or chorionic villus sampling.

Tazarotene

An antiacne drug; an antipsoriasis drug. Tazarotene (Tazorac) is a gel that is spread on the face to help keep the skin pores clean and acne free. Tazarotene works to treat psoriasis by reducing skin redness and inhibiting the formation of abnormal cells. Tazarotene is chemically related to vitamin A.

TB

See TUBERCULOSIS.

Tear duct, blocked

Blockage or narrowing of the tube that normally drains tears from a child's eyes. Many babies are born with the condition, usually because the membrane covering the ducts at birth fails to disappear. In older babies and children, blocked tear ducts most often result from an inflammation such as CONJUNCTIVITIS. Occasionally, a small cyst is the cause. In newborns who have blocked tear ducts, tears flow heavily from the eyes rather than draining normally through ducts into the nose and throat. (The eyes' tear ducts are

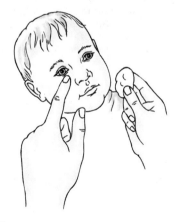

CLEARING A BLOCKED DUCT
To clear a baby's blocked tear duct, gentle massaging of the inner corner of the lower eyelid—using a small circular motion—several times a day helps open the duct. Any discharge can be wiped away with a moist washcloth or cotton ball.

T

located at the inner corners of the eyes, near the nose.) There may also be some discharge of mucus or pus. When tear duct obstruction is caused by infection, there may be redness, pain, and swelling in the eyes, in addition to excessive tears.

TREATMENT

If a bacterial infection has blocked the child's tear ducts, the pediatrician will prescribe an antibiotic. Otherwise, home care measures generally can relieve the problem. For example, massaging the lower eyelid in a gentle, circular motion, often helps open blocked ducts. A clean moist compress, cotton ball, or soft washcloth can be used to clear away discharge.

Blocked tear ducts in newborns usually clear up on their own or with massage by age 1. When blockages fail to respond to treatment, surgery may be necessary. While the person is under general anesthesia, the surgeon will insert a tiny probe into the tear duct to open the drainage system and empty the contents.

Tearing

Abnormal overflow of tears from the eye and down the cheek. In the healthy eye, tears are produced by the lacrimal glands in the upper eyelids and other glands in the conjunctiva, then they spread across the surface of the eyes and lubricate them at each blink.

Excess tears drain away through a duct that leads to the nose—the anatomical reason why crying often results in a stuffy nose.

Tearing results from either excessive tear production or inadequate

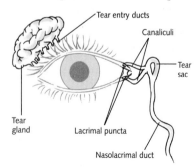

TEAR DRAINAGE
Tears produced in the tear glands next to either eye wash over the surface of the eyeball and either evaporate or drain through tiny openings in the eyelids into a duct that leads into the nose.

drainage. In adults, it can be caused by infection, irritation (from wind, chemicals, or pollutants, for example), foreign bodies, abrasions, allergies, inward growth of the eyelashes, or blockage of the tear duct (see DACRYOCYSTITIS).

Approximately 5 in every 100 infants is born with a tear duct that has failed to open and inflammation commonly results. In many cases the condition resolves on its own within a few months. If it does not, it can be repaired surgically. In some cases an artificial tear duct is created with a thin, flexible tube.

Tears

A liquid that lubricates the eyes, keeps them clean and moist, and helps prevent infection. The majority of tears are produced in the lacrimal glands, which are located in the upper eyelids, and other glands in the conjunctiva, and they spread across the eye in a film with each blink. Excess tears drain away through a duct that leads to the nose. Inadequate tear production results in DRY EYE; excess production or inadequate drainage, in TEARING.

The tear film consists of three layers. The outer, oily layer prevents evaporation and keeps the tears on the eye. The middle, watery layer nourishes the membranes and linings of eye and eyelids. The inner layer helps spread the watery layer across the eye and keep it adherent to the surface.

Technetium

A metallic element used in NUCLEAR MEDICINE in the preparation of radiopharmaceuticals such as radionuclides, which are used to diagnose various medical conditions.

Teeth

Hard structures set into the jaw and upper mouth that chew food and help form speech sounds.

Each tooth has three parts. The visible crown extends up from the line of the gum. The root, which represents most of the tooth's bulk, is bound into the bone by a tough, fibrous membrane. The neck is the narrow region between the crown and root. The surface of the crown is covered with enamel, which is the hardest substance in the body and

insensitive to touch or pain. Below the enamel lies the main part of the tooth called the dentin, which is less hard than the enamel and sensitive. The core of the crown, neck, and root is filled with a fibrous pulp richly supplied with nerves and blood vessels through the root canal. The tooth is partially encased in a bony socket.

Humans develop two sets of teeth. The 20 primary, or deciduous, teeth appear between the ages of 6 or 7 months and about 3 years. The front teeth (called incisors) are the first teeth to erupt. At about age 5 or 6, permanent or adult teeth begin to replace the primary teeth. By about 12 or 13 years of age, the permanent teeth are in place. The last four molars, the so-called wisdom teeth, appear in late adolescence or early adulthood, for a total of 32.

The teeth have different shapes that relate to their purposes. From the front to the back in an adult, there are eight incisors, four canines (bicuspids), eight premolars, and 12 molars. Teeth to the front of the mouth cut and slice, and those in the back grind.

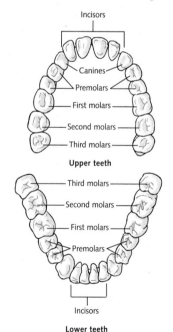

TYPES OF TEETH
The teeth are positioned in the mouth to accomplish different types of biting and chewing. The incisors and canines are shaped for biting and tearing, while the molars are flatter to grind and chew.

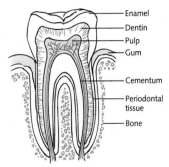

STRUCTURE OF A TOOTH
Enamel covers the surface of the tooth to the gum line. Dentin is the underlying hard part of the tooth, extending all the way through the root. It is covered below the gum by cementum, a substance harder than bone but softer than enamel. Under the dentin, the pulp contains nerves and blood vessels.

Teeth, care of

The combination of at-home routines and professional dental treatments to promote the good health of the teeth and surrounding tissues. The goal of taking care of the teeth is the prevention of TOOTH DECAY and PERIODONTAL DISEASE, both of which contribute to losing teeth. Various restorations (see RESTORATION, DENTAL) may be used by a dentist to replace lost teeth, but the natural teeth are essential to many vital body functions, and retaining them is important for maintaining optimum health.

Caring for the teeth involves maintaining good ORAL HYGIENE practices daily. This includes brushing the teeth at least twice daily with a FLUORIDE toothpaste, and dental flossing at least once a day using the technique recommended by a dentist or dental hygienist. See FLOSS, DENTAL. The use of DISCLOSING AGENTS to indicate the location of plaque (see PLAQUE, DENTAL) and target its removal is important to proper care of the teeth. Forming good oral hygiene habits at an early age is important. Tooth decay is one of the most common causes of infectious disease among children in the United States.

Poor oral habits that cause abrasion of the teeth, such as the overuse of toothpicks, holding a pipe stem between the teeth, and using the teeth to cut thread or break nutshells, should be avoided. Bruxism (teeth grinding) should be treated professionally. A healthy diet that is low in simple sugars should be followed.

Smoking and the use of tobacco products should be avoided. The use of a mouth guard during athletics and other activities that may pose a risk to the teeth and mouth is an important element in proper care of the teeth.

Professional dental care should begin soon after children have acquired all of their primary teeth. Regular dental examinations should be scheduled at recommended intervals. Toothaches may not be experienced until dental diseases and disorders have reached an advanced stage. For this reason, getting routine dental checkups twice a year even without pain or other symptoms is essential to taking good care of the teeth. Tooth decay, periodontal disease, and other disorders and diseases that affect the teeth, gums, and oral tissues should be treated at the earliest possible opportunity to prevent their progression to conditions that could result in the loss of teeth. Preventive care of the teeth, including professional cleanings, periodontic evaluations (see PERIODONTICS), dental scaling (see SCALING, DENTAL), and the use of dental sealants (see SEALANTS, DENTAL), should be maintained, as recommended by the dentist.

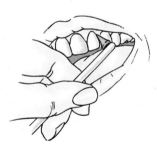

A FLEXIBLE RUBBER PICK
Massaging the gum line with a rubber dental pick helps remove debris and keep gums healthy.

Teeth, discolored

Stained, darkened, or yellowed teeth. The color of teeth may vary widely from one person to another. Discolored teeth may be due to hereditary factors. Yellowing of the teeth typically occurs with aging. Stains may be the result of habits that deposit color on the surface enamel of the teeth, such as smoking and tobacco use, which can permanently stain the teeth. Frequent drinking of coffee and tea, which contain tannin,

can etch stains into the tooth enamel. Children may have green stains on the primary teeth, typically on the top front teeth, caused by natural bacteria in the mouth. These stains tend to disappear within a few years. Environmental exposure to copper and iron dust, and medications that contain related metal salts may cause green or brown discoloration of the teeth. Tetracycline, an antibiotic drug, used during the second half of pregnancy when teeth are developing in the fetus, or when a child is 8 years old or younger, can produce gray, yellow, or brown discoloration to varying degrees. A mottled appearance on the surface of the teeth, including bands or spots of varying shades of white, yellow, brown, or black, may indicate FLUOROSIS (caused by the ingestion of excessive fluorides). Gray discoloration may be the result of dead tissue in the inner pulp (see PULP, DENTAL) of the tooth, a condition that requires ROOT CANAL TREATMENT.

Usually, discolored teeth present a problem that is primarily cosmetic, but discoloration may pose a risk to the enamel in the tooth and should be evaluated by a dentist. Depending on the severity of discoloration, the condition may be improved by a professional cleaning by the dentist, including coronal polishing which involves using an instrument that rotates a small rubber cup containing a mildly abrasive polishing paste against the surface of the teeth. A device that uses the mildly abrasive action of baking soda may also be used to remove tooth discoloration. Professional cleaning and polishing procedures may be performed by a dentist, a dental hygienist, or a dental assistant.

There are several cosmetic dentistry techniques that may be applied to improve the appearance of discolored teeth. Dental bleaching (see BLEACHING, DENTAL), under the supervision of a dentist, may help to lighten teeth. The use of dental bonding, composites, and veneers (see BONDING, DENTAL; VENEERS, DENTAL) can normalize and improve the appearance of more severely discolored teeth. Discolored teeth that are not strong enough to support these procedures may require artificial crowns (see CROWN, DENTAL) to correct the discoloration.

T

Teething

The gradual emergence of teeth in a baby or young child. Baby teeth start breaking through the gums at between 5 and 9 months of age. The two bottom front teeth usually come in first. Although the rate at which children teethe varies greatly, most have all 20 baby teeth by the age of 2½. Just before a tooth emerges, the gum directly above or below may be swollen or sore. A small bump can be felt where the new tooth is coming in. Babies are often fussy and irritable during the process. A one-piece teething ring or pacifier can help reduce the pain. Some teething products are frozen because the cold can be soothing. Home remedies include applying a cold, wet washcloth and rubbing the gums with a clean finger. The pediatrician may recommend acetaminophen to relieve pain. Commercial numbing products should be used with caution because they may cause a problem if swallowed.

Telangiectasia

Small, permanently dilated capillaries (small blood vessels) in the skin. Telangiectasias, which commonly appear on the nose and cheeks, cause redness. They can be symptoms of rosacea, elevated estrogen levels, liver disease, or collagen vascular disease. They may be treated cosmetically with lasers.

Temazepam

See BENZODIAZEPINES.

Temperature

The degree of heat in the body. A normal body temperature is about 98.6°F (37.0°C) but can range anywhere from 97.8°F (36.5°C) to 99.0°F (37.2°C). An abnormally increased body temperature, or fever, is a sign of illness. See also THERMOMETER.

Temporal arteritis

See ARTERITIS, GIANT CELL.

Temporal lobe epilepsy

See EPILEPSY, TEMPORAL LOBE.

Temporomandibular joint disorder (TMJ)

Also known as TMJ syndrome; see CLICKING JAW.

Tendinitis

The painful inflammation of the strong fibrous structures, called tendons, that connect muscles to bones. Tendinitis is usually caused by the tendon being stretched by overuse or injury or injured by repeated or prolonged pressure that produces friction between the tendon and bone tissue. Tendinitis most commonly occurs in joints such as the ankle, knee, and shoulder. People who are older may be more susceptible to the injuries that result in tendinitis as the tendons often become weaker with age. Athletes may be particularly vulnerable because of overuse of certain tendons. The symptoms include localized tenderness, possible swelling, and pain during an increased pace of activity. Diagnosis is made on the basis of physical examination and MRI (magnetic resonance imaging). Treatment may include rest, support, elevating and icing the affected area after the activity, physical therapy, and the use of nonsteroidal anti-inflammatory drugs (NSAIDs) to relieve pain and control inflammation and swelling. In serious cases, cortisone injections may provide relief. See also ACHILLES TENDINITIS; PATELLAR TENDINITIS.

Tendon

A fibrous cord that attaches a MUSCLE in place, often to a BONE or to cartilage. Tendons are strong but flexible connective tissue. They are made of dense masses of parallel elastic fibers, a structure that allows them to stretch in order to protect the muscles and ligaments from strain. Some tendons are simply short connectors to bone, but others, such as those visible in the back of the hand and the top of the foot, are quite long. Contraction of the muscle causes the tendon to pull on the bone or tendon to which it is attached, moving that part of the body. The tendons in the hands, wrists, and feet are enclosed in fibrous capsules and bathed in a fluid that helps the tendons move smoothly.

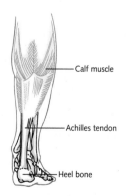

MUSCLE TO BONE
The Achilles tendon in the leg attaches the calf muscles to the heel bone. It can be felt by running a hand down the back of the ankle.

Tendon release

A surgical procedure for treating TRIGGER FINGER or other conditions involving restraint or binding of a tendon and its associated tissues. Tendon release is generally considered only when immobile joints are unresponsive to less invasive treatments, such as taking the nonsteroidal anti-inflammatory drugs (NSAIDs) aspirin or ibuprofen.

Tendon repair

The surgical reattachment of tendons that have been completely torn apart or severed as a result of excessive physical effort or injury. The Achilles tendon, or main tendon of the ankle, is most commonly injured in this way, but tendons in the forearm, hand, shoulder, and foot may also be torn or severed. Tendon repair should be performed as soon as possible for the best results. Tendons are highly elastic and held taut by tension; when they tear, the two cut ends pull away from each other quickly and may be difficult to retrieve and reattach. The distance between the two torn ends of tendon will determine the length of the surgical incision required to locate and connect them.

Tendon repair is usually accomplished by rejoining the two ends of tendon and sewing them together. In some instances, tissue may have to be taken from another tendon to repair the severed tendon. Following the procedure, the affected area is immobilized. Physical therapy may be prescribed as part of a recovery program. Passive exercise involving movement that does not put stress on the surgical site can help decrease the long-term stiffness that often results from tendon repair surgery.

Tendon transfer

Surgery to relocate or reposition a tendon. Tendons attach muscles to corresponding bones and transmit the forces of muscles that enable movement. Tendon transfer is performed to augment the function of muscle that has been impaired by a deformity, paralysis, or permanent injury.

Tenesmus

Persistent spasms of the rectum or bladder. Tenesmus is a common symptom of INFLAMMATORY BOWEL DISEASE and IRRITABLE BOWEL SYNDROME. It is also characterized by an urgent but ineffectual desire to empty the bowel or bladder.

Tennis elbow

An overuse sports injury (see SPORTS INJURIES) resulting in inflammation, strain, or minor tears in the tendons of the forearm muscles near the elbow. Tennis elbow is caused by repeated stress on this area of the arm, particularly the stress produced by sudden twisting movements of the forearm during a backhand tennis swing. The condition is also seen in electricians and carpenters. Extensor muscles in the forearm are attached to tendons that connect to the outer bump of the elbow. These extensor muscles are responsible for bending the wrist back.

Lateral epicondylitis is the medical term for the condition when the forearm muscles are extended in tennis playing. Medial epicondylitis is the condition when these muscles are flexed, as in a golf swing. In addition to backhand tennis swings and golf swings, continuous or repetitive rowing, throwing a ball (see also BASEBALL ELBOW), painting with a brush or roller, running a chain saw, and using manual screwdrivers and other hand tools may produce the same injury to the elbow.

SYMPTOMS AND DIAGNOSIS

The usual symptoms are tenderness when pressure is placed on the outer elbow, along with pain felt on the outer, bony bump of the elbow joint. Aching in the muscles at the outer side of the forearm often accompanies the pain in the soft tissues surrounding the elbow joint. Attempting to grasp objects may intensify the pain, and sometimes it becomes difficult to fully straighten the elbow. Tennis elbow is diagnosed by a phys-

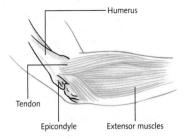

TENDINITIS IN THE FOREARM
When the tendon that attaches the extensor muscles in the forearm to the outer knob (epicondyle) of the bone of the upper arm (humerus) is inflamed, the elbow or forearm will hurt, especially when lifting, gripping, or carrying.

ical examination. X rays may be taken to rule out more serious bone or joint problems.

TREATMENT

When tennis elbow is mild, the best treatment may be limiting the amount of tennis playing or stopping entirely until the pain goes away. Learning to use a stable, neutral wrist position during sports and other activities may also be helpful. With persistent pain that becomes worse with time, consultation with a doctor specializing in sports medicine may become necessary. Anti-inflammatory medications and ice may help relieve symptoms. Physical therapy exercises may be recommended to help strengthen surrounding muscles. In some cases, corticosteroid injections may be considered. Surgery is a possible option for treating certain cases of tennis elbow.

Tenolysis

The surgical procedure for releasing a tendon from surrounding adhesions. A tendon is a tough band of fibrous connective tissue that unites muscle to bone and transmits the muscle's movement to bone. It is surrounded by a smooth sheath that allows it to glide freely. When a tendon is restricted, normal mobility is impaired. Tenolysis restores this function.

Tenosynovitis

An inflammation of the sheath of tissue and membrane that surrounds a tendon and aids in moving joints. Tenosynovitis often accompanies TENDINITIS. Most commonly affected are the tendons connecting muscles

to bones in the shoulder, elbow, wrist, fingers, hip, knee, or ankle. It is caused by injury or inflammation of a tendon or, in rare cases, by infection. Tenosynovitis is sometimes associated with rheumatoid arthritis, and in some cases, the cause is unknown. The condition may be caused by a bacterial infection, especially if there has been a puncture wound. This is a more medically serious form of tenosynovitis. If a joint feels hot as well as inflamed, emergency care should be sought, because this is an indication of infectious involvement in the synovium of the joint. The infection can cause permanent impairment to the affected tissues if not treated immediately with antibiotics.

Sometimes the inflammation causes the affected tissues to become visibly swollen as a result of fluid accumulation. There may be localized tenderness, difficulty moving a joint or straightening a finger, and severe or disabling pain with passive movement. There may be a crackling sound when the affected joint is moved. The typical symptom of a form of tenosynovitis called TRIGGER FINGER, which is caused by repetitive motions of the finger such as in keyboarding, is an inability to straighten the finger. That is followed by spontaneous, sudden straightening of the finger. As the condition worsens, the finger becomes more difficult to unlock.

The first line of treatment in the absence of infection is generally rest and stopping the activity that caused tenosynovitis. A resumption in activity tends to cause the condition to return. Ice may be applied, and painkilling and anti-inflammatory medications may become necessary to control pain and inflammation. If the symptoms are in the foot, a short-leg walking cast for 4 to 6 weeks may be helpful. In some cases, when more conservative approaches have failed, injections of the corticosteroid may be considered.

Tenotomy

The surgical division of a tendon. See TENDON REPAIR.

Tenovaginitis

See DE QUERVAIN DISEASE.

T

TENS

Transcutaneous electrical nerve stimulation. TENS is a type of therapy for pain relief. It uses electrical impulses to interfere with pain signals to the brain. With this technique, small electrodes are placed on the area of skin where there is pain. Electrical impulses are relayed to this area from a portable generator. There is usually a tingling sensation, but the degree of stimulation can be adjusted. After 30 minutes, pain is often reduced or relieved. TENS can be used along with other pain management strategies to relieve back or neck pain, arthritis pain, a pinched nerve, fibromyalgia, headache, menstrual cramps, sciatica, or shingles. Transcutaneous electrical nerve stimulation must be prescribed by a doctor. The portable units can be rented or purchased.

Teratogen

An agent or factor that produces abnormalities or deformities in a fetus. Teratogens usually fall into three categories: drugs and chemical agents; infectious agents; and radiation. Examples of teratogenic agents are alcohol, nicotine, caffeine, illegal drugs, hormones, radiation, pesticides, and some infections, such as the rubella virus. Certain over-the-counter drugs and medicines sold by prescription, such as isotretinoin (Accutane), can also harm the fetus. Teratogens have different effects, depending on the stage of the pregnancy. Some destroy the embryo or trigger a miscarriage, while others have a subtle impact that may not be noticed for years after the baby is born.

Teratoma

An abnormal growth, usually found in an ovary or testicle, formed from tissue that is not normally found in those organs. Teratomas can be benign or malignant and can consist of a mixture of tissues including cells from the EPITHELIUM, bone, hair, teeth, cartilage, or muscle.

Terazosin

A drug used to treat mild to moderate high blood pressure and a noncancerous prostate disease called benign prostatic hyperplasia (BPH). Terazosin (Hytrin) is an alpha blocker, a drug that blocks nerve endings. Terazosin lowers blood pressure by widening blood vessels and reducing the pressure within.

Terazosin is also used to treat BPH, a condition that can occur in men as they age. BPH can cause problems urinating, including the need to urinate frequently and the feeling of not being able to empty the bladder completely. Terazosin works by relaxing the muscles of the prostate and the opening to the bladder and increasing the flow of urine.

Terbinafine hydrochloride

One of the antifungal drugs. Terbinafine (Lamisil) is used to treat fungus infections of the scalp (ringworm), body, groin (called jock itch), feet (athlete's foot), fingernails, and toenails. As a cream, Terbinafine is spread on the skin to prevent the fungus from growing. It is taken as a tablet to treat infections of the nails and hair follicles.

Terconazole

An antifungal drug used to treat vaginal infections. Terconazole (Terazol 3, Terazol 7) is used to treat *Candida* (yeast) infections of the vagina. Terconazole works by preventing the fungus from growing and, thus, eradicating the yeast infection. It is available without prescription as a cream or suppository.

Terminal care

Care for a person with a limited time left to live. In terminal care, the emphasis shifts from finding a cure to maximizing the quality of the person's remaining life. Medical treatment consists primarily of relieving symptoms and pain. Terminal care may take place at home, in the hospital, or at a HOSPICE facility. Hospices are an increasingly popular option, as they offer a supportive, homelike environment as an alternative to spending the last weeks or months of life in a hospital. Hospice services may be provided in a hospice facility or in the person's home. In these facilities, in addition to medical care, there is access to emotional, social, and spiritual support. Grief counseling is usually provided for the family.

Termination of pregnancy

See ABORTION, ELECTIVE.

Testicle

One of the pair of oval glands that produce SPERM, the male reproductive cells, and the male sex hormone TESTOSTERONE. Also called testes, the testicles are located in the groin in a sac of skin called the scrotum. The male hormones secreted in the testicles, including testosterone, influence male characteristics, such as facial hair and a lower voice; sexual desire; and sexual function. These secretions are known collectively as androgen hormones. Muscle fibers originating from the groin surround the testicles. See REPRODUCTIVE SYSTEM, MALE.

Testicle self-examination

A procedure for a man or boy to check his own testicles for cancer. Since testicular cancer often develops without symptoms, regular self-examination is a preventive measure that can catch the disease early, when it is most curable. (See TESTICLE, CANCER OF THE.) Physicians recommend that males between the ages of 15 and 40 examine their testicles every month. The testicles are easiest to examine after a warm bath or shower. The heat relaxes the scrotum (the protective pouch between the legs at the base of the penis) and makes it easier to check the testicles, the male reproductive organs that produce sperm and the hormone testosterone.

HOW TO EXAMINE THE TESTICLES
The man or boy should stand in front of a mirror and check the skin of his scrotum for any changes or swelling. Next, he should raise his right leg by resting his foot on an elevated surface at about chair height. Then, he should place the thumbs of both hands below the right testicle and the middle and index fingers above. While pressing gently, he should roll the testicle between the fingers slowly and check its surface. It should feel firm, not hard, and smooth, without bumps. The man or boy should then locate the epididymis, a coil of small tubules at the back of the testicle. He should become familiar with its texture so that he does not mistake it for a lump. He should then raise the left leg and inspect the left testicle in the same way. It is normal for one testicle to be larger or lower than the other.

The man or boy should seek medical attention if an area feels bumpy and hard or if one of the testicles is swollen. Pain and swelling in the scrotum can indicate an infection. The presence of thin tubes above the testicle can indicate an abnormal collection of dilated veins. Those symptoms require consultation with a physician.

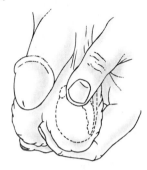

CHECKING FOR LUMPS
A man can examine his testicles by using both hands to gently roll each testicle between his thumb and fingers, checking for lumps. A healthy testicle will feel firm and smooth. Toward the back and top, the epididymis (a structure of coiled tubes) has a different texture and should not be confused with a lump. Many men find this examination to be most comfortable after a shower, when the skin of the scrotum is relaxed.

Testicle, cancer of the

Also called testicular cancer; a malignant tumor that begins in the testicle, one of the two organs located in the protective pouch between the legs of a boy or man. The testicles produce sperm cells and secrete the principal hormones (including testosterone) that control male sexuality and physical characteristics, such as facial hair, a deeper voice, and enlargement of the penis at puberty. Testicular cancer is rare, but it is the most common malignancy in men between 18 and 34 years old. The disease is highly curable, particularly when detected and treated early.

RISK FACTORS

The leading risk factor is an undescended testicle (see TESTICLE, UNDESCENDED.) In the fetus, the testicle normally develops inside the abdomen and descends into the scrotum shortly before birth. In a small number of boys, one or both testicles remain in the abdomen or descend only partway. Even if cryptorchidism (an

undescended testicle) is corrected surgically, a male who has had the condition remains at higher risk for cancer of the testicle.

Family history is also a risk factor. Men whose father or brother has had the disease are more likely to develop testicular cancer. Also, a man who has had cancer in one testicle has a higher than average risk of developing it in the other. Ethnic background plays a role as well. Caucasian Americans have a higher risk than do African Americans, Asian Americans, or Latin Americans. There is some evidence that infection with HIV (the human immunodeficiency virus), which causes AIDS (acquired immunodeficiency syndrome), is also a risk factor, but this connection has not been proven conclusively.

SYMPTOMS

The most common sign is painless enlargement of the testicle. The enlargement occurs gradually and may in time cause a sensation of heaviness or aching in the testicle and scrotum. Often, a hard lump can be felt. If the cancer has spread beyond the testicle, there may be pain in the back or discomfort in the abdomen. Certain rare testicular cancers can cause enlargement of breast tissue.

TYPES

A number of different kinds of malignant tumors can appear in the testicle. The vast majority are germ cell tumors, so named because they arise in the tissues that produce the sperm, or germ cells. Seminomas are the most common type of germ cell tumor. The others are known as nonseminomas. Malignancies can also begin in the supportive tissues of the testicle; these tumors are known as stromal tumors. Stromal tumors are much less common than germ cell tumors. In men older than age 50, cancer is less likely to originate in the testicle than to have spread from elsewhere in the body. A usual cause is cancer of the lymphatic system (lymphoma).

DIAGNOSIS AND TREATMENT

In addition to a physical examination, a doctor suspecting a man has testicular cancer may prescribe an ultrasound examination, which visualizes the organ by bouncing sound waves off it. The blood may also be tested to screen for certain proteins

and other substances that can indicate cancer. If the lump looks and feels "suspicious," the next step is to remove it and examine the tissue for cancer cells in the laboratory. In most cases, the entire testicle along with the tubule (vas deferens) that carries sperm cells from the testicle to the prostate gland is removed through an incision in the groin and then examined in the laboratory. Rarely, a sample of tissue is first taken and checked. If the tumor proves to be noncancerous, it may be removed surgically and the testicle returned to the scrotum.

Once a tumor of the testicle has been identified as cancer, follow-up tests are performed to see if the disease has spread. CT (computed tomography) scanning involves the use of rotating X rays to create a series of images from many angles to examine the lymph nodes in the groin and abdomen. If the physician suspects that the disease has spread or metastasized to more distant organs, chest X rays, bone scans, and other tests may be performed.

Follow-up treatment after removal of the testicle depends on the type of cancer and the degree to which it has spread. Early-stage cancer is usually treated with postsurgical radiation of the lymph nodes in the groin and the back of the abdomen. Seminomas are very sensitive to X rays; the dose of radiation needed to kill them is lower than for most other cancers. With nonseminoma germ cell cancers in adults, the lymph nodes in the back of the abdomen may also be removed. If the cancer has spread into the abdomen or into other organs, such as the lungs or brain, chemotherapy is used. In the case of stromal cancers, which usually do not spread beyond the testicle, radiation and chemotherapy are ineffective and are not used.

Complications depend on treatment. When only one testicle is removed, a man retains his ability to have erections and to father children. Radiation and chemotherapy produce temporary infertility; fertility usually returns within 2 years after treatment. Chemotherapy has other temporary side effects (such as hair loss, nausea, and vomiting) that disappear after the treatment ends. Surgical removal of the lymph nodes in the back of the abdomen can damage nerves that

T

TREATING TESTICULAR CANCER

In men between the ages of 15 and 34, testicular cancer is one of the most common forms of cancer. At the same time, death rates for this form of cancer have declined 70 percent since 1973, due to early detection and treatment. Surgical removal of a testicle is a common treatment for testicular cancer.

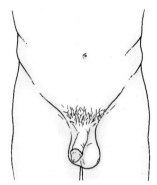

AN ENLARGED TESTICLE
An enlarged testicle may be a symptom of testicular cancer and should be reported to the physician as soon as it is noticed. Testicular cancer is highly curable, especially in the early stages.

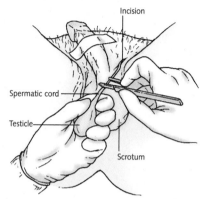

AN ORCHIECTOMY
For probable cancer, the testicle is removed through an incision in the groin. Nerves and veins leading to the testicle are clamped, and the testicle is separated from surrounding tissue and removed. A biopsy of the testicle is not usually done because cutting into the testicle can spread any existing cancer.

control ejaculation, potentially causing infertility. Some men undergoing this surgery have samples of their semen frozen beforehand in case they become infertile and want to have children later.

PREVENTION

Because the principal risk factors for cancer of the testicle are not within an individual's control, there are no specific prevention measures. The best strategy is to detect and treat the disease early, when testicular cancer is highly curable. Males who have cryptorchidism are generally advised to have the condition repaired surgically since a testicle in the scrotum is easier to monitor for cancer than is one in the abdomen or groin. Many physicians advise all men between 15 and 40 years old to inspect their testicles monthly and to seek medical attention promptly for changes in size, shape, or texture. See TESTICLE SELF-EXAMINATION.

Testicle, ectopic

A testicle that has strayed from the normal path of descent during development and lies in an abnormal posi-

tion outside the scrotum. The testicles are the organs found in the male scrotum (the pouch of protective skin between the legs). They produce sperm cells and the hormones responsible for male sexual characteristics, such as a deeper voice, facial hair, and enlarged genitals at puberty. In the fetus, the testicles develop in the abdomen and then descend into the scrotum shortly before birth. An ectopic testicle has descended, but into an abnormal position outside the scrotum. This condition differs from cryptorchidism, in which the testicle stops somewhere along the path of normal descent. An ectopic testicle is most often found under the skin in the groin. Rarely, it occurs near the anus, in the upper thigh, or at the base of the penis.

An ectopic testicle is usually treated surgically. The testicle and its blood supply are moved into the scrotum; more than one surgery may be needed to position the testicle correctly. In some cases, the ectopic testicle dies and must be removed. An artificial testicle can be placed in the scrotum for cosmetic purposes. Removal of one testicle does not

adversely affect the ability to father children or to have erections.

Testicle, pain in the

Aches or pains that begin in the testicles, the glands contained within the scrotum, which is the skin-covered pouch between the legs in a man. Sometimes, the discomfort radiates into the lower abdomen. Usually such aches and pains are not cause for alarm. However, severe pain from one side that comes on suddenly, particularly if accompanied by nausea or vomiting, requires immediate medical attention. It can arise from torsion of the testicle, a condition in which the normal blood supply to the testicle is cut off. Untreated torsion can cause the testicle to die and may require it to be removed. Pain in the testicle that results from MUMPS also requires medical attention. Other causes of pain in the testicle are injury, dilated veins in the scrotum, inflammation of the small tubules (epididymis) on the back of the testicle, hernia, or a stone in the lower end of the tube connecting the kidney to the bladder. Cancer is rarely a cause of pain in the testicle.

T

Testicle, retractile

A phenomenon found among boys before puberty in which one or both testicles are pulled up out of the scrotum during cold weather, excitement, or physical activity. The condition requires no treatment since a retractile testicle moves into normal position during puberty. The condition differs from cryptorchidism, in which the testicle fails to descend into the scrotum during development before birth and which often requires treatment.

Testicle, torsion of the

A twisting of the testicle on its blood supply, which blocks blood flow. Torsion usually affects only one testicle, and it typically causes sudden, severe pain accompanied by nausea and vomiting. The testicle quickly swells, the skin of the scrotum (the pouch between the legs containing the testicles) turns red, and the pain radiates into the abdomen. The condition is most common in adolescents and young men between 12 and 20 years of age. Immediate medical treatment is needed to prevent the death of the tissues in the testicles. In most cases, surgery is required to untwist the testicle and to attach it with surgical stitches to the wall of the scrotum; this prevents the condi-

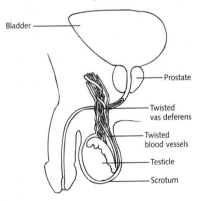

TWISTED TESTICLE
Torsion of the testicle is not only very painful, but dangerous because it cuts off the blood supply to the testicle. Immediate surgery is necessary to untwist the testicle and stitch it to the wall of the scrotum to prevent reoccurrence. The twisting of the vas deferens (the tube that carries sperm into the urethra during ejaculation) and blood vessels may occur after strenuous physical activity, or it may occur without any apparent cause.

tion from occurring again. Usually the surgeon also attaches the other testicle to the scrotal wall as well to eliminate the risk of torsion in that testicle. If torsion persists untreated for more than a few hours, the testicle may die and have to be removed. The remaining healthy testicle is sufficient to allow normal development into manhood, sexual activity, and the ability to father children.

Testicle, undescended

Failure of one or both testicles to descend into the scrotum (the protective pouch that hangs behind the penis) before birth. The condition is known as cryptorchidism. Normally,

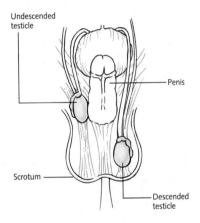

UNDESCENDED TESTICLE IN A NEWBORN
If the testicles have not dropped down by birth, they usually do so in the first 3 months of life. Rarely, surgery may be required to move the testicle down so that it will develop normally as the boy grows.

the testicles develop in the abdomen and then move down into the scrotum in the last 2 weeks before birth. In cryptorchidism, this process is incomplete at the time the baby is born, and one or both testicles have stopped in their normal descent, remaining outside the scrotum. The condition is common in premature infants and also occurs in some full-term babies. In most cases, the testicles descend into the scrotum within the first 3 months of life, and no treatment is required.

If cryptorchidism does not resolve on its own, surgery may be needed to locate the undescended testicle and move it into the scrotum. Treatment is usually successful.

Untreated cryptorchidism is likely to leave the man unable to father children in adulthood. The condition increases the risk of cancer of the testicle even when the testicle is placed into the scrotum.

Testicular feminization syndrome

The development of female sex characteristics in a male (see also PSEUDO-HERMAPHRODITISM). An affected individual is genetically male, with XY sex chromosomes, at the time of conception. Normally, in an XY fetus, male hormones called androgens cause male genitals to develop. However, in testicular feminization, the male fetus is unable to respond to the androgens produced, and the result is a fetus in whom female genitals are developed externally, even though male testes are developed internally, instead of a uterus and ovaries. People with the condition are infertile and cannot reproduce, although they otherwise function as normal females. The condition occurs in one in 20,000 individuals. The male testicles are usually present in the abdomen, where they are sometimes mistaken for hernias.

Testicular feminization, or the inability to use androgens in fetal development, is usually inherited from the mother, who carries a genetic error on one of her X chromosomes. About a third of all cases, however, are not inherited but stem from spontaneous mutations in the egg.

Testosterone

The primary male reproductive hormone, one of the ANDROGEN HORMONES, produced primarily within the cells inside the testicles. Testosterone circulates within the bloodstream and is critically important to the maintenance of male reproductive and sexual development and function. It has an important role in a man's bone and muscle growth, as well as in typical male physical characteristics, including facial hair, deepening of the voice, and increased muscle mass.

Testosterone is metabolized into different hormones at different sites in the body. An enzyme in the prostate and hair follicle cells of men converts testosterone into an androgen hormone many times more

T

potent than testosterone. In fat cells, testosterone may be converted into the female sex hormone estradiol. Some cells metabolize testosterone into less active or inactive steroid hormones.

The testosterone level seems to be controlled by changes in the time of day and the seasons and by a man's exposure to cycles of light and dark. As a result, the level of this hormone tends to be highest in the morning hours and in the spring and summer.

Methods for increasing the testosterone level naturally are not established. Synthetic supplementation of the hormone may be injected or absorbed through the skin by a patch when the testosterone level is abnormally low. This option is not recommended for men with a normal level. The athletic or sexual performance of men who already have normal levels of testosterone is not generally affected by taking additional testosterone. Taking supplemental doses of this hormone by men with normal testosterone levels is known to suppress testicular function, which can reduce a man's fertility.

Testicular failure may cause the testicles to stop producing testosterone. This condition may be caused by chromosome abnormalities present before birth, problems affecting sexual maturation, or damage to the testicles caused by disease, injury, or certain medications. The lack of testosterone can contribute to a man's INFERTILITY.

In very small amounts, testosterone is also produced in a woman's ovaries and adrenal glands. The hormone is involved in the sex drive of both men and women.

Tetanus

A bacterial disease that affects the nervous system. Tetanus, sometimes called lockjaw, is now a rare disease because of widespread immunization. The bacteria that cause the disease are found throughout the environment and are often seen in soil contaminated with animal manure. A person can contract tetanus by bacterial contamination of an open wound on the skin or mucous membrane. When the bacterium, *Clostridium tetani*, contaminates a wound, it produces a toxin called tetanospasmin, which attaches to nerves around the wound area. Inside the nerves, the toxin is transported to the brain or spinal cord, interfering with the normal activity of the nerves, especially those that signal muscle activity.

Tetanus occurs more commonly in older people and in agricultural workers who have greater contact with animal manure. Wounds that can lead to tetanus include burns, frostbite, abortion under unsanitary conditions, and illegal drug injections, such as "skin popping," which is when a person injects a drug right under the skin and not directly into a vein. Use of dirty or infected needles also can cause tetanus.

SYMPTOMS, DIAGNOSIS, AND TREATMENT

A cut or puncture injury susceptible to tetanus infection may be too minor to warrant medical evaluation, even after it has been contaminated. Symptoms of tetanus usually appear within 3 to 8 days after contamination, but may take as long as 3 weeks. More heavily contaminated wounds tend to produce earlier symptoms. Typically, the first sign of tetanus is muscular stiffness of the jaw, a symptom called TRISMUS, which is why the disease is known as lockjaw. The jaw stiffness is often followed by stiffness of the neck, difficulty swallowing or chewing, rigidity of abdominal muscles, spasms, profuse perspiration, and fever.

Complications from untreated tetanus can be severe, including spasm of the vocal cords or respiratory muscles that interferes with breathing, hypertension, abnormal heart rate, coma, systemic infection, clotting in the blood vessels of the lungs, pneumonia, and, ultimately, death. Mortality rates are highest among young children, people who are older, and intravenous drug abusers.

Tetanus may be suspected by a doctor if there is a history of a wound combined with characteristic symptoms such as muscle stiffness or spasm. The infective bacterium can be cultured from the wound in some cases, but it may not always be identified, so a diagnosis of tetanus can be missed.

If a person with suspected or confirmed tetanus has not had a tetanus toxoid booster within the previous 10 years, a single booster injection is given on the day the injury occurred, when possible. A booster may also be given if a wound is at high risk for tetanus and the last booster was administered more than 5 years before infection. If a person has not been previously immunized, he or she may be given tetanus immune globulin.

Tetanus infections are usually treated in an intensive care unit of a hospital. Antibiotics are given to destroy the tetanus bacteria, and antitoxin is administered to neutralize the toxin produced by the bacteria. Medications are generally given to control muscle spasms and to halt disturbances in heartbeat, blood pressure, and body temperature.

Tetany

An abnormal condition characterized by spasms of the arm and leg muscles. Tetany, a potentially life-threatening condition, is caused by a severe lowering in the calcium level, which may be due to a lack of vitamin D, HYPOPARATHYROIDISM (underactivity of the parathyroid glands), alkalosis (an abnormal state caused by excessive vomiting, hyperventilation, exposure to high altitudes), or the ingestion of alkaline salts. Tetany can also cause spasms of the larynx, resulting in breathing difficulties. Acute tetany may lead to respiratory obstruction requiring a TRACHEOSTOMY. The goal of treatment is to restore the calcium and associated mineral balances in the body.

Tetracaine

A topical anesthetic (medication applied directly to a site rather than injected) used to numb the eye and its surrounding membranes; the mucous membranes of the mouth, nose, throat; and skin. Tetracaine is also used for spinal anesthesia.

Tetracyclines

A class of antibiotics used to treat bacterial infections. Tetracyclines are used for many diseases, including Rocky Mountain spotted fever, typhus fever, and tick fevers; upper respiratory infections; pneumonia; and urinary tract infections. Tetracyclines are also used to treat severe acne; trachoma, a chronic eye infection; and conjunctivitis ("pink eye"). Tetracyclines are often prescribed for people who are allergic to penicillin. A woman who is pregnant should not take tetracycline. There are several different types of Tetracyclines.

DOXYCYCLINE

Doxycycline (Doryx, Monodox, Vibramycin) works by preventing bacteria from synthesizing protein. Doxycycline is effective against many organisms and is used to treat gonorrhea, syphilis, chlamydial infections, pelvic inflammatory disease, Lyme disease, and rickets and to prevent malaria.

MINOCYCLINE

Minocycline (Dynacin, Minocin) works to kill bacteria by preventing them from synthesizing protein. It is used to treat acne, syphilis, gonorrhea, cholera, urinary tract infections, and other bacterial infections.

OXYTETRACYCLINE

Oxytetracycline (Terramycin) is a tetracycline used to treat a wide variety of infections. It works by preventing bacteria from synthesizing protein and is used to treat middle ear infections, sexually transmitted diseases, bronchitis, pneumonia, and other infections.

TETRACYCLINE

Tetracycline (Achromycin V, Sumycin) works by preventing bacteria from synthesizing protein. Tetracycline is used to treat urinary tract infections, syphilis, Lyme disease, pelvic inflammatory disease, and other bacterial infections. As a cream or liquid preparation, tetracycline is used to treat acne and to prevent infection from minor skin abrasions.

Tetralogy of Fallot

A congenital defect of the heart, characterized by four abnormalities that result in inadequately oxygenated blood being pumped throughout the body.

Tetralogy of Fallot involves four defects in the structure of the heart: ventricular septal defect (a hole in the wall between the right and left ventricles); narrowing of the pulmonary valve; displaced aorta; and a thickening of the wall of the right ventricle.

Babies born with the defect have various symptoms, including difficulty feeding; failure to gain weight; slow growth; poor general development; bluish skin color, especially when agitated; and shortness of breath, which is made worse by exercise.

Treatment includes surgery to cor-

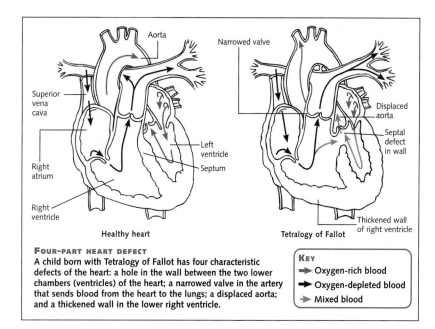

FOUR-PART HEART DEFECT
A child born with Tetralogy of Fallot has four characteristic defects of the heart: a hole in the wall between the two lower chambers (ventricles) of the heart; a narrowed valve in the artery that sends blood from the heart to the lungs; a displaced aorta; and a thickened wall in the lower right ventricle.

KEY
→ Oxygen-rich blood
→ Oxygen-depleted blood
→ Mixed blood

rect the defects in the heart, usually between ages 3 and 5. In severe cases, surgery may be performed earlier. Most cases can be surgically corrected, and the child will develop normally. Without surgery, death usually occurs around age 20.

About 10 percent of infants with Tetralogy of Fallot have the 22 gene deletion syndrome. All affected infants should be tested for this disorder using a specialized test of blood chromosome analysis.

Thai massage

An ancient form of massage therapy and bodywork practiced in Thailand for more than 2,500 years that combines elements of ACUPRESSURE, REFLEXOLOGY, stretching, and YOGA. In Thai massage, joints are loosened through manipulation, muscles are stretched, internal organs are toned, vitality is increased, and deep relaxation may be achieved. Thai massage is performed in a rhythmic and meditative way, with the goal of enabling both client and practitioner to achieve higher levels of consciousness. Thai massage is concerned with the whole body and focuses on the paths taken by energy.

Thalamus

A structure within the BRAIN that acts as a relay station for incoming and outgoing nerve impulses. Almost all

sensory information coming into the brain, except for the sense of smell, passes through the thalamus, and it is connected to the areas in the CEREBRUM that process sensory information and coordinate muscle movement. The thalamus helps to interpret sensory information and select a response to it, creates the feelings of pleasantness or unpleasantness associated with specific sensations, and regulates consciousness.

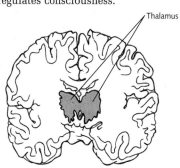

LOCATION OF THE THALAMUS
The two lobes of the thalamus lie deep in the forebrain. It is a mass of gray matter (nerve cell bodies) that relays information from many parts of the brain to the cerebral cortex.

Thalassemia

A group of genetic blood disorders that affect the production of one of the protein chains that forms the hemoglobin molecule. Thalassemia

T

exists in two types—alpha thalassemia and beta thalassemia—each of which is subdivided into three subtypes. Thalassemia minor, also called trait, is associated with a very mild anemia that cannot be corrected with iron supplements but has no other symptoms. Thalassemia intermedia causes moderately severe hemolytic anemia and requires regular medical care and occasional blood transfusions. Thalassemia major is a serious disease characterized by the inability to create enough normal hemoglobin to survive, calling for regular blood transfusions.

SYMPTOMS

Alpha thalassemia affects the formation of fetal and adult hemoglobin. Infants with alpha thalassemia major or intermedia suffer severe oxygen deprivation and are born with massive fluid accumulation. This type of the disorder usually affects only Southeast Asians.

Beta thalassemia minor, or trait, is associated only with mild incurable anemia, which may cause slight fatigue. A person with thalassemia trait is not at risk for developing a more severe form of the disease.

Beta thalassemia major is characterized by some or all of the following signs and symptoms: severe anemia; jaundice; enlarged spleen; fatigue; listlessness; reduced appetite; enlarged, fragile bones; facial malformations; growth problems; and increased susceptibility to infection. Children with untreated thalassemia major will die of the severe anemia that is characteristic of the condition.

TREATMENT AND RISK

People with thalassemia major require blood transfusions every 3 to 4 weeks to survive, while those with thalassemia intermedia may need only occasional transfusions. A side effect of regular transfusions is a buildup of excess iron in the organs of the body, especially the heart, liver, and pituitary gland. Excess iron buildup is treated with deferoxamine, a medication developed in the 1970s that binds with iron and allows it to be excreted. Before the medicine became available, people with thalassemia major were unlikely to live past their 20s, dying of an overload of iron.

The only cure for thalassemia is a bone marrow transplant, a treatment that is not without risk, particularly the risk that the transplant will be rejected.

Thalassemia is most common among people whose families come from Southeast Asia, southern China, the Middle East, the Mediterranean (Greece, Italy, Turkey), southern Asia, parts of North Africa, and some of the Pacific Islands. Males and females are equally at risk. Thalassemia trait can be passed from one parent to his or her children, but both parents must have thalassemia trait for any of their children to develop the disease. A simple blood test can identify people who are carriers of thalassemia trait, and prenatal tests can determine if a fetus has thalassemia.

Thalidomide

A drug used to treat skin sores associated with leprosy. Thalidomide (Thalomid) is a powerful drug that affects the immune system in ways that are not completely understood. It is used with other drugs to treat and prevent disfiguring skin sores associated with a complication of leprosy, called erythema nodosum leprosum.

Because thalidomide causes severe, life-threatening birth defects, its use is very limited; only registered doctors and pharmacists may prescribe or dispense the drug. A single dose of thalidomide can cause major birth defects, and the greatest risk to a fetus is during the first 2 months of pregnancy. A woman who is pregnant or could become pregnant, as well as her partner, should not use thalidomide. People who take thalidomide must participate in a special program called the "System for Thalidomide Education and Prescribing Safety (STEPS)," through which they are made thoroughly familiar with the drug and its risks. Women who take thalidomide must agree not to become pregnant, and men must agree not to make a partner pregnant while taking the drug.

Thallium

A radioisotope used in NUCLEAR MEDICINE that emits gamma rays and closely resembles potassium. Thallium 201 is used as a diagnostic imaging aid to evaluate the blood flow and viability of the heart muscle. When injected intravenously into the person to be scanned, the radioisotope enters healthy tissue quickly. Areas with poor blood flow and decreased blood supply, as well as tissue that has died because of insufficient blood supply, take up the thallium much more slowly and show up as "cold spots" on a nuclear scan.

A camera records the number of gamma rays the heart cells give off and displays an image. Healthy tissue, where the thallium has been taken up quickly and heavily, appears light on the image. Areas where there are damaged cells and where the uptake has been poor appear dark on the image. A sequence of two thallium scans can distinguish reversible damage caused by reduced blood flow to the heart muscle from cells that have been destroyed by lack of blood supply, an irreversible defect.

Theophylline

A bronchodilator; a drug used to treat symptoms of asthma, bronchitis, and emphysema. Theophylline (Aerolate, Theo-Dur, Theo-24, Uniphyl, and others) is one of the bronchodilators that works by relaxing muscles in the airways to allow more air into the lungs, by decreasing the sensitivity of the lungs to substances that cause inflammation, and by increasing diaphragm contractions, thereby drawing more air into the lungs. Theophylline is also available in combination with other drugs, such as guaifenesin, ephedrine, and phenobarbital, to treat the same symptoms.

Therapeutic

Beneficial or relating to a treatment.

Therapeutic recreation

A treatment service designed to rehabilitate people with disabling conditions or illnesses by reducing or eliminating the negative effects of their conditions. Therapeutic recreation restores or improves functioning and independence and provides recreation resources and opportunities. The goal of therapeutic recreation is to improve the health and well-being of people who are developmentally challenged. One example of therapeutic recreation might be adaptive versions of sports such as basketball for a person confined to a wheelchair.

Therapeutic touch

Healing techniques that may blend the laying on of hands, spirituality, and traditional Asian medical practices to increase the body's self-healing abilities. Therapeutic touch is a form of ENERGY MEDICINE used to unblock the life force energy. As currently practiced in the United States, therapeutic touch is a blend of ancient healing concepts from Indian and Chinese medicine and the religious practice of healing by the "laying on of hands." Therapeutic touch, or TT, is recognized as an official nursing skill in some countries, where it is considered an adjunct to conventional medical care.

Therapeutic touch does not necessarily involve physical contact but may be limited to the passing of the practitioner's hands 2 to 4 inches above a person's body. Practitioners believe that the treatments work by manipulating energy in and around people in a force field, clearing energy blockages and helping people restore their own curative energy. Therapeutic touch is also thought to relax the body, thereby helping it to function and heal more effectively. Craniosacral therapy is used to manipulate the tissues of the skull, spine, and pelvis to help people relax. Critics of therapeutic touch believe it is ineffective and has yet to be scientifically proven.

Therapy

See PSYCHOTHERAPY.

Thermometer

An instrument for measuring body TEMPERATURE. There are a variety of thermometers available. A person's temperature can be measured with an instrument placed in the mouth, rectum, or ear or under the arm. Rectal, ear, and armpit thermometers are particularly useful for measuring the temperatures of infants and toddlers. However, armpit thermometers may read 1°F lower than oral models, and rectal thermometers typically read 1°F higher.

The traditional thermometer consists of a sealed glass tube, marked in degrees of Celsius or Fahrenheit and containing liquid such as mercury or alcohol. The liquid rises or falls as it expands or contracts in response to changes in temperature. Newer digital thermometers are often easier to

read than traditional thermometers. Other innovations include disposable temperature strips that are placed on the forehead. However, there is some question about their reliability and accuracy. See Measuring body temperature, page 1206.

Thiamin

A nutrient that is essential for energy production from carbohydrates and for nerve and muscle function. See VITAMIN B.

Thiazolidinediones

A new class of oral drugs for the treatment of type 2 diabetes mellitus. They seem to work by decreasing the production of glucose by the liver and increasing the sensitivity of tissues to the presence of insulin. They restore the blood sugar level to normal without producing low blood sugar. Examples of this drug type include pioglitazone HCl (Actos) and rosiglitazone maleate (Avandia).

Thirst

The desire or need for water or other fluids. In healthy people, thirst indicates the body's need for fluid. A person who becomes dehydrated from exercise or illness may experience excessive thirst. See THIRST, EXCESSIVE.

Thirst, excessive

An abnormally increased desire or need for water or other drink. A person who becomes dehydrated (see DEHYDRATION) due to exercise or illness may experience excessive thirst. Excessive thirst, along with increased urination, is a common initial symptom of diabetes mellitus. See DIABETES MELLITUS, TYPE 2.

Thoracentesis

A procedure in which fluid is removed from the space around the lungs; also known as a pleural tap. Thoracentesis is performed to relieve the symptoms associated with fluid accumulation and to analyze the fluid for diagnostic purposes. In the procedure, which is performed under local anesthesia, the doctor uses a fine needle to draw out the fluid.

Thoracic outlet syndrome

A complex condition characterized by pain and abnormal sensations in

the hand, arm, shoulder, or neck. The thoracic outlet is located at the top of the rib cage, between the chest and neck. Compression of the nerves, veins, or arteries in this area may cause pain, numbness, tingling, muscular weakness, and atrophy. Inadequate blood flow may lead to bluish discoloration and swelling in the arm and hand. An affected person can also develop RAYNAUD DISEASE, in which exposure to the cold causes small arteries in the fingers to contract; this leads to paleness and ulceration of the fingers. Thoracic outlet syndrome may be caused by poor posture or anatomical abnormalities. The primary treatment is physical therapy. In some cases, surgery is necessary to correct the problem.

Thoracic surgeon

A doctor specially trained to perform general thoracic surgery. General thoracic surgery concentrates on surgical treatments for lung cancer, emphysema, swallowing problems related to the esophagus, cancer of the esophagus, and gastroesophageal reflux.

Thoracotomy

A surgical procedure to open the chest (THORAX). A thoracotomy is usually performed to allow a surgeon to operate on a diseased heart, lung, or other chest cavity organ. If lung cancer is suspected, opening the chest wall to take a tissue sample from the suspected tumor site may be necessary for diagnosis. A thoracotomy is also used in severe cases of EMPYEMA, an infection in the space surrounding the lungs. If medication and draining the infected fluid from the chest fail

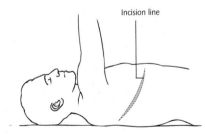

Incision line

LATERAL THORACOTOMY
A lateral thoracotomy provides the surgeon with access to the lungs and esophagus. An incision is made from the shoulder blade to the nipple, curving under the arm. The underlying muscles are divided to expose the ribs, and the ribs are separated. Sometimes, part of a rib is removed.

T

MEASURING BODY TEMPERATURE

There are a variety of methods for taking a person's body temperature. Two types of glass thermometers are available—the bulb of an oral thermometer is thin and long, while the bulb of a rectal thermometer is round (so as not to injure the walls of the rectum on insertion). Both types of glass thermometers have identical markings. Digital thermometers used to take ear or mouth temperature are fast and accurate but generally more expensive than glass thermometers. Armpit temperature, which can be obtained using either a glass or digital thermometer, provides the least accurate measurement but is the recommended method of obtaining a temperature from an uncooperative child or infants younger than 6 months.

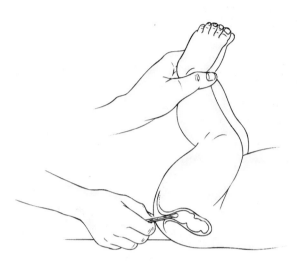

RECTAL THERMOMETER
The lubricated thermometer should be inserted ½ to 1 inch into the infant's rectum and held securely in place for 2 to 3 minutes.

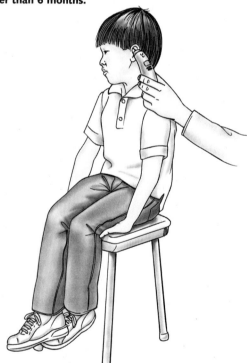

DIGITAL EAR THERMOMETER
Ear temperature is taken by inserting the thermometer into the ear and aiming the disposable tip toward the eardrum; digital thermometers usually beep when they display the person's body temperature.

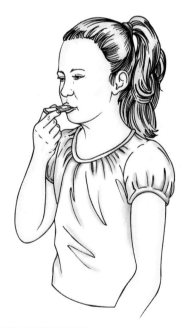

DIGITAL MOUTH THERMOMETER
The tip of a digital oral thermometer is placed under the tongue to determine temperature. The thermometer beeps when it is through recording and the reading appears on a digital display.

T

to stop the infection, a thoracotomy is performed. The length of the surgery and the hospital recovery period depend on the extent of the surgery and the condition of the person.

Thorax

The medical name for the chest, the region of the body that lies between the neck and the diaphragm muscle and is encased by the ribs. The main structures in the thorax are the heart, lungs, esophagus, aorta, and pulmonary arteries.

Thought

The result of the mind's cognitive or intellectual processes. In psychiatry, thoughts are distinguished from emotions or feelings, although the two areas are often connected. Thoughts can be key to the processes underlying certain emotional and mental disorders. See also COGNITIVE-BEHAVIORAL THERAPY.

Thought disorders

Abnormal thinking that is pathological, bizarre, or not based in reality. Common thought disorders include hallucinations (false perceptions in any of the senses based on no external reality, for example, hearing voices of the absent or dead), delusions (persistent, unshakable, and false beliefs held despite obvious evidence to the contrary), and confabulation (the invention of plausible fictions to account for gaps in memory). Thought disorders also include depersonalization (thinking that one's body is unreal, unfamiliar, floating, dead, changing in size, or being observed by the self from the outside), derealization (thinking that the environment is unreal and that one is separated from the surroundings), and word salad (a seemingly random, illogical mixture of words and sounds). A thought disorder may or may not be a sign of mental illness. Temporary feelings of depersonalization or derealization are normal and do not indicate mental illness. Persistent hallucinations are a key feature of SCHIZOPHRENIA, and delusions of persecution can be a symptom of PARANOIA. Some drugs may cause thought disorders.

Thrill

A vibration felt by doctors when examining the chest by touch (palpa-tion). Thrill can be a sign of abnormal blood flow in the heart caused by a defective valve.

Throat

The PHARYNX; muscular, membrane-lined passage that carries air from the nose to the trachea (windpipe) and food from the mouth to the esophagus. The throat is subdivided into the nasopharynx, (which lies above the soft palate), the oropharynx (between the soft palate and larynx), and laryngopharynx (which is behind the larynx and is continuous with the esophagus).

Throat cancer

A malignant tumor originating in the cells that cover the mucous membrane lining the THROAT. Throat cancer is also known as cancer of the pharynx. This cancer tends to penetrate the mucous membrane and muscle layers, spreading into surrounding tissue as it grows. It can spread to lymph nodes (see LYMPH NODE) in the neck and into the bloodstream and be carried to the lungs and other organs. Cancers near the mouth tend to remain localized unless they are not successfully treated. Cancers near the nose and in the lower throat may spread early before symptoms appear.

SYMPTOMS

A tumor growing in the pharynx can interfere with hearing, smell, taste, speech, and swallowing. Symptoms may include a mild, persistent sore throat or cold lasting for longer than 2 weeks; persistent cough; sudden hoarseness; or a change in the sound of the voice. The person may also experience difficulty swallowing; painful swallowing; coughing up blood with phlegm; blood in the SALIVA; a white patch in the mouth; ear pain or a blocked feeling in the ear; a hard lump in the throat or a lymph node in the neck; and swollen lymph nodes in the neck. A tumor located directly behind the nose may cause partial hearing loss, nasal obstruction, nosebleeds, ringing in the ears, and pain or pressure in the middle ear.

CAUSES

Although the cause of throat cancer is unknown, smokers are six times more likely than nonsmokers to develop this cancer. Almost everyone diagnosed with throat cancer is a smoker or ex-smoker. Smoking or chewing tobacco and excessive alcohol use are the major known risk factors. Cancers of the nasopharynx (the top area of the throat where it connects to the nasal passages) are associated with the Epstein-Barr virus, a type of herpesvirus that causes mononucleosis (see MONONUCLEOSIS, INFECTIOUS; VIRUSES.) The risk for throat cancer may be increased by the inhalation of coal or other mineral dust and by exposure to asbestos and diesel fumes. The use of wood-burning stoves seems to increase the risk of throat cancer, as does poor oral hygiene and frequent consumption of cured meats.

DIAGNOSIS AND TREATMENT

Abnormal growths in the upper area of the throat near the mouth may be visible to a doctor. Examination of the lower areas of the throat behind the nose and near the esophagus is done with mirrors or a lighted viewing tube, called a fiberoptic scope. All lesions, growths, or tumors are biopsied (meaning a sample of tissue is removed and analyzed for cancer), or a test for the Epstein-Barr virus is done. If cancer is present, imaging scans can help establish how widespread it is.

If the cancer has not spread beyond the lymph nodes, surgery can remove the abnormal growth entirely, and the cancer will go into remission. The surgery can be complex, however, depending on the location of the tumor and its stage of development. The impact of treatment on the person's speech and other essential functions is considered in determining the appropriate treatment.

If the cancer is in the area of the throat behind the nose, the person typically receives high-dose radiation to the head and neck, possibly after chemotherapy to shrink the tumors. If the growths are small and in the area of the throat near the mouth, they may be treated with radiation alone to avoid disfigurement and other complications. If the cancer does not respond to radiation treatments, surgery may become necessary. Sometimes chemotherapy is required before surgery, or RADIATION THERAPY may follow surgery. Tumors in the

Terms in small capital letters—for example, PHYSICAL THERAPY or PAGET DISEASE—indicate a cross-reference to another entry with more information.

T

lower throat usually require surgery, which may be preceded by chemotherapy or followed by radiation treatments. The part of the throat affected is removed, and reconstructive surgery is performed to reestablish the removed structures. When advanced throat cancer cannot be treated surgically, radiation therapy may help relieve symptoms and slow the progress of the spreading malignant tumor. Patients with throat cancer often need speech therapy after surgery to help them regain the ability to speak, swallow, and chew.

Laser surgery may be used to treat some throat cancers. This approach may be less risky and offer greater preservation of voice function and swallowing ability, as well as less potential for disfigurement. The decision to use laser surgery may depend on the stage of the throat cancer and its location. The laser beam is used as a cutting and sealing tool to precisely remove the cancerous tissue, following the margins of the tumor. Rather than making an incision, the surgeon uses special fiberoptic (see FIBEROPTICS) videoscopes and other devices to follow natural passageways, such as the mouth, to gain access to the tumor. The best candidates for laser surgery are those who have not previously been treated with radiation therapy and those with new cancer of the throat, as opposed to recurrent cancer. Chemotherapy and radiation treatments may be used with laser surgery to treat throat cancer.

Complications and side effects of radiation and chemotherapy may include nausea and vomiting, fatigue, hair loss and baldness, a reduced ability to resist infections, and, rarely, skin redness or blisters. Medications can help relieve the discomforts of some of these side effects. Support groups can help people with throat cancer cope with issues arising during the illness and recovery period.

Thrombectomy

A surgical procedure to remove a thrombus (blood clot) that has formed in a blood vessel and is blocking blood flow through it. The procedure is typically performed with a catheter (thin tube) tipped with an inflatable balloon. The catheter is inserted into the blood vessel above the clot, then the balloon is inflated. The catheter is drawn back out, pulling the thrombus with it.

Thrombocytopenia

A shortage of PLATELETS, blood cells that have a key role in clotting. The word comes from Greek roots meaning "shortage of clotting cells." Thrombocytopenia makes a person vulnerable to unusual bleeding, which can range from mild to severe. Symptoms include profuse blood loss after injury or surgery, a measleslike rash known as purpura (usually on the lower legs), nosebleeds, swollen joints, blood in vomit or feces, and heavy menstrual flow. Widespread bleeding, particularly in the digestive system or brain, can be life-threatening.

Thrombocytopenia is classified as idiopathic or secondary. Idiopathic thrombocytopenia usually arises from the body producing antibodies against its own platelets, which then attack and destroy them. This disease is also called autoimmune thrombocytopenic purpura. It occurs most often in children and young adults and affects males and females equally. In older adults, it is more likely to occur in women than in men.

Secondary thrombocytopenia is a complication of another disease. Possible causes include viral or bacterial infections, systemic lupus erythematosus, chronic lymphocytic leukemia, sarcoidosis, and cancer of the ovary. Drugs including chemotherapy agents (cancer-killing medications), quinidine, quinine, heparin, and rifampin can also cause the condition. Thrombocytopenia is a common, temporary complication of bone marrow transplant (see BONE MARROW TRANSPLANT, ALLOGENEIC; BONE MARROW TRANSPLANT, AUTOLOGOUS).

In children, idiopathic thrombocytopenia often resolves without treatment. In adults, the idiopathic form of the disease can be treated with corticosteroids (prednisone) or thrombopoietin, a substance that promotes the production of platelets. When medication does not work, the spleen may be removed surgically to reduce bleeding. Secondary thrombocytopenia is treated with therapy aimed at the underlying disease or by changing medication. If bleeding is severe, the person is given transfusions of platelets, to restore the blood's ability to clot, and red blood cells, to make up the lost blood. People who have undergone a bone marrow transplant receive platelet transfusions until platelet production by the transplanted marrow becomes sufficient.

Thrombocytosis

An increase in platelets, the blood elements that have a key role in clotting. In most cases, thrombocytosis is a physiological reaction to another condition, such as cancer, surgery (typically splenectomy), trauma or injury, severe infection, inflammatory disorders such as rheumatoid arthritis, iron-deficiency anemia, or recovery from thrombocytopenia (an abnormally low number of platelets). This kind of reactive thrombocytosis is usually temporary, and the person is free of symptoms. In older patients, however, it may lead to blood clots that precipitate a heart attack or stroke. Aspirin may be prescribed as a preventive medication. In a small number of cases, thrombocytosis is a sign of a disease known as essential thrombocytosis. See MYELOPROLIFERATIVE DISORDERS for more information about the disease and its treatment.

Thromboembolism

Blockage (embolism) of a blood vessel by a thrombus (blood clot) that has formed elsewhere in the body and has been carried through the bloodstream. A thromboembolism is the most common type of EMBOLISM.

Thrombolytic drugs

Drugs used to dissolve blood clots and to open blood vessels. Thrombolytic drugs are used in the treatment of blood clots within blood vessels in the heart and lungs and in clotting associated with hip replacement.

Vessel narrowed by fatty deposits   Vessel opened by drug treatment

EFFECTS OF "CLOT-BUSTERS"
Deposits of lipids (fats) and other fatty substances can build up inside blood vessels, narrowing the channel and increasing the chance that a blood clot will become lodged in the vessel. Thrombolytic drugs dissolve these deposits so that blood can flow more freely through the vessel.

Thrombolytic drugs are also used to prevent clotting when tubes are placed in the body. If given within 3 to 6 hours after a heart attack, the drugs help to increase survival.

Thrombolytic drugs are also known by other names, including anisoylated plasminogen-streptokinase activator complex (APSAC) and tissue-type plasminogen activator (t-PA, rt-PA). Examples of thrombolytic drugs include ALTEPLASE (Activase), re-teplase (Retavase), and STREPTOKINASE (Streptase).

Thrombophlebitis

Inflammation of a vein because of the formation of a blood clot (thrombus); also known as phlebitis. Thrombophlebitis usually develops in the veins of the legs and less commonly in the arms. If it affects the superficial veins, it can be treated with medications, such as analgesics to stop pain and anti-inflammatory drugs to reduce swelling. Support stockings help in some cases, as do elevating the leg and applying warm compresses. Thrombophlebitis affecting a deep vein is a more serious condition known as deep vein thrombosis and requires treatment with anticoagulants to prevent new clots and possibly thrombolytics to dissolve the clot. See THROMBOSIS, DEEP VEIN.

Thrombosis

The formation or presence of a blood clot inside a cavity of the heart or a blood vessel.

Thrombosis, deep vein

A blood clot in a large vein. Deep vein thrombosis usually occurs in the leg, less often in the arm or pelvic veins. The blood clot blocks the vein and prevents the flow of blood back to the heart, causing the blood to back up and resulting in swelling and pain or tenderness. There is a risk that a portion of the blood clot can break free, travel through the bloodstream, and lodge in the lungs, brain, heart, or other organ, where it can cause serious damage and even death. Deep vein thrombosis is most likely to occur when blood flow in deep veins is slow or stagnant or the vessel is injured. This occurs in persons who are confined to a chair or a bed for long periods, have undergone surgery

on the legs, have recently broken a bone in the lower extremities or have had a heart attack, or take birth control pills or estrogen. Cancer, obesity, chronic heart failure, and lack of exercise also increase the risk of deep vein thrombosis.

In most cases, deep vein thrombosis resolves through natural healing, as the blood clot dissolves and normal blood flow is restored. Hospitalization for initial treatment is usually required. Anticoagulants (such as heparin or warfarin) or antiplatelet drugs (such as aspirin) are used to prevent further clotting and prevent clots from traveling through the bloodstream. Analgesics may be needed to control pain. Bed rest, with the leg elevated and treated with warm, moist heat, may be advised. After the person returns home, anticoagulant or antiplatelet medication is often continued to decrease the risk of subsequent thromboses.

Thrombus

A blood clot that forms within a cavity of the heart or a blood vessel.

Thrush

A yeast infection of the mouth caused by *Candida* fungi, especially *Candida albicans.* Thrush is an infection involving the moist surfaces surrounding the lips, inside the cheeks, and on the tongue and palate.

Candida fungi are found throughout the environment. Thrush occurs when the normally prevalent organisms become overgrown under certain conditions, such as when a person is taking antibiotics. Antibiotic therapy can destroy the normal bacteria in the mouth, which upsets the balance of microbes and allows the *Candida* yeasts to grow and dominate. Thrush may also be triggered by viral upper respiratory diseases, infectious mononucleosis, or irritation of gums and other oral tissues caused by dentures. It can be contracted by close contact with infected people and can spread in child care settings.

Thrush generally flares up and then heals on its own, but it may cause serious and chronic infections in people with impaired immunity, chronic illness, or malnourishment. People who have an increased risk include those with diabetes mellitus,

older people, people using corticosteroids or other medications that suppress the immune system, and people who have cancer or HIV (human immunodeficiency virus) infection. It is very common in babies and newborns, who can contract the fungus during delivery when the mother has a vaginal yeast infection. The symptoms tend to appear within 7 to 10 days of infections that occurred during childbirth and delivery.

SYMPTOMS, DIAGNOSIS, AND TREATMENT
Creamy, white, curdlike patches appear inside the mouth, particularly on the tongue, roof of the mouth, back of the throat, and around the lips. The white material on the surface of the patches covers red, inflamed areas that may bleed slightly with contact. The corners of the mouth may be red, moist, and cracked. The typical thrush patches may be painful, and in infants, this can cause irritability and poor feeding. Any irregularity in the tissues inside an infant's mouth that prevents the infant from feeding normally should be checked by a doctor. In rare cases, the fungus that causes thrush can affect tissue in the esophagus and cause difficulty swallowing, which is a medical emergency.

Diagnosis of thrush is usually made by a physical examination of the mouth. If the patches bleed when gently scraped, the person probably has thrush. Patch scrapings may be tested in a laboratory if the preliminary diagnosis is in question. In infants, the diaper area may be examined to check for diaper rash caused by a *Candida* yeast infection.

Thrush is treated with antifungal medication, usually nystatin, clotrimazole, or fluconazole. When the infection is mild, a liquid or lozenge form of antifungal medication may be given. Most thrush infections are treated successfully and cured within 3 days of starting medication.

Thumb-sucking

A common habit that soothes, calms, and comforts an infant. Approximately nine of ten babies suck their thumbs or fingers at some point. A normal habit, thumb-sucking is an extension of rooting and sucking reflexes. Most children give up the

T

habit on their own by age 4. Thumb-sucking has the potential to distort the tooth alignment in the upper jaw and cause malformation of the roof of the mouth. If a child stops before age 5, the chances of damage are minimal. Thumb-sucking beyond age 5 requires the attention of a pediatrician or dentist. Once a child enters kindergarten, peer pressure discourages most daytime thumb-sucking. Only a child who continues thumb-sucking beyond age 5 ordinarily receives medical treatment. The doctor will review the situation to rule out any underlying emotional problems. All children eventually quit thumb-sucking on their own.

Thymus

A two-lobed organ of lymphatic tissue located under the top of the sternum (breastbone) near the end of the trachea (windpipe). The thymus is central to the IMMUNE SYSTEM and the development of white blood cells. One type of white blood cell, the T cell, is produced in the red bone marrow and matures in the thymus, from which its name derives. In a fetus just before birth and in newborns, the thymus is particularly large. It continues to grow throughout childhood, then declines in size and activity during adolescence. It begins to shrink after puberty. In adults the thymus is composed largely of fatty and fibrous tissue, and the organ's immune function slowly declines.

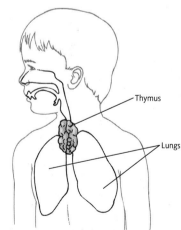

LOCATION OF THE THYMUS
The thymus lies just below the neck under the breastbone. It grows until puberty and then begins to shrink, returning to its weight at birth by the time a person is about 40 years old.

Thyroglossal cyst

An abnormality present at birth that produces a swelling in the neck. In a developing fetus, a small channel between the thyroid gland and the tongue is meant to close as the fetus grows. If this channel or parts of it remain in place or remain open when the infant is born, an abnormal channel between the thyroid gland and the tongue is created. A cyst can form around the channel, and the cyst causes swelling. If the thyroglossal cyst becomes infected, it can lead to formation of a thyroglossal fistula (abnormal passage between the cyst and the neck). Because of the chance of repeated infections, a cyst or fistula should be surgically removed.

Thyroid cancer

A cancerous tumor that develops in one or both lobes of the thyroid, the butterfly-shaped gland located below the Adam's apple at the front of the neck. Thyroid cancer is rare and affects women more than men. It can take one of four different forms. Three of these forms of cancer originate in the follicular cells of the gland, and one develops in the C cells. The C cells of the thyroid gland, sometimes called the parafollicular cells, produce calcitonin, which is a hormone that has a role in controlling the calcium and phosphate levels in the blood.

The follicular cells of the thyroid gland produce and store THYROXINE and the protein thyroglobulin. Thyroxine controls the breakdown of complex molecules to supply the body with energy in a process known as metabolism. Thyroxine also regulates the buildup of cells and tissues from less complex molecules.

The most prevalent form of thyroid cancer develops in the follicular cells and is called papillary carcinoma, or papillary adenocarcinoma. This is a slow-growing cancer that is usually present in only one of the lobes of the thyroid but, in some cases, may affect both lobes. Usually, papillary carcinomas are slow-growing tumors; however, in some individuals, the cancer is more aggressive and can spread rapidly. If papillary cancer spreads, it usually spreads to the lymph glands, which are located near the thyroid in the neck.

Follicular carcinoma, or follicular adenocarcinoma, is the second most common form of thyroid cancer. Like papillary carcinoma, it develops in the follicular cells. This type of thyroid cancer is considered more aggressive than papillary carcinoma and tends to grow into the blood vessels and spread from there to the lungs and bones, as well as to other body parts early in the course of the disease.

Papillary and follicular carcinoma are well-differentiated thyroid cancers because their superficial appearance is near that of normal thyroid tissue. When detected early and medically treated, the cure rate is more than 90 percent.

Anaplastic carcinoma, or undifferentiated thyroid cancer, is the rarest type of thyroid cancer and the most lethal. It is believed to develop in the follicular cells from existing papillary or follicular carcinoma. Anaplastic carcinoma is a fast-growing cancer that spreads aggressively to other parts of the body, especially to structures in the neck.

Medullary thyroid carcinoma, the only form of thyroid cancer to originate in the C cells, may spread to other areas of the body, particularly the lungs, liver, and lymph nodes, before symptoms are evident. This cancer produces and releases into the bloodstream excess amounts of two chemicals: the hormone calcitonin and the protein carcinoembryonic antigen. Medullary thyroid carcinoma takes two forms. Sporadic medullary thyroid carcinoma, which is not inherited, is the more common form and generally affects only one of the two lobes of the thyroid gland. Familial medullary thyroid carcinoma is an inherited disorder that can occur in several generations of the same family and takes several different forms. In general, medullary thyroid carcinoma has a good 10-year survival rate with timely treatment.

CAUSES
The exact cause of thyroid cancer is unknown. Some studies indicate that exposure to radiation may increase risks. This exposure can include high-dose radiation treatments early in life for acne or swollen adenoids, as well as exposure to nuclear fallout or to nuclear power plant accidents.

Thyroid cancer occurs more commonly in the populations of countries where the typical diet is low in iodine. The risk is higher among people with certain medical conditions such as Cowden disease (an inherited tendency to develop tissue overgrowths called hamartomas) and familial polyposis (an inherited predisposition to polyp growths in the bowel).

There is recent scientific evidence that gene mutations of DNA may have a role in certain types of thyroid cancer, especially papillary carcinoma, medullary thyroid carcinoma, and anaplastic carcinoma.

SYMPTOMS

A mass or a slow-growing lump in the neck is one of the symptoms of thyroid cancer. Other symptoms include a shooting pain in the neck area that spreads to the ears and a persistent cough that is resistant to treatment.

In some cases, a swollen lymph node may indicate the possibility of thyroid cancer. A hoarse voice may result from pressure on the nerve to the voice box caused by a tumor on the thyroid. If a thyroid tumor obstructs the windpipe, there may be difficulty swallowing or breathing.

DIAGNOSIS

During a physical examination, the neck will be felt to determine the size and condition of the thyroid gland and to check for the presence of nodules on the gland. The lymph nodes in the neck will also be examined for enlargement. If thyroid disorders including cancer are suspected, a doctor may order further diagnostic tests, particularly if a nodule is found on the thyroid gland.

The most conclusive diagnostic test for thyroid cancer is fine-needle aspiration of a thyroid nodule. Fine-needle aspiration is generally performed on an outpatient basis using a local anesthetic. When the area has been numbed, the doctor inserts a fine needle into the nodule on the thyroid and withdraws fluid and cells to be examined in a laboratory for indications of cancer. Usually the results of this procedure indicate that the nodule is benign (not cancerous). A very small percentage of fine-needle aspiration results indicate that cancer is definitely present. Sometimes further tests may be needed.

Although most people with thyroid cancer have a normal thyroid level,

testing is important to make sure hormone levels are normal.

When medullary thyroid carcinoma is suspected, a blood test for the level of the hormone calcitonin, which is produced by the C cells, may be performed. This is called a blood calcitonin test.

THYROID SCANNING allows a doctor to determine the spread of thyroid cancer. Ultrasound scans use sound waves instead of X rays to differentiate benign growths such as cysts and cystic tumors from cancerous growths such as solid tumors. CT SCANNING (computed tomography scanning) may be performed on the neck to view the thyroid from different angles. MRI (magnetic resonance imaging) uses radio waves and large magnets to produce computer-generated images of cross-sectional views of the thyroid and other structures in the neck area.

TREATMENT

Surgery is the main approach to the treatment of thyroid cancer. A surgeon removes all of the thyroid, including the cancerous cells and possibly other noncancerous parts of the thyroid. In most cases involving cancer, the entire thyroid gland and the lymph nodes in the area must be surgically removed. Radioactive iodine treatments may be used to destroy cancerous thyroid tissue remaining after surgery. CHEMOTHERAPY (injected or oral anticancer medication) and external beam RADIATION THERAPY (the use of high-energy rays to kill cancerous cells at the site of the cancer) are rarely used after surgical treatment for thyroid cancer.

When all of the thyroid gland is removed, thyroid hormone medication is taken orally for the rest of the person's life. This hormone therapy re-establishes normal metabolism and also suppresses the secretion of TSH (thyroid-stimulating hormone) by the pituitary gland. TSH tends to stimulate the development of remnant cancer cells.

Tumors can recur after treatment for thyroid cancer. Regularly scheduled evaluations are essential to detect these possible recurrences.

Thyroid function tests

Diagnostic procedures that measure the performance of the THYROID GLAND.

Thyroid function tests help diagnose disorders of the thyroid, including cancer. These tests can detect HYPERTHYROIDISM (overactivity of the thyroid gland) or HYPOTHYROIDISM (underactivity of the thyroid gland). The doctor may ask a person preparing to take a thyroid function test to temporarily stop taking thyroid medication before testing to provide a more accurate evaluation of the function of the gland.

Radiopharmaceuticals and nuclear scanning are used in two thyroid function tests. The iodine uptake test, which is generally performed on an outpatient basis, measures the ability of the thyroid to concentrate iodine. The thyroid requires iodine to produce the thyroid hormone THYROXINE. The test involves swallowing a small amount of radioactive iodine in capsule or liquid form. Within a set period after taking the iodine, which may be 6 hours or 24 hours (or at both intervals), the amount of iodine taken up by the thyroid is measured by a counting instrument placed over the neck.

THYROID SCANNING produces an image of the gland that may aid in an evaluation of its functioning. Radioactive iodine is taken orally or injected. A gamma camera, which produces an image on a screen, is then used to reveal the radioactive substance that has collected in the thyroid.

Blood tests that indicate hormone levels in the bloodstream may be used to evaluate the function of the thyroid gland. Tests for blood levels of the thyroid hormone thyroxine and the pituitary hormone TSH (thyroid-stimulating hormone) can reveal aspects of thyroid function.

Thyroid gland

The largest gland in the ENDOCRINE SYSTEM, located under the larynx (voice box) and wrapped around the top of the trachea (windpipe). The thyroid gland consists of two lobes, one on each side of the windpipe, joined by a piece of tissue called the isthmus.

The thyroid tissue has two types of cells capable of secretion called follicular cells and parafollicular cells (or C cells). Most of the thyroid is made up of follicular cells, which are arranged in the form of hollow folli-

T

LOCATION OF THYROID
The thyroid gland wraps around the top of the trachea (windpipe) in the neck. Levels of the hormones secreted by the thyroid are controlled by the thyroid-stimulating hormone released by the pituitary gland, which in turn is controlled by the hypothalamus.

Thyroid cartilage (Adam's apple)

Thyroid gland

Trachea

cles supported by a loose fibrous tissue richly supplied with blood vessels. The follicles produce a number of hormones. Two of these, thyroxine and triiodothyronine, are iodine-based compounds that regulate body metabolism (the chemical activity in cells that releases energy from nutrients or uses energy to create other needed components, such as proteins). Insufficient thyroid hormone production is known as HYPOTHYROIDISM; an overproduction of thyroid hormones causes HYPERTHYROIDISM. The hormones are involved in many aspects of growth, development, and daily activity. Another thyroid hormone, calcitonin, regulates the calcium level in the bloodstream. The functions of the thyroid are regulated by the pituitary gland and the hypothalamus.

Thyroid hormones

Chemicals produced in the thyroid gland and released directly into the bloodstream by the thyroid. There are two thyroid hormones contained in the follicles of the gland in combination with the protein thyroglobulin. The first is THYROXINE and is composed of the amino acid tyrosine containing four iodine atoms. The other thyroid hormone is triiodothyronine (or T3) and is made up of tyrosine with three iodine atoms.

The thyroid hormones regulate metabolism and growth and are stimulated by TSH (thyroid-stimulating hormone) from the pituitary gland. Excessive production of the thyroid hormones produces an elevated metabolism and heightened activity, resulting in HYPERTHYROIDISM (overactivity of the thyroid gland). Insufficiency of thyroid hormone produces HYPOTHYROIDISM (underac-

tivity of the thyroid gland), a condition characterized by a reduced metabolism and feelings of lethargy.

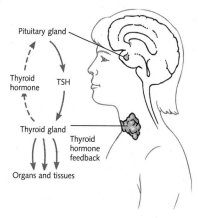

Pituitary gland

Thyroid hormone   TSH

Thyroid gland

Thyroid hormone feedback

Organs and tissues

THYROID HORMONE RESPONSE SYSTEM
The pituitary gland masterminds thyroid hormone activity by producing TSH (thyroid-stimulating hormone). TSH signals the thyroid glands to produce thyroid hormones. The pituitary gland detects even slight fluctuations in the level of thyroid hormones in the blood and adjusts production of TSH accordingly.

Thyroid nodule

A localized swelling in the THYROID GLAND. Thyroid nodules affect a small segment of the population, usually without symptoms. In rare instances, a thyroid nodule is an indication of THYROID CANCER. The nodules are more common in women but are more likely to be cancerous in men. Older people tend to develop nodules more often than younger people, and the nodules are more likely to be cancerous.

There are four types of thyroid nodules. The nodule may be a cyst filled with fluid, a benign (not cancerous) and degenerated ADENOMA, a slow-growing adenoma, or a cancerous

nodule. Usually, the remainder of the tissue in the thyroid gland is normal and thyroid function is not affected.

Several thyroid nodules sometimes develop in clusters forming a multinodular GOITER, a symptomless condition that occurs more commonly in older people. Cancer is rare in nodules associated with multinodular goiter, but it may be difficult to diagnose cancer in one nodule when many nodules are grouped together.

DIAGNOSIS
Because thyroid nodules are usually small, they do not exert pressure on other structures in the neck. As they are generally painless, the swelling may not be noticeable to the person with the nodule or by visual examination. The nodules are often discovered during routine physical examination. Benign thyroid nodules tend to be smooth, firm, and easily detected upon palpation of the neck. Cancerous nodules are usually hard. If the cancer has spread, the lymph nodes in the neck may be swollen. Further testing may be ordered to clarify a diagnosis of thyroid nodules.

Ultrasound scans can determine the size and location of the nodule and whether it is solid or contains fluid. If the nodule is a benign fluid-filled cyst, fine-needle aspiration (in which cells and fluid are drawn out of the nodule with a thin needle) often removes all or most of the fluid, and the cyst disappears.

THYROID SCANNING performed with the use of radioactive iodine may be implemented to provide diagnostic imaging of the nodule and the surrounding thyroid gland. Nodules that take up more iodine than the rest of the thyroid are called hot nodules. These may become overactive, produce excessive amounts of THYROXINE, and cause HYPERTHYROIDISM (overactivity of the thyroid gland). The nodules that do not take up radioactive iodine are called cold nodules. Cold nodules are more likely to be cancerous, but only a small percentage of cold nodules are thyroid cancers. Further tests, including biopsies, are often required to make a diagnosis.

TREATMENT
If a thyroid scan reveals a cold nodule, and further tests indicate that the nodule may be cancerous, the nodule will be surgically removed. If the cancer has spread to the lymph nodes

T

nearby in the neck, the lymph nodes must also be removed. Supplements of the thyroid hormone thyroxine must be taken for life after this surgery to prevent the formation of nodules on the remaining tissue.

Benign thyroid nodules are usually monitored regularly. They may be removed if they are growing, cause pressure on other neck structures, or are unsightly. If fluid-containing cysts return after fluid has been drawn out, they may be surgically removed.

Thyroxine medication may sometimes be taken to treat benign thyroid nodules. This hormone therapy is intended to inhibit the release of TSH (thyroid-stimulating hormone) from the pituitary and shrink the nodule. Thyroid nodules that contain fluid do not respond to thyroxine therapy.

Multinodular goiters may require surgical removal if they are large, grow, or interfere with breathing. Multinodular goiters are generally not treated with thyroxine as it is rare for thyroxine to shrink the nodules, and hyperthyroidism may result.

Thyroid scanning

A diagnostic procedure that generates an image of the thyroid gland. Thyroid scanning is one of several THYROID FUNCTION TESTS. The test is performed to determine the size, structure, and function of the thyroid gland and to diagnose the cause of an overactive thyroid. Thyroid scanning may be used to evaluate the activity or inactivity of a THYROID NODULE. It may also be used to determine the spread of THYROID CANCER.

Thyroid scanning is performed in conjunction with THYROID FUNCTION TESTS, one of which is called radioactive iodine uptake. Iodine is tagged with a radioisotope and injected into the person being tested. The thyroid gland absorbs the radioactive iodine, which highlights the gland on a scan. The person being tested lies facing upward with the neck extended. A camera detects the radioisotope that collects in the thyroid over a 20- to 30-minute period. An image of the thyroid tissue that has absorbed the radioactive iodine is produced and indicates a low or high intake of iodine by the gland. A low intake suggests an underactive thyroid gland or excessive supplementation of thyroid

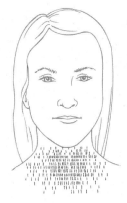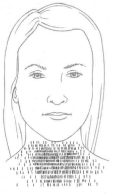

IMAGING THYROID ACTIVITY Part of thyroid function involves converting iodine into other chemical substances. This function can be measured by introducing radioactive iodine into the gland. In contrast with healthy thyroid activity, a scan of a hyperactive thyroid shows greatly increased activity required to convert the iodine.

Scan of healthy thyroid   Scan of hyperactive thyroid

medication. A high intake reveals an overactive thyroid gland. Thyroid scanning aids in evaluating thyroid function.

Thyroidectomy

Surgical removal of most or all of the thyroid gland. Thyroidectomy is performed to treat THYROID CANCER. It is generally followed with daily doses of thyroxine to prevent symptoms of hypothyroidism (underactivity of the thyroid gland).

Thyroiditis

Inflammation of the THYROID GLAND. Thyroiditis occurs in several different forms. The most common form of thyroiditis is HASHIMOTO THYROIDITIS. In Hashimoto thyroiditis, the thyroid becomes less efficient at converting iodine into the thyroid hormone THYROXINE. The gland then enlarges. Over time, production of TSH (thyroid-stimulating hormone) from the pituitary gland may increase to compensate, thyroxine levels drop, and HYPOTHYROIDISM (underactivity of the thyroid gland) results. Hashimoto thyroiditis is diagnosed by blood tests for thyroid antibodies. Depending on when thyroid hormone replacement therapy begins, the therapy prevents or corrects hypothyroidism and decreases the size of the thyroid or prevents it from enlarging.

In DE QUERVAIN DISEASE, the gland is tender and painful and swells rapidly. This form is less common than Hashimoto thyroiditis. The thyroid releases excessive amounts of thyroid hormone into the blood, causing HYPERTHYROIDISM (overactivity of the

thyroid gland). In response, the thyroid gland slows its uptake of iodine and produces less thyroid hormone so that the condition is resolved in a matter of weeks. The feelings of illness caused by de Quervain disease may require bed rest. One of the NONSTEROIDAL ANTI-INFLAMMATORY DRUGS (NSAIDs) may be recommended to reduce the inflammation in the gland. When the symptoms are prolonged, the medication cortisone may be prescribed to reduce inflammation, and thyroid hormones may be given to rest the overactive gland.

Silent thyroiditis is the least common form of this disease and usually occurs in young women after pregnancy. Diagnostic tests may indicate Hashimoto thyroiditis or de Quervain disease. Silent thyroiditis involves only a slight enlargement of the thyroid gland and frequently resolves within 3 months when the thyroid gland returns to normal. Medical treatment may involve BETA BLOCKERS to control rapid heart rates. Bed rest may be advised. In rare cases, permanent hypothyroidism results, and thyroid hormone replacement therapy becomes necessary.

Thyroid-stimulating hormone

See TSH.

Thyrotoxicosis

The general term for severe HYPERTHYROIDISM (overactivity of the thyroid gland). Thyrotoxicosis refers to the group of symptoms and physical changes associated with severe hyperthyroidism, regardless of the

T

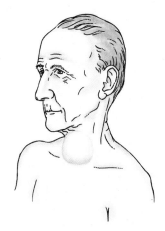

SEVERELY OVERACTIVE THYROID
In an older person, a condition called Plummer disease is the most common cause of an over-active thyroid, and a goiter (a swelling caused by an enlarged thyroid gland) is a typical symptom. In a younger person, the cause of thyrotoxicosis is usually Graves disease.

cause. Thyrotoxicosis is character-ized by nervousness, weakness, diffi-culty sleeping, increased appetite, restlessness, increased perspiration, muscle cramps, fatigue, excessive thirst, atrophy of muscles, tremor, menstrual irregularities, bulging eyes, unexplained weight loss, diarrhea, an intolerance to heat, an increased heart rate, and palpitations.

These symptoms are due to exces-sive production of the thyroid hor-mone THYROXINE, which leads to heightened metabolism. Tests and procedures including free thyroxine index, free triiodothyronine (or T3) blood level tests, radioactive iodine uptake tests, and TRH (thyrotropin-releasing hormone) tests may be given to diagnose thyrotoxicosis.

Thyrotoxicosis may be associated with GOITER and is sometimes a com-plication of GRAVES DISEASE. It can be fatal if congestive heart failure or PUL-MONARY EDEMA occur.

Thyrotropin-releasing hormone
See TRH.

Thyroxine
The principal metabolic hormone secreted by the thyroid glands; also known as T4. Thyroxine is produced in the thyroid gland by a synthesis of iodine with the amino acid tyro-sine. The thyroid gland requires

dietary iodine to produce thyroxine. Thyroxine molecules are composed of two joined tyrosine amino acids combined with four iodine atoms.

The synthesis and secretion of thy-roxine are regulated by TSH (thyroid-stimulating hormone), a hormone from the pituitary gland, and by thy-rotropin-releasing hormone (TRH), a hormone produced in the hypothala-mus. Thyroxine regulates the forma-tion of the two pituitary hormones.

Thyroxine is released by the thyroid in combination with the plasma protein globulin in the blood and dis-tributed to tissues that require the hormone in order to function. In the tissues, thyroxine is converted to tri-iodothyronine (T3) by removal of one iodine atom. Triiodothyronine is a more powerful hormone than thyrox-ine (see also THYROID HORMONES).

Thyroid hormone promotes the metabolism of glucose and fat by the liver and increases the release of cho-lesterol by the liver. It also regulates carbohydrate metabolism and the syn-thesis and breakdown of protein. In the digestive system, the hormone promotes the contractions of the smooth muscles and regulates the secretion of digestive juices. Thyrox-ine aids in the normal development, tone, and function of the muscles associated with the skeleton and the heart. Bone growth and regulation of the growth of the nervous system involve thyroxine; it also regulates the rate of oxygen use by the cells and the generation of body heat. Thyroxine is involved in fertility and the secretion of milk from the breasts of a lactating woman. Thyroid hormone also has a role in skin hydration, hair growth, and EXOCRINE GLAND secretions.

TIA
Also known as TRANSIENT ISCHEMIC ATTACK; a temporary loss of function in an area of the brain resulting from a reduced blood supply to the brain. A TIA is often a warning sign of an impending STROKE and requires eval-uation by a doctor. Medication or sur-gery may be indicated to prevent future TIAs and lessen the risk of developing a stroke.

Tibetan medicine
An ancient system of medical prac-tice that emphasizes the interdepend-ence of mind, body, and vitality for

mental and physical health. In Tibetan medicine, diagnosis involves listening to the person and examining his or her pulse, urine, and tongue—called the "three humors." Methods of therapy include diet, lifestyle mod-ification, HERBAL MEDICINE, and MOXI-BUSTION. Tibetan medicine is thought to be particularly successful in the treatment of chronic diseases, includ-ing arthritis, rheumatism, ulcers, asthma, eczema, anxiety, and various disorders of the nervous system.

Tic
A repetitive, rapid, sudden, and involuntary movement, spasm, or twitch that usually affects muscles in the face, neck, or shoulders, includ-ing the throat and voice. A person with a tic experiences the movement as irresistible but can suppress it for a limited period of time. Tics tend to worsen during periods of stress or focused concentration, such as public speaking or reading, and usually dis-appear during sleep. The action in a tic can be simple (for example, repeating a single word, grunting, or grimacing) or complex (for example, repeating phrases or sentences, jump-ing, or stamping the feet). Tics are common in children, particularly boys, and usually disappear as the child develops. As a result, tics are rare in adults. Tics can be precipitat-ed or worsened by stimulants, including medication used to treat attention deficit/hyperactivity disor-der in children. Tics are also a princi-pal feature of the neurological disor-der known as TOURETTE SYNDROME. The underlying cause of tics is unknown.

Tic douloureux
See TRIGEMINAL NEURALGIA.

Ticks and disease
The association of ticks as vectors of infection with the illnesses they may cause. Ticks are not technically insects, but are in the arachnid group, which also includes mites, spiders, and scorpions. Each tick has a single-segment body and harpoonlike barbs on its mouth that enable it to attach to a person for feeding on that person's blood. Other features of the tick, including a sticky substance it secretes and clinging, crablike legs, enhance the tick's ability to latch

TYPES OF TICKS
The very common American dog tick is found in the eastern states and California; it generally attacks only dogs. The wood tick is found in the western United States and may spread Rocky Mountain spotted fever, Colorado tick fever, and tularemia. The Lone Star tick is common in Texas and Louisiana and is associated with the spread of Rocky Mountain spotted fever.

American dog tick — ⅙ inch (4 mm)
Wood tick — 1/10 inch (2.5 mm)
Lone Star tick — ⅛ inch (3 mm)

PREVENTING OR TREATING TICK BITES

In any region that may be tick-infested and where temperatures exceed 40°F, it is wise to avoid direct contact with foliage, soil, leaf litter, and vegetation as much as possible. People who enjoy gardening, hiking, camping, hunting, or working outdoors or who need to spend time in the woods, brushy areas, or overgrown fields should take the following precautions against being bitten by ticks:

- Enclosed shoes, preferably boots reaching the ankle, will help protect the feet and lower legs. Pant legs should be tucked into boot tops; if shoes are worn, then heavy socks should also be worn and pant legs should be tucked into socks.
- Light-colored clothing made of tight-weave fabric offers the best protection from ticks. Long sleeves with fitted cuffs and long pants are preferable. Shirts should be tucked into pants.
- Repellent containing permethrin should be used on clothing when spending time in tick-infested areas. The repellent should be sprayed on clothing before it is worn and allowed to dry thoroughly before it is put on.
- A repellent containing DEET may be applied to exposed skin before spending time in tick-infested areas. Formulations containing up to 30 percent DEET are recommended for adults; 10 percent DEET formulations are appropriate for children. DEET repellents should be used sparingly as they may cause breathing difficulties, especially in children and in people with asthma.
- Clothing and exposed skin should be examined often during time spent outdoors, even when repellents are used. A thorough head-to-toe examination for ticks should be made after time spent outdoors.
- When hiking, staying on cleared, well-traveled trails and paths generally offers less exposure to tick populations than densely wooded areas. Sitting directly on the ground or on stone walls where there may be mice, chipmunks, and other small mammals that harbor ticks should be avoided.
- Long hair should be tied back or preferably tucked into a hat.
- Clothing worn outdoors in tick-infested areas should be laundered or spun in the hot cycle of a clothes dryer for at least 20 minutes to kill any clinging ticks.
- Bathing and shampooing are not completely effective at removing tenacious ticks, particularly deer tick nymphs, which are the size of a poppy seed, and even mature deer tick adults, which are only as big as a sesame seed.
- If a tick is found attached to the skin, these steps may be followed to remove it: Tweezers should be used to grasp the tick by its mouthparts where they enter the skin; care should be taken to avoid pulling the tick's body away from the head, leaving the head embedded in the skin, as the infectious organisms can be transmitted via the tick's head alone. When the tick's head is firmly grasped with tweezers, it should be pulled out steadily without jerking. Twisting, applying petroleum jelly, a hot match, or alcohol should be avoided as these techniques can increase the risk of transmitting infection. The tick should be placed in a container of alcohol when removed. A doctor can identify the species and its potential for causing disease. The bite wound should be thoroughly cleaned with disinfectant.
- It is important to remove ticks as soon as possible and not to panic. Infectious organisms are not usually transmitted until the tick has been feeding from 24 to 72 hours.

onto a person or animal. In addition to humans, potential hosts for ticks include all wild birds and mammals, as well as domestic pets.

Ticks can transmit infectious organisms from one host to another, and these organisms may cause disease in humans. Among the diseases caused by ticks are LYME DISEASE, ROCKY MOUNTAIN SPOTTED FEVER, RELAPSING FEVER, BABESIOSIS, and ehrlichiosis (see HUMAN GRANULOCYTIC EHRLICHIOSIS; HUMAN MONOCYTIC EHRLICHIOSIS). Lyme disease is the most frequently reported tick-borne disease, and Rocky Mountain spotted fever is the next most prevalent, although it occurs much more rarely than Lyme disease.

Ticks have a four-stage life cycle, lasting a year or more. An adult female can lay as many as 6,000 eggs in a single batch. The eggs hatch into six-legged larvae, which molt into eight-legged nymphs after at least one blood meal from a host person or animal. Some species molt more than once at this stage. In a final molting, the nymphs develop into eight-legged adults.

There are about 200 different species of ticks in the United States. Their habitats include the woods, beach grass, lawns, forests, and sometimes, urban areas. Deer ticks, the primary transmitters of two of the more prevalent tick-borne diseases, Lyme disease and ehrlichiosis, are found underneath leaf litter or clinging to low vegetation in shady, moist areas. Lawns, gardens, sheds, and old stone walls at the edge of woodlands are often inhabited by ticks.

Ticlopidine hydrochloride

A drug used to reduce the risk of stroke. Ticlopidine hydrochloride (Ticlid) is given to people known to be at risk for stroke, such as a person who has already had one. Ticlopidine prevents specific cells in the body (platelets) from clumping together to start forming a blood clot that could block blood flow to the brain, which is what causes a stroke.

Tietze syndrome
See COSTOCHONDRITIS.

Timolol
A beta blocker used to treat high blood pressure. Timolol (Blocadren) is also used to treat heart attacks and

arrhythmias. Timolol, in combination with the diuretic hydrochlorothiazide (Timolide), is used to lower blood pressure and decrease edema (swelling). By itself (Timoptic) or in combination with another drug (Cosopt), timolol is used as an eye drop to treat glaucoma and reduce pressure within the eye.

Tinea

A general term for a group of related skin infections caused by different species of fungi; or a fungal skin infection characterized by ring-shaped, red, scaly, or blistery patches. Fungi thrive in warm moist areas and cause tinea infections such as JOCK ITCH (tinea cruris) in the groin area and ATHLETE'S FOOT (tinea pedis) between the toes. Other locations of tinea include the body (tinea corporis), the face (tinea faciei), and scalp (tinea capitis). Tinea versicolor is a fungal infection characterized by a rash consisting of white or brown patches on the trunk.

CAUSES AND SYMPTOMS

Tinea can affect virtually any area of the skin. The different types of tinea take their names from the location of the infection or its appearance rather than the particular fungus that is the cause of the problem. Tinea infections are caused by moldlike fungi called dermatophytes.

The source of fungal infection can be the soil, an animal (such as a cat, dog, or rodent), or another person. Factors such as poor hygiene and immune deficiencies increase susceptibility to infection. In athlete's foot and jock itch, friction, moisture, sweating, and a lack of proper ventilation have a role. Teenagers and adult men are most susceptible to athlete's foot and jock itch, while tinea capitis most commonly affects children. The patchy discoloration of tinea versicolor is seen primarily in adolescents and young adults.

The most common symptoms of tinea are itching, redness, and a circular lesion with inflamed, spreading borders and a clear center. However, symptoms vary according to the site of the infection and its severity. For example, most cases of athlete's foot are characterized by a red, scaly, cracked rash between the toes. However, in some people, athlete's foot manifests as blistering or as redness and scaling on the soles and sides of the feet.

Symptoms of jock itch include itching of the groin and a scaly red skin rash with sharply defined borders. Usually the genitals are not involved, but there may be anal itching and discomfort. Jock itch often spreads in a circular rash, leaving normal-appearing skin in the center. In fungal infections of the scalp, swollen, tender masses of dandrufflike scales and broken stubbles of hair may develop.

DIAGNOSIS AND TREATMENT

To obtain proper treatment, it is essential to distinguish tinea from other skin problems such as dermatitis or psoriasis. Diagnosis is made through evaluating the appearance of the skin and tests such as a skin scraping. A small sample of skin is removed and examined under a microscope or is cultured in special media to detect possible fungus growth.

Simple cases of tinea respond well to treatment with antifungal creams or powders that contain clotrimazole, miconazole, econazole, or ciclopirox. Severe infections require oral antifungal medications such as terbinafine or itraconazole. Possible complications of tinea include secondary bacterial infections, which must be treated with antibiotics. It is also essential to keep the skin clean and dry. Good general hygiene can help prevent or control tinea infections.

Tinea versicolor

A fungal infection of the skin. Tinea versicolor is characterized by a rash consisting of scaly white and tan patches on the upper arms, chest, and back. The majority of people who develop the infection are teenagers or young adults. See TINEA.

Tinel sign

A diagnostic test in a doctor's physical examination involving the tapping of the skin over an injured area to elicit a tingling sensation from a nerve. The Tinel sign may be used by a physician as part of the procedure for diagnosing CARPAL TUNNEL SYNDROME. In this case, the skin of the wrist is tapped at the point where the tunnel compresses the nerve as it enters the palm. If carpal tunnel syndrome is present, this stimulus may elicit tingling in the nerve of the hand. The Tinel sign is also a valuable indication that an injured nerve is undergoing repair and beginning to regenerate.

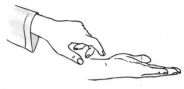

A TINGLING SENSATION
A doctor may lightly tap the skin over a particular nerve to see if it causes tingling farther along the length of the nerve. The so-called Tinel sign indicates injury to the nerve or the beginning of the recovery of an injured nerve.

Tingling

An abnormal, prickling feeling in the skin. Tingling may be a sign of damage or irritation to nerves in the affected area. It can also be a sign of poor circulation. It is a different problem than NUMBNESS, which suggests instead that the nerve is indeed damaged. A brief tingling sensation, as when a person's hand or foot "falls asleep," is not a cause for concern. However, a persistent tingling or PINS AND NEEDLES SENSATION may be caused by medical problems, such as nerve injury; lack of blood supply; diabetes mellitus, type 1 and type 2; thyroid problems; vitamin B12 (cyanocobalamin) deficiency; carpal tunnel syndrome; transient ischemic attack; stroke; or multiple sclerosis.

Tinnitus

The sensation of persistent or intermittent ringing, hissing, tinkling, whistling, roaring, buzzing, chirping, or other abnormal sounds in the ears or head in the absence of external sound. The tones may be single or multiple. The sensation can cause minimal discomfort or be severe and extremely disturbing. The condition, often described as ringing in the ears, is sometimes associated with hearing impairment. Subjective tinnitus is the term for head sounds heard only by the person with the condition. Objective tinnitus, caused by abnormalities in blood vessels around the outside of the ear or by muscle spasms (see SPASM), produces clicking or crackling sounds inside the middle ear that may be audible to others.

CAUSES

Most instances of tinnitus are due to damage to the microscopic endings of the hearing nerve in the inner ear. The damage may be associated with advancing age. Exposure to loud noise is the leading cause of tinnitus, which can cause hearing impairment as well. When tinnitus is caused by exposure to loud noise, it may occur gradually or it may occur suddenly at a high volume and be permanent.

Temporary tinnitus may result from a small plug of earwax. Otosclerosis (hardening of the middle ear bones) can cause tinnitus. Other possible causes include allergies, ear or sinus infections, a perforated eardrum (see EARDRUM, PERFORATED), jaw misalignment, high or low blood pressure, anemia, a tumor, disease in the cortex of the brain, diabetes mellitus, thyroid problems, cardiovascular disease, or injuries in the head and neck area.

DIAGNOSIS AND TREATMENT

Finding the specific cause of tinnitus may require extensive testing under the supervision of an otolaryngologist and an audiologist. The audiologist may perform a complete hearing evaluation, including AUDIOMETRY and other hearing tests. An otoacoustic emission test may be given to evaluate the actual structures that convert sound into nerve energy. Other tests may include X rays, imaging techniques, balance tests, and laboratory analysis. Ear infections, a perforated eardrum, and earwax buildup are treatable conditions, and treatment may stop tinnitus. However, in many cases, the cause of tinnitus cannot be determined, and treatment of symptoms is the focus of medical care. Medication to ease the associated stress, depression, and sleep disorders may be helpful.

If there is also hearing loss, a hearing aid set at a low level can reduce the level of sound and temporarily eliminate it for some individuals. A device called a tinnitus masker can be combined with a hearing aid or worn separately to produce a low-level, pleasant, neutral sound that can reduce or eliminate the perception of tinnitus. Sometimes the reduction or elimination of tinnitus continues for a short time after the masker is removed, a phenomenon called residual inhibition.

Therapy to help correct tinnitus sometimes focuses on the brain. Masking the noise may help reduce the discomfort from tinnitus. For example, tinnitus retraining therapy (TRT) involves wearing a small, low-level, white noise generator behind or in the ear, combined with intensive counseling to help a person learn to ignore or become accustomed to the sounds of tinnitus. The therapy has a success rate of about 80 percent. When tinnitus is related to temporomandibular joint disorder, or TMJ (see CLICKING JAW), a condition in which the joints, muscles, and ligaments of the jaw do not function properly, treatment of the condition may help eliminate the head noise.

Music can be played to mask the head noise. Concentration and relaxation exercises may reduce the intensity of tinnitus by helping to control muscle groups and circulation throughout the body.

Other self-help techniques to reduce the severity of tinnitus include avoiding exposure to loud noise; controlling high blood pressure under medical supervision; avoiding salt (which impairs blood circulation); getting regular exercise to improve circulation; and avoiding stimulants such as coffee, tea, cola, and tobacco (see TOBACCO CHEWING; SMOKING, TOBACCO). Support groups may help people cope with the associated stress of tinnitus.

Tirofiban

An anticoagulant drug to prevent formation of blood clots in blood vessels. Tirofiban (Aggrastat) works by interfering with the process by which blood clots, chiefly by inhibiting the clumping of platelets. In combination with HEPARIN, tirofiban is given as an injection both before and after open-heart surgery to prevent the formation of clots in blood vessels. It is also used to treat acute coronary syndrome, which is acute blood flow blockage in the heart.

Tissue

Any group of similar cells arranged to perform a particular function. The body consists of four types of tissue. Epithelial tissue forms the skin and mucous membranes that line organs and structures such as the respiratory system, the blood vessels, stomach, vagina, and intestine. Connective tissue, such as fat and tendons, supports and protects structures in the body. Muscle tissue, which has three distinct varieties (skeletal, smooth, and cardiac) helps move the limbs and forms much of the heart, lungs, and other internal organs. Nerve tissue, which makes up the cells called neurons, receives and conducts electrochemical impulses. The brain, spinal cord, and nerves are composed of nerve tissue.

Tissue plasminogen activator (t-PA)

See ALTEPLASE.

Tissue salts therapy

The use of certain minerals thought to promote health by correcting deficiencies at the cellular level. Tissue salts therapy, or the Schuessler biochemic system of medicine, was developed in the 1890s by a German doctor, scientist, and homeopath who identified 12 principal mineral salts he believed essential to health. In the Schuessler system, biochemic tissue salts are considered to be minerals in energy form, essential in cell formation and normally derived from organically grown plant foods eaten raw. Because of chemical additives and poor soil treatment, Schuessler believed the mineral and vitamin content of plant foods had diminished to levels inadequate for proper cell development. Symptoms of tissue salt deficiencies include signs of premature facial aging that are read by trained facial analysis therapists, who work out individual mineral replacement regimens for people, depending on their symptoms. The therapy is not clinically proven.

Tissue-typing

A laboratory test for identifying compatible tissue in prospective organ donors and recipients. Tissue-typing allows the transplant surgical team to determine the recipient best suited to receive a particular donor organ. Tissue-typing helps reduce the chances of rejection by closely matching the IMMUNE SYSTEM of the donor to that of the recipient.

The principal hurdle to successful transplant surgery is the immune system of the recipient. Designed to detect and destroy invading microorganisms and other foreign matter, the immune system treats the transplanted organ as an invader and attacks it.

T

Over time, the immune reaction can cause the body to reject the transplant. In kidney transplants, the most common type of transplant surgery, about five of every ten people who undergo the surgery experience rejection within 10 years.

Tissue-typing consists of identifying specific proteins, called antigens (see ANTIGEN), that reside on the surfaces of the white blood cells (LYMPHOCYTES). Together, these antigens make up the human leukocyte antigen (HLA) system. The HLA system plays a central role in helping the immune system distinguish the healthy cells of the body from those infected by invading microorganisms.

TMJ syndrome

Also known as temporomandibular joint disorder; see CLICKING JAW.

Tobacco chewing

Using tobacco that is not smoked but is placed in the mouth. When tobacco is chewed or placed between the cheek and gum, nicotine mixes with the saliva and enters the bloodstream through the mucous membrane lining the mouth. Smokeless tobacco produces the same nicotine drug response as tobacco smoking, but without the need to inhale smoke into the lungs. It is every bit as addictive as smoked tobacco.

In recent years, as the health effects of tobacco smoking have become more widely known, some smokers have turned to smokeless tobacco (snuff and chewing tobacco) as an alternative.

While smokeless tobacco reduces the risk of cancer of the respiratory tract associated with smoking, it poses serious health risks of its own. An increased risk of cancer of the mouth, particularly in the cheek and gum, is associated with smokeless tobacco. It is also linked to a higher incidence of cancer of the larynx, esophagus, and pancreas. In addition, smokeless tobacco can increase the growth of bacteria that cause dental cavities and also causes severe inflammation of the gums (periodontal disease), which can result in the loss of teeth.

Tobacco smoking

See SMOKING, TOBACCO.

Tobramycin

An antibiotic; one of the AMINOGLYCOSIDES. Tobramycin (TOBI) is administered by inhalation to treat cystic fibrosis. As eye drops, tobramycin (Tobrex) is used to treat bacterial infections of the eye. In the hospital, the drug is sometimes given intravenously to treat serious and life-threatening infections.

Tocopherol

See VITAMIN E.

Toe

One of the five digits of the foot, similar in skeletal structure to the FINGER. The toe consists of skin and connective tissue enclosing two or three joined bones called phalanges, which are connected by tendons to muscles in the foot and lower leg. The phalanges join at hinge joints, which are moved by tendons that flex or extend the toe. The main function of the toes is to help the body maintain balance and exert forward motion during walking or running.

Toenail, ingrown

See INGROWN TOENAIL.

Toilet training

Various methods for helping a child gradually achieve bowel and bladder control. Most children are not ready for toilet training until age 2, although it is also normal to begin a little later. Toilet training requires time, understanding, and patience on the part of parents. The process should be as natural and nonthreatening as possible.

The child must be physically and emotionally ready to toilet train. A child is physically prepared when he or she realizes when a diaper has been wet or soiled, can stay dry for 2 hours during the day, is dry after a nap, seems uncomfortable when a diaper is wet or soiled, asks for a diaper change, has regular bowel movements, can follow instructions, can use the potty-chair, and asks to wear underwear or use the potty-chair. Emotional readiness is apparent when a child is interested in the process and wants to participate in it. If a child appears uncooperative or reluctant, the process should be postponed till he or she is ready.

Training usually begins around age

Potty-seat   Potty-chair

POTTY-CHAIRS OR SEATS
For a small child just learning to use the toilet, a potty-chair (right) is easier to use than a regular toilet because the feet can rest on the floor. For a larger child, a potty-seat that fits over the toilet may also be helpful.

2 and takes about 4 months. During training, the child is reminded every hour to use the potty-chair. A potty-chair is easier for small children to use than a toilet because their feet can rest on the floor. Loose-fitting pants and underpants are recommended. Bowel training is ordinarily successful before bladder control. The child can learn to recognize the signs of an impending bowel movement in time to do something about it. Signs of urination are more urgent, and responding to them is more difficult. The child must also learn to relax the muscles that control the bowel and bladder. Nap and nighttime toilet training generally takes longer than daytime training. Most children have bowel and daytime urination under control by age 3 to 3½. Nighttime bladder control is generally achieved by 5 to 6 years of age. If bedwetting continues beyond age 6, a pediatrician or family doctor should be consulted.

Tolterodine tartrate

A drug used to relieve spasms of the bladder. Tolterodine tartrate (Detrol) tablets are used to treat symptoms associated with spasms of the bladder, such as frequent urination, urinary urgency, and urinary incontinence.

Tongue

The muscular, flexible organ on the floor of the mouth that functions in TASTE, chewing, SWALLOWING, and speaking. The tongue is formed by internal bands of striated muscle. External muscle attached to the bones of the mouth hold it in place. The surface of the tongue is covered with a mucous membrane dotted with structures called papillae. Taste buds located on the surface of the tongue detect sweet, salty, bitter, and acidic flavors and stimulate the salivary glands beneath the tongue to produce saliva. The tongue helps mix chewed food with saliva to start the process of digestion and helps consolidate chewed food in the mouth in preparation for swallowing. Positioning and movement of the tongue also are involved in speech production. Fissures or crevices on the tongue are common and usually are not cause for concern, although food can get caught in the fissures.

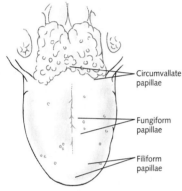

PROJECTIONS ON THE TONGUE
Tiny projections called papillae cover the tongue. Filiform (threadlike) papillae are the most numerous; they do not contain taste buds but sense the feel of food in the mouth. Fungiform (mushroomlike) papillae contain taste buds, as do the large circumvallate (wall-like) papillae at the back of the tongue.

Tongue cancer

A malignant tumor on the tongue that begins as a small lump or a thick, firm white patch. In time, the lump or patch becomes an ulcer with a firm, raised rim and a sensitive center that may bleed readily. This is a SQUAMOUS CELL CARCINOMA, meaning that when viewed under the microscope, the cells of the cancer are relatively flat, like skin cells. If left untreated, tongue cancer may spread throughout the mouth to the gums, floor of the mouth, lower jaw, and neck. Eventually, it can spread into other organs of the body, often the lungs. If the tumor enlarges, the tongue can become stiff and rigid. A large tumor can block the throat, interfering with normal speaking, swallowing, and breathing. It is one of the more serious forms of cancer that can occur in

the mouth. Tongue cancer occurs most often in people who use tobacco, consume large amounts of alcohol, or wear dentures. Tongue cancer generally affects people aged 50 or older, but it sometimes occurs, for unknown reasons, in young adults who are nonsmokers.

DIAGNOSIS AND TREATMENT
A dentist often detects the first signs of tongue cancer during a routine dental examination. A growth on the tongue that may be painless and lasts more than 10 to 20 days, becomes worse, or spreads rapidly should be examined by an otolaryngologist (a specialist in disorders of the ear, nose, and throat and related structures). The doctor will examine the tongue and mouth and possibly recommend a biopsy of the growth. The biopsy, performed under local anesthesia, involves the removal of a tissue sample for laboratory analysis.

Treatment is generally determined by an oncologist (cancer specialist), based on the stage or spread of the disease. Radiation therapy, chemotherapy, or surgery to remove the tumor may be recommended. A small tumor on the tongue may be removed with little effect on the tongue's function or the appearance of the mouth. If it is necessary to remove a larger portion of the tongue, lymph glands, or jaw during surgery, reconstructive surgery may be necessary to restore the function and appearance of these structures. Rarely, laser surgery may be done. Speech therapy can help patients adjust after treatment. Cancer support groups may help people cope during the treatment and recovery periods.

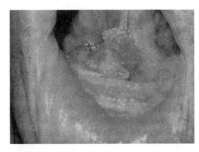

CANCER OF THE TONGUE
Smoking and drinking are known risk factors for tongue cancer. Squamous cell carcinoma, shown here, is by far the most common type of tongue cancer. Surgery for tongue cancer may affect swallowing and speech.

Tongue depressor

An instrument used to press down the tongue. A tongue depressor is a disposable, wooden, flat, sticklike device used by a doctor during a medical examination to press down the tongue so that the mouth and throat can be properly examined.

Tongue-tie

A condition present at birth in which the membrane under the tongue, called the frenulum, extends farther than usual toward the tip of the tongue, limiting forward and upward movement. The tongue tip is often notched and heart-shaped. The medical term for the condition is ankyloglossia. Tongue-tie is not usually considered a problem in healthy infants. However, if the restricted movement of the tongue interferes with a newborn's ability to suck, it may result in inadequate milk supply and low weight gain in the baby. In a breast-feeding mother, the nipples may become sore from the baby's struggle to suck. Frenotomy (surgical cutting of the frenulum) may be recommended. The condition does not cause problems beyond the first 2 to 3 years of life.

Tonometry

A test that measures pressure within the eyes. Tonometry is used to test for GLAUCOMA, a disease in which rising pressure inside the eyeball may impair vision.

There are three types of tonometry. In Schiøtz tonometry, the person being tested lies face up, and a drop of anesthetic is placed in each eye. While the person looks at a spot on the ceiling, the tonometer is placed on the surface of one eye, then the other, to measure the pressure. Applanation tonometry involves the use of the SLIT LAMP. Fluorescein dye is placed in the eyes, along with anesthetic drops. While the person being tested rests his or her head and chin on supports, the slit lamp is swung into place and the tonometer is brought into contact with the surface of the eye. The eye specialist looks through the slit lamp while he or she adjusts the tonometer. In air puff tonometry, a brief puff of air is blown into the eye while the person being tested stares straight ahead and a bright focused light is shined into the eye. The instrument reads the pressure from the change in light reflected off the cornea during the air puff. No anesthetic is needed. This method of tonometry is less accurate than the others, and it is performed less frequently than applanation tonometry.

Tonsillectomy

Surgical removal of the TONSILS as a treatment for severe, recurrent TONSIL-LITIS or for tonsils that obstruct the airway. A tonsillectomy is most commonly performed on children who are 6 or 7 years old. Because the tonsils and adenoids are now known to be important to the body's immune system, tonsillectomy is no longer recommended as a preventive treatment in children, nor is it considered a routine medical treatment for tonsillitis. Generally, if a child gets tonsillitis with high fever three or more times a year, the doctor will advise that tonsillectomy is also warranted.

The operation is also sometimes recommended when an abscess (collection of pus) develops on the tonsils or when a child has difficulty swallowing due to inflamed tonsils. Obstructed breathing due to enlarged tonsils may indicate the need for tonsillectomy. Such children will snore loudly and have obstructive SLEEP APNEA SYNDROME. In adults, tonsillectomy is usually performed only as a biopsy for cancer in the area of the tonsils or adenoids.

The adenoids (clusters of tissue above the soft palate) may become inflamed with tonsillitis and may sometimes be removed at the same time as the tonsils, a procedure called adenoidectomy. An ORTHODONTIST may recommend this procedure if mouth breathing due to enlarged adenoids results in malformations of the face and improper alignment of the teeth. Adenoidectomy may be helpful for chronic middle ear and eustachian tube problems.

The surgery is performed with the person under an anesthetic, usually with an overnight stay in the hospital. The person may be required to remain for up to 24 hours. Occasionally, bleeding or fever occurs after surgery; these complications, and other signs of infection, require immediate medical attention. After a tonsillectomy, a person may experience vomiting, swallowing problems, ear pain, or a sore throat that can last for 2 or more weeks after the operation.

Tonsillitis

An inflammation of the TONSILS, the two small masses of tissue at the back of the mouth, on both sides of the throat. Tonsillitis may occur intermittently and is caused by an infection, most commonly from viruses or the *Streptococcus* bacteria. The tonsils help filter out and fight bacteria and viruses that enter the body through the mouth and nose. When the tonsils become overwhelmed by infectious organisms, they become inflamed. Tonsillitis is a common childhood illness, most often affecting children between the ages of 5 and 10 years.

SYMPTOMS

Tonsillitis causes the tonsils to swell and become redder than usual. The tonsils may be observed by examining the inside of a child's open mouth with the tongue out. Attached to the back of the throat, the tonsils are located on either side of the uvula, the small appendage hanging from the back of the mouth's roof. The throat is usually sore, and the voice may be changed somewhat as a result of the swelling caused by tonsillitis. Swallowing may be uncomfortable or painful. The lymph nodes (see LYMPH NODE) in the neck may become swollen and tender. There may be fever, chills, coughing, headache, and foul-smelling breath. A white or yellow coating or white specks may appear on the tonsils within a few days of the onset of infection. If the infection becomes severe, a child may experience ear pain and have difficulty breathing. Breathing problems may lead to snoring and sleep problems. In babies, tonsillitis causes irritability and a hoarse or throaty cry. The infant may refuse feedings.

DIAGNOSIS AND TREATMENT

A doctor examines the tonsils and collects a sample of cells for laboratory analysis to identify the infectious agent. Antibiotics, such as penicillin, are prescribed to treat bacterial infections; symptoms usually disappear within 2 or 3 days. Bed rest, plenty of fluids and soft foods, and nonprescription painkillers, such as acetaminophen (not aspirin, which is associated with REYE SYNDROME in children) may relieve discomfort during recovery. In severe, recurrent, or resistant cases of tonsillitis, removal of the tonsils is recommended (see TONSILLECTOMY).

Tonsils

Small oval masses of lymphatic tissue in the mouth and throat (pharynx). Technically, there are three pairs of tonsils; they are located at the base of the tongue (lingual tonsils), in the throat just behind the tongue (palatine tonsils), and close to the opening of the nasal cavity into the pharynx (pharyngeal tonsils; also known as ADENOIDS). Tonsils are large in children, shrinking slowly after age 3. The pharyngeal tonsils disappear completely by adulthood, and the palatine tonsils decrease to the size of almonds. The tonsils filter and destroy infectious material entering the body through the mouth and nose. Invading bacteria or viruses can cause the tonsils to become inflamed, swollen, and painful to the touch—signs that they are doing their job and helping prevent further infection. In

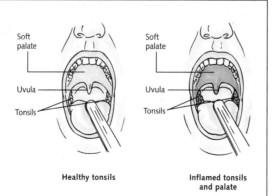

INFECTED TONSILS
The tonsils are visible on either side of the back of the throat. They are larger before about age 7, when they start to shrink. A child with tonsillitis has swollen, inflamed tonsils that are coated with pus. The swelling may interfere with breathing. The adenoids, which are clusters of tissue above the soft palate, may also become infected and need to be removed along with the tonsils.

Soft palate
Uvula
Tonsils

Soft palate
Uvula
Tonsils

Healthy tonsils

Inflamed tonsils and palate

the past, children's tonsils were removed almost routinely, but now surgery is used only in cases of repeated and severe infections. See TONSILLITIS; TONSILLECTOMY.

Tooth abscess

An accumulation of pus that is enclosed in the bone tissue at the tip of the root in a tooth. The cause of a tooth abscess is usually a bacterial infection in the pulp, which produces pus that drains out of the opening at the tip of the root. The infection may originate in untreated TOOTH DECAY or in dead pulp tissue inside the tooth. If there is bacteria in gum tissue that has severely receded or if bacteria remain in the gum surrounding the root of a tooth following a ROOT CANAL TREATMENT, the bacteria may produce an abscess.

SYMPTOMS AND TREATMENT

A tooth abscess causes persistent toothache or throbbing pain at the site. Biting and chewing often cause extreme pain. The side of the face may swell. In response to the infection, glands in the neck may become swollen and tender and there may be a fever.

If a tooth abscess is the result of a completely infected PERMANENT TOOTH located in the back of the jaw, or a PRIMARY TOOTH, the dentist may extract the tooth. In many cases, if enough tooth structure remains, the tooth can be saved by performing root canal treatment. If the abscess has not burst, the first stage of root canal treatment will be to create an opening into the pulp chamber, release the pressure created by the pus in the enclosed abscess, and relieve the pain. The dentist may leave an opening in the tooth to allow the abscess to drain before completing the root canal treatment at a later visit. If infected tissue outside the root of the tooth needs to be removed, this is accomplished in a procedure called an APICOECTOMY after completion of root canal treatment.

If an abscess is not treated promptly, it will begin to erode the bone at the tip of the root in the tooth. The erosion may extend toward the gum and form a narrow, pus-filled canal that causes swelling. If the abscess bursts, the canal carries the pus to an opening, called a FISTULA, on the surface of the gum. Foul-tasting pus

drains into the mouth, and the severe pain caused by the abscess is immediately relieved. At this stage, the infection can easily spread throughout the body, creating a feeling of general illness. A risk of BLOOD POISONING exists, and the infection will persist until treated with antibiotics.

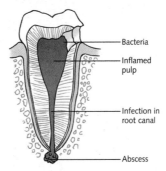

Bacteria

Inflamed pulp

Infection in root canal

Abscess

ABSCESSED TOOTH
If bacteria invade the pulp (soft inner tissue) of a tooth, the infection can produce pus that drains down into the root tip and accumulates there. The resulting tooth abscess is extremely painful. Left untreated, the infection will erode the bone. An abscess may be treated by root canal treatment or by pulling the tooth.

Tooth decay

The decalcification and disintegration of the structure of a tooth from plaque (see PLAQUE, DENTAL) and acid-producing food deposits on the TEETH. The acids dissolve the hard mineral enamel covering the surface of the teeth, creating a small hole, or cavity (see CAVITY, DENTAL), in the enamel. Tooth decay originates with this break in the protective outer layer of the tooth. If the small cavity is not treated, the acid continues to destroy the enamel until it has penetrated this layer and begins to damage the DENTIN below the enamel. Decay through the dentin allows bacteria to enter the inner area of the tooth, called the pulp chamber, which contains the pulp (see PULP, DENTAL) or nerve of the tooth. Ultimately, tooth decay can destroy the vital tissues at the core of a tooth and cause the tooth to die.

PREVENTION

Tooth decay is prevented by taking care of the teeth and following good ORAL HYGIENE practices, including brushing the teeth at least twice a day with a fluoride-containing toothpaste and using dental floss (see FLOSS, DENTAL) at least once a day.

Limiting starches and sugars in the diet is another way to prevent tooth decay. Sugary foods, such as sweetened soft drinks, candy, ice cream, cakes, and cookies, leave deposits on the teeth that interact with plaque to form acids that cause tooth decay. Starchy fruits and vegetables can also have this effect. It is important to remove the deposits these foods leave by brushing the teeth as soon as possible afterward.

Because pain may not be felt until tooth decay has progressed, regular dental checkups, at least every 6 months, are important. A dentist may recommend preventive techniques, including professional cleanings, fluoride treatments, and dental sealants (see SEALANTS, DENTAL) to help protect the teeth from tooth decay. Dental X rays are also needed to check under old fillings and in between teeth for decay.

TREATMENT

At a dental examination, the dentist will probe each tooth to check for signs of decay. The decay can be removed with a dental drill, and the tooth can be cleaned and filled with an amalgam or composite filling (see AMALGAM, DENTAL; BONDING, DENTAL). This prevents the decay from spreading, which can lead to the need for ROOT CANAL TREATMENT and, in cases of severe decay, TOOTH EXTRACTION.

Tooth eruption

The emergence of the PRIMARY TEETH and the PERMANENT TEETH as they appear above the gum line. Tooth eruption of the primary teeth generally begins with the bottom central incisors (the front teeth) when an infant is 6 months old and is completed when the second molars come in at the age of about 24 months. The primary teeth typically erupt in a fairly regular sequence from the front of the mouth to the back. They are shed in about the same sequence, with the first teeth to erupt being the first to be shed, usually starting at about the age of 6 or 7 years. At that age, the heavier, larger permanent teeth, which have developed within the gum below the primary teeth, usually begin to erupt. By the time a child is 11½ or 12 years old, he or she has often shed all the primary teeth and acquired most of the permanent teeth, with the exception of the

T

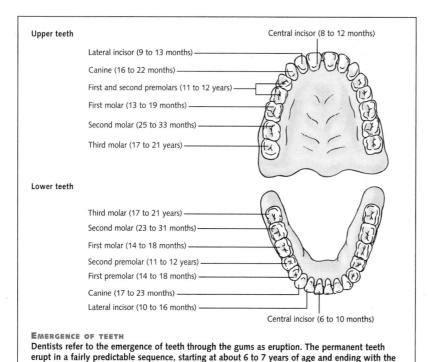

Upper teeth

Central incisor (8 to 12 months)
Lateral incisor (9 to 13 months)
Canine (16 to 22 months)
First and second premolars (11 to 12 years)
First molar (13 to 19 months)
Second molar (25 to 33 months)
Third molar (17 to 21 years)

Lower teeth

Third molar (17 to 21 years)
Second molar (23 to 31 months)
First molar (14 to 18 months)
Second premolar (11 to 12 years)
First premolar (14 to 18 months)
Canine (17 to 23 months)
Lateral incisor (10 to 16 months)
Central incisor (6 to 10 months)

EMERGENCE OF TEETH
Dentists refer to the emergence of teeth through the gums as eruption. The permanent teeth erupt in a fairly predictable sequence, starting at about 6 to 7 years of age and ending with the last wisdom teeth in the early 20s.

second and third molars (wisdom teeth).

Some pain may be experienced with the normal eruption of teeth. The pain may be caused by a loose primary tooth pinching the gum or by an erupting permanent tooth. If pain is intermittent and lasts for a week or more, there may be inflammation due to an impacted or partially impacted tooth (see IMPACTION, DENTAL). More prolonged pain may be experienced with the normal erupting of the first permanent molars or of the third molars, or wisdom teeth. Any pain in the area of the teeth or gums should be evaluated by a dentist.

Over-the-counter painkillers, such as acetaminophen, may be taken to manage the discomforts of erupting teeth until a dentist can be consulted. Aspirin should never be given to children younger than 18 years of age, because of the risk of their developing REYE SYNDROME, a rare but potentially fatal illness. Cold compresses or ice may be applied to help relieve the pain of erupting teeth. Topical ointments can be bought as over-the-counter drugs and applied for short-term pain relief.

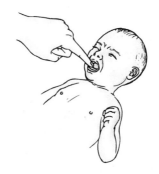

RELIEVING TEETHING PAIN
A baby may have some discomfort or pain when the primary teeth come in (erupt). If the pain is considerable, an over-the-counter painkiller applied to the baby's gums may provide short-term relief. Cold compresses or ice may also help. A child younger than 18 years should never take aspirin.

Tooth extraction

The removal of a tooth. Tooth extraction is generally performed by a dentist or oral surgeon because of TOOTH DECAY, severe fracture, dental impaction (see IMPACTION, DENTAL), overcrowding (see OVERCROWDING, DENTAL), or MALOCCLUSION (irregular alignment). Since the appearance and function of natural permanent teeth cannot be precisely duplicated, dentists prefer to try to save teeth rather than extract them. However, when the roots in a tooth cannot be repaired by ROOT CANAL TREATMENT and there is insufficient healthy structure remaining to support a dental crown (see CROWN, DENTAL), tooth extraction may be recommended. A tooth may also be extracted to correct a BITE that is interfering with the health or development of adjacent or opposing teeth. Other reasons for the procedure include a tooth that is impacted in the gum, teeth that have been loosened by advanced gum disease (see PERIODONTAL DISEASE), or a tooth that is obstructing normal TOOTH ERUPTION, usually of a permanent tooth. PRIMARY TEETH that have not been shed and are blocking the eruption of permanent teeth may require extraction by a dentist.

Tooth extraction is normally performed after the person is given local anesthesia, which numbs the tooth and surrounding gum. General anesthesia or an injected sedative may be used for a young child or an apprehensive adult when wisdom teeth are severely impacted or when several teeth need extraction.

After an extraction, a blood clot forms in the socket. This is the preliminary stage in a healing process that generally lasts about 2 months and allows new tissue and bone to develop at the site of the extracted tooth. The blood clot must be carefully protected to prevent a dry socket from forming. This occurs when the blood clot is prematurely dislodged. A dry socket is a painful condition that impedes normal healing. To prevent it, the socket should not be disturbed for 24 hours after the extraction. Disturbances may be caused by rinsing the mouth, probing with the tongue, or allowing food bits to accumulate in the socket. Drinking through straws, which creates suction in the mouth, and all tobacco use, which can contaminate the area, should also be avoided. If there is persistent bleeding from the socket, a sterile gauze pad should be placed in the socket and pressed on the site by clenching the jaws for 30 minutes.

High estrogen levels are associated with the incidence of dry socket. Women using oral contraceptives should attempt to schedule extractions during the last week of the cycle when their estrogen levels are relatively low.

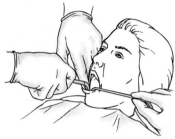

PULLING A TOOTH
If a tooth cannot be preserved, a dentist will use local anesthesia to numb the tooth and gum while the tooth is extracted. A tooth is usually pulled only if root canal treatment cannot save the tooth or if the tooth is impacted (trapped in the bone or gum tissue) or interfering with the emergence of other teeth.

Toothache

Pain experienced in a tooth or teeth. Mild toothaches and sensitivity to hot and cold food and beverages may be experienced following dental procedures that may have temporarily inflamed the nerves inside the tooth. If the discomfort increases or continues during a 4- to 6-week period, a dentist should be seen for an evaluation. When a toothache is transitory, periodic, and associated with sensitivity to hot or cold food or drinks, the cause may be minor gum recession, which exposes the CEMENTUM on the surface of the root and causes sensitivity. This discomfort may be improved by using special toothpaste for sensitive teeth and brushing with a soft toothbrush using an up-and-down, rather than horizontal, movement of the brush. If this is not helpful, a dentist should be consulted as the pain may be due to a loosened filling.

If sharp pain is experienced when biting down, or if there is lingering pain after exposure to hot or cold substances, the cause may be a loose filling, a crack in the tooth, or TOOTH DECAY. Decay that spreads through the enamel (the outer covering of a tooth) into the dentin (the inner tissue of a tooth) may reach some of the nerve endings in the tooth, resulting in a toothache. If the decay is untreated and continues to advance, it can penetrate the pulp chamber beneath the dentin. At this stage, the pulp, which contains the nerves, becomes infected. Extra white blood cells sent by the body to fight the infection enlarge the surrounding blood vessels and cause inflammation. Swollen tissues press against the nerves in the tooth and produce pain, which is exacerbated by the pressure of biting.

When a toothache is persistent and severe, highly sensitive to pressure or touch, and the surrounding gum is swollen, a TOOTH ABSCESS may be suspected. An abscess causes gum and bone tissue to become infected, which produces inflammation and pain. A dentist or ENDODONTIST should be consulted as soon as possible.

Toothaches generally indicate the need for a dental evaluation. In the interim, over-the-counter painkillers, such as acetaminophen or ibuprofen, may help to relieve discomfort. Aspirin should not be given to children younger than 18 years of age because of the risk of their developing REYE SYNDROME, a rare but potentially fatal condition. Oil of clove may provide relief from a toothache when it is applied to the tooth with a cotton swab. Other self-help procedures include rinsing the mouth with warm water and, if possible, using dental floss to clear away irritating food debris. A cold compress applied to the outside of the cheek may help to reduce swelling and pain.

Toothbrushing

Cleaning the teeth with a specially designed brush. Proper toothbrushing is an essential part of daily ORAL HYGIENE that helps to prevent TOOTH DECAY and PERIODONTAL DISEASE. Adults and children should brush their teeth at least twice a day to prevent these conditions, which can lead to the loss of primary teeth and permanent teeth. When food or beverages are consumed, bacteria in the saliva converts the solid food bits and liquids that remain clinging to the teeth into acids. If they are not removed, these acids can develop into sticky deposits, called plaque (see PLAQUE, DENTAL), that adhere to the enamel surface of the teeth (see ENAMEL, DENTAL) and eventually erode the protective mineralized tissue. This erosion results in decay, which causes cavities. Food debris on the teeth and plaque can also cause bad breath. Left in place on the teeth, plaque hardens into a deposit called calculus (see CALCULUS, DENTAL), or TARTAR. This hard deposit at the base of the teeth near the gums damages the gum tissue, which leads to periodontal disease and, without proper dental care, can cause the loss of teeth.

Toothpaste is an important part of toothbrushing because ingredients in the toothpaste increase the cleansing activity of brushing and help to remove some of the bacteria and plaque. Toothpaste that contains fluoride helps to strengthen the surface of the teeth. Fluoride toothpaste may be especially beneficial if the gums are receding, because exposed root surfaces are more vulnerable to decay than natural tooth crowns. The root surface, or cementum, can be reinforced by the fluoride in toothpaste. Toothpastes may carry promotional adjectives such as "tartar control," "baking soda," "plaque-fighting," "desensitizing," "whitening," and "natural." There may be benefits for some people to use these specialized ingredients, but certain elements in toothpaste may be inappropriate for, or even damaging to, individual dental and oral conditions. A dentist should be consulted regarding the best choice in toothpaste.

HOW TO BRUSH CORRECTLY

The head of the brush should be small enough to allow access to all the teeth easily. The bristles should be multitufted, soft nylon with rounded ends. Harder bristles tend to be abrasive and can wear down the teeth and injure the gums. A toothbrush should last 3 to 4 months. It should be replaced if the bristles

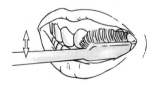

GOOD BRUSHING TECHNIQUE
For most people, toothbrushing is most effective when the toothbrush is held at about a 45-degree angle to the teeth. A small circular motion will move the brush down the surface of the teeth from the gum line to the chewing edge. Brushing back and forth over the teeth is not as effective, and it may actually wear down the gum. A thorough brushing of the teeth should include all the spaces between teeth and the tongue.

T

begin to break, flatten, or fall out. Toothbrushes should not be shared because they can become contaminated and spread gum disease or contagious diseases, such as the flu and the common cold.

Because the arrangement of the teeth, the nature of the bite, and the condition of the gums vary widely, each person should check with his or her dentist or dental hygienist regarding recommended brushing techniques. The basic technique involves placing the brush at a 45-degree angle against the crowns of teeth and using gentle circular movements over all the surfaces of several teeth at a time. Brushing back and forth across the teeth should be avoided as it may wear down the gum line, causing it to recede; this can expose the root surface and create sensitivity. The fronts and backs of teeth, the top chewing surfaces, the spaces between teeth, and the tongue should all be carefully brushed. A thorough brushing should take 3 to 4 minutes. It is preferable to brush meticulously for several minutes twice a day rather than to brush quickly with more frequency throughout the day.

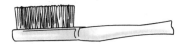

Standard toothbrush

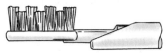

Electric toothbrush head

CHOOSING THE RIGHT BRUSH
A typical toothbrush is designed to be small enough to reach all of the teeth easily. The bristles are soft nylon with rounded ends, so that they do the job without wearing down the teeth or damaging delicate gum tissue. An electric toothbrush mechanically moves the head of the brush. The bristles of many brushes are arranged in alternating long and short tufts to reach between the teeth and up into the gum line.

Tophus

A deposit composed of needlelike crystals of a salt of uric acid that forms a chalky mass on the bones at the joints, most commonly the large joint of the big toe. Tophi result from HYPERURICEMIA, a condition caused by excessive amounts of uric acid in the blood. Hyperuricemia is caused by excess production or decreased excretion of uric acid. Although rare, tophi cause pain and swelling in the affected joint and can destroy the joint and the adjacent bone. See also GOUT.

TORCH syndrome

A rare congenital infection of a developing fetus or newborn caused by the infectious agents *Toxoplasma gondii*, RUBELLA virus, CYTOMEGALOVIRUS, and herpes simplex virus, types 1 and 2. Torch syndrome is associated with INTRAUTERINE GROWTH RETARDATION (IUGR) in the fetus. Each of the five infectious agents involved may produce abnormalities that vary according to other factors including the stage of fetal development during which the fetus became infected. The symptoms the syndrome may produce in a newborn baby include fever, sores in the mouth and feeding difficulties, enlargement of the liver and spleen, jaundice, hearing impairment, conjunctivitis and other eye abnormalities, and red or purple spots on the skin caused by small areas of bleeding under the skin. The heart, brain, and central nervous system may be involved.

Diagnosis of TORCH syndrome can be confirmed after symptoms appear and by identifying species-specific immunoglobulin M within 2 weeks of the baby's birth. Treatment depends on the infectious agents involved. It may include pyrimethamine with sulfadiazine to treat TOXOPLASMOSIS and acyclovir to treat herpesvirus infection. When congenital rubella and cytomegalovirus infections are involved, there is no specific medical treatment, and supportive care is given.

Torsemide

A diuretic, which is a drug used to treat high blood pressure. Torsemide (Demadex) reduces excessive amounts of water in the body (called edema), which is associated with conditions such as congestive heart failure, severe liver disease, and kidney disease. Torsemide acts on the kidney to increase urine flow; it is also used to treat congestive heart failure.

Torsion

Twisting of an object. Torsion is a factor in several medical conditions. For example, a torsion fracture, also called spiral fracture, refers to a bone that is broken because it has been twisted. Torsion also refers to the abnormal twisting of a testicle within the scrotum or of a loop of bowel in the abdomen; both conditions can prevent blood flow to those areas of the body, which can subsequently cause severe damage.

A condition called torsion dystonia is a postural disorder beginning in childhood at about 12 years old. In this debilitating disorder, affected children gradually become unable to perform the simplest of motor tasks and usually end up confined to wheelchairs.

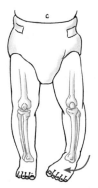

TWISTING OF THE LEG BONE
Intoeing, or the inward twisting of the tibia (lower leg bone) as a child learns to walk, is a completely normal stage of skeletal development during the first 2 years of life. If this twisting, or torsion, continues after that age, some doctors may recommend bracing or even surgery to correct the angle of the foot.

Torticollis

A muscle spasm in the neck that produces a contraction of several muscles pulling the head to one side in an unnatural position. Also called wryneck, torticollis causes pain and stiffness in the neck. The condition may be due to a physical injury of the neck muscles, to a twisted position of the neck during sleep, or to exposure from extreme cold (such as an air conditioner). Certain tranquilizers may cause torticollis. In newborn infants, it is sometimes caused by neck muscle damage following a difficult birth. In children, torticollis can be caused by infected, swollen glands in the neck. The condition is diagnosed by physical examination. In adults and older children, physical therapy, massage, application of heat, a supportive collar, and the use of painkilling medication may help control discomfort and restore function. This condition usually improves in 7 to 10 days without complications.

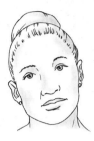

MUSCLE SPASM
In torticollis, a shortened or spasmodic muscle in the neck causes the head to tilt temporarily to one side.

Touch

One of the five SENSES. The sense of touch relates to the body's ability to sense touch, vibration, pressure, temperature, and pain. The skin, muscles, joints, tendons, and organs all have receptors that sense touch. These sensations are consciously perceived in the cerebrum, the largest and most developed part of the brain. The brain interprets these sensations variously as pleasing, displeasing, or neutral. Factors such as medication and brain injury can affect how a person interprets sensations.

Tourette syndrome

An inherited, neurological disorder characterized by involuntary movements (motor tics) and vocalizations (phonic or vocal tics). Other disorders related to Tourette syndrome (TS) include obsessive-compulsive disorder (OCD), attention deficit/hyperactivity disorder (ADHD), and chronic tic disorder.

SYMPTOMS

The symptoms of this disorder generally begin before the age of 21 years and continue throughout a person's lifetime. The severity of symptoms ranges from mild to severe and disabling. In most people, they are mild. The first signs of TS are usually facial tics, such as eye blinking. There may also be nose twitching and grimacing. In time, motor tics grow more extensive. They may come to include neck stretching, head jerking, foot stamping, and body twisting or bending.

Tics may be simple (as in eye blinking) or complex (as in a series of distinct patterns of successive movements).

The vocalizations of TS may include strange sounds and unacceptable words and phrases. A person with TS may repeatedly clear his or her throat, grunt, sniff, cough, bark, yelp, or shout. People may repeat the words of others (echolalia) or involuntarily shout obscenities (coprolalia).

DIAGNOSIS AND TREATMENT

Diagnosis is based on symptoms and medical history. Tests to confirm diagnosis may include CT (computed tomography) scanning, MRI (magnetic resonance imaging), electroencephalogram (EEG), and blood tests. There is no single medication to control TS. Drugs that may be helpful include haloperidol, pimozide, and clonidine. Other helpful measures include treatment of related behavioral disorders, psychotherapy, relaxation techniques, and biofeedback.

Tourniquet

A device used to stop severe bleeding. A tourniquet is usually made from a strong piece of cloth or bandage, wrapped around the blood pressure site nearest the wound but between the wound and the heart, and tightened by tying a knot or twisting it with a stick. Because the use of a tourniquet can be very dangerous, it should be used only when bleeding is life-threatening and uncontrollable by more conservative first aid.

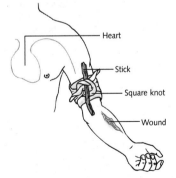

APPLYING A TOURNIQUET
As a last resort to stop bleeding, a tourniquet can be applied by wrapping a bandage twice around the limb above the wound, tied with a square knot. A stick can be tied on top of the knot and twisted to tighten the bandage until the bleeding stops. Then the stick is secured with more bandage, without loosening the tourniquet.

Toxemia

Contamination or poisoning of the blood by toxic material, usually from bacteria but also from chemicals or hormones. Toxemia is popularly known as blood poisoning. See SEPTICEMIA for more information on bacterial contamination of the blood.

Toxemia can also refer to a condition that can affect some women late in pregnancy. See ECLAMPSIA and PREECLAMPSIA for details.

Toxemia of pregnancy

Disorders characterized by high blood pressure, tissue swelling, and protein in the urine of a pregnant woman. Severe toxemia of pregnancy occurs in late pregnancy, can lead to ECLAMPSIA and coma, and is considered a medical emergency. See also PREECLAMPSIA.

Toxic shock syndrome

A rare disorder that mostly occurs in menstruating women who use tampons. This dangerous condition has also been noted in association with contraceptive sponges, diaphragms, cervical caps, and (rarely) in people with wound infections. Symptoms include a sudden high fever (a temperature of 102°F or higher), headache, sore throat, aching muscles, vomiting, diarrhea, dizziness and fainting, and a rash resembling sunburn, especially on the palms of the hands and soles of the feet. The initial flulike symptoms can progress rapidly to a serious illness that can be fatal.

Toxic shock syndrome is caused by strains of the *Staphylococcus* bacteria that are capable of producing certain toxins. Commonly, the bacteria enter the body on a tampon. A woman who experiences symptoms of toxic shock syndrome while using a tampon should remove it immediately and contact a doctor. A diagnosis is made by checking for the bacteria in blood samples and vaginal and cervical smears. Less common STAPHYLOCOCCAL INFECTIONS elsewhere in the body can also produce toxic shock syndrome. Immediate treatment with antibiotics and often hospitalization are needed. The patient may go into shock because the syndrome affects the mechanism that regulates blood pressure, which may drop quickly.

T

Prompt treatment stops the infection, and death is rare. However, toxic shock syndrome tends to recur in those who have had this disorder in the past. Women who have had it should not use tampons, cervical caps, or diaphragms.

Toxicity

The degree to which a substance is poisonous. Toxicity is a condition related to or caused by poisons or toxins and the quantitative effect of those substances on the human body. Some medications designed to improve or cure medical conditions may also have a level of toxicity that must be weighed against their benefits.

Toxin

A poisonous substance. Toxins are usually proteins produced by living cells or organisms that are capable of causing disease when released into body tissues. Toxins are commonly produced by microorganisms such as bacteria; examples include the microorganisms that cause anthrax, cholera, dysentery, diphtheria, and botulism.

Bacterial toxins typically do not cause symptoms until after a period of incubation has elapsed, during which time the organisms multiply until they are able to overwhelm leukocytes and antibodies that typically fight off infections. Disease occurs once the toxin reaches and affects body tissues. An exception to this can occur in the case of food poisoning, which can cause symptoms immediately because the toxin is consumed directly along with food.

Toxocariasis

An infection caused by the larvae of parasitic roundworms commonly found in the intestines of dogs and cats. Toxocariasis can take one of two forms known as ocular larva migrans and visceral larva migrans. The infection occurs most frequently in children, usually as a result of ingesting soil that has been contaminated with animal feces. In the United States, most cases of toxocariasis are associated with dogs, especially puppies. For this reason, having puppies dewormed before the shedding of roundworm larvae begins is important to preventing the infection in children.

SYMPTOMS, DIAGNOSIS, AND TREATMENT

Most infections are mild and may not produce noticeable symptoms. If symptoms are present, they may include abdominal pain, liver enlargement, headache, weakness, lethargy, coughing and wheezing, and fever. In some rare cases, toxocariasis can produce severe disease and death. The form of toxocariasis called ocular larva migrans causes an eye disease that can result in blindness. This occurs when a microscopic worm enters the eye, producing inflammation and scarring of the retina. Partial loss of vision may be permanent with this infection. Visceral larva migrans occurs as a result of severe or repeated toxocariasis. This form causes swelling of the body's organs and affects the central nervous system. The symptoms of this form of the infection are caused by the migration of the worms through the body and include fever, coughing, asthma, and pneumonia.

A blood test can be used to diagnose toxocariasis, but most people recover without specific therapy. The more severe form of the infection is treated with antiparasitic medications, usually in combination with anti-inflammatory medication. Ocular larva migrans is more difficult to treat; treatment generally consists of measures to prevent progressive damage to the eyes.

Toxoid

A form of a TOXIN that has been made harmless by chemical treatment. Toxoids are used in the preparation of vaccines. A toxoid retains its ability to combine with or stimulate the formation of antitoxin, or an antibody produced in the body in response to the presence of a toxin. Toxoids can be formed by applying heat or a chemical agent to the original toxin.

Examples of toxoids include those created from diphtheria and tetanus. Both diphtheria toxoid and tetanus toxoid are made inactive with formaldehyde and used as vaccine against the diseases. The vaccine is usually given to infants in combination with the pertussis (whooping cough) vaccine.

Toxoplasmosis

An infection caused by the single-celled parasite *Toxoplasma gondii*, which is widespread and carried by many people in the United States without symptoms. Toxoplasmosis occurs when the immune system cannot prevent the parasite from causing illness. The people most at risk for toxoplasmosis include congenitally infected infants, people who have AIDS (acquired immunodeficiency syndrome), people who have cancer, and people who have received bone marrow or heart transplants.

The infectious parasite that causes toxoplasmosis spends most of its life cycle in cats. An infected cat can shed millions of the parasites every day in its stool. The infection is easily transmitted to other animals sharing an environment with cats. Humans typically become infected in one of two ways: when they have direct contact with cat feces, as when changing cat litter, and accidentally swallow parasites that have contaminated their hands; or when they ingest undercooked pork, lamb, or venison meat from infected animals.

Once ingested, the *Toxoplasma* parasites multiply within the cells that line the human digestive tract. The parasites may spread to other organs and structures in the body, including the brain, skeletal muscles, heart muscle, eyes, lungs, and lymph nodes. The parasites' spread is eventually stopped by the immune system of a healthy person. Some parasites may remain in a dormant stage indefinitely, usually in the brain or the retina of the eye.

SYMPTOMS

The great majority of healthy people with normal immune defenses have no symptoms when they are infected with toxoplasmosis. If symptoms are present, they may include painless swelling of the lymph nodes, headache, malaise, fatigue, and low-grade fever. Less common symptoms may include muscle aches, sore throat, abdominal pain, a skin rash, or various symptoms related to nerve function.

In people who have AIDS or other forms of immune system impairment, the symptoms of toxoplasmosis are severe and related to brain function. They may include disturbances in mental functioning, disorientation, difficulty concentrating, or changes in behavior. There may also be disturbances in nerve function, includ-

FOCUS ON TOXOPLASMOSIS

Toxoplasmosis is typically transmitted when a person has direct contact with cat feces while changing a cat litter box (and accidentally swallows parasites that have contaminated the person's hands) or when a person eats undercooked pork, lamb, or venison meat from infected animals.

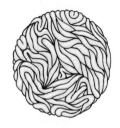

A TOXOPLASMA CYST
Under a microscope, a *Toxoplasma* cyst is sphere-shaped with interconnecting coils.

PREVENTING TOXOPLASMOSIS
A woman who is pregnant needs to be especially careful about hand washing after changing a cat's litter box. If she is infected with toxoplasmosis, she can pass the disease on to her fetus, who may be born with birth defects. A doctor can test a woman to see if she is immune to the infection. If the woman is immune, her fetus cannot become infected.

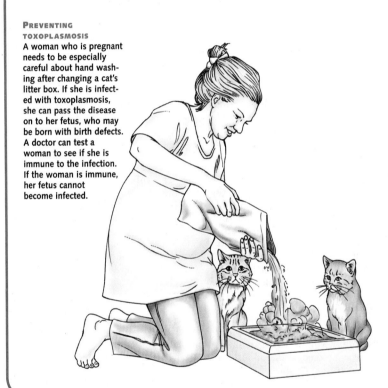

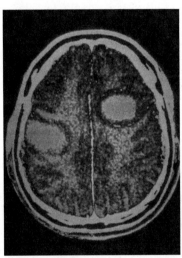

TOXOPLASMOSIS LESION
The ringlike lesion seen above in a CT (computed tomography) scan of the brain is typical. People with AIDS (acquired immunodeficiency syndrome) can become infected because their immune system is seriously weakened.

ing irregular movement, difficulty walking, difficulty speaking, and partial loss of vision. Fever, headache, and seizures may occur. If the infection affects the eyes, vision may be blurred, spots may appear in the field of vision, and the person's eyes may hurt and be extremely sensitive to light. If the lungs of a person with a weakened immune system are affected, shortness of breath, fever, a dry cough, coughing up blood, and respiratory failure can occur.

If a woman who is pregnant acquires toxoplasmosis within 6 to 8 weeks of becoming pregnant or during her pregnancy, her baby is at risk of being born with a congenital form of the disease. Congenital toxoplasmosis increases the risks of premature birth and fetal death. The baby may not have symptoms at birth, but signs of infection can be found in the infant's eyes during an eye examination. If there are symptoms in a newborn, they may include an abnormally small body, eye problems, atypical head size, seizures, jaundice, enlarged lymph nodes, abnormal bruising, skin rash, and developmental delays, sometimes including mental retardation.

DIAGNOSIS AND TREATMENT
If a person has symptoms of toxoplasmosis, a doctor will take a history to determine whether the person is taking medications that suppress the immune system or has a condition that causes immune system impairment, factors that can cause dormant *Toxoplasma* parasites to become active. Other inquiries may include a person's exposure to cats, particularly to pets that spend time outdoors and may eat small prey, and the person's usual diet, including the eating of raw or very rare meat.

During a physical examination, the

T

doctor will check for swollen glands, eye damage, and signs of brain involvement. CT SCANNING (computed tomography scanning) or MRI (magnetic resonance imaging) of the head may be done to look for evidence of ENCEPHALITIS. A blood test to identify antibodies to the *Toxoplasma* parasite is evaluated to determine blood levels of specific antibodies, which indicate the presence of acute infection or a past episode of infection. The diagnosis can be confirmed by the discovery of the parasites in samples of blood, body fluids, or infected tissues.

A woman who is pregnant may undergo ultrasonography (see ULTRASOUND, OBSTETRICAL) and AMNIOCENTESIS to diagnose congenital toxoplasmosis in the fetus. The newborn may undergo eye and neurologic examinations, CT scanning of the head, and a SPINAL TAP to obtain cerebrospinal fluid for laboratory analysis.

Treatment is usually unnecessary in a healthy person whose symptoms are not severe or persistent. If the eyes are affected, pyrimethamine may be prescribed in combination with sulfadiazine or clindamycin. People who have weakened immune systems are treated with a combination of medications to destroy the *Toxoplasma* parasite, including pyrimethamine, trimethoprim, sulfamethoxazole, sulfadiazine, and clindamycin. In cases of congenital toxoplasmosis in newborns, a combination of medications that may include pyrimethamine with sulfadiazine are given for a minimum of 1 year. A woman who is pregnant who develops toxoplasmosis can take prescription medications that reduce the risk of her fetus developing the infection. The type of medications and their scheduling depends on the woman's stage of pregnancy.

Trabeculectomy

An operation to facilitate drainage of fluid (aqueous humor) from the front of the eye. Trabeculectomy is used to treat GLAUCOMA, a disease in which rising pressure inside the eyeball impairs vision. After the person has been given a local anesthetic, the eye surgeon removes a small portion of the blocked drainage system (trabecular meshwork) to allow better flow of the aqueous humor out of the eye, reducing internal pressure. The procedure is safe, and those who under-

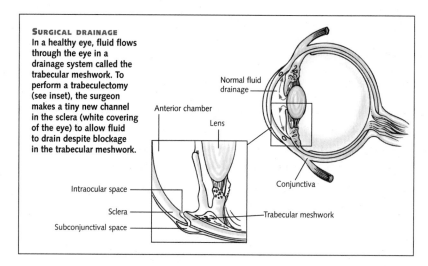

SURGICAL DRAINAGE
In a healthy eye, fluid flows through the eye in a drainage system called the trabecular meshwork. To perform a trabeculectomy (see inset), the surgeon makes a tiny new channel in the sclera (white covering of the eye) to allow fluid to drain despite blockage in the trabecular meshwork.

Normal fluid drainage

Anterior chamber

Lens

Conjunctiva

Intraocular space

Sclera

Trabecular meshwork

Subconjunctival space

go it often subsequently need less medication or no medication at all for glaucoma treatment. Trabeculectomy increases the risk of cataracts, and in some cases a second surgery is needed later to reopen the drain.

Trace elements

Minerals that are required by the body in very small quantities for good health. Trace elements include zinc, iodine, copper, chromium, sulfur, and selenium. Along with other nutrients, these minerals ensure that the body functions properly. A lack of any vitamin or mineral can lead to serious disorders.

Zinc and chromium deficiencies are often observed among older adults. Trace element deficiencies are probably more common than believed because few reliable clinical tests are available to detect most of them. A diet that lacks a variety of foods will likely be deficient in one or more trace elements because they are found in such small amounts in individual foods.

Tracer

A substance used to mark and indicate the course of a chemical or biological process inside the body. A radioactive tracer refers to an element (called a radioisotope) that has the same atomic number as another with a different atomic weight. Radioisotopes exhibit spontaneous decomposition, which gives off radiation in the form of gamma rays. These rays can be detected with special instruments. Radioactive tracers are attached

to biological compounds and injected into the body, where an image of their path can be produced.

Trachea

The windpipe, the airway that connects the pharynx (throat) with the bronchi, the two major tubes leading into the lungs. The trachea is about 4 inches long and slightly less than an inch in diameter. It begins at the larynx (voice box) and can be felt just under the skin below the larynx as a hard, ringed pipe. These rings are C-shaped cartilages that keep the trachea open and protect the airway against damage. The open area of the C-rings faces back toward the esophagus and is spanned by smooth muscle. This structure allows the trachea to stay open even as it flexes during swallowing. The interior of the trachea is lined with mucous membrane that helps trap tiny particles in inhaled air, thereby keeping the lungs and airway open. See RESPIRATORY SYSTEM.

Tracheoesophageal fistula

A silicone prosthetic tube placed in an opening from the upper end of the windpipe, or trachea, into the esophagus, enabling a person to speak following surgical removal of the voice box, or larynx, as a treatment for cancer of the larynx. This surgically implanted device, sometimes called a speech fistula, enables a person to learn to speak by using air forced into the mouth to create sounds and words. When the larynx is removed in a

T

procedure called LARYNGECTOMY, a person breathes through a STOMA (a surgical opening in the neck that keeps the airway open). The air breathed in through the stoma is forced through the tracheoesophageal fistula into the esophagus and up into the mouth. When a person blocks the tracheostomy opening with the thumb or finger, the air in the mouth is manipulated to form speech. Training is required to learn to speak using this technique, which is the most common method of restoring natural-sounding speech after a laryngectomy. The tracheoesophageal fistula is formed with a built-in, one-way valve system to prevent food and liquid from the mouth from entering the lungs. The valve requires changing and cleaning by the person who has the device. A tracheoesophageal fistula also may be caused by trauma or be present at birth. Surgical treatment is required.

Tracheostomy

A small opening, called a stoma, that is made by a TRACHEOTOMY, a surgical procedure through the neck and into the trachea, or windpipe. A tracheostomy usually involves the placement of a plastic tube into this opening to provide an airway and permit the removal of secretions from the lungs. The tube allows air to be pumped directly into the lungs and may be equipped with an inflatable cuff that makes speech possible by allowing air to pass over the vocal cords.

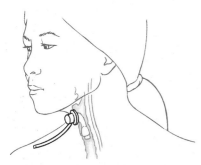

LIVING WITH A TRACHEOSTOMY
Breathing through a tracheostomy tube is difficult at first, but most patients adapt within a few days. If the tube is in place permanently or for a long time, most people can learn to talk with training and practice. A person is taught to take care of the tube at home and is encouraged to engage in normal activities.

A tracheostomy can become necessary as a result of diseases, conditions, or injuries that obstruct or interfere with breathing through the windpipe. These include long-term unconsciousness or coma, inherited abnormalities of the voice box or windpipe, severe injuries to the mouth or neck, a foreign body lodged in the airway, and the inhalation of a corrosive material, smoke, or steam. A tracheostomy may be temporary, in which case the tube is removed when no longer needed. Healing tends to take place quickly, and scarring is minimal. In some cases, the tube is permanent, and the tracheostomy remains open until it is advisable to perform surgical closure of the opening.

Tracheotomy

Surgery involving the insertion of a tube through the neck and into the windpipe to keep the airway open. Tracheotomy may be performed as a nonemergency surgical procedure to allow a person to use a VENTILATOR, or it may be done as an emergency, life-saving strategy when the windpipe is completely obstructed and breathing is not possible.

Trachoma

An eye infection caused by *Chlamydia trachomatis* bacteria. Trachoma causes inflammation of the cornea of the eye and clouding of vision. The eye becomes scarred, causing malformation of the eyelids and an abnormal inward growth of the eyelashes. The cornea, which is continually scraped by the eyelashes, hardens and becomes opaque, leading to a loss of vision. Trachoma, which is most prevalent in Africa and Asia, is the most common cause of blindness worldwide. It is common in hot, dry areas where there is insufficient water and hygiene is poor.

The infection is usually acquired by direct contact with the bacteria when contaminated fingers, cosmetics, towels, or bed linens touch the eye. The bacteria are sometimes spread by flies. In newborns, the infection may be contracted during passage through the birth canal when the mother has the vaginal infection CHLAMYDIA.

Trachoma is diagnosed by microscopic identification of the bacteria in scrapings from the eyes. Tetracycline

and erythromycin are the antibiotics used to treat the infection. If the eyelids are deformed, surgery is required to restore normal appearance and function.

Traction

A treatment procedure that uses a pulling force to prevent or reduce muscle spasm, to keep a joint or other body part stationary, or to hold the ends of broken bones in place. Skin traction is a form of traction that uses dressings, belts, halters, boots, or straps that may be attached to an arm, the head, a leg, or the pelvis. Skin traction is noninvasive and may be done at home under medical supervision. It is used to treat muscle injuries such as muscle spasm, some bone fractures, slipped disks, and arthritic conditions.

Skeletal traction is used for severe injuries that demand longer periods of immobilization. This form of traction requires a hospital stay. In the treatment of fractures, particularly of the thighbone, traction uses a pulley system of weights that are attached to the bone by a surgically implanted pin. The weights apply sufficient force to counteract the powerful thigh muscles and hold the bone fragments in a position of correct alignment while the fracture heals.

Trager approach

A form of massage designed to release deeply ingrained tension; a form of BODYWORK. The Trager approach is a form of gentle, rocking massage conducted by a therapist and combined with movement exercises called "mentastics," or mental gymnastics, intended to be performed by the person on his or her own. Trager bodywork is based on the idea that through a meditative state achieved by the therapist, the person receiving treatment can "hook up" with the subconscious mind of the therapist and transfer healing energy through massage. Based on the idea that discomfort, pain, and loss of physical function are symptoms of accumulated emotional stress and tension, Trager massage is intended to be a preventive therapy rather than a cure for specific ailments. It is used to help relieve back problems, treat physical injuries, and improve athletic performance.

T

Trait

Any genetically determined characteristic; an inherited condition without symptoms, such as sickle cell trait.

Tramadol

An analgesic that acts on the brain, tramadol (Ultram) treats moderately severe pain and is about one third as potent as morphine. Tramadol can impair the ability to drive.

Trance

A sleeplike state characterized by the partial or complete suspension of consciousness and motor activity. Trances may be associated with hypnosis, meditation, drugs, religious ecstasy, and dissociative disorders.

Tranquilizers

See ANTIPSYCHOTIC DRUGS; SEDATIVES.

Transcendental meditation (TM)

A simple program of MEDITATION for reducing stress. Transcendental meditation was originally developed for use by the poor in India by Maharishi Mahesh Yogi in the 1950s. It was adopted by the Beatles a decade later and thereafter became a popular activity among the affluent in the West. Followers of the TM movement believe that this method of meditation produces better health, reduces stress and related illnesses, increases energy and creative thinking, and manifests a younger biological age. TM is said by its followers to be effective in reducing anxiety, improving psychological health, and reducing substance abuse.

Transcendental meditation is taught by qualified teachers in seven steps, beginning with the assignment to each student of a secret mantra, a word or phrase repeated over and over by the practitioner to induce a meditative trance. Once learned, TM is practiced for 10 to 20 minutes twice each day to reduce stress and help develop full mental and physical potential. TM's promoters have made many claims for its unique ability to reduce blood pressure and heart

Terms in small capital letters—for example, PHYSICAL THERAPY or PAGET DISEASE—indicate a cross-reference to another entry with more information.

rate. Investigation of its effects on the body has demonstrated that they are identical to those of any form of meditation, including simple prayer and the saying of the rosary.

Transcutaneous electrical nerve stimulation

See TENS.

Transdermal patch

See SKIN PATCH.

Transesophageal echocardiogram

An ULTRASOUND image of the heart made by inserting a small device called a transducer into the esophagus (the tube that connects the throat to the stomach). An echocardiogram bounces ultrasound waves off the heart and into a machine that transforms the echoes into a computer-generated image. This allows doctors to see the heart while it is moving and to observe its main pumping chambers, the shape and thickness of the chamber walls, the valves, the outer covering, and the major vessels leading in and out of the heart. It is also possible to determine the volume and direction of blood flow through the heart. An echocardiogram is useful for assessing the size of the heart, its pumping strength, valve problems, damage to the heart muscle, abnormal blood flow patterns, structural abnormalities (such as enlargement of the heart, or cardiomegaly), and blood pressure in the artery leading to the lungs (pulmonary artery; see HYPERTENSION, PULMONARY). The advantage of a transesophageal echocardiogram over the

standard procedure, which involves placing the ultrasound transducer on the outside of the chest, is that it overcomes limitations of body size and shape and yields a particularly sharp image of the back portion of the heart.

To prepare for a transesophageal echocardiogram, a person must refrain from eating or drinking for 4 to 6 hours before the procedure. A tube is placed in a vein to administer a sedative, which relaxes the person and eliminates discomfort. The throat is sprayed with a numbing agent, and a thin tube with the transducer at its end is inserted into the esophagus and positioned close to the heart.

After the tube is removed, the person should refrain from eating or drinking for 2 hours to prevent choking until the numbing agent wears off. Complications are rare and are usually no more serious than a sore throat or difficulty in swallowing that goes away in 1 or 2 days.

Trans-fatty acids

Fats that are produced by the hydrogenation process that solidifies liquid oils for use in food products. Also known as trans fats, varying amounts of trans-fatty acids are present in stick margarine, crackers, cookies, doughnuts, and deep-fried foods. Like saturated fats, these substances contribute to increased levels of low-density lipoprotein cholesterol, promoting clogged arteries and increasing the risk of heart disease. Because of this, the Food and Drug Administration has proposed that the content of trans-fatty acids be included on the Nutrition Facts panel of food labels. See also FATS AND OILS.

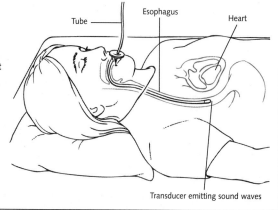

ALTERNATIVE METHOD For an echocardiogram, inserting a transducer into the esophagus (instead of moving it over the chest) brings it closer to the heart and therefore provides a clearer image. The person is conscious but heavily sedated for the procedure, which usually takes 60 to 90 minutes.

Tube

Esophagus

Heart

Transducer emitting sound waves

T

Transference

During therapy for emotional problems and mental illnesses, the person may show an unconscious tendency to direct feelings and attitudes connected with significant persons from childhood and adolescence, particularly parents, toward persons in the present, most often the therapist. Transference can be affectionate (positive) or hostile (negative). It is a key process in psychoanalysis, the method of psychotherapy based originally on the ideas of Sigmund Freud. Since the psychoanalyst is passive, traditionally seated in a chair taking notes while the patient lies on a couch or sits in a chair and talks, the patient transfers feelings onto the psychoanalyst as he or she articulates them. Achieving insight about the transferred feelings allows the patient to make progress in self-understanding.

Transfusion

A procedure for infusing blood or blood components into a person's bloodstream. The blood may come from a different person than the one who receives it, or it may have been taken in advance from the recipient and stored for use later (see AUTOLOGOUS BLOOD DONATION). Blood transfusion is a highly effective therapy that has saved the lives of many people, and it is used to treat many diseases.

BLOOD GROUP AND COMPATIBILITY
The first recorded blood transfusion was performed in the 16th century in France. Subsequent attempts often resulted in death. In the early 20th century, researchers discovered the reason for those deaths. Blood can be classified by groupings that determine whether a person can receive blood from a given donor. If blood from a person with one blood group (also known as blood type) is transfused into another person with a different blood group, antibodies in the recipient's blood recognize the donated blood as different and attack it, causing a transfusion reaction. Transfusion between people with the same blood group usually succeeds.

There are four principal blood groups: A, B, AB, and O. The blood groups are further divided by the presence or absence of the Rh factor (for rhesus, the name of the species of monkey in which the factor was discovered). Blood with the Rh factor is

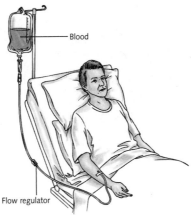

BLOOD COMPONENTS
Most transfusions consist of packed red blood cells, which have been separated from other blood components. The red blood cells contain hemoglobin, the protein that carries oxygen from the lungs to the rest of the body via the bloodstream.

Rh-positive (+); blood without it is Rh-negative (−). The most common blood group among Americans is O+, followed in order by A+, B+, O−, A−, AB+, B−, and AB−.

TYPES OF TRANSFUSION
Until approximately 40 years ago, almost all transfusions consisted of whole blood. Now blood is generally separated into its components, with different types of component transfusions used to meet different medical requirements.

When a person loses a large amount of blood because of bleeding from surgery or injury, he or she is likely to be given packed red blood cells. That is, the red blood cells are separated from the plasma (the liquid portion of the blood) and concentrated before transfusion.

In some circumstances, the volume of circulating blood falls because of a depletion of fluids, but there is little or no loss of red blood cells. This occurs with severe burns, crushing injury to a limb, peritonitis (inflammation of the lining of the abdomen), and some kidney and liver diseases. Plasma or serum albumin, which is made from plasma, is given in the transfusion.

People with bleeding disorders such as HEMOPHILIA receive clotting factors in a form known as cryoprecipitate, which is prepared from plasma. This kind of transfusion raises the concentration of the clotting fac-

tors the person is lacking and helps stop episodes of abnormal bleeding.

People who have undergone chemotherapy often have a deficient number of platelets, which can be transfused in concentrated form. Platelet transfusion is complicated by the fact that platelets survive only 5 days outside the body and must be transfused from donor to recipient promptly.

REACTIONS AND RISKS
Even when a blood transfusion has been carefully matched by blood group between donor and recipient, there is a risk that the recipient's immune system will contain antibodies against the donated red blood cells, platelets, or plasma. The immune system then attacks the donated blood, causing an immune reaction. The risk of immune reaction increases with each blood transfusion a person receives. The severity of an immune reaction varies. The symptoms of a minor reaction may be limited to itching and a low-grade fever. More severe symptoms include fever, shaking, chills, pain in the chest or lower back, pain at the site of the transfusion (usually the inside of the elbow or the back of the hand), shortness of breath, hives, discolored urine, and nausea or vomiting. In rare cases, the kidneys malfunction, blood clots occur in various sites in the body, and death may result.

Blood transfusions also carry a small risk of transferring blood-borne communicable disease. The diseases that can be transmitted include hepatitis, syphilis, malaria, cytomegalovirus, toxoplasmosis, and AIDS (acquired immunodeficiency syndrome). Donated blood is tested rigorously to minimize the risk of infection. Autologous blood transfusion eliminates the possibility of a new infection since the recipient receives his or her own blood. However, autologous transfusion is an option only for planned surgery and is not feasible for emergencies.

DONATION
Anyone can be a donor who is age 18 years or older, weighs at least 110 pounds, is not anemic, does not belong to certain AIDS high-risk groups, and has not had hepatitis, malaria, or certain other diseases. Even if all these conditions are met, taking certain medications may make a person ineligible to donate blood.

T

Donating blood is quick and painless. Since a new disposable needle is used for each donor, there is no risk of contracting blood-borne disease from donating blood.

The amount of blood withdrawn in a donation is usually 1 pint, which a healthy adult can spare without adverse consequences. A man has 10 to 12 pints of blood; a woman, 8 to 9. The body replaces the lost fluid within a few hours, and the number of red blood cells returns to normal in a few weeks. Donors can safely give blood every 8 weeks.

Transfusion, autologous

Using the previously donated and stored blood of a person during surgery to replace any blood that is lost as a result of the procedure. An autologous transfusion replaces a standard blood transfusion, in which blood from a donor other than the patient is used, avoiding any risk that the donor blood is infected.

Autologous transfusion has become more commonplace in the past few years because of concerns over the infectious risks of blood transfusion. The risks involve an adverse reaction by the patient to the donor blood, which can cause fever, shaking, chills, chest pain, low back pain, and other symptoms. In rare cases, shock, kidney failure, and death may occur. Although donor blood is tested carefully for compatibility before a transfusion, patients who have received numerous transfusions and been exposed to many different blood sources may be carrying antibodies that can cause an adverse reaction.

Another risk is infection with a contagious disease, particularly hepatitis and HIV (human immunodeficiency virus), the virus that causes AIDS (acquired immunodeficiency syndrome). Today, donor blood is tested for these diseases, making the risk of infection extremely rare. A person who opts for an autologous transfusion before surgery typically donates blood a couple of times in the weeks before the procedure. Assuming the patient is not anemic, up to 4 units of blood can be removed safely. The blood is then stored until the surgery. An autologous blood transfusion is more expensive than a standard blood transfusion because of the extra cost of labeling the blood, storing it, and having it ready on the day of surgery. Because of the advance preparation needed, an autologous blood transfusion is an option only for planned surgeries, as opposed to emergency procedures.

As an alternative, some surgeons now use a technique known as an intraoperative autologous transfusion. Blood is suctioned from bleeding in the surgical wound; then, it is filtered and returned to the patient through a needle in a vein. This technique is highly effective and will likely be used more frequently in the future, especially in surgeries that involve the cardiovascular system, orthopedic problems, and ectopic pregnancies. This technique is also useful in cases of red blood cell incompatibility and for people whose religious beliefs prevent them from receiving blood transfusions.

Transient ischemic attack

Also known as a TIA or a mini STROKE, a brain disorder caused by a temporary interruption of blood supply to the brain. A TIA is caused by reduced blood flow (ischemia). Ischemia may in turn be the result of ATHEROSCLEROSIS (narrowing of the arteries) or emboli (clots that travel and lodge in blood vessels). A TIA results in a temporary loss in brain functions that may last from several minutes to several hours. A TIA that lasts for more that 24 hours is a stroke.

Symptoms of a TIA usually occur rapidly. They may include numbness, tingling, weakness, speech difficulty, double vision, and loss of balance and coordination. Attacks are followed by full recovery. However, a transient ischemic attack may be a warning sign of the potential for a more serious stroke.

Diagnosis requires physical and neurological examination and other tests, including blood tests, CT (computed tomography) scanning or MRI (magnetic resonance imaging), ultrasound, and cerebral arteriogram. It is important to rule out other causes of symptoms, such as a tumor. The goal of treatment is to prevent a stroke from occurring. This means appropriate treatment of underlying disorders, such as hypertension (high blood pressure), heart disease, and diabetes mellitus. The doctor may also recommend aspirin or other medications to reduce clotting. Lifestyle changes such as reduced fat and salt in the diet are beneficial. If the doctor thinks a TIA is caused by a significant narrowing in the carotid artery, surgery may be recommended to reduce the risk of future stroke.

Transillumination

The inspection of an interior part of the body by means of the passage of a strong light through body tissues.

Translocation

The exchange of segments between chromosomes. This happens when both chromosomes are damaged or broken, and a repair is made that results in an abnormal rearrangement. If no genetic material is lost, the translocation is considered balanced and may have no noticeable effect. When material is lost, the translocation is considered unbalanced, and the result may be mental retardation or birth defects in the individual.

Transmissible

Capable of being passed along from one individual or species to another. Diseases can be transmissible, as can genetic traits.

Transplant surgery

A procedure in which a diseased organ or tissue is replaced with a healthy donor organ. The term usually refers to the surgical implantation of such organs as the heart and kidney. Transplant surgery is indicated for patients who have no other possible treatment options and who are likely to die or be seriously impaired without it. The list of organs that can be transplanted includes the cornea, heart, lungs, kidney, liver, pancreas, small intestine, and bone marrow. Tendons and teeth can also be transplanted.

Depending on the organ to be transplanted, the donor can be living or deceased. Hearts, corneas, livers, and pancreases for transplantation are removed from cadavers. Kidneys are also taken from cadavers, but they may also be removed from a consenting donor for transplantation.

Because of advances in surgical

TRANSPLANT OPERATIONS

In recent years technology has advanced so that many different types of organs can be transplanted successfully; even the very complex heart-lung surgery is possible today. In the early years of transplant surgery, progress was slow because recipients usually developed an immune response to the new tissues, but medications are now prescribed to help deal with that problem.

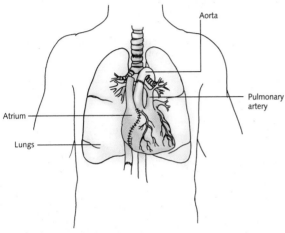

Aorta

Pulmonary artery

Atrium

Lungs

HEART-LUNG TRANSPLANT
Heart-lung transplantation, a relatively rare procedure, is most commonly used for a person who has life-threatening heart disease and lung disease that are difficult to treat.

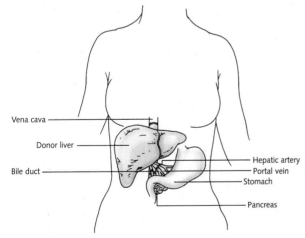

Vena cava

Donor liver

Bile duct

Hepatic artery
Portal vein
Stomach

Pancreas

LIVER TRANSPLANT
Liver transplantation is often considered for adults, and sometimes children, in end-stage liver disease. The liver is connected to the organs and blood vessels shown.

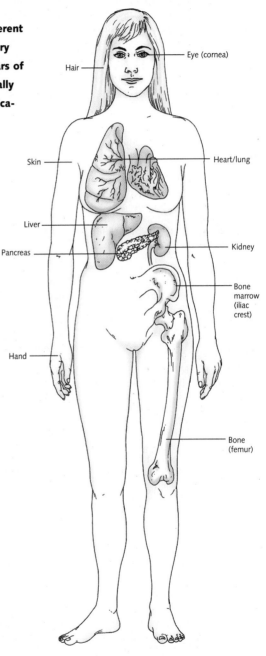

Hair

Eye (cornea)

Skin

Heart/lung

Liver

Pancreas

Kidney

Bone marrow (iliac crest)

Hand

Bone (femur)

POTENTIAL ORGANS FOR TRANSPLANT
A number of organs and tissues can be replaced with healthy donor organs, including the cornea, heart, lung, skin, hair, liver, kidney, pancreas, bone marrow, hand, and bone.

T

techniques, the challenge of transplant surgery is less in connecting the donated organ to the recipient than in managing the tendency of the body to reject the donor organ as a foreign invader. Before transplantation surgery, TISSUE-TYPING is performed to determine the best possible match between the donor and recipient (the more similar the tissue types of the two, the more likely the success of the transplant). Identical twins, for example, have identical tissue types and are highly compatible.

Powerful medications called immunosuppressant drugs are given to the recipient before and after the surgery and must be continued throughout life. These medications decrease the ability of the immune system to attack the transplanted organ as an invader. Since immunosuppressant drugs decrease the ability of the body to fight infection, the transplant recipient is at greater risk for various kinds of opportunistic bacterial and fungal infections. To reduce this risk, transplant recipients take preventive doses of medications targeted against these pathogens and also take precautions to avoid exposure to communicable diseases.

Transposition of the great vessels

A birth defect in which the positions of the pulmonary artery and the aorta are reversed. As a result, blood circulates to and from the body without picking up oxygen in the lungs. Babies born with transposition of the great vessels survive only if an abnormal connection, such as a hole between the two upper heart chambers (atrial septal defect), allows oxygen-rich blood to reach the body. Transposition of the great vessels can be repaired surgically. Long-term outlook depends on the severity of the defect, and lifelong medical follow-up is required.

Transsexualism

Acting and presenting oneself as a member of the opposite sex, combined with strong feelings of discomfort in one's physical sex, for a period of at least 2 years. This rare disorder appears in both children and adults. Children with the disorder want to be the opposite sex, express revulsion at their own genitals, dress in the

clothes of the opposite sex, and play games and pursue pastimes typical of the opposite sex. Transsexual boys prefer to be girls, and transsexual girls prefer to be boys. Adult male transsexuals typically want to be rid of their genitals, desire to live as a member of the opposite sex, believe their emotions and feelings are more like those of the opposite sex than their own sex, may be erotically oriented to either same-sex or opposite-sex relationships, and seek to rid themselves of the obvious characteristics of their sex by taking hormones, having facial hair removed, or seeking penile removal for sex-reassignment surgery. Both children and adult transsexuals tend to be socially isolated by peer pressure and rejection and experience depression and anxiety as a result.

The course of the disorder depends on when it begins. In boys, the disorder usually begins between 2 and 4 years of age and may be resolved by the time of adolescence. However, in a minority of cases the disorder continues into adulthood. These individuals usually seek sex-reassignment surgery as adults. If the disorder begins in late adolescence or adulthood, the degree of cross-gender identification is more changeable, and the individual is less likely to seek surgery as a solution. The course of the disorder in girls remains unclear.

The cause of gender-identity disorder is not fully understood. Theories linking the disorder to inherited abnormalities, imbalances in hormones, and defective maternal bonding in early childhood have been proposed. Treatment consists of family and individual psychotherapy. Sex-reassignment surgery is an option for some individuals, but emotional problems may continue after surgery.

Transvestism

Dressing in the clothing of the opposite sex as a way of becoming sexually excited, known popularly as "cross-dressing." The disorder occurs primarily among men who are generally heterosexual but may have had occasional homosexual encounters. Some men with the disorder wear only a single female garment, such as underwear or hose, under typical men's clothing. Others dress completely as women and wear makeup.

Transvestism may be a solitary activity connected with masturbation, or the individual may find other transvestites and associate with them. In a minority of cases, transvestism progresses to a deep-seated emotional dissatisfaction with one's current gender and a desire to become a member of the opposite sex (see GENDER-IDENTITY DISORDER). It may also be associated with sexual masochism.

Trastuzumab

A drug used to treat breast cancer that has spread (metastasized) to other parts of the body. Trastuzumab (Herceptin) may prevent the growth of breast tumors that produce extra amounts of a protein called HER2. Trastuzumab is used only to treat people whose breast tumors have been shown to produce extra amounts of this protein. The drug is given by injection.

Trauma

Injury, damage, wound, or shock. Trauma is used both to describe any physical injury caused by external force or violence, such as an automobile accident, and to describe psychological damage caused by distressing circumstances.

Common physical traumas include fractures, or broken bones, severe sprains, dislocations, and other serious bone and joint injuries. HEAD INJURIES, tooth loss, and eye injuries are also common traumas. Trauma emergencies are very serious, and the person should seek medical attention.

Trauma center

A hospital-based facility for the treatment of TRAUMA. Trauma centers are specialized facilities designed to provide diagnostic and therapeutic services to people who have sustained a severe injury, or trauma.

Trauma surgery

Specialized surgery used in emergency care of severe injuries. Trauma surgery is used in cases of extreme injury to provide immediate care to persons who have sustained complex and life-threatening injuries.

Traumatology

A branch of surgery used to treat TRAUMA. Traumatology is another name for trauma surgery.

Travel immunization

Vaccines for protection from disease for Americans traveling outside the United States. Travel immunization involves anticipating exposure to the infectious diseases endemic to a destination and the process of being vaccinated against those potential health hazards before a planned trip to a foreign country. IMMUNIZATION against a certain number of diseases is advisable when a person is planning a trip abroad. A person's immune status may be accurately determined, but when there is doubt about this, it is usually advisable to receive complete primary vaccinations or boosters as needed. Because many vaccines must be administered on a predetermined schedule, it is advisable to consult a physician regarding plans to travel outside the United States as far in advance of the departure date as possible. A vaccination schedule can be created that considers the destination, the traveler's overall health status and current immune status, the duration and type of travel planned, and the time available before departure.

There are distinctions among the vaccinations intended for travelers. To enter some countries, certain vaccinations may be required by law. The World Health Organization recommends certain vaccinations for general protection against specific diseases, and other kinds of vaccines are advised in certain circumstances involving travel to particular destinations at certain times of the year. Decisions about travel immunization should be made in consultation with a personal physician who is familiar with a person's medical history.

GENERALLY RECOMMENDED IMMUNIZATION BEFORE TRAVEL

Children younger than 2 years should be up-to-date on the following immunizations before travel abroad: measles, mumps, and rubella vaccine (MMR); diphtheria, tetanus, and acellular pertussis vaccine (DTaP); polio vaccine; *Haemophilus influenzae* type B vaccine (Hib); hepatitis B vaccine; and, for children who have not been infected with chickenpox, varicella vaccine.

Adults should review their health records to ensure that they have previously completed this primary series of vaccines and should also make sure they have received a booster dose of the adult tetanus-diphtheria vaccine (Td) within 10 years before planned travel. Individuals who were born in 1957 or later should consider a second dose of measles vaccine before travel abroad. Adult travelers to foreign destinations should also think about vaccinations against influenza and pneumococcal pneumonia, particularly if they are older than 65 years or at high risk for either disease.

SPECIFIC DESTINATIONS

People 18 years of age or older who have previously been vaccinated against polio should receive a single dose of polio vaccine before travel to the developing countries in southern, central, east, west, and northern Africa; the developing countries in eastern and southeastern Asia; the Middle East; the Indian subcontinent; and the new independent states of the former Soviet Union.

US travelers planning to visit parts of Africa and South America should be vaccinated against yellow fever. The hepatitis B vaccine should be given to adults and to any children who have not previously been vaccinated against hepatitis B who plan to live 6 months or longer in certain developing countries where they will have frequent close contact with the local population. The areas where there are high rates of hepatitis B include Southeast Asia; southern, central, east, west, and northern Africa; the Middle East; western and South Pacific islands; and the Amazon areas in South America.

It is generally recommended that travelers to foreign destinations other than Japan, Australia, New Zealand, northern and western Europe, and North America (outside Mexico) should receive either the hepatitis A vaccine or immune globulin (IG) injections, or both.

Typhoid vaccine is advisable for travelers who will spend time in the many areas of the world where there are precautions concerning food and water safety, particularly in developing nations where this is a known concern. Meningococcal vaccination is advised for people who plan to travel in sub-Saharan Africa and will have close contact with the local population during that area's dry season, which lasts from December through June. Long-term visitors to endemic areas should consider vaccination against Japanese encephalitis or tick-borne encephalitis. Cholera is a low risk to travelers from the United States, and vaccination against it is not generally advised. This should be discussed with a physician if relevant to an area of travel.

All vaccines mentioned can be safely received at the same time without diminished effectiveness, with the exception of cholera and yellow fever vaccines. A timely schedule of travel immunization can be designed with a physician.

The effectiveness of vaccination is decreased when IG is administered simultaneously with live-virus vaccines and varicella (chickenpox) vaccines. IG may be given at the same time but at different sites on the body with DTaP, IPV (inactive polio), Hib, hepatitis B, and hepatitis A vaccines.

TRAVEL IMMUNIZATION AND PREGNANCY

Most vaccines can be safely given to the appropriate-aged children of pregnant women and to breast-feeding mothers. Immunization during pregnancy has historically been avoided because of the potential risk of miscarriage and possible birth defects. This is a matter for discussion between a woman and her physician.

Some vaccines, such as the MMR and varicella (chickenpox) vaccines, should not be given to women when they are pregnant or may become pregnant within 3 months of the time of vaccination. If these women anticipate a significant risk of exposure to yellow fever or polio during travel to foreign countries, vaccination may be considered and should be discussed with a doctor. The risk of possible birth defects as a consequence of immunizations is decreased during the second and third trimesters of pregnancy.

An increased risk of complications from influenza exists for women during the second and third trimesters of pregnancy. The influenza vaccine is currently considered safe during any stage of pregnancy because it is an inactivated virus, but it is considered preferable to administer influenza vaccine during the second trimester because of the possibility of a coincidental miscarriage, which is more

T

common during the first trimester. This scheduling should be discussed with a physician.

The safety of cholera vaccination for pregnant women has not been established, but other inactivated viral or bacterial vaccines—including hepatitis A, hepatitis B, meningococcal, pneumococcal, the adult formulation of tetanus-diphtheria toxoid, and inactive polio vaccines—are considered safe during pregnancy as they are not known to pose a risk to the woman or her fetus.

Traveler's diarrhea

See DIARRHEA, TRAVELER'S.

Trazodone

One type of antidepressant. Trazodone (Desyrel) is used to treat depression or depression with anxiety. Trazodone works by changing the actions of certain brain chemicals to relieve symptoms such as sadness, fatigue, insomnia, and thoughts of suicide.

Treatment

A course of medical or surgical care. A physician designs a treatment plan for a person to cure or improve his or her condition. Types of care may include drug therapy, psychotherapy or counseling, surgery, or rehabilitation. Even when a medical problem cannot be reversed, it may be ameliorated by treatments to relieve pain and distress. In other cases, treatment consists of preventive or prophylactic measures to prevent a disease, disorder, or injury.

Trematode

A type of parasitic flatworm that includes the FLUKE. Trematodes can live in four different animal hosts in the course of their life cycle. During the first stage, pond snails are hosts to trematode eggs, which hatch inside the snail into tiny swimming trematodes that migrate out of the snail and into the pond water. They locate a tadpole host and burrow in, converting into a tough cyst that remains in the tadpole throughout the tadpole's life cycle. The tadpole undergoes metamorphosis to become a frog, and if there are many trematode cysts present, the frog may become deformed or grow extra legs. If the tadpole or frog is eaten by a garter

snake, the snake then eats the trematodes and becomes a host for the parasite. In the snake, the trematode develops from a cyst into an adult that lays eggs. The eggs are eliminated from the snake's intestines at the bottom of the pond, where aquatic snails feed. Trematode eggs on the plants and algae that the snails eat begin their life cycle again inside the snails. Trematodes enter the human body if people eat contaminated snails or drink contaminated water.

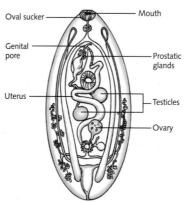

DISEASE-CAUSING FLATWORM
Trematodes are parasitic flatworms, also called flukes, that infect people worldwide. Many are hermaphroditic (containing both male and female tissue), which means that the infections they cause can be particularly long-lasting.

Trembling

Involuntary shaking or quivering, as with fear, cold, excitement, or weakness. Trembling may be a sign of physical illness or of an emotional problem, such as a panic disorder or depression.

Tremor

Involuntary, rhythmic muscle movement caused by alternate contraction and relaxation of the muscles. Tremor is the most common involuntary movement disorder. In many cases, it is a symptom of an underlying disease such as PARKINSON DISEASE. Other causes of tremor include MULTIPLE SCLEROSIS, stroke, head injury, alcohol or drugs, the effects of aging, and emotional disorders.

There are many different types of tremors. For example, resting tremors in Parkinson disease occur when limbs are fully supported against gravity and become less pronounced

with voluntary movement. Essential tremors occur as the only symptom and appear most often when the hands are being used. Proper evaluation of tremors is necessary because appropriate treatment depends on accurate clinical diagnosis. Tests to determine the cause include blood tests and CT (computed tomography) scanning or MRI (magnetic resonance imaging) of the brain. Some tremors respond to drug treatment.

Trephine

A surgical instrument used for cutting a circular hole. The trephine is used to cut a circular hole through bone, most commonly the skull during brain surgery. Another type of trephine is used to remove a circular section from the cornea, the outer covering of the eye.

Tretinoin

An antiacne skin cream. Retinoic acid, also known as tretinoin (Avita, Renova, Retin-A, Altinac) is a derivative of vitamin A that treats acne by preventing the formation of pimples. It is applied to the skin as a cream, gel, or liquid. Tretinoin is also available as an oral medication (Vesanoid) that is used to treat a form of leukemia. Tretinoin is also used to treat sun-damaged skin and some forms of skin cancer.

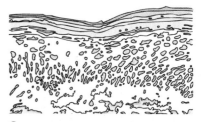

SKIN TREATMENT
Tretinoin works on sun-damaged skin by replacing older, damaged cells with newer cells and changing the way the body sloughs off old cells. A cross-section of skin treated with tretinoin shows dense proliferation of new cells growing up to replace and smooth cells on the surface.

TRH

Thyrotropin-releasing hormone; also known as protirelin or thyrotropin-releasing factor (TRF). TRH is a byproduct of the hypothalamus, which stimulates the pituitary gland to produce and release TSH (thyroid-stimulating hormone). TRH production in the hypothalamus is stimulated when blood levels of the thyroid hormone THYROXINE are low.

Trial, clinical

See CLINICAL TRIAL.

Triamcinolone

See CORTICOSTEROIDS.

Triamterene

A diuretic. Triamterene (Dyrenium, Maxzide) is used to reduce excessive amounts of water in the body associated with heart failure and to treat edema (swelling). Unlike some diuretics, triamterene does not cause the body to lose potassium.

Triazolam

See BENZODIAZEPINES.

Trichiasis

The growth of eyelashes inward, toward the eye, rather than outward. Trichiasis may affect all or part of an eyelid. The lashes can injure the clear outer covering of the eye (cornea), resulting in infection and possible vision loss. The condition can occur at any age and has a variety of possible causes. In children, a common cause is a congenital disorder that causes the lashes to grow vertically. Seen most often in children of Asian ancestry, the disorder is known as epiblepharon. Other causes include infection, particularly TRACHOMA or with the herpes simplex virus, autoimmune disorders, severe inflammation (for example, vernal KERATOCONJUNCTIVITIS), a complication of surgery, or burns from chemicals or heat. Trichiasis is treated surgically, either by removing the inward eyelashes and the follicles from which they grow or by repositioning the eyelids.

Trichinosis

A parasitic disease produced by eating undercooked or raw meat, usually pork or wild game, which contains the cysts of the parasitic roundworm called *Trichinella spiralis*. Trichinosis, also called trichinellosis, is an infestation of these roundworms that exists throughout the world, but is uncommon in the United States because of stringent regulations regarding animal feed and meat han-

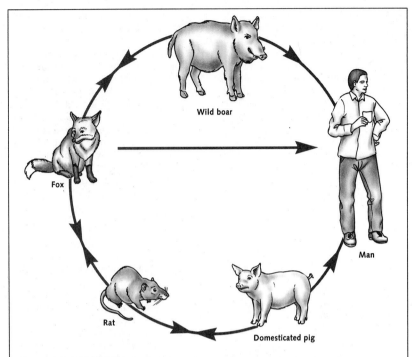

SPREAD OF TRICHINOSIS
Trichinosis is rare in the United States, but it can occur if a person eats wild game that is not well cooked. The infection can pass between both domestic and wild animals in feces. For example, a rat can infect a domestic pig, or one wild animal (for example, a fox) can infect another (a wild boar), which is then eaten by a person.

dling. It is most likely to occur in the United States when the meat of wild animals (such as bears), is not cooked thoroughly before it is eaten. Trichinosis develops when the worm cysts in the muscle tissue of infected animals are ingested. The cysts develop into adult roundworms in the human intestinal tract, where they produce many larvae that migrate to muscle tissue and form cysts.

SYMPTOMS, DIAGNOSIS, AND TREATMENT

Light infestations may not produce noticeable symptoms. Heavy infestations can cause severe symptoms and may result in heart failure. The early symptoms tend to occur in 1 or 2 days and are associated with cramping, nausea, vomiting, and diarrhea. Headache, fever, chills, cough, itchy skin, and fatigue may follow the start of infestation. Muscle pain occurs due to the inflammatory response to the presence of the worm larvae in muscle tissue. The pain may be especially intense when breathing, chew-

ing, or using the large muscles, and the diaphragm and rib muscles may be particularly painful. The person may have difficulty breathing, and muscle coordination may be impaired. During the larvae's migratory stage, there may be swelling in the face and around the eyes. If the larvae migrate to the heart muscle, it can become damaged or arrhythmias (abnormal heart rhythms or heart rate) may result.

If trichinosis is suspected, diagnostic tests including blood tests to identify the parasite and a muscle biopsy to locate *Trichinella* cysts may be performed. There is no treatment for this disease once the larvae have invaded the muscles. Nonprescription pain relievers such as aspirin, other nonsteroidal anti-inflammatory drugs, or acetaminophen may be used to relieve muscle pain. Mild to moderate infections usually improve within a few months. Fatigue, diarrhea, and weakness may persist for months afterwards.

T

Trichomoniasis

One of the common SEXUALLY TRANSMITTED DISEASES (STDs); caused by an infection in the vagina. Trichomoniasis can be transmitted to and from men by sexual contact. The infection can affect a man's urethra, usually without symptoms, and can be spread to other women via sexual intercourse. Use of a condom or other barrier method during sexual activity can help prevent spread of the infection. The infective protozoan can survive on moist surfaces for several hours, including washcloths, towels, underwear, bathing suits, and bed sheets. Women and children can acquire trichomoniasis by direct contact with one of these infected items. A woman who is pregnant can transmit the infection to her newborn during childbirth.

SYMPTOMS, DIAGNOSIS, AND TREATMENT

The organism that causes trichomoniasis can survive in a woman's vagina for years without symptoms. If symptoms are experienced, they may include a painful inflammation of the vagina, pain during sexual intercourse, redness and burning in the vagina, frequent and painful urination, abdominal pain, itching in the vagina and vulva, and an unusual vaginal discharge that has an odor and is yellow and frothy. These symptoms may increase in severity during a menstrual period. While symptoms in men are uncommon, they may include an unusual penile discharge, painful urination, inflammation and pain in the tip of the penis, and a tingling sensation inside the penis.

A doctor can test for trichomoniasis by taking a sample of secretions from the vagina or penis for laboratory evaluation.

Trichomoniasis is treated with antibiotics, usually metronidazole. While the infection is being treated, unprotected sexual activity should be avoided. Sex partners should be informed of the infection so they can seek medical testing and treatment. Care should be taken to wash all washcloths, towels, bathing suits, underpants, and bed linens that have been in direct contact with a woman's genitals or with her hands after she has touched her vagina. Reinfection can occur by contact with infected sex partners or contaminated personal items. Reinfection must be retreated.

Trichotillomania

Compulsive pulling and tearing out of the hair; the disorder is most common in females. A person with trichotillomania pulls out the hair on the head, which may take on a moth-eaten appearance. The eyebrows, eyelashes, or body hair can also be damaged. Dealing with the source of stress that underlies the compulsive behavior is the best treatment; antidepressants may be helpful.

Tricuspid insufficiency

Failure of the tricuspid valve of the heart to close tightly, causing it to regurgitate (leak); also known as tricuspid regurgitation. The tricuspid valve connects the right atrium (upper chamber) of the heart with the right ventricle (lower chamber). Leakage from the right ventricle back into the right atrium reduces the flow of blood to the lungs. The tricuspid valve usually leaks because of enlargement of the right ventricle, a condition that can result from a number of diseases, including pulmonary hypertension (abnormally high blood pressure in the blood vessels in the lungs). In addition, the tricuspid valve can be damaged by rheumatic fever.

If tricuspid insufficiency occurs in the absence of pulmonary hypertension, it often produces no symptoms and does not require treatment. If pulmonary hypertension is present, symptoms can include fatigue, weakness, decreased urine output, and swelling, particularly in the abdomen, feet, and ankles. Treatment of pulmonary hypertension or any other disease causing enlargement of the right atrium may resolve the tricuspid insufficiency. The valve may also be repaired or replaced surgically. See HEART VALVE SURGERY.

Trigeminal neuralgia

Also known as tic douloureux, a disorder of the trigeminal nerve that causes severe pain on one side of the face. When this major facial nerve is damaged or inflamed, sharp, stabbing pain can affect the cheek, lips, gums, or chin. A facial tic or twitching may accompany pain. Trigeminal neuralgia occurs mainly in people older than 50 years. This condition is rare in those younger than 50 years, except in cases of multiple sclerosis (a progressive disease of the central nervous system).

While an episode of trigeminal neuralgia is usually brief, it is also excruciating and debilitating. Pain may be triggered by touching, washing, shaving, eating, drinking, or exposure to cold air. Attacks often occur in clusters and over time may recur at shorter intervals. The pain of trigeminal neuralgia is difficult to control. Medications such as carbamazepine or phenytoin may be helpful. In some cases, surgery is necessary.

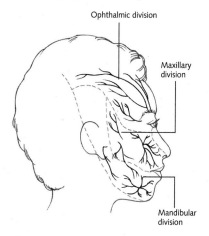

Ophthalmic division

Maxillary division

Mandibular division

BRANCHES OF THE TRIGEMINAL NERVE
The trigeminal nerve carries sensation from the face to the brain. Sensory branches travel to different sections of the face: ophthalmic, maxillary (upper jaw), mandibular (lower jaw). Treatment for trigeminal neuralgia may be directed at numbing or blocking parts of the nerve to stop pain signals.

Trigger finger

A locking of the finger in a bent position, caused by a constriction of the tendon sheath. Trigger finger is a form of TENOSYNOVITIS, an inflammation of the thin lining of the sheath that surrounds a tendon. Inflammation, usually due to overuse or trauma, causes narrowing of the sheath. A puncture wound can cause the tendon to become inflamed as a result of bacterial infection. Trigger finger may be treated with medications such as nonsteroidal anti-inflammatory drugs (NSAIDs) to relieve inflammation and swelling. If other treatments are ineffective, an injection of the corticos-

T

teroid cortisone may be considered. Surgical options include TENDON RELEASE.

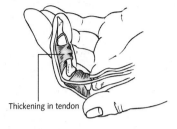

A LOCKED TENDON
If the slick sheath that covers the tendon in the finger becomes inflamed, a thickening or knot may develop in the tendon. When the person tries to straighten the affected finger, the knot stops the tendon from gliding into the extended position.

Thickening in tendon

Trigger point therapy

A form of massage therapy that relieves chronic pain by targeting trigger points, or accumulations of waste products surrounding nerve receptors. Trigger points form in muscles that have been overused or injured, thereby causing muscle tension and muscle shortening. A massage therapist practicing trigger point therapy works to flush toxins and calm the nerves, while the person breathes deeply to release tension. Trigger point therapy is used to relieve headache, stiff neck, carpal tunnel syndrome, tennis elbow, bursitis, back pain, and shin splints.

Triglycerides

A type of fat found in the blood and also the form in which excess fat is stored in tissue. Triglycerides constitute approximately 95 percent of fatty tissue. A high level of blood triglycerides increases the risk of heart disease, and excess body fat can lead to serious health problems such as high blood pressure, elevated CHOLESTEROL levels, atherosclerosis (arterial blockage by fat deposits), diabetes mellitus, and an increased risk of cancer. Most of the fats that Americans eat are triglycerides. When an individual consumes more calories than needed, the liver processes them into triglycerides, which are stored as fat in body tissue. When excess saturated fats are taken in, the liver produces cholesterol that circulates as lipoproteins in the blood. Finally, alcohol causes the

liver to produce more triglycerides and release them into the bloodstream.

MEASURING TRIGLYCERIDE LEVELS
Doctors often check triglyceride levels when evaluating blood cholesterol levels. Blood samples to measure triglyceride levels are taken after a 9- to 12-hour fast from food and drink (except water) because triglycerides normally increase after a meal. Triglyceride levels may also be affected by medications, alcohol, hormones, diet, and recent exercise. There is some controversy about what constitutes normal ranges of triglyceride levels. According to the National Institutes of Health, a level of 250 mg/dL (milligrams per deciliter) of blood is considered normal when blood cholesterol levels are also normal. A reading of 250 to 500 mg/dL is borderline high. A level of greater than 500 mg/dL is uncommon and is usually associated with other risk factors for heart disease or can be a risk factor for pancreatic disease. More than a single high reading is used to confirm that a person has a high triglyceride level before medical treatment is recommended. See also FATS AND OILS.

Trihexyphenidyl

See CO-TRIMOXAZOLE.

Trimethoprim

An antibacterial drug; an antibiotic. Trimethoprim is usually used in combination with sulfamethoxazole (Bactrim, Septra) to treat urinary tract infections, bronchitis, ear infections, traveler's diarrhea, and *Pneumocystis carinii* pneumonia (PCP). In eye drops, the combination of trimethoprim and polymyxin B (Polytrim) is used to treat bacterial infections of the eye.

Trismus

Spasm of the chewing muscles in the jaw. Trismus, also called lockjaw, may be caused by a variety of abnormal conditions or diseases. It is also a result of dental infections, drug reactions, jaw fracture, mumps, or severe strep throat. Usually, a person who has trismus cannot open the mouth more than about 1 inch. It is often the first symptom of TETANUS. Treatment varies, depending on the cause.

Trisomy

A state in which an individual or a cell carries an extra chromosome. Normally chromosomes exist in pairs; in trisomy, there are three copies of a given chromosome. In humans, trisomy occurs when a cell carries 47 chromosomes instead of 46. For example, in trisomy 21, which causes Down syndrome, there is an extra chromosome 21. Trisomy causes a higher rate of miscarriage.

Trisomy 13 syndrome

A genetic disorder involving an extra chromosome 13; hence, the individual has three copies of chromosome 13. Trisomy 13 syndrome is characterized by severe abnormalities in organs and features. Infants born with trisomy 13 syndrome tend to be small at birth and to have spells of interrupted breathing, or apnea, in early infancy. Trisomy 13 syndrome is associated with severe mental retardation, deafness, microcephaly (small head), and scalp defects. Brain malformations are common, and MYELO-MENINGOCELE, or protrusion of the spinal cord through the vertebrae, may occur. Polydactyly, or extra fingers or toes, and cleft lip and/or palate are often present, and the ears are abnormally shaped. Undescended testicles in boys and an abnormally shaped uterus in girls are sometimes seen.

Trisomy 13 syndrome occurs in one of 4,000 to 10,000 live births. Babies born to older mothers are at greater than normal risk for being born with the disorder. After birth, babies with the disorder are likely to have feeding problems, slow growth, seizures, scoliosis (or curvature of the spine), hypertension (high blood pressure), and kidney defects. About 90 percent of babies born with trisomy 13 syndrome will die by the age of 12 months.

Trisomy 18 syndrome

A genetic disorder involving an extra chromosome 18; hence, the individual has three copies of chromosome 18. Trisomy 18 syndrome is characterized by abnormal physical features, heart defects, and other organ malformations. Infants born with the syndrome are small, thin, and frail, and they fail to thrive. Babies with

T

the disorder may have microcephaly, or small heads; low-set, malformed ears; cleft lip and/or palate; short big toes that bend backward; absent or small thumbs; and clenched fists with the index finger overlapping the third and fourth fingers. Congenital heart defects occur in 90 percent of cases. Other associated conditions include spina bifida; scoliosis, or curvature of the spine; deafness; kidney defects; and severe mental retardation.

Trisomy 18 syndrome occurs in one of every 5,000 babies born. It is estimated that about half of the babies with trisomy 18 syndrome are stillborn. About 20 percent of babies born with the syndrome will die within 1 month, and 90 percent will die before the age of 12 months. Babies born to older mothers are at greater risk than normal for being born with the syndrome.

Trisomy 21 syndrome

DOWN SYNDROME; a genetic disorder involving an extra chromosome 21; hence, the affected individual has three copies of chromosome 21. Trisomy 21 syndrome is characterized by abnormal features, including a small skull, short nose with a flat bridge, and moderate to severe mental retardation. Trisomy 21 syndrome is associated with advanced maternal age.

Trophoblastic tumor

An abnormal growth arising from the trophoblast, the outer cell layer of a fertilized egg that develops into the placenta, which is the source of nutrition for the fetus. Trophoblastic tumors are curable with chemotherapy, even after they have metastasized or spread.

Tropical ulcer

A chronic, peeling sore due to unknown causes that is prevalent in wet, tropical regions. Tropical ulcers are moist, concave lesions that usually occur on the legs. Treatment usually consists of soap baths; over-the-counter wound ointments; or, if the ulcers do not respond to topical treatment, antibiotics.

Trovafloxacin mesylate

See FLUOROQUINOLONES.

Truss

A device worn to hold an intestine or other tissue in place when it protrudes through the abdominal wall. Trusses are also used to control the symptoms of a hernia in individuals who cannot have the operation to repair it for medical reasons or who refuse to have surgery.

Trypanosomiasis

A rare illness caused by the bite of an infected tsetse fly. Trypanosomiasis rarely occurs outside of affected regions in Africa. There are two types of trypanosomiasis, named after the regions where they occur: West African trypanosomiasis, also called Gambian sleeping sickness, is caused by the parasite *Trypanosoma brucei gambiense* and occurs in western and central Africa; East African trypanosomiasis is caused by the parasite *Trypanosoma brucei rhodesiense* and occurs in parts of eastern and central Africa including Uganda, Kenya, Tanzania, Malawi, Ethiopia, Zaire, Zimbabwe, and Botswana.

Tsetse flies carrying the West African form of infection inhabit forests and areas of thick shrubbery and trees near rivers and waterholes. Tourists in western and central Africa are not at great risk unless they spend long periods in rural areas. Few cases have been reported in the United States.

The East African tsetse flies are found in woodlands and savannas, away from human populations; people who work in or visit game parks in eastern or central Africa are at

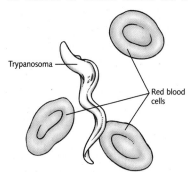

Trypanosoma

Red blood cells

greatest risk. There have been dozens of cases of East African trypanosomiasis in the United States since 1967, all occurring in travelers to Africa.

There is no vaccine or preventive medication for either form of trypanosomiasis. The infection can be diagnosed by identifying the parasite in blood samples or spinal fluid. Both forms of infection cause serious symptoms including fever, headache, irritability, extreme fatigue, swollen lymph nodes, aching muscles and joints, skin rash, progressive confusion, personality changes, slurred speech, seizures, and difficulty walking and talking; death can result if not promptly treated. East African trypanosomiasis can cause death within several weeks if untreated; the West African form may result in death within several months when not treated. Hospitalization and medication can effectively treat the infections if a correct diagnosis is made soon enough and treatment is begun early in the course of the illness. See also SLEEPING SICKNESS.

Tryptophan

An amino acid that is a building block of NIACIN and SEROTONIN. Tryptophan is important for maintaining normal levels of proteins and normal growth in infants. Good dietary sources include meats, poultry, fish, eggs, nuts, peanut butter, brewer's yeast, and wheat germ. Tryptophan deficiency is associated with a lowered serotonin level and a depressed mood. Tryptophan supplements are sometimes used by people who want to raise serotonin levels in their bodies or to improve sleep. However, doctors do not recommend them. Contaminated commercially produced tryptophan has caused death and injury.

TSH

Thyroid-stimulating hormone. TSH stimulates the production of the thyroid gland hormone THYROXINE and its release into the bloodstream. TSH secretion is regulated by TRH (thyrotropin-releasing hormone), a hormone produced by the hypothalamus. Secretion of TRH is stimulated or inhibited in response to blood levels of thyroxine and the metabolic rate of the body, which is regulated by thyroxine.

T

Tubal cannulation

A procedure used to open a FALLOPIAN TUBE blocked by scarring or narrowing, often where the blockage has prevented conception. In this procedure, a thin, flexible, balloon-tipped tube called a cannula is inserted into the blocked fallopian tube near its opening into the uterus. The procedure may be performed by using LAPAROSCOPY or HYSTEROSCOPY.

When hysteroscopy is used, the cannula is inserted through the vagina and cervix into the uterus through a hollow, flexible tube called a hysteroscope. Once it reaches the part of the fallopian tube that is blocked, the balloon is inflated to widen the tube so that eggs can pass through to the uterus.

OPENING A BLOCKED FALLOPIAN TUBE
To open a fallopian tube blocked by scar tissue, the doctor inserts a hollow instrument called a hysteroscope into the vagina, through the uterus, and into the fallopian tube to the site of the blockage. He or she then inserts a flexible tube called a cannula with a tiny balloon on the tip through the hysteroscope. The balloon is inflated to push open the walls of the narrowed tube; then the balloon is deflated and withdrawn.

Tubal ligation

A sterilization procedure for women in which the passage of eggs through the fallopian tubes is interrupted, using various methods. The goal is to block the eggs from traveling down the tubes to meet the sperm for fertilization. In the procedure, the tubes are looped and banded closed with rubber rings, pinched closed with metal or plastic clips, cut and tied off, or cauterized (burned) with an electric current and cut. A tubal ligation is commonly referred to as "tying the tubes," in reference to a method in which the surgeon ties sutures around the tubes. A tubal ligation is intended to be a permanent method of birth control, and reversal procedures are complicated and costly and may be unsuccessful. Therefore, sterilization is intended for women who are certain they will not want to become pregnant in the future. A tubal ligation is performed in a hospital with the patient usually under general anesthesia. Many women choose to have the procedure immediately after childbirth, when the uterus and fallopian tubes remain high in the abdomen and are easily reached through a small incision in the navel. The procedure is often done at the time of a cesarean delivery through the birth incision. By having a tubal ligation in conjunction with childbirth, a woman may be able to use the same anesthetic for labor, a cesarean section, and the sterilization. However, "regret" rates are higher among women who have an immediate postpartum tubal ligation than for those who have the procedure independent of pregnancy, possibly because the stress of pregnancy may influence the decision in the former.

METHODS OF TUBAL LIGATION
A tubal ligation is often done using laparoscopy, a surgical technique in which a laparoscope (a small viewing instrument) is inserted through an incision in the navel, allowing a surgeon to see inside the abdominal cavity. After general anesthesia has been administered, a hollow needle is inserted into the abdomen, and a harmless gas (usually carbon dioxide) is injected to inflate the abdominal cavity. The laparoscope is then inserted through an incision in the

STERILIZATION BY TUBAL LIGATION
Tubal ligation cuts off the fallopian tubes by one of several methods in order to prevent an egg from passing into the tubes to be fertilized. The procedure is usually done with laparoscopy, a surgical technique that requires only a small incision in the abdomen or navel. The surgeon can cut or seal off each tube by making a loop and closing it off with a rubber band; pinching the tube off with a clip; cauterizing (burning) and cutting; or tying and cutting.

Looped and banded · Pinched with a clip · Cauterized and cut · Tied and cut

T

navel. Using the laparoscope for guidance, a surgeon can locate and close off (ligate) the fallopian tubes.

A laparotomy, another surgical procedure used to perform a tubal ligation, requires a larger incision than a laparoscopy does. A laparotomy may be done when a woman has extensive scar tissue (adhesions) that would make it difficult to reach her fallopian tubes with a laparoscope. General anesthesia or spinal or epidural anesthesia is required for a laparotomy. During the procedure, a surgeon makes an incision about 2 to 3 inches long just above a woman's pubic hairline. Each fallopian tube is then lifted out and closed off.

ADVANTAGES AND DISADVANTAGES
A tubal ligation provides permanent and highly effective protection against pregnancy. It may help protect against ovarian cancer; it also avoids the side effects of hormonal contraception and does not interrupt sexual foreplay, as some barrier methods do. However, a tubal ligation is usually not reversible, provides no protection against most sexually transmitted diseases, and involves the risks associated with having general anesthesia and surgery.

Complications from tubal ligation procedures are rare, but may include infection, bleeding, or accidental injury to an adjacent organ or tissue during the procedure. A tubal ligation has a small failure rate, less than 1 percent, presumably due to incomplete blockage of the tubes. If pregnancy occurs, there is a higher risk of an ectopic (tubal) pregnancy.

Tubal pregnancy

A pregnancy that develops in a fallopian tube. The vast majority of ectopic pregnancies (pregnancies that start outside the uterus) take place in the fallopian tubes. Tubal pregnancies occur when a scarred or damaged fallopian tube is open enough to permit a sperm to reach an egg and fertilize it, but not enough to allow the fertilized egg to travel to the uterus. The fertilized egg gets stuck in the narrow part of the tube and grows there. Symptoms include a missed period, pelvic pain, or abnormal vaginal bleeding within the first 8 to 12 weeks of pregnancy. Pains can be sudden and severe, sharp, and stabbing. The woman may feel dizzy or

faint. Some women have no symptoms, or they may have light bleeding and assume they are miscarrying. Women with tubal pregnancies frequently do not realize they are pregnant.

Early detection of a tubal pregnancy is essential to prevent the rupture of the fallopian tube, which can be life-threatening. Diagnosis will be based on a vaginal examination, an ultrasound (see ULTRASOUND, OBSTETRICAL) to determine the location of the embryo, and blood tests to measure the level of the hormone HUMAN CHORIONIC GONADOTROPIN (HCG).

Treatment usually involves immediate surgery to remove the embryo and any damaged tissue in the fallopian tube. A laparoscope may be used to locate a tubal pregnancy and to remove it. If the fallopian tube is ruptured or bleeding, part or all of it is removed (see SALPINGECTOMY). Sometimes, surgery can be avoided by using a drug called METHOTREXATE, which breaks down the tissue of the abnormal pregnancy so that the woman's body can absorb it.

Tuberculin skin test

The injection of a small amount of testing fluid, called tuberculin, under the skin to see if a reaction develops and to determine whether TUBERCULOSIS, or TB infection, is present. Tuberculin skin tests, which are also referred to as Mantoux tests, are examined and measured 2 to 3 days after the injection. If the skin reaction is positive, other tests may be performed, such as a chest X ray, blood and urine tests, and a laboratory evaluation of a sputum culture.

Tuberculin skin tests are generally performed when a person has been exposed to someone with infectious tuberculosis. It takes several weeks after a person has been exposed and become infected for the immune system to react to the tuberculin skin test. For this reason, the first skin test of a person who has acquired the infection may be negative if the exposure to the infection was very recent. It may be necessary to perform a second skin test 10 to 12 weeks after the last occasion of exposure to a person with infectious disease. It is also used as a screening test for healthy people.

The tuberculin skin test can be given at a health department facility

or at a doctor's office. Testing is recommended for people who live with or are in close contact with a person who has infectious tuberculosis and for people who have HIV (human immunodeficiency virus) infection or other conditions that increase the risk of tuberculosis. TB infection is common in many countries in Latin America, the Caribbean, Africa, and Asia (except Japan). People who inject illicit drugs are at higher risk, and tuberculosis is common among people who live in homeless shelters, migrant farm camps, prisons, jails, and some nursing homes.

Tuberculosis

An infectious bacterial disease that usually affects the lungs. Tuberculosis, or TB, may also involve other parts of the body in up to one third of all cases. The lymph nodes, urinary tract, bones, joints, the membrane that covers the brain (called the meninges), and the membrane that covers the digestive organs (called the peritoneum) may be affected. The bacteria that cause tuberculosis are transmitted from one person to another via contaminated fluid droplets that become airborne when an infected person coughs, sneezes, laughs, or talks. TB is usually transmitted among family members or close associates living or working together in closed spaces over a long period. Transmission of the bacteria in an airplane is rare but has occurred. TB is not spread by contact with surfaces or objects that have been touched or used by an infected person.

Once the infected droplets are inhaled, they travel through the breathing passages deep into the lungs where a primary site of infection is established. Within 2 to 10 weeks, the infection is usually controlled by the body's immune system in most healthy adults who do not acquire active TB infection. When TB infection is not active, it cannot be spread by the person who has it.

Some TB bacteria usually remain dormant in the lungs over a lifetime even if active disease does not occur. In later years, the dormant bacteria can sometimes cause active TB infection if a person's immune system is impaired. People who take medications that suppress the immune system, as well as those who have cancer or HIV (human immunodeficiency

T

FOCUS ON TUBERCULOSIS

Tuberculosis is a highly infectious disease usually affecting the lungs. Symptoms include coughing, chest pain, shortness of breath, fever, sweating, and poor appetite. The disease has always been more common among people whose capacity to fight infection is diminished—the very old, the very young, and people who have debilitating diseases such as cancer.

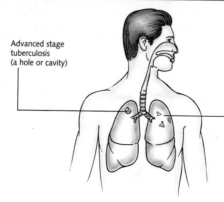

Advanced stage tuberculosis (a hole or cavity)

TUBERCULOSIS
Patches of infection form in the lungs in the early stages of tuberculosis. As the infection progresses, holes or cavities form in the lungs.

Early stage tuberculosis (patches of infection)

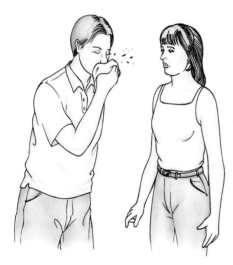

TUBERCULOSIS TRANSMISSION
Tuberculosis is transmitted when an infected person coughs or sneezes and expels the bacteria, which are then inhaled by another person.

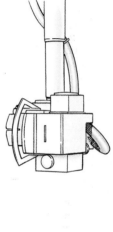
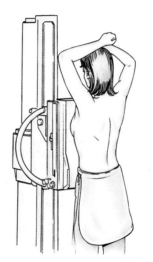

RECEIVING AN X RAY
Chest X rays are used to see if a person has tuberculosis and to determine the stage of tuberculosis infection.

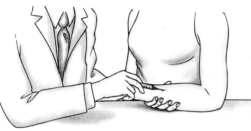

A SKIN TEST FOR POSSIBLE TUBERCULOSIS
To test for the presence of the tuberculosis bacteria, an injection is given just under the first layer of skin. Two or three days later the injection site is inspected for positive or negative results.

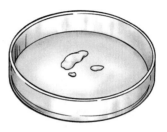

SPUTUM CULTURE TEST FOR TUBERCULOSIS
Expelled phlegm can also be tested for the presence of the tuberculosis bacteria.

T

virus) infection or are malnourished, are most at risk for acquiring active disease from the dormant bacteria. People with alcoholism and those who abuse intravenous illegal drugs are also at increased risk. This form of TB occurs most commonly in adults and may be referred to as postprimary pulmonary tuberculosis, adult-type tuberculosis, reactivation tuberculosis, or secondary tuberculosis. Large areas of the lung tissue can be destroyed by postprimary pulmonary tuberculosis. Cavities in the lungs eventually form where tissue has been destroyed, and these cavities become filled with TB bacteria and lung tissue debris.

There are two other forms of tuberculosis disease: primary pulmonary tuberculosis and extrapulmonary tuberculosis. Primary pulmonary tuberculosis involves a portion of the lungs and nearby lymph nodes. It occurs most often in infants and children, especially in developing countries where poor nutrition and inadequate medical care increase the risk. The infants' and children's immature immune systems are not strong enough to combat the primary TB infection under these conditions. In some children, the primary TB infection spreads from the lungs through the bloodstream to other areas of the body within 2 to 6 months, causing extrapulmonary tuberculosis.

SYMPTOMS AND DIAGNOSIS

A person with a primary tuberculosis infection generally has no symptoms of disease. The tuberculin skin test usually becomes positive within 3 months of contracting the infection. The symptoms associated with active TB infection vary depending on the specific form of disease.

More than half the children infected with primary pulmonary tuberculosis have no symptoms. Others may have a mild cough that persists, low-grade fever, night sweats, poor appetite, ongoing fatigue, and difficulty gaining weight.

Symptoms of postprimary pulmonary tuberculosis may include fever, night sweats, weight loss, poor appetite, weakness, general fatigue, and coughing. The cough eventually causes discolored mucus. As the disease becomes severe, coughing may produce blood, there may be short-

ness of breath, and severe breathing problems may develop.

Symptoms of extrapulmonary tuberculosis are related to the body areas affected by the infection. When the lymph nodes are involved, the glands become swollen without pain at the sides and base of the neck. The nodes may eventually drain a thick, foul-smelling liquid. If the bones and joints are affected, there may be a curvature of the spine, producing a hunchback, or pain and swelling of a knee or hip, usually resulting in a limp. If the urinary tract is involved, there may be side pain, frequent urination, pain or discomfort on urination, and blood in the urine.

Tuberculosis is diagnosed on the basis of physical symptoms and results of the skin test. If the skin test results are positive, a chest X ray will be evaluated for signs of active TB in the lungs. Sputum and other body fluids may be cultured and examined in a laboratory for TB bacteria. A PCR test (polymerase chain reaction test) may also be performed to determine the presence of TB bacteria in the blood and other body fluids.

TREATMENT, PROGNOSIS, AND PREVENTION

Tuberculosis is usually treated with isoniazid, which may be given in combination with a second drug. Some strains of TB bacteria are resistant to these first-line medications and are treated with "second-line" medications, including ethionamide, cycloserine, and ofloxacin. It may be necessary to take these medications for as long as 18 months.

A short hospital stay is sometimes required, after which the medication is continued at home. Once treatment is initiated, an infected person soon becomes noninfectious.

Tuberculosis can usually be cured by medication when the course of medication is followed for the full term, which may last as long as 6 months to 2 years. It is essential that TB medication be taken correctly and for the full term to prevent the bacteria from becoming resistant to the medication. Multidrug-resistant tuberculosis is a serious and dangerous form of TB infection that is much harder to treat and can be transmitted to others. Regular checkups during treatment, including testing of sputum speci-

mens, are important to assure the effectiveness of the therapy. Untreated, active TB infection causes death within 5 years in about half of all cases.

Prevention of tuberculosis in the United States is based on regular tubercular skin testing and treatment, when necessary, of people who live or work in high-risk environments. These include medical facilities, crowded or poorly ventilated institutions, long-term care facilities, prisons, and homeless shelters. If the skin tests show positive results, immediate treatment must be started to prevent the development of active TB infection and its spread to others. A vaccine against tuberculosis can be given to infants at birth in developing countries with high rates of TB.

Tuberosity

A rounded protuberance that is usually found on a bone at the point where muscles or ligaments are attached. Tuberosity describes the knob at the end of certain bones, such as the tuberosity at the upper end of the femur (thighbone).

Tuberous sclerosis

A genetic condition characterized by nodular tumors in the brain and other organs. Tuberous sclerosis (TS) develops before birth and continues to progress over the lifetime of the affected individual. Although TS can affect all systems of the body, the abnormal growths most commonly occur in the brain, heart, skin, and kidney. Other organs that can be affected include the eye, bone, lung, and liver. TS occurs in one in 10,000 individuals and leads to a variety of problems, including seizures, skin lesions, tumors, and mental retardation. The severity of the disease can vary widely.

TS is caused by an altered gene, TSC1 on chromosome 9. The faulty gene causes abnormal development of some cells in the body. The disease may be caused by an autosomal dominant gene, meaning that when one parent has TS, his or her children will have a 50 percent chance of having the condition. However, in 80 percent of cases, TS occurs as a spontaneous mutation, with neither parent having the disease.

SYMPTOMS

Symptoms of TS can vary from no signs of disease to severe symptoms involving one or more organs. The first symptom often may be patches of white skin, seen even on newborns, usually on the trunk and limbs. Older children with the disease develop a characteristic facial rash, particularly around the nose, chin, and cheeks. The rash begins as tiny red spots, which later become small lumps. Ninety percent of cases of TS include the rash among their symptoms.

Lesions in the brain (injuries caused by abnormal tumor growths) are responsible for the most severe symptoms of TS. For example, 86 percent of children with TS will have various types of epileptic seizures that are often difficult to control. Some children with TS will have mild to severe mental retardation. The degree of mental retardation is directly related to the early onset of seizures and the severity of the seizures. Behavior problems are common; some affected children are extremely overactive and may have difficulties sleeping, while others are autistic.

Symptoms involving other organs of the body are also possible. Tumors or cysts in the kidney are most often seen in adults and may cause severe bleeding and dysfunction. Growths in the heart are common in children with TS but rarely cause severe problems and tend to diminish as the child ages. Occasionally these growths in the heart are noted during prenatal ultrasound scanning.

TREATMENT

There is no cure for TS. Treatment is usually focused on the particular symptoms appearing in each case. Epilepsy is treated with anticonvulsant medication to try to control seizures. Skin problems can be treated with laser techniques. Behavioral problems and mental retardation require psychological and educational treatments.

People with mild cases of TS can lead full lives, with little loss of function. People with severe cases may be significantly disabled. Because the progression of the disease stops in adulthood, most affected individuals survive to live a normal life span.

Tubes in ears

See MYRINGOTOMY.

Tuboplasty

A surgical procedure used to open and sometimes to rebuild fallopian tubes (see FALLOPIAN TUBE), where blockage has prevented conception. In this procedure, a surgeon unblocks the tubes by using microsurgery or a balloon tuboplasty, in which a small balloon-tipped tube called a balloon catheter is inserted through the uterus and into the fallopian tube. The balloon is inflated to widen or unblock the fallopian tube. The balloon is then deflated, and the catheter is removed. The operation is used to create a passage for unfertilized eggs to move from the ovary through the fallopian tube to be fertilized and for fertilized eggs to migrate to the uterus. See TUBAL CANNULATION.

Tui-Na

Traditional Chinese massage techniques. Tui-na (pronounced "tway na") is a form of CHINESE MEDICINE that uses manual techniques to treat energy imbalances thought to cause disease. Along with acupuncture and herbology, tui-na is one of the major modalities of traditional Chinese medicine. The goal of tui-na is to remove obstructions to the flow of qi (life force energy, pronounced "chee") throughout the body; promote the circulation of both qi and blood; realign and mobilize the joints; heal soft tissue injuries; adjust internal organs; and help regulate the nerves.

Tularemia

An infectious disease caused by the bacterium *Francisella tularensis (F. tularensis)*, which is found worldwide in more than 100 species of wild animals, birds, and insects. Tularemia, an acute illness of humans marked by a high fever, is acquired by contact with an infected animal, most commonly a rabbit or tick.

The infection has two forms: the more common form, ulceroglandular tularemia has localized symptoms, and the more lethal typhoidal tularemia involves symptoms that may affect the whole body.

In ulceroglandular tularemia, *F. tularensis* enters the body via a cut or abrasion on the person's skin or by a tick or insect bite. The eyes may become infected as the result of contact with infectious material from contaminated hands. In other forms of tularemia, *F. tularensis* can be inhaled and affect the lungs or ingested and cause symptoms in the mouth and throat. The ingestion of organisms is one route of transmission for the typhoidal form of tularemia; in most cases of this illness, the means of transmission are unknown. Research is proceeding on the use of *F. tularensis* to spread tularemia as a form of bioterrorism.

Symptoms of ulceroglandular tularemia include ulcers at the infection site, enlarged lymph glands, headache, muscle pain, and fever. The illness can be effectively cured with antibiotic therapy. Tularemia, especially the typhoidal form, can cause death if it is not treated with appropriate antibiotics. A vaccine against tularemia is available and is recommended to people who are at high risk, including hunters and people who work with wild animals.

Tummy tuck

A surgical procedure to remove excess skin and fat from the abdomen and to tighten the muscles of the abdominal wall; known medically as an abdominoplasty. The procedure is most successful in individuals who are in good physical health but have a deposit of excess fat and loose skin in the abdomen. An example is a woman whose abdominal muscle and skin have been stretched permanently by multiple childbirths.

The time required for the surgery and the form of anesthesia used depend on the extent of the procedure. A complete tummy tuck, which involves the whole abdomen, takes 2 to 5 hours and is usually performed with the patient asleep under general anesthesia. The patient may go home the same day or stay in the hospital for one to several nights. A partial tummy tuck, which involves only the lower part of the abdomen, is often performed with local anesthesia and conscious sedation. The patient is awake, but relaxed and insensitive to pain.

In a complete tummy tuck, the surgeon makes a long incision that runs from one hipbone, down to just above the pubic area, and up and across to the other hipbone. Another incision separates the navel from the surrounding tissue to allow its position to be

T

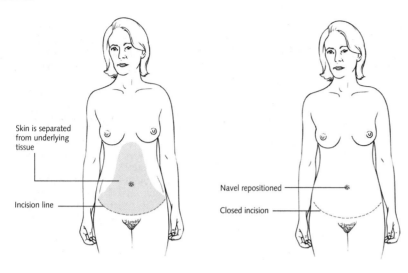

HOW A TUMMY TUCK IS PERFORMED
The surgeon makes a long incision that runs from the hip down to a point just above the pubic area and reaching to the other hipbone. A separate incision is made so that the navel can be moved. The skin is separated from the tissue, and the muscles of the abdomen are pulled closely together and stitched firmly in place. The skin is drawn down, the excess skin is trimmed away, and the navel is stitched in place at the new waistline.

moved in relationship to the skin. The skin is then separated from the underlying tissue, exposing the muscles of the abdomen. The muscles are pulled more closely together and stitched to hold them in place, firming the wall of the abdomen and narrowing the waist. The flap of skin is drawn down, the excess is cut way, and a new hole for the navel is made. The surgeon sutures the incision closed and attaches the navel to the new surrounding skin. Drain tubes may be placed in the wound, and dressings may be applied.

In a partial tummy tuck, the incision is smaller, and the skin is separated from the underlying tissue only up to the navel. The skin is then drawn down and trimmed, and the incision is sutured shut. This procedure moves the navel lower than its original position.

Full recovery from a tummy tuck takes an average of 10 weeks. Sutures are taken out in 10 to 14 days; if they are dissolvable, they will fall out in the same period. Some people, particularly those with strong abdominal muscles before surgery, can return to work within 2 weeks; others need 3 to 4 weeks for sufficient recovery.

The surgical scar seems to worsen during the first 3 to 6 months; then, it flattens out and lightens in color at 9 months to a year. The scar is permanent, but positioned so that it is out of sight even in a bathing suit. Results from a tummy tuck are long lasting, particularly in patients who watch their diet and exercise.

Complications can include excessive scarring, infection, and blood pooling under the skin (HEMATOMA).

Tumor

A new abnormal growth of tissue in which the reproduction of cells is uncontrolled and escalating. Typically, the more rapid the growth, the more abnormal the cells. Tumors, also called neoplasms, can be benign or malignant. Benign tumors, such as warts and moles, are clumps of cells that resemble the tissue from which they develop but have reproduced and multiplied faster than normal. The cells of benign tumors never spread to other parts of the body.

Malignant tumors do not remain in well-defined clumps, but spread to nearby tissues and organs. The tumor cells also spread along tissue surface and through blood and lymph systems to distant parts of the body.

Tumor suppressor genes

Genes that inhibit or stop cell growth and division. The products of tumor suppressor genes function in all parts of the cell. In the absence of functioning tumor suppressor genes, or when mutations have occurred in them, cell growth is unchecked, and the cells tend to divide at an uncontrolled rate, which is characteristic of cancer cells.

Mutations in tumor suppressor genes tend to be recessive; as a result, each paired gene must mutate in order for cancerous growth to occur.

TYPES OF TUMOR SUPPRESSOR GENES

A number of genes that prevent or hinder the formation of tumors have been identified. Below are known tumor suppressor genes and the tumors they are known to affect:

- DPC-4: pancreatic cancer
- NF1: neurofibromas and myeloid leukemia
- NF2: meningioma
- RB: bone, bladder, small cell lung, and breast cancers
- p53: various tumors (Mutations of this gene can cause tumors.)
- WT1: Wilms tumor of the kidney
- BRCA1: breast and ovarian cancers
- BRCA2: breast cancer

| Single cancerous cell | First doubling | Second doubling | Third doubling | Fourth doubling |

ABNORMAL TISSUE GROWTH
Tumor growth is measured by the time it takes for the number of cells present to double, which can vary between 1 month and 2 years. A tumor can usually be detected after 25 to 30 doublings. Cancerous cells usually do not have uniform nuclei, and they do not remain in regular clumps, but spread irregularly.

Tumor-lysis syndrome

A side effect of the rapid destruction and breakdown of a tumor, as with chemotherapy or radiation therapy, that can have dangerous, life-threatening effects. Certain bulky and fast-growing tumors that are very sensitive to treatment can shrink rapidly. The products of the breakdown of the tumor cells are rapidly released into the person's circulation, which can result in high levels of potassium that can affect the electrical rhythm of the heart or high levels of uric acid that can damage the kidneys. The syndrome should be anticipated and managed in advance to avoid harm to the person. Tumor-lysis syndrome is associated with non-Hodgkin lymphoma, leukemia, breast cancer, testicular cancer, and certain lung cancers.

Tunnel vision

Sight that lacks vision to the sides and is tightly restricted to the center of the visual field. A person with tunnel vision feels as if he or she is looking at the world through a narrow tube. Tunnel vision can be caused by a number of eye diseases, including RETINITIS PIGMENTOSA and advanced chronic GLAUCOMA. It can also be caused by tumors of the pituitary gland, by strokes, and by mercury poisoning.

Turf toe

An irritation of the joint at the base of the first, or big, toe, which is usually caused by the toe being bent backward or jammed against the ground. Turf toe occurs most frequently among people who play sports on hard surfaces, such as asphalt or artificial turf. Symptoms include pain and swelling of the toe and difficulty walking. Treatment consists of applying ice, taking pain relievers or anti-inflammatory medications, and elevating the foot. Avoiding playing sports on hard surfaces or wearing protective shoes can help prevent turf toe.

Turner syndrome

A chromosomal condition characterized by short stature and infertility in females. This genetic disorder is relatively common and affects approximately 1 of every 2,000 to 3,000 females. Turner syndrome is caused by a missing X chromosome; affected individuals have only 45 rather than the normal 46 chromosomes. The ovaries fail to develop, resulting in estrogen deficiency, which prevents development of secondary sexual characteristics, such as the breasts.

SYMPTOMS

Turner syndrome is associated with a number of symptoms and is usually suspected in newborn babies and children by the appearance of physical symptoms such as a "caved-in" chest and puffy hands and feet at birth, short stature, low hairline, drooping eyelids, and absent or retarded physical development at puberty, including the failure to menstruate.

Diagnosis is often made by physical examination, which reveals short stature and a short or webbed neck. Other findings may include heart defects and kidney abnormalities. Newborns typically are of normal size but may have excess skin around the neck and sweating of the hands and feet. The diagnosis is confirmed by chromosome analysis (see KARYOTYPING), if only 45 of the normal 46 chromosomes are found.

TREATMENT

There is no cure for Turner syndrome. Treatment is usually supportive and may include prescribing growth hormone for girls with the condition to improve growth rate and final adult height. Estrogen replacement therapy is usually started at age 12 or 13 to stimulate the development of secondary sex characteristics; it cannot, however, reverse the infertility associated with the syndrome. Women with Turner syndrome can sometimes become pregnant by having a donor egg implanted in the uterus. Cardiac surgery is sometimes required to correct heart defects. Small streaks of gonadal tissue may form in the place of ovaries and are at risk to become cancerous over time. Preventive surgical removal is often recommended.

Women and girls with Turner syndrome are subject to several health problems. These include heart defects, kidney abnormalities, and thyroid disorders. They are also at risk of developing high blood pressure, cataracts, arthritis, obesity, and diabetes mellitus. Most females with Turner syndrome are able to live full and satisfying lives.

Twelve-step program

A method of dealing with addiction that relies on self-help, peer counseling and support, abstinence, and spiritual awakening. The best-known twelve-step program is Alcoholics Anonymous (widely known as AA), founded by a recovered alcoholic in 1935. A number of similarly organized recovery groups follow much the same approach: Al-Anon (for the relatives and friends of people in recovery), Narcotics Anonymous, and Overeaters Anonymous. Many ideas and approaches from the twelve-step programs are used in individual counseling and clinic settings for the treatment of addiction.

FUNDAMENTAL CONCEPTS

All twelve-step programs have two general goals: accepting the need to abstain from the addicting substance or activity because of the person's powerlessness in the face of the addiction, and a willingness to take

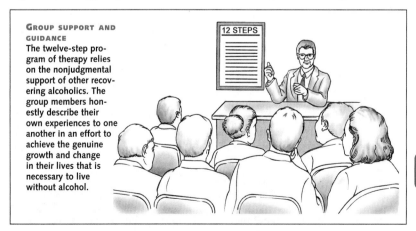

GROUP SUPPORT AND GUIDANCE
The twelve-step program of therapy relies on the nonjudgmental support of other recovering alcoholics. The group members honestly describe their own experiences to one another in an effort to achieve the genuine growth and change in their lives that is necessary to live without alcohol.

T

part in a twelve-step group as a way of maintaining sobriety. In a twelve-step program, addiction is considered a disease that needs curing, not a moral failing or a poorly controlled normal behavior. The person who is addicted has a physical and mental illness that makes it impossible for him or her to control the addiction. Thus, twelve-step programs do not seek to reduce drinking, drug use, or compulsive gambling—they aim for total abstinence. Twelve-step programs see addiction as an illness in and of itself, not the expression of some other malady, such as inadequate skills in managing stress or depression. Finally, support and counseling from other people recovering, rather than trained professionals, is a key aspect of all twelve-step programs. The recovering person tells the story of his or her recovery, describes the sobriety he or she has achieved through the twelve-step program, and invites newcomers into the group.

Twins

Two siblings resulting from the same pregnancy. Twins occur in about 1 percent of all births. Most twins are fraternal, meaning that each baby developed from a separate egg and sperm and has its own placenta and amniotic sac. Fraternal twins can be the same sex or different sexes, and they may not look alike. Identical twins are rare, occurring when one fertilized egg splits early in pregnancy and develops into two fetuses. Identical twins may share a single placenta, but each fetus usually has its own amniotic sac. They are always the same sex, with the same blood type, and they always look alike, with the same hair and eye colors. Some families are more likely than others to have twins, and women who take fertility drugs have a higher than average chance of having twins.

Twins are almost always diagnosed before delivery. Signs that a mother is carrying twins include a uterus that grows faster or larger than usual, the presence of more than one audible fetal heartbeat, and the mother's impression of more fetal movement than she might have experienced in previous pregnancies. When a twin pregnancy is suspected, ULTRASOUND SCANNING may be done to confirm it.

TYPES OF TWINS
Twins are usually fraternal, meaning that two eggs were fertilized by two sperm—so each fetus has different genetic material. Each fetus is enclosed within its own amniotic sac and nourished via its own placenta in the uterus. More rarely, twins are identical, meaning that a single fertilized egg has divided early in pregnancy. The resulting two fetuses have the same genetic material and may develop within one amniotic sac and share one placenta.

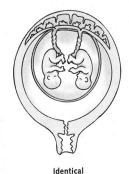
Identical

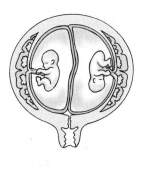
Fraternal

PRENATAL CARE
Women who are pregnant with twins need special prenatal care. They often see their medical caregiver more often than usual and have more prenatal tests. They need to eat about 2,700 calories per day, more than they would if they were carrying one baby. A woman carrying twins can expect to gain more weight than a woman with a single baby, about 35 to 45 pounds. Anemia is more common in women pregnant with twins, and they particularly must be careful to take prenatal vitamins, iron supplements, and folic acid as prescribed. A woman carrying twins often feels physically uncomfortable, because her uterus becomes much larger. She may need extra rest during the day, and she may need to restrict her activity or even to stay in bed for several weeks.

Twins can be delivered by vaginal delivery in some cases, although in others a CESAREAN SECTION may be required. The choice of delivery method will depend on the position and weight of each baby, as well as on the state of the mother's health and the health of the babies. In a vaginal delivery, labor may take longer with twins, especially the pushing stage (see MULTIPLE BIRTHS).

COMPLICATIONS
Certain complications are much more likely in twin pregnancies, including high blood pressure, anemia, preterm labor, premature rupture of membranes, and babies with low birth weight. Of these, preterm labor is the most serious, and any warning signs should be reported to the doctor immediately. Premature rupture of membranes, in which the membranes that hold the amniotic fluid break early in the pregnancy, is also very

serious and can lead to preterm labor and infection.

Sudden or extreme swelling of the face, feet, or legs may indicate high blood pressure appearing for the first time in pregnancy. Other signs include severe or constant headaches, blurred vision, pain in the upper right part of the abdomen, or sudden weight gain of more than a pound per day. Bed rest may be recommended for high blood pressure in pregnancy, and some women are hospitalized. In severe cases, the babies may have to be delivered early.

Twins are more likely to have growth problems such as INTRAUTERINE GROWTH RETARDATION (IUGR). Sometimes, one twin is much smaller than the other, which can be the result of one twin getting more blood than the other or having more amniotic fluid. Therefore, ultrasound is used to monitor each baby's growth and available amniotic fluid supply. The smaller baby is more likely to have problems during pregnancy and after birth.

Twins, conjoined

An extremely rare condition in which twins are physically joined at birth. The majority of conjoined twins are female; more than half are stillborn. Conjoined twins were once called Siamese twins, after Chang and Eng Bunker, the famous 19th century conjoined twins from then Siam (present-day Thailand). Twins may be joined at the head, chest, abdomen, or hip. Some of them share vital organs such as the heart or liver. In others, only umbilical blood vessels connect them. The care of conjoined twins and questions about separating them are extremely complicated. Many ethical dilemmas arise, such as when and if it

T

is ever appropriate to sacrifice one twin so that the other can survive.

Twitch

Involuntary movement of a muscle that produces a small, spasmlike jerk. Twitching can appear as restless legs, a tic (in the face, neck, or shoulders, including the throat and voice), or elsewhere in the body. A twitch can be a symptom of a nerve disorder, but occasional twitching is normal in healthy people.

Tympanometry

A test of the movement of the eardrum (tympanic membrane) to determine if there is fluid in the middle ear space and to measure the air pressure if there is no fluid. Tympanometry involves placing a soft plug snugly in the ear canal. The plug is connected to a tympanometer, a device that measures the eardrum's vibrations. The person being tested hears a low noise for a short time while the machine records how the eardrum responds to the sound. If there is fluid behind the eardrum's membrane, the membrane does not vibrate as it should, and hearing is usually impaired. Tympanometry is not a hearing test and cannot measure a person's ability to hear. Rather, it is a diagnostic tool used to determine a possible cause of hearing loss or impairment. The test is not painful; it requires the person being tested to hold his or her head still. See also OTITIS MEDIA.

Tympanoplasty

A surgical procedure to treat HEARING LOSS by repairing the eardrum (tympanic membrane) or by repairing or repositioning the tiny bones of the middle ear. Tympanoplasty is performed to eliminate an infection or repair a perforation of the eardrum and to repair the sound-transmitting structures of the middle ear. A number of disorders may warrant this operation, including conductive hearing loss caused by perforation of the eardrum and chronic or recurrent middle ear inflammation (OTITIS MEDIA), and infection due to a perforated eardrum (see EARDRUM, PERFORATED). Hearing tests, including AUDIOMETRY, are generally given in combination with other evaluations to help determine the need for tympanoplasty.

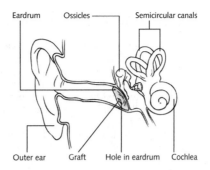

Grafting tissue

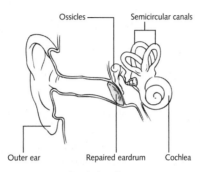

Repaired eardrum

REPAIRING THE EARDRUM
A surgical procedure called tympanoplasty is often done to repair an eardrum perforated by injury or severe infection. The eardrum is repaired or replaced using a tissue graft from other parts of the ear. The repaired eardrum can vibrate normally to conduct sound and adequately seals off the middle ear to reestablish normal pressure.

HOW TYMPANOPLASTY IS PERFORMED
If the eardrum is not perforated, the operation is generally performed under local anesthesia through the ear canal. If there is a perforation, the tympanoplasty may be performed as an incision behind the ear. The eardrum is repaired, and the diseased ear bones are repositioned or replaced. Tissue grafts may be used to replace or repair the eardrum. The tissue may be taken from the covering of muscle above the ear or the covering of ear cartilage. If the bones of the middle ear are diseased, they may be repositioned or replaced with a plastic prosthesis or with cartilage in order to achieve sound transmission to the inner ear.

Tympanoplasty is usually performed as an outpatient procedure. Side effects and complications may include VERTIGO, further hearing loss, drainage from the ear, jaw pain, and

TINNITUS. The surgeon should be notified if any of these symptoms are severe or if there is facial weakness or paralysis. After the procedure, a person is generally able to return to everyday activities in a week or so. While healing takes about 8 weeks, hearing improvement may take several months. The success rate of tympanoplasty in restoring normal hearing is high but may be related to the ability of the body to heal and the severity of the disease before surgery. If it is not possible to repair the eardrum and the bones of the middle ear at the same time, the eardrum is usually repaired first. The sound-transmitting mechanism can be reconstructed within 6 or more months of the initial operation.

Tympanum

The eardrum (tympanic membrane). The tympanum consists of a membrane in the ear canal between the outer ear and the middle ear. The eardrum resembles the head of a tiny

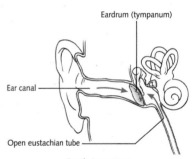

Equal air pressure

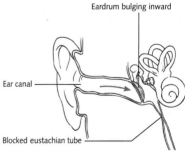

Unequal air pressure

PRESSURE IN THE EAR
The ear drum, or tympanum, is a membrane between the outer ear canal and the middle ear. Usually the pressure on both sides of the eardrum is equal, maintained by air coming into the middle ear via the eustachian tube. If congestion blocks the tube, pressure falls and the ear drum bulges inward, causing pain.

T

drum. Sound waves cause the tympanum to vibrate. These vibrations stimulate the eighth cranial nerve, which transmits these impulses to the brain where they are interpreted as sounds. See EAR.

Typhoid fever

A bacterial infection most commonly caused by *Salmonella typhi*. Typhoid fever, also called enteric fever, is spread by eating or drinking food or water contaminated by fecal matter containing infectious bacteria. Once ingested, the bacteria multiply in the blood and spread from the intestines through the bloodstream to the intestinal lymph nodes, the liver, and the spleen.

Early symptoms may include fever, malaise, and abdominal pain. The temperature tends to increase and may go as high as 103°F, often with severe diarrhea. Weakness, debilitating fatigue, delirium, and an ill physical appearance may follow. In about half of cases, a rash of small, pink, flat lesions called "rose spots" appears on the abdomen and chest, usually during the second week of fever. Other symptoms may include headache, loss of appetite, bloody stools, nosebleed, chills, confusion,

agitation, mood swings, attention deficit, and hallucinations. Adults, especially older adults, tend to have more severe disease with more complications than children. (See also SCARLET FEVER.) Complications may include intestinal hemorrhage or perforation, kidney failure, and PERITONITIS.

Typhoid fever is diagnosed by a blood culture taken during the first week of fever that shows the presence of the bacteria. Urine tests and blood tests for antibodies may also be performed. The illness is treated with antibiotics, intravenous fluids, and electrolytes given to combat dehydration. (See REHYDRATION FLUID, ORAL.) With treatment, the condition of a person with typhoid fever can improve within 5 days to 2 weeks.

Typhus

A group of bacterial diseases spread to people from insects such as lice, fleas, and mites. Typhus is caused by *Rickettsia* bacteria, which reproduce by entering a host cell and thriving on the host's metabolic processes. It may occur in epidemics when it is spread from one person to another by body lice. Fleas can become carriers of the disease by feeding on infected rats, opossums, or domestic cats. This

milder form of typhus is transmitted to humans when they are bitten by infected fleas. The secretion of the fleas contains the bacterial organism, which enters the body at the site of the flea bite, producing what is called murine or endemic typhus. Mites can transmit to humans a form of the disease called scrub typhus. Typhus is rare in the United States and occurs primarily in countries that have crowded living environments with heavy infestations of vermin.

The symptoms of typhus usually appear within 8 to 12 days of contact with infected insects. They may include headache, fever, nausea, cough, chest pain, and body aches. A sudden high fever and chills may follow, and a person with typhus may become delirious or fall into a stupor. Within a week, there may be a rash that first erupts on the trunk of the body, then spreads to the arms and legs. Typhus can last for several months and may be fatal if not treated. People who are older are most at risk. The bacteria can be detected and the disease diagnosed by blood tests. Typhus can be successfully treated with antibiotics. Once a person has been treated, the disease does not recur.

Ulcer

A sore or wound on the skin or a mucous membrane. A peptic ulcer is one that affects the mucous membrane lining the lower esophagus, stomach, or duodenum. See PEPTIC ULCER DISEASE.

Ulcerative colitis

See COLITIS.

Ulcer-healing agents

See ANTACIDS; HISTAMINE₂ BLOCKERS; PROTON PUMP INHIBITORS.

Ultrasound scanning

Also known as sonography or ultrasonography; a diagnostic screening technique that uses high-frequency sound waves transmitted from a wandlike instrument called a transducer into the body to create images of internal anatomical structures. The sound waves are reflected back as an echo that a computer translates into an image of the body area being examined.

WHY IT IS PERFORMED

Because ultrasound scanning does not involve exposure to ionizing radiation (as X rays do), it is a safe screening tool for many areas of the body. The technique can be safely used during pregnancy to assess the position, size, and gestational age of the fetus and the location of the placenta. Ultrasound scans can also reveal multiple pregnancies.

In children, the procedure may be used to examine organs and structures including the kidneys, the liver and spleen, the female pelvis, and the hips. Diagnostic screening of adults with ultrasound may be performed on these organs and structures as well as on the gallbladder, thyroid, parathyroid, ovaries, uterus, breasts, testicles, and prostate. The arteries and veins can also be evaluated by ultrasound scanning. Conditions leading to stroke, such as narrowing of the carotid arteries, can be detected by this technique.

Ultrasound scanning can serve as a

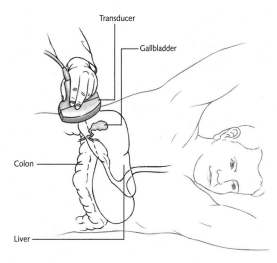

HAVING AN ULTRASOUND
A person getting an ultrasound scan (for example, of the gallbladder) lies on an examining table, and a technician runs a transducer over the area that is being examined. If the gallbladder contains gallstones, the solid stones will reflect sound waves differently than the bile fluid in the gallbladder.

guide for minimally invasive outpatient procedures including the insertion of small catheters to drain infections and thin-needle biopsies of tumors.

HOW IT WORKS

The sound waves used in ultrasound scanning are a higher frequency, or pitch, than can be heard by the human ear. When these sound waves are transmitted into the body by a transducer resting on a person's skin, they pass through tissue and are reflected back off internal structures, creating an echo. The echoes are received by the transducer and converted by an electronic instrument into electrical impulses, which are translated by a computer into a moving image that is produced on a monitor. The continuously changing images are recorded on videotape or film to be analyzed.

Solid-mass structures give off stronger ultrasound echoes and produce a brighter image on the monitor than fluid-filled areas. This allows abnormal growths in the body to be distinguished from normal tissue.

HOW IT IS PERFORMED

Ultrasound scanning is usually performed on an outpatient basis by a health care professional called a sonographer. If the scan is being performed on a woman who is in the early stages of pregnancy, she will be asked to drink several glasses of water about an hour before the scan. She will also be asked to refrain from urinating because a full urinary bladder allows for clearer visualization of the uterus and fetus.

For all ultrasound scanning, the person lies on an examining table, and a special water-soluble gel is applied to the skin area to be examined. The gel may feel cool to the skin. The transducer is placed on the skin, positioned over the internal organ or structure that will be scanned, and gently pressed against the area that has been lubricated with gel.

For certain examinations, a wandlike transducer may be inserted into the vagina or rectum. For example, in early pregnancy, insertion of the transducer into the vagina allows a closer view of the uterus and fetus. A rectal probe is helpful for assessing a man's prostate gland. Ultrasound scanning is generally considered painless and does not require special care after the procedure. See also DOPPLER ULTRASOUND.

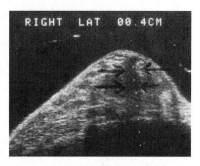

"READING" AN ULTRASOUND IMAGE
An ultrasound scan of a woman's breast shows the presence of a cyst, visible as a darker, more dense mass than the surrounding breast tissue (see arrows). The ultrasound scanner electronically converts sound waves bouncing off the internal structures into electrical impulses to form the image.

U

Ultrasound treatment

The use of sound waves to produce heat internally in an injured joint or muscle. Ultrasound treatment is a procedure used in PHYSICAL THERAPY. An ultrasound device is applied to the skin over the area that is to be treated. The sound waves produce heat in the internal structure being treated without producing a sensation of heat on the skin of the person being treated. This deep heat increases blood flow and promotes healing of the injury. Ultrasound treatment may be useful in a variety of musculoskeletal conditions.

Ultrasound, obstetrical

A test in which pictures of the developing fetus are made from sound waves. This painless and safe procedure is used in hospitals and many doctors' offices to determine the age and rate of growth of the fetus and its position in the uterus. Ultrasound can also be used to identify multiple pregnancies or a visible birth defect, and it is used to show the position of the placenta and amount of amniotic fluid. Certain procedures, such as AMNIOCENTESIS, CHORIONIC VILLUS SAMPLING, and fetal blood sampling, are guided by ultrasound. Most pregnant women in the United States will have at least one ultrasound examination during a pregnancy.

Ultrasound uses energy in the form of sound waves, sent out by a handheld instrument called a transducer that is moved along the woman's abdomen. The sound waves are reflected off the fetus and the mother's internal organs and are converted into an image on a monitor. In the very early stages of pregnancy, vaginal ultrasound may be used to see the fetus more clearly.

Ultrasound, vaginal

An imaging method used to detect abnormalities of the female reproductive system. Using energy in the form of sound waves, vaginal ultrasound produces an image of a woman's reproductive system on a video screen. During this painless procedure, a long, thin wand called a transducer is inserted into the vagina. The transducer sends out sound waves that are bounced off the

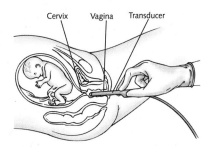

Cervix   Vagina   Transducer

VIEWING THE FETUS
Vaginal ultrasound, which can be used to examine the reproductive organs for a variety of reasons, may be done to check on the health of the fetus. The doctor inserts the small ultrasound transducer into the vagina, and the sound waves are converted into an electronic image that enables the doctor to get a clear image of the fetus.

ovaries, producing an image on the monitor. Doctors can then see if the size and shape of the ovary is normal, or they can examine a growth on the ovary, sometimes even ascertaining whether it is benign or malignant. Vaginal ultrasound is also used to determine the location of a pregnancy at a very early stage, particularly in order to diagnose an ectopic pregnancy.

Ultraviolet light

Invisible rays that produce the tanning and burning effects of sunlight (see SUN EXPOSURE, ADVERSE EFFECTS OF). Ultraviolet light is associated with SUNBURN, an increased risk of SKIN CANCER, premature aging of the skin, suppression of the immune system, and cataracts.

The ultraviolet light spectrum is divided into ultraviolet A (UVA) light, ultraviolet B (UVB) light, and ultraviolet C (UVC) light. Virtually no UVC reaches the surface of the Earth because it is absorbed by the ozone layer. The longer rays of UVA can penetrate windows and are also emitted by tanning beds. Although it has long been known that UVB causes superficial basal cell and squamous cell carcinomas, UVA may also contribute to cancer by penetrating deeper layers of skin and having a negative impact on the immune system. UVA also causes the brown spots, wrinkles, and sagging skin associated with premature aging of the skin.

The ultraviolet content of sunlight varies. It is more intense in places at higher elevations where it is not filtered out by clouds or haze. When ultraviolet light is reflected from water, sand, or snow, it can burn as severely as direct sunlight. Doctors recommend protecting the skin from ultraviolet light by minimizing sun exposure and using sunscreens on a regular basis. Sunglasses that provide UVA and UVB protection can help prevent cataracts.

Umbilical cord

A flexible tube connecting the abdomen of an embryo or fetus to the placenta inside the mother's womb. The umbilical cord is a flexible tube, frequently twisted into a spiral, through which nutrients are delivered to the embryo or fetus and

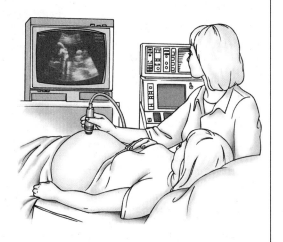

VIEWING THE FETUS
An abdominal ultrasound is a painless outpatient procedure that uses sound waves reflecting off the fetus to create an electronic image on a monitor as it is filmed. The pregnant woman lies on an examining table and a technician rubs a gel over her abdomen. (The ultrasound waves cannot penetrate air, and the gel eliminates air pockets between the transducer and the skin.) The technician then moves a wand called a transducer over the surface of the abdomen and watches the changing image on the monitor as it is filmed.

through which waste is expelled. The umbilical cord contains two arteries and one vein. The arteries carry blood without oxygen to the placenta, and the vein carries oxygen-rich blood to the fetus. At birth, the umbilical cord is clamped and cut.

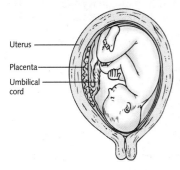

LIFELINE TO A FETUS
The umbilical cord delivers nutrients, including oxygen, to a fetus via the mother's bloodstream. The umbilical cord connects the fetus to the placenta, an organ in the uterus designed specifically to provide exchange between the bloodstreams of mother and fetus, without the blood actually mixing.

Umbilicus

The trace left behind on a baby's abdomen when the umbilical cord is cut. The umbilicus is commonly called the navel or the belly button.

Unconscious

The region of the mind that contains wishes, memories, fears, feelings, impulses, and ideas that cannot be accessed or expressed consciously. In the thinking of Sigmund Freud (see FREUDIAN THEORY), the unconscious contains feelings that have survived since infancy, including the sexual drive. Carl Jung maintained that the unconscious also contains inherited, universal, archaic archetypes that formed what he called the collective unconscious (see JUNGIAN THEORY).

Unconsciousness

A state of unawareness; the loss of the ability to respond. Unconsciousness, which is not the same as being asleep, involves being unable to respond to any stimuli. An unconscious person cannot cough or clear his or her throat, for example, which can lead to death if the airway is obstructed.

The symptoms of unconsciousness include unresponsiveness—the person does not respond when spoken to, touched, or otherwise stimulated. Any injury or major illness can cause unconsciousness, as can an overdose of drugs or medication (see OVERDOSE, DRUG; OVERDOSE, MEDICATION). Any unconscious person who does not regain consciousness right away must receive emergency medical assistance.

Brief episodes of unconsciousness, or FAINTING, can be caused by a low blood sugar level, standing too long in one place, or illness. If a person faints, bystanders should try to prevent him or her from falling. The person should lie face up on the floor, with the feet elevated about 12 inches, to promote the flow of blood to the brain. If the cause of unconsciousness is unknown, the person should not be moved in case there is a head, neck, or back injury.

Underage drinking

Consumption of alcohol by a person younger than the legal drinking age, which is 21 years old in most states and 18 in the remainder. Since alcohol is widely available, it is the drug most likely to be abused by adolescents, who often face peer pressure to drink illegally. It is estimated that as many as 7 of every 10 high school seniors have used alcohol during the previous month, even though such use is illegal. Overall, 5 to 7 of every 100 adolescents are alcoholics, and as many as 20 are problem drinkers who become intoxicated 6 or more times a year or have repeated, negative consequences as a result of drinking, such as arrest for driving while intoxicated, poor academic performance, or family conflicts. See ALCOHOL DEPENDENCE.

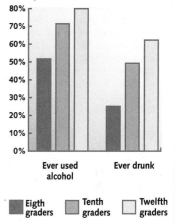

USE OF ALCOHOL BY US STUDENTS

In a 2000 survey, these percentages of eighth, tenth, and twelfth graders said they had used alcohol, or had become intoxicated or drunk, at some point in their lives.

Eigth graders / Tenth graders / Twelfth graders

Adapted from Monitoring the Future Survey 2000, National Institute on Drug Abuse.

Underbite

A form of MALOCCULSION (irregular alignment) in which the lower teeth are positioned in front of the upper teeth when the jaw is closed. An underbite is usually due to a person's heredity and may become a problem for cosmetic reasons. An underbite may also prevent opposing teeth from meeting properly when chewing, which can lead to the loosening of some teeth. An underbite is corrected with braces (see BRACES, DENTAL) as recommended by an orthodontist, who is a specialist in bite problems.

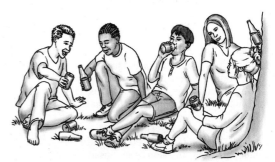

PROBLEM DRINKING
Peer pressure and a desire to belong is likely to be a factor in adolescent drinking. Parents can help teens resist social pressures by teaching them that they have a right to say no, to express their own opinions, to leave a situation that makes them uncomfortable, and to be responsible for their own actions.

U

Unsaturated fats

Dietary fats that come primarily from plants and fish rather than animal sources and are divided into two groups, polyunsaturated and monounsaturated. See FATS AND OILS.

Urea

A waste product found in the blood. Urea is normally filtered from the blood by the kidneys and then excreted in the urine. It is a nitrogen-containing by-product of the normal metabolism of protein in the liver and is the principal waste product in urine. The accumulation of urea in the blood, a condition called UREMIA, is an indication of KIDNEY FAILURE.

Uremia

An abnormal accumulation of UREA and other metabolic waste products in the bloodstream. Uremia is caused by impaired kidney function and occurs when the kidneys are unable to filter the waste product urea from the blood. It is a sign of kidney damage. Symptoms of uremia include nausea, vomiting, loss of appetite, hiccups, weakness, itching, and mental confusion.

Ureter

The tube that transports urine from each kidney to the bladder. Each ureter is made of fibrous connective tissue and smooth muscle. Urine flows down the ureters by means of gravity and peristalsis, a pumping action as contractions pass through the delicate muscle layers in the ureter walls. Each ureter enters the bladder through a passage in the bladder wall. See URINARY TRACT.

Ureteral colic

A usually severe pain in the back that occurs as the result of one or more KIDNEY STONES becoming trapped in a ureter (one of two tubes that transport urine from the kidneys to the bladder).

Ureterolithotomy

An operation to remove a stone from one of the tubes (ureters) connecting the kidney to the bladder. The surgery is done under general anesthesia through an incision. The ureter is opened, the stone is removed, and the ureter and the incision are closed with surgical stitches. A tube is often left in the wound to drain fluids during recovery. Ureterolithotomy usually requires a 4- or 5-day hospital stay, with full recovery in about 2 weeks.

Ureterolithotomy is rarely performed today, as ureteroscopy or extracorporeal shock wave lithotripsy (ESWL) is effective and easier. Ureteroscopy involves placing a small scope into the ureter and removing the stone; ESWL uses shock waves through the body to break the stone up. See LITHOTRIPSY.

Urethra

The narrow tube that transports urine from the bladder to be excreted by the body. In women, the urethra exits in front of the vaginal opening. In men, the urethra passes through the prostate to the penis and exits at its tip. In men the urethra also functions as the passage through which semen is ejaculated. The urethra in women is about 1¼ to 2 inches long; in men, it is about 8 inches long, which is probably why women experience far more URINARY TRACT infections than men.

Urethral dilation

A surgical procedure to widen an abnormally narrow urethra, the tube that carries urine from the bladder to the outside of the body. A narrow urethra in girls is a birth defect; in women, it results from injury to the urethra during childbirth. In men, narrowing usually results from injury. To perform dilatation, the urethra is lubricated; then, a very thin surgical instrument is passed along it to the bladder. Sometimes, a viewing device is used to allow the surgeon to see the inside of the urethra. Instruments of successively larger sizes are then introduced to stretch the narrowed area. Complications following the procedure include bleeding and pain.

Urethral discharge

Liquid, particularly pus, expelled from the body opening from which urine is normally excreted. The urethra is the tube that connects the bladder to the urinary opening. Urethral discharge is the most common complaint among males seeking medical attention for their genital and urinary organs. Discharge without blood typically indicates a sexually transmitted infection, such as gonorrhea or chlamydia. To determine what organism is causing the infection, the doctor collects a specimen of the discharge for examination in the laboratory. If an infection is found, antibiotic medication is then prescribed. Blood in the discharge may indicate a foreign body, abnormal narrowing of the urethra (urethral stricture), or a tumor. Examination is needed to determine the cause and treatment.

Urethral stricture

An abnormal narrowing of the tube (urethra) that carries urine from the bladder to the outside of the body. The problem is common in men but rare in women. Urethral stricture usually results from injury, sometimes as a side effect of surgery in the urinary tract, from infection, or from trauma to the pelvic region. Men who have a history of sexually transmitted diseases, frequent infections of the

WIDENING THE URETHRA
If the urethra is too narrow to allow normal passage of urine, either as the result of a birth defect or injury, it can be widened in a doctor's office. A very thin, curved instrument is inserted into the well-lubricated urethra, and then successively larger instruments are inserted to gently widen the tube.

Dilator
Public bone
Glans
Urethra
Testicle
Prostate
Bladder
Urethral dilators

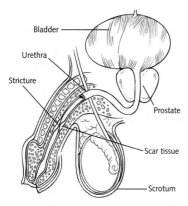

BLOCKAGE OF THE URETHRA
Urethral stricture, which almost always occurs in men, may result from injury, from surgery on the urinary tract, or from infection. The condition may be treated by dilating the urethra or with surgery to open a passage through the scar tissue.

urethra, or an enlarged prostate are at increased risk. Symptoms include pain on urination, difficulty in urinating or in retaining urine, a low urine stream and decreased urine output, an increased need to urinate frequently, blood in the semen or in the urine, pain in the lower abdomen or pelvis, discharge from the urethra, or swelling of the penis. Left untreated, urethral stricture can block urine flow and cause serious damage to the kidneys.

Diagnosis requires examination by a physician, laboratory tests of the urine for infectious organisms, and visual inspection of the urinary tract with a special viewing instrument. Treatment consists of widening the urethra with an expanding instrument (urethral dilation). If this is not successful, or if the stricture returns, surgery may be recommended. In the simplest cases, the operation consists of cutting through the narrowed tissue at the point of the stricture. In more complex situations, the narrow portion of the urethra is removed and reconstructed with a small piece of the person's skin or other material.

Urethral syndrome, acute

Irritation of the bladder that is not caused by an infection from a disease-causing organism. Also known as noninfectious cystitis, the condition is most common in women during the childbearing years; it rarely occurs in

men. Possible causes include bubble baths, feminine hygiene sprays, sanitary napkins, spermicidal jellies, and sexual intercourse. Acute urethral syndrome can also arise as a complication of radiation therapy for the pelvic region or as a side effect of anti-cancer medications (chemotherapy). Symptoms may include pressure in the lower pelvis; painful urination; frequent, urgent need to urinate; decreased ability to hold urine (incontinence); urination at night (nocturia); cloudy, bloody, or foul-smelling urine; pain during sexual intercourse; pain in the penis or the side below the ribs; fatigue; and chills. The condition is usually treated with medication to control symptoms and with dietary changes to avoid fluids that irritate the bladder, such as alcohol, caffeine, and citrus juices. Most cases of acute urethral syndrome improve or resolve over time.

Urethritis, nongonococcal

One of the SEXUALLY TRANSMITTED DISEASES (STDs); it causes an inflammation of the urethra. Nongonococcal urethritis (NGU) is similar in some ways to GONORRHEA, but is caused by an agent other than *Neisseria gonorrhoeae*, which is responsible for gonorrhea. NGU is usually due to infection with *Chlamydia* bacteria, but may also be caused by types of *Ureaplasma*, *Mycoplasma*, and *Trichomonas* bacteria and the herpes simplex virus. It occurs worldwide and is three times more common than gonorrhea in the United States.

There may not be symptoms of NGU, especially in women, or symptoms may be mild, usually much less severe than those associated with gonorrhea. The symptoms tend to begin slowly and intensify over a period of several days. In men, they may include a clear mucous discharge from the end of the urethra at the tip of the penis and redness around the urethra. Both men and women may experience frequent urination with pain or burning. If a woman's reproductive tract or rectum becomes involved, there may be a vaginal discharge, abnormal menstrual bleeding, and discomfort in the anal or rectal area.

Because the symptoms of NGU tend to be mild or nonexistent, an infected

person may not know to seek medical treatment. This can cause the infection to spread. In women, complications of untreated NGU include PELVIC INFLAMMATORY DISEASE (PID), a frequent and preventable cause of infertility in women. In men, the infection can spread, causing inflammation of the prostate gland and the epididymis. NGU is not known to be associated with male infertility.

NGU is diagnosed when the symptoms of urethral inflammation are present without having gonorrhea, as revealed by laboratory tests. The bacteria that cause NGU can be detected in the urine and in genital tract secretions of an infected person. Antibiotics can treat NGU successfully. Infected people should abstain from sexual activity until the infection has cleared. Sexual partners should be informed so that they may be tested and treated as necessary.

Urethrocele

A condition in which the urethra bulges into the vagina. A urethrocele most commonly occurs in women after childbirth has stretched the pelvic muscles supporting the vagina, rectum, and bladder. Symptoms may include a feeling of pressure or aching in the vagina, difficulty in urinating, and difficulty with penetration during sexual intercourse. Stress incontinence, when urine leaks out when a woman laughs or coughs, is also a common symptom.

A urethrocele is easily detected by a doctor during a routine pelvic examination. It is most likely to develop in a woman who has had a very large baby, many babies, or a long, difficult labor. Symptoms often develop after menopause, when loss of estrogen further weakens pelvic muscles. Practicing KEGEL EXERCISES (alternately contracting and relaxing pelvic floor muscles) may relieve symptoms. HORMONE REPLACEMENT THERAPY is often recommended to women who have completed menopause, to help reverse some of the weakening of pelvic support tissues. When symptoms are severe enough to interfere in

Terms in small capital letters—for example, PHYSICAL THERAPY or PAGET DISEASE—indicate a cross-reference to another entry with more information.

U

daily activities, urethroceles can be corrected with surgery in which the bladder is pushed upward and sewn into position. Incontinence, or urine leakage, can also be treated with medication or a plastic device called a pessary to restore prolapsed organs to their normal positions.

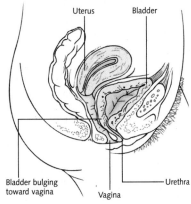

Uterus   Bladder

Bladder bulging toward vagina   Urethra

Vagina

A SAGGING URETHRA
If the pelvic muscles supporting a woman's bladder and urethra are weakened, the urethra can bulge down against the wall of the vagina. The woman may experience discomfort, difficulty urinating, leaking urine, or difficulty with intercourse. Pelvic exercises (Kegel exercises) may relieve these symptoms.

Uric acid

A component of blood and urine that is the end product of nucleic acid metabolism. Uric acid is an organic acid containing nitrogen. It is insoluble in water, and this can form solid crystals that lodge in the joints and skin, causing a painful condition called GOUT. Uric acid crystals can also form in the kidneys and cause kidney stones.

Uric acid comes from the natural breakdown of RNA (ribonucleic acid) and DNA (deoxyribonucleic acid). Large amounts of uric acid are found in certain foods, particularly red meats, organ meats such as liver and kidney, anchovies, and some shellfish. Normal amounts of uric acid remain dissolved in the blood and easily leave the body as waste, but high amounts of uric acid can accumulate and cause gout or kidney stones. Men older than 30, people who are overweight, people who drink alcohol frequently, and people who use diuretics to lower blood pressure are at greatest risk of developing gout.

Urinal

A receptacle for urine. A urinal is used for urination by a bedridden man.

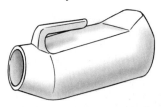

DISPOSABLE URINAL
Many hospitals use disposable urinals that reduce the risk of infection.

Urinalysis

A diagnostic tool that involves taking a sample of urine for chemical analysis in a laboratory. Urinalysis can reveal abnormal substances in urine that may indicate conditions, diseases, or other medical problems. White blood cells in the urine, for example, may reveal an infection in the body. Red blood cells can signal a tumor, a kidney stone, a kidney disorder, or a problem with the ureter or bladder. When bile is found in the urine, it may indicate liver disease. The presence of glucose in urine suggests diabetes mellitus.

WHAT A URINALYSIS CAN SHOW

A urinalysis may be done to detect alterations in the composition of normal urine. Urinalysis can help to check normal kidney function or to detect and diagnose urinary tract infections or other conditions.

- The presence of glucose in the urine is a typical sign of diabetes mellitus. The urine can be tested for acidity and ketones to confirm a suspected diagnosis of diabetes mellitus.
- Bacteria in the urine is a typical sign of cystitis, a bladder infection, or pyelonephritis, a kidney infection.
- Protein in the urine may be a sign of kidney damage or other disease.
- Bilirubin in the urine may be a sign of jaundice.
- Blood in the urine may be caused by a urinary tract infection, a kidney stone, a tumor, or some other abnormality.

Urinary diversion

A surgical procedure that changes the route urine follows from the kidney to the outside of the body. Urinary diversion is usually performed when the bladder must be removed because of cancer or a severe birth defect. A number of surgical operations can be performed, depending on the anatomy and health of the person.

Urinary diversion involves moving a small section of the large or small intestine from its usual location, implanting the tubes (ureters) that normally carry urine from the kidney to the bladder into one end of the section of intestine, and connecting the other end of the intestinal section to an opening (stoma) on the surface of the skin, usually near the navel. The patient wears a pouch taped to the skin to collect urine.

In another procedure, the ureters are implanted in the lower end of the large intestine close to the rectum. Urine is excreted along with the feces. In yet another type of operation, a reservoir is created from a section of intestine or stomach and connected either to the tube (urethra) that normally carries urine from the bladder out of the body or to a stoma on the skin surface. Since these substitute reservoirs can hold urine over a period of time, they are known as continent urinary diversions. The patient periodically empties the reservoir by inserting a thin rubber tube (catheter) or by urinating spontaneously.

Urinary diversion is a major abdominal operation that requires a hospital stay of several days and a lengthy recovery period at home. Complications during recovery can include abnormal bleeding, blood clots, and infection. Longer-term complications can include metabolic imbalance caused by the absorption of urine salts and other chemicals through the intestinal conduit or reservoir, infection or irritation of the stoma, calculi (stones) in the urinary tract, and infection of the kidneys. Psychological counseling before and after urinary diversion can help in dealing with potential emotional issues following surgery.

Urinary frequency

An abnormal increase in the number of times a person needs to urinate, often accompanied by greater urgency and discomfort or pain. Urinary fre-

U

quency can result from excessive fluid intake, particularly of alcoholic or caffeinated beverages; infection of the bladder; pregnancy; enlarged prostate gland; diabetes; calculi (stones) in the urinary tract; certain medications, such as diuretics; or radiation therapy for the lower pelvis. Treatment depends on the cause.

Urinary retention

Slow, hesitant, weak, or incomplete voiding of urine from the bladder. The condition may be sudden, accompanied by increasingly severe pain in the pelvis, or it may develop slowly and last over an extended period or become chronic. The person experiences little discomfort, but has great difficulty in starting the stream of urine, which is small and weak. Chronic urinary retention is often accompanied by constant dribbling of urine. The condition results from partial or complete blockage of the urinary tract by a calculus (stone), injury to the urine tube (urethral stricture), enlarged prostate gland, cancer of the prostate, birth defect, infection, or tumor. Left untreated, the condition can cause urine to back up into the kidneys and severely damage them. An examination by a doctor and various types of laboratory tests, such as analysis of the urine for infectious organisms or visual inspection of the urinary tract through X rays or a cystoscopy, are needed to establish the cause of the urinary retention. Treatment depends on the cause.

Urinary tract

The system of organs that filter out waste products and excess water from the bloodstream and expel it as a fluid called urine. The major structures within the urinary tract are the kidneys, the ureters, the bladder, and the urethra.

STRUCTURE

The kidneys are the pair of organs that perform the task of filtering blood. The kidneys are located in the back of the abdominal cavity, on either side of the spine, at about waist level. (The right kidney sits slightly lower than the left because of the position of the liver.) The kidneys are supplied with unfiltered blood by the two renal arteries, which branch off from the aorta (the major artery directing blood

from the heart to the rest of the body). Blood that has been filtered leaves the kidneys via the two renal veins, which flow into the inferior vena cava (the major vein that leads from the lower body to the heart).

Waste materials and excess fluid filtered out of the blood collect first in each kidney, in a system of collecting ducts and storage areas. This liquid substance, called urine, is composed of water, urea (the waste product), and sodium chloride. From each KID-NEY, a slender tube called a URETER transports the processed urine from the kidneys to the bladder. The bladder is a muscular sac that holds the urine until enough builds up for the body to excrete. When the bladder contracts, the urine flows into the urethra, a tube that passes out of the body. In a woman, the urethral opening is located just above the opening to the vagina; in a man, the urethra runs the length of the penis, and the opening is at the tip.

FUNCTION

As body cells consume nutrients and energy, chemical waste products begin to build up in the liver and throughout the body. These waste products, which could be toxic if they accumulated, must be removed. They are transported from the body to the kid-

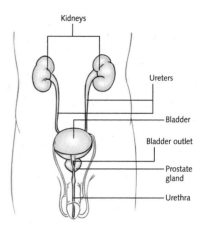

THE MALE URINARY TRACT
For both men and woman, the lower part of the urinary tract is located close to the reproductive organs. In a man, the urethra is about 8 inches long, running through the penis and opening at the tip. The male urethra serves as the passageway for semen from the reproductive organs, as well as the passageway for elimination of urine.

neys in the bloodstream. Excess amino acids and by-products such as ammonia are secreted into a substance called urea, which is excreted in the urine.

The tissue of the kidney is composed of microscopic filtering units called nephrons, which conserve protein (the structural element of body cells) but allow excess water, glucose, salts, and other by-products to flow into tubules. The tubules reabsorb essential nutrients, including glucose, but excrete fluid and wastes into the ureters. Urine flows from the urine down to the bladder as a result of both gravity and muscular contractions in the walls of the ureters. As urine collects in the bladder, the walls of the bladder stretch and trigger the reflexive (involuntary) urge to urinate. The reflex can be consciously controlled by signals from the brain. When the bladder contracts, urine is released into the urethra and flows out of the body.

Urinary tract infections

Bacterial infections affecting any part of the URINARY TRACT. Urinary tract infections occur more frequently in women than men, primarily because a woman's urethra is one-tenth the length of that of a man. Urinary tract infections are usually caused by bacteria such as *Escherichia coli*, which

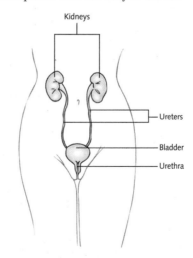

THE FEMALE URINARY TRACT
In both men and woman, the kidneys filter waste fluids from the blood. The ureters carry the fluid (urine) to the bladder to be held until it is released into the urethra for elimination. In a woman, the urethra is relatively short, and the opening lies just above the vaginal opening and close to the anus, making the urinary tract more susceptible to infection.

U

travel from the rectum to the urethra, bladder, and even to the kidneys. Symptoms include pain or a burning sensation while urinating, frequent urge to urinate, pressure in the lower part of the abdomen, blood in the urine, and foul-smelling urine. Additional symptoms such as high fever, vomiting, and back or abdominal pain may signal spread of the infection to the kidneys.

The most common urinary tract infection is of the bladder, or CYSTITIS. Infection of the urethra, or urethritis (see URETHRITIS, NONGONCOCCAL), often occurs at the same time. If bacteria travel up to the kidneys, they may cause PYELONEPHRITIS, a kidney infection. Diagnosis is made on the basis of the number of bacteria and white blood cells found in a urine sample. A pelvic examination may also be required. Treatment also includes antibiotics. Recurrent infections and kidney infections are more serious. The person may be referred to a urologist, a specialist who may perform intravenous pyelography, a special X ray of the urinary tract, or an X ray of the bladder to look for defects in the urinary tract that may be causing the infections.

Urinary tract infections in women can be prevented, chiefly by practicing good hygiene. Wiping from front to back after urinating or after a bowel movement, washing the area around the vagina and rectum daily, and washing those areas before and after sexual intercourse are recommended to prevent spread of bacteria into the urinary tract. Drinking plenty of fluids, particularly cranberry juice, helps flush out bacteria, as does emptying the bladder as soon as the urge to urinate occurs. Vitamin C makes the urine acidic, which discourages bacterial growth. Cotton underwear is preferred over other kinds, since synthetic fibers tend to trap moisture, which promotes bacterial growth.

Urination, painful

FOR SYMPTOM CHART
see Urination in men, painful or frequent, page 56
see Urination in women, painful or frequent, page 57

Discomfort or burning while voiding urine. Called dysuria, the problem is fairly common, and it typically

results from an infection in the urinary tract. Other, less typical causes include infection of the prostate gland (prostatitis), a calculus or stone in the urinary tract, or cancer of the cervix. Diagnosis requires a physical examination and laboratory tests of the urine to check for infectious organisms. Treatment depends on the cause. In the case of infection, antibiotics are prescribed. Pain medications may also be ordered by the doctor if the discomfort is severe.

Urine

Liquid waste produced by the kidneys, stored in the bladder, and excreted through the urethra. In humans, normal urine is a transparent, amber-colored fluid made up of water, urea, salt, and uric acid. Urine is about 96 percent water and 4 percent solid waste. The average amount of urine excreted by a person each day ranges from 40 to 80 ounces.

Abnormal urine contains substances not usually found in urine and is usually a sign of disease. Urine contains sugar in people with diabetes; the protein albumin in people with certain kidney diseases, such as Bright disease; bile pigments in people with jaundice; or possibly blood in people with kidney stones. Urine can also contain abnormal quantities of one or another of its normal components. See also CYSTITIS; URINARY TRACT INFECTIONS.

Urine tests

A series of laboratory studies done on a sample of urine to determine the health of the kidneys, bladder, and uri-

COMMON BLADDER-RELATED PROBLEMS		
SYMPTOM	**MEN OR WOMEN**	**POSSIBLE CAUSE**
Blood in the urine	Both	Calculus (stone in the kidney, ureter, or bladder)
	Both	Cystitis (bladder infection)
	Both	Tumor
	Men	Prostatitis (inflammation of the prostate gland)
Difficult urination	Women	Prolapsed uterus or vagina
	Men	Prostate gland enlargement
	Both	Medications
	Both	Stroke (nerve damage affecting bladder control)
Frequent urination	Both	Cystitis
	Both	Diabetes (glucose in urine)
	Women	Fibroid (benign tumor)
	Both	Incontinence
	Both	Medications
	Men	Prostate gland enlargement
	Both	Stroke
	Women	Urethritis (inflammation of urethra)
Painful urination	Both	Calculus (stone in kidney, ureter, or bladder)
	Women	Cancer of the cervix
	Both	Cystitis (bladder infection)
	Men	Prostate infection
	Women	Urethritis (inflammation of urethra)

nary tract or to gain information about overall body processes. The particular tests, usually called a urinalysis, depend on what the physician is investigating. If an infection of the bladder is suspected, the urine is tested for pus cells, bacteria, blood, and degree of acidity. Sugar (glucose) in the urine is a sign of diabetes, and protein in the urine can signal kidney disease.

Urologist

A physician who specializes in treating diseases of the urinary tract in both males and females and the reproductive system in males.

Urology

The branch of medicine that focuses on the urinary tract in both males and females and the reproductive system in males. See URINARY TRACT; REPRODUCTIVE SYSTEM, MALE.

Urticaria

See HIVES.

Uterine septum

A wall of tissue, or septum, that separates the uterus into two parts. If a woman is unable to achieve conception as a result, surgical intervention is sometimes used to correct this unusual defect. The surgeon removes the septum by using HYSTEROSCOPY.

Uterus

A hollow, muscular organ of the female reproductive system, located on top of the bladder in front of the rectum; also called the womb. In the event of PREGNANCY, the uterus holds the fetus until it is ready for birth.

The wall of the uterus is lined with ENDOMETRIUM, specialized tissue that builds up to nourish a fetus in case of pregnancy. In the absence of a pregnancy, this lining is shed each month in the cycle called MENSTRUATION. If a pregnancy does occur, a fertilized egg implants on the wall of the uterus and develops into a fetus. The uterus is remarkably elastic, able to expand to many times its original size to hold a fetus. Strong ligaments hold the organ in place, even if it is bearing considerable extra weight of a developing fetus. At the end of the pregnancy, the uterus returns to its usual size.

The neck of the uterus, the cervix, connects with the upper part of the vagina, which forms a passage out of the body. The cervix is actually cylindrical, with a small opening in the center. Menstrual fluids can pass out of the uterus through this opening. If sexual intercourse takes place, sperm cells can enter the small opening in the cervix and travel up through the uterus into the fallopian tubes. See REPRODUCTIVE SYSTEM, FEMALE.

Uterus, cancer of

Malignant tumors located in the uterus. Most uterine cancers are ADENOCARCINOMA, tumors involving cells in the uterine lining. Symptoms include abnormal bleeding, spotting, or discharge from the vagina in a steady or an intermittent flow. Cancer of the uterus is rare before age 40 and most often occurs in women between ages 60 and 75.

Cancer of the uterus is diagnosed by a number of tests, including ULTRASOUND SCANNING, ENDOMETRIAL BIOPSY, HYSTEROSCOPY, and D AND C. All of them can be performed in a doctor's office after the woman has been given local anesthesia, except for D and C, which is done in a hospital. A Pap smear is not a good test for cancer of the uterus because it identifies less than 50 percent of women who have uterine cancer.

Most women with cancer of the uterus will have both a HYSTERECTOMY and SALPINGO-OOPHORECTOMY, surgical removal of the uterus and ovaries. Some women will also require RADIATION THERAPY after surgery. CHEMOTHERAPY may be used to treat cancer that has spread to other organs. Women at risk for cancer of the uterus are those who are obese; do not ovulate regularly; often miss periods; have late menopause; have POLYCYSTIC OVARIAN SYNDROME or ENDOMETRIAL HYPERPLASIA; have had cancer of the ovary, breast, or colon; or have a close family member with cancer of the uterus. The risk for developing cancer can be lowered by reporting abnormal vaginal bleeding to the doctor immediately, having annual pelvic examinations, maintaining normal weight, and eating a low-fat, low-cholesterol, high-fiber diet.

Uterus, prolapse of

A condition in which the uterus is displaced and sags into or through the vagina. Prolapse occurs when the ligaments holding the uterus in place are

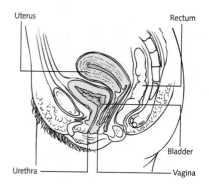

Normal position of uterus

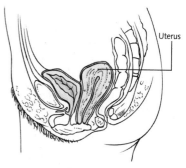

Prolapsed uterus

A DROPPED UTERUS
In some women, the ligaments supporting the uterus weaken as a result of aging or pregnancy, and the uterus drops from its normal position down against or even into the vagina. In severe cases, the uterus can sag down into the vaginal opening. The condition is fairly common after childbirth and after menopause. The prolapse can cause discomfort, backache, and incontinence.

stretched by pregnancy and childbirth or are weakened after menopause. Depending on the degree of prolapse, symptoms can include a lump or bulge in the vagina, a feeling of heaviness and discomfort, occasional backache, and stress incontinence, in which urine leaks when the woman coughs, laughs, or physically exerts herself. In a complete prolapse, most common in women over 70, the uterus bulges out of the vaginal opening.

Prolapse is common for a few months after childbirth and in later life. It may be uncomfortable and inconvenient, but poses little risk to general health. Women most at risk for developing prolapse are those who have had very large babies, who have had many pregnancies, who are obese, and who have fibroid tumors. Menopause with its reduced estrogen

U

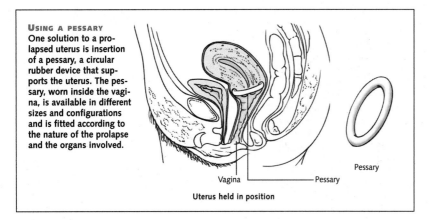

USING A PESSARY
One solution to a prolapsed uterus is insertion of a pessary, a circular rubber device that supports the uterus. The pessary, worn inside the vagina, is available in different sizes and configurations and is fitted according to the nature of the prolapse and the organs involved.

Vagina — Pessary
Pessary
Uterus held in position

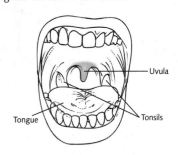

Uvula
Tongue
Tonsils

LOCATION OF THE UVULA
The uvula is visible in the back of the mouth where it hangs down from the middle of the soft palate.

levels can weaken the ligaments holding the uterus in place even further, and straining during a bowel movement can aggravate a prolapse. Prolapse of the uterus often accompanies CYSTOCELE, URETHROCELE, and RECTOCELE (prolapses of the bladder, urethra, and rectum).

Treatment of mild prolapse should include KEGEL EXERCISES to strengthen the pelvic muscles. Weight loss and a high-fiber diet to prevent constipation are also recommended. HORMONE REPLACEMENT THERAPY in women past menopause may strengthen supportive tissues. Insertion of a PESSARY can help support the uterus, while severe prolapse can be addressed with surgical procedures, including a HYSTERECTOMY.

Uterus, retroverted

Also called "tipped" uterus; a uterus that inclines downward and backward, lying close to the anal canal. This condition occurs in about 20 percent of women; in most cases, there are no symptoms, and no treatment is required. It can result from childbirth or after a disease such as a tumor or ENDOMETRIOSIS, which can cause displacement of the uterus. Some women experience dyspareunia (pain during sexual intercourse) or dysmenorrhea (pain during menstruation) as a result, and they may also have difficulty using tampons. Surgery to move the uterus forward can be performed if symptoms are severe.

UV light

See ULTRAVIOLET LIGHT.

Uveitis

Inflammation of the middle layer or uveal tract (uvea) of the EYE. The uvea lies between the sclera (the white outer covering of the eye) and the retina (the inner light-sensitive layer). It includes the iris (the colored part of the eye), the ciliary body (which lies behind the iris), and the choroid (which supports the retina). Since the uvea contains large numbers of blood vessels that nourish the eye, inflammation can threaten sight. The inflammation produces scars that correspond to areas of vision loss; the more scarring, the more loss.

Symptoms of uveitis may come on suddenly, or they may develop slowly. They include sensitivity to light, blurred vision, pain, and redness.

The disease has many possible causes, including infection by a virus (such as herpes or mumps), a fungus (such as histoplasmosis), or a parasite (such as toxoplasmosis, the most common cause of uveitis when present in infants at birth). Uveitis can also result from an injury to the eye or from autoimmune diseases such as rheumatoid arthritis and ankylosing spondylitis.

Treatment of uveitis consists of treatment of any underlying disease plus frequent use of corticosteroid and medicated eye drops. Sunglasses may be worn for comfort. Uveitis often recurs and may cause permanent damage to vision, even with treatment. Long-term use of corticosteroid eye drops and the inflammation from uveitis itself may lead to cataract formation and glaucoma.

Uvula

A small, fleshy mass in the mouth that hangs from the soft palate above the back of the tongue. The uvula is made of muscle and connective tissue and is covered by a mucous membrane. Although its exact function is not clear, it may have a role in clearing the mouth of secretions.

Uvulopalatopharyngoplasty

A procedure for surgically removing excess tissue at the back of the throat to expand the airway and improve certain sleep disorder symptoms such as obstructive sleep apnea (see SLEEP APNEA SYNDROME) and disruptive SNORING.

Obstructive sleep apnea is a potentially life-threatening disorder characterized by interruptions of breathing during sleep. Snoring is a major symptom of obstructive sleep apnea. Other conditions that may indicate a need for uvulopalatopharyngoplasty include restless sleep and sleep deprivation caused by breathing problems, associated debilitating daytime sleepiness, and cardiac arrhythmias (see ARRHYTHMIA, CARDIAC) associated with upper airway obstruction.

Before the procedure is recommended, a person is generally examined by an otolaryngologist (ear, nose, and throat specialist) to evaluate the cause of snoring. The examination may include the use of fiberoptic (see FIBEROPTICS) endoscopy. A person will usually be required to participate in a sleep study to evaluate his or her level of snoring and sleep apnea. Lifestyle changes to correct snoring and usually a breathing apparatus worn at night are often attempted before surgery is recommended.

HOW THE PROCEDURE IS DONE
Uvulopalatopharyngoplasty is performed under general anesthesia by a surgeon. The tissue removed during

U

the procedure may include tissue of the uvula, tonsils, and parts of the soft palate. A hospital stay of 1 to 3 days is usually required. Intravenous fluids are given until the person can take fluids by mouth. Pain medication is required. Possible side effects after the operation may include a sore throat, temporary airway obstruction due to swelling, and spitting up blood. People with severe sleep apnea are at great danger during and immediately after surgery and need intensive monitoring. Complications such as infection, bleeding from the mouth or nose, and the vomiting of fresh blood require immediate medical attention. Full recovery takes about 2 weeks.

While uvulopalatopharyngoplasty can usually decrease or eliminate snoring, it may not correct obstructive sleep apnea. It is difficult to predict what makes the procedure more effective in correcting sleep apnea in some people than in others. Full testing and evaluation before surgery may help determine a candidate's potential for postsurgery success.

LUAP AND SOMNOPLASTY

Laser-assisted uvulopalatoplasty, or LUAP, is an outpatient procedure, performed under local anesthesia, involving the use of a handheld laser device to remove tissue in the back of the throat. Anesthetic is sprayed over the back of the throat, the soft palate, tonsils, and uvula and injected into the muscle layer of the uvula. After the anesthesia has taken effect, the surgeon directs the laser beam through the open mouth to make vertical incisions in the soft palate on both sides of the uvula. The palate and uvula are shortened, which helps to eliminate the obstruction that has contributed to snoring. The procedure takes about 30 minutes. After having LUAP, a person can usually resume normal activities the next day. Side effects include a moderate to severe sore throat that can last 4 to 10 days and can be relieved by painkillers and anti-inflammatory medication. Depending on the severity of snoring, a person may require two to five sessions of LUAP, performed at intervals of 4 to 6 weeks.

The goal of LUAP is to eliminate snoring; it may not treat mild sleep apnea. It is not recommended for people with more severe sleep disorders.

Because the laser cannot reach enlarged tissues around the tonsils or along the wall of the throat, LUAP can only decrease the sound of severe snoring and may mask this symptom of sleep apnea. This presents the risk that the more serious condition will be difficult to diagnose or may go untreated.

Somnoplasty is a new and minimally invasive procedure for the treatment of snoring and obstructive sleep apnea. The operation is performed on an outpatient basis, using a needle electrode to emit radio waves. The radio waves shrink excess tissue surrounding the upper airway, including the soft palate and uvula, to correct snoring. The tissue at the base of the tongue may be treated in this way to correct sleep apnea. Somnoplasty may also be performed on the structures in the nose to treat chronic nasal obstruction.

U

V

Vaccination

The process of stimulating the body's ANTIBODY production and memory cells in the immune system by introducing substances that elicit these functions without actually causing the disease. Vaccination involves introducing an ANTIGEN designed to produce IMMUNITY to the disease associated with the antigen. The body develops active immunity after exposure to a pathogen has caused an illness. Vaccination mimics this process by exposing the body to the pathogen in an altered state that does not produce the illness, but stimulates production of antibodies that can defeat it. The goal of vaccination is to help the immune system develop long-term immunity to certain diseases. IMMUNIZATION is the successful outcome of vaccination. See also VACCINE; TRAVEL IMMUNIZATION.

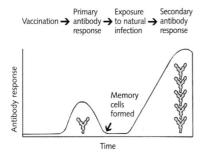

HOW VACCINATION WORKS
A vaccine is a modified organism that can be injected without causing harm. The person's immune system responds by forming antibody cells that "remember" the organism. When the person is exposed to the true disease, the memory cells produce a faster, stronger response that kills the potentially infecting organisms.

Vaccinations, childhood

Immunizations that protect children from a number of serious and contagious infections. DIPHTHERIA, PERTUSSIS (whooping cough), MEASLES, and POLIO once took the lives of thousands of children each year. Now regular vaccinations have virtually eradicated these childhood diseases, and they rarely occur in the United States.

Immunization increases children's resistance to infectious diseases by stimulating their immune systems to produce antibodies against disease-causing organisms. Because the digestive juices would destroy most vaccines if given orally, the majority of vaccinations are given by injection. Babies typically receive injections in the thigh, while older children usually receive them in the upper arm.

In most cases, children need a series of timely vaccinations to provide resistance. The first immunization induces the body to produce antibodies, while later shots boost the immune system and reinforce the protection. Vaccinations provide the maximum protection when children receive them on a specific schedule. Many vaccinations are given in the first 2 years of life. Because the presence of a mild illness does not interfere with the vaccine's ability to stimulate an IMMUNE RESPONSE, and because timing is important, a pediatrician or family physician will usually proceed with a scheduled vaccination for a child who has a minor illness or slight fever. A child who has a weakened immune system or a serious disease such as cancer may need to follow a different immunization schedule than that for a healthy child. Child care centers, schools, and camps usually require documentation that shows immunizations have been given on schedule.

TYPES OF VACCINATION

Children receive a scheduled series of vaccinations from birth until 16 years of age. Although vaccinations can cause reactions, they are usually mild. The risk of a child having a reaction is far lower than is the risk of getting a dangerous disease if the child is not immunized. The most common side effect is soreness or swelling at the site of injection. Serious reactions are rare.

■ **Diphtheria, tetanus, and pertussis** The combination diphtheria, tetanus, and pertussis (DTP) vaccination provides protection against three deadly infectious bacterial diseases. It is usually given in a series of five shots: at ages 2 months, 4 months, 6 months, 15 to 18 months, and 4 to 6 years. Booster shots for diphtheria and tetanus are recommended 10 years after the final childhood shot and every 10 years thereafter for life.

Common side effects include soreness at the injection site, fever, fussiness, and sleepiness. In rare cases, the DTP can cause excessive irritability or sleepiness, poor appetite, a high fever (above 103°F), or a seizure. A child who exhibits these symptoms requires a doctor's attention. A newer type of injection, DTaP, is the preferred form of the DTP vaccine because it causes fewer side effects. It contains substances that stimulate production of diphtheria and tetanus antibodies and a pertussis vaccine that contains elements of the pertussis bacteria rather than the whole cell. The DTP vaccine remains an acceptable alternative. Another vaccine preparation combines the diphtheria, tetanus, pertussis, and *Haemophilus influenzae* type B (Hib) into a single injection.

■ **Hepatitis B** The hepatitis B virus causes inflammation of the liver, which can lead to liver disease, liver cancer, and death. The vaccination is administered in a series of three shots: usually the first at birth or within an infant's first 2 months, the second between 1 and 4 months, and the third between 6 and 18 months. In addition to the hepatitis B vaccine, infants born to mothers infected with the virus need to receive hepatitis B immune globulin (antibodies) within 12 hours of birth. Older children who have not been vaccinated should receive the series of three injections beginning at age 9 or 10 years. The vaccine rarely causes any side effects.

■ **Polio** A disease that causes muscle pain and paralysis, polio was once very common in the United States. Because of widespread immunization, the illness has nearly disappeared. The polio vaccine is given in a series of four doses at ages 2 months, 4 months, between 6 and 18 months, and between 4 and 6 years. There are 2 types of polio vaccine: inactivated poliovirus vaccine (IPV) and oral poliovirus vaccine (OPV). IPV is given as an injection, while OPV is given orally. OPV was once more widely used because it is easier to give, but it is no longer recommended because it carries a slight risk of infecting the child with polio. IPV is recommended for all four doses.

■ **Haemophilus influenzae** *type B* This bacterium (Hib) causes several

SUGGESTED SCHEDULE OF CHILDHOOD VACCINATIONS

Vaccinations can protect children from hepatitis B, pertussis (whooping cough), diphtheria, tetanus (lockjaw), polio, measles, mumps, rubella (German measles), *Haemophilus influenzae* type b, and chickenpox. Immunizations should begin at birth, and all should be introduced by age 2, when a child needs the protection most. Most immunizations are given in a time-sensitive series of shots.

AGE	VACCINATION
Birth-2 months	Hepatitis B
1-4 months	Hepatitis B
2 months	DTaP, Hib, IPV
4 months	DTaP, Hib, IPV
6 months	DTaP, Hib
6-18 months	Hepatitis B, IPV
12-15 months	Hib, MMR
12-18 months	Chickenpox
15-18 months	DTaP
4-6 years	DTaP, IPV, MMR
11-16 years	Diphtheria, tetanus

KEY
DTaP — Diphtheria, tetanus, and acellular pertussis
Hib — *Haemophilus influenzae* type b
IPV — Inactivated poliovirus vaccine
MMR — Measles, mumps, rubella

types of dangerous infections: MENINGITIS, PNEUMONIA, and EPIGLOTTITIS. Immunization with one of the three available Hib vaccines makes children resistant to these infections. The vaccine is given in a series of three or four shots, depending upon which type is used, starting at age 2 months. Hib vaccinations have no serious side effects. Mild reactions may include soreness at the injection site, a slight fever, and fussiness; symptoms should subside within 48 to 72 hours.

■ *Measles, mumps, and rubella* Measles causes a high fever and rash and can lead to ear infections, croup, bronchitis, pneumonia, encephalitis, and, in rare cases, brain swelling. Mumps causes swelling and pain in the salivary glands and can spread to other organs such as the brain, testicles, and pancreas. Long-term complications may include infertility in males and HEARING LOSS. German measles, or rubella, does not usually cause serious problems for children. However, pregnant women who become infected with it risk having stillborn babies or babies with birth defects.

The combination measles, mumps, and rubella (MMR) vaccine is administered in two shots: the first at age 12 to 15 months and the second between the ages of 4 and 6 years. The second dose should be given by age 11 or 12 years at the latest. The most common side effect is a fever or rash 1 to 2 weeks following the vaccination. It may last a few days but is not contagious. Children who are allergic to eggs may not be able to have the MMR vaccination, which has an egg base. A skin test can determine whether the MMR is safe for a child. Children who have a weakened immune system or diseases such as cancer should not receive this vaccination. With a doctor's approval, children with HIV (human immunodeficiency virus) infection can be vaccinated. Because of the theoretical risk to the fetus, pregnant women should not get the MMR vaccination. However, there have been no reports of serious birth defects in women who were inadvertently immunized while they were pregnant.

■ *Chickenpox* Chickenpox begins with a mild fever and a skin rash, which progresses into fluid-filled blisters. Complications may include pneumonia and encephalitis. Chickenpox is a highly contagious disease that once affected most children in the United States by age 10. However, a chickenpox vaccine became available in 1995 that can prevent this viral infection or lessen its severity. The varicella zoster virus vaccine, or chickenpox vaccine, is given in a single dose to children 12 months or older. Older children who have not had chickenpox or been vaccinated for this virus can have the vaccination at any time. Children age 13 and older should receive two doses, given at least 4 weeks apart. The vaccination does not cause side effects in most children. There may be mild reactions such as soreness, swelling, redness, or stiffness at the injection site within 48 hours after the vaccination. In the following 3 weeks, a child may experience fatigue, fever, fussiness, nausea, or a mild rash. A vaccinated child with a rash may be contagious.

Vaccine

A preparation introduced into the body to stimulate antibodies, create immunity, and prevent disease. Vaccines contain antigens (see ANTIGEN) that are designed to stimulate an IMMUNE RESPONSE that will offer protection from specific diseases. A vaccine is composed of killed pathogens, such as viruses and bacteria, or weakened strains of microorganisms. These preparations are able to prompt the production of antibodies without causing the disease.

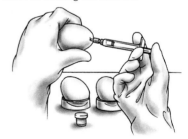

MAKING A VACCINE
To make a vaccine, scientists grow disease organisms and then alter them; for example, live chick eggs are injected with a virus. Some vaccines contain an inactivated virus, which has been treated chemically to make it noninfectious. Other vaccines contain a weakened form of the virus, which can still infect but is not dangerous.

V

Vacuum extraction

A procedure used when a vaginal delivery is difficult or prolonged, in which suction is used to pull the baby down the birth canal. A metal or plastic cap is attached to the baby's scalp and connected to a vacuum pump. Vacuum extraction is used instead of FORCEPS DELIVERY if the mother is exhausted or has a heart condition, or when the baby begins to show signs of FETAL DISTRESS. Vacuum extraction requires less pain medication than forceps delivery and may not require episiotomy, an incision in the opening of the vagina. If vacuum extraction is used, the baby's scalp may swell briefly, and there is some risk that the mother's vagina and cervix may be injured by the procedure.

Vagina

A muscular tube about 5 inches long that extends from the neck of the uterus to the outer genital area of a woman's body. The opening of the vagina is covered and protected by the labia majora and labia minora, the two pairs of lips in a woman's external genital area. The vagina's muscular walls have a ridged inner surface and are richly supplied with blood vessels.

As the passageway to the internal reproductive organs, the vagina has three functions: it provides an outlet for blood shed during menstruation, it accommodates a man's penis during sexual intercourse, and it is the canal through which a baby passes during CHILDBIRTH.

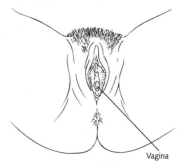

EXTERNAL VAGINAL OPENING
The external opening of the vagina, a tube leading to the uterus, is protected by two visible folds of skin on the outside of the body. The length of the vagina is ringed with muscle and lined with mucous membranes to maintain a moist environment and helpful bacteria that keep the area clean.

In a young girl, a membrane called the hymen lies just inside the vagina. This delicate membrane is easily torn, often by use of tampons or sexual activity. Once the hymen is broken, the remaining tissue becomes a ring around the vaginal wall. The vagina constantly produces secretions to maintain a moist environment and a balance of helpful bacteria. During sexual arousal, vaginal secretions increase to lubricate the vagina for intercourse. These secretions lessen after MENOPAUSE. See REPRODUCTIVE SYSTEM, FEMALE.

Vaginal bleeding

Abnormal bleeding from the vagina that is not part of the monthly period or bleeding during the period that is heavier than usual. In women of reproductive age, causes can include the use of birth control pills; problems with hormones produced by the ovaries or thyroid, pituitary, or adrenal glands; infections of the vagina, cervix, uterus, fallopian tubes, or ovaries, including sexually transmitted diseases; ectopic pregnancies; and miscarriage. Bleeding can also be caused by scars, tumors, fibroids, or other abnormal tissue on the uterus or cervix; cysts on the ovaries; or growths in the endometrium (the lining of the uterus).

Women who are approaching menopause may bleed irregularly as part of that process. Vaginal bleeding after menopause is most likely caused by benign or malignant tumors of the uterus or ovaries and requires a doctor's attention. At any age, vaginal bleeding can be caused by an injury to the vagina or reproductive tract during rape or surgery or by the presence of objects, such as a tampon forgotten in the vagina. Vaginal bleeding, along with fever, abdominal pain, or other vaginal discharge, may indicate the presence of an infection. Profuse vaginal bleeding may also occur in women taking blood thinning medications.

Evaluation of vaginal bleeding will depend on a woman's age and medical history. Diagnostic tests may include a pregnancy test, ultrasound, endometrial biopsy, and tests for the presence of specific hormones in the blood. Treatment depends on the cause of the bleeding.

Vaginal relaxation

The gradual weakening of pelvic muscles that permits prolapse of the uterus and allows other organs to bulge in the vagina. This weakening of the muscles is associated with childbirth, obesity, and loss of estrogen in women who have completed menopause. Symptoms include the bulging of the bladder (CYSTOCELE), urethra (URETHROCELE), rectum (RECTOCELE), or the uterus into the vagina, accompanied by feelings of pressure in the vagina and stress incontinence, in which urine leaks out when a woman sneezes, coughs, laughs, or is physically active.

Treatment usually consists of KEGEL EXERCISES to strengthen the pelvic muscles and, after menopause, HORMONE REPLACEMENT THERAPY, which can sometimes reverse the weakening of the muscles and ligaments supporting the uterus. In severe cases, a HYSTERECTOMY can be performed to correct prolapse. Surgeries can also be performed to correct cystocele, urethrocele, and rectocele.

Vaginal repair

Surgical repair or reconstruction of a vagina. In colporrhaphy, a prolapsed vaginal wall is repaired. More extensive surgery is performed after disease has necessitated surgical removal of the original vaginal tissue or when radiation has resulted in a loss of tissue. A reconstructed vagina is essential for a woman who wants to remain sexually active. Various surgical methods are used to restore the vagina, including one in which the skin of the labia is used to construct a new vagina.

Vaginal ultrasound

See ULTRASOUND, VAGINAL.

Vaginal vault prolapse

A condition in which the top of the vagina loses its support and drops, usually following a HYSTERECTOMY. The top of the vagina may drop partway into the lower vagina and remain there, or it may extend part or all the way through the vaginal opening. Symptoms include a feeling of heaviness in the vagina, aching in the lower abdomen or lower back, and bulging of organs against the vaginal wall. Most women with vaginal vault prolapse also have an ENTEROCELE (bulging of the intestines into the vaginal wall), and they may also have problems with bladder and bowel function.

The diagnosis of a vaginal vault prolapse will require a thorough pelvic examination. Treatment may include KEGEL EXERCISES to strengthen the pelvic muscles, a PESSARY, inserted into the vagina to support the pelvic organs, or surgery to try to correct the weakened pelvic support. The principal causes of vaginal vault prolapse are childbirth and aging, both of which weaken the tissues supporting the pelvic organs.

Vaginismus

An involuntary spasm of the muscles of the vagina, making sexual intercourse uncomfortable, difficult, or impossible. A woman with vaginismus may also be unable to tolerate a pelvic examination or the insertion of a tampon. Vaginismus tends to occur when a woman associates penetration with pain, and the resulting anxiety causes her vaginal muscles to tense. Traumatic sexual experiences of the past may predispose a woman to vaginismus. Sometimes, the painful experience may not have been particularly traumatic, such as the pain from chronic vaginitis, an inflammation of the vagina. Whatever the cause of the anxiety, it leads to muscular spasms that cause pain when penetration is attempted.

Treatment of vaginismus is best provided by a psychotherapist experienced with sexual disorders. A common approach involves exercises designed to teach the woman how to relax her vaginal muscles at will. Another treatment calls for the woman to lie quietly and insert one finger in her vagina for 5 minutes twice a day for 2 days, then to insert 2 fingers twice a day for 2 days, and so on. This combination of behavior therapy and psychotherapy has a high rate of success.

Vaginitis

A very common condition characterized by inflammation of the vagina. Symptoms include irritation, redness, or swelling of the vaginal tissues. Vaginitis can also cause a discharge, itching, odor, or a burn-

ing sensation. The most common cause of vaginitis is infection, but other causes include irritation from products like soaps and the lack of estrogen that accompanies menopause.

To diagnose vaginitis, a sample of the woman's vaginal discharge is viewed under a microscope. Treatment depends on the cause of the vaginitis and may include oral medication or a cream or gel to be applied to the vagina.

The risk of getting vaginitis can be reduced by using condoms during sexual intercourse, washing diaphragms and cervical caps carefully after each use, and abandoning the use of feminine hygiene sprays, deodorant tampons, and douches.

Vaginitis, atrophic

An inflammation of the vagina caused by degeneration of the vaginal tissue. Atrophic vaginitis is the most common cause of vaginal irritation in postmenopausal women. After menopause, as estrogen production decreases, the walls of the vagina become drier, thinner, less elastic, and more likely to bleed. Vaginal dryness can cause irritation, burning, or itching and a feeling of pressure, all of which may interfere with a woman's sexual enjoyment.

Treatment for atrophic vaginitis after menopause may include HORMONE REPLACEMENT THERAPY to restore estrogen levels. Hormonal creams, inserted vaginally, also alleviate local symptoms. Atrophic vaginitis during breast-feeding is only temporary and will correct itself in time. If the primary symptom is painful sexual intercourse, the use of a water-soluble lubricant may help. Regular sexual activity improves circulation in the vagina and helps to keep the tissues supple.

Vaginosis, bacterial

The most common vaginal infection; inflammation of the vagina caused by bacteria. Symptoms include an unpleasant or fishy odor, increased vaginal discharge, or itching, burning, or redness in the vaginal area. Bacterial vaginosis is caused by an overgrowth of one or more types of bacteria, all of which interact and proliferate, destroying healthy organisms. Women who are sexually active

are most likely to develop bacterial vaginosis, although it is not always a sexually transmitted disease.

Diagnosis requires a pelvic examination and microscopic laboratory analysis of the vaginal discharge. Treatment usually involves 5 to 7 days of antibiotics taken orally or inserted into the vagina as a suppository. Many doctors also treat the woman's sexual partner at the same time, to avoid reinfection after the couple resumes sexual intercourse, although this is controversial.

Vagotomy

A surgical procedure in which the vagus nerve is cut to reduce acid production in the stomach. The vagus nerve, a major nerve that extends from the brain to most of the other major organs, controls production of stomach acid in addition to many other activities. A vagotomy is performed when a peptic ulcer (see PEPTIC ULCER DISEASE) fails to respond to less invasive treatment or when complications, such as bleeding or obstruction, develop. The procedure is normally combined with a pyloroplasty (a surgical widening of the pylorus, the stomach outlet to the intestine). In some cases, a vagotomy is done with a partial GASTRECTOMY (surgical removal of part of the stomach).

A vagotomy is done in a hospital under general anesthesia. The surgeon cuts a number of the branches of the vagus nerve that stimulate the stomach. Nerve signals are thus prevented from stimulating acid secretion by the stomach lining. Reduction of acid reduces pain and inflammation, giving ulcers an opportunity to heal. In the accompanying pyloroplasty, the pylorus is cut and sewn, and the duodenum is widened, permitting stomach contents to pass through the duodenum more quickly. A pyloroplasty reduces the risk of impairing the ability of the stomach to empty properly, a possible complication of a vagotomy.

Valacyclovir hydrochloride

An antiviral drug. Valacyclovir hydrochloride (Valtrex) is used to treat the symptoms of herpes zoster (shingles), a viral infection of the skin, and to treat and prevent genital herpes infections. Valacyclovir hydrochloride will not eliminate shingles or genital herpes, but it helps relieve pain and discomfort and helps sores to heal faster.

Valerian

An herbal extract used as a mild sedative. Valerian can be prepared as a tea and as an extract or a tincture. Valerian is widely used in Europe and seems to help people fall asleep faster, although there is no scientific proof of this effect.

Valgus

Abnormally turned out. Valgus is an adjective used to describe a deformity in which a hand or foot is turned out from the center of the body, as with knock-knees.

Valproic acid

An anticonvulsant. Valproic acid (Depakene) is used either alone or with other anticonvulsants to control various types of seizure disorders, including epilepsy. A related drug called divalproex (Depakote) is used as an anticonvulsant, in migraine prevention, and as an antimania drug. Divalproex is metabolized to valproic acid in the body. The precise way in which these drugs work is not fully understood.

Valsalva maneuver

An exercise that is used as a diagnostic tool and as a treatment to correct abnormal heart rhythms and relieve chest pain. The Valsalva maneuver is the attempt to exhale while keeping the mouth and nose closed. Because the maneuver causes changes in blood pressure, doctors use the Valsalva maneuver to assess people they suspect have cardiovascular problems, such as fast heart rates. The maneuver is sometimes used with ECHOCARDIOGRAPHY, an ultrasound examination of the heart. Less frequently, the Valsalva maneuver is used to correct rapid heartbeats, to ease chest pain in people with mild cardiovascular disease, to relieve the symptoms of middle ear infection in children, and to help people with multiple sclerosis fully empty their bladders.

Valsartan

A drug used to treat high blood pressure. Valsartan (Diovan) is an angiotensin II inhibitor. The drug works by blocking the action of angiotensin II, a substance in the body that causes blood vessels to tighten, thereby raising the blood pressure. By relaxing the blood vessels, valsartan lowers blood pressure.

Valve

A structure found in some tubular body parts or organs that restricts the flow of fluid to a single direction. Valves are important to the function of the heart, the veins, and the lymphatic system. Valves consist of cusps, or flaps, fastened to the walls of the body part. When blood or lymph flows through the valves in the correct direction, the cusps stay close to the walls, but if the fluid flow is reversed, the cusps become filled with liquid and expand to fill the vessel, thereby blocking it.

In the heart, for example, there are four one-way valves that keep the blood flowing in a single direction. Blood entering the heart first passes through the tricuspid valve and then the pulmonary valve. After the blood returns from the lungs, it passes through the mitral or bicuspid valve and exits through the aortic valve.

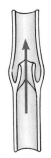 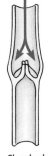

Opened valve   Closed valve

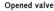

ONE-WAY FLOW
A valve in a vein opens when the muscles in the wall of the vein contract and cause pressure to build behind the valve. When the muscles relax and the pressure decreases, the valve closes and prevents backflow.

Valve replacement

See HEART VALVE SURGERY.

Valvotomy

An open-heart surgical procedure in which a damaged heart valve is cut in order to open it; also known as a valvulotomy. See HEART VALVE SURGERY for more information.

Valvular heart disease

Any dysfunction or abnormality affecting one or more of the valves that control blood flow into, out of, and within the heart. There are four valves in all: the mitral and aortic valves on the left side of the heart, and the pulmonic (or pulmonary) and tricuspid valves on the right side of the heart. Three fundamental kinds of problems can affect valves. Incompetence, or regurgitation, refers to valve leakage (see AORTIC INSUFFICIENCY; MITRAL INSUFFICIENCY; TRICUSPID INSUFFICIENCY). Narrowing or partial blockage of a valve is known as valvular stenosis (see STENOSIS, VALVULAR). Atresia is a serious condition in which a valve fails to develop properly and is closed at birth; it can affect any of the four valves. Prolapse refers to abnormal bulging of the valve when the heart contracts.

Valvuloplasty

A minimally invasive, nonsurgical procedure for treating stenosis (narrowing) of a heart valve; also known as balloon valvuloplasty. Valvuloplasty offers an alternative to open-heart surgery (see HEART VALVE SURGERY) for those whose symptoms are mild to moderate or who are considered poor candidates for major surgery.

Valvuloplasty is performed after injection of a local anesthetic, usually into the groin. The doctor makes a small incision into the numbed area to expose an artery or vein, then threads a catheter (thin tube) into the artery or vein. The catheter is guided through the blood vessel into the heart. When it reaches the narrowed valve, a balloon at the tip of the catheter is inflated to stretch and widen the narrowed valve. The balloon is then deflated and the catheter withdrawn.

Valvuloplasty is used most often with stenosis of the mitral valve (see MITRAL STENOSIS). The procedure is generally successful and is considered to pose minimal risks if the mitral valve is only mildly to moderately

V

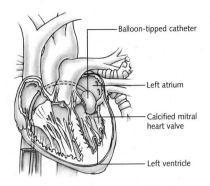

- Balloon-tipped catheter
- Left atrium
- Calcified mitral heart valve
- Left ventricle

WIDENING A VALVE
To perform valvuloplasty on the mitral valve, the surgeon guides a balloon-tipped catheter into a vein, through the heart and across the atrial septum (which separates the two atria), and then through the left atrium into the narrowed valve. When the balloon is inflated, it presses the valve leaflets apart and widens the opening.

narrowed. The recovery period after valvuloplasty is much shorter than that for open-heart surgery, requiring only a short hospital stay. There is some risk that the valve will narrow again, while in some cases, the opened valve leaks, allowing some blood to flow in the wrong direction.

Vancomycin
An antibiotic. Vancomycin (Vancocin) is used to treat diarrhea or colitis caused by a particular bacteria. Vancomycin is also used to treat heart valve disease, such as rheumatic fever or infections associated with artificial heart valves. It may also be used to prevent endocarditis (inflammation of the tissue lining the heart) in people at risk who are having dental work or surgery on the upper respiratory tract. Vancomycin is used in certain infections of the bone, skin, and tissues that might be resistant to other antibiotics.

Vaporizer
A device used to convert a liquid into aerosol so it can be inhaled or the air made moist. Vaporizers produce steam to moisten the air. Humidifiers break up water into fine droplets without the use of heat; they are used to moisten the air breathed by children with croup or other upper respiratory infections. Vaporizers called inhalers contain BRONCHODILATORS

and CORTICOSTEROIDS, drugs used in the treatment of asthma and other respiratory disorders.

Varicella
See CHICKENPOX.

Varices
Enlarged, twisted, winding veins, arteries, or lymphatic vessels; singular, varix. See VARICOSE VEINS.

Varicocele
Enlarged veins along the spermatic cord, or vas deferens, the tubular structure that suspends the testicles and transports sperm cells. Abnormal valves in the veins cause blood to back up and distend the veins, disrupting normal blood flow. Varicoceles often develop slowly and usually are painless. They are most likely to develop on the left side of the scrotum in men between ages 15 and 25. In an older man, the sudden appearance of a varicocele can be a sign of a kidney tumor affecting the renal vein and altering blood flow from the scrotum. Varicocele is a common cause of infertility among younger men.

Varicose veins
Enlarged, twisted, winding veins, usually close to the surface of the skin and visible as soft, bluish, bulging curves. Varicose veins are most likely to affect the feet and legs. The condition is common, occurring in one of ten adults, and it tends to worsen over time. Varicose veins may cause the legs to ache, and they can hemorrhage if injured. When deep veins are

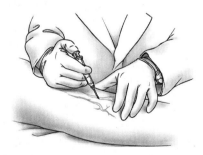

TREATING VARICOSE VEINS
Sclerotherapy involves injecting a solution into the vein that inflames the vessel, eventually shutting off the vein. This treatment does not correct the leaky valves that cause the problem.

involved, the leg may swell and skin ulcers can develop, usually near the ankles. The skin typically turns brown before a skin ulcer appears.

Women are approximately twice as likely as men to have varicose veins, often as a consequence of pregnancy. Pregnancy can stretch the valves in the veins so that they no longer prevent blood from flowing backward and pooling in response to gravity. Obesity and a history of THROMBOPHLEBITIS (inflammation of a vein because of blood clots) can have the same effect.

People with varicose veins should avoid sitting or standing for long periods. Elevating the legs at least 12 inches above the heart at the end of the day helps relieve swelling. Regular exercise is helpful, and losing weight reduces pressure on the legs. Support stockings or elastic bandages, which compress the varicose veins, may relieve discomfort. If an ulcer appears, it should be treated by a doctor to prevent infection and gangrene. Surgery to remove varicose veins or a skin ulcer is an option in severe cases. People with mild to moderate varicose veins can be treated with laser therapy or sclerotherapy (the injection of a solution into the veins that causes inflammation), which collapses the veins and prevents blood flow. Both laser therapy and sclerotherapy are outpatient procedures, and they have no significant effect on circulation in the leg.

Varus
Abnormally turned in. Varus is an adjective used to describe a deformity in which a hand or foot is turned in toward the center of the body, such as bowlegs or a type of clubfoot. The opposite of varus is VALGUS.

Vas deferens
In a man, the narrow, coiled tube that carries sperm released from the epididymis (a connecting duct) and testicles. The vas deferens passes through the prostate and joins with the urethra. Sperm and seminal fluid are passed through this duct into the urethra during ejaculation. The vas deferens, about 2 feet long, is also known as the spermatic cord. See REPRODUCTIVE SYSTEM, MALE.

V

Vascular dementia

A form of dementia caused by a series of small strokes (damage to the brain caused by interruption of its blood supply). It is the second most common form of dementia (a chronic brain disorder marked by confusion and memory loss) in older people. Vascular dementia is also known as multi-infarct dementia. High blood pressure is the primary risk factor for this problem. It affects slightly more men than women. Many people with dementia may have a combination of ALZHEIMER'S DISEASE and vascular dementia.

CAUSES

Strokes damage brain tissue. A stroke occurs when a blood vessel in the brain bursts or when a blood clot or fatty deposits called plaques block blood supply to the brain. Although the symptoms of a large stroke may be profound, the symptoms of a small stroke may be very slight. There may be only mild weakness in an arm or leg, slurred speech, or fleeting dizziness or confusion.

An abrupt onset of symptoms is characteristic of vascular dementia. The condition may progress in steps as each stroke occurs, in contrast with the continuing gradual progression of symptoms seen in Alzheimer's disease. In addition to confusion and short-term memory problems, vascular dementia's symptoms may include decreased judgment and understanding, disorientation, impaired speech, an inability to name objects, and difficulty concentrating. People who have vascular dementia may experience some improvement after a stroke but worsen after another stroke occurs.

DIAGNOSIS

No test provides a definitive diagnosis of vascular dementia. Diagnosis is based on a complete physical examination, a full medical history, and test results. During the examination, the doctor conducts a neurological examination to detect the presence of muscle weakness or numbness, slurred speech, and dizziness. A history of a stepwise progression or past strokes also suggests vascular dementia. Tests may include basic blood and urine analyses; neuropsychological testing that investigates memory, problem solving, and language in greater depth; and imaging studies of the brain, such as CT (computed

tomography) scanning or MRI (magnetic resonance imaging). The imaging studies may reveal areas of damaged brain tissue consistent with damage for strokes. Nevertheless, vascular dementia is sometimes difficult to distinguish from Alzheimer's disease. It is possible for an older person simultaneously to have vascular dementia and Alzheimer's disease.

TREATMENT

Treatment cannot reverse brain damage that has already taken place. However, treatment can reduce the risk of future strokes. High blood pressure and diabetes mellitus, type 2, two common risk factors for vascular dementia, can be helped by changes in diet and exercise and by medication. Sometimes, drugs to control high cholesterol and heart disease are prescribed, and aspirin may be recommended to prevent clots that can form in blood vessels and lead to a stroke. Older people who have vascular dementia may need considerable help with their daily routines. Community resources can be helpful in caring for them. State or AREA AGENCIES ON AGING can provide information on available services such as transportation, home-delivered meals, home health services, and adult day care programs (see DAY CARE, ADULT).

Vascular surgery

An operation on the blood vessels. Examples include CAROTID ENDARTERECTOMY and THROMBECTOMY.

Vasculitis

Inflammation of a blood vessel. Vasculitis can result from an allergic reaction to a drug or foreign substance (allergic vasculitis). Another cause is an inflammatory disease, such as rheumatoid arthritis or systemic lupus erythematosus, that scars blood vessels and can impair blood flow to a part of the body.

Vasectomy

An operation that makes a man permanently unable to father children (infertile) by cutting and sealing the small tubes that transport sperm cells from the testicles; also known as male sterilization. A vasectomy has no effect on sexual desire or on the ability to have an erection and ejaculate. A vasectomy is preferred as a method of family planning by many couples

who do not want children or who have completed their family because it is less traumatic and less costly than female sterilization and requires a shorter recovery time away from work. Although a vasectomy can sometimes be reversed later, it should be regarded as a permanent form of sterilization.

THE PROCEDURE

A vasectomy is a simple operation, usually performed in the office of the doctor or in an outpatient surgery setting. A local anesthetic is injected into the scrotum (the protective pouch between the legs containing the testicles) to make the surgical procedure pain-free. Then, the physician locates the tube (vas deferens) that carries sperm cells up from one of the testicles and makes a small incision to expose it. The vas deferens is cut, and the ends are tied off or closed with an instrument that uses electrical current to seal the tissues. The same procedure is repeated on the other vas deferens. The incisions in the scrotum are closed with small stitches, which are removed or dissolve within 5 to 7 days. The entire procedure typically takes from 20 to 30 minutes.

After surgery, the patient applies ice bags to the scrotum every 20 minutes to relieve swelling and pain. Bed rest is advised for the first 24 hours. The man wears an athletic supporter for several days and is usually comfortable enough to return to work in 2 or 3 days. Oral pain medications may be prescribed to control aching during the first few days of recovery. Some swelling or bruising is normal; it usually disappears within 2 to 3 weeks. Sexual intercourse can be resumed as soon as the man feels comfortable, usually within 1 week.

Serious complications are unusual. There is a small risk of infection, excessive bleeding during recovery, or blood collecting in the scrotum. In rare cases, the two ends of the vas deferens rejoin and fertility is restored.

A vasectomy has no effect on male hormone production, and any change in sexual attitudes is psychological rather than physical. The man continues to ejaculate normally since sperm cells make up only a fractional portion of the semen.

TESTING FOR INFERTILITY

A vasectomy does not result in imme-

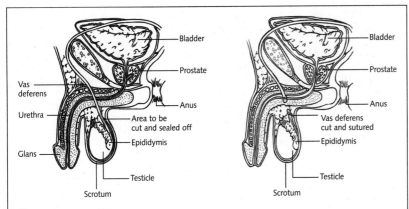

HOW VASECTOMY WORKS
In a vasectomy, each of the two vas deferens tubes is cut and sutured or clipped off, so sperm cannot leave the epididymis. Sex drive and ejaculation proceed normally, but the semen does not contain sperm. The sperm are absorbed by the testicles.

diate infertility because some sperm cells remain in the reproductive system, particularly in the reservoirs called the seminal vesicles, located near the prostate gland. Until these sperm cells are ejaculated or die, the man is still fertile. Usually it takes from 10 to 15 ejaculations, or a period of 4 to 6 weeks, to expel the last sperm cells. To ensure that none remain, the semen is checked (sperm count), beginning approximately 30 days after surgery. Until two consecutive counts reveal no sperm cells, the man and his partner should continue to use contraception.

REVERSAL

In some cases, a vasectomy can be reversed in a procedure known as a vasovasostomy. The operation is performed using a powerful microscope that allows the surgeon to see and repair the very small structures in the vas deferens. The procedure is usually performed in an outpatient setting. Most men who have a vasovasostomy are able to ejaculate sperm cells, but only approximately half of them are able to father a child. The most likely reason is that over time a man who has undergone vasectomy develops an immune response that is damaging to his own sperm cells. As a result, a vasovasostomy has the best chance of success when it is performed within 5 years of a vasectomy.

Vasoconstriction

The process by which a blood vessel narrows, slowing or stopping blood flow through it. The autonomic nerv-

ous system controls the smooth muscle in the blood vessel walls that constricts and dilates (widens) the blood vessel. The body uses vasoconstriction and vasodilation to help distribute blood to the different organs. Vasoconstriction can also result from medications such as oral decongestants, cold remedies, pseudoephedrine, and ergotamine (used to treat migraine headaches); caffeine; disease; and psychological states.

Vasodilation

The process by which blood vessels relax and widen, increasing blood flow through them. Certain medications used to treat hypertension (high blood pressure) achieve their effect through vasodilation. As the blood vessels relax, they offer less resistance to the flow of blood, and blood pressure drops.

Vasodilators

Drugs that widen blood vessels by relaxing their muscular walls. Vasodilators are used to treat congestive heart failure by dilating blood vessels to reduce the workload of the heart and by lowering blood pressure to increase the supply of oxygen and blood to the heart. These drugs are also used to treat high blood pressure.

ANGIOTENSIN-CONVERTING ENZYME (ACE) INHIBITORS

One group of vasodilators is called angiotensin-converting enzyme (ACE) inhibitors (see ANTIHYPERTENSIVES). These drugs block an enzyme needed

to produce a substance that causes blood vessels to constrict or tighten. ACE inhibitors that act as vasodilators include benazepril (Lotensin, Lotrel), captopril (Capoten), enalapril (Lexxel, Vasotec), fosinopril (Monopril), quinapril (Accupril), ramipril (Altace), and trandolapril (Mavik, Tarka).

ACE INHIBITOR AND HYDROCHLOROTHIAZIDE

An ACE inhibitor and a hydrochlorothiazide may be given as a combination drug, a vasodilator that combines an ACE inhibitor with a diuretic. The diuretic or "water pill" helps to reduce the amount of water and salt in the body by acting on the kidneys to increase urination. The combined drug is a vasodilator used to treat congestive heart failure. Examples include captopril and hydrochlorothiazide (Capozide), enalapril and hydrochlorothiazide (Vaseretic), and lisinopril and hydrochlorothiazide (Accuretic).

NITRATES

Nitrates are used to treat chest pain associated with angina. They work by relaxing or dilating blood vessels to increase the flow of blood and oxygen to the heart and heart muscle. These drugs are given under the tongue as long-acting tablets, as an ointment, or by transdermal (skin) patch. Examples are isosorbide dinitrate (Isordil, Sorbitrate) and NITROGLYCERIN (Nitro-Dur, Nitrolingual, Nitrostat).

OTHER VASODILATORS

Other drugs that act as vasodilators are used to treat congestive heart failure and high blood pressure. Examples include hydralazine and prazosin (Minipress, Minizide). These drugs work by relaxing blood vessels so blood can pass through them more freely, thus reducing blood pressure and the burden on the heart.

Epoprostenol (Flolan) is a prostaglandin, a vasodilator used to treat primary pulmonary hypertension, a disease in which high blood pressure occurs in the main artery carrying blood from the heart to the lungs. Epoprostenol works by relaxing blood vessels and increasing the supply of blood to the lungs, thereby reducing the workload of the heart.

Vasopressin

See ADH.

V

Vasospasm

The constriction or narrowing of blood vessels as a result of contraction of the smooth muscle in the blood vessel wall. Cerebral vasospasm is a common complication following a subarachnoid hemorrhage (bleeding into the space between the brain and the arachnoid membrane; see HEMORRHAGE, SUBARACHNOID). If the blood vessels in the brain narrow to the point of compromising blood flow, there is a greater risk of tissue damage and death.

Vasovagal attack

A temporary reaction marked by pale skin, nausea, sweating, slow heartbeat, and dropping blood pressure; often accompanied by a loss of consciousness. Vasovagal attack is also known as simple FAINTING, Gowers syndrome, and vasodepressor syncope. A vasovagal attack is rarely preceded by pain or squeezing in the chest or shortness of breath. The attack may have a variety of triggers, including standing at attention for long periods, standing up quickly, hypotension (low blood pressure), cardiac arrhythmia (abnormal heart rhythm), severe pain, sudden fright, medications or drugs (including alcohol, blood pressure medications, central nervous system depressants, and decongestants), strenuous coughing, strain during a bowel movement, or hyperventilation (rapid, shallow breathing). A person who experiences repeated vasovagal attacks should be examined by a doctor to determine the cause.

Vector

A public health term for a disease-carrying animal; arachnid, such as a tick; or insect, such as a mosquito that transmits pathogens to cause an infectious disease in a person. Vectors can transmit viruses, bacteria, protozoa, and worms from one host to another. The four most common diseases transmitted by infected vectors include ROCKY MOUNTAIN SPOTTED FEVER and LYME DISEASE, which are tick-borne, and MALARIA and DENGUE fever, which are carried by mosquitoes.

Vectors may transmit systemic infections of the blood from one host to another in a number of ways.

Infected ticks transmit Rocky Mountain spotted fever by injection from salivary glands while feeding on the skin of a human host. The pathogenic parasites, called rickettsiae, enter the bloodstream when they are rubbed or scratched into the skin at the site of the tick bite. These ticks are the reservoirs of the infectious agent, meaning they carry the parasite but have not acquired it from another host.

Lyme disease occurs when a tick becomes a vector for it by feeding on deer or wild rodents, which are reservoirs of the spirochete that causes the disease. The tick then transmits Lyme disease to a human host by feeding on the person. The person becomes infected via the tick's bite or by contact with the tick's feces.

Humans are the reservoirs for the pathogen that causes malaria, and the disease is spread from person to person when a particular species of mosquito becomes a vector and transmits the disease to a person. Malaria can also be acquired by a transfusion with infected blood or by congenital transferal of the infection.

Humans are the reservoirs of the type of virus that causes dengue fever. Certain species of mosquitoes acquire the viral pathogen from infected persons and then serve as vectors for the disease. The virus can be transmitted to the mosquitoes when they feed on an infected person within 5 days of appearance of symptoms in that person. Once infected, a mosquito continues to be infective throughout its 1- to 4-month life span.

Veganism

A strict form of VEGETARIANISM in which all animal products, such as eggs, dairy foods, gelatin, and honey are excluded, in addition to meats. A vegan diet consists of plant-based foods such as vegetables, fruits, grains, legumes, nuts, and seeds.

Vegetarianism

A diet that emphasizes plant rather than animal foods. There are three types of vegetarians: lacto-ovo-vegetarians, lacto-vegetarians, and vegans. Lacto-ovo-vegetarians continue to consume milk, cheese, yogurt, and eggs. Lacto-vegetarians consume milk, cheese, and yogurt but eat no

eggs. Vegans eat no animal products (see VEGANISM).

Some people follow vegetarian diets for health reasons, while others are motivated by religious or ethical beliefs. A balanced vegetarian diet offers a variety of health benefits. These include a reduced risk for health problems such as obesity, constipation, alcoholism, hypertension, coronary artery disease, diabetes, and gallstones. Vegetarian diets are rich in nutrients and fiber and low in saturated fat, which may also reduce the risk of certain types of cancer.

Individuals contemplating a vegetarian diet should see a doctor or registered dietician to obtain specific information about their individual nutrient and energy needs. For instance, vegetarian diets may be inappropriate for some older people because their bodies may no longer process nutrients efficiently enough. There are also special considerations during pregnancy, breast-feeding, and periods of growth. Iron, folic acid, and vitamin B12 supplements are necessary for vegetarians during pregnancy, and breast-fed infants may require supplementation of iron and vitamin D. It is especially important for infants, children, and teenagers to receive an adequate intake of calories, calcium, vitamin D, iron, and zinc.

A wide variety of foods and sufficient calories are necessary to ensure adequate nutrition and energy. (See also CALORIE REQUIREMENTS.) Vegetarians are generally advised to limit their intake of sweets and fatty foods and to consume no more than three to four egg yolks each week. The lack of protein from meat can be compensated for through soy products or a combination of grains, legumes, seeds, nuts, and vegetables. It is not necessary to consume all the different types of plant products in one meal, since the body has the capacity, although limited, to store amino acids.

Followers of veganism must be especially vigilant about their diets. When no dairy products are consumed, doctors recommend calcium supplements for children and pregnant or breast-feeding women. A vitamin D supplement is also necessary for those who consume no dairy products and have limited exposure to sunlight. Because vitamin B12 is present only in animal foods, doctors advise vegans to use fortified food sources (such as soy beverages and cereals). A VITAMIN B12 DEFICIENCY can result in serious health problems.

Vegetative state

A condition in which a person has lost cognitive neurological function and awareness of the environment, yet retains noncognitive or automatic functions and a sleep-wake cycle. Persistent vegetative states sometimes follow comas (see COMA); these are profound or deep states of unconsciousness that occur as outcomes of underlying illness or are caused by injury. People in vegetative states may appear somewhat normal; they may open their eyes and laugh or cry. However, they do not seem to understand or respond to commands.

Treatment of a person in a vegetative state includes balanced nutrition and the prevention of infections and pressure sores. Physical therapy may be used to prevent permanent muscular contractions and orthopedic deformities. The prognosis depends on the nature and cause of neurological damage. Some people regain a certain amount of awareness after a vegetative state. Others remain in this condition for many years without recovering. Pneumonia is the most common cause of death for those in a vegetative state.

Veins

Blood vessels that carry blood toward the heart. Veins complete the circula-

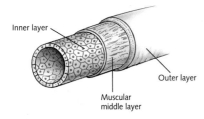

WALL OF THE VEINS
A vein returns blood to the heart, operating at lower pressure than an artery does. The wall can therefore be thinner, but it still has a muscular layer that pushes the blood along without the pumping action of the heart. Because they work at low pressure, many veins have valves to prevent backflow.

tion of the blood that begins in the arteries, which transport blood away from the heart. Veins begin as small vessels, called venules, that lie adjacent to capillaries and then join into successively larger vessels. The major veins, like the vena cava, are as thick as a finger. Like arteries, veins have three-layered walls, but they are thinner and less muscular. Unlike arteries, veins do not pulse. Rather, they depend on the movement of muscle surrounding them to push the blood along. Veins in the arms and legs, but not in the head, neck, or torso, have one-way valves that allow the blood to flow only in the right direction. See CARDIOVASCULAR SYSTEM.

Vena cava

Either of the two largest veins in the body. The superior vena cava starts at the top of the chest behind the lower edge of the right first rib and close to the breastbone. It carries blood returning from the head, neck, arms, and chest, entering the heart at the right atrium. The inferior vena cava transports blood from the legs, pelvis, and abdomen and enters the heart in the right atrium. It begins in the lower abdomen, passes in front of the spine, behind the liver, and through the diaphragm before entering the heart. See CARDIOVASCULAR SYSTEM.

Veneers, dental

Thin shells of ceramic material, usually porcelain, that are bonded to the front of teeth. Dental veneers correct surface irregularities or discoloration, brighten the color of teeth, and generally improve the appearance of teeth. The application of dental veneers is a technique offered by COSMETIC DENTISTRY. Veneers may be used to repair chipped teeth or to close spaces between teeth. Porcelain veneers cover the front and upper third of the back of the tooth.

Venereal disease

A group of infectious diseases that are spread through sexual contact. Venereal disease is an outdated term for SEXUALLY TRANSMITTED DISEASES (STDs).

Venipuncture

The puncture of a vein through the skin with a stylet or a steel needle attached to a syringe or catheter.

Venipuncture is performed to withdraw blood, instill a medication, start an intravenous infusion, or inject a radioactive substance for body imaging techniques. A convenient vein is chosen, usually from the inside of the elbow or back of the hand. The nurse or other health care worker cleans the puncture site with antiseptic and places a tourniquet around the upper arm to apply pressure. The veins below the tourniquet fill with blood, and the needle is inserted. During the procedure, the tourniquet is removed. If blood is being drawn, it is collected in an airtight bottle or syringe. Afterward, the needle is withdrawn, and the puncture site is covered to stop any bleeding.

Venlafaxine

An antidepressant; an antianxiety drug. Venlafaxine (Effexor) is used to treat depression in adults, as well as certain anxiety symptoms or disorders. Venlafaxine works by affecting neurotransmitters in the brain that are associated with depression.

Ventilation

A natural body function or a mechanical procedure that maintains the correct balance of oxygen and carbon dioxide in the body. Mechanical ventilation simulates human breathing with the use of a VENTILATOR when a person is not able to breathe independently. This provides for the exchange of gases between the lungs and the surrounding air, keeping the oxygen level in the blood high and the carbon dioxide level low.

Ventilator

A machine designed to provide proper gas exchange in the body, a process called VENTILATION, for people who are unable to breathe independently. Mechanical ventilators consist of a control panel for monitoring and adjusting the air delivery system and ventilation tubing connected to a humidifier and to the person receiving ventilation via an endotracheal tube, tracheostomy, or mask.

A ventilator delivers oxygen and venous carbon dioxide through the ventilation tubing. There are two types of ventilators now in use: volume ventilators, which deliver a preset volume of air in each cycle, and

V

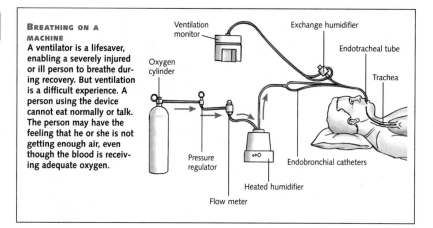

BREATHING ON A MACHINE
A ventilator is a lifesaver, enabling a severely injured or ill person to breathe during recovery. But ventilation is a difficult experience. A person using the device cannot eat normally or talk. The person may have the feeling that he or she is not getting enough air, even though the blood is receiving adequate oxygen.

pressure ventilators, which deliver air up to a preset pressure.

Ventilators are used by people who have respiratory failure; severe, chronic lung diseases; neuromuscular diseases; or other disorders. Their use extends life. Ventilators are commonly used in a hospital setting, and there are models that can be used in the home.

Ventral

In anatomy, on or of the front of the body or an organ; anterior. Ventral describes a position situated on or related to the front surface (the belly) of the body. The opposite of ventral is DORSAL.

Ventricle

A small functional space or cavity in an organ, particularly the HEART and BRAIN. In the heart, the two lower muscular chambers are called ventricles. They receive blood from the upper heart chambers and pump it to the lungs and to the rest of the body. The four ventricles of the brain are located in the lower center of the organ. They have a role in producing and circulating the cerebrospinal fluid that cushions the brain and spinal cord.

Ventricular ectopic beat

A heart rhythm abnormality in which the ventricles (lower chambers) of the heart contract before the atria (upper chambers); also known as premature ventricular contractions. Ventricular ectopic beat is a relatively common type of heart rhythm abnormality (arrhythmia). Some people with the

condition experience it as a wildly fast, galloping heartbeat (palpitations), which can be frightening and startling. In others, there are almost no symptoms.

Ventricular ectopic beat has a number of possible causes, including anxiety and stress, fatigue, alcohol, caffeine, and electrolyte imbalance from starvation, dehydration, or uncontrolled diabetes mellitus. Heart disease or damage from a past heart attack is another possible cause. A person experiencing frequent or worsening ventricular ectopic beats, particularly if accompanied by chest pain, should see a doctor to determine the cause of the condition.

If ventricular ectopic beats are caused by an underlying heart problem, treatment is directed at that disease. In others with troubling symptoms but without heart disease, eliminating the cause, if possible, is the best treatment. Medications, such as beta blockers, which block the stress response, may also be prescribed. In rare severe cases, a procedure called ABLATION THERAPY is used to eliminate the abnormal tissue causing the arrhythmia.

Ventricular fibrillation

Rapid, weak, uncontrolled quivering of the ventricles (lower chambers) of the heart, so that the heart pumps little or no blood. Ventricular fibrillation is a medical emergency requiring immediate attention. If a normal heartbeat cannot be reestablished within a few minutes, death will result. Defibrillation, which administers an electric shock to the heart, is

the necessary treatment for ventricular fibrillation.

Ventricular fibrillation strikes suddenly, sometimes preceded by feelings of light-headedness. Other warning symptoms can include a wildly galloping heartbeat (palpitations), fatigue, weakness, shortness of breath, and chest pain. The person faints because the oxygen supply to the brain is insufficient.

Anyone who survives an episode of ventricular fibrillation needs to be examined to determine its cause. Ventricular fibrillation is often the result of heart conditions such as coronary artery disease, heart valve disease, long QT syndrome, or congenital heart disease. Other causes include electrolyte imbalances in the blood caused by starvation, dehydration, or uncontrolled diabetes and drugs such as alcohol, cocaine, and caffeine. Treatment depends on the cause. Medications can be used to control heart rhythm. An electronic device that monitors the heart for arrhythmia and administers an electrical shock in the event of ventricular fibrillation (internal cardioverter DEFIBRILLATOR) may be implanted in the chest surgically.

Ventricular tachycardia

See TACHYCARDIA, VENTRICULAR.

Verapamil

A drug used to treat cardiac conditions and high blood pressure. Verapamil (Calan, Covera, Isoptin, Verelan) is used to treat angina (chest pain), certain kinds of arrhythmia (irregular heartbeat), and high blood pressure. Verapamil is also used to prevent headaches caused by high blood pressure. Calcium channel blockers, including verapamil, work by blocking the movement of calcium into the cells of the heart and blood vessels to relax the blood vessels and increase the blood and oxygen supply to the heart.

Vernix

A greasy, white coating covering the skin of the newborn. The vernix protects the skin of the fetus while inside the uterus.

Verruca

See WART.

Version

A procedure used to reposition a fetus in the uterus to prevent a BREECH DELIVERY. If a fetus is in a breech presentation (buttocks-first or feetfirst, instead of headfirst) after the 36th week of pregnancy, external version may be used to turn the head of the fetus downward. The doctor applies slow steady pressure by manipulating the fetus through the mother's abdominal wall, which is known as external version. Internal version, in which the doctor reaches inside the uterus, is rarely used.

Version is usually successful for a mother who has had babies before and whose abdominal walls have previously been stretched, and in pregnancies in which sufficient amniotic fluid is available to turn the baby around. Version is not used in pregnancies that involve oligohydramnios (insufficient amniotic fluid), placenta previa (placenta covering the cervix), or premature rupture of the membranes or in mothers who have previously had a CESAREAN SECTION. Fetuses believed to be unusually small or to have birth defects should not be turned.

Vertebra

One of the ringlike bones that make up the SPINE or vertebral column. Each vertebra is a uniquely shaped, asymmetrical bone, consisting of an oval body around a central canal. The SPINAL CORD passes through this canal. Extending from the back of each vertebra are bony projections called processes. Nerves passing into and out of the spinal cord pass through the open spaces between the processes. A cushion of fibrous cartilage with a gelatinous center, called a disk, lies between each of the vertebrae except the first two below the skull and the last two structures of the spine, the sacrum and coccyx (tailbone). The disks allow each vertebra to move as a unit, giving the spine some flexibility even as it remains rigid enough to protect the spinal column. Joints on the back side of the vertebrae add to the spine's range of movement and allow a person to stand erect.

Vertebrobasilar insufficiency

A narrowing or partial blockage of either of the two arteries leading into the BRAIN stem and cerebellum.

Vertebrobasilar insufficiency results in temporary attacks of vertigo, double vision, jerky eye movements, slurred speech, and muscle weakness. Fatty deposits (plaque) or blood clots are the usual causes of the blockage.

Vertigo

FOR SYMPTOM CHART
see Dizziness, page 36

The sensation of loss of balance, unsteadiness, disorientation, dizziness, or faintness produced by an illusion of movement. When a person experiences the external world as though it were spinning or moving around him or her, the condition is called objective vertigo; if the person experiences the feeling his or her body is revolving in space, it is called subjective vertigo.

Vertigo is often accompanied by nausea, vomiting, headache, or sweating. Usually there is no change in mental status. It is not a disease in itself, but rather a symptom of a disorder, usually in the organs of balance in the inner ear.

CAUSES AND TREATMENT
The mechanism of balance is complicated, involving the coordination of impulses from the ear, the eyes, the legs, and the soles of the feet. The organ of balance, called the vestibular labyrinth, is in the inner ear. If the inner structure of one ear is not functioning correctly, or if the inner ear fluids are overstimulated (as happens when a person spins around quickly, then stops), the brain may receive incorrect nerve impulses and send messages to the eyes causing them to move back and forth quickly. This rapid eye movement makes the surroundings appear to spin or makes a person feel as though he or she is spinning, which creates the sensation of dizziness or vertigo. Many of the situations and disorders that cause vertigo are mild and temporary. Some medications may cause vertigo. Dizziness is often experienced by older people.

Sometimes an inflammation, infection, or other disorder of the semicircular canals of the labyrinth can be responsible. An inflammation of the labyrinth, called LABYRINTHITIS, may be accompanied by hearing problems, called aural vertigo, which include deafness and ringing in the ear. When ear infections cause vertigo, the dizziness tends to come on suddenly and be experienced briefly and intermittently, usually for no longer than a few weeks. Leaking of inner ear fluid into the middle ear can cause vertigo; this is called perilymphatic fistula and may be caused by a head injury or sudden changes in atmospheric pressure, or it may be a complication of ear surgery. Sometimes, the leak stops without medical intervention; if not, exploratory surgery may become necessary to repair it. MENIERE DISEASE, a disorder in the pressure of inner ear fluids, may be the cause of ongoing episodes of vertigo. Tumors that develop on the balance nerve or the hearing nerve can cause vertigo with accompanying HEARING LOSS and TINNITUS (ringing or similar sound in the ears or head). These tumors can be removed at an early stage when diagnosed soon enough. In rare instances, diseases of the cerebral cortex, eye muscles, or cerebellum are responsible for vertigo.

Treatment of vertigo depends on the cause. Many of the underlying disorders producing vertigo can be medically or surgically treated. If an otolaryngologist (ear, nose, and throat specialist) cannot find an identifiable underlying cause, medication may be prescribed to stabilize the balancing mechanism in the inner ear. Surgery on the ear may be an option when medical treatment fails. One conservative operation attempts to provide control of the abnormal fluid pressure in the inner ear.

Vertigo, benign positional

Abrupt, short episodes of dizziness precipitated by a change in the position of the head or body. Benign positional vertigo is caused by small crystals of calcium carbonate that have collected within a part of the inner ear. These crystals, called otoliths, are debris from structures in the ear that have been damaged. The damage may be caused by head injury or an infection or other disorder of the inner ear or may be the result of aging. In half of all cases, the cause is unknown. Benign positional vertigo, also called benign paroxysmal positional vertigo, or BPPV, produces intermittent symptoms that may include lightheadedness, loss of balance, and nausea in

V

addition to dizziness. Rapid, involuntary eye movements may accompany the dizziness. Specific activities that cause BPPV vary from one person to another: the dizziness may be caused by rolling over in bed or getting out of bed; tilting the head back to look up; or using an over-the-head, bonnet-style hair dryer such as those used in beauty salons. Episodes of BPPV may appear intermittently for several weeks, then disappear before returning again. Recovery usually takes 3 months.

DIAGNOSIS AND TREATMENT

An otolaryngologist or neurologist usually diagnoses benign positional vertigo based on a person's history, a physical examination, and the evaluation of the results of hearing tests and tests of the vestibular system (system in the inner ear responsible for balance, posture, and the body's orientation in space). The doctor may check blood pressure with the person lying down and sitting up. Rapid eye movements may be monitored by caloric testing (see CALORIC TEST). If there is suspicion of a stroke or brain tumor, MRI (magnetic resonance imaging) will be used in the diagnosis. If BPPV is due to conditions affecting both ears, diagnosis and treatment are more challenging.

Treatment may be postponed

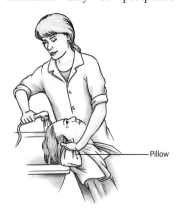

PREVENTING VERTIGO
Vertigo (a symptom rather than a disorder) involves the mechanism of balance, which is centered in the inner ear. Older people often experience vertigo as a result of medication or other factors. The sensation of dizziness may occur only in certain positions, as when the head is down or one ear is down. The sensation may go away when the head is repositioned with a towel or pillow. Sometimes doctors advise not raising the head too quickly or getting up too quickly.

because symptoms often decrease in intensity or disappear within 6 months. The nausea may be controlled with motion sickness medication. Various physical maneuvers and exercises may be performed with a physician's guidance to relieve symptoms: the Semont maneuver involves rapid changes in movement from lying on one side to the other; the Epley maneuver involves sequential movements of the head into different positions. The goal of both sets of exercises is to move the debris out of the sensitive back part of the ear to a less sensitive location. A person being treated for BPPV performs these maneuvers in a doctor's office and is given specific instructions on modifying everyday activities as these activities relate to head and body position. The modifications in movement must be implemented between office visits to control the symptoms of BPPV. The Semont and Epley maneuvers are effective at resolving this form of vertigo most of the time. When they are not successful, a doctor may recommend further exercises, which can be done at home with the doctor's guidance. If these maneuvers or exercises do not eliminate symptoms, surgery on the back of the ear may be recommended.

Vesicle

A small pouch, sac, or hollow organ. Vesicles typically are filled with fluid, as in a blister; the seminal vesicles (located behind the bladder in males) contribute fluid to the ejaculate. A skin vesicle is generally less than half a centimeter (a quarter of an inch) in diameter.

Vestibulitis

Recurring inflammation of the area of the external genitals just outside the vagina. Vestibulitis occurs most often in sexually active women of childbearing age. The most common symptoms are a burning sensation around the opening of the vagina and extreme pain during sexual intercourse. Some women find it painful to insert tampons. Vestibulitis is known to disappear suddenly, only to reappear a few months later. It can become chronic and persistent and is sometimes so painful that women are unable to engage in sexual activity.

The most common causes of vestibulitis are chemical irritants, including soap, deodorant, shampoo, bubble bath, and fabric softener. Some women have a reaction to panty hose or underwear not made of cotton. Depending on the source of the inflammation, treatment may include antibiotics or other medication. Severe cases may not respond to medication, and the inflamed tissue may be removed with laser surgery or traditional surgery. Women with vestibulitis may be tested for the HUMAN PAPILLOMAVIRUS because evidence suggests that vestibulitis may be associated with the virus, a sexually transmitted disease that causes genital warts and may heighten the risk for cancer of the cervix.

Viability

The ability to continue living. A fetus is said to be viable when it can live and develop under normal conditions outside the uterus.

Vibrational medicine

The use of resonance to promote health. In vibrational medicine, different frequencies of sound waves are used to help restore balance to the body. Vibrational medicine is a form of ALTERNATIVE MEDICINE based on the idea that all matter vibrates to a precise frequency and that imbalances or blockages can be corrected with resonant vibration. Practitioners use different kinds of music, media, and vibrational modalities to activate the nervous system and assist the body's own healing mechanism to restore health. See ENERGY MEDICINE.

Villus

One of many tiny hairlike or finger-like vascular projections on certain mucous membranes in the body. Villi are present in all three sections of the small intestine, but are largest and most numerous in the duodenum and jejunum (the first and second parts), where most of the absorption of food takes place. See also CHORIONIC VILLI.

Villous adenoma

An abnormal growth of the mucosa of the large intestine. Villous adenomas are slow-growing tumors that become soft and spongy in texture. They are potentially malignant.

Violence

The physical attack or abuse of one person by another. Violence may include many forms of aggressive behavior, including very excited action, displays of rage, and the use of physical force to combat unwanted activities. Crimes of violence are defined as those that involve physical force for the purpose of violating, damaging, or abusing another person. See ASSAULT; BATTERY; VIOLENCE, FAMILY; RAPE; VIOLENCE, SCHOOL; and VIOLENCE, STREET.

Violence, family

The physical attack or abuse of one family member by another; also called domestic violence. Violence that occurs in families includes partner abuse (see ABUSE, PARTNER), child abuse (see, ABUSE, CHILD), and child neglect. All of these acts are crimes. Family violence can consist of physical abuse, sexual abuse, verbal abuse, emotional abuse, or threats.

As defined in the law, child abuse is any form of harm to, or neglect of, a child by another person, including another child. The abuse of a child can be performed physically, emotionally, sexually, and verbally. Such abuse must be performed deliberately. As a general rule, parents are held responsible for abuse of their children, and if they are aware that another person is abusing their child and they do not report it to authorities, they are committing a crime.

Child neglect and abandonment is another form of family violence. Child neglect includes lack of adequate nutrition, shelter, or supervision. The outright abandonment of a child is also considered a crime.

Abuse of older family members is another type of family violence. Elder abuse may be physical, emotional, or verbal; neglect is another form of abuse of older family members (see ABUSE, OF OLDER PEOPLE).

Violence, school

Extreme aggressive behavior occurring in a school setting. School violence includes different types of criminal behavior, ranging from theft, property offenses, and vandalism to homicide of teachers and other students. High levels of school violence are not confined to urban schools but take place at suburban and rural

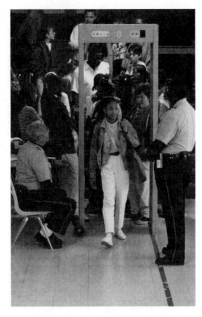

PREVENTING SCHOOL VIOLENCE
Metal detectors can reduce the number of weapons brought into schools, but they cannot prevent violence. They may be useful as part of a larger program that provides instruction in conflict resolution and anger management, as well as counseling for troubled students. Some educators believe that metal detectors offer a false sense of security, divert attention from the underlying causes of violence, and create an atmosphere of distrust.

schools as well. School violence has been a matter of concern since the 1950s: one study determined that between 1950 and 1975, misbehavior in the school setting shifted from violence against property to violence against persons, sometimes with fatal consequences.

In 1999, two students shot and killed 15 people, including themselves, at Columbine High School in Littleton, Colorado. Other high-profile school shootings have taken place since that time, leading to a national discussion on ways to improve school safety through better communication and finding ways to identify and help deeply troubled students.

Violence, street

Organized aggressive behavior usually committed by members of adolescent gangs. Street violence is a public health problem in more than 800 of the largest US cities, where as many as 35 percent of high school dropouts and 5 percent of elementary school

---

EARLY WARNING SIGNS OF SCHOOL VIOLENCE

One outcome of a national discussion on ways to improve school safety is to help educators, parents, and students to try to identify the early warning signs of school violence, which include the following:

- Social withdrawal
- Excessive feelings of isolation and being alone
- Excessive feelings of rejection
- Being a victim of violence
- Feelings of being picked on and persecuted
- Low school interest and poor academic performance
- Expression of violence in writings and drawings
- Uncontrolled anger
- Patterns of impulsive and chronic hitting, intimidating, and bullying behaviors
- History of discipline problems
- History of violent and aggressive behavior
- Intolerance for differences and prejudicial attitudes
- Drug use and alcohol use
- Affiliation with gangs
- Inappropriate access to, possession of, and use of firearms
- Serious threats of violence

Adapted with permission of US Department of Education from "Early warning, timely response: A guide to safe schools," 2002.

---

children are affiliated with street gangs. Membership in a street gang increases the person's risk of violent death by 60 percent. Firearms are used in 80 to 95 percent of all gang-related homicides.

Viremia

The presence of a virus or viruses in the blood, which may be detected by laboratory analysis of a blood sample and indicates a viral infection.

Virginity

The state of being a virgin, or a person who has not yet engaged in SEXUAL INTERCOURSE. Although the term is more frequently applied to women, it can apply to either sex.

Virilism

A condition caused by the excessive production of the male hormones,

ANDROGEN HORMONES. Virilism results in the development of secondary male sexual characteristics in girls or women or in the fetus before birth, causing sexual abnormalities in newborns.

Androgen hormones are adrenal hormones that regulate body functions. They are produced normally in girls and women, but if one or both of the adrenal glands become enlarged or overactive, the excess androgen hormones result in masculine characteristics.

Congenital adrenal hyperplasia (see ADRENAL HYPERPLASIA, CONGENITAL) causes enlargement of the adrenal gland that is present at birth. Adrenal tumors are rarely the cause of virilism but, in some cases, it may be caused by a benign (not cancerous) tumor called an adrenal ADENOMA or a cancerous tumor called an adrenal carcinoma. In women, an ovarian tumor may cause virilism.

SYMPTOMS
Virilization in women may cause growth of facial hair, deepening of the voice, and a prominent Adam's apple. Menstrual cycles may also be disrupted.

In newborn girls with virilism, external sex organs may show a combination of male and female organs, a condition called female PSEUDOHERMAPHRODITISM. Infant boys may have enlarged external sex organs that develop at an abnormal rate.

DIAGNOSIS AND TREATMENT
To diagnose virilism, blood tests are evaluated in a laboratory to measure the concentration of different hormones, possible abnormal hormone patterns, and whether the disorder is caused by problems with the adrenal glands or the ovaries. If a tumor is suspected, DIAGNOSTIC IMAGING may be used to observe the glands, and a biopsy may be performed to examine tissue samples under a microscope.

When virilism is caused by adrenal hyperplasia, which has no cure, it is treated daily with glucocorticoids, usually PREDNISONE for adults and hydrocortisone (see CORTICOSTEROIDS) for infants. Surgery to normalize the appearance of the sex organs may be necessary for girls with pseudohermaphroditism. If a tumor is causing virilism, treatment will depend on the type of tumor. Benign tumors may be surgically removed. Cancerous tumors are generally treated with a combination of surgery, chemotherapy, and radiation therapy. In some cases, the adrenal gland and surrounding tissues must be removed.

Virility
The capability of a man to procreate, or produce children. The term "virility" is also used more generally to refer to masculinity or manly strength and vigor.

Virilization
The development of masculine characteristics in a woman. Virilization is caused by an overproduction of the male sex hormones, ANDROGEN HORMONES, either by the ovaries or by the adrenal glands. Especially in postmenopausal women, the disorder may be due to ovarian cancer, resulting in the secretion of too much androgen hormone by the tumor. Virilization may cause excessive body hair growth, deepening of the voice, increased muscle mass, and acne. In premenopausal women, menstrual periods may cease. Synthetic gonadotropin-releasing hormone (GNRH) may be administered to treat some forms of virilization caused by an ovarian tumor.

Virion
A complete, potentially virulent virus particle, consisting of an RNA (ribonucleic acid) or DNA (deoxyribonucleic acid) core with a protein layer. A virion is the infective form of a virus.

Virology
The branch of science that studies viruses.

Virulence
The capacity of a microorganism to overcome the body's immune system and other defenses and cause disease. Virulence is increased when disease-causing agents have special characteristics, called virulence factors, which contribute to the agent's ability to survive in the human body. Certain signals can sometimes control the growth of the virulence factors; for example, oxygen, pH, and temperature levels and the concentration of ions are among the signals that influence the virulence factors of bacteria.

Viruses
Infectious ultramicroscopic microorganisms that are found in virtually all life forms, including humans, animals, plants, fungi, and bacteria. Viruses vary in size, but all are too small to be seen by a light microscope. Their size can range from 20 to 100 times smaller than bacteria. Each viral unit, or VIRION, consists of a strand of nucleic acid, which consists of either ribonucleic acid (RNA) or deoxyribonucleic acid (DNA) and is enclosed in a protein shell of one or two layers, called a capsid. Some viruses are coated with another layer called a viral envelope. No virus contains both RNA and DNA, a characteristic that distinguishes viruses from all living cells, including bacteria, which contain both RNA and DNA.

VIRAL REPRODUCTION
Individual virus units are not cells and are not themselves made up of cells, and when they exist outside of cells, they are inert. Viruses are parasites because they are not independently capable of vital activities, such as growth, metabolism, and reproduction. A virus has to invade living cells and take over their internal processes in order to survive and reproduce. Viruses are not considered free-living because they cannot reproduce outside of a living cell. When viruses enter living cells, they are able to reproduce by taking over the living cells and redirecting cell functions.

In order to enter a cell, a virus must first attach itself to the cell's surface. This is possible only if the cell has specific protein receptor sites for the particular virus on the surface of the host cell. While many different types of infections are caused by viruses, a particular virus can attack only the tissues and organs of the human body that have the unique receptor sites for that specific virus. For example, structures and tissues in the respiratory tract have receptor sites for the virus that causes the most common infectious disease in the United States, the common cold (see COLD, COMMON).

The virus needs certain components of the cell in order to reproduce. Once inside a cell, a virus particle is broken down by enzymes in the cell and in some cases by enzymes carried within the virus. This process allows the virus to release its genetic material into the host cell. The genetic material guides the reproduction of the virus, which allows the virus to replicate itself and form complete, new virus particles.

These particles take over the host cell, which becomes swollen with the new particles. When the particles are released individually, they may cause only minor damage to the cell. If they are released all at the same time, they can cause the cell to burst open and die. In the course of reproduction, viruses use the reproductive and metabolic parts of the living cells they have invaded. This disruption of normal cell function can produce the symptoms of disease. In some cases, viruses can be present in the body without causing any illness.

VIRAL INFECTIONS
The response of the human body to this invasion by a virus depends on several factors, which have a role in whether the virus causes an insignificant infection or results in a fatal disease. The factors that influence the severity of the illness include the amount of infecting virus to which the body's cells have been exposed, the site of the virus's entry, the number and kinds of cells that have been infected, the nature of the interaction between the cell and the virus, and the person's resistance to the virus. People with weakened immune systems are at a high risk for severe and fatal viral infections because their body's defenses are impaired.

Viruses are found worldwide in all climates and among all human populations. Because different viruses affect different tissues, structures, and organs in varying ways, they produce different kinds of illness. Influenza, rabies, smallpox, mumps, measles, herpes simplex, polio, AIDS (acquired immunodeficiency syndrome), and warts are all among the diseases caused by viruses. Within the major virus groups, there are sometimes a number of distinct types. There are 110 distinct types of the rhinovirus that causes the common cold; humans are susceptible to all types of rhinovirus. The adenovirus includes 32 different types, 7 of which commonly infect humans. There are eight distinct types of herpesvirus, one of which causes chickenpox. The same major virus group that causes parainfluenza also causes mumps and measles.

TESTS AND TREATMENTS FOR VIRAL INFECTIONS
Detecting the presence of a virus in a person who is ill may involve one of several different approaches. Immunoassays (see IMMUNOASSAY) are the most common method for detecting viruses in a blood sample. These tests detect specific antibodies in the blood to the particular virus causing the infection. Another kind of test, which is used to detect antibodies to the AIDS virus, uses antigens (fragments of disease-causing, protein substances that trigger the body's immune response; see ANTIGEN) to detect the presence of antibodies produced by the body to fight the infecting virus. The enzyme-linked immunosorbent assay (see ELISA TEST) is an efficient diagnostic tool that uses prepared antigens to detect antibodies to a specific virus.

Viruses cannot be easily cultured, so indirect methods are sometimes used to detect them. One such diagnostic technique uses active cells grown in a solution of nutrients. When blood or other body fluid samples are added to the cells, they cause changes in the cells that can be associated with the presence of specific viruses in the blood or body fluids. In some cases, the cells will adhere to each other, which is known as agglutination.

Viruses are difficult to treat medically because they reproduce so quickly. Also, because they incorporate their own genetic material into the genetic material of the host cell, medications that are intended to destroy a virus may also destroy the living cell the virus has invaded. Most antiviral medications function by inhibiting the reproduction of the virus. They are formulated to have a structure that is similar to the chain of substances, called nucleosides, contained in a virus's genetic material. These antiviral medications are called nucleoside analogues. During its reproduction, a virus mistakenly uses these analogues instead of its own nucleosides. This disrupts the viral replication process and halts the progression of the infection. ACYCLOVIR,

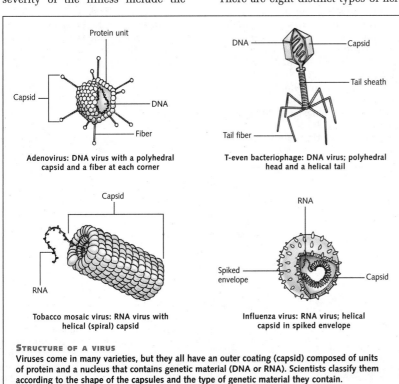

Protein unit

Capsid

DNA

Fiber

Adenovirus: DNA virus with a polyhedral capsid and a fiber at each corner

DNA

Capsid

Tail sheath

Tail fiber

T-even bacteriophage: DNA virus; polyhedral head and a helical tail

Capsid

RNA

Tobacco mosaic virus: RNA virus with helical (spiral) capsid

RNA

Spiked envelope

Capsid

Influenza virus: RNA virus; helical capsid in spiked envelope

STRUCTURE OF A VIRUS
Viruses come in many varieties, but they all have an outer coating (capsid) composed of units of protein and a nucleus that contains genetic material (DNA or RNA). Scientists classify them according to the shape of the capsules and the type of genetic material they contain.

which is used to treat herpes simplex and herpes zoster (shingles), and ZIDOVUDINE (AZT), which is a treatment for HIV (human immunodeficiency virus), are nucleoside analogues. Because these medications are designed to interfere in the virus's replication, they are most effective when taken preventively or at a very early stage of viral infection. Other antiviral medications are designed to prevent viruses from penetrating host cells. The medication for preventing influenza, amantadine, serves this function.

Viscera

The internal organs of the body. The viscera consist of the large internal organs found in the three major cavities of the body—the head, the chest or thorax, and the abdomen. However, the term "viscera" usually refers to the organs found in the abdomen, such as the stomach and the intestines.

Viscosity

Thickness and stickiness of a liquid. Viscosity is a physical property of fluids that causes them to resist flowing freely.

Vision

The ability to perceive the visual features of objects, such as color, shape, size, detail, depth, and contrast. Vision occurs when the eyes and brain work together.

Light enters the eye through the cornea (the clear outer covering of the eye), which, along with the lens, focuses it on the retina (the light-

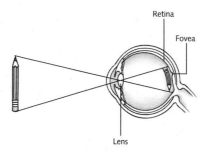

INVERTED IMAGE ON RETINA
Light rays coming into the eye are focused by the lens onto the retina, which receives the image accurately but upside down. The brain interprets the image right side up.

sensitive layer at the back of the eye). The retina contains nerve cells known as rods and cones that respond to different aspects of light. Cones perceive color and are sensitive to detail. Rods are insensitive to color, but very responsive to dim light and movement. Since the retina has many more rods than cones, the eye can see even in darkness, but it perceives color and detail best in bright light.

The electrical signals generated by the retina pass through the optic nerve, which connects directly into the brain and follows a pathway leading to the visual cortex in the back of the brain. The visual cortex makes sense of the incoming visual information. Since the eye contains only one lens, the image it receives is upside down. The brain puts it right-side up once again. It also joins the images of both eyes to provide depth perception and binocular vision.

Vision tests

A variety of examinations used to determine how well a person can see. Vision tests may be administered individually or in a battery of examinations, and they are often combined with physical examination of the eye. See EYE, EXAMINATION OF.

VISUAL ACUITY

Sharpness (acuity) of sight is commonly measured with the Snellen chart, which displays letters arranged in lines of decreasing size. The person is asked to read the letters on the line that can be seen by people with perfect vision from 20 feet away. If he or she can do this, he or she is said to have 20/20 vision. If vision is less sharp—if, for example, he or she can read at 20 feet that which a person with normal vision can read at 60 feet—he or she has 20/60 vision.

Near vision, for reading and other close work, is assessed with a chart held approximately 14 inches from the face. The person is asked to read the sentences on the chart with each individual eye or with both eyes open. Difficulty indicates a deficiency in near vision.

REFRACTION

If vision is less than 20/20 and needs correction, this examination is performed to determine the correct prescription for glasses or contact lenses. Sitting in a chair, the person looks through a special device (Phoroptor) at an eye chart approximately 20 feet away. The Phoroptor contains lenses of various strengths that can be moved into the line of view. As the specialist tries different lenses, he or she asks whether the eye chart is more or less clear. Information from the refraction test helps the specialist to diagnose what kind of vision error the person has and to prescribe glasses or contact lenses of the right type and strength to correct the error.

BLIND SPOTS

A test for blind spots is performed with the Amsler grid, which looks like a piece of paper with dark lines forming a square grid around a dot in the center. The grid is held at a comfortable reading distance with one eye covered while the person focuses on the center dot. The test is then repeated with the other eye covered. Blurring of the grid or distortion of its lines into wavy, fuzzy, or missing

PATH OF VISUAL IMPULSES
Receptor cells on the retinas receive visual stimuli and send impulses along the optic nerves to an intersection in the brain where some nerve fibers cross so that both sides of the brain receive impulses from both eyes. The signals enter the thalamus and are relayed to the visual cortex, which interprets the combined signals as one three-dimensional image.

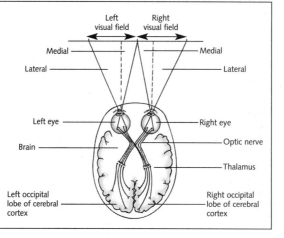

TYPES OF VISION TESTS

Several different methods are used by eye specialists to test a person's vision. The eye doctor often examines not only how well a person sees, but also how healthy the interior of the eye appears to be.

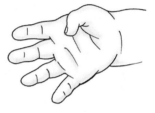

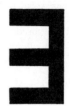

RANDOM E OPTOTYPES
Also referred to as the tumbling E eye test, random E forms are used to measure the visual acuity (sharpness of the central portion of vision) of small children and people who are unable to read. The person being tested responds to what is seen by extending his or her fingers in the direction of the E form being "read."

HUMPHREY TEST
This test is administered to measure peripheral vision (the outer portion of the field of vision). While focusing on a red light in the center field of vision, people undergoing testing indicate whether they see flashing lights in their peripheral fields of vision.

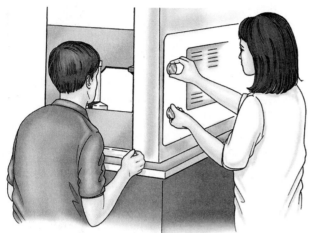

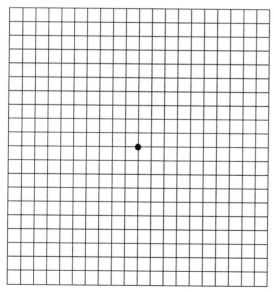

AMSLER GRID
A grid of evenly spaced vertical and horizontal lines with a dot in the center is used to test the macula. If areas of the grid appear to be distorted or missing or if the lines appear wavy, macular degeneration may be diagnosed.

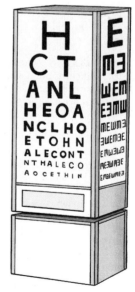

SNELLEN CHART
Lines of letters of decreasing size, usually viewed during an eye test at a distance of 20 feet, help eye specialists measure visual acuity.

areas of vision can indicate a common age-related vision loss called MACULAR DEGENERATION or other abnormalities of the macula.

COLOR PERCEPTION

In the standard test for COLOR BLINDNESS, the person is asked to identify symbols composed of primary-color dot patterns superimposed on a background of randomly mixed colors. The person covers one eye, and the tester shows him or her the symbols one after another. The test is then repeated for the other eye. If color vision is normal, the symbol is obvious. But if the person cannot distinguish certain colors, the symbols are difficult or impossible to recognize. The test results can be used to determine the type and degree of color blindness.

VISUAL FIELD

The visual field test checks how well the eyes can see throughout the full range of vision. In the computerized version of this test, the person places his or her chin on a stand in front of a computerized screen. Every time a light is seen, he or she presses a button. The printout reveals the range of vision, which is useful for detecting the degree of impairment of vision on either side of the head that characterizes early GLAUCOMA.

Vision, loss of

See BLINDNESS.

Visual acuity

The ability to distinguish details and shapes. Measurement of visual acuity is part of a standard eye examination. See EYE, EXAMINATION OF.

Visual field

The ability of the eye to perceive objects to the side of central vision. A normal visual field is 180 degrees, or a half-circle. The visual field is measured as part of a standard eye examination. In the simplest form of this test (confrontational visual field), the eye specialist sits in front of the person being tested, who covers one eye. The specialist moves his or her hand from the side to the center of the field of vision and asks the person being tested to report when he or she can first see the movement. The same test is repeated for the other eye. In the

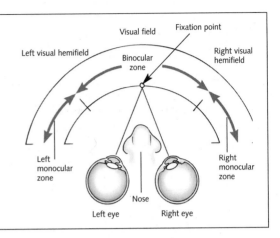

VIEW FROM BOTH EYES
When both eyes are focused on an object, the view seen by both eyes without moving the head is called the visual field. Each half (hemifield) has a monocular zone, in which light enters only one eye because the nose blocks the other eye. In the central binocular zone, light strikes both eyes.

Visual field — Fixation point
Left visual hemifield
Right visual hemifield
Binocular zone
Left monocular zone
Right monocular zone
Nose
Left eye   Right eye

automated test, the person being tested sits in front of a concave dome and focuses on an object or light in its center. One eye is covered. A computer program flashes small lights at various positions within the dome, and the person being tested presses a button whenever he or she sees a flash. The test is repeated for the other eye. The perimetry device prints out a chart that maps the visual field and reveals blind spots or other abnormalities.

Visual field testing is useful for diagnosing and evaluating diseases that can limit or impair the field of vision, such as glaucoma, multiple sclerosis, stroke, or a tumor in the brain.

Visual field defect

A blind spot or area within the normal range of vision. Visual field defects caused by migraine are temporary; most others are persistent. Visual field defects have a number of possible causes. Overall narrowing of the range of vision can be caused by GLAUCOMA (abnormal pressure within the eye) or inflammation of the optic nerves in SYPHILIS. A blind spot in the center of vision may come from swelling in the center of the optic nerve (see OPTIC DISC EDEMA) or an abnormality of the macula. Defects in the interior of the visual field can be caused by poisoning (with wood alcohol or quinine, for example), diseases that attack the optic nerve (such as multiple sclerosis), nutritional deficiencies, and diseases of the blood vessels, primarily atherosclerosis. Defects that affect one half or one quarter of the visual field in each eye

are usually caused by strokes or tumors in the brain.

Visualization

The use of the imagination to heal; using the mind to communicate with the body. Visualization uses imagery to relieve pain, speed healing, and promote mental and physical health. Many athletes use visualization to help perform in competition. Images can be visual, auditory, sensory (touch), olfactory (smell), and gustatory (taste). Imagery has been used as a healing tool in many of the world's cultures and religions for centuries. Today it is used as an adjunctive or complementary therapy for people with cancer.

Through such techniques as creative visualization, which seeks to harness mental energy to achieve positive goals, the imagination is used to combat stress, tension, and anxiety by replacing negative thoughts with positive ones. Applied to medical concerns, such techniques are used to help with chronic pain by minimizing it, such as by imagining a painful area of the body surrounded by ice and becoming numb.

In practice, people are able to achieve a profoundly relaxed state while gaining insight and control during the disease process.

Vital sign

A critical measurement of function. Vital signs include blood pressure, temperature, pulse rate, and respiratory rate. In the hospital, health care providers monitor a person's vital signs to assess how well his or her body is functioning.

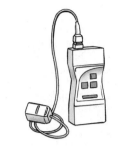

Pulse oximeter

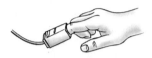

Sensor attachment

TAKING A PULSE
A device called a pulse oximeter provides a simple, accurate way to take a person's pulse from the pulse point at the end of the index finger. The person—from infant to adult—inserts his or her index finger into a sensor attachment and the device provides a digital read-out of the strength and rate of the pulse and the oxygen level in the bloodstream.

Vitamin A

Retinol, a fat-soluble vitamin important for healthy eyes, skin, hair, and mucous membranes. Vitamin A is also essential for proper growth and reproduction, as well as normal bone development. Carotenes, which are building blocks of vitamin A, are antioxidant chemicals that prevent changes that damage cells. Studies are ongoing to determine whether antioxidants help reduce the risk of heart disease and certain types of cancer. BETA-CAROTENE, a carotene found in plants, is converted into vitamin A by the liver. Retinoids, a group of compounds that are structurally related to retinol, function like vitamin A and are used in the treatment of various skin diseases and digestive ailments.

Good dietary sources of vitamin A include fish-liver oil, egg yolks, milk, cheese, and butter. Low-fat milk and ready-to-eat cereals are also fortified with vitamin A. Vitamin A can be derived from carotenes in fruits and vegetables. Beta-carotene is found in orange produce such as carrots, cantaloupe, papaya, sweet potatoes, and pumpkin; dark green, leafy vegetables such as spinach and kale; and deep yellow vegetables such as winter squash. Because vitamin A and beta-carotene can be destroyed in foods, preparation is important. To retain vitamins, serve raw fruits and vegetables; cover and refrigerate all produce (except sweet potatoes and winter squash); steam vegetables; and avoid frying foods, as vitamin A can be lost in fat.

A deficiency of vitamin A results in night blindness. It may also cause dry eyes, eye and respiratory infections, skin problems, and slow growth and bone deformities in children. Conditions that may increase the body's need for vitamin A include cystic fibrosis, chronic diarrhea, serious injury, liver disease, malabsorption, pancreatic disease, and chronic illness.

BETA-CAROTENE SUPPLEMENTS

Some studies have suggested that beta-carotene supplements provide health benefits that are different from those of vitamin A. Scientists are investigating the role that these supplements have in illnesses ranging from heart disease to cancer, as well as the impact they may have on aging. While some research is promising, other studies show no benefit. One study showed an increase of lung cancer in persons taking a beta-carotene supplement. As a result, experts remain divided on beta-carotene supplements. The safest source of this nutrient is foods.

Vitamin B

A group of water-soluble vitamins important to good health. B vitamins have a variety of roles. They help the body metabolize carbohydrates, fats, and protein and build red blood cells and are important to nerve and muscle function. A combination of folic acid (a B vitamin) and vitamins B6 and B12 can reduce the blood level of HOMOCYSTEINE, an amino acid that, when elevated, is associated with an increased risk of diseases related to the heart and blood vessels.

Good dietary sources of B vitamins include meats, dairy products, nuts, grains, and leafy green vegetables. Because B vitamins dissolve in water and can easily be lost from foods, preparation is important. B vitamins can be retained by serving raw fruits and vegetables, steaming foods briefly with a minimal amount of water, cooking potatoes in their skins, and refrigerating juices and keeping them no longer than 2 or 3 days.

Fruits and vegetables should not be soaked in water. B deficiency diseases depend on which B vitamin is missing. For example, folic acid deficiency in pregnant women increases the risk that a fetus's nervous system will not develop properly, while niacin deficiency results in pellagra, a nutritional disorder. A lack of B vitamins can cause anemia.

TYPES OF B VITAMINS

Among the B vitamins are the chemical substances thiamin, riboflavin, cobalamin, niacin, pyridoxine, folic acid, and biotin.

■ *Vitamin B1* Thiamin is essential for energy production from carbohydrates and nerve and muscle function, including function of the heart muscle. Vitamin B1 also helps the body metabolize glucose. Good dietary sources of B1 or thiamin include pork, low-fat milk, low-fat cheese, eggs, peas, potatoes, and whole-grain and enriched breads and cereals. A deficiency of thiamin can lead to symptoms such as loss of appetite, depression, and memory loss.

■ *Vitamin B2* Riboflavin is important in the metabolism of carbohydrates, fats, and protein. It helps to provide energy and maintain healthy skin. Good dietary sources of B2 or riboflavin include liver, kidney, low-fat milk, low-fat cheese, leafy green vegetables, lean meats, eggs, nuts, peas, beans, and whole-grain and enriched breads and cereals. A deficiency of riboflavin may lead to fatigue and changes the appearance of the lips and tongue.

■ *Vitamin B3* Niacin (nicotinic acid) improves blood circulation by dilating arteries and is important to a healthy skin, gastrointestinal tract, nervous system, and sex hormones. Niacin is also a key element in the metabolism of nutrients such as carbohydrates that yield energy. Good dietary sources of B3 or niacin include meats, poultry, fish, eggs, nuts, peanut butter, brewer's yeast, and wheat germ. A niacin deficiency can lead to symptoms such as weakness, fatigue, insomnia, irritability, tension, depression, nausea, vomiting, headaches, skin rashes, and tender gums. Severe deficiency causes pellagra, a disease characterized by dermatitis, diarrhea, and dementia.

■ *Vitamin B6* Pyridoxine assists the body to use protein. It is essential for

V

the formation of hemoglobin, promotes a healthy heart and blood vessels, helps regulate the nervous system, maintains healthy skin, and is important to a healthy pregnancy. Good dietary sources of B6 or pyridoxine include poultry, fish, eggs, whole-grain breads and cereals, peas, beans, liver, and low-fat dairy products. Vitamin B6 deficiency causes an anemia that is similar to iron-deficiency anemia but cannot be corrected with iron supplements.

■ *Folic acid* Sometimes called vitamin B9, folic acid is essential to growth and cell repair and is usually available in food as folate. Folic acid is important to a healthy pregnancy and cardiovascular function. Good dietary sources of folic acid include leafy green vegetables, liver, mushrooms, oatmeal, peanut butter, red beans, soybeans, and wheat germ. Adults require at least 0.4 milligrams (400 micrograms) of folic acid daily. Requirements are at least double during pregnancy. Folic acid deficiency can lead to severe birth defects such as spina bifida, megaloblastic anemia, and elevated blood levels of homocysteine.

■ *Vitamin B12* Cyanocobalamin is essential to the development of red blood cells. B12 is important to a healthful pregnancy, cardiovascular health, and normal function of nerves. Dietary sources of cyanocobalamin include liver, meat, dairy products, fish, and legumes. Consequently, vegetarians sometimes develop a VITAMIN B12 DEFICIENCY. A deficiency can also occur because of a lack of intrinsic factor, a substance produced in the stomach that is necessary for the body to absorb B12. In the absence of adequate intrinsic factor, B12 cannot be absorbed by the intestine and instead passes out of the body as waste. This results in pernicious anemia (see ANEMIA, PERNICIOUS). Symptoms of this disease include fatigue, dizziness, ringing in the ears, pale skin, a fast heart rate, an enlarged heart, loss of appetite, weight loss, diarrhea, cramping, numbness and tingling in the extremities, muscle weakness, depression, confusion, and irritability. Treatment is with lifelong injections of vitamin B12.

> 📖 Terms in small capital letters—for example, PHYSICAL THERAPY or PAGET DISEASE—indicate a cross-reference to another entry with more information.

■ *Other B vitamins and related substances* Vitamin B5 (pantothenic acid) helps in production of energy and synthesis of body compounds. BIOTIN, also known as vitamin H, aids the action of various enzymes in cells. Its roles include constructing proteins from amino acids, breaking down fats, and forming new fatty acids and glucose. Choline is important to liver function, heart health, physical performance, and nerve function. Inositol is involved in cell membrane health.

Vitamin B complex
See VITAMIN B.

Vitamin B12
See VITAMIN B.

Vitamin B12 deficiency
The absence or decreased ability of the body to absorb vitamin B12, resulting in an insufficient amount of B12 to meet the body's needs. It is almost always due to the inability of the intestine to absorb the vitamin. A B12 deficiency can cause pernicious anemia (see ANEMIA, PERNICIOUS), a disease in which red blood cells are abnormally formed. It can result from diets that entirely exclude animal products. Pernicious anemia is most common in people from northern Europe and in African Americans. B12 deficiency is also associated with various autoimmune disorders, especially those involving the thyroid, parathyroid, and adrenal glands. This deficiency can also develop if stomach acid is not produced in sufficient amounts. Many adults older than age 65 may not produce enough stomach acid and, thus, absorb insufficient B12. Acid helps to change the vitamin into a form in which it can be absorbed.

Vitamin B12 is a key factor in the development of red blood cells. When foods rich in B12 such as liver, meats, dairy products, and legumes are digested, vitamin B12 bonds to intrinsic factor, a chemical produced by parietal cells in the stomach lining that is essential to the absorption of B12. When parietal cells atrophy or shrink, they make less intrinsic factor, and B12 cannot be absorbed by the intestine; it instead passes out of the body as waste.

Symptoms of pernicious anemia

and B12 deficiency relate to three body systems: the hematopoietic system (which is responsible for the formation of red blood cells), the gastrointestinal system, and the nervous system. Decreased numbers of red blood cells (anemia) can result in fatigue, dizziness, ringing in the ears, pale skin, a fast heart rate, and an enlarged heart. Gastrointestinal symptoms include loss of appetite, weight loss, diarrhea, and cramping. Left untreated, nervous system manifestations, such as numbness and tingling in the extremities, muscle weakness, depression, cognitive impairment, confusion, and irritability, may develop.

Occasionally conditions other than atrophied parietal cells lead to poor B12 absorption. These may include Celiac disease, Crohn disease, Whipple disease, intestinal worms, structural defects of the intestinal system, conditions that require surgical removal of the stomach, poisoning with corrosive substances, and tuberculosis. Underlying causes of B12 deficiency require appropriate treatment. Treatment of pernicious anemia is with lifelong injections of B12, since the lack of intrinsic factor limits the ability of oral supplements to be absorbed. Other forms of B12 deficiency that do not involve lack of intrinsic factor may be treated with oral supplements.

Vitamin C
Ascorbic acid, a water-soluble vitamin involved in fat metabolism, the development of connective tissue, biosynthesis of neurotransmitters, immune function, wound healing, and iron absorption. Vitamin C is necessary for healthy bones, teeth, and skin. This vitamin is also an antioxidant, which means that it destroys free radicals before they can enter and damage cells. Studies are ongoing to determine whether antioxidants help reduce the risk of heart disease and certain types of cancer. A deficiency of vitamin C can lead to scurvy, a condition characterized by fatigue, muscle weakness, joint and muscle aches, bleeding gums, and a rash on the legs.

Numerous fresh fruits and vegetables are rich in vitamin C. These include citrus fruits such as oranges, lemons, limes, and grapefruit; green vegetables such as broccoli and kale; berries, tomatoes, potatoes, and green peppers. Juices and cereals are often fortified with vitamin C. Preparation is important because vitamin C can be readily lost from foods. It dissolves in water and can be destroyed by heat and oxygen. To retain vitamin C, serve raw fruits and vegetables, steam foods in a minimal amount of water for a short time, cook potatoes in their skins, refrigerate prepared juices and keep them for no longer than 2 or 3 days, and do not store or soak fruits and vegetables in water.

In the 1970s, Nobel laureate Linus Pauling suggested that megadoses of vitamin C could be used to treat cancer, lower cholesterol levels, and relieve common cold symptoms. Research has not borne out these claims. Large doses of vitamin C can cause diarrhea. In some people, they can also cause or aggravate gout and lead to kidney stones.

Vitamin D

Cholecalciferol, a fat-soluble vitamin essential for the formation of bones and teeth and for the absorption of calcium and phosphorus. A deficiency of vitamin D causes bone diseases such as rickets and osteoporosis. Good dietary sources of vitamin D include organ meats, fish liver oils, egg yolks, and saltwater fish such as salmon, sardines, and herring. Because relatively small amounts of vitamin D are naturally available, milk, dairy products, cereals, and breads are usually fortified with it. Exposure to sunlight also enables the skin to manufacture vitamin D. As little as 10 minutes of exposure to sunlight may produce sufficient quantities of vitamin D. Because of the high risks of skin cancer associated with exposure to sunlight, however, exposure should be closely monitored.

Vitamin E

Tocopherol, a fat-soluble vitamin that helps form red blood cells, muscles, and lung and nerve tissue. Vitamin E is also important in reproduction and is an antioxidant chemical that may prevent damaging changes in cells. Studies are ongoing to determine whether ANTIOXIDANTS help to reduce the risk of heart disease and certain types of cancer.

Vitamin E is composed of eight related compounds: four tocopherols and four tocotrienols. Alpha toco-

pherol is the main type of vitamin E in the body. Foods such as vegetable oils, whole grains, wheat germ, nuts, and leafy green vegetables are good sources of vitamin E. Most ready-to-eat cereals are also fortified with vitamin E. Because this vitamin can be readily lost from foods, preparation is important. Using whole-grain flours, storing foods in airtight containers, and avoiding exposing foods to light can help retain vitamin E.

Several epidemiologic studies have linked vitamin E supplements with a reduced rate of heart disease. Some doctors recommend that people take a vitamin E supplement (200 to 800 international units, or IU, a day) for cardiovascular and other benefits. Because large doses may be harmful, however, it is important not to exceed these dosages. People who are taking anticoagulant drugs need to be careful, since large doses of vitamin E can increase the risk of spontaneous bleeding.

Vitamin K

A fat-soluble vitamin essential for blood clotting. It may also have a role in the health of the skeleton by preserving the strength of bones. Good dietary sources of vitamin K include leafy green vegetables such as spinach, lettuce, and cabbage; liver; egg yolks; cauliflower; grain products; potatoes; fruits; low-fat milk; and low-fat cheese. Little of this vitamin is lost in cooking. Vitamin K is also synthesized by bacteria that normally reside in the large intestine. Prolonged use of antibiotics can lead to a vitamin K deficiency if dietary intake is not increased to compensate for the reduced amounts from intestinal bacteria. Vitamin K deficiency can result in spontaneous bleeding and serious and potentially fatal bleeding in the event of an injury. High doses of vitamin E can increase this problem. Vitamin K is routinely administered to newborns to prevent bleeding problems.

Vitamin K–dependent coagulation factors

Blood-clotting substances that require VITAMIN K to form blood clots. Vitamin K deficiency can result in spontaneous bleeding. If there is a severe deficiency, even a minor wound can cause serious and potentially fatal

bleeding. Vitamin K–dependent coagulation factors are factor II (also known as prothrombin), factor VII, factor IX, and factor X.

Vitamin supplements

Usually nonprescription preparations that contain one or more vitamins (see also MULTIVITAMIN). Vitamin supplements are typically taken to compensate for vitamin deficiencies in the diet. Taking vitamin supplements is not as effective as getting vitamins by eating a balanced diet that includes a variety of foods, especially whole grains, fruits, and vegetables. Vitamin supplements do not offset the health risks associated with high fat intake, refined sugars, and overeating. However, they can benefit people with nutritionally inadequate diets, such as older people who often eat too little. Supplements can help women who are breast-feeding, pregnant, or planning to become pregnant; people with a chronic illness; or vegetarians and individuals who are on low-calorie diets. Doctors prescribe supplements for individuals with true vitamin deficiencies, although such cases are rare. Before beginning a regimen of vitamin supplements, an individual should consult a physician to discuss nutritional needs. Large doses of some vitamins can cause toxic effects.

Vitamins

Complex chemical compounds that the body cannot manufacture but are essential for good health. Vitamins regulate chemical processes in the body and are essential to immune system maintenance. They have a role in both maintaining health and preventing disease. A deficiency of vitamins leads to a wide range of diseases, from birth defects (most often due to folic acid deficiency) to scurvy (caused by a lack of vitamin C).

Vitamins can be water-soluble or fat-soluble. Water-soluble vitamins dissolve in water and mix easily in the blood. The body is able to store only small amounts of these vitamins, most of which are excreted in urine and sweat. Consequently, these vitamins must be replaced daily. The water-soluble vitamins are vitamin C and the B complex vitamins—including thiamin (B1), riboflavin (B2), niacin (B3), pyridoxine (B6), cyanocobalamin (B12), folic acid, and biotin. The fat-soluble vitamins—A, D, E, and K—are found in fats and oils in foods. They are stored in the body's fat cells. If a person takes too many fat-soluble vitamins, the vitamins can build up in the body and have harmful effects.

Vitiligo

A skin disorder characterized by patches of white skin due to loss of pigment cells (melanocytes). Many people report pigment loss shortly after emotional stress or sunburn. Although its exact cause remains unknown, vitiligo is believed to have an autoimmune component. That is, for unknown reasons, the body manufactures antibodies that destroy its own melanocytes. Although most people with vitiligo are generally in good health, they are at greater risk of developing thyroid dysfunction, vitamin B12 deficiency, diabetes, and alopecia areata (a temporary loss of hair in patches). Vitiligo affects all races and sexes equally and most commonly occurs between the ages of 20 and 30. Although there is no cure for vitiligo, treatments are available.

SYMPTOMS

Any part of the body may be affected. Common sites of pigment loss are around the eyes, nose, and mouth; on the hands and genitals; and at sites of injury. The hair that grows in areas affected by vitiligo may turn white, or there may be premature graying of the hair.

Vitiligo may appear in a segmental pattern where depigmented patches are limited to one segment of the body. Segmental vitiligo is more common in childhood and rarely spreads. Generalized involvement, in which depigmentation occurs on various parts of the body in a symmetric pattern, is more common. There is no way to predict whether vitiligo will spread. Lesions may remain stable for years or progress rapidly. Some people experience further depigmentation after emotional or physical stress.

DIAGNOSIS AND TREATMENT

Vitiligo is diagnosed according to the appearance of the skin. Blood tests may be ordered to measure thyroid function, check for anemia, and detect other autoimmune conditions.

Treatment of vitiligo involves trying

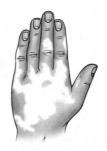

LOSS OF PIGMENTATION
Vitiligo causes white patches on the skin, more commonly on areas of the body that have been exposed to the sun. Vitiligo may appear in different patterns—in limited areas, only on one side of the body, or on many parts of the body. It may spread rapidly after a time of stress or slowly over a period of years.

to restore normal pigment to the affected areas (repigmentation) or to destroy the remaining pigment (depigmentation). Treatment depends on the severity of the disease. Widespread white patches can affect physical appearance and emotional state. Treatment includes topical corticosteroids and the drug psoralen plus ultraviolet A (PUVA), which is a form of PHOTOTHERAPY (treatment with light). PUVA is the most beneficial treatment for vitiligo. Psoralen is an agent that maximizes the effect of ultraviolet light on the skin, promoting PHOTOSENSITIVITY (heightened sensitivity to the sun). It can be taken orally or applied topically to the skin. Unfortunately, long-term treatment increases the risk of skin cancer. In addition, possible side effects include sunburn, blistering, and darkening of the treated skin. Surgical therapies for vitiligo include skin grafts, tattooing, and melanocyte transplants.

Depigmentation is another option for persons with vitiligo involving more than half of their bodies. Chemicals are used to fade the rest of the skin to match the white patches. Some people use makeup to camouflage depigmented patches. Because depigmented areas are sensitive to the sun, they should be protected with a sunblock. Finally, since vitiligo can lead to psychological problems such as depression, many people benefit from counseling.

Vitrectomy

An operation in which the normally clear, jellylike liquid (vitreous) inside the eye is removed and replaced with

a salt solution. The surgery is performed when large amounts of blood have leaked into the vitreous and clouded the vision or to treat retinal disorders. The surgeon makes a small incision in the white (sclera) of the eye and inserts an instrument that draws out the cloudy vitreous and replaces it with the clear salt solution. Vitrectomy can be performed under local or general anesthesia and may require an overnight hospital stay. The eye is red and irritated for a few days to weeks following the surgery, and a shield may be worn to protect the eye until healing is complete. Vision following a vitrectomy can be greatly improved.

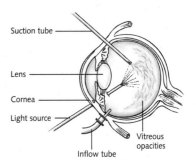

CLEARING CLOUDED VISION
Vitrectomy is an advance in eye surgery in which vitreous humor that has been clouded with blood is suctioned out and replaced with a clear salt solution. The procedure makes more space in the eye and clears the vision.

Vitreous hemorrhage

Bleeding into the clear, jellylike liquid (vitreous) inside the eye. In small amounts, blood clouds vision; larger amounts lead to a mass of red or

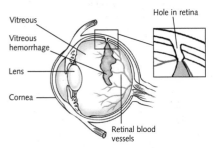

BLEEDING IN THE EYE
Bleeding from a blood vessel into the vitreous (clear gel in the eyeball) causes poor vision. The bleeding may result from a number of problems, including diabetic retinopathy, high blood pressure, a tear in the retina, or an unknown cause.

black lines and very dark vision. If the blood is not absorbed on its own, vitreous hemorrhage is treated with VITRECTOMY to replace the vitreous with a clear salt solution. Once the view inside the eye is good enough, laser surgery (see PHOTOCOAGULATION) may be performed to cause the abnormal bleeding vessels to regress.

Vitreous humor

The transparent jellylike substance that fills the eyeball. The vitreous humor, which is also called the vitreous body, is located behind the lens of the eye, between the lens and the retina. In medicine, the term "humor" refers to a fluid or semifluid.

Vivisection

Operating surgically on live animals for research purposes. Vivisection has traditionally been used by scientists to learn more about physiological and pathological processes. For example, vivisection might be used to observe the effects of certain drugs on a beating heart. The animal is anesthetized before the operation begins.

Over time, as humane societies have questioned the need for using live animals for research, vivisection has come to refer to any experimentation on live animals. In the United States, the Animal Welfare Act of 1970 sets limits on the use of animals in laboratories.

VLDL

Very-low-density lipoprotein. VLDL is a type of lipid and protein complex made by the liver and transported in the blood. Elevated levels of VLDL in blood are associated with high triglyceride levels, a buildup of plaque in the arteries, and an increased risk of atherosclerosis and heart disease. See CHOLESTEROL.

Vocal cord nodules

Noncancerous growths of the epithelium (mucous membrane covering) on the surface of the VOCAL CORDS. The vocal cords are folds of mucous membrane draped over a ligament and muscle that extend from the wall of the larynx (voice box). The nodules are usually located on both sides of the vocal cords. The most common symptom is hoarseness and, possibly, a breathy sound to the voice. The nodules are the result of irritation and

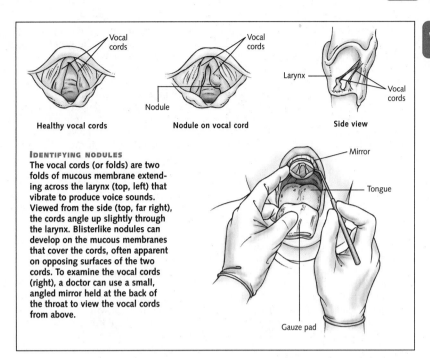

Healthy vocal cords   **Nodule on vocal cord**   **Side view**

IDENTIFYING NODULES
The vocal cords (or folds) are two folds of mucous membrane extending across the larynx (top, left) that vibrate to produce voice sounds. Viewed from the side (top, far right), the cords angle up slightly through the larynx. Blisterlike nodules can develop on the mucous membranes that cover the cords, often apparent on opposing surfaces of the two cords. To examine the vocal cords (right), a doctor can use a small, angled mirror held at the back of the throat to view the vocal cords from above.

inflammation of the mucous membrane, typically caused by excessive use, prolonged overuse, or misuse of the voice. Professional singers tend to have vocal cord nodules, and sometimes children acquire them from extended or frequent screaming. The nodules may also occur as the result of a single overuse of the voice, such as yelling at a sports event. The strain on the vocal cords causes the inflamed membrane tissue to become fibrous and hardened, producing small, rounded masses of tissue that protrude from the vocal cords.

DIAGNOSIS AND TREATMENT

An otolaryngologist (ear, nose, and throat specialist) can diagnose vocal cord nodules by examining the vocal cords with a lighted viewing instrument. Speech therapy to teach a person how to avoid voice behaviors that aggravate or cause the formation of the nodules is the first line of treatment. Resting the voice by using it as little as possible for several weeks may help to shrink the nodules. If rest and therapy are not successful, the nodules may be surgically removed, but with ongoing misuse, overuse, or abuse of the voice, they tend to return. For this reason, therapy to retrain speech patterns is usually recommended both before and after surgery.

Vocal cord paralysis

The inability of one or both VOCAL CORDS (folds of mucous membrane in the larynx) to move because of damage to the nerves or the brain. The opening and closing of the vocal cords has a vital role in speech, swallowing, and breathing. Any impairment in their capacity for movement can affect any or all of these essential functions.

SYMPTOMS AND CAUSES

If the movement of one fold is impaired, it cannot move in unison with the other fold. The impairment may cause a loss of the normal voice quality or hoarseness; speaking may require significant effort and sound weak and breathy. The person may cough or choke while eating and drinking because the folds do not close completely when a person swallows. When both folds are impaired, they tend to remain close to the midline of the larynx. This bilateral paralysis can compromise the airflow through the throat and restrict or block normal breathing.

Vocal cord paralysis is most often the result of an injury to the nerve that controls the muscles of the larynx. The injury can be caused by physical injury to the nerve or compression during intubation (insertion of a breathing tube into the trachea to allow breathing), or it can be a complication of surgery or a result of other causes. Sometimes, an injury to the brain or a brain disease or disorder, such as a stroke, can impair this nerve's function and produce paralysis. A mechanical obstruction may also produce impairment to the vocal cords' movement. The cartilage that attaches the vocal folds may become locked in place and restrict movement of the folds. Accumulated scar tissue can also prevent the vocal folds from moving normally.

TREATMENT

If one of the vocal cords is immobilized, the condition may be treated with surgery, implants, or injections. The surgical procedure, called medialization thryoplasty and performed under local anesthesia, is considered effective and painless. It involves making a small incision through the skin near the larynx, removing a small piece of the cartilage, and inserting a small block of silicone into the cartilage to help promote the closing of the vocal folds. Another procedure involves an implant of bioactive material (a material that can affect living tissue), which stimulates cartilage growth and helps correct the defect. The procedure involving injections introduces small amounts of material into the affected vocal fold that pushes the fold inward toward the center of the larynx so it can meet the other fold and produce sound. The materials used for injection include autologous fat (fat tissue taken from the body of the person having the procedure).

If both vocal cords are paralyzed, treatment is directed toward opening the airway and restoring breathing. This condition may be corrected by TRACHEOSTOMY (an opening from the trachea to the surface of the neck to permit airflow) or by transverse cordotomy (a procedure in which a small portion of tissue from one or both vocal cords is removed). When there is serious blockage of breathing, a cordectomy (surgical removal of the vocal cords) may be performed. Another treatment for bilateral vocal cord paralysis is called a posterior cricoid split, which involves splitting the surrounding cartilage and inserting a cartilage graft to enlarge the airway opening. Another new procedure, called laryngeal pacing, involves implanting a small device to coordinate the opening of the vocal folds as air passes through them.

Vocal cords

Two folds of mucous membrane overlying two vocal ligaments in the larynx (voice box) that vibrate to produce the sounds of speech. The cords are attached at the front to the inner surface of the thyroid cartilage (Adam's apple). Muscles attached to the vocal cords alter their length and tension. As air expelled from the lungs passes through them, the folds can be opened, closed, and vibrated to vary the sound produced. The sounds are further modified by the tongue, teeth, and lips to produce speech. See SPEECH MECHANISM.

Most of the time the vocal cords lie apart, forming a triangle-shaped opening through which air for breathing passes. The cords also close automatically during swallowing to prevent food from going down the trachea instead of the esophagus.

Voice box

See LARYNX.

Voice, loss of

FOR SYMPTOM CHART
see Hoarseness or voice loss, page 31

An inability of the larynx (voice box) to produce normal speech. A person can lose his or her ability to speak when the nerve supply that normally pushes the two vocal cords together is damaged or destroyed. This nerve loss may be due to a stroke, throat cancer or its treatments, an injury to the throat or neck, or other conditions. Sometimes there is no identifiable cause. When the vocal cords are unable to close, the voice cannot be projected, and the sound is lost. Usually, when it becomes impossible to speak, breathing is also restricted, and there is a risk of choking when swallowing. When the loss of voice is severe and prolonged, surgery may be required. Under local anesthesia, this operation involves the surgical implantation of a device that adds volume to an impaired vocal cord and restores sound production. By trying a variety of different sized devices and asking the person to speak, the doctor determines what size device to insert, and a person's natural speaking voice is restored. See also VOCAL CORD PARALYSIS.

Volkmann contracture

A contraction of the muscles that suppresses the flow of blood to an extremity, most commonly the hand. It is usually a complication of elbow or forearm fractures causing a severe deformity and paralysis of the hand or wrist. A surgical procedure may be needed if conservative therapy fails.

Volvulus

A condition in which a loop of the intestine becomes knotted or twisted. Volvulus can obstruct the passage of intestinal contents. (See INTESTINE, OBSTRUCTION OF.) As gas and feces become trapped, the abdomen becomes swollen, and pain and vomiting result. If the blood supply is cut off, gangrene (death of tissue) may develop.

Volvulus is usually diagnosed through imaging studies such as X rays. When the problem develops in the small intestine, only surgery provides a definitive diagnosis. However, volvulus most frequently occurs in the S-shaped sigmoid portion of the colon. Doctors are frequently able to treat this condition through SIGMOIDOSCOPY. In this procedure, a flexible, lighted tube is inserted through the anus into the colon. The intestine is untwisted, and obstructed gas and feces are released. In recurrent cases of volvulus in the sigmoid colon, or when the problem develops elsewhere in the intestine, more extensive abdominal surgery may be required.

Vomiting

FOR SYMPTOM CHART
see Nausea or vomiting, page 46

The forceful, involuntary ejection of stomach contents through the mouth. Unless vomiting is recurrent, prolonged, painful, or contains blood (see VOMITING BLOOD), it is usually not a sign of serious disease. Vomiting can be a symptom of many minor disorders, such as elevated hormone levels during pregnancy or gastroenteritis (inflammation of the stomach and intestines as a result of infection).

Doctors advise individuals with

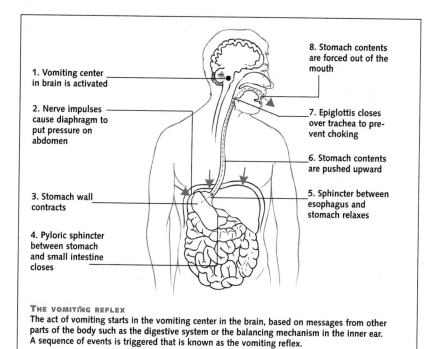

1. Vomiting center in brain is activated

2. Nerve impulses cause diaphragm to put pressure on abdomen

3. Stomach wall contracts

4. Pyloric sphincter between stomach and small intestine closes

8. Stomach contents are forced out of the mouth

7. Epiglottis closes over trachea to pre- vent choking

6. Stomach contents are pushed upward

5. Sphincter between esophagus and stomach relaxes

THE VOMITING REFLEX
The act of vomiting starts in the vomiting center in the brain, based on messages from other parts of the body such as the digestive system or the balancing mechanism in the inner ear. A sequence of events is triggered that is known as the vomiting reflex.

nausea and vomiting to eat nothing until symptoms subside. To prevent dehydration, small amounts of nonalcoholic fluids, such as water or weak tea, should be consumed. After 24 hours, a normal diet can be resumed. If vomiting is violent or persistent, medical attention should be sought. This type of vomiting may be a sign of a more serious underlying disorder such as an intestinal obstruction; it can also cause a tear in the esophagus. Severe vomiting can be treated with rectal suppositories or injection of an antiemetic drug.

Vomiting blood

A symptom of a disorder in the digestive tract. Also known as hematemesis, vomiting blood can result from excessive vomiting or consumption of alcohol. It is also symptomatic of potentially life-threatening internal bleeding and should not be ignored. Blood in vomit can be red or resemble coffee grounds. An individual who vomits blood should call a doctor. If other symptoms, such as chills, sweating, weakness, or dizziness, are present, immediate medical attention is required.

Bleeding in the digestive tract occurs when blood vessels in its walls become damaged. Internal bleeding

and vomiting may develop as a complication of PEPTIC ULCER DISEASE. Vomiting blood may also occur in the advanced stages of STOMACH CANCER when a tumor erodes a blood vessel. Severe GASTRIC EROSION (a superficial raw area in the mucous membrane that lines the stomach) may also cause bleeding and blood in the vomit. Severe cases of vomiting blood, such as those associated with CIRRHOSIS (a severe liver disease), require blood transfusions and surgery.

Vomiting in pregnancy

Nausea and vomiting in pregnancy are attributed to changing hormone levels. Typical of the first trimester of pregnancy, nausea and vomiting

may last into the second trimester. Because these symptoms occur more often in the morning, they are often called "morning sickness." However, the nausea of pregnancy can occur at any time of day. A woman should not take medication for morning sickness without first consulting her doctor. To lessen or avoid episodes of nausea and vomiting, doctors recommend that pregnant women eat bland foods such as crackers, drink ample fluids, and avoid greasy and highly seasoned foods. Nonpharmacological treatments using acupressure or biofeedback can help. In severe cases in which morning sickness endangers a woman's health, medicine may be prescribed to stop the vomiting.

von Willebrand disease

An inherited chronic bleeding disorder. von Willebrand disease (VWD) is the most common inherited bleeding disorder, affecting up to 3 percent of the population. It is a platelet disorder caused by a defect in a clotting factor known as von Willebrand factor, a protein essential for the formation of blood clots. Deficient or absent von Willebrand factor impairs the aggregation of platelets at the site of a wound, which delays or prevents the formation of blood clots needed to stop bleeding. Factor VIII, a substance in the blood that is necessary for coagulation, may be reduced in people with VWD because von Willebrand factor serves as a carrier for factor VIII.

SYMPTOMS AND CAUSES
Symptoms may vary in severity from person to person. While the severest form of the disease is rare, many milder forms are much more common. A key symptom in childhood is

---

AVOIDING NAUSEA AND VOMITING WHILE PREGNANT

Women report relief from these measures:

- Arising from bed slowly, sitting on the edge of the bed for a few minutes to accustom the body to being upright
- Eating a few crackers (kept on the nightstand) upon awakening
- Eating dry toast, crackers, or a peeled apple every few hours throughout the day
- Drinking plenty of liquids between meals, but avoiding any that are very hot or very cold
- Sipping ginger ale or ginger tea
- Avoiding foods that are fried, greasy, or highly seasoned

V

nosebleeds that are severe enough to require visits to a doctor or emergency department. Women and girls will experience very heavy menstrual flow. Other symptoms include a tendency to bruise easily, blood in the urine or the stool, and heavy bleeding after surgery or tooth extraction.

Unlike people with hemophilia, people with VWD do not usually bleed into joints and muscles. Because it is a disorder of the platelets, VWD causes bleeding into mucous membranes of the mouth, nose, intestine, or uterus.

HOW VWD IS INHERITED

Unlike hemophilia, VWD is not sex-related; both girls and boys are at risk. VWD is a dominant genetic disorder. If a parent has a defective gene for von Willebrand factor, there is a 50 percent chance that each of his or her children will be affected. If both parents have the defective gene, their children will have a 25 percent chance of not having VWD, a 50 percent chance of having a single defective gene and mild disease, or a 25 percent chance of having two defective genes, resulting in severe disease. Genetic counseling and testing are recommended to individuals with a family history of the disorder.

TREATMENT

Many people with VWD must take a drug that stimulates release of von Willebrand factor and factor VIII from the walls of the blood vessels. Transfusion of plasma or cryoprecipitate, a concentrate of clotting factor derived from human blood, may also be used. People with VWD must avoid taking drugs such as aspirin that might worsen bleeding.

Voyeurism

A mental illness characterized by seeking and watching unsuspecting people undress, become naked, or engage in sexual activity. Also known as peeping, voyeurism serves as a way for the person with the disorder to become sexually excited. He or she may masturbate while watching or later while engaging in a fantasy about what has been seen. In extreme form, voyeurism becomes the person's only sexual activity. Voyeurism usually begins before age 15, lasts at least 6 months, and is much more common in males than females. Voyeurism tends to continue through-out life.

Vulva

The external female genitals. See REPRODUCTIVE SYSTEM, FEMALE.

Vulva, cancer of the

Malignant tumors involving women's external genitalia. Cancer of the vulva is relatively rare and usually occurs in women older than 50, although younger women can develop it, too. Most cancer of the vulva (90 percent) is squamous cell carcinoma, a type of skin cancer, and another 5 percent is melanoma, another type of skin cancer. The most common symptom of cancer of the vulva is persistent itching. Lumps may appear on the labia, or outer lips, on the inner labia, the clitoris, or the perineum (the area between the anus and the vagina). Burning, pain, discharge, or bleeding may also occur. If the cancer has become invasive, a large mass may develop on the vulva or the groin. When the cancer is a melanoma, it usually appears on the clitoris and the outer labia, as brown, black, or blue-black lumps or patches.

DIAGNOSIS AND TREATMENT

Diagnosis of cancer of the vulva includes a thorough pelvic examination and a biopsy. Sometimes, the doctor also uses colposcopy to examine the vagina and cervix closely, to find out how far the cancer has spread. Because cancer of the vulva often occurs simultaneously with other genital cancers, a PAP SMEAR generally is done.

Treatment depends on the extent of the disease. If the area of cancerous tissue is small, a cream containing a chemotherapy agent can be applied directly to the vulva. Larger areas of cancerous tissue may need to be surgically removed by vulvectomy. The affected area can also be removed by laser surgery, which is more painful but generally involves less scarring. If the cancer has spread to the lymph nodes, the doctor usually recommends radiation therapy after surgery.

Vulvar dystrophy

A condition in which the skin of the vulva, or external female genitalia, becomes either abnormally thickened or thinned out. Dystrophy occurs when tissues do not function or develop properly because they are inadequately nourished. Vulvar dys-

trophy is most common after menopause, when a drop in the estrogen level can cause changes in the skin. Symptoms include itching and discomfort; the skin may be abnormally thin or thick, red or white, and it can sometimes become blistered.

Diagnosis requires a biopsy to rule out cancer and identify the type of dystrophy. Treatment usually includes topical testosterone creams, although some women do not respond well to the creams and may need to have some skin removed from the vulva. Vulvar dystrophy is usually a recurrent condition that requires long-term treatment.

Vulvectomy

Surgical removal of the vulva, or external female genitalia, and the lymph nodes in the groin. A vulvectomy is the most common and effective treatment for cancer of the vulva. A simple vulvectomy involves removal of the skin and some underlying fatty tissue. In a radical vulvectomy, all the tissue down to the muscle layer is removed. The urethral opening, the rectum, and most of the vagina are generally preserved. Skin grafts can be used to reconstruct some of the vulva, although results may not be ideal.

Laser surgery may be an alternative to vulvectomy, leading to more postoperative pain but less scarring. Sexual intercourse is possible after a vulvectomy, although some women are not able to achieve orgasm because so much of the sexually sensitive skin has been removed from the clitoris.

Vulvitis

Inflammation of the vulva, or external female genitalia. Vulvitis typically involves redness, swelling, and itching of the labia and other parts of the vulva. Vulvitis is itself a symptom that can result from many different diseases, infections, allergies, and chemical irritants, such as perfumed soap and spray, or laundry detergent. Stress, poor hygiene, inadequate diet, and insufficient rest can all increase a woman's chance of having vulvitis.

Vulvitis is usually not life-threatening, except when it is associated with cancer of the vulva. It can be extremely uncomfortable and inconvenient to a woman because the itching can be severe and can be made worse by scratching and washing. If vulvitis becomes chronic, scaly whitish sore patches may develop on the skin along with blisters that burst and crust over. A foul-smelling vaginal discharge is also possible.

Diagnosis requires a pelvic examination and various tests to rule out serious conditions and diseases. Blood tests and urine tests, and sometimes tests for sexually transmitted diseases, may be done. A biopsy may be performed if sores suggesting cancer of the vulva are present. Treatment may simply involve soothing baths with baking soda or warm boric acid compresses. Hydrocortisone creams can be used without prescription to relieve itching, although long-term use can aggravate the skin. Keeping the genital area cool, dry, and clean is recommended to help control irritation. If vulvitis does not respond to these measures, a doctor will need to evaluate and treat it. HORMONE REPLACEMENT THERAPY may help women who have completed menopause and whose irritation is from a lack of estrogen. See also VESTIBULITIS; VULVA, CANCER OF THE.

Vulvovaginitis

Inflammation of the vulva (the external female genitalia) and the vagina. Symptoms include redness, itching, and soreness of the vulva and the vagina, sometimes accompanied by vaginal discharge.

Vulvovaginitis can occur at any age. It can be caused by infectious agents, such as yeast; a skin allergy to wool, nylon, or laundry products; pinworms; and, in the case of children, bed-wetting. Repeated sexual intercourse over short periods can also lead to vulvovaginitis. Diagnosis can usually be made by microscopic examination of a sample of vaginal discharge. Treatment can range from soothing baths and improved personal hygiene to vaginal antibiotic creams. Women with recurrent vulvovaginitis should avoid chemical irritants and using tampons at least for a few months.

W

W

Waist-to-hip ratio

A tool used in the assessment of fat distribution and health risk. In people who are overweight, the risk for heart disease and other medical problems depends not only on excess weight but on how and where fat is stored. Waist-to-hip ratio is calculated by measuring waist and hip circumferences and then dividing waist measurement by hip measurement.

The waist-to-hip ratio indicates whether a person carries more weight around the waist (an apple shape) or around the hips and thighs (a pear shape). Apple-shaped individuals are generally at higher risk for many diseases. They tend to have elevated levels of harmful low-density lipoprotein (LDL) cholesterol, which causes fatty plaque deposits to accumulate on artery walls. Storing fat around the waist puts people at a greater risk of high blood pressure, cardiovascular disease, cancer, and diabetes. Regardless of how the fat is distributed, overweight people are at equally high risk of other complications such as sleep apnea and osteoarthritis. See also BODY MASS INDEX; BIOELECTRIC IMPEDANCE ANALYSIS.

Waldenström macroglobulinemia

An uncommon cancer affecting bone marrow cells in which abnormal cells that resemble both lymphocytes (white blood cells) and plasma cells produce an abnormal protein, an immunoglobulin known as IgM. The protein causes weakness, fatigue, drowsiness, pale skin, a tendency to bleed easily, fever, weight loss, dizziness, headaches, and enlarged lymph nodes. People with a large concentration of IgM can develop hyperviscosity, a thickening of the blood, which can result in sluggish blood flow and may cause stroke or congestive heart failure.

Waldenström macroglobulinemia progresses slowly with a median survival rate of 5 years. It behaves like MULTIPLE MYELOMA, arising in the bone marrow and causing bone defects. Diagnosis is made by microscopic examination of the bone marrow and blood serum. Treatment involves chemotherapy. People who have blood hyperviscosity need to be treated with plasmapheresis, a procedure that filters out concentrations of unwanted substances from the blood. This cancer chiefly occurs in men older than 60.

Walking aids

Assistive devices, such as walkers, crutches, canes, and prostheses, that enable individuals whose walking ability is limited to walk. Walking aids help them cope with muscle weakness, poor flexibility, poor balance, degenerative diseases, or injuries that make it difficult to get around. The purpose of walking aids is to help people preserve their mobility with as much comfort and stability as possible. If prescribed by a physician, Medicare and Medicaid partially cover the cost of some walking aids. To determine whether an individual can benefit from a walking aid such as a cane or walker, a doctor usually refers him or her to a physical therapist. The physical therapist evaluates a person's balance, strength, and range of movement and makes recommendations accordingly. Once a walking aid is selected and acquired, the therapist rechecks the size and fit to ensure correct and safe mobility and instructs the person on how to use the aid properly. See also WHEELCHAIR; PROSTHESIS.

THE RIGHT SIZE AND FIT

Walking aids must be the right size and fit. Walkers are adjustable and can be fitted according to a person's height, weight, physical disabilities, and environment. For good traction and grip, the bottom tips of walkers, canes, and crutches should be made of flat flexible rubber or plastic. Length of a walking aid is critical for comfortable walking. The tops of canes and walkers should meet the crease at the wrist; the elbows should bend at a 20- to 30 degree angle. A cane is for someone whose impairment is on one side and should be held in the hand of the person's unaffected side. Crutches should be of a length that allows the arms to bend at the elbows 15 to 20 degrees. Handles that are contoured are more comfortable than rounded ones.

Walking, delayed

Not developing the ability to walk within the normal age range. Although

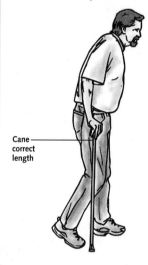

Cane correct length

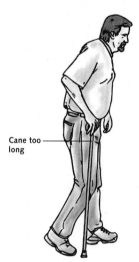

Cane too long

LENGTH OF A CANE
A wooden cane is cut to length, but a metal one can be adjusted. The appropriate length for a cane or walking stick varies by an individual's height; if the cane is too long, it feels unstable to the person using it.

WALKING AIDS

People whose walking is limited can use walking aids to improve their stability and safely increase their mobility. The selection of a device is based on the person's type of impairment and whether one or both sides of the body are affected. A doctor or physical therapist can determine which aid best helps address the problem. For example, people with single-leg injuries commonly use full-length crutches, while people recovering from strokes often require the upper body support of elbow crutches. Walkers are good for people who are weak on both sides or have poor balance. Well-fitting shoes with rubber soles and low heels are recommended to be worn when using any walking aid.

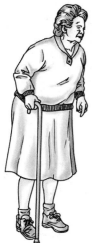

SOME STABILITY: CANE

A cane can help people who are slightly unsteady and whose weakness is on one side. A wooden cane is cut to length, but a metal one can be adjusted. Frequent users may prefer the "swan neck" cane that directs body weight from the wrist to the cane shaft. The cane's single point is not as stable as other aids, but its small size is practical on stairs.

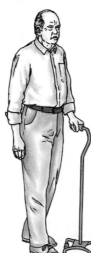

MEDIUM STABILITY: QUAD CANE

People whose impairment is on one side get more balance control with a quad cane, also called a footed cane. Its four legs increase the cane's stability; the wider the distance between the feet, the more stable the cane. It can be awkward in narrow places like stairs, but its contoured handle is easier to hold than the hook handle of normal canes.

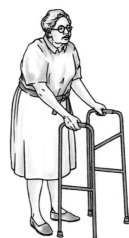

SUBSTANTIAL STABILITY: WALKER

Walkers can help those with generalized weakness or impairment on one or both sides who lack balance. Four adjustable legs and twin handgrips support half the person's weight. The person picks up the walker, places it one step ahead, and walks into it.

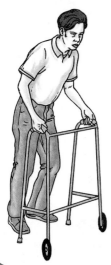

SUBSTANTIAL STABILITY: WALKER WITH WHEELS

A person who cannot lift the frame or does not have good standing balance can use a walker with wheels, which requires no lifting. As the walker is rolled forward, its rear legs drag. Pushing the rear legs down stops it. A wheeled walker is difficult on thick carpets and requires the stability and vigor to keep up with it.

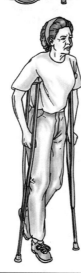

TEMPORARY SUPPORT: CRUTCHES

Crutches require significant upper body strength and are best for fit individuals who need to stay off an injured leg or foot while it heals.

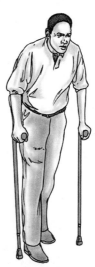

UPPER BODY SUPPORT: ELBOW CRUTCHES

Individuals who experience chronic weakness due to stroke or other illnesses can augment the muscles of the upper body with elbow crutches.

each child has his or her own particular rate of development, babies normally become able to bear some weight on their legs by 7 months. A child who cannot walk by the age of 18 months is generally considered delayed in motor or movement development (see DEVELOPMENTAL DELAY).

Of the developmental abilities, motor skills are the least linked to intelligence. A physical cause such as cerebral palsy or spina bifida is more likely to be the cause of delayed walking than a mental problem. In cerebral palsy, the longer the delay in walking, the more severe the neurological damage. Other factors such as a lack of stimulation in a child's environment can contribute to a delay in walking. If cerebral palsy, spina bifida, and lack of stimulation have been ruled out, the cause may be neuromuscular. See also ABUSE, CHILD; FAILURE TO THRIVE.

A complete medical and developmental evaluation is necessary for children who cannot walk at 18 months of age. Consultation with a developmental pediatrician, a doctor who specializes in such problems, may be involved. Depending on the diagnosis, treatment may include physical or occupational therapy. Therapists can evaluate children's abilities, define appropriate goals, and teach parents beneficial exercises to practice with their children. After the age of 3, children who have developmental disabilities are legally entitled to special education in preschools and schools.

Warfarin

An anticoagulant drug. Warfarin (Coumadin) is used to prevent blood clots. It is also used to prevent or treat blood clots that may form in a blood vessel or in the lungs. It may be prescribed to prevent blood clots associated with certain heart conditions or to people with a heart valve replacement. Warfarin may be used after a heart attack to prevent blood clots from forming anywhere in the body. Warfarin can reduce the risk of death, another heart attack, or a stroke following a heart attack.

Warfarin works by decreasing the ability of the blood to clot, thereby preventing the formation of dangerous clots in the blood vessels. Warfarin cannot dissolve clots that have already formed, but it can prevent existing clots from getting larger and causing serious problems. Although warfarin is often called a "blood thinner," it does not actually thin the blood.

Wart

A rough, infectious, skin-colored bump caused by a virus in the human papillomavirus family. There are more than 70 types of warts. The typical wart is a bump, but some warts are small, hard, and flat. They are contagious and can be passed from person to person through direct contact. Warts may grow anywhere on the body but most frequently occur on the hands, feet, and face. Common warts usually occur on the fingers and hands. Periungual warts occur around the nails; subungual warts occur under the nails. Plantar warts occur on the soles of the feet. Juvenile warts (also known as flat or plane warts) are smooth, flat warts that

TYPES OF WARTS

Warts are benign growths that occur anywhere on the skin or mucous membranes. Warts are contagious and are caused by direct or indirect contact with the human papillomavirus.

PLANTAR WARTS
Plantar warts occur most often on the soles of the feet and tend to grow inward. These warts are often very thick and callused. Plantar warts may develop into cluster, or mosaic, warts and become very resistant to treatment.

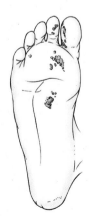

A WART ON A FINGER
A typical wart is a raised lump, which appears most often on the tops of the fingers and hands. Warts may be pink, tan, or the same color as the person's skin.

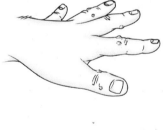

GENITAL WARTS
Genital warts, condyloma acuminta, vary from tiny, shiny lesions to large, cauliflower-shaped lesions. They can extend into the internal organs and should always be examined by a physician. Genital warts on a small child may be the result of sexual abuse or of contact with an adult who has warts on his or her hands.

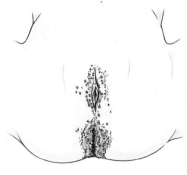

occur primarily in children but also can occur in adults. GENITAL WARTS (also known as condylomas) are infectious warts that occur around and on the genitals and anus.

Diagnosis of warts is based on their appearance. Some warts are unsightly and cause emotional discomfort. Plantar warts on the bottom of the feet can be painful. It is important to consult a dermatologist when there is a change in the appearance of a wart or if there is pain, bleeding, or ulceration.

Approximately two thirds of warts disappear on their own within 2 years. However, new warts may continue to develop in the meantime. Treatment can be difficult; multiple treatment sessions may be necessary. Over-the-counter topical remedies include salicylic acid and lactic acid, which must be applied on a daily basis for several weeks. Stronger prescription medications are available to remove persistent or recurrent warts. In-office treatments include CRYOSURGERY (freezing with liquid nitrogen), electrodesiccation (burning with an electric current delivered through a probe), and LASER SURGERY.

Genital warts require treatment because they are sexually transmitted. They may be treated with liquid nitrogen, podophyllin, interferon injections, prescription topical medications, or laser. Because they can be sexually transmitted, protection must be used during intercourse with a person who has genital warts. Women with a history of genital warts or exposure to partners with genital warts should have annual Pap smears since some types of human papillomavirus are linked to cervical cancer.

Water intoxication

Also known as overhydration, an abnormal increase in the volume of water in the body. Infants younger than 1 month are especially susceptible to overhydration. In adults, water intoxication is most common in people with impaired kidney function and may occur in hospitals when more water-producing fluids are administered than a person can assimilate or excrete. In people whose kidneys and other organs are functioning properly, water intoxication is rarely caused simply by drinking too much water. Symptoms of water intoxication include nausea, vomiting, diarrhea, bloating, headache, muscle twitches, seizures, restlessness, dizziness, disorientation, and stupor. Left untreated, water intoxication can result in coma and death. Treatment focuses on immediate cessation of water intake. Sometimes, anticonvulsants and intravenous infusions of serum sodium are administered. Infants (especially in the first month of life) receive sufficient water from breast milk or formula, and supplementing with additional water can be dangerous.

Water pollution

See POLLUTION, WATER.

Waterborne infection

Illness that is acquired by contact with or ingestion of water contaminated with disease-causing organisms and microorganisms. Waterborne infections may be contracted when people drink or swim in water containing agents, such as bacteria, that produce disease. Water contamination is most commonly caused by the presence of infected human or animal feces or urine. In the case of waterborne infection with SALMONELLA, the infective organisms, which have been ingested by drinking contaminated water, invade and multiply in the gastrointestinal tract, causing GASTROENTERITIS, enteric fever, SEPTICEMIA, salmonellosis, PARATYPHOID FEVER, and TYPHOID FEVER.

Some waterborne infections are contracted by swimming in contaminated water. GIARDIASIS is caused by a protozoon that lives in the small intestines of infected humans and some wild animals and is shed in the feces. Water that is contaminated with human sewage or with infected animal feces can transmit the disease to people who drink the water. CRYPTOSPORIDIOSIS is caused by a waterborne parasitic pathogen and can result in a life-threatening, choleralike disease in people with impaired immune systems. This parasite has been known to escape the filtration systems of public drinking water systems and infect large numbers of people. The pathogen that causes the illness is difficult to destroy, and there is no known cure for the infection it causes.

Escherichia coli, or E. COLI, primarily known as a food-borne infectious agent, can cause infection if people swim in or ingest water contaminated with the bacteria. Waterborne *E. coli* infections have occurred among swimmers in natural lakes and even chlorinated pools in the United States. LEPTOSPIROSIS may be contracted by swimming in slow-moving, warm waters that have been contaminated by infected animals, including reptiles, rodents, livestock, and dogs, that shed the bacterium *Leptospira* in their urine. SHIGELLOSIS is a waterborne infection that is caused by a form of intestinal bacteria and can be acquired by swimming in water that has been exposed to fecal contamination. A potentially fatal from of MENINGITIS can be produced by microbes found in standing water, such as the water in unfiltered small bathing pools.

Recommendations for protection against waterborne infections that may be acquired from swimming include heeding "no swimming" postings by local health departments for natural bodies of water; requesting records of chlorination, cleaning, and treatment schedules of public swimming pools; avoiding the ingestion of water while swimming; emptying and cleaning shallow baby pools daily; and preventing diapered children from entering public swimming areas.

Waterhouse-Friderichsen syndrome

A form of SEPTICEMIA (blood poisoning) caused by meningococcal bacteria that causes hemorrhaging of the person's adrenal tissue. This serious but very rare condition causes bleeding into the adrenal glands, which leads to adrenal failure and shock. The condition is almost always fatal unless the person is immediately hospitalized and treated.

Watering eye

See TEARING.

Weakness

Lack of strength or vigor. Weakness is the state or quality of being without strength, firmness, or power.

W

Weaning

Usually in infancy, the gradual transition from breast or bottle to drinking from a cup and eating solid foods. Weaning is a natural step in growing up. There is no right or wrong time to make this transition, and often it is easiest to let the child control the timing of the process. Most doctors recommend introducing solid foods around 6 months of age and weaning babies from the breast or bottle after the first birthday. Breast milk or formula should be given to babies until the digestive system matures. After age 1 year, cow's milk can be introduced to the child.

WEANING FROM BREAST TO BOTTLE

Many breast-feeding mothers begin to wean babies between 4 and 7 months. As they enter the second half of the first year, babies are beginning to explore their environments and learn new skills. This is a natural time to introduce the bottle and cup. As children grow older and continue to nurse, they may grow increasingly attached to the breast and find it hard to give up. Babies often find changes in routine confusing and upsetting. Consequently, a breast-feeding infant may object to a bottle the first few times it is offered. Because of the mother's close association with breast-feeding, it is helpful for a caregiver other than the mother to introduce the bottle.

Although the timing varies, a baby can be weaned from breast to bottle over the course of 2 weeks. At first, one bottle of formula should be substituted for a breast-feeding each day. On the third day, the bottle can be used for two feedings. By the fifth day, the baby can take three to four bottle feedings per day. The last breast-feeding to be replaced with a bottle should be the one at bedtime. Many mothers prefer to take a more leisurely approach to weaning. Some continue a combination of bottle and breast-feeding throughout the first year. Breast-feeding provides a special closeness between mother and child. Bottle feeding has the advantage of allowing the father to participate in feeding. For infant and mother alike, weaning from the breast involves emotional adjustments. As a baby adapts to the bottle, extra cuddling and stroking can compensate for lost skin-to-skin contact.

WEANING TO A CUP

The older infant, 8 to 10 months of age, is usually ready for a cup. However, for some infants, a cup can be introduced as early as the fifth month. A training cup with two handles and a lid with a spout will minimize spillage. At first, cups should be given at one meal a day and should contain only water. This way, when a baby plays with the cup or throws it, little nutrition is lost.

Signs that a baby is ready for the cup may include looking around while drinking from the bottle or nursing; mouthing the nipple without sucking; or trying to get free before a feeding is complete. Most babies treat the cup as a toy for at least the first few weeks, and it may take 6 months before a baby is willing to take all liquids from the cup. As a baby gradually adapts to the cup, the final bottle or breast-feeding is the bedtime one. Babies often resist surrendering this evening source of comfort. The transition can be smoothed by replacing formula or milk with a bottle of water at bedtime and eventually switching to a cup of water. Babies with teeth should not be put to bed with a bottle of milk or juice. That practice can lead to baby bottle tooth decay, in which milk or juice pools in the mouth and causes serious tooth decay. Breast milk or formula is all the nutrition a baby needs for the first 6 months. Around this age, solid foods can be introduced. See also FEEDING, INFANT.

Wegener granulomatosis

A condition believed to be an autoimmune disorder that produces inflammation of the blood vessels that damages the walls of the small and medium-sized arteries and capillaries. Wegener granulomatosis is a potentially life-threatening form of VASCULITIS. The normal blood supply to tissues near the arteries is disrupted, which causes injury and destruction in the parts of the body affected. The disease process is called granulomatosis because characteristic islands of inflamed cells (called granulomas) located in the tissues involved in the disease are revealed by microscopic examination. Without treatment, Wegener granulomatosis is always fatal. It occurs most commonly in a person's 40s or 50s and affects men and women with equal frequency.

It is not known what triggers the mechanisms that cause Wegener granulomatosis. One immune protein that attacks the body, called an autoantibody, has been discovered and seems to be associated with the disease process. This autoantibody is called antineutrophil cytoplasmic antibody, or ANCA.

SYMPTOMS, DIAGNOSIS, AND TREATMENT

The lungs, the kidneys, the upper airways, including the sinuses, windpipe, and nose, are usually affected by Wegener granulomatosis. In 60 to 80 percent of people with Wegener granulomatosis, chronic nasal and sinus problems produce sinusitis, sinus pain, persistent nasal congestion and runny nose with discolored nasal discharge, recurrent nose bleeds, and sores or crusting inside the nose. When the lungs become involved, respiratory illness develops with chest discomfort, shortness of breath, wheezing, and a cough that may bring up blood. There may be other symptoms including malaise, fever, weakness and fatigue, weight loss, night sweats, joint pain, and muscle aches.

Kidney involvement occurs in approximately 75 percent of people with Wegener granulomatosis. Other organs of the body that may become involved include the eyes, ears, skin, joints, and nerves. The eyes may be painful and red, and a person may have a burning sensation in the eyes, but rarely with decreased vision or double vision. Leg swelling can occur; the person may have an earache and experience hearing loss as well. Symptoms that appear on the skin include red or purple patches, small blisters, ulcers, or small nodules. The joints may become swollen, and there may be swelling of the gums and ulcers on the tonsils.

A preliminary diagnosis is based on a medical history of persistent symptoms of sinusitis, respiratory tract infection, or respiratory allergies and a complete physical examination. Wegener granulomatosis is usually suspected when common respiratory symptoms do not respond to treatment. Diagnostic tests may include a complete blood cell count, erythrocyte sedimentation rate, measurements of blood urea nitrogen (BUN) and creatinine levels, a urinalysis, a chest X ray, and a CT (computed tomography) scan or X ray of the sinuses. To confirm the diagnosis, a biopsy sample may need to be taken from an affected tissue in the sinuses, lung, or kidney. Blood tests for ANCA assist in making the diagnosis.

Treatment is usually based on two medications, the corticosteroid prednisone to reduce inflammation and a low-dose of oral cyclophosphamide, which suppresses immune activity. Prednisone is discontinued as symptoms improve, while cyclophosphamide is generally taken for about 1 year. This regimen can offer improvement or remission to about 90 percent of people with the disease. This medication can produce serious and injurious side effects, including cancer risks. In some cases, less toxic alternatives may be recommended. The antibiotic combination trimethoprim-sulfamethoxazole may be effective in helping people with Wegener granulomatosis remain in remission.

Typically, the disease requires at least 2 years of treatment and monitoring from the time of diagnosis. Without appropriate medical treatment, Wegener granulomatosis may cause a rapid death. Treatment can promote long-term remission, but relapses are often common.

Weight

The quality or quantity of being heavy; the amount a thing weighs. Weight is the effect of gravity, or the downward pressure of a body under the influence of gravity; therefore, weight constitutes a measure of the force of gravity. Weight is proportional to the amount of matter in a body.

Weight is also a system of units for measuring heaviness or mass. In the United States, weight is chiefly expressed in pounds and ounces.

Weight gain

FOR SYMPTOM CHART
see Weight gain, page 60

An accumulation of body weight, usually a result of consuming more calories than the body burns off. Weight gain is a major problem in the United States, where more than half the population is OVERWEIGHT or obese (see OBESITY). Excess weight is associ-

ated with serious weight-related problems such as HYPERTENSION (high blood pressure), elevated CHOLESTEROL levels, cardiovascular disease, diabetes, stroke, and cancer. It has been linked with colon and prostate cancer in men and with breast, uterine, and endometrial cancer in women. Other concerns include back pain, sleep apnea (a potentially life-threatening condition in which individuals stop breathing for short periods during sleep), gallstones, osteoarthritis, heartburn, gout, and varicose veins. Studies have shown that heavier people generally have a shorter life expectancy. Excess weight is associated with an increase in emotional and psychological problems.

Weight loss

FOR SYMPTOM CHART
see Weight loss, page 62

A reduction in body weight. Weight loss requires that a person take in fewer calories than are needed to maintain his or her weight. (See also OBESITY.) Being OVERWEIGHT is associated with health problems including heart disease, high blood pressure, diabetes, and a higher risk for cancer. Overweight people can benefit from even a modest weight loss of 10 to 20 pounds. For example, weight loss can help reduce blood pressure and cholesterol levels.

Before beginning a weight-loss plan, individuals should consult a physician or a registered dietician (RD). Nine of 10 dieters gain back lost weight within 5 years. A safe weight-loss plan, and one that is most likely to keep excess pounds from returning, is based on a balanced, nutritious eating plan and regular exercise. Doctors warn against popular or fad diets, or herbal drugs, which can pose dangerous health risks. Fluctuating in weight due to fad diets, or yo-yo dieting, can increase an individual's risk of heart disease. Successful weight loss usually results from a gradual change in eating and exercise habits that need to continue through life to maintain the weight loss. Both the calorie and fat contents of food must be considered. Excess calories are stored as body fat. But even a low-calorie diet is not necessarily low in fat. Portion size is also key, because large serv-

ings of even low-calorie or low-fat foods can lead to weight gain.

In order to shed pounds, doctors recommend that people who are overweight (10 to 20 percent more than average) eat 500 calories a day less than the amount needed to meet a person's daily energy needs. Those who are obese (more than 20 percent overweight) should consume 750 calories less per day than needed. Specific dietary recommendations might include cutting back on total fat intake and replacing saturated fats with unsaturated ones, eliminating certain fatty foods or those with "empty calories" (see CARBOHYDRATES), opting for low-fat or skim dairy products, eating large amounts of vegetables and salads, choosing only small portions of fish and lean meats, and drinking 8 glasses of water a day.

EXERCISE AND WEIGHT LOSS
A sensible weight loss plan is one that emphasizes slow, gradual loss based on healthful eating and exercise. Gradually increasing the amount or intensity of physical activity expedites weight loss because people lose weight when they burn more calories than they take in. To promote weight loss, exercise does not have to be intense. Moderate or low intensity exercise such as walking can be effective if it is done for at least 30 minutes daily or for 10-minute periods 3 times daily.

Strength training also is recommended for weight loss because the amount of muscle determines the amount of energy needed daily. Muscle uses more energy than any other tissue, even while resting. Moderate gains in the amount of muscle can make a difference and can be achieved by anyone, regardless of age. Strength training also helps strengthen bones and may protect against osteoporosis. Doctors recommend that individuals get 30 to 45 minutes of cardiovascular or aerobic exercise at least 3 times a week to promote healthy functioning of the heart and blood vessels. Walking and swimming are good examples of this type of exercise, which elevates the heart rate. In addition to its contribution to weight loss, exercise lowers blood pressure, reduces cholesterol levels, and strengthens the heart and bones. It is also a natural stress reliever and helps promote sleep.

W

Weight training

The use of free weights or weight machines to increase muscular strength. Weight training also increases bone strength and may help prevent bone loss associated with aging. To build strength in the muscles, the weights lifted must offer a challenge to a person's present muscular strength. The ideal weight is one that painlessly exhausts the muscles after 20 repetitions of the same exercise. Lighter weights will build muscle endurance but will have less effect on strength. Proper technique is important to preventing injuries when lifting weights. A certified professional instructor or trainer should demonstrate how to lift free weights or use weight machines correctly when a person begins a weight-lifting program. See also EXERCISE, RESISTANCE; EXERCISE, STRENGTHENING.

Weight-bearing exercise

See EXERCISE, WEIGHT-BEARING.

Weil disease

An infection or parasitic disease produced by the bacteria *Leptospira*. Weil disease is a severe form of LEPTOSPIROSIS that is characterized by severe dysfunction of the liver and kidneys. The infection causes excessive bleeding within the body and is potentially fatal. It is contracted by ingesting or swimming in water contaminated with the infected urine of wild and domestic animals (rats, cats, dogs) who shed the bacteria in their urine. Treatment consists of administering penicillins, tetracyclines, chloramphenicol, or erythromycin.

Well-being

A person's sense of being in good physical and emotional health. A sudden lack of well-being can be a sign of disease.

Werdnig-Hoffmann disease

A rare genetic disease of the motor neurons of the spinal cord, characterized by wasting muscles and progressive weakness. Werdnig-Hoffmann disease is one of the three major types of childhood-onset spinal muscular atrophy, a group of inherited neuromuscular diseases, and is also known as severe infantile spinal muscular atrophy. Werdnig-Hoffmann disease usually develops in utero, before the baby is born, and may result in a lack of fetal movement during the last months of pregnancy. The disease is caused by a defect in a single gene on chromosome 5, a defect that results in the uncontrolled death of anterior horn cells in the spinal column. The premature death of these cells severely limits the affected individual's ability to move his or her muscles voluntarily. In most cases, the defective gene must be inherited from both parents for a child to develop the disease. One in 40 people is a carrier of the defective gene, and one in 6,000 live births is affected by some form of spinal muscular atrophy.

SYMPTOMS
Babies born with Werdnig-Hoffmann disease have HYPOTONIA, or diminished muscle tone, generalized weakness, difficulties feeding and swallowing, and breathing problems. These symptoms may first become evident during pregnancy, at the time of birth, or during the first 6 months of life. Infants with the disease may lack head control; they may be unable to roll over or support their weight; and they may tend to lie still, with little or no movement. They may also be susceptible to the development of respiratory infections, such as pneumonia, or to the development of other complications that can lead to life-threatening abnormalities during the first months of life.

For babies born with Werdnig-Hoffmann disease who appear normal for a few months after birth, the disorder may develop and progress more slowly.

DIAGNOSIS AND TREATMENT
Diagnosis is made on the basis of a family medical history and a thorough physical examination. Tests to evaluate enzyme levels, such as creatine kinase in the blood and biopsy of muscle tissues are sometimes used to differentiate this disease from other neuromuscular disorders. Electromyogram (EMG) may be used to measure muscle contractions. DNA testing to detect the abnormal gene can now be performed on a blood sample. The same type of testing permits prenatal diagnostics using amniocentesis or chorionic villus sampling.

Treatment is directed at symptoms. Physical and respiratory therapies are important, even when the affected babies are quite young. Techniques associated with chest physiotherapy, a means of clearing the lungs of mucus, are required, because babies with Werdnig-Hoffmann disease are usually unable to cough effectively. Tube feeding may be required when the baby's ability to swallow is inadequate. Babies may be helped to breathe by using devices such as the Port-a-Lung, which uses external ventilation to create negative pressure to set the breathing rate.

Because of the progressive nature of the disease, the associated overall weakness, and the constant risk of repeated respiratory infection, the prognosis or outcome for this disease is not very favorable. Most children with acute Werdnig-Hoffmann disease die by age 2. In milder cases, however, the weakness will progress more slowly. Some children may learn to walk with the help of bracing, and they may even survive to adulthood. In milder cases as well as more severe ones, the cause of death is usually pneumonia or another respiratory infection.

Wernicke encephalopathy

Also known as Wernicke disease, a life-threatening brain disorder characterized by confusion, an unsteady gait, and abnormal eye movements. Wernicke encephalopathy most commonly occurs in chronic alcoholics as a result of vitamin B1 (thiamin) deficiency. (Less frequently, a deficiency of this vitamin is associated with other factors, such as excessive vomiting or kidney dialysis.) Wernicke encephalopathy can involve damage to nerves throughout the body. Left untreated, it results in death.

SYMPTOMS
Symptoms of Wernicke encephalopathy include confusion, memory loss, inattention, delirium, disorientation, and drowsiness. Poor balance and coordination result in an unsteady gait, making walking difficult. Often there are abnormal eye movements, such as double vision and jerking of the eyes.

Wernicke encephalopathy is often accompanied or followed by KORSAKOFF PSYCHOSIS (also known as Korsakoff syndrome). Korsakoff psychosis involves the impairment of memory and cognitive skills; its hallmark symptom is confabulation, or the concoction of detailed, realistic stories about situations or experiences in order to compensate for gaps in memory. The combination of Wernicke encephalopathy and Korsakoff psychosis is known as WERNICKE-KORSAKOFF SYNDROME.

DIAGNOSIS AND TREATMENT

To diagnose Wernicke encephalopathy, doctors look for a history of chronic alcohol use. Examination may reveal gait and eye problems, abnormal reflexes, neuropathy, muscle weakness, low blood pressure and body temperature, and malnourishment. Blood tests can confirm problems such as malnourishment and elevated alcohol levels.

Prompt administration of vitamin B1 is essential to the treatment of Wernicke encephalopathy. Without this treatment, the disorder can progress to stupor, coma, and death. Hospitalization is usually required to bring the initial symptoms under control. The results of treatment vary from person to person. In some people, problems such as poor coordination and abnormal vision are slowed or stopped. However, when Wernicke encephalopathy is accompanied by Korsakoff psychosis in Wernicke-Korsakoff syndrome, symptoms such as memory loss and impairment of cognitive skills may be permanent. Following treatment, a person must abstain from all alcohol use and follow a nutritious diet.

Wernicke-Korsakoff syndrome

A life-threatening brain disorder caused by vitamin B1 (thiamin) deficiency. The most common cause of vitamin B1 deficiency is malnutrition as a result of chronic alcohol use or alcoholism. Less commonly, a deficiency of this vitamin is associated with excessive vomiting or kidney dialysis. Wernicke-Korsakoff syndrome is composed of two separate disorders: WERNICKE ENCEPHALOPATHY (also known as Wernicke disease) and KORSAKOFF PSYCHOSIS (also known as Korsakoff syndrome). Wernicke encephalopathy is a brain disorder characterized by confusion, abnormal eye movements, and an unsteady gait. The symptoms of Korsakoff psychosis are the impairment of memory

and cognitive skills; a hallmark of this syndrome is confabulation, or the concoction of detailed, realistic stories about situations or experiences in order to compensate for gaps in memory.

SYMPTOMS

Wernicke-Korsakoff syndrome most commonly affects people between ages 40 and 80 years. Its onset is gradual. The symptoms of Wernicke encephalopathy often precede those of Korsakoff psychosis. These include confusion, memory loss, inattention, delirium, disorientation, and drowsiness. Often there are abnormal eye movements, such as double vision, twitching, and eyelid drooping. Poor balance and coordination result in an unsteady gait, making walking difficult. Other possible symptoms include hand tremor, facial paralysis, muscle atrophy, tingling, numbness, and a malnourished appearance.

The symptoms of Korsakoff psychosis may accompany or follow those of Wernicke encephalopathy. This condition involves a loss of cognitive skills, such as the ability to think abstractly or solve problems. Profound memory loss leads to confabulation, in which people concoct elaborate fictions to make up for facts they can no longer recall. The symptoms of alcohol withdrawal sometimes accompany those of Wernicke encephalopathy and Korsakoff psychosis. See ALCOHOL DEPENDENCE.

DIAGNOSIS AND TREATMENT

To diagnose Wernicke-Korsakoff syndrome, doctors look for a history of chronic alcohol use. Examination may reveal gait and eye problems, abnormal reflexes, neuropathy, muscle weakness, low blood pressure and body temperature, and malnourishment. Blood tests can confirm the diagnosis.

Hospitalization is usually required to bring initial symptoms under control. Prompt administration of vitamin B1 is essential to the treatment of Wernicke encephalopathy. Without this treatment, the disorder can progress to stupor, coma, and death. However, vitamin B1 is less successful in controlling the symptoms of Korsakoff psychosis. While problems such as poor coordination and abnormal vision may be slowed or stopped, memory loss and impairment of

cognitive skills may be permanent. Following treatment, a person must abstain from all alcohol use and follow a nutritious diet.

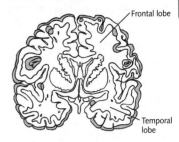

Frontal lobe

Temporal lobe

LOSS OF BRAIN TISSUE

A deficiency of the B vitamin thiamin reduces the body's ability to metabolize glucose to supply the brain, resulting in a loss of brain tissue. The damage is generally evident by changes in appetite, emotional response, and memory. The color shows the grey matter that is lost.

West Nile virus

A recently identified virus that first appeared in North America in 1999 and caused severe cases of encephalitis and hundreds of deaths. The death rate is more than 10 percent for people sick enough to be hospitalized. West Nile virus was first reported in Africa in 1937. It is transmitted to humans by mosquito bites. During the summer, these mosquitoes can infect horses, humans, birds, and squirrels. The majority of the infections (80 percent) do not cause symptoms. Mild infections cause fever, fatigue, enlarged lymph nodes, eye pain, stomach pain, muscle ache, and headache. A very delicate rash may be found in children. Rarely, people have muscle weakness, arm and leg paralysis, confusion, and coma. Diagnosis of West Nile virus is made through blood tests; there is no specific antiviral therapy, but insect repellant can reduce mosquito bites.

Wheal

See HIVES.

Wheelchair

A chair mounted on large wheels and used by disabled or injured persons and either self-powered, pushed by others, or battery operated. Wheelchairs are available for people with quadriplegia, paraplegia, and amputated limbs. There are specialized wheelchairs for playing sports.

Wheezing

The musical, high-pitched, whistling sound of air passing over a partial obstruction in the airways. Wheezing is caused by an impediment to airflow in the airways. Asthma is the most common cause of recurrent wheezing. Other diseases, such as CHRONIC OBSTRUCTIVE PULMONARY DISEASE (COPD), can cause a narrowing of the airways that results in wheezing. A localized narrowing of the airways may be caused by the presence of a tumor. Alternatively, there may be a foreign particle, such as a piece of food, lodged in an airway. Wheezing can also be a temporary event that many people experience for unknown or medically insignificant reasons, such as a transitory response to exposure of an airborne irritant.

A doctor can hear wheezing sounds as a person inhales and exhales during a physical examination of the chest with a stethoscope. In some cases, pulmonary function tests may be needed to determine the extent of airway obstruction or narrowing and to evaluate treatment possibilities.

Whiplash

An injury to the cervical vertebrae (neck bones) or adjacent soft tissues (muscles, ligaments, disks, and tendons) that occurs from a sudden, accelerated, jerking movement of the head and neck or by a rapid back and forth movement of the head or the neck. This may happen to the passenger of a car as the result of an unexpected, forcible rear impact or head-on collision. Whiplash causes pain and stiffness in the neck. It is generally treated with anti-inflammatory and pain-relieving medication and often improves with time. In some cases, a rigid collar covered with soft material, called a cervical collar, is worn around the neck to support the bones and soft tissue injured by whiplash. Physical therapy, including deep heat and traction, is also prescribed.

Whipple disease

See INTESTINAL LIPODYSTROPHY.

Whipple operation

A surgical procedure to remove cancer in the head of the PANCREAS. The operation is named after Allen Whipple, the American surgeon who first developed the procedure.

In certain kinds of pancreatic cancer, a tumor develops in the head of the organ, near where it joins with the small intestine below the stomach. Such a tumor often causes jaundice by blocking the common bile duct; this prevents secretions produced by the liver and stored in the gallbladder from entering the small intestine. In a minority of cases of this kind of cancer, the Whipple operation may remove the tumor successfully by taking out all or most of the pancreas. However, since the pancreas is closely associated with the duodenum (the first section of the small intestine) and since the two organs share the same blood supply, it must be removed as well.

HOW IT IS DONE

After the person is asleep under general anesthesia and pain-free, the abdomen is opened, and most or all of the pancreas is removed, depending on the extent of the cancer. The nearby portion of the stomach, the duodenum, the gallbladder, and the distal common bile duct are also removed. The remaining sections of the stomach and common bile duct are joined directly to the next section of the small intestine, the jejunum. If any of the pancreas remains, it too is joined to the jejunum to provide its juices to the digestive system. If the entire pancreas is removed, the person is treated with medication to replace the insulin and the digestive enzymes that are removed with it.

OUTLOOK

The Whipple operation can remove only localized cancers. If the disease has spread, the likelihood of success is diminished. Cancer of the pancreas is aggressively invasive and commonly spreads before it is diagnosed.

Whipworm infestation

Infestation with the nematode *Trichuris trichiura*, called the human whipworm. Whipworm infestation is also called trichuriasis. It usually occurs in tropical areas with inadequate sanitation standards. In the United States, whipworm infestation occurs in some southern states. Whipworms are the third most common nematode to infest humans.

The eggs of the nematodes, or roundworms, are found in the soil. They are transmitted to humans when food or a person's hands come in contact with contaminated soil and the worms are ingested. Adult whipworms live in the human colon where the females lay eggs. The eggs are passed from the body with the stool. In 15 to 30 days, the eggs become infective. After they are ingested, the eggs hatch in the small intestine and release larvae that mature into adult whipworms. The adult worms then become attached to the mucous lining of the colon throughout their life span, which lasts about 1 year. The females lay their eggs in the colon within 60 to 70 days of the infestation.

SYMPTOMS, DIAGNOSIS, AND TREATMENT

A person with whipworm infestation does not usually have symptoms. Heavy infestations may cause gastrointestinal problems and sometimes

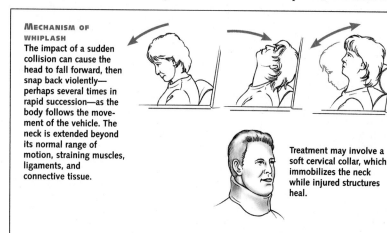

MECHANISM OF WHIPLASH
The impact of a sudden collision can cause the head to fall forward, then snap back violently— perhaps several times in rapid succession—as the body follows the movement of the vehicle. The neck is extended beyond its normal range of motion, straining muscles, ligaments, and connective tissue.

Treatment may involve a soft cervical collar, which immobilizes the neck while injured structures heal.

slowed growth. If symptoms occur, they may include abdominal pain, diarrhea, and rectal prolapse.

The infestation is diagnosed by identifying the worm eggs in the feces under a microscope. In mild cases, it may be difficult to detect the eggs. Examination of the mucous membrane of the rectum either directly or by proctoscopy may help identify adult worms. Antiworm medications, including mebendazole and albendazole, are generally prescribed to treat whipworm infestation.

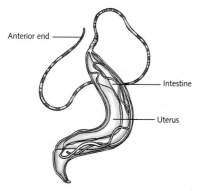

PARASITIC ROUNDWORM
A whipworm, so named for its long, whiplike tail, is about 1/25 of an inch (1 mm) long. The whipworm lives in the large intestine, and the female lays from 3,000 to 20,000 eggs per day. The eggs pass from the body in stool.

White matter
Brain tissue containing myelinated nerve fibers. MYELIN, the substance covering nerve fibers that acts as insulation, gives the tissue its white color. White matter carries information between the nerve cells in the brain and the spinal cord. White matter is found in the inner portion of the cerebrum where thought and higher brain function take place.

White matter is differentiated from gray matter, the cortex of the brain containing nerve cell bodies.

Whitehead
A small, hard, painless, white blemish that may appear in clusters on the cheeks, nose, and chin. See ACNE.

Whitlow, herpetic
An intensely painful infection of the hand that causes blisters on one or more fingers, usually on the palm-side surface of the finger segment closest to the finger tip. Herpetic whitlow is most commonly caused by herpes simplex virus 1, but may also be due to herpes simplex virus 2. The infection is transmitted when a person's hands make contact with body fluids infected with the herpesvirus. The virus usually gains entry to the bloodstream through a break in the skin of the hands, often a torn cuticle. Herpetic whitlow is an occupational hazard among doctors, dentists, and other health care workers. In other adults, the infection generally is caused by exposure of the hands to genital herpes. Children may become infected by thumb- or finger-sucking that exposes skin breaks on the hands and fingers to herpes infections of the lips and mouth.

SYMPTOMS, DIAGNOSIS, AND TREATMENT
Diagnosis is generally based on an examination of symptoms and a history indicating exposure or previous infection. The physical symptoms of intense localized pain and swelling, with the characteristic blister or cluster of blisters on a finger or fingers, indicate a diagnosis of herpetic whitlow. The infection may spread to the area under the fingernail, and there may be swollen glands. A physical examination may reveal herpes infections in the oral or genital regions. A clinical history generally reveals a recent fever or feelings of malaise that preceded the finger lesion by a few days. Previous, similar eruptions in the same finger may indicate a recurrent or reactivated infection.

Diagnostic testing may include the Tzanck test, which uses a smear from material scraped from the base of a blister. A viral culture of fluid from the blisters is considered the most sensitive test for herpetic whitlow.

The infection usually improves and may not require medical treatment. Painful symptoms may be treated in many cases. Sometimes, the blisters may be medically treated by a physician to relieve pain and swelling. The antiviral medication acyclovir may be beneficial.

WHO
See WORLD HEALTH ORGANIZATION.

Whooping cough
See PERTUSSIS.

Will, living
One type of advance directive (see ADVANCE DIRECTIVES) signed by a person for the purpose of establishing a set of instructions to health care professionals that specifies what medical care the person wants in the event he or she is unable to communicate his or her wishes about an end-of-life decision. It is called a living will because the person makes his or her own choices while still alive. In a DURABLE POWER OF ATTORNEY for health care, another form of advance directive, the person authorizes someone else to make medical decisions if and when he or she is unable to make them.

Living wills are authorized by statutes in all states. In most states, the law recognizes the basic language of a living will that has been developed by medical associations and other experts to provide for various choices a person may make about the circumstances under which extraordinary means to sustain life should be continued or withdrawn. Living wills offer people the opportunity to designate the kind of medical treatment and life-sustaining procedures they do and do not wish to receive if they are unable to express their wishes. These procedures may include measures such as mechanical ventilation and artificial feeding.

A DO-NOT-RESUSCITATE ORDER may be part of a living will.

Williams syndrome
A rare genetic condition associated with mental retardation, heart and blood vessel problems, and characteristic facial features. Williams syndrome is caused by a mutation of a gene on chromosome 7, which is responsible for creating elastin, a protein that provides strength and elasticity to the walls of blood vessels. Williams syndrome is estimated to occur in 1 of every 20,000 births. Most cases occur as a result of spontaneous mutation, although parent-to-child transmission can also happen. A person with the syndrome has a 50 percent chance of passing it on to each of his or her children.

SYMPTOMS
The most commonly observed symptoms of Williams syndrome are mild to moderate mental retardation and

characteristic facial features. These include prominent lips with an open mouth; a long philtrum (the line between the upper lip and the nose); low nasal bridge; and puffiness around the eyes. Teeth may be absent or have defective tooth enamel; and the iris of the eye may have an irregular, starlike pattern, particularly in children with blue or green eyes. The facial features associated with Williams syndrome become more prominent with age.

Heart and blood vessel problems associated with the syndrome include abnormalities caused by a defect in the connective tissues. Examples include a narrowing of the aorta (supravalvular aortic stenosis) and narrowing of the pulmonary arteries that carry blood to the lungs (pulmonary artery stenosis). Some children with Williams syndrome have elevated blood levels of calcium, or hypercalcemia, which can cause extreme irritability and colic-like symptoms, including spasms of abdominal pain and crying.

Babies with Williams syndrome are often born postterm (after the due date), have lower birth weight than normal, and gain weight slowly during the first few years of life. They are often diagnosed with failure to thrive. Adults will be slightly smaller than average. Children with Williams syndrome are characteristically over friendly and unafraid of strangers. They tend to be more interested in socializing with adults than with other children, have especially strong language skills, and are extremely polite.

TREATMENT
The most immediate health concerns are the heart and blood vessel problems, which will be treated according to specific diagnosis. Lifelong regular monitoring of heart function will be necessary, since narrowing of the arteries may worsen over time. High blood pressure can occur and may need treatment. For people with hypercalcemia, which can occur at any age, the diet must be adjusted to reduce calcium intake. Developmental disability should be addressed through special education programs and vocational training. Speech therapy and behavioral counseling may be required.

Wilms tumor

A cancerous tumor of the kidneys that occurs mainly in children. Wilms tumor is the most common type of kidney tumor in children; the cause is not known. The tumor may develop in fetal tissue, but the peak incidence is in 3-year-olds. It is associated with certain congenital defects such as urinary tract abnormalities and enlargement of one side of the body. There is an increased incidence of Wilms tumor among siblings and twins, and there may be a contributing genetic factor. Although it generally remains localized, the tumor can become large and spread to other tissues. It is usually diagnosed through ULTRASOUND SCANNING. Treatment may require radical NEPHRECTOMY.

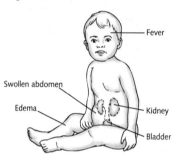

SIGNS OF WILMS TUMOR
Wilms tumors can be hard to find early in infants or very young children; they sometimes grow without causing pain. The first sign is usually a large lump in the belly and perhaps a swollen abdomen that parents may notice. Some children may have abdominal pain, fever, bloody urine, or swelling in the legs.

Wilson disease

An inherited disease in which copper accumulates in several organs of the body, particularly the brain, eyes, kidney, and liver. Most people are able to excrete excess copper, which is present in most foods. People with Wilson disease cannot excrete copper, and copper begins to accumulate immediately after birth, producing symptoms that usually show up in late adolescence. Essentially it is a disease of copper poisoning. Symptoms include jaundice, abdominal swelling, vomiting of blood, and abdominal pain. Some people have neurological symptoms, such as difficulty walking, talking, and swallowing. Symptoms of depression are sometimes present. Women with Wilson disease may have irregular menstrual periods, multiple miscarriages, or infertility.

If Wilson disease is not diagnosed and treated, it will be fatal. Liver damage can occur before symptoms are present, and people with the condition may seem to be in good health even when they are not. Diagnosis can be made with blood and urine tests, eye tests, and liver biopsy. Treatment consists of administering penicillamine, a medication that removes excess copper and blocks its further accumulation. The medication must be taken for life. People with the disease will also need to follow a diet low in copper, which means avoiding shellfish, mushrooms, nuts, chocolate, liver, and dried fruit. With treatment, individuals can fully recover.

Wilson disease is caused by a defective gene, ATP7B, on chromosome 13. It is an autosomal recessive disease and must be inherited from both parents. Whenever Wilson disease is diagnosed, the affected individual's blood relatives should also be screened for the disease.

Wired jaws

An immobilization technique to hold broken jaw bones in place and allow them to heal in the proper position. A fractured jaw is wired because its structure prevents it from being held in place with a plaster cast. Jaw fractures generally require 4 to 6 weeks, or longer, to heal. During the healing period, the wires may be removed in stages as the healing progresses. An antibiotic may be prescribed when the jaws are wired to prevent infection. Jaws are sometimes wired in the course of reconstructive surgical procedures or in cases of surgery for weight control. A person with a wired jaw must consume a liquid or semiliquid diet.

Wisdom tooth

The third molar, or the last back tooth in the upper and lower jaws. Generally, there are four wisdom teeth: one on each side of the upper jaw and one on each side of the lower jaw. Many people have fewer than four. Wisdom teeth are the last of the PERMANENT TEETH to erupt, usually when a person is between the ages of 17 and 23 years. They do not always erupt properly and tend to become impacted. Not all wisdom teeth cause problems but dental impaction (see

THE THIRD MOLARS
The four so-called wisdom teeth are actually the third molars, or the last back teeth on either side in the upper and lower jaws. They usually emerge through the gums in the late teen years or early 20s. In many people, there is not room in the jaw for the wisdom teeth, and they either remain trapped in the bone or gum or emerge only partially. A buried, or impacted, wisdom tooth is often surgically removed to prevent infection and overcrowding of the other teeth.

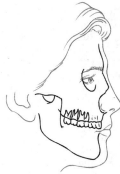

Normal position of
upper wisdom tooth

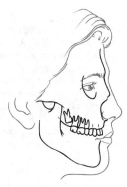

Impacted wisdom tooth

IMPACTION, DENTAL) of these back molars is fairly common. There is often insufficient space in the dental arch for the last back teeth to develop and emerge from the gums after all the permanent teeth are in place.

If a wisdom tooth has not fully erupted by the time a person is 25 years old, the tooth is generally considered to be impacted. When a wisdom tooth emerges only partially, infection-producing bacteria may gather in the area of the irritated gum tissue. The site of an incompletely erupted wisdom tooth may also be at risk for developing cysts and tumors. An impacted wisdom tooth can cause infections, PERIODONTAL DISEASE, and cavities, which may produce pain and swelling in the jaw and at the site of the impaction. If TOOTH DECAY in a wisdom tooth progresses to produce a dental abscess, the lymph glands may become swollen and symptoms associated with the common cold may be experienced. If an impacted or partially impacted wisdom tooth is suspected, a dental evaluation should be sought.

REMOVAL OF WISDOM TEETH

A dentist may recommend the extraction of a wisdom tooth before symptoms appear. Potential irregularities in the development of wisdom teeth can be detected early on with dental X rays. The goal of early removal is to prevent future infections and possible injury to the adjacent teeth, particularly the second molars, which are located directly in front of the wisdom teeth and may be loosened when the wisdom teeth begin to enlarge and press against them. Another reason for removing wisdom teeth before they show signs of impaction is to create more space in

the jaw for the correction of BITE problems and overcrowding.

Wisdom teeth are generally removed by a dentist or an oral surgeon as an office procedure using a form of dental anesthesia. The operation involves removing the gum tissue and bone that cover the tooth, stripping connective tissue away from the tooth and bone, removing the wisdom tooth, and suturing the gum to close the remaining opening. As with all tooth extractions, the removal of a wisdom tooth involves a small risk of a dry socket forming. This condition may occur within 5 days of the extraction with symptoms including persistent or increased pain and, possibly, an earache. Treatment of a dry socket by a dentist generally includes sterile packing with a topical anesthetic, which can relieve discomfort within a few hours. Oral medications not containing aspirin may be prescribed to reduce pain.

Withdrawal method

See COITUS INTERRUPTUS.

Withdrawal syndrome, alcohol

The physical and psychological symptoms that result when an individual dependent on alcohol suddenly stops drinking. See ALCOHOL DEPENDENCE; DELIRIUM TREMENS.

Withdrawal syndrome, opiates

The physical and psychological symptoms that result when someone dependent on morphine, heroin, or a related drug stops using the substance. Symptoms vary in intensity and duration with the drug and with

the habitual dosage before withdrawal. The syndrome begins 6 to 12 hours after the last dose. Symptoms during the first 24 hours include restlessness, watering of the eyes, runny nose, yawning, heavy sweating, goose bumps, restless sleep, and dilation of the pupils. As time passes, these symptoms become more severe. There may also be severe aches in the back, abdomen, and legs; muscle spasms and twitching, including cramps in the abdomen and legs; kicking; hot and cold flashes; loose stools; inability to sleep; nausea and vomiting; profuse discharge from the nose; and moderate elevation in body temperature, blood pressure, respiratory rate, and heart rate.

Typically these symptoms peak between 36 and 72 hours after withdrawal and gradually diminish. Withdrawal symptoms usually end in 5 to 7 days, although craving for the drug may continue for months. Opiate withdrawal is usually treated in a clinical setting (see DETOXIFICATION) by administering controlled doses of the synthetic opiate methadone to reduce symptoms, then decreasing the methadone dosage over time.

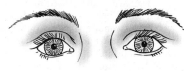

Normal pupils

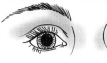

Dilated pupils

A VISIBLE SIGN
A prominent sign of withdrawal from opiates (such as heroin, morphine) is dilation (widening) of the pupils. The first signs of withdrawal become evident 6 to 12 hours after the last dose of the drug.

Wolff-Parkinson-White syndrome

Episodes of rapid heart rate caused by an extra, abnormal pathway between the upper and lower parts of the heart; also known as pre-excitation syndrome. In the healthy heart, the electrical signals that trigger a heartbeat follow a specific route from the atria (upper chambers) to the ventricles (lower chambers). In Wolff-Parkinson-White syndrome, the electrical signals instead travel along an accessory pathway known as the Kent bundle. This can cause the heart to beat abnormally fast, more than 100 beats per minute (tachycardia). Other symptoms can include lightheadedness, palpitations (an uncomfortably rapid heart rate), and syncope (fainting). Symptoms vary in severity from person to person, ranging from nonexistent to disabling.

Wolff-Parkinson-White syndrome is thought to be congenital (present at birth). Most people with symptoms first experience them between ages 11 and 50. The syndrome may become dormant, only to recur later in life. In some cases, it resolves on its own, as the Kent bundle loses its ability to conduct electrical signals. A small number of people with Wolff-Parkinson-White syndrome are at risk for ventricular fibrillation, an uncontrolled heartbeat that is fatal without prompt emergency treatment.

Most people with Wolff-Parkinson-White syndrome have no other heart problem. The remainder have MITRAL VALVE PROLAPSE (MVP), cardiomyopathy (impaired heart muscle function), or Ebstein anomaly, a rare condition in which the tricuspid valve is deformed and misplaced.

If Wolff-Parkinson-White syndrome causes no symptoms, treatment is not needed. When symptoms are present, medication that coordinates the electrical signals of the heart is sometimes successful in controlling episodes of tachycardia. Another approach involves a minimally invasive procedure (see ABLATION THERAPY) that destroys the abnormal conduction pathway. In rare cases, open-heart surgery is used.

Womb

The uterus. See REPRODUCTIVE SYSTEM, FEMALE.

Word blindness

Loss of the ability to understand written language as a result of brain damage (also known as ALEXIA).

World Health Organization

A specialized agency of the United Nations established in 1948 to serve as the directing and coordinating authority in international health; also known as WHO. According to the WHO constitution, the organization's objective is to help all people achieve the highest level of health, which is defined as complete mental, social, and physical well-being, not simply the absence of disease or disability.

Some 200 nations are members of the WHO Assembly, which meets yearly, elects the executive committee of 31 individuals, and sets the organization's policy. Headquartered in Geneva, Switzerland, WHO maintains regional organizations for Southeast Asia, the eastern Mediterranean, Europe, Africa, North America, South America, and the western Pacific.

Through its staff, WHO offers member nations advisory services in such areas as malaria, influenza, smallpox, tuberculosis, sexually transmitted diseases, HIV (human immunodeficiency virus), mother and child health, nutrition, chemical safety, population planning, and sanitation. The organization showcases demonstrations around the world to exhibit and evaluate the use of modern techniques to improve health and combat diseases. WHO's technical staff members gather and publish data on disease and public health, standardize pharmaceutical names and laboratory methods, and pursue research on parasitic and viral diseases.

Wound

FOR FIRST AID
see Bleeding, page 1315
see Cuts and scrapes, page 1318

Any break or opening in the skin or a mucous membrane, such as the inside of the mouth or nose. A wound may come from a physical injury, or it may result from the incision that is used in surgery to open and repair a part of the body. Other types of wounds include cuts, punctures, and tears.

Wound infection

FOR FIRST AID
see Cuts and scrapes, page 1318

Bacterial contamination of broken skin. Wound infections occur when bacteria enter an opening in the skin and produce inflammation. In some cases, serious skin disorders including impetigo, erysipelas, and cellulitis occur. These infections are generally caused by streptococcal or staphylococcal bacteria. The surface layers of the skin are most commonly involved, but some wound infections, such as cellulitis and streptococcal impetigo, can affect deeper tissues.

Some wound infections can produce serious medical conditions, particularly if the bacteria that enter the wound penetrate so deeply into the skin that there is no oxygen supply. This condition is referred to as an anaerobic wound infection. If the wounds are infected with the bacterium *Clostridium* and an anaerobic infection develops, the condition may progress to myonecrosis, or gas gangrene. In severe cases, this type of infection can lead to shock, toxic delirium, and death within several days of the infection.

Another potentially serious wound infection, also caused by clostridial bacteria, is TETANUS. People who do not have immunity to tetanus infection are susceptible if they receive a cut, bite, or puncture wound. Spores of the bacteria that cause tetanus can occur almost anywhere, but are usually found in the soil. If these spores infect the deeper parts of a wound where no oxygen is present, they germinate and produce a toxin that interferes with the nerves that control muscles.

Treatment for tetanus includes the use of an antibody, human tetanus immunoglobulin, and a tetanus antitoxin. A small number of tetanus cases are reported yearly in the United States. The infection can be fatal, even with antibiotic treatment, but this is very rare in the United States. Developing countries have more incidents of tetanus and more deaths from the infection.

Tetanus is prevented by routine immunization as one part of the DPT (diphtheria, pertussis, tetanus) injection given to most school-aged children in the United States. The booster shot should be repeated every 10 years.

People who have diabetes mellitus must take special care to seek medical attention for prevention of wound infection, particularly in the feet. An associated condition called

Preventing wound infection

Most cuts, scrapes, and other minor wounds do not require a trip to the emergency department or even a visit to a doctor. Proper self-care can prevent the risk of infection or other complications. Following are guidelines for treating wounds:

- If bleeding from a wound does not stop soon after the injury, gentle pressure should be applied using a clean cloth or bandage. If bleeding persists or if the blood spurts from the wound, emergency medical care should be sought.
- Any area where skin is broken must be thoroughly cleaned and kept clean. Wounds should be rinsed with clean water. Soap and water should be used to clean the area surrounding the wound itself; this area around the wound may also be cleaned with hydrogen peroxide, iodine, or an iodine-containing cleanser. These cleansers should not come in contact with the open area of the wound. Dirt or debris may be removed from the wound with tweezers cleaned with alcohol; if dirt is deeply embedded in a wound, a doctor should be seen.
- An over-the-counter, topical antibiotic cream or ointment applied to a wound can help prevent bacterial infection and help the wound site close. Although exposure to the air speeds healing, covering a wound with a clean bandage protects the injured skin and prevents exposure to harmful bacteria. Skin openings, including broken blisters that are draining, should be kept covered until a scab forms.
- If the edges surrounding a wound are gaping, jagged, or do not meet, surgical tape may be used to hold the edges closed. If this cannot be accomplished easily, medical care is necessary. Proper closure of a wound helps prevent bacterial contamination and minimizes scarring.
- Wounds should be tended on a daily basis with repeated cleaning, use of a topical antibiotic, and fresh bandaging. The process should also be repeated whenever the bandage becomes wet or dirty. People who are allergic to bandage adhesives may use adhesive-free bandages or sterile gauze with paper tape.
- Vigilance helps stop infection before it becomes serious. A doctor should be consulted if redness, draining, warmth, or swelling occur near a wound or if the person has increased pain, fever, or chills.

diabetic neuropathy causes a loss of sensation and diminished circulation that can lead to wounds that are vulnerable to infection and slow healing. These wounds must be treated quickly to prevent the need for amputation.

Wrinkle

Skin damage that ranges from a fine line to a deep furrow. Wrinkles have two primary causes: aging and sun exposure (see SUN EXPOSURE, ADVERSE EFFECTS OF). Over years, the skin becomes thinner and produces less oil. Collagen and elastin, fibrous proteins in the dermis (the middle layer of skin), normally provide skin with strength and elasticity. However, these fibers weaken with age. Repeated sun exposure also damages fibers, leading to premature wrinkling and sagging. Smoking too can damage collagen.

A variety of drugs and procedures are used to reduce the appearance of fine lines and deeper wrinkles. In addition to simple over-the-counter moisturizers containing sunscreen, helpful topical products include retinol, tretinoin (a vitamin A derivative) and alpha-hydroxy acids (naturally occurring acids in fruit and milk). Higher concentrations of alpha-hydroxy acids are used in a CHEMICAL PEEL. Other medical procedures include botulinum toxin injections or COLLAGEN INJECTIONS that make wrinkles temporarily disappear, DERMABRASION (removal of the surface layer of skin by high-speed sanding), LASER RESURFACING, and traditional cut-and-stitch plastic surgery. See also FACE-LIFT.

While medications and surgery can reduce wrinkles, doctors caution that certain risks are involved. Tretinoin cream and alpha-hydroxy acids may cause irritation and redness of the skin. Some people have allergic reactions to collagen injections, and this type of treatment usually must be repeated every few months. Laser and surgical procedures have more lasting benefits, but afterward there is considerable bruising, scabbing, and swelling. There is also a small risk of scarring and, in the case of traditional cosmetic or plastic surgery, nerve damage. Finally, it is important before undergoing surgery to have realistic expectations of what can and cannot be accomplished.

Wrist

The region where the hand joins the arm. The wrist is a complex arrangement of joints between eight wrist bones (carpals in two rows of four bones each), the two bones of the lower arm (radius and ulna), and the five bones in the palm (metacarpals). This structure gives the wrist flexibility to move in a variety of directions and ways. The tendons that control the actions of the fingers pass through the wrist from the muscles in the lower arm that control them. Also passing across the wrist are the arteries and nerves supplying the muscles, bones, and skin of the hand and fingers.

Wristdrop

A type of paralysis in which there is an inability to extend or lift the wrist. This is caused by damage to the radial nerve. It is also referred to as Saturday night palsy because it occurs when a person hangs his or her arm over a chair, thereby compressing the radial nerve as it travels through the upper arm.

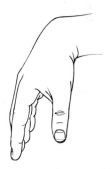

RADIAL NERVE DAMAGE
A loss of function in the radial nerve to the hand can cause an inability to extend the wrist or fingers. The damage to the nerve is usually at a point in the armpit or upper arm. Splinting the wrist into a straight position may restore nerve function.

Wryneck

See TORTICOLLIS.

X chromosome

The female sex chromosome. The X chromosome is one of two chromosomes (X and Y), appearing in pairs, that determine sex in humans and most animals. The female pair includes two X chromosomes, while the male pair consists of one X and one Y chromosome.

X rays

Electromagnetic waves that have a shorter wavelength than light and can penetrate the body to form an image on film or a digital screen. X rays are generated by an electrical current that passes through an X-ray tube and produces a beam of ionizing radiation that can pass through the body part being examined. This process creates an image of internal body structures called a RADIOGRAPH. "X ray" is also the term for the image or for an examination with X rays.

Because soft body structures are less dense, a greater amount of radiation passes through them, and more radiation reaches the film (the film is exposed to larger amounts of X rays). Soft body tissues appear dark on X-ray film. Because bones are more dense than soft tissue, they absorb more of the radiation, and a lesser amount passes through them. Bones leave the film only slightly exposed and appear light or white on the X-ray film.

WHY IT IS PERFORMED

X rays, formerly known as roentgen rays, are performed on different parts of the body for various diagnostic purposes. A chest X ray may be performed to look for evidence of pneumonia, tumors, or fluid or to evaluate the size of the heart. Chest X rays are usually performed before major surgery as part of screening, but they are no longer given as a part of routine checkups.

X rays of the abdomen are usually done to determine the cause of acute abdominal pain. They also may be helpful for locating a swallowed foreign object, an intestinal obstruction, or a perforation in the digestive tract.

A myelogram is an X ray of the spine that uses a contrast medium injected into the spinal fluid to outline the spinal cord. It is usually done to check for damaged disks in people with lower back pain. An arthrogram is an X ray of the inside of a joint (usually the knee or hip) that uses contrast medium injected into the joint to make the image clearer. Arthrograms are usually done to detect a tear in the cartilage or other joint abnormality. In some X-ray procedures, a contrast medium containing iodine is injected into a vein or artery; in other procedures, a contrast medium such as barium is ingested to help outline internal structures.

A fluoroscope, a device that is equipped with a fluorescent screen, may be used to produce moving images of the body while the examination is taking place. The images can be recorded on videotape or as still pictures for evaluation. A fluoroscope may be used to examine the function of the gastrointestinal tract, the respiratory system, and the bladder.

Mammography uses special X-ray equipment to help detect breast cancer. Dental X rays may be performed to detect cavities and other problems with the teeth and gums.

HOW X RAYS ARE DONE

X-ray examinations are generally performed in a radiology department of a hospital or in an outpatient clinic. A woman undergoing a mammogram will be told not to use deodorant, body powders, or lotions under the arms or on the chest before the procedure because these products can interfere with the image. If soft internal structures are being examined (such as the intestines or blood vessels), a contrast medium such as barium or an iodine-based compound may be ingested or injected for better definition of these structures.

The person being examined is positioned against a cassette holding the film, or the person may be asked to hold the cassette holding the film against the body part being studied. A lead shield may be placed over other parts of the body to reduce their exposure to the X rays.

The X-ray unit is aligned over the part of the body to be examined. The technician moves away from the area to activate the X-ray unit and to avoid exposing himself or herself to unnecessary radiation. It is important that the person being examined remain as motionless as possible as the X ray is taken to prevent the images from being blurred.

After an X-ray examination, a person can resume normal activities. If a contrast medium was used, it is important that the person consume extra fluids to enhance the prompt excretion of the contrast medium.

TYPES OF X RAYS
X rays can image the human head in different ways, enabling doctors to view internal structures for a variety of purposes. An X ray of the human skull shows the condition of and relationship between the bones and teeth, including dental fillings. An angiogram is an X ray image of the blood vessels of the head after they have been injected with a contrast medium; malformation of the veins is visible. A CT (computed tomography) scan of the head, which images a thin section, clearly shows a brain tumor as a dense mass.

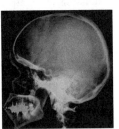
X ray of skull

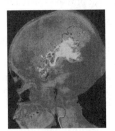
Angiogram of head

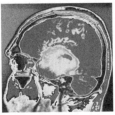
CT scan of head

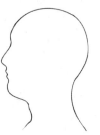
Orientation of images

X rays, dental

A diagnostic dental tool that involves electromagnetic radiation to create photographic images of the teeth, mouth, jaw, and related structures. X rays pass through softer tissues, such as the skin of the cheek and the gums, and are absorbed by denser structures, such as teeth and bone. When dental X rays are taken as part of a dental examination, they allow the dentist to observe parts of the teeth and mouth that cannot be seen visually. X rays can show hidden surfaces of the teeth where tooth decay may be located because the radiation passes through the softer decay tissue and makes it appear darker on film. X rays can reveal infections, abscesses, impactions, cysts, and some tumors. They may also be helpful in detecting the existence or stage of PERIODONTAL DISEASE.

At the initial dental examination, a dentist may require dental X rays of the entire mouth to assess conditions and possible problems. These baseline X rays may be compared with newer X rays at a later time to evaluate the status of oral conditions. There are three categories of dental X rays. The first category provides highly detailed images of small areas in the mouth. These are called periapical and bitewing X rays, which are taken by using X-ray film inserted into a plastic holder that is held between the teeth. Periapical X rays reproduce an image of a root structure in a tooth and surrounding bone, as well as the possible presence of

cysts or abscesses. Bitewing X rays are typically used to detect hidden decay between the teeth and under old fillings. The second category of dental X rays is panoramic radiographs, which involve a special machine that reproduces a single image of all the top and bottom teeth and parts of the jawbone, offering a comprehensive view of dental conditions. This kind of dental X ray is generally used to examine the growth and development of teeth in children, to evaluate the condition of the jawbone in people who have lost teeth, and to detect fractures and abnormalities in the jaw. The third category of dental X rays, usually used by orthodontists for teeth in children, is called a cephalometric X ray. The images reproduced by this technique reveal the relationship of the teeth to the skull and allow the orthodontist to observe changes due to growth and to evaluate evolving conditions that may affect treatment.

SAFETY CONCERNS

Much greater amounts of radiation than are commonly used in dentistry have been implicated in genetic disorders and cancer risks. Dental X rays use a small amount of radiation directed at the mouth for a fraction of a second. Dental X rays are considered safe procedures. During panoramic or cephalometric X-ray exposure, a dentist may use a lead collar to shield the thyroid gland of the person from exposure, since this gland is especially sensitive to radiation. As a safeguard, lead aprons may be used

during all dental X-ray procedures. To minimize exposure to radiation, dentists tend to use only the most current and safest X rays—and only when necessary.

Xanthelasma

A XANTHOMA (a yellow-orange bump beneath the surface of the skin) on the eyelids representing cholesterol deposits. Xanthelasmas are typically not associated with an elevated blood cholesterol level. Although they may be cosmetically disturbing, xanthelasmas are benign (not cancerous) and painless. If the growths become bothersome, they can be surgically removed or treated with applications of trichloroacetic acid.

Xanthoma

A yellow-orange nodule (solid mass of tissue) with sharply defined borders beneath the surface of the skin. Xanthomas commonly appear on the elbows, hands, feet, knees, and buttocks. Growths range in size from small to more than 3 inches in diameter. Although they may be cosmetically disturbing, xanthomas are benign (not cancerous) and painless. They most frequently affect people with elevated blood lipid levels or genetic lipoprotein disturbances. The goal of treatment is to manage underlying disorders, which may include diabetes, cirrhosis, or hypercholesterolemia. Once triglyceride and cholesterol levels are under control, the development of xanthomas will be reduced. If the growths become bothersome, they can be surgically removed. See also CHOLESTEROL.

Xanthomatosis

A condition in which fatty deposits accumulate in the brain, skin, internal organs, and tendons. Fat deposits that accumulate in the linings of the blood vessels (ATHEROSCLEROSIS) can narrow blood vessels and impair the blood supply to the body's organs.

Xenograft

A procedure in which tissue from a donor is grafted or transplanted into another species. The only xenograft now done routinely in medicine involves the heart valves of pigs to replace diseased human heart valves. Pigs are used as donor animals because their internal organs are

---

IMAGING THE TEETH AND GUMS
Dental X rays provide the dentist with highly detailed images of small areas of the mouth or comprehensive views of the position of the teeth in the jaws. The periapical image shows the root structure of a tooth, gum, and surrounding bone, useful to find cysts or abscesses. A bitewing image shows the crowns of the teeth and helps the dentist locate decay hidden between or within teeth. The panoramic image reveals all the teeth and bones of the jaw, which is useful in examining general development of teeth and detecting abnormalities.

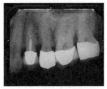
Periapical X ray

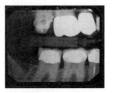
Bitewing X ray

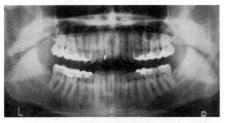
Panoramic X ray

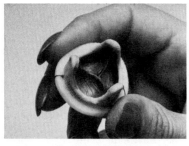

A HEART VALVE FROM A DONOR PIG
The only xenograft (transplantation of tissue from another species) done regularly is the replacement of a person's diseased heart valve with the heart valve from a pig. A valve from a pig is useful because it is about the same size as a human valve and needs only slight modification. A xenograft is difficult because the immune system recognizes the pig valve as foreign tissue and tries to reject it.

approximately the same size as human organs. Since pigs are raised for meat and leather, using them as donors for humans poses few ethical problems. Apart from heart valve replacement, xenografts remain highly experimental. Work is now being done, for example, on the technique for possible use in therapies for Parkinson disease, diabetes, and Huntington chorea.

Xenografts pose difficult challenges. Since the donor is of another species, the IMMUNE SYSTEM tries to attack and reject the heart valve. There is also the risk that animal viruses may be transferred to humans and cause new strains of disease. If these challenges can be overcome, xenografts offer the potential to increase the number of available donor organs dramatically.

Xeroderma pigmentosum

A very rare inherited disease that causes extreme sensitivity to all sources of ultraviolet light, especially sunlight. Many people with xeroderma pigmentosum (XP) can get unusually severe sunburns after only short periods of exposure to the sun, and most develop many freckles at an early age. In XP, cells lose the ability to repair damage to their DNA, usually from ultraviolet light. Exposure to the sun leads to changes in the skin and the freckles, including irregular dark spots, thin skin, excessive dryness, rough patches, and skin cancer. These changes often begin in infancy and are almost always present before age 20. Skin cancers may develop before age 10, usually on the face, the eyes, lips, and tip of the tongue. All three common types of skin cancer—basal cell carcinoma, squamous cell carcinoma, and melanoma—occur much more often in people with XP. Melanoma can be fatal if it is not removed before it has spread to internal organs; and basal cell and squamous cell carcinomas can destroy skin and underlying tissues.

The eyes of people with XP are also extremely sensitive to the sun and may easily become bloodshot, irritated, and clouded. Growths, both cancerous and noncancerous, may occur on the eyes. Other medical problems that may occur include deafness, poor coordination, spastic muscles, and developmental delay. XP has no cure. Treatment includes protection from ultraviolet light, frequent skin and eye examinations, and the prompt removal of any cancerous growths.

Xeroderma pigmentosum is inherited as a recessive trait: both parents must have the defective gene for their children to inherit the condition. It is a very rare condition, with fewer than 1,000 known cases worldwide.

Xerophthalmia

Abnormal dryness and thickening of the exposed outer layer of the eye as a result of a deficiency of vitamin A (beta-carotene) in the diet or as a result of disease. Xerophthalmia can lead to serious vision loss, which begins with difficulty seeing in dim light (night blindness) and progresses to ulceration of the clear covering of the eye (cornea). Xerophthalmia from vitamin A deficiency is a leading cause of blindness among children in developing countries.

Xerostomia

See DRY MOUTH.

X-linked characteristic

A trait associated with a gene carried on the X chromosome. Whether dominant or recessive, any trait associated with a gene on the X chromosome will always be expressed in males, who have only one X chromosome.

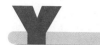

Y chromosome

The male sex chromosome. The Y chromosome is one of two chromosomes (X and Y), appearing in pairs, that determine sex in humans and most animals. The male pair consists of one X and one Y chromosome, while the female pair includes two X chromosomes.

Yawning

Involuntary deep inhalation of air with the mouth open. Although its exact purpose is unclear, yawning frequently occurs at the same time as stretching and is usually caused by drowsiness, fatigue, or boredom. It is also often caused by suggestion—if an individual sees another person yawning, he or she may yawn as well. Repeated yawning is usually a sign of drowsiness, but it may also be a sign of depression.

Yeast infections

The most common form of vaginal infection. Yeast infections, also known as candidiasis, are caused by an overgrowth of a fungus commonly present in the vagina. Principal symptoms are intense itching, burning, and redness in the vaginal area. A thick, white, cottage cheese–like discharge is frequently present. Some women with yeast infections experience pain during sexual intercourse, while others have burning sensations when they urinate.

Diagnosis is made by physical examination and microscopic examination of a sample of the discharge. The doctor may prescribe suppositories or creams to be used in the vagina or oral medication. Over-the-counter medications are available but should not be used by women who have never had a yeast infection diagnosed by a doctor and are unfamiliar with its symptoms. Women who have diabetes, who are obese, or who are taking antibiotics or birth control pills are at greatest risk for yeast infections. Each of those factors can alter the chemical balance of the vagina, allowing the fungus to grow.

Yellow fever

A viral infection that varies in severity and occurs in two forms. Urban yellow fever is acquired when a person is bitten by a certain species of mosquito that has been infected by previously feeding on an infected person. Jungle yellow fever, also called sylvatic yellow fever, is transmitted by mosquitoes that have fed on infected wild primates. The illness is principally found in central Africa and in South and Central America.

SYMPTOMS

Yellow fever can be very mild with symptoms limited to fever and headache within 48 hours of infection, or it can be severe. There may be a sudden onset of symptoms including high fever (temperature of 102°F to 104°F), flushing, headache, and a rapid pulse that slows on the second day of symptoms. Common symptoms of yellow fever include nausea, vomiting, constipation, headache, severe prostration, restlessness, irritability, and muscle pains, particularly in the neck, back, and legs. In mild cases, the symptoms improve within 1 to 3 days and do not recur. When the illness is more severe, there is a remission of symptoms that lasts for several hours or several days and occurs within 5 days of the start of the illness. The fever then recurs, the pulse remains slow, and other symptoms appear, including jaundice and internal bleeding, which causes black vomit. These symptoms may last as long as a week. Very severe cases cause delirium, seizures, and coma, resulting in death.

DIAGNOSIS, TREATMENT, AND PREVENTION

Yellow fever can be definitively diagnosed by laboratory evaluation of blood samples that reveal the presence of the virus or increased antibodies to fight the virus. Treatment is supportive and directed toward relieving the major symptoms and correcting imbalances of fluids and electrolytes. Medication to ease nausea and control vomiting may be given. Transfusions may be necessary.

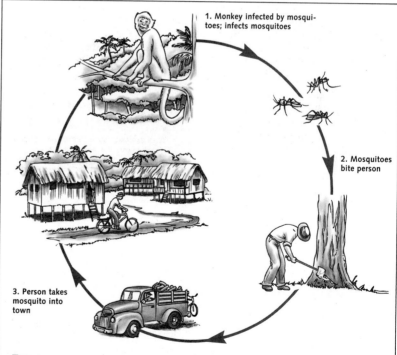

TRANSMITTING YELLOW FEVER
In the wild, the yellow fever virus passes between mosquitoes and monkeys. A person can be bitten by an infected mosquito. A uninfected mosquito can acquire the virus by biting an infected person, and the person can also carry an infected mosquito into an inhabited environment, where the mosquito bites others.

Y

Although the disease occurs rarely in travelers, visitors must meet requirements for vaccination against yellow fever before entering most countries where it is endemic, for example, India. The vaccine is a live virus vaccine that provides immunity for 10 years. It cannot be given to women who are pregnant or breast-feeding, people with a hypersensitivity to eggs (the vaccination is prepared in embryonated eggs), infants younger than 6 months (because of a risk of viral encephalitis), and people with weakened immune systems.

Yin and yang

An ancient Chinese world view based on the belief that all things have aspects that oppose each other yet are independent. Applied to medicine, yin and yang express certain qualities and characteristics of different organs and processes of the body; moreover, health is viewed as a state of relative balance of the opposing forces of yin and yang. In this view, whenever a condition of prolonged excess or deficiency of either yin or yang occurs, disease is the result. Yin is associated with the body's solid organs, such as heart, lungs, kidneys, liver, and spleen; the front, lower half, and right side of the body; long-term pain; intellectualism; and introversion. Yang corresponds to hollow organs in the body, such as the gallbladder, stomach and intestines, and bladder; the surface of the body; the back, upper half, and left side of the body; acute pain; extroversion; and physicality. See also CHINESE MEDICINE.

Yoga

An ancient holistic Indian system of disciplined exercise and breathing associated with meditation; a philosophy and way of life. Yoga includes a set of exercises with proven health benefits that have been shown to lower high blood pressure; lower respiratory rate; increase cardiac efficiency; reduce stress; and improve sleep. The goal of yoga exercises, or postures, is to stretch muscle groups in the body while gently squeezing internal organs. Breathing techniques are practiced before and during exercise to help focus the mind.

Through controlled breathing, prescribed postures, and meditation, yoga seeks to enhance the life force ("prana") in order to achieve a state of balance and harmony between body and mind. The meditative nature of yoga calms and focuses the mind. Yoga can be a useful relaxation technique, and may be beneficial to persons coping with chronic pain. There are many types of yoga, each one emphasizing different techniques designed to achieve the same goal—unifying body, mind, and spirit. Yoga has a significant role in holistic health systems. See also MIND-BODY MEDICINE.

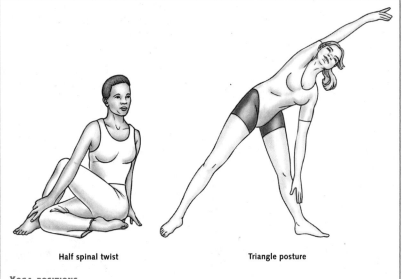

Half spinal twist   Triangle posture

YOGA POSITIONS
Yoga exercises such as the half spinal twist and triangle posture are designed to stretch and lengthen muscles and to gently compress internal organs to promote circulation. Controlled breathing techniques are an important part of the exercises.

Z

Zafirlukast

An antiasthma drug. Zafirlukast (Accolate) is a type of medication called a leukotriene receptor antagonist that is used by people with mild to moderate asthma to decrease symptoms and the number of acute asthma attacks. It works by inhibiting leukotrienes, substances in the body that are associated with the inflammation and tightening of airway muscles in the lung that are characteristic of asthma. Zafirlukast cannot relieve an asthma attack that has already started.

Zalcitabine (ddC)

An antiviral drug; an AIDS (acquired immunodeficiency syndrome) drug. Zalcitabine, or ddC (Hivid), is used alone or in combination with other drugs in the treatment of the infection caused by HIV (human immunodeficiency virus). Zalcitabine (ddC) cannot cure or prevent HIV infection or AIDS, although it can keep HIV from reproducing, and it seems to slow the destruction of the immune system by the virus, which may delay development of problems associated with AIDS.

Zaleplon

A drug used for the short-term treatment of insomnia. Zaleplon (Sonata) is a central nervous system depressant that causes drowsiness. Zaleplon works rapidly and should be taken right before going to bed. It works for a only short time and can be used if a person wakes up during the night.

Zanamivir

An antiviral drug. Zanamivir (Relenza) is used to treat influenza virus A and B (flu) in people who have had symptoms such as weakness, headache, fever, cough, and sore throat for less than 2 days. Zanamivir cannot prevent flu, nor can it keep a person from spreading the virus to others, but it seems to decrease the duration and severity of the flu by 1 or 2 days. Zanamivir is breathed in through a special inhaler.

Zenker diverticulum

An abnormal pouch of tissue that forms at the juncture of the pharynx (lower part of the throat) and the esophagus (the muscular tube that connects the throat to the stomach). Zenker diverticulum is a common type of ESOPHAGEAL DIVERTICULUM.

The diagnosis is usually made through an upper gastrointestinal (GI) series (an X-ray procedure also called a barium swallow). Zenker diverticulum may not require treatment. However, because it is possible for food to become trapped in the diverticulum and inhaled, doctors often recommend surgery to correct the problem.

Zidovudine

An antiviral medication; an AIDS (acquired immunodeficiency syndrome) drug. Zidovudine (Retrovir), also known as AZT, is used with other drugs to treat the infection caused by HIV (human immunodeficiency virus). Zidovudine is also used to help prevent pregnant women who have HIV from passing the virus to their babies during pregnancy or at birth.

Zidovudine works by helping to keep HIV from reproducing, which slows the destruction of the immune system by the virus. It cannot cure or prevent HIV infection or AIDS. Some side effects include nausea, headache, and insomnia. Serious side effects are possible.

ZIFT

Zygote intrafallopian transfer; an ASSISTED REPRODUCTIVE TECHNOLOGY in which zygotes are placed in a fallopian tube, usually by LAPAROSCOPY. The initial steps are similar to IN VITRO FERTILIZATION (IVF), in which the eggs are retrieved and then fertilized in vitro (outside the body). The resulting zygotes are transferred into a fallopian tube so that cell division of the early embryo occurs in a natural environment. As IVF success rates have improved, the need for ZIFT has declined. ZIFT is not often performed because it requires an additional surgical procedure over and above the procedures required for IVF.

Zileuton

An antiasthma drug. Zileuton (Zyflo) is a type of antiasthma drug called a leukotriene inhibitor, used by people with mild to moderate asthma to decrease symptoms and the number of acute asthma attacks. Zileuton cannot relieve an asthma attack that has already started. It works by inhibiting leukotrienes, substances in the body that are associated with the inflammation and tightening of airway muscles in the lung that are characteristic of asthma.

Zinc

A mineral that is essential for cell production, normal growth and development, tissue repair and growth, and production of sperm and testos-

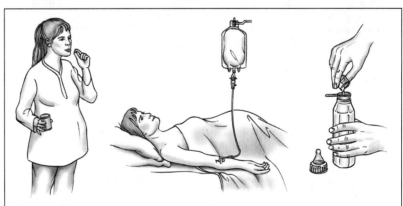

PROTECTING A FETUS OR NEWBORN FROM HIV
An HIV-positive pregnant woman can take zidovudine (AZT) orally and reduce the risk of passing the infection along to her fetus by two thirds. She can be given AZT intravenously to prevent transmission during delivery. AZT in liquid form can be added to infant formula to additionally reduce the risk of infection of a child born to an HIV-positive mother.

terone. Zinc is found in meats, poultry, eggs, milk, yogurt, oysters, nuts, legumes, and whole-grain cereals. There is some evidence that zinc supplements may shorten the duration of cold symptoms.

Zolmitriptan

An antimigraine drug. Zolmitriptan (Zomig) is used to treat severe migraine headaches. Zolmitriptan cannot prevent migraine but can only ease a migraine headache that is already occurring. Zolmitriptan relieves symptoms that are associated with migraine, including nausea, vomiting, and sensitivity to light and sound. It is thought to work by narrowing blood vessels in the brain that cause the pain.

Zolpidem

A drug used to treat insomnia. Zolpidem (Ambien) is a central nervous system depressant that causes drowsiness. Zolpidem should be used only for short-term treatment of insomnia, usually limited to 2 weeks or less. It should not be taken by children younger than 18 years or by women who are breast-feeding.

Zone therapy

A form of pressure point massage of the feet and hands designed to reduce and relieve pain. Zone therapy is based on the idea that the body is divided into 10 equal energy channels: five on each side and each containing its own "bioelectrical energy" that travels from the toes to the brain to the fingers. Pain relief is achieved by pressing the joints of toes and fingers in the appropriate zone. Zone therapy is used by chiropractors and osteopaths who, whenever possible, prefer not to use pain-relieving drugs. See REFLEXOLOGY.

Zoonosis

A type of disease that occurs in animals and may be passed from animals (usually mammals) to humans. Zoonotic diseases occur more commonly and tend to be more serious in developing countries, especially in tropical areas. Zoonosis can also occur in domestic animals in the United States. RABIES is a zoonosis that can be transmitted from an infected dog or cat to a person bitten by the animal, which has usually become infected after being bitten by an infected wild animal. The rabies vaccine protects pets from becoming infected.

TOXOPLASMOSIS is a disease carried by cats that feed on small rodents and then shed the cysts in their stool. The illness is dangerous to unborn babies and to people with weakened immune systems. Most puppies contract roundworm infestations (see ROUNDWORMS) from their mothers and carry the worm's eggs in their stool. Puppies can transmit the worms to humans, especially children, who handle the puppies. Roundworms usually cause mild infections in humans, but they have the potential for producing severe illness. Skin infections including RINGWORM and SCABIES can be carried by cats and dogs and transmitted to people.

Ticks can transmit disease to animals and to people. These arachnids acquire disease by feeding on infected wild mammals or birds. People who are bitten by infected ticks can acquire diseases including ROCKY MOUNTAIN SPOTTED FEVER and LYME DISEASE. See also TICKS AND DISEASE.

Some zoonoses are viral diseases: ENCEPHALITIS is transmitted by mosquitoes to humans from infected birds, rodents, bats, and rabbits. Hantavirus may be transmitted by the bites of infected deer mice and other rodents or by inhaling airborne dust particles from their feces. Fungal disease may also be zoonotic. Histoplasmosis occurs in humans who have contact with soil contaminated with the feces of infected bats or birds.

BUBONIC PLAGUE occurs in humans as a result of contact with infected rodents and fleas that have fed on them. TULAREMIA is contracted by humans via ingestion or inhalation of, or physical contact with, the waste products of infected wild animals, birds, and certain snakes. Bovine spongiform ENCEPHALOPATHY (BSE), also called MAD COW DISEASE, is a fatal disease caused by ingesting the meat from infected cattle. Other zoonoses include LEPTOSPIROSIS, BRUCELLOSIS, salmonellosis, campylobacteriosis, PSITTACOSIS, and ANTHRAX. See also ANIMALS, DISEASES FROM.

Z-plasty

A surgical technique to make a scar less noticeable by partially removing and repositioning it. The technique also helps relieve tension on the skin caused by a scar that has contracted as it healed.

The scar is removed, and incisions are cut on each side to create small triangular flaps of skin. Rearranging the flaps at a new angle to cover the old scar area and then connecting them with fine sutures creates the Z pattern that gives the technique its name. The sutures are removed within a few days. A Z-plasty is usually performed as an outpatient procedure with local anesthesia.

Zygote

The fertilized egg; the cell formed by fertilization, or the union of a male sex cell (sperm) and the female sex cell (ovum). The zygote has yet to undergo cleavage, or division, and is a single cell with a full set of genetic material. As instructed by the genetic material within it, the zygote develops into an embryo.

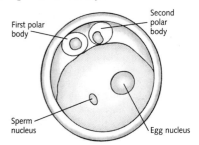

Egg and sperm

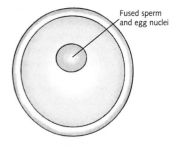

Zygote

FUSION OF SPERM AND EGG
A zygote is formed when a sperm penetrates an egg, and the nucleus of the sperm (which carries 23 chromosomes) and the nucleus of the egg (which carries 23 chromosomes) fuse. The resulting cell has one nucleus with 46 chromosomes—a unique combination of genetic material.

Zygote intrafallopian transfer

See ZIFT.

Resources

First aid

Sample legal form

Self-help organizations

HIPAA and confidentiality of patients' health information

First aid

In serious emergencies, first-aid treatment in the first few minutes can save a life. If you know what to do and can act quickly and calmly before medical help arrives, you will be helping the injured or sick person and medical personnel when they arrive on the scene. When the injury or illness is minor, knowing what to do can save needless visits to the doctor or hospital. So how do you know if you are dealing with a true medical emergency or a minor injury that can be handled at home?

This special First Aid section is designed to help you quickly assess the situation and, if appropriate, provide immediate help for everything from back injuries to food poisoning to stroke. Entries are arranged alphabetically. The main entries and their sections are listed with page numbers so that you can find immediate help and, in some cases, helpful step-by-step illustrations to show you what to do. Each first-aid procedure listed will most often have even more detailed information in the alphabetical encyclopedia of medicine.

In general, if a person has no pulse, is breathing with difficulty or not at all, is unconscious, or is bleeding severely, you or someone on the scene of the accident or injury needs to call 911 or your local emergency number. No severely injured or ill person should be moved without trained help unless that person's life is in immediate danger. Make sure the person is covered, but loosen any tight or constricting clothing. See page 1328 for administering CPR. See page 1318 if someone is choking (Heimlich maneuver), and see page 1315 for severe bleeding.

First Aid topics

BACK INJURIES ■ 1314

BITES AND STINGS ■ 1314
    Animal bites / 1314
    Human bites / 1314
    Insect bites and stings / 1314
    Spider bites / 1314
    Tick bites / 1315

BLEEDING ■ 1315

BRUISES ■ 1316

BURNS ■ 1316
    First-degree burns / 1316
    Second-degree burns / 1316
    Third-degree burns / 1316
    Chemical burns / 1316
    Electrical burns / 1316

CHILDBIRTH ■ 1317

CHOKING (HEIMLICH MANEUVER) ■ 1318

CUTS AND SCRAPES ■ 1318

DEHYDRATION ■ 1319

DIABETIC COMA ■ 1319

DIARRHEA ■ 1319

DISLOCATIONS ■ 1319

EAR INJURIES ■ 1319
    Earache / 1319
    Foreign object inside the ear / 1320
    Frostbitten ears / 1320

EYE INJURIES ■ 1320
    Foreign objects in the eye / 1320
    Chemical burns of the eye / 1320
    Blows to the eye / 1321
    Eye infection / 1321
    Cuts to the eye / 1321

FAINTING ■ 1321

FEVER ■ 1321

FISHHOOK INJURIES ■ 1322

FOOD POISONING ■ 1322
    Botulism / 1322
    Escherichia coli (E. coli) infections / 1322
    Mushroom poisoning / 1323
    Salmonella poisoning / 1323
    Staphylococcus poisoning / 1323

FRACTURES (BROKEN BONES) ■ 1323

FROSTBITE ■ 1324

HEAD INJURIES ■ 1324

HEART ATTACK ■ 1325

HEAT CRAMPS ■ 1325

HEAT EXHAUSTION ■ 1326

HEAT STROKE ■ 1326

HYPERVENTILATION ■ 1326

HYPOGLYCEMIA ■ 1326

HYPOTHERMIA ■ 1327

POISONING ■ 1327

POISONING, CARBON MONOXIDE ■ 1327

RAPE/SEXUAL ASSAULT ■ 1327

RESUSCITATION (CPR) ■ 1328
    Airway / 1328
    Breathing / 1328
    Circulation / 1329

SEIZURES ■ 1329

SHOCK ■ 1329
    Anaphylactic shock / 1330
    Shock from severe injury / 1330
    Insulin shock / 1330
    Septic shock / 1330
    Streptococcal toxic shock–like syndrome / 1330
    Toxic shock syndrome / 1330

SPLINTERS ■ 1331

STRAINS AND SPRAINS ■ 1331

STROKE ■ 1332

SUNBURN ■ 1333

Back injuries

You should never move a person with a severe back injury without direction or assistance from a trained medical person unless the injured person is in danger from a fire, explosion, or any other life-threatening situation. If the injury is serious, any movement of the back could cause paralysis or even death. The person may not be able to move his or her arms, fingers, legs, feet, or toes or may have tingling, numbness, or pain in the back, neck, or down the arms or legs. Call the local emergency number (911) and keep the person still and warm while you wait for medical help to arrive.

Bites and stings

Bites and stings can range from mild to extremely serious and even fatal. Animal bites can cause serious infections, and many can be avoided. Never tease, provoke, or surprise an animal. Insect stings usually cause only local reactions, such as redness and swelling, but they can be life-threatening if the person is allergic to the insect's venom.

ANIMAL BITES

If an animal bites you, clean the wound with a solution of 1 percent povidone iodine or with soap and running water for at least 5 minutes or more to wash out any contamination. Do not put any medication or antiseptics in the wound. Put a sterile bandage or clean, dry cloth over the wound. If it is bleeding, apply pressure to the wound for 5 minutes or until the bleeding stops. Seek medical attention, particularly if the bite is on the face, neck, or hands, where it can become infected. About one half of all cat bites cause infection. If skin tissue, such as part of an ear or a nose, is bitten off, take the skin with you to the doctor's office or hospital. If the animal that has bitten you is suspected of having rabies, notify the local police, health department, or animal warden so that the animal can be observed and evaluated for rabies.

HUMAN BITES

Any human bite that breaks the skin needs immediate medical attention since infection from bacteria or viruses may contaminate the wound, leading to serious infections. As with animal bites, human bites should be washed thoroughly for 5 minutes or more to wash out any contaminants. Do not put medication or antiseptic in the wound, which should be bandaged with a clean, dry cloth. Medical help should be sought promptly.

INSECT BITES AND STINGS

Most insect bites cause local reactions, such as redness and swelling, but some can be life-threatening if the person is allergic to the insect's venom. Stings from insects, such as bees, hornets, and wasps, can also cause pain, itching, and burning. If the insect has left a stinger inside your skin, carefully remove it by gently scraping the skin with a dull knife blade, the edge of a credit card, or your fingernail. Do not use tweezers because this may cause more venom to enter your body. The area should be washed with soap and water, and you should place a cold compress on the sting and take an oral antihistamine to help ease symptoms.

Rarely, an allergic reaction to insect stings can be life-threatening. Anaphylactic shock is a total body allergic reaction. Call 911 for help or get the person or yourself to the closest emergency department if the reaction is severe (including difficulty breathing, hives, swelling of the lips or tongue, weakness, or dizziness).

SPIDER BITES

Black widow spider bites can be harmful to young children, elderly people, and chronically ill people. The bite can cause redness and swelling and pinpricklike pain followed by a dull ache in 20 to 40 minutes. Profuse sweating, nausea, vomiting, muscle cramps, rigid back and abdomen, difficulty breathing, weakness, and swelling at the site may also be present.

The brown recluse spider causes similar redness and pain at the bite site (and occasionally a small blister), but also destroys tissue, causing a skin ulcer. Mild fever, muscle aches, and joint pains may develop within 3 days. Call 911 or take the person to the nearest hospital for immediate evaluation and care.

Tarantula bites are not usually as serious as those of the black widow spider or the brown recluse spider. Symptoms include severe itching, mild pain at the site of the bite, and a severe, painful wound a few days after the bite. If you are bitten, pull off the spider hairs with adhesive or cellophane tape, wash the area with soap and water, and place ice wrapped in a cloth on the bite area. Elevate the affected part of the body above the level of the heart, and take an oral antihistamine or a pain reliever.

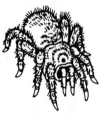

Tarantula

TICK BITES

Ticks can transmit disease-causing organisms from animals to people. The greatest risk for tick bites is May through August. A tick should be removed from the skin very carefully, preferably while wearing rubber gloves. Use tweezers to grasp the tick's head and mouth and pull it out gently but firmly so it stays in one piece. Wash your hands thoroughly with soap and water, and see your doctor. Your doctor may do a blood test to see if you have a Lyme disease infection and to offer follow-up care when appropriate.

Bleeding

In an injury or accident, blood may flow from a vein or an artery or both. Severe bleeding can be serious (call 911 or get to the closest hospital), but most incidents of bleeding are helped by applying direct pressure to the site. Use a thick, clean compress, such as a cloth, handkerchief, towel, undershirt, or strips from a sheet. Apply steady pressure and keep the injured limb elevated, if possible. Although direct pressure may cause some pain, it is usually all that is necessary to stop the bleeding. Cover the wound with a bandage.

Pressure points on the body
Apply pressure to pressure points only if bleeding does not stop after elevating an injured limb and applying direct pressure to the wound itself. Pressing the artery that supplies blood to the wound firmly against the underlying bone can help. Apply pressure only until the bleeding stops. The circled areas on the arteries show the places to apply pressure to control bleeding in specific injured areas of the body. Pressure points are shown on one side of the body only, but arteries and pressure points are the same on both sides of the body.

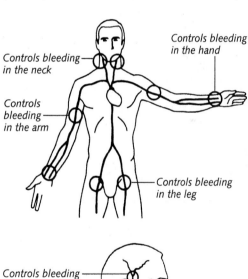

Controls bleeding in the neck

Controls bleeding in the hand

Controls bleeding in the arm

Controls bleeding in the leg

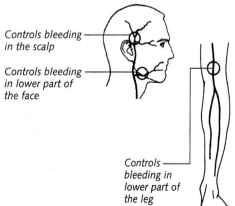

Controls bleeding in the scalp

Controls bleeding in lower part of the face

Controls bleeding in lower part of the leg

Bruises

Bruises occur when a fall or blow causes bleeding into the tissues beneath the skin. Bruises usually fade and change color, disappearing without any treatment in a week to 10 days. Bruises on the head or the shin, where the bone is just under the skin, may swell quite a bit. Place ice wrapped in a cloth over the bruise for about 10 minutes, using steady pressure

Burns

The primary objectives of first aid for serious burns are to relieve the pain, prevent infection, and prevent or treat the person for shock. It is important to first try to decrease the temperature of the burned area, which will help prevent further heat injury to the skin and tissues.

Treating a burn
To lower the temperature of the burned area and stop further skin damage, immediately put the burned area under cool running water or apply cool-water compresses until the pain subsides.

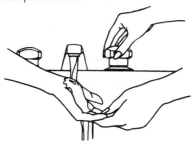

Elevate a burned area
Cover the burn with a nonfluffy sterile or clean bandage to prevent infection. If the burn is on your leg, for example, and the burn is serious, elevate the wrapped leg or foot above your heart to keep blood flowing freely throughout the body and to lessen swelling.

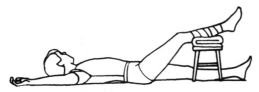

FIRST-DEGREE BURNS

First-degree burns are caused when contact with hot water, steam, or the sun results in the outside layer of the skin being injured. Symptoms include pain, mild swelling, and redness without blisters. If you burn your finger, for example, immediately put it under cool running water or apply a clean, cool, wet compress until the pain decreases. The burn should be covered with a clean bandage, not with butter or grease.

SECOND-DEGREE BURNS

Second-degree burns cause injury to the layers of skin beneath the surface of the body. A serious sunburn, spilled hot liquids, and burns from gasoline can cause second-degree burns and may take up to 3 weeks to heal. The burned area should be cooled as quickly as possibly with cool water until the pain lessens. The purpose of the first aid is to decrease the temperature of the burned skin to limit tissue damage.

THIRD-DEGREE BURNS

Third-degree burns destroy all layers of the skin. Fire, electrical burns, and prolonged contact with hot substances are common causes of third-degree burns. Call 911 or your local emergency number or take the person to the nearest hospital emergency department.

CHEMICAL BURNS

Quickly flush the burned area with a large amount of running water for 5 to 10 minutes. Continue to flush the area with water while removing clothing from the burned area. Cover the burn with a cool, wet dressing, and seek immediate medical attention.

ELECTRICAL BURNS

Electrical burns may appear slight on the surface of the skin but can be severe to underlying tissue. Ordinary household appliances are the cause of most electrical burns, but the burns are seldom serious or fatal. There may not be any signs of external injury, but electrical burns can cause significant internal damage. If you are the first person to help someone who has been electrocuted, however, be careful to avoid touching the person until that person is not in direct contact with the electric current. All electrical burns require immediate medical attention. Call 911 or your local emergency number.

Removing someone from a live wire

Be extremely careful to avoid being electrocuted yourself. Stand on something dry, wear dry gloves if possible, and push the person away from the wire with a dry board, stick, or non-metal tool—or pull the person away with a dry rope looped around the person's arm or leg.

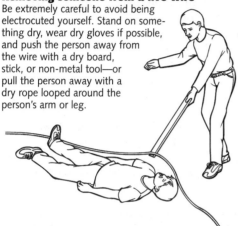

Childbirth

Sometimes childbirth occurs before the due date or labor proceeds more quickly than is typical. If the contractions are 2 to 3 minutes apart and the woman feels the need to push, the baby's head is visible, or the woman cannot get to the hospital in time to deliver, you may find yourself assisting in the childbirth.

If a clean sheet is available, place it on the bed or surface. Try to make the area warm. Wash your hands with soap and water. If possible, sterilize a pair of scissors or a knife with boiling water. Have the woman lie on her back with her knees bent, her feet flat, and her knees and thighs wide apart. Birth is imminent when you see the baby's head. Once the head and shoulders emerge, support the baby's head, but do not pull. The rest of the baby's body will slide out.

Hold the baby with its head lower than its feet, and turn the head sideways to allow fluid to drain from the mouth and nose. Wipe fluid from both, but if breathing does not start within 1 minute, give artificial res-

piration. Wait until the umbilical cord stops pulsating before cutting it. Tie a tight knot with a clean string (preferably sterilized) at least 4 inches from the baby's navel and another knot 2 to 4 inches away. Cut the cord between the two knots with the sterilized scissors or knife.

Within 20 minutes after the baby is born, the placenta (afterbirth) will usually emerge. If bleeding seems heavy, gently massage the woman's lower abdomen until help arrives.

Preparing for delivery

Place clean sheets on the bed. If a bed is not available, place clean cloths, clothes, or newspapers under the mother's hips and thighs on the floor, leaving room for the birth of the baby. Have the mother lie on her back with her knees bent, her feet flat, and her knees and thighs wide apart.

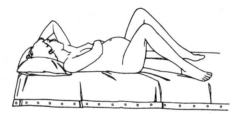

After the delivery

After the baby is born, hold the baby with his or her head lower than the feet so that secretions can drain from the infant's lungs, mouth, and nose. Support the head and body with one hand while grasping the baby's legs and ankles with the other hand.

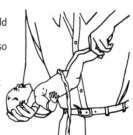

Tying the umbilical cord

To cut the umbilical cord, tie a clean string around the cord at least 4 inches from the baby's body. Tie a tight square knot so that circulation is cut off in the cord. Use a second piece of string to tie another tight square knot 6 to 8 inches from the baby (2 to 4 inches from the first knot). Cut the cord between the two ties.

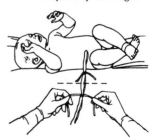

First Aid

Choking (Heimlich maneuver)

The Heimlich maneuver (abdominal thrust) is the method of choice to use when a person is choking. Do not use back blows unless the abdominal thrust is not effective in dislodging the foreign object from the windpipe. A person who is choking will grasp his or her neck and be unable to talk.

Classic maneuver
If the person cannot speak, cough, or breathe, stand behind the person and place your fist with the thumb side against his or her stomach just above the navel and below the ribs and breastbone. Hold your fist with your other hand and give several quick, forceful upward thrusts. This maneuver increases pressure in the abdomen, which pushes up the diaphragm. It may be necessary to repeat this 6 to 10 times.

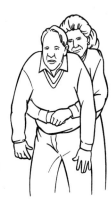

Prone position
If the person is unconscious or becomes unconscious, place the person on his or her back on a rigid surface, such as the ground. Open the person's airway by extending the head backward. Place the palm of your hand on the person's forehead and the fingers of your other hand under the bony part of the chin. Attempt to give mouth-to-mouth resuscitation. (See page 1328.) If unsuccessful, begin the Heimlich maneuver by putting the heel of one hand on the person's stomach slightly above the navel and below the ribs. Put your free hand on top of your other hand to provide additional force. Give several quick forceful downward and forward thrusts toward the head.

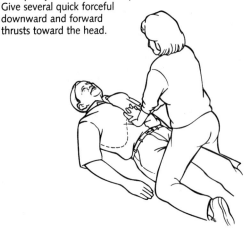

Cuts and scrapes

If a cut is bleeding heavily and the bleeding cannot be stopped after a few minutes of applying pressure to the site, this is a medical emergency and you should get to the closest hospital.

Slight bleeding from a cut or a scrape usually stops on its own within a few minutes. Make sure the cut is washed with warm, soapy water and rinsed thoroughly. If the bleeding does not stop, press a gauze pad or clean cloth firmly over the wound for about 5 to 10 minutes. If the cut is deep, irregular, or on the face or the edges gape and cannot easily be pulled together with bandaging tape, it is best to seek medical help. With any cut or puncture, you should consult with your doctor about whether you need a tetanus shot or antibiotics.

ROLLER GAUZE BANDAGES

A circular bandage is the easiest to apply. It is used on areas that do not vary much in width, such as the wrist, toes, and fingers.

1. Anchor the bandage by placing the end at a slight angle and making several circular turns to hold the end in place. Do not wrap it too tightly.

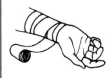

2. Make additional circular turns by overlapping the preceding strip by about three fourths of its width. Continue circling in the same direction until the dressing is completely covered.

3. To secure the bandage, cut the gauze with scissors or a knife and apply adhesive tape or a safety pin to the bandage.

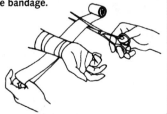

Dehydration

Dehydration, a lack of adequate water in the body, is a medical emergency and can be fatal. Common in infants and elderly people, severe dehydration can occur with vomiting, excessive heat and sweating, diarrhea, or a lack of food or fluid intake. Symptoms of dehydration include extreme thirst, tiredness, light-headedness, abdominal or muscle cramping, dry mouth, and restlessness. A person who is suspected of being dehydrated in extremely hot weather should be moved to a shady or cool area and given water, flat carbonated beverages, an electrolyte-replacement drink, liquid gelatin, or clear broth. If symptoms persist, the person should seek prompt medical attention.

Diabetic coma

Diabetic coma is a life-threatening condition that can occur in people who have diabetes mellitus when the level of the sugar-regulating hormone, insulin, is too low in their blood. Insulin levels may become low when people do not eat properly or miss an injection of insulin or because of infection. Symptoms of diabetic coma come on gradually and include extreme thirst; warm and dry skin; drowsiness; fruity-smelling breath; deep, rapid breathing; dry mouth and tongue; nausea with upper abdominal discomfort; vomiting; confusion; frequent urination; and fast heart rate. Call 911 or your local emergency number, or take the person to the closest hospital.

Diarrhea

Frequent, loose, watery bowel movements (diarrhea) have many causes, most commonly food poisoning, certain medications, viral and bacterial infections, and emotional stress. If the diarrhea is not severe and the person is drinking liquids, the body will replace lost fluids. But if the person cannot or will not drink liquids or is vomiting, replacement of fluids will be impossible and dehydration can occur. Stomach cramping, tiredness, thirst, and blood streaks in or on stools may also be present. A liquid diet (clear broth, flat carbonated beverages, liquid gelatin, electrolyte-replacement drinks) is recommended to replace lost fluids and some body chemicals. If diarrhea persists longer than a day or two, or if urine decreases in frequency and amount, seek medical attention immediately.

Dislocations

A dislocation occurs when the end of a bone is displaced from its joint; it usually is caused by a fall or a blow to the bone. Common areas of dislocations include the shoulder, hip, elbow, fingers, thumb, and kneecap. Symptoms of dislocation include swelling, deformity, pain, discoloration, tenderness, and numbness. If you think you have a dislocated joint, immobilize the area with a splint, pillow, or sling, and get to the nearest hospital.

Ear injuries

All ear injuries, whether earaches, foreign objects inside the ear, or frostbitten ears, should be considered serious, and prompt medical attention should be sought because of the possibility of hearing loss. Symptoms of ear injury include bleeding from inside the ear canal, pain, hearing loss, and dizziness.

EARACHE
One of the most common causes of pain in the ear is an infection of the outer ear caused by a fingernail scratch. Prolonged

First Aid

swimming or swimming in contaminated water also can cause "swimmer's ear." Earaches in the middle ear can follow respiratory infections when germs in the nose and throat move through the eustachian tube to the middle ear. If pain does not go away, you should see a doctor, who may prescribe medication.

FOREIGN OBJECT INSIDE THE EAR

Children often put objects, such as peas, beans, beads, and cotton balls, in their ears. Sometimes, insects get trapped inside the ear. All small objects trapped inside the ear need medical attention for removal.

FROSTBITTEN EARS

Frostbite is freezing of parts of the body by exposure to very cold temperatures. Frostbite occurs when ice crystals form in the fluid inside cells of the skin and other tissues, with the ears being affected more than other parts. Symptoms of frostbite include redness and pain, white or grayish yellow skin, coldness and numbness, blisters, and, in the later stages, an absence of pain. If you think your ears are frostbitten, cover them with extra clothing or a warm cloth. Do not rub the ears, but try to rewarm the ears with warm compresses. Seek medical help immediately.

Eye injuries

FOREIGN OBJECTS IN THE EYE

A foreign object in the eye can cause intense pain, burning, tearing, redness, or sensitivity to light. If the object is embedded in the eye, gently cover both eyes (because when one eye moves, so does the other) with a sterile dressing and tape it tightly in place without applying pressure. Immediately seek medical attention. Transport the person lying flat on his or her back if possible.

If the object is resting or floating on the eye or inside the eyelid, wash your hands before examining the eye. Do not allow the person to rub the eye or remove contact

lenses. Gently pull the upper eyelid over the lower lid for a moment to cause tears to flow. This may wash out the particle. If that does not work, fill a medicine dropper with water and squeeze water over the eye (or use a shower, low-pressure hose, or pitcher of water) to flush out the particle. If the object is still there, lift the lids and if the object is visible, gently lift it out with a moist clean cloth or tissue. If the particle remains, gently cover the affected eye with a clean compress and seek medical attention promptly.

REMOVING A PARTICLE FROM THE EYE

1. To remove a particle resting on the inside of the upper lid, have the person look down as you hold the lashes of the upper eyelid and pull the eyelid upward.

2. While holding the eyelid, place a cotton-tipped swab across the back of the lid and flip the eyelid backward over it.

3. Carefully remove the particle with a moistened, clean cloth or tissue.

CHEMICAL BURNS OF THE EYE

Chemical burns of the eye are very serious and may lead to blindness if immediate action is not taken. Acids, drain cleaner, bleach, and other cleaning solutions are some chemical agents that can burn the eye. Speed in removal of the chemical agent is vital as damage can occur within 1 to 5 minutes.

If the person wears contact lenses, they should be removed immediately and the eyes flushed with large quantities of cool, running water for at least 10 minutes to rinse out the chemical agent. If water is not available, milk can be used. With the person's head under a faucet (or shower, low-pressure hose, or pitcher of water) and eyes open, allow the water to run from the inside corner of the eye outward to prevent the chemical from getting into the unaffected eye. If both eyes are affected, alternate between eyes. Be sure to lift the eyelids so the water reaches all affected areas. As an alternative, have the person submerge the eyes in a bowl of water and move the eyelids up and down. After rinsing the affected eye, cover with a sterile gauze pad or clean cloth and tape the pad or cloth in place with the eye closed. The person should not rub the eye. Medical treatment should be sought at the nearest emergency department.

BLOWS TO THE EYE

Any injury resulting from a direct blow to the eye requires medical attention, even if the injury does not appear serious, because there could be internal bleeding. A black eye takes roughly 2 to 3 weeks to clear up.

If the person is wearing contact lenses, do not remove them. A physician should remove the person's contact lenses as soon as possible. Apply a cold compress to the eye, and have the person lie down with eyes closed and head elevated. Seek immediate medical attention.

EYE INFECTION

There are several different types of eye infections, but if you have pain, redness, blurred vision, or itching, you should see a doctor who will diagnose and treat the condition. Some eye problems can be treated at home. A stye, an inflammation of the glands on the edge of the eyelid, can usually be treated with warm compresses, but if it persists, medical care should be sought. Conjunctivitis, also called pinkeye, is a contagious infection that needs to be treated with prescribed medication, so a trip to the doctor is in order. Symptoms include redness or pinkness in the white portion of the eye and a discharge, sometimes sticky, from the eye.

CUTS TO THE EYE

Any cuts to the eye or eyelid can be very serious and could lead to blindness if immediate action is not taken. Do not remove contact lenses; a physician should remove them as soon as possible. Gently cover both eyes (because when one eye moves, so does the other) with a sterile dressing and tape it tightly in place without applying pressure. Immediately seek medical attention. Transport the person lying flat on his or her back if possible.

Fainting

Fainting is a brief loss of consciousness caused by a reduced blood supply to the brain. A fainting episode is usually over within a few minutes and is rarely, in itself, serious, except when a person faints and is not breathing. Then you need to call 911 or your local emergency number. Sometimes fainting occurs during the first 5 days of hot weather, before a person's body adjusts to the heat. Symptoms include pale, cool, and wet skin; light-headedness or dizziness; nausea; restlessness; and frequent yawning. If you feel faint, lie down with your legs elevated about a foot, or sit down and slowly bend your body so that your head is between your knees. If you think the spell is caused by hot weather, get to a cool place and drink plenty of fluids to prevent dehydration.

Fever

A fever is your body's way of telling you that something is wrong, usually that an infection is present. You should always call your doctor if a fever changes from slight (99°F to 100°F) to high (104°F) and persists. That is true for a child as well, who should be seen by a doctor without delay if the high fever persists. If you have a persistent fever and no obvious reasons for it, do not take any medication to reduce the fever because it can mask the symptoms or give you a false sense of well-being. Most mild fevers respond well to aspirin (but do not give aspirin to children younger than 18 years), acetaminophen, ibuprofen, or naproxen.

Fishhook injuries

A fishhook caught in the body is a common injury. The fishhook should be removed by a doctor if possible. If only the point of the hook and not the barb entered the skin, you can remove the hook by carefully pulling it out. Never attempt to remove a fishhook caught in the eye or face. Seek medical help immediately.

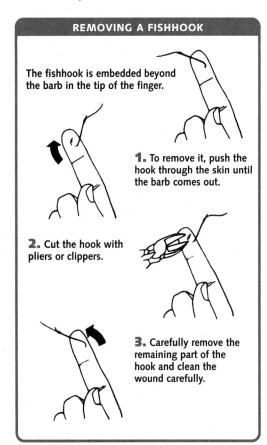

REMOVING A FISHHOOK

The fishhook is embedded beyond the barb in the tip of the finger.

1. To remove it, push the hook through the skin until the barb comes out.

2. Cut the hook with pliers or clippers.

3. Carefully remove the remaining part of the hook and clean the wound carefully.

Food poisoning

If several people become ill with similar symptoms at about the same time after eating the same food, suspect food poisoning. Or you may suspect food poisoning if one person becomes ill after eating food no one else has eaten. Food poisoning typically begins suddenly, usually with stomach pain, vomiting, and diarrhea within 48 hours of eating the tainted food. Most cases are the result of contamination of food by bacteria or viruses.

BOTULISM

The most serious form of food poisoning, botulism is a true medical emergency because it is often fatal. Botulism most often occurs after eating improperly home-canned foods but can also occur after eating store-bought frozen foods, including pot pies, asparagus, green beans, and peppers. Botulism has also been found in seafood, including salmon, seal, walrus, and whale meat. Symptoms, which appear within 6 to 72 hours, include dry mouth, dizziness, headache, blurred vision, muscle weakness, and difficulty swallowing, talking, and breathing. If you suspect botulism, get to the nearest hospital immediately.

ESCHERICHIA COLI (E. COLI) INFECTIONS

Escherichia coli, often associated with eating contaminated ground beef, can cause severe, bloody diarrhea and abdominal cramps that can be fatal. Other possible causes include unpasteurized milk or milk products and unpasteurized fruit juice. Some outbreaks of *E. coli* infections have been linked to contaminated soil, sand, modeling clay, and leaking of a soiled diaper into a swimming pool. Severe infections with *E. coli* can damage the kidneys, heart, lungs, and central nervous system. Children under 5 years and the elderly are at the highest risk for severe infection. Seek prompt medical attention if you think you may have an *E. coli* infection.

MUSHROOM POISONING

Mushroom poisoning occurs after a person eats wild mushrooms. Symptoms, which can appear within minutes to more than 24 hours later, depend on the type of mushroom eaten, but often include abdominal pain, diarrhea, vomiting, difficulty breathing, sweating, dizziness, hallucinations, seizures, hepatitis, and muscle spasms. Seek medical attention immediately.

SALMONELLA POISONING

Salmonella poisoning usually occurs during the summer after eating fresh foods that have been contaminated with *Salmonella* bacteria. Foods most commonly affected include eggs, milk, raw meats, raw poultry, and raw fish. Salmonella poisoning can be very serious in infants, young children, elderly people, and chronically ill people. *Salmonella* bacteria can be destroyed by cooking foods properly. Symptoms of poisoning include abdominal cramps, diarrhea, fever, chills, vomiting, headache, weakness, and watery or foul smelling stools. See a doctor for proper diagnosis and treatment.

STAPHYLOCOCCUS POISONING

Staphylococcus poisoning occurs most often from eating foods that have not been properly refrigerated. The most common foods affected include meats, poultry, eggs, milk, cream-filled bakery goods, salami, sausage, ham, tongue, and tuna and potato salads. Staphylococcus poisoning can cause abdominal cramps, nausea, vomiting, and diarrhea, usually within 1 to 6 hours after eating the contaminated food. Seek medical attention if the symptoms persist for more than 1 day or if symptoms become severe.

Fractures (broken bones)

A break or crack in a bone is called a fracture, which may be closed or open. A broken bone that does not come through the skin is a closed fracture; an open fracture has an open wound that extends down to the bone or the bone sticks out through the skin. An open break is usually more serious because of severe bleeding and the greater possibility of infection. If you think you have broken a bone, do not move, especially if the injury is on the head, neck, or spine. If a person has a head injury, neck pain, or tingling or paralysis in the arms or legs, do not move the person—suspect a broken neck or spinal injury. If you or someone with you has a closed break, try to immobilize the broken bone and splint it to keep it from moving, thereby easing pain and preventing the break from becoming worse. If the fracture is severe or is an open break, call 911 or your local emergency number.

SPLINTING FOR KNEE-CAP INJURY

If the leg is numb below the level of the injury, if the person is unable to walk or extend the leg, if the skin under the toenail is blue, or if the person has an open wound, get to the nearest hospital emergency department. If the person does not have any of these symptoms, you should try to immobilize the leg before transporting the person to the hospital or doctor's office.

1. Gently straighten the person's injured leg, if necessary. Place a padded board at least 4 inches wide underneath the injured leg. The board should be long enough to reach from the person's heel to the buttocks. Place extra padding under the ankle and knee.

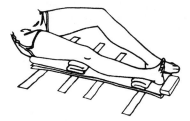

2. Tie the splint in place at the ankle, just below and above the knee, and at the thigh. Do not tie over the kneecap.

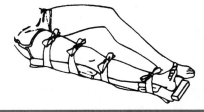

First Aid

Any suspected fracture needs to be evaluated by a doctor. After immobilizing a broken bone, take the person immediately to a hospital emergency department.

1. Carefully place the lower arm at a right angle to the person's chest with the palm facing toward the chest and the thumb pointing upward.

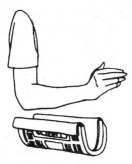

2. Apply a padded splint on each side of the lower arm, or use folded, padded newspapers or magazines wrapped under and around both sides of the arm. The splint should reach from the elbow to well beyond the wrist. Tie the splint in place above and below the break.

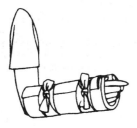

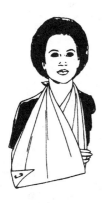

3. Support the lower arm with a wide sling tied around the neck. The sling should be placed so that the fingers are slightly higher (3 to 4 inches) than the level of the elbow.

Frostbite

Frostbite is the freezing of parts of the body by exposure to very low temperatures and occurs when ice crystals form in the fluid of skin and other tissue cells. Most often the toes, fingers, nose, and ears are affected. You are more susceptible to frostbite when exposed to cold, windy weather after consuming alcohol or if you get your skin wet while out in such weather.

In you think you have frostbite, cover the frozen areas with extra clothing or a warm cloth. Hands or fingers can be put under the armpits for extra warmth. Promptly seek shelter and remove wet, cold, and constricting clothing from the frostbitten area. Rewarm the frostbitten area using lukewarm water for a half hour, or if you cannot use warm water, gently wrap the frostbitten areas in blankets or other warm, dry materials. Put sterile gauze or a clean towel between your fingers and toes to keep them separated, and, if possible, elevate the affected parts. Do not try to rewarm the skin with stoves or heaters. When the skin returns to its normal color and feeling comes back, you can stop the warming process. After feeling comes back, move the affected parts to increase circulation and then seek medical attention promptly.

Head injuries

All head injuries must be taken seriously because they can result in brain or spinal cord damage or even death. If a person is found unconscious, assume a head and neck injury has occurred until medical personnel determine otherwise. Most head injuries are caused by a fall, a blow to the head, a collision, or stopping suddenly, as in an automobile collision. Anyone with a head injury may also have a neck injury. Symptoms may include cuts or bruises on the scalp, unconsciousness, confusion, or drowsiness; bleeding from the nose, ear, or mouth; pale or reddish face; headache; vomiting; seizures; pupils of unequal size; difficulty speaking; change in pulse rate; and restlessness or confused behavior. Call 911 or your local emergency number and keep the person lying down, quiet, and comfortably warm until medical help arrives. Do not give the person anything by mouth. Control serious bleeding by compressing the affected area.

IMMOBILIZING A BROKEN NECK

1. Carefully wrap a towel, sweater, newspaper, or some other cushioned item, about 4 inches wide, around the person's neck, keeping the head as still as possible.

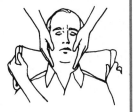

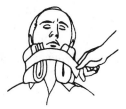

2. Tie the wrap in place, being careful not to interfere with the person's breathing.

3. If the person is being rescued from an automobile or from water, place a board behind the person's head and neck to avoid twisting the neck when moving the person. The board should extend at least to the person's buttocks. If possible, tie the board to the person's body around the forehead and under the armpits. Move the person slowly and gently.

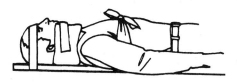

Heart attack

A heart attack is a life-threatening emergency. A heart attack occurs when there is not enough blood and oxygen reaching a portion of the heart because of narrowing or obstruction of the arteries that supply the heart muscle. A prolonged lack of blood and oxygen can cause part of the heart muscle to die, or it can trigger an abnormal heartbeat that can be fatal. The sooner a person having a heart attack receives medical treatment, the less damage the heart is likely to undergo and the better the prognosis. Symptoms include central chest pain or chest tightness that is constant, severe, and crushing (not sharp) and lasts for several minutes; chest pain that moves to either arm or shoulder or to the neck, jaw, mid-back, or stomach; profuse sweating; nausea and vomiting; extreme weakness; anxiety and fearfulness; pale skin; blue fingernails and lips; extreme shortness of breath; and dizziness or fainting. If aspirin is available and the person is not allergic to it, give the person one tablet to help prevent the formation of blood clots. Call 911 or your local emergency number and get help immediately. See also RESUSCITATION, page 1328.

Heat cramps

Heat cramps are muscle pains, spasms, and possibly seizures that are caused by the loss of salt from the body because of profuse sweating—usually brought on by strenuous activity in the heat. Typically, the stomach and leg muscles are affected first. Heat cramps may also be symptoms of heat exhaustion. If you have heat cramps, sit quietly in a cool place. You may sip a sports drink, clear juice, or cool salt water (¼ to ½ teaspoon of table salt or two to four 10-grain salt tablets dissolved in 4 cups of water). Do not take undissolved salt tablets. Try to drink half a glass of liquid every 15 minutes for 1 hour. Stop drinking fluids if vomiting occurs, and seek medical attention.

First Aid

Heat exhaustion

Heat exhaustion can occur after prolonged (about 3 to 5 days) exposure to high temperatures and high humidity. Symptoms include above normal body temperature, pale and clammy skin, heavy sweating, tiredness or weakness, headache, nausea, cramps, vomiting, fainting, and a fast heart rate. Seek shade or a cooler area and lie down. Raise your feet 8 to 12 inches and loosen your clothing. You may try drinking a sports drink, clear juice, or cool salt water (¼ to ½ teaspoon of table salt or two to four 10-grain salt tablets dissolved in 4 cups of water). Place cool wet cloths on your forehead and body, use a fan to cool yourself, or place ice packs on the neck, armpits, and groin. If symptoms are severe, worsen, or last longer than 1 hour, seek medical attention promptly.

Heat stroke

Heat stroke (also called sunstroke) is a life-threatening medical emergency. It is a disturbance in the body's heat-regulating system caused by an extremely high body temperature and the body's inability to cool itself. Heat stroke can cause a very high body temperature, rapid and strong pulse, unconsciousness or confusion, fast breathing, vomiting and diarrhea, seizures, and incoordination.

If you think someone has heat stroke, undress the person and get the person into a tub of cool water if possible. Otherwise, the person can be cooled with water, fanning, and ice packs applied to the person's neck, armpits, and groin. Continue treatment until the body temperature is lowered to 101°F or 102°F. The person should not take aspirin, acetaminophen, or other pain relievers or drink alcoholic beverages or stimulants (such as coffee or tea). After the temperature has lowered, dry off the person and place the person in front of a fan or air conditioner. Take the person to the nearest hospital emergency department or call your local emergency number.

Hyperventilation

Hyperventilation is breathing faster and more deeply than normal because of tension or emotional upset. The person feels as if he or she is not getting enough air into the lungs. Because of feeling out of breath, the person increases breathing in an attempt to take in more air. As rapid breathing continues, the level of carbon dioxide in the blood is lowered, causing muscle tightness in the throat and chest, which further aggravates the symptoms. A person may feel light-headed and may have numbness and tingling in the hands and feet and around the mouth and lips, tightness in the throat, muscle twitching, and difficulty getting a deep, "satisfying" breath. A seizure may occur. Encourage a person who is hyperventilating to relax and try to breathe slowly and easily. Breathing into a paper bag may be helpful. Seek medical attention if breathing does not return to normal. The person should see a doctor to determine the underlying cause of the hyperventilation.

Hypoglycemia

Hypoglycemia occurs when a person has an abnormally low level of glucose (sugar) in the blood. It may be caused by taking too much insulin, alcohol use, or drug effects. Not eating a regular meal, especially breakfast, can also cause the condition. Symptoms include bizarre behavior, amnesia, seizures, profuse sweating, tremors, and a fast heart rate. If the person is becoming lethargic but is relatively alert, give him or her a candy bar or glass of juice. If a person has hypoglycemia caused by oral antidiabetic medications, the person should seek medical attention (in addition to eating candy or drinking juice) because the low blood sugar level can be present for several hours.

Hypothermia

Hypothermia is chilling of the entire body to a temperature of less than 95°F. Hypothermia may be caused by immersion in very cold water, prolonged exposure to extremely cold weather, or wearing damp clothing in very cold conditions. Symptoms can include shivering, numbness, drowsiness or sleepiness, muscle weakness, dizziness, nausea, low body temperature, unconsciousness, a weak, slow pulse, and large pupils.

If hypothermia occurs, call 911 or your local emergency number. Maintain an open airway for the person, and restore breathing and circulation if necessary. (See page 1328.) Bring the person into a warm room and remove any wet clothes. Have the person lie down, and wrap him or her in blankets, towels, or additional clothes. If the person is conscious, give warm, nonalcoholic beverages, and check for and treat frostbite.

Poisoning

If you think you or someone with you has ingested poisonous chemicals, call the poison center, hospital emergency department, a doctor, or 911 (or your local emergency number) for instructions before doing anything. Never induce vomiting without first talking to a medical specialist. And do not give another liquid to try to neutralize the poison. When calling for help, give the person's age and the name of the poison and state how much was swallowed, when the poison was swallowed, whether the person has vomited, and how much time it will take to get the person to a medical facility.

Poisoning, carbon monoxide

Carbon monoxide, a colorless, odorless, tasteless gas, is a common cause of poisoning death. Most accidental cases occur in the home during the winter months when people are sleeping; these cases can be prevented by installing electronic carbon monoxide detectors on each floor of your home. The gas is also present in the exhaust of motor vehicles. Sources in the home include faulty forced-air gas furnaces, unventilated space heaters, poorly ventilated fireplaces, and cooking indoors with grills meant for outdoors. If you think someone has carbon monoxide poisoning, get the person into fresh air and call 911 or your local emergency number immediately.

Rape/sexual assault

Rape is usually defined as forced vaginal or anal intercourse, oral sex, or penetration with an object. Sexual assault is a term used in many states instead of rape. If you have been raped, call the police immediately to report the crime. Next, call a relative, friend, or rape hotline. Then call your doctor or get to the closest hospital emergency department.

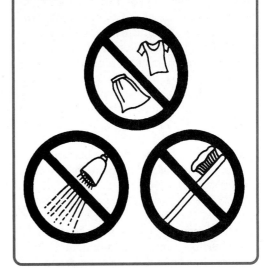

IF A RAPE HAS OCCURRED

Do not allow the person who has been raped to change clothes, take a shower, or brush his or her teeth.

Do not take a shower, bathe, wash, brush your teeth, or eat or drink anything. The doctor will want to take samples from your mouth, vagina, and rectum to test for and treat sexually transmitted infections such as chlamydia, gonorrhea, syphilis, and HIV (human immunodeficiency virus). The police will most likely want to collect physical evidence of the assault for prosecution. Special sexual assault counseling will be available.

Resuscitation (CPR)

Resuscitation is the attempt to restore breathing and, if necessary, blood circulation in a person. This is done by mouth-to-mouth, mouth-to-nose, or mouth-to-mouth-and-nose respirations and by chest compressions.

Cardiopulmonary resuscitation (CPR) is a basic life-support technique used for a person who is not breathing and whose heart may have stopped beating. CPR involves opening and clearing the person's airway (by tilting the head backward and lifting the chin), restoring breathing (by mouth-to-mouth, mouth-to-nose, or mouth-to-mouth-and-nose resuscitation), and restoring blood circulation (by external chest compressions). A simple method of remembering the order of action to take in an emergency (the person is not breathing or his or her heart is not beating) is ABC, which stands for Airway, Breathing, and Circulation—the three basic steps in CPR. You need to open and clear the person's airway, restore breathing, and restore blood circulation.

AIRWAY
Make sure the airway is clear. Listen for signs of breathing and air escaping. Feel for the pulse.

BREATHING
Pinch the person's nose shut, take a breath, seal your lips around the mouth, and blow. Your breath contains enough oxygen for the person's needs.

MOUTH-TO-MOUTH RESUSCITATION

Here is a summary of the four steps to restore breathing in a person who has stopped breathing.

1. Make sure the person is on a hard, flat surface. Quickly clear the mouth and airway of foreign material.

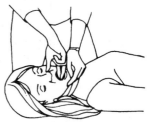

2. Tilt the person's head backward by placing the palm of your hand on his or her forehead and the fingers of your other hand under the bony part of the chin.

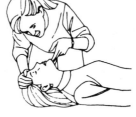

3. Pinch the person's nostrils with your thumb and index finger. Take a deep breath. Place your mouth tightly over the person's mouth (mouth and nose for an infant younger than 1 year). Give two full breaths.

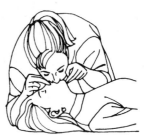

4. Stop blowing when you notice the person's chest expanding. Remove your mouth from the person's mouth and turn your head toward the person's chest, so that your ear is over his or her mouth. Listen for air being exhaled. Watch for the person's chest to rise and fall. Repeat the breathing procedure.

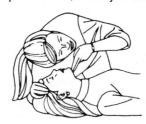

POSITION FOR CHEST COMPRESSIONS

In emergency situations, restoring circulation for the person is essential for survival, and chest compressions, outlined below, should be attempted.

1. Make sure the person is lying on a hard, flat surface, with the head at the same level as the rest of the body or slightly lower. If possible, slightly elevate the legs, which will help blood flow back to the heart. Kneel near the person's chest, and, with two fingers, locate his or her rib cage on the side closest to you. Move your fingers up to where the ribs meet the breastbone. Place the heel of your other hand two finger-widths above your fingers.

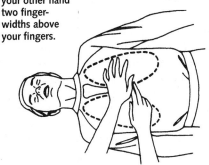

2. Remove your fingers from the notch of the breastbone and put them on top of your other hand. Interlace the fingers of both hands. Do not allow your fingers to rest on the ribs: press down with the heel of your hand only.

3. While kneeling, position your shoulders directly over the person so that all of your weight is applied, through the heel of your hand, onto the person's chest. Straighten your arms and lock your elbows. Use your arms to exert pressure. Push down on the chest 15 times to a depth of about 2 inches. Let the chest rise after each compression. Pinch the person's nostrils shut and blow two slow, full breaths into the person's mouth so that the chest rises. Repeat the cycle of 15 compressions and two breaths until you have performed four complete cycles. Check to see if the person's pulse has returned.

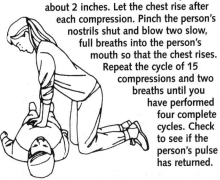

CIRCULATION

If breathing does not restart and you cannot detect a pulse or heart beat, start cardiac compression. Press with the heel of one hand placed on top of the other. The pressure should be applied at the lower part of the breastbone, at a rate of about 80 compressions per minute, with two breaths given after every 15 compressions.

AUTOMATED EXTERNAL DEFIBRILLATOR

Portable defibrillators are lifesaving devices used on commercial airplanes, in airports, and in other community settings to treat sudden cardiac arrest, a condition triggered by an electrical malfunction of the heart. Defibrillation can restore a person's normal heart rhythm if administered within the first few minutes following cardiac arrest. The AED device, approved by the Food and Drug Administration, is battery operated and allows a trained responder to place two pads on the person's chest to deliver an electrical shock that triggers a normal heart rhythm to resume. The American Heart Association estimates that as many as 100,000 deaths could be prevented yearly through prompt use of defibrillators.

Seizures

Seizures, or convulsions, result from a disturbance in the electrical activity of the brain, which causes a series of uncontrollable muscle movements. Seizures, which usually last from 1 to 2 minutes and can be caused by many conditions, injuries, or diseases, may cause the person to be totally or partially unconsciousness; breathing may also stop temporarily. A seizure is a medical emergency unless the person having it is known to have epilepsy and is being treated for it. Even then, if the seizure lasts more than 5 minutes, call 911 or your local emergency number, or get the person to a doctor.

Shock

Shock is a life-threatening situation in which the body's vital functions, such as breathing and heartbeat, are seriously

First Aid

threatened by not enough blood reaching body tissues in the lungs, the brain, and the heart. Shock can be caused by a serious injury, a heart attack, spinal injury, persistent vomiting or diarrhea, perforation of an organ, poisoning, a severe allergic reaction, or a bacterial infection in the blood. If you suspect a person is in shock, call 911 or your local emergency number or take the person to the nearest hospital.

ANAPHYLACTIC SHOCK

Anaphylactic shock is caused by a life-threatening allergic reaction to an insect sting, a medication, or food. Symptoms can include weakness, coughing and wheezing, difficulty breathing, severe itching or hives, stomach cramps, nausea and vomiting, anxiety, a bluish tinge to the skin, dizziness, collapse, unconsciousness, and a weak pulse. Call 911 or your local emergency number if you suspect anaphylactic shock. If the person has a known allergy, he or she may have an anaphylaxis emergency kit, which will include an injection of adrenaline. If the kit is not available, an oral antihistamine, such as diphenhydramine (Benadryl), may be of some use. But the person needs to get medical assistance immediately.

SHOCK FROM SEVERE INJURY

Shock can occur with injuries that result in a heavy loss of blood or too little oxygen reaching the lungs. Symptoms from a severe injury can include pale or bluish and cool skin, moist and clammy skin, overall weakness, rapid pulse, increased rate of breathing, restlessness, anxiety, unusual thirst, vomiting, sunken eyes, blotchy or streaked skin, and, in severe cases, unconsciousness. With any case of shock, it is best to call 911 or your local emergency number and to try to keep the person calm while waiting for help.

INSULIN SHOCK

Insulin shock can occur in people who have diabetes mellitus when there is too little glucose (sugar) in the blood. The condition arises when the person takes too much insulin or eats too little food after taking insulin or other antidiabetic medications. Symptoms of insulin shock, which can come on suddenly, include hunger, pale and sweaty skin, excited or belligerent behavior, and shallow breathing. If the person is unconscious, seek medical attention immediately. If the person is conscious, give him or her food containing sugar, such as fruit juice, sweetened drinks, honey, or just sugar in water.

SEPTIC SHOCK

Septic shock is a life-threatening condition in which the body's tissues and vital organs are unable to use nutrients from the blood. This form of shock is brought on by an infection in the bloodstream, usually caused by bacteria. Septic shock can cause light-headedness, fainting, and weakness. If you think you have septic shock, call 911 or your local emergency number or get to the nearest hospital emergency department.

STREPTOCOCCAL TOXIC SHOCK–LIKE SYNDROME

Streptococcal toxic shock–like syndrome is a severe infection that is fatal in about one third of the people who have it. The infection is caused by a virulent form of streptococcal bacteria, which is sometimes referred to as "flesh-eating bacteria" because the skin and muscle can be destroyed rapidly. Symptoms include sudden fever, shaking chills, muscle pain, confusion, fast heart rate, pain in the arms or legs, vomiting, headache, mild redness of the skin, or a local rash that progresses into blisters or develops a bluish color. Emergency medical treatment is required.

TOXIC SHOCK SYNDROME

Toxic shock syndrome is a serious, rare infection caused by staphylococcal bacteria. Toxins produced by the bacteria enter the bloodstream and are spread throughout the body. Toxic shock syndrome restricts the supply of oxygenated blood that reaches body tissues, which can be fatal. Toxic shock syndrome was previously associated with the use of high-absorbency tampons (no longer on the market). Most cases now are caused by packing around wounds, such as nosebleeds; the wound becomes infected for unknown reasons. Symptoms include sudden fever, vomiting, diarrhea, light-headedness or dizziness, aching muscles and joints, headache, weak pulse, fainting, weakness, and rash. If you think you have toxic shock syndrome or suspect it in someone else, call 911 or your local emergency number or go to the nearest hospital emergency department.

Splinters

A splinter (also called a sliver) can be a small piece of wood, glass, or other material that becomes lodged under the surface of the skin, usually on a finger or in the foot. Make sure you wash your hands and the area around the splinter before trying to remove it. Then, follow the steps outlined in the illustration. If you cannot remove the splinter, it is best to see a doctor.

REMOVING A SPLINTER

1. Before trying to remove a splinter, wash the area with soap and water. Then, take a sewing needle and tweezers and sterilize the instru- 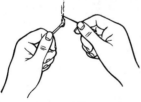 ments by holding them over an open flame or by placing them in boiling water for about 5 minutes.

2. If the splinter is sticking out of the skin, gently pull it out with the tweezers at the same angle at which it entered. If the splinter is not sticking out but is not deeply lodged, 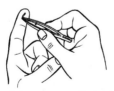 gently loosen the skin around the splinter with the needle and carefully remove the splinter with the tweezers. Squeeze the wound gently to allow slight bleeding to help wash out germs, or rinse the site under running water for at least 5 minutes. If the splinter is deeply embedded, seek medical help.

Strains and sprains

A strain is caused by pulling or overexerting a muscle. Back strains are common injuries that cause a dull pain in the affected muscle that worsens with movement. There may also be swelling. Rest the affected area immediately and apply ice (wrapped in a towel) or a cold compress to the area (30 minutes on, 30 minutes off) to decrease swelling during the first 24 hours after the injury. After 24 hours, apply warm, wet compresses to the area. Try to elevate the

Rest and ice
Treat a sprain with RICE: Rest, Ice, Compression, and Elevation. First, rest the ankle or wrist, preferably raised and on a cushion, with a bag of ice (wrapped in a towel) over the sore or swollen portion.

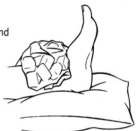

Compression
Rolling a bandage around a swollen or sore ankle helps keep the injured part from moving and helps keep down swelling. Be careful not to make the bandage too tight.

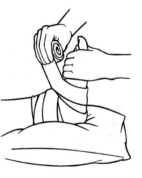

Elevation
Keeping an injured leg or ankle elevated keeps blood flowing freely throughout the body and helps to lessen swelling.

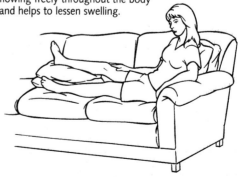

APPLYING A FIGURE-EIGHT BANDAGE

A figure-eight bandage is useful for the ankle, wrist, or hand. Be careful not to wrap the bandage too tightly.

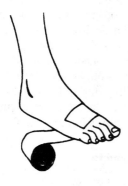

1. To make the figure eight, bring the bandage across and under the foot, diagonally across the top of the foot, around the ankle, down across the top of the foot, and under the arch.

2. Continue these figure-eight turns, with each turn overlapping the preceding turn at about three fourths of its width. Bandage until the foot (not the toes), ankle, and lower part of the leg are covered. Secure the bandage with a clip or safety pin. Keep the toes exposed to help avoid circulation problems.

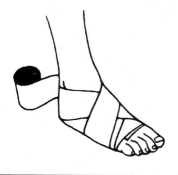

strained area above the level of the heart. Seek medical attention if the pain or swelling is severe.

A sprain is an injury to the ligaments, those strong, flexible bands of fibrous tissue that bind bones together and support the joints. A ligament may be stretched or completely torn. A sprain is usually caused by overextending or twisting a limb beyond its normal range of movement. Symptoms include a popping sound or tearing sensation at the time of the injury and pain when trying to move the injured part. The joint may be swollen and tender to the touch, and there may be black and blue discoloration of the skin around the injured area. If you are uncertain whether an injury is a sprain or a broken bone, treat it as a broken bone and see a doctor immediately. If the ankle or knee is sprained, place cold packs over the area (30 minutes on, 30 minutes off) for the first 12 to 24 hours to decrease swelling. Do not use heat or hot water soaks for the first 24 hours after the injury. Apply a supporting bandage, pillow, or blanket to splint the injury, and keep the injured leg elevated above the level of the heart. Avoid walking. After 24 hours, apply heat to the area and soak it in warm water periodically for several minutes at a time.

If the wrist, elbow, or shoulder is sprained, place the injured arm in a sling. For a wrist injury, apply a supporting bandage but loosen it if swelling increases. Place cold packs or a small ice bag wrapped in a cloth over the affected area for the first 24 hours. Do not use heat or hot water soaks during the first 24 hours following the injury. Seek medical care to rule out a broken bone.

Stroke

A stroke is caused by an interruption in blood flow to part or all of the brain. If you suspect a stroke, call 911 or your local emergency number immediately because the sooner treatment is received, the more successful it will be in preventing or reversing any brain damage.

Symptoms of a stroke include a sudden headache or sudden paralysis, weakness, or numbness on one side of the body. The corner of the mouth may droop, and the person may have slurred speech or loss of speech. Other symptoms include mental confusion, dizziness, or unconsciousness; a fall due to sudden weakness; impaired or double vision; pupils of different size; difficulty breathing, chewing, talking, and swallowing; loss of bladder or bowel control; and a strong, slow pulse.

After medical help is sought, try to maintain an open airway for the person, and

restore breathing and circulation if necessary. See Resuscitation (CPR) on page 1328. Do not give fluids or food to the person, and try to keep the person warm and quiet as you apply cool cloths to the person's head.

STROKE SYMPTOMS? GET HELP NOW!

If you think you or someone near you may be having a stroke, call 911 or your local emergency number without delay. The sooner treatment starts, the more successful you will be in preventing or reversing any possible brain damage.

Stroke symptoms typically occur suddenly, and include weakness or numbness of the face, arm, or leg; severe headache; vision trouble; confusion, trouble speaking or difficulty understanding; or trouble walking, dizziness, loss of balance, or loss of coordination.

Sunburn

Sunburn is usually a first-degree burn of the skin caused by overexposure to the sun, especially in people with fair complexions. Prolonged sun exposure can cause second-degree burns. The peak hours for sunburn, when the ultraviolet rays from the sun are most harmful, are between 10 AM and 3 PM. Sunburn symptoms include redness, pain, mild swelling, blisters, and itching.

If you get sunburned, put cool water on the affected area. If the sunburn is severe, submerge the area under cold water until the pain is relieved. Placing cold, wet towels on the affected area is also helpful. Elevate the affected area, and, if possible, apply sterile bandages on severely sunburned areas. For severe sunburn, seek medical attention. Do not use medications or home remedies on severe sunburns.

First Aid

Sample legal form

In the event you lose the ability to make health care decisions for yourself, advance directives give you the opportunity to specify how you would like those decisions made. A living will and durable power of attorney for health care are the two most commonly prepared advance directives. A living will typically specifies the type of medical care you want if you lose the ability to make your own decisions. It is called a living will because it takes effect while you are still living. Durable power of attorney for health care names another person, such as a wife, husband, partner, son, daughter, or friend, as your authorized agent to make medical decisions for you if you lose the ability to make them for yourself. It is possible to combine a living will and durable power of attorney for health care into a single document, as in the sample form provided here.

This health care advance directive form was designed by the American Medical Association (AMA), the American Bar Association (ABA), and the American Association of Retired Persons (AARP). Even though it has been created to comply with laws in all 50 states, it may not meet the specific legal requirements of each particular state. This is not legal advice and should not be construed as such. Therefore, while legal counsel is not required to prepare an advance directive, you may wish to contact an attorney regarding the law in your state.

Health Care Advance Directive

Caution: This health care advance directive is a general form provided for your convenience. While it meets the legal requirements of most states, it may or may not fit the requirements of your particular state. Many states have special forms or special procedures for creating health care advance directives. Even if your state's law does not clearly recognize this document, it may still provide an effective statement of your wishes if you cannot speak for yourself.

PART 1: APPOINTMENT OF HEALTH CARE AGENT

Section 1: Health Care Agent

Print your full name here as the "principal" or creator of the health care advance directive.

Print the full name, address and telephone number of the person (age 18 or older) you appoint as your health care agent. Appoint only a person with whom you have talked and whom you trust to understand and carry out your values and wishes.

Many states limit the persons who can serve as your agent. If you want to meet all existing state restrictions, do not name any of the following as your agent, since some states will not let them act in that role:

- *Your health care providers, including physicians*
- *Staff of health care facilities or nursing facilities providing your care; guardians of your finances (also called conservators)*
- *Employees of government agencies financially responsible for your care*
- *Any person serving as agent for ten or more persons*

_____

I, Principal

hereby appoint

_____

    Health Care Agent's Name

_____

    Address

_____

    Home Telephone Number   Work Telephone Number

as my agent to make health and personal care decisions for me as authorized in this document.

Section 2: Alternate Agents

It is a good idea to name alternate agents in case your first agent is not available. Of course, only appoint alternates if you fully trust them to act faithfully as your agent and you have talked to them about serving as your agent. Print the appropriate information in this paragraph. You can name as many alternate agents as you wish, but place them in the order you wish them to serve.

If I revoke my Agent's authority; or my Agent becomes unwilling or unavailable to act; or if my agent is my spouse and I become legally separated or divorced, I name the following (each to act alone and successively, in the order named) as alternates to my Agent:

_____

A. First Alternate Agent

_____

Address

_____

Telephone

_____

B. Second Alternate Agent

_____

Address

_____

Telephone

Section 3: Effective Date and Durability

This sample document is effective if and when you cannot make health care decisions. Your agent and your doctor determine if you are in this condition. Some state laws include specific procedures for determining your decision-making ability. If you wish, you can include other effective dates or other criteria for determining that you cannot make health care decisions (such as requiring two physicians to evaluate your decision-making ability). You also can state that the power will end at some later date or event before death.

In any case, you have the right to revoke or take away the agent's authority at any time. To revoke, notify your agent or health care provider orally or in writing. If you revoke, it is best to notify in writing both your agent and physician and anyone else who has a copy of the directive. Also destroy the health care advance directive document itself.

By this document, I intend to create a health care advance directive. It is effective upon, and only during, any period in which I cannot make or communicate a choice regarding a particular health care decision. My agent, attending physician, and any other necessary experts should determine that I am unable to make choices about health care.

Section 4: Agent's Powers

This grant of power is intended to be as broad as possible. Unless you set limits, your agent will have authority to make any decision you could make to obtain or stop any type of health care. Even under this broad grant of authority, your agent still must follow your wishes and directions, communicated by you in any manner now or in the future. To specifically limit or direct your agent's power, you must complete section 6 in Part II of the advance directive.

I give my agent full authority to make health care decisions for me. My agent shall follow my wishes as known to my agent either through this document or through other means. When my agent interprets my wishes, I intend my agent's authority to be as broad as possible, except for any limitations I state in this form. In making any decision, my agent shall try to discuss the proposed decision with me to determine my desires if I am able to communicate in any way. If my agent cannot determine the choice I would want, then my agent shall make a choice for me based upon what my agent believes to be in my best interests.

Unless specifically limited by section 6, below, my agent is authorized as follows:

A. To consent, refuse, or withdraw consent to any and all types of health care. Health care means any care, treatment, service or procedure to maintain, diagnose or other-wise affect an individual's physical or mental condition. It includes, but is not limited to, artificial respiration, nutritional support and hydration, medication and cardiopul-monary resuscitation;

B. To have access to medical records and information to the same extent that I am entitled, including the right to disclose the contents to others as appropriate for my health care;

C. To authorize my admission to or discharge (even against medical advice) from any hospital, nursing home, residential care, assisted-living or similar facility or service;

D. To contract on my behalf for any health-care-related service or facility on my behalf, without my agent incurring personal financial liability for such contracts;

E. To hire and fire medical, social service, and other support personnel responsible for my care;

F. To authorize, or refuse to authorize, any medication or procedure intended to relieve pain, even though such use may lead to physical damage, addiction, or hasten the moment of (but not intentionally cause) my death;

G. To make anatomical gifts of part or all of my body for medical purposes, authorize an autopsy, and direct the disposition of my remains, to the extent permitted by law;

H. To take any other action necessary to do what I authorize here, including (but not limited to) granting any waiver or release from liability required by any hospital, physician, or other health care provider; signing any documents relating to refusals of treatment or the leaving of a facility against medical advice; and pursuing any legal action in my name at the expense of my estate to force compliance with my wishes as determined by my agent, or to seek actual or punitive damages for the failure to comply.

PART 2: INSTRUCTIONS ABOUT HEALTH CARE

Section 5: My Instructions about End-of-Life Treatment

The subject of end-of-life treatment is particularly important to many people. In this paragraph, you can give general or specific instructions on the subject. The different paragraphs are options. Choose only one, or write your desires or instructions in your own words (in the last option). If you are satisfied with your agent's knowledge of your values and wishes and you do not want to include instructions in the form, initial the first option and do not give instructions in the form.

Any instructions you give here will guide your agent. If you do not appoint an agent, they will guide any health care providers or surrogate decision makers who must make a decision for you if you cannot do so yourself. The instruction choices in the form describe different treatment goals you may prefer, depending on your condition.

Initial only one of the following statements:

No Specific Instructions. My agent knows my values and wishes, so I do not wish to include any specific instructions here. _____

Directive to Withhold or Withdraw Treatment. Although I greatly value life, I also believe that at some point, life has such diminished value that medical treatment should be stopped, and I should be allowed to die. Therefore, I do not want to receive treatment, including nutrition and hydration, when the treatment will not give me a meaningful quality of life. I do not want my life prolonged…

…if the treatment will leave me in a condition of permanent unconsciousness, such as with an irreversible coma or a persistent vegetative state. _____

…if the treatment will leave me with no more than some consciousness and in an irreversible condition of complete, or nearly complete, loss of ability to think or communicate with others. _____

…if the treatment will leave me with no more than some ability to think or communicate with others, and the likely risks and burdens of treatment outweigh the expected benefits. Risks, burdens and benefits include consideration of length of life, quality of life, financial costs, and my personal dignity and privacy. _____

Directive to Receive Treatment. I want my life to be prolonged as long as possible, no matter what my quality of life. _____

Directive in Your Own Words *If you would like to state your wishes about end-of-life treatment in your own words instead of choosing one of the options provided, you can do so in this section. Since people sometimes have different opinions on whether nutrition and hydration should be refused or stopped under certain circumstances, be sure to address this issue clearly in your directive. Nutrition and hydration means food and fluids given through a nasogastric tube or tube into your stomach, intestines, or veins, and does not include nonintrusive methods such as spoon feeding or moistening of lips and mouth.*

Some states allow the stopping of nutrition and hydration only if you expressly authorize it. If you are creating your own directive, and you do not want nutrition and hydration, state so clearly.

Directive about End-of-Life Treatment in My Own Words:

Section 6: Any Other Health Care Instructions or Limitations or Modifications of My Agent's Powers

In this section, you can provide instructions about other health care issues that are not end-of-life treatment or nutrition and hydration. For example, you might want to include your wishes about issues like nonemergency surgery, elective medical treatments or admission to a nursing home. Again, be careful in these instructions not to place limitations on your agent that you do not intend. For example, while you may not want to be admitted to a nursing home, placing such a restriction may make things impossible for your agent if other options are not available.

You also may limit your agent's powers in any way you wish. For example, you can instruct your agent to refuse any specific types of treatment that are against your religious beliefs or unacceptable to you for any other reasons. These might include blood transfusions, electroconvulsive therapy, sterilization, abortion, amputation, psychosurgery, or admission to a mental institution, etc. Some states limit your agent's authority to consent to or refuse some of these procedures, regardless of your health care advance directive.

Be very careful about stating limitations, because the specific circumstances surrounding future health care decisions are impossible to predict. If you do not want any limitations, simply write in "No limitations."

Section 7: Protection Of Third Parties Who Rely on My Agent

In most states, health care providers cannot be forced to follow the directions of your agent if they object. However, most states also require providers to help transfer you to another provider who is willing to honor your instructions. To encourage compliance with the health care advance directive, this paragraph states that providers who rely in good faith on the agent's statements and decisions will not be held civilly liable for their actions.

No person who relies in good faith upon any representations by my agent or alternate agent(s) shall be liable to me, my estate, my heirs or assigns, for recognizing the agent's authority.

Section 8: Donation of Organs at Death

In this section, you can state your intention to donate bodily organs and tissues at death. If you do not wish to be an organ donor, initial the first option. The second option is a donation of any or all organs or parts. The third option allows you to donate only those organs or tissues you specify. Consider mentioning the heart, liver, lung, kidney, pancreas, intestine, cornea, bone, skin, heart valves, tendons, ligaments, and saphenous vein in the leg. Finally, you may limit the use of your organs by crossing out any of the four purposes listed that you do not want (transplant, therapy, research or education). If you do not cross out any of these options, your organs may be used for any of these purposes.

Upon my death: (Initial one)

_____ I do not wish to donate any organs or tissue, or

_____ I give any needed organs, tissues, or parts, or

_____ I give only the following organs, tissues, or parts: (please specify) _____

_____

My gift (if any) is for the following purposes: (Cross out any of the following you do not want)

Transplant

Research

Therapy

Education

Section 9: Nomination of Guardian

Appointing a health care agent helps to avoid a court-appointed guardian for health care decision making. However, if a court becomes involved for any reason, this paragraph expressly names your agent to serve as guardian. A court does not have to follow your nomination, but normally it will honor your wishes unless there is good reason to override your choice.

If a guardian of my person should for any reason need to be appointed, I nominate my agent (or his or her alternate then authorized to act), named above.

Section 10: Administrative Provisions

These items address miscellaneous matters that could affect the implementation of your health care advance directive.

____ (All apply)

____ I revoke any prior health care advance directive.

____ This health care advance directive is intended to be valid in any jurisdiction in which it is presented.

____ A copy of this advance directive is intended to have the same effect as the original.

Signing the Documents

Required state procedures for signing this kind of document vary. Some require only a signature, while others have very detailed witnessing requirements. Some states simply require notarization.

This form is likely to be far more complex than your state law requires because it combines the formal requirements from virtually every state. Follow it if you do not know your state's requirements and you want to meet the signature requirements of virtually every state.

First, sign and date the document in the presence of two witnesses and a notary.

By signing here, I indicate that I understand the contents of this document and the effect of this grant of powers to my agent.

I sign my name to this health care advance directive on this day ____ of ____

_____
My Signature

_____
My Name

_____
My Current Home Address

Your witness should know your identity personally and be able to declare that you appear to be of sound mind and under no duress or undue influence.

To meet the different witnessing requirements of most states, do not have the following people witness your signature:

Anyone you have chosen to make health care decisions on your behalf (agent or alternate agents).

Your treating physician, health care provider, health facility operator, or an employee of any of these.

Insurers or employees of your life/health insurance provider.

Anyone financially responsible for your health care costs.

Anyone related to you by blood, marriage, or adoption.

Anyone entitled to any part of your estate under an existing will or by operation of law, or anyone who will benefit financially from your death. Your creditors should not serve as witnesses.

If you are in a nursing home or other institution, a few states have additional witnessing requirements. This form does not include witnessing language for this situation. Contact a patient advocate or an ombudsman to find out about the state's requirements in these cases.

Witness Statement

I declare that the person who signed or acknowledged this document is personally known to me, that he/she signed or acknowledged this health care advance directive in my presence, and that he/she appears to be of sound mind and under no duress, fraud, or undue influence.

I am not: the person appointed as agent by this document, the principal's health care provider, an employee of the principal's health care provider, financially responsible for the principal's health care, related to the principal by blood, marriage, or adoption, and, to the best of my knowledge, a creditor of the principal/or entitled to any part of his/her estate under a will now existing or by operation of law.

Witness #1

_____
Signature

_____
Print Name   Telephone

_____
Residence Address

Notarization

Witness #2

_____

Signature

_____

Print Name   Telephone

_____

Residence Address

Second, have your signature notarized. Some states permit notarization as an alternative to witnessing. Doing both witnessing and notarization is more than most states require, but doing both will meet the execution requirements of most states. This form includes a typical notary statement, but it is wise to check state law in case it requires a special form of notary acknowledgment.

Notarization

_____

STATE of

_____

County of

_____

on this day of

The said known to me (or satisfactorily proven) to be the person named in the foregoing instrument, personally appeared before me, a Notary Public, within and for the State and County aforesaid, and acknowledged that he or she freely and voluntarily executed the same for the purposes stated therein.

My Commission Expires   _____

NOTARY PUBLIC

Adapted by permission from *Medicolegal Forms With Legal Analysis*, AMA Press, 1999.

Self-help organizations

A number of institutes and associations help people cope with their particular health care concerns. The following list provides the names, phone numbers, and Web site addresses of a variety of such organizations.

AGING

National Institute on Aging (NIA)
(800) 222-2225
http://www.nih.gov/nia

American Association of Retired Persons (AARP)
(800) 424-3410
http://www.aarp.org

Eldercare Locator
(800) 677-1116
http://www.eldercare.gov

ALCOHOL AND DRUG ABUSE

Alcoholics Anonymous
(212) 870-3400
http://www.alcoholics-anonymous.org

American Council on Alcoholism
(800) 527-5344
http://www.aca-usa.org

National Clearinghouse for Alcohol and Drug Information
(800) 729-6686
http://www.health.org

National Council on Alcoholism and Drug Dependence
(800) 622-2255
http://www.ncadd.org

ALZHEIMER'S DISEASE

Alzheimer's Association
(800) 272-3900
http://www.alz.org

Alzheimer's Disease Education and Referral Center
(800) 438-4380
http://www.alzheimers.org

ARTHRITIS

Arthritis Foundation
(800) 283-7800
http://www.arthritis.org

National Institute of Arthritis and Musculoskeletal and Skin Diseases Information Clearinghouse
(877) 22-NIAMS
http://www.niams.nih.gov

BLOOD DISORDERS

Cooley's Anemia Foundation
(800) 522-7222
http://www.cooleysanemia.org

Sickle Cell Disease Association of America
(800) 421-8453
http://www.sicklecelldisease.org

BURNS

Phoenix Society for Burn Survivors
(800) 888-2876
http://www.phoenix-society.org

CANCER

American Cancer Society
(800) 227-2345
http://www.cancer.org

National Cancer Institute
(800) 422-6237
http://www.nci.nih.gov

Y-ME National Breast Cancer Organization
(800) 221-2141
http://www.y-me.org

CHILDREN
American Academy of Pediatrics
(847) 228-5005
http://www.aap.org

National Center for Missing and
Exploited Children
(800) THE-LOST (24 hour hotline)
http://www.missingkids.com

Notmykid Inc.
(602) 652-0163
http://www.notmykid.org

Parents of Chronically Ill Children
(202) 619-0257
http://www.dhhs.org/children

CHRONIC FATIGUE SYNDROME
CFIDS Association of America
(800) 442-3437
http://www.cfids.org

CYSTIC FIBROSIS
Cystic Fibrosis Foundation
(800) 344-4823
http://www.cff.org

DENTISTRY
American Dental Association
(312) 440-2500
http://www.ada.org

DIABETES
American Diabetes Association
(800) 342-2383
http://www.diabetes.org

Juvenile Diabetes Foundation
(800) JDF-CURE
http://www.jdf.org

DISABILITIES
National Information Center for
Children and Youth with Disabilities
(800) 695-0285
http://www.nichcy.org

American Association of People with
Disabilities
(800) 840-8844
http://www.aapd.com

DOWN SYNDROME
National Down Syndrome Society
(800) 221-4602
http://www.ndss.org

EYE PROBLEMS
American Academy of Ophthalmology
(415) 561-8500
http://www.aao.org

American Council of the Blind
(800) 424-8666
http://www.acb.org

American Foundation for the Blind
(800) 232-5463
http://www.afb.org

Foundation Fighting Blindness
(800) 683-5555
http://www.blindness.org

National Association for Parents of
Children with Visual Impairments
(800) 562-6265
http://www.spedex.com/napvi/

National Eye Institute
(301) 496-5248
http://www.nei.nih.gov

FAMILY PLANNING
The Alan Guttmacher Institute
(212) 248-1111
http://www.agi-usa.org

Planned Parenthood
(800) 230-PLAN
http://www.plannedparenthood.org

GENERAL
American Association of Family
Physicians
(800) 274-2237
http://www.familydoctor.org

American Medical Association
(312) 464-5000
http://www.ama-assn.org

HEADACHE
National Headache Foundation
(800) 843-2256
http://www.headaches.org

HEARING PROBLEMS
American Speech-Language-Hearing
Association
(800) 638-8255
http://www.asha.org

Deafness Research Foundation
(800) 535-3323
http://www.drf.org

HEART AND CIRCULATION DISORDERS
American Heart Association
(800) 242-8721
http://www.americanheart.org

National Heart, Lung, and Blood
Institute
(800) 575-WELL
http://www.nhlbi.nih.gov

HIV INFECTION AND AIDS
CDC National HIV/AIDS Hotline
(800) 342-2437
http://www.cdc.gov

Gay Men's Health Crisis
(800) 243-7692
http://www.gmhc.org

HIV/AIDS Treatment Information
Service
(800) 448-0440
http://www.hivatis.org

HUNTINGTON CHOREA
Huntington's Disease Society of
America
(800) 345-HDSA
http://www.hdsa.org

LEARNING DISABILITIES
The International Dyslexia Association
(800) ABCD123
http://www.interdys.org

National Center for Learning
Disabilities
(888) 575-7373
http://www.ncld.org

LIVER DISEASE
American Liver Foundation
(800) 465-4837
http://www.liverfoundation.org

LUNG DISEASE
American Academy of Allergy,
Asthma and Immunology
(800) 822-2762
http://www.aaaai.org

American Lung Association
(800) 586-4872
http://www.lungusa.org

National Heart, Lung, and Blood
Institute
(800) 575-WELL
http://www.nhlbi.nih.gov

LUPUS
Lupus Foundation of America
(800) 558-0121
http://www.lupus.org

LYME DISEASE
Lyme Disease Foundation
(800) 886-LYME (24-hour free hotline)
http://www.lyme.org

MENTAL HEALTH
Depression and Bipolar Support
Alliance
(800) 826-3632
http://www.dbsalliance.org

National Alliance for the Mentally Ill
888-999-NAMI
http://www.nami.org

National Foundation for Depressive
Illness
(800) 239-1265
http://www.depression.org

National Mental Health Association
(800) 969-6642
http://www.nmha.org

MENTAL RETARDATION
American Association on Mental
Retardation
(800) 424-3688
http://www.aamr.org

**MUSCULOSKELETAL
DISORDERS**
American College of Rheumatology
(404) 633-3777
http://www.rheumatology.org

NEUROLOGICAL DISORDERS
The ALS Association
(800) 782-4747
http://www.alsa.org

National Institute of Neurological
Disorders
(301) 496-5751
http://www.ninds.nih.gov

National Spinal Cord Injury
Association
(800) 962-9629
http://www.spinalcord.org

United Cerebral Palsy Associations
(800) USA-5UCP
http://www.ucpa.org

OSTEOPOROSIS
National Osteoporosis Foundation
(800) 223-9994
http://www.nof.org

PARKINSON DISEASE
National Parkinson Foundation
(800) 327-4545
http://www.parkinson.org

PREGNANCY AND CHILDBIRTH
America's Crisis Pregnancy Helpline
(888) 467-8466
http://www.thehelpline.org

SAFETY
Consumer Product Safety Commission
(800) 638-2772
http://www.cpsc.gov

National Highway Traffic Safety
Association
(800) 424-9393
http://www.nhtsa.dot.gov

National Safety Council
(800) 621-7619
http://www.nsc.org

**SEXUALLY TRANSMITTED
DISEASES**
National STD Hotline of the CDC
(800) 227-8922
http://www.ashastd.org

SKIN
American Academy of Dermatology
(847) 330-0230
http://www.aad.org

SPINA BIFIDA
Spina Bifida Association of America
(800) 621-3141
http://www.sbaa.org

STROKE
National Stroke Association
(800) 787-6537
http://www.stroke.org

SURGERY
American College of Surgeons
(312) 202-5000
http://www.facs.org

TRAVEL
CDC Travel Information Hotline
(404) 332-4559
(888) 232-2388
http://www.cdc.gov/travel

URINARY DISORDERS
National Kidney Foundation
(800) 822-9010
http://www.kidney.org

HIPAA and confidentiality of patients' health information

The Department of Health and Human Services (HHS) issued new regulations in 2003 under the Health Insurance Portability and Accountability Act (HIPAA). The new regulations, known as the HIPAA Privacy Rules, establish federal confidentiality protections for patient health information that is gathered by doctor's offices, hospitals, long term care facilities, and other health care providers. HHS issued the fact sheet reprinted below to explain the Privacy Rules to consumers and inform them of their rights under the law.

PROTECTING THE PRIVACY OF PATIENTS' HEALTH INFORMATION

Overview: The first-ever federal privacy standards to protect patients' medical records and other health information provided to health plans, doctors, hospitals and other health care providers took effect on April 14, 2003. Developed by the Department of Health and Human Services (HHS), these new standards provide patients with access to their medical records and more control over how their personal health information is used and disclosed. They represent a uniform, federal floor of privacy protections for consumers across the country. State laws providing additional protections to consumers are not affected by this new rule.

Congress called on HHS to issue patient privacy protections as part of the Health Insurance Portability and Accountability Act of 1996 (HIPAA). HIPAA included provisions designed to encourage electronic transactions and also required new safeguards to protect the security and confidentiality of health information. The final regulation covers health plans, health care clearinghouses, and those health care providers who conduct certain financial and administrative transactions (e.g., enrollment, billing and eligibility verification) electronically. Most health insurers, pharmacies, doctors and other health care providers were required to comply with these federal standards beginning April 14, 2003. As provided by Congress, certain small health plans have an additional year to comply. HHS has conducted extensive outreach and provided guidance and technical assistant to these providers and businesses to make it as easy as possible for them to implement the new privacy protections. These efforts include answers to hundreds of common questions about the rule, as well as explanations and descriptions about key elements of the rule. These materials are available at http://www.hhs.gov/ocr/hipaa.

PATIENT PROTECTIONS

The new privacy regulations ensure a national floor of privacy protections for patients by limiting the ways that health plans, pharmacies, hospitals and other covered entities can use patients' personal medical information. The regulations protect medical records and other individually identifiable health information, whether it is on paper, in computers or communicated orally. Key provisions of these new standards include:

■ *Access to Medical Records* Patients generally should be able to see and obtain copies of their medical records and request corrections if they identify errors and mistakes. Health plans, doctors, hospitals, clinics, nursing homes and other covered entities generally should provide access [to] these records within 30 days and may charge patients for the cost of copying and sending the records.

■ *Notice of Privacy Practices* Covered health plans, doctors and other health care providers must provide a notice to their patients [about] how they may use personal medical information and their rights under the new privacy regulation. Doctors, hospitals and other direct-care providers generally will provide the notice on the patient's first visit following the April 14, 2003, compliance date and upon request. Patients generally will be asked to sign, initial or otherwise acknowledge that they received this notice. Health plans generally must mail the notice to their enrollees by April 14 and again if the notice changes significantly. Patients also may ask covered entities to restrict the use or disclosure of their information beyond the practices included in the notice, but the covered entities would not have to agree to the changes.

■ *Limits on Use of Personal Medical Information* The privacy rule sets limits on how health plans and covered providers may use individually identifiable health information. To promote the best quality care for patients, the rule does not restrict the ability of doctors, nurses and other providers to share information needed to treat their patients. In other situations, though, personal health information generally may not be used for purposes not related to health care, and covered entities may use or share only the minimum amount of protected information needed for a particular purpose. In addition, patients would have to sign a specific authorization before a covered entity could release their medical information to a life insurer, a bank, a marketing firm, or another outside business for purposes not related to their health care.

■ *Prohibition on Marketing* The final privacy rule sets new restrictions and limits on the use of patient information for marketing purposes. Pharmacies, health plans, and other covered entities must first obtain an individual's specific authorization before disclosing their patient information for marketing. At the same time, the rule permits doctors and other covered entities to communicate freely with patients about treatment options and other health-related information, including disease-management programs.

■ *Stronger State Laws* The new federal privacy standards do not affect state laws that provide additional privacy protections for patients. The confidentiality protections are cumulative; the privacy rule will set a national "floor" of privacy standards that protect all Americans, and any state law providing additional protections would continue to apply. When a state law requires a certain disclosure—such as reporting an infectious disease outbreak to the public health authorities—the federal privacy regulations would not preempt the state law.

■ *Confidential Communications* Under the privacy rule, patients can request that their doctors, health plans and other covered entities take reasonable steps to ensure that their communications with the patient are confidential. For example, a patient could ask a doctor to call his or her office rather than home, and the doctor's office should comply with that request if it can be reasonably accommodated.

■ *Complaints* Consumers may file a formal complaint regarding the privacy practices of a covered health plan or provider. Such complaints can be made directly to the covered provider or health plan or to HHS' Office for Civil Rights (OCR), which is charged with investigating complaints and enforcing the privacy regulation. Information about filing complaints should be included in each covered entity's notice of privacy practices. Consumers can find out more information about filing a complaint at http://www.hhs.gov/ocr/hipaa or by calling (866) 627-7748.

HEALTH PLANS AND PROVIDERS

The privacy rule requires health plans, pharmacies, doctors and other covered entities to establish policies and procedures to protect the confidentiality of protected health information about their patients. These requirements are flexible and scalable to allow different covered entities to implement them as appropriate for their businesses or practices. Covered entities must provide all the protections for patients cited above, such as providing a notice of their privacy practices and limiting the use and disclosure of information as required under the rule. In addition, covered entities must take some additional steps to protect patient privacy:

■ *Written Privacy Procedures* The rule requires covered entities to have written privacy procedures, including a description of staff that has access to protected information, how it will be used, and when it may be disclosed. Covered entities generally must take steps to ensure that any business associates who have access to protected information agree to the same limitations on the use and disclosure of that information.

■ *Employee Training and Privacy Officer* Covered entities must train their employees in their privacy procedures and must designate an individual to be responsible for ensuring the procedures are followed. If covered entities learn an employee failed to follow these procedures, they must take appropriate disciplinary action.

PUBLIC RESPONSIBILITIES

In limited circumstances, the final rule permits—but does not require—covered entities to continue certain existing disclosures of health information for specific public responsibilities. These permitted disclosures include: emergency circumstances; identification of the body of a deceased person, or the cause of death; public health needs; research that involves limited data or has been independently approved by an Institutional Review Board or privacy board; oversight of the health care system; judicial and administrative proceedings; limited law enforcement activities; and activities related to national defense and security. The privacy rule generally establishes new safeguards and limits on these disclosures. Where no other law requires disclosures in these situations, covered entities may continue to use their professional judgment to decide whether to make such disclosures based on their own policies and ethical principles.

■ *Equivalent Requirements for Government* The provisions of the final rule generally apply equally to private sector and public sector covered entities. For example, private hospitals and government-run hospitals covered by the rule have to comply with the full range of requirements.

OUTREACH AND ENFORCEMENT

HHS' Office for Civil Rights (OCR) oversees and enforces the new federal privacy regulations. Led by OCR, HHS has issued extensive guidance and technical assistance materials to make it as easy as possible for covered entities to comply with the new requirements. Key elements of OCR's outreach and enforcement efforts include:

■ *Guidance and Technical Assistance Materials* HHS has issued extensive guidance and technical materials to explain the privacy rule, including an extensive, searchable collection of frequently asked questions that address major aspects of the rule. HHS will continue to expand and update these materials to further assist covered entities in complying. These materials are available at http://www.hhs.gov/ocr/hipaa/assist.html

■ *Conferences and Seminars*. HHS has participated in hundreds of conferences, trade association meetings and conference calls to explain and clarify the provisions of the privacy regulation. These included a series of regional conferences sponsored by HHS, as well as many held by professional associations and trade groups. HHS will continue these outreach efforts to encourage compliance with the privacy requirements.

■ *Information Line* To help covered entities find out information about the privacy regulation and other administrative simplification provisions of the Health Insurance Portability and Accountability Act of 1996, OCR and HHS' Centers for Medicare & Medicaid Services have established a toll-free information line. The number is (866) 627-7748.

■ *Complaint Investigations* Enforcement will be primarily complaint-driven. OCR will investigate complaints and work to make sure that consumers receive the privacy rights and protections required under the new regulations. When appropriate, OCR can impose civil monetary penalties for violations of the privacy rule provisions. Potential criminal violations of the law would be referred to the U.S. Department of Justice for further investigation and appropriate action.

■ *Civil and Criminal Penalties* Congress provided civil and criminal penalties for covered entities that misuse personal health information. For civil violations of the standards, CR may impose monetary penalties up to $100 per violation, up to $25,000 per year, for each requirement or prohibition violated. Criminal penalties apply for certain actions such as knowingly obtaining protected health information in violation of the law. Criminal penalties can range up to $50,000 and one year in prison for certain offenses; up to $100,000 and up to five years in prison if the offenses are committed under "false pretenses"; and up to $250,000 and up to 10 years in prison if the offenses are committed with the intent to sell, transfer or use protected health information for commercial advantage, personal gain or malicious harm.

Note: All HHS press releases, fact sheets and other press materials are available at http://www.hhs.gov/news

Index

Note: Page numbers in *italics* indicate illustrations and charts.

A

Abacavir, 98
Abdomen, 98, *98*
  acute, 98, *98*
    nausea or vomiting, 46
  aneurysm, 167
  paracentesis, 952
  retroperitoneal fibrosis, 1073
  situs inversus, 1123
Abdominal pain, 98-99
  afterbirth, 125
  diarrhea, 34
  nausea or vomiting, 46
  symptom chart, 14-15
Abdominoplasty. *See* Tummy tuck.
Abduction, 99
Ablation, 99
Ablation therapy, 99
  atrial fibrillation, 207
  cardiac arrhythmia, 192
  endometrial, 509
Abortion, 99-101
  elective, 99-100
  missed, 100
  spontaneous, 100
  threatened, 100-101
Abrasion, 101
Abreaction, 101
Abscess, 101
  of Bartholin glands, 229
  of bone, 261
  of brain, 271
  of breast, 276, 287
  epidural, 517
  lancing, 768
  of liver, 799
  peritonsillar, 64, 975
  spinal, 101
  subphrenic, 1175
  of tooth, 1221
Absence seizure, 101, 178
Absorption, 101-102
Abstinence, 102
Abuse, 102-106
  of child, 102-103, 105-106, 1275
  drugs, 477-480, *479*
  emotional, 102, 103-104

of older people, 104-105
of partner, 105
sexual, 105-106
Acanthosis nigricans, 106, *106*
Acarbose, 106
Accident prevention, 106-107, *107*
Accommodation, 107, *107*
  presbyopia, 1016
Accreditation, 107
ACE inhibitors. *See* Antihypertensives.
Acetaminophen, 107, 154, 220
  pain management, 945-946
Acetylcholine, 107
Acetylsalicylic acid. *See* Aspirin.
Achalasia, 108
Achilles tendinitis, 108, *108*
Achlorhydria, 108
Achondroplasia, 108-109, 1123-1124
Acid, 109
Acid reflux. *See* Esophageal reflux.
Acid-base balance, 109
Acidosis, 109
  renal tubular, 1062
Acne, 109-111, *110*
  adapalene, 116
  Agent Orange, 125
  benzoyl peroxide, 234
  self-care, *109*
  stages of, *110*
  treatment, 111, 234
    isotretinoin, 743
Acoustic neuroma, 111-112, *112*
Acoustic trauma, 112-113, 492, 635, *112*
Acquired immunodeficiency syndrome. *See* AIDS. *See also* HIV.
Acromegaly, 113-114, 939, 1190, *113*
Acroparesthesia, 114
Acrophobia, 114
ACTH, 114, 409
  in Addison disease, 116-117
Acting out, 114
Actinic keratosis, 114
Actinomycosis, 114
Acupressure, 114, 355

pain management, 947
Acupuncture, 114-116, 142, 355, *115, 116*
  ear, 116
  moxibustion, 862, *355*
  pain management, 947
Acute, 116
Acyclovir, 116
ADA. *See* Americans with Disabilities Act.
Adapalene, 116
ADD. *See* Attention Deficit/Hyperactivity Disorder.
Addiction, 116, *116*
  sexual, 1108
Addison disease, 116-117, *117*
  autoimmunity, 212
Adduction, 117, *117*
Adenitis, 117
Adenocarcinoma, 117
Adenoidectomy, 117-118
Adenoids, 118, *117*
Adenoma, 118
  acromegaly, 113
  polyposis, familial, 1006
  villous, 1274
Adenomatosis, 118
Adenomyosis, 118, *118*
Adenosine deaminase deficiency, 76
Adenosine diphosphate. *See* ADP.
Adenosine triphosphate. *See* ATP.
Adenovirus, 118-119
Adequate Intake, 466
ADH, 119
ADHD. *See* Attention deficit/hyperactivity disorder.
Adhesions, 119
Adhesive otitis media, 119
Adipose tissue, 119, *119*
Adjustment disorder, 119-120
Adjuvants, 120
Adolescence, 120-121, 1035
  drug abuse, 479
  growth, 618-620, *619*
ADP, 121
Adrenal glands, 121-122, *122*
  adenoma, 118
  failure of, 121

pheochromocytoma, 982
tumors, 122-123
Adrenal congenital hyperplasia,
122, 135, *122*
virilism, 1276
Adrenaline. *See* Epinephrine.
Adrenocorticotropic hormone. *See*
ACTH.
Adrenogenital syndrome, 122, 123
Advance directives, 123-124
do not resuscitate order, 123-124
legal aspects, 124
living will, 123, 802, 1299
power of attorney, durable, 123
Adverse drug reactions, 124
Aerobic, 124, *124*
Aerodontalgia, 124
Aerophagia. *See* Air swallowing.
Aerospace medicine, 124
Affect, 125
Affective disorders, 125
AFP test, 125
Afterbirth, 125
Afterpains, 125
Agar, 125
Age spots, 125
Agenesis, 125
Agent, 125
Agent Orange, 125-126
Ageusia, 126
Aggregation, 126
Aggression, 126
Aging, 126
antiaging therapies, 174-175
and exercise, 531, 533
See also Older people.
Agitation, 126
Agnosia, 126-127
Agonal, 127
Agonist, 127
Agoraphobia, 127, 184
Agraphia, 127
AIDS, 127-129, 1110, 1111, *129*
cytomegalovirus retinitis, 434
drugs. *See* Alitretinoin; Non-
nucleoside reverse transcrip-
tase inhibitors; Protease
inhibitors; Zalcitabine
Zidovudine.
related cancers, 129
genetic factors, 75
herpesvirus B, 684

infections, *129*
opportunistic, 921
timeline, *128*
toxoplasmosis, 1226-1228, *1227*
weight loss, 62
Air ambulance, 129-130, *129*
Air bags, 130, 312-313, *130*
Air pollution. *See* Pollution, air.
Air swallowing, 130
Air traveling, barotrauma, 228-229
Airway, 130
chronic obstructive pulmonary
disease, 366-368
reactive disease, 1053-1054, *1053*
uvulopalatopharyngoplasty,
1260-1261
Akathisia, 130
Akinesia, 130
Al-Anon, 130-131
Albinism, 131
Albumin, 131
Albuminuria, 131
Albuterol sulfate, 131
Alcohol
dependence, 131-133, *132*
versus abuse, 132
and abuse of older people,
104
addiction, 116
and child abuse, 103
physical effects of, 442, *132*
screening test for alcoholism,
132
withdrawal symptoms, 133,
133
fetal alcohol syndrome, 556
hangover, 628
intoxication, 133-134, *134*
and older people, 131
Alcoholics Anonymous (AA), 130,
133, 135, 848, 1247-1248, *1247*
group therapy, 481
Alcoholism, 135
aversion therapy, 214
and depression, 32
drunk driving, 481-482
and duodenal ulcers, 485
hepatitis, 661
hoarseness or voice loss, 31
Korsakoff psychosis, 763-764
self-screening test, 1100

sleep problems, 55
underage drinking, 1253
withdrawal syndrome, 1303
Aldosterone, 121-122, 135, 409,
699, 849
Aldosteronism, 135
Alendronate sodium, 135, 243
Alexander technique, 135, 260
Alexia, 135, 1302
Alienation, 135
Alignment, dental, 135
Alimentary tract, 135-136
Alitretinoin, 129, 136
Alkali, 136
Alkaloids, 136
Allergen, 136
anaphylaxis, 155
immunotherapy, 711
sensitization, 1102
Allergic alveolitis, 144
Allergic reaction, 136, *136*
allergy response, *138, 676*
to anesthesia, 163
angioedema, 169
antihistamines as treatment, 180
asthma, 200
bee stings, 232
childhood rash, 51
contact dermatitis, 397-398, *398*
to foods, 572-573
hay fever, 629-630
Henoch-Schönlein purpura,
659-660
histamine, 672
insect stings, 243, 244
patch test, 959, *959*
rhinitis, 1077-1078
scratch test, 1095
skin test, 1127, 1129
swallowing difficulty, 64
Allergies, 136-139
Allergist, 139
Allograft, 139
Allopathy, 139
Allopurinol, 139
Aloe, 139
Alopecia, 139-140, *139*
Alpha blockers, 140-141, *140*
Alpha 1-antitrypsin deficiency,
140, 503
Alpha-fetoprotein (AFP) test. *See*
AFP test.

Alpha-tocopherol, 141
Alprazolam. *See* Benzodiazepines.
ALS, 141-142, 806, 860, *141*
Alteplase, 142
Alternative medicine, 142-143, *142*
    See also specific therapies by
    name.
Altitude sickness, 143
Aluminum, 143
Alveolectomy, 1143
Alveoli, 143, 807
Alveolitis, 144
    bagassosis, 223
Alveoloplasty, 144
Alzheimer's disease, 85-86, 144-146,
    145
    and alcoholism, 131
    apraxia, 190
    brain scanning, 85-86, *86*
    dementia, 443, *443*
    genetic factors, 75
    medications, 145
    neuropsychological testing, 900
Amalgam, dental, 146
    filling, 564-565
Amaurosis fugax, 146, *146*
Ambidexterity, 146
Amblyopia, 146-147, *147*
Ambulance, 147
    air, 129-130
Ambulatory surgery, 147
Amebiasis, 147-148, *147*
    in travelers, 148
Amebic dysentery, 147, 148
Amelogenesis imperfecta, 148
Amenorrhea, 148, 841
American Medical Association
    (AMA), 148-149
American Sign Language, *437*
Americans with Disabilities Act
    (ADA), 149
Amino acids, 149
Aminoglycosides, 149
Amiodarone hydrochloride, 149
Amitriptyline, 946
Ammonia, 149-150
Amnesia, 150
Amnio infusion, 150
Amniocentesis, 150-151, *150*
    birth defects, 242
    chromosomal abnormalities, 365
    prenatal screening, 597

rH incompatibility, 654
Amniotic fluid, 157
    hydramnios, 687
    meconium, 830
    oligohydramnios, 916
    polyhydramnios, 1005
Amniotomy, 157
Amoxicillin. *See* Penicillins.
Amphetamines
    addiction to, 478
    for ADHD, 209
Amphotericin B, 151
Ampicillin. *See* Penicillins.
Amplifying devices, 199, *200*
Amprenavir, 151
Amputation, surgical, 151
    phantom limb pain, 981
    stump, 1174
Amsler grid, 151, 1278, *1279*
Amyloidosis, 151-152
    Addison disease, 116
Amyotrophy, 152
Anabolic steroids, 152, *152*
Anaerobic, 152, *152*
Anal dilation, 152, *152*
Anal discharge, 152
Anal fissure, 152-153, 267
    constipation, 26
Anal fistula, 153
Anal pain or itching, symptom
    chart, 17
Anal sex, 153
Anal stenosis, 153
Anal stricture. *See* Anal stenosis.
Analgesia, 153-154
    pain management, 945
    patient-controlled, 153, 961, *153*
Analgesics, 153-154, *154*
Analysis, scientific, 154
Anaphylactic reaction, 154-155, *154*
    childhood rash, 51
Anaphylactoid purpura, *See*
    Henloch-Schonlein purpura.
Anaphylaxis, 137, 155-156, 1114,
    155
    bee venom, 233
    first aid, 1330
Anastomosis, 156
    ileal pouch–anal, 707
Anastrozole, 156
Anatomy, 156
Androgen hormones, 122, 156, 1107,
    156

testosterone, 1201-1202
    virilism, 1275-1276
Androgens, 156
Andrology, 156
Anemia, 157-160, *157*
    aplastic, 157-158
    Cooley, 158, *158*
    dizziness, 36, 37
    Fanconi, 158
    hemolytic, 158-159
    iron-deficiency, 159, 741, *159*
    megaloblastic, 159
    pernicious, 159-160, 976, 1282
    sickle cell. *See* Sickle cell anemia.
    sideroblastic, 160
Anencephaly, 160
Anesthesia, 160-167
    ambulatory, 161
    caudal block, 332
    dental, 161
    epidural, 161-162, *161*
    general, 162-163, *162*
    inhalation, 163
    intravenous, 163
    local, 163-164, *164*
    pain management, 945-946
    pediatric, 164-165, *164*
    regional, 165, 1059, *165*
        brachial plexus block, 268
    saddle block, 1086
    side effects, *161*
    spinal, 165-166, *166*
    types, *160*
Anesthesiologist, 166
Anesthesiology, 166
Anesthetics, 166-167
Aneurysm, 167, *167*
    aortic, 167
    cerebral, 167
Angina, 167-169, *168*
    atherosclerosis, 205
    balloon angioplasty, 225
    chest pain, 24, 348
    ischemia, 742
    ischemic heart disease, 642
    Ludwig, 806
    types, 168
Angioedema, 169
Angiogenesis, 169
Angiogram, 169
Angiography, 169-170, *170*
    brain, 273

kidney, 759
lung, 809
Angioma, 170
cherry, 348
Angioplasty, balloon. *See* Balloon
angioplasty.
Angiotensin, 170
Angiotensin II receptor antagonists,
180
Angiotensin-converting enzyme
(ACE) inhibitors. *See* Antihyper-
tensives.
Anhidrosis, 170-171
Animals
brucellosis, 295
diseases from, 171
experimentation, 171
organ transplants, 93
Anisometropia, 1219
Ankle
arthroscopic surgery, 195
symptom chart, 18-19
tarsal tunnel syndrome,
1191-1192
Ankyloglossia. *See* Tongue-tie.
Ankylosing spondylitis, 171-172,
171
back pain, 220
spondylarthropathy, 1153
Ankylosis, 172
Anodontia, 172
Anomaly, 172
Anorexia nervosa, 172-173, *173*
adolescents, 120
body image, 259
Anorgasmia. *See* Orgasm, lack of.
Anosmia, 173
Anovulation. *See* Ovulation, lack of.
Anoxia, 173
Antabuse, 471
Antacids, 173, *173*
Antagonist, 173
Antepartum hemorrhage, 173-174
Antepartum testing. *See* Prenatal
testing.
Anterior, 174
Anthrax, 174, 1310
animal-transmitted, 171
Anthroposophical medicine, 174
Antiaging therapies, 174-175
Antianxiety drugs, 175
addiction to, 477

Antiarrhythmics, 175
Antibiotics, 175-176, *175*
aminoglycosides, 149
cephalosporins, 337
fluoroquinolones, 570
macrolides, 817
penicillins, 175, 966
sulfa drugs, 1178-1179
tetracyclines, 1202-1203
Antibody, 176-177, 709-710
in allergies, 136-137
anticardiolipin, 177
monoclonal, 78, 177, *78*
Anticholinergic agents, 177
Anticoagulants, 177, *177*
Anticonvulsants, 177-178
Antidepressants, 178
Antidiuretic hormone. *See* ADH.
Antidote, 178
Antiemetics, 178
Antiepileptic agents. *See*
Anticonvulsants.
Antifreeze poisoning, 178-179
Antifungal drugs, 179
Antigen, 179, 709-710
in allergies, 136-137
autoimmune disorders, 211-212
histocompatibility, 672
Antihistamines, 179-180, *179*
Antihypertensives, 180, 205, *180*
aortic stenosis, 185
atherosclerosis, 205
beta blockers, 180, 234-235, *235*
calcium channel blockers, 180,
305
coughing, 30
diuretics, 180
Antimicrobial agents, 180
Antineoplastons, 180-181
Antioxidants, 181
antiaging therapy, 175
Anti-Parkinson drugs, 181
Antipsychotic drugs, 181
Antipyretic drugs, 181
Antireflux surgery, 181-182
Antiseptics, 182
Antiserum, 182
Antisocial personality disorder.
See Personality disorders.
Antitoxin, 182
Antituberculosis drugs, 182-183
Antivenin, 183

Anuria, 183
Anus, 183
cancer of, 183
ileal pouch-anal anastomosis, 707
imperforate, 183
Anxiety, 183
free-floating, 582
separation, 1103
Anxiety disorders, 183-184, 583
generalized anxiety disorder, 184
obsessive-compulsive disorder,
184, 913-914
panic disorders, 184
phobia, 184
posttraumatic stress disorder, 184
sleep problems, 54
weight loss, 63
Anxiolytics. *See* Antianxiety drugs.
Aorta, 184
coarctation of, 374, 642, *374*
Aortic insufficiency, 184-185
Aortic stenosis, 185, *185*
chest pain, 348
Aortic valve, 645-647
stenosis, 1161
Aortitis, 186
Aortography, 186
Apert-Crouson disease. *See* Cranio-
facial dysostosis.
Apgar score, 186, *186*
Aphakia, 186, *186*
Aphasia, 186-187, *187*
Apheresis, 187, 254
Aphonia, 187
Aphrodisiac, 187
Apicoectomy, 187-188, *187*
Apitherapy. *See* Bee venom and
bee products, therapeutic.
Aplasia, 188
Aplastic anemia, 157-158
Apnea, 188
Apolipoprotein, 188
Aponeurosis, 188, *188*
Apoptosis, 188
Appendectomy, 188
Appendicitis, 188-189
abdominal pain, 14
acute abdomen, 98
Appendix, 189, *189*
Appetite, 189-190
loss of, 189
in older people, 189-190

stimulants, 189
suppressants, 189
Applied kinesiology, 190
Apraxia, 190
Arachnoiditis, 190
Arcus senilis, 190
Area Agencies on Aging, 190
Arm, fractured, 190-191, *190*
Armpit, 215
Aromatherapy, 191
Arousal, 191
Arrhenoblastoma, 191
Arrhythmia, cardiac, 191-192, *191*
Arsenic, 192
Art therapy, 192
Arteries, 192-193, *192*
    hardening of, 204, 628
Arteriole, 193
Arteriosclerosis, 193, *193*
Arteriovenous fistula, 193
Arteriovenous malformation, 193
Arteritis, 193
    giant cell, 193
Arthralgia, 193-194
Arthritis, 194, *194*
    See also Osteoarthritis;
        Rheumatoid arthritis.
    back pain, 220
    hallux rigidus, 626
    hip pain, 43
    human growth hormone, 174
    Lyme disease, 812-813
    paraffin bath, 952
    psoriatic, 1031
    Reiter syndrome, 1060
    spondylarthropathy, 1153
Arthrodesis, 194
Arthrogram, 194
Arthrography, 194-195
Arthroplasty. *See* Joint replacement.
Arthroscopic surgery, 195, *195*
Arthroscopy. *See* Arthroscopic
    surgery.
Artificial coloring agent, 59
Artificial insemination, 195, *195*
Artificial kidney, 196
Artificial respiration, 196, *196*
    drowning, 476
Artificial sweeteners, 196
Asbestos, 196
    and lung cancer, 808
Asbestosis, 196-197, 486

Ascariasis, 197
Ascites, 197
Ascorbic acid. *See* Vitamin C.
Aseptic technique, 197
Aspartame, 196, 197
Asperger disorder, 198, 979
Aspergillosis, 198, *198*
Asphyxia, 198
Aspiration, 198
Aspirin, 198
    Reye syndrome, 1074
Assault, 198
    sexual, 198-199, *199*
Assay, 199
Assisted living facility, 199, 804
Assisted reproductive technology,
    199
    artificial insemination, 195, *195*
    infertility treatments, 723
    in vitro fertilization, 714, *714*
    ZIFT, 1309
Assistive listening devices, 199-200,
    199, 200
Astereognosis, 126, 200
Asthma, 200-202, *201*
    cardiac, 202
    prevention of, *202*
    status asthmaticus, 1160-1161
Astigmatism, 202-203, 398, *203*
Aston-patterning, 203
Astringents, 203
Astrocytoma, 203
Asymptomatic, 203
Asystole, 203
Ataxia, 203
    Friedreich, 582
Atelectasis, 203-204
Atenolol. *See* Beta blockers.
Atherectomy. *See* Balloon angio-
    plasty.
Atheroma, 204
Atherosclerosis, 204-206, *204*
    cholesterol, 360
    coronary artery disease, 406
    hyperlipidemias, 691-692
    plaque, 991
    RIND, 1080
Athetosis, 206, 740
Athlete's foot, 206, 451
Atlas of the body, 65-72
    digestive system, 69
    endocrine and lymphatic systems,
        72

heart and circulatory system, 68
muscular system, 66
nervous system, 67
reproductive systems, male and
    female, 70
skeletal system, 65
urinary systems, male and female,
    71
Atmospheric pressure, aerodontal-
    gia, 124
Atony, 206
ATP, 206
Atresia, 206
Atrial fibrillation, 192, 206-207, *206*
    cardioversion, 321
Atrial flutter, 207-208, *208*
Atrial natriuretic peptide, 208
Atrial septal defect, 642, 1103-1104,
    1103
    See also Septal defect, atrial.
Atrium, 208
Atrophy, 208
Atropine, 208
Attending physician, 208
Attention deficit/hyperactivity
    disorder, 208-209, 779, *209*
    in adults, 208
    art therapy, 192
    autism, 211
Audiologist, 210
Audiology, 210
Audiometry, 210, *210*
Aura, 210, 1098
    headache, 38
Auranofin, 210
Auricular therapy. *See* Acupuncture,
    ear.
Autism, 210-211, 979
    aversion therapy, 214
Autoclave, 211, *211*
Autoimmune disorders, 211-213,
    710, *212*
    Addison disease, 116
    collagen diseases, 383
    CREST syndrome, 419
    dermatomyositis, 451
    gene therapy, 76
    Goodpasture syndrome, 612, *612*
    Graves disease, 614-615
    Hashimoto thyroiditis, 629
    Lupus erythematosus, systemic,
        810

multiple sclerosis, 868-869, *868*
pemphigoid, bullous, 965
progressive systemic sclerosis, 1019
sarcoidosis, 1090
Wegener granulomatosis, 1294-1295
Autologous blood donation, 213
Autologous bone marrow transplant. *See* Bone marrow transplant.
Automatism, 213
Autonomic nervous system, 213, 271, *213*
Autopsy, 213-214, *214*
Autosomal dominant traits, 214
Autosomal recessive traits, 214
Avascular necrosis of femoral head, 214
Aversion therapy, 214
Aviation medicine, 214
AVM. *See* Arteriovenous malformation.
Avoidant personality disorder. *See* Personality disorders.
Avulsed tooth, 215, *215*
Axilla, 215, *215*
Axillary lymph node dissection, 215
Axons, 899
Ayurveda, 215-216, *216*
Azithromycin, 216
Azoospermia, 216
AZT. *See* Zidovudine.

B

B cell, 217, 709, 814-815, *217*
Babesiosis, 217
Babinski reflex, 217, *217*
Baby bottle tooth decay, 217-218, 1017, *218*
Baby teeth. *See* Primary teeth.
Bach flower remedies, 218
Bacilli, 218
Bacitracin zinc, 218
Back injuries, first aid, 1314
Back pain, 218-221
diskography, 470
exercises, *219*
lifting, *220*
spinal injury, 1150

Backache, symptom chart, 20-21
Baclofen, 221
Bacteremia, 221
Bacteria, 221-222, *221*
flesh eating, 222, *222*
Bacterial infections, *222*
Bacterial vaginosis. See Vaginosis, bacterial.
Bacteriology, 222
Bacteriuria, 222
Bad breath, 222-223
Bagassosis, 223, 486
Baker cyst, 223
Balance, 223
Balanitis, 223
penis problems, 49
Baldness, 139-140, *139*
Ballismus, 223, 740
Balloon angioplasty, 223-225, 641, 643, *224*
Balloon catheter, 225, *225*
Balloon valvuloplasty. *See* Valvuloplasty.
Bandage, 225, *225*
Barbiturates, 226
addiction to, 477
anesthesia, 163
butalbital compound, 3011
Bariatric surgery, 226-227, *226*
Barium enema, 227-228, *227*, *228*
Barium swallow, 228, *228*
Barodontalgia, 124
Barotrauma, 228-229, *229*
aviation medicine, 214
Eustachian tube, 530
Bartholin glands, 229, *229*
Bartonelliosis. *See* Cat-scratch disease.
Basal body temperature (BBT), 229
Basal cell carcinoma, 229-230, 1127-1128, *230*
Basal ganglia, 230
Baseball elbow, 230, 515
Baseball finger, 231, *231*
Basophils, 252
Battery, 231
BCG vaccination, 231
Becaplermin, 231
Beclomethasone. *See* Corticosteroids.
Becker muscular dystrophy, 873

Beckwith-Wiedemann syndrome, 817, 939
Bed bath, 231
Bed rest, 231
Bedpan, 231
Bedridden, 231
Bedsores. *See* Pressure sores.
Bed-wetting, 231-232, *232*
Bee pollen, 232
Bee stings, 232, 243
Bee venom and bee products, therapeutic, 233
Behavior therapy, 233
adolescents, 120-121
Alzheimer's disease, 145-146
attention deficit/hyperactivity disorder, 209
autism, 210-211
automatism, 213
aversion therapy, 214
compulsive, 392
Belching, 233, *233*
Bell palsy, 233-234, 542
Benazepril hydrochloride. *See* Antihypertensives.
Bends. *See* Decompression sickness.
Benign, 234
Benign familial tremor, 234
Benign prostatic hyperplasia. *See* Prostate, enlarged.
Benzodiazepines, 226, 234
Benzoyl peroxide, 111, 234
Bereavement, 234, 509
Beriberi, 234
Berylliosis, 234, 486
Beta2 antagonists, 1156
Beta blockers, 180, 234-235, *235*
Beta-carotene, 235
Bezoar, 235
BIA. *See* Bioelectric impedance analysis.
Bier block, 165
Bifocal, 235
Bigeminy, 235
Biguanides, 235
Bilateral, 235
Bile, 235-236
Bile acids
sequestrants, 361-362
Bile duct, 236, *236*
cancer, 236

obstruction, 236, 237
    gallstones, 588-589
Bilharziasis, 1092
Biliary atresia, 236-237
Biliary cirrhosis, 237
Biliary colic, 237
Biliary system, 237
Bilirubin, 237-238, 253, 689-690
Billroth operation, 238
Binet test, 238
Bioavailability, 238
Biochemistry, 238
Bioelectric impedance analysis, 238
Biofeedback, 238, *238*
    bruxism, 296
    pain management, 947, *947*
Biological therapy, 308
Biomechanical engineering, 238
BioMEMS, 81
Bionic people, 88-93
Biopsy, 239, *239*
    brain tumor, 274
    breast, stereotactic, 1162-1163
    breast cancer, 276, *277*
    endometrial, 510
    jejunal, 745
    kidney, 757-758
    liver, 799
    needle, 890, *890*
    renal, 1062
    skin, 1127
Biorhythms, 239
Bioterrorism, 239, *240*
Biotherapeutic agents, 239
Biotin, 239
Bipolar disorder, 239, 241
    depression, 33
Bird fancier's lung, 144
Birth, 241
    multiple, 865, 867
Birth canal, 241, *241*
Birth control. *See* Contraception.
Birth defects, 241-242
Birth rate, 242, *242*
Birth weight, 242
Birthing centers, 242
Birthmark, 242, 649
    port-wine stain, 1007, *1007*
Births, multiple. *See* Twins;
  Multiple births.
Bisacodyl, 242
Bisexuality, 242-243

Bismuth, 243
Bisoprolol. *See* Beta blockers.
Bisphosphonates, 243
Bite, 243, *243*
Bites and stings, 243
    animal, 243-244, *243*
    first aid, 1314, *1315*
    human, 244
    insect, 244
    reptile, 244-245, *244, 245*
    spider, 245, *245*
    tick, 245-246, *246, 1215*
Bitolterol, 246
Black cohosh, 246
Black hairy tongue, 246
Blackhead, 246, *110*
Blackout, 246
Bladder, 246-247, *246*
    cancer, 246-247, *247*
        cystectomy, 430
    cystitis, 421
    cystourethrocele, 432
    exstrophy, 535-536
    infection, 15
    irritable, 741
    and bowel management, 246
    muscular control of, *717*
    tumors, 247
Blastomycosis, 247-248
Bleaching, dental, 248, 410, *248*
Bleeding, 248-249, 254, *249*
    See also Hemorrhage.
    anal pain, 17
    breakthrough, 275
    disorders, 248-249
    first aid, 1315
    gums. *See* Periodontal disease.
    hemostasis, 659
    menstruation, 841
    metrorrhagia, 845
    rectal, 1055
    threatened abortion, 100-101
    transfusion, 1231-1232, *1231*
    vaginal, 1264
    von Willebrand disease,
        1287-1288
Blepharitis, 249
Blepharoplasty. *See* Eyelid surgery.
Blepharoptosis, 249, 541, *249*
Blepharospasm, 249-250, *250*
Blind loop syndrome, 250
Blind spot, 250, 1278

Blindness, 250-251
    visual impairment aids, *251*
Blister, 251-252, *252*
    fever, 560
Blocking, 252
Blood, 252-258
    cells, 252-253, *253*
    clotting, 253
    donation, 254
    in feces, 553
    gases, 254, 256
    groups, 252, 254, 257
    loss, 254
    platelets, 992
    products, 255-256
    transfusion, 257, 1231-1232, *257,
        1231*
Blood cell count, complete. *See*
    CBC (complete blood cell count).
Blood count, 253-254, 256
Blood culture, 427
Blood loss, 254
Blood poisoning, 254
    bacteremia, 221
Blood pressure, 254-255, *254*
    See also Antihypertensives.
    classification, *695*
    cuff, 255, *255*
    diastolic, 465
    hypertension, 694-696
    prehypertension, 694, 1014,
        695, 696
    systolic, 1187
Blood smear, 256
Blood tests, 256-257
Blood urea nitrogen. *See* Kidney
    function tests.
Blood vessels, 257, 320
    broken, 291
    defects, 249
    transposition of great vessels, 1234
Blood volume, 704
Blood-brain barrier, 257, 269, *257*
Bloodless surgical techniques, 258,
    258
Blow-out fracture, 258, *258*
Blurred vision, 258-259
Blushing, 259, 571
BMI. *See* Body mass index.
Board-and-care homes, 804
Body image, 259, 296
Body mass index, 259-260, *259*

overweight, 939
waist-to-hip ratio, 1290
Body piercing, 260, *260*
Bodywork, 260, 1081
Boil, 260, 314, *260*
Bolus, 261
Bonding, 261
dental, 261, 564-565
Bone, 261
abscess, 261
cancer, 261-262
hip pain, 43
cyst, 262
graft, 262
imaging, 263
knee pain, 44
loss, 263
malunion, 823
nonunion, 905
skeletal system, *65*
spur, 1157, *1157*
See also Fracture.
Bone density testing, 262, 444
Bone graft, 262
Bone imaging, 263
Bone loss, 263
Bone marrow, 263-265
biopsy, 263
transplant, *264*
allogeneic, 263-265, *264*
aplastic anemia, 158
autologous, 213, 265
graft-versus-host disease,
613, *613*
stem cell replacement, 92
Bone scan, 265, *65*
Booster, 265
Borborygmi, 265-266
Borderline personality disorder. *See*
Personality disorders.
Bottle-feeding, 266, *266*
Botulinum toxin, type A, 266, *266*
Botulism, 176, 266-267, *266*
first aid, 1322
Bougie, 267, *267*
Bovine spongiform encephalopa-
thy, 819, 1310
Bow legs, 267
Bowel, 267
and bladder management, 246
sounds, 267
Bowel movements, abnormal, 267
Bowen disease, 267-268, 1157, *268*

Braces
dental, 268
orthodontic appliances, 924-925,
925
orthopedic, 268
bow legs, 267
Brachial plexus, 268
Brachial plexus block, 165, 268
pain management, 946
Brachialgia, 268
Brachytherapy, 268-269
prostate cancer, 1023
Bradycardia, 269
pulse, 1044
Bradykinesia, 269
Brain, 269-274, *270, 336*
abscess, 271
aneurysm, 167
basal ganglia, 230
cerebral thrombosis, 338-339, *339*
damage, 271
evoked responses, 530
functions of, *67*
gray matter, 616
hemorrhage, 271, 656-658
hypothalamus, 702-703, *703*
imaging, 271-273, *272*
meninges, 836
organic disorder, 924
sensory cortex, 1102-1103
stroke, 1171, 1173, *1172*
tumor, 273-274
aphasia, 186
dizziness, symptom chart,
36-37
headache, symptom chart,
38-40
Brain death, 271, 438
Brain stem, 273, *273*
Bran, 274, *274*
Branchial cleft abnormalities,
274-275
Braxton Hicks contractions, 275
BRCA, 275
Breakthrough bleeding, 275
Breast, 275-284, *274*
abscess, 276
enlargement, 278-279, *279*
fibroadenoma, 561, *561*
fibrocystic, 562, *562*
gynecomastia, 621
lift, 279-280, *280*
lump, 280

nipple, 903
paget disease, 943
pain or lumps, symptom chart,
22-23
reconstruction, 281-283, *282*
reduction, 283-284, *283*
self-examination, 284, *285*
stereotactic biopsy, 1162-1163
Breast cancer, 276-278, *276, 277*
biopsy, *277*
BRCA, 275, 278
mastectomy, 827-828, *827*
oncogenes, 917
See also Mammogram.
Breast cancer genes. *See* BRCA.
Breast milk, 280
Breast pump, 281, *281*
Breast-feeding, 284-287, *286*
Breath, shortness of, 287
Breathing, 287-288, 807
artificial respiration, *863*
exercises, 287, *287*
orthopnea, 926
problems, 287-288
stridor, 1171
tachypnea, 1189
Breathlessness. *See* Dyspnea.
Breech delivery, 241, 288, *289*
cesarean section, 343
Breech presentation, 288
Bridge, dental, 290, *290*
Brimonidine, 290
Brittle bones, 290-291
Broca aphasia, 186
Broken blood vessels, 291
Broken tooth, 291
Bronchi, 807, 1068
obstructive airways disease,
914-915
Bronchiectasis, 291
Bronchioles, 291
Bronchiolitis, 291-292
Bronchitis, 292-293, *292*
chest pain, 24
chronic obstructive pulmonary
disease, 366
coughing, 29
Bronchoconstriction in asthma, 200
Bronchodilators, 293, *293*
Bronchopneumonia, 294
Bronchopulmonary dysplasia, 294,
294
Bronchoscopy, 294-295, *295*

Bronchospasm, 295
Bronchus, 295
Brucellosis, 295, 1310
Bruise, 295, 1316
Bruit, 295
Bruxism, dental, 295-296, 1195
Bubonic plague, 296
Budd-Chiari syndrome, 296
Buerger disease, 296
Bulimia, 296-297
    adolescents, 120
    body image, 259
Bulk-forming laxatives, 777
Bulla. See Blister.
Bumetanide, 297
BUN. See Kidney function tests.
Bundle branch block, 297, *297*
    bradycardia, 269
Bunion, 297-298
Buphthalmos, 298, *298*
Bupivacaine, 164
Buprenorphine, 298
Bupropion, 298
Burkitt lymphoma, 129, 298
    oncogenes, 917
Burning tongue, idiopathic, 298
Burns
    chemical, 298
    classification, *300*
    electrical, 298-299, *299*
    to eye, 538
    first aid, 1316-1317
    heat, 299
    scalds, 1091
Burping. See Belching.
Burr hole, 299, 418, *419*
Bursa, 299
    Baker cyst, 223
Bursitis, 299, 301
    hip pain, 43
Buspirone, 301
Butalbital compound, 301
Bypass surgery, 301-303, *302*
    for angina, 169
    ischemic heart disease, 643
Byssinosis, 303, 486

C

CA-125 test, 304
C-reactive protein, 304

Cachexia, 304
Cadaver, 304
Cadmium poisoning, 304
Café au lait spots, 304
    neurofibromatosis, 898
Caffeine
    headache, 40
    sleep problems, 55
CAGE test, 1100
Calciferol, 304
Calcification, 304
    dental, 304
Calcinosis, 304
Calcitonin, 304
    osteoporosis, 932
Calcium, 304-305, 849
    for adolescents, 120
    and bone loss, 263
Calcium channel blockers, 305
Calculus
    dental, 305, *305*
    urinary tract, 305-306, *306*
Caliper splint, 306
Callus
    bony, 306
    skin, 307
Caloric test, 307
Calorie, 307
Calorie requirements, 307-308
Calorimetry, 308
Calve-Perthes disease. See Osteo-
    chondrosis.
Campylobacter, 308
Cancer, 308-311, *309-310*
    hereditary risk factors for, 311
    metastasis, 843, *843*
    oncogenes, 917
    screening, 311
    See also parts of the body by
    name.
Candidiasis. See Yeast infections.
Canker sore, 312
Cannabis compounds, 312, 478
Cannula, 312
Cap, dental. See Crown, dental.
Capecitabine, 312
Capgras syndrome, 312
Capillary, 312
Capitation, 312, 683
Caplan disease, 994
Caplet, 312
Capsaicin, 312
    pain management, 946

Capsule, 312
Capsulitis, adhesive. See Frozen
    shoulder.
Captopril. See Antihypertensives.
Car restraints, 312-313, 353
Carbamazepine, 313
Carbamide peroxide, 313
Carbohydrates, 313-314, 468, *313*
    absorption, 101-102
    glucose, 607
Carbon dioxide, 314
    shortness of breath, 287
Carbon monoxide poisoning, 999
    first aid, 1327
Carbon tetrachloride, 314
Carbuncle, 314
Carcinogen, 314
Carcinogenesis, 314
Carcinoid syndrome, 314-315
Carcinoma, 315
Carcinomatosis, 315
Cardiac arrest, 315
    hypoxia, 271
Cardiac output, 315, 639
Cardiac rehabilitation, 315
Cardiac stress testing, 315-317, *316*
Cardiologist, 317
Cardiology, 317
Cardiomegaly, 317
Cardiomyopathy, 317-318
    postpartum, 1008
Cardiopulmonary resuscitation
    (CPR), 319, 1070, *319*
    anaphylaxis, 155
    artificial respiration, 196
    drowning, 476
Cardiorespiratory fitness, 319-320
Cardiothoracic surgery, 320
Cardiovascular fitness, 320
Cardiovascular surgeon, 320
Cardiovascular system, 320-321, *321*
    fitness, 320
    See also Blood; Blood vessels.
Cardioversion, 321-322, *322*
Caregiving for older people, 322-
    324, *323, 324*
    abuse, 104
    Area Agencies on Aging, 190
Caries
    bottle. See Baby bottle tooth
    decay.
    dental. See Cavity, dental.

Carisoprodol, 324, 870
Carotene, 324, 1281
Carotid artery, 324-325, *325*
Carotid endarterectomy, 325, *325*
  atherosclerosis, 206
Carpal tunnel syndrome, 325, 327, 1063
  grip, 617
  numbness or tingling, 48
  Tinel sign, 1216
  wrist protection, *326*
Carrier, 327
Cartilage, 327, *327*
  chondrosarcoma, 363
  knee pain, 44
Cartilage-hair hypoplasia, 1124
Carvedilol, 180
Case manager, 327
Case-control studies, 327
Cast, 327-328, *328*
Castration, 328
Cat-scratch disease, 328
Catalepsy, 328
Cataplexy, 328
  narcolepsy, 883-884
Cataract, 328-329, *91, 329*
  aphakia, 186, *186*
  blindness, 250
  night blindness, 902
  surgery, 329-330, *329*
  vision loss or impairment, 41
Catatonia, 330
Catharsis, 330
Cathartics, 330
Catheter, 330
  balloon, 225, *225*
Catheter-related infections, 332
Catheterization
  access sites, *651*
  cardiac, 330-331
    angiography, 169
    coronary artery disease, 408
  urinary, 331-332, *331*
Cats, toxoplasmosis, 1226-1228, *1227*
Cauda equina, 332
  syndrome, 332
Caudal, 332
Caudal block, 332
Causalgia, 332
Caustic, 332
  ingestion. *See* Poisoning,

swallowed caustics.
Cauterization, 332
Cavernous sinus thrombosis, 332
Cavity, dental, 324, 332-333, *333*
CBC (complete blood cell count), 333
CCU. *See* Coronary care unit.
CD4 cell, 333
CDC. *See* Centers for Disease Control and Prevention.
Cecum, 333, 467
Cefaclor, 333
Cefadroxil. *See* Cephalosporins.
Cefixime. *See* Cephalosporins.
Cefpodoxime. *See* Cephalosporins.
Cefprozil. *See* Cephalosporins.
Ceftazidime. *See* Cephalosporins.
Ceftibuten. *See* Cephalosporins.
Ceftriaxone sodium. *See* Cephalosporins.
Cefuroxime. *See* Cephalosporins.
Celecoxib, 333
Celiac disease, 333-334
  diarrhea, 35
  feces, 553
  gluten, 608
  malabsorption, 820
  weight loss, 62
Cell, 334-335, *334*
  division, 335
Cell death, programmed, 188
Cellulitis, 335
Celsius scale, 335, *335*
Cementum, 335
Centers for Disease Control and Prevention, 335
  bioterrorism, 239
  reportable diseases, 1064
Central nervous system, 335-336, *335, 336*
  brain, 269
  tabes dorsalis, 1188
Centrifuge, 336
Cephalexin, 336
Cephalhematoma, 336-337
Cephalosporins, 337
Cerclage, cervical, 337
Cerebellum, 337, *337*
Cerebral contusion, 337
Cerebral hemorrhage. *See* Hemorrhage, cerebral.
Cerebral palsy, 337-338, *338*

Cerebral thrombosis, 338-339, *339*
Cerebrospinal fluid, 339
  hydrocephalus, 687-688
  lumbar puncture, 806
Cerebrovascular accident, 339
Cerebrovascular disease, 339
Cerebrum, 339-340, *340*
Certificate of need, 340
Certification board, 340
Cerumen. *See* Earwax.
Cervical cap, 340, 401, *340*
Cervical dysplasia, 341
Cervical intraepithelial neoplasia. *See* CIN.
Cervical osteoarthritis, 341. *See also* Osteoarthritis.
Cervical polyps, 341
Cervical rib, 341
Cervicitis, 341-342
  breakthrough bleeding, 275
Cervix, 342, *342*
  cancer of, 342-343, *343*
  culture of, 427
  incompetence. *See* Incompetent cervix.
  LEEP, 780, *780*
  Pap smear, 951, *951*
  polyps, 341
Cesarean section, 343-344, *343*
  breech delivery, 288
Cetirizine. *See* Antihistamines.
Chagas disease, 344, 954
Chakra balancing, 344, 425, 513
Chalazion, 344, *344*
Chancre, 344
  syphilis, 1186
Chancroid, 344-345
Charcoal, 345
Charcoal, activated, 345, 503
Charcot joint, 345
Charcot-Marie-Tooth disease, 345
Checkup, 345
Cheilitis, 345-346
Chelating agents, 346
Chelating therapy, 346
  penicillamine, 965-966
Chemical burns, first aid, 1316, 1320
Chemical peel, 346-347, *347*
  for acne, 111
  actinic keratosis, 114
Chemical poisoning, 999

Chemonucleolysis, 347
Chemotherapy, 347-348, *347, 348*
Cherry angiomas, 348
Chest pain, 348-349, *349*
  and heart attack, *349*
  first aid, resuscitation (CPR), 1328
  symptom chart, 24-25
Chest tube, 349
Chest x-ray, 349, *349*
Chewing tobacco, 349-350
Cheyne-Stokes, 350
Chickenpox, 350
  rash, 50, 52
  vaccination, 1263
Chilblains. *See* Pernio; Cold injury.
Child abuse. *See* Abuse, child.
Child development, 350-353
  milestones, *351*
  theories, 352-353
Childbirth, 353, 1064
  anesthesia, 167
  cesarean section, 343-344, *343*
  emergency, 353
  episiotomy, 520, *520*
  first aid, 1317
  malpresentation, 823
  maternal mortality, 828-829
  midwife, 847
  natural, 886
  pudendal block, 1038
  puerperal sepsis, 1038
  vacuum extraction, 1264
  version, 1273
Child safety seats, 313, 353, *354*
Children
  anesthesia, 164-165, *164*
  art therapy, 192
  asthma, 200
  avascular necrosis of femoral
    head, 214
  baby bottle tooth decay, 217-218
  bed-wetting, 231-232
  car seats, 313, 353, *354*
  development, 350-353
  failure to thrive, 544-545
  growth, 618-620, *619*
  knock-knees, 763
  pedophilia, 963
  rehabilitation, 961-962, *961*
  toilet training, 1218
  vaccination, 1262-1263
Chinese medicine, 353, 355, 428,
  1060, *355*

herbal medicine, 664-666
  ma huang, 817
  moxibustion, 862, *355*
  Qigong, 1047
  T'ai chi, 1189, *1189*
  Tui-Na, 1245
Chinese restaurant syndrome, 355
Chiropractic, 355-356, *356*
  applied kinesiology, 190
  manipulation, 825
  network, 356
Chlamydia, 356, 964, 1110
Chloasma, 356
Chlorpheniramine maleate, 356
Chlorzoxazone, 870
Choking, 356-357, *357*
  first aid, 1317
Cholangiocarcinoma, 357
Cholangiopancreatography, 357
Cholangitis, 357
  biliary atresia, 237
Cholecalciferol, 1283
Cholecystectomy, 357, 359, *358*
Cholecystitis, 359
  chest pain, 348
  gallstones, 588-589
Cholecystography, 359
  biliary colic, 237
Cholera, 359-360
Cholescintigraphy, 360
Cholestasis, 360
Cholesteatoma, 360
Cholesterol, 360-361, *361*
  bile, 236
  lowering drugs, 361-362, *362*
  in obesity, 913
Cholestyramine resin, 362
Cholinergic drugs, 987
Cholinesterase inhibitors, 145
Chondritis, 362
Chondrocalcinosis, 362
Chondromalacia, 362-363
Chondromatosis, 363
Chondrosarcoma, 363
Chordee, 363
Chorea, 363, 740
Choreoathetosis, 363
Chorioamnionitis, 363
Choriocarcinoma, 363
Chorionic villi, 363
Chorionic villus sampling,
  363-365, *364*

birth defects, 242
Choroidal melanoma. *See* Eye
  tumors.
Christian Science, 364, 545
Christmas disease, 544
Chromium, 364, 849
Chromium picolinate, 364
Chromosomes, 334, 365
  abnormalities, 364-365, 441, *365*
  analysis, 752
  karyotyping, 752
  Klinefelter syndrome, 762
  mosaicism, 860
  sex, 1106-1107, *1106*
  trisomy syndromes, 1239-1240
  tuberous sclerosis, 1244-1245
Chromotherapy. *See* Color therapy.
Chronic, 365
Chronic care facility, 365-366
Chronic fatigue syndrome, 366
Chronic obstructive lung disease.
  See Chronic obstructive
  pulmonary disease.
Chronic obstructive pulmonary dis-
  ease, 366-368, 405, *367*
  emphysema, 503
  wheezing, 1298
Cidofovir, 368
Cigarettes. *See* Smoking, tobacco.
Cilia, 368
Cilostazol, 368
Cimetidine, 368
CIN, 368
Ciprofloxacin. *See* Fluoro-
  quinolones.
Circadian rhythm, 368
Circulatory system. *See* Cardio-
  vascular system.
Circumcision, male, 368-369, *369*
Cirrhosis, 369, *369*
  alcoholic, 800
  esophageal varices, 526
  weight gain, 60
Cisapride, 369
Cisplatin, 370
Citalopram, 370
Clarithromycin, 370
Claudication, 370
  atherosclerosis, 205
  ischemia, 742
Claustrophobia, 370
Clavicle, 384. *See also* Collarbone.
Clawhand, 370, *370*

Cleft lip and palate, 370-371, 441, *371*
Clicking jaw, 296, 371, 1196, *371*
Clinical trial, 371-372
Clitoridectomy, 372, 555
Clitoris, 372, 1064, *372*
Clomiphene citrate, 372, 723, 940
Clonazepam. *See* Benzodiazepines.
Clone, 372, *373*
Clonidine, 372
Cloning, 1054-1055, *76, 373*
Clonus, 372
Clopidogrel bisulfate, 372
Closed-caption service, 199
Clostridium difficile, 372, 374
Clotrimazole, 374
Clotting factors, 256
Clubbing, 374
Clubfoot. *See* Talipes.
Cluster headache, 632
Coagulation, disseminated intravascular (DIC), 249
Coal dust, 994
Coarctation of aorta, 374, *374*
COBRA-EMTALA, 374
Cocaine. *See* Crack cocaine.
Cocaine Anonymous, 481
Coccidioidomycosis, 374-375
Coccydynia, 375
Coccygodynia. *See* Coccydynia.
Cochlea, 375
    acoustic trauma, 112
    ototoxicity, 936
Cochlear implant, 375-376, 713, *93, 376*
Codeine, 376
Codependence, 376
Coffee enemas, 376-377
Cognitive-behavioral therapy, 377
Cohort study, 377
Coinsurance, 377
Coitus, 377
Coitus interruptus, 377
Colchicine, 377
Cold injury, 378, *378*
Cold remedies, 378-379
Cold sore, 379, 560, *379*
Cold, common, 379-381, *380, 381*
    coughing, 28
    headache, 39
    parainfluenza, 952
    rhinitis, 1077-1078

sore throat, 1142
Colectomy, 381, *381*
Colestipol hydrochloride, 381
Colic, 381-382, *382*
    biliary, 236, 237
    and child abuse, 103
    renal, 1062
    ureteral, 1254
Colitis, 382-383, *383*
    anal discharge, 152
    bowel movements, 267
    enterostomy, 514
    pseudomembranous, 1030
    rectal bleeding, 1055
Collagen, 383
    aging, 126
    brittle bones, 290
    diseases, 383
    Ehlers-Danlos syndrome, 498-499
    injections, 383-384, *384*
    in skeletal dysplasia, 1124
Collar, orthopedic, 384
Collarbone, 384
Colles fracture, 384, *384*
Colon, 384-385, 467, 737
    cleansing, 385
    hemicolectomy, 651
    Hirschsprung disease, 671-672
    irritable. *See* Irritable bowel syndrome.
    megacolon, 832, *832*
    pseudo-obstruction, 1029
    spastic. *See* Irritable bowel syndrome.
Colon and rectal surgeon, 385
Colon cancer, hereditary nonpolyposis, 385
Colon, cancer of the, 385-386, *385*
    colectomy, 381, *381*
    iron-deficiency anemia, 159
    weight loss, 62
Colonoscopy, 386, *387*
    versus barium enema, 227
    colon cancer, 386
    virtual, 84
Color blindness, 388, 1280
Color therapy, 388
Color vision, 388, *388*
Colorado tick fever, 388-389
Colorectal cancer, anal pain, 17
Colostomy, 381, 386, 389, *390*

Colostrum, 280, 389
Colposcopic biopsy, 389
Colposcopy, 389
Coma, 389
    diabetic, 462, 1319
Commensal, 389
Commode, 389
Common cold. *See* Cold, common.
Communicable disease, 389
Community health. *See* Public health.
Compartment syndrome, 389, 391
Complementary medicine, 143, 391
    See also Alternative medicine.
Complex, 391
Compliance, 391
Complication, 391
Composite, dental. *See* Bonding, dental.
Compress, 391
Compression fracture, 391-392, *392*
Compression syndrome, 392
    carpal tunnel syndrome, 325
Compulsive behavior, 392
Computed tomography. *See* CT scanning.
Concentration, 392
Conception, 392, *393*
Concussion, 392, *392*
    headache, 38
Conditioning, 392-393, 399-400
Condom, 393
    penis problems, 49
Condyloma. *See* Human papillomavirus.
Condyloma acuminatum, 393-394
Condyloma latum, 394
Cone biopsy, 394
Confabulation, 394
Confidentiality, 394-395
Confusion in older people, 395
Congenital, 395
Congenital, hypothyroidism, 395
Congestive heart failure. *See* Heart failure, congestive.
Conjunctiva, 395
Conjunctivitis, 395-396, *396*
Conn syndrome, 135
Connective tissue disease, mixed, 396

Conscious sedation, 396-397
  See also Anesthesia.
Consciousness, 397
  blackout, 246
  coma, 389
  dizziness symptom chart, 36-37
  drowsiness, 477
  fainting, 545, *545*
Consensual sex, 397
Constipation, 397, 553
  abdominal pain, 98
  anal pain, 17
  and diarrhea, 34
  symptom chart, 26-27
  weight loss, 62
Contact dermatitis, 397-398
Contact lenses, 398-399, *399*
Contact tracing, 399
Contagious, 399
Continuing care retirement communities. *See* Long-term care
  facility.
Contraception, 399-401, *400*
  barrier methods, 399-401, *400*
  cervical cap, 340, 401, *340*
  coitus interruptus, 377
  condom, 399-400
  cramps or pain, 16
  diaphragm, 401
  emergency postcoital, 401
  hormonal methods, 401-402,
    401
  oral mestranol and northin-
    drone, 842
  other methods, 402-403, *403*
  postcoital, 1007-1008
  safer sex, 1086
  sponge, 401
Contraceptive, 403
  foam and jelly, 403
  implant, 403
Contraction stress test, 404, 1015
  fetal monitoring, 558
Contractions, uterine, 404
Contracture, 404
  Dupuytren, 486
Contraindication, 404
Contrast medium, 404
  angiography, 169-170
  barium enema, 227, 228
  biomedical imaging, 80-81
  digital subtraction angiography,
    468

Controlled substance, 404
Contusion, 295, 337, 404
  See also Bruise.
Convalescence, 404
Conversion disorder, 404-405
Convulsion, 405. *See also* Seizure.
Cooley anemia. *See* Anemia, Cooley.
COPD. *See* Chronic obstructive
  pulmonary disease.
Copper, 405, 849
  Wilson disease, 1300
Cor pulmonale, 405
  asthma, 202
Cordotomy, 405
Cornea, 405, 536, *405*
  refractive surgery, 1059
Corneal abrasion, 405
Corneal implants, stem cell
  research, 79
Corneal reflex, 1057
Corneal transplant. *See*
  Keratoplasty, penetrating.
Corneal ulcer, 398, 406
Coronary artery bypass grafting
  (CABG). *See* Bypass surgery.
Coronary artery disease, 406-408,
  407
  angina, 168
  bypass surgery, 301-303, *302*
  cardiomyopathy, 317
Coronary care unit, 408
Coronary heart disease. *See*
  Coronary artery disease.
Coronary thrombosis, 408-409
Coroner, 409
Corpus luteum cyst, 409
Corpuscle, 409
Corset, 409
Corticosteroid hormones, 409
Corticosteroids, 409
Corticotropin. *See* ACTH.
Corticotropin-releasing hormone.
  See CRH.
Cortisol, 121-122, 409, 410
Cortisone. *See* Corticosteroids.
Cosmetic dentistry, 410-411, *410*
Cosmetic surgery, 411, *411*
Costochondritis, 411
Co-trimoxazole, 411
Cough, 411-412, *720*
  chronic, 412
  smoker's, 412

Cough remedies, 378-379, 412
Counseling, genetic, 596-597
Counseling, psychological, 413
  marital, 826
Couples therapy, 413
COX-2 inhibitors, 154
Coxa vera, 413, *413*
Coxsackievirus, 414
Crab lice, 414-415, *414*
Crack cocaine, 415, *415*
Cradle cap, 415
  childhood rash, 51
Cramp, 415-416, *415*
  heat, 647
  writer's, 416
Cranberry, 416
Cranial nerves, 416, *417*
Craniofacial dysostosis, 416, *416*
Craniopharyngioma, 416, 418
Craniosacral technique. *See*
  Visualization.
Craniosynostosis, 418
Craniotomy, 418-419
Cranium, 419
Creatinine. *See* Kidney function
  tests.
Creatine clearance. *See* Kidney
  function tests.
Creative visualization. *See*
  Visualization.
Cremation, 419
Crepitus, 419
CREST syndrome, 419, 1019
Creutzfeldt-Jakob disease, 419,
  1134
CRH, 419
Crib death. *See* Sudden infant
  death syndrome.
Cricothyroidotomy, 419-420, *419*
Crisis intervention, 420
Critical, 420
Critical care, 420, *420*
Crohn disease, 420-421, 724-725, *421*
  stem cell research, 79
Cromolyn sodium, 421
Crossbite, 421
Cross-dressing, 1234
Crossed eyes. *See* Strabismus.
Crossmatching, 421-422
Cross-tolerance, 422
Croup, 422, *422*
Crouzon disease. *See* Craniofacial
  dysostosis.

Crowding, dental. *See* Over-crowding, dental.
Crown, dental, 422-423, *423*
Cruciferous vegetables, 423, *423*
Crush syndrome, 423
Crutch palsy, 423
Crying, in infants, 424, *424*
Cryopreservation, 424
Cryosurgery, 424-425
    Bowen disease, 268
Cryotherapy, 425
Cryptococcosis, 425
Cryptorchidism. *See* Testicle, undescended.
Cryptosporidiosis, 425, *425*
    opportunistic infection, 921
    waterborne, 1293
Cryptosporidium, 425
Crystal therapy, 425-426
C-section. *See* Cesarean section.
CT scanning, 80, 426-427, *426*
    bone imaging, 263
    brain, 273
    kidney, 759-760
    liver and gallbladder, *69*
    lung, 809
Culture, 427-428, *427*
Cunnilingus, 428
Cupping, 428, *355*
Cure, 428
Curet, 428, *428*
Curettage, 428. *See also* D and C.
    ablation, 99
    abortion, 99, 100
    actinic keratosis, 114
    basal cell carcinoma, 230
    Bowen disease, 268
    dental, 428
Cushing syndrome, 428-429, *429*
    weight gain, 60
Cusps, dental, 429
Cutaneous, 429
Cutdown, 429
Cuts and scrapes, first aid, 1318
Cutting and burning. *See* Self-mutilation.
CVS. *See* Chorionic villus sampling.
Cyanide, 429
Cyanocobalamin, 429, 1282
Cyanosis, 429-430
Cybernetics, 89

Cyborg, 88
Cyclobenzaprine, 430
Cycloplegia, 430
Cyclosporine, 430
Cyclothymia, 430
Cyst, 430
    Baker, 223
    Bartholin glands, 229
    bone, 262
    breast pain, 22
    dermoid, 451
    epidermal, 516
    kidney, 758-759
    marsupialization, 826
    ovarian, 936-937, *936*
    pilonidal, 987
    polycystic kidney disease, 1003-1004
    sebaceous, 1097
    thyroglossal, 1210
Cystectomy, 430
Cystic fibrosis, 430-431, *430*
    bronchiectasis, 291
Cystitis, 431
    abdominal pain, 15
    urine discoloration, 58
Cystocele, 431, *431*
Cystography, voiding 431
Cystometrogram, 431-432
Cystoscopy, 432
    bladder cancer, 247
Cystotomy, 432, *432*
Cystourethrocele, 432, 1073, *432*
Cytokines, 433
Cytologist, 433
Cytology, 433, *433*
Cytomegalic viral retinitis, 433
Cytomegalovirus, 433-434, 1111
    retinitis, 433, 434
Cythopathologist, 434
Cytopathology, 434, *434*
Cytoplasm, 334

D

D and C, 435, *435*
D and E, 435
    abortion, 99
    elective, 100
Dacryocystitis, 435-436, *435*
Danazol, 436
Dandruff, 436

Dapsone, 436
Date rape, 436
Day care, adult, 436, *436*
    Alzheimer's disease, 144-146
    Area Agencies on Aging, 190
Day treatment program, 436
De Morgan spots. *See* Cherry angiomas.
de Quervain disease, 436, 1197
Deafness, 436-437, 635, *437*
Death, 437-438
    medical ethics, 529
    sudden, 1176
    sudden infant, 1176
Death certificate, 438
Death rate, 438
Debility, 438
Debridement, 438, *438*
Decalcification, dental, 438
Decerebrate, 438
Deciduous teeth, 438
Decoding devices, 199
Decompression sickness, 438-439
Decompression, spinal cord, 439
Decongestant drugs, 439, *439*
    for common cold, 378
    ephedrine, 515
    phenylpropanolamine, 982
Decorticate, 439
Decubitus ulcers. *See* Pressure sores.
Deductible, 439
Deer. *See* Lyme disease.
Defecation, 439-440
Defense mechanisms, 440, *440*
Defibrillation, 440-441
    atrial fibrillation, 207
    cardioversion, 321
    ventricular fibrillation, 192, 1272
Defibrillator, 440-441, *441*
    implantable, 80
Defoliant poisoning, 441
Deformity, 441
Degeneration, 441
Degenerative joint disease, 927
    See also Osteoarthritis.
Dehiscence, 441
Dehydration, 441
    first aid, 1319
Dehydroepiandrosterone. *See* DHEA.
Déjà vu, 441
Deletion 22q syndrome, 441

Delirium, 441-442
Delirium tremens, 442
Delivery
   breech, 288, *289*
   cesarean, 343
   forceps, 579, *579*
   vacuum extraction, 1264
   vaginal, 241, 442
Delusion, 442-443
Dementia, 443, *443*
   Alzheimer's disease, 144-146
   Lewy body, 789
   neuropsychological testing, 900
   Pick disease, 986
   vascular, 1268
Demyelination, 443
Dendrites, 899
Dendritic ulcer. *See* Herpes
   keratitis.
Dengue, 443-444
Densitometry, 444
Density, 444
Dental assistant, 444
Dental dam, 444
Dental examination, 444-445, *445*
Dental hygienist, 445
Dental implants, 90
   See also Implants, dental.
Dental laboratory technician, 445
Dental x rays. *See* X rays, dental.
Dentin, 445
Dentist, 445
Dentistry , 445
   aerodontalgia, 124
   alignment, 135
   alveoloplasty, 144
   amalgam, 146
   avulsed tooth, 215
   bleaching, 248, 1195
   bonding, 261
   calculus, 305
   cosmetic, 410-411, *410*
   crown, 422-423
   curettage, 428
   decalcification, 438
   deciduous teeth, 438
   fillings, 564-565
   gingival pocket, 998
   gingivectomy, 601
   impaction, 711-712
   impression, 713
   inlays, 728

   onlay, 918
   oral and maxillofacial surgeon,
      921
   overbite, 938, *938*
   periodontal disease, 971-972
   permanent teeth, 975-976
   plaque, 991
   primary teeth, 1017-1018
   prosthodontics, 1028
   pulpitis, 1043
   reimplantation, 1060
   resorption, 1066
   restoration, 1069-1070
   retainer, 1070
   root canal treatment, 1081-1082,
      1082
   scaling, 1091, *1091*
   sealants, 1096
   splinting, 1153
   supernumerary teeth, 1180-1181
   tooth care, 1195
   underbite, 1253
   veneers, 1271
   wisdom tooth, 1300-1301
Dentition, 445
Dentures, 445-446, *446*
Deoxyribonucleic acid, 446
Dependence, 446-447
Depersonalization, 447
Depilatories, 623
Depression, 447-448
   adolescents, 121
   alcoholism, 133
   bipolar disorder, 239, 241
   bowel movements, 267
   in older people, 448
   postpartum, 1008-1009
   sleep problems, 54
   symptom chart, 32-33
   weight gain, symptom chart,
      60-61
   weight loss, symptom chart,
      62-63
   See also Personality disorders.
Depressor, tongue, 1219
Derealization, 448-449
Dermabrasion, 449, *449*
   for acne, 111
Dermatitis, 449
   artefacta, 449
   atopic, 449-450
   contact, 397-398, *398*
      plants, 991

   herpetiformis, 450
   seborrheic, 1097
Dermatofibroma, 450
Dermatographism, 450
Dermatologist, 450
Dermatology, 450-451
Dermatomycosis, 451
Dermatomyositis, 451
Dermatophyte infections, 451
Dermis, 1126-1127
Dermoid cyst, 451
DES. *See* Diethylstilbestrol.
Desensitization, 451
Desensitization, allergy, 451
Designer drugs, 451
Desipramine, 451
Desmoid tumor, 452
Desogestrel. *See* Estradiol.
Desoximetasone. *See* Corticosteroids.
Detergent worker's lung, 144
Detoxification, 452, 481
Detoxification programs, 452
Developmental delay, 452-453, *453*
Developmental disorders, perva-
   sive, 453
DEXA. *See* Dual-energy X-ray
   absorptiometry.
Dexamethasone, 453
Dextroamphetamine, 453
Dextrocardia, 453
Dextromethorphan hydrobromide,
   453
Dextrose, 453
DHEA, 453
   antiaging therapy, 175
Diabetes, gestational, 461-462,
   599-600
Diabetes insipidus, 453-454, *454*
   ADH, 119
Diabetes mellitus, 454-461
   acidosis, 109
   atherosclerosis, 205
   autoimmunity, 212
   coma, 462, *462*
   gene therapy, 77
   glucose metabolism, 607-608
   hyperglycemia, 691
   hypoglycemia, 700
   insulin, 731-732
   insulin shock, 1115, 1330
   insulin-dependent. *See* Diabetes
      mellitus, type 1.

nephropathy, 893-894, *894*
non–insulin-dependent. See
  Diabetes mellitus, type 2.
numbness or tingling, 48
retinopathy, 250, 463,
  1072-1073, *1073*
type 1, 454-457, *456*
type 2, 457-461, *460*
urination problems, 56, 57
weight loss, 62
Diabetic coma, 462
Diabetic retinopathy, 250, 463,
  1072-1073, *1073*
Diagnosis, 463
Diagnosis-related group. See DRG.
Diagnostic imaging, 463
Dialysis, 463
  machine, 463
  peritoneal, 973, 975, *974*
  See also Hemodialysis
Dialyzer. *See* Dialysis machine.
Diaper rash, 50, 463-464
Diaphoresis, 464
Diaphragm muscle, 464, *464*
Diaphragm, contraceptive, 49, 401,
  464
Diarrhea, 464-465, 553
  abdominal pain, 98
  anal pain, 17
  and constipation, 27
  E. coli, 464-465, 490
  first aid, 1319
  rehydration fluid, 1060
  symptom chart, 34-35
  traveler's, 465, 1236
  weight loss, 62
Diastolic blood pressure, 465
Diathermy, 465
Diathesis, 465
Diazepam. *See* Benzodiazepines.
Diclofenac sodium. *See*
  Nonsteroidal anti-inflammatory
  drugs.
Dicloxacillin. *See* Penicillins.
Didanosine (ddI), 465
Diet
  balanced, 465-466
  constipation, 26
  and diabetes mellitus, 459
  fad, 544
  fiber, 560-561
  Food Guide Pyramid 573-575,
  574

Gerson therapy, 599
low-fat, *551*
macrobiotics, 817
Mediterranean, 831-832
phytochemicals, 986
renal, 1062
vegetarianism, 1270-1271
Dietary assessment, 466
Dietary reference intakes, 466, 476
Dietetics, 466
Diethylstilbestrol, 466
Dietitian, registered, 466
Differentiation, 466
Diffusion, 466
Diflunisal, 466-467
Digestion, 467
Digestive system, 467-468, *467,*
  468
  atlas, *69*
Digital scanners, 73
Digital subtraction angiography,
  468
Digoxin, 468
Dilation, 468
Dilation and curettage. See D and C.
Dilation and evacuation. See D
  and E.
Dilator, 468
Diltiazem. *See* Calcium channel
  blockers.
Dimenhydrinate, 468
Diphenhydramine, 468
Diphtheria, 468-469
  vaccination, 1262
Diplopia. *See* Double vision.
Disability, 469-470, *469*
Discharge, 470
Disclosing agents, 470
Disinfectants, 470
Disk prolapse. *See* Slipped disk.
Disk, intervertebral, 470
  back pain, 220
Diskography, 470
Dislocation, joint, 470
  first aid, 1319
Disorientation, 470
Displacement, 470
Dissociative disorders, 470-471
  fugue, 585
  multiple personality disorder,
  867-868
Distal, 471

Disulfiram, 471
Diuretics, 180, 471
Divalproex. *See* Valproic acid.
Diverticular disease, 471-472, *472*
  abdominal pain, 99
  colectomy, 381, *381*
  constipation, 26
Diverticulitis, 471
  acute abdomen, 98
Diverticulosis, 471
Diving medicine, 472
  decompression sickness,
  438-439
Dizziness, 472, 1273
  symptom chart, 36-37
DNA, 335, 446, 595, 596, 909
  See also Deoxyribonucleic acid.
  fingerprinting, 472
  forensic testing, 473
  Human Genome Project,
  683-684
  paternity testing, 960
  recombinant, 1054-1055
DNR. *See* Advance directives;
  Do-not-resuscitate order (DNR).
Do-not-resuscitate order (DNR),
  473, 1299
Docetaxel, 473
Docusate sodium, 473
Dofetilide, 473
Donepezil, 473
  for Alzheimer's disease, 145
Dong Quai root, 473
Donor, 473
  uniform card, *473*
Dopamine, 473
Doppler ultrasound, 473-474
  of kidney, 759
Dorsal, 474
Dorzolamide, 474
Dose, 474
Double vision, 474
Double-blind, 474
Douche, 474
Down syndrome, 474-475, 841,
  1240, *365*
  amniocentesis, 150
  heart disease, 641
  microcephaly, 845
Doxazosin, 475
Doxepin, 475
Doxycycline, 475

Drain, surgical, 475
Dream analysis, 475
Dreaming, 475-476
  analysis, 475
Dressings, 476, *476*
Dressler syndrome, 476
DRG, 476
DRIs. *See* Dietary reference
  intakes.
Drip, postnasal, 1008
Dronabinol, 476
Drooling, 476
Drop attack, 476
Drowning, 476
  dry, 477
Drowsiness, 477
Drug, 477
  abuse, 477, *479*
  addiction, 477-480, *478*
  and abuse of older people, 104
  and child abuse, 103
  and depression, 32
  approval process, 480
  dependence. *See* Drug addic-
    tion.
  eruption, 480
  generic, 596
  investigational, 740
  orphan, 924
  overdose, 938-939
  over-the-counter, 939, *1120*
  proprietary name, 1020
  resistance, 1066
  sensitivity, 480
  smart, 1136
  and sports, 1155-1156, *1156*
  testing. *See* Drug approval
    process.
  treatment programs, 480-481,
    481
  trial. *See* Clinical trial.
Drunk driving, 481-482, *482*
Dry eye, 482
Dry mouth, 482-483
  bad breath, 222-223
DSA. *See* Digital subtraction
  angiography.
DSM-IV, 483
DTaP vaccination, 483
DTs. See Delirium tremens.
Dual diagnosis, 483
Dual-energy X-ray absorptiometry

(DEXA), 483, *484*
  bone density testing, 262, 263,
    484
  osteopenia, 930
  osteoporosis, 931
Duchenne muscular dystrophy,
  872
Duct, 483
Dumping syndrome, 483
Duodenal contents culture, 427
Duodenal ulcer, 483, 485, *485*
  abdominal pain, 14, 98
Duodenitis, 485-486
Duodenum, 486, *486*
Dupuytren contracture, 486
Dura mater, 269
Durable power of attorney, 486
Dust diseases, 486-487
  asbestosis, 196-197, 486
  farmer's lung, 548-549
  pneumoconiosis, 994
  silicosis, 1121
Dust mites, 487
Dwarfism, 1123-1124
DXA. *See* Dual-energy X-ray
  absorptiometry.
Dyes
  in angiography, 170
  fluorescein, 569-570
  Gentian violet, 598
  See also Contrast medium.
Dying, care of the. *See* End-of-life
  care.
Dysarthria, 487
Dyscalculia, 779
Dysentery, 488
Dysequilibrium, 488
Dysgraphia, 779, *779*
Dyshidrotic eczema, 488
Dyskinesia, 488
Dyslexia, 488, 779
Dysmenorrhea, 488, 841
Dyspareunia, 488
Dyspepsia, 488, 717
Dysphagia. *See* Swallowing
  difficulty.
Dysphasia, 488
Dysphonia. *See* Hoarseness.
Dysphoria, 488
Dysplasia, 488-489
Dyspnea, 489, *489*
Dysthymia, 489
Dystonia, 489

Dystrophy, 489
Dysuria. *See* Urination.

E

E. coli, 176, 490, 524, *490*
  first aid, 1322
  food poisoning, 577, *577*
  waterborne, 1293
E. coli diarrhea. *See* Diarrhea,
  E.coli.
Ear, 490-491, *491*
  discharge from, 491
  eustachian tube, 530
  examination of, 491-492
  foreign body in, 492
  injuries, first aid, 1319-1320
  labyrinthitis, 766-767
  otic preparations, 933
  pinning back of. *See* Otoplasty.
  swimmer's, 1184
  See also Hearing.
Earache, 492
Eardrum, perforated, 492-493
Earwax, 493, 635, *493*
  syringing of the ears, 1187
Eating disorders, 493
  See also Anorexia nervosa;
    Bulimia; Weight loss.
  pica, 986
Eaton-Lambert syndrome, 493
Ebola virus, 493-494
Ecchymosis, 494
ECG, 494-495, *495*
Echinacea, 495
Echocardiogram, 495, *495*
Echocardiography, 495
  transesophageal, 1230
Echolalia, 496
Eclampsia, 496
ECT, 496
Ecstasy, 451
Ectoparasite, 496
Ectopic
  heartbeat, 496-497
  pregnancy, 98, 100-101, 497,
    497
Ectropion, 497-498, 541, *497*
Eczema. *See* Dermatitis.
Edema, 498, *498*
  optic disc, 921
  pulmonary, 1039, 1067

EEG. *See* Electroencephalogram.
Efavirenz, 498
Efficacy, drug, 498
Effusion, 498
  joint, 498
Egg, 498
  implantation, 713
  infertility, 721-723
Ego, 498, 582
Ehlers-Danlos syndrome, 498-499
Eisenmenger complex, 499
Ejaculation, 499
  premature, 1014
Ekbom syndrome, 1069
EKG. *See* ECG.
Elbow
  arthroscopic surgery, 195
  baseball, 230, 515
  epicondylitis, 515
  golfer's, 609-610
  nursemaid, 909-910, *909*
  tennis, 1197
Eldercare locator, 190
Electra complex, 499
Electric shock, 1114-1115
Electric shock treatment. *See* ECT.
Electrical burns, first aid, 1316
Electroacupuncture. *See*
  Homeopathy.
Electrocardiogram, 499
Electrocardiography, 494-495, 499,
  495
Electrocautery, 499, *499*
Electroconvulsive therapy. *See* ECT.
Electrodiagnostic studies, 499-500
Electroencephalogram, 498, 500,
  500
Electrolysis, 500, 623
  hair removal, 623
Electrolyte, 500
Electromyogram, 500
Electromyography, 500
Electrophoresis, 500
Elephantiasis, 500-501
ELISA test, 501
Ellis-van Creveld syndrome, 1124
Embolectomy, 501
Embolism, 501-502, *501*
  pulmonary, 809, 1039-1040,
  1040
Embolization, therapeutic, 502
Embolus, 502

Embryo, 502, *502*
  agenesis, 125
  medical ethics, 529
  transfer, 502
Emergency, 502-503
  childbirth. *See* Childbirth,
    emergency.
  department, 503
  medical technician (EMT), 503,
    953
  physician, 503
Emery-Dreifuss dystrophy, 873
Emesis, 503
Emetics, 503
EMG. *See* Electromyography.
Emotional deprivation, 503
Emotional problems, 503
Empathy, 503
Emphysema, 503-504, *504*
  smoking effects, 1139
  subcutaneous, 504
Empirical treatment, 504
Employee assistance program (EAP),
  504, *505*
Empyema, 505
EMT. See Emergency medical
  technician (EMT).
Emulsion, 505
Enabling, 505
Enalapril, 180, 505
Enamel
  dental, 505-506
  hypoplasia, 702
Encephalitis, 506, 1310
  herpes, 667
  hypoxia, 271
Encephalomyelitis, 506
Encephalopathy, 506-507
Encopresis, 507
Endarterectomy, 507
Endemic, 507
Endocarditis, 507, *507*
Endocrine glands. *See* Endocrine
  system.
Endocrine system, 507-508, *508*
  atlas, *72*
Endocrinologist, 508
Endocrinology, 508
Endodontics, 508
Endodontist, 508
End-of-life care, 508-509, *509*
Endogenous, 509

Endometrial ablation, 509
Endometrial biopsy, 510
Endometrial cancer, 510
Endometrial hyperplasia, 510
Endometrial polyp, 510, 511
Endometrioma, 511
Endometriosis, 511, *511*
  cramps or pain, 16
  infertility, 721
Endometritis, 511
Endometrium, 512, *510*
Endorphins, 512
Endoscope, 512
Endoscopic retrograde cholan-
  giopancreatography. *See* ERCP.
Endoscopy, 512, *512*
Endothelium, 512
Endotoxin, 512
Endotracheal tube, 512-513
End-stage renal disease. *See*
  Kidney failure.
Enema, 513
  barium, 227-228
  coffee, 376-377
Energy, 513
Energy medicine, 513, *513*
Energy requirements. *See* Calorie
  requirements.
Engagement, 514
Enkephalins, 514
Enlarged prostate. *See* Prostate,
  enlarged.
Enophthalmos, 514
Enoxaparin sodium, 514
ENT. *See* Otolaryngologist.
Entacapone, 514
Enteric fever. *See* Typhoid fever.
Enteritis. *See* Crohn disease.
Enterocele, 514
Enteroclysis, 514
Enterocolitis, necrotizing, 889-890
Enterostomy, 514
Enterotoxin, 514
Entropion, 514-515, *514*
Enuresis, 515
  nocturnal, 231
Environment, global warming, 605
Environmental medicine, 515, *515*
Enzyme, 515
Enzyme-linked immunosorbent
  assay. *See* ELISA test.
Enzyme therapy, 515

Eosinophils, 252
Ependymoma, 515
Ephedra, 665
Ephedrine, 515
Epicondylitis, 515
Epidemic, 515
Epidemiology, 515-516
Epidermal cyst, 516
Epidermis, 516, 1126
Epidermolysis bullosa, 516
Epididymal cyst. See
   Spermatocele.
Epididymis, 516-517, 1065, 516
Epididymitis, 516-517
Epidural abscess, spinal, 517
Epidural block, childbirth, 167
Epiglottis, 64, 517, 517
Epiglottitis, 517, 517
Epilepsy, 517-519, 518
   anticonvulsants, 177-178
   autism, 211
   seizures, 1097-1099
   status epilepticus, 1161
   temporal lobe, 519
Epinephrine, 519
   anesthesia, 164
Epiphora, 519
Epiphysis, slipped capital femoral,
   519-520, 519
Episcleritis, 520, 520
Episiotomy, 520, 520
Epispadias, 520-521, 521
Epistaxis, 907
Epithelium, 521
Epstein-Barr virus, 521
ERCP, 521, 523, 521
Erectile dysfunction, 523, 1066,
   1109, 522
   penile implant, 966
   sildenafil citrate, 1121
Erection, 523
Ergocalciferol. See Calciferol.
Ergometer, 523
Erhlichiosis
   human granulocytic, 684
   human monocytic, 684-685
Erikson, Erik, 352-353
Erogenous zones, 523
Eroticism, 523
Erysipelas, 523
Erythema infectiosum. See Fifth
   disease.

Erythema multiforme. See Drug
   eruption.
Erythema nodosum, 523-524, 523
Erythrocyte, 524
Erythrocyte sedimentation rate.
   See ESR.
Erythroderma, 524, 524
Erythromycin, 524
   and sulfisoxazole, 1179
Erythropoietin, 524
Esalen massage, 524
Eschar, 524
Escherichia coli. See E. coli.
Esophageal atresia, 524
Esophageal dilation, 524-525
Esophageal diverticulum, 525, 525
Esophageal spasm, 526
Esophageal stricture, 526
Esophageal varices, 237, 526-527,
   527
Esophageal reflux, 525-526, 526
   abdominal pain, 14
chest pain, 24, 348
   heartburn, 647
   hiatal hernia, 669
Esophagectomy, 527
Esophagitis. See Esophageal reflux.
Esophagogastroduodenoscopy.
   See Gastroscopy.
Esophagogastrostomy. See
   Gastroscopy.
Esophagogram, 228, 527
Esophagoscopy. See Gastroscopy.
Esophagus, 467, 527-528, 527
   cancer of the, 64, 528
   Mallory-Weiss syndrome,
   821-822
Esotropia, 528
ESR, 528
Estradiol, 528
Estriol, 528
Estrogen, 528, 1065, 1107
and breast cancer, 277
   conjugated, 528-529
   in menopause, 838-839
   and osteoporosis, 931
   replacement therapy, 680-681
Estrone. See Estrogen.
Etanercept, 529
Ethanol. See Alcohol.
Ether, 163
Ethics, medical, 529, 791

Ethnic factors
   antihypertensives, 180
   diabetes mellitus, 458
   Tay-Sachs disease, 1193
   See also Sickle cell anemia.
Ethylene diaminetetraacetic acid
   (EDTA), 346
Ethylene glycol 529
   antifreeze poisoning, 178-179,
Etiology, 529
Etretinate, 529
Euphoria, 529-530
Eustachian tube, 530
   adhesive otitis media, 119
   otitis media, 933
Euthanasia, 530
Euthyroid, 530
Eversion, 530
Evoked responses, 530
Ewing sarcoma, 530-531
Examination, physical, 531, 532
Excision, 531
Excoriation, 531
Exemestane, 531
Exercise, 531
   aerobic, 533, 124
   and aging, 531, 533
   anaerobic, 533
   benefits of, 531
   breathing, 287, 287
   Kegel, 753, 753
   pelvic floor, 964
   pulmonary function, 1041
   range-of-motion, 1052
   resistance, 533, 1066, 533
   and sleep problems, 55
   strengthening, 534, 534
   stress testing, 533
   stretching, 568
   weight loss, 62
   weight-bearing, 534, 1296, 534
Exfoliation, 534
Exfoliative dermatitis. See
   Erythroderma.
Exhibitionism, 534
Exocrine gland, 534-535
Exophthalmos, 535, 535
   vision loss or impairment, 41
Exostosis, 535
Exotoxin, 535
Exotropia, 535
Expectorants, 535
Expectoration, 535

Expiration, 535
Exploratory surgery, 535
Explosive disorder, 535
Exstrophy of the bladder, 535-536
Extrapyramidal system, 536
Extrinsic factor deficiency, 544
Extradural hemorrhage. *See*
    Hemorage, epidural.
Extrapyramidal system, 536
Extrovert, 536
Exudate, 536
Eye, 536, *537*
    drops, 536, *536*
    examination of, 539-540, *540*
    foreign body in, 538
    injury, 536, 538
        first aid, 1320-1321
    prosthetic, 540
    tumors, 538-539
    See also disease or condition by
        name.
Eye movements
    nonrapid (NREM), 1130
    rapid (REM), 1130
Eyelash, trichiasis, 1237
Eyelid, 536
    blepharitis, 249
    blepharoptosis, 249, *249*
    blepharospasm, 249-250
    chalazion, 344
    drooping, 541
    ectropion, 497-498
    entropion, 514-515, *514*
    meibomianitis, 832
    surgery, 540-541, *541*
    tarsorrhaphy, 1192
    tumors, 539

F

Fabry disease, 542
Face-lift, 542, *543*
Facial palsy, 542.
    See also Bell palsy.
Facial spasm, 544
Facies, 544
Factitious disorder, 544
Factor VII deficiency, 544
Factor VIII deficiency, 544,
    1287-1288
Factor IX deficiency, 544
Fad diets, 544

Fahrenheit scale, 544, *544*
Failure to thrive, 544-545
Fainting, 545, 1253, 1270, *545*
    first aid, 1321
    symptom chart, dizziness, 34-35
Faith healing, 545-546
Fallen arches. *See* Flat feet.
Fallopian tube, 546, *546*
    cannulation, 1241
    ligation, 1241-1242, *1241*
    pregnancy, 1242
    salpingo-oophorectomy, 1089
    tuboplasty, 1245
Fallout, 546
Falls, in older people, 546-547,
    547
False memory, 547-548
False teeth, 548
Famciclovir, 548
Familial, 548
Familial hypercholesterolemia,
    548
Familial Mediterranean fever, 548
Family medicine, 548
Family physician, 548
Family therapy, 548
Family violence, 1275
Famotidine, 548
Fanconi anemia. *See* Anemia,
    Fanconi.
Fantasy, 548
Farmer's lung, 548-549
Farsightedness, 549, *550*
Fascia, 549
Fasciculation, 549
Fasciitis, 549
Fasciotomy, 549
    necrotizing, 890
Fasting, 549, *549*
Fat
    body, 551, *551*
    waist-to-hip ratio, 1290
Fatigue, 551
    Chronic fatigue syndrome, 366
Fats and oils, 551-552
    absorption, 101-102
    hydrogenated, 688
    monounsaturated, 552, 858
    saturated, 1090
    trans-fatty acids, 1230
    unsaturated, 361, 1254
Fatty acids, 552

FDA. *See* Food and Drug
    Administration.
Febrile seizures. *See* Seizure,
    febrile.
Fecal impaction, 552
Fecal incontinence, 716
Fecalith, 552
Fecal-occult blood test, 267, 311,
    386, 552, 915
Feces, 552-553
    abnormal, 553
    blood in the, 553
    diarrhea, 464-465, 553
    steatorrhea, 1161
Feeding, infant, 553
    burping, *554*
Feldenkrais method, 553
Fellatio, 553
Felodipine, 553, 555
Female
    genital mutilation, 555
    puberty stages, *1036*
    reproductive system, *70,*
        1064-1065, *1065*
    sex hormones. *See* Estrogen;
        Progestin.
    urinary tract, *71*
    X chromosome, 1304
Femur
    avascular necrosis, 214
    slipped capital epiphysis,
        519-520, *519*
Fentanyl, 555
Ferrous sulfate, 555
Fertility, 555
    See also GnRH; Ovulation
        stimulants.
Fertilization, 555, 714, 1064, 1065,
    70, 555, 714-715
    in vitro, 199
        assisted hatching, 629
        sperm extraction, 1146
FESS, 555-556, *556*
Fetal alcohol syndrome, 133, 556
    microcephaly, 845
Fetal distress, 556-557
Fetal monitoring, 556-558, *557*
Fetal tissue research, 558
Fetishism, 558
Fetus, 558
    development of, *558*
    intrauterine growth retardation,
        739

umbilical cord, 1252-1253
Fever, 558-560, *560*
   first aid, 1321-1322
Fever blister, 560
Feverfew, 560
Fexofenadine, 560
Fiber
   dietary, 560-561
   constipation, 26
   flatulence, 568
Fiberoptics, 561
Fibric acid derivatives, 362
Fibrillation, 561
   atrial, 206-207, *206*
   ventricular, 192, 1272
Fibrinolysis, 561
Fibroadenoma, 561, *561*
   breast, 280
Fibrocystic breasts, 562, *562*
   breast pain or lumps, 22
Fibroid, uterine, 562, *562*
Fibroma, 562-563
Fibromyalgia, 563, *563*
   back pain, 220
Fibrosarcoma, 563
Fibrosis, 563
   interstitial, of lung, 735
   pulmonary, 1040-1041
   retroperitoneal, 1073
Fifth disease, 563-564
   childhood rash, 50
Fight-or-flight response, 564
Filariasis, 564
Filgrastim, 564
Filling, dental, 564-565, *545*
Film badge, 565
Financial abuse, 104
Finasteride, 565
Finger, 565
   baseball, 231, *231*
   joint replacement, 748
   trigger, 1238-1239
Fingernail, paronychia, 958
Fingerprint, 565
First aid, 1312-1333
   See also specific conditions.
Fishhook injuries, first aid, 1322,
   1322
Fissures, anal, 152-153
Fistula, 565, *565*
   arteriovenous, 193
   tracheoesophageal, 1228-1229

Fitness, 565-566, *567*
   testing, 566
Fixation, 566
Flail chest, 566, *566*
Flat feet, 566
Flatulence, 566
Flatus. *See* Flatulence.
Flatworm, 568, 569, 1236
Flesh eating bacteria, 222, 1330
Flexibility training, 568
Floaters, 568, *568*
Floppy infant, 568-569
Floss, dental, 569, *569*
Flow cytometry, 569
Flu, 569, 725-726
Fluconazole, 569
Fluctuant, 569
Fluke, 569, 801, 956, 1236, *569*
Fluocinolone, 569
Fluorescein, 569-570
   angiogram, 570, 817
Fluoridation, 570
Fluoride, 570, 849, *570*
Fluoride toothpaste, 223, 1195
Fluoroquinolones, 570
Fluorosis, 570-571, 1195
Fluoxetine, 571
Flurbiprofen. *See* Nonsteroidal
   anti-inflammatory drugs.
Flush, 571
Flutamide, 571
Fluticasone, 571
Fluvastatin sodium, 571
Fluvoxamine maleate, 571
Folic acid, 571, 1282
Folic acid deficiency, 571
Follicle, 572
Follicle-stimulating hormone.
   See FSH.
Folliculitis, 572
Fomite, 572
Fontanelle, 418, 572, 1141, *572*
Food. *See* Diet, balanced; Nutrition.
Food additives, 572
Food allergy, 137, 572-573
   anaphylaxis, 155
Food and Drug Administration,
   573
Food Guide Pyramid, 573-575,
   910, *574*
Food intolerance, 575
Food poisoning, 575-577, *576*
   E. coli, 577, *577*

first aid, 1322-1323
   seafood, 577-578
Food-borne infection, 578
Food-drug interactions, 578
Foot, 578-579, *579*
   fallen arches, 546, 566
   hallux valgus, 626, *626*
   hammer toe, 627
   metatarsalgia, 844
   reflex points, *1059*
   syndactyly, 1185
Footdrop, 579
Foramen, 579, *579*
Forceps, 579, *579*
   delivery, 579
Forebrain, 269, 271
Foreign body
   in ear, 492
   in eye, 538, 540
Forensic medicine, 579-580, *580*
Foreplay, 580
Foreskin, 580, *580*
Formaldehyde, 580
Formula, chemical, 580
Formulary, 580
Fosinopril, 580
Fracture, 580-581, *581*
   ankle or foot, 18
   arm, 190-191, *190*
   blow-out, 258
   cast, 327-328, *328*
   compression, 391-392, *392*
   dental, 581
   first aid, 1323, *1323, 1324*
   hip, 42, 670-671
   jaw, 745
   leg, 780-781
   March, 825
   Monteggia, 858-859
   nose, 907
   Pott, 1010
   rib, 1079
   skull, 1130, *1130*
   stress, 1171
Fragile X syndrome, 581-582, 841,
   582
Freckle, 582
Free-floating anxiety, 582
Frenulum, 1219
Freud, Sigmund, 352, 583
   dream analysis, 475
   psychoanalysis, 1032

Freudian theory, 582-583
  Electra complex, 499
  neurosis theory, 900-901
  Oedipus complex, 916
  subconscious, 1175
  unconscious, 1253
Friedreich ataxia, 583, 1151
Frontal lobe syndrome, 583
Frostbite, 583-584, *584*
  first aid, 1324
Frottage, 584
Frozen section, 584
Frozen shoulder, 585
Fructose, 585
Frustration, 585
FSH (follicle stimulating hor-
  mone), 585, 1107
  hypogonadism, 700-701
  infertility, 723
Fugue, 585
Functional endoscopic sinus
  surgery. *See* FESS.
Functional improvement, 585
Fundoplication, 585-586, *586*
Fungal infections. *See* Mycosis.
Fungi, 586
Furosemide, 586
Furuncle. *See* Boil.
Fusion for back pain, 221

G

G6PD deficiency, 157-158, 587
GABA, 587
Gabapentin, 587
Gag reflex, 1057
Gait, 587, *587*
Galactorrhea, 587
Galactosemia, 587
Gallbladder, 587-588, 738
  cancer, 588
  nausea or vomiting, 47
Gallium scan, 588
Gallstones, 588-589, *589*
  acute abdomen, 98
  bile, 236
Gambling, addictive, 589-590, *590*
Gamete, assisted reproductive tech-
  nology, 199, 601
Gamete intrafallopian transfer.
  See GIFT.

Gamma globulin, 590, 699-700
Gamma knife radiosurgery, 590
Ganciclovir, 590
Ganglion, 590
Gangrene, 590-591
Ganser syndrome, 591
Garlic, 591
Gas exchange, alveoli, 143
Gas, toxic, inhalation, 728
Gastrectomy, 591, *591*
  Bilroth operation, 238
Gastric, 1166-1167
  See also Stomach.
Gastric contents culture, 427
Gastric erosion, 591-592
Gastric lavage. *See* Stomach
  pumping.
Gastric ulcer, 485, 592, 1167, 1251
  abdominal pain, 14
Gastritis, 592-593
  nausea or vomiting, 46
Gastroenteritis, 593
  abdominal pain, 14
  diarrhea, 35
  nausea or vomiting, 46
Gastroenterologist, 593
Gastroenterology, 593
Gastroesophageal reflux disease
  (GERD). *See* Esophageal reflux.
Gastrointestinal (GI) series,
  593-594
Gastrointestinal system. *See*
  Alimentary tract; Digestive system.
Gastrointestinal tract. *See*
  Digestive system.
Gastrojejunostomy, 594, *594*
Gastroplasty, 226
Gastroscopy, 394
Gastrostomy, 594
Gatekeeper, 594
Gaucher disease, 594-595
Gauze, 595
Gay, 595
G-CSF, 595
Gem therapy. *See* Crystal therapy.
Gemfibrozil, 595
Gender identity disorder, 595,
  1034
Gene, 595-596, *595*
  tumor suppressor, 1246
Gene mapping, 596, 683, *73, 75*
Gene therapy, 596, *77*

General anesthesia. *See*
  Anesthesia, general.
Generalized anxiety disorder.
  See Anxiety disorders.
Generic drugs, 596
Genetic code, 596
Genetic counseling, 596-597
Genetic disorders, 597
  See also disorders by name.
Genetic engineering, 76-77, 1054
Genetic screening, 597
Genetics, 597
  See also Twenty-first century
    medicine, 73-96
    behavioral, 597-598
    markers, bone marrow trans-
      plant, 265
Genital herpes. *See* Herpes, geni-
  tal; Sexually transmitted diseases.
Genital ulceration, 598
Genital warts, 598
Genitalia, 598
  mutilation of female, 555
Genotype, 598
Gentamicin, 598
Gentian violet, 598
Geographic tongue, 598, *598*
Geriatric care manager, 598
Geriatric medicine, 598-599, *599*
Geriatrician, 599
Germ, 599
Germ cell tumor, 599
German measles. *See* Rubella.
Gerontologist, 599
Gerontology, 599
Gerson therapy, 599
Gerstmann-Straussler-Scheinker
  disease, 1134
Gestalt theory, 599
Gestation, 599
Gestational diabetes, 599-600
Gestational trophoblastic disease,
  600
GI series. *See* Gastrointestinal
  (GI) series.
Giant cell arteritis. *See* Arteritis,
  giant cell.
Giardiasis, 600-601, *601*
  waterborne, 1293
GIFT, 601
Gigantism, 939, 1190
Gilbert disease, 601

Gingiva, 601
Gingivectomy, 601
Gingivitis. *See* Periodontal
  disease.
Ginkgo biloba, 601-602, 665, 912
Ginseng, 602
Gland, 602
Glands, swollen, 602
Glass eye. *See* Eye, prosthetic.
Glasses, 602
Glaucoma, 602-605, *604*
Glioblastoma multiforme, 605
Glioma, 605
Glipizide. *See* Sulfonylurea.
Global warming, 605
Globulin, 605
Globus hystericus, 605
Glomangioma. *See* Glomus tumor.
Glomepiride. *See* Sulfonylurea.
Glomerulonephritis, 605-606, *606*
  Goodpasture syndrome, 612
Glomerulosclerosis, 606
Glomerulus, *71, 757*
Glomus tumor, 606
Glossectomy, 606
Glossopharyngeal nerve, 606
Glottis, 606
Glucagon, 606, *606*
Glucocorticoids. *See* Corticosteroids.
Glucosamine-chondroitin, 607, 912
Glucose, 607, *607*
  See also Diabetes mellitus, type 1;
    Diabetes mellitus, type 2
  metabolism, 607-608, *607*
  meter, 608
  tolerance test, 608
Glucose-6-phosphate dehydroge-
  nase deficiency. *See* G6PD defi-
  ciency.
Glucosidase inhibitors, and dia-
  betes mellitus, 460
Glue sniffing, 608
Gluten, 608
  intolerance. *See* Celiac disease.
Gluten-sensitive enteropathy. *See*
  Celiac disease.
Glyburide, 608
Glycemic index, 608
Glycerol, 608
Glycogen, 608
Glycosuria, 608
GM-CSF, 608-609

GnRH, 609
Goiter, 609, *609*
  hyperthyroidism, 697
Gold compounds, 609
Golfer's elbow, 609-610, *610*
Gonadotropin hormones, 610
Gonadotropin-releasing hormone.
  See GnRH.
Gonads, 610
Gonioscopy, 610-611, *610, 611*
Gonorrhea, 611, 964, 1110
  anal pain, 17
Good Samaritan laws, 611-612
Goodpasture syndrome, 612, *612*
Goserelin, 612
Gout, 612-613, *613*
  ankle or foot problems, 18
  arthritis, 194
  hip pain, 42
  knee pain, 45
  pseudogout, 1029
Gout therapies, 613
G6PD deficiency, 587
Grafting, 613
  bone, 262
  skin, 1129
Graft-versus-host disease, 613, *613*
  bone marrow transplant, 265
Gram stain, 613
Grand mal seizure, 613
Granulation tissue, 613
Granulocyte, 613
Granuloma, 613-614
  annulare, 614
  inguinale, 614
  pyogenic, 1046
Graves disease, 614-615, 1214, *615*
  autoimmunity, 212
  eye, 615
  hyperthyroidism, 697
  vision loss or impairment, 41,
    615
Gravida, 615-616
Gray matter, 616
Greenhouse effect, 605, 616, *616*
Grieving, 234, 616, *616*
Grip, 616-617
Griseofulvin, 617
Groin, 617, *727*
  lump in the, 617
  strain, 617, *617*
Group A streptococcus infection,
  617

Group therapy, 617
Growing pains, 618
Growth
  childhood, 618-620, *619*
  intrauterine retardation, 739
Growth hormone, 618
  and sports, 1156
  short stature, 1115
  tall stature, 1190
Guaifenesin, 620
Guillain-Barré syndrome, 620, *620*
Guilt, 620
Gulf War syndrome, 620
Gum, 620
  bleeding, 249
  gingival hyperplasia, 693-694
Gumma, 621
Gynecologist, 621
Gynecology, 621
Gynecomastia, 621

H

H. pylori, 622, *622*
  duodenal ulcers, 485
Habituation, 622
Haemophilus influenzae, 622
  vaccination, 1262-1263
Hair, 622-623, *623*
  alopecia, 139-140
  hirsutism, 672
  pubic, 1038
  removal, 623-624, *623, 624*
  transplant, 624-625, *624, 625*
  trichotillomania, 1238
Halitosis. *See* Bad breath.
Hallucination, 625
Hallucinogenic drugs, 625-626
Hallux, 626, *626*
  rigidus, 626
  valgus, 626
Haloperidol, 626-627
Halothane. *See* Anesthesia, inhalation.
Hamartoma, 627
HAMAs (human antimouse antibodies), 78
Hammer toe, 627, *627*
Hamstring pull, 627
Hand, 627, *627*
  polydactyly, 1004-1005, *1005*
  syndactyly, 1185

Hand-foot-and-mouth disease, 627-628
  coxsackievirus, 414
Hangover, 628
Hansen disease. *See* Leprosy.
Hantavirus infection, 628, *628*
  animal-transmitted, 171
Hardening of the arteries. *See* Atherosclerosis.
Hashimoto thyroiditis, 629
Hatching, assisted, 629
Hatha yoga, 629
Hay fever, 629-630, *630*
  rhinitis, 1077-1078
HCG. *See* Human chorionic gonadotropin.
HDL. *See* Cholesterol.
Head
  banging, 630-631
  injuries, 631, *631*
    brain damage, 271
    first aid, 1324-1325, *1325*
    headache, 38
    nausea or vomiting, 46
  lag, 632
Head and neck cancer, 630
Headache, 632-634, *633*
  migraine, 847-848
  symptom chart, 38-40
Healing, 634
Healing touch. *See* Energy medicine; Therapeutic touch.
Health, 634
Health care, in the home. *See* Home health care.
Health food, 634
Health law, 634
Health maintenance organization. *See* HMO.
Hearing, 634-635, 939
  aids, 635, *636*
  hyperacusis, 689
  loss, 635, 637
    barotrauma, 228-229
    in older people, 637
    otosclerosis, 935, *935*
    tests. *See* Audiometry.
    tinnitus, 1216-1217
  sense of, 1101-1102
Hearing protection, 113, *112*
Heart, 637-639, *638*
  artificial, 647
  bypass surgery, 301-303, *302*

cardiomegaly, 317
cardiomyopathy, 317-318
dextrocardia, 453
long QT syndrome, 803-804
murmur, 644
open-heart surgery, 918
pericarditis, 970-971, *970*
transplant, 644-645
valvular stenosis, 1161-1162
Heart and circulatory system
  atlas, *68*
  diseases of, *407*
Heart attack, 639-641, 1325, *640*
  chest pain, 24
  cholesterol, 360
  dizziness, 36
  first aid, 1325
  infarction, 719
  ischemia, 742
  resuscitation, 1070, *1070*
Heartbeat
  arrhythmia, 191-192, *191*
  asystole, 203
  bradycardia, 269
  bundle branch block, 297, *297*
  ectopic, 496-497
  long QT syndrome, 803-804
  pacemaker, 943, *944*
  pulse, 1043-1044, *1043*
  Stokes-Adams syndrome, 1165
  tachycardia, 1188
Heart block, 641
Heart disease
  congenital, 641-642
  genetic research, 77
  hormone replacement therapy, 680
    hypertension, 695
    ischemic, 642-643
    valvular, 1266
Heart failure
  congestive, 643-644, *643*
    ankle or foot problems, 18
    aortic insufficiency, 184-185
    aortic stenosis, 185
    asthma, 202
    atrial fibrillation, 207
    coughing, 28, 30
    digoxin, 468
    shortness of breath, 287
    urination problems, 56, 57
    weight gain, 60
Heart murmur, 644

Heart rate, 644
  prenatal care, 1015
  Wolff-Parkinson-White syndrome, 1301-1302
Heart rhythm
  ventricular ectopic beat, 1272
Heart transplant, 644-645
Heart valve, 645-647, *646*
Heart valve surgery, *646*
  ablation, 99
Heartburn, 647
  abdominal pain, 14
  chest pain, 24, 348
  surgical treatment, *586*
Heart-lung machine, 647
Heart-lung transplant, 647
Heat
  cramps, 647
    first aid, 1325
  disorders, 647-648
  exhaustion, 647, 648, 1326, *648*
  stroke, 647-648, 1326, *648*
  treatment, 648-649
Heimlich maneuver, 196, 357, 649, 1070, 1318, *649, 1318*
  drowning, 476
Helicobacter pylori. See H. pylori.
Hellerwork. *See* Rolfing.
Helmets, sports, 649
Hemangioblastoma, 649
Hemangioma, 649, *649*
Hemarthrosis, 649-650
Hematemesis. *See* Vomiting blood.
Hematocrit, 650
Hematologist, 650
Hematology, 650
Hematoma, 650, *650*
Hematopoietic progenitor cells, 650
Hematospermia, 650
Hematuria, 650, *650*
Heme, 650-651
Hemianopia, 651
Hemiballismus, 651
Hemicolectomy, 651
Hemiparesis, 651
Hemiplegia, 651
Hemizygote, 651
Hemochromatosis, 651
Hemodialysis, 463, 651, 653, *651-652*
  See also Dialysis.
HIPAA, 1347-1350

Hemodialyzer. *See* Dialysis machine.
Hemoglobin, 252, 653
Hemoglobin C, 653-654
Hemoglobinopathy, 653-654
  prenatal screening, 597
Hemoglobinuria, 654
Hemolysis, 654
Hemolytic anemia, 158-159
Hemolytic disease of newborn, 654
Hemolytic-uremic syndrome, 655
Hemophilia, 655-656, *249, 655*
  diathesis, 465
  gene therapy, 77
  transfusion, 1231-1232, *1231*
Hemophilia A, 544
Hemophilia B, 544
Hemorrhage, 656, 1315
  antepartum, 173-174
  brain, 271
    dizziness, 37
    headache, 38
  cerebral, 656, *656*
  epidural, 656-657, *657*
  hypertensive, 696-697
  intracerebral. *See* Hemorrhage, cerebral.
  intraventricular, 657, 739, *657*
  postpartum, 1009
  retinal, 1071
  subarachnoid, 167, 657-658, 1174, *657*
  subconjunctival, 1174-1175
  subdural, 1175
  vitreous, 1284-1285, *1284*
Hemorrhoidectomy, 658
Hemorrhoids, 267, 658-659, 1055, *658*
  anal pain, 17
  constipation, 26
  removal of, 658, *658*
Hemosiderosis, 659
Hemostasis, 659
Hemothorax, 659, *659*
  chest tube, 349
Henoch-Schönlein purpura, 659-660
Heparin, 660, *660*
Hepatectomy
  partial, 660
  total. *See* Liver transplant.

Hepatic, 660
Hepatitis, 660-661
  A, 661-662
  alcoholic, 800
  B, 662, *662*
    vaccination, 1262
  C, 662-663
  chronic active, 664
  D, 663
  E, 663-664
  nausea or vomiting, 47
  nonalcoholic steatohepatitis, 800, 904
  viral, 664
Hepatoma, 664
Hepatomegaly, 664
Herbal medicine,
Herbal remedies, 664-666, *665*
  black cohosh, 246
  for common cold, 379
  feverfew, 560
  ginkgo biloba, 601-602
  ginseng, 602
  kava, 752
  Ma huang, 817
  Saw palmetto, 1090
  St. John's wort, 1158
  Tibetan medicine, 1214
  valerian, 1266
Hereditary nonpolyposis colon cancer (HNPCC), 385
Heredity, 666
  autosomal dominant traits, 214
  autosomal recessive traits, 214
  See also Chromosomal abnormalities; Chromosomes.
Heritability, 666
Hermaphroditism, 666
  pseudo, 1029-1030
Hernia, 666, *666*
  hiatal, 669-670, *669*
  strangulation, 1168-1169
Herniated disk. *See* Slipped disk.
Herniorrhaphy, 666
Herpangina, 666-667
Herpes
  B virus, 667, 684
  encephalitis, 667
  genital, 667-668, 1110
    penis problems, 49
  gestationis, 667
  keratitis, 667

  orolabial, 668-669, *669*
  roseola infantum, 1083
  Whitlow, herpetic, 1299
  zoster. *See* Shingles.
Heterosexuality, 669
Heterozygote, 669
HGE. *See* Human granulocytic ehrlichiosis.
HHV-8. *See* Human herpesvirus 8.
Hiatal hernia, 669-670, *669*
  abdominal pain, 14
  chest pain, 24, 348
Hib vaccine, 670
Hiccup, 670, *670*
HIDA scan, 670
Hidradenitis, 670
High blood pressure, 670
Hip, 670
  arthritis, 194
  avascular necrosis of femoral head, 214
  congenital dislocation of, 670
  fractured, 670-671, *671*
  joint replacement, 748-749, *749*
  osteochondrosis, 929
  pain, symptom chart, 42-43
  snapping, 671
Hippocratic oath, 671
Hirschsprung disease, 671-672
Hirsutism, 672
Histamine, 672
  in allergies, 137
  asthma, 200
Histamine$_2$ blockers, 672
Histocompatibility antigens, 672
Histologist, 672
Histology, 673
Histopathology, 673
Histoplasmosis, 673
History-taking, 673
Histrionic personality disorder, 673, 977
HIV, 673-676, *675,* 1110, 1111. *See also* AIDS.
Hives, 676, *676*
  childhood rash, 51
HLA types, 676
HME. *See* Human monocytic ehrlichoiosis.
HMG. *See* Human menopausal gonadotropin.

HMO, 676
HNPCC. *See* Colon cancer,
   hereditary nonpolyposis.
Hoarseness, 676-677
   symptom chart, 31
Hodgkin disease, 677, 815
   Agent Orange, 125
Holistic medicine, 677, 1308
Holter monitor, 677-678, *678*
Homatropine hydrobromide, 678
Home health care, 678, *678*
   for older people, 678-679, *678*
Home pregnancy tests, 679
Homeopathy, 679
Homeostasis, 679
Homocysteine, 679
   and folic acid, 571
Homocystinuria, 679
Homosexuality, 679-680
Homozygote, 680
Hookworm infestation, 680, *680*
Hormone replacement therapy,
   680-681, *681*
   and breast cancer, 277, 278
   breast pain, 23
   and dementia, 681
   and heart disease, 680
   and osteoporosis, 931
Hormone therapies, alternative, 681
Hormones, 681-682
Horn, cutaneous, 682, *682*
Horner syndrome, 682
Hospice, 508-509, 682, 804, *509*
Hospitals, types of, 682-683
Host, 683
Hot flashes, 683
HPV. *See* Human papillomavirus.
HRT. *See* Hormone replacement
   therapy.
HSG. *See* Hysterosalpingogram.
Human antihuman antibodies, 78
Human bites, 244
   first aid, 1314
Human chorionic gonadotropin
   (HCG), 683
   home pregnancy tests, 679
Human Genome Project, 74-75,
   596, 683-684
Human granulocytic ehrlichiosis,
   684
Human growth hormone, antiaging
   therapies, 174-175

Human herpesvirus 8, 684
Human immunodeficiency virus.
   See HIV.
Human menopausal gonadotropin,
   684
Human monocytic ehrlichiosis,
   684-685
Human papillomavirus, 685-686
Humidifier lung, 144, 686
Huntington chorea, 686
Huntington disease. *See*
   Huntington chorea.
Hurler syndrome, 686
Hydatid disease, 686-687
Hydatidiform mole, 687
Hydralazine, 687
Hydramnios, 687
Hydrocele, 687, *687*
Hydrocephalus, 687-688, *688*
   prenatal scanning, 84
Hydrochloric acid, 688
Hydrochlorothiazide, 688, 1269
Hydrocodone, 688
Hydrocortisone. *See* Cortico-
   steroids.
Hydrogen sulfide poisoning,
   999-1000
Hydrogenated fats and oils, 688
Hydronephrosis, 688
Hydrops, 688
Hydroquinone, 688
Hydrotherapy, 688-689, *688*
Hydroxychloroquine sulfate, 689
Hydroxyzine, 689
Hygiene, 689
Hymen, 689
   imperforate, 712
Hyoid, 689, *689*
Hyperacidity, 689
Hyperactivity, 689
Hyperacusis, 689
Hyperaldosteronism. *See* Aldostero-
   nism.
Hyperalimentation. *See* Parenteral
   nutrition.
Hyperbaric injuries. *See*
   Decompression sickness.
Hyperbaric oxygen treatment, 689
Hyperbilirubinemia, 689-690
Hypercalcemia, 690
Hypercholesterolemia, 690, *690*
   familial, 548

Hyperemesis, 690-691
   gravidarum, 691
Hyperglycemia, 691
   See also Diabetes mellitus, type 1;
      Diabetes mellitus, type 2.
Hypergonadism, 691
Hyperhidrosis, 691
Hyperkeratosis, 691
Hyperlipidemias, 691-692
Hypernephroma. *See* Renal cell
   carcinoma.
Hyperopia. *See* Farsightedness.
Hyperosmotics, 777
Hyperparathyroidism, 692-693,
   693
Hyperplasia, 693
   endometrial. *See* Endometrial
      hyperplasia.
   gingival, 693-694
Hyperpyrexia, 647, 694
Hypersensitivity, 694
Hypersplenism, 694
Hypertension, 255, 694-696, *696*
   atherosclerosis, 205
   classification, *695*
   coronary artery disease, 406
   dizziness, 36
   genetic research, 77
   in obesity, 913
   prehypertension, 1014
   pulmonary, 696, 1042
   renal vascular, 1063, *1063*
   urination problems, 56, 57
Hypertensive hemorrhage, 696-697
Hyperthermia, 559, 697
   malignant, 163, 697
Hyperthyroidism, 697, 1212, 1213
Hypertonia, 697
Hypertrophy, 697
Hyperuricemia, 698
Hyperventilation, 698
   first aid, 1326
   shortness of breath, 287
Hyphema, 698, *698*
Hypnosis, 698, 848
Hypnotic drugs, 698
   addiction to, 477
   and anesthesia, 163
Hypoaldosteronism, 699
Hypochondriasis, 699, 1142
Hypochondroplasia, 1124
Hypogammaglobulinemia, 699-700

Hypoglycemia, 700
  See also Diabetes mellitus, type
    1; Diabetes mellitus, type 2
  first aid, 1326
Hypogonadism, 700-701, 762
Hypohidrosis, 701
Hypomania, 701
Hypoparathyroidism, 701
Hypophysectomy, 701, *701*
Hypopituitarism, 701-702
Hypoplasia, 702
  enamel, 702
Hypoplastic left heart syndrome,
  702
Hypospadias, 702
Hypotension, 702
  postural, 1010
Hypothalamus, 702-703, *703*
Hypothermia, 703, *703*
  first aid, 1327
Hypothyroidism, 703-704, 1212
  congenital, 395
  myxedema, 882
  prenatal screening, 597
  weight gain, 60
Hypotonia, 704
  in infants, 704
Hypovolemia, 704
Hypoxia, 704
  aviation medicine, 214
Hysterectomy, 705, *705*
Hysteria, 705-706
Hysterosalpingogram, 706
Hysteroscopy, 706, *706*

I

Iatrogenic, 707
Ibuprofen, 707
ICD. *See* Defibrillator.
Ichthyosis vulgaris, 707
ICSI, 707
Icterus, 707
Id, 707
Idiopathic, 707
Idiopathic thrombocytopenic
  purpura. *See* ITP.
Ileal pouch–anal anastomosis, 707,
  707
Ileitis. *See* Crohn disease.
Ileostomy, 707-708, *708*
Ileum, 708

Ileus, paralytic, 708
Illness, 708
Illusion, 708
Imaging
  MRI, 80, 862, 865, *866*
  radiology, 907, 1051
  See also CT Scanning; X rays;
    Twenty-first century medicine,
    73-96
Imipramine, 708
  pain management, 946
Immobility, 708
Immune globulins, 708-709
Immune response, 709
Immune serum globulin. *See*
  Immunoglobulins.
Immune system, 709-710, *709*
  lymphocytes, 814-815
  T cells, 1188
Immune system disorders, 710
Immunity, 710
Immunization, 710-711
Immunoassay, 711
Immunoglobulin A nephropathy,
  894
Immunoglobulins, 711
Immunologist, 711
Immunology, 711
Immunosuppressants, 1189
Immunotherapy, allergen, 711
Impaction, dental, 711-712, *712*
Impairment, 712
Imperforate anus. *See* Anus,
  imperforate.
Imperforate hymen, 712
Impetigo, 712
  childhood rash, 51
Impingement syndrome, 947
Implant, 712-713
  cochlear, 375-376, *376*
  dental, 713, *713*
  hormonal, 402, 403
  intraocular lens, 739
  lens, 782
  after mastectomy, 828
  nerve stimulators, 91
  penile, 966, *966*
Implantable bone conduction hear-
  ing device. *See* Cochlear implant.
Implantation, egg, 713
Impotence, 523, 713
Impression, dental, 713
Impulse noise, 112

In situ, 714, *714*
In vitro fertilization, 714, *714-715*
In vivo, 714
Incest, 714, 716
Incidence, 716
Incision, 716
Incompetent cervix, 716, *716*
Incontinence
  fecal, 716
  urinary, 716-717
Incubation period, 717
Indigestion, 717-718
Indinavir, 718
Indomethacin. *See* Nonsteroidal
  anti-inflammatory drugs.
Induction agents, 718
Induction of labor, 718
Infant mortality, 718, *718*
Infantile spasms, 719
Infants
  bronchopulmonary dysplasia,
    294, *294*
  crying, 424, *424*
  failure to thrive, 544-545
  febrile seizures, 1098-1099, *1098*
  feeding, 553
  floppy, 568-569
  growth, 618-620, *619*
  head banging, 630-631
  hemolytic disease of newborn,
    654
  hypotonia, 704
  kernicterus, 755-756
  mortality rates, 718, *718*
  neonatal intensive care,
    891-892, *891*
  newborn screening, 1095
  premature birth, 1014
    retinopathy, 1072
  shaken baby syndrome, 1112
  stillbirth, 1165
  sudden infant death syndrome,
    1176
  thumb-sucking, 1209-1210
Infarction, 719
  myocardial, 639
  pulmonary, 1042
Infection, 719, 721, *720*
  congenital, 719, 721
  nosocomial, 907-908
  opportunistic, 920-921, 954
  respiratory tract, 1069
  waterborne, 1293

See also Bacteria; Bacteria,
  flesh-eating; fungal infections;
  Retrovirus; Rotavirus;
  Sexually transmitted diseases;
  Viruses.
Infectious disease, 721
Infectious mononucleosis. *See*
  Mononucleosis, infectious.
Inferiority complex, 721
Infertility, 721-723, 1110
  artificial insemination, 195,
    195
  assisted reproductive technology,
    199
  surrogate motherhood, 1181
  treatments, 723-724, *723*
Infestation, 724, *724*
Infiltrate, 724
Inflammation, 724
  C-reactive protein, 304
Inflammatory bowel disease,
  724-725
  diarrhea, 34
  stem cell research, 79
Infliximab, 725
Influenza, 725-726
  coughing, 28
  headache, 39
Informed consent, 529
  for research, 726
  for surgery or treatment, 726, *726*
Infrared, 726
Ingrown toenail, 726-727, *727*
Inguinal, 727, *727*
Inhalants, 477, 727, *727*
Inhalation, 727-728
  smoke, 728, *728*
  toxic gas, 728
Inhaler, 202, 728
Inheritance, 728
Inhibin, 728
Inhibition, 728
Injection, 728
  types, *729*
Inkblot test. *See* Rorschach test.
Inlay, dental, 728
Inoculation, 730
Inoperable, 730
Inorganic, 730
Inpatient treatment, 730
Insanity, 730
Insects and disease, 730, *730*

Insect bites and stings, 243-244,
  730, *730*
  allergies to, 137, 243
  anaphylaxis, 155
  childhood rash, 51
  first aid, 1314
Insecurity, 730
Insemination, artificial, 723, 731,
  731
  sperm bank, 1146
  surrogate motherhood, 1181
Insight, 731
Insoluble fiber. *See* Fiber, dietary.
Insomnia, 731, 1131
  fatal familial, 1134
Inspiration, 731
Instinct, 731
Institutionalization, 731
Insulin, 731-732, *732*
  See also Diabetes mellitus type
    1; Diabetes mellitus type 2
  antibodies, 732
  and glucagon, 606
  and glucose, 607
  pump, 732
  resistance, 732
  shock, 1115, 1330
Insulinlike growth factor, 732-733
Insulinoma, 733
Insurance
  long-term care, 805
  nursing home, 910
Integrative medicine, 733
Intelligence, 733-734
Intelligence tests, 734
  Binet test, 238
Intensive care. *See* Critical care.
Intensive care unit, 734
Intercostal, 734
Intercourse, painful, 734
Interferons, 734-735
Interleukins, 735, *735*
Intermediate care facility, 735
Intermittent explosive disorder.
  See Explosive disorder.
Intern, 735
Internal medicine, 735
Internist, 735
Interstitial fibrosis of lung, 735
Interstitial fluid, 735-736
Interstitial nephritis. *See* Nephritis,
  interstitial.

Interstitial radiation therapy. *See*
  Brachytherapy.
Intertrigo, 736
Intervention studies, 736
Intestinal lipodystrophy, 736
Intestine, 736-737
  blind loop syndrome, 250
  large, 737
  Meckel diverticulum, 830
  obstruction, 737-738, *737*
    abdominal pain, 14
    borborygmi, 266
    constipation, 26
  small, 736-737
    ileostomy, 707-708, *708*
    paralytic ileus, 708
  resection, 1135
  transplant, 1135
  tumors of, 738
  volvulus, 1286
  See also diseases by name.
Intoeing, 738
Intolerance, 738
Intoxication, alcohol, 133-134
Intracavitary therapy, 738
Intracerebral hemorrhage. *See*
  Hemorrhage, cerebral.
Intracorneal ring, 738-739
Intractable, 739
Intracytoplasmic sperm injection.
  See ICSI.
Intraductal papilloma, 739
Intraocular lens implant. *See*
  Cataract surgery.
Intraocular pressure, 739
Intrauterine device (IUD), 401-403,
  739, 744, *744*
  and infertility, 722
Intrauterine growth retardation,
  739
Intravenous anesthesia. *See*
  Anesthesia, intravenous.
Intravenous pyelography, 739, *739*
Intraventricular hemorrhage. *See*
  Hemorrhage, intraventricular.
Introvert, 740
Intubation, 740
Intussusception, 740, *740*
Investigational drug, 740
Involuntary movements, 740
Iodine, 740, 849, *740*
Ion, 740

Ipecac, 503, 740-741
Ipratropium, 741
IQ, 741
Irbesartan, 741
Iridectomy, 741
Iridology, 741
Iridotomy, 741
Iris, 536, 741
Iron, 741, 849
    for adolescents, 120
    ferrous sulfate, 555
    hemosiderosis, 659
Iron-deficiency anemia, 159, *159*
Irradiation, 741
Irrigation, wound, 741
Irritable bladder, 741
Irritable bowel syndrome, 742
    constipation, 27
    diarrhea, 34
Irritable colon. *See* Irritable bowel
    syndrome.
Ischemia, 742
    cardiomyopathy, 317
    heart disease and, 642-643
    RIND, 1080
    stroke, 1171, 1173, *1172*
Isoflurane, 742
Isolation, 742-743
Isoniazid, 743
Isopropyl alcohol, 743
Isosorbide dinitrate, 743
Isotretinoin, 111, 743
Itching. *See* Pruritis.
    anal, 17
ITP, 743-744
Itraconazole, 744
IUD, 744, *744*
IUGR. *See* Intrauterine growth
    retardation.
IVF. *See* In vitro fertilization.
IVP. *See* Intravenous pyelography.

J

Japanese medicine, 1060, 1112
Jaundice, 745
    bile, 236
    biliary atresia, 236-237
    biliary cirrhosis, 237
    icterus, 707
    neonatal intensive care, 892

phototherapy, 984-985
    urine discoloration, 58
Jaw, 745
    dislocated, 745
    fractured, 745
    orthognathic surgery, 925-926,
        926
    prognathism, 1019
    trismus, 1239
    wired, 1300
Jealousy, morbid, 745
Jejunal biopsy, 745
Jejunum, 745
Jet lag, 214, 745-746
Jock itch, 451, 746
Jogger's nipple, 746
Joint, 746, 748, *746*
    ankylosing spondylitis, 171-172
    aspiration, 746, 748, *746*
    inflammation, knee pain, 45
    injection, 748, *748*
    neuropathic, 900
    osteoarthritis, 927, *928*
    reduction, 1056
    replacement, 89, 748, *88*
        for arthritis, 194
        finger, 565, 748
        hip, 748-749, *749*
        knee, 749-750
    rheumatoid arthritis, 1076-1077
    subluxation, 1175, *1175*
    synovium, 1185
    types, *747*
Joule, 750
Jugular vein, 750, *750*
Jumper's knee, 750
Jung, Carl, 1253
Jungian theory, 750
Juvenile rheumatoid arthritis,
    750-751, *751*

K

Kala-azar, 781-782
Kaposi sarcoma, 129, 136, 752
    herpesvirus B, 684
Kartagener syndrome, 752
Karyotyping, 364, 752
Kasai procedure, biliary atresia,
    237
Kava, 752
Kawasaki disease, 752-753, *753*

Kegel exercises, 753-754, *753*
Keloid, 754, *754*
Keratin, 754
Keratitis, 754
Keratoacanthoma, 754
Keratoconjunctivitis, 754
Keratoconjunctivitis sicca. *See*
    Dry eye.
Keratoconus, 754, *754*
Keratopathy, 754
    ultraviolet, 754-755
Keratoplasty
    conductive, 755
    penetrating, 755
Keratosis, 755
    actinic, 114
    pilaris, 755
    seborrheic, 1097
Keratotomy, radial, 1048-1049
Kerion, 755
Kernicterus, 755-756
Ketoacidosis, 109, 756
Ketoconazole, 179, 756
Ketorolac, 756
Ketosis, 756
Kidney, 756-757, *757*
    abdominal pain, 14
    acidosis, 109
    anuria, 183
    artificial, 196, 463
    biopsy, 757-758, *758*
    cancer, 758
    cyst, 758-759
    failure, 759
    function tests, 759
    glomerulonephritis, 605-606,
        606
    glomerulosclerosis, 606
    hydronephrosis, 688
    hypertension, 695
    imaging, 759-760, *759*
    polycystic, 761-762, 1003-1004,
        761
    pyelography, 1044-1045
    stones, 760-761, 1045, *760*
    transplant, 761, *761*
    urination problems, 56, 57, 59
    Wilms tumor, 1300
    weight gain, 60
Kilocalorie, 762
Kilojoule, 762
Kinesiology, applied naprapathy,
    883

Kleptomania, 762
Klinefelter syndrome, 365, 762
Klumpke paralysis, 762
Knee, 762-763, *763*
   arthroscopic surgery, 195
   artificial, 90
   Baker cyst, 223
   replacement, 749-750
   Osgood-Schlatter disease, 926-927
   osteonecrosis, 930
   pain, symptom chart, 44-45
   patellar tendinitis, 959-960
   runner's, 1084-1085
Kniest syndrome, 1124
Knock-knees, 763, *763*
Koilonychia, 763
Koplik spots, 763
Korsakoff psychosis, 763-764, 1296
Kuru, 1134
Kyphoscoliosis, 764
Kyphosis, 764, *764*
   orthopedic brace, 268

L

La Leche League, 765
Labetalol, 765
Labia, 765, 1064, *765*
Labile, 765
Labor, 765-766, *766*
   afterbirth, 125
   amniotomy, 157
   Braxton Hicks contractions, 275
   breech delivery, 288
   induction of, 718
   oxytocin, 941-942
   preterm, 1017
   stages of, *766*
   uterine contractions, 404
   See also Placenta.
Labyrinthitis, 766-767, *767*
   balance, 223
   dizziness, 37
   nausea or vomiting, 47
Laceration, 767
Lacrimal apparatus, 767
Lacrimal gland, 767
Lactase deficiency, 767
Lactation, 767
Lactic acid, 767
Lactobacillus, 767-768
Lactose, 768

intolerance, 768
   malabsorption, 820
Lactulose, 768
Lagophthalmos, 768
Laminectomy, 768
   for back pain, 221
Lamivudine, 768
Lance, 768
Lancet, 768
Language, 1145
Lanolin, 768
Lansoprazole. *See* Proton pump
   inhibitors.
Laparoscopic surgery, 182, 768,
   770, *770*
   tools for, *769*
Laparoscopy, 770
Laparotomy, exploratory, 770
   appendicitis, 188-189
Larva migrans, 770-771
Laryngeal papilloma, 771
Laryngectomy, 771, *771*
Laryngitis, 771-772, *772*
   hoarseness or voice loss, 31
Laryngocele, 772
Laryngomalacia, 772
Laryngoscopy, 772, *772*
Laryngospasm, 772
Larynx, 772-773, 1068, *773*
   cancer of, 773, *773*
      hoarseness or voice loss, 31,
      676
   papilloma, 771
Laser, 773
Laser in-situ keratomileusis.
   See LASIK.
Laser surgery, 774-775, *775*
Laser resurfacing, 773-774, *774*
LASIK, 775-776, 1049
Lassa fever, 776
Latanoprost, 776
Lateral, 776
Lavage, gastric. *See* Stomach
   pumping.
Laxatives, 267, 776-777
Lazy eye. *See* Amblyopia.
LDL, 360-362, 777
Lead poisoning, 777
Learning, 777-778
   behavior therapy, 233
   brain scanning, 87, *87*
Learning disabilities, 778-779, *779*

dyslexia, 488
   neuropsychological testing, 900
Leech, 780, *780*
LEEP, 780, *780*
Leflunomide, 780
Left heart syndrome, hypoplastic,
   702
Leg
   fractured, 780-781
   shortening of, 781
   ulcer, 780
Legal forms, sample, 1335-1343
Legg-Calvé-Perthes disease. *See*
   Osteochondrosis.
Legionnaires disease, 781
Leiomyoma, 781
Leishmaniasis, 781-782, *782*
Lens, 536, 782
   dislocation, 782
   implant. *See* Cataract surgery.
Lentigo. *See* Age spots.
Leprosy, 782-783
   thalidomide, 1204
Leptin, 783
Leptospirosis, 783, 1310
   animal-transmitted, 171
   waterborne, 1293
Lesbianism, 783
Lesion, 783
Lethargy, 783
Leukemia, 308, 783-785, *784*
   acute lymphoblastic, 785
   acute myelogenous, 785-786
   chronic lymphocytic, 786-787
   chronic myeloid, 787, 879
   graft-versus-host disease, 613,
     613
   hairy cell, 787
   oncogenes, 917
Leukocyte, 787-788
Leukoencephalopathy, progressive
   multifocal, 788
Leukopenia, 788
Leukoplakia, 788
Leukorrhea, 788
Leuprolide acetate, 788
Levamisole, 788
Levodopa and carbidopa, 788-789
Levofloxacin, 789
Levonorgestrel, 789
Levothyroxine, 789
Lewy body dementia, 146, 789

LH, 789, 1107
  hypogonadism, 700-701
  infertility, 723
LH-RH, 789
Libido, 789
Lice, 724, 789-790, 956, 1111, *789*
  head, 789-790
  nit, 903
  pediculosis, 963
  pubic, 1038
Licensure, medical, 790
Lichen
  planus, 780
  sclerosus, 156, 790
  simplex, 790
Lichenification, 790
Licorice root, 790
Lidocaine, 164
Life expectancy, 126, 790-791, *790*
Life support, 791
  advance directives, 123-124
Ligament, 791
  injuries, knee, 44, 791-792, *791*
Ligation, 792
Ligature, 792
Light treatment. *See* Phototherapy.
Lightning injuries, 792, *793*
Limb, artificial, 89-90, 792, 794
Limb-girdle dystrophy, 873
Limbic system, 794
Limp, 794
Linkage analysis, neurofibromato-
  sis, 898
Lip, 794
  cancer, 794
Lipid-lowering agents. *See*
  Cholesterol-lowering drugs.
Lipids, 795
  in blood, 256
  cholesterol, 360
  hyperlipidemias, 691-692
  and lipoprotein metabolism,
  794-795
Lipodystrophy, insulin, 795
Lipoma, 795
Lipoprotein, 406, 795
  cholesterol, 361
Liposarcoma, 795
Liposuction, 795-796, *795-796*
Lipreading, 796
Lisinopril, 796-797
Lisp, 797

Listeriosis, 797
Lithium, 797
Lithotomy position, 797
Lithotripsy, 797-798, *798*
Live cell therapy, 798
Livedo reticularis, 798
Liver, 467, 736, 798-799, *799*
  abscess, 799
  bile duct, 236
  biopsy, 799
  cancer, 799-800
  cirrhosis of the. *See* Cirrhosis.
  disease, alcoholic, 800
  failure, 800-801
  function tests, 801
  Hepatitis, 660-661
  lobectomy, 802, *802*
  organ donation, 923
  scan, 801
  spots, 125
  steatohepatitis, nonalcoholic,
  904
  transplant, 801-802
Liver cell therapy, 175
Liver fluke, 801
Living will, 123, 802
LLETZ. *See* LEEP.
Lobe, 802
Lobectomy
  liver, 802, 802
  lung, 802-803, *803*
Lobotomy, prefrontal, 803, 1034
Local anesthesia. *See* Anesthesia,
  local.
Lochia, 803
Lockjaw. *See* Tetanus; Trismus.
Locomotor, 803
Loiasis, 803
Long QT syndrome, 803-804
Long-term care facility, 199, 804-805
Long-term care insurance, 805
Loop electrosurgical excision
  procedure. *See* LEEP.
Loose bodies, 805
Loperamide, 805
Loracarbef. *See* Cephalosporins.
Loratadine, 805
Lorazepam. *See* Benzodiazepines.
Lordosis, 805-806, *805*
Losartan, 806
Lou Gehrig disease. *See* ALS.

Lovastatin, 806
Ludwig angina, 806
Lumbar, 806, *806*
Lumbar puncture, 806-807, *807*
Lumbosacral spasm, 807
Lumen, 807
Lumpectomy, 277, 807
  axillary lymph node dissection,
  215, *215*
Lumps
  breast, 22-23, 277, 287
  in groin, 617
Lung, 807, *807*
  collapsed, 809
  function, peak flow meter, 961
  hemothorax, 659, *659*
  imaging, 809
  lobectomy, 802-803, *803*
  pleura, 992
  postural drainage, 1009-1010,
  1009
  surfactant, 809, 1181
  thoracentesis, 1205
  transplantation, 809, *809*
  See also Pulmonary; Respiratory
  system.
Lung disease
  alveolitis, 144
  asbestosis, 196-197
  aspergillosis, 198
  bagassosis, 223
  berylliosis, 234
  cancer, 808-809, *808*
  coughing, 28, 30
  oncogenes, 917
  small cell carcinoma,
  1134-1135
  COPD. *See* Chronic obstructive
  pulmonary disease.
  cystic fibrosis, 430-431
  disease, chronic obstructive. *See*
  Chronic obstructive pulmonary
  disease.
  humidifier lung, 686
  interstitial fibrosis, 735
  Kartagener syndrome, 752
  occupational lung disease, 915
  pneumoconiosis, 994
  pulmonary hypertension, 696
  tumors. *See* Lung cancer.
  Wegener granulomatosis,
  1294-1295

Lupus erythematosus
    discoid, 809-810, *810*
    systemic, 810, *810*
Lupus pernio, 810
Luteinizing hormone. *See* LH.
Luteinizing hormone-releasing hor-
    mone. *See* LH-RH.
Luxated tooth, 811
Lyme disease, 176, 244, 245, 366,
    811-813, *812*
    babesiosis, 217
Lymph node, 813, *813*
Lymphadenitis, 813
Lymphadenopathy, 813
Lymphangioma, 813
Lymphangitis, 813
Lymphatic system, 814, *814*
    atlas, *72*
Lymphocytes, 814-815
    B cells, 217, 709, 814-815, *217*
    T cells, 1188
Lymphogranuloma venereum, 815
Lymphoma, 308, 815-816, *815*
    Agent Orange, 125
    Burkitt, 298
    non-Hodgkin, 129
Lynch syndrome, 816
Lysis, 816
    of adhesions, 816

M

Ma huang, 817
Macrobiotics, 817, *911*
Macrocephaly, 817
Macroglossia, 817
Macrolides, 817
Macular degeneration, 151, 819,
    1280, *818*
    blindness, 251
    vision loss or impairment, 41
Macule, 819
Mad cow disease, 819, 1310
Magnesium, 819, 849
Magnet therapy, 819, *819*
Magnetic resonance angiography.
    See MRI.
Magnetic resonance cholangiopan-
    creatography. *See* MRI.
Magnetic resonance imaging.
    See MRI.

Magnetic resonance spectroscopy.
    See MRI.
Malabsorption syndrome, 819-820
    blind loop syndrome, 250
    diarrhea, 35
Maladjustment, 820
Malalignment, 820
Malar flush, 820
Malaria, 820-821, 954, *821*
Male
    puberty stages, *1037*
    reproductive system, *70,*
        1065-1066, *1066*
    sex hormones. *See* Androgen
        hormones.
    urinary tract, 56, 1257, *71, 1257*
    Y chromosome, 1307
Malformation, congenital, 821
Malignant, 821
Malignant melanoma. *See* Mela-
    noma, malignant.
Mallet finger. *See* Baseball finger.
Mallet toe, 821
Mallory-Weiss syndrome, 821-822
Malnutrition, 822
Malocclusion, 135, 243, 421,
    822-823, *822*
    bruxism, 295
    underbite, 1253
Malpractice, 823
Malpresentation, 823, *823*
MALToma, 823
Malunion, 823
Mammary gland. *See* Breast.
Mammogram, 276, 823-824, *823,*
    824
Managed care, 824
    HMO, 676
    PPO, 1010
Mandible, 824
Mandible, orthopedic reposition-
    ing appliance, 824
Mandibulofacial dysostosis,
    824-825, *825*
Manganese, 849
Mania, 239, 241, 825
Manic-depressive illness, 825
    See also Depression.
Manipulation, 825
    pain management, 947
Manometry, 825
Mantoux test. *See* Tuberculin
    skin test.

Manual lymph drainage, 825
MAOIs. *See* Monoamine oxidase
    inhibitors.
Marasmus, 825
March fracture, 825
Marfan syndrome, 825-826, 855
Marijuana addiction, 478
Marine animal stings, 1165, *1166*
Marital counseling, 826
Marsupialization, 826
Masculinization, 826
Massage, 826
Massage therapy, 216, 260, 355,
    826-827, *826*
    Alexander technique, 135
    pain management, 947
    reflexology, 1057, 1059
    shiatsu, 1112
    Swedish massage, 1184
    Thai, 1203
    trigger point, 1239
Mast cell, 827, *827*
    in allergic response, *827*
Mastectomy, 277, 827-828, *827*
    axillary lymph node dissection,
        215, *215*
Mastitis, 276, 286, 828
    breast pain, 22
Mastocytosis, 828
Mastoidectomy, 828
Mastoiditis, 828
Mastopexy, 279-280, *280*
Masturbation, 828
Maternal mortality, 828-829, *829*
McArdle disease, 829
Meals-on-Wheels, 105
Measles (rubeola), 506, 829-830,
    1084
    rash, 50, 52
    vaccination, 1263
Meatus, 830
Mebendazole, 830
Meckel diverticulum, 830
Meclizine hydrochloride, 830
Meconium, 830
Medial, 830
Mediastinoscopy, 830
Mediastinum, 830
Medicaid, 830,
Medical examiner, 830-831
Medical records, 831
    confidentiality, 394-395

Medicare, 831, *831*
  home health care, 678
  long-term care, 805
Medication. *See* Drug and see also
  individual drug by name.
Meditation, 143, 215-216, 831, 848
  transcendental, 1230
Mediterranean diet, 831-832
Mediterranean fever, familial, 548
Medroxyprogesterone, 832
Medulla, 832
Medulla oblongata, 832
Medulloblastoma, 832
Mefloquine hydrochloride, 832
Megacolon, 832, *832*
Megaloblastic anemia, 159
Megavitamin therapy, 143
Megestrol, 832
Meibomianitis, 832
Meigs syndrome, 832
Meiosis, 335, 364, 832-833
Melanin, 833, 986
Melanoma
  choroidal, 364
  of eye, 539
  malignant, 125, 229, 833,
    1128-1129, *833, 834*
  oncogenes, 917
  spitz nevus, 1152
  sun exposure, 1179
Melanosis coli, 833
Melasma, 833
Melatonin, 833-834, 912
Melena, 834
Membrane, 834
Memory, 834-835
  in Alzheimer's disease, 144-146,
    145
  amnesia, 150
  disabilities, 779
  false, 547-548
  loss, 835
  loss of, in older people, *835*
Menarche, 835
Meniere disease, 634, 835-836, *836*
  balance, 223
  dizziness, 36
  nausea or vomiting, 47
Meninges, 269, 836
Meningioma, 274, 836
Meningitis, 836-837, *837*
Meningocele, 837

Meningomyelocele, 837
Meniscal tears, 837-838, *838*
Meniscectomy, 838, *838*
Meniscus, 838, *838*
Menopause, 838-839, 1065
  hormone replacement therapy,
    680-681
  hot flashes, 683
  night sweats, 902
  osteoporosis, 930-932
  premature, 839
Menorrhagia. *See* Menstruation.
Menstruation, 839, *840*
  abdominal pain, 15
  adenomyosis, 118
  breakthrough bleeding, 275
  disorders of, 839-841
  irregular, 841
  oligomenorrhea, 916
  symptom chart, 16
  weight gain, 60
Mental illness, 841
Mental retardation, 841
Mental status examinations, 841
Meralgia paresthetica, 841-842
Mercury, 842
Mesalamine, 842
Mesentery, 842, *842*
Mesothelioma, 842
  asbestosis, 197
Mesothelium, 842
Mestranol and norethindrone, 842
Metabolic disorders, 842-843
Metabolism, 842-843
  inborn errors of, 843
Metabolite, 843
Metaphysis, 843
Metaplasia, 843
Metastasis, 843, *843*
Metatarsalgia, 844
Metformin hydrochloride, 844
Methadone maintenance, 844
Methamphetamine hydrochloride,
  844
Methanol, 844
Methocarbamol, 870
Methotrexate, 844
Methoxsalen, 844
Methyl alcohol. *See* Methanol.
Methylphenidate, 844
Methylprednisolone. *See*
  Corticosteroids.

Metoclopramide, 844-845
Metoprolol, 845
Metronidazole, 845
Metrorrhagia, 845
Miconazole, 845
Microalbuminuria, 845
Microangiopathy, 845
Microbe, 845
Microbiology, 845
Microcephaly, 845
Microorganism, 845
Microprocessor technology, 90
Microscope, 845-846, *846*
Microsurgery, 846, *846*
Microvascular angina, 168
Micturition, 846
Middle-ear effusion, persistent.
  See Otitis media.
Midlife crisis, 846-847
Midwife, 847
Migraine, 632, 847-848
  aura, 210
  headache, 38
Milia, 848
Milk, breast, 280
Milk-alkali syndrome, 848
Mind-body medicine, 848
Mineralocorticoids, 848-849
Minerals, 849-850
Mineral supplements, 848
Mineralization, dental, 848
Mineralocorticoid, 848-849
Minilaparotomy, 850
Minipills, 850
Minnesota Multiphasic Personality
  Inventory (MMPI), 978
Minocycline, 850, 1203
Minoxidil, 850
Miosis, 850
Miscarriage, 100, 850-851, *851*
  chromosomal abnormalities, 364
  incompetent cervix, 716, *716*
Misoprostol, 851
Mites, dust, 487
Mitochondria, 334, 851-852
Mitochondrial diseases, 851-852
Mitosis, 335, 852
Mitral valve, 645-647, *854*
  insufficiency, 852
  prolapse, 852, 855
  stenosis, 852, 1162, *853*
Mittelschmerz, 855

Mobility, 855
Mohs surgery, 855, *855*
    basal cell carcinoma, 230
    Bowen disease, 268
    squamous cell carcinoma, 1158
Molar pregnancy, 855
Mold, 855-856
Molecule, 856, *856*
Mole, 855-856, *856*
Molluscum contagiosum, 856-857,
    1111
Molybdenum, 849
Monamine oxidase inhibitors, 857
Monarthritis, 857
Monckeberg arteriosclerosis, 193
Moniliasis, 857
Monitoring
    fetal, 556-558, *557*
Monoamine oxidase inhibitors,
    178, 857
Monoclonal antibody. *See* Antibody,
    monoclonal.
Monocytes, 252
Monogamy, 857
Mononucleosis, infectious, 857-858
Monoparesis, 858
Monosodium glutamate. *See* MSG.
Monounsaturated fats, 552, 858
Monteggia fracture, 858-859
Montelukast, 859
Mood, 859
Morbidity, 859
Morning sickness, 859
Morning-after pill, 401, 859
Morphea, 859
Morphine sulfate, 163, 859
Mortality rate, 859
    zinfant, 718, *718*
    maternal, 828-829, *829*
Morton neuroma, 859-860
Mosaicism, 860
Motility, sperm, 1146
Motion sickness, 860
    seasickness, 1096
Motor neuron disease, 860-861, *860*
Mouth, 467, 861, *861*
    cancer. *See* Oral cancer.
    guard, 861, *861*
    ulcer, 861
Mouth-to-mouth resuscitation, 862,
    863
Movement, 862, *864*

generation of, *864*
    involuntary, 740
Movement disorder, 862
Moxibustion, 115, 862, *355*
MRA, 862
MRCP. *See* MRI.
MRI, 80, 862, 865, *81, 866*
MRS. *See* MRI.
MS. *See* Multiple sclerosis.
MSG, 865
Mucocele, 865
Mucopolysaccharidosis, 865
Mucous membrane, 865
Mucus, 865
Multi-infarct dementia. *See*
    Vascular dementia.
Multiple births, 865, 867
Multiple chemical sensitivity, 867
Multiple myeloma, 867
Multiple personality disorder,
    867-868, 1153
Multiple sclerosis, 868-869, *868*
    stem cell research, 79
Multivitamin, 869
Mumps, 869, *869*
    vaccination, 1263
Munchausen syndrome, 869-870
Mupirocin, 870
Murmur. *See* Heart murmur.
Muscle, 870, *871, 874*
    cardiac, 870
    skeletal, 870
    smooth, 870
    spasm, 872
    strain, 1168
    strength training, 1169
Muscle relaxants, 221
Muscular atrophy, progressive,
    1019
Muscular dystrophy, 489, 872-873,
    873
    atony, 206
Muscular system, 873, *874*
    atlas, *66*
Musculoskeletal system, 873, *874*
    fitness, 873, 875
Mushroom picker's disease, 144
Mushroom poisoning, 1000,
    first aid, 1323
Music therapy, 1142
Mutagen, 875
Mutation, 875
Mutism, 875

Myalgia, 875
    back pain, 220
Myasthenia gravis, 875-876, *876*
Mycetoma, 876
Mycology, 876
Mycoplasma, 876
Mycoplasma pneumonia, 996-997
Mycosis, 876
Mycosis fungoides,876
Mydriasis, 876
Myectomy, 876
Myelin, 876-877, 1299, *877*
Myelitis, 877
Myelocele, 877
Myelodysplastic syndrome,
    877-878
Myelofibrosis with myeloid meta-
    plasia, 878, 879-880
Myelography, 878
    back pain, 220
Myeloid leukemia, oncogenes, 917
Myelomeningocele, 878
Myelopathy, 878-879
Myeloproliferative disorders,
    879-880
Myiasis, 880
Myocardial infarction, 880, *880*. *See*
    also Heart attack.
Myocarditis, 880
Myoclonic seizures, 178, 880
Myoclonus, 880
Myofascial pain disorder, 880-881
Myoglobin, 881
Myoma. *See* Fibroid, uterine.
Myomectomy, 881
Myopathy, 881
Myopia. *See* Nearsightedness.
Myositis, ossificans, 881
Myotonia, 881
Myringitis, bullous, 881
Myringoplasty, 881-882
Myringotomy, 882, *882*
Myxedema, 882
Myxoma, 882

N

Nabumetone. *See* Nonsteroidal anti-
    inflammatory drugs.
Nafarelin acetate, 883
Nail, 883, *883*

Naloxone, 883
Naltrexone hydrochloride, 883
Naprapathy, 883
Naproxen. *See* Nonsteroidal anti-
  inflammatory drugs.
Narcissism, 883, 977
Narcolepsy, 883-884, 1131
Narcotics, 154, 884, *154*
  addiction to, 478
  anesthesia, 163
  self-screening tests, 1100
Narcotics Anonymous, 481, 1247
Nasal congestion, 884
Nasal discharge. *See* Rhinitis.
Nasal obstruction. *See* Rhinitis.
Nasal polyps, 884
Nasal turbinates, 885
NASH. *See* Nonalcoholic steato-
  hepatitis.
Nasogastric tube, 885
Nasopharyngeal culture, 427
Nasopharynx, 885, 905
  cancer of, 885-886
National Institute of Occupational
  Safety and Health (NIOSH), 886
National Institutes of Health (NIH),
  886
Natural childbirth, 241, 886
  birthing centers, 242
Natural family planning, 886-887
Natural healing, 143
Naturopathy, 887
Nausea, 887
  antiemetics, 178
  symptom chart, 46-47
Navel, 887
  piercing, 260
Nearsightedness, 887, 902, *888*
  radial keratotomy, 1048-1049
  refractive surgery, 1059
Nebulizer, 887
  for asthma, 202
Neck, 887-888, *888*
  dissection, radical, 888-889
  injuries, 889, *889*, *1325*
  rigidity, 889
  stiff, 1163, 1165
  torticollis, 1224-1225
Necrolysis, toxic epidermal, 889
Necrophilia, 889
Necrosis, 889
Necrotizing enterocolitis, 889-890

Necrotizing fasciitis group A, 890
Needle aspiration, 890
Needle biopsy, 890
Needle localization, 890, *890*
Nefazodone, 891
Neglect
  of child, 102
  of older people, 104
Nelfinavir mesylate, 891
Nematodes, 680, 891, 1298-1299,
  891
Neologism, 891
Neomycin, 891
Neonatal intensive care, 891-892,
  891
Neonate, 892
Neonatologist, 892
Neonatology, 892
Neoplasia, 892
Nephrectomy, 892, *892*
Nephritis, 892-893
Nephrocalcinosis, 893
Nephrolithotomy, 893, *893*
Nephron, 893, *71*, *893*
Nephropathy
  analgesic, 893
  diabetic, 893-894, *894*
  IgA, 894
Nephrosclerosis, 894, *894*
Nephrosis, 894
Nephrostomy, 894
Nephrotic syndrome, 894-895
  weight gain, 60
Nerve, 895. See also Nervous
  system.
  block, 895, *895*
  entrapment, 895
  carpal tunnel syndrome, 325
  implantable stimulators, 91
  injuries, 895, *895*
Nerve gas, 895
Nerve growth factor, 895
Nerve injuries, 895, *895*
Nervous breakdown, 896
Nervous habit, 896
Nervous system, 896
  atlas, *67*
  autonomic, 213, *213*
  brain, 269
  central, 335-336
  parasympathetic, 956
  peripheral, 973

  spinal cord, 1149, *1149*
  sympathetic, 1185
Neural tube defect, 896, *897*
Neuralgia, 896
Neurapraxia, 896
Neurasthenia, 896
Neuritis, 896-897
Neuroblastoma, 897
Neurodermatitis, 897
Neuroendocrinology, 897-898, *897*
Neurofibromatosis, 311, 898
  acoustic neuroma, 111
Neurologist, 898
Neurology, 898
Neuroma, 899
  acoustic, 111-112, *112*
  Morton, 859-860
Neuron, 899-900, *899*
  synapse, 1185
Neuropathic joint, 900
Neuropathology, 900
Neuropathy, 900, *900*
  numbness or tingling, 48
Neuropsychiatry, 900
Neuropsychological testing, 900
Neurosis, 900-901
Neurosurgery, 901
Neurosyphilis, 901
Neurotoxin, 901
Neurotransmitter, 901
Nevirapine, 901
Nevus, 856, *834*, *856*. See also Mole.
Newborn, 901
NGU. *See* Urethritis, nongonococ-
  cal.
Niacin (nicotinic acid), 362, 901,
  912, 963, 1281
Nicardipine hydrochloride, 901
Nickel, 901-902
Nicotine
  addiction, 1137
  gum, 902
  patch, 902
  skin patch, 1129
Nicotinic acid, 901
Nifedipine, 902
Night blindness, 902
Night sweats, 902
Night terror, 902
Nightmare, 902
Nipple, 903
Nit, 724, 903

Nitrates, 168, 1269
Nitrites, 903
Nitrofurantoin, 903
Nitrogen, 903
Nitroglycerin, 903
Nitrosamines, 903
Nitrous oxide, 163
Nizatidine, 903
Nocardiosis, 903-904
Nocturia, 904
Nocturnal emission, 904
Node, 904
Nodule, 904
    cold, 904
    hot, 904
    rheumatoid, 1077, *1077*
    surfer's, 1181
    thyroid, 1212-1213, *1213*
    vocal cord, 1285
Noise pollution, 1002-1003
Nonalcoholic steatohepatitis, 904
Nonconsensual sex, 904
Nongonococcal urethritis.
    See Urethritis, nongonococcal.
Non-Hodgkin lymphoma, 815, 816
Noninvasive, 904
Nonnucleoside reverse transcriptase
    inhibitors (NNRTIs), 129, 904
Nonprescription drugs, 904
Nonsteroidal anti-inflammatory
    drugs, 153-154, 904-905
Nonstress test, 905, 1015
Nonunion, 905
Norepinephrine, 121-122, 905
Nortriptyline, 178, 905
Nose, 905-906, 1068, *906*
    broken, 907
    reshaping, 906-907, *906*
Nosebleed, 907, *907*
Nosocomial infections, 907-908
NSAIDs. *See* Nonsteroidal anti-
    inflammatory drugs.
Nuclear medicine, 81-82, 907-908,
    908
Nucleic acids, 909
Nucleus, 334, 909
Numbness, 909, 957
Nurse, 909
Nurse anesthetist, 909
Nurse practitioner, 909
Nursemaid elbow, 909-910, *909*
Nurse-midwife, 910

Nursing. *See* Breast-feeding.
Nursing facility, 910
Nursing home. *See* Long-term care
    facility.
Nutrient, 910
Nutrition, 910
    parenteral, 957
    supplements, 911-912, *911*
Nutrition Labeling and Education
    Act, 910-911, *910*
Nutritional medicine, 911, *911*
Nutritional supplements, 911-912,
    911, 912
Nystagmus, 912
Nystatin, 912

O

Obesity, 913, 939
    bariatric surgery, 226-227, *226*
    body mass index, 259-260
    and diabetes mellitus, 458
    weight gain, 61
Obesity-hypoventilation syndrome,
    913
Obsessive-compulsive disorder,
    184, 913-914, 977, *914*
Obstretrician, 914
Obstetrics, 914
Obstructive airways disease,
    914-915
Occlusion, 915
    dental, 135, 243
Occult, 915
Occult blood test, fecal. *See* Fecal-
    occult blood test.
Occupational health, 915
Occupational lung disease, 915
    silicosis, 1121
Occupational medicine, 915
Occupational safety, 106
Occupational therapy, 915, *915*
    pediatric, 962
OCT. *See* Oxytocin challenge test.
Octreotide, 915-916
Oculogyric crisis, 916
Oedipus complex, 391, 916
Ofloxacin. *See* Fluoroquinolones.
Olanzapine, 916
Older people
    abuse of, 104-105, 1275

alcohol, 131
Alzheimer's disease, 144-146, *145*
appetite, loss of in, 189-190
Area Agencies on Aging, 190
Caregiving for older people,
    322-324.
confusion in, 395
depression in, 448
falls in, 546-547, *547*
hearing loss in, 637
home health care for, 678-679
memory loss in, 835
sleep problems in, 54, 1132
taste, loss of in, 1192
Oligodendroglioma, 916
Oligohydramnios, 157, 916
Oligomenorrhea, 916
Oligospermia, 916
Oliguria, 916
Omentum, 916
Omeprazole, 916
Onchocerciasis, 916-917
Oncogenes, 917
Oncologist, 917-918
Oncology, 917-918
Oncology, surgical, 918
Ondansetron hydrochloride, 918
Onlay, dental, 918
Onycholysis, 918
Onychomycosis, 918
Oocyte, 918
Oophorectomy, 918
Open-heart surgery, 918
Operating room, 918, *919*
Operation, 920, *921*
Ophthalmologist, 920
Ophthalmology, 920
Ophthalmoplegia, 920
Ophthalmoscope, 920
Opiates, withdrawal syndrome,
    1303
Opioids. *See* Narcotics.
Opportunistic infection, 920-921,
    954
Optic atrophy, 921
Optic disc edema, 921
Optic neuritis, 921
Optical coherence tomography,
    83, *83*
Optician, 921
Optometrist, 921
Oral, 921

Oral cancer, 921-922
Oral contraceptives. *See* Contraception, hormonal methods.
Oral hygiene, 922, 1195
Oral and maxillofacial surgeon, 921
Oral sex, 922
  cunnilingus, 428
  fellatio, 553
Oral surgery, 922
Orbit, 922
Orbital fracture, 922-923
Orbital tumor, 539
Orchiectomy, 923
Orchiopexy, 923
Orchitis, 923, *923*
Order of protection, 923
Organ, 923
Organ donation, 923-924
Organic, 924
Organic brain disorder, 924
Organism, 924
Orgasm, 924, 1109
  lack of, 924
Orlistat, 924
Orphan drugs, 924
Orthodontic appliances, 924-925, *925*
Orthodontics, 925
Orthodontist, 925
Orthognathic surgery, 925-926, *926*
Orthopedic surgery, 926
Orthopedics, 926
Orthopedist, 926
Orthopnea, 926
Orthoptics, 926
Orthotics, 926, *926*
Os, 926
Oseltamivir, 926
Osgood-Schlatter disease, 926-927
Osmosis, 927
Ossicle, 927
Ossification, 927
Osteitis, 927
Osteitis deformans. *See* Paget disease.
Osteoarthritis, 194, 927, *928*
Osteochondritis dissecans, 927, 929
Osteochondroma, 929
Osteochondrosis, 929
Osteodystrophy, 929
Osteogenesis imperfecta. *See*

Brittle bones.
Osteogenic sarcoma. *See* Osteosarcoma.
Osteoid osteoma, 929
Osteomalacia, 929-930
  hyperparathyroidism, 692
Osteomyelitis, 930
Osteonecrosis, 930
Osteopathic medicine, 930
Osteopenia, 930
Osteopetrosis, 930
Osteophyte, 930, *930*
Osteoporosis, 930-932, *931, 932*
  and aging, 126
  bone density testing, 262
  bone loss, 263
  hormone replacement therapy, 681
  hyperparathyroidism, 692
Osteosarcoma, 262, 932
Osteosclerosis, 932
Osteotomy, 932, *932*
Ostomy, 932-933, *933*
Otalgia. *See* Earache.
Otic preparations, 933
Otitis externa. *See* Swimmer's ear.
Otitis externa, malignant, 933
Otitis media, 634, 933-934
  adhesive, 119
Otolaryngologist, 934
Otolaryngology, 934
Otoplasty, 934-935, *935*
Otorhinolaryngology, 935
Otorrhea. *See* Ear, discharge from.
Otosclerosis, 634, 635, 935, *935*
Otoscopy, 935-936, *935, 936*
Ototoxicity, 936
Outpatient treatment, 936
Ovarian cyst, 936-937, *936*
Ovary, 937, *937*
  cancer of, 937-938
  CA-125 test, 304
  hypogonadism, 700-701
  Meigs syndrome, 832
  oophorectomy, 918
  polycystic ovarian syndrome, 1004, *1004*
Overbite, 243, 938, *938*
Overcrowding, dental, 938, *938*
Overdose
  drug, 938-939, *938*
  medication, 939
Overgrowth syndromes, 939

Over-the-counter drugs (OTC). *See* Nonprescription drugs.
Overuse injury, 1063
Overweight, 939
Ovulation, 939, 1065, *940*
  basal body temperature (BBT), 229
  lack of, 940
  stimulants, 940
Ovum, 940, *940*
Oxaprozin, 940
Oxidation, 940
Oximetry, 940-941
Oxycodone, 941
Oxygen, 941
Oxygen, supplemental, 941
Oxygen free radicals, 181, 941
Oxytocin, 941-942
  and abortion, 100
  challenge test, 404, 942
Ozena. *See* Rhinitis, atrophic.
Ozone, 942

P

PABA. *See* Para-aminobenzoic acid
Pacemaker, 943, *944*
  cardiac arrhythmia, 192
Paclitaxel, 943
Paget disease, 943, *943*
  bone cancer, 262
  of the breast, 943
  of the vulva, 943, 945
Pain, 945. *See also* Symptom charts.
Pain management, 945
  acute, 945-946
  chronic 946-947
Painful arc syndrome, 947, 1083
Palate, 947
Palliative care, 947, *947*
Pallor, 947
Palpate, 947
Palpitations, 947-948
Palsy, 940, 948
  facial, 542
Pancreas, 736, 948, *948*
  cancer of the, 949, *949*
  transplant, 948-949, *949*
Pancreatectomy, 949-950
Pancreatitis, 950

Pandemic, 950
Panic attack, 950
Panic disorder, 184, 950-951
Pantothenic acid, 951
Pap smear, 951, *951*
Papilla, 951
Papilledema, 952
Papilloma, 952
   cutaneous, 1129
   intraductal, 739
   laryngeal, 771
Papillomavirus, human. *See*
   Human papillomavirus.
Papule, 952, 1046
Para-aminobenzoic acid, 952
Paracentesis, 952, *952*
Paraffin bath, 952
Parainfluenza virus, 952
Paralysis, 952-953, *953*
   hemiplegia, 651
   Klumpke, 762
   ophthalmoplegia, 920
   periodic, 953
   sleep, 1132
   spastic, 1143
   vocal cord, 1285-1286
Paramedic, 953
Paraneoplastic syndrome, 953
Paranoia, 953-954, 977
Paraparesis, 954
Paraphilia, 954, 1033-1034
Paraphimosis, 954
Paraplegia, 954, *954*
Parapsychology, 954
Parasite, 954, 956
   life cycle, *821*
   transmission of, *955*
Parasitology, 956
Parasomnia, 956, 1131
Parasympathetic nervous system,
   956
Parathion, 956
Parathyroid glands, 692-693, 956,
   956
   hypoparathyroidism, 701
   removal of, 957
   tumor, 956-957
Parathyroid hormone, 956
Parathyroidectomy, 957
Paratyphoid fever, 957
Parenchyma, 957
Parenteral nutrition, 957

Paresis, 957
Paresthesia, 957
Parietal, 957
Parkinson disease, 957-958, *957*
   stem cell research, 79, 92
Parkinsonism, 958
Paronychia, 958
Parotid glands, 958, *958*
Paroxetine, 958
Paroxysm, 958
Parturition, 958-959
Parvovirus. *See* Fifth disease.
Passive smoking, 959, *959*
Passive-aggressive personality dis-
   order. *See* Personality disorders.
Pasteurization, 959
Patch test, 959, *959*
Patellar tendinitis, 959-960
Paternity testing, 960
Pathogen, 960
Pathogenesis, 960
Pathognomonic, 960
Pathologist, 960
Pathologist, forensic, 960
Pathology, 960
   anatomical, 960, *960*
   surgical, 960
Pathophysiology, 961
Patient-controlled analgesia. *See*
   Analgesia, patient-controlled.
PCB, 961
PCOD. *See* Polycystic ovarian
   syndrome.
Peak flow meter, 961
Peau d'orange, 961
Pediatrician, 962
Pediatric rehabilitation, 961-962,
   961
Pediatrics, 962
Pediculosis, 963
Pedophilia, 106, 963
Peduncle, 963
Pellagra, 963
Pelvic examination, 963, *963*
Pelvic floor exercises. *See* Kegel
   exercises.
Pelvic inflammatory disease, 964,
   1110
   cervicitis, 341-342
   infertility, 722
Pelvic pain, 964-965

Pelvimetry, 965
Pelvis, 965
Pemoline, 965
Pemphigoid, bullous, 965
Pemphigus vulgaris, 965
Penicillamine, 965-966
Penicillins, 175, 966
Penile implant, 966, *966*
Penile warts, 966-967
Penis, 967, 1065, *967*
   balanitis, 223
   cancer of, 967, *967*
   chordee, 363
   foreskin, 580, *580*
   orchitis, 923, *923*
   paraphimosis, 954
   Peyronie disease, 980, *980*
   phimosis, 982
   priapism, 1017
   problems of the, symptom chart,
     49
Pentamidine, 967
Pepsin, 967-968, *968*
Peptic ulcer disease, 968-969, *969*
Perception, 969, 1101
Percussion, 969-970, *969*
Percutaneous umbilical cord
   sampling, 970
Perforation, 970
Pergolide, 970
Pericarditis, 970-971, *970*
Pericardium, 971
Pericoronitis, 971
Perimenopause, 971
Perimetry, 971
Perinatal, 971
Perinatologist, 971
Perinatology, 971
Perineum, 971
Period, menstrual. *See*
   Menstruation.
Periodontal disease, 144, 971-972,
   972
Periodontics, 972-973
Periodontist, 972-973
Periodontitis. *See* Periodontal
   disease.
Periosteum, 261, 973
Periostitis, 973
Peripheral nervous system, 973
Peripheral vascular disease, 973
Peristalsis, 973, *973*

Peritoneal dialysis, 973-974, *974*
Peritoneum, 975
Peritonitis, 975
   abdominal pain, 14
   acute abdomen, 98
Peritonsillar abscess, 975
Permanent teeth, 975-976, *976*
Permethrin, 976
Pernicious anemia. *See* Anemia,
   pernicious.
Pernio, 976, *378*
Peroneal muscular atrophy, 976
Personality, 976
Personality disorders, 976-978
Personality tests, 978
Perspiration, 691, 701, 978, 1005
Perthes disease. *See* Osteochon-
   drosis.
Pertussis, 978-979
   vaccination, 1262
Pervasive developmental disorder,
   979
Pessary, 979, *979, 1260*
Pesticide poisoning, 979
PET scanning, 979-980
Petechiae, 980
Petit mal, 101, 980, 1098
Peutz-Jeghers syndrome, 980
Peyronie disease, 980, *980*
pH, 980
Phacoemulsification, 91-92
Phagocyte, 980-981
Phantom limb pain, 981
Pharmacokinetics, 981
Pharmacology, 981
Pharyngitis. *See* Sore throat.
Pharyngoesophageal diverticulum,
   981
Pharynx, 981, 1068, *981*
   cancer of, *See* Throat cancer.
Phenazopyridine, 981
Phenobarbital, 981
Phenotype, 981-982
Phentermine, 982
Phenylalanine, 982
Phenylketonuria. *See* PKU.
Phenylpropanolamine, 982
Phenytoin sodium, 982
Pheochromocytoma, 982
Pheromone, 982
Phimosis, 982
Phlebitis. *See* Thrombophlebitis.

Phlebotomy, 983
Phlegm, 983
Phobia, 983
Phocomelia, 983
Phonological disorder, 983
Phosphates, 983
Phospholipids, 983
Phosphorus, 849, 983
Photocoagulation, 983
Photophobia, 984
Photorefractive keratectomy, 984,
   1059
Photosensitivity, 984
Phototherapy, 984-985, 1044
Physiatrist, 985
Physiatry, 985
Physical examination. *See* Examina-
   tion, physical.
Physical medicine and rehabilita-
   tion, 985, *985*
Physical therapy, 985-986, *985*
Physician, 986
Physiology, 986
Phytochemicals, 986
Pica, 159, 986
Pick disease, 146, 986
PID. *See* Pelvic inflammatory
   disease.
Pigeon toes. *See* Intoeing.
Pigmentation, 986-987
Pill, birth control. *See*
   Contraception, hormonal methods.
Pilocarpine, 987
Pilonidal sinus, 987
Pimple, 987, *110*
Pinched nerve, 987
Pineal gland, 987, *987*
Pinguecula, 987
Pink eye. *See* Conjunctivitis.
Pinna, 987
Pins and needles sensation, 987
Pinworm infestation, 956, 987-988,
   988
Piroxicam, 988
Pituitary gland, 271, 701-702, 988,
   988
Pituitary tumors, 988-989
Pityriasis alba, 989
Pityriasis rosea, 989
PKU, 989
   prenatal screening, 84,1015
Placebo, 989
Placenta, 989-990, *990*

   abruption, 990
   afterbirth, 125
   previa, 174, 990, *990*
   retained, 990
Plague, 171, 990-991
Planned Parenthood, 991
Plantar wart, 991
Plants
   phytochemicals, 986
   poisonous, 991, 999-1000, *1000*
Plaque, 991
   dental, 991
Plasma, 252, 253, 991
Plasma cells, 991
Plasma proteins, 991
Plasmapheresis, 991
Plasminogen activator, 992
Plastic surgeon, 992
Plastic surgery, 992
Platelets, 252-254, 256, 992
   thrombocytopenia, 1208
Play therapy, 992
Pleura, 992
Pleural effusion, 992-993, *992*
Pleurisy, 993
Plexus, 993
Plication, 993, *993*
Plummer-Vinson syndrome, 993
PMS. *See* Premenstrual syndrome.
Pneumaturia, 993-994
Pneumoconiosis, 994
Pneumocystis pneumonia, 994
Pneumonectomy, 994-995, *995*
Pneumonia, 995-997, *996*
   bacterial, 996
   mycoplasmal, 996-997
   pneumocystis, 994
   viral, 996
Pneumonitis, 997-998, *997*
Pneumothorax, 997-998, *997*
Pocket, gingival, 998
Podiatrist, 998
Podiatry, 998
Poison, 999
Poison center, 999
Poison ivy, 998-999, 1000, *999*
Poisoning
   carbon monoxide, 999, *999*
   chemical, 999
   first aid, 1322, 1327
   food, 1322
   hydrogen sulfide, 999-1000

lead, 777
mushroom, 1000, *1000*
plant, 1000, *1000*
swallowed caustics, 1001
Polarity therapy, 1001
Polio, 1001-1002, *1002*
postpolio syndrome, 1009
vaccination, 1262
Poliomyelitis. *See* Polio.
Pollen, 1002
Pollution
air, 1002
noise, 904, 1002-1003
water, 1003, *1003*
Polyarthritis, 1003
Polychondritis, relapsing, 1003
Polycystic kidney disease,
761-762, 1003-1004, *761*
Polycystic ovarian syndrome,
1004, *1004*
Polycythemia, 879, 1004
Polydactyly, 1004-1005, *1005*
Polydipsia, 1005
Polyhidrosis, 1005
Polyhydramnios, 157, 1005
Polymyxin B sulfate, 1005
Polymyalgia rheumatica, 1005
back pain, 218
Polymyositis, 1005-1006
Polymyxin B sulfate, 1005
Polyp, 1006
Polypectomy, 1006
Polypharmacy, 1006
Polyposis, familial, 1006-1007
Polyuria, 1007
Pore, 1007
Porphyria, 1007
Port-wine stain, 242, 1007, *1007*
Positron emission tomography
scanning. *See* PET scanning.
Postcoital contraception. *See*
Contraception, hormonal methods.
Posterior, 1008
Postmaturity, 1008
Postmortem examination. *See*
Autopsy.
Postnasal drip, 1008
Postoperative care, 1008, *1008*
Postpartum cardiomyopathy, 1008
Postpartum depression, 1008-1009
Postpartum hemorrhage, 1009
Postpolio syndrome, 1009

Posttraumatic stress disorder, 184,
1009
Postural drainage, 1009-1010, *1009*
Postural hypotension. *See* Hypo-
tension.
Posture, 1010
Potassium, 849, 1010
Pott fracture, 1010
Power of attorney, 1010
durable, 123, 486
PPO, 1010
Prader-Willi syndrome, 1010
Pravastatin, 1010
Precancerous, 1011
Preconception counseling. *See*
Genetic counseling.
Predisposing factors, 1011
Prednisolone, 1011
Prednisone, 1011
Preeclampsia, 1011
Preferred provider organization.
See PPO.
Pregnancy, 1011, 1013, *1012*
amniocentesis, 150-151, *150*
choriocarcinoma, 363
eclampsia, 496
ectopic, 497, 722, *497*
fetal alcohol syndrome, 556
fetal monitoring, 556-558, 557
and folic acid, 571
gestational diabetes, 461-462
gestational trophoblastic disease, 600
gravida, 615-616
herpes gestationis, 667
hyperemesis gravidarum, 691
miscarriage, 850-851
molar, 855
morning sickness, 859
multiple, 865, 867, 1013-1014
nausea or vomiting, 46
nonstress test, 905
placenta, 989
polyhydramnios, 1005
postmaturity, 1008
prenatal care, 1014-1015
prenatal ultrasound, 84, *84*
quickening, 1047
Rh incompatibility, 1074-1075
smoking effects, 1013
surrogate motherhood, 1181
tests, 1013, 1015, *1013*
toxemia, 1225

toxoplasmosis, 1226-1228, *1227*
travel immunization, 1235-1236
tubal, 1242
ultrasound, obstetrical, 1252
urination problems, 57
vomiting, 1287
weight gain, 61
Pregnancy tests, home, 679
Prehypertension, 1014, *695*
Preleukemia. *See* Myelodysplastic
syndrome.
Premature birth, 1014
lung surfactant, 1181
Premature ejaculation, 1014, 1109
Premature ovarian failure, 1014
Premenstrual syndrome, 841, 1014
Prenatal care, 1014-1015
Prenatal screening, 84, *84*
Prenatal testing, 1015
Preoperative care, 1015-1016
Prepuce, 580, 1016, *580*
Presbycusis. *See* Hearing loss in
older people.
Presbyopia, 107, 1016
Preservatives, 1016
Pressure, intraocular, 739
Pressure points, 1016, *1016*
Pressure sores, 1016-1017, *1016*
Preterm labor, 1017
Prevalence, 1017
Priapism, 1017
Primary, 1017
Primary care physician, 1017
Primary teeth, 1017-1018, *1018*
Prinzmetal angina, 168
PRK. *See* Photorefractive keratec-
tomy.
Procainamide hydrochloride, 1018
Procaine, 164, 1018
Prochlorperazine, 1018
Procidentia, 1018
Proctitis, 1018
Proctoscopy, 1018
Prodrome, 1018
Progeria, 1018
Progesterone, 1018-1019, 1065,
1107
Progestin, 1019
Prognathism, 925-926, 1019, *926*
Prognosis, 1019
Progressive muscular atrophy,
1019

Progressive systemic sclerosis, 1019
Prolactin, 1019-1020
Prolactinoma, 1020
Prolapse, 1020
  disk. *See* Slipped disk.
  mitral valve, 645-647
  uterine, 1259-1260
  rectal, 1055
  vaginal vault, 1264-1265
Prolotherapy, 1020
Promethazine, 1020
Pronation, 1020
Prophylactic, 1020
Propoxyphene, 1020
Propranolol, 1020
Proprietary name, 1020
Proprioception, 1020, *1020*
Proptosis. *See* Exophthalmos.
Prostaglandins, 1021
Prostate gland, 1021, 1065, *1021*
  surgical removal, 1025-1026, *1026*
Prostate, cancer of the, 1021-1024, *1022*
  leuprolide acetate, 788
Prostate, enlarged, 1024-1025, *1024*
  urination problems, 56, 58
Prostatectomy, 1025-1026, *1026*
Prostate-specific antigen (PSA) test, 1026-1027
Prostatitis, 1027
  infertility, 721
Prosthesis, 1027-1028, *1027*
Prosthodontics, 1028
Protease inhibitors, 1028
Protein synthesis, 1028
Proteins, 468, 1020, 1028
Proteinuria, 759, 1028
Proteus syndrome, 939
Proton pump inhibitors, 485, 1028
Protozoa, 1028, *1028*
Proximal, 1028
Prurigo, 1029
Pruritus, 1029
Pseudarthrosis, 1029
Pseudodementia, 1029
Pseudoephedrine, 1029
Pseudofolliculitis. *See* Shave bumps.
Pseudogout, 1029
Pseudohermaphroditism, 1029-1030

Pseudomembranous colitis, 1030
Pseudo-obstruction, 1029
Pseudotumor cerebri, 1030
Psittacosis, 1030, 1310
Psoriasis, 1030-1031, *1030*
Psoriatic arthritis, 1031, *1031*
Psyche, 1031
Psychiatric hospital, 1031
Psychiatrist, 1031
Psychiatry, 1031
Psychoanalysis, 1032
  transference, 1231
Psychoanalyst, 1032
Psychoanalytic theory, 1032
Psychogenic, 1032
Psychological counseling. *See* Counseling, psychological.
Psychological testing, 1032
Psychologist, 1032
Psychology, 1032
Psychometry, 1032
Psychoneuroimmunology (PNI), 1032-1033
Psychoneurosis, 1033
Psychopathology, 1033
Psychopharmacology, 1033
Psychosexual disorders, 1033-1034
Psychosis, 1034
Psychosomatic, 1034
Psychosurgery, 1034-1035
Psychotherapist, 1035
Psychotherapy, 848, 1035
Psychotropic drugs. *See* Antipsychotic drugs.
Psyllium, 1035
Pterygium, 1035, *1035*
PTH. *See* Parathyroid hormone.
Ptosis, 249, 541, 1035
Puberty, 1035, 1038, *1036-1037*
  breast development, 275
  female, 1065, *1036*
  growth, 618-620, *619*
  male, 1065, *1037*
  sexual characteristics, secondary, 1108
Pubes, 1038
Pubic lice, 1038
Public health, 1038
PUBS. *See* Percutaneous umbilical cord sampling.
Pudendal block, 162, 1038
Puerperal sepsis, 1038

Puerperium, 1038-1039
Pulling teeth. *See* Tooth extraction.
Pulmonary edema, 1039
Pulmonary embolism, 1039-1040, *1040*
Pulmonary fibrosis, 1040-1041
Pulmonary function tests, 1041-1042
Pulmonary hypertension. *See* Hypertension, pulmonary.
Pulmonary hypertension, primary, 696, 1042
Pulmonary infarction, 1042
Pulmonary insufficiency, 1042-1043
Pulmonary rehabilitation, 1043
Pulmonary disease, chronic obstructive. *See* Chronic obstructive pulmonary disease.
Pulp, dental, 1043
Pulpectomy, 1043
Pulpitis, 1043
Pulpotomy, 1043
Pulse, 1043-1044, *1043*
Puncture wounds, 1044
Pupil, 1044
Purpura, 1044, *1044*
Purulent, 1044
Pus, 1044, 1181
Pustules, 1044
PUVA, 1044
Pyelography, 739, 1044-1045, *739, 1044*
Pyelolithotomy, 1045
Pyelonephritis, 1045
Pyloric stenosis, 1045, *1045*
Pyloroplasty. *See* Vagotomy.
Pyoderma gangrenosum, 1046
Pyogenic granuloma, 1046
Pyorrhea. *See* Periodontal disease.
Pyramidal system, 1046
Pyrexia, 1046
Pyrogen, 1046
Pyromania, 1046
Pyuria, 1046

Q fever, 1047
Qi (chee), 355, 428, 513
Qigong, 513, 1047
Quackery, 1047
Quadriparesis, 1047

Quadriplegia. *See* Paralysis.
Quarantine, 1047
Quickening, 1047
Quinapril, 1047
Quinidine, 1047
Quinine, 1047

R

Rabies, 1048, 1310, *1049*
  animal-transmitted, 171
  immune globulin, human, 1048
Rad, 1048
Radial keratotomy, 1048-1049
Radiation, 1049
Radiation sickness, 1049-1050
Radiation therapy, 308, 1050-1051,
  1050
  breast cancer, 278
  prostate cancer, 1023
Radiculopathy, 1051
Radioactivity, 1051
Radiograph, 1051
Radiography, 1051
Radioisotope scanning, 1051
Radiologist, 1051
Radiology, 907, 1051
  See also X ray.
Radiolucent, 1051
Radionics, 1051-1052
Radionuclide scanning, 81-82,
  908-909
Radiopharmaceuticals, 1052
Radon, 1052
  lung cancer, 808
Raloxifene, 1052
Ramipril, 1052
Range-of-motion exercises, 1052
Ranitidine, 1052
Rape, 106, 198, 1052-1053
  first aid, 1327
Rash, 1053, *1053*
  shingles, 1113-1114
  symptom chart
    in adults, 52-53
    in infants and children, 50-51
Raynaud disease, 1053
  numbness or tingling, 48
Raynaud phenomenon, 1053
RDIs. *See* Reference Daily Intakes.
Reactive airway disease, 1053-1054,

1053, 1054
Reading, 778
Reagent, 1054
Rebound headache, 632
Receptors, 1054
  sensory, 969
Recombinant DNA, 1054-1055,
  1054
Recommended Dietary Allowances,
  466
Recovery room, 1008
Rectocele, 1055
Rectum, 467, 1055
  bleeding, 1055
  cancer of the, 1055-1056
  examination, 1055
  proctitis, 1018
  prolapse, 1055, *1055*
Red blood cells, 252, 255
  hemolysis, 654
  polycythemia, 1004
  spherocytosis, hereditary, 1147
Red eye, 1056
Reduction, 1056
Reed-Sternberg cells, 815
Reference daily intakes, 1056
Referred pain, 1056-1057, *1056*
Reflex, 1057, *1057*
  infant, *1058*
  primitive, 1057
Reflex sympathetic dystrophy, 1057,
  1115
Reflexology, 260, 1057, 1059, *1059*
  Thai massage, 1203
Reflux. *See* Esophageal reflux.
Refraction, 1059, 1278
Refractive surgery, 1059
Regional anesthesia. *See* Anesthesia.
Regional enteritis. *See* Crohn
  disease.
Regression, 1059
Regurgitation, 1059
Rehabilitation, 1059-1060
  cardiac, 315, 641
  pediatric, 961-962, *961*
  physical medicine and, 985
  pulmonary, 1043
  See also Physical therapy.
Rehydration fluid, oral, 1060
Reiki, 1060, *826*
Reimplantation, dental, 1060
Reiter syndrome, 1060, 1089

autoimmunity, 212
back pain, 220
spondylarthropathy, 1153
Relapse, 1060
Relapsing fever, 1061
Relaxation techniques, 1061, *1061*
REM sleep, 475, 1061
  in menopause, 838
  nightmares, 902
Remission, 1061
Renal. *See also* Kidney.
  biopsy, 1062
  colic, 1062
  diet, 1062
  failure, 759
  transplant, 761, *761*
  tubular acidosis, 1062
  vascular hypertension, 1063,
    1063
Renal cell carcinoma, 1062, *1062*
Renin, 1063
Repetitive strain injury, 1063-1064,
  1063
  carpal tunnel syndrome, 325
Reportable diseases, 1064
Reproduction, sexual, 1064, *1064*
Reproductive systems, 498
  female, 1064-1065, *1064,1065*
  male, 1065-1066, *1066*
Reptile bites, 244-245, *244*
Research study. *See* Clinical trial.
Resection, 1066
Resident, 1066
Residential care facility, 1066
Resistance exercises. *See* Exercise.
Resistance, drug, 1066
Resorcinol, 111
Resorption, dental, 1066
Respiration, 252, 1066-1067, *1067*
  artificial, 196, *196*
Respirator, 1067, *1067*
Respiratory arrest, 1067
  hypoxia, 271
Respiratory distress syndrome,
  1015, 1067-1068
  neonatal intensive care, 892
  oxygen therapy, 294
Respiratory system, 1068-1069, *1068*
  failure, 1068
  function tests, 1068
  infections, 952, 1069
  lung, 807-808, *807*

therapy, 1069
Respiratory therapy, 1069
    COPD, 367
    postural drainage, 1009-1010,
        1009
Respiratory tract infection, 1069
    See also Cold, common.
Respite care, 104, 1069
Restless leg syndrome, 1069, 1131
Restoration, dental, 1069-1070
Resuscitation, 1070, *1070*
    cardiopulmonary, 319, *319*
    first aid, 1328-1329, *1328*
    mouth-to-mouth, 862
    portable, *196*
Retainer, dental, 1070
Reticulocyte, 1070
Retina, 536, 1070
    blind spot, 250
    detachment, 41, 1070-1071, *1071*
    hemorrhage, 1071
    macular degeneration, 817-819,
        818
Retinal artery occlusion, 1070
    vision loss or impairment, 41
Retinal vein occlusion, 1071
Retinitis, 1072
    cytomegalovirus, 433, 434
Retinitis pigmentosa, 1072
Retinoblastoma. *See* Eye tumors.
Retinoic acid, 1072
Retinoids, 1072
Retinol, 1281
Retinopathy, 1072
    diabetic, 1072-1073, *1073*
    of prematurity, 1072
Retractor, 1073, *1073*
Retrobulbar optic neuritis. *See* Optic
    neuritis.
Retroperitoneal fibrosis, 1073
Retropubic suspension, 1073-1074
Retrovirus, 1074, 1134
Rett syndrome, 979, 1074
Reversible ischemic neurologic
    deficit. *See* RIND.
Reye syndrome, 198, 1074
Rh immune globulin, 1074
Rh incompatibility, 257, 654, 1015,
    1074-1075
    missed abortion, 100
    stillbirth, 1165
Rhabdomyolysis, 1075

Rhabdomyosarcoma, 1075
Rheumatic fever, 1075-1076,
    1075,1076
Rheumatism, 1076
Rheumatoid arthritis, 194,
    1076-1077, *1076, 1077*
    ankle or foot problems, 18
    ankylosing spondylitis, 171
    autoimmunity, 212
    hip pain, 42
    juvenile, 750-751, 1077, 1165,
        751
        bow legs, 267
        nodules, 1077, *1077*
        Sjögren syndrome, 1123
        synovitis, 1185
    See also Osteoarthritis.
Rheumatoid spondylitis, 1077
Rheumatologist, 1077
Rheumatology, 1077
Rhinitis, 1077-1078, *1078*
    allergic, 1078
    atrophic, 1078-1079
Rhinophyma, 1079
Rhinoplasty. *See* Nose reshaping.
Rhinorrhea, 1079
Rhythm method, 402, 886-887
Ribavirin, 1079
Riboflavin, 1079, 1281
Ribonucleic acid (RNA), 595, 596,
    909, 1079, 1080, *1081*
    antiaging therapy, 175
    retrovirus, 1074
Ribosomes, 334
Ribs, 1079
    fracture, 1079, *1079*
RICE, 1079, 1155, 1331, *1331*
    knee pain, 44
Rickets, 1079-1080, *1080*
    bow legs, 267
Rifampin, 182-183, 1080
Rigidity
    muscle, 1080
    Parkinson's disease, 958
Rigor, 1080
Rigor mortis, 1080
Riluzole, 1080
Rimantadine hydrochloride, 1080
RIND, 1080
Ring, intracorneal, 738-739
Ringing in ears. *See* Tinnitus.

Ringworm, 1080
Risk factors, 1080
Risperidone, 1080
Ritodrine, 1080
Rituximab, 1080
River blindness, 250
RNA, 1080, *1081*
Robotic surgery, 73, *94-96*
Rocky Mountain spotted fever, 244,
    245, 1081
Roe vs. Wade, 99
Rofecoxib, 1081
Rolfing, 203, 260, 1081, *1081*
Root canal treatment, 1081-1082,
    1221, *1082*
    apicoectomy, 187-188, *187*
Ropivacaine, 164
Rorschach test, 1082
Rosacea, 1079, 1082-1083
Roseola infantum, 1083
    childhood rash, 50
Rosiglitazone maleate, 1083
Rotator cuff disease, 1083
    swimmer's shoulder, 1184
    tendinitis, 1083, *1083*
Rotavirus, 1083
Roundworms, 197, 1083-1084,
    1310, *1084*
    larva migrans, 770-771
    strongyloidiasis, 1173-1174
    toxocariasis, 1226
Rubella, 1084, *1084*
    rash, 50, 52
    vaccination, 1263
Rubeola. *See* Measles.
Runner's knee, 1084-1085
Running injuries, 1085, *1085*
Rupture, 1085

Sac, 1086
Saccharin, 196, 1086
Sacralization, 1086
Sacroilitis, 1086
Sacrum, 1086
SAD. *See* Seasonal affective disorder.
Saddle block. *See* Anesthesia,
    spinal.
Sadomasochism, 1086, *1086*
Safer sex, 1086

Safety belts, 312
Saline, 1086
Saliva, 467, 1086-1087
  excess, 1087
Salivary glands, 1087, *1087*
  sialadenitis, 1116
  Sjögren syndrome, 1123
  stones, 1087
  tumors, 1087
Salmeterol, 1087
Salmonella infections, 176,
  1088-1089, 1310, *1088*
  poisoning, first aid, 1323
  prevention of infection, *1088*
  waterborne, 1293
Salpingectomy, 1089
Salpingitis, 1089
Salpingostomy, 1089
Salpinoophorectomy, 1089
Salsalate, 1089
Salt, 1089
Saquinavir mesylate, 1089-1090
Sarcoidosis, 1090
  lupus pernio, 810
Sarcomas, 308, 1090
SARS. *See* Severe acute respiratory
  syndrome.
Saturated fats, 551, *1090.*
Saw palmetto, 1090
Scabicides, 1090-1091
Scabies, 1091, *1091*
Scalds, 1091
Scaling, dental, 1091, *1091*
Scalp, 1091
Scalpel, 1092, *1092*
Scaphoid, 1092
Scar, 1092
Scarlet fever, 1092
Schistosome, 1092
Schistosomiasis, 1092
Schizophrenia, 1092-1093
  body image, 259
  mutism, 875
  neuropsychological testing, 900
  See also Personality disorders.
School violence, 1275
Schuessler biochemic system. *See*
  Tissue salts therapy.
Schwannoma, 898
Sciatica, 1093
Scirrhous, 1093-1094
Sclera, 536, 1094

Scleritis, 1094
Scleroderma, 1094
  progressive systemic sclerosis,
    1019
  Sjögren syndrome, 1123
  spondylarthropathy, 1153
Scleromalacia, 1094
Sclerosis, 1094
Scoliosis, 1094-1095, *1094*
  brachialgia, 268
  neurofibromatosis, 898
  orthopedic brace, 268
Scopolamine, 1095
Scorpion stings, 1095
Scotoma, 1095
Scratch test, 137, 1095
Screening, 1095
  for cancer, 311
  genetic, 597
  glaucoma, 603
  newborns, 1095
  phenylketonuria, 989
Scrofula, 1095
Scrotum, 1096
  hydrocele, 687, *687*
Scuba-diving medicine. *See* Diving
  medicine.
Scurvy, 1096
Seafood poisoning, 577-578
Sealants, dental, 1096
Seasickness, 1096
Seasonal affective disorder (SAD),
  792, 1086, 1096
Seat belts, 1096-1097, *354*
Sebaceous cyst. *See* Epidermal cyst.
Sebaceous glands, 1097
  blackhead, 246
Seborrhea, 1097
Seborrheic dermatitis, 50, 52, *1097*
Seborrheic keratosis, 1097, *1097*
Sebum, 1097
Secondary, 1097
Secondhand smoke. *See* Passive
  smoking.
Secretion, 1097
Sedation, 1097
Sedation, conscious. *See* Conscious
  sedation.
Sedatives, 1097
  addiction to, 477
  sleep problems, 55
Sedimentation test, 256
Seizures, 517-519, 1097-1098, 1329

absence, 101
anticonvulsants, 177-178
aura, 210
cerebral aneurysm, 167
drop attack, 476
febrile, 552,1098-1099,
  1098,1099
first aid, 1329
grand mal, 613
infantile spasms, 719
Selective serotonin reuptake
  inhibitors (SSRI), 178, 1099, *1099*
Selegiline, 1099
Selenium, 849-850, 912, 1099-1100
Self-esteem, 1100
Self-help organizations, 1344-1345
Self-image, 1100
Self-mutilation, 1100
Self-screening test, 1100, *1100*
Semen, 1100
  analysis, 1101, *1101*
  blood in, 650
Seminoma, 1101
Sensate focus technique, 1101
Sensation, 1101-1102, *1102*
  abnormal, 1102
Senses, 969, 1101-1102
Sensitive teeth. *See* Dentin.
Sensitization, 136, 137, 1102
Sensory cortex, 1102-1103
Sensory deprivation, 1103
Sensory integration dysfunction, 779
Separation anxiety, 1103
Sepsis, 1103
Septal defect
  atrial, 1103-1104, *1103*
  ventricular, 1104, *1103*
Septic shock, 1104
  bacteremia, 221
  first aid, 1330
Septicemia, 254, 1104-1105, *1104*
  Waterhouse-Friedrichsen
    syndrome, 1293
Septum, 1105
  deviated, 1105, *1105*
  perforated, 1105
  uterine, 1259
Sequela, 1105
Sequestration, 1105
Serology, 1106
Serotonin, 1106
  SSRI drugs, 1099

Sertraline, 178, 1106
Serum, 1106
Serum sickness, 1106
Severe acute respiratory syndrome, 1106
Sex, 1106, *1107*
Sex change, 1106
Sex chromosomes, 365, 1106-1107, *1106*
Sex determination, 1107
Sex drive, 1107
Sex education, 1107
  adolescents, 121
Sex hormones, 1107
  anabolic steroids, 152, *152*
  androgens, 156
  progesterone, 1018-1019
Sex therapy, 1108
Sexual abuse, 105-106, *105*
Sexual addiction, 116, 1108
Sexual assault. *See* Assault, sexual; Rape.
  first aid, 1327-1328
Sexual characteristics, secondary, 1108
Sexual desire, inhibited, 1108
Sexual dysfunction, 1033, 1108-1109
Sexual intercourse, 1064, 1109
  safer sex, 1086
Sexual orientation, 1109
  bisexuality, 242-243
  heterosexuality, 669
  homosexuality, 679-680
  transsexualism, 1234
Sexual response, 1109-1110
  orgasm, 924
Sexuality, 1110
Sexually transmitted diseases, 1110-1112, *1111*
  anal sex, 153
  Chlamydia, 356
  condyloma acuminatum, 393-394
  epididymitis, 516-517
  genital herpes, 667-668
  gonorrhea, 611
  granuloma inguinale, 614
  infertility, 722
  lymphogranuloma venereum, 815
  molluscum contagiosum, 856-857
  parasites, 954

safer sex, 1086
salpingitis, 1089
syphilis, 1186-1187, *1186*
trichomoniasis, 1238
urethritis, nongonococcal, 1255
  See also AIDS.
Sezary syndrome, 1112
Shaken baby syndrome, 102, 1112
Shave bumps, 623, 1029, 1112
Shiatsu, 1112
Shigellosis, 1112-1113
  waterborne, 1293
Shin splints, 1113,*1113*
Shingles, 1113-1114, *1114*
Shivering, 1115
Shock
  anaphylactic, 1114
  bee stings, 232
  electric, 1114-1115, *1114*
  first aid, 1329-1330
  insulin, 1115, *1115*
  physiological, 1115
  septic, 1104
  spinal, 1115
Short stature, 1115
Shortening of leg, 781
Shortness of breath. *See* Breath, shortness of.
Shoulder
  anatomy, 1124
  arthroscopic surgery, 195
  dislocation, 1115
  frozen, 585
  rotator cuff, 1083, *1083*
  separation, 1115
  swimmer's, 1184
Shoulder-hand syndrome, 1115
Shunt, 1116, *1116*
Shy-Drager syndrome, 1116
Sialadenitis, 1116
Sibling rivalry, 1116-1117, *1116*
Sibutramine, 1117
Sick building syndrome, 1117
Sick sinus syndrome, 1117
  bradycardia, 269
Sickle cell anemia, 160, 654, 1117-1118, *1119*
  blindness, 251
  prenatal screening, 597
Sickle cell trait, 1118
Side effect, 1118, 1120
Sideroblastic anemia, 160

SIDS. *See* Sudden infant death syndrome.
Sight, 1120
Sigmoid colon, 1120
Sigmoidoscopy, 311, 1120-1121, *1120*
  colon cancer, 386
  polyposis, familial, 1006
SIL, 1121
Sildenafil citrate, 1121
Silica dust, 994
Silicone, 1121
Silicosis, 486, 1121
Simethicone, 1121
Simvastatin, 1121-1122
Sinew. *See* Tendon.
Single photon emission computerized tomography, 1144, *80*
  See also SPECT.
Sinoatrial node, 637
Sinus, 1122
  sinus facial, 1122, *1122*
Sinus bradycardia, 1122
Sinus tachycardia, 1122
Sinusitis, 38, 632, 1122-1123
  headache, 39
  Wegener granulomatosis, 1294-1295
Situs inversus, 1123
Sitz bath, 1123
Sjögren syndrome, 1123
  autoimmunity, 212
Skeletal muscle injury. *See* Rhabdomyolysis.
Skeletal system, 1124-1126, *1125*
  atlas, 65
  cartilage, 327, *327*
  dysplasia, 1123-1124
Skeleton. *See* Skeletal system.
Skier's thumb, 1126
Skilled care facility, 804, 1126
Skilled nursing facility. *See* Long-term care facility.
Skin, 1126-1127, *1126*
  allergy, 137, 1127
  biopsy, 1127
  cancer, 114, 1127-1129
    basal cell, 229-230, *230*
  graft, 1129
  ichthyosis vulgaris, 707
  impetigo, 712
  keratosis, 755

laser resurfacing, 773-774
and muscle flap, 1127
patch, 1129, *1129*
peau d'orange, 961
psoriasis, 1030-1031, *1030*
sun exposure, 1179
tag, 1129, *1129*
tests, 1129
tuberculin test, 1242
See also Cosmetic surgery; sunscreens.
Skull, 1129-1130, *1130*
anatomy, 1124
fracture, 1130, *1130*
Sleep, 1130-1131
deprivation, 1131, *1131*
in older people, 1132, *1132*
paralysis, 1132
Sleep apnea syndrome, 188, 1131
asthma, 202
obesity-hypoventilation syndrome, 913
Sleep disorders, 54, 1131-1132,
1132
insomnia, 731
narcolepsy, 883-884
night terror, 902
parasomnia, 956
symptom chart, 54-55
Sleeping sickness, 954, 1133, 1240
Sleepwalking, 1133
automatism, 213
Sling, 1133
Slipped disk, 1133-1134, 1150, *1134*
backache, 20
Slit lamp, 1134, *540*
Slow virus diseases, 1134
Small cell carcinoma, 1134-1135
Small-bowel
resection, 1135
series, 1135
transplant, 1135
Small intestine, 467
Smallpox, 1135
Smart drugs, 1136
Smear, 1136
Smell, 969, 1101-1102, 1136-1137,
1136
anosmia, 173
Smoke inhalation. *See* Inhalation,
smoke.
Smoking, tobacco, 1137-1140, *1139*

addiction, 116
and aging, 126
angina, 168
asbestosis, 197
and atherosclerosis, 205
aversion therapy, 214
bad breath, 223
and bronchitis, 293
and cancer, *311*
cessation, 1129, 1137, *1138*
COPD, 366
coughing, 29, 30
and depression, 33
and duodenal ulcers, 485
and Goodpasture syndrome, 612
hoarseness or voice loss and, 31
and lung cancer, 808
and nasopharyngeal cancer, 885
passive, 959,
and weight gain, 61
Snails and disease, 1140, *955*
Snakebite, 1140
Sneezing, 1140
Snellen chart, 1140, *1279*
Snoring, 1140-1141, *1140, 1141*
somnoplasty, 1142
Sobriety, 1141
Sodium, 850, 1141
Soft spot, infant, 572, 1141
Soft-tissue injury, 1141
Soiling. *See* Encopresis.
Solar plexus, 1141
Soluble fiber. *See* Fiber, dietary.
Solvent abuse. *See* Inhalants.
Somatic, 1141
Somatization disorder, 1141-1142
Somatoform disorders, 1142
Somatotype, 1142
Somnoplasty, 1142
Sonohysterogram, 1142
Sore throat, 1142
swallowing difficulty, 64
Sores, pressure, 1016-1017
Sotos syndrome, 939
Sound therapy, 1142
Soy, 1142-1143, *1143*
Space medicine. *See* Aerospace
medicine.
Sparfloxacin. *See* Fluoroquinolones.
Spasm, 1143
esophageal, 526
facial, 544

infantile, 719
lumbosacral, 807
muscle, 872
tetany, 1202
vaginismus, 1265
Spastic colon. *See* Irritable bowel
syndrome.
Spastic paralysis, 1143
Spasticity, 1143
Spatulate, 1143
Specialist, 1143
Specimen, 1143
SPECT, 80-81, 1144
Speculum, 1144
Speech, 1144
blocking, 252
disorders, 1144
dysarthria, 487
mechanism, 1144-1145, *1145*
stuttering, 1174
therapy, 1145-1146
voice loss, 1286
See also Autism; Child development.
Speech therapy, pediatric, 962
Sperm, 1146, *70, 1146*
artificial insemination, 195, *195*
assisted reproductive technolo-
gy, 199
bank, 1146
count, 1146
extraction, 1146
ICSI (intracytoplasmic sperm
injection), 707
infertility, 721-723
motility, 1146
oligospermia, 916
Sperm bank, 1146
Spermatocele, 1146, *1146*
Spermatozoa, 1146, *1146, 1147*
Spermicides, 402, 1147
SPF. *See* Sun protection factor.
Spherocytosis, hereditary, 1147
Sphincter, 1147, *1147*
artificial, 1147
Sphincterotomy, 152, 1147-1148
Sphygmomanometer, 255, 1148
Spider bites, 243, 245, *245*
first aid, 1314-1315
Spider veins, 1148
Spina bifida, 242, 1148-1149, *1148*
meningomyelocele, 837

myelomeningocele, 878
Spinal anesthesia. *See* Anesthesia, spinal.
Spinal column, *335*
  anatomy, 1124
Spinal cord, 1149, *1149*
  abscess, 101
  decompression, 439
  fusion, 1150, *1150*
  injury, 1150
  injuries, stem cell replacement, 92
  meninges, 836
  myelopathy, 878-879
  radiculopathy, 1051
  Werdnig-Hoffmann disease, 1296
Spinal muscular atrophy, 860
Spinal stenosis, back pain, 220, 1150-1151, *1150*
Spinal tap, 806, 1151
Spine, 1151, *1151*
  injury, 1150
  scoliosis, 1094-1095, *1094*
  slipped disk, 1133-1134
  spondylolisthesis, 1154
  stenosis, 1150-1151, *1150*
  vertebra, 1273
Spinocerebellar degeneration, 583, 1151
Spirituality and healing, 1151
Spirochete, 1152
Spirometry, 1041, 1152
  asthma, 200
Spironolactone, 180, 1152
Spitz nevus, 1152
Spleen, 1152, *1152*
  hypersplenism, 694
Splenectomy, 1152-1153
Splenomegaly, 1153
Splicing, gene, 77
Splint, 1153
Splinters, 1153
  first aid, 1331, *1331*
Splinting, dental, 1153
Split personality, 1153
Spondylarthropathy, 1153
Spondylitis, 1153-1154
Spondylolisthesis, 1154, *1154*
  back pain, 220, 221
Spondylolysis, 1154
Spondylosis, 1154

Sponge, contraceptive, 401
Sporotrichosis, 1154
Sports
  and drugs, 1155-1156, *1156*
  helmets, 649
  mouth guard, 861
Sports injuries, 1154-1155, *1155*
  baseball elbow, 230
  baseball finger, 231
  golfer's elbow, 609-610
  knee ligaments, 791-792
  runner's knee, 1084-1085
  self-care, *1155*
  shin splints, 1113
  shoulder separation, 1115
  skier's thumb, 1126
  swimmer's ear, 1184
  tennis elbow, 1197
Sports medicine, 1155
Sprain, 1156-1157
  ankle or foot, 18
Sprue. *See* Celiac disease.
Sprue, tropical, 1157
Spur, 1157, *1157*
Sputum, 1157
Sputum culture, 427
Squamous cell carcinoma, 1114, 1128, 1157-1158, *1157, 1158*
  Bowen disease, 267-268
Squamous intraepithelial lesion. *See* SIL.
SSRI drugs. *See* Selective serotonin reuptake inhibitor drugs.
St. John's wort, 1158
Stable, 1158
Stage, 1158
Staining, 1158
Stammering. *See* Stuttering.
Stanford-Binet Intelligence Scale, 734
Stapedectomy, 1158, *1159*
Staphylococcal infections, 175-176, 1159, *1160*
  first aid, 1323
  prevention of, *1160*
Staples, surgical, 1159, *1159*
  stomach, 1167
Starch. *See* Carbohydrates.
Starvation, 1159-1160
Stasis, 1160
Statins, 361
Statistics

medical, 1160
  vital, 1160
Status asthmaticus, 1160-1161
Status epilepticus, 1161
  hypoxia, 271
Stavudine (d4T), 1161
STDs. *See* Sexually transmitted diseases.
Steatohepatitis, nonalcoholic, 664, 800, 904
Steatorrhea, 1161
Steele-Richardson-Olszewski syndrome, 1161
Stem cells, 1161
  bone marrow transplant, 263, *92*
  research, 79, 92-93, *79*
Stenosis
  aortic, 642
  heart valve, 645
  pulmonary, 642
  pyloric, 1045, *1045*
  spinal, 1150-1151
  subglottic, 1175
  valvular, 1161-1162
Stent, 641, 1162, *1162*
  for angina, 169
  atherosclerosis, 205
Stereotactic
  breast biopsy, 1162-1163
  imaging, 82-83, *83*
  brain tumor, 274
  surgery, 1163, *1164*
Sterility, 1163
Sterilization, 403, 1163
  female. *See* Tubal ligation.
  male. *See* Vasectomy.
Sternum, 1163
Steroids. *See* Anabolic steroids; Androgens; Corticosteroids; and Sports, drugs in.
Stethoscope, 1163, *1163*
Stevens-Johnson syndrome. See Drug eruption.
Stiff neck, 1163, 1165
Stiffness, 1165
Still disease, 1165
Stillbirth, 1165
Stimulants, 1165
Stimulus, 1165
Stingray injury, 1166
Stings, bee. *See* Bee stings.
  marine, 1165, *1165*

scorpion, 1095
St. John's wort, 1158
Stokes-Adams syndrome, 1165
Stoma, 1166
  colectomy, 381, 386, *381*
Stomach, 467, 1166
  bariatric surgery, 226-227, *226*
  cancer, 1166-1167
  weight loss, 62
  erosion, 591-592
  fundoplication, 585-586, *586*
  imaging, 1167
  pumping, 1167
  pyloric stenosis, 1045, *1045*
  stapling, 1167
  ulcer, 592, 1167
  abdominal pain, 14, 98
Stomatitis, 1167
Stones
  kidney, 760-761
  salivary gland, 1087
  See also Gallstones.
Stool, 1167
  culture, 427
  softeners, 777, 1167-1168
  See also Constipation; diar-
    rhea.
Strabismus, 147, 535, 1168, *1168*
  albinism, 131
Strains, 1168
  first aid, 1331-1332, *1331*
Strangulation, 1168-1169
Strangury, 1169
Strapping, 1169
Strawberry nevus. *See* Hemangioma.
Street violence, 1275
Strength training, 1169, 1295
Strep throat, 1169, *1169*
Streptococcal infections, 176, 617,
  1169-1170, 1169, *1170*
  erysipelas, 523
  bacteria, flesh eating, 222, *222*
  pneumonia, 996
  rheumatic fever, 1075-1076, *1076*
  scarlet fever, 1092
Streptococcal toxic shock-like
  syndrome, 1330
Streptokinase, 1170
Stress, 1170-1171
Stress fracture, 1171
Stress incontinence, 1073
Stress testing, cardiac, 315-317,
  533, *316*

Stretch marks, 1171
Stretcher, 1171
Stretching exercise, 568
Striae atrophicae. *See* Stretch
  marks.
Stricture, 1171
Stricture, esophageal, 526
Stridor, 1171
Stroke, 1171, 1173, *1172, 1173*
  aphasia, 186
  atony, 206
  brain hemorrhage, 656-658
  cerebral aneurysm, 167
  dizziness, 36
  first aid, 1332-1333
  heat, 647-648
  hemiparesis, 651
  hypertension, 695
  numbness or tingling, 48
Strongyloidiasis, 1173-1174
Structural integration. *See* Rolfing.
Stuffy nose. *See* Rhinitis.
Stump, 1174
Stupor, 1174
Sturge-Weber syndrome, 1174
Stuttering, 1174
Stye, 1174
Subacute, 1174
Subarachnoid hemorrhage. *See*
  Hemorrhage, subarachnoid.
Subarachnoid space, 269
Subclinical, 1174
Subconjunctival hemorrhage,
  1174-1175
Subconscious, 1175
Subcutaneous, 1175
Subdural hemorrhage, 1175
  dizziness, 37
  vision loss or impairment, 41
Subglottic stenosis, 1175
Sublimation, 1175
Subluxation, 1175, *1175*
Subphrenic abscess, 1175
Substrate, 1175
Succimer, 346. *See* Chelating agents.
Sucralfate, 1175
Sucralose. *See* Artificial sweeteners.
Sucrose, 1176
Suction, 1176, *1176*
Sudden death, 1176
Sudden infant death syndrome,
  1176, *1176*
Sudeck atrophy, 1176-1177

Suffocation, 1177, *1177*
Sugar, 1177, *1177*
Suicide, 1177-1178
  adolescents and, 121
  physician-assisted, 530
  risk factors for, 447
  threatened, 1178, *1178*
  warning signs, *1178*
Sulfa drugs, 1178-1179
Sulfamethoxazole. *See* Co-trimoxa-
  zole.
Sulfasalazine, 1179
Sulfonamides. *See* Sulfa drugs.
Sulfonylurea, 1179
  and diabetes mellitus, 459-460
Sulfur, 1179
Sulindac, 1179
Sullivan, Harry Stack, 352
Sumatriptan, 1179
Sun
  exposure, adverse effects of,
    1179, 1303
  age spots, 125
  protection factor, 1179
Sunburn, 1179-1180
  first aid, 1333
Sunscreens, 952, 1180, *1180*
Sunstroke. *See* Heat stroke.
Superego, 582, 1180
Superficial, 1180
Superinfection, 1180
Supernumerary teeth, 1180-1181,
  938
Supination, 1181
Supplements
  dietary, ferrous sulfate, 555
  nutritional, 911-912
  vitamin, 1283
Support groups, 848
Suppository, 1181
Suppuration, 1181
Suprarenal glands. *See* Adrenal
  glands.
Supraspinatus syndrome. *See*
  Rotator cuff disease.
Surfactant, 1181
Surfer's nodules, 1181, *1181*
Surgeon, 1181
Surgery, 1181
Surgical procedures. *See* procedure
  by name.
Surgicenter. *See* Ambulatory sur-
  gery.

Surrogate motherhood, 1181
Susceptibility, 1181-1182
Suture, 1182
Suturing, 1182, *1182*
Swab, 1182
Swallowing, 108, 1182, *1182*
    belching, 233, *233*
    chest pain, 24
    difficulty, 1182-1183, *1182*
    Plummer-Vinson syndrome, 993
    symptom chart, 64
Swayback, 805
Sweat glands, 1183
Sweating, 978, 1183, *1183*
    anhidrosis, 170-171
Swedish massage, 1184
Sweeteners, artificial. *See* Artificial
    sweeteners.
Swimmer's ear, 491, 635, 1184,
    1184
Swimmer's shoulder, 1184
Sympathectomy, 1184-1185
Sympathetic nervous system, 1185
    Sudeck atrophy, 1176-1177
Sympathomimetic amines, 1156
Symptom, 1185
Symptom charts, 12-64
Synapse, 1185
Syncope, 1185
Syndactyly, 1185, *1185*
Syndrome, 1185
Synovectomy, 1185
Synovitis, 1185
    toxic, 1185
Synovium, 1185
Syphilis, 1186-1187, *1186*
    gumma, 621
Syringe, 1187, *1187*
Syringing of the ears, 1187
Syrinx, 1187
System, 1187
Systemic, 1187
Systemic lupus erythematosus. *See*
    Lupus eyrthematosus, systemic.
Systolic blood pressure, 1187

T

T cells, 709-710, 814-815, 1188
    Sezary syndrome, 1112
Tabes dorsalis, 1188
Tachycardia, 192, 1188

angina, 168
    cardioversion, 321
    paroxysmal supraventricular,
        1188
    pulse, 1044
    ventricular, 1188-1189
Tachypnea, 1189
Tacrine, 1189
    for Alzheimer's disease, 145
Tacrolimus, 1189
Tag, skin. *See* Skin tag.
T'ai chi, 513, 1189, *1189*
Talipes, 1189-1190, *1190*
Talk therapy, 1190
Tall stature, 1190
    acromegaly, 113, *113*
Tamazepam, 1196
Tamoxifen, 1190, *1190*
Tampon, 1190
Tamponade, 1190
Tamsulosin, 1190
Tannin, 1191
Tantrum, 1191
Tapeworm infestation, 686-687, 956,
    1191, *1191*
Tarsal tunnel syndrome, 1191-1192
Tarsalgia, 1192
Tarsorrhaphy, 1192
Tartar, 1192
Taste, 969, 1101-1102, 1192, *1192*
    ageusia, 126
    loss of in older people, 1192,
        1192
Tattooing, 1192-1193
Tay-Sachs disease, 1193, *1193*
    prenatal screening, 597
Tazarotene, 1193
TB. *See* Tuberculosis.
Tear duct, blocked, 1193-1194,
    1193
Tearing, 1194, *1194*
Tears, 536, 1194
    meniscal, *837*
Technetium, 1194
Technology and medicine. *See*
    Twenty-first century medicine,
    73-96
Teeth, 1194, *1194*, *1195*
    abscess, 1221
    aerodontalgia, 124
    amelogenesis imperfecta, 148
    anodontia, 172
    apicoectomy, 187-188

avulsed, 215, *215*
    baby bottle decay, 217-218
    bad breath, 222-223
    bite, 243
    broken, 291
    bruxism, 295-296
    care of, 1195, *1195*
    cavity, 332-333, *333*
    cementum, 335
    cosmetic dentistry, 410-411, *410,
        411*
    deciduous, 438
    dental alignment, 135
    dental amalgam, 146
    discolored, 1195
    eruption, 1221-1222
    extraction, 1222
    false, 548
    impaction, 711-712
    luxated, 811
    malocclusion, 822-823, *822*
    orthodontic appliances, 924-925,
        925
    overbite, 938, *938*
    pericoronitis, 969-970
    permanent, 975-976, 1221-1222,
        976
    primary, 1017-1018, 1221-1222,
        1018
    pulp, 1043
    resorption, 1066
    root canal treatment, 1081-1082,
        1082
    supernumerary, 1180-1181
    wisdom, 1300-1301
Teething, 1196
Telangiectasia, 1196
Temazepam. *See* Benzodiazepines.
Temperature, 1196
    basal body, 229
Temporal arteritis. *See* Arteritis,
    giant cell.
Temporal lobe epilepsy. *See*
    Epilepsy, temporal lobe.
Temporomandibular joint disorder
    (TMJ). *See* Clicking jaw.
    bruxism, 296
    myofascial pain disorder,
        880-881
Tendinitis, 1063, 1196
    hip pain, 42, 43
    knee pain, 44
    rotator cuff, 1083

swimmer's shoulder, 1184
See also RICE (first aid).
Tendon, 1196, *1196*
 release, 1196
 repair, 1196
 transfer, 1196-1197
Tenesmus, 1197
Tennis elbow, 515, 1197, *1197*
Tenolysis, 1197
Tenosynovitis, 1197, 1238
Tenotomy. *See* Tendon repair.
Tenovaginitis. *See* de Quervain
 disease.
TENS (transcutaneous electrical
 nerve stimulation), 1198, 1230
 pain management, 946
Tension headache, 632
Teratogen, 1198
Teratoma, 1198
Terazosin, 1198
Terbinafine hydrochloride, 1198
Terconazole, 1198
Terminal care, 1198
Testicles, 1065, 1198
 cancer, 1199-1200, *1200*
 ectopic, 1200
 hypergonadism, 691
 hypogonadism, 700-701
 pain, 1200
 retractile, 1201
 self-examination, 1198-1199,
 1199
 torsion of the, 49, 1201, *1201*
 undescended, 1201, *1201*
Testicular feminization syndrome,
 1201
Testosterone, 1107, 1201-1202
 antiaging therapy, 175
Tetanus, 1202
 body piercing, 260
 vaccination, 1262
 wound infection, 1302-1303
Tetany, 1202
Tetracaine, 1202
Tetracyclines, 1202-1203
Tetralogy of Fallot, 642, 1203, *1203*
Thai massage, 260, 1203
Thalamus, 271, 1203, *1203*
Thalassemia, 158, 1203-1204
Thalidomide, 1204
 phocomelia, 983
Thallium, 1204

Theophylline, 1204
 for asthma, 202
Therapeutic, 1204
 recreation, 1204
 touch, 1205
Therapy. *See* Psychotherapy.
Thermometer, 1205, *1206*
Thiamin, 1205, 1281
Thiazolidinediones, 1205
Thigh, osteoid osteoma, 929
Thirst, 1205
 excessive, 1205
 polydipsia, 1005
Thoracentesis, 1205
Thoracic outlet syndrome, 1205
Thoracic surgeon, 1205
Thoracotomy, 1205, 1207, *1205*
Thorax, 1207
Thought, 1207
Thought disorders, 1207
Throat, 1207
 cancer, 1207-1208
 culture, 427
 sore, 1142
 symptom charts, coughing,
 28-30; hoarseness or voice loss,
 31
Thrombectomy, 1208
Thromboangiitis obliterans, 296
Thrombocytes, 252-253
Thrombocytopenia, 249, 1208
Thrombocytopenic purpura,
 idiopathic, 743-744
Thrombocytosis, 1208
 essential, 879
Thromboembolism, 1208
Thrombolytic drugs, 1208-1209,
 1208
 streptokinase, 1170
Thrombophlebitis, 1209
 hip pain, 43
Thrombosis
 cerebral, 338-339, *339*
 coronary, 408-409
 deep vein, 1209
Thrombus, 1209
Thrush, 1209
Thumb, skier's, 1126
Thumb-sucking, 1209-1210
Thymus, 1210, *1210*
Thyroglossal cyst, 1210
Thyroid gland, 1211-1212, *1212*

cancer, 1210-1211
 function tests, 1211
 goiter, 609, *609*
 Graves disease, 614-615
 Hashimoto thyroiditis, 629
 hormones, 697, 1212, *1213*
 hyperthyroidism, 697
 nodules, 1212-1213,
 normal scan, *72*
 scanning, 1213, *1213*
Thyroidectomy, 1213
Thyroiditis, 1213
 Hashimoto, 629
 hyperthyroidism, 697
Thyroid-stimulating hormone. *See*
 TSH.
Thyrotoxicosis, 1213-1214, *1214*
Thyrotropin-releasing hormone.
 See TRH.
Thyroxine, 703, 1212, 1214
TIA. *See* Transient ischemic attack.
Tibetan medicine, 1214
Tic, 1214
Tic douloureux. *See* Trigeminal
 neuralgia.
Ticks and disease, 1214-1215,
 1310, *1215*
 animal-transmitted, 171
 babesiosis, 217
 bites, 245-246, *246, 1215*
 Colorado tick fever, 388-389
 ehrlichiosis, 684
 first aid, 1315
 Lyme disease, 811-813, *812*
 relapsing fever, 1061
 Rocky Mountain spotted
 fever, 1081
Ticlopidine hydrochloride, 1215
Tietze syndrome. *See* Costochon-
 dritis.
Timolol, 1215-1216
Tinea, 206, 1216
Tinea versicolor, 1216
Tinel sign, 1216, *1216*
Tingling, 957, 1216, *1216*
Tinnitus, 112, 492, 1216-1217
 barotrauma, 228
Tirofiban, 1217
Tissue, 1217
Tissue plasminogen activator
 (t-PA), 992, 1040
Tissue salts therapy, 1217

Tissue-typing, 1217-1218
TMJ syndrome. *See* Clicking Jaw.
Tobacco. *See* Smoking cessation;
  Smoking, tobacco.
  chewing, 1218
  coughing, 29
Tobramycin, 1218
Tocopherol. *See* Vitamin E.
Toe, 1218
  turf, 1247
Toenail, ingrown. *See* Ingrown
  toenail.
Toilet training, 1218, *1218*
Tolerable Upper Intake Level (UL),
  466
Tolterodine tartrate, 1218
Tongue, 1218-1219, *1219*
  burning, 298
  cancer, 1219, *1219*
  depressor, 1219
  geographic, 598, *598*
  macroglossia, 817
Tongue-tie, 1219
Tonometry, 1219-1220
Tonsillectomy, 1220
Tonsillitis, 1220, *1220*
Tonsils, 1220-1221
Tooth abscess, 1221, *1221*
Tooth decay, 1221
  baby bottle, 1017
  filling, 564-565
Toothache, 1223
Toothbrushing, 1223-1224, *1223*
Tooth eruption, 1221-1222, *1222*
Tooth extraction, 1222-1223, *1223*
Tophus, 1224
TORCH syndrome, 1224
Torsemide, 1224
Torsion, 1224, *1224*
  testicular, 1201, *1201*
Torticollis, 1224-1225, *1225*
Total parenteral nutrition, 957
Touch, 969, 1101-1102, 1225
  therapeutic, 1205
Tourette syndrome, 209, 1225
Tourniquet, 1225, *1225*
Toxemia, 1225
  of pregnancy, 1225
Toxic shock syndrome, 1225-1226
  first aid, 1330-1331
Toxicity, 1226
Toxin, 1226

bacterial, 222
Toxocariasis, 1226
Toxoid, 1226
Toxoplasmosis, 1226-1228, 1310,
  1227
  opportunistic infection, 921
Trabeculectomy, 259, 1228, *1228*
Trace elements, 1228
Tracer, 1228
Trachea, 807, 1068, 1228
Tracheoesophageal fistula,
  1228-1229
Tracheostomy, 1229, *1229*
Tracheotomy, 1229
Trachoma, 1229
  blindness, 250
Traction, 1229
  for back pain, 220
Trager approach, 260, 1229
Trait, 1230
Tramadol, 946, 1230
Trance, 1230
Tranquilizers. *See* Antipsychotic
  drugs; Sedatives.
Transcendental meditation, 1230
Transcutaneous electrical nerve
  stimulation. *See* TENS.
  for back pain, 220
Transdermal patch. *See* Skin
  patch.
Transesophageal echocardiogram,
  1230, *1230*
Trans-fatty acids, 551-552, 1230
Transference, 1231
Transfusion, 1231-1232, *1231*
  autologous, 1232
Transient ischemic attack, 1214,
  1232
  anticoagulants, 177
  dizziness, 36
  numbness or tingling, 48
  RIND, 1080
Transillumination, 1232
Translocation, 1232
Transmissible, 1232
Transplant surgery, 1232-1234,
  1233
  bone marrow, *92, 264*
    allogeneic, 263-265
    autologous, 265
  graft-versus-host disease, 613, *613*
  hair, 624-625, *624*

heart, 644-645, *93*
heart-lung, 647
kidney, 761
liver, 801-802
lung, 809, *809*
organ, 93
pancreas, 948-949, *949*
renal, 1062
small bowel, 1135
stem cells, 1161
tissue-typing, 1217-1218
xenograft, 1305-1306
Transposition of the great vessels,
  642, 1234
Transsexualism, 1234
Transvestism, 1234
Trastuzumab, 1234
Trauma, 1324
  acoustic, 112-113, *112*
  amnesia, 150
  aphasia, 186
  brain damage, 271
  to eye, 538
  surgery, 1234
Trauma center, 1234
Traumatology, 1234
Travel immunization, 1235-1236
Traveler's diarrhea. *See* Diarrhea,
  traveler's.
Trazodone, 178, 1236
Treacher Collins syndrome, 824
Treatment, 1236
  See also Drug; Radiation thera-
    py; Surgery; treatments by name.
Trematode, 1236, *1236*
Trembling, 1236
Tremors, 740, 1236
Trephine, 1236
Tretinoin, 111, 1236, *1236*
TRH, 214, 1236-1237
Trial, clinical. *See* Clinical trial.
Triamcinolone. *See* Corticosteroids.
Triazolam. *See* Benzodiazepines.
Triamterene, 1237
Trichiasis, 1237
Trichinosis, 956, 1237, *1237*
Trichloroethylene, 166
Trichobezoars, 235
Trichomoniasis, 1238
Trichotillomania, 1238
Tricuspid valve, 645-647
  insufficiency, 1238

stenosis, 1162
Tricyclic antidepressants, 178
Trigeminal neuralgia, 1238, *1238*
Trigger finger, 1238-1239, *1239*
Trigger point therapy, 1239
Triglycerides, 1239
Trihexyphenidyl. *See* Co-trimoxazole.
Trimethoprim, 1239
Trismus, 1239
Trisomy, 1239
Trisomy 13 syndrome, 365, 1239
Trisomy 18 syndrome, 365, 1239-1240
Trisomy 21 syndrome, 1240
Trophoblastic tumor, 1240
Tropical spastic paraparesis, 1134
Tropical ulcer, 1240
Trovafloxacin mesylate. *See* Fluoroquqinolones.
Truss, 1240
Trypanosomiasis, 1240, *1240*
Tryptophan, 1240
TSH, 1212, 1240
Tubal cannulation, 1241, *1241*
Tubal ligation, 403, 1241-1242, *1241*
Tubal pregnancy, 1242
Tuberculin skin test, 1242
Tuberculosis, 176, 1242, 1244, *1243*
　acute abdomen, 98
　Addison disease, 116
　BCG vaccination, 231
　coughing, 29, 30
　urine discoloration, 58
　weight loss, 62
Tuberosity, 1244
Tuberous sclerosis, 311, 1244-1245
Tubes in ears. *See* Myringotomy.
Tuboplasty, 1245
Tui-Na, 1245
TUIP (transurethral incision of prostate), 1025
Tularemia, 1245
　animal-transmitted, 171
Tummy tuck, 1245-1246, *1246*
Tumor suppressor genes, 1246
Tumor-lysis syndrome, 1247
Tumor, 308, 1246, *1246. See also* specific disease.

Tunnel vision, 1247
Turbinates, nasal, 885
Turf toe, 1247
Turner syndrome, 365, 1247
TURP (transurethral resection of prostate), 1023, 1025
Twelve-Step Program, 130, 135, 481, 1247-1248, *1247*
Twenty-first century medicine, 73-96
　biomedical imaging, 80-87
　　brain function, 85-87, *85-87*
　　nuclear medicine, 81-82, *81*
　　optical coherence tomography, 83, *83*
　　PET scan, 82, *82*
　　prenatal scanning and in utero surgery, 84, *84*
　　SPECT, *80*
　　stereotactic imaging, 82-83, *83*
　　virtual colonoscopy, 84
　bionic people, 88-93
　　cataract surgery, 91-92, *91*
　　joint replacement, 89, *88*
　　nerve stimulators, implantable, 91
　　organ transplants, 93, *93*
　　prosthetic limbs, 89-90, *89-90*
　　stem cell replacement therapy, 92-93, *92*
　genetics, 74-79, *74-75*
　　gene splicing, 77
　　genetic engineering, 76-77, *76*
　　monoclonal antibodies, 78, *78*
　　stem cell research, 79, *79*
　　therapeutic proteins, 77-78, *77*
　surgical techniques, 94-96
　　image-guided surgery, 95, *95*
　　robotic surgery, 74
　　virtual surgery, 96, *96*
Twins, 1248, *1248*
　conjoined, 1248-1249
Twitch, 1249
Tylenol, 107
Tympanometry, 1249
Tympanoplasty, 1249, *1249*
Tympanum, 1249-1250, *1249*
Typhoid fever, 176, 1250
Typhus, 1250

U

Ulcerative colitis, 382-383, 724-725. *See also* Colitis.
　cholangitis, 357
　diarrhea, 34
Ulcer-healing agents. *See* Antacids; Histamine blockers; Proton pump inhibitors.
Ulcers, 1251
　abdominal pain, 98
　and alcoholism, 133
　backache, 21
　chest pain, 348
　corneal, 406
　duodenal, 483, 485
　gastric, 592
　genital, 598
　and Helicobacter pylori, 622
　and iron-deficiency anemia, 159
　mouth, 861
　peptic, 968-969, *968*
　stomach, 1167
　stress, 1171
　tropical, 1240
Ulcer, leg, 780
Ultrasound scanning, 1251-1252, *1251*
　fetal monitoring, 558
　kidney, 759
　lung, 809
　obstetrical, 99, 1252, *1252*
　AFP test, 125
　birth defects, 242
　threatened abortion, 100
　prenatal, 84, *84*
　treatment, 1252
Ultraviolet light, 1252
Umbilicus, 1253
Umbilical cord, 1252-1253, *1253*
　blood sampling, 970
　placenta, 989
　prolapse, 823
Unconscious, 582, 1253
Unconsciousness, 1253
Underage drinking, 1253, *1253*
Underarm, 215
Underbite, 243, 1253
Unsaturated fats, 1254
Urea, 253, 1254
Uremia, 1254

Ureter, 1254
Ureteral colic, 1254
Ureterolithotomy, 1254
Urethra, 1065, 1254
 culture of, 427
 dilation, 1254, *1254*
 discharge, 1254
 hypospadias, 702
 stricture, 1254-1255, *1255*
Urethral syndrome, acute, 1255
Urethritis
 nongonococcal, 904, 1255
 penis problems, 49
Urethrocele, 1255-1256, *1256*
Uric acid, 1256
 gout, 612-613
Urinal, 1256, *1256*
Urinalysis, 1256, *1256*
Urinary tract, 1257, *1257*
 abdominal pain, 15
 atlas, *71*
 calculus, 305-306, *306*
 catheterization, 331-332, *331*
 infections, 1257-1258
Urination
 incontinence, 716-717
 nocturia, 904
 oliguria, 916
 painful, 1258
 polyuria, 1007
Urine, 1258
 culture, 427
 diversion, 1256
 frequency, 1256-1257
 retention, 1257
 tests, 1258-1259
Urologist, 1259
Urology, 1259
Uterine septum, 1259
Urticaria. *See* Hives.
Uterus, 1064, 1259
 cancer of, 1259
 fibroids, 562, *562*
 hysterectomy, 705, *705*
 hysteroscopy, 706, *706*
 prolapse of, 1259-1260, *1259, 1260*
 retroverted, 1260
UV light. *See* Ultraviolet light.
Uveitis, 1260
Uvula, 1260, *1260*
Uvulopalatopharyngoplasty, 1260-1261

V

Vaccination, 1262, *1262*
 childhood, 1262-1263, *1263*
Vaccines, 710-711, 1263, *1263*
 BCG (Bacille Calmette-Guerin), 231
 DTaP (diphtheria, tetanus, pertussis), 483, 711
 hepatitis B, 662
 Hib, 670
 rubella, 1084
 travel immunization, 1235-1236
Vacuum aspiration, 100
Vacuum extraction, 1264
Vagina, 1064, 1264, *1264*
 Bartholin gland disease, 229, *229*
 bleeding, 1264
 hymen, 689
 leukorrhea, 788
 prolapse, 1264-1265
 rectocele, 1055
 repair, 1264
 vault prolapse, 1264-1265
 vestibulitis, 1274
Vaginismus, 1265
Vaginitis, 1265
 atrophic, 1265
Vaginosis, bacterial, 222, 1265
Vagotomy, 1265
Valacyclovir hydrochloride, 1265-1266
Valerian, 1266
Valgus, 1266
Valproic acid, 1266
Valsalva maneuver, 1266
 for barotrauma, 229
Valsartan, 1266
Valves, 1266, *1266*
 heart, 645-647, *646*
Valvotomy, 1266
Valvular heart disease, 1266
Valvuloplasty, 1266-1267, *1267*
 balloon, 225
Vancomycin, 1267
Vaporizer, 1267, *381*
Varicella. *See* Chickenpox.
Varices, 1267
 esophageal, 526-527, *527*
Varicocele, 1267
 infertility, 721, 723
Varicose veins, 1267, *1267*

ankle or foot problems, 18
Varus, 1267
Vas deferens, 1065, 1267
Vascular dementia, 1268
Vascular surgery, 1268
Vasculitis, 1268
 Wegener granulomatosis, 1294-1295
Vasectomy, 403, 1268-1269, *1269*
Vasoconstriction, 1269
Vasodilation, 1269
 for cardiomyopathy, 318
Vasodilators, 1296
Vasopressin. *See* ADH.
Vasospasm, 1270
Vasovagal attack, 1270
Vector, 1270
Veganism, 1270
Vegetables, cruciferous, 423, *423*
Vegetarianism, 1270-1271
 and iron-deficiency anemia, 159
Vegetative state, 1271
Veins, 1271, *1271*
Vena cava, 1271
Veneers, dental, 410, 1271
Venereal disease, 1271
Venipuncture, 1271
Venlafaxine, 1271
Ventilation, 808, 1271-1272
 mechanical, for anaphylaxis, 155
Ventilators, 791, 1271, *1272*
Ventricle, 1272
 ectopic beat, 1272
 fibrillation, 1272
 tachycardia, 1271
Ventricular fibrillation, 641
 angina, 168
Ventricular septal defect, 641-642
Ventricular tachycardia, 192
Verapamil, 1272
Vernix, 1272
Verruca. *See* Wart.
Version, 1273
 external, breech delivery, 288
Vertebra, 1273
Vertebrobasilar insufficiency, 1273
Vertigo, 1273
 benign positional, 1273-1274, *1274*
 Meniere disease, 835-836
Vesicle, 1274
Vestibulitis, 1274
Viability, 1274

Vibrational medicine, 1274
Villus, 1274
Villous adenoma, 1274
Violence, 1275, *1275*
Viral infections
   chickenpox, 350
   coughing, 28
   dengue, 443-444
   Ebola, 493-494
   hantavirus, 628
   hepatitis, 664
   herpes, 667-669
   molluscum contagiosum, 856-857
   mumps, 869, *869*
   opportunistic, 920-921
   papillomavirus, 685-686
   parainfluenza, 952
   pneumonia, 996
   poliomyelitis, 1001-1002
   respiratory tract, 1069
   shingles, 1113-1114
   West Nile, 1297
   yellow fever, 1307-1308, *1307*
Viremia, 1275
Virginity, 1275
Virilism, 1275-1276
Virility, 1276
Virilization, 1276
Virion, 1276
Virology, 1276
Virtual surgery, 96, *96*
Virulence, 1276
Viruses, 1276-1278, *1277*
   infections, 1277-1278
   structure of, 1277
Viscera, 1278
Viscosity, 1278
Vision, 969, 1278, *1278*
   albinism, 131
   amaurosis fugax, 146
   amblyopia, 146-147, *147*
   Amsler grid, 151, *1279*
   astigmatism, 202-203, *203*
   blurred, 258-259
   cataract, 328-329
   color blindness, 388
   farsightedness, 549, 550
   glaucoma, 602-605, *604*
   loss or impairment, 41
   macular degeneration, 817-819
   nearsightedness, 887, *888*
   ophthalmology, 920

   perimetry, 971
   retina, 1070
   sense of, 1101-1102
   Snellen chart, 1140, *1279*
   tests, 1278, *1279*
Visual acuity, 539-540, 1278, 1280
Visual field, 1280, *1280*
   tunnel vision, 1247
Visualization, 1280
Vital sign, 1280, *1281*
Vitamin A, 235, 912, 1072, 1281
   and blindness, 251
Vitamin B, 1281-1282
Vitamin B1, 234, 1281, 1297
Vitamin B2, 1079, 1281
Vitamin B3, 901, 963, 1281
Vitamin B5, 951
Vitamin B6, 1281-1282
Vitamin B12, 159-160, 429, 1282
Vitamin C, 1282-1283
   scurvy, 1096
Vitamin D, 1283
   and bone loss, 263
   bow legs, 267
   and osteomalacia, 929-930
Vitamin E, 141, 1283
Vitamin H, 239
Vitamin K, 1283
Vitamins, 1283-1284
   absorption of, 102
Vitiligo, 1284, *1284*
   phototherapy, 984
Vitrectomy, 1284, *1284*
Vitreous hemorrhage, 1284-1285,
   1284
Vitreous humor, 1285
Vivisection, 1285
VLDL, 1285
Vocal cords, 1286
   hoarseness or voice loss, 31, 676
   nodules, 1285, *1285*
   paralysis, 1285-1286
   subglottic stenosis, 1175
Voice, loss of, 1286
   symptom chart, 31
Voice box. *See* Larynx.
Volkmann contracture, 1286
Volvulus, 1286
Vomiting, 1286-1287, *1287*
   blood, 1287
   hyperemesis, 690-691

   Ipecac, 740-741
von Recklinghausen disease, 898
von Willebrand disease, 248,
   1287-1288
Voyeurism, 1288
Vulva, 1064
   cancer of the, 1288
   dystrophy, 1288
   Paget disease, 943
Vulvectomy, 1288
Vulvitis, 1288-1289
Vulvovaginitis, 1289

W

Waist-to-hip ratio, 1290
Waldenström macroglobulinemia,
   1290
Walking, delayed, 1290-1292
Walking aids, 1290, *1290*, *1291*
Warfarin, 1292
Warts, 1292-1293, *1292*
   genital, 17, 49, 598
   human papillomavirus (HPV),
   685-686
   penile, 966-967
   plantar, 991
Water
   intoxication, 1293
   molecule, *856*
   pollution, 1003
   therapy, 688-689
Waterborne infections, 1293
Waterhouse-Friedrichsen syn-
   drome, 1293
Watering eyes. *See* Tearing.
Weakness, 1293
Weaning, 1294
Wechsler Intelligence tests, 734
Wegener granulomatosis, 1294-1295
Weight, 1295
Weight gain, 60-61, 1295
Weight loss, 62-63, 913, 1295
Weight training, 1296
Weight-bearing exercise. *See*
   Exercise, weight-bearing.
Weil disease, 1296
   animal-transmitted, 171
Well-being, 1296
Werdnig-Hoffmann disease, 860,
   1296

Wernicke aphasia, 186
Wernicke encephalopathy, 1296-1297, *1297*
Wernicke-Korsakoff syndrome, 133, 506, 1297
West Nile virus, 1297
Wheal. *See* Hives.
Wheelchair, 1297
Wheezing, 288, 1298
Whiplash, 1298, *1298*
Whipple disease. *See* Intestinal lipodystrophy.
Whipple operation, 1298
Whipworm infestation, 1298-1299, *1299*
White blood cells, 252, 255
White matter, 1299
Whitehead, 1299
Whitlow, herpetic, 1299
WHO. *See* World Health Organization.
Whooping cough. *See* Pertussia. breathing problems, 288
Will, living, 1299
Williams syndrome, 1299-1300
Wilms tumor, 1300, *1300*
Wilson disease, 1300
Wired jaw, 1300
Wisdom tooth, 1300-1301, *1301*
Withdrawal method. *See* Coitus interruptus.
Withdrawal syndrome
    alcohol, 133, 1301, *133*
    opiates, 1303, *1303*
Wolff-Parkinson-White syndrome, 1301-1302
Womb. *See* Reproductive system, female.
Wood alcohol, 844
Word blindness, 1302
World Health Organization, 1302
Wounds
    bleeding, first aid, 1315
    botulism, 266
    culture of, 427
    cuts and scrapes, first aid, 1318
    infection, 1302-1303, *1303*
Wrinkle, 1303
Wrist, 1303
Wristdrop, 1303, *1303*
Writer's cramp, 416
Wryneck. *See* Torticocllis

X

X chromosome, 1304, 1306
    Turner syndrome, 1247
X rays, 1304, *1304*
    bone imaging, 263
    chest, 349, *349*
    dental, 1305, *1305*
    gastrointestinal series, 593-594
    See also Imaging; Radiology.
Xanthelasma, 539, 1305
Xanthoma, 1305
Xanthomatosis, 1305
Xenograft, 1305-1306, *1306*
Xeroderma pigmentosum, 1306
Xerophthalmia, 1306
Xerostomia. *See* Dry mouth.
X-linked characteristic, 1306

Y

Y chromosome, 1307
Yawning, 1307
Yeast infections, 1307
    cryptococcosis, 425
Yellow fever, 1307-1308, *1307*
Yin and yang, 1308
Yoga, 215, 216, 513, 848, 1308, *1308*
    hatha, 629
    Thai massage, 1203

Z

Zafirlukast, 1309
Zalcitabine (ddC), 1309
    AIDS treatment, 129
Zalepion, 1309
Zanamivir, 1309
Zenker diverticulum, 1309
Zidovudine, 1309, *1309*
    AIDS treatment, 129
ZIFT (zygote intrafallopian transfer), 1309
Zileuton, 1309
Zinc, 850, 1309-1310
Zolmitriptan, 1310
Zolpidem, 1310
Zone therapy, 1310

reflexology, 1057, 1059
Zoonosis, 1310
    Q fever, 1047
    See also Animals, diseases from; Brucellosis; Hantavirus infection; Plague; Rabies; Ticks and disease; Toxoplasmosis.
Z-plasty, 1310
Zygote, 1310, *1310*
    assisted reproductive technology, 199
    intrafallopian transfer. *See* ZIFT.

Illustration sources

5: ©American Medical Association
65 (top): P. Berndt/Custom Medical Stock Photo
65 (bottom): Educational Images/ Custom Medical Stock Photo
66: ©Frank Lane Picture Agency/CORBIS
69: ©CNRI/ Phototake
70 (top): ©Don W. Fawcett/ Photo Researchers, Inc.
70 (bottom): ©Ken Wagner/Phototake
71 (top): ©Lester V. Bergman/CORBIS
71 (bottom): ©Dennis Kunkel/Phototake
72: SIU BioMed/Custom Medical Stock Photo
73 (top): ©G. Tompkinson/Photo Researchers, Inc.
73 (bottom): Photograph by Bobbi Bennett/Courtesy of Computer Motion
74: photolibrary.com/Index Stock
75 (both): ©Roger Ressmeyer/CORBIS
76 (left): Richard Carson/Reuters/ TimePix
76 (right): Fernand Ivaldi/Getty Images
77: ©J. Dowdalls/Photo Researchers, Inc.
78 (left): ©Jacob Halaska/Index Stock
78 (right): ©Dan McCoy/Rainbow/ PictureQuest
79 (left): R. Rawlins PhD/Custom Medical Stock Photo
79 (right): ©G. Tompkinson/ Photo Researchers, Inc.
80: Custom Medical Stock Photo
81 (top): SIU BioMed/Custom Medical Stock Photo
81 (bottom): R. D'Amico/Custom Medical Stock Photo
82: ©Hank Morgan/Photo Researchers, Inc.
83 (top left): © Roger Ressmeyer/CORBIS
83 (top right): © Lief Skoogfors/CORBIS
83 (both, bottom): Courtesy of LightLab Imaging, LLC. All rights reserved.
84 (left): ©Marigaux/ Photo Researchers, Inc.
84 (right): Max Aguilera-Hellweg/TimePix
85 (both): Wellcome Department of Cognitive Neurology/Science Photo Library/ Custom Medical Stock Photo
86 (top and middle): ©ISM/ Phototake
86 (bottom): Steve Liss/TimePix
87 (top left): Michael Newman /Photo Edit
87 (top right): Laura Dwight/ Photo Edit
87 (bottom): Bill Aron/Photo Edit
88: ©M. Kulyk/Photo Researchers, Inc.
89: PMRH/Photo Researchers, Inc.
90 (left): ©Richard T. Nowitz/Science Source/Photo Researchers, Inc.
90 (right): ©Yoav Levy/Phototake
91: ©Laurent/ Photo Researchers, Inc.
92 (left): ©Simon Fraser/Photo Researchers, Inc.

92 (right): ©Richard T. Nowitz/ Science Source/ Photo Researchers, Inc.
93 (top): Reuters/ TimePix
93 (bottom): Photo courtesy of Cochlear Ltd.
94: Photograph by Bobbi Bennett/ Courtesy of Computer Motion
95 (top right): Courtesy of Intuitive Surgical
95 (top left): ©EURELIOS/Phototake
96 (top right): ©Geoff Tompkinson/Photo Researchers, Inc.
96 (bottom left): Courtesy of Intuitive Surgical
136 (top): ©Oliver Meckes/Photo Researchers, Inc.
136 (bottom): ©PhotoDisc
142 (both): ©PhotoDisc
203 (both): ©PhotoDisc
214: A. Glauberman/Science Source Photo/ Photo Researchers, Inc.
222: Yvonne Hemsey/Liaison/ Getty Images
230: Custom Medical Stock Photo
252: ©Phototake/Picture Quest
306: Courtesy of EDAP TMS, SA, 4/6 rue du Dauphine, Vaulx-en-Velin, France 69120.
343 (both): Dr. E. Walker/Science Photo Library/Photo Researchers, Inc.
365: ©Biophoto Associates/Science Source Photo/Photo Researchers, Inc.
369: Public Health Image Library
373: Roslin Institute
378: ©Dr. P. Marazzi/Photo Researchers, Inc.
379: Reprinted with permission from the American Academy of Dermatology. All rights reserved.
425: Courtesy of Dr. Jeffrey Melton/ Chicago, Illinois
484: CORBIS
580: Newsmakers/Getty
646 (left): ©Nathan Benn/Stock Boston, Inc./ Picture Quest
646 (middle): ©Klaus Guldbrandsen/ Science Photo Library/Photo Researchers, Inc.
646 (right): Photo courtesy of ON-X valves
688: ©PhotoDisc
759: ©Biophoto Associates/Science Source Photo/Photo Researchers, Inc.
780: ©Astrid and Hanns-Friedler Michler/Science Photo Library/Photo Researchers, Inc.
814: Lymph node illustration by John Bavosi/Science Photo Library/Photo Researchers, Inc.
818: (both): National Eye Institute, National Institutes of Health
846: Public Health Image Library

908: ©Elscint/Science Photo Library/ Photo Researchers, Inc.
932 (both): Prof. P. Motta/Department of Anatomy/University "La Sapienza." Rome/Science Photo Library/ Photo Researchers, Inc.
960 (top): ©Biophoto Associates/Science Source Photo/Photo Researchers, Inc.
960 (bottom): Public Health Image Library
1031: Reprinted with permission from the American Academy of Dermatology. All rights reserved.
1044: CNRI/Science Photo Library/Photo Researchers, Inc.
1073 (both): National Eye Institute, National Institutes of Health
1075 (both): Astrid and Hanns-Frieder Michler/Science Photo Library/Photo Researchers, Inc.
1077 (top): Princess Margaret Rose Orthopaedic Hospital/Science Photo Library/Photo Researchers, Inc.
1078: ©EyeWire
1106 (both): CNRI/Science Photo Library/ Photo Researchers, Inc.
1116 (bottom): ©PhotoDisc
1219: Reprinted with permission from the American Academy of Dermatology. All rights reserved.
1227: ©Phototake/ Picture Quest
1251: ©Alexander Tsiaras/ Science Source Photo/Photo Researchers, Inc.
1262: Figure reprinted from Immunology, 4th edition, Roitt, page 1.11, Copyright 1997, with permission from Elsevier.
1275: ©PhotoDisc
1304 (top left): ©Science Photo Library/ Photo Researchers, Inc.
1304 (top right): ©Lunagrafix, Inc./Photo Researchers, Inc.
1304 (bottom left): Howard Sochurek/ ©CORBIS-Stock Market
1305 (all): © PhotoDisc
1306: SIU/ Custom Medical Stock Photo